369 0291557

D1336874

RETINA

RETINA

Editor-In-Chief

Stephen J. Ryan MD

President, Doheny Eye Institute, Los Angeles, CA, USA

Volume One

Part 1 Retinal Imaging and Diagnostics

Edited by
SriniVas R. Sadda MD

Part 2 Basic Science and Translation to Therapy

Edited by
David R. Hinton MD

Volume Two

Medical Retina

Edited by
Andrew P. Schachat MD and **SriniVas R. Sadda** MD

Volume Three

Part 1 Surgical Retina

Edited by
C. P. Wilkinson MD and **Peter Wiedemann** MD

Part 2 Tumors of the Retina, Choroid, and Vitreous

Edited by
Andrew P. Schachat MD

Editor-In-Chief
Stephen J. Ryan MD
President, Doheny Eye Institute, Los Angeles, CA, USA

RETINA

FIFTH EDITION

Volume Two

Medical Retina

Edited by
Andrew P. Schachat MD
Vice Chairman
Cole Eye Institute
Cleveland Clinic Foundation
Cleveland, OH, USA

SriniVas R. Sadda MD
Associate Professor of Ophthalmology
Doheny Eye Institute
Associate Professor
Department of Ophthalmology
Keck School of Medicine
University of Southern California
Los Angeles, CA, USA

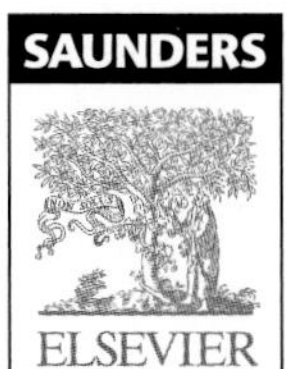

London New York Oxford St Louis Sydney Toronto

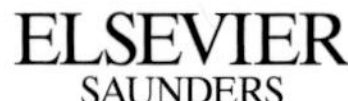

First edition 1989
Second edition 1994
Third edition 2001
Fourth edition 2006
Fifth edition 2013

British Library Cataloguing in Publication Data

Retina.
1. Retina–Diseases. 2. Retina–Surgery. 3. Retina–Physiology.
I. Ryan, Stephen J., 1940-617.7'35-dc23
ISBN-13: 9781455707379

Ebook ISBN: 9781455737802
Printed in China
Last digit is the print number: 9 8 7 6 5 4 3 2 1

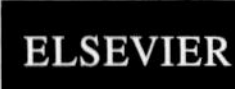

Senior Content Strategist: Russell Gabbedy
Content Development Specialist: Nani Clansey
Content Coordinator: Emma Cole/Trinity Hutton/Sam Crowe/Humayra Rahman
Project Manager: Caroline Jones
Design: Miles Hitchen
Illustration Manager: Jennifer Rose
Illustrator: Antbits
Marketing Manager: Helena Mutak
Cover image photographer: Tamera Schoenholz, CRA, OCT-C

Contents

Volume Two

Medical Retina

Edited by Andrew P. Schachat and SriniVas R. Sadda

Section 1: Retinal Degenerations and Dystrophies

Section 2: Retinal Vascular Disease

Section 3: Choroidal Vascular/Bruch's Membrane Disease

Section 4: Inflammatory Disease/Uveitis

Inflammation

Infections

 **Indicates additional online content at www.expertconsult.com**

Video Table of Contents

Section 6: Ocular Tumors

Section 7: Miscellaneous

Contributors

Michael Abràmoff MD, PhD
Associate Professor
Retina Service
Department of Ophthalmology and Visual Sciences
Biomedical Engineering, and Electrical and Computer Engineering
University of Iowa
Iowa City, IA, USA
Chapter 6

Gary W. Abrams MD
The David Barsky MD Professor and Chair
Department of Ophthalmology
Wayne State University
Director, Kresge Eye Institute
Detroit, MI, USA
Chapter 108

Anita Agarwal MD
Associate Professor of Ophthalmology
Retina, Vitreous and Uveitis
Vanderbilt Eye Institute
Nashville, TN, USA
Chapter 129

Everett Ai MD
Director, Ophthalmic Diagnostic Center
California Pacific Medical Center
San Francisco, CA, USA
Chapter 1

Lloyd M. Aiello MD
Director Emeritus
Beetham Eye Institute
Joslin Diabetes Center
Boston, MA, USA
Chapter 48

Lloyd Paul Aiello MD, PhD
Professor of Ophthalmology
Harvard Medical School
Vice Chair, Centers of Excellence
Harvard Department of Ophthalmology
Medical Director of Ophthalmology
Brigham & Women's Hospital
Section Head, Eye Research
Vice President of Ophthalmology
Director, Beetham Eye Institute
Joslin Diabetes Center
Boston, MA, USA
Chapter 48

Daniel M. Albert MD, MS
RRF Emmett A. Humble Distinguished Director of the UW Eye Research Institute
F.A. Davis and Lorenz E. Zimmerman Professor
Department of Ophthalmology and Visual Sciences
University of Wisconsin-Madison
Madison, WI, USA
Chapter 138

Mathew W. Aschbrenner MD
Instructor in Ophthalmology and Visual Science
Department of Ophthalmology and Visual Sciences
Washington University School of Medicine
St Louis, MO, USA
Chapter 119

Marcos Ávila MD
Professor
Head of the Department of Ophthalmology
Federal University of Goias
Goiânia, GO, Brazil
Chapter 86

G. William Aylward FRCS, FRCOphth, MD
Consultant Vitreoretinal Surgeon
Moorfields Eye Hospital
London, UK
Chapter 105

Matthew Bedell MD
Clinical Research Fellow
Department of Ophthalmology
Shiley Eye Center
University of California, San Diego
La Jolla, CA, USA
Chapter 46

Rubens Belfort Jr MD, PhD, MBA
Head Professor of Ophthalmology
Department of Ophthalmology
Federal University of São Paulo
São Paulo, Brazil
Chapter 85

Jean Bennett MD, PhD
F.M. Kirby Professor of Ophthalmology
Professor of Cell and Developmental Biology
Department of Ophthalmology
Scheie Eye Institute
University of Pennsylvania Perelman School of Medicine
Research Scientist
Center for Cellular and Molecular Therapeutics
The Children's Hospital of Philadelphia
Philadelphia, PA, USA
Chapter 34

Chris Bergstrom MD, OD
Assistant Professor of Ophthalmology
Emory University Eye Center
Emory University School of Medicine
Atlanta, GA, USA
Chapter 133

Cagri G. Besirli MD, PhD
Fellow
Retina and Uveitis
Department of Ophthalmology and Visual Sciences
University of Michigan
Ann Arbor, MI, USA
Chapter 73

Pramod S. Bhende MS
Senior Consultant
Department of Vitreoretinal Surgery
Sankara Nethralaya
Nungambakkam, Chennai, India
Chapter 109

Susanne Binder MD
Professor
Department of Ophthalmology
Rudolph Foundation Hospital (Rudolfstiftung)
Vienna, Austria
Chapter 111

Alan C. Bird MD
Emeritus Professor
Department of Ophthalmic Genetics
Institute of Ophthalmology
University College London
London, UK
Chapter 64

Barbara A. Blodi MD
Professor of Ophthalmology and Visual Sciences
University of Wisconsin School of Medicine and Public Health
Madison, WI, USA
Chapter 48

Mark S. Blumenkranz MD
Professor and Chair
Department of Ophthalmology
Stanford University
Palo Alto, CA, USA
Chapter 39, Chapter 67

H. Culver Boldt MD
Professor of Ophthalmology
Department of Ophthalmology
University of Iowa
Iowa City, IA, USA
Chapter 145

Norbert Bornfeld MD
Professor
Center for Ophthalmology
University Hospital of Essen
Essen, Germany
Chapter 148

Ferdinando Bottoni MD, FEBO
Staff Member
Eye Clinic
Department of Clinical Science Luigi Sacco
Sacco Hospital, University of Milan
Milan, Italy
Chapter 2

Michael E. Boulton PhD
Professor
Department of Anatomy and Cell Biology
University of Florida
Gainesville, FL, USA
Chapter 24

Sara J. Bowne PhD
Faculty Associate, Human Genetics Center
Division of Epidemiology
Human Genetics and Environmental Sciences
School of Public Health
The University of Texas Health Science Center at Houston
Houston, TX, USA
Chapter 31

Milam A. Brantley Jr MD, PhD
Assistant Professor
Ophthalmology and Visual Sciences
Vanderbilt Eye Institute
Vanderbilt University
Nashville, TN, USA
Chapter 22

Neil M. Bressler MD
The James P. Gills Professor of Ophthalmology
Chief of the Retina Division
Wilmer Eye Institute
Johns Hopkins University School of Medicine
Baltimore, MD, USA
Chapter 65, Chapter 66

Susan B. Bressler MD
The Julia G. Levy, PhD Professor of Ophthalmology
Wilmer Eye Institute
Johns Hopkins University School of Medicine
Baltimore, MD, USA
Chapter 65, Chapter 66

Andreas Bringmann PhD
Associate Professor
Department of Ophthalmology and Eye Hospital
University of Leipzig
Leipzig, Germany
Chapter 17

Daniel A. Brinton MD
Assistant Clinical Professor
Department of Ophthalmology
University of California, San Francisco
San Francisco, CA, USA
Chapter 103

Gary C. Brown MD, MBA
Chief and Attending Surgeon
Retina Service, Wills Eye Institute
Professor of Ophthalmology
Jefferson Medical College
Philadelphia, PA
Chief Medical Officer
Center for Value-Based Medicine
Flourtown, PA, USA
Chapter 59, Chapter 152

Justin C. Brown MD
Medical and Surgical Retinal Fellow
The Wilmer Eye Institute
Johns Hopkins Hospital
Baltimore, MD, USA
Chapter 92

Simon Brunner MD
Professor of Ophthalmology
Department of Ophthalmology
Rudolph Foundation Hospital (Rudolfstiftung)
Vienna, Austria
Chapter 111

Ronald A. Bush PhD
Staff Scientist
Section on Translational Research on Retinal and Macular Degeneration
National Institute of Deafness and Other Communication Disorders
National Institutes of Health
Bethesda, MD, USA
Chapter 37

Dingcai Cao PhD
Associate Professor
Department of Ophthalmology and Visual Sciences
University of Illinois at Chicago
Chicago, IL, USA
Chapter 10

Antonio Capone Jr MD, PhD
Clinical Professor
Oakland University/William Beaumont Hospital School of Medicine
Auburn Hills, MI
Professor, European School for Advanced Studies in Ophthalmology
Lugano, Switzerland
Partner, Associated Retinal Consultants
Royal Oak, MI
Director. Vision Research Foundation
Novi, MI, USA
Chapter 137

David Carruthers MBBS, PhD, FRCP
Consultant Rheumatologist
Birmingham City Hospital
Birmingham, UK
Chapter 80

Jerry D. Cavallerano OD, PhD
Optometrist
Beetham Eye Institute
Joslin Diabetes Center
Associate Professor
Department of Ophthalmology
Harvard Medical School
Boston, MA, USA
Chapter 48

Usha Chakravarthy MD, PhD
Professor of Ophthalmology and Vision Science
The Queen's University
Consultant in Ophthalmology
The Belfast Health and Social Care Trust
Belfast, UK
Chapter 94

Chi-Chao Chan MD
Chief, Immunopathology Section
Laboratory of Immunology
Chief, Histology Core
National Eye Institute
National Institutes of Health
Bethesda, MD, USA
Chapter 25

Waiman Chan MBBS(HK), MRCP(UK), FRCS(Edin), FRCP(Edin), FRCOphth(HK), FRCOphth(UK), FHKAM (Ophthalmology)
Consultant
Department of Ophthalmology
Hong Kong Sanatorium & Hospital
Hong Kong
Chapter 72

Steven Charles MD
Clinical Professor of Ophthalmology
University of Tennessee
College of Medicine
Memphis, TN, USA
Chapter 101

David G. Charteris MD
Consultant Vitreoretinal Surgeon
Moorfields Eye Hospital
London, UK
Chapter 29

Dong Feng Chen MD, PhD
Associate Professor
Schepens Eye Research Institute
Department of Ophthalmology
Harvard Medical School
Boston, MA, USA
Chapter 33

Jeannie Chen PhD
Professor
Department of Cell and Neurobiology
Zilkha Neurogenetic Institute
Keck School of Medicine
University of Southern California
Los Angeles, CA, USA
Chapter 14

Youxin Chen MD
Professor
Department of Ophthalmology
Peking Union Medical College Hospital
Beijing, PR China
Chapter 91

Carol Yim Lui Cheung PhD
Research Scientist
Singapore Eye Research Institute
Singapore
Adjunct Assistant Professor
Office of Clinical Sciences
Duke-NUS Graduate Medical School
Durham, NC, USA
Chapter 49

Emily Y. Chew MD
Chief of Clinical Trials
Deputy Director
Division of Epidemiology and Clinical Applications
National Eye Institute
National Institutes of Health
Bethesda, MD, USA
Chapter 52, Chapter 55, Chapter 130

Allen Chiang MD
Fellow in Vitreoretinal Surgery
Retina Service
Wills Eye Institute
Philadelphia, PA, USA
Chapter 103

Michael F. Chiang MD
Professor of Ophthalmology
Professor of Medical Informatics and Clinical Epidemiology
Oregon Health & Science University
Portland, OR, USA
Chapter 61, Chapter 62

Ian J. Constable FRANZCO, FRCSE, DSc (Hon)
Professor of Ophthalmology
Lions Eye Institute
University of Western Australia
Perth, Australia
Chapter 107

Gabriel Coscas MD, FEBO
Professor Emeritus of Ophthalmology
Department of Ophthalmology
University of Paris-East Créteil Val de Marne
Créteil, Paris, France
Chapter 30

Alan F. Cruess MD, FRCSC
Professor and Head
District Chief, Capital Health
Department of Ophthalmology and Visual Sciences
Dalhousie University
Halifax, Nova Scotia, Canada
Chapter 131

Emmett T. Cunningham Jr MD, PhD, MPH
Director, The Uveitis Service
California Pacific Medical Center
San Francisco, CA
Adjunct Clinical Professor of Ophthalmology
Stanford University School of Medicine
Stanford, CA
West Coast Retina Medical Group
San Francisco, CA, USA
Chapter 1

Christine A. Curcio PhD
Professor of Ophthalmology
University of Alabama School of Medicine
Birmingham, AL, USA
Chapter 20

Stephen P. Daiger PhD
TS Matney Professor of Environmental and Genetic Sciences
Human Genetics Center
Division of Epidemiology
Human Genetics and Environmental Sciences
School of Public Health
The University of Texas Health Science Center at Houston
Houston, TX, USA
Chapter 31

Bertil E. Damato MD, PhD, FRCOphth
Honorary Professor
Ocular Oncology Service
Royal Liverpool University Hospital
Liverpool, UK
Chapter 147

Janet L. Davis MD, MA
Professor of Ophthalmology
University of Miami Miller School of Medicine
Miami, FL, USA
Chapter 87

Matthew D. Davis MD
Emeritus Professor of Ophthalmology and Visual Sciences
University of Wisconsin School of Medicine and Public Health
Madison, WI, USA
Chapter 48

Shelley Day MD
Clinical Assistant Professor of Ophthalmology
Stanford University School of Medicine
Palo Alto, CA, USA
Chapter 153

Patrick De Potter MD, PhD
Professor of Ophthalmology
Chairman
Ophthalmology Department
Cliniques Universitaires St-Luc
Catholic University of Leuven
Brussels, Belgium
Chapter 58

Marc D. de Smet MDCM, PhD, FRCSC, FRCOpth
Professor of Ophthalmology
University of Amsterdam
Amsterdam, The Netherlands
Director of the Retina and Inflammation Unit
Center for Specialized Ophthalmology
Clinique de Montchoisi
GSMN Medical Networks
Lausanne, Switzerland
Chapter 112

Alastair K. Denniston PhD, MRCP, FRCOphth
Clinical Lecturer
Academic Unit of Ophthalmology
University of Birmingham
Birmingham, UK
Chapter 80

Ranjit S. Dhaliwal MD, FRCSC, FACS
Ophthalmologist
Adjunct Faculty
Department of Ophthalmology
Queen's University School of Medicine
Kingston, Ontario, Canada
Consultant Retinal Specialist and Founder
Retina Consultants, PC (The Retina Eye Center)
Augusta, GA, USA
Chapter 134, Chapter 155

Xiaoyan Ding MD, PhD
Associate Professor
Department of Retina
Zhongshan Ophthalmic Center
Sun Yat-sen University
Guangzhou, PR China
Chapter 41

Diana V. Do MD
Associate Professor of Ophthalmology
The Wilmer Eye Institute
Johns Hopkins University School of Medicine
Baltimore, MD, USA
Chapter 124, Chapter 155

Guorui Dou MD, PhD
Professor
Department of Ophthalmology
Xijing Hospital
Fourth Military Medical University
Xi'an, PR China
Chapter 16

William A. Dunn Jr PhD
Professor and Interim Chairman
Department of Anatomy and Cell Biology
University of Florida College of Medicine
Gainesville, FL, USA
Chapter 24

Justis P. Ehlers MD
Staff Physician
Retina Service
Cole Eye Institute
Cleveland Clinic Foundation
Cleveland, OH, USA
Chapter 70, Chapter 120

Michael Engelbert MD, PhD
Attending Physician and Research Assistant Professor
Department of Ophthalmology
New York University School of Medicine
New York, NY, USA
Chapter 55

Lisa J. Faia MD
Vitreoretinal Surgery Fellow
Associated Retinal Consultants
William Beaumont Hospital
Royal Oak, MI, USA
Chapter 114

Benedetto Falsini MD
Associate Professor of Ophthalmology
Department of Ophthalmology
Università Cattolica del S. Cuore,
Rome, Italy
Chapter 37

Amani A. Fawzi MD
Associate Professor of Ophthalmology
Northwestern University, Feinberg School of Medicine
Chicago, IL, USA
Chapter 44

Sharon Fekrat MD, FACS
Associate Professor
Vitreoretinal Surgery
Department of Ophthalmology
Duke Eye Center
Chief of Ophthalmology
Durham Veterans Affairs Medical Center
Durham, NC, USA
Chapter 54

Steven E. Feldon MD
Director, Flaum Eye Institute
Professor and Chair
Department of Ophthalmology
University of Rochester
Rochester, NY, USA
Chapter 12

Rodrigo A. Brant Fernandes MD
Research Associate
Doheny Eye Institute
Keck School of Medicine
University of Southern California
Los Angeles, CA, USA
Chapter 126

Henry A. Ferreyra MD
Assistant Clinical Professor
Department of Ophthalmology
Shiley Eye Center
University of California, San Diego
La Jolla, CA, USA
Chapter 46

Deborah A. Ferrington PhD
Associate Professor
Department of Ophthalmology
University of Minnesota
Minneapolis, MN, USA
Chapter 32

Frederick L. Ferris III MD
Director
Division of Epidemiology and Clinical Applications
Clinical Director,
National Eye Institute
National Institutes of Health
Bethesda, MD, USA
Chapter 47

Paul T. Finger MD
Clinical Professor of Ophthalmology
New York University School of Medicine
Director
The New York Eye Cancer Center
New York, NY, USA
Chapter 149

Steven K. Fisher PhD
Research Professor
Neuroscience Research Institute
Professor Emeritus
Molecular, Cellular and Developmental Biology
University of California, Santa Barbara
Santa Barbara, CA, USA
Chapter 29

Gerald A. Fishman MD
Director
Pangere Center for Inherited Retinal Diseases
The Chicago Lighthouse for People Who Are Blind or Visually Impaired
Professor Emeritus of Ophthalmology
Department of Ophthalmology and Visual Sciences
UIC Eye Center
Chicago, IL, USA
Chapter 43

Monika Fleckenstein MD
Ophthalmology Specialist
Department of Ophthalmology
University of Bonn
Bonn, Germany
Chapter 4

Harry W. Flynn Jr MD
Associate Professor of Ophthalmology
The J. Donald M. Gass Distinguished Chair in Ophthalmology
Bascom Palmer Eye Institute
Miami, FL, USA
Chapter 87

Andrew C. Fok MBChB, FRCS
Resident Specialist
Department of Ophthalmology
Hong Kong Eye Hospital
Kowloon, Hong Kong
Chapter 72

Wallace S. Foulds CBE, MD, ChM, DSc, FRCS, FRCOphth
Emeritus Professor of Ophthalmology
University of Glasgow
Glasgow, Scotland
Senior Consultant
Singapore Eye Research Institute
Singapore
Chapter 147

William R. Freeman MD
Professor of Ophthalmology
Director of the Jacobs Retina Center
Department of Ophthalmology, Shiley Eye Center
University of California, San Diego
La Jolla, CA, USA
Chapter 81

Aurélien Freton MD
Clinical Assistant Professor
Department of Ophthalmology
Saint Roch Hospital
Nice, France
Chapter 149

Martin Friedlander MD, PhD
Professor
Department of Cell Biology
The Scripps Research Institute
Division of Ophthalmology
Department of Surgery
Scripps Clinic
La Jolla, CA, USA
Chapter 35

Laura J. Frishman PhD
Moores Professor, Vision Sciences
College of Optometry
University of Houston
Houston, TX, USA
Chapter 7

Arthur D. Fu MD
Clinical Professor of Ophthalmology
California Pacific Medical Center
San Francisco, CA, USA
Chapter 1

Carlos Alexandre de Amorim Garcia Filho MD
Post Doctoral Associate
Department Of Ophthalmology
Bascom Palmer Eye Institute
University of Miami Miller School of Medicine
Miami, FL, USA
Chapter 3

Enrique Garcia-Valenzuela MD, PhD
Clinical Assistant Professor
Department of Ophthalmology
University of Illinois Eye and Ear Infirmary
Consulting Staff, Vitreo-Retinal Surgery
Midwest Retina Consultants, SC
Parkside Center
Park Ridge, IL, USA
Chapter 108

Alain Gaudric MD
Professor of Ophthalmology
Hôpital Lariboisière
Paris Diderot University
Paris, France
Chapter 117

Mary Gayed MBChB MRCP(UK)
Academic Clinical Fellow
Rheumatology
Division of Immunity and Infection
Birmingham Medical School
Birmingham, UK
Chapter 80

Mohamed A. Genead MD
Ophthalmologist and Retinal Specialist
Pangere Center for Hereditary Retinal Diseases
The Chicago Lighthouse for People Who Are Blind or Visually Impaired
Chicago, IL, USA
Chapter 43

Heinrich Gerding MD
Professor of Ophthalmology
Department of Ophthalmology
Pallas Clinic
Olten, Switzerland
Chapter 136

Andrea Giani MD
Ophthalmologist, Vitreo-Retinal Service
Eye Clinic
Department of Clinical Science Luigi Sacco
Sacco Hospital
University of Milan
Milan, Italy
Chapter 2

Morton F. Goldberg MD
Joseph E. Green Professor of Ophthalmology
Director Emeritus
Wilmer Ophthalmological Institute
Department of Ophthalmology
Johns Hopkins University School of Medicine
Baltimore, MD, USA
Chapter 57

Dan S. Gombos MD
Associate Professor
Chief, Section of Ophthalmology
Department of Head and Neck Surgery
The University of Texas
MD Anderson Cancer Center
Houston, TX, USA
Chapter 128

Lingam Gopal MS, FRCS
Consultant
Vitreo-retinal Services
Sankara Nethralaya
Medical and Vision Research foundations
Chennai, India
Chapter 109

Caroline Gordon MD, FRCP
Professor of Rheumatology
School of Immunity and Infection
College of Medical and Dental Sciences
The Medical School
University of Birmingham
Birmingham, UK
Chapter 80

Hiroshi Goto MD
Professor and Chairman
Department of Ophthalmology
Tokyo Medical University
Tokyo, Japan.
Chapter 75

Evangelos S. Gragoudas MD
Charles Edward Whitten Professor of Ophthalmology
Harvard Medical School
Director of Retina Service
Massachusetts Eye & Ear Infirmary
Boston, MA, USA
Chapter 146

Maria B. Grant MD
Professor
Department of Pharmacology and Therapeutics
University of Florida, Gainesville
Director of Translational Research
Department of Ophthalmology
Gainesville, FL, USA
Chapter 18

W. Richard Green MD (posthumously)
Former Independent Order of Odd Fellows
Professor of Ophthalmology
Professor of Pathology Eye
Pathology Laboratory
Johns Hopkins University School of Medicine
Baltimore, MD, USA
Chapter 21

Ronald G. Gregg PhD
Professor of Biochemistry and Molecular Biology
Professor of Ophthalmology and Visual Sciences
Director, Center for Genetics and Molecular Medicine
University of Louisville
Louisville, KY, USA
Chapter 15

Zdenek Gregor FRCS (Eng), FRCOphth
Consultant Vitreoretinal Surgeon
Moorfields Eye Hospital
London, UK
Chapter 116

Giovanni Gregori PhD
Assistant Research Professor
Department of Ophthalmology
University of Miami
Miller School of Medicine
Miami, FL, USA
Chapter 3

Kevin Gregory-Evans MD, PhD, FRCS, FRCOphth
Julia Levy BC Leadership Chair in Macular Research
Professor in Ophthalmology
Department of Ophthalmology and Visual Sciences
University of British Columbia Eye Care Centre
Vancouver, BC, Canada
Chapter 40

Seanna Grob MD, MAS
Clinical Research Fellow
Department of Ophthalmology
Shiley Eye Center
University of California, San Diego
La Jolla, CA, USA
Chapter 46

Carl Groenewald MD
Consultant Ophthalmologist
St Paul's Eye Unit
Royal Liverpool University Hospital
Liverpool, UK
Chapter 147

Hans E. Grossniklaus MD, MBA
F. Phinizy Calhoun Jr Professor of Ophthalmology
Director, L.F. Montgomery Pathology Laboratory
Director, Ocular Oncology and Pathology Service
Department of Ophthalmology
Emory University School of Medicine
Atlanta, GA, USA
Chapter 142

Sandeep Grover MD
Assistant Professor of Ophthalmology
Director, Inherited Retinal Diseases & Electrophysiology
University of Florida College of Medicine
Jacksonville, FL, USA
Chapter 43

Vamsi K. Gullapalli MD, PhD
Associate
Coastal Bend Retina
Corpus Christi, TX, USA
Chapter 125

Aditi Gupta MS, DNB
Clinical Fellow
Department of Vitreoretinal Services
Sankara Nethralaya
Chennai, India
Chapter 50

Rudolf F. Guthoff MD
Head
University Eye Department
University of Rostock
Rostock, Germany
Chapter 9

Paul Hahn MD, PhD
Fellow
Vitreoretinal Surgery
Department of Ophthalmology
Duke Eye Center
Durham, NC, USA
Chapter 54

Julia A. Haller MD
Ophthalmologist-in-Chief
Professor and Chair
Department of Ophthalmology
Jefferson Medical College
William Tasman, MD Endowed Chair in Ophthalmology
Wills Eye Institute
Philadelphia, PA, USA
Chapter 56

J. William Harbour MD
Director, Center for Ocular Oncology
Assistant Professor of Ophthalmology
Washington University School of Medicine
St Louis, MO, USA
Chapter 128

Christos Haritoglou MD
Professor
Department of Ophthalmology
Ludwig Maximilians University
Munich, Germany
Chapter 127

Mary E. Hartnett MD, FACS
Associate Professor of Ophthalmology
Department of Ophthalmology
University of North Carolina
Chapel Hill, NC, USA
Chapter 95

Barbara S. Hawkins PhD
Professor Emeritus
Professor of Ophthalmology, School of Medicine
Professor of Epidemiology, Bloomberg School of Public Health
Johns Hopkins University
Baltimore, MD, USA
Chapter 70, Chapter 94, Chapter 150

Shikun He MD
Associate Professor
Department of Ophthalmology
Doheny Eye Institute
University of Southern California
Los Angeles, CA, USA
Chapter 33

Martina C. Herwig MD
Professor, Department of Ophthalmology
Emory University School of Medicine
Atlanta, GA, USA
Professor, Department of Ophthalmology
University of Bonn
Bonn, Germany
Chapter 142

Florian M.A. Heussen MD
Resident Physician
Department of Ophthalmology
Charité – University Medicine Berlin
Berlin, Germany
Chapter 60

David R. Hinton MD
Gavin S. Herbert Professor of Retinal Research
Professor of Pathology and Ophthalmology
Keck School of Medicine
University of Southern California
Los Angeles, CA, USA
Chapter 16, Chapter 35

Frank G. Holz MD, FEBO
Professor and Chairman
Department of Ophthalmology
University of Bonn
Bonn, Germany
Chapter 4

Samuel K. Houston MD
Resident Physician
Department of Ophthalmology
Bascom Palmer Eye Institute
University of Miami Miller School of Medicine
Miami, FL, USA
Chapter 145

Yan-Nian Hui MD
Professor
Department of Ophthalmology
Xijing Hospital
Fourth Military Medical University
Xi'an, PR China
Chapter 97

Mark S. Humayun MD, PhD
Professor of Ophthalmology
Biomedical Engineering, Cell and Neurobiology
Keck School of Medicine
University of Southern California
Associate Director of Research
Doheny Eye Institute
Los Angeles, CA, USA
Chapter 36, Chapter 38, Chapter 126

Yasushi Ikuno MD
Associate Professor
Department of Ophthalmology
Osaka University Graduate School of Medicine
Osaka, Japan
Chapter 68, Chapter 113

David Isaac MD
Assistant Professor
Department of Ophthalmology
Federal University of Goias
Goiânia, GO, Brazil
Chapter 86

Tatsuro Ishibashi MD, PhD
Professor and Chairman
Department of Ophthalmology
Graduate School of Medical Sciences
Kyushu University
Fukuoka City, Japan
Chapter 68

Douglas A. Jabs MD, MBA
Professor and Chair
Department of Ophthalmology
Mount Sinai School of Medicine
New York, NY, USA
Chapter 78

Glenn J. Jaffe MD
Professor of Ophthalmology
Chief, Vitreoretinal Service
Director, Duke Reading Center
Durham, NC, USA
Chapter 79

Lee M. Jampol MD
Louis Feinberg Professor in Ophthalmology
Northwestern University
Chicago, IL, USA
Chapter 76

Leonard Joffe MD, FCS(SA), FRCSEd
Clinical Professor
Department of Ophthalmology
University of Arizona
Tucson, AZ, USA
Chapter 135

Mark Johnson PhD
Professor
Departments of Biomedical Engineering, Mechanical Engineering, and Ophthalmology
Northwestern University
Evanston, IL, USA
Chapter 20

Mark W. Johnson MD
Professor and Director of Retina Service
Department of Ophthalmology and Visual Sciences
Kellogg Eye Center
University of Michigan
Ann Arbor. MI, USA
Chapter 73

Robert N. Johnson MD
Clinical Professor of Ophthalmology
California Pacific Medical Center
San Francisco, CA, USA
Chapter 1

Antonia M. Joussen MD, PhD, FEBO
Professor
Department of Ophthalmology
Charité, University Medicine Berlin
Berlin, Germany
Chapter 28

Karina Julian MD
Senior Instructor
Ophthalmology
Austral University School of Medicine
Buenos Aires, Argentina
Chapter 112

J. Michael Jumper MD
Retina Service Chief
California Pacific Medical Center
San Francisco, CA, USA
Chapter 1

Peter K. Kaiser MD
Professor of Ophthalmology
Cleveland Clinic Lerner College of Medicine
Cleveland, OH, USA
Chapter 53

Anselm Kampik MD
Chairman
Department of Ophthalmology
Ludwig Maximilians University
Munich, Germany
Chapter 127

Robert Katamay MD
Research Fellow
Laboratory of Immunology
National Eye Institute
National Institutes of Health
Bethesda, MD, USA
Chapter 27

Christine N. Kay MD
Assistant Professor
Department of Ophthalmology
University of Florida
Gainesville, FL, USA
Chapter 6

Pearse A. Keane MD, MRCOphth, MRCSI
Clinical Lecturer in Ophthalmic Translational Research
NIHR Biomedical Research Centre for Ophthalmology
Moorfields Eye Hospital NHS Foundation Trust
UCL Institute of Ophthalmology
London, UK
Chapter 5

M. Cristina Kenney MD, PhD
Professor
Director of Research
Gavin Herbert Eye Institute
Ophthalmology Research Laboratories
University of California, Irvine
Irvine, CA, USA
Chapter 32

Khizer R. Khaderi MD
Neuro-Ophthalmology Fellow
Doheny Eye Institute
Keck School of Medicine
University of Southern California
Los Angeles, CA, USA
Chapter 93

Mohamad A. Khodair MD, PhD
Lecturer
Robertwood Johnson Medical School
New Brunswick, NJ, USA
Chapter 125

Ivana K. Kim MD
Assistant Professor, Department of Ophthalmology
Harvard Medical School, Retina Service
Massachusetts Eye and Ear Infirmary
Boston, MA, USA
Chapter 146

Tae Wan Kim MD, PhD
Assistant Professor
Department of Ophthalmology
Seoul National University
Seoul, South Korea
Chapter 123

Bernd Kirchhof MD, PhD
Professor and Chairman
Department of Ophthalmology, University of Cologne
Cologne, Germany
Chapter 95, Chapter 121

Barbara E.K. Klein MD, MPH
Professor
Department of Ophthalmology and Visual Sciences
University of Wisconsin, School of Medicine and Public Health
Madison, WI, USA
Chapter 45

Ronald Klein MD MPH
Professor
Department of Ophthalmology and Visual Sciences
University of Wisconsin School of Medicine and Public Health
Madison, WI, USA
Chapter 45

Lazaros Konstantinidis MD
Professor
Vitreoretinal Department
St Paul's Eye Unit
Royal Liverpool University Hospital
Liverpool, UK
Chapter 118

Igor Kozak MD, PhD
Assistant Clinical Professor
Department of Ophthalmology
Shiley Eye Center
University of California, San Diego
La Jolla, CA, USA
Chapter 81

Baruch D. Kuppermann MD
Professor of Ophthalmology and Biomedical Engineering
University of California, Irvine
The Gavin Herbert Eye Institute
University of California, Irvine
Irvine, CA, USA
Chapter 38

Leanne T. Labriola DO
Clinical Assistant Professor of Ophthalmology
Medical Retina Service
University of Pittsburgh School of Medicine
Pittsburgh, PA, USA
Chapter 9

Timothy Y. Lai MD, FRCS, FRCOphth
Honorary Clinical Associate Professor
Department of Ophthalmology and Visual Sciences
The Chinese University of Hong Kong
Hong Kong
Chapter 72

Dennis S. Lam MD, FRCOphth
S.H. Ho Professor and Chairman
Department of Ophthalmology and Visual Sciences
The Chinese University of Hong Kong
Hong Kong
Chapter 72

Linda A. Lam MD
Assistant Professor of Ophthalmology
Doheny Eye Institute
Keck School of Medicine
University of Southern California
Los Angeles, CA, USA
Chapter 69

Maurice B. Landers III MD
Professor of Ophthalmology
Department of Ophthalmology
University of North Carolina
Chapel Hill, NC, USA
Chapter 95

Anne Marie Lane MPH
Instructor in Ophthalmology
Harvard Medical School
Research Associate
Retina Service
Massachusetts Eye & Ear Infirmary
Boston, MA, USA
Chapter 146

Erin B. Lavik ScD
Elmer Lindseth Associate Professor of Biomedical Engineering
Case Western Reserve University
Cleveland, OH, USA
Chapter 38

James F. Leary PhD
SVM Professor of Nanomedicine
Professor of Basic Medical Sciences and Biomedical Engineering
Department of Basic Medical Sciences
Weldon School of Biomedical Engineering
Purdue University
West Lafayette, IN, USA
Chapter 36

Sun Young Lee MD, PhD
Clinical Instructor
Doheny Eye Institute
Keck School of Medicine
University of Southern California
Los Angeles, CA, USA
Chapter 98

Thomas C. Lee MD
Director, Retina Institute
The Vision Center
Children's Hospital Los Angeles
Associate Professor of Ophthalmology
Director, Surgical Retina Fellowship
Doheny Eye Institute
Keck School of Medicine
University of Southern California
Los Angeles, CA, USA
Chapter 61, Chapter 128

Loh-Shan B. Leung MD
Postdoctoral Fellow
Department of Ophthalmology
Stanford University
Palo Alto, CA, USA
Chapter 67

David A. Lewis MD
Ocular Pathology Fellow
Department of Ophthalmology
University of Wisconsin
Madison, WI, USA
Chapter 138

Geoffrey P. Lewis PhD
Research Biologist
Neuroscience Research Institute
University of California, Santa Barbara
Santa Barbara, CA, USA
Chapter 29

Anita Leys MD, PhD
Professor of Ophthalmology
Department of Medical Retina
Department of Ophthalmology
Catholic University of Leuven
Leuven, Belgium
Chapter 58

Xiaoxin Li MD
Professor of Ophthalmology
People's Eye Centre of People's Hospital
Peking University
Beijing, PR China
Chapter 71

Sandra Liakopoulos MD
Professor
Department of Ophthalmology
University of Cologne
Cologne, Germany
Chapter 60

Chang-Ping Lin MD, PhD
Professor
Department of Ophthalmology
Changhua Christian Hospital
Kaohsiung, Changhua, Taiwan
Chapter 96

Phoebe Lin MD, PhD
Vitreoretinal Surgical Fellow
Department of Ophthalmology
Duke University
Durham, NC, USA
Chapter 79

David T. Liu FRCOphth, FRCS, MSc
Associate Professor
Department of Ophthalmology and Visual Sciences
The Chinese University of Hong Kong
Hong Kong
Chapter 72

Nikolas J.S. London MD
Fellow in Vitreoretinal Surgery
Wills Eye Institute
Philadelphia, PA, USA
Chapter 56

Brandon J. Lujan MD
Associate
West Coast Retina
San Francisco, CA, USA
Chapter 1

Yan Luo MD, PhD
Professor
State Key Laboratory of Ophthalmology
Zhongshan Ophthalmic Center
Sun Yat-sen University
Guangzhou, PR China
Chapter 41

Gerard A. Lutty PhD
G. Edward and G. Britton Durell Professor of Ophthalmology
Wilmer Ophthalmological Institute
Johns Hopkins Hospital
Baltimore, MD, USA
Chapter 18, Chapter 57

Robert MacLaren FRCOph, MD, PhD
Nuffield Laboratory of Ophthalmology
University of Oxford
John Radcliffe Hospital
Oxford, UK
Chapter 121

Steven Madreperla MD
Associate
Retina Associates of New Jersey
Teaneck, NJ, USA
Chapter 125

Albert M. Maguire MD
Associate Professor of Ophthalmology
Department of Ophthalmology
Scheie Eye Institute
University of Pennsylvania Perelman School of Medicine
Investigator, Center for Cellular and Molecular Therapeutics
Retina Specialist, Pediatric Ophthalmology
The Children's Hospital of Philadelphia
Philadelphia, PA, USA
Chapter 34

Martin A. Mainster PhD, MD, FRCOphth
Luther and Ardis Fry Professor Emeritus of Ophthalmology
University of Kansas School of Medicine
Kansas City, KS, USA
Chapter 90

Nancy C. Mansfield (posthumously)
Family Counselor and Patient Ombudsman
The Retinoblastoma Centre
Children's Hospital of Los Angeles
Los Angeles, CA, USA
Chapter 128

Arnold M. Markoe MD
Professor and Chairman Emeritus
Department of Radiation Oncology
University of Miami, Miller School of Medicine
Miami, FL, USA
Chapter 145

Michael F. Marmor MD
Professor of Ophthalmology
Stanford University School of Medicine
Byers Eye Institute at Stanford
Palo Alto, CA, USA
Chapter 19

Daniel F. Martin MD
Barbara & A. Malachi Mixon III Institute
Chair of Ophthalmology
Chairman
Cole Eye Institute Cleveland Clinic
Cleveland, OH, USA
Chapter 67

Stephen C. Massey PhD
Elizabeth Morford Chair and Research Director
Ophthalmology and Visual Sciences
The University of Texas Medical School at Houston
Houston, TX, USA
Chapter 15

Maureen A. McCall PhD
Professor
Department of Ophthalmology and Visual Sciences
University of Louisville
Louisville, KY, USA
Chapter 15

Tara A. McCannel MD, PhD
Assistant Professor
Director of Ophthalmic Oncology Center
Department of Ophthalmology
The Jules Stein Eye Institute
University of California, Los Angeles
Los Angeles, CA, USA
Chapter 139, Chapter 140

J. Allen McCutchan MD, MSc
Professor of Medicine
Department of Medicine
Division of Infectious Diseases
University of California, San Diego
La Jolla, CA, USA
Chapter 81

H. Richard McDonald MD
Clinical Professor of Ophthalmology
California Pacific Medical Center
Director, Vitreoretinal Fellowship Program
California Pacific Medical Center
Director, San Francisco Retina Foundation
San Francisco, CA, USA
Chapter 1

Milap P. Mehta MD, MS
Oculoplastics Fellow
Department of Ophthalmology
Cole Eye Institute
Cleveland Clinic
Cleveland, OH, USA
Chapter 144

Petra Meier MD
Associate Professor
Department of Ophthalmology
University of Leipzig
Leipzig, Germany
Chapter 115

Shannath Merbs MD, PhD
Associate Professor of Ophthalmology and Oncology
Wilmer Eye Institute
Johns Hopkins University School of Medicine
Baltimore, MD, USA
Chapter 141

Travis A. Meredith MD
Sterling A. Barrett Distinguished Professor
Chairman
Department of Ophthalmology
University of North Carolina
Chapel Hill, NC, USA
Chapter 122

Carsten H. Meyer MD
Professor of Ophthalmology
Department of Ophthalmology
Pallas Clinic
Olten, Switzerland
Chapter 136

William F. Mieler MD
Professor and Vice-Chairman
Director, Residency Training
Department of Ophthalmology and Visual Sciences
University of Illinois at Chicago
Chicago, IL, USA
Chapter 89

Joan W. Miller MD
Chair & Henry Willard Williams Professor of Ophthalmology
Department of Ophthalmology
Harvard Medical School
Chief of Ophthalmology
Massachusetts Eye and Ear Infirmary
Massachusetts General Hospital
Boston, MA, USA
Chapter 26

Rukhsana G. Mirza MD
Assistant Professor in Ophthalmology
Northwestern University
Chicago, IL USA
Chapter 76

Sayak K. Mitter MTech
Graduate Student
Department of Anatomy and Cell Biology
University of Florida
Gainesville, FL, USA
Chapter 24

Robert A. Mittra MD
Vitreoretinal Surgeon
Vitreoretinal Surgery
Minneapolis, MN, USA
Chapter 89

Yozo Miyake MD, PhD
Chairman of the Board of Directors
Aichi Medical University
Aichi, Japan
Chapter 8

Carlo Montemagno PhD
Dean
College of Engineering and Applied Science
Geier Professor of Engineering Education
University of Cincinnati
College of Engineering
Cincinnati, OH, USA
Chapter 36

Ala Moshiri MD, PhD
Retina Fellow
Department of Ophthalmology
Wilmer Eye Institute
Johns Hopkins University School of Medicine
Baltimore, MD, USA
Chapter 92

Prithvi Mruthyunjaya MD
Assistant Professor of Ophthalmology
Department of Vitreoretinal Surgery and Ocular Oncology
Duke University Eye Center
Durham, NC, USA
Chapter 54, Chapter 153

Cristina Muccioli MD, PhD
Associate Professor of Ophthalmology
Department of Ophthalmology
Federal University of São Paulo
São Paulo, Brazil
Chapter 85

Robert F. Mullins PhD
Associate Professor
Department of Ophthalmology and Visual Sciences
The University of Iowa
Iowa City, IA, USA
Chapter 42

Toshinori Murata MD, PhD
Professor and Chairman
Department of Ophthalmology
School of Medicine
Shinshu University
Matsumoto Nagano, Japan
Chapter 68

A. Linn Murphree MD
Professor of Ophthalmology and Pediatrics
Keck School of Medicine
University of Southern California
Los Angeles, CA, USA
Chapter 128

Robert P. Murphy MD
Private Practitioner
Retina Group of Washington
Fairfax, VA, USA
Chapter 52

Philip I. Murray PhD, FRCP, FRCS, FRCOphth
Professor of Ophthalmology
Academic Unit of Ophthalmology
School of Immunity and Infection
College of Medical and Dental Sciences
University of Birmingham
Birmingham and Midland Eye Centre
Sandwell and West Birmingham Hospitals NHS Trust
City Hospital
Birmingham, UK
Chapter 80

Timothy G. Murray MD, MBA
Professor
Department of Ophthalmology
Bascom Palmer Eye Institute
Miami, FL, USA
Chapter 145

Manish Nagpal, MS, DO, FRCS(UK)
Vitreoretinal Consultant
Retina Foundation
Shahibag, Ahmedabad
Gujarat, India
Chapter 107

Perumalsamy Namperumalsamy MS, FAMS
Professor of Ophthalmology
Retina-Vitreous Service
Aravind Eye Hospital and Postgraduate Institute of Ophthalmology
Madurai, India
Chapter 82, Chapter 83

Sumit K. Nanda MD
Clinical Associate Professor
Department of Ophthalmology
University of Oklahoma
Oklahoma City, OK, USA
Chapter 108

Quan Dong Nguyen MD, MSc
Associate Professor of Ophthalmology
Wilmer Eye Institute
Johns Hopkins University School of Medicine
Baltimore, MD, USA
Chapter 78, Chapter 124

Robert B. Nussenblatt MD, MPH
Chief
Laboratory of Immunology
National Eye Institute
Associate Director (Clinical Director)
NIH Center for Human Immunology
Acting Scientific Director
National Center for Complementary and Alternative Medicine
National Institutes of Health
Bethesda, MD, USA
Chapter 27, Chapter 77

Kean T. Oh MD
Assistant Professor of Ophthalmology
Department of Ophthalmology
University of North Carolina
Chapel Hill, NC, USA
Chapter 95

Masahito Ohji MD
Professor and Chairman
Department of Ophthalmology
Shiga University of Medical Science
Otsu, Japan
Chapter 113

Kyoko Ohno-Matsui MD
Associate Professor
Department of Ophthalmology and Visual Sciences
Tokyo Medical and Dental University
Tokyo, Japan
Chapter 68

Daniel Palanker PhD
Associate Professor
Department of Ophthalmology and Hansen Experimental Physics Laboratory
Stanford University
Stanford, CA, USA
Chapter 39

Purnima S. Patel MD
Assistant Professor of Ophthalmology
Emory University School of Medicine
Atlanta Veterans Affairs Medical Center
Atlanta, GA, USA
Chapter 51

Anna C. Pavlick MD
Associate Professor
New York University Comprehensive Cancer Center
New York University School of Medicine
New York, NY, USA
Chapter 149

David M. Peereboom MD
Associate Professor of Medicine
Cleveland Clinic Lerner College of Medicine
The Rose Ella Burkhardt Brain Tumor and Neuro-Oncology Center
Solid Tumor Oncology
Cleveland, OH, USA
Chapter 156

Mark E. Pennesi MD, PhD
Assistant Professor of Ophthalmology
Casey Eye Institute
Oregon Health and Science University
Portland, OR, USA
Chapter 40

Jay S. Pepose MD, PhD
Professor of Clinical Ophthalmology and Visual Sciences
Washington University School of Medicine
St Louis, MO, USA
Chapter 88

Julian D. Perry MD
Director
Orbital and Oculoplastic Surgery
Cole Eye Institute
Cleveland Clinic Foundation,
Cleveland, OH, USA
Chapter 144

Carmen A. Puliafito MD, MBA
Dean
Keck School of Medicine
May S and John Hooval Dean's Chair in Medicine
Professor of Ophthalmology and Health Management
Doheny Eye Institute
University of Southern California
Los Angeles, CA
Voluntary Professor of Ophthalmology
Bascom Palmer Eye Institute
University of Miami
Miami, FL, USA
Chapter 3

Polly A. Quiram MD, PhD
Pediatric Retina Specialist
Vitreoretinal Surgery
Minneapolis, MN, USA
Chapter 137

Rajiv Raman MS, DNB
Consultant
Department of Vitreo-Retinal Services
Sankara Nethralaya
Chennai, India
Chapter 50

Rajeev S. Ramchandran MD
Assistant Professor
Retinal Services
Flaum Eye Institute
University of Rochester Medical Center
Rochester, NY, USA
Chapter 12

Haripriya Vittal Rao PhD
Chennai, India
Chapter 24

Narsing A. Rao MD, PhD
Preceptor of Ophthalmology and Pathology
Universidade Federal de Minas Gerais
Belo Horizonte, MG, Brazil
Chapter 74, Chapter 75, Chapter 84

P. Kumar Rao MD
Associate Professor of Ophthalmology and Visual Sciences
Department of Ophthalmology
School of Medicine
Washington University in St. Louis
St. Louis, MO, USA
Chapter 75

Sivakumar R. Rathinam MNAMS, PhD
Professor of Ophthalmology
Head of Uveitis Service
Uveitis Service
Aravind Eye Hospital & Postgraduate Institute of Ophthalmology
Madurai, India
Chapter 82

Franco M. Recchia MD
Associate Professor of Ophthalmology and Visual Sciences
Chief, Retina Division
Director, Fellowship in Vitreoretinal Diseases and Surgery
Vanderbilt Eye Institute
Vanderbilt University School of Medicine
Nashville, TN, USA
Chapter 110

Kristin J. Redmond MD
Instructor
Department of Radiation Oncology and Molecular Radiation Sciences
Johns Hopkins University School of Medicine
Baltimore, MD, USA
Chapter 151

Thomas A. Reh PhD
Professor
Department of Biological Structure
Institute for Stem Cells and Regenerative Medicine
University of Washington
Seattle, WA, USA
Chapter 13

Andreas Reichenbach MD
Full Professor
Department of Pathophysiology of Neuroglia
Paul Flechsig Institute of Brain Research
University of Leipzig
Leipzig, Germany
Chapter 17

Robert Ritch MD
Shelley and Steven Einhorn Distinguished Chair
Surgeon Director and Chief
Glaucoma Services
The New York Eye and Ear Infirmary
New York, NY
Professor of Ophthalmology
New York Medical College
Valhalla, NY, USA
Chapter 36

Philip J. Rosenfeld MD, PhD
Professor of Ophthalmology
Bascom Palmer Eye Institute
Miami, FL, USA
Chapter 3, Chapter 67

Gary S. Rubin PhD
Helen Keller Professor of Ophthalmology
UCL Institute of Ophthalmology
London, UK
Chapter 11

Humberto Ruiz-Garcia MD
Retina Specialist
Clinica Santa Lucia
Universidad de Guadalajara
Guadalajara, Mexico
Chapter 5

Stephen J. Ryan MD
President, Doheny Eye Institute
Professor, University of Southern California
Los Angeles CA, USA
Chapter 98

SriniVas R. Sadda MD
Associate Professor of Ophthalmology
Doheny Eye Institute
Associate Professor
Department of Ophthalmology
Keck School of Medicine
University of Southern California
Los Angeles, CA, USA
Chapter 5, Chapter 51, Chapter 60

Alfredo A. Sadun MD, PhD
Professor of Ophthalmology
Doheny Eye Institute
Keck School of Medicine
University of Southern California
Los Angeles, CA, USA
Chapter 93

Taiji Sakamoto MD, PhD
Professor and Chair
Department of Ophthalmology
Kagoshima University Graduate School of Medical and Dental Sciences
Kagoshima, Japan
Chapter 68

Alapakkam P. Sampath PhD
Associate Professor
Zilkha Neurogenetic Institute
Department of Physiology and Biophysics
University of Southern California School of Medicine
Los Angeles, CA, USA
Chapter 14

Andrew P. Schachat MD
Vice Chairman
Cole Eye Institute
Cleveland Clinic Foundation
Cleveland, OH, USA
Chapter 70, Chapter 130, Chapter 134, Chapter 150, Chapter 151, Chapter 155, Chapter 156

Steffen Schmitz-Valckenberg MD, FEBO
Professor
Department of Ophthalmology
University of Bonn
Bonn, Germany
Chapter 4

Stephen G. Schwartz MD, MBA
Associate Professor of Clinical Ophthalmology
Department of Ophthalmology
Bascom Palmer Eye Institute
University of Miami Miller School of Medicine
Medical Director
Bascom Palmer Eye Institute at Naples
Naples, FL, USA
Chapter 87

Adrienne W. Scott MD
Assistant Professor of Ophthalmology
Wilmer Eye Institute
Baltimore, MD, USA
Chapter 57

Jerry Sebag MD, FACS, FRCOphth, FARVO
Professor of Clinical Ophthalmology
VMR Institute
Huntington Beach, CA, USA
Chapter 21

Johanna M. Seddon MD, ScM
Professor of Ophthalmology
Tufts University School of Medicine
Director of Ophthalmic Epidemiology & Genetics Services
Turfs Medical Center,
Boston, MA, USA
Chapter 63, Chapter 139, Chapter 140

H. Nida Sen MD, MHSc
Director
Uveitis and Ocular Immunology Fellowship Program
National Eye Institute
National Institutes of Health
Bethesda, MD
Associate Clinical Professor
Department of Ophthalmology
The George Washington University
Washington DC, USA
Chapter 77

Yasir Jamal Sepah MBBS
Research Fellow
Retinal Imaging Research and Reading Center
Wilmer Eye Institute
Johns Hopkins University School of Medicine
Baltimore, MD, USA
Chapter 78

Sanjay Sharma BSc, MD, FRCS, MSc (Epid), MBA
Professor of Ophthalmology and Epidemiology
Director, Cost Effective Ocular Health Policy Unit
Queen's University
Kingston, Ontario, Canada
Chapter 59, Chapter 131, Chapter 152

Tarun Sharma MS, FRCS Ed, MBA
Director
Shri Bhagwan Mahavir Vitreoretinal Services
Sankara Nethralaya
Chennai, India
Chapter 50, Chapter 109

Shwu-Jiuan Sheu MD
Chair
Department of Ophthalmology
Kaohsiung Veterans General Hospital
Professor
National Yang-Ming University
Taipei, Taiwan
Chapter 102

Carol L. Shields MD
Professor of Ophthalmology
Thomas Jefferson University Hospital
Co-Director, Oncology Service
Wills Eye Institute
Philadelphia, PA, USA
Chapter 56, Chapter 132, Chapter 135, Chapter 143, Chapter 152

Jerry A. Shields MD
Director
Oncology Service
Wills Eye Institute
Professor of Ophthalmology
Thomas Jefferson University Hospital
Philadelphia, PA, USA
Chapter 132, Chapter 135, Chapter 143, Chapter 152

Kei Shinoda MD, PhD
Associate Professor
Department of Ophthalmology
Teikyo University School of Medicine
Tokyo, Japan
Chapter 8

Dhananjay Shukla MS, MAMS
Professor of Ophthalmology
Consultant, Retina-Vitreous Service
Aravind Eye Hospital and Postgraduate Institute
Tamil Nadu, India
Chapter 83

Paul A. Sieving MD, PhD
Director
National Eye Institute
National Institutes of Health
Bethesda, MD, USA
Chapter 37

Paolo A.S. Silva MD
Instructor in Ophthalmology
Harvard Medical School
Associate Surgeon
Brigham and Women's Hospital
Attending Staff
Beth Israel Deaconess Medical Center
Staff Ophthalmologist
Assistant Chief of Telemedicine
Beetham Eye Institute
Joslin Diabetes Center
Boston, MA, USA
Chapter 48

Claudio Silveira MD, PhD
Professor of Ophthalmology
Clinica Silveira
Erechim, RS, Brazil
Chapter 85

Arun D. Singh MD
Professor of Ophthalmology
Director, Department of Ophthalmic Oncology
Cole Eye Institute, Cleveland Clinic Foundation
Cleveland, OH, USA
Chapter 144, Chapter 156

Sylvia B. Smith PhD, FARVO
Professor of Cellular Biology/Anatomy, Ophthalmology and Graduate Studies
Basic Science Co-Director, Vision Discovery Institute
Medical College of Georgia
Augusta, GA, USA
Chapter 23

Wendy M. Smith MD
Clinical Fellow
Uveitis and Ocular Immunology
National Eye Institute
National Institutes of Health
Bethesda, MD, USA
Chapter 25

Lucia Sobrin MD, MPH
Assistant Professor of Ophthalmology
Massachusetts Eye and Ear Infirmary
Harvard Medical School
Boston, MA, USA
Chapter 63

Akrit Sodhi MD, PhD
Assistant Professor
Retina Division
Wilmer Eye Institute
Johns Hopkins University
Baltimore, MD, USA
Chapter 141

Elliott H. Sohn MD
Assistant Professor
Department of Ophthalmology
University of Iowa Hospitals and Clinics
Iowa City, IA, USA
Chapter 42

Gisèle Soubrane MD, PhD, FEBO, FARVO
Consultant Professor
Department of Ophthalmology
University of Paris-East Créteil Val de Marne
Créteil, Paris, France
Chapter 30

Leigh Spielberg MD
Ophthalmology Resident
Rotterdam Eye Hospital
Rotterdam, The Netherlands
Chapter 58

Sunil K. Srivastava MD
Staff Physician
Cole Eye Institute
Cleveland Clinic Foundation
Cleveland, OH, USA
Chapter 133

Oliver Stachs PhD
Physicist
Department of Ophthalmology
Faculty of Medicine
University of Rostock
Rostock, Germany
Chapter 9

Giovanni Staurenghi MD
Professor of Ophthalmology
Chairman Eye Clinic
Department of Clinical Science Luigi Sacco
Sacco Hospital
University of Milan
Milan, Italy
Chapter 2

Paul Sternberg Jr MD
G.W. Hale Professor and Chair
Vanderbilt Eye Institute
Associate Dean for Clinical Affairs
Vanderbilt School of Medicine
Assistant Vice Chancellor for Adult Health Affairs
Vanderbilt Medical Center
Nashville, TN, USA
Chapter 22, Chapter 110, Chapter 129

Edwin M. Stone MD, PhD
Professor
Department of Ophthalmology
University of Iowa
Iowa City, IA, USA
Chapter 42

Ilene K. Sugino MA
Principal Research Associate
Institute of Ophthalmology and Visual Sciences
New Jersey Medical School
University of Medicine and Dentistry
Newark, NJ, USA
Chapter 125

Lori S. Sullivan PhD
Faculty Associate, Human Genetics Center
Division of Epidemiology
Human Genetics and Environmental Sciences
School of Public Health
The University of Texas Health Science Center
Houston, TX, USA
Chapter 31

Paul Sullivan MBBS, MD, FRCOphth
Consultant Ophthalmic Surgeon
Director of Education
Moorfields Eye Hospital
London, UK
Chapter 100

Jennifer K. Sun MD, MPH
Assistant Professor of Ophthalmology
Harvard Medical School
Chief, Center for Clinical Eye Research and Trials
Staff Ophthalmologist
Beetham Eye Institute
Joslin Diabetes Center
Boston, MA, USA
Chapter 48

Janet S. Sunness MD
Medical Director
Richard E. Hoover Low Vision Rehabilitation Services
Greater Baltimore Medical Center
Baltimore, MD, USA
Chapter 92

Ramin Tadayoni MD, PhD
Professor
Department of Ophthalmology,
Hôpital Lariboisière
Paris, France
Chapter 117

Shibo Tang MD, PhD
Professor
Department of Retina
Zhongshan Ophthalmic Center
Sun Yat-Sen University
Guangdong, PR China
Chapter 41

Hiroko Terasaki MD, PhD
Professor and Chair
Department of Ophthalmology
Nagoya University Graduate School of Medicine
Nagoya, Japan
Chapter 102

Matthew A. Thomas MD
Clinical Professor of Ophthalmology
The Retina Institute
Washington University
St Louis, MO, USA
Chapter 119

John T. Thompson MD
Assistant Professor
The Wilmer Institute
Johns Hopkins University
Baltimore, MD, USA
Chapter 99

Gabriele Thumann MD
Professor
Department of Ophthalmology
RWTH Aachen University
Aachen, Germany
Chapter 16

Cynthia A. Toth MD
Professor
Department of Ophthalmology and Biomedical Engineering
Duke Universtiy
Durham, NC, USA
Chapter 120

Michael T. Trese MD
Clinical Professor of Biomedical Sciences
Eye Research Institute
Oakland University
Rochester, MI
Chief of Pediatric and Adult Vitreoretinal Surgery
William Beaumont Hospital
Royal Oak, MI, USA
Chapter 114

Julie H. Tsai MD
Assistant Professor
Department of Ophthalmology
SUNY-Stony Brook
Stony Brook, NY, USA
Chapter 84

Mary E. Turell MD
Ophthalmic Oncology Fellow
Cole Eye Institute
Cleveland Clinic
Cleveland, OH, USA
Chapter 156

Patricia L. Turner MD
Clinical Associate Professor of Ophthalmology
University of Kansas School of Medicine
Kansas City, KS, USA
Chapter 90

Nitin Udar PhD
Project Scientist
Department of Ophthalmology
University of California, Irvine
Irvine, CA, USA
Chapter 32

J. Niklas Ulrich MD
Assistant Professor
Department of Ophthalmology
University of North Carolina at Chapel Hill
Chapel Hill, NC, USA
Chapter 122

Russell N. Van Gelder MD, PhD
Boyd K. Bucey Memorial Chair
Professor and Chair
Department of Ophthalmology
Adjunct Professor
Department of Biological Structure
University of Washington
Seattle, WA, USA
Chapter 88

Jan C. van Meurs MD, PhD
Professor
The Rotterdam Eye Hospital and Erasmus University
Rotterdam, The Netherlands
Chapter 121

Daniel Vítor Vasconcelos-Santos MD, PhD
Preceptor of Ophthalmology and Pathology
Universidade Federal de Minas Gerais
Belo Horizonte, MG, Brazil
Chapter 74

Demetrios G. Vavvas MD, PhD
Chief Resident in Ophthalmology
Massachusetts Eye and Ear Infirmary
Massachusetts General Hospital
Boston, MA, USA
Chapter 26

G. Atma Vemulakonda MD
Assistant Professor
Vitreoretinal Surgery and Disease
Department of Ophthalmology
University of Washington
Seattle, WA, USA
Chapter 88

Hao Wang MD
Ophthalmologist and Vitreoretinal Specialist
Capital Region Retina
Albany, NY, USA
Chapter 125

Yusheng Wang MD, PhD
Professor
Department of Ophthalmology
Xijing Hospital
Fourth Military Medical University
Xi'an, PR China
Chapter 16, Chapter 97

James D. Weiland PhD
Associate Professor
Ophthalmology and Biomedical Engineering
University of Southern California
Los Angeles, CA, USA
Chapter 126

Richard G. Weleber MD, FACMG
Professor of Ophthalmology and Molecular and Medical Genetics
Casey Eye Institute
Department of Ophthalmology
Oregon Health and Science University
Portland, OR, USA
Chapter 40

Moody D. Wharam Jr MD, FACR, FASTRO
Professor of Radiation Oncology
Department of Radiation Oncology and Molecular Radiation Sciences
The Sidney Kimmel Comprehensive Cancer Center
Johns Hopkins CRB II
Baltimore, MD, USA
Chapter 151

Louisa Wickham FRCOphth, MD, MSc
Consultant Vitreoretinal Surgeon
Moorfields Eye Hospital
London, UK
Chapter 29, Chapter 116

Peter Wiedemann MD
Professor of Ophthalmology
Department of Ophthalmology
University of Leipzig, Faculty of Medicine
Leipzig, Germany
Chapter 97, Chapter 115

Henry E. Wiley MD
Staff Clinician
Division of Epidemiology and Clinical Applications
National Eye Institute
National Institutes of Health
Bethesda, MD, USA
Chapter 47

C. P. Wilkinson MD
Chairman
Department of Ophthalmology
Greater Baltimore Medical Center
Professor, Department of Ophthalmology
Johns Hopkins University
Baltimore, MD, USA
Chapter 106

David J. Wilson MD
Thiele-Petti Chair
Department of Ophthalmology
Director, Casey Eye Institute
Oregon Health and Science University
Portland, OR, USA
Chapter 154

Thomas J. Wolfensberger MD, PD, MER
Associate Professor
Vitreoretinal Department
Jules Gonin Eye Hospital
University of Lausanne
Lausanne, Switzerland
Chapter 28, Chapter 118

David Wong MBChB (Liverpool), FRCS (Eng), FRCP (UK), FRCOphth
Chair Professor
Eye Institute
The University of Hong Kong
Hong Kong
Chapter 104

Ian Y. Wong MBBS (HKU), MMed (Singapore), MRCS (Edinburgh), FCOphthHK, FHKAM (Oph)
Assistant Professor
Eye Institute
The University of Hong Kong
Hong Kong
Chapter 104

Tien Yin Wong MD, PhD
Director
Singapore Eye Research Institute
Professor
Department of Ophthalmology
National University Health System
Kent Ridge, Singapore
Chapter 49

David M. Wu MD, PhD
Clinical Instructor
Doheny Eye Institute
Keck School of Medicine
University of Southern California
Los Angeles, CA, USA
Chapter 44

Yanors Yandiev MD
Professor
Department of Ophthalmology and Eye Hospital
University of Leipzig
Leipzig, Germany
Chapter 97

Chang-Hao Yang MD, PhD, EMBA
Associate Professor of Ophthalmology
Department of Ophthalmology
National Taiwan University Hospital
Taipei, Taiwan
Chapter 96

Chung-May Yang MD
Professor
Department of Ophthalmology
National Taiwan University Hospital
National Taiwan University College of Medicine
Taipei, Taiwan
Chapter 96

Lawrence A. Yannuzzi MD
Professor of Clinical Ophthalmology
Columbia University Medical School
Vice-Chairman, Director
Retinal Research Center
Manhattan Eye, Ear and Throat Hospital
President of the Macula Foundation Inc.
New York, NY, USA
Chapter 55

Miho Yasuda MD
Assistant Professor
Department of Ophthalmology
Graduate School of Medical Sciences
Kyushu University
Fukuoka, Japan
Chapter 68

Po-Ting Yeh MD
Lecturer
Department of Ophthalmology
National Taiwan University College of Medicine
Taipei, Taiwan
Chapter 96

Zohar Yehoshua MD, MHA
Assistant Research Professor
Department of Ophthalmology
University of Miami
Miller School of Medicine
Miami, FL, USA
Chapter 3

Glenn Yiu MD, PhD
Clinical Fellow in Ophthalmology
Department of Ophthalmology
Massachusetts Eye and Ear Infirmary
Harvard Medical School
Boston, MA, USA
Chapter 33

Young Hee Yoon MD, PhD
Professor and Chair
Department of Ophthalmology
Asan Medical Center
University of Ulsan College of Medicine
Seoul, South Korea
Chapter 102

Hyeong Gon Yu MD, PhD
Professor
Department of Ophthalmology
Seoul National University
Seoul, South Korea
Chapter 123

Alex Yuan MD, PhD
Ophthalmologist
Cole Eye Institute
Cleveland Clinic
Cleveland, OH, USA
Chapter 53

Marco A. Zarbin MD, PhD
Alfonse A. Cinotti, MD/Lions Eye Research Professor
Chair
Institute of Ophthalmology and Visual Science
New Jersey Medical School
Newark, NJ, USA
Chapter 36, Chapter 67, Chapter 125

Jun Jun Zhang MD
Professor
Department of Ophthalmology
West China Hospital, Sichuan University
Chengdu, PR China
Chapter 46

Kang Zhang MD, PhD
Professor of Ophthalmology and Human Genetics
Director, Institute for Genomic Medicine
Department of Ophthalmology
University of California, San Diego
La Jolla, CA
Shiley Eye Center
UCSD Zhang Lab
La Jolla, CA, USA
Chapter 46

Mingwei Zhao MD
Professor of Ophthalmology
Department of Ophthalmology
People's Hospital
Peking University
Beijing, PR China
Chapter 91

Peng Zhou MD, PhD
Attending Ophthalmologist
Department of Ophthalmology
Eye and ENT Hospital
Fudan University
Shanghai, PR China
Chapter 33, Chapter 91

List of Video Contributors

Gary W. Abrams MD
The David Barsky, M.D. Professor and Chair
Department of Ophthalmology
Wayne State University
Director, Kresge Eye Institute
Detroit, MI, USA

Everett Ai MD
Director, Ophthalmic Diagnostic Center
California Pacific Medical Center
San Francisco, CA, USA

J. Fernando Arevalo MD FACS
Chief of Vitreoretinal Division
Senior Academic Consultant
The King Khaled Eye Specialist Hospital
Riyadh, Kingdom of Saudi Arabia
Adjunct Professor of Ophthalmology Wilmer Eye Institute
The Johns Hopkins University
Baltimore, MD, USA

Jose Garcia Arumi MD
Professor
Instituto Microcirugia Ocular
Universidad Autonoma
Barcelona, Spain

G. William Aylward FRCS, FRCOphth, MD
Consultant Vitreoretinal Surgeon
Moorfields Eye Hospital
London, UK

Jean Bennett MD, PhD
F.M. Kirby Professor of Ophthalmology
Professor of Cell and Developmental Biology
Department of Ophthalmology
Scheie Eye Institute
University of Pennsylvania Perelman School of Medicine
Research Scientist
Center for Cellular and Molecular Therapeutics
The Children's Hospital of Philadelphia
Philadelphia, PA, USA

Susanne Binder MD
Professor
Department of Ophthalmology
Rudolph Foundation Hospital
Vienna, Austria

Vicente Martinez Castillo MD
Department of Ophthalmology
Vall d'Hebron Hospital
Barcelona, Spain

Stanley Chang MD
KK Tse and Ku The Ying Professor
Department of Ophthalmology
Columbia University
New York, NY, USA

Martin Charles MD
Professor of Medicine
Centro Oftalmologico Dr Charles
Buenos Aires, Argentina

Lawrence P. Chong MD
VMR Institute
Huntington Beach, CA, USA

Carl Claes MD
Head of VR Surgery
ST Augustinus
Antwerp, Belgium

Ian J. Constable FRANZCO, FRCSE, DSc (Hon)
Professor of Ophthalmology
Lions Eye Institute
University of Western Australia
Perth, Australia

Lyndon da Cruz MBBS, MA, FRCOphth, PhD, FRACO
Consultant Ophthalmic Surgeon
Moorfields Eye Hospital
Vitreo-Retinal Service
London, UK

Bertil E. Damato MD, PhD, FRCOphth
Honorary Professor
Ocular Oncology Service
Royal Liverpool University Hospital
Liverpool, UK

Arthur D. Fu MD
Clinical Professor of Ophthalmology
California Pacific Medical Center
San Francisco, CA, USA

Enrique Garcia-Valenzuela MD, PhD
Vitreo-Retinal Surgery
Midwest Retina Consultants, S.C.
Clinical Assistant Professor of Ophthalmology
University of Illinois Eye & Ear Infirmary
Parkside Center
Park Ridge, IL, USA

Alain Gaudric MD
Professor of Ophthalmology
Hôpital Lariboisière
Université Paris-Diderot
Paris, France

Andre Vieira Gomes MD, PhD
Colaborator Professor
Department of Ophthalmology
University of Sao Paulo
Sao Paulo, Brazil

Christine R Gonzales MD
Assistant Professor of Ophthalmology
Jules Stein Eye Institute
University of California Los Angeles School of Medicine
Los Angeles, CA, USA

Zdenek Gregor FRCS (Eng) FRCOphth
Consultant Vitreoretinal Surgeon
Moorfields Eye Hospital
London, UK

Stratos Gotzaridis MD
Director of Retinal Services
Athinaiki General Hospital
Athens, Greece

Heinrich Heimann MD
Consultant Ophthalmic Surgeon
St Paul's Eye Unit
Royal Liverpool University Hospital
Liverpool, UK

Nancy M. Holekamp MD
Associate Clinical Professor
Department of Ophthalmology and Visual Science
Washington University School of Medicine
Barnes Retina Institute
St. Louis, MO, USA

Jason Hsu MD
Clinical Instructor
Retina Service of Wills Eye Institute
Thomas Jefferson University
Philadelphia, PA, USA

Mark S. Humayun MD, PhD
Professor of Ophthalmology
Biomedical Engineering, Cell and Neurobiology
Keck School of Medicine of the University of Southern California
Associate Director of Research,
Doheny Eye Institute
Los Angeles, CA, USA

Yasushi Ikuno MD
Associate Professor
Department of Ophthalmology
Osaka University Graduate School of Medicine
Osaka, Japan

Timothy L Jackson MB. ChB, PhD, FRCOphth
Honorary Consultant Ophthalmic and Retinal Surgeon
Department of Ophthalmology
King's College Hospital
London, UK

Glenn J. Jaffe MD
Professor of Ophthalmology
Chief, Vitreoretinal Service
Director
Duke Reading Center
Durham, NC, USA

Robert N. Johnson MD
Clinical Professor of Ophthalmology
California Pacific Medical Center
San Francisco, CA, USA

J. Michael Jumper MD
Retina Service Chief
California Pacific Medical Center
San Francisco, CA, USA

Bernd Kirchhof MD, PhD
Professor and Chairman
University Eye Department Cologne
Koln, Germany

Allan E Kreiger MD
Professor, Department of Ophthalmology
The Jules Stein Eye Institute
Los Angeles, CA, USA

Anthony Kwan
Queensland Eye Institute in the Brisbane Region,
Queensland Ophthalmic Surgeons
Brisbane, QLD, Australia

Henry C. Lee MD
Barnes Retina Institute
Washington University School of Medicine
St. Louis, MO, USA

Jennifer I. Lim MD
Professor of Ophthalmology and Visual Sciences
Lions of Illinois Eye Research Institute
University of Illinois at Chicago
Chicago, IL, USA

Albert M. Maguire MD
Associate Professor of Ophthalmology
Department of Ophthalmology
Scheie Eye Institute
University of Pennsylvania Perelman School of Medicine
Investigator
Center for Cellular and Molecular Therapeutics
Retina Specialist
Pediatric Ophthalmology
The Children's Hospital of Philadelphia
Philadelphia, PA, USA

H. Richard McDonald MD
Clinical Professor of Ophthalmology
California Pacific Medical Center
Director, Vitreoretinal Fellowship Program
California Pacific Medical Center
Director, San Francisco Retina Foundation
San Francisco, CA, USA

Petra Meier MD
Assistant Professor
Klivik und Poliklinik fur Augen
Leipzig, Germany

Jan C. van Meurs MD PhD
Professor
The Rotterdam Eye Hospital and Erasmus University
Rotterdam, the Netherlands

Virgilio Morales-Canton MD
Chief of the Retina Department
Asociacion para Evitar la Ceguera
Hospital Dr. Luis Sanchez Bulnes
Mexico City
Professor
Universidad Nacional Autonoma de Mexico
Mexico City, Mexico

Prithvi Mruthyunjaya MD
Assistant Professor of Ophthalmology
Department of Vitreoretinal Surgery and Ocular Oncology
Duke University Eye Center
Durham, NC, USA

Manish Nagpal MS, DO, FRCS(UK)
Vitreo Retinal Consultant
Retina Foundation
Ahmedabad, Gujarat, India

Yoshitaka Nakashima MD
Department of Ophthalmology
Hospital das Clinicas
University of Sao Paulo
Sao Paulo, Brazil

Sumit K. Nanda MD
Clinical Associate Professor
Department of Ophthalmology
University of Oklahoma
Oklahoma City, Oklahoma, USA

Yusuke Oshima MD, PhD
Associate Professor
Department of Ophthalmology
Osaka University Graduate School of Medicine
Suita, Osaka, Japan

Ehab N EL Rayes MD PhD
Professor
Retina Department
Institute of Ophthalmology
Cairo, Egypt

Franco M. Recchia MD
Associate Professor of Ophthalmology and Visual Sciences
Chief, Retina Division
Director, Fellowship in Vitreoretinal Diseases and Surgery
Vanderbilt Eye Institute
Vanderbilt University School of Medicine
Nashville, TN, USA

Kourous A. Rezaei MD
Associate Professor
Illinois Retina Associates, S.C
Rush University Medical Center
Harvey, IL, USA

Stanislao Rizzo MD
Director U.O. Chirurgia Oftalmica
Azienda Ospedaliero Universitaria Pisana
Pisa, Italy

Abdulaziz Adel Rushood MD
Vitreoretinal Fellow
Department of ophthalmology
King Fahad Hospital of the University,
Al-Khobar, Saudi Arabia

Michael Samuel MD
Attending Surgeon, Retina Service
Wills Eye Hospital
Thomas Jefferson University
Philadelphia, PA, USA

V Sivagnanavel MD
Department of Ophthalmology
Kings College Hospital
University of London,
London, UK

Raymond N Sjaarda MD
Retina Specialist
Baltimore, MD, USA

Eduardo C de Souza MD
Ophthalmologist
Federal University of Santa Catarina
Florianopolis, Santa Catarina, Brasil

Marcin Stopa MD PhD
Consultant, Department of Ophthalmology
Poznan University of Medical Sciences
Poznan, Poland

Paul Sullivan MBBS, MD, FRCOphth
Consultant Opthalmic Surgeon
Director of Education
Moorfields Eye Hospital
London, UK

Hiroko Terasaki MD, PhD
Professor and Chair
Department of Ophthalmology
Nagoya University Graduate School of Medicine
Nagoya, Japan

John T. Thompson MD
Assistant Professor
The Wilmer Institute
Johns Hopkins University
Baltimore, MD, USA

Cynthia A. Toth MD
Professor
Department of Ophthalmology and Biomedical Engineering
Duke Universtiy
Durham, NC, USA

Michael T. Trese MD
Clinical Professor of Biomedical Sciences
Eye Research Institute
Oakland University
Rochester, MI
Chief Pediatrid and Adult Vitreoretinal Surgery
William Beaumont Hospital
Royal Oak, MI, USA

Peter Wiedemann MD
Professor of Ophthalmology
Department of Ophthalmology
University of Leipzig Faculty of Medicine
Leipzig, Germany

Andre J. Witkin MD
Assistant Professor
Department of Ophthalmology
Tufts University School of Medicine
Boston, MA, USA

Young Hee Yoon MD, PhD
Professor and Chair
Department of Ophthalmology
Asan Medical Center
University of Ulsan College of Medicine
Seoul, South Korea

Dedication

The original and all subsequent editions of *RETINA* are dedicated to the clinicians and scientists who have contributed to the education in our field of medical students, residents, and fellows, and especially to retina specialists and all ophthalmologists who participate in continuing medical education. We recognize that we are all students and committed to lifelong learning, especially in our field of retina.

The Second Edition included a special dedication to **Ronald G. Michels (1942–1991),** who was vitally involved in the planning of the original edition and in the recruitment of our initial team of editors and authors. Ron was an enthusiastic and talented leader in vitreoretinal surgery. His teaching and innovations had a major impact on the other editors of *RETINA* specifically and on the entire field of ophthalmology generally. We are thankful for the privilege of having known and worked with Ron.

For the Third Edition we offered an additional special dedication to **A. Edward Maumenee (1913–1998)**, a true giant who influenced virtually every field and subspecialty in ophthalmology. While most of his later contributions involved anterior segment surgery, his original observations regarding macular degeneration provided a basis for subsequent clinical and research investigations in this area. As a gifted teacher, relentless investigator, and treasured mentor, Ed inspired the editors and many authors of this textbook, as well as a multitude of academicians and clinicians around the world. He was the Professors' Professor.

For the Fourth Edition we added a special dedication to **Arnall Patz (1920–2010)**, who was an editor of the original edition. Arnall was a pioneer and leader in the establishment of the field of medical retina. He founded the Retinal Vascular Center at the Wilmer Institute and, subsequently, he became the Director of the Wilmer Institute. He trained many of today's leaders in the field and many contributing authors to *RETINA*. Arnall was an inspiration for the multitude of retinal specialists around the world.

For this present edition we wish to stress the development of knowledge and the contribution of the international community of retinal specialists. From the time of the First Edition in 1989 – more than 20 years ago – we have benefited from the rapid evolution of science – basic and clinical – in all fields related to biology and medicine, and especially in relation to ophthalmology and our chosen specialty of retina. The evolution of knowledge and contributions of colleagues from around the world have shown that there are no borders; the free exchange of information directly benefits our patients in the prevention of the most common forms of blindness caused by retinal diseases. Thus, it is wholly appropriate that this Fifth Edition of *RETINA* is dedicated to the **international community of retinal clinicians and educators**.

Foreword

"In the fields of observation, chance favors the prepared mind."
Louis Pasteur

In science and medicine, it is said that the doubling time for information is two and a half years. By this measure, information regarding the retina and the intimately interactive brain has increased more than four-fold since the most recent edition of *RETINA* in 2006.

Related to the retina and the visual system, the massive increase in knowledge extends from the approximately 125 million rod and cone photoreceptors in each eye, through the hierarchical circuitry of the inner retina to nearly one-third of the 100 trillion neurons in the human brain that participate in vision. Also embracing the glial and vascular structures, retinal pigment epithelium and contiguous vitreous and choroid, new retina-related information is derived from genetics and the Human Genome Project, basic sciences such as neurobiology and immunology, applied disciplines including pharmacology and bioengineering, as well as the emerging sciences of regenerative medicine and nanotechnology.

Assimilating this wealth of discovery, the Editor-in-Chief, Stephen J. Ryan MD, and Editors of *RETINA* are to be commended for maintaining the focus on information that is essential to clinical medicine and retina specialty practice through:

Volume 1 Retinal imaging and diagnostics, basic science, genetics, and translation to therapy;
Volume 2 Retinal degeneration and dystrophy, vascular disease, and chorioretinal inflammatory disease; and
Volume 3 Retinal surgery, complicated forms of retinal detachment, vitreous surgery, and tumors of retina, choroid, and vitreous.

Authors of the 156 chapters in the three volumes are internationally recognized leaders of biomedical science and medical–surgical ophthalmology. Each chapter is authoritatively presented with the central purpose of providing current, evidence-based and clinically relevant information. Authorship by outstanding clinician–scientists is extremely important, because the value of *RETINA* stems in large part from the scholarship, content selection, and clinical experience of the chapter authors.

In this Internet era with widespread electronic communication and data access, *RETINA* serves at least two purposes. First, it presents an organized framework for the vast amount of retina-related data and builds the "prepared mind" for clinical examination, ancillary testing, diagnosis, and treatment of retinal abnormalities. Second, *RETINA* is a peer-created reference for specific information regarding retinal, choroidal, and vitreal diagnostics, abnormalities, and therapies. As a comprehensive framework of organized information and an authoritative resource, *RETINA* is requisite to sustained competence in retinal clinical research and retinal specialty practice.

Bradley R. Straatsma MD, JD
Jules Stein Eye Institute
David Geffen School of Medicine at UCLA
University of California, Los Angeles, CA, USA

Preface

Retinal specialists, both clinicians and scientists, share a fascination with the retina, a unique tissue. The retina forms the anatomic and physiologic basis for the gift of sight and accounts for over 35% of the neurons entering and exiting the human brain.

In the 21st century we are fortunate to be in the middle of the most exciting scientific revolution in the history of man. We all anticipate that this revolution in biomedicine and our present "century of biology" predict a bright future for our specialty of retina.

It is helpful to recall that although there had long been a fascination with the eye and sight, and prior speculation regarding the retina, it was not until the 19th century that modern ophthalmology and the study of the retina truly began. Everyone in our field points with pride to the revolution brought about by von Helmholtz in 1850 with his introduction of his innovative ophthalmoscope in Berlin. Great contributions in ophthalmology and descriptions of the retina followed, particularly in Europe. In the 20th century, ophthalmologists from the United States joined in these contributions. Further advances in this 21st century, with important contributions from every continent – Asia, Latin America, North America, Australia, Africa, and Europe – have continued at breakneck speed with the full expectation that the entire world will participate in this expansion of our knowledge of the retina and retinal diseases.

As scientific knowledge explodes, it is often at the interface of different disciplines and of science and clinical observation that great contributions are made. Ophthalmology is fortunate to be at the forefront of the interaction of engineering, biology, and medicine. From the time the laser was invented in 1960, the specialty of ophthalmology was the earliest adapter, with clinical applications developed within 10 years.

While we can see a logical progression over the five editions of *RETINA*, if one steps back to the publication of the first edition in 1989, the progress in science since that time has truly been breathtaking. It is remarkable to recall the vigorous debate as to the chances of success of sequencing the human genome, whereas now with the advent of high throughput whole genomic and epigenomic analyses we have entered a new era in discovering the genetic basis of retinal disease.

In revising *RETINA* for the Fifth Edition, we now begin Volume 1 with imaging, where there is a veritable revolution underway. The human eye cannot resolve what advanced imaging technologies including ocular coherence tomography (OCT) can detect. This is followed by the basic sciences, which have been updated to include not only the fundamentals of retinal anatomy and physiology, but also recent advances in cell injury, genetics (both nuclear and mitochondrial) and epigenetics, and their translation to novel therapies that encompass stem cells, neuroprotection, gene therapy, nanotechnology, and drug delivery to the posterior segment.

One constant is that the second volume remains devoted to medical retina. Tremendous progress has been made in retinal vascular diseases such as diabetic retinopathy and with treatments for certain consequences of age-related macular degeneration. Around the time of the publication of the First Edition, the understanding of molecular mechanisms of angiogenesis was in its infancy; this edition documents how intravitreal pharmacotherapy has become standard care for the leading blinding retinal diseases. These diseases and treatments are stressed in Volume 2.

Volume 3 addresses both surgical diseases and the oncology section. Human retina is a direct outgrowth of the forebrain and, therefore, is the most accessible part of the brain for neuroscience studies. Many of us consider the retina to be aesthetically the most beautiful tissue in nature. We hope the reader will enjoy and appreciate the major revisions to the figures and illustrations throughout the text. The new edition includes 20 new chapters and 1304 new figures.

Thus, this Fifth Edition features a significant reorganization as well as a tremendous consolidation – for example, one chapter in this new edition has replaced what were previously five chapters in the Fourth Edition. At the same time, we have added whole new chapters in every section of the book. The field of retina is so broad and the contribution of knowledge is so rapid that we cannot be comprehensive, but we have attempted to weight the content to match the needs of the wide array of our readers worldwide. The authors have updated their references, as the reader will note; most chapters include references from 2011.

We have many authors from around the world contributing to this Fifth Edition, who are recognized for their leadership in retina throughout the world.

As a truly international multi-authored text, there are multiple literary styles. The editors have worked to provide a level of conformity and scientific balance to preserve accuracy and knowledge as of 2012 without sacrificing the originality and style of the individual authors.

The editors gratefully acknowledge the support of many of the faculty and staff of the Wilmer Eye Institute and the Doheny Eye Institute and many eye institutions from around the world who have contributed immensely to the completion of this project. Timothy Hengst, whose artistic talent is displayed in the illustrations, contributed substantially to the quality of these volumes. We thank the office staffs of the individual authors and editors and, in particular, Joy Roque, who contributed tremendously to this effort. We have enjoyed working with Elsevier and, specifically, Russell Gabbedy, Nani Clansey, and Caroline Jones and their staff, who share our commitment to the highest standards of quality for *RETINA*.

S.J.R.
A.P.S.
C.P.W.
D.R.H.
S.R.S.
P.H.W.

For additional online content visit http://www.expertconsult.com

Chapter 40

Retinitis Pigmentosa and Allied Disorders

Kevin Gregory-Evans, Mark E. Pennesi, Richard G. Weleber

Retinitis pigmentosa (RP) is the term used for a group of disorders that are characterized by inherited, progressive dysfunction, cell loss, and eventual atrophy of retinal tissue. Initial involvement of photoreceptors leads to subsequent damage to inner retinal cells. Eventually there is widespread atrophy of several, if not most, layers of the retina. Consequent visual impairment usually manifests initially as night blindness and visual field loss. Ultimately, in most cases, there is central visual dysfunction. Both rods and, in most types, cones are abnormal early in the disorder. The age of onset of visual impairment in the different types of RP ranges from infancy to late adulthood. The eventual visual burden from retinal dystrophy ranges from regional visual field loss, unnoticed by the patient, to severe, profound concentric loss of the peripheral visual field (tunnel vision). Varying degrees of loss of central macular function can occur at any age but are more frequent in advanced stages.

The term "retinitis pigmentosa" implies that inflammation is a prominent part of the pathophysiology of the condition. Although a role of inflammation at some level in the retina is still discussed, RP is not considered a primary inflammatory disease. Vascular permeability is greater in eyes of patients with RP and trauma or surgery is accompanied by a greater incidence and severity of inflammation. Through the years, many terms have been used to describe RP, including "tapetoretinal degeneration" (by Leber in 1916), "primary pigmentary retinal degeneration," "pigmentary retinopathy," and "rod–cone dystrophy."

RP may be seen in isolation (typical RP) or in association with systemic disease (syndromic RP). The prevalence of typical RP is approximately 1:5000 worldwide. In Maine, USA, the prevalence of typical RP has been found to be 1:5200, and the birth incidence of those who will eventually be affected with RP has been calculated as 1:3500.[1] The prevalence of RP has been found to be 1:7000 in Switzerland,[2] 1:4016 in China,[3] and 1:4500 in Israel.[4] The highest frequency of occurrence, 1 in 1878, is among the Navajo Indians.[5] The prevalence of syndromic RP is less well documented. The prevalence of Usher syndrome (RP with congenital deafness) is estimated to be 1:6000.[6]

The clinical aspects and basic science of RP and allied disorders are extensively documented in the published literature. A recent literature search (June 2011) using Medline found over 6800 articles on RP alone. Numerous scholarly reviews have been written, many of which are cited in previous versions of this chapter. Because the field is changing so rapidly, we recommend current reviews through major electronic journals as the best mean of obtaining the most recent information.

EARLY HISTORY

The first description of the fundus findings and the use of the term "retinitis pigmentosa" are attributed to Donders in 1855 and 1857.[7–9] However, the diagnosis of complicated night blindness (presumably RP) has probably existed in all cultures for hundreds, if not thousands, of years. Ovelgün, in 1744, made observations on familial complicated hemeralopia (or night blindness), which probably represented RP.[9] Shortly after the discovery of the ophthalmoscope by Helmholtz in 1851, van Trigt[10] in 1853 and Ruete[11] in 1854 described cases that most assuredly were RP.

TYPICAL RETINITIS PIGMENTOSA

Clinical features

Nyctalopia

Difficulty with vision at night (night blindness) is one of the two hallmark symptoms of RP. Patients with typical RP usually attribute the beginning of night vision difficulties to the first or second decade of life. In some patients, especially those living in an urban setting, night vision problems may not be apparent until ocular disease is at an advanced stage. Tanino and Ohba[12] noted that the onset of symptoms of RP, most commonly nyctalopia, occurred at a median age of 10.7 years in autosomal recessive disease and 23.4 years in autosomal dominant disease. The symptom of nyctalopia should not be confused with the symptom of blurred vision with night myopia or uncorrected refractive error. People with RP have a narrowing of the visual field in the dark and may describe getting easily disoriented on dimly lit evenings when others are able to see adequately. Becoming accident-prone, especially at night, is a highly suggestive symptom.

Night blindness is not pathognomonic of RP and can be a feature of other retinal disorders, such as congenital stationary night blindness and age-related macular degeneration. Deteriorating night vision can also be a prominent feature of other ocular disease, such as high myopia.

Visual field loss

The second hallmark feature or symptom of RP is an insidious, progressive loss of peripheral visual field. In some patients, especially those with severe disease beginning in childhood, this may be manifested as a progressive contraction of the visual field (see also Perimetry under Psychophysical findings). Loss of peripheral vision can be detected in early disease with small, dim test targets (Fig. 40.1). For many types of RP, field deficits are usually found first, and are most severe, in the superior visual field (Fig. 40.2). This reflects the early involvement of the

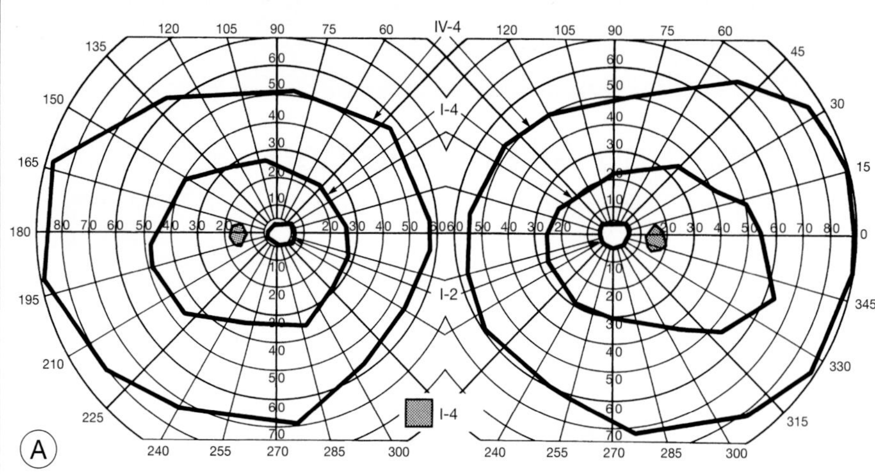

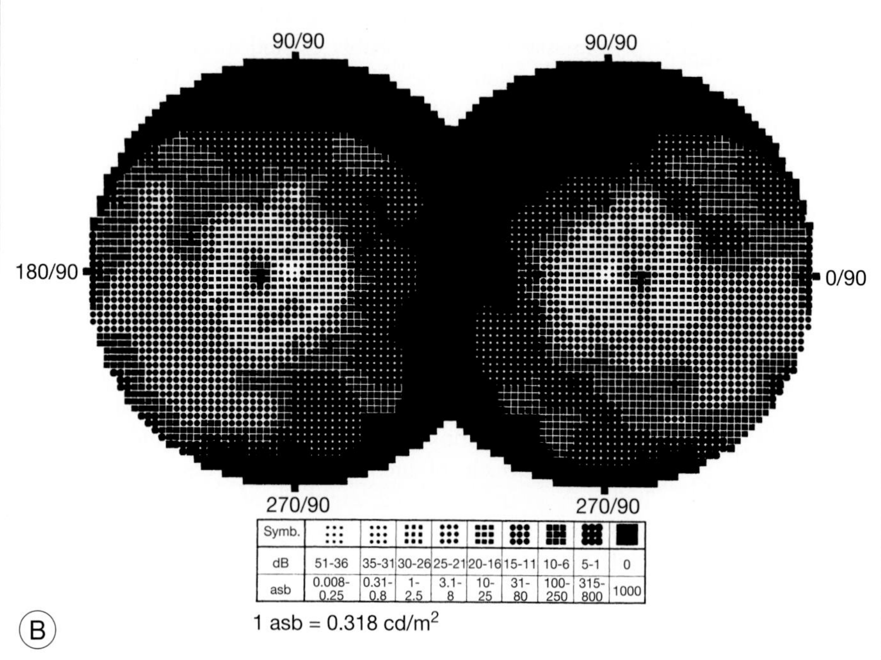

Symb.									
dB	51-36	35-31	30-26	25-21	20-16	15-11	10-6	5-1	0
asb	0.008-0.25	0.31-0.8	1-2.5	3.1-8	10-25	31-80	100-250	315-800	1000

1 asb = 0.318 cd/m^2

Fig. 40.1 (A) Goldmann kinetic visual fields in a 27-year-old woman with autosomal dominant retinitis pigmentosa. Note that the visual field is full to the IV-4-e test target but that isopters are contracted for smaller and dimmer test targets. No scotomas were plotted. (In this and all subsequent kinetic perimetric visual fields, although not specified on the illustration, all isopters were measured with the e setting.) (B) Octopus static perimetric fields for the same patient (combined programs 23 and 34). Note the overall decrease in retinal sensitivity in the mid and far periphery, with patchy areas of greater loss of sensitivity. The electroretinogram was profoundly abnormal with no detectable rod-mediated responses and very small (10–15 μV) prolonged residual cone responses. The 40-minute dark-adapted retinal threshold was elevated 2.8 log units above the normal mean.

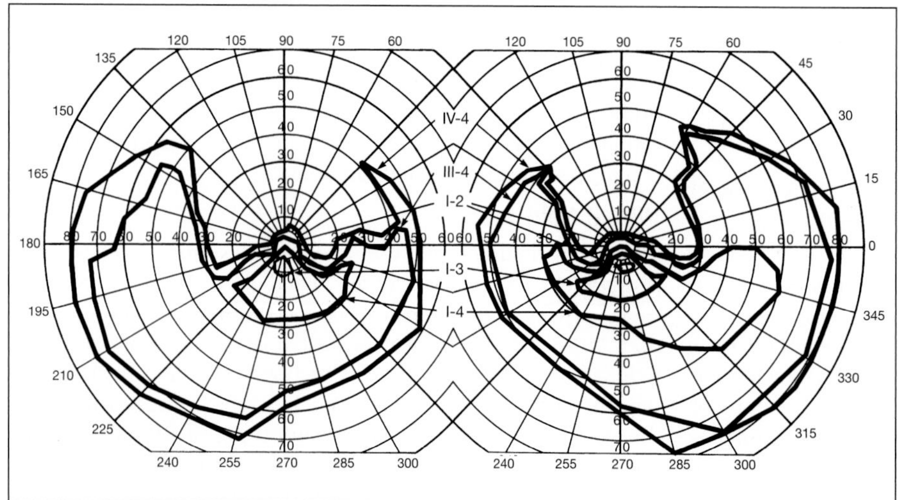

Fig. 40.2 Goldmann kinetic perimetry showing visual field loss, which is greatest in the upper field, in a 27-year-old man with high myopia and X-linked retinitis pigmentosa. Note that the smaller test target isopters are contracted inferiorly as well, suggesting relative decreased retinal sensitivity in the inferior fields. The electroretinogram (ERG) showed subnormal, prolonged rod responses with even more subnormal, prolonged cone responses, suggesting a cone–rod ERG pattern.

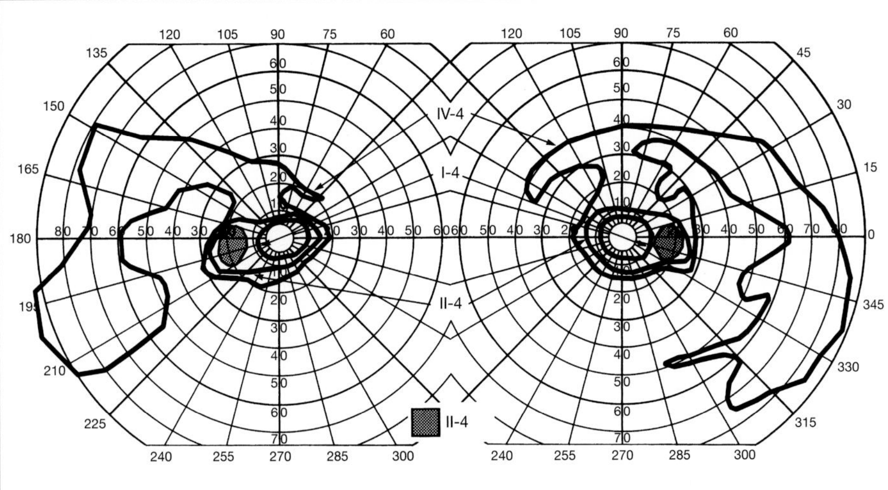

Fig. 40.3 Goldmann kinetic perimetry for an 18-year-old man with autosomal recessive retinitis pigmentosa associated with posterior column ataxia (same patient as Fig. 40.15A and brother of patient in Fig. 40.21). Visual acuity was 20/30, J1, right eye, and 20/50, J2, left eye.

inferior retina in RP. Occasionally the visual field loss will be greater temporally, nasally, or inferiorly (Fig. 40.3). See the section on Perimetry for specifics about testing the visual field.

In a group of patients with several types of RP, Berson et al.[13] found that overall about 4.6% of the remaining visual field was lost per year. Massof et al.[14,15] found that, in most forms of generalized RP, the kinetic visual field shrank approximately 50% over 4.5 years. Massof and Finkelstein[15] argue that the time course for field loss in all major genetic and functional classes of RP is nearly identical if one corrects for the critical age, which is defined as the age when visual field loss is first detected by a test target of given size and brightness. In conjunction with this concept, they have proposed a two-stage hypothesis for the natural course of RP. The first stage is a predisposition for retinal degeneration, such as genetic or environmental factors, which would be different for the separate types of RP and possibly among individuals. The second stage involves the actual retinal degeneration, which proceeds on its own internal time course and which would be common to most forms of RP.

In general, there is a strong tendency for the visual field loss to be symmetric between the two eyes.[14,15] A notable exception to this is the phenotype expressed in female carriers of X-linked RP. In this situation, the distribution of mutant photoreceptors in the retina is determined by lyonization (X-chromosomal inactivation). This is a random event determining which genes of the two X chromosomes (the normal or mutant copy) are expressed in a particular cell. This leads not only to unusual, irregular patterns of visual field loss in individual eyes but also to quite striking differences in field loss between the two eyes.[16] However, even in these cases the visual fields usually correspond quite closely to the fundus appearance, with the greater visual field loss in the eye with greater pigmentary abnormalities.

In typical RP the rate of progression of visual field loss is usually slow and relentless, with changes best appreciated when observed over many years or even decades. However, the visual fields may change dramatically over a few months or years. A patient may not notice what may be a striking loss of peripheral visual field if the central field remains clear. As the visual field reaches the stage of "tunnel vision," the patient usually becomes acutely aware of subsequent change with time. This often leads the patient to the conclusion that the rate of degeneration is accelerating. In the USA, statutory legal blindness results when the remaining central visual field measures 20° or less horizontally in the better eye, using the III-4-e test target on a Goldmann perimeter.[17] In the UK, most RP patients, with normal acuity, would be registered as partially sighted ("gross field defect"). Legal blindness occurs when fields become "very contracted" – a stage at which acuity loss has also usually occurred (www.dh.gov.uk/assetRoot/04/07/48/48/04074848.doc).

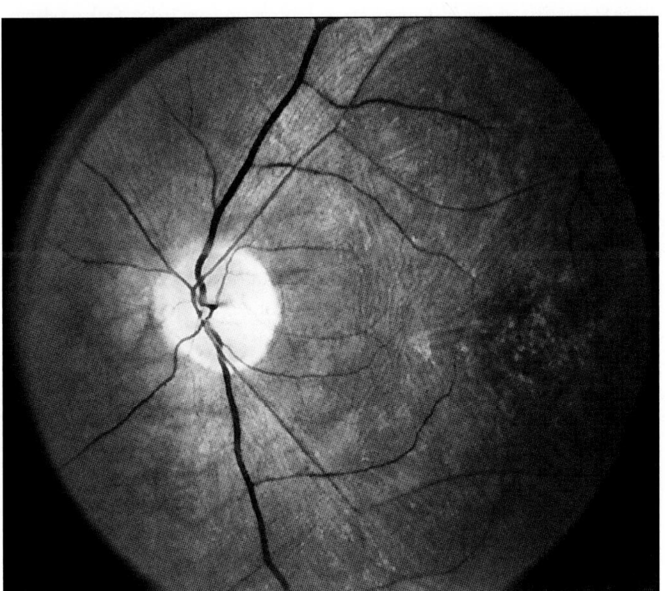

Fig. 40.4 Posterior pole of the left eye of a 33-year-old man with Bardet–Biedl syndrome from homozygosity for the common Met390Arg mutation of *BBS1*, demonstrating preretinal fibrosis with wrinkling of the internal limiting membrane. The acuity was 20/400. The maculae developed atrophic lesions over the next 5 years with further reduction of visual acuity.

Central vision loss

There is a common misconception in RP (documented in older texts) that the central vision will remain good until most, if not all, the peripheral field is lost. Central visual function can, however, be seriously affected early in typical RP, while significant peripheral field remains.[18] Cystoid macular edema (CME),[19] diffuse retinal vascular leakage,[20] macular preretinal fibrosis[21] (Fig. 40.4), and retinal pigment epithelial (RPE) defects in the macula or fovea[22,23] can occur early in the disease. Macular edema is the topic of a section on treatment of RP later in this chapter.

To a considerable extent, the likelihood of retaining "good vision" (central acuity) to a given age in life depends on the specific inheritance type of RP. Patients with regional ("sector") RP may retain good visual acuity all their life. Patients with autosomal dominant RP (adRP) are more likely than patients with autosomal recessive (arRP) or X-linked RP to retain good acuity beyond 60 years of age.[13] Marmor, in his study of visual loss in adRP and arRP,[26] found that when visual acuity began to fail, it generally dropped to 20/200 within 4–10 (median 6) years. Patients with X-linked RP are usually blind (acuity 20/200 or worse) by 30–40 years of age.[13,24,25] A good prognostic sign of retention of central acuity is electroretinograph (ERG) amplitudes remaining quite large (e.g., greater than 100 μV).[26]

Color vision defects

In general, color vision in typical RP remains good until the visual acuity is 20/40 or worse. Color vision may fail early in cases where central cones appear to be abnormal from the beginning. In such cases, pericentral scotomas encroach very close to fixation early in the disease. These patients, even though they show a rod–cone loss on ERG, may show impressive color vision defects even when peripheral vision is relatively good.

Photopsia and other symptoms

Many patients with RP at some time during the course of their disease have light flashes, or photopsias. These are reported as occurring in the midperipheral field of vision, often adjacent to areas of relative or absolute scotomas. These photopsias are described as tiny, blinking or shimmering lights or as a coarse, sparkling graininess to vision. The phenomenon is similar to that reported by patients with ophthalmic migraine except that, although retinal disease involvement expands over the years, the photopsias are generally stationary within the field. Also, unlike ophthalmic migraine, the photopsias may be continuous rather than episodic. As the scotomas become denser over the years, the photopsias decrease and finally disappear. In a retrospective survey of symptoms and findings in 500 patients with RP, Heckenlively et al.[27] reported light flashes in 170 (35%). Since 8 patients in this series had retinal detachments, the symptom of light flashes must be considered an indication for careful fundus examination.

The cellular or tissue correlates that underlie photopsias in RP are unknown but may include photoreceptor dysfunction, neurite sprouting, aberrant synapse formation, and secondary remodeling of the retina, all of which occur as sequelae of photoreceptor degeneration (see section on Cell and tissue biology: Histopathology, for further discussion).

Fundus appearance

The classically described fundus appearance of RP includes attenuated retinal vessels, mottling and granularity of the RPE, bone spicule intraretinal pigmentation, and optic nerve head pallor (Fig. 40.5). In general, when ophthalmoscopically detectable abnormalities of the fundus are present, there is a high degree of symmetry between the two eyes and fundus pigmentation is often greater in the midperiphery (Fig. 40.6). In advanced disease, atrophy of the RPE and choriocapillaris leads to fundus pallor and larger choroidal vessels become visible (Fig. 40.7). In some forms of RP and allied disorders, sufficient atrophy of the retina and choroid will occur during the late stages of the disease that the fundus appearance overlaps with certain of the primary choroidal atrophies (Fig. 40.7).[28] As the disease advances to late stages, vessel attenuation can become so severe that the retinal vessels appear thread-like (Fig. 40.8).

Almost all forms of RP go through a stage where the retina appears either normal or nearly normal, even though relative scotomas may be evident on visual field testing or areas of decreased retinal threshold may be present on static perimetry. Patients who have very early RP without fundus pigmentary abnormalities are often diagnosed as having RP sine pigmento or paucipigmentary RP. This is no longer considered a specific subtype of RP but a stage through which many, if not most, patients with RP pass. The sine pigmento stage may exist for decades before typical RP signs appear. For patients with high myopia and RP, the typical fundus features of high myopia may delay the appreciation of other retinal abnormalities (Fig. 40.9).

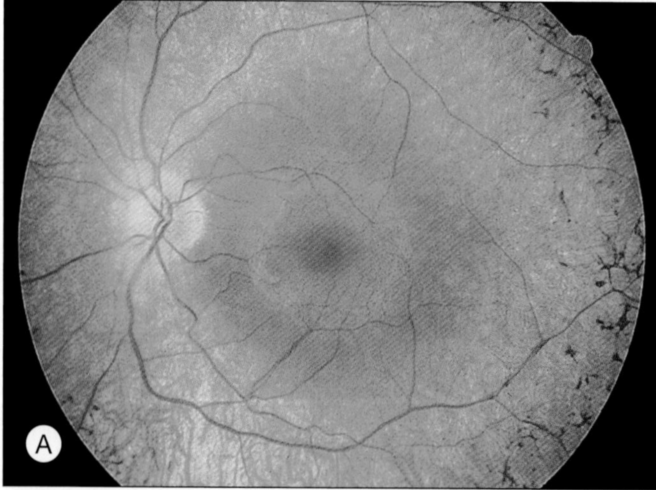

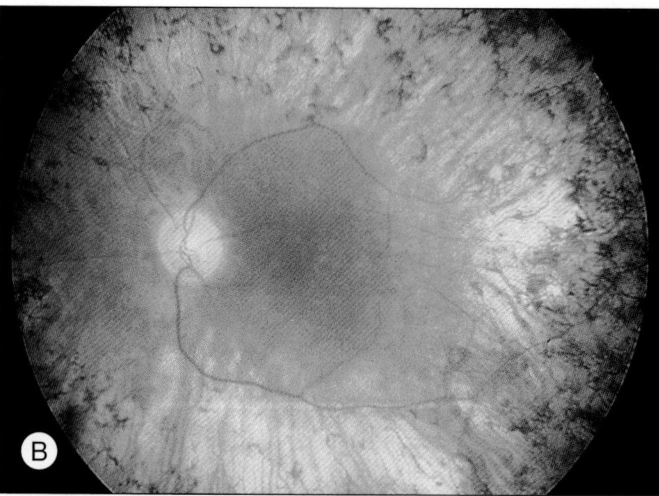

Fig. 40.5 (A) Fundus appearance of the left eye of a 13-year-old girl with autosomal recessive retinitis pigmentosa. Visual acuity was 20/20 but visual field was constricted to 20° diameter with the III-4-e test target. (B) Advanced autosomal dominant retinitis pigmentosa in the left eye of a 57-year-old man from the Pro347Leu mutation of rhodopsin. Visual acuity was 20/100 right eye and 20/200 left eye and visual field constricted to 18° in both eyes with the III-4-e target.

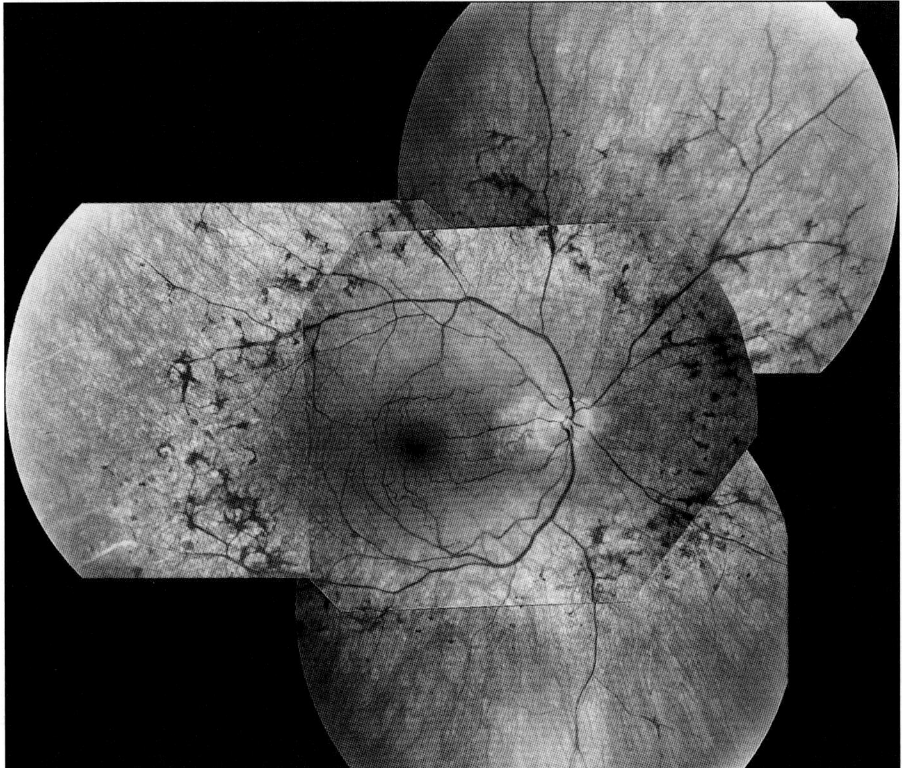

Fig. 40.6 Fundus appearance of the right eye of a 40-year old patient with rhodopsin Pro23His retinitis pigmentosa. Areas of fundus changes correlated well with kinetic visual fields, performed at 39 years of age, as shown in Figure 40.19.

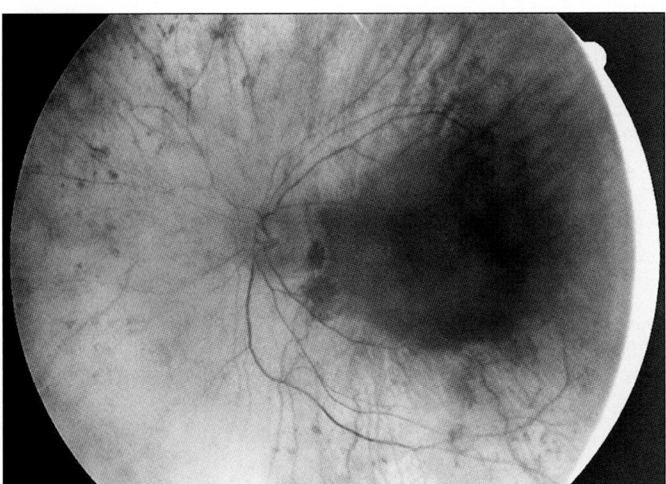

Fig. 40.7 Fundus appearance of the left eye of a 75-year-old patient with advanced rhodopsin Pro23His retinitis pigmentosa. This patient is the father of the patient whose visual field is shown in Figure 40.19 and whose fundus appearance is shown in Figure 40.6.

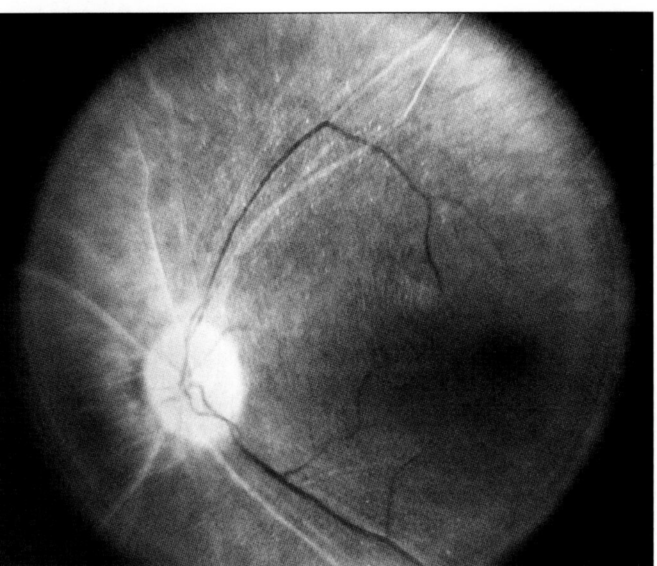

Fig. 40.8 Thread-like retinal vessels, pale, waxy optic discs, epiretinal fibrosis, and mottling of the retinal pigment epithelium in the left eye of a 10-year-old girl with advanced retinal degeneration in Alström disease. (Reproduced with permission from Millay RH, Weleber RG, Heckenlively JR. Ophthalmologic and systemic manifestations of Alström's disease. Am J Ophthalmol 1986;102:482–90.)

When fundus abnormalities are evident, the earliest features are attenuation of retinal vessels and the appearance of fine mottling or granularity of the RPE in the mid and far periphery (Fig. 40.10). Spectral-domain optical coherence tomography (SD-OCT) imaging demonstrates that retinal thickness is decreased, particularly for outer layers, outside the macula and in areas of

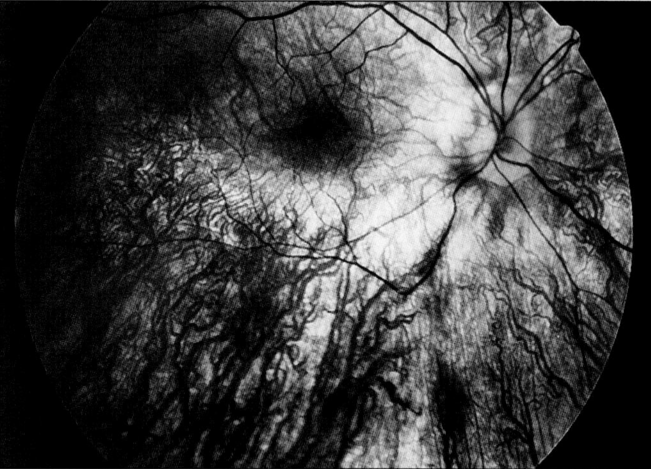

Fig. 40.9 Fundus of a 27-year-old man with high myopia and X-linked retinitis pigmentosa (same patient as in Fig. 40.2). Sparse but definite bone spicules were present in the inferior mid and far periphery. Discs showed a myopic tilt with peripapillary chorioretinal atrophy. The retinal pigment epithelium was diffusely hypopigmented.

abnormal pigmentation with bone spicules.[29,30] The macular region may exhibit increased luster, abnormal highlights, or wrinkling, suggesting either macular edema or early epiretinal membrane formation or preretinal fibrosis.[19,22] In advanced stages, patients with RP may exhibit atrophic macular lesions (Fig. 40.11) that simulate what some authors have called (perhaps inappropriately so) "macular coloboma."

Intraretinal, bone spicule pigment formations represent migration of pigment into the retina from disintegration of RPE cells with accumulation in the interstitial spaces surrounding retinal vessels. This process occurs most prominently at the junctions of vessels producing perivascular pigmentary cuffing and spicule-shaped deposits. The loss of pigment within the pigment epithelial cells often produces an overall gray, desaturated appearance to the retina with greater visibility of underlying choroidal vessels through the more transparent pigment epithelium. Eventually, the normal salmon-pink color of the entire mid and far peripheral fundus is replaced by dense bone spicule pigmentary formations. Heckenlively[31] has described several patients with advanced RP with preservation of the RPE in a para-arteriolar distribution. Porta and colleagues[32] described two additional cases. Van den Born et al.[33] reported a large consanguineous family with preserved periarteriolar RP and confirmed the autosomal recessive inheritance. Almost all these patients were hyperopic. The gene for this form of RP (termed RP12) has been found to be the human homolog *CRB1* of the *Drosophila crumbs* gene.

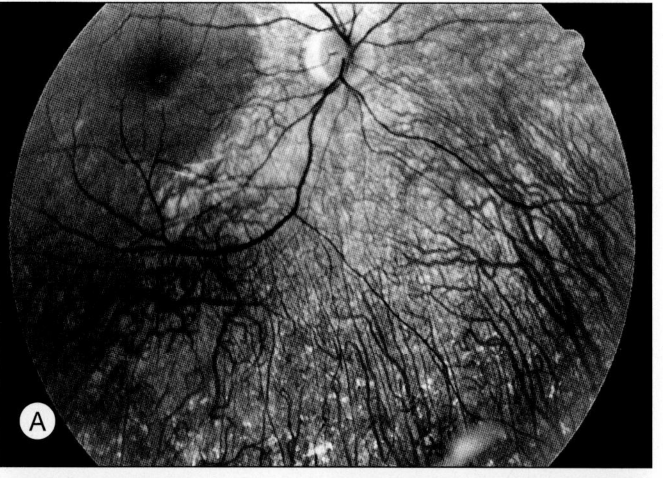

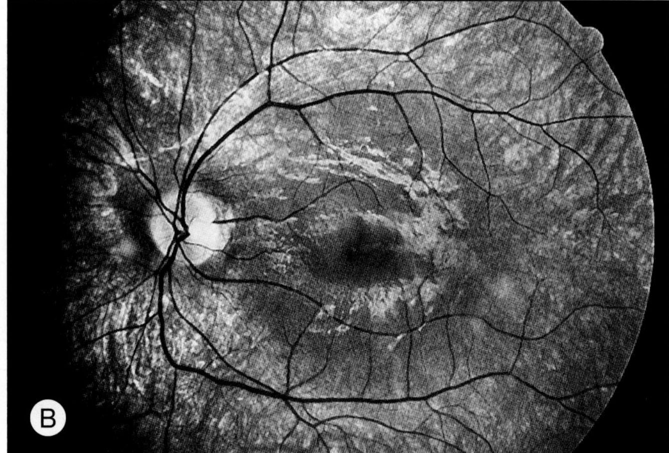

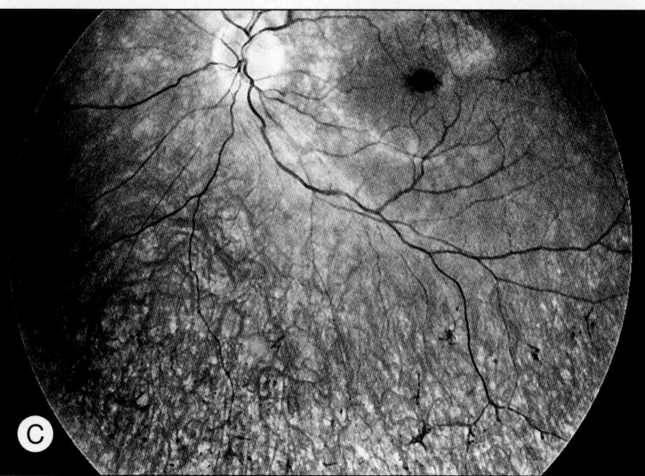

Fig. 40.10 Fundus findings of early simplex retinitis pigmentosa at age 7 years (A), simplex retinitis pigmentosa at age 9 years (B), and autosomal dominant retinitis pigmentosa at age 14 years (C). Note midperipheral pigment dispersion in A and C and wrinkling of internal limiting membrane in B.

In some patients abnormal pigmentation and atrophy are confined to one area of the retina. Such an appearance is termed "sector RP," a diagnosis that undoubtedly represents a heterogeneous group of disorders characterized by marked regionality of disease. Sector RP is discussed in further detail in the section Subdivision by distribution of retinal involvement or fundus appearance, below. However, since many patients with generalized disease present with localized pigmentary changes with regional functional loss, sector RP must always remain a provisioinal diagnosis until an adequate period of observation has occurred.

A yellowish-white metallic tapetal-like reflex or sheen can occasionally be observed in women who are carriers for the X-linked form of RP[34] (Fig. 40.12) and rarely in young males with early disease[35–37] (Fig. 40.13). With time, regional or diffuse mottling and atrophy of the RPE eventually replace the tapetal-like sheen. At least one form of dominant RP can show a tapetal-like reflex limited to the foveal and parafoveal region (Fig. 40.14). No histopathologic assessment has yet identified the source of a tapetal-like reflex. Cideciyan and Jacobson[38] suggested that abnormal cones are the sources of the tapetal reflex. Berendschot et al.,[39] using spectral fundus reflectance, confirmed that outer segments of peripheral photoreceptor cells are the source of the abnormal reflex but that this abnormality was not confined to cones. The carrier state for X-linked RP appears to be a slowly progressive retinal dystrophy in its own right, with a patchy distribution of affected retina as determined by lyonization.[40,41] A number of studies have reported that the ERG is abnormal in most X-linked RP carriers.[16,42–45] A tapetal-like reflex is not pathognomonic of X-linked RP but has also been reported in occasional cases of X-linked retinoschisis,[46] and Oguchi disease.[47]

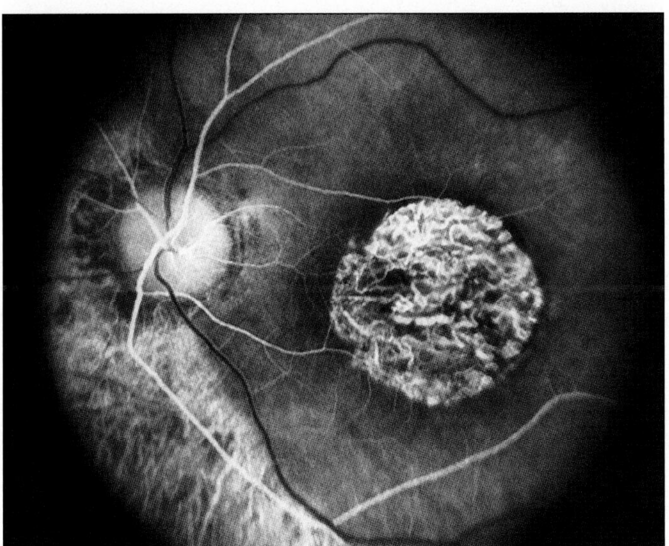

Fig. 40.11 Early-phase fluorescein angiogram frame of the left eye of a 44-year-old woman with autosomal dominant retinitis pigmentosa and bilateral atrophic macular lesions. Visual acuity was 20/300 right eye and 20/200 left eye.

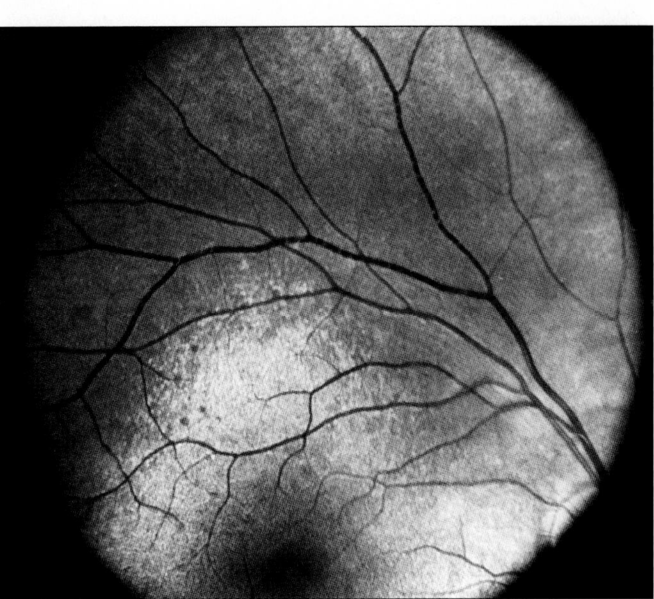

Fig. 40.13 Tapetal-like yellow-white reflex in a 13-year-old boy with X-linked retinitis pigmentosa.

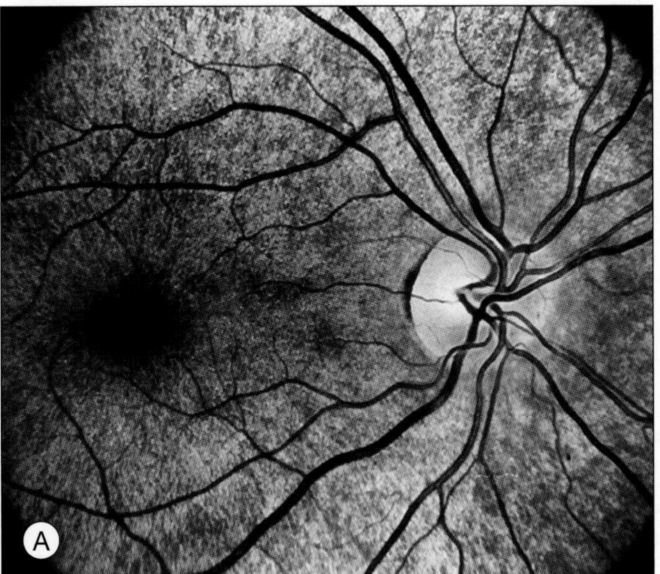

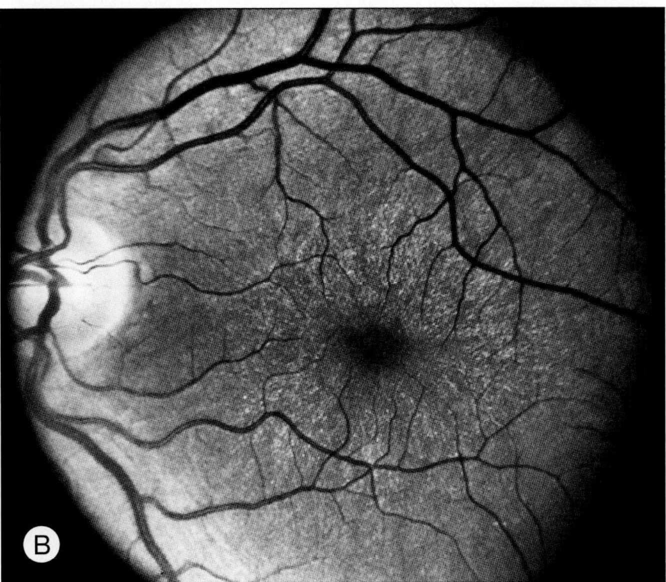

Fig. 40.12 Golden granular tapetal-like sheen or reflex in 20-year-old (A) and 44-year-old (B) carriers for X-linked retinitis pigmentosa.

The optic disc may be normal in early RP, show a waxy fullness with hyperemia, or appear waxy and pale (Fig. 40.15A). A "golden ring" or yellowish-white halo can often be seen surrounding the optic disc in early RP (Fig. 40.15B). As disease progresses, this golden ring is replaced with peripapillary mottling, hyperpigmentation, and atrophy of the RPE (Fig. 40.15C). The optic nerve head cup-to-disc ratio has been reported to be significantly smaller in RP patients of all types (0.19 compared to 0.35 in normal subjects).[48] In advanced disease, dense optic nerve head pallor results, in part from optic atrophy and

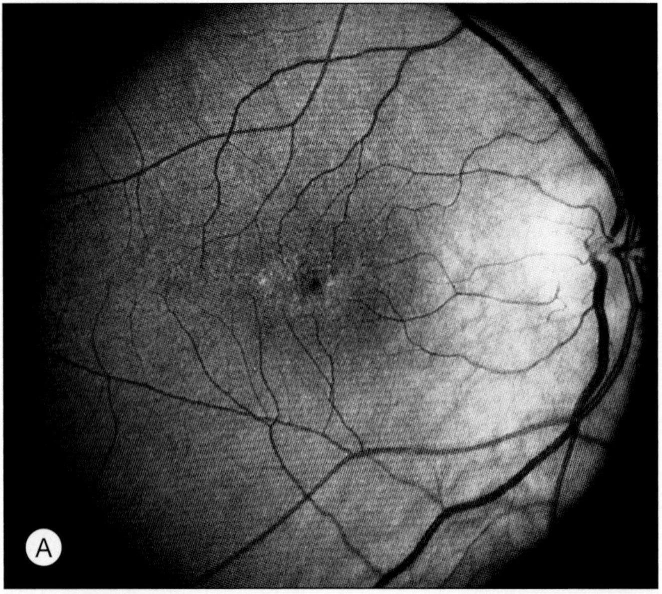

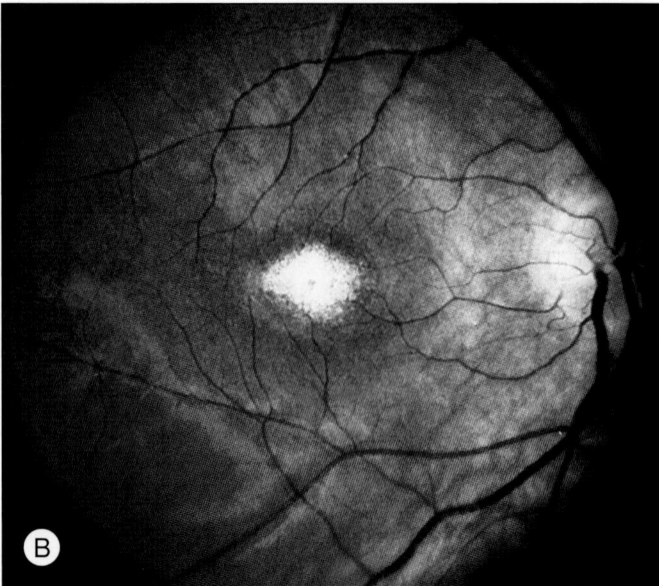

Fig. 40.14 Tapetal-like golden foveal reflex in an 11-year-old boy with autosomal dominant retinitis pigmentosa. Left (A) and right (B) stereo pair of right macula. In these and all stereo pairs for both eyes, the bright sheen was only visible in the photograph obtained through the nasal half of the pupil. This marked orientation dependency is similar to that seen in crystalline structures and may result from deformations of the outer photoreceptor segments.

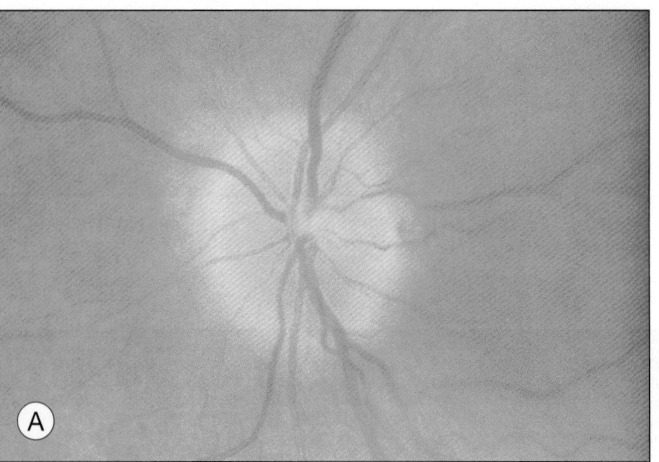

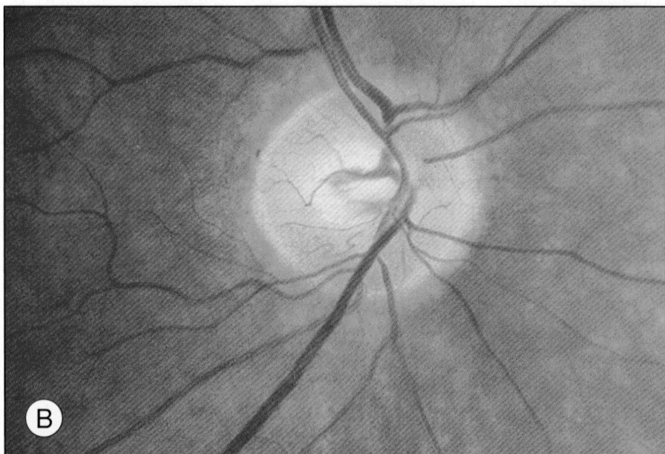

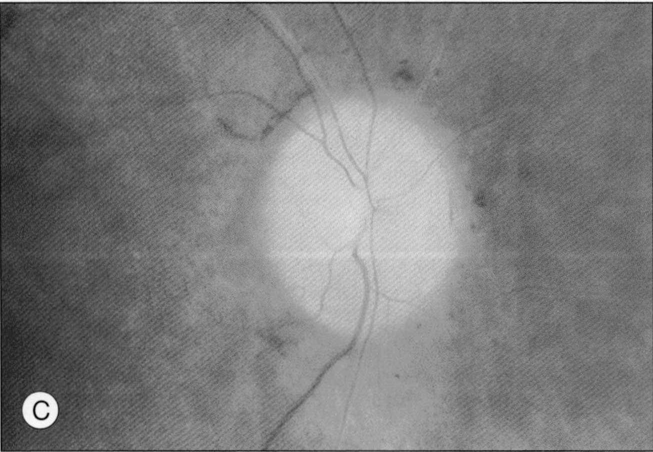

Fig. 40.15 Optic discs in an 18-year-old man with autosomal recessive retinitis pigmentosa as part of posterior-column ataxia and retinitis pigmentosa syndrome (A) (same patient as in Fig. 40.3), a 32-year-old man (B), and his 55-year-old father (C), both of whom have autosomal dominant retinitis pigmentosa. The disc in A shows peripapillary chorioretinal pallor, or the "golden ring" sign, that is characteristic of early retinitis pigmentosa. Note that the disc is nearly normal in the son (B), but shows severe waxy pallor in the father (C).

in part from gliosis overlying the discs.[21] Drusen-like globular excrescences may develop on the optic nerve or adjacent retina (Fig. 40.16). These have been mistaken for astrocytic hamartomas[49] and are consistent with disc drusen due to aberrant axoplasmic transport.[50,51] In a survey of 117 RP patients,[52] 10% were found to have clinically apparent optic nerve head drusen. Edwards et al.[53] suggested that this phenomenon is particularly common in RP associated with Usher syndrome type 1.

Flynn et al.[54] found that the presence or absence of macular RPE defects is of significant prognostic importance with regard to retention of visual acuity over the next 5 years. Specifically, the absence of macular lesion was associated with only one line of acuity loss over the 5-year period, whereas bull's-eye or geographic atrophy lesions were associated with a predicted acuity loss of three to four lines. The authors emphasize the importance of this type of information for prognostic counseling of patients with RP regarding the likelihood of preservation of visual acuity. Other maculopathies associated with RP include cellophane maculopathy, macular hole (complications of CME),[55] and a single report of RP with central serous retinopathy.[56]

Vitreous abnormalities

The most common abnormality of the vitreous in RP is the presence of fine, dust-like pigmented cells released from degeneration of the RPE. In patients with RP, complete posterior detachment of the vitreous, "cotton-ball" opacities, interwoven filaments in the retrocortical space, and spindle-shaped vitreous condensations are seen more frequently than in normal subjects.[57,58] A single case is reported of vitreous opacity so dense that vitrectomy was required.[59] Vitreous abnormalities related to peripheral retinal ischemia and preretinal neovascularization have been reported in rare cases of adRP and arRP.[60] Uncommonly, a peripheral Coats-like retinal vasculopathy with lipid exudations and serous retinal elevation can be seen in RP[61–63] (Fig. 40.17). Unlike idiopathic Coats syndrome, the retinal vasculopathy seen in RP is usually bilateral, shows no sex predilection, and typically occurs in older patients. Coats-like disease is seen in 3.6% of RP cases[64] and has been reported with adRP,[62,63] arRP[33] but not X-linked inheritance[63] (although see Fig. 40.17). Coats-like changes that occur in children[64,65] may change over a relatively short period of months to years, must be monitored carefully, and may need to be considered for laser or cryocoagulation. Vitreous hemorrhage related to preretinal neovascularization has also been described in rare cases.[60,66] Retinal edema in some cases may be caused by inflammation resulting from the degeneration of outer retina.[60,67]

Anterior-segment abnormalities

Cataracts are frequent anterior-segment complications of RP. The prevalence of cataracts in RP patients aged 20–39 years varied with the inheritance type, being roughly 52% for autosomal dominant, 39% for recessive, and 72% for X-linked cases.[68] The incidence of cataracts in RP is highly age-dependent.[68,69] The most frequent type of cataract is a posterior subcapsular lens opacity, which occurs in 35–51% of patients.[69,70] One study has suggested that posterior subcapsular opacities are most commonly associated with autosomal dominant inheritance (51%),[69,70] whereas another has suggested a more common association with X-linked inheritance.[71] Although keratoconus has been claimed to be more frequent among patients with RP,[72] the occurrence of keratoconus in typical juvenile- or adult-onset RP is extremely rare in our experience. Glaucoma, especially primary open angle glaucoma, is also allegedly more frequent in RP.[73] Sector RP appears to be associated with hyperopia and angle closure glaucoma.[74] Because of the other abnormalities of the disc and fundus and because of the already abnormal visual fields, the diagnosis and management of glaucoma are quite challenging in RP patients.

Refractive status

High myopia and astigmatism are frequently associated with RP.[68,75]

Psychophysical findings

Perimetry

Assessment of visual field is an important aspect of the management of RP. This is an invaluable tool in the diagnosis of RP, as well as being the most reliable method of quantifying real

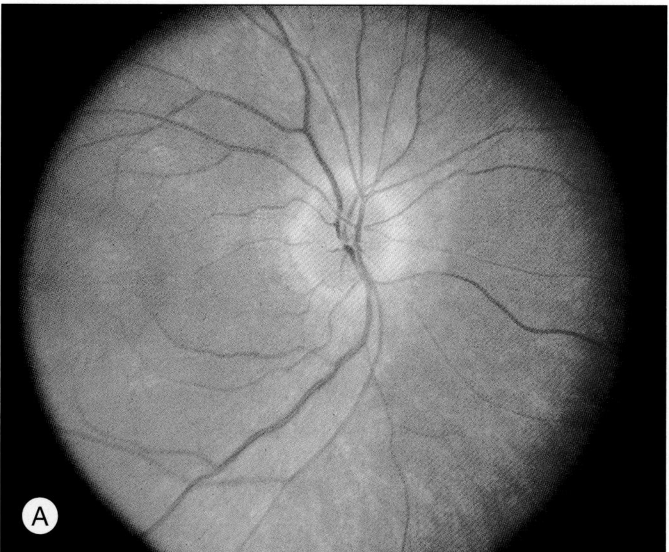

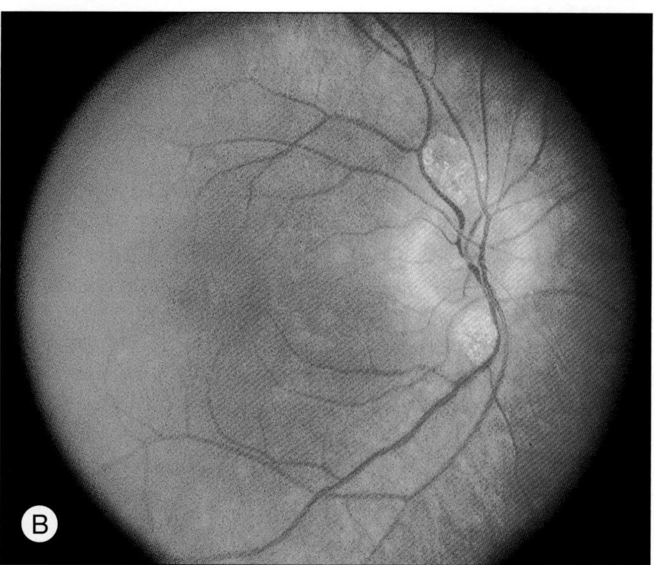

Fig. 40.16 Optic discs in the right eye of a patient with type 1 Usher syndrome (retinitis pigmentosa and prelingual deafness) at age 16 (A) and 25 (B), demonstrating development of peripapillary drusen.

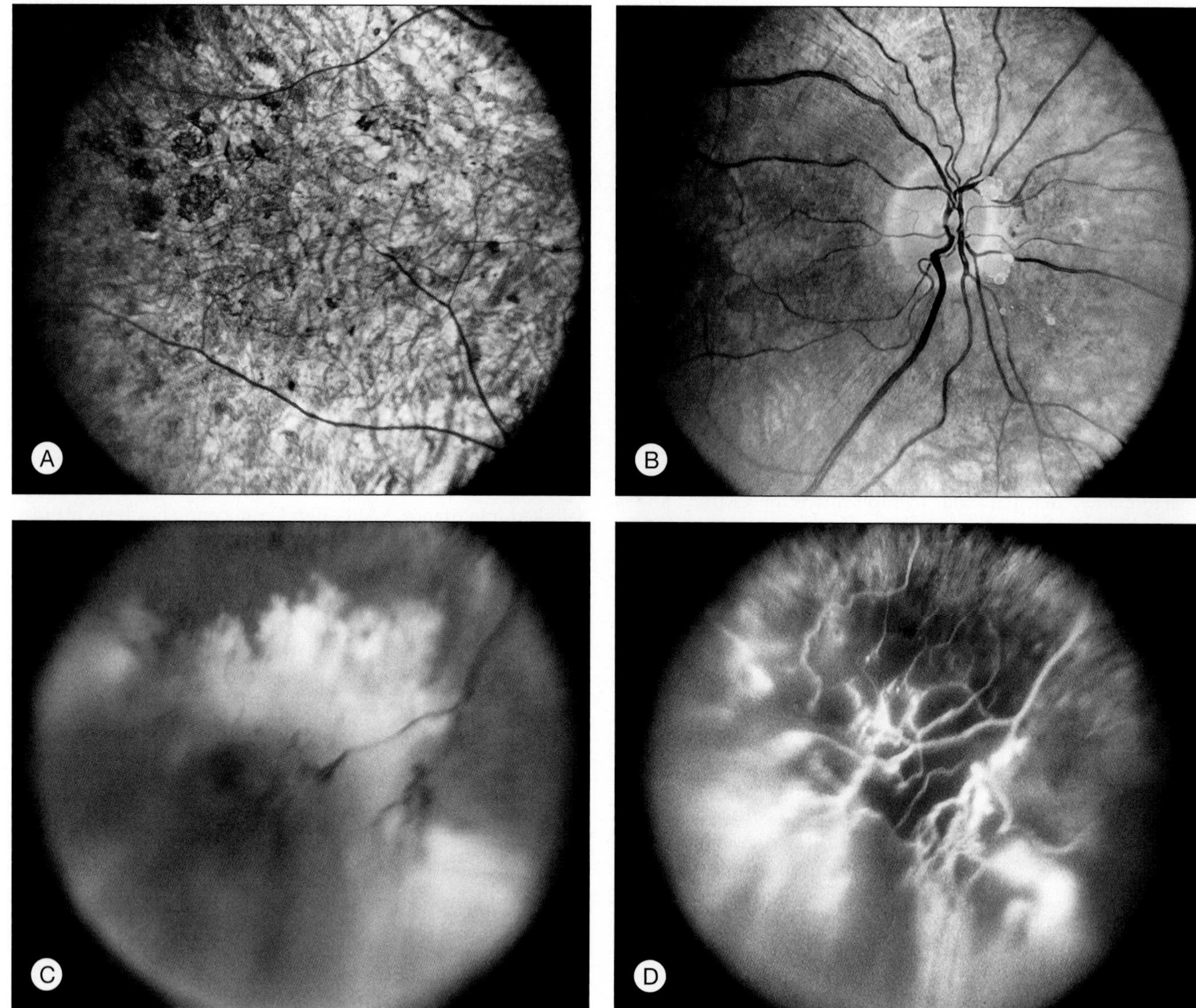

Fig. 40.17 Coats disease in the right eye (A, temporal retina; B, posterior pole; C and D, inferotemporal retina) of a 33-year-old man with retinitis pigmentosa that is probably X-linked. Note also peripapillary retinal drusen nasal to the disc. Visual acuity was 20/30–, J8, right eye, and 20/25–, J3, left eye.

change in visual deficit. It should be remembered when assessing the results of visual field testing that the reproducibility of visual fields is significantly less in patients with RP than in normal subjects. Kinetic visual fields tested on separate days by the same examiner varied by 5–6% in normal subjects but by 11–13% in patients with RP (intraobserver variation); variability between examiners for the same patient was 4–6% for normal subjects but 10–16% for patients with RP (interobserver variation).[76]

In the great majority of cases of RP, the earliest defects of the visual field, on kinetic perimetry, are relative scotomas in the midperiphery, between 30 and 50° from fixation (Fig. 40.18). These enlarge, deepen, and coalesce to form a ring of visual field loss. These midperipheral depressions of retinal sensitivity are readily documented as decreased retinal thresholds on static perimetry. As ring scotomas enlarge toward the far periphery, islands of relatively normal visual field remain, usually temporal but occasionally inferior or nasal (Fig. 40.19). The peripheral islands or remnants of visual field are often lost before the central field contracts sufficiently to qualify the individual as legally blind.

Kinetic visual field testing has traditionally been performed with the manual Goldmann perimeter. Recent advances have occurred in both kinetic and static perimetry. Semiautomated kinetic perimetry,[77] as implemented on the Octopus 101 and 900 perimeters (Haag-Streit, Köniz, Switzerland) (Fig. 40.20) automatically documents the testing and enables quantification of field by measurement of isopter area. A new fast thresholding algorithm, known as German adaptive thresholding estimation (GATE),[78] has enabled another advance in perimetry, that of full-field static perimetry to assess the entire visual field in a time frame comparable to that required to test the central 30° field with the Standard 4-2-1 strategy (Fig. 40.20) (Weleber et al., 2012, in preparation). The static threshold data from such testing can be modeled as sensitivity values into a three-dimensional hill of vision from which the magnitude and extent of the total visual field can be determined as a volumetric measurement (Weleber et al. 2011, in preparation).

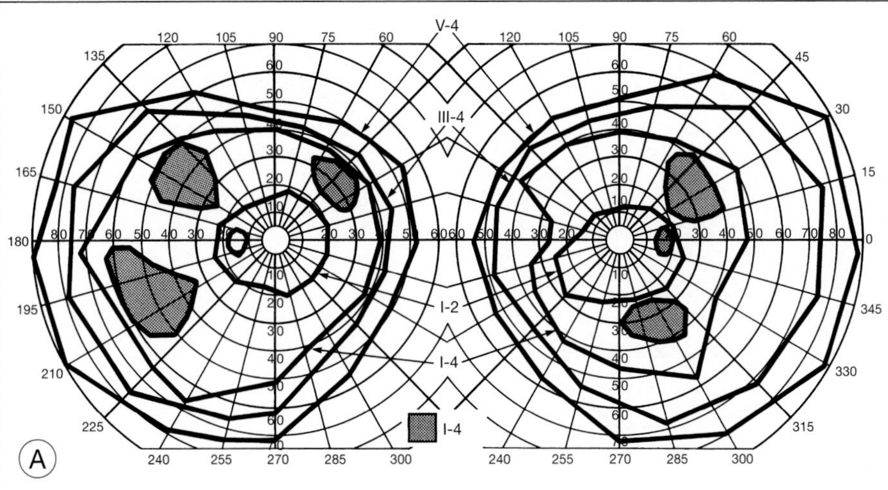

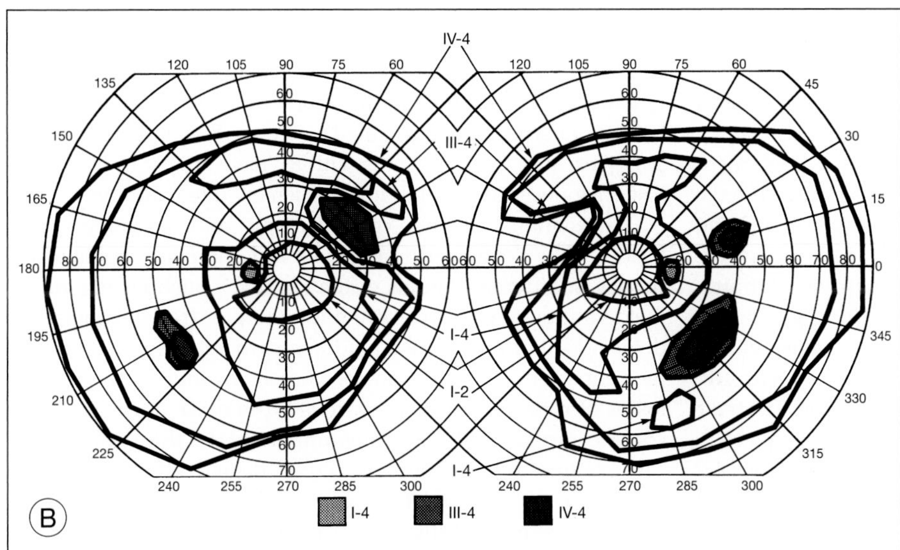

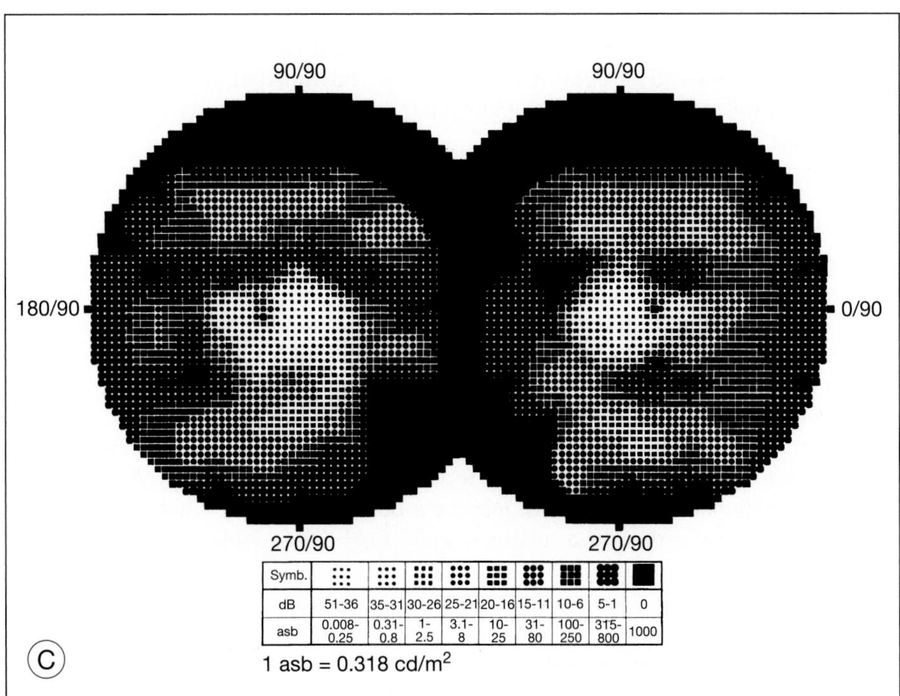

Fig. 40.18 Goldmann kinetic perimetry for a patient with autosomal dominant retinitis pigmentosa from the Pro23His mutation of rhodopsin at age 41 (A) and 47 years (B). (C) Octopus static (combined programs 23 and 34) perimetry using stimulus size III for the patient at age 47. Note enlargement and deepening of midperipheral scotomas and overall correlation of static visual field with detailed kinetic perimetry.

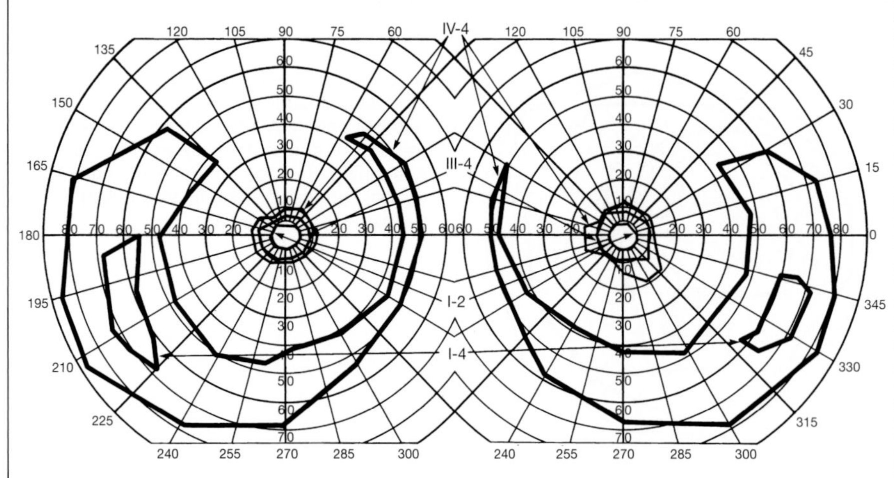

Fig. 40.19 Goldmann kinetic perimetry for a 36-year-old patient with retinitis pigmentosa from the Pro23His mutation of rhodopsin. Dense ring scotomas have broken through to the periphery superiorly, leaving a central field of 25° in diameter and only an incomplete annulus of peripheral vision in each eye. The fundus appearance of this patient at 40 years of age is shown in Figure 40.6.

If an RP patient is driving a motor vehicle, regular visual field assessments are mandatory and should be undertaken at least every 2 years. Most centers perform kinetic visual fields using a Goldmann perimeter for clinical evaluation and for assessment for driving and for disability. Almost all patients with RP have to restrict their driving at night and eventually stop driving altogether. Periodic assessment of full-field kinetic perimetry helps to provide patients with knowledge of their visual limitations and when to restrict and eventually stop driving.

Two-color static perimetry has been shown to be a useful tool in assessing the dark-adapted visual fields of patients with RP. Using this technique, Massof and Finkelstein[79–81] found that their patients with RP could be divided into two groups: (1) type I RP, which is associated with early diffuse loss of rod sensitivity relative to cone sensitivity and childhood-onset nyctalopia; and (2) type II RP, associated with regional and combined loss of both rod and cone retinal sensitivity and adult-onset nyctalopia. No patients have been observed to change from one type to the other.[82] No families have been reported that contain both types I and II in the same sibship.[15] An excess of type II RP over the type I form has been reported in simplex disease. Analysis of subgroups within simplex and multiplex RP suggest that a sizable proportion of type II patients may represent sporadic or acquired disease, and not true RP.[83]

Arden et al.[84] studied a series of cases of adRP both with ERGs and psychophysically with scotopic static thresholds. They found that the preservation of sizable rod responses on the ERG correlated perfectly with the Massof type II classification. Absence of rod ERG did not always indicate type I disease, and both types were seen in this group. Lyness et al.[85] reported clinical, psychophysical, and ERG findings in 104 patients (from 44 families) with adRP. Subgroup D (13 patients in four families) had diffuse loss of rod function and night blindness before the age of 10. Subgroup R (28 patients in 13 families) had regional loss of rod function, and most of these patients were unaware of night blindness until after the age of 20. Both groups had regional loss of cone functions. In the R group the rod-mediated ERG was usually present and substantial, whereas in the D group the rod ERG was undetectable. Although not identical, the D group bears similarities to Massof type I, and the R group bears similarities to type II. These studies suggest that the two types or groups may represent different pathophysiologic subtypes of RP. It should be emphasized, however, that a large proportion of patients (27 of the 44 families studied by Lyness et al.[85]) could not be incorporated into the D- versus R-type classification, partly because many patients with RP have almost undetectable ERG responses at presentation, which is quite common.

The techniques of two-color scotopic static perimetry have been further developed to evaluate rod and cone retinal sensitivities in different regions of the retina.[86,87] Such testing allows the definition of which class of photoreceptor (rod or cone) is the determinant of retinal threshold in a particular region or area of the retina. This has allowed the characterization of the relative losses of rods and cones in various types of RP associated with specific mutations.[88,89] Equally important to the definition of early retinal abnormalities in retinal degenerations, two-color perimetry can be used for monitoring disease therapy or for testing hypothesis of disease pathophysiology. For example, the abnormal, thickened Bruch's membrane, which acts as a diffusion barrier between the retina and choroid, has been proposed as a major factor leading to night blindness in Sorsby's fundus dystrophy.[90] The return of rod function after oral vitamin A supplements (50 000 IU/day) was elegantly recorded using these techniques.[90]

Dark adaptometry

Normal subjects, when placed in the dark after exposure to a strong adapting light, will rapidly reduce their retinal psychophysical threshold using their cone system, reaching a plateau in about 5 minutes. Thereafter rod adaptation slowly increases, and rods determine retinal thresholds for another 3 log units of sensitivity before a second plateau occurs at about 30 minutes of dark adaptation. Patients with RP, when tested with dark adaptometry, may show elevation of the cone segment, the rod segment, or both, to varying degrees (Fig. 40.21). Also, in some patients there may be a delay in reaching what eventually for them is a relatively good final dark adaptation rod threshold[91] (Fig. 40.22).

Time course analysis of dark adaptometry has been performed in patients with adRP and prolonged dark adaptation is associated with rhodopsin mutations Thr17Met, Pro23His, Gly106Arg, and Thr58A.[88,89,92] The most characteristic feature of the Pro23His genotype was prolonged dark adaptation, which was present in all patients regardless of their stage of disease.[89] Jacobson et al.[88]

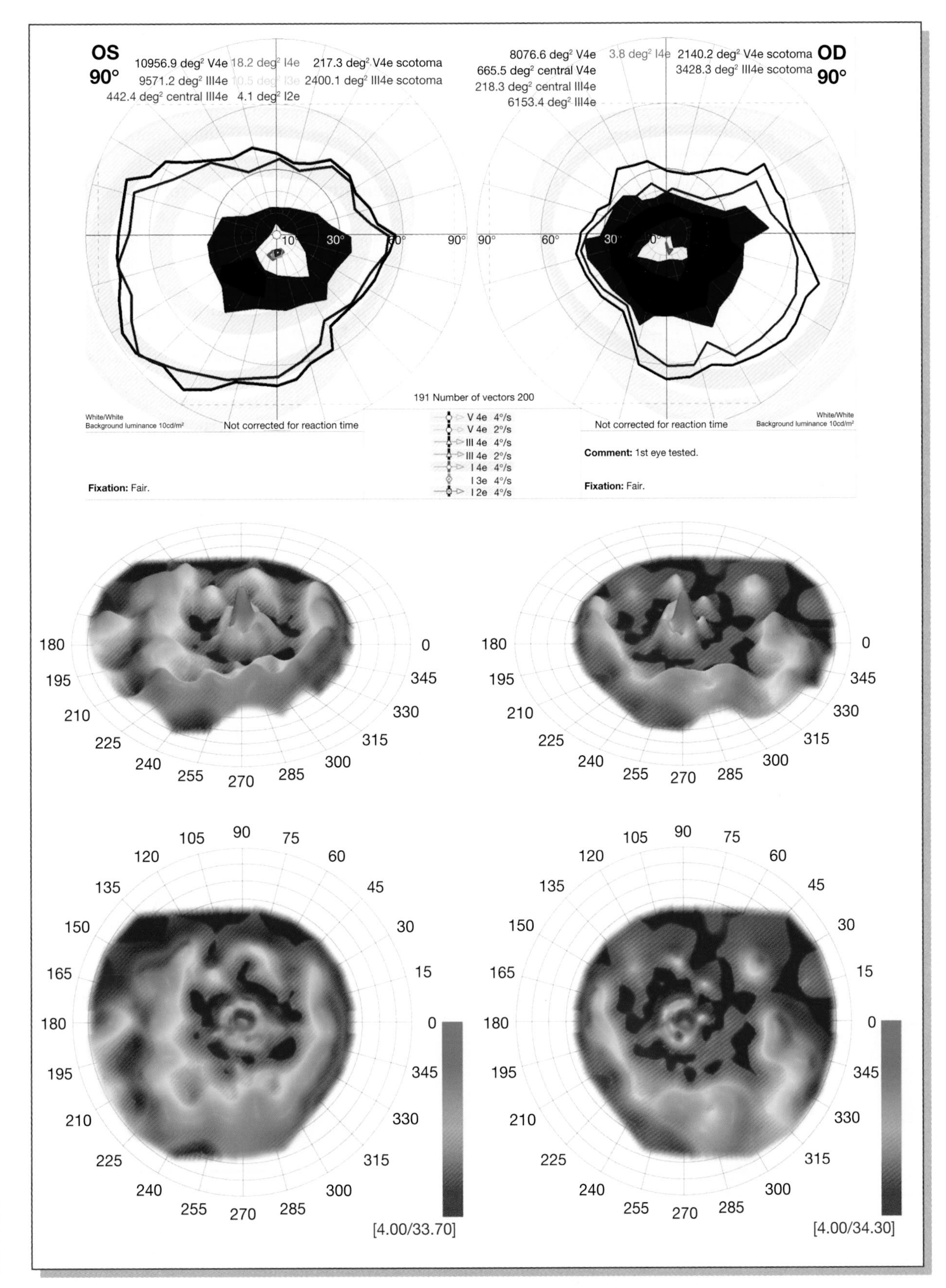

Fig. 40.20 Semiautomated kinetic perimetry in a 27-year-old woman with retinitis pigmentosa (top). The shaded areas depict the normal range for the isopters for the test targets presented. Three-dimensional (3D) model of the hill of vision for full-field static perimetry for this same subject (middle in tilted view, below in face view) using the size V test target and the German adaptive thresholding estimation thresholding algorithm.[78] The volume of this model, which was 40.2 dB-sr OD and 28.0 DB-sr OS (compared to a normal 112.5 dB-sr for a normal), reflects the magnitude and extent of the visual field for this subject. Thus, this patient has 35.7% OD and 24.9% OS of expected field volume for his age. Note that the 3D model provides much more topographical information on the location of the defects in the field of vision than does the kinetic perimetry. This is the same patient whose fundus autofluorescence image for the left eye is shown in Figure 40.29A.

also reported prolonged rod dark adaptation in patients with Thr58Arg and Thr17Met mutations of rhodopsin. Indeed, prolonged rod dark adaptation appears to be a characteristic finding of virtually all rhodopsin mutations. These studies suggest that each of these mutations produces specific abnormalities in the rate of reactions within the rods that limit the recovery of scotopic sensitivity. For patients with regional forms of RP from other causes, zones of more normally functioning retina may allow reasonably good final rod thresholds (Fig. 40.22). Minor abnormalities in cone thresholds are more likely to result in complaints of poor dark adaptation than mild to moderate elevation of rod thresholds. One study has indicated that abnormalities in the normal interactions between rods and cones may underlie the symptoms of poor night vision in some patients rather than isolated rod deficits.[93]

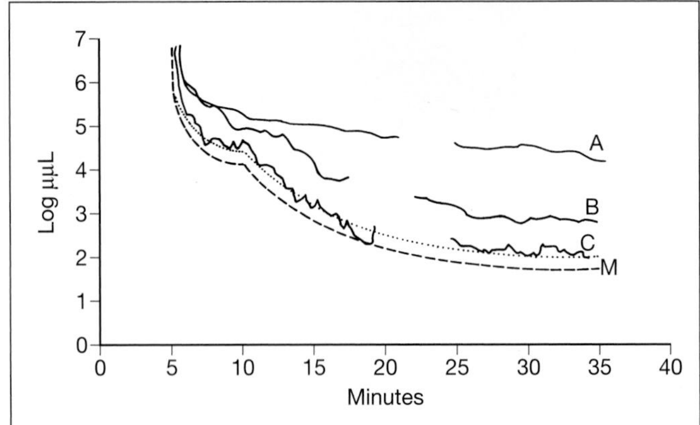

Fig. 40.21 Dark adaptometry showing marked elevation of both cone and rod thresholds with little or no cone–rod break in an 18-year-old woman, broken solid curve (A), with autosomal recessive retinitis pigmentosa and large-fiber sensory peripheral neuropathy (sister of patient shown in Figs 40.3 and 40.15A). Mild elevation of cone threshold with greater elevation of rod threshold in a 15-year-old young woman with Bardet–Biedl syndrome, broken solid curve (B). Borderline normal cone and rod segments in a 15-year-old young woman with type 2 Usher syndrome, broken solid curve (C). Dashed curve (M) is mean for normals aged 10–20 years.

Retinal densitometry (fundus reflectometry)

Retinal densitometry is a technique whereby, to deduce effective photoreceptor photopigment density, measurements are made of the difference between light shone into the eye and light reflected out of the eye. These measurements can be made and compared at different retinal loci, at different times, or against a retinal standard. From these data, estimates can be made of the rates of photopigment regeneration. Retinal densitometry has been performed on patients with RP by several investigators using a variety of techniques.[94–97] Rhodopsin levels were found to be reduced in all patients, but rhodopsin bleaching and regeneration kinetics have been normal. Van Meel and van Norren[98] found subnormal cone pigment levels in all patients studied and found prolonged cone pigment regeneration in eight of 12 patients with RP.

The losses of retinal sensitivity in RP in some patients are believed to relate to loss of quantum catch by the reduction of rhodopsin levels in the retina.[94,95] A reduction of rhodopsin level to one-tenth of normal, for example, would be expected to be associated with a 10-fold elevation in the rod threshold. These calculations are only estimates, however. In vitamin A deficiency, the elevation of the rod threshold is much greater than predicted by the reduction in rhodopsin levels.[95] Perlman and Auerbach[99] described a group of patients with RP who, when

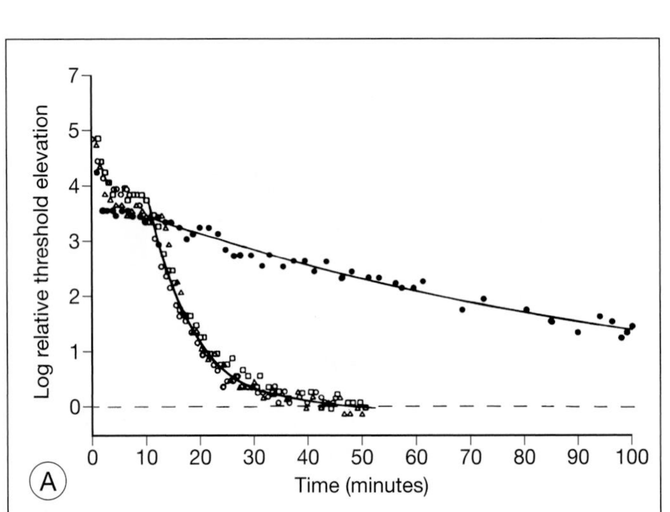

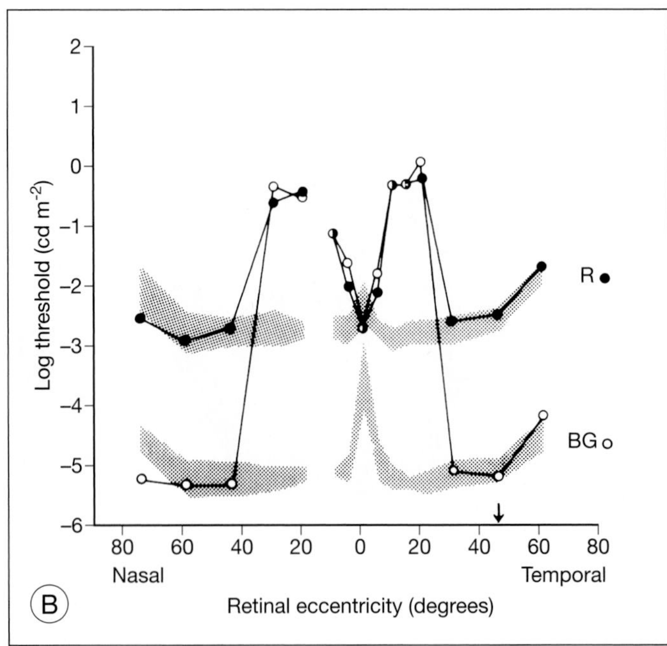

Fig. 40.22 (A) Delayed achievement of final dark adaptation threshold in a patient with autosomal dominant retinitis pigmentosa. Filled circles are data from the patient; open triangles, circles, and squares are from three normals. The time constant for reduction of the rod retinal threshold by a factor of 1/2.718 of the threshold at the beginning of the curve was 8.5 minutes for the normal data and 101.6 minutes for the patient. Measurements were taken from a point approximately 45° temporal to the fovea. (B) Retinal thresholds measured at different points of retinal eccentricity for the same patient as in A, showing zones of elevated thresholds in nasal and temporal midperiphery with lower thresholds centrally and more peripherally. The shaded regions represent the range of absolute thresholds for the long- (R) and middle-wavelength (BG) test flashes for 5 normal subjects. (The point used for A is noted with an arrow in B.) (Reproduced with permission from Alexander KR, Fishman GA. Prolonged rod dark adaptation in retinitis pigmentosa. Br J Ophthalmol 1984;68:561–9.)

studied with retinal densitometry, were found to have elevations of rod thresholds greater than what would be expected purely on the basis of reductions of rhodopsin levels. Kemp et al.[100] found that 4 patients with type II (regional) adRP had elevations of retinal threshold that could be explained solely by loss of quantum catch from reductions of rhodopsin levels in the retina. However, 5 patients with type I (diffuse) adRP had elevations of threshold that were much greater than expected on the basis of loss of rhodopsin and quantal absorption for the reduction of rhodopsin levels observed.[100] These studies provide evidence suggesting that the two classifications represent different pathophysiologic entities. Others have studied patients with defined mutations of rhodopsin. Kemp et al.[89] have shown that, for patients with the Pro23His mutation of rhodopsin, rhodopsin levels are decreased below normal by amounts that indicate that rod sensitivity loss is determined by the reduced ability to absorb light. Similar findings were reported for patients with rhodopsin Thr17Met, Thr58Arg, and Gln344ter.[88]

Fulton and Hansen[97] have reported reflectometry results on a mother and three daughters whose RP appeared to have a sectoral distribution. Elevations of retinal threshold were greater than those predicted by reductions of rhodopsin seen on densitometry measurements, suggesting that the dysfunction was central to the photoreceptor outer segments.

Electrophysiology

Karpe[101] in 1945 first reported that the ERG was "extinguished" in RP. The standing, or resting, potential of the eye was first described by DuBois-Reymond in 1849. Riggs[102] in 1954 was the first to report that the resting potential was decreased in pigmentary degeneration of the eye. Arden et al.[103] in 1962 developed the currently widely used technique for measurement of the light-induced rise of the resting potential of the eye (the electro-oculogram (EOG)), which is considered a function of the RPE. Fast oscillations of the resting potential can be recorded, and these offer another measure of RPE function.[104] Gouras[105] in 1970 based clinical ERG on the use of Ganzfeld stimulation. Standardized conditions and assessment protocols have now been established for electrodiagnostic investigations.[106,107]

Electrodiagnostic responses in an RP patient can range from normal to undetectable. In general, more sizable responses are seen with younger patients or at earlier stages of disease. Most patients with advanced RP have undetectable responses (typically less than 10 μV) to single-flash, nonaveraged techniques.[105] Computer averaging, however, can usually detect small ERG responses in even moderately advanced stages.[13,108] In studying the natural course of RP, Berson et al.[13] found that patients lost an average of 16–18.5% per year of remaining ERG amplitude to bright white flashes (a mixed rod–cone response).

Many studies have compared ERG responses in the different RP inheritance types. Tanino and Ohba[12] and Berson,[109] using conventional techniques, found that the ERG is more likely to be recordable in older patients with adRP than arRP. Berson et al.[13] have also shown that progressive ERG loss of amplitude over a 3-year period is least in adRP. Birch and Fish[110] found that the rate of progression of rod loss, as indicated by the half-saturation coefficient of the rod stimulus–response curve, varied among the inheritance groups. This ranged from 0.3 log unit/year in elevation of rod threshold in X-linked RP to 0.12 log unit/year elevation in adRP.

Agreement exists that the cone-mediated implicit times can be significantly prolonged in various forms of RP. Berson[111] has also stressed the importance of delays in the implicit time for cone-mediated 30-Hz flicker responses. Berson and colleagues[112,113] found that the cone-mediated b-wave implicit time in their patients was characteristically prolonged in adRP with reduced penetrance but not in completely penetrant adRP. Sandberg et al.[114] suggested that this was due to an abnormal contribution of extrafoveal cones in adRP with incomplete penetrance. This may be due to abnormal cone light adaptation or a disturbance of normal rod–cone interactions.

Histopathologic study has indicated that, in RP, a postreceptor deficit may contribute to macular dysfunction.[115] ERG study has confirmed this. Falsini et al.[116] have assessed 8–10-Hz focal ERGs in 22 simplex and recessive RP cases. They found a loss of fundamental and second harmonic components and an increase in the fundamental-to-second harmonic ratio. This was interpreted as suggesting that both inner and outer retinal abnormalities contribute to visual deficit. Cideciyan and Jacobson[117] have documented electronegative b-waves in some cases of RP. This finding was seen with abnormalities of on/off components of cone ERGs and reduced oscillatory potentials[117] and was interpreted as indicative of significant inner retinal abnormalities in these RP cases.

Models of analysis of the ERG have been developed that attempt to isolate from the ERG the photoreceptor and bipolar contributions, specifically the original components of Granit's model of the cat ERG, termed P3 and P2[118] (Fig. 40.23A). These analysis methods have been developed to quantify the visual deficit attributable to outer and inner retinal disease (Fig. 40.23B–D). P3 is the corneal-negative response of photoreceptor outer segments that contributes to the a-wave of the Ganzfeld ERG. The analysis involves subjecting the leading edge of the a-wave of the ERG at a range of intensities to a mathematical curve-fitting algorithm[119–121] (Fig. 40.23C) using equations that describe the kinetics of rod phototransduction activation.[122] The method of Hood and Birch[123] allows for estimation of two variables: S, which is a sensitivity factor, and R_{mp3}, which is the maximum amplitude. Such analysis can determine whether phototransduction is affected in a given disease.

P2 is the bipolar cell-derived component of the rod-isolated b-wave. The P2 component of the rod b-wave, derived from bipolar cells, can be isolated from the full-frequency ERG, using an algorithm whereby the P3 is first calculated for a given series of intensities, after which the P3 is subtracted from the series of rod responses[124,125] (Fig. 40.23D). This gives a much better estimate of the ON bipolar contribution to the b-wave, especially for patients in whom the ON bipolar cells are more affected than the photoreceptors.[124]

Application of these techniques to 15 patients with RP has shown that, for P3 analysis, all patients had significantly reduced values of R_{mp3}, indicating effective loss or damage of rods, and a wide spectrum of values for S.[126] Three patients had normal values for S. Four RP patients had subnormal S values but normal local retinal psychophysical thresholds in some regions of their retina. The rest had abnormal S values and abnormal visual fields with globally reduced thresholds. The rod b-wave amplitudes to a range of intensities for these RP patients were fitted with the Michaelis–Menten equation, generating the parameters K_{bw} (the semisaturation intensity, which is a sensitivity function) and V_{max} (the maximum amplitude). For all patients,

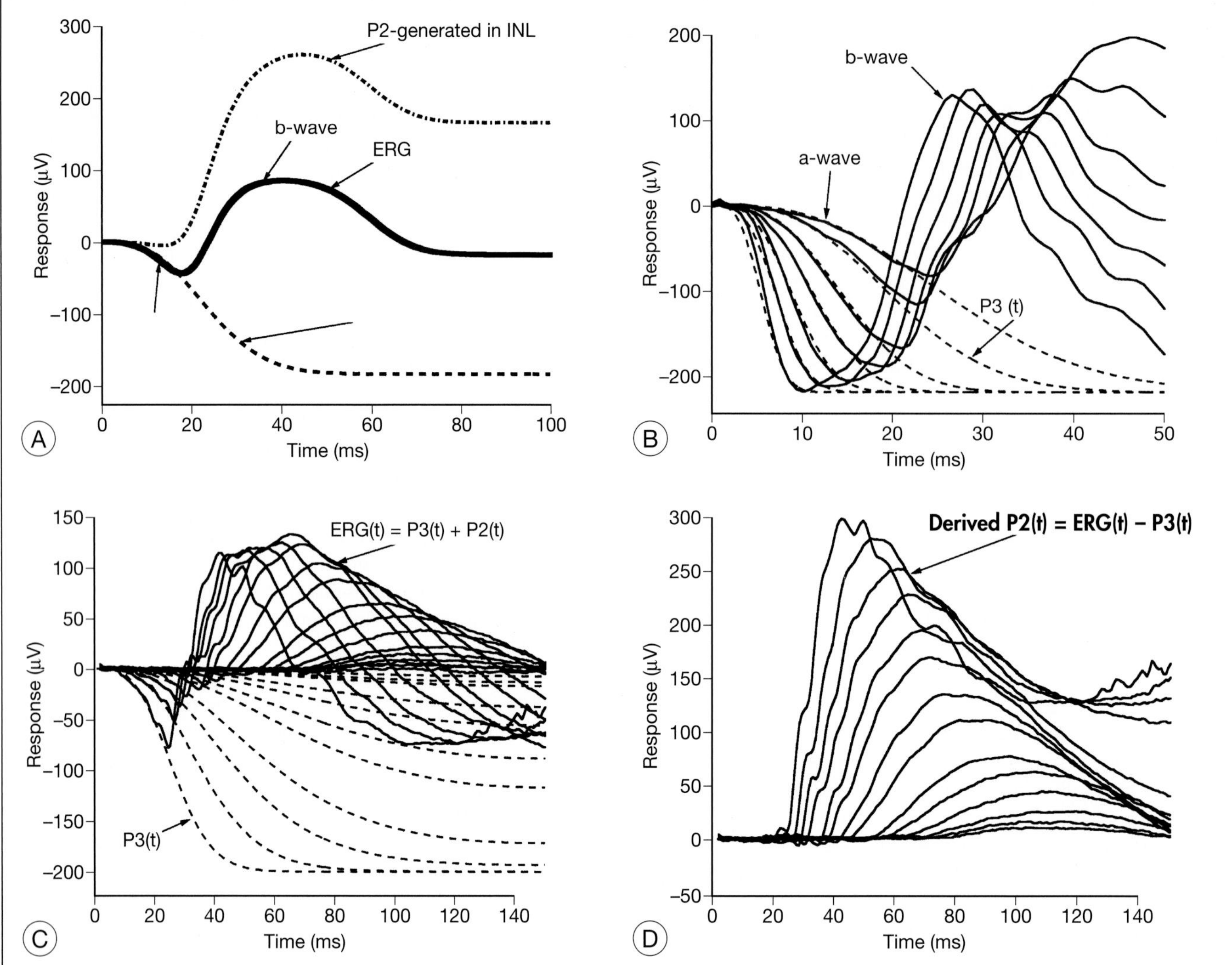

Fig. 40.23 (A) Simplified illustration of the retinal elements of the rod electroretinogram (ERG: upper left) based on Granit's model of the cat ERG. The b-wave of the corneal ERG (solid line) is the summation of a negative P3 generated by photoreceptors and a positive P2 generated in the inner layers of the retina. (B) The solid curves (upper right) are the scotopic ERG responses elicited by a high-intensity series of flashes from a normal subject. The dashed curves are the predicted P3 responses from a model of the receptor response fitted to the leading edge of the a-wave. (C) The solid curves (lower left) are records from a normal subject to a series of brief flashes, up to about 2 log scotoma td-s in energy, with the underlying P3 (rod receptor) responses shown as the dashed curves. (D) The curves (lower right) are the derived P2 responses obtained by computer subtraction of the P3 responses from the ERGs. INL, inner nuclear layer. (Modified with permission from Hood DC, Birch DG. A computational model of the amplitude and implicit time of the b-wave of the human ERG. Visual Neurosci 1992;8:107–26.)

the changes in K_{bw} and V_{max} followed the changes seen in S and R_{mp3}.[126] Hood and Birch[123] studied rod phototransduction in 11 patients with RP and four with cone–rod dystrophy (CRD). Their findings, which were similar to those above, supported the conclusion that the activation stage of rod phototransduction is affected in some forms of RP and CRD but not all.

Supernormal and delayed derived P2 responses were found by Hood et al.[127] when they applied modeling analysis to an unusual retinal dystrophy, first reported by Gouras et al.[128] in 1983 as "cone dystrophy, nyctalopia, and supernormal rod responses." Although Gouras et al.[128] initially attributed this dystrophy to an abnormality in receptor cyclic guanosine monophosphate (cGMP) activity, P3 and P2 modeling by Hood et al.[127] showed that the delays in the rod and cone b-wave were not caused by the speed or amplification of phototransduction but resulted from delays beyond the outer segments involving a delay in activation of the inner nuclear layer activity. This disorder was subsequently clinically and electrophysiologically defined as the enhanced S-cone syndrome (ESCS)[129,130] and was later shown to result from mutation of the gene *NR2E3*.[131]

Paradigms have been developed to study the kinetics of rod transduction deactivation.[132] This technique uses a bright conditioning flash followed by a probe flash. The recovery of the amplitude of the response to the probe, which is presented at varying intervals after the conditioning flash, provides a measure of the return to baseline of the response to the conditioning flash and, hence, the kinetics of transduction deactivation. The authors conclude that the lifetime of activated rhodopsin in normal human rods is 2.3 seconds. This technique has been applied to humans with the Pro23His rhodopsin mutation, demonstrating a reduction of the gain of activation and marked slowing of deactivation of rhodopsin (by a factor of at least 5).[132] Animal models of RP, for example, transgenic mice expressing the mutant Pro23His rhodopsin gene, have also demonstrated increases in the half-maximal recovery period, $T_{50\%}$, indicating abnormally prolonged recovery from the conditioning flash.[133]

Analysis of the a-wave leading edge has also recently shown that in RP, the efficiency of cone phototransduction is affected very early, even in some patients in whom the sensitivity of rod phototransduction is normal. X-linked inheritance seemed to be associated with greater phototransduction abnormalities in cones and rods at a younger age than seen in other modes of inheritance.[134]

Multifocal ERG techniques have been developed whereby, through patterned stimulation of the retina cross-correlated with recording of the ERG responses from a corneal electrode, very small ERG responses can be obtained from precisely localized regions of the retina[135–137] (Fig. 40.24). Multifocal ERGs can be seen in advanced RP where the 30-Hz flicker response is barely detectable[138] (Fig. 40.25). Hood and Li[137] have shown that, in RP, amplitudes of ERG responses do not correspond as well as b-wave implicit times with the retinal sensitivity as measured by static perimetry (Fig. 40.26). This is most evident with the regional or sectoral types of RP. Thus the b-wave implicit time appears to reflect early involvement of the disease process in regions of the retina that still have relatively good retinal sensitivity. Robson et al.[139] compared pattern ERG changes in RP patients with abnormalities of fundus autofluorescence (FAF). In such patients, pattern ERG responses suggested that visual loss was attributable to dysfunction rather than cell death.

In general, the EOG is abnormal in diffuse hereditary rod–cone degenerations of the retina.[140] In typical RP, the slow and fast light-induced oscillations of the resting potential are usually decreased simultaneously early in the disease (Fig. 40.27). In some patients the fast oscillations of the resting potential are diminished earlier than the slow oscillation.[104] In others the fast oscillations of the EOG are more preserved than the slow oscillation, a finding that also occurs in Best vitelliform macular dystrophy.[104,141] In most cases of RP the EOG is abnormal when the ERG is abnormal.

Imaging modalities in RP

Fundus photography/fluorescein angiography

Documentation by fundus photography can assist in monitoring changes in patients with RP. Fluorescein angiography in patients with RP will demonstrate hyperfluorescence in areas of RPE atrophy and can highlight areas of CME (Fig. 40.28). However, fluorescein angiography has largely been supplanted by OCT for detecting cystoid maculopathy. In addition, concerns about light exposure accelerating certain forms of RP in animal models have prompted many ophthalmologists to exercise caution in obtaining excessive photographs.[142]

In many cases of mild to moderate RP, fluorescein angiography reveals transmission defects of the RPE with later diffuse leakage.[143] In 78 of 82 patients with RP, Newsome[144] found extravasation of dye from perifoveal capillaries in only a few patients but frequent abnormalities of the blood–retinal barrier at the level of the RPE. Such angiographically significant CME can often be seen at an early stage of disease in young patients who still retain good vision (20/25 or better). Macular edema is a significant cause of early loss of visual acuity in RP.[144,145]

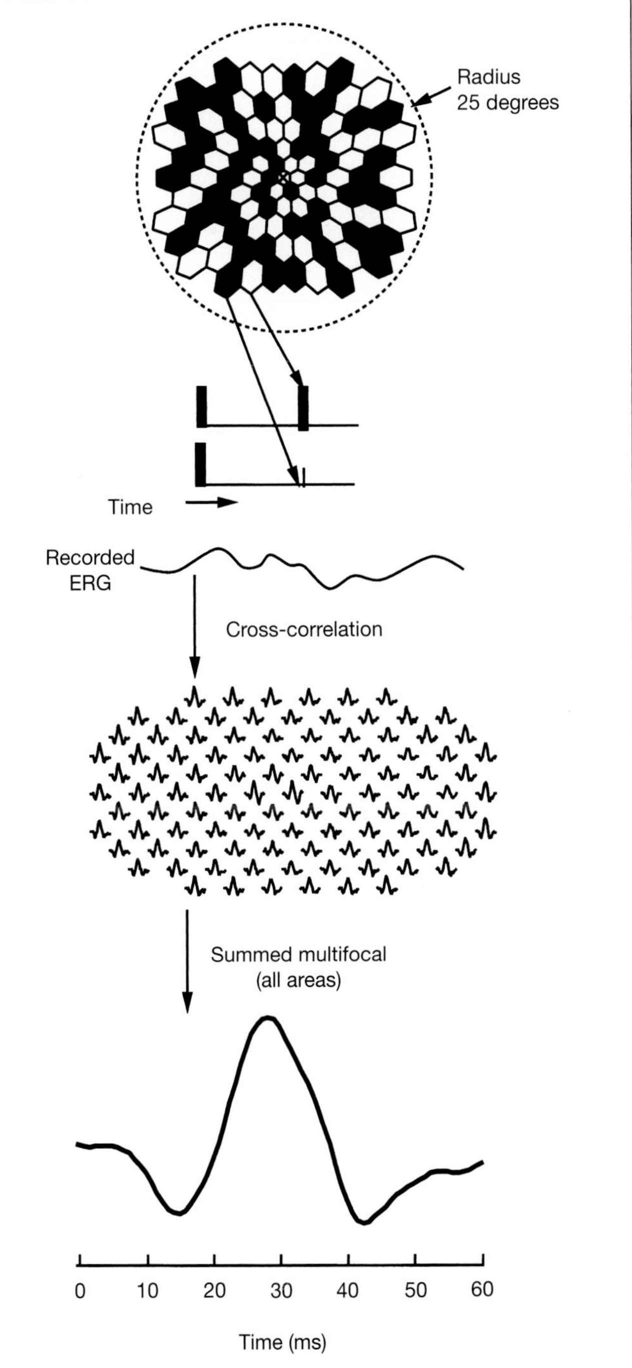

Fig. 40.24 Schematic of multifocal paradigm. The stimulus consists of a pattern of 103 hexagons contained within a 50° diameter area. The subject fixates on the center of the pattern, while the hexagons undergo changes from black to white and from white to black according to a mathematical sequence that allows the stimulation of various local areas of the retina to be cross-correlated with the electroretinogram (ERG) continuously recorded from the cornea. Within a few minutes (typically 4–8 minutes), one can record tiny submicrovolt ERGs corresponding to the changing pattern of each hexagon of the stimulus pattern. (Modified with permission from Hood DC, Seiple W, Holopigian K, et al. A comparison of the components of the multifocal and full-field ERGs. Visual Neurosci 1997;14:533–44.)

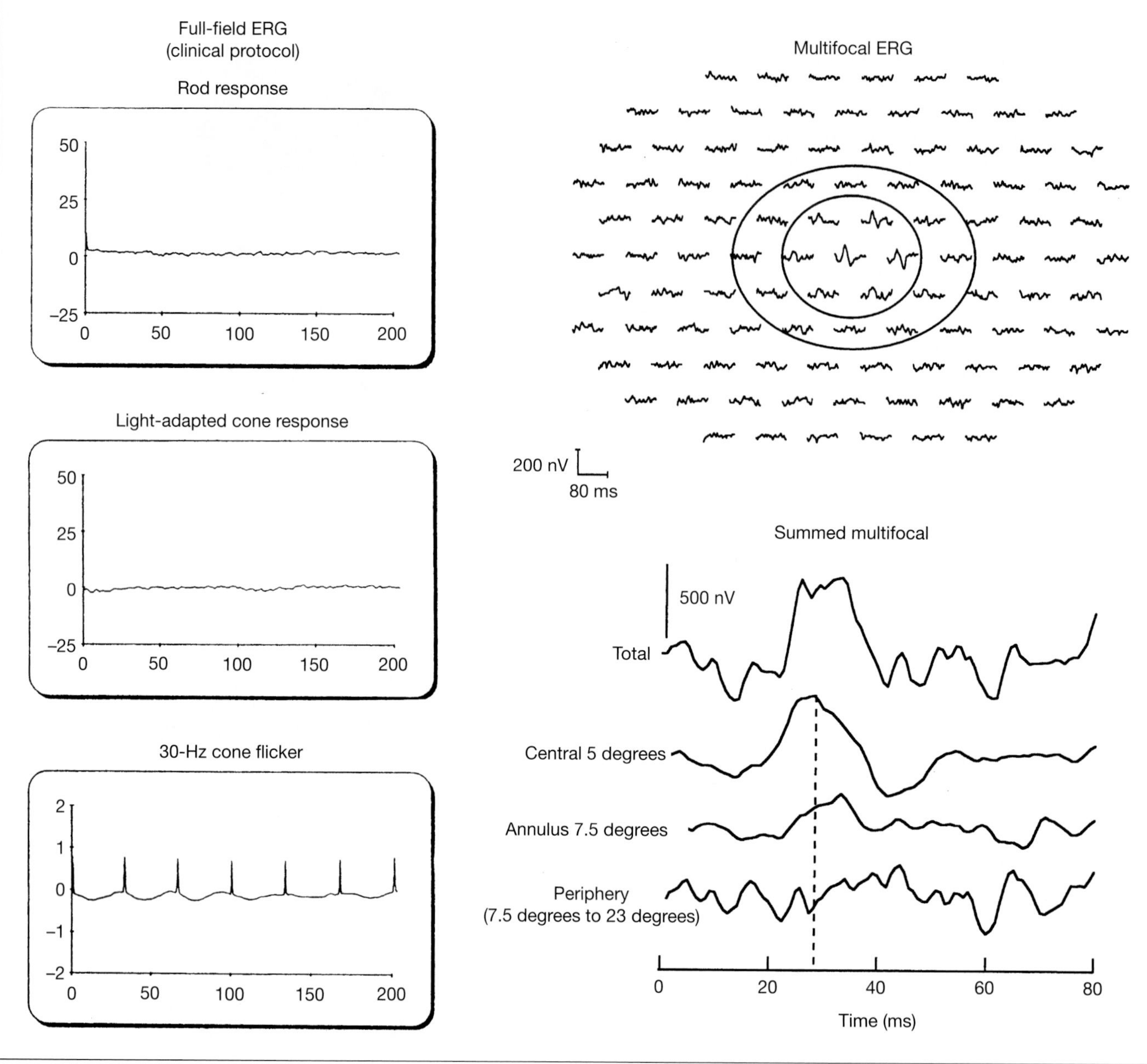

Fig. 40.25 Full-field clinical electroretinogram (ERG) protocol (left) and multifocal ERG (right) from a patient with retinitis pigmentosa. The full-field ERG showed no discernible rod or light-adapted cone response to single flash and a barely detectable 0.2-μV response to 30-Hz flicker response. However, sizable ERGs were detected within the central fields using the multifocal ERG technique. (Courtesy of D.C. Hood and D.G. Birch.)

Autofluorescence

FAF utilizes a scanning laser ophthalmoscope to stimulate intrinsically autofluorescent molecules of lipofuscin to visualize the RPE.[146] Studies from patients with RP have shown that lack of signal on FAF correlate well with areas of RPE atrophy, while areas of increased FAF can be seen in areas with persistent macular edema as well as within areas of surviving retina.[147] Most RP patients demonstrate a perifoveal ring (Fig. 40.29) of increased autofluorescence within the macula, which denotes the border between functional and dysfunctional retina (see Chapter 4, Autofluorescence).[139,147–149] The border of the parafoveal ring of increased autofluorescence has been shown to correlate with functional status as measured by pattern ERG, multifocal ERG, scotopic fine matrix mapping, and microperimetery.[150,151] In addition, areas outside the ring have been correlated with the loss of outer nuclear layer thickness and disruption of the inner-segment–outer-segment (IS/OS) junction on OCT.[152,153] Near-infrared autofluorescence (NIA) has also been used to image melanin present in the apical tips of the RPE.[154] Similar to FAF, rings with increased NIA are seen in patients with RP.[155] Combined NIA and blue light FAF imaging suggest that the presence of NIA may correlate better with preserved cone function, while blue light FAF indicates only preservation of RPE cells.[155]

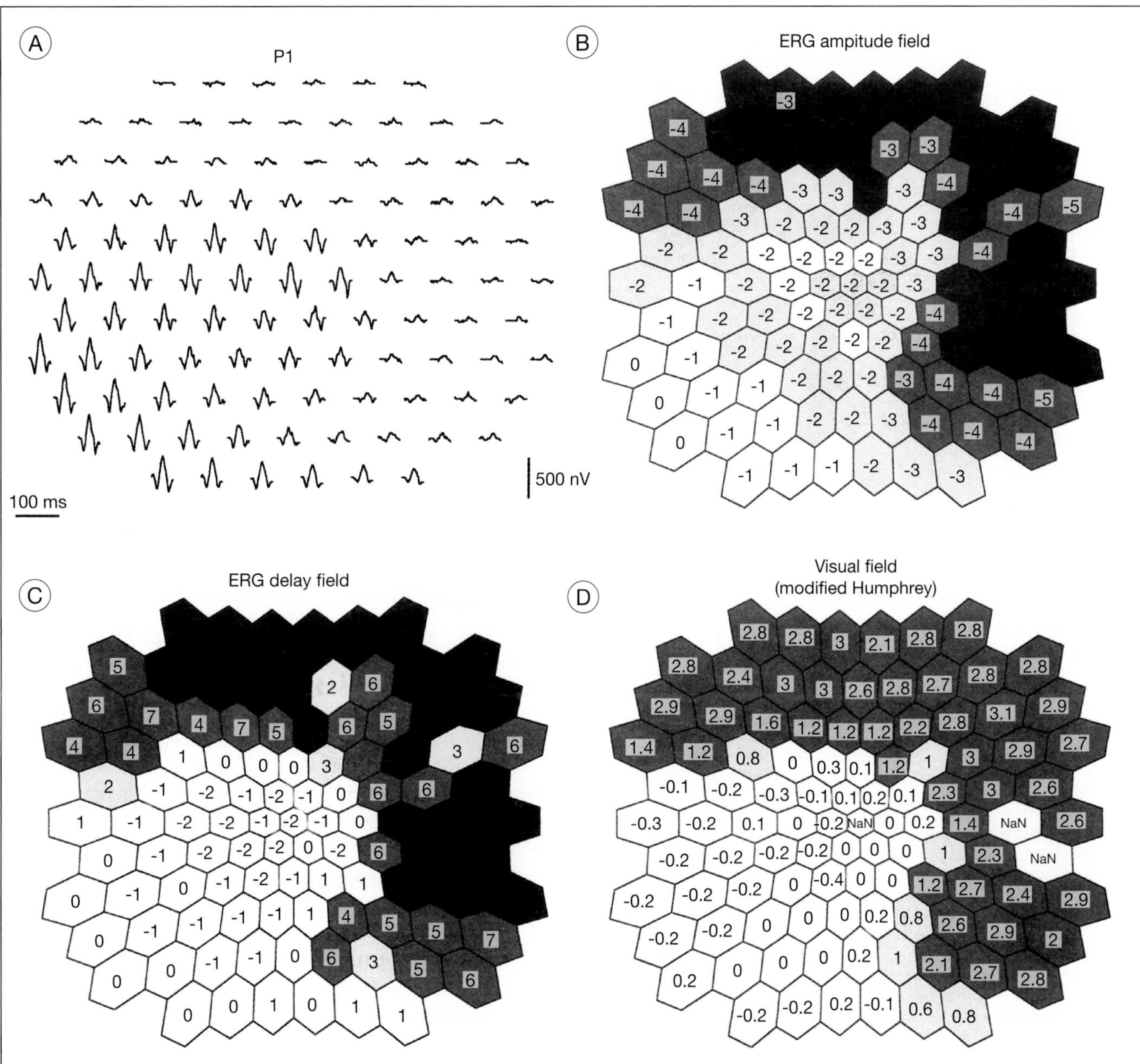

Fig. 40.26 (A) Multifocal electroretinograms (ERGs) from the right eye of a patient (P1) with autosomal recessive retinitis pigmentosa. The amplitude of the responses was decreased throughout the retina. However, this subject's disease was regional in distribution with marked preservation of function centrally and inferotemporally. (B) ERG amplitude loss field (in SD from normal) for the same subject calculated by subtracting the mean trough-to-peak amplitude for the controls from the trough-to-peak amplitude for the patient's response at each location. These differences were rounded and expressed in units of 100 nV. The clear regions indicate a decrease in amplitude of less than 162 nV (< −2 SD); the light-gray regions signify a decrease between 162 and 324 nV (−2 to −4 SD); and the darkest gray regions signify a decrease greater than 324 nV (> −4 SD). The black hexagons indicate that the response amplitude did not meet the criterion value of 90 nV. (C) ERG delay field for same subject, showing that regions that had subnormal amplitudes could be either normal or delayed in implicit time. The numbers in the hexagons were calculated by subtracting the mean implicit time for the controls from the implicit time for the patient's response at each location. The numbers in these fields are rounded to the nearest millisecond for presentation. The black hexagons indicate that the response amplitude did not meet the criterion value of 90 nV. The clear regions signify that the delay was less than 1.7 ms (< +2 SD); the light-gray regions signify that the delay was between 1.7 and 3.4 ms (+2 to +4 SD); and the darkest gray regions signify that the delay was greater than 3.4 ms (> +4 SD). (Note that, since the numbers in these figures have been rounded, the same delay, for example, 2 ms, can appear as clear or as light gray depending on whether it was less than or greater than 1.7 ms.) (D) Modified Humphrey visual field thresholds for the corresponding hexagons using a 40-minute size target on a background luminance of 10 cd/m^2. The number at each point is the log of the ratio of the patient's threshold to the mean threshold of the control group for that point. The clear regions signify that the patient's threshold at that point was within 0.5 log unit (< +2 SD) of the mean; the light-gray regions signify values between 0.5 and 1.0 log unit (+2 to +4 SD); and the dark-gray signify values greater than 1.0 log unit (> 4 SD). The regions designated NaN include the central point (which the Humphrey system does not allow to be measured with a custom program) and two points that fall within the blind spot of normals. Note that ERG delay field was a better predictor of visual field threshold loss than the ERG amplitude field. (Reproduced with permission from Hood DC, Holopigian K, Greenstein V et al. Assessment of local retinal function in patients with retinitis pigmentosa using the multi-focal ERG technique. Vis Res 1998;38:163–79.)

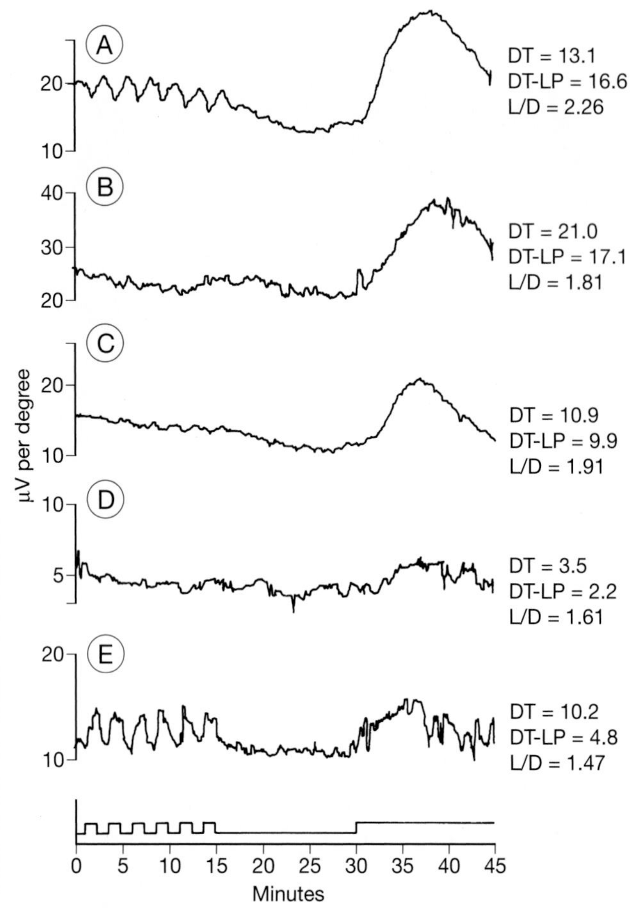

Fig. 40.27 Electro-oculogram (EOG) in (A) a normal subject; (B) a 24-year-old man with autosomal dominant retinitis pigmentosa; (C) a 25-year-old woman with autosomal recessive retinitis pigmentosa (case 3); (D) a 30-year-old man with retinitis punctata albescens (case 12); and (E) a 35-year-old woman with autosomal recessive pericentral retinitis pigmentosa. The event marker line below the tracings indicates "on" (up) or "off" (down) in regard to the 68 cd/m^2 background light in the Ganzfeld stimulator. The ordinate is the indirectly measured amplitude of the corneofundal or standing potential of the eye (in microvolts per degree of fixation shift), as generated by alternating fixation between two red light-emitting diode fixation lights 30° apart. During the first 15 minutes of testing, the light alternates between dark and light periods of 75 seconds each to stimulate the so-called fast oscillations of the standing potential of the eye. The dark trough (DT) is the lowest point in the standing potential during the second 15 minutes of total darkness. During the third 15-minute period the background light is on continuously, stimulating a slow light-induced rise in the standing potential to a light peak (LP) 7–8 minutes later. As retinitis pigmentosa progresses, the light-induced rise of the resting potential (DT-LP), especially as indicated by the light-to-dark ratio (L/D), decreases. Note that, in all patients except E, the slow oscillation, as evidenced by the L/D ratio, is more preserved than the fast oscillations. (Reproduced with permission from Weleber RG. Fast and slow oscillations of the electro-oculogram in Best's macular dystrophy and retinitis pigmentosa. Arch Ophthalmol 1989;107:530–7.)

Optical coherence tomography

OCT has become one of the most utilized imaging modalities for studying retinal disease in the past several years. Ultrahigh-resolution OCT and SD-OCT have been used to study retinal structures in patients with RP.[156,157] In these patients, such studies have demonstrated decreased thickness of the outer nuclear layer and loss of the external limiting membrane and IS/OS junctions. Loss of outer nuclear layer thickness or of the IS/OS has been correlated with visual defects measured by visual fields, microperimetry, or multifocal ERG.[29,158–160] SD-OCT is especially useful for detecting CME (Fig. 40.30) or epiretinal membranes, which are common features in patients with RP.[161] The ability to detect CME by OCT ring often eliminates the need for fluorescein angiography.

Adaptive optics scanning laser ophthalmoscopy

Traditional imaging modalities cannot resolve individual retina cells due to the optical limits imposed by the cornea and lens which create higher-order aberrations resulting in image blur.[162] A combination of adaptive optics with flood illumination or scanning laser ophthalmoscopy can compensate for these factors and provide imaging of individual cone photoreceptors.[163] Adaptive optics studies from patients with both CRD and RP have demonstrated increased cone spacing as well as qualitative areas where cone profiles could not be identified.[164–166] Recent advances have now enabled imaging of rod photoreceptors and foveal cones.[167] The ability to quantify cone photoreceptors has already been studied in one treatment trial for RP[168] and will undoubtedly play a role in future studies.

Classification

The ideal classification system would subdivide RP on the basis of molecular and biochemical abnormality and correlate this with useful, if not characteristic, clinical features. Despite the explosion of molecular genetic information that has become available in the past 15 years, a unified subclassification system that can be used by clinicians, cell biologists, and molecular geneticists is still far off. Because of this, the different ways of classifying RP listed below are all still valid. The one used by an individual depends on that person's area of interest.

Subdivision by inheritance type

The most useful subclassification of RP both in clinical and research setting is still subdivision on the basis of mode of inheritance. Typical RP can be inherited as an arRP, adRP, or X-linked recessive trait (X-linked RP). Although mitochondrial inheritance is associated with pigmentary retinopathy, typical nonsyndromic RP has yet to be reported with this type of inheritance. The percentage of each inheritance type has been found to vary from author to author and with country of origin of the study. Despite the fact that typical RP is always genetic, a lack of family history of retinal disease is often reported. Studies around the world have found that no other affected family member can be identified in 15–63% of cases. Such cases are labeled "simplex RP." Averaging results from different studies suggests that 35% of RP patients in the USA, 42% in the UK, and 48% in China are simplex. It is assumed that large proportions of these cases represent recessive inheritance. Jay[169] has estimated that no more than 70% of simplex cases are autosomal recessive.

Subdivision by age of onset

Early-onset RP may be subdivided into congenital and childhood-onset forms. Timing of onset of blindness, by the patient's parent(s), and the occurrence of nystagmus (usually suggestive of a congenital disease) can be used to differentiate between congenital and early-onset cases. Occasionally, a member of a family with otherwise typical RP may present in late infancy or early childhood, while other affected members present anywhere from the end of the first decade to the third decade. arRP

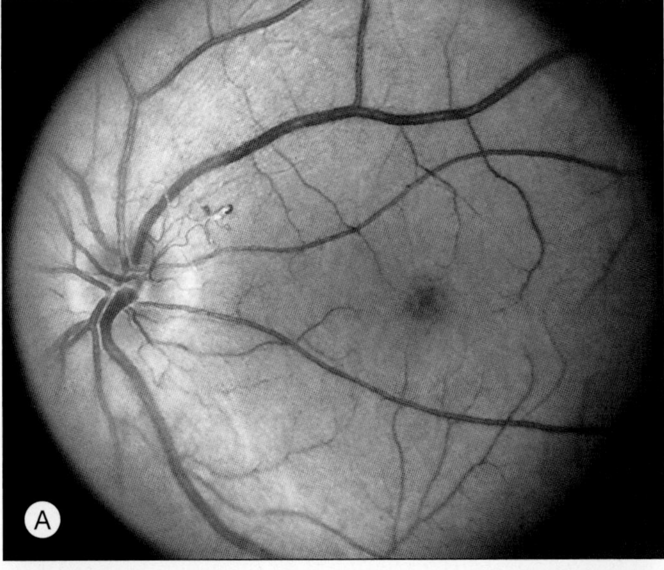

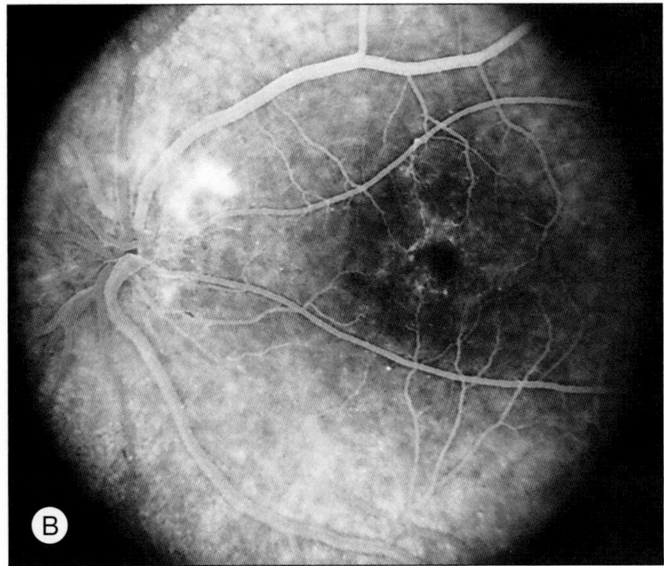

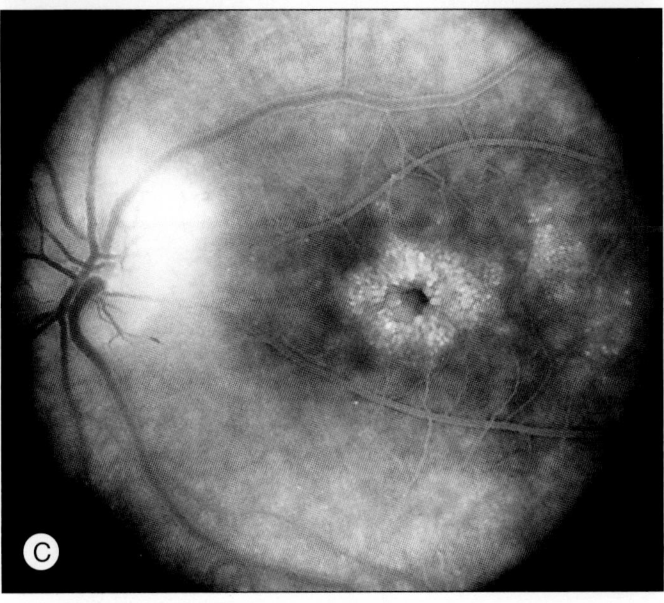

Fig. 40.28 Fundus appearance (A) and fluorescein angiograms (B and C) of the left eye of a patient with presumed autosomal recessive retinitis pigmentosa at 26 years of age. Note the vascular abnormality superotemporal to the disc, vascular leakage, and cystoid macular edema on the fluorescein angiogram.

is usually more consistent in the age of presentation among affected siblings.

The most common age for presentation of symptoms and subsequent diagnosis of RP is in the first three decades of life – juvenile-onset and early adult-onset RP. All three inheritance types may present in such a fashion. Often, children with juvenile-onset disease function quite well at home but have great difficulties navigating strange environments. Reliable testing of visual fields may be possible in some children as young as 6 or 7 years of age. Perimetry indicative of progression or improvement of visual field deficits should, however, be interpreted with caution in this age range.

Adult-onset and late-onset forms of RP are not uncommon but often go unrecognized as a retinal dystrophy. Some of these retinal degenerations may have a nongenetic basis, but those that are genetic are usually autosomal recessive.

Subdivision by molecular defect

The expanding discovery of gene mutations associated with forms of RP is leading to an ever-increasing understanding of these entities at the molecular level. We now recognize that a mutant allele for a gene can behave in different ways, depending on where the sequence change resides within the gene and the status of the other allele. Gene mutations that produce no gene product (so-called null alleles) may exhibit autosomal recessive inheritance, if one good copy of the gene is sufficient to produce enough product to maintain normal function. Null alleles can also be associated with dominant inheritance from haploinsufficiency if one good copy of the gene cannot produce enough product to maintain normal function. Dominant inheritance can be seen with "dominant-negative" alleles, where multiple products of the wild-type gene must normally interact to form a multimeric protein complex or supramolecular structure. Missense mutations can also behave as a dominant trait by producing a "toxic gain of function" whereby the mutant protein disables normal gene regulation to downregulate gene expression of the normal copy. Dominant inheritance can also occur if the mutant gene product eithers fails to bind or binds too tightly to another gene product, disabling normal regulation pathways or important biochemical systems. Eventually, information on

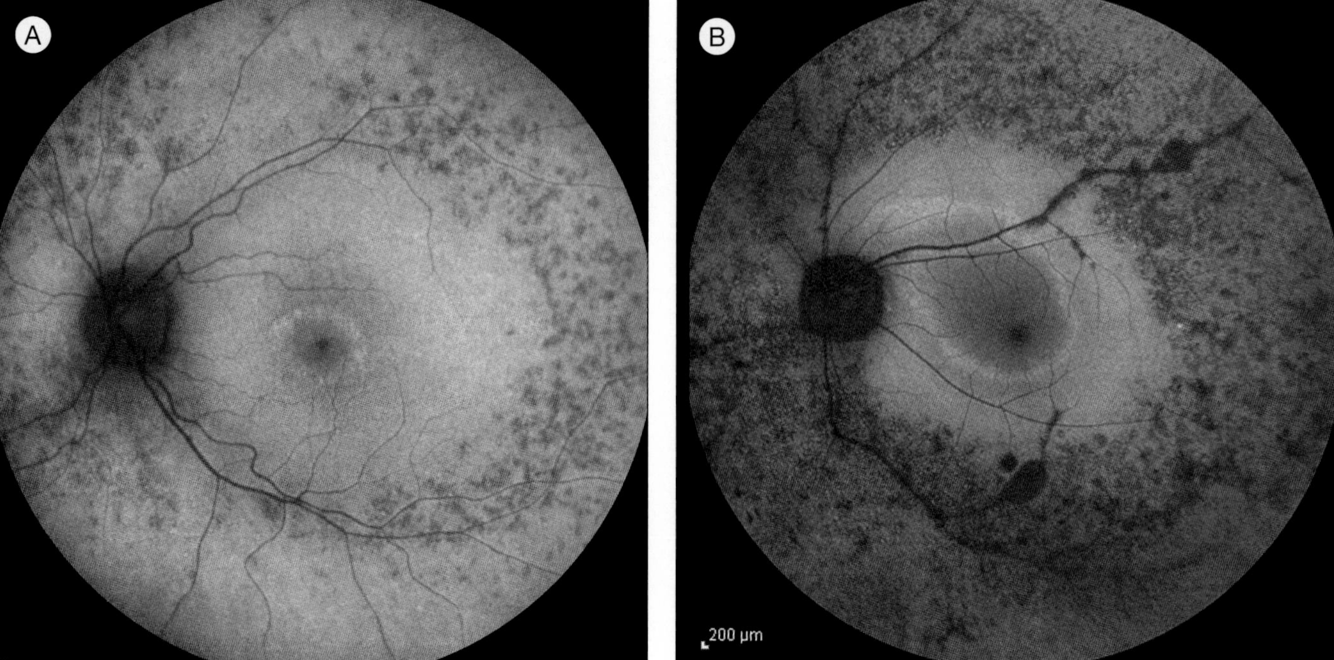

Fig. 40.29 Fundus autofluorescence image of left eye of patient with early retinitis pigmentosa (A) and more advanced retinitis pigmentosa (B) showing in each eye a central ring of hyperfluorescence and a region of mottled hypofluorescence in the region along the arcades.

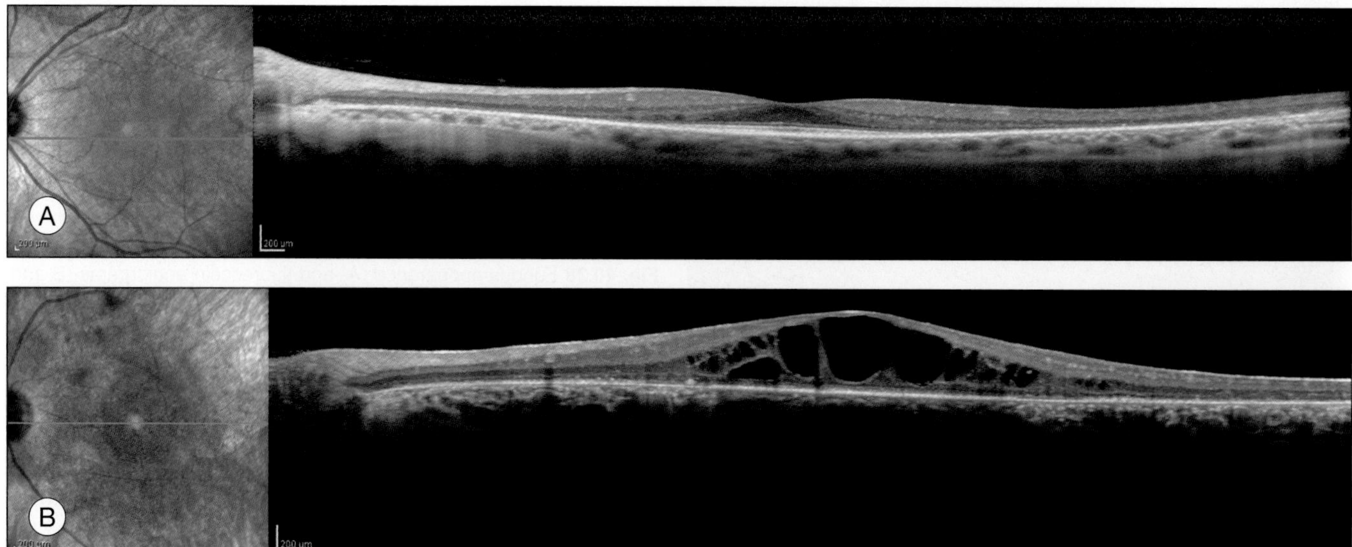

Fig. 40.30 Spectral-domain optical coherence tomography of a patient with retinitis pigmentosa without cystoid macular edema (A) and with cystoid macular edema (B). Note the loss of outer retinal structures, such as the inner-segment–outer-segment junction outside the fovea in both patients.

both the gene and the specific mutation or combination of mutations at each allele will be essential for optimum care. Additionally, as more information is discovered on modifiers of genetic diseases, molecular information will be needed on the status of these genes as well.

Since patients rarely present with information on the specific gene mutation for their disease, a classification based on molecular genetic defect will not entirely supplant the need to consider subdivisions of RP on clinical or psychophysical grounds. However, such molecular information will aid immensely in defining the true spectrum and natural history of specific types of RP. This refinement of classification will be particularly useful for prognostic counseling. The ability to detect the presence of the gene defect by examining DNA taken from a blood sample will allow earlier and more accurate diagnosis, facilitate genetic counseling, open the way for prenatal diagnosis, and eventually guide the patient toward specific gene defect-related therapies. Schemes for molecular classification of RP are given later in this text.

Subdivision by distribution of retinal involvement or fundus appearance

A number of recognizable fundus appearances have been seen in certain cases of RP. RP sine pigmento – RP without signs of intraretinal pigmentation – is one. In almost all cases these represent early RP. In the early stages of RP, fine, whitish, punctate lesions in the mid and far periphery at the level of the RPE can be seen. This fundus appearance is similar to that seen in retinitis punctata albescens.[170] White lesions or dots deep in the retina can be seen with RP in younger members of families with older affected members who have typical findings of RP. A myriad of tiny, irregularly shaped, gray-white, deep retinal lesions (Fig. 40.31) associated with lifelong stationary night blindness, minimally attenuated retinal vessels, and absence of pigment clumps or bone spicules are characteristic of fundus albipunctatus. Bilateral central scotomas can be present in later years. History of slow progressive visual loss with the macular atrophic degeneration is suggestive of the fleck retinal degeneration known as retinitis punctata albescens.[171] However, differentiation of fundus albipunctatus from retinitis punctata albescens can be difficult. Macular atrophic lesions have been reported by Miyake and colleagues to occur also in fundus albipunctatus.[172–174]

Sector and sectoral retinitis pigmentosa

Sector RP, first described by Bietti[175] in 1937, refers to a specific subtype of RP. This is characterized by pigmentary changes limited to one or two quadrants, visual field defects usually only in the regions of retinal pigmentation, relatively good ERG responses, and minimal or no extension of the retinal area involved with time.

Patients may be minimally symptomatic. The area of retinal involvement is usually an arcuate swathe of retina just below the macula. In later years this involved region of the fundus may show almost a total regional atrophy of choroid and retina.[176] Occasionally the nasal retina[177] or inferior and nasal retina is involved.[176] Rarely, sector RP has been reported as affecting the temporal or superior quadrants.[178] True sector RP can be either autosomal dominant or autosomal recessive.[176] Although sector RP has been reported with mutations of the rhodopsin gene[179,180] and with mutations of *USH1C*,[181] sporadic or isolated cases of sector retinal degeneration are common and may possibly result from nongenetic causes.

Massof and Finkelstein[79] have shown in autosomal dominant sector RP that the absolute retinal thresholds are elevated throughout the retina, including the fovea. Rods and cones appear to be equally affected. Over a period of years, the visual field defects worsen. Overall, however, visual prognosis is good. Using a combination of testing modalities, Fleckenstein et al.[151] studied the FAF associated with various forms of retinal dystrophy, including one case with sector RP. Microperimetry disclosed that the ring of hyperfluorescence sharply delineated the areas of severe impairment of sensitivity. In cases of true sector RP, the ERG demonstrates relative preservation of amplitudes, with mild to moderate subnormalities of both rod- and cone-mediated responses with normal implicit times.[177] One form of sector RP appears to be associated with angle closure glaucoma.[74]

Most cases of RP that begin or present in a sectoral distribution are, in fact, merely the sectoral presentation of what will become with time a more diffuse disease. One notable example of this is the brother of the patient shown in Figures 40.3 and 40.15A, who presented with a strikingly sectoral phenotype in association with rhodopsin Pro23His RP. Although he had poor night vision from age 17, he began to notice areas of blindness in his upper visual fields at age 30 years. The diagnosis of RP was made at age 42 years. At age 50, his best-corrected visual acuity was 20/20 J1 in each eye. His visual fields (Fig. 40.32) showed dense superior loss but good preservation of inferior field. Fundus appearance (Fig. 40.33) showed inferior and nasal pigmentary changes in the right eye and well-demarcated inferior sectoral changes in the left eye. The Ganzfeld ERG at age 51 showed small but measurable rod responses, markedly subnormal scotopic bright flash responses, and modestly subnormal photopic cone responses; rod and cone implicit times were normal. The 45-minute dark-adapted rod psychophysical threshold was elevated about 0.5 log unit above normal in each eye. His acuity remains normal, and he was able to drive a car both during the day and at night until his mid-60s. This patient illustrates the phenotypic variability that can be evident with the age of onset of symptoms, varying from early adulthood to the fifth decade

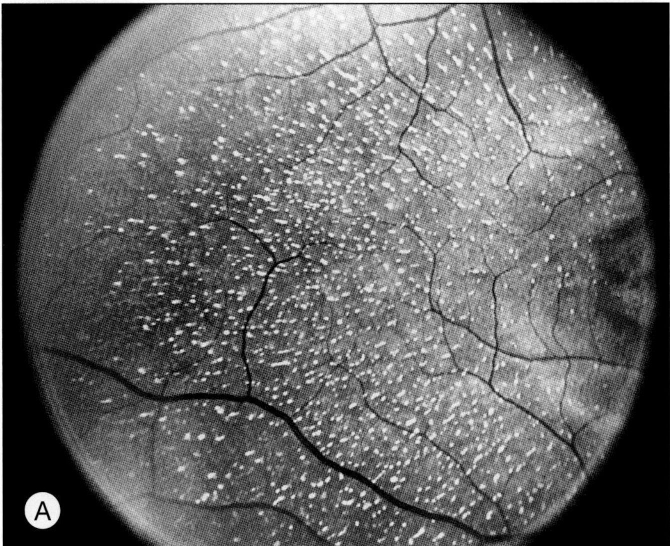

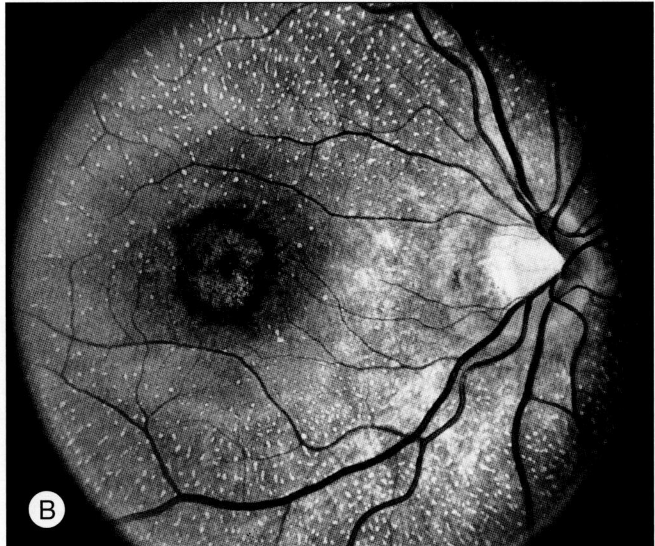

Fig. 40.31 Temporal raphe (A) and posterior pole (B) of fundus of the patient with either fundus albipuncata or retinitis punctata albescens at age 30. Myriads of discrete white dots are present throughout the retina and the macula has a bull's-eye atrophic lesion.

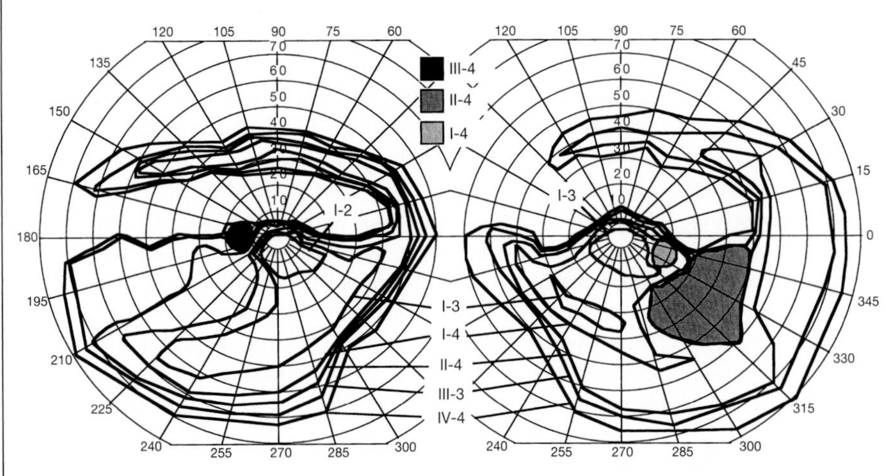

Fig. 40.32 Goldmann perimetry for a 51-year-old patient with autosomal dominant sectoral retinitis pigmentosa from the Pro23His mutation of rhodopsin. Note that the major visual field defect is superior.

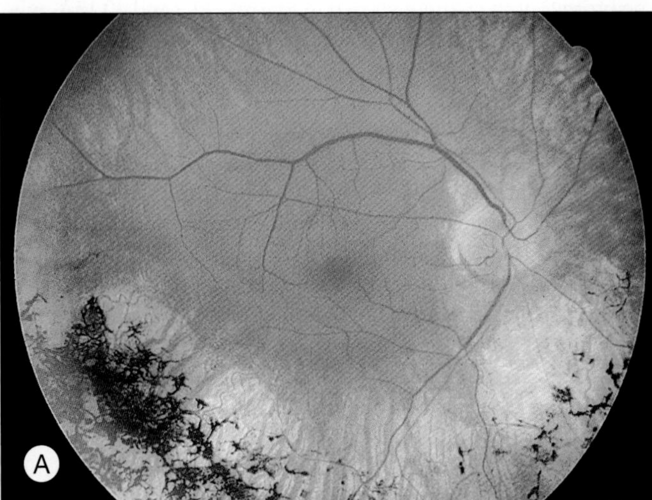

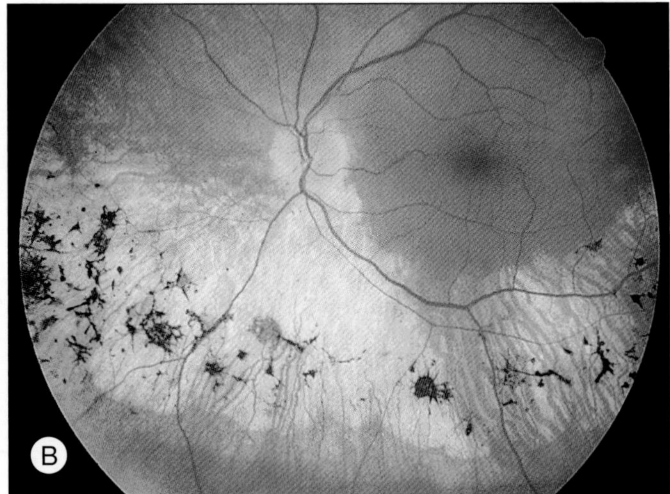

Fig. 40.33 Fundus appearance of the right (A) and left (B) eyes of the 51-year-old patient with autosomal dominant sectoral retinitis pigmentosa from the Pro23His mutation of rhodopsin. Note the discrete border between affected and normal-appearing retina and how well the fundus appearance correlates with the visual field in Figure 40.32.

of life. The normal implicit times for rod and cone responses for his case are unusual but are consistent with the sectoral nature of the expression of his disease.

Pericentral retinitis pigmentosa

Pericentral RP is a special phenotype whereby the loss of visual field typically occurs between 5 and 15° (Fig. 40.34) from fixation rather than between 20 and 40° from fixation, as is seen more commonly. Retinal diseases may commence inferiorly (Fig. 40.35), with commensurate superior field loss leading to the misconclusion that this is a form of sector RP. Pericentral RP is an important subtype because, as the areas of depressed field deepen, coalesce, and enlarge, they encroach more on the central region of seeing field and, thus, create greater disability at an earlier stage of disease.[182] Eventually, as the central region of retina becomes progressively smaller or if the macula develops cystoid edema or atrophic changes, the visual acuity can decrease rapidly from relatively good acuity to less than 20/400. Pericentral RP can occur in many genetic forms of RP and can even be seen in relatives whose other affected family members have a different pattern or a more limited form of disease (Fig. 40.36), suggesting that modifying genes, other ocular conditions (e.g., high myopia), or environmental factors may contribute to this phenotype. Pericentral RP can occur as an autosomal recessive or dominant trait. Selmer et al.[183] reported a Norwegian family with autosomal dominant pericentral retinal dystrophy associated with a novel mutation of the gene *TOPORS*.

Unilateral or extremely asymmetrical retinitis pigmentosa

The vast majority of cases of so-called unilateral RP are acquired rather than genetic unilateral disease. The most common form of unilateral pigmentary retinopathy that is refered to as unilateral RP is diffuse unilateral subacute neuroretinitis or DUSN. This will be covered in the section on Differential diagnosis: pseudoretinitis pigmentosa.

Extremely asymmetrical RP of genetic etiology can occur in two instances. One is the carrier state for X-linked RP. Lyonization, or X-chromosomal inactivation,[40] occurs close in time to lateralization during embryogenesis. Thus, if the number of cells undergoing inactivation of the X-chromosomes that contain the normal gene for RP is uneven at the time of lateralization and, by chance occurrence, a greater number of those cells are directed to one side of the developing embryo, the carrier will express an

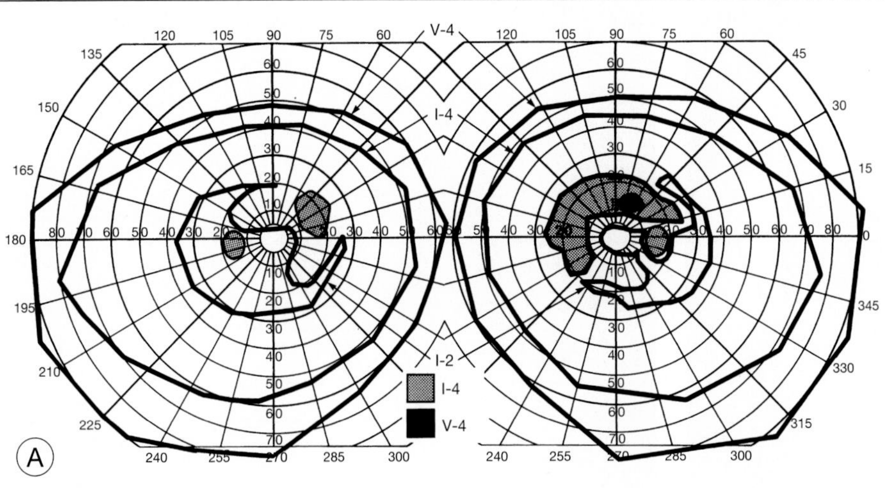

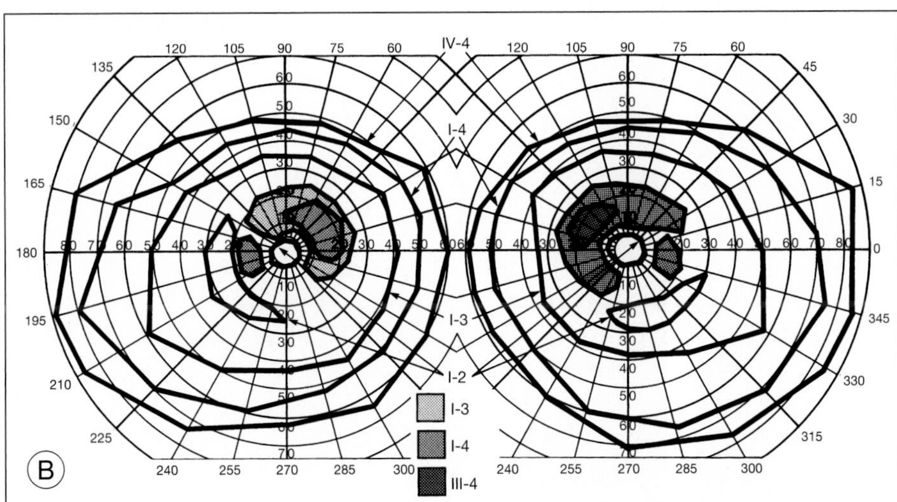

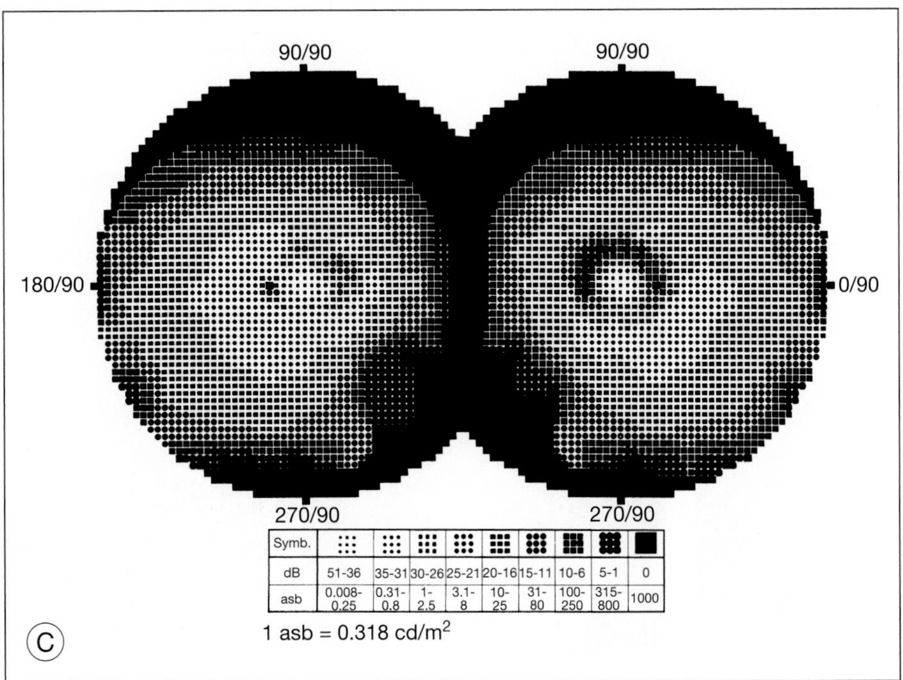

Fig. 40.34 Goldmann kinetic perimetry of a woman with pericentral retinitis pigmentosa at 51 (A) and 54 years of age (B) and Octopus static (combining programs 23 and 34) perimetry (C) at 54 years of age. Although the defect was greater in the superior visual field, the nasal scotoma extends into the inferior field. By 65 years of age a dense, complete ring scotoma was present with a small window of central field remaining, which within a year thereafter was lost, reducing her visual acuity to 20/400.

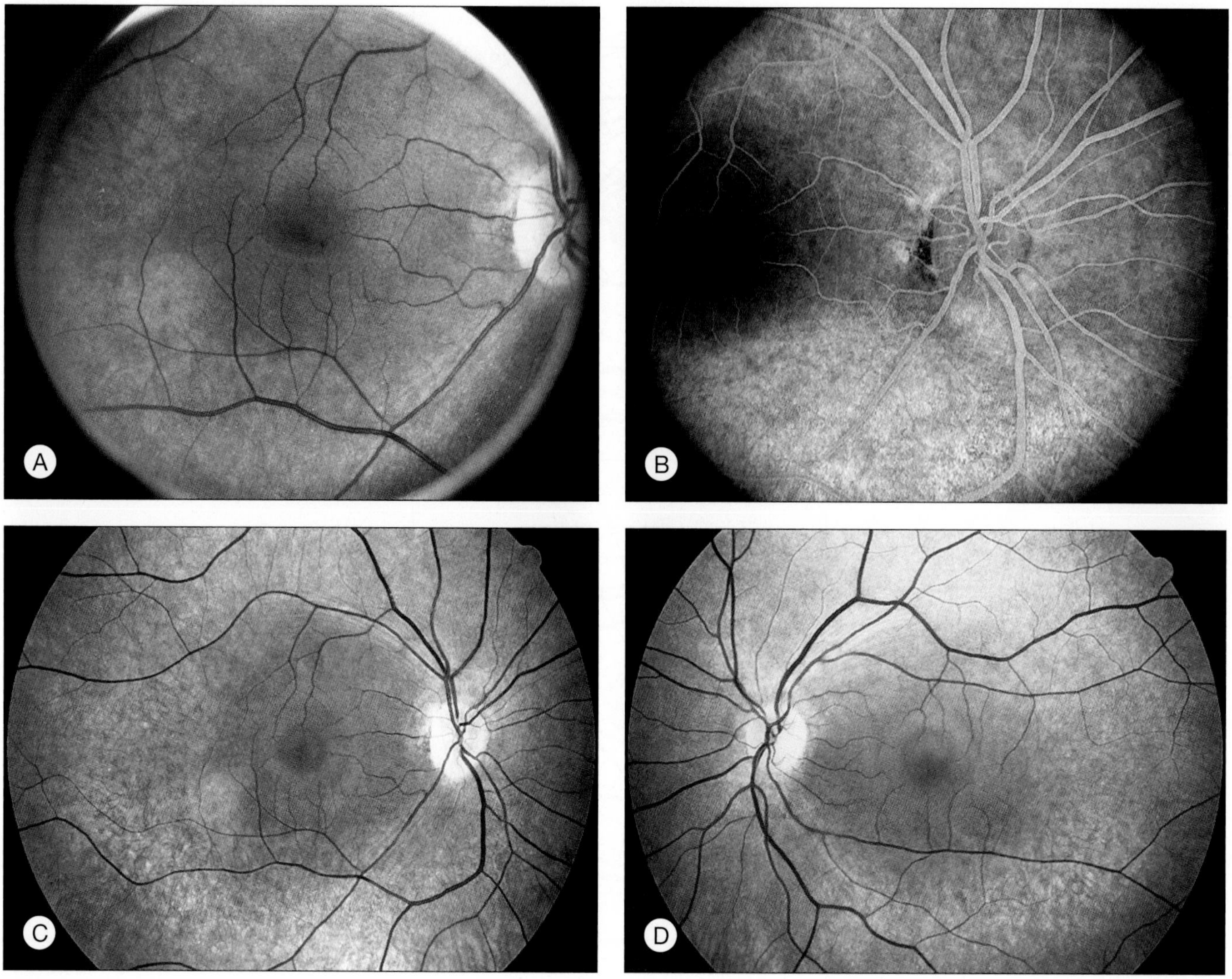

Fig. 40.35 Fundus appearance (A) and fluorescein angiogram (B) of the right eye of patient at age 51 years, and right (C) and left (D) fundi at 54 years.

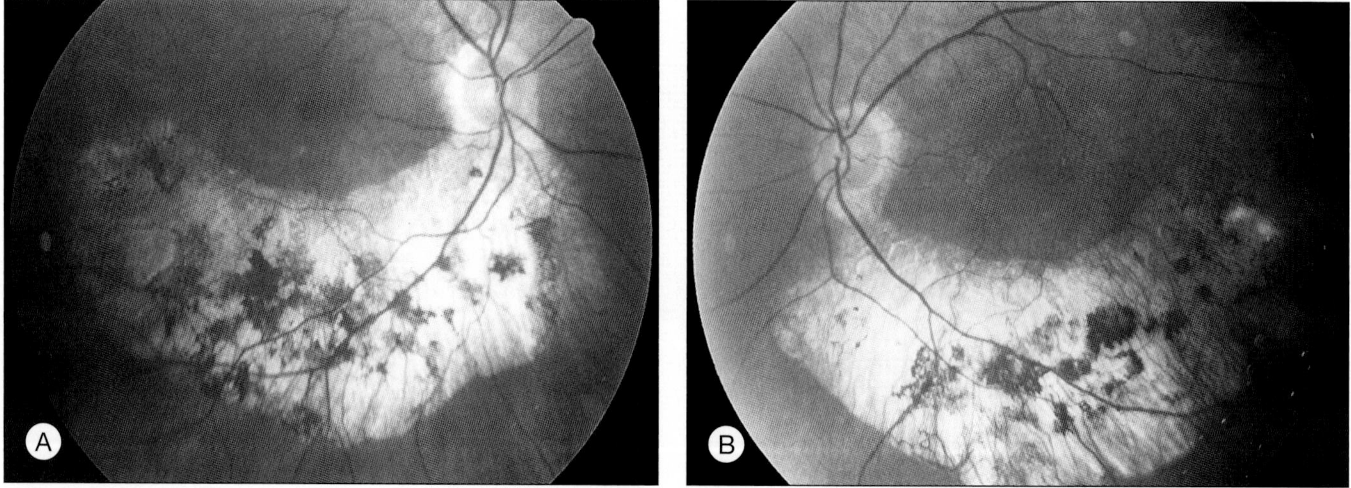

Fig. 40.36 Right (A) and left (B) fundi of the 81-year-old father of the patient presented in Figures 40.29 and 40.30. His condition was considered as a form of sector retinitis pigmentosa but his daughter's disease fit the phenotype for pericentral retinitis pigmentosa.

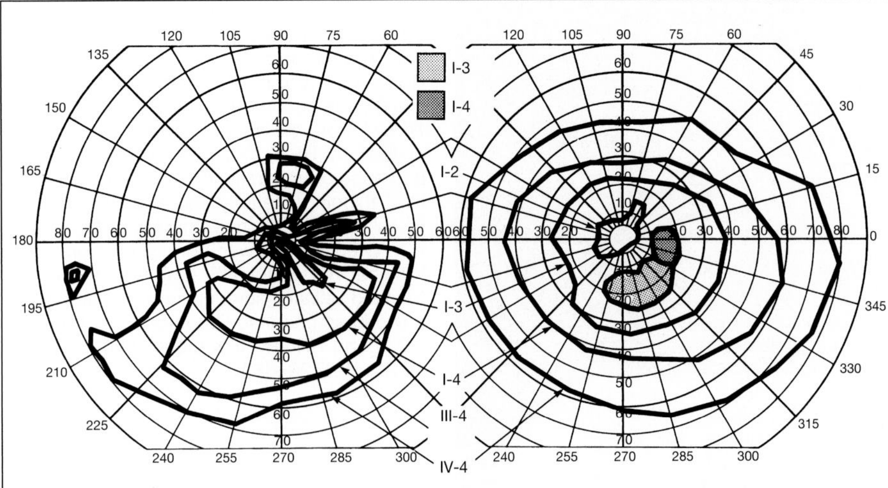

Fig. 40.37 Goldmann kinetic perimetry for the 64-year-old carrier of X-linked retinitis pigmentosa, whose fundus appearance is shown in Figure 40.38. She had mild, lifelong difficulty with night vision that was stable. The vision in her left eye began to fail as a young adult. At 64 years of age, the visual acuity was 20/25 OD and 20/60 OS, with −5.00 +1.00 axis 120° OD and −9.75 +0.75 axis 105° OS. Color vision was normal on the right and markedly disturbed on the left (AOHRR plates). Note the inferior arcuate defect in the right eye and severe irregular superior field loss in the left eye. The electroretinogram was moderately subnormal (OD) and severely abnormal (OS).

extremely asymmetrical phenotype with asymmetrical field loss (Fig. 40.37) and pigmentary changes (Fig. 40.38). The second mechanism by which unilateral RP can occur as a genetic trait is through somatic mosaicism of a dominant gene for RP. This mechanism has been reported as the cause of unilateral RP in a patient with somatic mosaicism of *RP1*.[184]

COMPLICATED RETINITIS PIGMENTOSA

Systemic associations

Most cases of RP are not associated with manifestations outside the eye. Patients with RP have been reported to have a greater than normal risk for thyroid disease.[185] Of 670 respondents to a questionnaire mailed to patients with RP, 7.3% reported mild and 1.3% reported severe thyroid conditions.[186,187] Several studies have reported immunologic abnormalities for patients with RP.[188] We suspect, however, that many of the psychiatric and other systemic associations with RP are either coincidental or epiphenomena.

However, approximately 30% of all patients with RP might experience mild to severe hearing loss as adults.[189] It is unknown what proportion of these are in fact cases of Usher syndrome and what proportion is coincidental or a feature of other genes associated with RP. Zito et al.[190] reported RP with a sensorineural and conductive hearing loss, recurrent ear infections, sinusitis, and chronic recurrent respiratory tract infections in a family with a 845–846delTG mutation of *RPGR*. This and other reports of similar systemic features in X-linked RP from mutation of *RPGR* may be related to the ubiquitous expression of elsewhere in the body. Kenna et al.[191] reported a large nonconsanguineous Irish family with a progressive pigmentary retinopathy (RP), deafness beginning in the third decade of life, and a subclinical myopathy, identified by skeletal muscle biopsy, electromyography, and electrocardiography. Mansergh et al.[192] identified a C12258A mutation in the mitochondrial gene *MTTS2* in this family; RetNet (http://www.sph.uth.tmc.edu/Retnet/home.htm) lists this mutation as affecting the serine tRNA 2 (AGU/C), nt 12207–12265.

Usher syndrome

Usher syndrome is defined as autosomal recessive deafness (most commonly congenital) with retinopathy indistinguishable from typical RP. Although first described by von Graefe in 1858, credit is given to the British ophthalmologist Charles Usher for the appreciation that this condition was familial and represented a distinct entity.[193] He also recognized the existence of at least two types on the basis of severity of hearing loss, age of onset, and rate of vision loss. Usher syndrome is the most common of the syndromes associated with RP and accounts for about 18% of all patients with RP.[194] Although the prevalence has been estimated at between 1.8 and 6.2 cases per 100 000,[195,196] a more recent study found the population prevalence to be 1 : 6000.[6] Usher syndrome accounts for 50% of those persons in the USA who are both deaf and blind.[196,197] The Usher Consortium has recommended specific clinical criteria for the diagnosis of Usher syndrome.[198]

Usher syndrome can be divided clinically into three major groups. The two most frequent forms are type 1, with profound congenital sensorineural deafness and resultant prelingual deafness or severe speech impairment, vestibular symptoms, and childhood-onset retinopathy, and type 2, with congenital partial, nonprogressive deafness, absence of vestibular symptoms, and milder, later-onset retinopathy.[199] The least common is type 3 Usher syndrome, which is characterized by progressive deafness starting late in the second to fourth decades, adult-onset retinopathy, and hypermetropic astigmatism.[200–202] Another variant, Hallgren syndrome, was defined as congenital progressive deafness, vestibular ataxia, and retinopathy.[203] The validity of this as an entity distinct from Usher type 1 has been questioned.[199] Approximately 3–6% of those persons with profound prelingual deafness have type 1 Usher syndrome.[197] Piazza et al.,[204] in a study of 106 patients with Usher syndrome, found that 33% had type 1 and 67% had type 2 disease. No type 3 cases were identified. Most cases of type 3 disease are of Finnish descent.[205] As many as 40% of Usher syndrome cases are classified as type 3 in Finnish[202] and Ashkenazi Jewish[206] populations.

One of the earliest signs of type 1 Usher syndrome is vestibular dysfunction, which in infancy can manifest as a delay in motor development in children and in adulthood as a nonprogressive ataxia.[199] Occasional ataxia is present in type 2 disease and has been attributed to cerebellar atrophy.[199] Because of vestibular dysfunction, almost all children with type 1 Usher syndrome fail to walk before the age of 18 months.[207] Patients with type 1 Usher syndrome almost invariably report onset of nyctalopia later, by

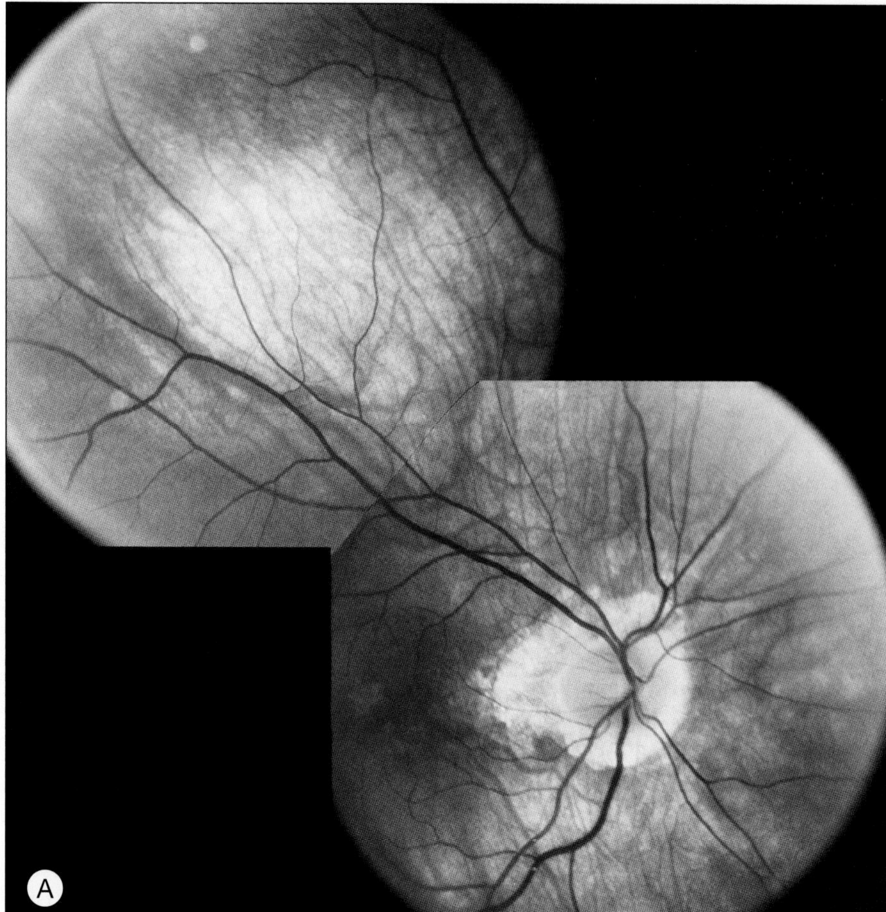

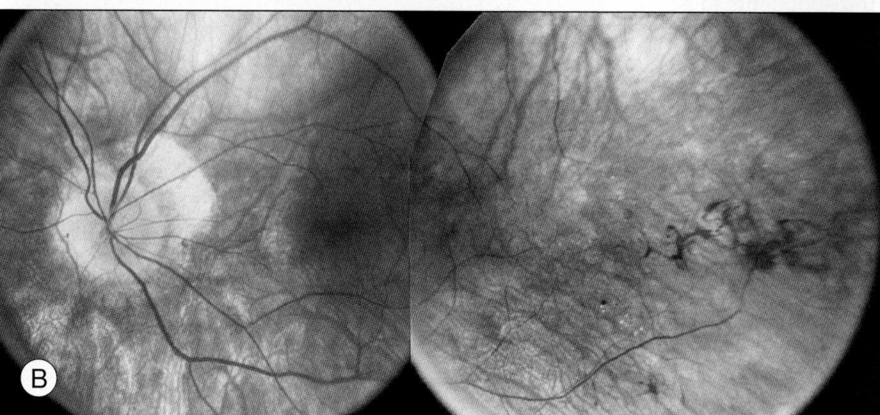

Fig. 40.38 Posterior pole and superotemporal retina of the right eye (A) and posterior pole and temporal retina of the left eye (B) of a 64-year-old carrier of a 2-bp insertion in codon 99 of the RP3 gene *RPGR*. Note the areas of retinal pigment epithelium (RPE) atrophy around the discs and superotemporally in the right eye and RPE thinning inferiorly and nasally with bone spicule pigmentation temporally in the left eye. (Reproduced with permission from Weleber RG, Butler NS, Murphey WH, et al. X-linked retinitis pigmentosa associated with a two base-pair insertion in codon 99 of the RP3 gene *RPGR*. Arch Ophthalmol. 1997;115:1429–35.)

age 15 years, whereas type 2 and type 3 patients report onset of nyctalopia over a greater range, up to the early 30s.[199,208] Visual acuity appears to be better retained in older patients with type 2 Usher syndrome, as compared to type 1.[204] The cumulative percentage of patients retaining 20/40 visual acuity or better at age 29 was 69% for type 1 and 94% for type 2. For retention of 20/80 visual acuity at age 29, the figures were 89% for type 1 and 98% for type 2. Approximately 77% of type 1 patients and 95% of type 2 patients maintained 20/200 visual acuity at age 40. Foveal lesions were seen on fluorescein angiogram more frequently and at an earlier age in type 1 (14 of 35 with a mean age of 34.4 years) as compared with type 2 (19 of 71 with a mean age of 42.9 years). No difference in the prevalence of posterior subcapsular cataracts was noted between the two types in this study (roughly 50% in each).[204] No comparable figures are available for type 3 disease. The ERG is often profoundly abnormal to undetectable by nonaveraging techniques in all types.

The dual impairments of deafness and severe visual impairment in all Usher syndrome patients necessitate a great deal of educational and sociopsychologic interventions to help them to maintain independence and productivity.[209,210]

Cochlear implantation in profoundly deaf children has been successful in allowing these children to enter the world of the hearing. In order that the parents understand the importance of cochlear implantation, we believe that all infants with profound congenital deafness should be screened for Usher syndrome.

Usher syndrome can only be reliably diagnosed in infancy and early childhood through the ERG.[207] Because receptive and expressive language is most closely correlated with the precocity of cochlear implantation, the diagnosis of Usher syndrome should be established as early as feasible to optimize speech therapy.[207]

The diagnosis of Usher syndrome is missed in two common situations. The first is early disease, in which bone spicule retinal pigmentation is not yet visible, and the second is in the patient with retinal disease that is described as fine pigment clumping and is misdiagnosed as rubella retinopathy. When the diagnosis is suspected, Usher syndrome must be confirmed with an ERG. Other syndromes that can be associated with deafness and pigmentary retinopathy must also be contemplated when considering a diagnosis of Usher syndrome. These include infantile Refsum disease (IRD: also called infantile phytanic acid storage disease), adult Refsum disease, Cockayne syndrome, Bardet–Biedl syndrome (BBS), Alström disease, Flynn–Aird syndrome, Friedreich ataxia, and Kearns–Sayre syndrome.

DIFFERENTIAL DIAGNOSIS – PHENOCOPIES OF RETINITIS PIGMENTOSA

Many other inherited retinal conditions may be confused with RP. These can be conditions confined to the retina or have associated systemic manifestations that may or may not be apparent at the time of examination. Misdiagnosis is common and causes the greatest problem in pediatric practice. Such phenocopies can usually be differentiated from RP on detailed retinal investigation and a thorough survey for systemic signs in the patient and relatives. This differentiation is important because it has a great bearing on the genetic and prognostic counseling given to the family. A great deal of anxiety and social problems can be avoided, for example, in families with BBS if problems of obesity are predicted for a child who might otherwise be labeled as having an eating disorder as a result of the psychologic stress of blindness. When confronted with inherited retinal disease, especially when associated with systemic manifestations, the reader is encouraged to consult the phenotype catalog of Online Mendelian Inheritance in Man (OMIM), which is available at http://www.ncbi.nlm.nih.gov/omim.

Cone–rod and cone dystrophy

In the later stages of disease, many retinal dystrophies (e.g., choroideremia, Stargardt macular dystrophy, Sorsby fundus dystrophy, and others) involve the entire retina and can be confused with RP. Of these other retinal dystrophies, CRD is the one that is most frequently confused with RP.

CRD is characterized by early loss of visual acuity and color vision, with subsequent progressive peripheral visual field loss. There is little literature on the prevalence of CRD, although it has been suggested that the disease may be relatively common.[211] Moreover, some patients otherwise labeled as having RP may have a greater involvement of cones than rods. One study of 278 RP patients with recordable ERGs and fields large enough for rod threshold measurements reported that 41% had a cone–rod-type ERG deficit.[27] Macular pigmentation and atrophy precede variable degrees of peripheral pigmentary abnormality in CRD. In early disease, before peripheral field deficits or peripheral retinal abnormalities are apparent, a diagnosis of macular or cone dystrophy may be made.[211] Peripheral retinal bone spicule pigmentation, in later disease, may resemble that seen in classic RP. Often the midperipheral retina is relatively spared or affected late in the evolution of disease.[212,213]

With such potential for diagnostic confusion, it has been suggested that a diagnosis of CRD should be made on the basis of marked reduction or absence of cone ERG responses in the presence of quantitatively less reduction in rod responses.[214] However, this definition includes a range of phenotypes, and early attempts have subclassified CRD on the basis of fundus appearance[215] or visual field deficits.[216] Two studies have attempted to subclassify CRD on the basis of dark-adapted static threshold profiles[217] or differences in ERG responses.[218] Yagasaki and Jacobson[217] tested 14 autosomal recessive and simplex CRD cases using full-field ERGs, dark adaptometry, and modified perimetric techniques. They suggested that a subclassification could be based on three distinct patterns of visual field loss. Type 1 case had central rod and cone functional loss, eccentric fixation, mild peripheral photoreceptor dysfunction, and slow progression. Type 2 was described as more severe, with a central scotoma, eccentric fixation, more cone than rod functional loss in the periphery, and relatively normal midperipheral fields. Subjects classified as type 3 had central fixation, no measurable cone function, and patchy rod function loss. Szlyk and coworkers[218] studied 33 CRD patients, and reviewed the records of a further 150, and described four functionally distinct subtypes. Subjects were subdivided into type 1 (less rod than cone dysfunction) and type 2 (equal cone and rod dysfunction) on the basis of quantitative ERG responses. These groups were further subdivided into type a (cone thresholds more elevated centrally, rod thresholds more peripherally) or b (matching areas of cone and rod threshold elevation mostly peripherally) on the basis of pattern of field loss and threshold elevation.

There is a tendency for the visual field defects in CRD to begin in the pericentral region between 5 and 30° from fixation.[216] Many nonretinal conditions have been documented in association with CRD in certain patients, including optic nerve head atrophy and telangiectasia,[215,216] high myopia,[219] and macular coloboma.[220] Also, there have been associations with spinocerebellar ataxia,[221] dental ameliogenesis imperfecta,[222] alopecia,[223] and hypertrichosis.[224] In the vast majority of cases, however, CRD is identified as the only genetic disease.

Autosomal dominant, recessive, and X-linked inheritance patterns of inheritance have been described, as well as simplex cases implying genetic heterogeneity.[225] Recent molecular genetic studies have identified 16 different genomic regions, each of which contains a CRD-causing gene (Table 40.1).

In the early stage of disease, an isolated cone dystrophy may be difficult to distinguish from a CRD. CRD can be associated with mutations in the gene *GUCY2D* for guanylate cyclase-activating protein-1 (GCAP-1)[226] and cone dystrophy (COD3) has been associated with the functionally related gene *GUCA1A* encoding GCAP-1.[227,228] GCAPs play an important role in regulating the function of RETGC-1 in a calcium-dependent manner, but the reason why defects of these proteins result in degeneration limited to cones is difficult to explain. One suggested explanation focuses on the interactions of the defect of GCAPs at different levels of calcium.[228]

Text continued on page 794

Table 40.1 Genetic mutations associated with typical retinitis pigmentosa and its phenocopies

Disease	Inheritance	Genome locus	Gene/protein	Reference
Retinitis pigmentosa				
RP	AR	1p36.1	*DHDDS*	785
RP32	AR	1p21.2	–	786
RP	AR	1p21.1	*ABCA4*	787
RP12	AR	1q31.3	*CRB1*	788
RP18	AD	1q21.2	*HPRP3*	497
RP	AR	1q32.2	*FLVCRI*/AXPC1	789
RP	AR	2p23.2	*ZNF513*	790
RP54	AR	2p23.2	*C2ORF71*	791
RP28	AR	2p15	*FAM161A*	792
RP33	AD	2q11.2	*SNRNP200*	793
RP26	AR	2q31.3	*CERKL*	794
RP	AR	3q12.3	*IMPG2*/SPARCAN	795
RP38	AR	2q13	*MERTK*	441
RP	AD	3q21.1	*RHO* Pro23His	396
RP	AR	3q21.1	*RHO*	479
RP40	AR	4p16.3	*PDE6B*	796
RP	AR	4p15.32	*PROML1*	797
RP	AR	4p15.33	*CC2D2A*	798
RP49	AR	4p12	*CNGA1, CNCG*	432
RP29	AR	4q32	–	799
RP	AR	4q32.1	*LRAT*	798
RP	AR	5q33.1	*PDE6A*	800
RP14	AR	6p21.31	*TULP1*	240
RP7	AD	6p21.2	*RDS*	420
RP25	AR	6q12	*EYS*/SPAM	801
RP42	AD	7p14.3	*KLHL7*	398
RP9	AD	7p14.3	*PAP1,* PIM1K	428
RP10	AD	7q32.1	*IMPDH1*	802
RP1	AD	8q12.1	*ORP1*	803
RP	AR	8q12.3	*TTPA*	804
RP31	AD	9p21.1	*TOPORS*	805
RP	AR	10q11.22	*RBP3,* IRBP	806
RP44	AR	10q23.1	*RGR*	807
RP	Digenic	11q12.3	*ROM1*	459

Table 40.1 Genetic mutations associated with typical retinitis pigmentosa and its phenocopies—Cont'd

Disease	Inheritance	Genome locus	Gene/protein	Reference
RP27	AD	14q11.2	*NRL*	425
RP22	AR	16p12.3	–	808
RP	AR	15p26.1	*RLBP1*, CRALBP	809
RP45	AR	16q13	*CNGB1*	810
RP13	AD	17p13.3	*PRPF8*	811
RP30	AD	17q25.3	*FSCN2*	428
RP	AR	17q25.3	*PDE6G*	812
RP17	AR	17q23.2	*CA4*	813
RP36	AR	17q25.1	*PRCD*	814
RP11	AD	19q13.42	*PRPF31*	815
RP	AD	20q13.33	*PRPF6*	816
RP	AR	20p13	*IDH3B*	817
RP23	XL	Xp22	–	818
RP6	XL	Xp21.3-p21.2	–	819
RP3	XL	Xp11.4	*RPGR*	447
RP2	XL	Xp11.23	*RP2*	820
RP24	XL	Xq26-q27	–	821
Usher syndrome				
USH1B	AR	11q13.5	*MYO7A*/myosin VIIa	472
USH1C	AR	11p15.1	*DFNB18*/harmonin	822
USH1D	AR	10q22.1	*CDH23*/*cadherin23*	464
USH1E	AR	21q21	–	823
USH1F	AR	10q21.1	*PCDH15*/ procad.15	469
USH1G	AR	17q25.1	*USH1G*/SANS	824
USH1H	AR	10q21.1	–	825
USH2A	AR	1q41	*USH2A*/usherin	472
USH2B	AR	3p24.2-p23	–	826
USH2C	AR	5q14.3	*VLGR1*/mass1	827
USH2D	AR	9q32	*DFNB31*/whirlin	828
USH3A	AR	3q25.1	*USH3A*/clarin-1	474
RP + deafness	Maternal	mtDNA	*MT-TH*	829
RP + deafness	Maternal	mtDNA	*MT-TS2*	193
RP + deafness	Maternal	mtDNA	*MT-TP*	830

Continued

Table 40.1 Genetic mutations associated with typical retinitis pigmentosa and its phenocopies—Cont'd

Disease	Inheritance	Genome locus	Gene/protein	Reference
Bardet–Biedl syndrome				
BBS1	AR	11q13	*BBS1*	831
BBS2	AR	16q12.2	*BBS2*	832
BBS3	AR	3p11.2	*ARL6*	833
BBS4	AR	15q24.1	*BBS4*	834
BBS5	AR	2q31	*BBS5*	835
BBS6	AR	20p12.2	*MKKS*	291
BBS7	AR	4q27	*BBS2L1*	836
BBS8	AR	14q32.11	*TTC8*	837
BBS9	AR	7p14.3	*PTHB1*	838
BBS10	AR	12q21.2	*FLJ23560*	839
BBS11	AR	9q33.1	*TRIM32*	840
BBS12	AR	4q27	*FLJ35630*	841
BBS13	AR	17q22	*MKS1*	842
BBS14	AR	12q21.32	*CEP290*	843
Leber congenital amarausis				
LCA1	AR	17p13.1	*GUCY2D*	844
LCA2	AR	1p31.2	*RPE65*	845
LCA3	AR	14q24.1	*SPATA7*	846
LCA4	AR	17p13.2	*AIPL1*	847
LCA5	AR	6q14.1	*LCA5*	848
LCA6	AR	14q11.2	*RPGRIP1*	849
LCA9	AR	1p36	–	850
LCA10	AR	12q21.32	*CEP290*	260
LCA12	AR	1q32.3	*C1ORF36*	851
LCA	AR	14q24.1	*RDH12*	852
LCA	AR	1q31.3	*CRB1*	853
LCA	AR	14q24,1	*RDH12*	854
LCA	AR	4q32.1	*LRAT*	855
LCA	AR	19q13.32	*CRX*	856
Cone–rod dystrophy				
CORD1	–	18q21-q21	–	857
CORD4	–	17q	–	858
CORD 5	AD	17p13.2	*PITPNM3*	859
CORD6	AD	17p13.1	*GUCY2D*	860

Table 40.1 Genetic mutations associated with typical retinitis pigmentosa and its phenocopies—Cont'd

Disease	Inheritance	Genome locus	Gene/protein	Reference
CORD7	AD	6q13	*RIMS1*	861
CORD8	AR	1q23.1	–	862
CORD9	AR	8p11.23	*ADAM9*	863
CORD10	AD	1q22	SEMA4A	864
CORD11	AD	19q13.3	*RAX2*	865
CORDX3	XL	Xp11.23	CACNA1F	865
CRD	AD	6p21.2	*RDS*	866
CRD	AD	6p21.1	*GUCA1A*	227
CRD	AD	6p21.1	*GUCA1B*	108
CRD	AD	17q11.2	UNC119, *HGR4*	868
CRD	AR	2q11	CNNM4/ACDP4	869
CRD	AR	2q11	*LOC619531*	870
CRD	AR	10q23.1	*CDH21*	871
Refsum disease				
Refsum	AR	6q23.3	*PEX7*	872
Refsum	AR	7q21.2	*PEX1*	873
Refsum	AR	8q21.13	*PXMP3*	874
Refsum	AR	10p13	*PHYH/PAHX*	875
Batten disease				
Infantile onset	AR	1p32	*CLN1*,PPT1	876, 877
Late infantile onset	AR	11p15.5	*CLN2*,TPP1	878
Juvenile onset	AR	16p12.1	*CLN3*	879
Adult onset	AR	1p32	*CLN1*,PPT1	880
Finnish variant	AR	13q21.1	*CLN5*	881
Joubert syndrome				
Joubert	AD	6q23.3	*ATXN7*	882
Joubert	AR	9q34.3	*INPP5E*	883
Joubert	AR	11p12	CORS2, JBTS2	884
Joubert	AR	12q21.32	*CEP290*	885
Joubert	AR	16q12.2	*RPGRIP1L*	886
Joubert	XL	Xp22.2	*OFD1*	887
RP + ataxia + acne	AR	10q23.33	*RBP4*	888
RP + ataxia	AR	1q32.3	*FLVCR1*/AXPC1	789
RP + ataxia	AR	8q12.3	*TTPA*	889

Continued

Table 40.1 Genetic mutations associated with typical retinitis pigmentosa and its phenocopies—Cont'd

Disease	Inheritance	Genome locus	Gene/protein	Reference
RP + ataxia	AD	3p14.1	*ATXN7*	890
RP + ataxia	Maternal	mtDNA	*MT-ATP6*	891
Senior Loken syndrome				
Senior Loken	AR	1p36.31	*NPHP4*/SLSN4	892
Senior Loken	AR	2q13	*NPHP1*/SLSN1	893
Senior Loken	AR	3q13.33	*NPHP5*/SLSN5	894
Senior Loken	AR	3q22.1	*NPHP3*/SLSN3	895
Senior Loken	AR	9q31.1	INVS/NPHP2	896
Abetalipoproteinemia	AR	4q23	*ABL, MTTP*	897
Fundus albipunctatus	AR	12q12-q14	*RDH5*	134
Fundus albipunctatus	AR	15q26	*RLBP1*	898
Retinitis punctata albescens	AR	3q21.1	*RHO*	899
Retinitis punctata albescens	AD	6P21.2	*RDS*	420
Retinitis punctata albescens	AR	15q26.1	*RLBP1* CRALBP	434
Alstrom syndrome	AR	2p13.1	*ALMS1*/ALSS	900
Oguchi disease	AR	2q37.1	*SAG*	901
Enhanced S cone	AR	15q23	*NR2E3*	902, 903
Hallervorden–Spatz syndrome	AR	20p13	*PANK2*	904

AR, autosomal recessive; AD, autosomal dominant.

Leber congenital amaurosis/severe early childhood onset retinal dystrophy (SECORD)

Leber congenital amaurosis (LCA) is not a single entity but a group of disorders due to mutation of at least 16 different genes. The disorder is characterized by severe visual impairment or blindness from infancy. The vast majority of cases are autosomal recessive, although rare dominant families have been reported, all of which, when molecularly characterized, have been found to result from 1- and 2-bp deletions of *CRX*.[229,230] Cases of LCA are often confused with early-onset RP, especially sporadic cases. In 1869, Theodor Leber originally described children with the condition as severely visually impaired before age 1 year, with nystagmus, poor pupillary reflexes, either normal or abnormal fundus appearance, and an autosomal recessive inheritance pattern.[231] In 1954, Franceschetti and Dieterlé[232] described a profoundly abnormal or absent ERG that has since become a requirement for the diagnosis of LCA. Eye-rubbing – the oculodigital sign – is a common association.[233]

Foxman and colleagues[234] and Heckenlively and Foxman[235] have subdivided LCA into two types. Uncomplicated LCA is described as congenital blindness, nystagmus, and high hyperopia with extinguished ERG responses.[235-237] Complicated LCA is used to group together cases of LCA associated with other ocular or systemic features.[235] Fulton et al.[238] studied 36 patients with LCA and did not find that hyperopia predicted an uncomplicated course. More likely, it is the lifelong extreme defect of vision combined with the hyperopia normally present during early infancy that interferes with the emetropization process, leaving the child with high hyperopia.

In 1916, Leber wrote that in his experience the disorder that he originally described in infants (that now carries his name) merged into a continuum with children who presented later in early childhood, without the history of nystagmus or poor papillary responses from birth.[239] These cases typically presented at age 4–5 and had extremely poor vision by 30 years of age. Several names have been used for children presenting this second phenotype, including juvenile and early-onset RP,[234] childhood-onset severe retinal dystrophy,[240] early-onset severe retinal dystrophy,[241] and SECORD.[242]

Most patients with LCA or SECORD show either a normal fundus appearance or only subtle RPE granularity and mild vessel attenuation. Retinal abnormalities that have been described in LCA include so-called macular coloboma,[243,244] "salt and pepper" retinopathy,[245] retinitis punctata albescens,[246] and nummular pigmentation.[247] LCA is often associated with keratoconus.[248] Elder[249] evaluated 35 children with LCA and found a prevalence of keratoconus of 29%. The author suggested that keratoconus is not a consequence of the eye-rubbing frequently seen in LCA but may be due to other genetic factors.[249]

Systemic associations are commonly made. Several reports describe the association of LCA with deafness,[250] renal anomalies,[251] infantile cardiomyopathy (this case was later reclassified by Russell-Eggitt et al.[252] as Alström syndrome), hepatic dysfunction,[253] and skeletal abnormalities.[247,253] Neurologic abnormalities are the most common association and have been reported in 17–37% of LCA cases.[245,254] Nickel and Hoyt[255] have suggested that mental retardation is secondary to the visual impairment, although we believe this is unlikely to account for the severe intellectual impairment that can occur.[256] More recent studies suggest that up to 20% of LCA children without associated anomalies will develop mental retardation.[257,258] It is unknown whether these cases represent undiagnosed systemic disorders or a genetic subtype or subtypes of LCA. To date, none of the molecularly defined types of LCA are associated with mental retardation or neurodevelopmental degeneration. Walia et al.[259] studied 169 patients with LCA and 27 patients with early childhood-onset RP and found that the visual acuity varied widely among those with mutations of *RPE65*, *RDH12*, and *CRB1* whereas *AIPL1*, *CUCY2D*, *CRX*, and *RPGRIP* gene mutations were associated with severely decreased visual acuity commencing within the first year of life. Patients with either *RPE65* or *CRB1* mutations had progressive vision loss with age; those with onset of symptoms after infancy had better visual acuity. The gene *CEP290* is not only a frequent cause of LCA[260] but also is associated with the Joubert spectrum of diseases and with nephronophisis.

Unfortunately, unless other diagnoses are considered and the correct tests are performed, several other entities can be confused with LCA,[261] including IRD,[262,263] congenital stationary night blindness,[264] early infantile neuronal ceroid lipofuscinosis (INCL; Hagberg–Santavuori syndrome),[265,266] and any of several renal–retinal syndromes (Loken–Senior syndrome and Saldino–Mainzer syndrome).[251,267–269] There is the suggestion that the original report by Leber may have included cases of INCL.[270] Although, in the past, LCA has been considered synonymous with infantile blindness and a "flat ERG," LCA should be thought of as a clinical/electrophysiologic sign rather than a distinct pathologic entity. In the context of systemic anomalies, such misdiagnosis can be avoided if LCA is considered a diagnosis of exclusion.

Bardet–Biedl syndrome

Bardet[271] in 1920 described a patient with retinopathy, polydactyly, and congenital obesity. Biedl[272] in 1922 added the fourth and fifth cardinal features, mental retardation and hypogenitalism, of the disorder now known as BBS. A similar syndrome to BBS had been described by Laurence and Moon[273] in 1866, and Hutchinson[274] in 1900. As well as retinopathy and mental retardation, they described paraplegia as a prominent feature without polydactyly or obesity. Some authors classified all these cases together under the term "Laurence–Moon–Bardet–Biedl syndrome" until Ammann[275] in 1970 reasserted the separation of the two syndromes. The controversy continued, however, with some authors still recommending the combined term.[276,277] Most ophthalmologists today consider the features of Laurence–Moon within the spectrum of BBS. Beales et al. refined the diagnostic criteria in 1999 and proposed that the phenotype in the patients be renamed "polydactyly-obesity-kidney-eye syndrome."[278] The prevalence has been placed at 1 in 160 000 in Switzerland.[275] Farag and Teebi[279] have found that BBS is more prevalent among the consanguineous Arab population of Kuwait and among the Bedouin, where the estimated minimum prevalence was 1 in 13 500.[280] Because of a founder effect, the prevalence of BBS in Newfoundland is approximately 1 in 17 500.[281]

Importantly, the retinopathy in BBS differs from typical RP in that visual acuity fails early in the course of the disease and usually the fundus shows little pigmentary dispersion until later stages. Macular lesions and atrophy of the RPE or choriocapillaris often develop early and prominently as the disease progresses.[282] These macular abnormalities may include macular wrinkling, preretinal membrane formation, and leakage on fluorescein angiogram from paramacular capillaries. When detectable, the ERG may show a rod–cone loss or, in many cases, even within the same family, a cone–rod loss pattern, the latter of which has led authors to call the retinal dystrophy in BBS a cone–rod retinal degeneration.[214,283,284] The absence of pigmentary deposits has also led to the retinopathy in BBS being called RP sine pigmento, or, when patchy whitish RPE lesions are evident, retinitis punctata albescens.[282] The onset of night blindness is recognized by a mean age of 8.5 years and legal blindness by a mean age of 15.5 years.[194] Approximately 73% of patients reach legal blindness status by age 20 years and 86% by the age of 30 years.[282]

Incomplete manifestation of the five cardinal features is the rule rather than the exception in BBS. Prosperi et al.[285] estimated from previous reports that 40–45% of cases are incomplete. Another study of 102 cases showed only 24 with the complete syndrome.[286] Schachat and Maumenee[283] reviewed BBS and related disorders and suggested that at least four of the five cardinal features, of which retinopathy must be one, must be present to establish the diagnosis conclusively. Pigmentary retinopathy is reported in 90–100%[281,283] of cases, with ERG responses being abnormal in all cases. Most agree that mental retardation, which has been reported in 85–87% of cases,[283] is not an essential feature of this syndrome. Green et al.[281] found only 13 of 32 patients had mental retardation. When encountered, mental retardation is mild in slightly over 50% of cases.[282] Indeed, intelligence has been reported to be above normal in some patients. Although the tendency for obesity seems nearly universal, some patients have been able to control their weight by dieting and exercise. Polydactyly is present in 75% of cases, is postaxial, and may involve any or all extremities.[283] Syndactyly or brachydactyly is present in 14.4% of patients.[282] Both have been considered as equivalents of polydactyly with reference to determining the number of cardinal features present.[281,282,287] Hypogenitalism is present in roughly half of patients over the age of 15. Infertility is particularly prominent in male BBS patients,[284] although in our experience rare patients do remain fertile and father children. Vaginal atresia,[288] urogenital sinuses, uterine and ovarian hypoplasia,[288] and congenital hydrometrocolpos[289] have been described in female BBS patients. Many of these patients, however, have also met the cardinal diagnostic features (hydrometrocolpos and polydactyly) for McKusick–Kaufman syndrome, which is now recognized as having significant phenotypic overlap with the much more frequent disorder BBS.[290–292]

Of nonocular abnormalities not considered cardinal features of BBS, renal abnormalities are the most common, having been reported in 19 of 21 autopsied patients.[293] Hurley et al.[294] have observed radiologic abnormalities of the renal parenchyma or collecting system in 11 of 11 patients. Since renal disease can be severe enough to lead to uremia and death, Churchill et al.[276]

have argued for renal disease to be considered the sixth cardinal feature of BBS. Pagon et al.[295] reported a BBS child with renal failure and hepatic fibrosis. Cardiac abnormalities were identified on ultrasound in 50% of patients from Bedouin families.[296] Deafness is uncommonly associated with BBS, occurring in approximately 5% of patients.[283] Occasional cases with Hirschsprung disease have been described.[297] Croft and Swift[298] suggested that even heterozygotes have an increased frequency of obesity, hypertension, diabetes mellitus, and renal disease.

Only subtle phenotypic differences between the different linkage types have been reported, the most striking of which was the finding of taller affected offspring compared with their parents in BBS1 families. Affected subjects in the BBS2 and BBS4 groups were significantly shorter than their parents. Carmi et al.[299] have shown that polydactyly of all four limbs seems associated with BBS3, whereas it is confined to the hands in BBS4. Early-onset obesity seems common in families with BBS4, whereas obesity is not associated with BBS2.[299] No confirmation of these correlations between phenotype and linkage loci has been reported with limited studies of molecularly confirmed genetic types of BBS.

In our experience, BBS fails to be recognized more frequently than any other syndrome associated with retinopathy, with the exception of the juvenile form of neuronal ceroid lipofuscinosis (NCL). This is either because patients are not asked about previously surgically corrected polydactyly or because the polydactyly is considered an isolated congenital birth defect unrelated to the manifest retinopathy.

Refsum syndromes

Refsum's name has been associated with two rare, autosomal recessive, peroxisomal diseases associated with progressive neurologic deficit, deafness, liver disease, skeletal abnormalities, and a pigmentary retinopathy. One, IRD, is a disorder of peroxisomal biogenesis that presents during infancy. The other, adult (or classical) Refsum disease, is a disorder of a single peroxisomal enzymatic function that presents as an early-to-middle-life adult-onset disease. Peroxisomes are cytoplasmic single-membrane-bound organelles present in almost all eukaryotic cells. They contain a number of enzymes such as catalases, hydroxylases, and oxidases involved in many oxidative reactions. Serum phytanic acid levels are elevated, either moderately (infantile form) or dramatically (adult form).

Infantile Refsum disease

IRD was first reported in 1982 by Scotto et al.[300] in infants presenting with craniofacial malformation, severe hypotonia, psychomotor retardation, bleeding episodes, liver dysfunction by 6 months of age, and severe deafness within the first year of life. The ophthalmic manifestations were reported in 1984[262] to include nystagmus, poor vision, retinal degeneration with white flecks evident in the midperipheral retina (leopard spots) that fade and are replaced by coarse pigment clumping, optic atrophy, and eventually cataract. The ERG is profoundly abnormal early in the disease and can be electronegative.[262,263] Abnormalities of general peroxisomal biogenesis and function, similar to that seen with Zellweger syndrome and neonatal adrenoleukodystrophy, were identified in IRD and it is now classified as a milder variant of Zellweger syndrome (reviewed by Pennesi and Weleber[263]). The disease is often fatal by the second or third decade of life.[262,263]

Adult-onset Refsum disease

This autosomal recessive disease, also called heredopathia atactica polyneuritiformis, was first described in 1946[301] with the ophthalmic features reviewed by Refsum in 1977.[302] This disease has been recently reviewed by Pennesi and Weleber.[263] The earliest symptoms in adult-onset Refsum syndrome are ataxia, weakness in the extremities, and nyctalopia presenting in later childhood. Progressive peripheral neuropathy and peripheral muscle wasting usually follow this and cardiac conduction defects occur in early adulthood. Other common findings include paresthesia, anosmia, deafness, dry skin and ichthyosis, epiphyseal dysplasia, spondylitis, and kyphoscoliosis.

Ocular features include cataract, miosis with poor pupil dilation, and retinopathy. Nyctalopia in the second decade of life is followed by peripheral field defects. A pigmentary retinopathy is not evident until the third decade. ERG responses are severely abnormal or unrecordable at all ages.

Phytanic acid levels in blood and urine are always very high due to a deficiency of phytanic acid oxidation. Protein levels in the cerebrospinal fluid are also characteristically elevated. Rather than a deficit of peroxisome biogenesis, as is seen in IRD, a specific peroxisomal enzyme, phytanoyl-coenzyme A hydroxylase, is deficient and inactivating mutations of the gene *PAHX*, also called *PHYH*, as well as mutations of the PTS2 receptor have been identified in Refsum syndrome patients.[303,304]

Restriction of dietary phytanic acid (which is present in dairy products and ruminant fat) can limit progression of disease and often improve the ichthyosis, neurologic deficits, and cardiac disease. There is limitation without improvement of visual or auditory deficits.[305,306]

Neuronal ceroid lipofuscinosis (Batten's disease)

The NCLs are a group of progressive neurodegenerative disorders characterized by accumulation of complex storage material within lysosomes. An extensive review by Mole and Williams is available at the website for GeneReview.[307] This class of conditions is the commonest neurodegenerative disorder to affect children, with a collective incidence worldwide of about 1:12500 live births.[308] Characteristically, severe psychomotor deterioration eventually leads to a vegetative state, seizures, visual failure from retinal degeneration, and premature death.[309] Four classic forms exist: three childhood-onset forms, which are all autosomal recessive, and one adult-onset form, which may be autosomal recessive or dominant:

1. An infantile-onset form (INCL, *CLN1*), also called Haltia–Santavuori disease, Hagberg–Santavuori disease, or simply the Finnish form. This usually manifests at 8–24 months of age with severe psychomotor retardation, blindness, and microcephaly.[310]
2. A late infantile-onset form (LINCL, *CLN2*), also called Jansky–Bielschowsky disease. This condition manifests at 2–4 years of age with ataxia, loss of speech, regression of development milestones, seizures, and later loss of vision.[311–313]
3. A juvenile-onset form (JNCL, *CLN3*), also called Batten–Mayou syndrome, Spielmeyer–Vogt disease, or Spielmeyer–Sjögren syndrome, which manifests at 4–8 years of age with visual acuity loss that progresses to loss of virtually all

useful vision over a year or two.[309,314,315] The fundus appearance on presentation includes attenuated retinal vessels, a bull's-eye maculopathy, and fine pigmentary changes (Fig. 40.39).

4. The adult-onset disorder (ANCL, *CLN4*), also called Kufs disease,[316] usually manifests as a motor disturbance without visual symptoms or findings. Although Kufs disease is believed to be an autosomal recessive trait, autosomal dominant inheritance has been described.[317]

In addition, as many as 15 atypical forms have been described, some of which may be allelic to certain of the classical forms.[318] One of the variant forms (vLINCL, *CLN5*) occurs essentially only in the Finnish population and shows linkage to a site (13q22) distinct from the three classic forms of childhood NCL.[319] In Europe, the term "Batten disease" is often used collectively for all forms of NCL.[320,321]

INCL has an incidence of 1 in 13 000–20 000 in Finland, 1 in 50 000 in Scandinavia, and 1 in 100 000 worldwide.[309,322] LINCL has a frequency of 0.46 per 100 000 in Germany.[323] JNCL has an incidence of 1 in 21 000 in Finland and a frequency of 0.71 per 100 000 in Germany.[323]

The visual failure in the three classic childhood forms (numbers 1–3 above) involves central vision first and eventually results in profound visual loss, often with complete blindness, within a few years. The ERG becomes abnormal early in the course of all these disorders and within a few years is usually totally abolished to standard single-flash recording techniques. Goebel[309] states that the ERG becomes flat (undetectable to standard techniques) for LINCL between ages 3 and 4 years and for JNCL between 5 and 7 years of age. Visual symptoms and abnormalities on electrophysiologic testing are rare and even then occur late in the course of Kufs disease.[316]

Recent studies have examined the ERG in patients with INCL, LINCL, and JNCL.[265,266] The ERG is abnormal early in the course of all three disease types. For patients with INCL, rod responses were severely subnormal; the scotopic ERG to the 0.6 log cd-s/m² stimulus was normal for the a-wave and profoundly subnormal for the b-wave, indicating that the earliest manifestation of this disease appears not to affect phototransduction directly. Instead, this result was interpreted as an effect on neurotransmission from proximal photoreceptors to ON bipolar cells. This appeared to occur from one of three possible sites: (1) a disturbance of proximal photoreceptor function that interfered with presynaptic neurotransmission; (2) a disturbance of the postsynaptic plate region; or (3) some other effect on the bipolar cells, with subsequent reduction of the generation of the b-wave. The ERGs of three patients with LINCL were different in showing nearly normal rod amplitudes, mildly prolonged rod implicit times, and severely subnormal, prolonged cone responses. Patients with more advanced stages of LINCL had a greater deficit of the b-wave than a-wave, suggesting development of loss of effective transmission of the signal from photoreceptor inner segments to bipolar cells. Unlike the ERG in either INCL or JNCL, the rod responses in early LINCL were only mildly subnormal and prolonged but with much more preserved amplitude, even though cone responses were severely subnormal and prolonged. Three patients with JNCL had a third ERG phenotype (Fig. 40.40) with essentially no discernible rod responses and severely subnormal cone responses with normal to prolonged implicit times. The maximum scotopic a-waves in all three JNCL cases were subnormal, indicating loss of effective outer segments.

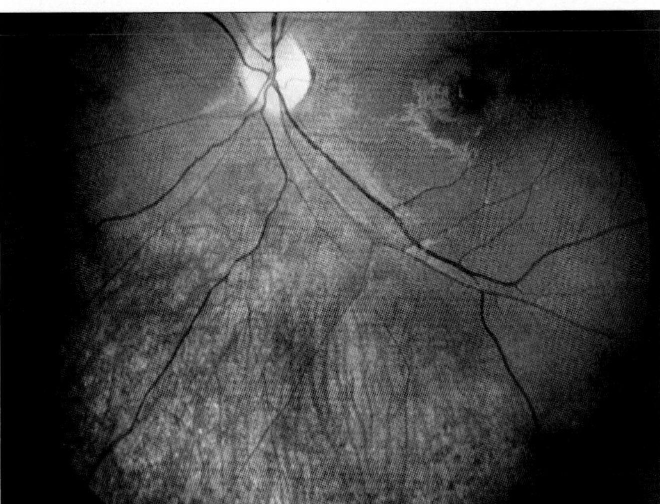

Fig. 40.39 Fundus appearance of the left eye of a girl with juvenile-onset neuronal ceroid lipofuscinosis at 6 years of age. Attenuated retinal vessels, bull's-eye maculopathy, and peripheral fine pigment clumping were evident.

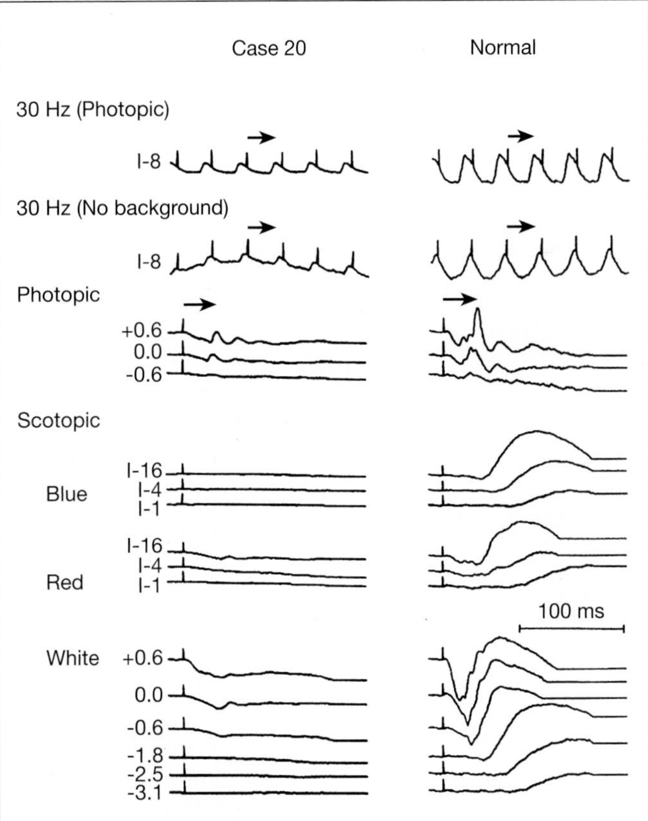

Fig. 40.40 Electoretinogram responses of a 6-year-old girl with juvenile-onset neuronal ceroid lipofuscinosis (Batten disease) (left) compared with those of a normal subject (right). Note the absence of rod responses to the dark-adapted white light (–1.8 log cd-s/m²) and blue I-16 stimuli. The scotopic response to +0.6 log cd-s/m² white light was electronegative in configuration with greater loss of the b-wave than the a-wave amplitude.

The b-wave responses, however, were even more subnormal, creating an electronegative configuration. Oscillatory potentials were profoundly subnormal. The greater disturbance of the b-wave than that of the a-wave for patients with JNCL is consistent with the inner retinal localization of the *CLN3* gene product, which appears localized to mitochondria of Müller cells, inner retinal neurons, and the inner segments (but not the outer segments) of photoreceptors.[324]

All forms of NCL show accumulation of storage material that is autofluorescent, sudanophilic, and periodic acid–Schiff-positive within lysosomes in neurons and other cells. Because of its osmophilic nature and appearance on light microscopy, the storage material resembles ceroid and lipofuscin, but actually it is a complex mixture of lipoproteins and other hydrophobic peptides. The lipoprotein deposits within cells on electron microscopy take on characteristic patterns that are used for diagnosis and classification. Granular inclusions are seen in INCL, Kufs disease, and some atypical forms of JNCL. Curvilinear inclusions predominate in LINCL (with occasional to rare fingerprint inclusions). Fingerprint inclusions are seen in JNCL (with occasional to rare curvilinear inclusions).[325,326]

Historically the diagnosis of this group of disorders has been established by looking for inclusion bodies in cells from brain biopsy or full-thickness rectal biopsy.[327,328] Skin or bulbar conjunctival biopsies typically show fingerprint inclusions (Fig. 40.41), which have been valuable in establishing the diagnosis.[324,325] Buffy-coat leukocytes can be used but may include a wider range of inclusions that may represent other storage disorders, such as the mucopolysaccharidoses.[329,330] Fingerprint and tubular inclusions on electron microscopy of lymphocytes have been seen in children with LINCL and JNCL. These can also be seen in carriers of these conditions.[331,332] Rapola et al.[328] were unable to determine reliably the presence or absence of electron microscopic inclusions in lymphocytes from patients with INCL. Muscle biopsy may represent the best approach to ultrastructural diagnosis for ANCL.[333] However, since skeletal muscle fibers show only the curvilinear type of inclusions on electron microscopy, one cannot use muscle biopsy to differentiate the specific types of NCL.[334] Brain biopsies are no longer justifiable for establishment of the diagnosis of NCL.

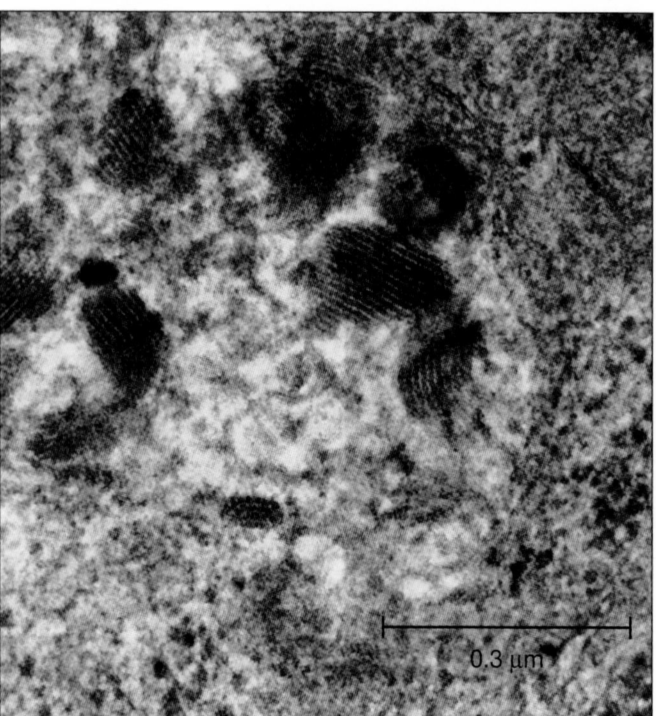

Fig. 40.41 Electron microscopy of endothelial cells from conjunctival biopsy taken from an 8-year-old girl with Batten disease. Fingerprint inclusions were numerous, but one field showed curvilinear inclusions as well.

DIFFERENTIAL DIAGNOSIS: PSEUDORETINITIS PIGMENTOSA

To some extent, damage to the retina produces nonspecific symptoms and signs. This is especially true of panretinopathies. A number of acquired conditions can cause extensive chorioretinal atrophy that is difficult to distinguish from advanced RP. In such situations, specific details of the history or asymmetry of disease may be the most important differentiating factors. The accounts below summarize the acquired conditions most commonly confused with RP. More extensive descriptions of some of these are given elsewhere in the text.

Retinal inflammatory diseases

Rubella retinopathy

The most common ocular manifestation of congenital rubella, rubella retinopathy,[335] is occasionally confused with RP. This confusion is especially likely in children with congenital deafness and a pigmentary retinopathy that are erroneously thought to represent both congenital rubella retinopathy and deafness rather than Usher syndrome. Uncommonly, the converse occurs, and the pigmentary disturbance of rubella retinopathy in a child with deafness triggers the suspicion or even the presumptive diagnosis of RP. Rubella retinopathy is one of the most characteristic manifestations of congenital rubella.[336] Rubella retinopathy may take any of several forms. In some, the macula is the only site of abnormality, with a speckling of fine pigment granules. In others, pigmentary changes can extend further into the peripheral retina. Usually the correct diagnosis can be established by a combination of clinical features and ERG, which is only mildly abnormal in rubella retinopathy but will be, almost invariably, severely abnormal in Usher syndrome. Rubella retinopathy is a disease that is capable of mild progressive increase in pigmentary changes[337] or the development of clinically significant subretinal neovascularization.[338]

Syphilis

Congenital or acquired syphilis can present as a pigmentary retinopathy that may appear similar in some respects to advanced RP,[339] but careful examination usually establishes the correct diagnosis. Interstitial keratitis is commonly seen in congenital syphilis, and the pigmentary retinal changes are more varied and patchy. Usually the pigment deposits are clumps or large patches of black pigment associated with chorioretinal scars; typical bone spicule pigment formations are uncommon. The posterior pole may be as involved as the periphery. There may be evidence of past or present overlying vitreous reaction or uveitis. Acquired syphilis can also present with a diffuse retinal involvement.[339]

Infectious retinitis

Rarely, toxoplasmosis or herpes infections of the retina may leave a pigmentary retinopathy that poses a diagnostic challenge. These entities usually produce extensive full-thickness chorioretinal scars but may in certain areas produce only mottling and granularity of the RPE. Usually, randomly arranged patches of severe retinopathy exclude a diagnosis of RP. ERG is usually only minimally affected in postinfectious retinopathies, unless extensive areas of retina are severely damaged, in which case the ERG will be accordingly decreased in amplitude.

Autoimmune paraneoplastic retinopathy

Several reports have documented the existence of severe panretinal degeneration as a remote effect of cancer, usually either small-cell (oat-cell) carcinoma of the lung[340,341] or small-cell undifferentiated cervical carcinoma.[342] In several cases the vision loss preceded the diagnosis of the cancer.[271] Cancer-associated retinopathy (CAR) can progress rapidly or slowly with loss of vision over a period of months or years. ERG responses are usually severely abnormal. The fundus appearance may be normal even when the ERG is extinguished and the vision severely decreased. The first autoantigen in the human retina identified with a CAR is recoverin.[343,344] Antibodies to retinal enolase have also been reported in CAR.[345,346]

A paraneoplastic form of night blindness associated with "shimmering lights" and a characteristic ERG has been reported with malignant melanoma and has been called melanoma-associated retinopathy (MAR).[347,348] The scotopic ERG to maximum-intensity flash has a "negative" configuration, identical to that seen with congenital stationary night blindness. The a-wave amplitude is normal, and the b-wave amplitude is severely subnormal, distinguishing this form of paraneoplastic retinopathy from CAR. Alexander et al.[349] found a defect in the ON response of the ERG, reflecting abnormal rod neurotransmission to depolarizing bipolar cells.

It has been suggested that in MAR there is a selective loss of function subserved by magnocellular cells with preservation of midget type 1 parvocellular cell function.[350] We have seen a patient with acquired night blindness and a negative-configuration ERG typical for congenital stationary night blindness associated with an anaplastic squamous cell carcinoma of the nasopharynx (WT Shults and RG Weleber, unpublished observations, 1991). Other acquired cases of visual symptoms, field loss, and electronegative-configuration ERGs have been reported in the absence of either melanoma or other discernible cancer but with serum antiretinal antibodies that specifically labeled the inner plexiform layer of cadaver retina by indirect immunoperoxidase testing.[351] Presumably, these patients have produced an antibody to an antigen that is similar (by molecular mimicry) to one found in normal retina, producing the disturbance of retinal function and electrophysiology.

Drug toxicity (see Chapter 89, Drug toxicity)

Thioridazine

This phenothiazine has been linked to severe, blinding retinal toxicity. In general, phenothiazines bind to melanin and concentrate in the uveal tract and RPE.[352,353] The retinal toxicity of thioridazine is believed to result from the presence of a piperidyl group. Thioridazine can cause a pigmentary retinopathy that can be confused with RP (in its early stages) or choroideremia (in its later stages).[354] In most patients with thioridazine retinopathy the drug has been taken at doses higher than 800 mg/day.[355]

The earliest symptoms include blurring of central vision, poor night vision, and a brownish discoloration to the vision. Early toxicity produces fine, deep retinal pigment posterior to the equator, which becomes coarser as the condition progresses. Large "signal" plaques of pigment deposition occur late. The characteristic appearance of advanced thioridazine retinopathy is diffuse, patchy atrophy of choriocapillaris, RPE, and overlying retina, simulating the fundus appearance of early choroideremia.[356] The ERG may show decreased amplitudes of both cone- and rod-mediated responses; responses of both a-waves and b-waves are subnormal.

Chlorpromazine

This drug has been reported to produce a pigmentary retinopathy when taken at high doses for prolonged periods.[357] The pigmentary retinopathy does not significantly affect retinal function, and the retinopathy appears to regress when the drug is stopped.

Chloroquine

Similar to the phenothiazines, chloroquine, if taken over a prolonged period, binds to melanin and causes a toxic retinal degeneration. Very few cases have been reported with patients taking a total dose of less than 300 g.[358] Early in the course of toxicity the ERG, EOG, and visual fields can be normal, although in late, severe toxicity, they can become markedly abnormal.[359,360] In advanced chloroquine retinopathy, unlike RP, the dark adaptometry may be either normal or only minimally abnormal.[359] The typical picture of advanced chloroquine toxicity is that of a bull's-eye maculopathy, although pigmentary changes with bone spicule formations can occur in the mid and far periphery.[279,360]

Hydroxychloroquine

This drug has mostly supplanted chloroquine usage for rheumatoid arthritis and systemic lupus erythematosus. However, toxicity can occur with chronic usage and the current recommendation is periodic ophthalmological examination with static permetric visual fields (Humphrey field analyzer 10–2 or 24–2) when the duration of usage is over 5 years, particularly if the dosage is greater than 6.5 mg/kg per day.[361] The multifocal ERG appears to be a useful diagnostic tool to help differentiate pericentral visual field loss due to hydroxychloroquine from that due to optic nerve or other causes.[362]

Quinine

Retinopathy due to oral ingestion of quinine is usually a consequence of large doses taken either during a suicide attempt or to abort a pregnancy. Often, the diagnosis is aided by the history of acute loss of vision and the finding of characteristic pallor and edema of the retina early, with later development of attenuation of retinal vessels and optic nerve head pallor.[363,364] At this stage, quinine toxicity may be misdiagnosed as RP sine pigmento.[363] The ERG in quinine toxicity is usually of a "negative" configuration, with far greater depression of the scotopic b-wave than a-wave.[365,366]

Pigmented paravenous retinochoroidal atrophy

Pigmented paravenous retinochoroidal atrophy (PPRCA) was first described in 1937 as retinochoroiditis radiata.[367] PPRCA is a pigmentary retinopathy that is currently poorly understood but probably represents an acquired response pattern to an infectious or inflammatory disease.[176,368-373] It has been reported in association with meningoencephalitis,[370] tuberculosis,[176,368,370,371] syphilis,[176,372] and rubeola.[374,375] In most, the fundus appearance is first noticed on a routine examination. Three small pedigrees with PPRCA have been described.[376-378] These may, however, represent examples of infectious factors clustering in families rather than true genetic cases. As the name implies, the pigmentary changes are closely associated in distribution with retinal veins (Fig. 40.42). Most cases are relatively stable over time, although progression has been reported in one case.[379,380] ERG responses are only mildly to moderately abnormal, if at all,[176,368,381-383] but the EOG is usually affected, often significantly.[382]

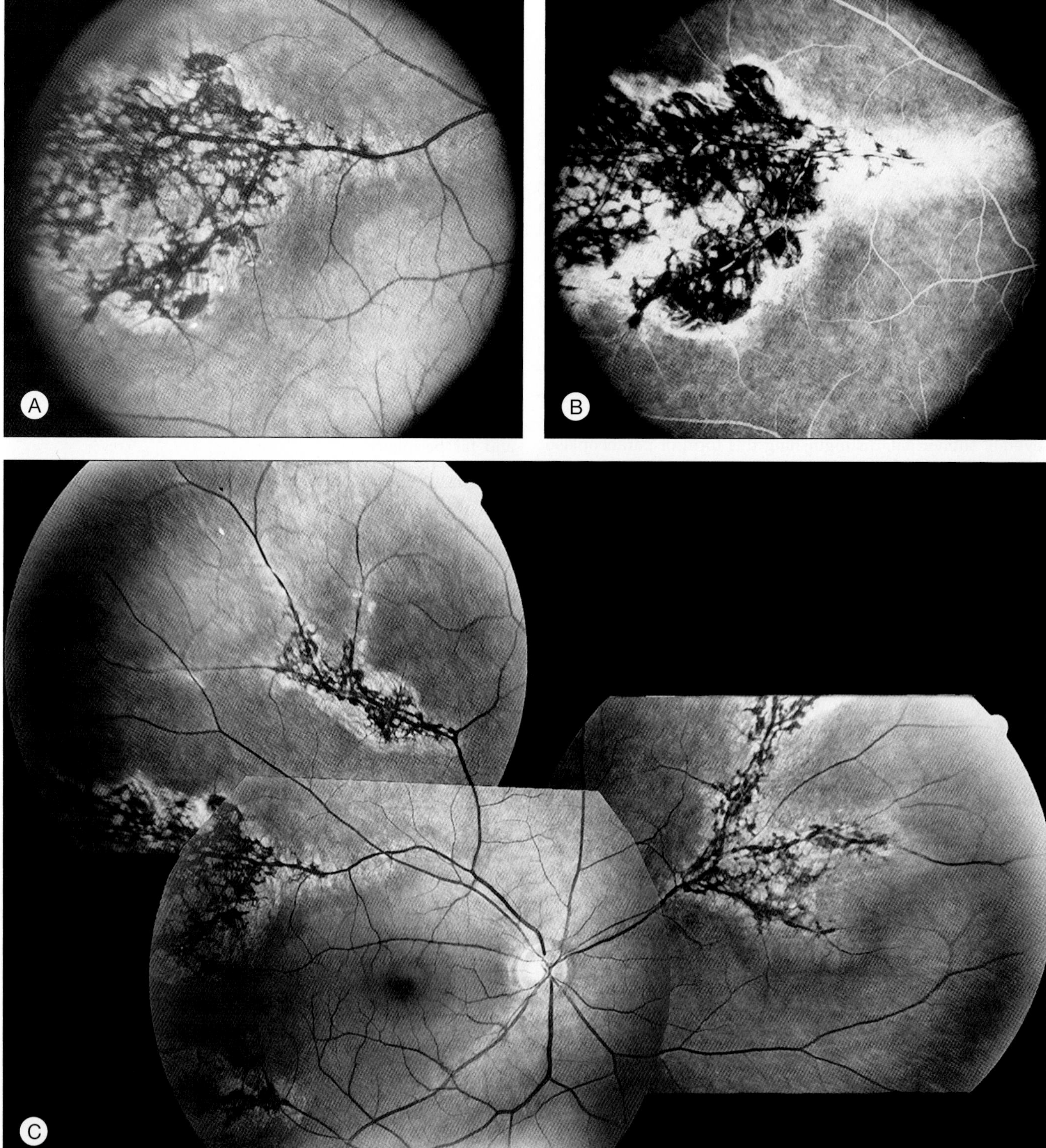

Fig. 40.42 Fundus appearance (A) and fluorescein angiogram (B) of the right eye of a 33-year old patient with pigmented paravenous retinochoroidal atrophy and the fundus appearance of the right eye at age 41 (C).

Traumatic retinopathy

Traumatic retinopathy is probably the commonest acquired retinopathy that is confused with RP and may, with DUSN, account for many previously misnamed cases of "unilateral RP." The RPE and retina have only a limited range of responses to a traumatic insult. One of these is regional or generalized loss of the RPE with migration of melanin into the retinal layers where it accumulates along vessels, especially at branching points, creating a bone spicule pattern. Thus patients with past traumatic injury to an eye can present with a fundus appearance in the traumatized eye that mimics RP.[384]

Diffuse unilateral subacute neuroretinitis

DUSN is the term now used for the disorder previously called "unilateral wipe-out syndrome,"[385] and "unilateral RP."[176] True unilateral inherited RP does not exist, except as an example of extreme lyonization of retinal involvement in a carrier of X-linked RP. DUSN is believed to result from the panretinal degeneration that takes place in eyes that have been infected by any of several possible worms. The raccoon nematode (*Baylisascaris procyonis*)[386,387] has been incriminated, but other worms such as *Toxocara canis*[388] have been suspected. Cases have been seen mainly in the USA and Caribbean, but a few cases have also been reported from Brazil[388] and Germany.[389] Cuhna de Souza et al.[390] described the first instance of bilateral acute neuroretinitis with documentation of the nematode in both eyes.

At the time of initial visual disturbance, the retina may either appear normal or show early signs of retinal degeneration (mottling, edema, narrowing of retinal vessels). Occasionally, one can see an elevated gliotic mass in the mid or far periphery that may represent the encased worm. The visual field often shows abnormalities early in the course of the disease, but these are usually patchy. With time, the visual function usually deteriorates in the affected eye but remains normal in the fellow eye. Eventually the retina develops pigmentary clumping and scarring reminiscent of advanced RP (Fig. 40.43). The pigmentary abnormalities within the retina in some patients may take the form of accumulation of medium to coarse clumps of pigment rather than bone spicules. ERG recordings show clinically significant abnormalities in the affected eye only. Retinal laser photocoagulation has been used in cases where the fundal view is clear.[385] Vitrectomy with surgical removal of the subretinal nematode has been achieved,[388] and oral tiabendazole or ivermectin is indicated when vitritis obscures retinal detail.[391]

Grouped pigmentation of the retina

Grouped pigmentation of the retina, also called "bear-track" pigmentation, is a benign congenital condition in which round and irregularly shaped lesions representing RPE hypertrophy are scattered throughout the retina[392] (Fig. 40.44). The condition does not appear to be hereditary. Usually the differentiation of this condition from more significant pigmentary retinopathies presents little difficulty. Retinal function and electrophysiologic tests are normal.

Grouped pigmentation of the retina should be differentiated from multiple patches of congenital hypertrophy of the RPE, which are associated with familial adenomatous polyposis or Gardner syndrome.[393]

BASIC SCIENCE

Molecular biology

Molecular genetics

Retinal dystrophy research in the past decade has been the subject of many important discoveries in molecular genetics. This occurred because of the well-publicized advances in the methodology of investigating the human genome. Especially important were the development of molecular genetic markers (DNA polymorphisms identified throughout the genome), polymerase chain reaction methodology, and ever easier DNA sequencing for mutation screening.

Using molecular genetic analysis, 14 specific genes have been associated with adRP, 29 with arRP (with three more loci), two specific genes associated with X-linked RP (along with three more loci), and one with digenic inheritance. Further genetic mutations are now being identified. For those interested in the most recent gene assignments and localizations, a list of cloned and mapped genes causing retinal degenerations or allied disorders has been compiled by Dr. Stephen P. Daiger and is accessible on the internet at the following address: www.sph.uth.tmc.edu/Retnet/.

Autosomal dominant RP genes

In rod photoreceptors, rhodopsin is the light-absorbing, conjugated photopigment found in outer-segment discs. It is composed of an apoprotein opsin molecule covalently bound to 11-*cis*-retinal (Figs 40.45 and 40.46).[394] Incident light induces isomerization of the retinal and decay through a sequence of spectrally defined photoproducts. These light-induced changes result in a number of conformational changes in the opsin molecule, exposing G-protein-binding sites. A cascade of reactions (the phototransduction cascade; Fig. 40.47) is then set in motion and results in closing cGMP-dependent cation channels and relative transmembrane hyperpolarization.[395]

McWilliam et al.[396] were the first to detect linkage of adRP with an anonymous marker on the long arm of chromosome 3q. Shortly thereafter, Dryja et al.[397] reported a mutation of codon 23 (Pro23His) of the rhodopsin gene mapping to chromosome 3q (Fig. 40.45). A mutation in the third exon of rhodopsin, Met207Arg, has been found in the Irish family originally linked to chromosome 3q.[398]

It has been estimated that rhodopsin mutation accounts for approximately 25% of adRP.[399] In the USA, rhodopsin Pro23His is by far the most common of all rhodopsin mutations, being found in 12–15% of all American families with adRP.[400] It is interesting that the Pro23His mutation has rarely been reported anywhere else in the world.[401] In fact, the mutation rate of the rhodopsin gene appears to vary with ethnic background. For instance, frequencies of *RHO* mutations in Asian populations, such as Japanese (5.9%),[402] Chinese (2.0%–5.6%),[403] Indian (2.0%),[404] and Korean (2.0%),[405] are lower than that in the USA,[400] and Europe.[406]

From the occurrence of a rare, intron 1 polymorphism in all patients with Pro23His adRP, it has been suggested that all persons with this mutation may have originated from a single-mutation founder.[407] The phenotype associated with rhodopsin Pro23His is best described as Massof type II[79] or R-type RP.[84,85] Most rhodopsin adRP phenotypes have in fact been described as type II or R-type disease,[408–410] with a minority of mutations associated with type I or D-type disease.[411,412]

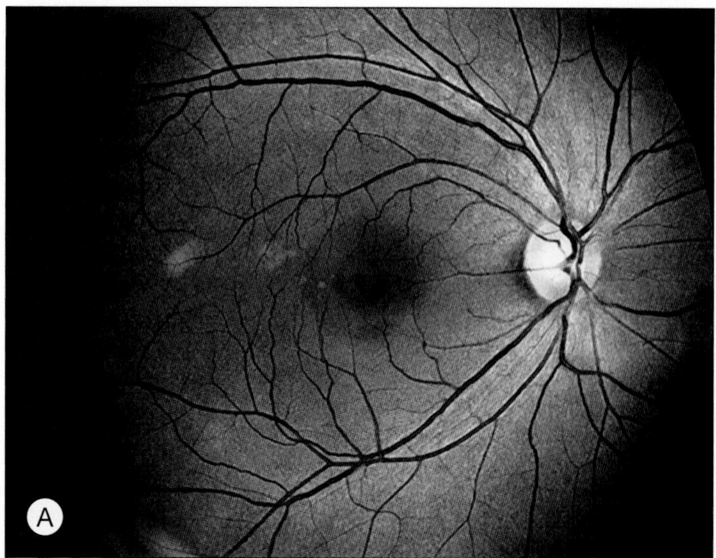

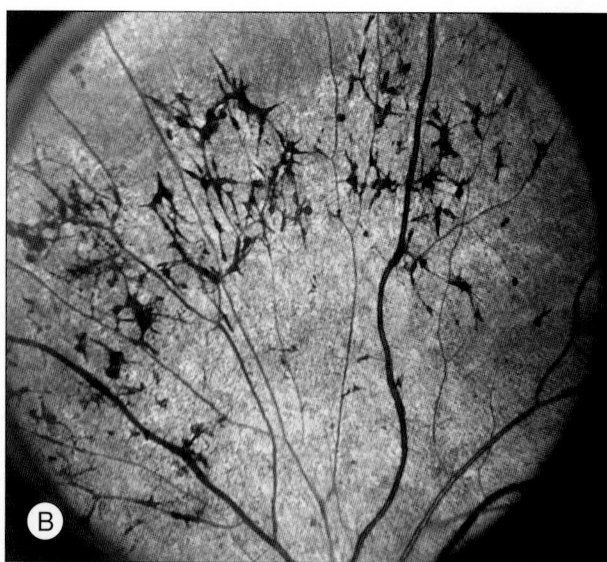

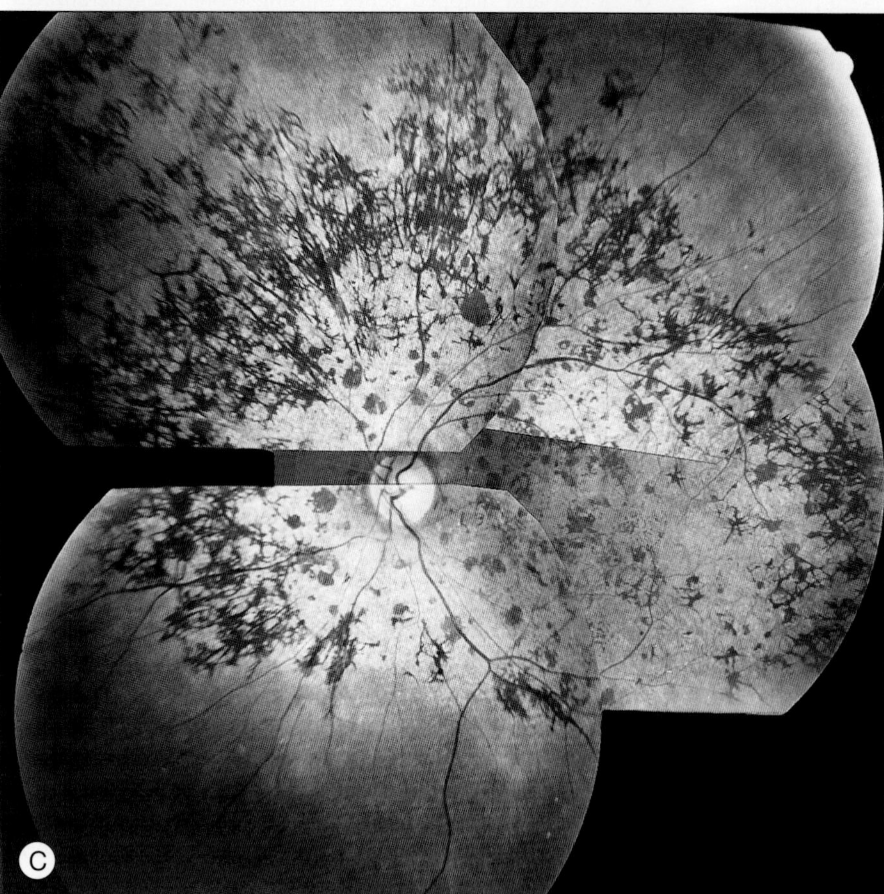

Fig. 40.43 Right (A) and left (B) fundi of the patient with diffuse unilateral subacute neuroretinitis at age 35 and left fundus (C) at age 45.

Pro347Leu is the next most frequent mutation of rhodopsin, accounting for approximately 5% of 148 adRP families in one series.[413] This form of adRP is a more severe, diffuse phenotype, with comparatively smaller visual fields with more ERG deficit than that seen in cases of Pro23His adRP.[414] The ophthalmologic findings of patients with Gly106Arg mutation of the rhodopsin gene[408] appear to be variable in expression, with patients rarely having normal cone and low-normal rod ERGs, a finding quite unusual among patients with RP. Sieving et al.[415] have reported the evaluations of seven affected members of a large family with a Gly90Asp rhodopsin mutation and described the condition for this family as autosomal dominant congenital nyctalopia, to distinguish it from typical RP.

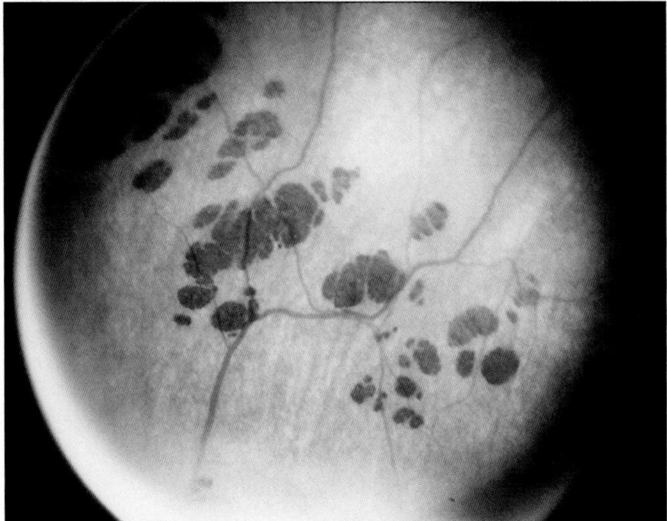

Fig. 40.44 Grouped pigmentation ("bear tracks") of the retina. (Reproduced with permission from Buettner H. Congenital hypertrophy of the retinal pigment epithelium. Am J Ophthalmol 1975;79:177–89.)

Sandberg et al.[416] have reported clinical details on patients with 27 different dominant rhodopsin mutations. They suggested that severity of disease, measured by visual acuity, visual field diameter, dark-adapted sensitivity, and ERG amplitudes, increased with increasing codon number (Fig. 40.46). Berson et al.[417] have suggested that the rate of progression of RP from mutation of rhodopsin is correlated with the site of mutation and that other modifying factors, genetic or environmental, may influence phenotypic expression. A "constant equivalent light" model has been proposed for the severe adRP phenotype associated with rhodopsin codon 296 mutation. Lys296 is the chromophore-opsin attachment site and is also involved in holding the opsin in an inactive conformation. Theoretically this would lead to overstimulation of the phototransduction cascade, a situation similar to constant light exposure. This situation is known to lead to photoreceptor cell death.[418] This explanation has been questioned, however, because the opsin appears to be inactivated by phosphorylation and arrestin binding in Lys-296Glu transgenic mice.[419]

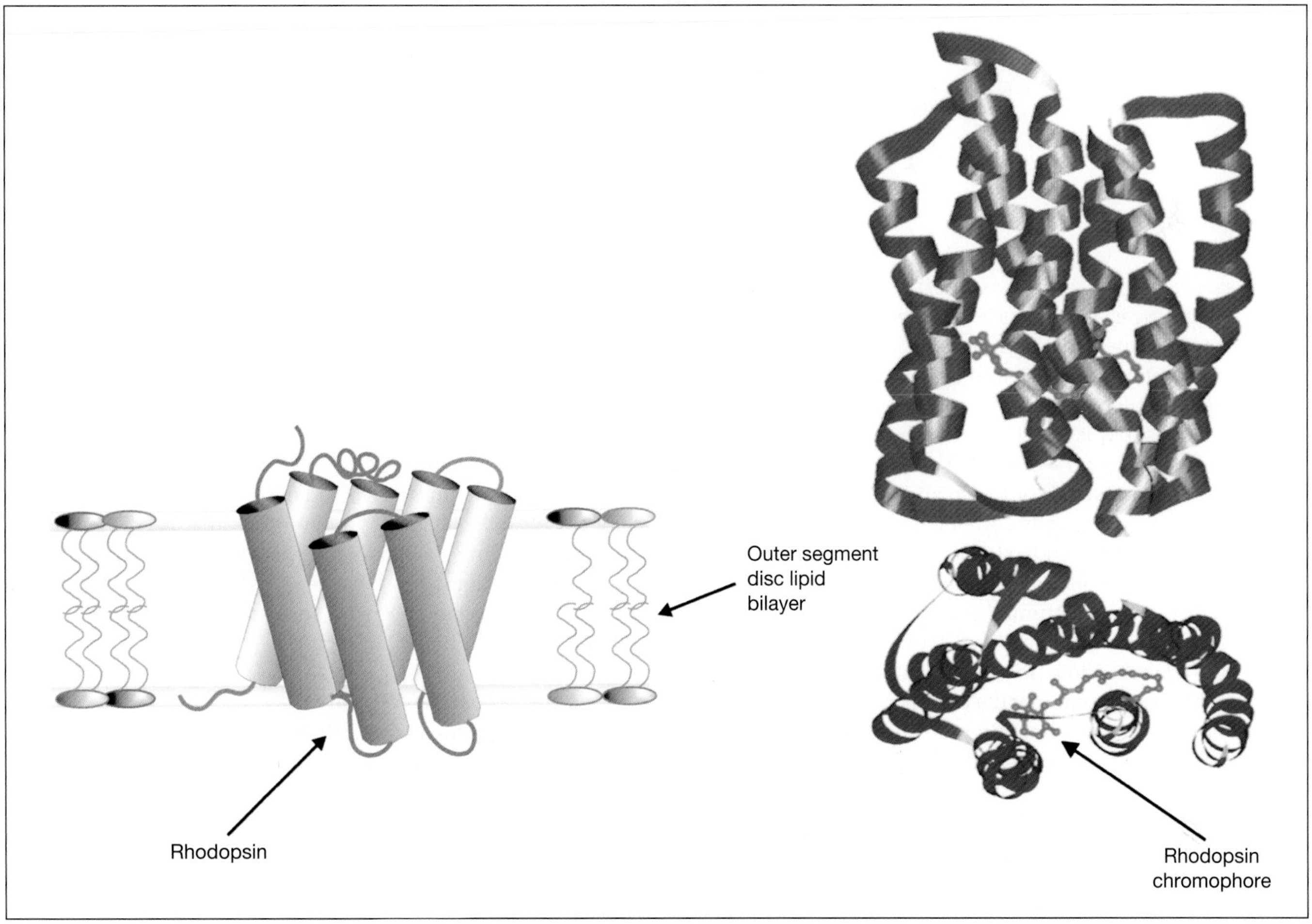

Fig. 40.45 Diagrammatic representations of rhodopsin protein. Left, Positioning of rhodopsin within the rod outer-segment disc membrane. Right, Three-dimensional representation of rhodopsin illustrating the central localization of the retinaldehyde chromophore. (Courtesy of Dr. D. Farrens.)

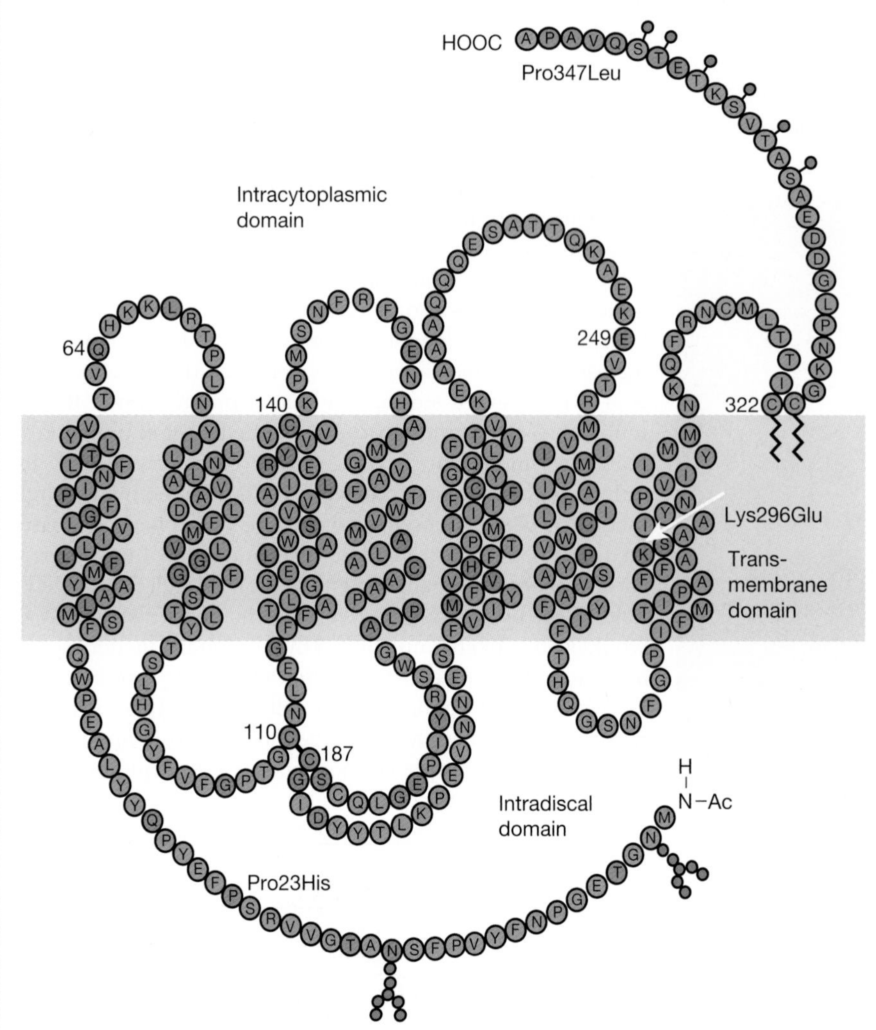

Fig. 40.46 Diagrammatic representation of rhodopsin. Amino acids mutated in retinitis pigmentosa are highlighted in red. There is a disulfide bridge important for the tertiary structure between the cysteines (C) at codons 110 and 187; palmitoylation sites exist at the cysteines at codons 322 and 323. The lysine (K) at codon 296 is the site of binding of retinal to rhodopsin; the glutamic acid (E) at codon 113 is the counter ion for the lysine at codon 296.

The *peripherin/rds* gene was first associated with RP in 1991,[420,421] and over 39 sequence variants have been associated with a range of autosomal dominant phenotypes, including RP, macular dystrophy, CRD, central areolar choroidal dystrophy, fundus flavimaculatus, and pattern dystrophy.[422] Most are missense mutations, but it is unlikely that *peripherin/rds* mutations account for more than 5% of adRP.[423] These reports do however represent the first instance of which an animal model of RP has been found to have a directly correlated human disease counterpart. Much of what we understand to be the role of peripherin/RDS in human photoreceptors (Figs 40.48–40.50) comes from initial studies on this naturally occurring mouse model (rds), which has a 10-kb insert in codon 230 of the disease gene, creating a null allele.[424] From this work and more recent human studies, it has been found that the peripherin/*rds* molecule accumulates in the rims of photoreceptor outer-segment discs and plays an important role in disc morphogenesis and stability.[425]

Bessant et al.[426] reported a large family with adRP previously linked to chromosome 14q11 that is associated with a Ser50Thr mutation of *NRL*. The gene product NRL is a retinal-specific DNA-binding transcription factor that interacts with the cone–rod homeobox transcription factor CRX to promote and regulate transcription of rhodopsin and other retinal genes. The Ser50Thr NRL mutation, when coexpressed with CRX in transfection experiments, produced a marked increase in transactivation of the rhodopsin promoter, producing excessive transcription of rhodopsin. Other families with adRP have been reported with NRL mutations.[427]

A rare but remarkable regional (type II) phenotype with graded disease severity (variable expressivity) has been reported associated with mutations in *PIM1*, on chromosome 7p.[428] This encodes a protein kinase involved in transcriptional control. The gene *FSCN2*, which encodes a photoreceptor-specific paralog of the actin-bundling protein fascin, with presumptive cytoskeletal formation functions, has been reported with autosomal dominant RP.[429] A common *FSCN2* mutation, 208delG, appears to account for 3.3% of adRP in Japan.[429]

Autosomal recessive RP genes

Phenotypes associated with arRP loci can occur at any age, often tend to be early-onset and severe, and are usually consistent within a family.

The third phototransduction cascade protein (Fig. 40.48), cGMP phosphodiesterase (PDE), has been associated with a number of phenotypes.[430] PDE is a holoenzyme consisting of two large subunits α and β, which become enzymatically active when the two γ subunits are removed by activated transducin. Many nonsense and missense mutations of the α and β subunits

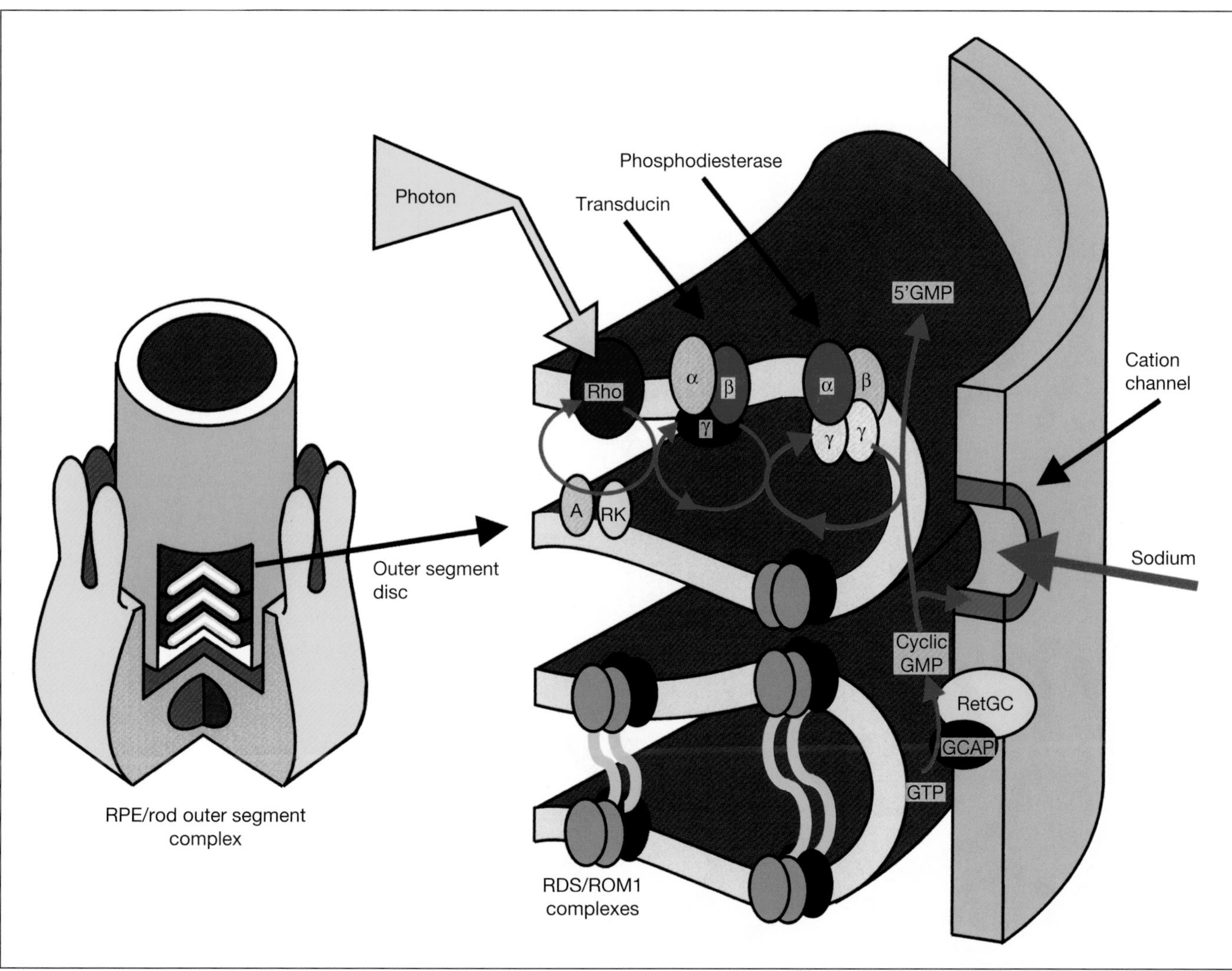

Fig. 40.47 Diagrammatic representation of the retinitis pigment epithelium (RPE)–rod complex. Phototransduction and the role of rds/ROM-1 protein complexes in maintaining outer-segment discs are illustrated. Rho, rhodopsin; A, arrestin; RK, rhodopsin kinase; RetGC, retinal guanylate cyclase; GCAP, guanylate cyclase-activating protein; GMP, guanosine monophosphate.

of PDE (gene symbols *PDE6A* and *PDE6B,* respectively) have been associated with arRP, with the *PDE6A* mutations representing null alleles. No mutation of the PDEγ subunit gene, *PDEG,* has yet been associated with human retinal disease. This might be due to the fact that *PDEG* has an exceptionally low mutation rate, that in humans the gene is expressed in other vital tissues and is lethal in utero, or the function of the mutant PDEγ may be taken over by some other protein. Most PDEβ subunit mutations associated with arRP are found in the C-terminal half of the molecule, which contains the catalytic domain. These mutations presumably directly affect the enzymatic activity of the protein. The His258Asp mutation, however, is near the N-terminal portion adjacent to the PDEγ-binding domain. This mutation has been reported in a Danish family associated with an autosomal dominant congenital stationary night blindness. It has been postulated that this mutation impedes complete inactivation of PDE in dark-adapted rod photoreceptors. This would result in rod desensitization and an inability to transduce at low light levels.[431]

Activated PDE hydrolyses intracellular cGMP. This second-messenger molecule is generated from guanosine triphosphate by membrane-bound and soluble guanylate cyclase.[432] Increased intracellular cGMP leads to relative opening of membrane-bound cGMP-gated cation channels and cell hyperpolarization. The cGMP-gated cation channels are composed of three subunits, α, β, and γ. Mutations (usually null alleles) of the gene for the α subunit (*CNGA1*) have been associated with arRP.[433]

Recovery of active rod opsin, for further phototransduction, involves the regeneration of the 11-*cis* retinaldehyde chromophore from the *all-trans* isomer. In part, this process involves a cellular retinaldehyde-binding protein (CRALBP), which binds and promotes 11-*cis* retinol oxidation to 11-*cis* retinaldehyde in the RPE.[434,435] A homozygous R150Q mutation of the gene for CRALBP (*RLBP1*) has been associated with childhood-onset arRP.[435] Nyctalopia was evident by 3–4 years of age. Optic atrophy, vascular attenuation, macular atrophy, and peripheral white dots without classic bone spicule pigmentation were reported. Mutations of *RLBP1* have also been reported in autosomal recessive retinitis punctata albescens,[436] Bothnia dystrophy,[437] and Newfoundland rod–cone dystrophy.[438]

The tubby-like protein (TULP) gene family includes *TUB,* the human homolog of the mouse *tub* gene, *TULP1,* and *TULP2,* and

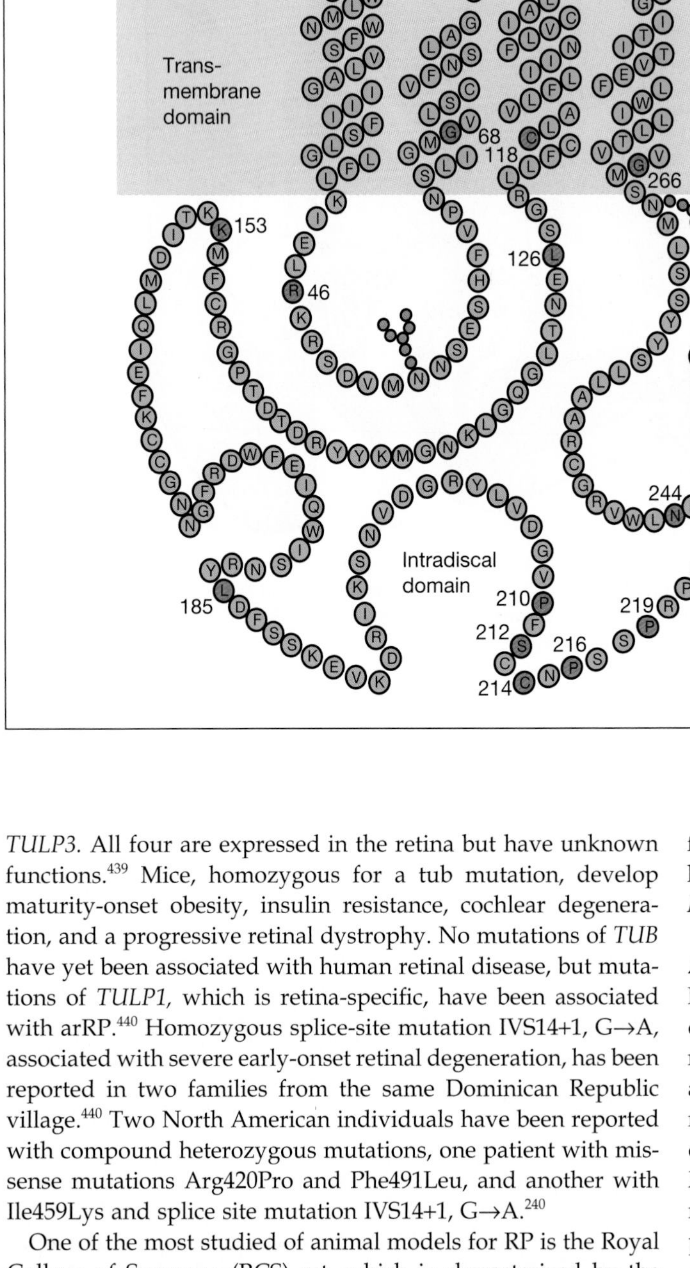

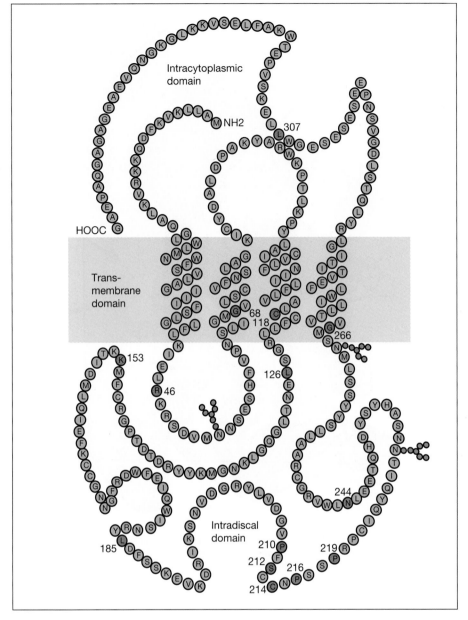

Fig. 40.48 Diagrammatic representation of peripherin/RDS protein. Amino acids mutated in retinitis pigmentosa are highlighted in red. Both the carboxyl-terminus and acetylated amino-terminus are cytoplasmic. Morphogenesis of the disc rims appears to involve interactions among tetramers of the large second intradiscal loop.

TULP3. All four are expressed in the retina but have unknown functions.[439] Mice, homozygous for a tub mutation, develop maturity-onset obesity, insulin resistance, cochlear degeneration, and a progressive retinal dystrophy. No mutations of *TUB* have yet been associated with human retinal disease, but mutations of *TULP1*, which is retina-specific, have been associated with arRP.[440] Homozygous splice-site mutation IVS14+1, G→A, associated with severe early-onset retinal degeneration, has been reported in two families from the same Dominican Republic village.[440] Two North American individuals have been reported with compound heterozygous mutations, one patient with missense mutations Arg420Pro and Phe491Leu, and another with Ile459Lys and splice site mutation IVS14+1, G→A.[240]

One of the most studied of animal models for RP is the Royal College of Surgeons (RCS) rat, which is characterized by the inability of outer segments shed by photoreceptors to be recognized and phagocytized by RPE, leading to retinal degeneration. Mutations in the receptor tyrosine kinase gene *Mertk* have been found to underly the defect in the RCS rat.[441] Patients with arRP have been reported with mutations of the human ortholog *MERTK*.[442]

X-linked RP genes

Positional cloning in X-linked RP at the RP3 locus has led to the discovery of mutations in *RPGR* (RP GTPase regulator).[443] A number of mutations have now been described. Detailed clinical assessments of families with a number of mutations[444,445] have revealed severe, early-onset RP in hemizygotes and variable disease in heterozygotes, as has been typically described in X-linked RP. All the affected males have shown evidence of both rod and cone ERG loss consistent with the expression of the gene product of *RPGR* in both classes of photoreceptor. On the basis of poorer ERG responses in hemizygotes and severe symptoms and clinical findings in heterozygotes, Andréasson et al.[446] have suggested that microdeletion mutation of exons 8 through 10 is a more severe disease than that seen with splice site mutations.

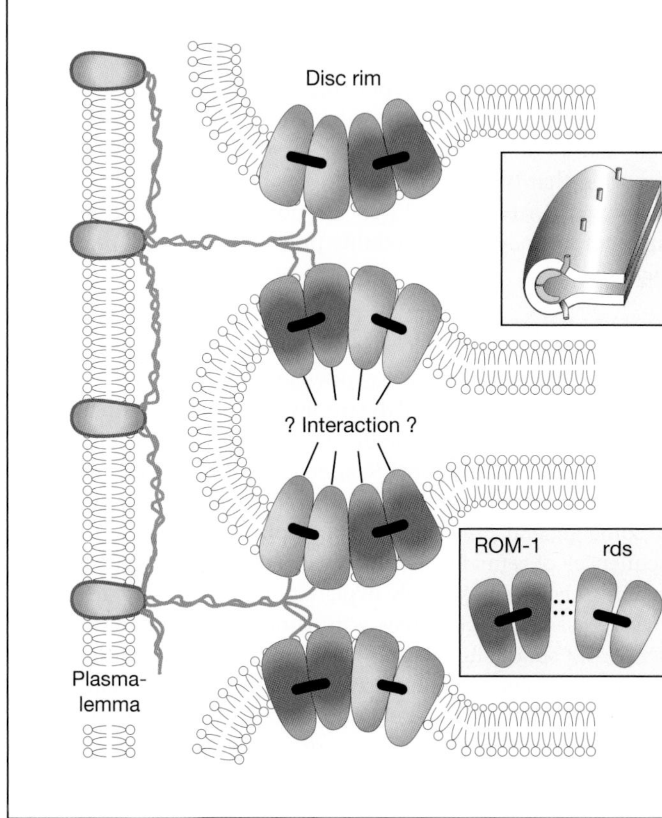

Fig. 40.49 rds/ROM-1 interactions at the disc rim, showing the homodimers of rds and ROM-1 forming tetramers by noncovalent bonds. These tetramers, which may represent the extracellular margin templates of Corless and Fetter, appear to interact across the intradiscal space at the rim margin to form the terminal loop complex (upper inset). (Reproduced with permission from Weleber RG. Phenotypic variation in patients with mutations in the peripherin/*RDS* gene. Digit J Ophthalmol 1999;5:1–8.)

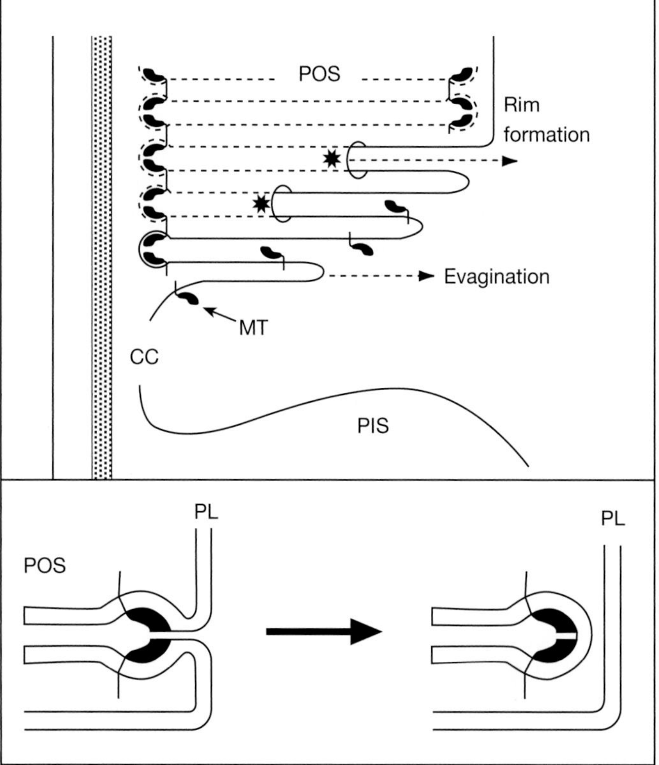

Fig. 40.50 Schematic illustration of the template theory of disc morphogenesis proposed by Corless and Fetter. Disc morphogenesis begins as a plate-like evagination from the plasma membrane in the region of the connecting cilium. The extracellular margin templates (MT) become aligned and assemble to form the terminal loop complexes that Corless and Fetter believe represent the primary morphogen of the disc rims. The asterisk denotes the leading edge of disc rim closure. CC, connecting cilium; POS, photoreceptor outer segment; PIS, photoreceptor inner segment; PL, plasmalemma. (Reproduced with permission from Weleber RG. Phenotypic variation in patients with mutations in the peripherin/*RDS* gene. Digit J Ophthalmol 1999;5:1–8.)

Despite a strong association between the tapetal-like reflex and the X-linked RP carrier state, this has been documented in few patients carrying an *RPGR* mutation.[445]

The predicted RPGR protein contains some sequence homology to RCC1 (regulator of chromosome condensations), which is a guanine nucleotide exchange factor for the small nuclear GTPase Ran. This enzyme is essential for nucleocytoplasmic transport, although it might also be involved in other cellular activities. Other proteins with homology to RCC1 (e.g., ARF1) appear to be guanine nucleotide exchange factors for non-Ran GTPases. These enzymes are involved in protein trafficking through the Golgi apparatus. This has led to the proposition that the RPGR protein may have a similar function in intracellular trafficking.

Although studies suggested that 70–90% of X-linked pedigrees are linked to the RP3 locus, mutations of *RPGR* were initially identified in only about 10–20% of families with X-linked RP.[443,446,447] Recently, however, another retina-enriched transcript, called the ORF15 transcript, was discovered, which utilizes exons 1–13 as before but utilizes exon 14 through part of intron 15 as a large terminal exon (termed the ORF15 exon). This ORF15 exon has accounted for the remainder of families linked to RP3.[448] Mutations of *RPGR* can result in other phenotypes, including CRD,[449] cone dystrophy,[373] and even macular dystrophy.[450]

A disease gene has also been identified at the RP2 locus.[451] Most of the mutations cause truncation of the gene product.[452] Mutations of this gene, termed *RP2,* account for approximately 8–10% of families of X-linked RP.[453] The gene product has homology with human cofactor C, a protein involved in the ultimate step of β-tubulin folding, suggesting that this gene may act as a chaperone or in some way be involved in the structure or function of the cilium of photoreceptors.[451,452] Together, mutations of *RP2* and *RPGR* account for the vast majority of cases of X-linked RP and the RP phenotypes associated with these genes have been reported as clinically indistinguishable from one another or, at most, to show modest differences.[454]

Digenic inheritance and RP

In rod photoreceptors, two peripherin/*rds* molecules form homodimers that bind noncovalently to homodimers of the glycoprotein ROM-1[455,456] (Fig. 40.49). In cones, peripherin/rds homodimers form tetramers with homodimers of either ROM-1 or a homolog.[457] These tetramers may represent the "extracellular marginal templates" described by Corless and Fetter[458] (Fig. 40.50) that are crucial to the creation and structural integrity of the disc rim.

In a few families, three *rds* point mutations – Leu185Pro, Arg13Trp, and Leu45Phe[459] – have been seen in association with

ROM-1 mutations. The affected compound heterozygotes had a severe RP phenotype. This type of inheritance has been termed digenic and highlights the important structural relationship between RDS and ROM-1 in the architecture of the rod photoreceptor. Despite studies around the world, very few RP families have been found to exhibit this phenomenon. Putative mutations of *ROM-1* in isolation have been reported in some small families.[460] As yet, isolated *ROM-1* mutations are not convincingly associated with retinal disease.[423]

Usher syndrome molecular genetics

Molecular genetic linkage analysis has shown that not only are the three clinical subtypes of Usher syndrome genetically distinct but also that there is notable genetic heterogeneity. Currently 15 chromosomal loci have been linked to Usher syndrome and 12 of the associated disease genes have been identified (Table 40.1). The most severe and most common subtype, USH1B, has been associated with mutations of myosin VIIA (*MYO7A*).[461] Mutation of *MYO7A* can also cause nonsyndromal deafness of either recessive (DFNB2) or dominant (DFNA22) type.

Four other genes have been discovered for type 1 Usher syndrome. The gene for USH1C encodes harmonin, a novel PDZ domain containing protein that functions in the organization and assembly of larger protein complexes for cell adhesion, signal transduction, and intracellular transport.[462] Mutations in the ear-specific exons of the gene for harmonin also cause nonsyndromic recessive deafness (DFNB18).[463] The gene for USH1D is *CDH23*, which encodes cadherin 23, a novel member of a class of intercellular adhesion proteins.[464] Mutations in *CDH23* also cause autosomal recessive nonsyndromic deafness (DFNB12).[465] CDH23 is expressed in the cochlea and retina and mutations in the mouse ortholog cause disorganization of inner-ear stereocilia and deafness in the *waltzer* mouse animal model.[466] Two of the harmonin PDZ domains interact with MYO7A and CDH23, indicating that these three proteins form a complex important for organization, maintenance, and function of stereocilia in the cochlea.[467,468] The gene for USH1F is *PCDH15*, which encodes protocadherin 15.[469] Mutations in *PCDH15* have also been reported in nonsyndromic recessive deafness (DFNB23).[470] PCDH15 localizes to stereocilia in inner-ear hair cells and to the photoreceptors of the retina and is presumed to be essential for homeostasis. Mutation of the murine homolog causes vestibular dysfunction and deafness in the *Ames waltzer* mouse.[471] USH1G encodes the protein SANS, which is a novel scaffold protein gene that is expressed in retina and cochlea and is associated with harmonin within stereocilia.[472] Thus, it appears that many of the genes for type 1 Usher syndrome (MYO7A, harmonin, CDH23, and SANS) function together in a complex essential for determining and maintaning cohesion of the stereocilia of the cochlea.[472]

The commonest gene association with type 2 Usher syndrome (*USH2A*) has recently been identified,[473] and encodes a protein called usherin that has motifs that show homology to thrombospondin, laminin epidermal growth factor, and fibronectin type III. This indicates that the gene product may function as a cellular adhesion molecule or as a component of the basal lamina and extracellular matrix. Although discovered first in patients with type 2 Usher syndrome, a Cys759Phe mutation of *USH2A* was found in approximately 4.5% of 224 patients with arRP without hearing loss.

The gene for type 3 Usher syndrome (*USH3A*) was first reported as encoding a 120-amino-acid protein in 2001 by Joensuu et al.[474] A common termination mutation, Y100X, accounts for the majority of mutant alleles in Finnish cases.[474] The gene product, clarin-1, is believed to have a role in hair cell and photoreceptor cell synapses.[475] Pennings et al. have reported that type *USH3A* mutations can produce disease that mimics either type 1 or 2 Usher syndrome and that the fundus appearance may mimic retinitis punctata albescens or RP sine pigmento.[476]

Protein chemistry

Considerable information has now accumulated on the molecular consequences of retinal dystrophy gene mutation. In turn that has led to a much deeper understanding of the molecular physiology of the human retina. Readers are directed to a number of significant reviews on the subject.[477,478]

Some general principles can be applied to the molecular consequences of retinal gene mutation. Deficiency of gene product seems to be the most likely explanation for recessive disease. In two recessive RP pedigrees with rhodopsin mutations (a nonsense and splice site mutation) for example, the aberrant alleles theoretically encode nonfunctional rhodopsin.[479,480] Haploinsufficiency is unlikely to be important in dominant rhodopsin disease though, because carriers of at least one apparently null allele have been shown to be phenotypically normal.[480] Mutant rhodopsin expression in COS cells has shown that mutations in the intradiscal domain adversely influence normal rhodopsin folding.[481] Autosomal dominant mutations within the rhodopsin transmembrane helices still cause misfolding, but to a much lesser effect, and have a more profound effect on retinal binding.[482] In vitro studies have shown that mutant rhodopsin can accumulate within the rough endoplasmic reticulum of rod photoreceptors.[483] This could lead to inhibition of transport of the wild-type rhodopsin to the cytoplasmic membrane and loss of function and might explain pathogenesis in some cases of retinal dystrophy with rhodopsin mutations. However, different results in rhodopsin expression in in vitro studies in nonmammalian models and mammals have suggested that the true relevance of this mechanism in humans is as yet unproved. Truncation of the rhodopsin protein due to mutation of codon,[345,484] for example, is associated with expression of mutant and wild-type rhodopsin in the plasma membrane of tissue culture cells but leads to accumulation of the mutant in the rough endoplasmic reticulum in transgenic mice. The effect in humans is unknown.

Abnormal pre-mRNA splicing

Proteins encoding three RP genes, *PRPF8* (RP13), *PRPF31* (RP11), and *PRPF3* (RP18), have been associated with RNA splicing. RNA splicing is an essential process that removes intron sequences from pre-mRNA. This is carried out by the spliceosome, a high-molecular-weight ribonucleoprotein complex.[485] The vast majority of pre-mRNA introns (designated the U2 type) are spliced by the major spliceosome, which is composed of five uridine-rich small nuclear ribonucleoproteins, or snRNPs, termed U1, U2, U4, U5, and U6. Each snRNP is the central component of a protein complex that also contains seven Sm or Sm-like proteins, which are assembled by the so-called SMN (survival of motor neurons) protein. In addition to the Sm and Sm-like proteins, snRNPs also contain 3–10 particle-specific proteins.[486] The major spliceosome also contains a poorly defined number of other non-snRNP protein factors. The minor spliceosome is responsible for splicing a rare class of pre-mRNA introns, called the U12 type.[485] Minor spliceosomes contain the U5 snRNP and four nonabundant snRNPs: U11, U12, U4atac, and U6atac.

The *PRPF8* gene (chromosome 17p13.3) encodes precursor RNA processing factor 8 (PRPF8). The yeast homolog, Prp8p, is a U5 snRNP factor that is first required for assembly of the U4/U6 and U5 tri-snRNP[487] and then for facilitating the binding of the tri-snRNP to the 50 and 30 splice sites.[488] It functions as the catalytic core of the spliceosome, either by facilitating formation of the core and/or by stabilizing RNA interactions.[489] Seven different missense mutations of *PRPF8*, all clustered within a 14-codon stretch in the last exon, have been identified in five RP13-linked families.[490] *PRPF8* mutations are associated with early-onset adRP with diffuse retinal involvement and a severe prognosis in comparison with other forms of adRP.[490,491] Individuals experience night blindness beginning between 4 and 10 years of age and constricted visual field as teenagers.[491] Classic midequatorial bone spicule pigmentation is seen by middle age.[491] Typically, individuals are registered as blind or partially sighted by age 30.[490] *PRPF31* (chromosome 19q13.4) encodes protein 61K, the putative ortholog of the yeast pre-mRNA splicing factor Prp31p.[492] Protein 61K is specific to the U4/U6 snRNP and is required for pre-mRNA splicing in vitro.[493] Protein 61K participates in the formation of the tri-snRNP, possibly by physically tethering the U5 snRNP to the U4/U6 snRNP.

Haploinsufficiency appears to be the mechanism underlying the photoreceptor degeneration in the majority of alleles of the *PRPF31* gene associated with RP because most of these alleles are predicted to be protein truncation mutations. Families with *PRPF31* mutations are unique in showing bimodal expressivity of the phenotype, with asymptomatic carriers who have both affected parents and affected children.[494,495] Symptomatic individuals experience night blindness and loss of visual field in their teenage years and are typically registered as blind by their 30s.[494] Evans et al. suggested that the bimodal expressivity seen in these pedigrees may be explained by a second allelic genetic factor influencing phenotype. This idea was taken further by McGee et al.,[496] who confirmed that penetrance of the *PRPF31* mutations may be influenced in trans by otherwise silent *PRPF31* alleles or by a closely linked locus on the wild-type chromosome, because a statistically significant correlation was found between the development of RP in a carrier and the inheritance of the region around RP from the noncarrier parent.[496] Vithana et al.[492] have demonstrated that asymptomatic patients inherit a different wild-type allele to the one inherited by their symptomatic siblings. The third of the three known pre-mRNA splicing factors associated with adRP is encoded by the *PRPF3* gene (chromosome 1q21.1).[497] PRPF3 protein associates with the U4/U6 snRNP during pre-mRNA splicing.[498] Mutations in its yeast ortholog, Prp3p, cause instability of the U4/U6 snRNP and prevent assembly of the tri-snRNP, thereby preventing splicing.[499] Two different missense mutations have been identified in three individuals and three families.[499] Affected individuals suffer night blindness toward the end of the first decade of life.[497] Visual field defects are seen by the fourth decade of life but the central field remains relatively spared. A few patients progress to total blindness by age 80.

Several mechanisms have been proposed to account for the fact that mutations in these three, ubiquitously expressed, splicing factor genes only cause adRP and not a more widespread abnormality. The loss of one functional copy of these splice factor genes may affect only rods because of their unusually high requirement for protein synthesis and, consequently, for pre-mRNA splicing.[500] Alternatively, the adRP-associated mutations may decrease the rate at which spliceosome activation occurs,[501] making activation the rate-limiting step in rod photoreceptors but not other cells. Finally, it has also been suggested that the retina-specific phenotype may occur as a result of an unidentified retina-specific splicing cofactor that interacts with all three of these splicing factor proteins.[496]

RPGR interactome

An interactome is a complex representation of functional interactions between molecules either within a cell or within the organism as a whole. Often such interactomes reveal important interactions between molecules that at first would not appear to be functionally related. In this way, the functional consequences of genetic mutation can be predicted without the need for lengthy experimentation. An RPGR interactome has also been proposed.[502] RPGR is a component of centrioles, ciliary axonemes, and microtubular transport complexes, although its precise function is unknown. It colocalizes with RPGRIP1 at the axonemes of connecting cilia in rod and cone photoreceptors[503] by binding to RPGRIP1. This localization is lost in Rpgrip1 knockout (KO) mice. Rpgr KO mice develop a slow retinal degeneration, with features resembling a cone–rod degeneration – cone photoreceptors degenerate faster than rods and there is partial mislocalization of cone opsins.[504] Some residual Rpgr^{ORF15} expression has been reported in this model.[505] RPGR has been shown to co-immunoprecipitate in retinal extracts with a number of different axonemal, basal body, and microtubular transport proteins.[505] These include nephrocystin-5 and calmodulin, which localize to photoreceptor-connecting cilia; the microtubule-based transport proteins, kinesin II (KIF3A, KAP3 subunits), dynein (DIC subunit), SMC1, and SMC3; and two regulators of cytoplasmic dynein, p150Glued and p50-dynamitin, which tether cargoes to the dynein motor. Inhibition of dynein by overexpressing p50-dynamitin abrogates the localization of RPGR^{ORF15} to basal bodies. RPGRORF15 can be co-immunoprecipitated from retinal extracts with other basal body proteins, including NPM, IFT88, 14-3-3ε, and γ-tubulin.[502,505] RPGR^{ORF15} and RPGRIP1 co-localize at centrosomes in a wide variety of nonciliated cells and at basal bodies in ciliated cells. Both proteins are core components of centrioles and basal bodies.[502] In summary, RPGRORF15 appears to have a role in microtubule-based transport to and from the basal bodies and within photoreceptor axonemes, perhaps concerned with movement of cargoes between IS and OS. RPGRORF15 is predominantly expressed in photoreceptor connecting cilia and basal bodies but expression has also been reported in OS in some species,[506] although this has been disputed.[503] RPGR is also expressed in the transitional zone of motile cilia in the epithelial lining of human bronchi and sinuses (RPGR^{ex1-19} only) and within the human and monkey cochlea.[503,507–509]

Ush interactome

The USH genes encode proteins of different classes and families, including motor proteins, scaffold proteins, cell adhesion molecules, and transmembrane receptor proteins. In vitro direct interaction studies between USH proteins and also localization studies in mouse models have however suggested functional relationships between these proteins such that an "USH interactome" has been proposed.[510] In these studies, it should be noted, however, that although all the USH mouse models show severe hearing loss and vestibular dysfunction, only the Ush2A$^{-/-}$ mouse, shows signs of RP.[511] From such work, a "multiprotein scaffold complex" model has been proposed for harmonin, whirlin, and sans. There is also evidence that harmonin and whirlin can bind all other components of the USH network, including cadherin 23, protocadherin 15, usherin, VLGR1, and myosinVIIA.[467,507,512]

Myosin VIIa has also been found to interact with sans 11 and protocadherin 15.[468] Such findings suggest that the USH proteins form a transmembrane network that regulates hair bundle morphogenesis, particularly the growing stereocilia or the kinocilium, and may also have a role in the mechanoelectrical signal transduction and synaptic function of mature hair cells.[513] In the USH interactome model, it is proposed that the extracellular interstereocilia links are anchored intracellularly by the scaffold proteins, harmonin and whirlin, through direct binding to the actin cytoskeleton or through other proteins, including myosin VIIa.[467,507,514,515]

Additionally, it has been shown that the association of other proteins with the USH complex (through harmonin) may function in determining cell polarity and cell–cell interactions.[516] Also Myo7a is believed to use long filaments of actin as tracks along which to transport other USH complex molecules.[517] In photoreceptors, proteins of the USH interactome are localized in the connecting cilium and may participate in the ciliary transport, but are also arranged at the interface between the inner segment and the connecting cilium where they control cargo passage. USH protein complexes may also provide mechanical stabilization to membrane calycal processes and the connecting cilium.[518] Studies of coexpression of USH1 and USH2 proteins also show accumulation at synaptic endings of photoreceptor cells, indicating that they are organized in an USH protein network there.[519]

Bardet–Biedl syndrome and the "BBSome"

Recently it has been proposed that many of the proteins encoded by Bardet–Biedl genes form complexes, e.g., BBS1, BBS2, BBS4, BBS5,BBS7, BBS8 and BBS9 - the "BBSome."[520] The complex is important in the function of primary cilia, nonmotile projections found in numerous cell types. In particular, BBSome complexes are thought to play a central role in vesicular trafficking of membrane proteins within cilia. The BBSome binds to Rab8, a GTP/GDP exchange factor involved in docking and fusion of rhodopsin carrier vesicles in the connecting cilium of photoreceptors.[521] It is also known that other Bardet–Biedl genes, e.g., BBS3 (Arl6), form functional relationships with this BBSome.[522] Others appear to function as chaperones, e.g., BBs6, BBS10, and BBS12, and in protein ubiquitination (BBS11/TRIM32).[523]

Abnormal intracellular trafficking

An increasingly important consequence of retinal disease gene mutation has been the concept of abnormal intracellular trafficking.[400,524] For instance, another rod damage in rhodopsin mutants is often associated with mutant rhodopsin accumulating in the outer segment.[400,525,526] It is thought that this interferes with normal phototransduction and triggers apoptotic cell death. It has been shown in transgenic mice that mutant rhodopsin is only transported to the rod outer segment when the C-terminal region of the molecule is intact.[527] This observation has been corroborated in human eyes.[528]

Cell death pathways

A prevalent proposition in the last decade has been that, since many different gene mutations result in a similar clinical outcome (RP), there must be a "final common cell death pathway" precipitated by these mutations.[529] Apoptosis, the first cell death biochemical pathway linked to RP, characteristically appears histologically as a rounding up of the cell, reduction of cellular volume, chromatin condensation, and finally engulfment by resident phagocyte. Apoptosis is triggering of intrinsic and (to some extent) extrinsic pathways involving activation of caspases which can be subclassified into both initiator (2, 8, 9, 10) and effector (3, 6, 7) molecules. Studies with caspase inhibitors, however, have often produced only marginal neuroprotection in RP models.[530,531] Other studies have highlighted that caspase-independent inducers of cell death such as apoptosis-inducing factor, calpains, and poly(ADP-ribose) polymerases 1 are activated during retinal degeneration.[532]

Previously, necrosis had not been considered a significant part of retinal degeneration. This passive, unregulated form of cell death is now considered to be inducible by regulated signal transduction pathways such as those mediated by RIP kinases.[532] Such necroptosis may play a role in RP.[532,533] Apoptosis and necroptosis mechanisms may act together or may form alternate pathways.

Cell and tissue biology

Histopathology

Early histopathologic studies found that the first degenerative abnormalities in RP occur in the photoreceptors. As more and more animal model histopathologic correlates of specific human genetic mutations become available, our knowledge of both outer and inner retinal changes in RP is leading to new concepts for therapy.[477,534]

Photoreceptor abnormalities

The earliest histologic sign of retinal dystrophy is shortening of rod outer segments (Fig. 40.51).[535] With progression of disease, rod outer segments become more severely shortened, and eventually whole cells are lost. This is reflected in reduced numbers of nuclei in the outer nuclear layer. Rod cell loss is usually seen initially in the midperiphery. In certain cases cell loss is initially seen in the inferior retina. This is a typical finding in cases with rhodopsin mutation Pro23His.[179] In such cases there is a corresponding altitudinal field defect. Interestingly, a similar pattern of photoreceptor loss is seen in transgenic Pro23His mutant mice. In this model, if mutant mice were dark-reared, the resultant retinal degeneration was more uniform across the retina and was significantly milder.[536] This suggests that limiting light exposure in patients with this mutation may moderate the progression of disease.

Using immunocytochemistry and antirhodopsin antibodies, extensive studies have been undertaken of cytopathologic abnormalities in photoreceptors. In normal rods, rhodopsin is concentrated in the outer segments. In a number of rhodopsin-mutant animal models, abnormal localization of mutant rhodopsin has been seen,[537] and this has also been seen in human eyes.[538,539] Such observations have led to interesting hypotheses as to how mutant protein may damage photoreceptors.[540] It has been proposed that certain mutant rhodopsin molecules accumulate in the endoplasmic reticulum or Golgi apparatus in the inner segment and lead to cell death by interfering with the function

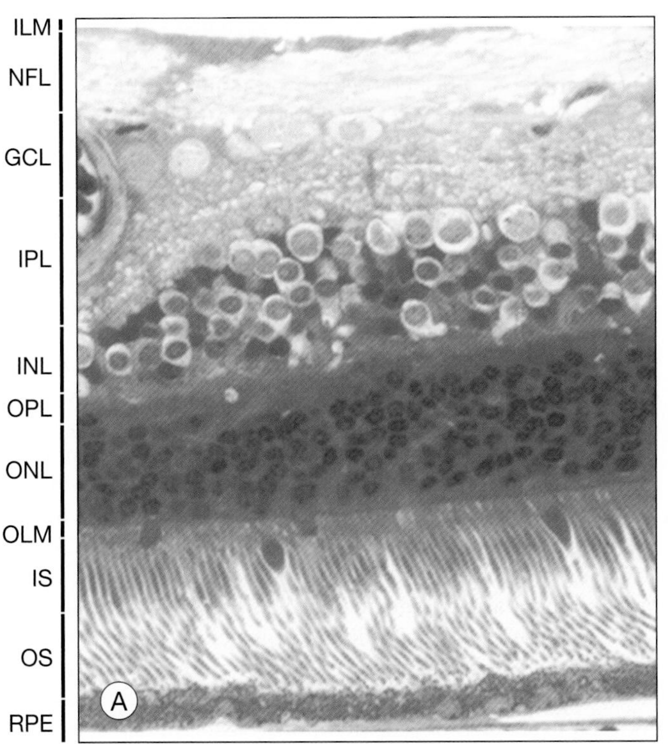

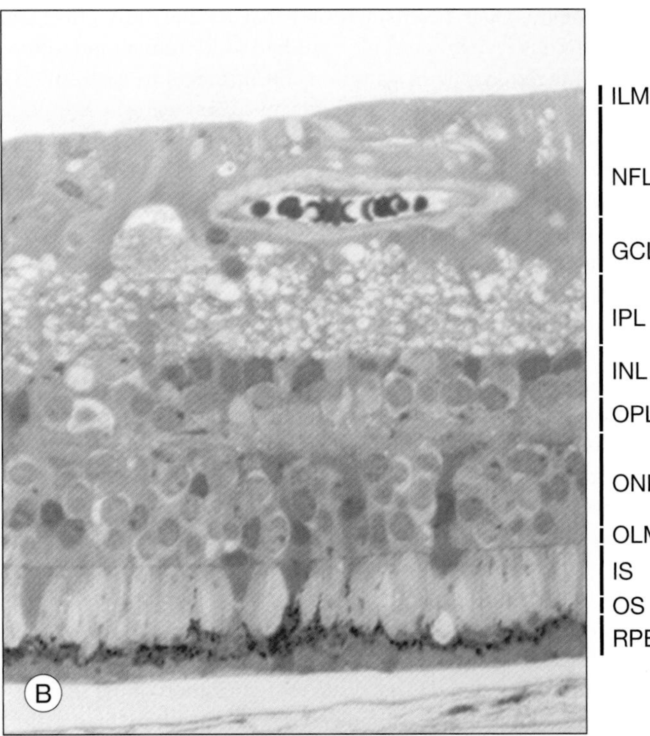

Fig. 40.51 Light micrograph from a normal eye (A) and an eye with retinitis pigmentosa (B). Richardson methylene blue/azure II stain. Note marked loss of outer segments in retinitis pigmentosa. ILM, internal limiting membrane; NFL, nerve fiber layer; GCL, ganglion cell layer; IPL, inner plexiform layer; INL, inner nuclear layer; OPL, outer plexiform layer; ONL, outer nuclear layer; OLM, outer limiting membrane; IS, inner segments and OS, outer segments of rod and cone layer; RPE, retinal pigment epithelium (×60). (Courtesy of A.H. Milam.)

of these organelles. Clearly, though, there are species differences in the cytopathologic effects of particular mutations. In transgenic Pro347Ser mice, rhodopsin is seen to accumulate in extracellular vesicles attached to rod inner segments.[541] Alternatively, in the transgenic Pro347Ser pig, rhodopsin accumulates in the inner segments.[542,543] Such aberrant accumulation of rhodopsin in the inner segment has not, however, been seen in human cases of Pro347Ser.

Clarke et al.[544,545] studied 11 different animal models of outer retinal dystrophy. These authors noted that the kinetics of photoreceptor death fit an exponential model. This in turn suggests three important features: (1) the risk of death is constant throughout the lifetime of each mutant photoreceptor; (2) each mutant photoreceptor is at the same risk of death as every other mutant photoreceptor (other things being equal); (3) the time at which death will occur is random and independent of the time of death of other photoreceptors. The regional variation in photoreceptor death in RP is not inconsistent with the feature of equal risk because local geographic factors may be superimposed on the equal risk of death of all the photoreceptors, resulting in a higher risk in certain parts of the retina. In the animal model studies, the same region of the retina was always examined, eliminating any effect of regional variation. The identification of these three characteristics of outer retinal dystrophies is important for at least two reasons. First, exponential kinetics refutes the major alternative model of photoreceptor death, the cumulative damage model, in which the risk of death increases with time (akin to the risk of death in an aging population of people) and the cell death kinetics are sigmoidal, not exponential. Second, the recognition that mutant photoreceptors are at a constant risk of death requires that biochemical mechanisms proposed to underlie the photoreceptor death must explain both the exponential kinetics as well as other major characteristics of the disease. For example, this may mean that, for all the different gene mutations, probably only a few pathways triggering apoptotic cell death are relevant to photoreceptor degeneration.[546]

Outer retinal disease

After photoreceptor cell death, the RPE becomes detached from Bruch's membrane and migrates into the neurosensory retina. The subretinal space is abolished. Accumulation of RPE cells in a cuff around retinal vessels leads to bone spicule pigmentation.[547] Bruch's membrane thickening has also been recorded under degenerate RP retina. In late-onset RP, material has been seen to accumulate between the RPE and the inner collagenous layer of Bruch's membrane.[548–550] This material was periodic acid–Schiff-positive and contained lipid, calcium, and iron. Choriocapillaries underlying areas of debrided RPE undergo atrophy.[551]

Inner retinal pathology

Reactive changes have been reported in all cell types in the inner retina subsequent to photoreceptor cell death. Müller cells undergo reactive gliosis.[552,553] In advanced RP, entangled, thickened Müller cell processes result in extensive scarring in the remaining retina. Glial fibrillary acidic protein-positive astrocytes undergo reactive hyperplasia. This growth of astrocytes contributes to the pallor of the optic nerve head and epiretinal membrane formation.[554,555] Microglia migration into the outer retina has been documented in the RCS rat model of retinal dystrophy,[556] but the human and pathophysiologic significance of this is unknown.

Previously it has been suggested that RP has little effect on ganglion cells.[557,558] Stone et al.[115] studied 41 RP retinas and found significant reductions in ganglion cell numbers in each inheritance type of RP. The most significant losses were in X-linked RP and adRP. Transneuronal degeneration[534,559] has been the explanation for this phenomenon. Compression of cell bodies by retinal vessels[560] and inner retinal ischemia has also been proposed as causes for ganglion cell loss. Inner retinal ischemia, a consequence of pigment epithelium perivascular cuffing,[547] may in part also explain the optic nerve head pallor that is observed clinically.[561]

More recent publications have expanded on the details of the anomalous remodeling and the misguided attempts at repair that take place within the retina in retinal degenerations following death and loss of the photoreceptors.[562,563] The changes appear in response to the stress of injury and cell death and progress through three stages: (1) the primary insult to the photoreceptors, which results in their dysfunction (and produces visual symptoms); (2) death of photoreceptors that ablates the sensory retina, by initial photoreceptor stress, phenotype deconstruction, and cell death of other cell types, through bystander effects or loss of trophic support; and (3) a protracted period of global remodeling and large-scale reorganization of the remaining neural retina.[564] These attempts at repair result in three major tranformations: (1) the reactive hypertrophy of Müller cells and the formation of a distal glial seal that essentially isolates the remaining neuroretina from the surviving RPE/choroids; (2) apparent neuronal migration along glial surfaces to ectopic sites; and (3) the establishment of aberrant rewiring through a complex formation of neurite fasicles, new synaptic foci, and aberrant connections within the retina.[561] It is also now known that bipolar and horizontal cells in particular undergo significant morphological changes and changes in neurotransmitter receptor expression in response to outer retinal degeneration.[564] RP triggers permanent loss of bipolar cell glutamate receptor expression, though spontaneous iGluR-mediated signaling by amacrine and ganglion cells. It has been proposed that rod bipolar cell dendrite switching likely triggers new gene expression patterns and may impair cone pathway function.[565] These changes may place constraints on the concepts of cell or tissue transplantation or implantation of artificial retinas for regaining sight in advanced retinal degenerations.

Cellular remodeling and vascular changes

In the slowly degenerating dystrophic retina, peripheral rods sprout long, axon-like processes that can extend as far as the inner limiting membrane.[535,566] These neurites have been found in rhodopsin mutant eyes and in cases of X-linked RP. They are found in areas of marked cell death but have yet to be seen in the macula. Neurite processes bypass bipolar and horizontal cell synapses to become closely associated with hypertrophied Müller cell processes (Fig. 40.52). Neurites aggregate to form fascicles that arborize at the inner plexiform layer to form beaded processes under the inner limiting membrane. Although numerous vesicles similar to those seen in synapses are found in neurites, true synaptic connections have yet to be identified. Immunocytochemistry has shown that rhodopsin photopigment accumulates within neurites. It is still unknown whether these processes fulfill any functional role. Rod neurite sprouting does not seem to occur in dystrophic mouse models of RP. This suggests that the process occurs in retinas that undergo protracted degeneration over years, rather than rapid degeneration over weeks to months that is typical of mouse models of retinal dystrophy. Such models therefore may not be suitable in retinal transplantation studies ultimately intended to justify human studies. The environment in which it is intended to re-establish synaptic contact between transplanted rods and second-order neurons must be very different in dystrophic mice as compared with humans.[566] Thus, models of RP in larger animals, such as the transgenic pig,[542,567] are necessary.

Cone degeneration may occur early or late in RP. The evolution of cone changes is similar to that seen in rods. Cytoplasmic densification, axon elongation, and eventual reduction in number of cell bodies indicative of cell death follow initial cone outer-segment shortening. In the peripheral retina,

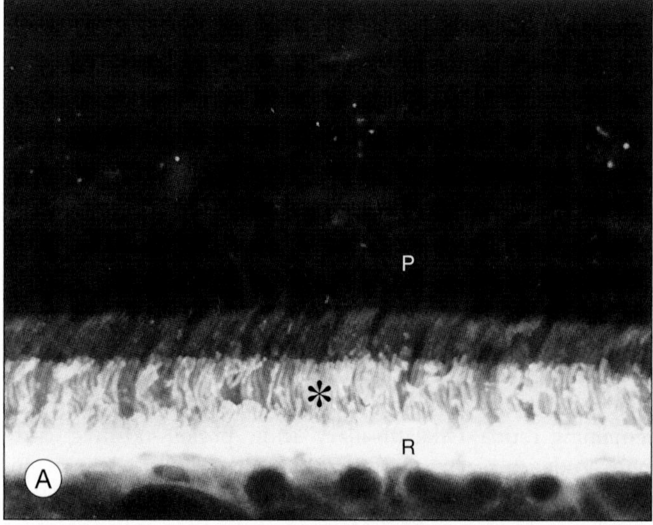

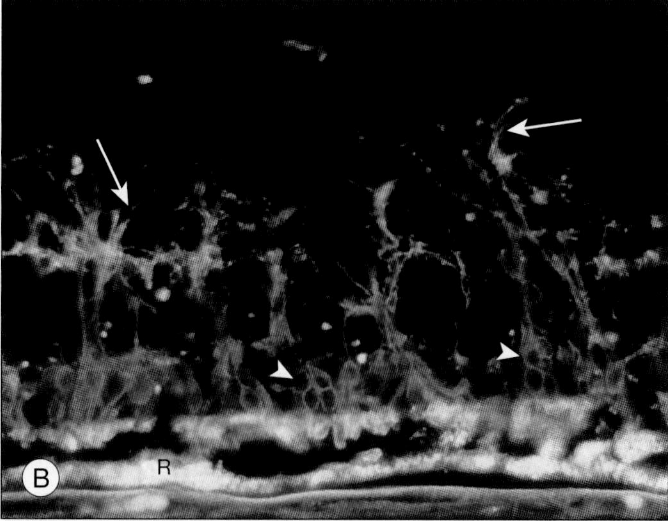

Fig. 40.52 Rhodopsin immunofluorescence in the retina in a normal (A) and a Q64ter rhodopsin mutant retinitis pigmentosa (B) subject. In the normal retina, rhodopsin immunolabeling is confined to the rod outer segments (asterisk). In the retinitis pigmentosa eye, rhodopsin is seen delocalized to processes (rod neurites) extending into the inner retina (arrows). R, Retinal pigment epithelium; P, photoreceptor somata (×230). (Courtesy of A.H. Milam.)

shortened cone outer segments become surrounded by pyramidal-shaped RPE processes.[568] Cones do not, however, undergo neurite sprouting to the extent seen in rods. In some RP eyes, peripheral cones occasionally evolve limited projections.[535,566] In an RP eye with a rhodopsin 64ter mutation, enlarged cone axons that extended into the inner plexiform layer were noted.[535] If cell death has been extensive, a monolayer of cone somata is still evident in the macula. A cell survival factor specifically elaborated by rods but important for cones has been discovered.[569] This factor, termed rod-derived cone viability factor, is a truncated thioredoxin-like protein that holds promise for the generation of potential new treatment possibilities for RP.

Retinal vascular abnormalities can be a prominent feature in cases of RP. Perivascular cuffing[547] and arteriolar attenuation are common features of advanced disease. Retinal blood flow decreases in advanced RP.[570] This may be caused by this perivascular cuffing, which constitutes migrated pigment epithelium and deposited extracellular matrix, or it may be a phenomenon secondary to reduced metabolic need. Reduced cell density in the degenerating retina may lead to a reduced metabolic demand and therefore reduced flow.[570]

In a few RP patients, changes in retinal permeability can lead to exudative retinal detachment (Coats-like disease).[63] This can be associated with peripheral retinal telangiectasia.[571] Peripheral retinal ischemia and preretinal neovascularization have also been reported.[60] Histopathologic evaluations of these vascular changes in humans however have only been reported from eyes that were already at the endstage of disease.

GENETIC CONSULTATION

A diagnosis of RP always implies genetic disease. Therefore, once a diagnosis is suspected, further patient management is carried out within the special context of genetic consultation.[572] This can be subdivided into three areas: (1) diagnosis; (2) genetic counseling; and (3) management of therapeutic options. The first steps in the management of a patient with RP are to establish an accurate diagnosis and a mode of inheritance. Both involve the traditional methods of history-taking and clinical examination. Clinical investigations and molecular genetic diagnosis can augment information gathered in this way. The patient whose diagnosis brought the family to the attention of physicians is called the proband or propositus.[189]

A complete, detailed pedigree is an essential part of the workup before informed genetic counseling can begin. Examination of other family members may be essential not only to establish the correct diagnosis but also to gain a better appreciation of the range and extent of the manifestation shown by other family members and the expected rate of progression. For some retinal dystrophies, such as Usher syndrome and BBS, the inheritance, autosomal recessive in these examples, can be accurately predicted on the basis of the diagnosis. For others, such as typical RP, the family workup may be the only way an inheritance subtype may be uncovered.

The scope for molecular genetic diagnosis is clearly opening up and a number of centers around the world now offer molecular diagnostic testing for a growing number of RP genes. A list of laboratories can be obtained through www.genetests.org. For other genes, molecular diagnosis can only be obtained through research laboratories.

Counseling family groups

Genetic counseling may be defined as a communication process that deals with the human problems associated with the occurrence, or risk of genetic disease, in a family. After a diagnosis has been made, the first important issue is to determine who should undertake the genetic counseling of an RP patient. Traditionally, this has been done by the ophthalmologist who establishes the diagnosis. With the recent advances in RP research, however, many ophthalmologists now refer such patients to specialist ophthalmologists who are more actively involved in the field. Recently it has been suggested that counseling should be undertaken by clinical medical geneticists, genetic counselors, or genetic nurses. This is in recognition of skills not formally within the training of ophthalmologists. There is increasing awareness of the need for more than just simple passing on of information about disease pathophysiology, mode of inheritance, and therapeutic options during the counseling process. The single most common patient complaint about genetic counseling is that the consultant does not address the problems that really concern the patient,[573] which are more often psychologic and social problems than specific details of disease. One of the most psychologically stressful periods in the life of an RP patient consists of the events surrounding the diagnosis of RP. Michie et al.,[574] in a survey of patients undergoing counseling, found that 50% expected direct advice, 30% expected help in making decisions, and 50% wanted simple reassurances about how the disease would affect their and their family's lives. The RP patient is often more concerned about how to cope, now that driving is prohibited because of peripheral field loss, than what actual percentage of field remains. No clinical trials have been undertaken to determine the best way to undertake the counseling of RP patients, but, with the promise of future advances in genetic therapeutics, this is certainly an area that will change dramatically within the next decade.

A major principle of genetic counseling has been that it should be nondirective and supportive. However, it has been conceded that, to some extent, this is an ideal rather than a practical aim.[574,575] Most RP patients, for example, those who are given options to choose whether to undergo cataract surgery, act on the recommendation of the consulting physician. Similarly, many patients are influenced by the manner of presentation of risks and options for family planning. Reproductive counseling should always present the various options in as nondirective a manner as possible.

Predictions of severity of disease can be influenced by a number of non-Mendelian factors that are becoming more recognized in ophthalmic genetic variable expressivity (variation in severity)[576] and incomplete penetrance (disease gene carriers who are not symptomatic)[494] is particularly common in autosomal dominant disease. Digenic inheritance[459] (i.e., symptomatic individuals heterozygous for mutations in two separate genes) can also influence the predictions of severity. Other non-Mendelian influences, such as meiotic drive,[577] anticipation,[578] and imprinting,[579] may also be relevant to predictions of disease severity in particular families.

After the discussion of symptoms and prognosis for vision with the patient, issues dealing with risk to the patient's children arise. Mode of inheritance will have already been assessed. An autosomal dominant trait with affected members in each generation and male-to-male transmission would imply a 50% risk to the offspring of affected individuals. In autosomal recessive families, in which both parents are carriers, each child of those parents has a 25% risk of being affected, irrespective of the number of children already affected. An affected individual with an autosomal recessive disease has a small risk of having an affected offspring, depending on the frequency of carrier state in the population. Inheritance of autosomal recessive traits is influenced by traditions of consanguinity in the community. Information on such traditions should be sought, since consanguinity can be common in various populations.

Classically, X-linked traits are only symptomatic in affected males (hemizygotes). However, female carriers of X-linked RP can be symptomatic even with minimal fundus abnormality.[580] Affected males cannot transmit the abnormal gene to their sons, but all daughters will be carriers (obligate heterozygotes). The variability and spectrum of clinical expression in heterozygotes are attributed to lyonization, the random inactivation of one of the two X chromosomes, with the extent of disease depending on the relative proportion of activity for the parental X chromosome that carries the mutant gene.[40,41] Rarely, because of extremes of lyonization, a carrier for an X-linked disorder, such as X-linked RP or choroideremia, may be moderately to severely affected.

A common problem is the assessment of risk to offspring in simplex cases for which no family history of disease or limited pedigree information is available. In such cases the risk to offspring is likely quite small (e.g., <5%) unless the proposed union is consanguineous.

With the advent of molecular diagnosis, the possibility of prenatal diagnosis with the option of selective termination is becoming more of a reality in ophthalmic genetic disease.[581–583] Prevailing opinion and current law relating to prenatal diagnosis with subsequent termination of an affected fetus vary from country to country. In the UK, it is considered justifiable if two registered medical practitioners perceive the handicap as severe (the Abortion Act 1967 and Human Fertilization and Embryology Act 1990). A similar situation exists in Germany, with the restriction that termination be undertaken before 22 weeks' gestation (Strafgesetzbuch para. 218 and 218a abs. 3, amended 1995). No laws in the USA specifically forbid prenatal diagnosis for an ocular disorder with subsequent termination of an affected fetus, but in practice it has been rarely, if ever, done, at least for risk of a retinal dystrophy. In Ireland prenatal diagnosis for selective termination of pregnancy is prohibited. A definition of "severe" handicap is often not given. Childhood-onset recessive RP might be considered "severe," whereas adult-onset pattern retinal dystrophy might not. Between these two extremes, opinion is divided and greatly depends on the definition of "severe handicap" as understood by the patient, the family, and the attendant practitioners.

In terms of ophthalmic genetic counseling, it is required to explain the severity of probable visual handicaps in terms that are understandable to the patient (e.g., relating loss of ability to read and to the extent of restriction of mobility rather than predicting probable Snellen visual acuity). To some extent comparisons can be made to the experience of another older affected family member. Many visually impaired individuals, despite severe visual deficit, are surprisingly well adjusted and lead highly productive lives. Such families may perceive the handicap as milder than would an outside observer, and support for affected children within these families may be so great that the risk of passing on the disease is not perceived as a large burden. When discussing such matters the practitioner needs to be particularly sensitive to racial, religious, and social influences. For instance, termination is rarely acceptable to Catholics or Muslims.[584]

No study has yet attempted to assess the requirements for prenatal diagnosis in ophthalmic genetics in the USA, although such studies have been undertaken in Europe. Members of the German Retinitis Pigmentosa Society participated in a questionnaire survey on attitudes toward prenatal diagnosis of RP.[585] Of the 414 respondents, 64% thought that prenatal diagnosis was appropriate. A similar study in Sweden found that 60% had a positive attitude toward prenatal diagnosis.[586] Both studies found that, although most people would accept an offer of prenatal diagnosis, this did not imply that they would then proceed with the termination of an affected pregnancy. In the former study, over 32% responded that they would disagree with termination if the child were destined to be blind soon after birth, and 61% would decline if the onset of blindness would occur in adulthood. The latter study also found that, although prenatal diagnosis would be used, over 30% would not use this information to decide on termination. These attitudes were expressed even though the fetus is subjected to risk during such tests. However, despite the theoretical possibilities and some evidence to suggest a modicum of patient need, we are not aware of much demand for prenatal diagnosis of RP in the USA or UK.

The families of those with genetic diseases need to know their options for family planning. The most frequently considered options are proceeding with childbearing with the knowledge and acceptance of the risk, deciding against having children, and delaying childbearing with the hope of future options not yet available. If the mother is not a carrier for either a dominant or X-linked trait, parents who wish to have a normal child may consider artificial insemination from a normal donor. Other options that will become increasingly available are forms of prefertilization gamete selection (particularly applicable for traits inherited from the male) and a procedure referred to as preimplantation genetic diagnosis, which involves in vitro fertilization with implantation of only an embryo for which a cell taken from the 6–8-cell blastomere stage has been analyzed molecularly and has been shown not to carry the mutation in question. (Removal of a single cell at this stage appears to be tolerated by the embryo without consequence.)

A great deal of information is given to patients in genetic counseling sessions. For this reason, it should be normal practice to plan a number of visits rather than try to complete the process at one consultation. Also, a formal letter explaining the major points should be sent to the family members who attended the counseling session.

Support services

Patients can benefit greatly from appropriate referral to local, regional, or national agencies that provide services and support to the visually impaired. These services may be for visually impaired individuals in general or to those specifically afflicted with RP. All patients should be offered referral. Coordination by social services personnel familiar with working with the visually handicapped is appropriate. This is particularly true when dealing with issues such as integrating the visually impaired child into the school system or coordinating vocational rehabilitation training.[587]

Specific societies for RP patients have been established in many countries. In the USA there is the Foundation Fighting Blindness, which was formerly called the Retinitis Pigmentosa Foundation (7168 Columbia Gateway Drive, Suite 100, Columbia, MD 21046, USA. Tel: +1 (800) 683-5555+. www.blindness.org/). In the UK there is RP Fighting Blindness (PO Box 350, Buckingham, MK18 1GZ, UK. Tel: +44 01280 821334+, Fax: +44 1 712723862. info@rpfightingblindness.org.uk). In Canada, there is The Foundation Fighting Blindness Canada (890 Yonge Street, 12th Floor, M4W 3P4, Ontario, Toronto, Tel: ++ 14163604200, Fax: ++14163600060. www.ffb.ca). Addresses of some other RP societies are given below. The most updated addresses of RP societies in other countries may be found at www.retina-international.org/.

For deaf and blind RP patients the following contacts might be appropriate: in the USA, Helen Keller National Center, 141 Middle Neck Road, Sands Point, NY 11050, USA. Tel: +1 516944 8900. In the UK, Sense, Sense Head Office, 101 Pentonville Road, London N1 9LG. Tel: +44 0845127 0060. Fax: +44 0845127 0061. info@sense.org.uk).

For problems of visual handicap in general, in the USA, Commissions for the Blind have been established in each state to help in vocational training of blind adults. State and regional programs for the visually impaired child also exist. In the UK, patients may be referred to the Royal National Institute of Blind People (RNIB), 105 Judd Street, London, WC1H 9NE, UK. Tel: +44020 7388 1266. www.rnib.org.uk/).

TREATMENT

A major fallacy in the management of RP is the common assertion that the condition is untreatable; it is more accurate to say that RP is incurable. The patient with RP can always be helped (treated), and after diagnosis, it is no longer acceptable to dismiss such patients with "I can't do anything for you." It should not be forgotten that aiding the patient to become adjusted to RP by supplying useful information and support can do a great deal of good. Other major options to consider as appropriate include careful refraction, cataract extraction when indicated, treatment of macular edema, and referral for low-vision aids.

It is mandatory to ensure that the patient has appropriate correction of refractive error and access to low-vision aids. The night vision aid is a monocular, handheld device that amplifies low-level illumination to help patients with defective night vision see under dim illumination conditions.[588] Although such devices may be useful in specific instances, a wide-angle, powerful flashlight is usually more effective and far less expensive than the night vision aid.[589] Those interested in more information about night scopes and other visual aids specifically for the RP patient should contact their national RP society (see above).

Limiting ocular light exposure is a common theme in attempts to limit progression of RP.[590] This theory has been tested in several small clinic trials. In one study, a single patient with adRP and another with arRP were tested by occluding one eye with an opaque shell for 6–8 hours/day for 5 years.[591] However, no significant difference was seen between the covered and uncovered eyes with respect to visual acuity, visual fields, fundus examination and photography, or ERG. In a similar study, 12 patients with RP wore tinted contact lens for several years in one eye. The covered eye demonstrated a trend towards less visual field loss than the uncovered eye, but these results have not been replicated in a larger trial.

Periodic visual field examinations with compassionate explanation of visual field defects can help patients appreciate the rate of progression and hence plan for future disability. Furthermore, regular examinations can help to ensure that the patient is referred to specific community and legal support agencies where appropriate. Explanation of statutory visual requirements for driving will help patients who are still driving to plan for when this will no longer be possible. Reassurance that the changes seen are typical or usual for patients with RP often allays fears that they are losing visual function at a rate faster than expected.

Cataract extraction

Patients with RP often develop cataracts that are visually significant. Cataract surgery should be considered and recommended in many of these cases. The most frequent cataract type seen is a posterior subcapsular lens opacity (35–51% of adult RP patients).[69–71] The greatest benefit from cataract surgery seems to occur in patients with posterior subcapsular opacities rather than other types of cataract.[592] Clinical examination of the macula, including high-resolution OCT, may help to assess the potential for improvement of acuity. Examination of the macula in the fellow eye can be helpful but is not an infallible assessor of potential in the cataract eye.[593] Laser interferometry[594] and the potential acuity meter may help to determine whether cataract extraction will improve vision. A 2-week trial of mydriasis may also help in this assessment.[70] Most RP patients with a cataract that warrants surgery are younger (approximately 35 years of age) than comparable cataract patients without other ocular disease.[70,595]

Studies have suggested significant improvement in acuity in appropriate patients after cataract extraction. Bastek et al.[70] reported that 83% of 30 RP eyes improved by two lines on the Snellen chart. Over 50% of patients improved to 20/50 or better. Newsome et al.[595] studied 26 RP and Usher patients undergoing cataract extraction and found that visual acuity improved in 22. Two studies of RP patients undergoing cataract surgery have emphasized phacoemulsification extraction and posterior-chamber intraocular lens.[592,596] Both reported results comparable with those published for cataract patients without other ocular disease. RP patients do not seem to be more predisposed to anterior- or posterior-segment complications,[595,596] except for posterior capsular opacification,[596] anterior capsulorrhexis contracture,[596,597] and possible dislocation of the intraocular lens from loss of zonular support.[597,598] Because the eyes of patients with RP are more prone to inflammation from intraocular surgery, particularly if manipulation of the iris is required, topical steroids and nonsteroidal anti-inflammatory medication should be used for a longer extent following cataract surgery in patients to prevent the occurrence of CME. Anterior capsular contracture following cataract surgery should be treated promptly with radial relaxing incisions using the yttrium aluminum garnet laser.[599] Augmented use of corticosteroids is recommended to protect the remaining posterior pole from postoperative CME.

If surgery is planned, the patient must realize that any improvement in central acuity will not be associated with improvement in visual field[70,596,600] and that the cataract surgery will in no way affect the expected rate of progression of the disease.[595] It is important for patients to have a realistic expectation for visual improvement before surgery.

Macular edema

CME can significantly reduce visual acuity in patients with RP.[144,145] Loss of central vision is especially problematic for these patients who may have already lost significant peripheral vision. The prevalence of CME has been reported to be 11–70% in patients with nonsyndromic RP, with most studies reporting an incidence around 20%,[601–606] while the incidence of CME in patients with Usher syndrome has been found to range from 8 to 60%.[607–609] The wide variability in incidence is likely due to varying definitions of significant CME, the development of newer technologies such as OCT, which more effectively detect CME, as well as population differences between the studies. Some reports suggested a higher incidence in autosomal dominant and recessive forms of RP and a lower incidence in X-linked forms, but other studies have demonstrated no difference.[67,161,604,605]

The exact origin of CME in RP is unclear and is likely multifactorial. Low-grade inflammation may lead to the breakdown of the blood–retinal barrier resulting in leakage from retinal or choroidal vessels.[610–614] Decreased pumping efficiency of RPE cells could also result in the accumulation of fluid in the macula.[615] The presence of antiretinal antibodies, such as antienolase and anticarbonic anhydrase, has been correlated with the occurrence of CME.[616–618] Epiretinal membranes are an additional source for CME and have been noted to be more prominent in patients with RP.[606] Cataract surgery can induce CME or worsen already present edema, raising concern in RP patients who frequently have posterior subcapsular cataracts. However, Jackson et al.[596] reported that most patients with RP who underwent cataract extraction benefited significantly and that the rate of CME was lower than expected.

CME in RP has traditionally been described as a nonleaking CME, which was detectable with careful stereoscopic fundus examination but showed little leakage on fluorescein angiography. The detection of CME in patients with RP has evolved and OCT, specifically SD-OCT, now appears to be the most sensitive method.[604,619–621] Hajali and Fishman[604] demonstrated that, even in patients with no fundoscopic evidence, the rate of CME in at least one eye using SD-OCT was 32%.

While OCT is quite sensitive in detecting the presence of CME, the relationship between retinal thickness and visual acuity can be difficult. Thickness measurements can be confounded by the fact that patients with RP usually have significant parafoveal cell loss. Several studies have shown conflicting results between the relationship of visual acuity and central thickness on OCT.[603,619,620] In a larger study, Sandberg et al.[605] found that visual acuity was inversely related to retinal thickness at the foveal center as well as independently related to parafoveal thickness. Additionally, the presence of the IS/OS junction by OCT seems to be a more reliable indicator of visual potential.[156,602,622,623]

A number of treatment methods for CME in RP have been attempted, including vitrectomy,[624] laser grid photocoagulation,[625] intravitreal,[626,627] or systemic steroids,[628] and anti-vascular endothelial growth factor (VEGF) agents.[629–631] However, the most effective agents to date have been the carbonic anhydrase inhibitors (CAIs).[615,632] When assessing the results of treatment of CME in RP, it should be remembered that CME may improve spontaneously with no intervention.[144,633]

Laser photocoagulation is a commonly used, effective treatment for the exudative, Coats-like retinopathy that is sometimes seen in RP.[63,65] While treatment of grid photocoagulation for CME has been reported,[625] Heckenlively[633] has challenged the wisdom of treating, in a destructive manner, any retina within the central field in patients with RP.

CAIs, both oral and topical, remain the mainstay of treatment for CME in RP. Cox et al.[615] first undertook a prospective crossover study using oral acetazolamide. Four of six RP patients showed a significant, reproducible improvement in macular edema. A similar effect on visual acuity was found by Fishman et al.,[632] who undertook a similar study design in 12 RP patients over a 2-week period. Grover et al.[634] found that, while a topical CAI, dorzolamide, provided improvement in angiographic macular edema and subjective visual function, visual acuity did not improve. They concluded that oral acetazolamide was a more effective treatment. A repeat study with a larger cohort measured the OCT changes in RP patients with CME treated with topical dorzolamide.[635] They demonstrated that 13 out of 15 patients had reduced macular edema following treatment with topical dorzolamide. Rebound macular edema has been reported with continued use of CAIs.[635–637] Recently, Thobani et al.[638] have shown that a vacation from CAI therapy in patients with rebound phenomenon can restore the efficacy of these medicines.

A practical treatment approach is to start with a topical CAI, such as dorzolamide, three times a day and proceed to an oral CAI if no improvement is seen. It can take several months before a treatment effect is observed.[637] For acetazolamide, an induction dose of 500 mg/day, followed by a maintenance dose of 250 mg/day, is recommended. Side-effects, such as loss of appetite, fatigue, hand tingling, renal stones, and anemia, are major problems that often limit the length of time RP patients will tolerate treatment with acetazolamide. Because of these adverse side-effects, Fishman et al.[639] have assessed the efficacy of methazolamide 50 mg/day, another CAI with milder side-effects. Although they found improvement in macular edema in 9 of 17 patients, the improvements in both subjective and objective visual acuity were disappointing. It was concluded that acetazolamide was the more effective treatment.

A number of authors have noted that improvement in objective (Snellen acuity) and subjective vision may not correlate with angiographic changes.[632,639,640] This may occur because angiographic changes correlate more with permeability in retinal vessels, and the major effect of CAIs may be to increase fluid passage through the RPE. It was also proposed that improving extrafoveal sensitivity might explain why many patients report subjective improvement in vision without supportive improvement in Snellen acuity. Chen et al.[641] studied the psychophysical effects of 500 mg/day acetazolamide on CME in one adRP patient. Despite little improvement in acuity (one Snellen line), a significant improvement in macular edema and extrafoveal retinal sensitivity, as measured by scotopic-threshold fine-matrix mapping, was seen. Overall, the best way to monitor the effectiveness of acetazolamide treatment is through the subjective report of the patient rather than relying on visual acuity assessment or angiography.

Intravitreal injections of triamcinolone have been used in refractory cases of CME not responsive to CAIs. These injections provide temporary resolution of macular thickening and can result in improved acuity.[601,626,627,642] Steroids have the benefit of delivering an anti-inflammatory effect, which may counteract autoimmune antibodies, but also provide an antiangiogenic effect, which may reduce vascular leakage. One distinct disadvantage of intravitreal steroids is that the effect is limited and repeat injections would likely be needed. Subsequent injections increase the risk of accelerating the development of cataracts, inducing glaucoma, or causing endophthalmitis.

The anti-VEGF agents, pegaptanib sodium (Macugen), ranibizumab (Lucentis), and bevacizumab (Avastin), have been used to treat CME in small series of patients with RP.[629–631,643] While these agents appear effective in some patients at reducing macular thickness and improving vision, there are legitimate concerns that the chronic use of these agents may exacerbate the vascular attenuation that is already present in patients with RP.[644] These agents should likely be reserved for patients with CME that is refractory to other treatments.

Vitamin A supplements

Vitamin A supplements effectively treat retinopathies that are associated with vitamin A deficiency resulting from intestinal malabsorption or defective transport, such as occurs in Bassen–Kornzweig syndrome (abetalipoproteinemia).[645] Between 1984 and 1991 a randomized, double-masked, prospective study was undertaken by Berson et al.[646] to determine the effects of oral vitamin A (retinyl palmitate) and E (DL-α-tocopherol) on the course of the more common form of RP. Patients with typical RP or Usher syndrome type 2 were assigned to one of four treatment groups: (1) 15000 IU/day of vitamin A; (2) 15000 IU/day of vitamin A plus 400 IU/day of vitamin E; (3) trace amounts of both vitamins; or (4) 400 IU/day of vitamin E.

Ninety-five percent[598] of 601 adult patients completed at least 4 years of follow-up. Although no significant difference occurred for the slow loss of visual field with time, the authors found that the two groups receiving 15000 IU/day of vitamin A had, on average, a slightly slower rate of decline of cone ERG amplitudes. Interestingly, the two groups receiving 400 IU/day of vitamin E were found to be 42% more likely to have a decline in amplitude of 50% or more from baseline. No significant change in visual acuity was found between the two groups. It was speculated that the apparent adverse effect of vitamin E could result from secondary interference with vitamin A absorption. The authors recommended that most adult RP patients take vitamin A (retinyl palmitate) in 15000 IU/day supplements under the supervision of an ophthalmologist and avoid high-dose supplemental vitamin E, such as the 400 IU/day vitamin E used for this trial.[647]

This study and its recommendation were controversial and led to a series of articles on the significance of this work on clinical practice.[648–651] In particular a number of issues were raised.[652,653] The positive outcome of vitamin A use was only reported in terms of reduced decline of 30 Hz, and to some extent 0.5 Hz, flash amplitudes. No improvement in psychophysical visual parameters, perceivable by patients, was detected. It has been suggested that the changes in cone ERG responses, rather than being a positive effect of vitamin A, might be caused by effects on background noise and were misinterpreted by idiosyncracies of the methodology. With reference to this possibility, it should be remembered that very-low-amplitude responses (as little as 0.12 μV) were being recorded in the RP patients. No adverse effects of vitamin use were found in the cases studied. Side-effects such as increased intracranial pressure, hepatomegaly, bone disease in the young, and elevated blood lipids can, however, occur with this dose of vitamin A.[654] In addition, large doses of supplemental vitamin A are considered by many to be teratogenic, leading to congenital abnormalities such as cardiac defects and cleft palate.[655,656] One survey found that, among babies born to women who took more than 10000 IU of preformed vitamin A per day in the form of supplements, an estimated one infant in 57 had a malformation attributable to the supplement.[657] Thus supplemental vitamin A at the 15000 IU/day dose is of particular concern in women of childbearing potential. The argument was made that greater benefit needed to be proven before recommending the use of vitamin A in RP.[653] Additional concerns have been reported about increased risk of osteoporosis from high-dose vitamin A supplementation.[658–661]

Although no serious problems of safety in the recommended dose were encountered in the above-mentioned study, the long-term safety of taking high-dose vitamin A supplements for many decades is uncertain. Questions raised about the toxicity to the liver of high-dose vitamin A supplements,[662] and the fact that similar beneficial results of such high-dose supplements of vitamin A on RP have yet to be reproduced, led ophthalmologists in many parts of the world to adopt the view that vitamin A may be of marginal benefit, at best, in patients with RP and that this must be weighed against the somewhat uncertain risks associated with its use.[648]

Sibulesky et al.[663] have reported no clinical symptoms or signs of liver toxicity in 146 otherwise healthy adults 18–54 years of age with RP who took 15000 IU/day of vitamin A for ≤12 years. Berson still advocates supplemental vitamin A as beneficial for most patients with RP, particularly those with the Pro23His mutation of rhodopsin (E.L. Berson, personal communication, 2004). If patients elect to take supplemental vitamin A, they should be periodically monitored for hepatic toxicity, warned of the teratogenic risk for pregnancies, and monitored for osteoporosis. If patients have initiated its use on their own, it is recommended that they undergo regular assessment of vitamin A levels and liver function tests.

Docosahexaenoic acid supplements

Docosahexaenoic acid (DHA) is an abundant lipid in photoreceptors, accounting for 30–40% of lipids in rod photoreceptor outer segments.[664] DHA levels are reduced in plasma,[665] erythrocytes,[666,667] and sperm[668] of selected patients with RP. DHA synthesis appears to be impaired in at least some patients with X-linked RP.[669] Long-term supplementation of 400 mg/day DHA resulted in a 2.5-fold elevation of mean plasma DHA levels but was not associated with any significant adverse effects.[670] A trial of oral supplementation with 400 mg/day DHA for 4 years for patients with X-linked RP demonstrated a correlation of preservation of cone ERG with red blood cell DHA level, suggesting that supplementation may be of possible benefit for patients.[671]

Lutein supplements

Lutein and zeaxanthin are macular pigments that cannot be synthesized in the body and must be derived from dietary sources. Evidence suggests that, in quail, macular pigments convey protection from oxidative damage and light-induced photoreceptor cell death.[672] A study of oral supplementation with 20 mg/day lutein for 6 months demonstrated increased macular pigment in 50% of subjects with RP or Usher syndrome but no change in central vision.[673] The long-term effects of such supplementation are unknown.

Clinical trial of DHA supplementation

Berson and colleagues[674] in 2004 reported the results of a 4-year randomized, double-masked trial of 221 patients with RP who were given either 1200 mg/day of supplemental DHA or a placebo capsule. Because of the results of the previous trial of vitamin A, both the treated and the control groups were also given 15000 units of vitamin A palmitate per day. The primary outcome measure was the total point score for the Humphrey 30–2 visual fields and secondary outcome measures were the total point score for the combined 30–2 and 30–60–1 kinetic visual fields and the 30-Hz ERG amplitudes. Of the original 221 patients, 208 completed the 4-year trial. No significant differences in decline of visual field sensitivity or ERG amplitudes were seen between the treated and control groups. The conclusion of this trial was that, in patients receiving 15000 IU/day of vitamin A, the addition of 1200 mg/day did not, on average, slow the course of field or ERG amplitude loss from PR.

A second report by the same authors described further evaluations of the data from subcohort analyses of the original study of DHA supplementation.[675] These evaluations focused on the finding that, of the patients entering the study, some were naive to vitamin A whereas others were already taking supplemental vitamin A. In the subcohort analyses of these two groups, those participants who were naive to vitamin A who received supplemental DHA and vitamin A were found to have a slower course of disease (slower decline in visual sensitivity and ERG amplitudes, at $P = 0.01$ and $P = 0.03$, respectively) for the first 2 years of monitoring during the trial compared to the control group, who were taking vitamin A at the time of entry into the study; no similar slowing was observed for the cohort already taking vitamin A when given DHA supplementation. For years 3 and 4, there was no significant benefit for either subcohort. However, dietary omega-3 fatty acid for the vitamin A control group was inversely correlated to loss of visual sensitivity over the 4 years of the trial (test for trend, $P = 0.05$) and similarly the duration of vitamin A supplementation prior to entry into the study was inversely correlated to the rate of decline in ERG amplitude ($P = 0.008$). The authors interpreted these findings of the subcohort analyses to be sufficient to make the recommendation that patients who are taking vitamin A should supplement their diet with DHA and those who are not taking vitamin A should take it as well as supplement their diet with additional DHA.

Clinical trials of lutein supplementation

In 2010, Berson et al.[676] reported a trial of supplementation of lutein for patients with RP. In the same issue, an editorial was published by Massof and Fishman,[677] entitlted "How strong is the evidence that nutritional supplements slow the progression of retinitis pigmentosa?" This article examined the evidence from the earlier trials on vitamin A as well as the current trials on DHA and lutein supplementation. The authors note that none of the studies produced simple, clearcut benefits with primary analyses. Only when the original study was divided in a post hoc fashion into subcohorts was there any significance. The study's Data and Safety Monitoring Committee reported in a letter to the editor that there was no difference between the vitamin A group and the control group or between the A + E and the control group and argued that much of the originally reported significant differences was a consequence of pooling of data and could be attributed to early and consistently large differences between the vitamin E and all of the other groups.

With regard to the 2004 DHA supplementation study, Massof and Fishman[677] point out that no significance was obtained in analysis of the primary outcome data ($P = 0.88$) and there was no difference between treatment and control groups for any of the secondary outcomes (rate of loss of 30/60–2 Humphrey field analyzer total point score, 30 Hz ERG $\log_e$ amplitude, and logMAR visual acuity). When subcohort analyses were applied to the data. a significance was found for years 1 and 2, but not years 3 and 4.

Based on the subcohort analyses of these in the first study, Berson and colleagues[646] recommended that patients with RP consume 15000 IU/day of vitamin A palmitate to slow the progression of disease. Based on the subcohort analyses of the second study, the authors concluded that supplementary DHA facilitates and hastens the benefit of high-dose vitamin A in the first 2 years of treatment.

Massof and Finkelstein[677] then presented two important issues regarding these trials: (1) the misinterpretation of outcomes because of incorrect assumptions built into the data analyses, such as linear decline over time when this assumption may not hold true; and (2) the question of how much weight should be placed on clinical practice recommendations that are drawn from secondary subcohort analyses, which disrupt and unbalance the initial design of the study. Finally, the authors discuss the concept of the clinical trial as a special class of study that is highly formal in design, structure, and execution and is motivated by a clinical question that, when resolved, will set the new standard for clinical practice. They conclude that the primary outcome, which is agreed on in advance and which is the heart of the study design, should render the verdict of the trial. Secondary analyses are useful to mine for potential other factors that may be operative and may lead into useful future studies but should not dictate the standard of patient care.

PURPORTED "CURES" FOR RP

During consultation, RP patients often raise difficult questions on information and validation of less conventional therapies that have received media coverage or which they have read about on the internet. An online survey of patients with RP revealed that 95% of respondents had tried at least one form of complementary and alternative medicine for treatment of their RP, including acupuncture, massage, yoga, aromatherapy, mind–body therapies, and herbal therapies.[678] Some patients reported improvements in subjective visual acuity, although there have not been any controlled scientific studies to assess vision with these treatments.

While many of the above-mentioned therapies are well intentioned and likely do provide some stress relief for patients, there exist other regimens, especially on the internet, that claim to improve vision significantly in patients with RP. Testimonials from successfully "treated" patients often support such claims, but few objective data are provided. Such regimens usually have little scientific basis for their claims and often lead to great disappointment for patients.

Ophthalmologists involved in the care of RP patients are obliged to dissuade patients from subjecting themselves to the risks of unsubstantiated therapies and should warn patients that the pursuit of false hope can lead to significant emotional trauma and economic loss.[679]

Many unconventional treatments for RP have been proposed for many years. These have included therapeutic beestings,[680] vasodilators,[681] and injections of placental tissues.[682] In Russia, RP patients have been treated with intramuscular or peribulbar injections of ENCAD, an RNA extract of yeast.[683] A number of studies by outside agencies have, however, discredited this as an effective treatment for either halting or reversing RP.[684,685]

Patients attending a clinic in Cuba undergo electric stimulation to the head, shoulders, and feet for 21 days; their blood is also drawn, ozonated, and reinjected on multiple days. A surgical procedure is then undertaken to transplant a flap of retrobulbar fat, with blood vessels, into a scleral pocket in the posterior globe. Some patients are also given oral vasodilator drugs and vitamins. Berson et al.[686] evaluated 10 RP patients over a 6–8-month period before and after they had undergone treatment in Cuba. Visual function testing, including assessment of acuity, visual field, and ERG changes, found no beneficial effect to the treatment. More worrisome was the fact that the magnitude of mean decline in ERG amplitude and visual field relative to those reported in other studies suggested that the intervention was associated with a worsening of the course of the disease. Similar poor results for this treatment have been published by others.[687,688] Diplopia requiring surgical correction has also been seen as a complication.[687,689] These reports conclude that this treatment protocol is of no benefit to RP patients.

Two studies have examined acupuncture for treatment of vision loss in RP and, while both studies reported impressive results, neither study was randomized nor had a control group where patients receive "sham" acupuncture with needles placed at nontraditional locations, thus raising questions about the validity of the data.[690,691] Determining whether or not acupuncture has value in preserving vision in RP will require larger, well-controlled randomized studies.

The previous studies looked at a heterogeneous population of RP patients, but there is evidence that light exposure may play an important role in a subset of RP patients, specifically those with adRP caused by class B1 rhodopsin mutations.[692] These patients can demonstrate greater loss in the inferior retina compared with the superior retina, which has been attributed to increased light exposure from above.[179,693] Additionally, both canine and rodent models of adRP have demonstrated retinal degeneration that can be slowed by dark rearing and is worsened with exposure to bright light.[142,537,694–698] Therefore, although a direct relationship between light exposure and progression in RP has not been established, it seems reasonable to recommend patients (especially those with autosomal dominant forms of RP) to wear tinted lenses when outside. Moreover, care should be taken when examining these patients to avoid unnecessary light exposure from photographic or surgical procedures.

Tinted lenses may provide comfort outdoors, and, for some patients with RP, may provide subjective vision improvement, although more controlled subjective studies are needed.[699] Lenses with special tints, such as the Corning 550 lens, are appreciated as being subjectively better than ordinary sunglasses by some patients with RP, particularly those with a cone–rod pattern of dysfunction. We recommend that patients find an optician willing to allow an adequate trial period before purchasing these rather expensive tinted glasses.

Future management

Much of the work on new therapeutic strategies for RP depends on animal models. Many such models are already available. Both transgenic[700] and KO[701] rodent models of retinal dystrophy exist and, at the moment, are the most popular models for work in therapeutics. These have advantages over naturally occurring examples of retinal dystrophy of unknown genetic cause, in that the underlying molecular genetic defect can be chosen. For example, all work on disease due to mutant rhodopsin is based on such constructs, since, prior to 2002, no rhodopsin mutant animals, apart from humans, had been found in nature. The usefulness of these constructed rodent models is, however, limited by differences in the constitutional makeup of the rodent as compared to the human eye. The most pertinent differences are in the number and distribution of photoreceptors in the retina, especially cones, the absence of a true macula, and the fact that rodent eyes are much smaller than human globes.

By far the greatest visual handicap in human RP is caused by secondary loss of cone function.[567] The identification of a rod-derived cone viability factor offers hope for future therapeutic strategies to preserve cone survival and function in human RP.[569] It has also been suggested that cone death in RP is often a secondary phenomenon, due to the oxidative stress induced by primary rod death.[702] Antioxidant therapies, most notably *N*-acetylcysteine, have recently been shown to preserve cones in mouse models of RP.[703]

Further validation of such therapies will however require larger animals than the mouse or rat. Unfortunately, rodent retinas have sparse, evenly distributed cone photoreceptors and so reflect the human situation only to a limited extent. The rodent eye is also very small, approximately 3–6 mm diameter, compared to a human globe (approximately 24 mm diameter) and the rodent lens is relatively large, almost filling the internal cavity of the globe. These two mechanical factors severely limit the usefulness of rodents in the evaluation of surgical techniques on the eye. Petters et al.[542] have developed a transgenic porcine animal model of RP that expresses a mutated rhodopsin gene (Pro347Leu). The pig eye is much more comparable in constitution and size (approximately 22 mm diameter) to the human eye. Although the pig also does not have a formed macular region, the number and gross distribution of cones are much more similar to human retina.[567] Other large animals of value to retinal degeneration work include the Briard dog (*RPE65* mutation),[704] the T4R rhodopsin mutant dog,[705] and the Siberian husky (*RPGR* mutation).[706]

Gene therapy

As a target for genetic manipulation, the retina has some advantages. Target cells (usually photoreceptors) are more directly accessible than in most tissues, and the effects of manipulations can be directly observed. The cell population is static and nondividing. Once appropriate expression is obtained, it will be theoretically effective indefinitely.

The consequences of genetic mutation can be divided into two categories: (1) those abnormalities that lead to loss of function (e.g., most autosomal recessive disease, the majority of X-linked disorders, and some dominant conditions); and (2) those that lead to extra (usually detrimental) function (often seen in dominant disease). Examples of this are the deficits caused by PDE deficiency in autosomal recessive PDEβ mutations,[707] and the theoretical gain of function in some rhodopsin mutations in adRP.[483] Recognizing which is relevant to the disease process of interest is the starting point of any gene therapy strategy, since dramatically different methods will be employed. In "loss-of-function"-type disease, replacing the mutant may be sufficient for cure. In "gain-of-function"-type disease it would be more appropriate to block, or "switch off," the disease gene (e.g., with complementary, antisense oligonucleotides).

The main problems associated with gene therapy in the retina are delivery of genetic material to cells and appropriate expression of that material in the target without adverse effects. Of the various gene transfer vectors used (e.g., ligand–DNA conjugates, DNA-loaded liposome vesicles, electroporation), adenovirus and adeno-associated virus have been the most extensively studied. Transfection with adeno and adeno-associated virus[708] can be nonspecific. Intravitreal injection of adenovirus frequently leads to widespread expression in the lens, ciliary body, and retina.[709] Subretinal injection leads to more confined gene expression.[710] Other major problems associated with the use of adenovirus are host immune response and theoretical problems of inhibition of host cell protein synthesis and neoplastic transformation. Adjuvant use of immunosuppressives is being studied to try to reduce immune responses.[711]

Landmark gene therapy studies in human human retinal degeneration were undertaken in 2007.[712,713] A recombinant AAV-2 vector was used by Bainbridge et al.[712] to deliver a human RPE65 cDNA driven by elements of the endogenous RPE65 promoter in cases of LCA. Maguire et al.[713] used an AAV-2 vector with a constitutive promoter to drive RPE65 transgene expression and reported objective evidence of improved retinal function (e.g., by pupillometry) in all 3 patients. Both groups reported improvement in subjective measures of visual acuity in 4 of the 6 participants in both trials. Maguire et al.[713] reported improvement in pupillometry. Neither group reported improvement in retinal function on ERG. After subretinal injection Bainbridge et al.[712] reported one case of macular hole. Further follow-up has suggested stable clinical benefits and no unexpected complications.[714,715]

An innovative approach to the treatment of autosomal dominant disease has involved the use of hammerhead ribozymes.[716] Dominant disease is often associated with (adverse) gain of function by the mutant gene or a dominant-negative effect of the mutant allele's gene product. For example, mutant protein may accumulate in the Golgi apparatus or otherwise fail to be transported to the normal site within the cell, resulting in cell dysfunction and death. Mutant mRNA may accumulate in the nucleus, inhibiting normal mRNA maturation. If the mutant gene can be effectively suppressed by attacking its mRNA, the remaining wild gene may be sufficient for normal cell function. Ribozymes are RNA enzymes that induce sequence-specific cleavage of targeted RNA. In this way ribozymes can be designed to be mutation-specific and so destroy mutant RNA. "Proof of principle" for ribozyme therapy for Pro23His transgenic rats has been demonstrated.[717] In vivo expression in this rhodopsin mutant model is achieved by transduction with an rAAV incorporating a rod opsin promoter of either a hammerhead or hairpin ribozyme that targets the mutant message. The expression of the mutant-specific ribozyme and its effect on reduction of mutant mRNA significantly slowed the course of disease for 3 months. In a more recent innovation, Georgiadis et al.[718] used a virally transferred miRNA-based hairpin to silence peripherin/RDS in murine retina.

Another interesting gene therapy approach for dominant RP mutations is combined gene knock-down and gene addition therapy. Rather than targeting specific alleles, which in the case of rhodopsin would require targeting over a hundred different alleles, both endogenous rhodopsin alleles, regardless of whether mutated or not, are downregulated by siRNA technology, while at the same time, a codon-modified rhodopsin cDNA that is not sensitive to siRNA interference is added by AAV-mediated gene transfer.[719]

Cell therapy (see Chapter 35, Stem cells and cellular therapy, and Chapter 125, Transplantation frontiers)

Tissue transplantation into the eye was first undertaken just over 100 years ago.[720] It is only recently, though, that cell therapeutics have become sufficiently understood to justify attempts to treat RP. Work in 1988[721] showed that transplanting normal RPE cells into the subretinal space of the RCS rat, an animal model of autosomal recessive retinal dystrophy, rescued photoreceptors in the immediate vicinity of the transplant. Such photoreceptor rescue in the RCS rat has also been documented using human fetal RPE cells,[722] nonfetal human RPE,[723] and most recently using human induced pluripotent stem cell-derived RPE.[724] Long-term effectiveness requires adjunctive immunosuppression (e.g., with cyclosporine).[722] Although most efforts in RPE transplantation have been directed toward macular diseases such as age-related macular degeneration,[725-727] this methodology may be useful in RP due to RPE-specific mutations.[728,729] Current tissue transplantation work in RP though is focused on replacing lost photoreceptors. Cells from three different sources lead this work: (1) adult-derived human stem cells; (2) human embryonic stem cells; and (3) human-induced pluripotent stem cells.

A number of sources have been targeted for adult-derived stem cells, including bone marrow[730] and adult brain-derived neural progenitor cells,[731] but with very limited success. Others have focused on stem cell sources within the eye itself. A number of researchers have highlighted the potential for Müller glial cells to dedifferentiate, proliferate, and produce new retinal neurons and glia.[732,733] In addition, considerable interest has emerged in stem cells derived from the epithelium of the ciliary body.[734,735] However more recent studies have questioned the potential of these cells for retinal regeneration.[736] More promising work has been undertaken using embryonic stem cells. These cells have been differentiated in vitro into photoreceptor-like cells[737] as well as RPE.[727,729] Currently, though, these techniques have proven time-consuming, labor-intensive, and of low yield. Despite these technical limitations for widespread application, subretinal injection of ESC-derived photosensitive cells has been shown to restore visual function in CRX-deficient mice, as detected by ERG.[738]

Overcoming many of the ethical limitations and sourcing difficulties of using embryonic stem cells, the most intensively discussed stem cell source is induced pluripotent stem cells.[739,740] "Reprogramming" of adult, differentiated cells to recapture their pluripotency allows for versatile tissue regeneration from a plentiful source without immunogenic difficulties. Both mouse and human iPS cells have been induced to differentiate into retinal progenitor cells in vitro.[741] Very recent work has shown histological evidence that iPS-derived rhodopsin expressing cells can integrate into the iodoacetic acid-damaged pig retina.[742] Further studies are required to show long-term retinal integration and functional benefits.

Another interesting approach in cell therapy has been to use cells not for their potential to regenerate lost cells but as a way to deliver therapeutic molecules long-term to the degenerating retina. This may be as an innate ability of the cells or by using cells genetically modified to deliver therapeutic molecules. Mesenchymal stem cells[743] have proven neuroprotective effects and have been used in animal models, demonstrating neuroprotective effects in the retina after subretinal injection[744] and injection in the systemic circulation.[745] Mouse embryonic stem cells have been genetically modified to secrete glial-derived neurotrophic factor. A neuroprotective effect was reported with these cells after intravitreal injection in a rat rhodopsin mutant.[746]

Apoptosis/neuroprotection

It has been shown that, in animal models of a number of retinal dystrophies, photoreceptor cell death occurs by a common mechanism known as apoptosis, or programmed cell death.[747,748] Apoptosis is an alternative mode of cell death to necrosis and is part of normal cell turnover during embryogenesis (termed histogenetic cell death), as well as playing an important role in disease pathology. Apoptosis is biochemically characterized by cleavage of DNA at internucleosomal sites. Such DNA fragmentation can be observed at the single cell level by in situ labeling of apoptotic cell nuclei using a histochemical technique known as TUNEL (*T*dT-mediated d*U*TP-biotin *n*ick *e*nd *l*abeling).[748] Microscopically, apoptosis can be seen as cytoplasmic and nuclear condensation and fragmentation of cells into membrane-bound structures (apoptotic bodies). Inflammation and scarring do not occur.[747,748]

In animal models of RP, such as the rd, rds, the RCS rat and rhodopsin mutant transgenic mice, apoptotic photoreceptor nuclei have been observed during normal retinal development and in periods of retinal degeneration.[747–749] The molecular triggering of apoptosis in the retina is a tightly controlled process that reflects the balance of proapoptotic versus antiapoptotic factors.[750] Due to the complexity and number of signals involved in the apoptotic cascade, there are many points for potential therapeutic intervention. One strategy has been to try and influence the balance of the proteins in the Bcl-2 family to tip the scale away from a commitment to apoptosis. For example, overexpression of the antiapoptotic protein, Bcl-2, in the retina of several rodent models of RP was able to slow photoreceptor degeneration.[751,752] In a converse strategy, reducing the levels of the proapoptotic proteins, Bax and Bak, protected photoreceptors in a light damage model.[753] However, not all studies have shown a protective effect of the overexpression of Bcl-2 or Bcl-X_L[754] and it has been suggested that alteration of Bcl-2 levels may actually be detrimental to cell survival.[755]

Elevated levels of calcium have long been known to play an integral role in photoreceptor degeneration in RP by triggering apoptosis.[756] Attempts to block calcium influx into photoreceptors to elicit neuroprotection have resulted in conflicting results. Administration of calcium channel blockers, such as dilitiazem, in animal models of retinal degeneration has exhibited neuroprotection in some studies,[757, 758, 759] but other studies have demonstrated no effect.[760] More recently, there have been reports that the calcium channel blocker, nilvadipine, can provide a protective effect in animal models of retinal degeneration. One small study in patients with RP demonstrated that nilvidapine reduced visual field loss in RP patients treated with nilvadipine.[761] Larger-scale clinical trials are needed to confirm these results.

A different strategy to eliciting photoreceptor protection in RP is to block mediators of apoptosis further downstream, such as the caspase proteins. Increased caspase activity has been detected in photoreceptors undergoing apoptosis in animal models of RP.[762] Intraocular injection of caspase-3 inhibitors or ablation of caspase-1 has been shown to decrease photoreceptor death in some, but not all, animal models of retinal degeneration.[763,764] However, such therapies have yet to be translated into human studies and it is now realized that there are also noncaspase-dependent pathways that mediate apoptosis.[765] Another alternative approach is to deliver endogenous neurotrophic factors, which elicit cell protection by preventing apoptosis via multiple mechanisms. Through direct injection, viral-mediated delivery, nanoparticles, and encapsulated cell technology, a variety of different neurotrophic factors have been delivered in animal models of retinal degeneration, including basic fibroblast growth factor,[766,767] brain-derived neurotrophic factor,[768] ciliary neurotrophic factor (CNTF),[769,770] and glial-derived neurotrophic factor.[746,771] In spite of the success of these agents in animal models, few have yet to be translated into the clinic setting.

An exception to this has been CNTF, which in humans has been delivered using encapsulated cell technology.[770] Animal models treated with CNTF have demonstrated protection of the photoreceptor cell bodies, but have also demonstrated no improvement and sometimes a worsening in the ERG as well as a decrease in vision. It appears that CNTF downregulates proteins involved in rod phototransduction in a dose-dependent manner, leading to a tradeoff between prolonged cell survival at the cost of immediate decreased vision.[772] Phase II studies aimed at eliciting visual or morphological preservation have been completed and results are expected soon.

Electronic prosthesis (artificial retina)

In 1929, Foerster showed that, if the occipital pole is electrically stimulating the occipital pole, the subject will perceive "light" (phosphine).[773] In 1969, Potts and Inoue[774] also demonstrated that external electrical stimulation of the eye itself can also elicit the perception of light and a cortical response in patients with advanced RP. These results indicate that at least some retinal ganglion cells and more central elements of the visual system retain function, even in very advanced RP. These studies form the basis for developing an electronic prosthesis in RP. Four different approaches are being studied. Subretinal implants are placed under the retina (between the degenerate photoreceptors and the RPE) and input into second-order neurons or ganglion cells. Epiretinal implants lie on the retina–vitreous interface and stimulate ganglion cells. Optic nerve implants stimulate the axons of ganglion cells and cortical implants are implanted intracranially to stimulate the visual areas of the brain.

Currently the most promising trials are in retinal prosthetics. The Boston Retinal Implant Project has developed a subretinal prosthesis consisting of a miniaturized, hermetically sealed device connecting to additional equipment attached to the sclera. The device is currently undergoing animal studies only.[775]

A number of epiretinal devices have undergone trials in human subjects. The Argus II is an epiretinal ocular prosthesis secured to the eye with a retinal tack. In a group of 22 subjects it was demonstrated that there was significant improvement in recognizing letters and improved spatial-motor tasks but with limited visual field.[776] Recently, the Argus II device was cleared by regulatory bodies in Europe to become commercially available for patients. The learning retinal implant system includes an extraocular retinal encoder (mounted on a spectacle frame) with wireless conection to an intraocular epiretinal stimulator.[777] Trials in 20 RP patients reported phosphenes visible during stimulation.[778] The EPI-RET3 implant also consists of an extraocular and intraocular component. An extraocular camera fitted to spectacle frames transmits images wirelessly to a receiver placed in the anterior vitreous. This receiver in turn stimulates an epiretinal implant via a connecting microcable. The EPI-RET3 implant started human trials in 2007 when it was implanted in 6 patients for 4 weeks. The implant was tolerated with moderate postoperative inflammation, and the position of the implants remained stable until removal.[779]

A number of excellent reviews have been written on this subject.[780,781] The major issues facing development of these devices are inner retinal cell viability, stimulus threshold, signal encoding, power requirements, biocompatibility, encapsulation, and the best way of testing these implants.

For online acknowledgments visit **http://www.expertconsult.com**

REFERENCES

1. Bunker CH, Berson EL, Bromley WC, et al. Prevalence of retinitis pigmentosa in Maine. Am J Ophthalmol 1984;97:357–65.
2. Ammann F, Klein D, Franceschetti A. Genetic and epidemiological investigations on pigmentary degeneration of the retina and allied disorders in Switzerland. J Neurol Sci 1965;2:183–96.
3. Hu D. Genetic aspects of retinitis pigmentosa in China. Am J Med Genet 1982;12:51–6.
4. Merin S, Auerbach E. Retinitis pigmentosa. Surv Ophthalmol 1976;20: 303–46.
5. Heckenlively J, Friederich R, Friederich R, et al. Retinitis pigmentosa in the Navajo. Metab Pediatr Ophthalmol 1981;5:201–6.
6. Kimberling WJ, Hildebrand MS, Shearer AE, et al. Frequency of Usher syndrome in two pediatric populations: Implications for genetic screening of deaf and hard of hearing children. Genet Med 2010;12:512–6.
7. Donders FC. Torpeur de la rétine congénital e héréditarie. Ann Ocul (Paris) 1855;34:270–3.
8. Donders FC. Beiträge zur pathologischen Anatomie des Auges. II. Pigmentbildung in der Netzhaut. Graefes Arch Opthalmol 1857;3:139–50.
9. Ovelgün. Nyctalopia haerediotria. Acta Physico Med (Nuremburg) 1744;7: 76–7 obs. 28.
10. van Trigt AC. De oogspiegel. Nederlandisch Lancet's Gravenhage 1852–1853; 3rd Series (2nd J.B.):417–509.
11. Ruete CGT. Bildliche Darstellung der Krankheiten des menschlichen Auges. Leipzig: Teubner; 1854.
12. Tanino T, Ohba N. Studies on pigmentary retinal dystrophy. II. Recordability of electroretinogram and the mode of inheritance. Jpn J Ophthalmol 1976; 20:482–6.
13. Berson EL, Sandberg MA, Rosner B, et al. Natural course of retinitis pigmentosa over a three-year interval. Am J Ophthalmol 1985;99:240–51.
14. Massof RW, Benzschawel T, Emmel T, et al. The spread of retinal degeneration in retinitis pigmentosa. Invest Ophthalmol Vis Sci 1984;25(Suppl):196.
15. Massof RW, Finkelstein D. A two-stage hypothesis for the natural course of retinitis pigmentosa. Adv Biosci 1987;62:29–58.
16. Jacobson SG, Yagasaki K, Feuer WJ, et al. Interocular asymmetry of visual function in heterozygotes of X-linked retinitis pigmentosa. Exp Eye Res 1989;48:679–91.
17. Department of Health Education and Wefare. Disability operational policy and procedures, informational digest. Code A2.01b, Special senses and hearing, listing of impairments, part A-2.00A3. Washington, D.C.: US Government Printing Office; 1979.
18. Grover S, Fishman GA, Anderson RJ, et al. Visual acuity impairment in patients with retinitis pigmentosa at age 45 years or older. Ophthalmology 1999;106:1780–5.
19. ffytche TJ. Cystoid maculopathy in retinitis pigmentosa. Trans Ophthalmol Soc U K 1972;92:265–83.
20. Geltzer AI, Berson EL. Fluorescein angiography of hereditary retinal degenerations. Arch Ophthalmol 1969;81:776–82.
21. Hansen RI, Friedman AH, Gartner S, et al. The association of retinitis pigmentosa with preretinal macular gliosis. Br J Ophthalmol 1977;61:597–600.
22. Fishman GA, Fishman M, Maggiano J. Macular lesions associated with retinitis pigmentosa. Arch Ophthalmol 1977;95:798–803.
23. Fishman GA, Magianno J, Fishman M. Foveal lesions seen in retinitis pigmentosa. Arch Ophthalmol 1977;95:1993–6.
24. Fishman GA. Retinitis pigmentosa. Visual loss. Arch Ophthalmol 1978;96: 1185–8.
25. Jay B, Bird A. X-linked retinitis pigmentosa. Trans Am Acad Ophthalmol Otolaryngol 1973;77:OP-641–51.
26. Marmor MF. The electroretinogram in retinitis pigmentosa. Arch Ophthalmol 1979;97:1300–4.
27. Heckenlively JR, Yoser SL, Friedman LH, et al. Clinical findings and common symptoms in retinitis pigmentosa. Am J Ophthalmol 1988;105:504–11.
28. Weleber RG, Francis PJ. Degeneration and atrophy of the choroid. In: Tasman W, Jaeger EA, editors. Duane's clinical ophthalmology: 2005 CD-ROM edition. Philadelphia: Lippincott Williams & Wilkins; 2005. p. 1–26.
29. Hood DC, Ramachandran R, Holopigian K, et al. Method for deriving visual field boundaries from OCT scans of patients with retinitis pigmentosa. Biomed Opt Express 2011;2:1106–14.
30. Hood DC, Lin CE, Lazow MA, et al. Thickness of receptor and post-receptor retinal layers in patients with retinitis pigmentosa measured with frequency-domain optical coherence tomography. Invest Ophthalmol Vis Sci 2009;50: 2328–36.
31. Heckenlively JR. Preserved para-arteriolar retinal pigment epithelium (PPRPE) in retinitis pigmentosa. Br J Ophthalmol 1982;66:26–30.
32. Porta A, Pierrottet C, Aschero M, et al. Preserved para-arteriolar retinal pigment epithelium retinitis pigmentosa. Am J Ophthalmol 1992;113:161–4.
33. van den Born LI, van Soest S, van Schooneveld MJ, et al. Autosomal recessive retinitis pigmentosa with preserved para-arteriolar retinal pigment epithelium. Am J Ophthalmol 1994;118:430–9.
34. Falls HF, Cotterman CW. Choroidoretinal degeneration: a sex-linked form in which heterozygous women exhibit a tapetal-like retinal reflex. Arch Ophthalmol 1948;40:685–703.
35. Goodman G, Ripps H, Siegel IM. Sex-linked ocular disorders: trait expressivity in males and carrier females. Arch Ophthalmol 1965;73:387–98.
36. Heckenlively JR. X-linked recessive retinitis pigmentosa (X-linked pigmentary retinopathy). In: Heckenlively JR, editor. Retinitis pigmentosa. Philadelphia: JB Lippincott; 1988. p. 162–87.
37. Heckenlively JR, Weleber RG. X-linked recessive cone dystrophy with tapetal-like sheen. A newly recognized entity with Mizuo–Nakamura phenomenon. Arch Ophthalmol 1986;104:1322–8.
38. Cideciyan AV, Jacobson SG. Image analysis of the tapetal-like reflex in carriers of X-linked retinitis pigmentosa. Invest Ophthalmol Vis Sci 1994;35: 3812–24.
39. Berendschot TTJM, DeLint PJ, van Norren D. Origin of tapetal-like reflexes in carriers of X-linked retinitis pigmentosa. Invest Ophthalmol Vis Sci 1996;37: 2716–23.
40. Lyon MF. The William Allan memorial award address: X-chromosome inactivation and the location and expression of X-linked genes. Am J Hum Genet 1988;42:8–16.
41. Szamier RB, Berson EL. Retinal histopathology of a carrier of X-chromosome-linked retinitis pigmentosa. Ophthalmology 1985;92:271–8.
42. Berson EL, Rosen JB, Simonoff EA. Electroretinographic testing as an aid in detection of carriers of X-chromosome-linked retinitis pigmentosa. Am J Ophthalmol 1979;87:460–8.
43. Arden GB, Carter RM, Hogg CR, et al. A modified ERG technique and the results obtained in X-linked retinitis pigmentosa. Br J Ophthalmol 1983;67: 419–30.
44. Fishman GA, Weinberg AB, McMahon TT. X-linked retinitis pigmentosa: clinical characteristics of carriers. Arch Ophthalmol 1986;104:1329–35.
45. Peachey NS, Fishman GA, Derlacki DJ, et al. Rod and cone dysfunction in carriers of X-linked retinitis pigmentosa. Ophthalmology 1988;95:677–85.
46. Miyake Y, Terasaki H. Golden tapetal-like fundus reflex and posterior hyaloid in a patient with X-linked juvenile retinoschisis. Retina 1999;19:84–6.
47. Noble KG, Margolis S, Carr RE. The golden tapetal sheen reflex in retinal disease. Am J Ophthalmol 1989;107:211–7.
48. Rajacich GM, Parelhoff ES, Heckenlively JR. The cup-disc ratio in retinitis pigmentosa subgroups. Invest Ophthalmol Vis Sci 1982;22(Suppl):55.
49. De Bustros S, Miller NR, Finkelstein D, et al. Bilateral astrocytic hamartomas of the optic nerve heads in retinitis pigmentosa. Retina 1983;3:21–3.
50. Novack RL, Foos RY. Drusen of the optic disc in retinitis pigmentosa. Am J Ophthalmol 1987;103:44–7.
51. Spencer WH. Drusen of the optic disk and aberrant axoplasmic transport. The XXXIV Edward Jackson memorial lecture. Am J Ophthalmol 1978;85:1–12.
52. Grover S, Fishman GA, Brown Jr J. Frequency of optic disc or parapapillary nerve fiber layer drusen in retinitis pigmentosa. Ophthalmology 1997;104: 295–8.
53. Edwards A, Grover S, Fishman GA. Frequency of photographically apparent optic disc and parapapillary nerve fiber layer drusen in Usher syndrome. Retina 1996;16:388–92.
54. Flynn MF, Fishman GA, Anderson RJ, et al. Retrospective longitudinal study of visual acuity change in patients with retinitis pigmentosa. Retina 2001;21: 639–46.
55. Giusti C, Forte R, Vingolo EM. Clinical pathogenesis of macular holes in patients affected by retinitis pigmentosa. Eur Rev Med Pharmacol Sci 2002;6:45–8.

56. Dorenboim Y, Rehany U, Rumelt S. Central serous chorioretinopathy associated with retinitis pigmentosa. Graefes Arch Clin Exp Ophthalmol 2004; 242:346–9.
57. Takahashi M, Jalkh A, Hoskins J, et al. Biomicroscopic evaluation and photography of liquefied vitreous in some vitreoretinal disorders. Arch Ophthalmol 1981;99:1555–9.
58. Vingolo EM, Giusti C, Forte R, et al. Vitreal alterations in retinitis pigmentosa: biomicroscopic appearance and statistical evaluation. Ophthalmologica 1996; 210:104–7.
59. Hong PH, Han DP, Burke JM, et al. Vitrectomy for large vitreous opacity in retinitis pigmentosa. Am J Ophthalmol 2001;131:133–4.
60. Uliss AE, Gregor ZJ, Bird AC. Retinitis pigmentosa and retinal neovascularization. Ophthalmology 1986;93:1599–603.
61. Grizzard WS, Deutman AF, Pinckers AJ. Retinal dystrophies associated with peripheral retinal vasculopathy. Br J Ophthalmol 1978;62:188–94.
62. Spallone A, Carlevaro G, Ridling P. Autosomal dominant retinitis pigmentosa and Coats'-like disease. Int Ophthalmol 1985;8:147–51.
63. Khan JA, Ide CH, Strickland MP. Coats'-type retinitis pigmentosa. Surv Ophthalmol 1988;32:317–32.
64. Pruett RC. Retinitis pigmentosa: Clinical observations and correlations. Trans Am Ophthalmol Soc 1983;81:693–735.
65. Kim RY, Kearney JJ. Coats-type retinitis pigmentosa in a 4-year-old child. Am J Ophthalmol 1997;124:846–8.
66. Naoi N, Fukiyama J, Sawada A. Retinitis pigmentosa with recurrent vitreous hemorrhage. Acta Ophthalmologica Scand 1996;74:509–12.
67. Spalton DJ, Bird AC, Cleary PE. Retinitis pigmentosa and retinal oedema. Br J Ophthalmol 1978;62:174–82.
68. Berson EL, Rosner B, Simonoff E. Risk factors for genetic typing and detection in retinitis pigmentosa. Am J Ophthalmol 1980;89:763–75.
69. Heckenlively J. The frequency of posterior subcapsular cataract in the hereditary retinal degenerations. Am J Ophthalmol 1982;93:733–8.
70. Bastek JV, Heckenlively JR, Straatsma BR, et al. Cataract surgery in retinitis pigmentosa patients. Ophthalmology 1982;89:880–4.
71. Fishman GA, Anderson RJ, Lourenco P. Prevalence of posterior subcapsular lens opacities in patients with retinitis pigmentosa. Br J Ophthalmol 1985;69: 263–6.
72. Franceschetti A, François J, Babel J. Tapetoretinal degeneration and keratoconus. In: Franceschetti A, François J, Babel J, editors. Chorioretinal heredodegenerations. Springfield, Ill: Charles C Thomas; 1974. p. 855–9.
73. Franceschetti A, François J, Babel J. Glaucoma. In: Franceschetti A, François J, Babel J, editors. Chorioretinal heredodegenerations. Springfield, Ill: Charles C Thomas; 1974. p. 851–2.
74. Omphroy CA. Sector retinitis pigmentosa and chronic angle-closure glaucoma: a new association. Ophthalmologica 1984;189:12–20.
75. Sieving PA, Fishman GA. Refractive errors of retinitis pigmentoa patients. Br J Ophthalmol 1978;62:163–7.
76. Ross DF, Fishman GA, Gilbert LD, et al. Variability of visual fields measurements in normal subjects and patients with retinitis pigmentosa. Arch Ophthalmol 1984;102:1004–10.
77. Nowomiejska K, Vonthein R, Paetzold J, et al. Comparison between semiautomated kinetic perimetry and conventional Goldmann manual kinetic perimetry in advanced visual field loss. Ophthalmology 2005;112:1343–54.
78. Schiefer U, Pascual JP, Edmunds B, et al. Comparison of the new perimetric GATE strategy with conventional full-threshold and SITA standard strategies. Invest Ophthalmol Vis Sci 2009;50:488–94.
79. Massof RW, Finkelstein D. Vision threshold profiles in sector retinitis pigmentosa. Arch Ophthalmol 1979;97:1899–904.
80. Massof RW, Finkelstein D. Rod sensitivity relative to cone sensitivity in retinitis pigmentosa. Invest Ophthalmol Vis Sci 1979;18:263–72.
81. Massof RW, Finkelstein D. Subclassifications of retinitis pigmentosa from two-color scotopic static perimetry. Doc Ophthalmol Proc Series 1981;26: 219–25.
82. Massof RW. Psychophysiological subclassifications of retinitis pigmentosa. In: LaVail MM, Hollyfield JG, Anderson RE, editors. Retinal degeneration, experimental and clinical studies. New York: Alan R Liss; 1985. p. 91–107.
83. Massof RW, Finkelstein D, Boughman JA. Genetic analysis of subgroups within simplex and multiplex retinitis pigmentosa. Birth Defects 1982;18: 161–6.
84. Arden GB, Carter RM, Hogg CR, et al. Rod and cone acitivity in patients with dominantly inherited retinitis pigmentosa: comparisons between psychophysical and electroretinographic measurements. Br J Ophthalmol 1983;67: 405–18.
85. Lyness AL, Ernst W, Quinlan MP, et al. A clinical, psychophysical, and electroretinographic survey of patients with autosomal dominant retinitis pigmentosa. Br J Ophthalmol 1985;69:326–39.
86. Ernst W, Faulkner DJ, Hogg CR, et al. An automated static perimeter/adaptometer using light emitting diodes. Br J Ophthalmol 1983;67:431–42.
87. Jacobson SG, Voigt WJ, Parel J-M, et al. Automated light- and dark-adapted perimetry for evaluating retinitis pigmentosa. Ophthalmology 1986;93: 1604–11.
88. Jacobson SG, Kemp CM, Sung C-H, et al. Retinal function and rhodopsin levels in autosomal dominant retinitis pigmentosa with rhodopsin mutations. Am J Ophthalmol 1991;112:256–71.
89. Kemp CM, Jacobson SG, Roman AJ, et al. Abnormal rod dark adaptation in autosomal dominant retinitis pigmentosa with proline-23-histidine rhodopsin mutation. Am J Ophthalmol 1992;113:165–74.
90. Jacobson SG, Cideciyan AV, Regunath G, et al. Night blindness in Sorsby's fundus dystrophy reversed by vitamin A. Nat Genet 1995;11:27–32.
91. Alexander KR, Fishman GA. Prolonged rod dark adaptation in retinitis pigmentosa. Br J Ophthalmol 1984;68:561–9.
92. Moore AT, Fitzke FW, Kemp CM, et al. Abnormal dark adaptation kinetics in autosomal dominant sector retinitis pigmentosa due to rod opsin mutation. Br J Ophthalmol 1992 8;76:465–9.
93. Arden GB. Rod–cone interactions in night-blinding disease. Jpn J Ophthalmol 1987;31:6–19.
94. Highman VN, Weale RA. Rhodopsin density and visual threshold in retinitis pigmentosa. Am J Ophthalmol 1973;75:822–32.
95. Ripps H, Brin KP, Weale RA. Rhodopsin and visual threshold in retinitis pigmentosa. Invest Ophthalmol Vis Sci 1978;17:735–45.
96. Faulkner DJ, Kemp CM. Human rhodopsin measurement using a t.v.-based imaging fundus reflectometer. Vision Res 1984;24:221–31.
97. Fulton AB, Hansen RM. The relation of rhodopsin and scotopic retinal sensitivity in sector retinitis pigmentosa. Am J Ophthalmol 1988;105: 132–40.
98. van Meel GJ, van Norren D. Foveal densitometry in retinitis pigmentosa. Invest Ophthalmol Vis Sci 1983;24:1123–30.
99. Perlman I, Auerbach E. The relationship between visual sensitivity and rhodopsin density in retinitis pigmentosa. Invest Ophthalmol Vis Sci 1981;20: 758–65.
100. Kemp CM, Jacobson SG, Faulkner DJ. Two types of visual dysfunction in autosomal dominant retinitis pigmentosa. Invest Ophthalmol Vis Sci 1988;29: 1235–41.
101. Karpe G. The basis of clinical electroretinography. Acta Ophthalmol (Copenh) 1945;23(Suppl):1–114.
102. Riggs LA. Electroretinography in cases of night blindness. Am J Ophthalmol 1954;38:70–8.
103. Arden GB, Barrada A, Kelsey JH. New clinical test of retinal function based on the standing potential of the eye. Br J Ophthalmol 1962;46:449–67.
104. Weleber RG. Fast and slow oscillations of the electro-oculogram in Best's macular dystrophy and retinitis pigmentosa. Arch Ophthalmol 1989;107: 530–7.
105. Gouras P. Electroretinography: some basic principals. Invest Ophthalmol 1970;9:557–69.
106. Marmor MF. An updated standard for clinical electroretinography. Arch Ophthalmol 1995;113:1375–6.
107. Marmor MF, Fulton AB, Holder GE, et al. ISCEV Standard for full-field clinical electroretinography (2008 update). Doc Ophthalmol Adv Ophthalmol 2009; 118:69–77.
108. Andréasson SOL, Sandberg MA, Berson EL. Narrow-band filtering for monitoring low-amplitude cone electroretinograms in retinitis pigmentosa. Am J Ophthalmol 1988;105:500–3.
109. Berson EL. Retinitis pigmentosa and allied disease: applications of electroretinographic testing. Int Ophthalmol 1981;4:7–22.
110. Birch DG, Fish GF. Rod ERGs in retinitis pigmentosa and cone–rod degeneration. Invest Ophthalmol Vis Sci 1987;28:140–50.
111. Berson EL. Electrical phenomena in the retina. In: Moses RA, Hart WM, editors. Adler's physiology of the eye: clinical application. 8 ed. St Louis: CV Mosby; 1987. p. 506–67.
112. Berson EL, Simonoff EA. Dominant retinitis pigmentosa with reduced penetrance: further studies of the electroretinogram. Arch Ophthalmol 1979;97: 1286–91.
113. Berson EL, Gouras P, Gunkel RD, et al. Dominant retinitis pigmentosa with reduced penetrance. Arch Ophthalmol 1969;81:226–34.
114. Sandberg MD, Effron MH, Berson EL. Focal cone electroretinograms in dominant retinitis pigmentosa with reduced penetrance. Invest Ophthalmol Vis Sci 1978;17:1096–101.
115. Stone JL, Barlow WE, Humayun MS, et al. Morphometric analysis of macular photoreceptors and ganglion cells in retinas with retinitis pigmentosa. Arch Ophthalmol 1992;110:1634–9.
116. Falsini B, Iarossi G, Porciatti V, et al. Postreceptoral contribution to macular dysfunction in retinitis pigmentosa. Invest Ophthalmol Vis Sci 1994;35: 4282–90.
117. Cideciyan AV, Jacobson SG. Negative electroretinograms in retinitis pigmentosa. Invest Ophthalmol Vis Sci 1993;34:3253–63.
118. Granit R. The components of the retinal action potential in mammals and their relation to the discharge of the optic nerve. J Physiol (Lond) 1933;77: 207–39.
119. Breton ME, Quinn GE, Schueller AW. Development of electroretinogram and rod phototransduction response in human infants. Invest Ophthalmol Vis Sci 1995;36:1588–602.
120. Hood DC, Birch DG. A quantitative measure of the electrical activity of human rod photoreceptors using electroretinography. Vis Neurosci 1990;5: 379–87.
121. Hood DC, Birch DG. The a-wave of the human electroretinogram and rod receptor function. Invest Ophthalmol Vis Sci 1990;31:2070–81.
122. Lamb TD, Pugh Jr EN. A quantitative account of the activation steps involved in phototransduction in amphibian photoreceptors. J Physiol 1992;449: 749–57.
123. Hood DC, Birch DG. Rod phototransduction in retinitis pigmentosa: estimation and interpretation of parameters derived from the rod a-wave. Invest Ophthalmol Vis Sci 1994;35:2948–61.
124. Hood DC, Birch DG. A computational model of the amplitude and implicit time of the *b*-wave of the human ERG. Vis Neurosci 1992;8:107–26.

125. Hood DC, Birch DG. *b*-wave of the scotopic (rod) electroretinogram as a measure of the activity of human on-bipolar cells. J Opt Soc Am A 1996;13:623–33.
126. Shady S, Hood DC, Birch DG. Rod phototransduction in retinitis pigmentosa: distinguishing alternative mechanisms of degeneration. Invest Ophthalmol Vis Sci 1995;36:1027–37.
127. Hood DC, Cideciyan AV, Halevy DA, et al. Sites of disease action in a retinal dystrophy with supernormal and delayed rod electroretinogram *b*-waves. Vision Res 1996;36:889–901.
128. Gouras P, Eggers HM, MacKay CJ. Cone dystrophy, nyctalopia, and supernormal rod responses: a new retinal degeneration. Arch Ophthalmol 1983; 101:718–24.
129. Marmor MF, Jacobson SG, Foerster MH, et al. Diagnostic clinical findings of a new syndrome with night blindness, maculopathy and enhanced S cone sensitivity. Am J Ophthalmol 1990;110:124–34.
130. Jacobson SG, Marmor MF, Kemp CM, et al. SWS (blue) cone hypersensitivity in a newly identified retinal degeneration. Invest Ophthalmol Vis Sci 1990; 31:827–38.
131. Haider NB, Jacobson SG, Cideciyan AV, et al. Mutation of a nuclear receptor gene, *NR2E3*, causes enhanced S cone syndrome, a disorder of retinal cell fate. Nat Genet 2000;24:127–31.
132. Birch DG, Hood DC, Nusinowitz S, et al. Abnormal activation and inactivation mechanisms of rod transduction in patients with autosomal dominant retinitis pigmentosa and the Pro-23-His mutation. Invest Ophthalmol Vis Sci 1995;36:1603–14.
133. Goto Y, Peachey NS, Ziroli NE, et al. Rod phototransduction in transgenic mice expressing a mutant opsin gene. J Opt Soc Am A 1996;13:577–85.
134. Tzekov RT, Locke KG, Hood DC, et al. Cone and rod ERG phototransduction parameters in retinitis pigmentosa. Invest Ophthalmol Vis Sci 2003;44: 3993–4000.
135. Sutter EE, Tran D. The field topography of ERG components in man – I. The photopic luminance response. Vis Res 1992;32:433–46.
136. Bearse MA, Sutter EE, Lerner L. Imaging retinal damage with the multi-input electroretinogram. In: Vision science and its applications. Technical Digest Series. Washingon, DC: Optical Society of America; 1994. p. 358–61.
137. Hood DC, Li J. A technique for measuring individual mulifocal ERG records. OSA TOPS 1997;11:33–41.
138. Hood DC, Seiple W, Holopigian K, et al. A comparison of the components of the multifocal and full-field ERGs. Vis Neurosci 1997;14:533–44.
139. Robson AG, El-Amir A, Bailey C, et al. Pattern ERG correlates of abnormal fundus autofluorescence in patients with retinitis pigmentosa and normal visual acuity. Invest Ophthalmol Vis Sci 2003;44:3544–50.
140. Arden GB, Fojas MR. Electrophysiological abnormalities in pigmentary degenerations of the retina. Arch Ophthalmol 1962;68:369–89.
141. Weleber RG, Eisner A. Retinal function and physiological studies. In: Newsome DA, editor. Retinal dystrophies and degenerations. New York, NY: Raven Press; 1988. p. 21–69.
142. Cideciyan AV, Jacobson SG, Aleman TS, et al. In vivo dynamics of retinal injury and repair in the rhodopsin mutant dog model of human retinitis pigmentosa. Proc Natl Acad Sci USA 2005;102:5233–8.
143. Spalton DJ, Bird AC, Cleary PE. Retinitis pigmentosa and retinal oedema. Br J Ophthalmol 1978;62:174–82.
144. Newsome DA. Retinal fluorescein leakage in retinitis pigmentosa. Am J Ophthalmol 1986;101:354–60.
145. Fetkenhour CL, Choromokos E, Weinstein J, et al. Cystoid macular edema in retinitis pigmentosa. Trans Am Acad Ophthalmol Otolaryngol 1977;83: OP-515–21.
146. von Ruckmann A, Fitzke FW, Bird AC. Distribution of fundus autofluorescence with a scanning laser ophthalmoscope. Br J Ophthalmol 1995;79: 407–12.
147. Robson AG, Egan CA, Luong VA, et al. Comparison of fundus autofluorescence with photopic and scotopic fine-matrix mapping in patients with retinitis pigmentosa and normal visual acuity. Invest Ophthalmol Vis Sci 2004; 45:4119–25.
148. Popovic P, Jarc-Vidmar M, Hawlina M. Abnormal fundus autofluorescence in relation to retinal function in patients with retinitis pigmentosa. Graefes Arch Klin Exp Ophthalmol 2005;243:1018–27.
149. Robson AG, Saihan Z, Jenkins SA, et al. Functional characterisation and serial imaging of abnormal fundus autofluorescence in patients with retinitis pigmentosa and normal visual acuity. Br J Ophthalmol 2006;90:472–9.
150. Robson AG, Michaelides M, Saihan Z, et al. Functional characteristics of patients with retinal dystrophy that manifest abnormal parafoveal annuli of high density fundus autofluorescence; a review and update. Doc Ophthalmol Adv Ophthalmol 2008;116:79–89.
151. Fleckenstein M, Charbel Issa P, Fuchs HA, et al. Discrete arcs of increased fundus autofluorescence in retinal dystrophies and functional correlate on microperimetry. Eye 2009;23:567–75.
152. Robson AG, Tufail A, Fitzke F, et al. Serial imaging and structure-function correlates of high-density rings of fundus autofluorescence in retinitis pigmentosa. Retina 2011;31:1670–9.
153. Lima LH, Cella W, Greenstein VC, et al. Structural assessment of hyperautofluorescent ring in patients with retinitis pigmentosa. Retina 2009;29: 1025–31.
154. Aleman TS, Cideciyan AV, Sumaroka A, et al. Retinal laminar architecture in human retinitis pigmentosa caused by Rhodopsin gene mutations. Invest Ophthalmol Vis Sci 2008;49:1580–90.
155. Kellner U, Kellner S, Weber BH, et al. Lipofuscin- and melanin-related fundus autofluorescence visualize different retinal pigment epithelial alterations in patients with retinitis pigmentosa. Eye 2009;23:1349–59.
156. Witkin AJ, Ko TH, Fujimoto JG, et al. Ultra-high resolution optical coherence tomography assessment of photoreceptors in retinitis pigmentosa and related diseases. Am J Ophthalmol 2006;142:945–52.
157. Lim JI, Tan O, Fawzi AA, et al. A pilot study of Fourier-domain optical coherence tomography of retinal dystrophy patients. Am J Ophthalmol 2008;146: 417–26.
158. Wolsley CJ, Silvestri G, O'Neill J, et al. The association between multifocal electroretinograms and OCT retinal thickness in retinitis pigmentosa patients with good visual acuity. Eye 2009;23:1524–31.
159. Lupo S, Grenga PL, Vingolo EM. Fourier-domain optical coherence tomography and microperimetry findings in retinitis pigmentosa. Am J Ophthalmol 2011;151:106–11.
160. Fischer MD, Fleischhauer JC, Gillies MC, et al. A new method to monitor visual field defects caused by photoreceptor degeneration by quantitative optical coherence tomography. Invest Ophthalmol Vis Sci 2008;49:3617–21.
161. Hajali M, Fishman GA, Anderson RJ. The prevalence of cystoid macular oedema in retinitis pigmentosa patients determined by optical coherence tomography. Br J Ophthalmol 2008;92:1065–8.
162. Liang J, Williams DR. Aberrations and retinal image quality of the normal human eye. J Opt Soc Am A Opt Image Sci Vis 1997;14:2873–83.
163. Roorda A, Romero-Borja F, Donnelly Iii W, et al. Adaptive optics scanning laser ophthalmoscopy. Opt Express 2002;10:405–12.
164. Duncan JL, Zhang Y, Gandhi J, et al. High-resolution imaging with adaptive optics in patients with inherited retinal degeneration. Invest Ophthalmol Vis Sci 2007;48:3283–91.
165. Wolfing JI, Chung M, Carroll J, et al. High-resolution retinal imaging of cone–rod dystrophy. Ophthalmology 2006;113:1019 e1.
166. Choi SS, Doble N, Hardy JL, et al. In vivo imaging of the photoreceptor mosaic in retinal dystrophies and correlations with visual function. Invest Ophthalmol Vis Sci 2006;47:2080–92.
167. Dubra A, Sulai Y, Norris JL, et al. Noninvasive imaging of the human rod photoreceptor mosaic using a confocal adaptive optics scanning ophthalmoscope. Biomed Opt Express 2011;2:1864–76.
168. Talcott KE, Ratnam K, Sundquist SM, et al. Longitudinal study of cone photoreceptors during retinal degeneration and in response to ciliary neurotrophic factor treatment. Invest Ophthalmol Vis Sci 2011;52:2219–26.
169. Jay, M. On the heredity of retinitis pigmentosa. Br J Ophthalmol 1982;66: 405–16
170. Dryja TP. Molecular genetics of Oguchi disease, fundus albipunctatus, and other forms of stationary night blindness: LVII Edward Jackson Memorial Lecture. Am J Ophthalmol 2000;130:547–63.
171. Franceschetti A, François J, Babel J. Retinitis punctata albescens. In: Franceschetti A, François J, Babel J, editors. Chorioretinal heredodegenerations. Springfield, Ill: Charles C Thomas; 1974. p. 222–31.
172. Miyake Y, Shiroyama N, Sugita S, et al. Fundus albipunctatus associated with cone dystrophy. Br J Ophthalmol 1992;76:375–9.
173. Nakamura M, Miyake Y. Macular dystrophy in a 9-year-old boy with fundus albipunctatus. Am J Ophthalmol 2002;133:278–80.
174. Nakamura M, Hotta Y, Tanikawa A, et al. A high association with cone dystrophy in fundus albipunctatus caused by mutations of the *RDH5* gene. Invest Ophthalmol Vis Sci 2000;41:3925–32.
175. Bietti G. Su alcune forme atipiche o rare di degenerazione retinica (degenerazioni tappeto-retiniche e quadri morbosi similari). Boll Oculist 1937;16: 1159–244.
176. Krill AE. Incomplete rod–cone degenerations. In: Krill AE, editor. Krill's hereditary retinal and choroidal diseases. New York, NY: Harper & Row; 1977. p. 577–643.
177. Berson EL, Howard J. Temporal aspects of the electroretinogram in sector retinitis pigmentosa. Arch Ophthalmol 1971;86:653–65.
178. Deutman AF. Rod–cone dystrophy: primary, hereditary, pigmentary retinopathy, retinitis pigmentosa. In: Krill AE, editor. Krill's hereditary retinal and choroidal diseases. New York, NY: Harper & Row; 1977. p. 479–576.
179. Heckenlively JR, Rodriguez JA, Daiger SP. Autosomal dominant sectoral retinitis pigmentosa: two families with transversion mutation in codon 23 of rhodopsin. Arch Ophthalmol 1991;109:84–91.
180. Audo I, Friedrich A, Mohand-Said S, et al. An unusual retinal phenotype associated with a novel mutation in RHO. Arch Ophthalmol 2010;128: 1036–45.
181. Saihan Z, Le Quesne Stabej P, Robson AG, et al. Mutations in the Ush1c gene associated with sector retinitis pigmentosa and hearing loss. Retina 2011;31: 1708–16.
182. de Crecchio G, Alfieri MC, Cennamo G, et al. Pericentral pigmentary retinopathy: long-term follow-up. Eye 2006;20:1408–10.
183. Selmer KK, Grondahl J, Riise R, et al. Autosomal dominant pericentral retinal dystrophy caused by a novel missense mutation in the TOPORS gene. Acta ophthalmol 2010;88:323–8.
184. Mukhopadhyay R, Holder GE, Moore AT, et al. Unilateral retinitis pigmentosa occurring in an individual with a germline mutation in the RP1 gene. Arch Ophthalmol 2011;129:954–6.
185. Whitcup SM, Iwata F, Podgor MJ, et al. Association of thyroid disease with retinitis pigmentosa and gyrate atrophy. Am J Ophthalmol 1996;122:903–5.
186. Cowan CL, Grimes PE, Chakrabarti S, et al. Retinitis pigmentosa associated with hearing loss, thyroid disease, vitiligo, and alopecia areata. Retina 1982;2: 84–8.

187. Boughman JA. Personal communication, January 28, 1988 1988.
188. Newsome DA. The immune system in retinitis pigmentosa. In: LaVail MM, Hollyfield JG, Anderson RE, editors. Retinal degeneration: experimental and clinical studies. New York: Alan R Liss; 1985. p. 75–90.
189. Boughman JA, Caldwell RJ. Assessment of clincial variables and counseling needs in patients with retinitis pigmentosa. Am J Med Genet 1982;12: 185–93.
190. Zito I, Downes SM, Patel RJ, et al. *RPGR* mutation associated with retinitis pigmentosa, impaired hearing, and sinorespiratory infections. J Med Genet 2003;40:609–15.
191. Kenna P, Mansergh F, Millington-Ward S, et al. Clinical and molecular genetic characterisation of a family segregating autosomal dominant retinitis pigmentosa and sensorineural deafness. Br J Ophthalmol 1997;81:207–13.
192. Mansergh FC, Millington-Ward S, Kennan A, et al. Retinitis pigmentosa and progressive sensorineural hearing loss caused by a C12258A mutation in the mitochondrial MTTS2 gene. Am J Hum Genet 1999;64:971–85.
193. Usher CH. On the inheritance of retinitis pigmentosa, with notes of cases. R Lond Ophthalmol Hosp Rep 1914;19:130–236.
194. Koenig R. Bardet–Biedl syndrome and Usher syndrome. Dev Ophthalmol 2003;37:126–40.
195. Hope CI, Bundey S, Proops D, et al. Usher syndrome in the city of Birmingham – prevalence and clinical classification. Br J Ophthalmol 1997;81: 46–51.
196. Boughman JA, Vernon M, Shaver KA. Usher syndrome: definition and estimate of prevalence from two high-risk populations. J Chronic Dis 1983;36: 595–603.
197. Vernon M. Usher's syndrome – deafness and progressive blindness: Clinical cases, prevention, theory, and literature review. J Chronic Dis 1969;22: 133–51.
198. Smith RJH, Berlin CI, Hejtmancik JF, et al. Clinical diagnosis of the Usher syndromes. Usher Syndrome Consortium. Am J Med Genet 1994;50:32–8.
199. Fishman GA, Kumar A, Joseph ME, et al. Usher's syndrome: ophthalmic and neuro-otologic findings suggesting genetic heterogeneity. Arch Ophthalmol 1983;101:1367–74.
200. Davenport SLH, Omenn GS. The heterogeneity of Usher syndrome. International Congress Series, publication 426 abstract 215. Amsterdam, Excerpta Medica Foundation, 1977, p. 87–8.
201. Pakarinen L, Karjalainen S, Simola KOJ, et al. Usher's syndrome type 3 in Finland. Laryngoscope 1995;105:613–7.
202. Pakarinen L, Tuppurainen K, Laippala P, et al. The ophthalmological course of Usher syndrome type III. Int Ophthalmol 1996;19:307–11.
203. Merin S, Abraham FA, Auerbach E. Usher's and Hallgren's syndromes. Acta Genet Med Gemellol (Roma) 1974;23:49–55.
204. Piazza L, Fishman GA, Farber M, et al. Visual acuity loss in patients with Usher's syndrome. Arch Ophthalmol 1986;104:1336–9.
205. Sankila E-M, Pakarinen L, Kääriäinen H, et al. Assignment of an Usher syndrome type III (USH3) gene to chromosome 3q. Hum Mol Genet 1995;4: 93–8.
206. Ness SL, Ben-Yosef T, Bar-Lev A, et al. Genetic homogeneity and phenotypic variability among Ashkenazi Jews with Usher syndrome type III. J Med Genet 2003;40:767–72.
207. Loundon N, Marlin S, Busquet D, et al. Usher syndrome and cochlear implantation. Otol Neurotol 2003;24:216–21.
208. Matthews TW, Poliquin J, Mount J, et al. Is there genetic heterogeneity in Usher's syndrome? J Otolaryngol 1987;16:61–6.
209. Szlyk JP, Fishman GA, Alexander KR, et al. Relationship between difficulty in performing daily activities and clinical measures of visual function in patients with retinitis pigmentosa. Arch Ophthalmol 1997;115:53–9.
210. Tamayo ML, Rodriguez A, Molina R, et al. Social, familial and medical aspects of Usher syndrome in Colombia. Genetic Counseling 1997;8:235–40.
211. Krill AE, Deutman AF, Fishman M. The cone degenerations. Doc Ophthalmol 1973;35:1–80.
212. Evans K, Duvall-Young J, Fitzke FW, et al. Chromosome 19q cone–rod retinal dystrophy. Arch Ophthalmol 1995;113:195–201.
213. Rabb MF, Tso MOM, Fishman GA. Cone–rod dystrophy: a clinical and histopathologic report. Ophthalmology 1986;93:1443–50.
214. Berson EL, Gouras P, Gunkel RD. Progressive cone–rod degeneration. Arch Ophthalmol 1968;80:68–76.
215. Heckenlively JR, Martin DA, Rosales TO. Telangiectasia and optic atrophy in cone–rod degenerations. Arch Ophthalmol 1981;99:1983–91.
216. Krauss HR, Heckenlively JR. Visual field changes in cone–rod degenerations. Arch Ophthalmol 1982;100:1784–90.
217. Yagasaki K, Jacobson SG. Cone–rod dystrophy: phenotypic diversity by retinal function testing. Arch Ophthalmol 1989;107:701–8.
218. Szlyk JP, Fishman GA, Alexander KR, et al. Clinical subtypes of cone–rod dystrophy. Arch Ophthalmol 1993;111:781–8.
219. Mäntyjärvi M, Tuppurainen K. Progressive cone–rod dystrophy and high myopia in a Finnish family. Acta Ophthalmol (Copenh) 1989;67:234–42.
220. Heckenlively JR, Foxman SG, Parelhoff ES. Retinal dystrophy and macular coloboma. Doc Ophthalmol 1988;68:257–71.
221. Aleman TS, Cideciyan AV, Volpe NJ, et al. Spinocerebellar ataxia type 7 (*SCA7*) shows a cone–rod dystrophy phenotype. Exp Eye Res 2002;74: 737–45.
222. Jalili IK, Smith NJD. A progressive cone–rod dystrophy and amelogenesis imperfecta: a new syndrome. J Med Genet 1988;25:738–40.
223. Samra D, Abraham FA, Treister G. Inherited progressive cone–rod dystrophy and alopecia. Metab Pediatr Syst Ophthalmol 1988;11:83–5.
224. Jalili IK. Cone–rod congenital amaurosis associated with congenital hypertrichosis: an autosomal recessive condition. J Med Genet 1989;26:504–10.
225. Moore AT. Cone and cone–rod dystrophies. J Med Genet 1992;29:289–90.
226. Kelsell RE, Gregory-Evans K, Payne AM, et al. Mutations in the retinal guanylate cyclase (RETGC-1) gene in dominant cone–rod dystrophy. Hum Mol Genet 1998;7:1179–84.
227. Payne AM, Downes SM, Bessant DA, et al. A mutation in guanylate cyclase activator 1A (*GUCA1A*) in an autosomal dominant cone dystrophy pedigree mapping to a new locus on chromosome 6p21.1. Hum Mol Genet 1998;7: 273–7.
228. Wilkie SE, Li Y, Deery EC, et al. Identification and functional consequences of a new mutation (E155G) in the gene for GCAP1 that causes autosomal dominant cone dystrophy. Am J Hum Genet 2001;69:471–80.
229. Sohocki MM, Sullivan LS, Mintz-Hittner HA, et al. A range of clinical phenotypes associated with mutations in *CRX*, a photoreceptor transcription-factor gene. Am J Hum Genet 1998;63:1307–15.
230. Rivolta C, Berson EL, Dryja TP. Dominant Leber congenital amaurosis, cone–rod degeneration, and retinitis pigmentosa caused by mutant versions of the transcription factor CRX. Hum Mutat 2001;18:488–98.
231. Leber T. Ueber Retinitis pigmentosa und angeborene Amaurose. Graefes Arch Clin Exp Ophthalmol 1869;15:1–25.
232. Franceschetti A, Dieterlé P. Importance diagnostique et pronostique de l'électrorétinogramme (ERG) dans les dégénérescences tapéto-rétiniennes avec rétrécissement du champ visuel et héméralopie. Confinia Neurol 1954; 14:184–6.
233. Franceschetti A. Rubeola pendant la grossesse et cataracte congenitale chez l'enfant, accompagnée du phenomène digito-oculaire. Ophthalmologica 1947; 114:332–9.
234. Foxman SG, Heckenlively JR, Bateman JB, et al. Classification of congenital and early onset retinitis pigmentosa. Arch Ophthalmol 1985;103:1502–6.
235. Heckenlively JR, Foxman SG. Congenital and early-onset forms of retinitis pigmentosa. In: Heckenlively JR, editor. Retinitis pigmentosa. Philadelphia: JB Lippincott; 1988. p. 107–18.
236. Foxman SG, Wirtschafter JD, Letson RD. Leber's congenital amaurosis and high hyperopia: a discrete entity. In: Henkind P, editor. Acta XXIV International Congress of Ophthalmology. Philadelphia: JB Lippincott; 1982. p. 55–8.
237. Wagner RS, Caputo AR, Nelson LB, et al. High hyperopia in Leber's congenital amaurosis. Arch Ophthalmol 1985;103:1507–9.
238. Fulton AB, Hansen RM, Westall CA. Development of ERG responses: the ISCEV rod, maximal and cone responses in normal subjects. Doc Ophthalmol 2003;107:235–41.
239. Leber T. Die Krankheiten der Netzhaut. In: Saemish T, editor. Graefe Handbuch der gesamten Augenheilkunde. 2nd ed. Leipzig, Germany: W. Engelman; 1916. p. 1076–225.
240. Hagstrom SA, North MA, Nishina PM, et al. Recessive mutations in the gene encoding the tubby-like protein TULP1 in patients with retinitis pigmentosa. Nat Genet 1998;18:174–6.
241. Lorenz B, Gyürüs P, Preising M, et al. Early-onset severe rod–cone dystrophy in young children with *RPE65* mutations. Invest Ophthalmol Vis Sci 2000; 41:2735–42.
242. Weleber RG, Michaelides M, Trzupek KM, et al. The phenotype of severe early childhood onset retinal dystrophy (SECORD) from mutation of RPE65 and differentiation from Leber congenital amaurosis. Invest Ophthalmol Vis Sci 2011;52:292–302.
243. Leighton DA, Harris R. Retinal aplasia in association with macular coloboma, keratoconus and cataract. Clin Genet 1973;4:270–4.
244. Margolis S, Scher BM, Carr RE. Macular colobomas in Leber's congenital amaurosis. Am J Ophthalmol 1977;83:27–31.
245. François J. Choroideremia (progressive chorioretinal degeneration). Int Ophthalmol Clin 1968;8:949–64.
246. Edwards WC, Price WD, McDonald Jr R. Congenital amaurosis of retinal origin (Leber). Am J Ophthalmol 1971;72:724–8.
247. Schroeder R, Bets MB, Maumenee IH. Leber's congenital amaurosis: retrospective review of 43 cases and a new fundus finding in two cases. Arch Ophthalmol 1987;105:356–9.
248 Flanders M, Lapointe ML, Brownstein S, et al. Keratoconus and Leber's congenital amaurosis: a clinicopathological correlation. Can J Ophthalmol 1984; 19:310–4.
249. Elder MJ. Leber congenital amaurosis and its association with keratoconus and keratoglobus. J Pediatr Ophthalmol Strabismus 1994;31:38–40.
250. Lambert SR, Kriss A, Taylor D, et al. Follow-up and diagnostic reappraisal of 75 patients with Leber's congenital amaurosis. Am J Ophthalmol 1989;107: 624–31.
251. Senior B, Friedmann A, Braudo JL. Juvenile familial nephropathy with tapetoretinal degeneration. Am J Ophthalmol 1961;52:625–33.
252. Russell-Eggitt IM, Clayton PT, Coffey R, et al. Alström syndrome. Report of 22 cases and literature review. Ophthalmology 1998;105:1274–80.
253. Ehara H, Nakano C, Ohno K, et al. New autosomal-recessive syndrome of Leber congenital amaurosis, short stature, growth hormone deficiency, mental retardation, hepatic dysfunction and metabolic acidosis. Am J Med Genet 1997;71:258–66.
254. Alström CH, Olson OA. Heredoretinopathia congenitalis monohybrida recessiva autosomalis. Hereditas 1957;43:1–177.
255. Nickel B, Hoyt CS. Leber's congenital amaurosis: Is mental retardation a frequent associated defect? Arch Ophthalmol 1982;100:1089–92.

256. Weinstein JM, Gleaton M, Weidner WA, et al. Leber's congenital amaurosis: relationship of structural CNS anomalies to psychomotor retardation. Arch Neurol 1984;41:204–6.
257. Schuil J, Meire FM, Delleman JW. Mental retardation in amaurosis congenita of Leber. Neuropediatrics 1998;29:294–7.
258. Casteels I, Spileers W, Demaerel P, et al. Leber congenital amaurosis – differential diagnosis, ophthalmological and neuroradiological report of 18 patients. Neuropediatrics 1996;27:189–93.
259. Walia S, Fishman GA, Jacobson SG, et al. Visual acuity in patients with Leber's congenital amaurosis and early childhood-onset retinitis pigmentosa. Ophthalmology 2010;117:1190–8.
260. den Hollander AI, Koenekoop RK, Yzer S, et al. Mutations in the CEP290 (NPHP6) gene are a frequent cause of Leber congenital amaurosis. Am J Hum Genet 2006;79:556–61.
261. Weleber RG. Infantile and childhood retinal blindness: a molecular perspective (the Franceschetti lecture). Ophthalm Genet 2002;23:71–97.
262. Weleber RG, Tongue AC, Kennaway NG, et al. Ophthalmic manifestations of infantile phytanic acid storage disease. Arch Ophthalmol 1984;102: 1317–21.
263. Pennesi ME, Weleber RG. Peroxisomal disorders. In: Traboulsi EI, editor. Genetic diseases of the eye. Oxford: Oxford University Press; 2011. p. 663–96.
264. Weleber RG, Tongue AT. Congenital stationary night blindness presenting as Leber's congenital amaurosis. Arch Ophthalmol 1987;105:360–5.
265. Weleber RG. The dystrophic retina in multisystem disorders: the electroretinogram in neuronal ceroid lipofuscinoses. Eye 1998;12:580–90.
266. Weleber RG, Gupta N, Trzupek KM, et al. Electroretinographic and clinicopathologic correlations of retinal dysfunction in infantile neuronal ceroid lipofuscinosis (infantile Batten disease). Mol Genet Metab 2004;83:128–37.
267. Loken AC, Hanssen O, Halvolsen S, et al. Hereditary renal dysplasia and blindness. Acta Paediatr 1961;50:177–94.
268. Otto EA, Loeys B, Khanna H, et al. Nephrocystin-5, a ciliary IQ domain protein, is mutated in Senior–Loken syndrome and interacts with RPGR and calmodulin. Nat Genet 2005;37:282–8.
269. Stone EM, Cideciyan AV, Aleman TS, et al. Variations in NPHP5 in patients with nonsyndromic Leber congenital amaurosis and Senior–Loken syndrome. Arch Ophthalmol 2011;129:81–7.
270. Pinckers AJL. Leber's congenital amaurosis as conceived by Leber. Ophthalmologica 1979;179:48–51.
271. Bardet G. Sur un syndrome d'obésité infantile avec polydactylie et rétinite pigmentaire (contributions à l'étude des formes cliniques de l'obésité hypophysaire). Paris: University of Paris; 1920.
272. Biedl, A. Ein Geschwisterpaar mit adiposgenitaler Dystrophie. Dtsch Med Wochenschr 1922;48:1630.
273. Laurence JZ, Moon RC. Four cases of retinitis pigmentosa occurring in the same family and accompanied by general imperfections of development. Ophthalmic Rev 1866;2:32–41.
274. Hutchinson J. Slowly progressive paraplegia and disease of the choroids with defective intellect and arrested sexual development in several brothers and a sister. Arch Surg (Lond) 1900;11:118–22.
275. Ammann F. Investigations cliniques et genetiques sur le syndrome de Bardet–Biedl en Suisse. J Genet Hum 1970;18(Suppl):1–310.
276. Churchill DN, McManamon P, Hurley RM. Renal disease: a sixth cardinal feature of the Laurence–Moon–Biedl syndrome. Clin Nephrol 1981;16:151–4.
277. Rizzo III JF, Berson EL, Lessell S. Retinal and neurological findings in the Laurence–Moon–Bardet–Biedl phenotype. Ophthalmology 1986;93:1452–6.
278. Beales PL, Elcioglu N, Woolf AS, et al. New criteria for improved diagnosis of Bardet–Biedl syndrome: results of a population survey. J Med Genet 1999;36:437–46.
279. Farag TI, Teebi AS. Bardet–Biedl and Laurence–Moon syndromes in a mixed Arab population. Clin Genet 1988;33:78–82.
280. Farag TI, Teebi AS. High incidence of Bardet Biedl syndrome among the Bedouin. Clin Genet 1989;36:463–5.
281. Green JS, Parfrey PS, Harnett JD, et al. The cardinal manifestations of Bardet–Biedl syndrome, a form of Laurence–Moon–Biedl syndrome. N Engl J Med 1989;321:1002–9.
282. Klein D, Ammann F. The syndrome of Laurence–Moon–Bardet–Biedl and allied diseases in Switzerland: clinical, genetic and epidemiological studies. J Neurol Sci 1969;9:479–513.
283. Schachat AP, Maumenee IH. The Bardet–Biedl syndrome and related disorders. Arch Ophthalmol 1982;100:285–8.
284. Heckenlively JR. RP syndromes. In: Heckenlively JR, editor. Retinitis pigmentosa. Philadelphia: JB Lippincott; 1988. p. 221–52.
285. Prosperi L, Cordella M, Bernasconi S. Electroretinography and diagnosis of the Laurence–Moon–Bardet–Biedl syndrome in childhood. J Pediatr Ophthalmol 1977;14:305–8.
286. Warkany J, Frauenberger GS, Mitchell AG. Heredofamilial deviations: I. The Laurence–Moon–Biedl syndrome. Am J Dis Child 1937;53:455–70.
287. Bell J. The Laurence–Moon syndrome. In: Penrose LS, editor. The treasury of human inheritance. Cambridge: Cambridge University Press; 1958. p. 51–96.
288. Stoler JM, Herrin JT, Holmes LB. Genital abnormalities in females with Bardet–Biedl syndrome. Am J Med Genet 1995;55:276–8.
289. Mehrotra N, Taub S, Covert RF. Hydrometrocolpos as a neonatal manifestation of the Bardet–Biedl syndrome. Am J Med Genet 1997;69:220.
290. David A, Bitoun P, Lacombe D, et al. Hydrometrocolpos and polydactyly: a common neonatal presentation of Bardet–Biedl and McKusick–Kaufman syndromes. J Med Genet 1999;36:599–603.
291. Katsanis N, Beales PL, Woods MO, et al. Mutations in *MKKS* cause obesity, retinal dystrophy and renal malformations associated with Bardet–Biedl syndrome. Nat Genet 2000;26:67–70.
292. Schaap C, ten Tusscher MP, Schrander JJ, et al. Phenotypic overlap between McKusick–Kaufman and Bardet–Biedl syndromes: are they related? Eur J Pediatr 1998;157:170–1.
293. Bauman ML, Hogan GR. Laurence–Moon–Biedl syndrome. Am J Dis Child 1973;126:119–26.
294. Hurley RM, Dery P, Nogrady MB, et al. The renal lesion of the Laurence–Moon–Biedl syndrome. J Pediatr 1975;87:206–9.
295. Pagon RA, Haas JE, Bunt AH, et al. Hepatic involvement in the Bardet–Biedl syndrome. Am J Med Genet 1982;13:373–81.
296. Elbedour K, Zucker N, Zalzstein E, et al. Cardiac abnormalities in the Bardet–Biedl syndrome: echocardiographic studies of 22 patients. Am J Med Genet 1994;52:164–9.
297. Islek I, Kucukoduk S, Erkan D, et al. Bardet–Biedl syndrome: delayed diagnosis in a child with Hirschsprung disease. Clin Dysmorphol 1996;5:271–3.
298. Croft JB, Swift M. Obesity, hypertension, and renal disease in relatives of Bardet–Biedl syndrome sibs. Am J Med Genet 1990;36:37–42.
299. Carmi R, Elbedour K, Stone EM, et al. Phenotypic differences among patients with Bardet–Biedl syndrome linked to three different chromosome loci. Am J Med Genet 1995;59:199–203.
300. Scotto JM, Hadchouel M, Odievre M, et al. Infantile phytanic acid storage disease, a possible variant of Refsum's disease: three cases, including ultrastructural studies of the liver. J Inherit Metab Dis 1982;5:83–90.
301. Refsum S. Heredopathia atactica polyneuritiformis: a familial syndrome not hitherto described. Acta Pyschiatr Scand Suppl 1946;38:1–303.
302. Refsum S. Heredopathia atactica polyneuritiformis: phytanic acid storage disease (Refsum's disease) with particular reference to ophthalmological disturbances. Metabol Ophthalmol 1977;1:73–9.
303. Jansen GA, Ofman R, Ferdinandusse S, et al. Refsum disease is caused by mutations in the phytanolyl-CoA hydroxylase gene. Nat Genet 1997;17: 190–3.
304. Jansen GA, Waterham HR, Wanders RJ. Molecular basis of Refsum disease: sequence variations in phytanoyl-CoA hydroxylase (PHYH) and the PTS2 receptor (PEX7). Hum Mutat 2004;23:209–18.
305. Hansen E, Bachen NI, Flage T. Refsum's disease. Eye manifestations in a patient treated with low phytol low phytanic acid diet. Acta Ophthalmol 1979;57:899–913.
306. Djupesland G, Flottorp G, Refsum S. Phytanic acid storage disease: hearing maintained after 15 years of dietary treatment. Neurology 1983;33:237–40.
307. Mole SE, Williams RE. Neuronal ceroid-lipofuscinosis. GeneReviews. Available online at: http://www.genetests.org 2010 (updated Mar 2 2010).
308. Rider JA, Rider DL. Batten disease: past, present and future. Am J Med Genet [Suppl] 1988;5:21–6.
309. Goebel HH. The neuronal ceroid-lipofuscinoses. Semin Pediatr Neurol 1996;3:270–8.
310. Santavuori P, Vanhanen S-L, Sainio K, et al. Infantile neuronal ceroid-lipofuscinosis (INCL): diagnostic criteria. J Inherit Metab Dis 1993;16:227–9.
311. Bielschowsky M. Über spät-infantile familiäre amaurotische Idiotie mit Kleinhirnsymptomen. Dtsch Zschr Nervenheilk 1913;50:7–29.
312. Janský J. Dosud nepopsaný prípad familiárni amaurotické idiotie komplikované s hypoplasii mozeckovou. Sb Ved Pr Lek Fak Karlovy 1908;9: 165–96.
313. Goebel HH, Gerhard L, Kominami E, et al. Neuronal ceroid-lipofuscinosis – late-infantile or Jansky-Bielschowsky type – revisited. Brain Pathol 1996;6: 225–8.
314. Zeman W, Donahue S, Dyken P, et al. The neuronal ceroid-lipofuscinosis (Batten–Vogt syndrome). In: Vinken PJ, Bruyn GW, editors. Handbook of clinical neurology. Amsterdam: North Holland; 1970. p. 588–679.
315. Zeman W. Batten disease: ocular features, differential diagnosis and diagnosis by enzyme analysis. Birth Defects Orig Artic Ser 1976;12:441–53.
316. Kufs H. Über einen Fall von spätester Form der amaurotischen Idiotie mit dem Beginn im 42 und Tod im 59 Lebens-jahre in klinischer, histologischer und Vererbungs-pathologischer Beziehung. Z ges Neurol 1931;137:432–48.
317. Boehme DH, Cottrell JC, Leonberg SC, et al. A dominant form of neuronal ceroid-lipofuscinosis. Brain 1971;94:745–56.
318. Dyken P, Wisniewski K. Classification of the neuronal ceroid-lipofuscinoses: expansion of the atypical forms. Am J Med Genet 1995;57:150–4.
319. Tyynelä J, Suopanki J, Santavuori P, et al. Variant late infantile neuronal ceroid-lipofuscinosis: pathology and biochemistry. J Neuropathol Exp Neurol 1997;56:369–75.
320. Batten FE. Cerebral degeneration with symmetrical changes in the maculae in two members of a family. Trans Ophthalmol Soc UK 1903;23:386–90.
321. Batten FE. Family cerebral degeneration with macular change (so-called juvenile form of family amaurotic idiocy). Q J Med 1914;7:444–54.
322. Jongen PJH, Gabreëls FJM, Schuurmans Stekhoven JH, et al. Early infantile form of neuronal ceroid lipofuscinosis. Clin Neurol Neurosurg 1987;89: 161–7.
323. Claussen M, Heim P, Knispel J, et al. Incidence of neuronal ceroid-lipofuscinoses in West Germany: variation of a method for studying autosomal recessive disorders. Am J Med Genet 1992;42:536–8.
324. Katz ML, Gao C-L, Prabhakaram M, et al. Immunochemical localization of the Batten disease (CLN3) protein in retina. Invest Ophthalmol Vis Sci 1997;38: 2375–86.
325. Libert J. Diagnosis of lysosomal storage diseases by the ultrastructural study of conjunctival biopsies. Pathol Annu 1980;15:37–66.

326. Arsenio-Nunes ML, Goutieres F, Aicardi J. An ultramicroscopic study of skin and conjunctival biopsies in chronic neurological disorders of childhood. Ann Neurol 1981;9:163–73.
327. Lake BD. The differential diagnosis of the various forms of Batten disease by rectal biopsy. Birth Defects Orig Artic Ser 1976;12:441–53.
328. Rapola J, Santavuori P, Savilahti E. Suction biopsy of rectal mucosa in the diagnosis of infantile and juvenile types of neuronal ceroid-lipofuscinosis. Hum Pathol 1984;15:352–60.
329. Markesbery WR, Shield LK, Egel RT, et al. Late-infantile neuronal ceroid-lipofuscinosis: an ultrastructural study of lymphocyte inclusions. Arch Neurol 1976;33:630–5.
330. Schwendemann G. Lymphocyte inclusions in the juvenile type of generalized ceroid-lipofuscinosis. An electron microscopic study. Acta Neuropathol 1976;36:327–38.
331. Dolman CL, MacLeod PM, Chang E. Skin punch biopsies and lymphocytes in the diagnosis of lipidoses. Can J Neurol Sci 1975;2:67–73.
332. Brod RD, Packer AJ, Van Dyk HJ. Diagnosis of neuronal ceroid lipofuscinosis by ultrastructural examination of peripheral blood lymphocytes. Arch Ophthalmol 1987;105:1388–93.
333. Dom R, Brucher JM, Ceuterick C, et al. Adult ceroid-lipofuscinosis (Kufs' disease) in two brothers. Retinal and visceral storage in one; diagnostic muscle biopsy in the other. Acta Neuropathol 1979;45:67–72.
334. Becker K, Goebel HH, Svennerholm L, et al. Clinical, morphological, and biochemical investigations on a patient with an unusual form of neuronal ceroid-lipofuscinosis. Eur J Pediatr 1979;132:197–206.
335. Cooper LZ, Krugman S. Clinical manifestations of postnatal and congenital rubella. Arch Ophthalmol 1967;77:434–9.
336. Hanshaw JB, Dudgeon JA, Marshall WC. Viral Diseases of the fetus and newborn. 2nd ed. Philadelphia: WB Saunders; 1985.
337. Menne K. [Congenital rubella retinopathy – a progressive disease.] Klin Monatsbl Augenheilkd 1986;189:326–9.
338. Slusher MM, Tyler ME. Rubella retinopathy and subretinal neovascularization. Ann Ophthalmol 1982;14:292–4.
339. Heckenlively JR. Secondary retinitis pigmentosa (syphilis). Doc Ophthalmol Proc Series 1977;13:245–55.
340. Sawyer RA, Selhorst JB, Zimmerman LE, et al. Blindness caused by photoreceptor degeneration as a remote effect of cancer. Am J Ophthalmol 1976; 81:606–13.
341. Thirkill CE, Roth AM, Keltner JL. Cancer-associated retinopathy. Arch Ophthalmol 1987;105:372–5.
342. Keltner JL, Roth AM, Chang RS. Photoreceptor degeneration. Possible autoimmune disorder. Arch Ophthalmol 1983;101:564–9.
343. Polans AS, Buczylko J, Crabb J, et al. A photoreceptor calcium binding protein is recognized by autoantibodies obtained from patients with cancer-associated retinopathy. J Cell Biol 1991;112:981–9.
344. Polans AS, Witkowska D, Haley TL, et al. Recoverin, a photoreceptor-specific calcium-binding protein, is expressed by the tumor of a patient with cancer-associated retinopathy. Proc Natl Acad Sci USA 1995;92:9176–80.
345. Adamus G, Aptsiauri N, Guy J, et al. The occurrence of serum autoantibodies against enolase in cancer-associated retinopathy. Clin Immunol Immunopathol 1996;78:120–9.
346. Borgstrom MK, Riise R, Tornqvist K, et al. Anomalies in the permanent dentition and other oral findings in 29 individuals with Laurence–Moon–Bardet–Biedl syndrome. J Oral Pathol Med 1996;25:86–9.
347. Berson EL, Lessell S. Paraneoplastic night blindness with malignant melanoma. Am J Ophthalmol 1988;106:307–11.
348. Boeck K, Hofmann S, Klopfer M, et al. Melanoma-associated paraneoplastic retinopathy: case report and review of the literature. Br J Dermatol 1997; 137:457–60.
349. Alexander KR, Fishman GA, Peachey NS, et al. 'On' response defect in paraneoplastic night blindness with cutaneous malignant melanoma. Invest Ophthalmol Vis Sci 1992;33:477–83.
350. Wolf JE, Arden GB. Selective magnocellular damage in melanoma-associated retinopathy: comparison with congenital stationary nightblindness. Vision res 1996;36:2369–79.
351. Mizener JB, Kimura AE, Adamus G, et al. Autoimmune retinopathy in the absence of cancer. Am J Ophthalmol 1997;123:607–18.
352. Potts AM. The reaction of uveal pigment in vitro with polycyclic compounds. Invest Ophthalmol 1964;3:405–16.
353. Potts AM. Further studies concerning the accumulation of polycyclic compounds on uveal melanin. Invest Ophthalmol 1964;3:399–404.
354. Meredith TA, Aaberg TM, Willerson WD. Progressive chorioretinopathy after receiving thioridazine. Arch Ophthalmol 1978;96:1172–6.
355. Hamilton JD. Thioridazine retinopathy within the upper dosage limit. Psychosomatics 1985;26:823–4.
356. Miller 3rd FS, Bunt-Milam AH, Kalina RE. Clinical-ultrastructural study of thioridazine retinopathy. Ophthalmology 1982;89:1478–88.
357. Mathalone MB. Eye and skin changes in psychiatric patients treated with chlorpromazine. Br J Ophthalmol 1967;51:86–93.
358. Marks JS. Chloroquine retinopathy: is there a safe daily dose? Ann Rheum Dis 1982;41:52–8.
359. Krill AE, Potts AM, Johanson CE. Chloroquine retinopathy. Investigation of discrepancy between dark adaptation and electroretinographic findings in advanced stages. Am J Ophthalmol 1971;71:530–43.
360. Michaelides M, Stover NB, Francis PJ, et al. Retinal toxicity associated with hydroxychloroquine and chloroquine: risk factors, screening, and progression despite cessation of therapy. Arch Ophthalmol 2011;129:30–9.
361. Marmor MF, Carr RE, Easterbrook M, et al. Recommendations on screening for chloroquine and hydroxychloroquine retinopathy: a report by the American Academy of Ophthalmology. Ophthalmology 2002;109:1377–82.
362. Maturi RK, Yu M, Weleber RG. Multifocal electroretinographic evaluation of long-term hydroxychloroquine users. Arch Ophthalmol 2004;122:973–81.
363. Francois J, De Rouck A, Cambie E. Retinal and optic evaluation in quinine poisoning. Ann Ophthalmol 1972;4:177–85.
364. Handelman IL, Robertson JE, Weleber RG. Retinal toxicity of theraputic agents. Toxicol Cut Ocular Toxicol 1983;2:131–52.
365. Brinton GS, Norton EW, Zahn JR, et al. Ocular quinine toxicity. Am J Ophthalmol 1980;90:403–10.
366. Hommer K. [On quinine poisoning of the retina. With a remark on experimental chloroquine poisoning.] Klin Monatsbl Augenheilkd 1968;152: 785–804.
367. Brown TH. Retino-choroiditis radiata. Br J Ophthalmol 1937;21:645–8.
368. Noble KG, Carr RE. Pigmented paravenous chorioretinal atrophy. Am J Ophthalmol 1983;96:338–44.
369. Krill AE. Krill's hereditary retinal and choroidal diseases. Clinical characteristics. New York: Harper and Row; 1977.
370. Breageat P, Amalric P. Postmeningoencephalitis bilateral paravenous chorioretinal degeneration. In: Henkind P, Shimizu K, Blodi FC, et al. editors. Acta XXIV International Congress of Ophthalmology. Philadelphia: JB Lippincott; 1983.
371. Takei Y, Harada M, Mizuno K. Pigmented paravenous retinochoroidal atrophy. Jpn J Ophthalmol 1977;21:311–7.
372. Chi HH. Retinochoroiditis radiata. Am J Ophthalmol 1948;31:1485–7.
373. Yang Z, Peachey NS, Moshfeghi DM, et al. Mutations in the RPGR gene cause X-linked cone dystrophy. Hum Mol Genet 2002;11:605–11.
374. Foxman SG, Heckenlively JR, Sinclair SH. Rubeola retinopathy and pigmented paravenous retinochoroidal atrophy. Am J Ophthalmol 1985;99: 605–6.
375. Peduzzi M, Guerrieri F, Torlai F, et al. Bilateral pigmented paravenous retino-choroidal degeneration following measles. Int Ophthalmol 1984;7: 11–4.
376. Noble KG. Hereditary pigmented paravenous chorioretinal atrophy. Am J Ophthalmol 1989;108:365–9.
377. Skalka HW. Hereditary pigmented paravenous retinochoroidal atrophy. Am J Ophthalmol 1979;87:286–91.
378. Traboulsi EI, Maumenee IH. Hereditary pigmented paravenous chorioretinal atrophy. Arch Ophthalmol 1986;104:1636–40.
379. Pearlman JT, Heckenlively JR, Bastek JV. Progressive nature of pigmented paravenous retinochoroidal atrophy. Am J Ophthalmol 1978;85:215–7.
380. Karmous-Benailly H, Martinovic J, et al. Antenatal presentation of Bardet-Biedl syndrome may mimic Meckel syndrome. Am J Hum Genet 2005;76:3.
381. Hirose T, Miyake Y. Pigmentary paravenous chorioretinal degeneration: fundus appearance and retinal functions. Ann Ophthalmol 1979;11:709–18.
382. Lessel MR, Thaler A, Heilig P. ERG and EOG in progressive paravenous retinochoroidal atrophy. Doc Ophthalmol Adv Ophthalmol 1986;62:25–9.
383. Miller SA, Stevens TS, Myers F, et al. Pigmented paravenous retinochoroidal atrophy. Ann Ophthalmol 1978;10:867–71.
384. Bastek JV, Foos RY, Heckenlively J. Traumatic pigmentary retinopathy. Am J Ophthalmol 1981;92:621–4.
385. Gass JD, Braunstein RA. Further observations concerning the diffuse unilateral subacute neuroretinitis syndrome. Arch Ophthalmol 1983;101:1689–97.
386. Goldberg MA, Kazacos KR, Boyce WM, et al. Diffuse unilateral subacute neuroretinitis: morphometric, serologic, and epidemiologic support for Baylisascaris as a causative agent. Ophthalmology 1993;100:1695–701.
387. Kazacos KR, Raymond LA, Kazacos EA, et al. The raccoon ascarid. A probable cause of human ocular larva migrans. Ophthalmology 1985;92:1735–44.
388. de Souza EC, Nakashima Y. Diffuse unilateral subacute neuroretinitis. Report of transvitreal surgical removal of a subretinal nematode. Ophthalmology 1995;102:1183–6.
389. Naumann GO, Knorr HL. DUSN occurs in Europe. Ophthalmology 1994;101:971–2.
390. de Souza EC, Abujamra S, Nakashima Y, et al. Diffuse bilateral subacute neuroretinitis: first patient with documented nematodes in both eyes. Arch Ophthalmol 1999;117:1349–51.
391. Gass JD, Callanan DG, Bowman CB. Oral therapy in diffuse unilateral subacute neuroretinitis. Arch Ophthalmol 1992;110:675–80.
392. Buettner H. Congenital hypertrophy of the retinal pigment epithelium. Am J Ophthalmol 1975;79:177–89.
393. Traboulsi EI, Maumenee IH, Krush AJ, et al. Congenital hypertrophy of the retinal pigment epithelium predicts colorectal polyposis in Gardner's syndrome. Arch Ophthalmol 1990;108:525–6.
394. Dratz EA, Hargrave PA. The structure of rhodopsin and the rod outer segment disc membrane. Trends Biochem Sci 1983;8:128–31.
395. Bitensky MW, Wheeler DA, Yamazaki A. Cyclic-nucleotide metabolism in vertebrate photoreceptors – a remarkable analogy and an unraveling enigma. Curr Topics Membrane Transport 1981;15:237–71.
396. McWilliam P, Farrar GJ, Kenna P, et al. Autosomal dominant retinitis pigmentosa (ADRP): localization of an ADRP gene to the long arm of chromosome 3. Genomics 1989;5:619–22.
397. Dryja TP, McGee TL, Reichel E, et al. A point mutation of the rhodopsin gene in one form of retinitis pigmentosa. Nature 1990;343:364–6.
398. Farrar GJ, Findlay JBC, Kumar-Singh R, et al. Autosomal dominant retinitis pigmentosa: a novel mutation in the rhodopsin gene in the original 3q linked family. Hum Mol Genet 1992;1:769–71.

399. Friedman JS, Ray JW, Waseem N, et al. Mutations in a BTB-Kelch protein, KLHL7, cause autosomal-dominant retinitis pigmentosa. Am J Hum Genet 2009;84:792–800.
400. Sung C-H, Davenport CM, Hennessey JC, et al. Rhodopsin mutations in autosomal dominant retinitis pigmentosa. Proc Natl Acad Sci U S A 1991;88:6481–5.
401. Marmor MF. Fundus albipunctatus: a clinical study of the fundus lesions, the physiologic deficit, and the vitamin A metabolism. Doc Ophthalmol Adv Ophthalmol 1977;43:277–302.
402. Kawano H, Hotta Y, Fujiki K, et al. [A study on the rhodopsin gene in Japanese retinitis pigmentosa - screening of mutation by restriction endonucreases and frequencies of DNA polymorphisms.] Nihon Ganka Gakkai Zasshi 1995;99:1151–7.
403. Chan WM, Yeung KY, Pang CP, et al. Rhodopsin mutations in Chinese patients with retinitis pigmentosa. Br J Ophthalmol 2001;85:1046–8.
404. Gandra M, Anandula V, Authiappan V, et al. Retinitis pigmentosa: mutation analysis of RHO, PRPF31, RP1, and IMPDH1 genes in patients from India. Mol Vision 2008;14:1105–13.
405. Kim KJ, Kim C, Bok J, et al. Spectrum of rhodopsin mutations in Korean patients with retinitis pigmentosa. Mol Vision 2011;17:844–53.
406. van Soest S, Westerveld A, de Jong PTVM, et al. Retinitis pigmentosa: defined from a molecular point of view. Surv Ophthalmol 1999;43:321–34.
407. Dryja TP, McGee TL, Hahn LB, et al. Mutations within the rhodopsin gene in patients with autosomal dominant retinitis pigmentosa. N Engl J Med 1990;323:1302–7.
408. Fishman GA, Stone EM, Gilbert LD, et al. Ocular findings associated with a rhodopsin gene codon 106 mutation: glycine-to-arginine change in autosomal dominant retinitis pigmentosa. Arch Ophthalmol 1992;110:646–53.
409. Fishman GA, Stone EM, Sheffield VC, et al. Ocular findings associated with rhodopsin gene codon 17 and codon 182 transition mutations in dominant retinitis pigmentosa. Arch Ophthalmol 1992;110:54–62.
410. Kranich H, Bartowski S, Denton MJ, et al. Autosomal dominant "sector" retinitis pigmentosa due to a point mutation predicting an Asn-15-Ser substitution of rhodopsin. Hum Mol Genet 1993;2:813–4.
411. Berson EL, Rosner B, Sandberg MA, et al. Ocular findings in patients with autosomal dominant retinitis pigmentosa and rhodopsin, proline-347-leucine. Am J Ophthalmol 1991;111:614–23.
412. Restagno G, Maghtheh M, Bhattacharya S, et al. A large deletion at the 3′ end of the rhodopsin gene in an Italian family with a diffuse form of autosomal dominant retinitis pigmentosa. Hum Mol Genet 1993;2:207–8.
413. Berson EL, Rosner B, Sandberg MA, et al. Ocular findings in patients with autosomal dominant retinitis pigmentosa and a rhodopsin gene defect (Pro-23-His). Arch Ophthalmol 1991;109:92–101.
414. Oh KT, Longmuir R, Oh DM, et al. Comparison of the clinical expression of retinitis pigmentosa associated with rhodopsin mutations at codon 347 and codon 23. Am J Ophthalmol 2003;136:306–13.
415. Sieving PA, Richards JE, Naarendorf F, et al. Dark-light: model for nightblindness from the human rhodopsin Gly-90 → Asp mutation. Proc Natl Acad Sci U S A 1995;92:880–4.
416. Sandberg MA, Weigel-DiFranco C, Dryja TP, et al. Clinical expression correlates with location of rhodopsin mutation in dominant retinitis pigmentosa. Invest Ophthalmol Vis Sci 1995;36:1934–42.
417. Berson EL, Rosner B, Weigel-DiFranco C, et al. Disease progression in patients with dominant retinitis pigmentosa and rhodopsin mutations. Invest Ophthalmol Vis Sci 2002;43:3027–36.
418. Robinson PR, Cohen GB, Zhukovsky EA, et al. Constitutively active mutants of rhodopsin. Neuron 1992;9:719–25.
419. Li T, Franson WK, Gordon JW, et al. Constitutive activation of phototransduction by K296E opsin is not a cause of photoreceptor degeneration. Proc Natl Acad Sci U S A 1995;92:3551–5.
420. Farrar GJ, Kenna P, Jordan SA, et al. A three-base-pair deletion in the peripherin-*RDS* gene in one form of retinitis pigmentosa. Nature 1991;354:478–80.
421. Kajiwara K, Hahn LB, Mukai S, et al. Mutations in the human retinal degeneration slow gene in autosomal dominant retinitis pigmentosa. Nature 1991;354:480–3.
422. Weleber RG. Phenotypic variation in patients with mutations in the peripherin/RDS gene. Dig J Ophthalmol 1999;5:1–8.
423. Dryja TP, Hahn LB, Kajiwara K, et al. Dominant and digenic mutations in the *peripherin/RDS* and *ROM1* genes in retinitis pigmentosa. Invest Ophthalmol Vis Sci 1997;38:1972–82.
424. Ma J, Norton JC, Allen AC, et al. Retinal degeneration slow (rds) in mouse results from simple insertion of a t haplotype-specific element into protein-coding exon II. Genomics 1995;28:212–9.
425. Arikawa K, Molday LL, Molday RS, et al. Localization of peripherin/rds in the disk membranes of cone and rod photoreceptors: relationship to disk membrane morphogenesis and retinal degeneration. J Cell Biol 1992;116:659–67.
426. Bessant DA, Payne AM, Mitton KP, et al. A mutation in NRL is associated with autosomal dominant retinitis pigmentosa. Nat Genet 1999;21:355–6.
427. DeAngelis MM, Grimsby JL, Sandberg MA, et al. Novel mutations in the NRL gene and associated clinical findings in patients with dominant retinitis pigmentosa. Arch Ophthalmol 2002;120:369–75.
428. Keen TJ, Hims MM, McKie AB, et al. Mutations in a protein target of the Pim-1 kinase associated with the RP9 form of autosomal dominant retinitis pigmentosa. Eur J Hum Genet 2002;10:245–9.
429. Wada Y, Abe T, Takeshita T, et al. Mutation of human retinal fascin gene (*FSCN2*) causes autosomal dominant retinitis pigmentosa. Invest Ophthalmol Vis Sci 2001;42:2395–400.
430. Farber DB. From mice to men: the cyclic GMP phosphodiesterase gene in vision and disease. The Proctor Lecture. Invest Ophthalmol Vis Sci 1995;36:263–75.
431. Gal A, Orth U, Baehr W, et al. Heterozygous missense mutation in the rod cGMP phosphodiesterase beta-subunit gene in autosomal dominant stationary night blindness. Nat Genet 1994;7:551.
432. Yau KW. Phototransduction mechanism in retinal rods and cones. The Friedenwald Lecture. Invest Ophthalmol Vis Sci 1994;35:9–32.
433. Dryja TP, Finn JT, Peng Y-W, et al. Mutations in the gene encoding the α subunit of the rod cGMP-gated channel in autosomal recessive retinitis pigmentosa. Proc Natl Acad Sci U S A 1995;92:10177–81.
434. Saari JC, Bredberg DL, Noy N. Control of substrate flow at a branch in the visual cycle. Biochemistry 1994;33:3106–12.
435. Maw MA, Kennedy B, Knight A, et al. Mutation of the gene encoding cellular retinaldehyde-binding protein in autosomal recessive retinitis pigmentosa. Nat Genet 1997;17:198–200.
436. Morimura H, Berson EL, Dryja TP. Recessive mutations in the RLBP1 gene encoding cellular retinaldehyde-binding protein in a form of retinitis punctata albescens. Invest Ophthalmol Vis Sci 1999;40:1000–4.
437. Burstedt MS, Forsman-Semb K, Golovleva I, et al. Ocular phenotype of Bothnia dystrophy, an autosomal recessive retinitis pigmentosa associated with an R234W mutation in the *RLBP1* gene. Arch Ophthalmol 2001;119:260–7.
438. Eichers ER, Green JS, Stockton DW, et al. Newfoundland rod–cone dystrophy, an early-onset retinal dystrophy, is caused by splice-junction mutations in *RLBP1*. Am J Hum Genet 2002;70:955–64.
439. Hagstrom SA, Duyao M, North MA, et al. Retinal degeneration in *tulp1–/–* mice: vesicular accumulation in the interphotoreceptor matrix. Invest Ophthalmol Vis Sci 1999;40:2795–802.
440. Banerjee P, Kleyn PW, Knowles JA, et al. *TULP1* mutation in two extended Dominican kindreds with autosomal recessive retinitis pigmentosa. Nat Genet 1998;18:177–9.
441. D'Cruz PM, Yasumura D, Weir J, et al. Mutation of the receptor tyrosine kinase gene Mertk in the retinal dystrophic RCS rat. Hum Mol Genet 2000;9:645–51.
442. Gal A, Li Y, Thompson DA, et al. Mutations in *MERTK*, the human orthologue of the RCS rat retinal dystrophy gene, cause retinitis pigmentosa. Nat Genet 2000;26:270–1.
443. Meindl A, Dry K, Herrmann K, et al. A gene (*RPGR*) with homology to the *RCC1* guanine nucleotide exchange factor is mutated in X-linked retinitis pigmentosa (RP3). Nat Genet 1996;13:35–42.
444. Fujita R, Buraczynska M, Gieser L, et al. Analysis of the *RPGR* gene in 11 pedigrees with the retinitis pigmentosa type 3 genotype: paucity of mutations in the coding region but splice defects in two families. Am J Hum Genet 1997;61:571–80.
445. Jacobson SG, Buraczynska M, Milam AH, et al. Disease expression in X-linked retinitis pigmentosa caused by a putative null mutation in the *RPGR* gene. Invest Ophthalmol Vis Sci 1997;38:1983–97.
446. Andréasson S, Ponjavic V, Abrahamson M, et al. Phenotypes in three Swedish families with X-linked retinitis pigmentosa caused by different mutations in the *RPGR* gene. Am J Ophthalmol 1997;124:95–102.
447. Buraczynska M, Wu W, Fujita R, et al. Spectrum of mutations in the *RPGR* gene that are identified in 20% of families with X-linked retinitis pigmentosa. Am J Hum Genet 1997;61:1287–92.
448. Vervoort R, Lennon A, Bird AC, et al. Mutational hot spot within a new RPGR exon in X-linked retinitis pigmentosa. Nat Genet 2000;25:462–6.
449. Demirci FY, Rigatti BW, Wen G, et al. X-linked cone–rod dystrophy (locus COD1): identification of mutations in RPGR exon ORF15. Am J Hum Genet 2002;70:1049–53.
450. Ayyagari R, Mandal MN, Karoukis AJ, et al. Late-onset macular degeneration and long anterior lens zonules result from a CTRP5 gene mutation. Invest Ophthalmol Vis Sci 2005;46:3363–71.
451. Schwahn U, Lenzner S, Dong J, et al. Positional cloning of the gene for X-linked retinitis pigmentosa 2. Nat Genet 1998;19:327–32.
452. Rosenberg T, Schwahn U, Feil S, et al. Genotype–phenotype correlation in X-linked retinitis pigmentosa 2 (RP2). Ophthalmic Genet 1999;20:161–72.
453. Bader I, Brandau O, Achatz H, et al. X-linked retinitis pigmentosa: *RPGR* mutations in most families with definite X linkage and clustering of mutations in a short sequence stretch of exon ORF15. Invest Ophthalmol Vis Sci 2003;44:1458–63.
454. Flaxel CJ, Jay M, Thiselton DL, et al. Difference between RP2 and RP3 phenotypes in X linked retinitis pigmentosa. Br J Ophthalmol 1998;83:1144–8.
455. Goldberg AF, Loewen CJ, Molday RS. Cysteine residues of photoreceptor peripherin/rds: role in subunit assembly and autosomal dominant retinitis pigmentosa. Biochemistry 1998;37:680–5.
456. Travis GH, Sutcliffe JG, Bok D. The retinal degeneration slow (rds) gene product is a photoreceptor disc membrane-associated glycoprotein. Neuron 1991;6:61–70.
457. Moritz OL, Molday RS. Molecular cloning, membrane topology, and localization of bovine rom-1 in rod and cone photoreceptor cells. Invest Ophthalmol Vis Sci 1996;37:352–62.
458. Corless JM, Fetter RD. Structural features of the terminal loop region of frog retinal rod outer segment disk membranes: III. Implications of the terminal

loop complex for disk morphogenesis, membrane fusion, and cell surface interactions. J Comp Neurol 1987;257:24–38.
459. Kajiwara K, Berson EL, Dryja TP. Digenic retinitis pigmentosa due to mutations at the unlinked peripherin/*RDS* and *ROM1* loci. Science 1994;264: 1604–8.
460. Bascom RA, Liu L, Heckenlively JR, et al. Mutation analysis of the ROM1 gene in retinitis pigmentosa. Hum Mol Genet 1995;4:1895–902.
461. Adato A, Weil D, Kalinski H, et al. Mutation profile of all 49 exons of the human myosin VIIA gene, and haplotype analysis, in Usher 1B families from diverse origins. Am J Hum Genet 1997;61:813–21.
462. Bitner-Glindzicz M, Lindley KJ, Rutland P, et al. A recessive contiguous gene deletion causing infantile hyperinsulinism, enteropathy and deafness identifies the Usher type 1C gene. Nat Genet 2000;26:56–60.
463. Ouyang XM, Xia XJ, Verpy E, et al. Mutations in the alternatively spliced exons of USH1C cause non-syndromic recessive deafness. Hum Genet 2002; 111:26–30.
464. Bolz H, von Brederlow B, Ramirez A, et al. Mutation of CDH23, encoding a new member of the cadherin gene family, causes Usher syndrome type 1D. Nat Genet 2001;27:108–12.
465. Bork JM, Peters LM, Riazuddin S, et al. Usher syndrome 1D and non-syndromic autosomal recessive deafness DFNB12 are caused by allelic mutations of the novel cadherin-like gene CDH23. Am J Hum Genet 2001;68: 26–37.
466. Di Palma F, Holme RH, Bryda EC, et al. Mutations in Cdh23, encoding a new type of cadherin, cause stereocilia disorganization in waltzer, the mouse model for Usher syndrome type 1D. Nat Genet 2001;27:103–7.
467. Boeda B, El-Amraoui A, Bahloul A, et al. Myosin VIIa, harmonin and cadherin 23, three Usher I gene products that cooperate to shape the sensory hair cell bundle. EMBO j 2002;21:6689–99.
468. Siemens J, Kazmierczak P, Reynolds A, et al. The Usher syndrome proteins cadherin 23 and harmonin form a complex by means of PDZ-domain interactions. Proc Natl Acad Sci USA 2002;99:14946–51.
469. Ahmed ZM, Riazuddin S, Bernstein SL, et al. Mutations of the protocadherin gene PCDH15 cause Usher syndrome type 1F. Am J Hum Genet 2001; 69:25–34.
470. Ahmed ZM, Riazuddin S, Ahmad J, et al. PCDH15 is expressed in the neurosensory epithelium of the eye and ear and mutant alleles are responsible for both USH1F and DFNB23. Hum Mol Genet 2003;12:3215–23.
471. Alagramam KN, Murcia CL, Kwon HY, et al. The mouse Ames waltzer hearing-loss mutant is caused by mutation of Pcdh15, a novel protocadherin gene. Nat Genet 2001;27:99–102.
472. Weil D, El-Amraoui A, Masmoudi S, et al. Usher syndrome type I G (USH1G) is caused by mutations in the gene encoding SANS, a protein that associates with the USH1C protein, harmonin. Hum Mol Genet 2003;12:463–71.
473. Eudy JD, Weston MD, Yao S, et al. Mutation of a gene encoding a protein with extracellular matrix motifs in Usher syndrome type IIa. Science 1998;280: 1753–7.
474. Joensuu T, Hämäläinen R, Yuan B, et al. Mutations in a novel gene with transmembrane domains underlie Usher syndrome type 3. Am J Hum Genet 2001;69:673–84.
475. Adato A, Vreugde S, Joensuu T, et al. USH3A transcripts encode clarin-1, a four-transmembrane-domain protein with a possible role in sensory synapses. Eur J Hum Genet 2002;10:339–50.
476. Pennings RJ, Fields RR, Huygen PL, et al. Usher syndrome type III can mimic other types of Usher syndrome. Ann Otol Rhinol Laryngol 2003;112: 525–30.
477. Berger W, Kloeckener-Gruissem B, Neidhardt J. The molecular basis of human retinal and vitreoretinal diseases. Prog Retin Eye Res 2010;29:335–75.
478. Hosch J, Lorenz B, Stieger K. RPGR: role in the photoreceptor cilium, human retinal disease, and gene therapy. Ophthalm Genet 2011;32:1–11.
479. Rosenfeld PJ, Cowley GS, McGee TL, et al. A *null* mutation in the rhodopsin gene causes rod photoreceptor dysfunction and autosomal recessive retinitis pigmentosa. Nat Genet 1992;1:209–13.
480. Rosenfeld PJ, Hahn LB, Sandberg MA, et al. Low incidence of retinitis pigmentosa among heterozygous carriers of a specific rhodopsin splice site mutation. Invest Ophthalmol Vis Sci 1995;36:2186–92.
481. Liu X, Garriga P, Khorana HG. Structure and function in rhodopsin: correct folding and misfolding in two point mutants in the intradiscal domain of rhodopsin identified in retinitis pigmentosa. Proc Natl Acad Sci U S A 1996;93:4554–9.
482. Garriga P, Liu X, Khorana HG. Structure and function in rhodopsin: correct folding and misfolding in point mutants at and in proximity to the site of the retinitis pigmentosa mutation Leu-125 →?Arg in the transmembrane helix C. Proc Natl Acad Sci U S A 1996;93:4560–4.
483. Sung C-H, Schneider BG, Agarwal N, et al. Functional heterogeneity of mutant rhodopsins responsible for autosomal dominant retinitis pigmentosa. Proc Natl Acad Sci U S A 1991;88:8840–4.
484. Apfelstedt-Sylla E, Kunisch M, Horn M, et al. Ocular findings in a family with autosomal dominant retinitis pigmentosa and a frameshift mutation altering the carboxyl terminal sequence of rhodopsin. Br J Ophthalmol 1993;77: 495–501.
485. Hastings ML, Krainer AR. Functions of SR proteins in the U12-dependent AT-AC pre-mRNA splicing pathway. Rna 2001;7:471–82.
486. Will CL, Luhrmann R. Spliceosomal UsnRNP biogenesis, structure and function. Curr Opin Cell Biol 2001;13:290–301.
487. Brown JD, Beggs JD. Roles of PRP8 protein in the assembly of splicing complexes. EMBO J 1992;11:3721–9.
488. Teigelkamp S, Newman AJ, Beggs JD. Extensive interactions of PRP8 protein with the 5′ and 3′ splice sites during splicing suggest a role in stabilization of exon alignment by U5 snRNA. EMBO J 1995;14:2602–12.
489. Collins CA, Guthrie C. The question remains: is the spliceosome a ribozyme? Nat Struct Biol 2000;7:850–4.
490. McKie AB, McHale JC, Keen TJ, et al. Mutations in the pre-mRNA splicing factor gene *PRPC8* in autosomal dominant retinitis pigmentosa (RP13). Hum Mol Genet 2001;10:1555–62.
491. Greenberg J, Goliath R, Beighton P, et al. A new locus for autosomal dominant retinitis pigmentosa on the short arm of chromosome 17. Hum Mol Genet 1994;3:915–8.
492. Vithana EN, Abu-Safieh L, Allen MJ, et al. A human homolog of yeast pre-mRNA splicing gene, PRP31, underlies autosomal dominant retinitis pigmentosa on chromosome 19q13.4 (RP11). Mol Cell 2001;8:375–81.
493. Makarova OV, Makarov EM, Liu S, et al. Protein 61K, encoded by a gene (PRPF31) linked to autosomal dominant retinitis pigmentosa, is required for U4/U6*U5 tri-snRNP formation and pre-mRNA splicing. Embo J 2002;21: 1148–57.
494. Evans K, Al-Maghtheh M, Fitzke FW, et al. Bimodal expressivity in dominant retinitis pigmentosa genetically linked to chromosome 19q. Br J Ophthalmol 1995;79:841–6.
495. Moore AT, Fitzke F, Jay M, et al. Autosomal dominant retinitis pigmentosa with apparent incomplete penetrance: a clinical, electrophysiological, psychophysical, and molecular genetic study. Br J Ophthalmol 1993;77:473–9.
496. McGee TL, Devoto M, Ott J, et al. Evidence that the penetrance of mutations at the RP11 locus causing dominant retinitis pigmentosa is influenced by a gene linked to the homologous RP11 allele. Am J Hum Genet 1997;61: 1059–66.
497. Chakarova CF, Hims MM, Bolz H, et al. Mutations in HPRP3, a third member of pre-mRNA splicing factor genes, implicated in autosomal dominant retinitis pigmentosa. Hum Mol Genet 2002;11:87–92.
498. Horowitz DS, Kobayashi R, Krainer AR. A new cyclophilin and the human homologues of yeast Prp3 and Prp4 form a complex associated with U4/U6 snRNPs. Rna 1997;3:1374–87.
499. Anthony JG, Weidenhammer EM, Woolford JL, Jr. The yeast Prp3 protein is a U4/U6 snRNP protein necessary for integrity of the U4/U6 snRNP and the U4/U6.U5 tri-snRNP. Rna 1997;3:1143–52.
500. Baehr W, Chen CK. RP11 and RP13: unexpected gene loci. Trends Mol Med 2001;7:484–6.
501. Kuhn AN, Reichl EM, Brow DA. Distinct domains of splicing factor Prp8 mediate different aspects of spliceosome activation. Proc Natl Acad Sci USA 2002;99:9145–9.
502. Murga-Zamalloa C, Swaroop A, Khanna H. Multiprotein complexes of retinitis pigmentosa GTPase regulator (RPGR), a ciliary protein mutated in X-linked retinitis pigmentosa (XLRP). Adv Exp Med Biol 2010;664:105–14.
503. Hong DH, Pawlyk B, Sokolov M, et al. RPGR isoforms in photoreceptor connecting cilia and the transitional zone of motile cilia. Invest Ophthalmol Vis Sci 2003;44:2413–21.
504. Hong DH, Pawlyk BS, Shang J, et al. A retinitis pigmentosa GTPase regulator (RPGR)-deficient mouse model for X-linked retinitis pigmentosa (RP3). Proc Natl Acad Sci USA 2000;97:3649–54.
505. Khanna H, Hurd TW, Lillo C, et al. RPGR-ORF15, which is mutated in retinitis pigmentosa, associates with SMC1, SMC3, and microtubule transport proteins. J Biol Chem 2005;280:33580–7.
506. Mavlyutov TA, Zhao H, Ferreira PA. Species-specific subcellular localization of RPGR and RPGRIP isoforms: implications for the phenotypic variability of congenital retinopathies among species. Hum Mol Genet 2002;11:1899–907.
507. Adato A, Michel V, Kikkawa Y, et al. Interactions in the network of Usher syndrome type 1 proteins. Hum Mol Genet 2005;14:347–56.
508. Iannaccone A, Wang X, Jablonski MM, et al. Increasing evidence for syndromic phenotypes associated with RPGR mutations. Am J Ophthalmol 2004;137:785–6; author reply 6.
509. Wright AF, Shu X. X-linked retinal dystrophies and microtubular functions within the retina. Ophthalmol Res 2007:257–67.
510. Saihan Z, Webster AR, Luxon L, et al. Update on Usher syndrome. Curr Opin Neurol 2009;22:19–27.
511. Liu X, Bulgakov OV, Darrow KN, et al. Usherin is required for maintenance of retinal photoreceptors and normal development of cochlear hair cells. Proc Natl Acad Sci USA 2007;104:4413–8.
512. Pan L, Yan J, Wu L, et al. Assembling stable hair cell tip link complex via multidentate interactions between harmonin and cadherin 23. Proc Natl Acad Sci USA 2009;106:5575–80.
513. Yan D, Liu XZ. Genetics and pathological mechanisms of Usher syndrome. J Hum Genet 2010;55:327–35.
514. Delprat B, Michel V, Goodyear R, et al. Myosin XVa and whirlin, two deafness gene products required for hair bundle growth, are located at the stereocilia tips and interact directly. Hum Mol Genet 2005;14:401–10.
515. Muller U. Cadherins and mechanotransduction by hair cells. Curr Opin Cell Biol 2008;20:557–66.
516. Yan D, Li F, Hall ML, et al. An isoform of GTPase regulator DOCK4 localizes to the stereocilia in the inner ear and binds to harmonin (USH1C). J Mol Biol 2006;357:755–64.
517. Rhodes CR, Hertzano R, Fuchs H, et al. A Myo7a mutation cosegregates with stereocilia defects and low-frequency hearing impairment. Mamm Genome 2004;15:686–97.
518. Roepman R, Wolfrum U. Protein networks and complexes in photoreceptor cilia. Subcell Biochem 2007;43:209–35.

519. Reiners J, Nagel-Wolfrum K, Jurgens K, et al. Molecular basis of human Usher syndrome: deciphering the meshes of the Usher protein network provides insights into the pathomechanisms of the Usher disease. Exp Eye Res 2006; 83:97–119.
520. Jin H, Nachury MV. The BBSome. Curr Biol 2009;19:R472–3.
521. Nachury MV, Seeley ES, Jin H. Trafficking to the ciliary membrane: how to get across the periciliary diffusion barrier? Annu Rev Cell Dev Biol 2010;26:59–87.
522. Jin H, White SR, Shida T, et al. The conserved Bardet–Biedl syndrome proteins assemble a coat that traffics membrane proteins to cilia. Cell 2010;141: 1208–19.
523. Locke M, Tinsley CL, Benson MA, et al. TRIM32 is an E3 ubiquitin ligase for dysbindin. Hum Mol Genet 2009;18:2344–58.
524. Schulein R. The early stages of the intracellular transport of membrane proteins: clinical and pharmacological implications. Rev Physiol Biochem Pharmacol 2004;151:45–91.
525. Chinchore Y, Mitra A, Dolph PJ. Accumulation of rhodopsin in late endosomes triggers photoreceptor cell degeneration. PLoS Genet 2009;5:e1000377.
526. Deretic D, Williams AH, Ransom N, et al. Rhodopsin C terminus, the site of mutations causing retinal disease, regulates trafficking by binding to ADP-ribosylation factor 4 (ARF4). Proc Natl Acad Sci USA 2005;102:3301–6.
527. Chen J, Makino CL, Peachey NS, et al. Mechanisms of rhodopsin inactivation in vivo as revealed by a COOH-terminal truncation mutant. Science 1995;267:374–7.
528. Sung CH, Tai AW. Rhodopsin trafficking and its role in retinal dystrophies. Int Rev Cytol 2000;195:215–67.
529. Luthert PJ, Chong NH. Photoreceptor rescue. Eye 1998;12:591–6.
530. Danesh-Meyer HV, Levin LA. Neuroprotection: extrapolating from neurologic diseases to the eye. Am J Ophthalmol 2009;148:186–91 e2.
531. Yoshizawa K, Kiuchi K, Nambu H, et al. Caspase-3 inhibitor transiently delays inherited retinal degeneration in C3H mice carrying the rd gene. Graefes Arch Clin Exp Ophthalmol 2002;240:214–9.
532. Murakami Y, Miller JW, Vavvas DG. RIP kinase-mediated necrosis as an alternative mechanisms of photoreceptor death. Oncotarget 2011;2:497–509.
533. Sancho-Pelluz J, Arango-Gonzalez B, Kustermann S, et al. Photoreceptor cell death mechanisms in inherited retinal degeneration. Mol Neurobiol 2008;38:253–69.
534. Milam AH, Li Z-Y, Fariss RN. Histology of the human retina in retinitis pigmentosa. Prog Retin Eye Res 1998;17:175–205.
535. Milam AH, Li Z-Y, Cideciyan AV, et al. Clinicopathologic effects of the Q64ter rhodopsin mutation in retinitis pigmentosa. Invest Ophthalmol Vis Sci 1996; 37:753–65.
536. Naash ML, Peachey NS, Li ZY, et al. Light-induced acceleration of photoreceptor degeneration in transgenic mice expressing mutant rhodopsin. Invest Ophthalmol Vis Sci 1996;37:775–82.
537. Roof DJ, Adamian M, Hayes A. Rhodopsin accumulation at abnormal sites in retinas of mice with a human P23H rhodopsin transgene. Invest Ophthalmol Vis Sci 1994;35:4049–62.
538. Milam AH, Jacobson SG. Photoreceptor rosettes with blue cone opsin immunoreactivity in retinitis pigmentosa. Ophthalmology 1990;97:1620–31.
539. Li ZY, Jacobson SG, Milam AH. Autosomal dominant retinitis pigmentosa caused by the threonine-17-methionine rhodopsin mutation: retinal histopathology and immunocytochemistry. Exp Eye Res 1994;58:397–408.
540. Daiger SP, Sullivan AS, Rodriguez JA. Correlation of phenotype with genotype in inherited retinal degeneration. Behav Brain Sci 1995;18:452–67.
541. Li T, Snyder WK, Olsson JE, et al. Transgenic mice carrying the dominant rhodopsin mutation P347S: evidence for defective vectorial transport of rhodopsin to the outer segments. Proc Natl Acad Sci USA 1996;93:14176–81.
542. Petters RM, Alexander CA, Wells KD, et al. Genetically engineered large animal model for studying cone photoreceptor survival and degeneration in retinitis pigmentosa. Nat Biotechnol 1997;15:965–70.
543. Li ZY, Wong F, Chang JH, et al. Rhodopsin transgenic pigs as a model for human retinitis pigmentosa. Invest Ophthalmol Vis Sci 1998;39:808–19.
544. Clarke G, Collins RA, Leavitt BR, et al. A one-hit model of cell death in inherited neuronal degenerations. Nature 2000;406:195–9.
545. Clarke G, Lumsden CJ, McInnes RR. Inherited neurodegenerative diseases: the one-hit model of neurodegeneration. Hum Mol Genet 2001;10:2269–75.
546. Pacione LR, Szego MJ, Ikeda S, et al. Progress toward understanding the genetic and biochemical mechanisms of inherited photoreceptor degenerations. Annu Rev Neurosci 2003;26:657–700.
547. Li ZY, Possin DE, Milam AH. Histopathology of bone spicule pigmentation in retinitis pigmentosa. Ophthalmology 1995;102:805–16.
548. Meyer KT, Heckenlively JR, Spitznas M, et al. Dominant retinitis pigmentosa. A clinicopathologic correlation. Ophthalmology 1982;89:1414–24.
549. Duvall J, McKechnie NM, Lee WR, et al. Extensive subretinal pigment epithelial deposit in two brothers suffering from dominant retinitis pigmentosa. A histopathological study. Graefes Arch Clin Exp Ophthalmol 1986;224: 299–309.
550. Brosnahan DM, Kennedy SM, Converse CA, et al. Pathology of hereditary retinal degeneration associated with hypobetalipoproteinemia. Ophthalmology 1994;101:38–45.
551. Del Priore LV, Kaplan HJ, Hornbeck R, et al. Retinal pigment epithelial debridement as a model for the pathogenesis and treatment of macular degeneration. Am J Ophthalmol 1996;122:629–43.
552. Eisenfeld AJ, Bunt-Milam AH, Sarthy PV. Muller cell expression of glial fibrillary acidic protein after genetic and experimental photoreceptor degeneration in the rat retina. Invest Ophthalmol Vis Sci 1984;25:1321–8.
553. Milam AH, De Leeuw AM, Gaur VP, et al. Immunolocalization of cellular retinoic acid binding protein to Muller cells and/or a subpopulation of GABA-positive amacrine cells in retinas of different species. J Comp Neurol 1990;296:123–9.
554. Sastry SM, Li ZY, Milam AH. Epiretinal membranes in retinitis pigmentosa. Invest Ophthalmol Vis Sci 1996;37:4789.
555. Szamier RB. Ultrastructure of the preretinal membrane in retinitis pigmentosa. Invest Ophthalmol Vis Sci 1981;21:227–36.
556. Thanos S, Moore S, Hong Y-M. Retinal microglia. Prog Retin Eye Res 1996;15:331–61.
557. Flannery JG, Farber DB, Bird AC, et al. Degenerative changes in a retina affected with autosomal dominant retinitis pigmentosa. Invest Ophthalmol Vis Sci 1989;30:191–211.
558. Santos A, Humayun MS, de Juan E, Jr., et al. Preservation of the inner retina in retinitis pigmentosa. A morphometric analysis. Arch Ophthalmol 1997;115: 511–5.
559. Newman NM, Stevens RA, Heckenlively JR. Nerve fibre layer loss in diseases of the outer retinal layer. Br J Ophthalmol 1987;71:21–6.
560. Villegas-Perez MP, Vidal-Sanz M, Lund RD. Mechanism of retinal ganglion cell loss in inherited retinal dystrophy. Neuroreport 1996;7:1995–9.
561. Gartner S, Henkind P. Pathology of retinitis pigmentosa. Ophthalmology 1982;89:1425–32.
562. Marc RE, Jones BW, Watt CB, et al. Neural remodeling in retinal degeneration. Prog Retin Eye Res 2003;22:607–55.
563. Jones BW, Watt CB, Frederick JM, et al. Retinal remodeling triggered by photoreceptor degenerations. J Comp Neurol 2003;464:1–16.
564. Marc RE, Jones BW, Anderson JR, et al. Neural reprogramming in retinal degeneration. Invest Ophthalmol Vis Sci 2007;48:3364–71.
565. Puthussery T, Taylor WR. Functional changes in inner retinal neurons in animal models of photoreceptor degeneration. Adv Exp Med Biol 2010;664: 525–32.
566. Li Z-Y, Kljavin IJ, Milam AH. Rod photoreceptor neurite sprouting in retinitis pigmentosa. J Neurosci 1995;15:5429–38.
567. Gregory-Evans K, Weleber RG. An eye for an eye: New models of genetic ocular disease. Nature Biotechnology 1997;15:947–8.
568. Bunt-Milam AH, Saari JC, Klock IB, et al. Zonulae adherentes pore size in the external limiting membrane of the rabbit retina. Invest Ophthalmol Vis Sci 1985;26:1377–80.
569. Leveillard T, Mohand-Said S, Lorentz O, et al. Identification and characterization of rod-derived cone viability factor. Nat Genet 2004;36:755–9.
570. Grunwald JE, Maguire AM, Dupont J. Retinal hemodynamics in retinitis pigmentosa. Am J Ophthalmol 1996;122:502–8.
571. Ward MM, Puthussery T, Vessey KA, et al. The role of purinergic receptors in retinal function and disease. Adv Exp Med Biol 2010;664:385–91.
572. Harris HJ. Personal view – genetic counselling – does the terminology matter? Br Med J 1997;315:1241–2.
573. Korsch BM, Negrete VF. Doctor-patient communication. Sci Am 1972;227: 66–74.
574. Michie S, Marteau TM, Bobrow M. Genetic counselling: the psychological impact of meeting patients' expectations. J Med Genet 1997;34:237–41.
575. Clarke A. Is non-directive counselling possible? Lancet 1991;338:998–1001.
576. Kim RY, Fitzke FW, Moore AT, et al. Autosomal dominant retinitis pigmentosa mapping to chromosome 7p exhibits variable expression. Br J Ophthalmol 1995;79:23–7.
577. Evans K, Fryer A, Inglehearn C, et al. Genetic linkage of cone–rod retinal dystrophy to chromosome 19q and evidence for segregation distortion. Nat Genet 1994;6:210–3.
578. Richards RI, Holman K, Friend K, et al. Evidence of founder chromosomes in fragile X syndrome. Nat Genet 1992;1:257–60.
579. Magenis RE, Toth-Fejel S, Allen LJ, et al. Comparison of the 15q deletions in Prader–Willi and Angelman syndromes: specific regions, extent of deletions, parental origin, and clinical consequences. Am J Med Genet 1990;35:333–49.
580. Bird AC. X-linked retinitis pigmentosa. Br J Ophthalmol 1975;59:177–99.
581. Evans K, Gregory CY, Fryer A, et al. The role of molecular genetics in the prenatal diagnosis of retinal dystrophies. Eye 1995;9:24–8.
582. Redmond RM, Graham CA, Kelly ED, et al. Prenatal exclusion of Norrie's disease. Br J Ophthalmol 1992;76:491–3.
583. van den Hurk JAJM, van de Pol TJR, Molloy CM, et al. Detection and chracterization of point mutations in the choroideremia candidate gene by PCR-SSCP analysis and direct DNA sequencing. Am J Hum Genet 1992;50:1195–202.
584. Mehta L, Young ID. Attitudes of Asian families to genetic counselling. J Med Genet 1985;22:413.
585. Pawlowitzki IH, Ruther K, Brunsmann F, et al. Acceptability of prenatal diagnosis for retinitis pigmentosa. Lancet 1986;2:1394–5.
586. Furu T, Kaariainen H, Sankila EM, et al. Attitudes towards prenatal diagnosis and selective abortion among patients with retinitis pigmentosa or choroideremia as well as among their relatives. Clin Genet 1993;43:160–5.
587. Bothe N, Hetzer R. Ophthalmic disorders and job measures of adults with late onset of visual handicap. Klin Monatsbl Augenheilkd 1992;200:237–41.
588. Berson EL, Mehaffey L, Rabin AR. A night vision device as an aid for patients with retinitis pigmentosa. Arch Ophthalmol 1973;90:112–6.
589. Morrissette DL, Marmor MF, Goodrich GL. An evaluation of night vision mobility aids. Ophthalmology 1983;90:1226–30.
590. Berson EL. Light deprivation for early retinitis pigmentosa: a hypothesis. Arch Ophthalmol 1971;85:521–9.
591. Berson EL. Light deprivation and retinitis pigmentosa. Vision res 1980;20: 1179–84.

592. DelBeato P, Tanzilli P, Grenga R, et al. It is useful to perform cataract surgery in retinitis pigmentosa patients? Invest Ophthalmol Vis Sci 1997;38:868.
593. Marmor MF. Visual loss in retinitis pigmentosa. Am J Ophthalmol 1980; 89:692–8.
594. Kogure S, Iljima H. Preoperative evaluation by laser interferometry in cataractous eyes with retinitis pigmentosa. Jpn J Ophthalmol 1993;37:282–6.
595. Newsome DA, Stark Jr WJ., Maumenee IH. Cataract extraction and intraocular lens implantation in patients with retinitis pigmentosa or Usher's syndrome. Arch Ophthalmol 1986;104:852–4.
596. Jackson H, Garway-Heath D, Rosen P, et al. Outcome of cataract surgery in patients with retinitis pigmentosa. Br J Ophthalmol 2001;85:936–8.
597. Hayashi K, Hayashi H, Matsuo K, et al. Anterior capsule contraction and intraocular lens dislocation after implant surgery in eyes with retinitis pigmentosa. Ophthalmology 1998;105:1239–43.
598. Lee HJ, Min SH, Kim TY. Bilateral spontaneous dislocation of intraocular lenses within the capsular bag in a retinitis pigmentosa patient. Korean J Ophthalmol 2004;18:52–7.
599. Davison JA. Capsule contraction syndrome. J Cataract Refract Surg 1993; 19:582–9.
600. Pierrottet C, Carrara M, Orzalesi N. Cataract surgery in retinitis-pigmentosa. Invest Ophthalmol Vis Sci 1995;36:S810.
601. Ozdemir H, Karacorlu M, Karacorlu S. Intravitreal triamcinolone acetonide for treatment of cystoid macular oedema in patients with retinitis pigmentosa. Acta Ophthalmol Scand 2005;83:248–51.
602. Oishi A, Otani A, Sasahara M, et al. Photoreceptor integrity and visual acuity in cystoid macular oedema associated with retinitis pigmentosa. Eye (Lond) 2009;23:1411–6.
603. Adackapara CA, Sunness JS, Dibernardo CW, et al. Prevalence of cystoid macular edema and stability in oct retinal thickness in eyes with retinitis pigmentosa during a 48-week lutein trial. Retina 2008;28:103–10.
604. Hajali M, Fishman GA. The prevalence of cystoid macular oedema on optical coherence tomography in retinitis pigmentosa patients without cystic changes on fundus examination. Eye (Lond) 2009;23:915–9.
605. Sandberg MA, Brockhurst RJ, Gaudio AR, et al. Visual acuity is related to parafoveal retinal thickness in patients with retinitis pigmentosa and macular cysts. Invest Ophthalmol Vis Sci 2008;49:4568–72.
606. Grigoropoulos VG, Emfietzoglou J, Nikolaidis P, et al. Optical coherence tomography findings in patients with retinitis pigmentosa and low visual acuity. Ophthalm Surg Lasers Imaging 2010;41:35–9.
607. Walia S, Fishman GA, Hajali M. Prevalence of cystic macular lesions in patients with Usher II syndrome. Eye (Lond) 2009;23:1206–9.
608. Tsilou ET, Rubin BI, Caruso RC, et al. Usher syndrome clinical types I and II: could ocular symptoms and signs differentiate between the two types? Acta Ophthalmol Scand 2002;80:196–201.
609. Schwartz SB, Aleman TS, Cideciyan AV, et al. Disease expression in Usher syndrome caused by VLGR1 gene mutation (USH2C) and comparison with USH2A phenotype. Invest Ophthalmol Vis Sci 2005;46:734–43.
610. Kuchle M, Nguyen NX, Martus P, et al. Aqueous flare in retinitis pigmentosa. Graefes Arch Clin Exp Ophthalmol 1998;236:426–33.
611. Vinores SA, Kuchle M, Derevjanik NL, et al. Blood–retinal barrier breakdown in retinitis pigmentosa: light and electron microscopic immunolocalization. Histol Histopathol 1995;10:913–23.
612. Mallick KS, Zeimer RC, Fishman GA, et al. Transport of fluorescein in the ocular posterior segment in retinitis pigmentosa. Arch Ophthalmol 1984;102: 691–6.
613. Fishman GA, Cunha-Vaz J, Salzano T. Vitreous fluorophotometry in patients with retinitis pigmentosa. Arch Ophthalmol 1981;99:1202–7.
614. Cunha-Vaz JG, Travassos A. Breakdown of the blood-retinal barriers and cystoid macular edema. Surv Ophthalmol 1984;28(Suppl):485–92.
615. Cox SN, Hay E, Bird AC. Treatment of chronic macular edema with acetazolamide. Arch Ophthalmol 1988;106:1190–5.
616. Heckenlively JR, Jordan BL, Aptsiauri N. Association of antiretinal antibodies and cystoid macular edema in patients with retinitis pigmentosa. Am J Ophthalmol 1999;127:565–73.
617. Wolfensberger TJ, Aptsiauri N, Godley B, et al. [Antiretinal antibodies associated with cystoid macular edema.] Klin Monbl Augenheilkd 2000;216:283–5.
618. Heckenlively JR, Solish AM, Chant SM, et al. Autoimmunity in hereditary retinal degenerations. II. Clinical studies: antiretinal antibodies and fluorescein angiogram findings. Br J Ophthalmol 1985;69:758–64.
619. Chung H, Hwang JU, Kim JG, et al. Optical coherence tomography in the diagnosis and monitoring of cystoid macular edema in patients with retinitis pigmentosa. Retina 2006;26:922–7.
620. Hirakawa H, Iijima H, Gohdo T, et al. Optical coherence tomography of cystoid macular edema associated with retinitis pigmentosa. Am J Ophthalmol 1999;128:185–91.
621. Stanga PE, Downes SM, Ahuja RM, et al. Comparison of optical coherence tomography and fluorescein angiography in assessing macular edema in retinal dystrophies: preliminary results. Int Ophthalmol 2001;23:321–5.
622. Oishi A, Nakamura H, Tatsumi I, et al. Optical coherence tomographic pattern and focal electroretinogram in patients with retinitis pigmentosa. Eye (Lond) 2009;23:299–303.
623. Sandberg MA, Brockhurst RJ, Gaudio AR, et al. The association between visual acuity and central retinal thickness in retinitis pigmentosa. Invest Ophthalmol Vis Sci 2005;46:3349–54.
624. García-Arumí J, Martinez V, Sararols L, et al. Vitreoretinal surgery for cystoid macular edema associated with retinitis pigmentosa. Ophthalmology 2003; 110:1164–9.
625. Newsome DA, Blacharski PA. Grid photocoagulation for macular edema in patients with retinitis pigmentosa. Am J Ophthalmol 1987;103:161–6.
626. Saraiva VS, Sallum JM, Farah ME. Treatment of cystoid macular edema related to retinitis pigmentosa with intravitreal triamcinolone acetonide. Ophthalmic Surg Lasers Imaging 2003;34:398–400.
627. Scorolli L, Morara M, Meduri A, et al. Treatment of cystoid macular edema in retinitis pigmentosa with intravitreal triamcinolone. Arch Ophthalmol 2007;125:759–64.
628. Forte R, Pannarale L, Iannaccone A, et al. Cystoid macular edema in retinitis pigmentosa - clinical and functional evaluation of patients treated with deflazacort. Invest Ophthalmol Vis Sci 1994;35:1958.
629. Artunay O, Yuzbasioglu E, Rasier R, et al. Intravitreal ranibizumab in the treatment of cystoid macular edema associated with retinitis pigmentosa. J Ocul Pharmacol Ther 2009;25:545–50.
630. Melo GB, Farah ME, Aggio FB. Intravitreal injection of bevacizumab for cystoid macular edema in retinitis pigmentosa. Acta Ophthalmol Scand 2007;85:461–3.
631. Yuzbasioglu E, Artunay O, Rasier R, et al. Intravitreal bevacizumab (Avastin) injection in retinitis pigmentosa. Curr Eye Res 2009;34:231–7.
632. Fishman GA, Gilbert LD, Fiscella RG, et al. Acetazolamide for treatment of chronic macular edema in retinitis pigmentosa. Arch Ophthalmol 1989;107: 1445–52.
633. Heckenlively JR. Grid photocoagulation for macular edema in patients with retinitis pigmentosa. Am J Ophthalmol 1987;104:94–5.
634. Grover S, Fishman GA, Fiscella RG, et al. Efficacy of dorzolamide hydrochloride in the management of chronic cystoid macular edema in patients with retinitis pigmentosa. Retina 1997;17:222–31.
635. Grover S, Apushkin MA, Fishman GA. Topical dorzolamide for the treatment of cystoid macular edema in patients with retinitis pigmentosa. Am J Ophthalmol 2006;141:850–8.
636. Apushkin MA, Fishman GA, Grover S, et al. Rebound of cystoid macular edema with continued use of acetazolamide in patients with retinitis pigmentosa. Retina 2007;27:1112–8.
637. Genead MA, Fishman GA. Efficacy of sustained topical dorzolamide therapy for cystic macular lesions in patients with retinitis pigmentosa and usher syndrome. Arch Ophthalmol 2010;128:1146–50.
638. Thobani A, Fishman GA. The use of carbonic anhydrase inhibitors in the retreatment of cystic macular lesions in retinitis pigmentosa and X-linked retinoschisis. Retina 2011;31:312–5.
639. Fishman GA, Gilbert LD, Anderson RJ, et al. Effect of methazolamide on chronic macular edema in patients with retinitis pigmentosa. Ophthalmology 1994;101:687–93.
640. Orzalesi N, Pierrottet C, Porta A, et al. Long-term treatment of retinitis pigmentosa with acetazolamide. A pilot study. Graefes Arch Clin Exp Ophthalmol 1993;231:254–6.
641. Chen JC, Fitzke FW, Bird AC. Long-term effect of acetazolamide in a patient with retinitis pigmentosa. Invest Ophthalmol Vis Sci 1990;31:1914–8.
642. Kim JE. Intravitreal triamcinolone acetonide for treatment of cystoid macular edema associated with retinitis pigmentosa. Retina 2006;26:1094–6.
643. Querques G, Prascina F, Iaculli C, et al. Intravitreal pegaptanib sodium (Macugen) for refractory cystoid macular edema in pericentral retinitis pigmentosa. Int Ophthalmol 2009;29:103–7.
644. Salom D, Diaz-Llopis M, Garcia-Delpech S, et al. Intravitreal ranibizumab in the treatment of cystoid macular edema associated with retinitis pigmentosa. J Ocul Pharmacol Ther 2010;26:531–2.
645. Gouras P, Carr RE, Gunkel RD. Retinitis pigmentosa in abetalipoproteinaemia: effects of vitamin A. Invest Ophthalmol 1971;10:784–93.
646. Berson EL, Rosner B, Sandberg MA, et al. A randomized trial of supplemental vitamin A and vitamin E supplementation for retinitis pigmentosa. Arch Ophthalmol 1993;111:761–72.
647. Berson EL, Rosner B, Sandberg MA, et al. A randomized trial of vitamin A and vitamin E supplementation for retinitis pigmentosa. Arch Ophthalmol 1993;111:1465–6.
648. Marmor MF. Letter to the editor. Arch Ophthalmol 1993;111:1460–1.
649. Clowes D. Letter to the editor. Arch Ophthalmol 1993;111:1461–2.
650. Fielder AR, Marshall J. Letter to the editor. Arch Ophthalmol 1993;111:1463.
651. Bird AC. Retinal photoreceptor dystrophies: LI. Edward Jackson Memorial Lecture. Am J Ophthalmol 1995;119:543–62.
652. Massof RW, Finkelstein D. Editorial: Supplemental vitamin A retards loss of ERG amplitude in retinitis pigmentosa. Arch Ophthalmol 1993;111:751–4.
653. Massof RW, Finkelstein D. Vitamin A supplementation for retinitis pigmentosa. Arch Ophthalmol 1993;111:1458–9.
654. Bauernfeind JC. The safe use of vitamin A: A report of the International vitamin A consultative group. Washington, D.C: The Nutrition Foundation; 1980 1980.
655. Bendich A, Langseth L. Safety of vitamin A. Am J Clin Nutr 1989;49:358–71.
656. Evans K, Hickey-Dwyer MU. Cleft anterior segment with maternal hypervitaminosis A. Br J Ophthalmol 1991;75:691–2.
657. Rothman KJ, Moore LL, Singer MR, et al. Teratogenicity of high vitamin A intake. N Engl J Med 1995;333:1369–73.
658. Melhus H, Michaelsson K, Kindmark A, et al. Excessive dietary intake of vitamin A is associated with reduced bone mineral density and increased risk for hip fracture. Ann Intern Med 1998;129:770–8.
659. Feskanich D, Singh V, Willett WC, et al. Vitamin A intake and hip fractures among postmenopausal women. Jama 2002;287:47–54.
660. Michaelsson K, Lithell H, Vessby B, et al. Serum retinol levels and the risk of fracture. N Engl J Med 2003;348:287–94.

661. Lips P. Hypervitaminosis A and fractures. N Engl J Med 2003;348:347–9.
662. Geubel AP, De Galocsy C, Alves N, et al. Liver damage caused by therapeutic vitamin A administration: estimate of dose-related toxicity in 41 cases. Gastroenterology 1991;100:1701–9.
663. Sibulesky L, Hayes KC, Pronczuk A, et al. Safety of <7500 RE (<25000 IU) vitamin A daily in adults with retinitis pigmentosa. Am J Clin Nutr 1999;69:656–63.
664. Fliesler SJ, Anderson RE. Chemistry and metabolism of lipids in the vertebrate retina. Prog Lipid Res 1983;22:79–131.
665. Gong J, Rosner B, Rees DG, et al. Plasma docosahexaenoic acid levels in various genetic forms of retinitis pigmentosa. Invest Ophthalmol Vis Sci 1992;33:2596–602.
666. Schaefer EJ, Robins SJ, Patton GM, et al. Red blood cell membrane phosphatidylethanolamine fatty acid content in various forms of retinitis pigmentosa. J lipid res 1995;36:1427–33.
667. Hoffman DR, Uauy R, Birch DG. Red blood cell fatty acid levels in patients with autosomal dominant retinitis pigmentosa. Exp Eye Res 1993;57: 359–68.
668. Connor WE, Weleber RG, DeFrancesco C, et al. Sperm abnormalities in retinitis pigmentosa. Invest Ophthalmol Vis Sci 1997;38:2619–28.
669. Hoffman DR, DeMar JC, Heird WC, et al. Impaired synthesis of DHA in patients with X-linked retinitis pigmentosa. J Lipid Res 2001;42:1395–401.
670. Wheaton DH, Hoffman DR, Locke KG, et al. Biological safety assessment of docosahexaenoic acid supplementation in a randomized clinical trial for X-linked retinitis pigmentosa. Arch Ophthalmol 2003;121:1269–78.
671. Hoffman DR, Locke KG, Wheaton DH, et al. A randomized, placebo-controlled clinical trial of docosahexaenoic acid supplementation for X-linked retinitis pigmentosa. Am J Ophthalmol 2004;137:704–18.
672. Thomson LR, Toyoda Y, Langner A, et al. Elevated retinal zeaxanthin and prevention of light-induced photoreceptor cell death in quail. Invest Ophthalmol Vis Sci 2002;43:3538–49.
673. Aleman TS, Duncan JL, Bieber ML, et al. Macular pigment and lutein supplementation in retinitis pigmentosa and Usher syndrome. Invest Ophthalmol Vis Sci 2001;42:1873–81.
674. Berson EL, Rosner B, Sandberg MA, et al. Clinical trial of docosahexaenoic acid in patients with retinitis pigmentosa receiving vitamin A treatment. Arch Ophthalmol 2004;122:1297–305.
675. Berson EL, Rosner B, Sandberg MA, et al. Further evaluation of docosahexaenoic acid in patients with retinitis pigmentosa receiving vitamin A treatment: subgroup analyses. Arch Ophthalmol 2004;122:1306–14.
676. Berson EL, Rosner B, Sandberg MA, et al. Clinical trial of lutein in patients with retinitis pigmentosa receiving vitamin A. Arch Ophthalmol 2010;128: 403–11.
677. Massof RW, Fishman GA. How strong is the evidence that nutritional supplements slow the progression of retinitis pigmentosa? Arch Ophthalmol 2010; 128:493–5.
678. Kiser AK, Dagnelie G. Reported effects of non-traditional treatments and complementary and alternative medicine by retinitis pigmentosa patients. Clin Exp Optom 2008;91:166–76.
679. Weleber RG. The Cuban experience. False hope for a cure for retinitis pigmentosa. Arch Ophthalmol 1996;114:606–7.
680. Potok A. Ordinary daylight: portrait of an artist going blind. New York: Holt, Rinehart and Winston; 1980.
681. Biro I. Therapeutic experiments in cases of retinitis pigmentosa. Br J Ophthalmol 1939;23:332–42.
682. Gordon DM. The treatment of retinitis pigmentosa with special reference to the Filatov method. Am J Ophthalmol 1947;30:565–80.
683. Katznelson LA, Khoroshilova-Maslova IP, Eliseyeva RF. A new method of treatment of retinitis pigmentosa/pigmentary abiotrophy. Ann Ophthalmol 1990;22:167–72.
684. Birch DG, Anderson JL, Fish GE. Longitudinal measures in children receiving ENCAD for hereditary retinal degeneration. Doc Ophthalmol Adv Ophthalmol 1991;77:185–92.
685. McManus EH, Hartenstine DL, Laties AM, et al. Summary of exchange visit to Helmholtz Institute of Ophthalmology. Bethesda, Maryland: National Eye Institute; 1983.
686. Berson EL, Remulla JF, Rosner B, et al. Evaluation of patients with retinitis pigmentosa receiving electric stimulation, ozonated blood, and ocular surgery in Cuba. Arch Ophthalmol 1996;114:560–3.
687. Berger RW, Haase W, Gerding H. Original papers: Ocular motility disorders after surgery for retinitis pigmentosa 'Cuba-therapy'. Strabismus 1995;3: 13–20.
688. Hetland JG. [Management of retinitis pigmentosa. 8 patients treated for retinitis pigmentosa/Usher syndrome in Cuba.] Tidsskr Nor Laegeforen 1994; 114:1515–6.
689. Bacal DA, Rousta S, Hertle RW, et al. Restrictive strabismus after ocular surgery for retinitis pigmentosa in Cuba. Arch Ophthalmol 1997;115:930–1.
690. Reddy NS, Fouzdar NM. Role of acupuncture in the treatment of 'incurable' retinal diseases. Ind J Ophthalmol 1983;31(Suppl):1043–6.
691. Wu XW, Tang YZ. [Study on treatment of retinitis pigmentosa with traditional Chinese medicine by flicker electroretinogram.] Zhongguo Zhong Xi Yi Jie He Za Zhi 1996;16:336–9.
692. Paskowitz DM, LaVail MM, Duncan JL. Light and inherited retinal degeneration. Br J Ophthalmol 2006;90:1060–6.
693. Cideciyan AV, Hood DC, Huang Y, et al. Disease sequence from mutant rhodopsin allele to rod and cone photoreceptor degeneration in man. Proc Natl Acad Sci USA 1998;95:7103–8.
694. Vaughan DK, Coulibaly SF, Darrow RM, et al. A morphometric study of light-induced damage in transgenic rat models of retinitis pigmentosa. Invest Ophthalmol Vis Sci 2003;44:848–55.
695. Organisciak DT, Darrow RM, Barsalou L, et al. Susceptibility to retinal light damage in transgenic rats with rhodopsin mutations. Invest Ophthalmol Vis Sci 2003;44:486–92.
696. Naash MI, Hollyfield JG, Al-Ubaidi MR, et al. Simulation of human autosomal dominant retinitis pigmentosa in transgenic mice expressing a mutated murine opsine gene. Proc Natl Acad Sci U S A 1993;90:5499–503.
697. Walsh N, van Driel D, Lee D, et al. Multiple vulnerability of photoreceptors to mesopic ambient light in the P23H transgenic rat. Brain Res 2004;1013: 194–203.
698. Bicknell IR, Darrow R, Barsalou L, et al. Alterations in retinal rod outer segment fatty acids and light-damage susceptibility in P23H rats. Mol Vision 2002;8:333–40.
699. Eperjesi F, Fowler CW, Evans BJ. Do tinted lenses or filters improve visual performance in low vision? A review of the literature. Ophthalm Physiol Opt 2002;22:68–77.
700. Naash MI, Al-Ubaidi MR, Hollyfield JG, et al. Simulation of autosomal dominant retinitis pigmentosa in transgenic mice. In: Anderson RE, Hollyfield JG, LaVail MM, editors. Retinal degenerations. New York: Plenum Press; 1993. p. 201–10.
701. Humphries MM, Rancourt D, Farrar GJ, et al. Retinopathy induced in mice by targeted disruption of the rhodopsin gene. Nat Genet 1997;15:216–9.
702. Shen J, Yang X, Dong A, et al. Oxidative damage is a potential cause of cone cell death in retinitis pigmentosa. J Cell Physiol 2005;203:457–64.
703. Lee SY, Usui S, Zafar AB, et al. *N*-Acetylcysteine promotes long-term survival of cones in a model of retinitis pigmentosa. J Cell Physiol 2011;226: 1843–9.
704. Veske A, Nilsson SE, Narfström K, et al. Retinal dystrophy of swedish Briard/ Briard-beagle dogs is due to a 4-bp deletion in RPE65. Genomics 1999;57: 57–61.
705. Kijas JW, Cideciyan AV, Aleman TS, et al. Naturally occurring rhodopsin mutation in the dog causes retinal dysfunction and degeneration mimicking human dominant retinitis pigmentosa. Proc Natl Acad Sci USA 2002;99: 6328–33.
706. Zhang Q, Acland GM, Wu WX, et al. Different *RPGR* exon ORF15 mutations in *Canids* provide insights into photoreceptor cell degeneration. Hum Mol Genet 2002;11:993–1003.
707. Farber DB. From mice to men: the cyclic GMP phosphodiesterase gene in vision and disease. Invest Ophthalmol Vis Sci 1995;36:263–75.
708. Ali RR, Reichel MB, Thrasher AJ, et al. Gene transfer into the mouse retina mediate by an adeno-associated viral vector. Hum Mol Genet 1996;5: 591–4.
709. Mashhour B, Couton D, Perricaudet M, et al. In vivo adenovirus-mediated gene transfer into ocular tissues. Gene Ther 1994;1:122–6.
710. Li T, Adamian M, Roof DJ, et al. In-vivo transfer of a reporter gene to the retina mediated by an adenoviral vector. Invest Ophthalmol Vis Sci 1994; 35:2543–9.
711. Hoffman LM, Maguire AM, Bennett J. Cell-mediated immune response and stability of intraocular transgene expression after adenovirus-mediated delivery. Invest Ophthalmol Vis Sci 1997;38:2224–33.
712. Bainbridge JW, Smith AJ, Barker SS, et al. Effect of gene therapy on visual function in Leber's congenital amaurosis. N Engl J Med 2008;358:2231–9.
713. Maguire AM, Simonelli F, Pierce EA, et al. Safety and efficacy of gene transfer for Leber's congenital amaurosis. N Engl J Med 2008;358:2240–8.
714. Cideciyan AV, Hauswirth WW, Aleman TS, et al. Human RPE65 gene therapy for Leber congenital amaurosis: persistence of early visual improvements and safety at 1 year. Hum Gene Ther 2009;20:999–1004.
715. Simonelli F, Maguire AM, Testa F, et al. Gene therapy for Leber's congenital amaurosis is safe and effective through 1.5 years after vector administration. Mol Ther 2010;18:643–50.
716. Haseloff J, Gerlach WL. Simple RNA enzymes with new and highly specific endoribonuclease activities. Nature 1988;334:585–91.
717. Lewin AS, Drenser KA, Hauswirth WW, et al. Ribozyme rescue of photoreceptor cells in a transgenic rat model of autosomal dominant retinitis pigmentosa. Nat Med 1998;4:967–71.
718. Georgiadis A, Tschernutter M, Bainbridge JW, et al. AAV-mediated knockdown of peripherin-2 in vivo using miRNA-based hairpins. Gene Ther 2010;17:486–93.
719. Stieger K, Lorenz B. Gene therapy for vision loss – recent developments. Discov Med 2010;10:425–33.
720. Bok D. Retinal transplantation and gene therapy. Present realities and future possibilities. Invest Ophthalmol Vis Sci 1993;34:473–6.
721. Li LX, Turner JE. Inherited retinal dystrophy in the RCS rat: prevention of photoreceptor degeneration by pigment epithelial cell transplantation. Exp Eye Res 1988;47:911–7.
722. Little CW, Castillo B, DiLoreto DA, et al. Transplantation of human fetal retinal pigment epithelium rescues photoreceptor cells from degeneration in the Royal College of Surgeons rat retina. Invest Ophthalmol Vis Sci 1996; 37:204–11.
723. Castillo BVJ, del Cerro M, White RM, et al. Efficacy of nonfetal human RPE for photoreceptor rescue: A study in dystrophic RCS rats. Exp Neurol 1997;146:1–9.
724. Carr AJ, Vugler AA, Hikita ST, et al. Protective effects of human iPS-derived retinal pigment epithelium cell transplantation in the retinal dystrophic rat. PLoS One 2009;4:e8152.

725. Algvere PV, Berglin L, Gouras P, et al. Transplantation of fetal retinal pigment epithelium in age-related macular degeneration with subfoveal neovascularization. Graefes Arch Clin Exp Ophthalmol 1994;232:707–16.
726. Du H, Lim SL, Grob S, et al. Induced pluripotent stem cell therapies for geographic atrophy of age-related macular degeneration. Semin Ophthalmol 2011;26:216–24.
727. Lu B, Malcuit C, Wang S, et al. Long-term safety and function of RPE from human embryonic stem cells in preclinical models of macular degeneration. Stem Cells 2009;27:2126–35.
728. Wang NK, Tosi J, Kasanuki JM, et al. Transplantation of reprogrammed embryonic stem cells improves visual function in a mouse model for retinitis pigmentosa. Transplantation 2010;89:911–9.
729. Lund RD, Wang S, Klimanskaya I, et al. Human embryonic stem cell-derived cells rescue visual function in dystrophic RCS rats. Cloning Stem Cells 2006;8:189–99.
730. Kicic A, Shen WY, Wilson AS, et al. Differentiation of marrow stromal cells into photoreceptors in the rat eye. J Neurosci 2003;23:7742–9.
731. Pressmar S, Ader M, Richard G, et al. The fate of heterotopically grafted neural precursor cells in the normal and dystrophic adult mouse retina. Invest Ophthalmol Vis Sci 2001;42:3311–9.
732. Fischer AJ, Reh TA. Potential of Muller glia to become neurogenic retinal progenitor cells. Glia 2003;43:70–6.
733. Fischer AJ, Bongini R. Turning Muller glia into neural progenitors in the retina. Mol neurobiol 2010;42:199–209.
734. Tropepe V, Coles BL, Chiasson BJ, et al. Retinal stem cells in the adult mammalian eye. Science 2000;287:2032–6.
735. Coles BL, Angenieux B, Inoue T, et al. Facile isolation and the characterization of human retinal stem cells. Proc Natl Acad Sci USA 2004;101:15772–7.
736. Cicero SA, Johnson D, Reyntjens S, et al. Cells previously identified as retinal stem cells are pigmented ciliary epithelial cells. Proc Natl Acad Sci USA 2009;106:6685–90.
737. Reh TA, Lamba D, Gust J. Directing human embryonic stem cells to a retinal fate. Methods Mol Biol 2010;636:139–53.
738. Lamba DA, Gust J, Reh TA. Transplantation of human embryonic stem cell-derived photoreceptors restores some visual function in Crx-deficient mice. Cell Stem Cell 2009;4:73–9.
739. Takahashi K, Yamanaka S. Induction of pluripotent stem cells from mouse embryonic and adult fibroblast cultures by defined factors. Cell 2006;126: 663–76.
740. Lamba DA, McUsic A, Hirata RK, et al. Generation, purification and transplantation of photoreceptors derived from human induced pluripotent stem cells. PLoS One 2010;5:e8763.
741. Hirami Y, Osakada F, Takahashi K, et al. Generation of retinal cells from mouse and human induced pluripotent stem cells. Neurosci Lett 2009;458:126–31.
742. Zhou L, Wang W, Liu Y, et al. Differentiation of induced pluripotent stem cells of swine into rod photoreceptors and their integration into the retina. Stem Cells 2011;29:972–80.
743. Joe AW, Gregory-Evans K. Mesenchymal stem cells and potential applications in treating ocular disease. Curr Eye Res 2010;35:941–52.
744. Lu B, Wang S, Girman S, et al. Human adult bone marrow-derived somatic cells rescue vision in a rodent model of retinal degeneration. Exp Eye Res 2010;91:449–55.
745. Wang S, Lu B, Girman S, et al. Non-invasive stem cell therapy in a rat model for retinal degeneration and vascular pathology. PLoS One 2010;5:e9200.
746. Gregory-Evans K, Chang F, Hodges MD, et al. Ex vivo gene therapy using intravitreal injection of GDNF-secreting mouse embryonic stem cells in a rat model of retinal degeneration. Mol Vis 2009;15:962–73.
747. Chang GQ, Hao Y, Wong F. Apoptosis: final common pathway of photoreceptor death in rd, rds, and rhodopsin mutant mice. Neuron 1993;11:595–605.
748. Tso MO, Zhang C, Abler AS, et al. Apoptosis leads to photoreceptor degeneration in inherited retinal dystrophy of RCS rats. Invest Ophthalmol Vis Sci 1994;35:2693–9.
749. Portera-Cailliau C, Sung C-H, Nathans J, et al. Apoptotic photoreceptor cell death in mouse models of retinitis pigmentosa. Proc Natl Acad Sci U S A 1994;91:974–8.
750. Cottet S, Schorderet DF. Mechanisms of apoptosis in retinitis pigmentosa. Curr Mol Med 2009;9:375–83.
751. Nir I, Kedzierski W, Chen J, et al. Expression of Bcl-2 protects against photoreceptor degeneration in retinal degeneration slow (rds) mice. J Neurosci 2000;20:2150–4.
752. Eversole-Cire P, Concepcion FA, Simon MI, et al. Synergistic effect of Bcl-2 and BAG-1 on the prevention of photoreceptor cell death. Invest Ophthalmol Vis Sci 2000;41:1953–61.
753. Hahn P, Lindsten T, Lyubarsky A, et al. Deficiency of Bax and Bak protects photoreceptors from light damage in vivo. Cell Death Different 2004;11: 1192–7.
754. Joseph RM, Li T. Overexpression of Bcl-2 or Bcl-XL transgenes and photoreceptor degeneration. Invest Ophthalmol Vis Sci 1996;37:2434–46.
755. Quiambao AB, Tan E, Chang S, et al. Transgenic Bcl-2 expressed in photoreceptor cells confers both death-sparing and death-inducing effects. Exp Eye Res 2001;73:711–21.
756. Frasson M, Sahel JA, Fabre M, et al. Retinitis pigmentosa: rod photoreceptor rescue by a calcium-channel blocker in the rd mouse. Nat Med 1999;5: 1183–7.
757. Frasson M, Sahel JA, Fabre M, et al. Retinitis pigmentosa: rod photoreceptor rescue by a calcium-channel blocker in the rd mouse. Nat Med 1999;5:1183–7.
758. Sanges D, Comitato A, Tammaro R, et al. Apoptosis in retinal degeneration involves cross-talk between apoptosis-inducing factor (AIF) and caspase-12 and is blocked by calpain inhibitors. Proc Natl Acad Sci USA 2006;103: 17366–71.
759. Vallazza-Deschamps G, Cia D, Gong J, et al. Excessive activation of cyclic nucleotide-gated channels contributes to neuronal degeneration of photoreceptors. Eur J Neurosci 2005;22:1013–22.
760. Pawlyk BS, Li T, Scimeca MS, et al. Absence of photoreceptor rescue with D-*cis*-diltiazem in the rd mouse. Invest Ophthalmol Vis Sci 2002;43: 1912–5.
761. Nakazawa M. Effects of calcium ion, calpains, and calcium channel blockers on retinitis pigmentosa. J Ophthalmol 2011;2011:292040.
762. Liu C, Li Y, Peng M, et al. Activation of caspase-3 in the retina of transgenic rats with the rhodopsin mutation s334ter during photoreceptor degeneration. J Neurosci 1999;19:4778–85.
763. Bode C, Wolfrum U. Caspase-3 inhibitor reduces apototic photoreceptor cell death during inherited retinal degeneration in tubby mice. Mol Vision 2003;9: 144–50.
764. Samardzija M, Wenzel A, Thiersch M, et al. Caspase-1 ablation protects photoreceptors in a model of autosomal dominant retinitis pigmentosa. Invest Ophthalmol Vis Sci 2006;47:5181–90.
765. Doonan F, Donovan M, Cotter TG. Caspase-independent photoreceptor apoptosis in mouse models of retinal degeneration. J Neurosci 2003;23:5723–31.
766. Faktorovich EG, Steinberg RH, Yasumura D, et al. Photoreceptor degeneration in inherited retinal dystrophy delayed by basic fibroblast growth factor. Nature 1990;347:83–6.
767. Sakai T, Kuno N, Takamatsu F, et al. Prolonged protective effect of basic fibroblast growth factor-impregnated nanoparticles in royal college of surgeons rats. Invest Ophthalmol Vis Sci 2007;48:3381–7.
768. Gauthier R, Joly S, Pernet V, et al. Brain-derived neurotrophic factor gene delivery to muller glia preserves structure and function of light-damaged photoreceptors. Invest Ophthalmol Vis Sci 2005;46:3383–92.
769. Li Y, Tao W, Luo L, et al. CNTF induces regeneration of cone outer segments in a rat model of retinal degeneration. PLoS One 2010;5:e9495.
770. Sieving PA, Caruso RC, Tao W, et al. Ciliary neurotrophic factor (CNTF) for human retinal degeneration: phase I trial of CNTF delivered by encapsulated cell intraocular implants. Proc Natl Acad Sci U S A 2006;103:3896–901.
771. McGee Sanftner LH, Abel H, et al. Glial cell line derived neurotrophic factor delays photoreceptor degeneration in a transgenic rat model of retinitis pigmentosa. Mol Ther 2001;4:622–9.
772. Wen R, Song Y, Kjellstrom S, et al. Regulation of rod phototransduction machinery by ciliary neurotrophic factor. J Neurosci 2006;26:13523–30.
773. Foerster O. Beitriige zur Pathophysiologie der Sehbahn und der Sehsphare. J Psychol Neuro, Lpz 1929;39:463–85.
774. Potts AM, Inoue J. The electrically evoked response (EER) of the visual system. II. Effect of adaptation and retinitis pigmentosa. Invest Ophthalmol 1969;8: 605–12.
775. Rizzo 3rd JF, Wyatt J, Loewenstein J, et al. Perceptual efficacy of electrical stimulation of human retina with a microelectrode array during short-term surgical trials. Invest Ophthalmol Vis Sci 2003;44:5362–9.
776. Ahuja AK, Dorn JD, Caspi A, et al. Blind subjects implanted with the Argus II retinal prosthesis are able to improve performance in a spatial-motor task. Br J Ophthalmol 2011;95:539–43.
777. Javaheri M, Hahn DS, Lakhanpal RR, et al. Retinal prostheses for the blind. Ann Acad Med Singapore 2006;35:137–44.
778. Hornig R, Zehnder T, Velikay-Parel M, et al. The IMI retinal implant system. In: Humayun MS, Chader G, Weiland JD, editors. Artificial sight: basic research, biomedical engineering, and clinical advances. New York: Springer-Verlag; 2007. p. 111–28.
779. Roessler G, Laube T, Brockmann C, et al. Implantation and explantation of a wireless epiretinal retina implant device: observations during the EPIRET3 prospective clinical trial. Invest Ophthalmol Vis Sci 2009;50:3003–8.
780. Normann RA, Greger B, House P, et al. Toward the development of a cortically based visual neuroprosthesis. J Neural Eng 2009;6:035001.
781. Freeman DK, Rizzo 3rd JF, Fried SI. Encoding visual information in retinal ganglion cells with prosthetic stimulation. J Neural Eng 2011;8:035005.
782. Millay RH, Weleber RG, Heckenlively JR. Ophthalmologic and systemic manifestations of Alstrom's disease. Am J Ophthalmol 1986;102:482–90.
783. Hood DC, Holopigian K, Greenstein V, et al. Assessment of local retinal function in patients with retinitis pigmentosa using the mulit-focal ERG technique. Vision Res 1998;38:163–79.
784. Weleber RG, Butler NS, Murphey WH, et al. X-linked retinitis pigmentosa associated with a two base-pair insertion in codon 99 of the RP3 gene *RPGR*. Arch Ophthalmol 1997;115:1429–35.
785. Zelinger L, Banin E, Obolensky A, et al. A missense mutation in DHDDS, encoding dehydrodolichyl diphosphate synthase, is associated with autosomal-recessive retinitis pigmentosa in Ashkenazi Jews. Am J Hum Genet 2011;88:207–15.
786. Zhang Q, Zulfiqar F, Xiao X, et al. Severe autosomal recessive retinitis pigmentosa maps to chromosome 1p13.3-p21.2 between D1S2896 and D1S457 but outside ABCA4. Hum Genet 2005 Sep;28:1–10.
787. Martínez-Mir A, Paloma E, Allkimets R, et al. Retinitis pigmentosa caused by a homozygous mutation in the Stargardt disease gene *ABCR*. Nat Genet 1998;18:11–2.
788. den Hollander AI, ten Brink JB, de Kok YJ, et al. Mutations in a human homologue of Drosophila crumbs cause retinitis pigmentosa (RP12). Nat Genet 1999;23:217–21.

789. Rajadhyaksha AM, Elemento O, Puffenberger EG, et al. Mutations in FLVCR1 cause posterior column ataxia and retinitis pigmentosa. Am J Hum Genet 2010;87:643–54.
790. Li L, Nakaya N, Chavali VR, et al. A mutation in ZNF513, a putative regulator of photoreceptor development, causes autosomal-recessive retinitis pigmentosa. Am J Hum Genet 2010;87:400–9.
791. Collin RW, Safieh C, Littink KW, et al. Mutations in C2ORF71 cause autosomal-recessive retinitis pigmentosa. Am J Hum Genet 2010;86:783–8.
792. Bandah-Rozenfeld D, Mizrahi-Meissonnier L, Farhy C, et al. Homozygosity mapping reveals null mutations in FAM161A as a cause of autosomal-recessive retinitis pigmentosa. Am J Hum Genet 2010;87:382–91.
793. Zhao C, Bellur DL, Lu S, et al. Autosomal-dominant retinitis pigmentosa caused by a mutation in SNRNP200, a gene required for unwinding of U4/U6 snRNAs. Am J Hum Genet 2009;85:617–27.
794. Tuson M, Marfany G, Gonzalez-Duarte R. Mutation of *CERKL*, a novel human ceramide kinase gene, causes autosomal recessive retinitis pigmentosa (RP26). Am J Hum Genet 2004;74:128–38.
795. Bandah-Rozenfeld D, Collin RW, Banin E, et al. Mutations in IMPG2, encoding interphotoreceptor matrix proteoglycan 2, cause autosomal-recessive retinitis pigmentosa. Am J Hum Genet 2010;87:199–208.
796. McLaughlin ME, Sandberg MA, Berson EL, et al. Recessive mutations in the gene encoding the ß-subunit of rod phosphodiesterase in patients with retinitis pigmentosa. Nat Genet 1993;4:130–4.
797. Maw MA, Corbeil D, Koch J, et al. A frameshift mutation in prominin (mouse)-like 1 causes human retinal degeneration. Hum Mol Genet 2000;9:27–34.
798. Ruiz A, Kuehn MH, Andorf JL, et al. Genomic organization and mutation analysis of the gene encoding lecithin retinol acyltransferase in human retinal pigment epithelium. Invest Ophthalmol Vis Sci 2001;42:31–7.
799. Noor A, Windpassinger C, Patel M, et al. CC2D2A, encoding a coiled-coil and C2 domain protein, causes autosomal-recessive mental retardation with retinitis pigmentosa. Am J Hum Genet 2008;82:1011–8.
800. Huang SH, Pittler SJ, Huang X, et al. Autosomal recessive retinitis pigmentosa caused by mutations in the α subunit of rod cGMP phosphodiesterase. Nat Genet 1995;11:468–71.
801. Abd El-Aziz MM, Barragan I, O'Driscoll CA, et al. EYS, encoding an ortholog of *Drosophila* spacemaker, is mutated in autosomal recessive retinitis pigmentosa. Nat Genet 2008;40:1285–7.
802. Kennan A, Aherne A, Palfi A, et al. Identification of an IMPDH1 mutation in autosomal dominant retinitis pigmentosa (RP10) revealed following comparative microarray analysis of transcripts derived from retinas of wild-type and Rho(-/-) mice. Hum Mol Genet 2002;11:547–58.
803. Pierce EA, Quinn T, Meehan T, et al. Mutations in a gene encoding a new oxygen-regulated photoreceptor protein cause dominant retinitis pigmentosa. Nat Genet 1999;22:248–54.
804. Yokota T, Shiojiri T, Gotoda T, et al. Retinitis pigmentosa and ataxia caused by a mutation in the gene for the α-tocopherol-transfer protein. N Engl J Med 1996;335:1770–1.
805. Chakarova CF, Papaioannou MG, Khanna H, et al. Mutations in TOPORS cause autosomal dominant retinitis pigmentosa with perivascular retinal pigment epithelium atrophy. Am J Hum Genet 2007;81:1098–103.
806. den Hollander AI, McGee TL, Ziviello C, et al. A homozygous missense mutation in the IRBP gene (RBP3) associated with autosomal recessive retinitis pigmentosa. Invest Ophthalmol Vis Sci 2009;50:1864–72.
807. Morimura H, Saindelle-Ribeaudeau F, Berson EL, et al. Mutations in *RGR*, encoding a light-sensitive opsin homologue, in patients with retinitis pigmentosa. Nat Genet 1999;23:393–4.
808. Finckh U, Xu S, Kumaramanickavel G, et al. Homozygosity mapping of autosomal recessive retinitis pigmentosa locus (RP22) on chromosome 16p12.1-p12.3. Genomics 1998;48:341–5.
809. Burstedt MS, Sandgren O, Holmgren G, et al. Bothnia dystrophy caused by mutations in the cellular retinaldehyde-binding protein gene (RLBP1) on chromosome 15q26. Invest Ophthalmol Vis Sci 1999;40:995–1000.
810. Bareil C, Hamel CP, Delague V, et al. Segregation of a mutation in CNGB1 encoding the beta-subunit of the rod cGMP-gated channel in a family with autosomal recessive retinitis pigmentosa. Hum Genet 2001;108:328–34.
811. van Lith-Verhoeven JJ, van der Velde-Visser SD, Sohocki MM, et al. Clinical characterization, linkage analysis, and PRPC8 mutation analysis of a family with autosomal dominant retinitis pigmentosa type 13 (RP13). Ophthalmic Genet 2002;23:1–12.
812. Dvir L, Srour G, Abu-Ras R, et al. Autosomal-recessive early-onset retinitis pigmentosa caused by a mutation in PDE6G, the gene encoding the gamma subunit of rod cGMP phosphodiesterase. Am J Hum Genet 2010;87:258–64.
813. Alvarez BV, Vithana EN, Yang Z, et al. Identification and characterization of a novel mutation in the carbonic anhydrase IV gene that causes retinitis pigmentosa. Invest Ophthalmol Vis Sci 2007;48:3459–68.
814. Nevet MJ, Shalev SA, Zlotogora J, et al. Identification of a prevalent founder mutation in an Israeli Muslim Arab village confirms the role of PRCD in the aetiology of retinitis pigmentosa in humans. J Med Genet 2010;47:533–7.
815. Vithana EN, Abu-Safieh L, Pelosini L, et al. Expression of *PRPF31* mRNA in patients with autosomal dominant retinitis pigmentosa: a molecular clue for incomplete penetrance? Invest Ophthalmol Vis Sci 2003;44:4204–9.
816. Tanackovic G, Ransijn A, Ayuso C, et al. A missense mutation in PRPF6 causes impairment of pre-mRNA splicing and autosomal-dominant retinitis pigmentosa. Am J Hum Genet 2011;88:643–9.
817. Hartong DT, Dange M, McGee TL, et al. Insights from retinitis pigmentosa into the roles of isocitrate dehydrogenases in the Krebs cycle. Nat Genet 2008;40:1230–4.
818. Hardcastle AJ, Thiselton DL, Zito I, et al. Evidence for a new locus for X-linked retinitis pigmentosa (RP23). Invest Ophthalmol Vis Sci 2000;41:2080–6.
819. Ott J, Bhattacharya S, Chen JD, et al. Localizing multiple X chromosome-linked retinitis pigmentosa loci using multilocus homogeneity tests. Proc Natl Acad Sci U S A 1990;87:701–4.
820. Schwahn U, Lenzner S, Dong J, et al. Positional cloning of the gene for X-linked retinitis pigmentosa 2. Nat Genet 1998;19:327–32.
821. Gieser L, Fujita R, Göring HH, et al. A novel locus (RP24) for X-linked retinitis pigmentosa maps to Xq26–27. Am J Hum Genet 1998;63:1439–47.
822. Verpy E, Leibovici M, Zwaenepoel I, et al. A defect in harmonin, a PDZ domain-containing protein expressed in the inner ear sensory hair cells, underlies Usher syndrome type 1C. Nat Genet 2000;26:51–5.
823. Chaib H, Kaplan J, Gerber S, et al. A newly identified locus for Usher syndrome type I, USH1E, maps to chromosome 21q21. Hum Mol Genet 1997;6:27–31.
824. Kikkawa Y, Shitara H, Wakana S, et al. Mutations in a new scaffold protein Sans cause deafness in Jackson shaker mice. Hum Mol Genet 2003;12:453–61.
825. Astuto LM, Bork JM, Weston MD, et al. CDH23 mutation and phenotype heterogeneity: a profile of 107 diverse families with Usher syndrome and nonsyndromic deafness. Am J Hum Genet 2002;71:262–75.
826. Hmani M, Ghorbel A, Boulila-Elgaied A, et al. A novel locus for Usher syndrome type II, USH2B, maps to chromosome 3 at p23–24.2. Eur J Hum Genet 1999;7:363–7.
827. Weston MD, Luijendijk MW, Humphrey KD, et al. Mutations in the VLGR1 gene implicate G-protein signaling in the pathogenesis of Usher syndrome type II. Am J Hum Genet 2004;74:357–66.
828. Ebermann I, Lopez I, Bitner-Glindzicz M, et al. Deafblindness in French Canadians from Quebec: a predominant founder mutation in the USH1C gene provides the first genetic link with the Acadian population. Genome Biol 2007;8:R47.
829. Crimi M, Galbiati S, Perini MP, et al. A mitochondrial tRNA(His) gene mutation causing pigmentary retinopathy and neurosensorial deafness. Neurology 2003;60:1200–3.
830. Da Pozzo P, Cardaioli E, Malfatti E, et al. A novel mutation in the mitochondrial tRNA(Pro) gene associated with late-onset ataxia, retinitis pigmentosa, deafness, leukoencephalopathy and complex I deficiency. Eur J Hum Genet 2009;17:1092–6.
831. Mykytyn K, Nishimura DY, Searby CC, et al. Identification of the gene (BBS1) most commonly involved in Bardet–Biedl syndrome, a complex human obesity syndrome. Nat Genet 2002;31:435–8.
832. Nishimura DY, Searby CC, Carmi R, et al. Positional cloning of a novel gene on chromosome 16q causing Bardet- Biedl syndrome (BBS2). Hum Mol Genet 2001;10:865–74.
833. Chiang AP, Nishimura D, Searby C, et al. Comparative genomic analysis identifies an ADP-ribosylation factor-like gene as the cause of Bardet–Biedl syndrome (BBS3). Am J Hum Genet 2004;75:475–84.
834. Riise R, Tornqvist K, Wright AF, et al. The phenotype in Norwegian patients With Bardet–Biedl syndrome With mutations in the *BBS4* gene. Arch Ophthalmol 2002;120:1364–7.
835. Young TL, Penney L, Woods MO, et al. A fifth locus for Bardet–Biedl syndrome maps to chromosome 2q31. Am J Hum Genet 1999;64:900–4.
836. Badano JL, Ansley SJ, Leitch CC, et al. Identification of a novel Bardet–Biedl syndrome protein, BBS7, that shares structural features with BBS1 and BBS2. Am J Hum Genet 2003;72:650–8.
837. Riazuddin SA, Iqbal M, Wang Y, et al. A splice-site mutation in a retina-specific exon of BBS8 causes nonsyndromic retinitis pigmentosa. Am J Hum Genet 2010;86:805–12.
838. Nishimura DY, Swiderski RE, Searby CC, et al. Comparative genomics and gene expression analysis identifies BBS9, a new Bardet–Biedl syndrome gene. Am J Hum Genet 2005;77:1021–33.
839. Stoetzel C, Laurier V, Davis EE, et al. BBS10 encodes a vertebrate-specific chaperonin-like protein and is a major BBS locus. Nat Genet 2006;38:521–4.
840. Chiang AP, Beck JS, Yen HJ, et al. Homozygosity mapping with SNP arrays identifies TRIM32, an E3 ubiquitin ligase, as a Bardet–Biedl syndrome gene (BBS11). Proc Natl Acad Sci USA 2006;103:6287–92.
841. Stoetzel C, Muller J, Laurier V, et al. Identification of a novel BBS gene (BBS12) highlights the major role of a vertebrate-specific branch of chaperonin-related proteins in Bardet–Biedl syndrome. Am J Hum Genet 2007;80:1–11.
842. Kyttälä M, Tallila J, Salonen R, et al. MKS1, encoding a component of the flagellar apparatus basal body proteome, is mutated in Meckel syndrome. Nat Genet 2006;38:155–7.
843. Baala L, Audollent S, Martinovic J, et al. Pleiotropic effects of CEP290 (NPHP6) mutations extend to Meckel syndrome. Am J Hum Genet 2007;81:170–9.
844. Perrault I, Rozet JM, Calvas P, et al. Retinal-specific guanylate cyclase gene mutations in Leber's congenital amaurosis. Nat Genet 1996;14:461–4.
845. Gu S, Thompson DA, Srikumari CRS, et al. Mutations in *RPE65* cause autosomal recessive childhood-onset severe retinal dystrophy. Nat Genet 1997;17:194–7.
846. Wang H, den Hollander AI, Moayedi Y, et al. Mutations in SPATA7 cause Leber congenital amaurosis and juvenile retinitis pigmentosa. Am J Hum Genet 2009;84:380–7.
847. Sohocki MM, Bowne SJ, Sullivan LS, et al. Mutations in a new photoreceptor-pineal gene on 17p cause Leber congenital amaurosis. Nat Genet 2000;24:79–83.

848. den Hollander AI, Koenekoop RK, Mohamed MD, et al. Mutations in LCA5, encoding the ciliary protein lebercilin, cause Leber congenital amaurosis. Nat Genet 2007;39:889–95.
849. Dryja TP, Adams SM, Grimsby JL, et al. Null *RPGRIP1* alleles in patients with Leber congenital amaurosis. Am J Hum Genet 2001;68:1295–8.
850. Keen TJ, Mohamed MD, McKibbin M, et al. Identification of a locus (LCA9) for Leber's congenital amaurosis on chromosome 1p36. Eur J Hum Genet 2003;11:420–3.
851. Friedman JS, Chang B, Kannabiran C, et al. Premature truncation of a novel protein, RD3, exhibiting subnuclear localization is associated with retinal degeneration. Am J Hum Genet 2006;79:1059–70.
852. Janecke AR, Thompson DA, Utermann G, et al. Mutations in RDH12 encoding a photoreceptor cell retinol dehydrogenase cause childhood-onset severe retinal dystrophy. Nat Genet 2004;36:850–4.
853. den Hollander AI, Heckenlively JR, van den Born LI, et al. Leber congenital amaurosis and retinitis pigmentosa with Coats-like exudative vasculopathy are associated with mutations in the crumbs homologue 1 (*CRB1*) gene. Am J Hum Genet 2001;69:198–203.
854. Perrault I, Hanein S, Gerber S, et al. Retinal dehydrogenase 12 (*RDH12*) mutations in leber congenital amaurosis. Am J Hum Genet 2004;75:639–46.
855. Thompson DA, Li Y, McHenry CL, et al. Mutations in the gene encoding lecithin retinol acyltransferase are associated with early-onset severe retinal dystrophy. Nat Genet 2001;28:123–4.
856. Freund CL, Wang Q-L, Chen S, et al. *De novo* mutations in the *CRX* homeobox gene associated with Leber congenital amaurosis. Nat Genet 1998;18:311–2.
857. Warburg M, Sjö O, Tranebjaerg L, et al. Deletion mapping of a retinal cone-rod dystrophy: assignment to 18q211. Am J Med Genet 1991;39:288–93.
858. Kylstra JA, Aylsworth AS. Cone-rod retinal dystrophy in a patient with neurofibromatosis type 1. Can J Ophthalmol 1993;28:79–80.
859. Köhn L, Kadzhaev K, Burstedt MS, et al. Mutation in the PYK2-binding domain of PITPNM3 causes autosomal dominant cone dystrophy (CORD5) in two Swedish families. Eur J Hum Genet 2007;15:664–71.
860. Kelsell RE, Gregory-Evans K, Payne AM, et al. Mutations in the retinal guanylate cyclase (RETGC-1) gene in dominant cone–rod dystrophy. Hum Mol Genet 1998;7:1179–84.
861. Johnson S, Halford S, Morris AG, et al. Genomic organisation and alternative splicing of human *RIM1*, a gene implicated in autosomal dominant cone–rod dystrophy (CORD7)(small star, filled). Genomics 2003;81:304–14.
862. Ismail M, Abid A, Anwar K, et al. Refinement of the locus for autosomal recessive cone–rod dystrophy (CORD8) linked to chromosome 1q23-q24 in a Pakistani family and exclusion of candidate genes. J Hum Genet 2006;51: 827–31.
863. Parry DA, Toomes C, Bida L, et al. Loss of the metalloprotease ADAM9 leads to cone–rod dystrophy in humans and retinal degeneration in mice. Am J Hum Genet 2009;84:683–91.
864. Abid A, Ismail M, Mehdi SQ, et al. Identification of novel mutations in the SEMA4A gene associated with retinal degenerative diseases. J Med Genet 2006;43:378–81.
865. Wang QL, Chen S, Esumi N, et al. QRX, a novel homeobox gene, modulates photoreceptor gene expression. Hum Mol Genet 2004;13:1025–40.
866. Bech-Hansen NT, Naylor MJ, Maybaum TA, et al. Loss-of-function mutations in a calcium-channel alpha1-subunit gene in Xp11.23 cause incomplete X-linked congenital stationary night blindness. Nat Genet 1998;19:264–7.
867. Nakazawa M, Kikawa E, Chida Y, et al. Asn244His mutation of the peripherin/RDS gene causing autosomal dominant cone–rod degeneration. Hum Mol Genet 1994;3:1195–6.
868. Kobayashi A, Higashide T, Hamasaki D, et al. HRG4 (UNC119) mutation found in cone–rod dystrophy causes retinal degeneration in a transgenic model. Invest Ophthalmol Vis Sci 2000;41:3268–77.
869. Parry DA, Mighell AJ, El-Sayed W, et al. Mutations in CNNM4 cause Jalili syndrome, consisting of autosomal-recessive cone–rod dystrophy and amelogenesis imperfecta. Am J Hum Genet 2009;84:266–73.
870. Michaelides M, Bloch-Zupan A, Holder GE, et al. An autosomal recessive cone-rod dystrophy associated with amelogenesis imperfecta. J Med Genet 2004;41:468–73.
871. Henderson RH, Li Z, Abd El Aziz MM, et al. Biallelic mutation of protocadherin-21 (PCDH21) causes retinal degeneration in humans. Mol Vision 2010;16:46–52.
872. van den Brink DM, Brites P, Haasjes J, et al. Identification of PEX7 as the second gene involved in Refsum disease. Am J Hum Genet 2003;72:471–7.
873. Reuber BE, Germain-Lee E, Collins CS, et al. Mutations in PEX1 are the most common cause of peroxisome biogenesis disorders. Nat Genet 1997;17: 445–8.
874. Shimozawa N, Tsukamoto T, Suzuki Y, et al. A human gene responsible for Zellweger syndrome that affects peroxisome assembly. Science 1992;255: 1132–4.
875. Jansen GA, Wanders RJ, Watkins PA, et al. Phytanoyl-coenzyme A hydroxylase deficiency – the enzyme defect in Refsum's disease. N Engl J Med 1997;337:133–4.
876. Vesa J, Hellsten E, Verkruyse LA, et al. Mutations in the palmitoyl protein thioesterase gene causing infantile neuronal ceroid lipofuscinosis. Nature 1995;376:584–7.
877. Schriner JE, Yi W, Hofmann SL. cDNA and genomic cloning of human palmitoyl-protein thioesterase (PPT), the enzyme defective in infantile neuronal ceroid lipofuscinosis. Genomics 1996;34:317–22.
878. Sleat DE, Donnelly RJ, Lackland H, et al. Association of mutations in a lysosomal protein with classical late-infantile neuronal ceroid lipofuscinosis. Science 1997;277:1802–5.
879. Munroe PB, Mitchison HM, O'Rawe AM, et al. Spectrum of mutations in the Batten disease gene, CLN3. Am J Hum Genet 1997;61:310–6.
880. van Diggelen OP, Thobois S, Tilikete C, et al. Adult neuronal ceroid lipofuscinosis with palmitoyl-protein thioesterase deficiency: first adult-onset patients of a childhood disease. Ann Neurol 2001;50:269–72.
881. Savukoski M, Klockars T, Holmberg V, et al. CLN5, a novel gene encoding a putative transmembrane protein mutated in Finnish variant late infantile neuronal ceroid lipofuscinosis. Nat Genet 1998;19:286–8.
882. Dixon-Salazar T, Silhavy JL, Marsh SE, et al. Mutations in the AHI1 gene, encoding jouberin, cause Joubert syndrome with cortical polymicrogyria. Am J Hum Genet 2004;75:979–87.
883. Bielas SL, Silhavy JL, Brancati F, et al. Mutations in INPP5E, encoding inositol polyphosphate-5-phosphatase E, link phosphatidyl inositol signaling to the ciliopathies. Nat Genet 2009;41:1032–6.
884. Valente EM, Marsh SE, Castori M, et al. Distinguishing the four genetic causes of Jouberts syndrome-related disorders. Ann Neurol 2005;57:513–9.
885. Valente EM, Silhavy JL, Brancati F, et al. Mutations in CEP290, which encodes a centrosomal protein, cause pleiotropic forms of Joubert syndrome. Nat Genet 2006;38:623–5.
886. Arts HH, Doherty D, van Beersum SE, et al. Mutations in the gene encoding the basal body protein RPGRIP1L, a nephrocystin-4 interactor, cause Joubert syndrome. Nat Genet 2007;39:882–8.
887. Coene KL, Roepman R, Doherty D, et al. OFD1 is mutated in X-linked Joubert syndrome and interacts with LCA5-encoded lebercilin. Am J Hum Genet 2009;85:465–81.
888. Seeliger MW, Biesalski HK, Wissinger B, et al. Phenotype in retinol deficiency due to a hereditary defect in retinol binding protein synthesis. Invest Ophthalmol Vis Sci 1999;40:3–11.
889. Yokota T, Shiojiri T, Gotoda T, et al. Retinitis pigmentosa and ataxia caused by a mutation in the gene for the alpha-tocopherol-transfer protein. N Engl J Med 1996;335:1770–1.
890. David G, Abbas N, Stevanin G, et al. Cloning of the SCA7 gene reveals a highly unstable CAG repeat expansion. Nat Genet 1997;17:65–70.
891. Lamminen T, Majander A, Juvonen V, et al. A mitochondrial mutation at nt 9101 in the ATP synthase 6 gene associated with deficient oxidative phosphorylation in a family with Leber hereditary optic neuroretinopathy. Am J Hum Genet 1995;56:1238–40.
892. Mollet G, Salomon R, Gribouval O, et al. The gene mutated in juvenile nephronophthisis type 4 encodes a novel protein that interacts with nephrocystin. Nat Genet 2002;32:300–5.
893. Saunier S, Calado J, Benessy F, et al. Characterization of the NPHP1 locus: mutational mechanism involved in deletions in familial juvenile nephronophthisis. Am J Hum Genet 2000;66:778–89.
894. Estrada-Cuzcano A, Koenekoop RK, Coppieters F, et al. IQCB1 mutations in patients with leber congenital amaurosis. Invest Ophthalmol Vis Sci 2011;52: 834–9.
895. Olbrich H, Fliegauf M, Hoefele J, et al. Mutations in a novel gene, NPHP3, cause adolescent nephronophthisis, tapeto-retinal degeneration and hepatic fibrosis. Nat Genet 2003;34:455–9.
896. Otto EA, Schermer B, Obara T, et al. Mutations in INVS encoding inversin cause nephronophthisis type 2, linking renal cystic disease to the function of primary cilia and left-right axis determination. Nat Genet 2003;34: 413–20.
897. Narcisi TM, Shoulders CC, Chester SA, et al. Mutations of the microsomal triglyceride-transfer-protein gene in abetalipoproteinemia. Am J Hum Genet 1995;57:1298–310.
898. Yamamoto H, Simon A, Eriksson U, et al. Mutations in the gene encoding 11-*cis* retinol dehydrogenase cause delayed dark adaptation and fundus albipunctatus. Nat Genet 1999;22:188–91.
899. Souied E, Soubrane G, Benlian P, et al. Retinitis punctata albescens associated with the Arg135Trp mutation in the rhodopsin gene. Am J Ophthalmol 1996;121:19–25.
900. Hearn T, Renforth GL, Spalluto C, et al. Mutation of ALMS1, a large gene with a tandem repeat encoding 47 amino acids, causes Alstrom syndrome. Nat Genet 2002;31:79–83.
901. Nakazawa M, Wada Y, Tamai M. Arrestin gene mutations in autosomal recessive retinitis pigmentosa. Arch Ophthalmol 1998;116:498–501.
902. Haider NB, Jacobson SG, Cideciyan AV, et al. Mutation of a nuclear receptor gene, NR2E3, causes enhanced S cone syndrome, a disorder of retinal cell fate. Nat Genet 2000;24:127–31.
903. Coppieters F, Leroy BP, Beysen D, et al. Recurrent mutation in the first zinc finger of the orphan nuclear receptor NR2E3 causes autosomal dominant retinitis pigmentosa. Am J Hum Genet 2007;81:147–57.
904. Hayflick SJ, Westaway SK, Levinson B, et al. Genetic, clinical, and radiographic delineation of Hallervorden–Spatz syndrome. N Engl J Med 2003;348: 33–40.

Chapter 41

Hereditary Vitreoretinal Degenerations

Shibo Tang, Xiaoyan Ding, Yan Luo

Hereditary vitreoretinal degeneration, also known as hereditary vitreoretinopathy, is classically characterized by early-onset cataracts, vitreous anomalies, coarse fibrils and membranes, and retinal detachment. Genetic and clinical advances in the last two decades have enabled a reassessment of the essential criteria that define this group of conditions. More recently, these conditions have been defined as the presence of congenital abnormalities of the vitreous, including severe degeneration or maldevelopment, early-onset progressive cataracts, and an increased predisposition to rhegmatogenous retinal detachment.[1] Additional ocular and systemic features may be present, depending on the underlying cause.

Since many vitreoretinal degenerations are autosomal dominant, high variability in severity and expression is common both within and between families, so examination of more than one family member is often necessary to reach the correct diagnosis. Molecular genetic studies have demonstrated a correlation between the clinical features of the disease and the underlying gene mutation. Thus, the clinician is able to predict which gene is involved within a family and provide appropriate counseling and management. Failure to recognize a syndromic cause of a childhood retinal detachment can lead to vision loss not only in the patient, but also in other siblings, that could have been avoided.

In this chapter, we discuss five main types of vitreoretinopathies: (1) snowflake vitreoretinal degeneration; (2) X-linked juvenile retinoschisis; (3) the chromosome 5q vitreoretinopathies (e.g., Wagner syndrome); (4) chondrodysplasias with vitreoretinal degeneration (e.g., Stickler syndrome); and (5) enhanced S-cone syndrome (ESCS)/Goldmann–Favre vitreotapetoretinal degeneration. Several additional vitreoretinal degenerations are also summarized, including autosomal dominant neovascular inflammatory vitreoretinopathy (ADNIV) and autosomal dominant vitreoretinochoroidopathy (ADVIRC). We review the common features of vitreoretinal degenerations and highlight those features that can be used to distinguish them from each other clinically. Lattice degeneration and familial exudative vitreoretinopathy are not discussed in this chapter. Table 41.1 summarizes the main features of these disorders. Note that a given patient need not have all of the listed features. The pattern of clinical findings, rather than a specific feature, is the best strategy to make the diagnosis.

SNOWFLAKE VITREORETINAL DEGENERATION

General features

The term "snowflake vitreoretinal degeneration" (SVD) was originally coined by Hirose et al.[2] in 1974, who described an American family of European extraction with early-onset cataracts, fibrillar vitreous degeneration, vascular sheathing, peripheral minute crystalline-like deposits, and retinal detachment. The condition received its name from the minute crystalline-like deposits that can be seen by contact lens biomicroscopy in some patients.[2] The vitreous degeneration is fibrillar to a variable extent; the bands of condensed vitreous fibrils may obscure fundus details and peripheral condensations of vitreous on the retinal surface can be observed. Radial or circumferential lattice degeneration is not observed. The average spherical equivalent is –2.90 D, indicating moderate myopia. Other distinguishing features include a dysmorphic optic nerve head that appears flat and often without a cup. Peripapillary vascular sheathing and atrophy, as well as waxy pallor, may be present.

Clinical findings

Ocular features

There were 31 individuals in the Hirose family enrolled in the original study in 1974 (13 affected individuals, 14 unaffected individuals, and 4 unaffected spouses). The 13 subjects diagnosed with SVD ranged from 12 to 85 years of age, with clinical features such as early-onset cataract, fibrillar vitreous degeneration, vascular sheathing, and retinal detachment.[2] The inheritance pattern was autosomal dominant, and no obligatory carriers of the snowflake trait were found to be normal. After about 20 years, Lee et al.[3] restudied 6 of these 13 patients and identified additional clinical features, including corneal guttata (4 out of 5 patients) and optic nerve head dysplasia (the exact number of affected individuals was not recorded). Early-onset cataracts (5 out of 6), fibrillar vitreous degeneration (6 out of 6), and peripheral retinal abnormalities (5 out of 6), including minute crystalline-like deposits called snowflakes (4 out of 6), were common. Compared to other hereditary vitreoretinal degenerations, there was a relatively low rate of retinal detachment, occurring in 1 of the 6 examined family members.[3] Orofacial features, early-onset hearing loss, and arthritis that are typical of Stickler syndrome were absent. Thus, the clinical

Table 41.1 Features of hereditary vitreoretinal degenerations

Name	Snowflake vitreoretinal degeneration	X-linked retinoschisis	Wagner syndrome	Stickler syndrome	Enhanced S-cone syndrome/ Goldmann–Favre vitreotapetoretinal degeneration/	Autosomal dominant vitreoretinochoroidopathy
Abbreviation	SVD	XLRS	WGN1	STL1/STL2	ESCS/GFV	ADVIRC
Inheritance	Autosomal dominant	X-linked recessive	Autosomal dominant	Autosomal dominant or recessive	Autosomal recessive	Autosomal dominant
Genetic loci	2q36	Xp22.1	5q13–14	12q13.11,1p21, 6q12-q14,1p33-p32, 20q13.3	15q23	11q13
Genes	*KCNJ13*	*RS1*	*CSPG2*	*COL2A1, COL11A1* *COL9A1, COL9A2, COL9A3*	*NR2E3*	*VMD2*
Prevalence	Less than 1:10 000	1: 15000–1:30000	Less than 1:1 000 000	1:10 000	Less than 1:1 000 000	Rare
Refraction/ motility	Myopic	Axial hyperopia, strabismus	Moderate myopic, pseudostrabismus with positive-angle κ	High myopic Astigmatism	Variable, myopic	Variable
Visual acuity	Not usually affected	Vision loss: average visual acuity in young adults is around 20/70	Deteriorates slowly after age of 20 due to posterior chorioretinal atrophy	Usually good unless affected by retinal detachment or foveal atrophy	Poor centrally and peripherally	Usually good unless affected by retinal detachment or foveal retinoschisis
Anterior segment	Corneal guttae Presenile cataract	Neovascular glaucoma	Anterior chamber dependent, typical dot-like cortical cataracts, glaucoma	Presenile cataracts with characteristic curved cortical distribution, lentis ectopia	Usually normal	Usually normal, but dysgenesis and congenital cataract reported
Vitreous	Fibrillar vitreous degeneration	Vitreous hemorrhage	Vitreous syneresis, posterior strands and veils in the vitreous cavity	Vitreous syneresis and band formation, membranous vitreous veils in type I, fibrillar vitreous in type II	Usually normal, may be degenerated in GFV	Normal to fibrillar degeneration, cells

Continued

Table 41.1 Features of hereditary vitreoretinal degenerations—Cont'd

Name	Snowflake vitreoretinal degeneration	X-linked retinoschisis	Wagner syndrome	Stickler syndrome	Enhanced S-cone syndrome/ Goldmann–Favre vitreotapetoretinal degeneration/	Autosomal dominant vitreoretinochoroidopathy
Optic nerve	Dysmorphic optic nerve head, flat appearance, absent cup, waxy pallor	Optic atrophy	Optic atrophy, optic nerve dysmorphism	Usually normal	Usually normal	May have neovascularization
Macula	Usually normal	Foveal schisis, foveal ectopia	Foveal ectopia	Usually normal	Cystoid changes, loss of normal retinal lamellae	May have macular edema or atrophy
Retinal vessels	Parapapillary sheathing, radial perivascular degeneration	Lie in either the outer or inner leaf or cross through the schisis cavity	Abnormal retinal vessel architecture (inverted papilla), perivascular pigmentation, and sheathing	Sclerosing of retinal vessels	Pigmentary degeneration along the arcades	Preretinal neovascularization
Retinal detachment	20%	5–20%	Infrequent	50–60%	Uncommon	Infrequent
Periphery	Minute inner retinal crystals, focal RPE degeneration, vitreous condensations	Peripheral retinoschisis	Chorioretinal atrophy	Peripheral chorioretinal degeneration	Peripheral degeneration with clumped pigment may be present	A sharply demarcated, circumferential, peripheral retinal degeneration from ora serrata to a posterior margin anterior to the equator is typical
Systemic features	None	None	None	Cleft palate Hearing loss Arthritis Midface hypoplasia Epiphyseal dysplasia Osteoarthritis	None	None
ERG	Reduced in late stages	Selective b-wave reduction	Reduced in late stages, the amplitudes of the b-waves are generally better preserved than those of the a-waves	Usually normal	Enhanced S cone Phenotype to undetectable	Normal or depressed Arden ratio with variable reduction

RPE, retinal pigment epithelium; ERG, electroretinogram.

findings were not typical of Stickler syndrome or chromosome 5q retinopathies, suggesting SVD may be a distinct form of vitreoretinal degeneration.

According to the dominant features present on fundoscopic examination, SVD has been classified into four stages: (1) extensive white with pressure; (2) snowflake degeneration; (3) sheathing of retinal vessels and fundus pigmentation; and (4) further pigmentation and disappearance of the peripheral retinal vessels. Hejtmancik et al. classified the clinical features of SVD into subgroups of congenital and progressive abnormalities.[4] The congenital abnormalities include optic nerve head dysmorphism with fibrillar degeneration of the vitreous. Progressive ocular features include corneal guttae and peripheral retinal degeneration within which minute crystalline deposits, referred to as snowflakes, might be seen. These characteristics distinguish SVD from other vitreoretinal degenerations.

Using Hejtmancik's genetic studies, it is evident that although the term "snowflake" has been used in reports of other families, they do not appear to be the same condition according to the clinical criteria and/or genetic evaluation. Moreover, the proportion of patients diagnosed with non-syndromic Stickler syndrome that ultimately share a common genetic basis with SVD patients is currently unknown, thus the real prevalence of SVD to date is difficult to estimate. So far, there is only one family reported in the literature with a case history similar to the classic description of SVD. This family was reported by Pollack and colleagues[5,6] and showed an autosomal dominant vitreoretinal degeneration with minute crystalline-like dots, probably similar to the Hirose family. A distinguishing feature of this family, however was the appearance of neovascular tufts in the temporal periphery in 4 of the 9 affected members of the middle generation.[6] Two other reports have described subjects with SVD. Robertson et al.[7] reported familial clustering of granular deposits 100–200 μm in diameter in 10 patients from four families, which was described as snowflake degeneration of the retina in 1982. The deposits were evenly distributed about the circumference of the eye near the equatorial fundus. Smaller crystalline deposits were observed between the granular deposits. However, findings of vitreoretinal degeneration, such as early-onset cataract, severe vitreous degeneration, and retinal detachment, were not observed. The granular deposits are also not similar to those in patients with *COL2A1* mutations causing Stickler syndrome.[2,3] Chen and colleagues[8] reported a family with vitreoretinal degeneration in 1986, but they were distinguished from the Hirose family by nyctalopia, poor visual acuity, annular scotomas, and attenuated retinal vessels. They may also have shown different-appearing deposits compared to the classical SVD description.[2] Unfortunately, these two families have not been subject to genetic analysis.

Molecular genetics of SVD

Jiao et al.[9] re-examined the family and localized the mutation to chromosome 2q36. Molecular genetic investigation excluded the known locations of genes causing vitreoretinal degeneration,[3] and a novel gene location was subsequently identified. One of the authors (XD) studied the location of Kir7.1 (the protein product of *KCNJ13*) in the retina, and found that it is bound to the inner limiting membrane and the retinal pigment epithelium, which suggests that the mutation could affect development of the vitreous through alteration of Müller cell function.[4] The mutation in *KCNJ13* demonstrates that classic vitreoretinal degeneration can arise from gene mutations that are not structural components of the vitreous. Alteration in potassium transport provides a mechanism for the electrophysiological abnormalities seen in these patients, but further study is required for a precise explanation. The condition arises due to a mutation in *KCNJ13* disrupting the selective transport of potassium through the channel.[4] Thus, SVD can be clinically and genetically confirmed as a unique form of vitreoretinal degeneration.

Visual psychophysics

Kinetic perimetry shows peripheral defects, which are more pronounced in the superior field.[10] Flicker perimetry reveals abnormalities undetected by kinetic perimetry and dark adaptation tests show elevated rod thresholds, except during the early stage of the disease.

Electrophysiology

The scotopic b-wave of the electroretinogram (ERG) elicited by dim light is low in amplitude and may be almost extinguished in late stages of the disease. The photopic b-wave and the photopic flicker responses may show decreased amplitudes in some patients. The electro-oculographic light peak–dark trough ratio is abnormal in only a few patients.

Differential diagnosis

Gene identification in SVD-like families is the gold standard in the diagnosis of SVD. Clinical diagnosis of SVD is difficult, as the clinical manifestation overlaps with other types of vitreoretinal degeneration. The key distinguishing features are fibrillar degeneration of the vitreous, optic nerve dysmorphism, peripheral areas of retinal pigment epithelial degeneration, corneal guttae, and retinal crystalline-like spots. It is unknown if the discrete crystalline-like spots characteristic of the Hirose family are specific indicators of the underlying gene, or a rare manifestation of vitreoretinal degeneration unique to a few families. Severe fibrillar degeneration of the vitreous also can be seen in type II Stickler syndrome (*COL11A1*). Corneal guttae may also be a diagnostic feature of SVD in some pedigrees. Abnormal optic nerve heads and posterior sheathing of the retinal vessels are also suggestive. The optic disc is always flat and without a cup, and nasal deviation of the vessels, waxy pallor, and peripapillary atrophy may also be present.

Stickler syndrome type I

This is the most common form of vitreoretinal degeneration. Mutations leading to haploinsufficiency of the collagen 2A1 (*COL2A1*) gene cause Stickler syndrome type I (STL1, MIM 108300). These patients have a vitreous degeneration characterized by a unique vitreous appearance vestigial vitreous gel occupying the immediate retrolental space and no discernible gel in the central vitreous cavity. The expression of syndromic features, including hearing loss, facial dysmorphism, and joint pain, exhibits variability both between and within families.[11]

Stickler syndrome type II

Mutations leading to haploinsufficiency of the collagen 11A1 (*COL11A1*) gene cause Stickler syndrome type II (STL2, MIM 604841). Unlike *COL2A1* disease, these mutations lead to a fibrillar vitreous degeneration with limited and random fibrils throughout the vitreous cavity.[12–14] In some cases, severe fibrillar degeneration of the vitreous can also be seen.

Marshall syndrome

Mutations altering intron–exon splicing of the *COL11A1* gene lead to Marshall syndrome (MIM 154780), distinguished from SVD and Stickler syndrome by a more pronounced facial dysmorphism and lower frequency of retinal detachment.[15,16] Membranous vitreous veils and radial lattice have also been noted in patients with Marshall syndrome.[17]

Wagner syndrome

Wagner syndrome (MIM 143200) is caused by noncoding mutations that are thought to affect the splicing of chondroitin sulfate proteoglycan-2 (*CSPG2*), the gene encoding versican.[18,19] These mutations may lead to disease through abnormal ratios of versican isoforms. The distinguishing features of Wagner syndrome are pseudostrabismus, thickened and partially detached posterior hyaloids with an empty vitreous cavity, variable degeneration of the retina and choroid, and the absence of systemic manifestations.[20] The absence of nyctalopia, posterior chorioretinal atrophy, and tractional retinal detachment distinguishes Wagner syndrome from other chromosome 5q vitreoretinopathies such as Jansen syndrome and erosive vitreoretinopathy (ERVR).

Goldmann–Favre vitreotapetoretinal degeneration

Patients with Goldmann–Favre vitreotapetoretinal degeneration have nonrecordable ERGs and central and/or peripheral retinoschisis. This is in contrast to patients with snowflake degeneration, who have fairly good ERG responses and absence of central or peripheral retinoschisis.[21]

Management

At this time, no specific management is available, and there are no established guidelines for prophylactic therapy. As the risk of retinal detachment is 20% and cataract surgery of early-onset lens opacification can be difficult due to vitreous liquefaction, family members should be examined to determine if they carry the condition. Affected patients should be educated about cataract and retinal detachments and examined regularly. Children should be given special attention because of cataract-induced refractive problems and their frequent failure to recognize and/or report retinal detachment symptoms.

Common issues in the management of hereditary vitreoretinal degenerations are described below:

1. Cataract surgery is difficult in these patients due to lack of vitreous support during surgery, and should be performed by experienced surgeons with specific experience with vitrectomized eyes that behave similarly. Microinvasive 23- or 25-gauge infusion cannulae via the pars plana are beneficial for maintaining the intraocular pressure.
2. Glaucoma can occur, usually after cataract surgery, and should be monitored and treated using established methods.
3. Prophylactic cryopexy is performed by some groups, while peripheral laser retinopexy is favored by others. Although a randomized trial has yet to be published comparing the two methods, a recent report using cryopexy is the most comprehensive study to date.[22] Ang et al. found that, in patients with type I Stickler syndrome, the prevalence of RD was significantly less in bilateral 360° prophylactic cryotherapy than that in untreated patients, suggesting that prophylactic cryotherapy may be substantially beneficial.[22]
4. Retinal detachments are also common and should be managed using standard vitrectomy-based approaches, including vitrectomy, artificial posterior vitreous detachment, and release of peripheral traction, perfluorocarbon-mediated retinal reattachment, scleral buckle, laser retinopexy, and tamponade with gas or silicone oil.

THE CHROMOSOME 5Q RETINOPATHIES: WAGNER SYNDROME, JANSEN SYNDROME, EROSIVE VITREORETINOPATHY, AND RELATED CONDITIONS

General features

The chromosome 5q retinopathies include Wagner syndrome, ERVR, and Jansen syndrome. Jansen syndrome and ERVR share clinical and allelic features with Wagner syndrome. Knowledge of the chromosome 5q retinopathies has expanded greatly over the past few years, along with the identification of the responsible genes for the allelic syndromes. It is not possible to easily identify a pathological mutation for the above syndromes due to the difficulties in determining splicing defects in large complex genes. Even so, recent genetic and clinical advances enable a reassessment of the essential criteria which define this group of diseases.

Wagner syndrome is characterized by an optically empty vitreous with avascular vitreous strands and veils, moderate myopia, presenile cataracts, and retinal degeneration with atrophy.[23] Stickler syndrome is also associated with craniofacial abnormalities and a progressive arthropathy.[24] Wagner syndrome and Stickler syndrome were once incorrectly considered as one entity: the Wagner–Stickler syndrome.

Wagner syndrome is an autosomal dominant genetic disorder first mapped to chromosome 5q13–14 in 1995. A mutation in the chondroitin sulfate proteoglycan 2 gene (*CSPG2*), now named *VCAN*, encoding for the versican protein, was found in 2005.[20,25,26] *VCAN* is the only gene currently associated with Wagner syndrome and ERVR.[19,27] Autosomal dominant Stickler syndrome is an inherited progressive disorder of the collagen connective tissues and is associated with the mutation of extracellular matrix collagen genes, such as *COL2A1, COL11A, COL11A2,* and *COL9A1*.[24,28–30]

Jansen syndrome was described as vitreoretinal and lenticular degeneration associated with retinal detachments in the absence of nonocular findings. However, the disease gene for the original Jansen family was demonstrated to be linked to the same region of chromosome 5q14[31] where genes for Wagner syndrome and ERVR were located.[25]

ERVR also displays an autosomal dominant inheritance pattern and shares some clinical features with Wagner syndrome. The critical region of the genetic defect underlying ERVR was found to overlap with the critical region for Wagner syndrome, 5q13-q14.[19]

Clinical findings

Ocular features

Wagner syndrome is characterized by an optically empty vitreous with equatorial avascular vitreous veils. Additional features include its early-onset, moderate myopia, and typical

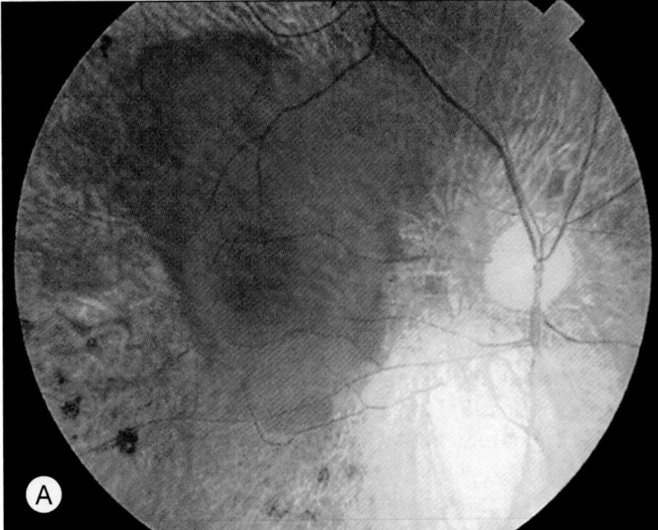

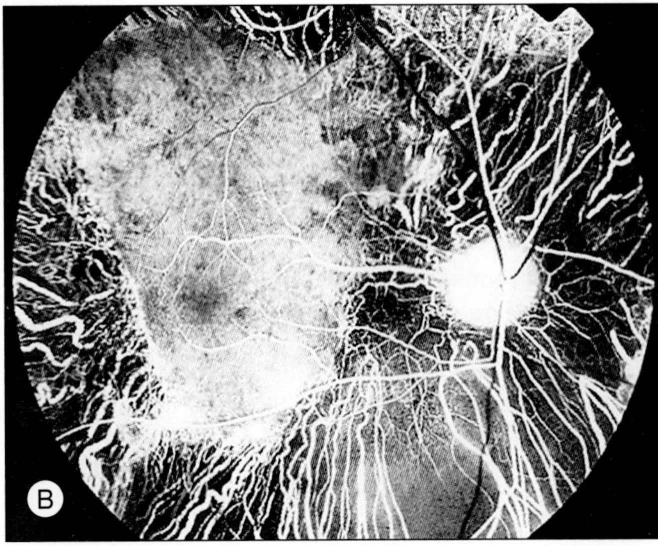

Fig. 41.1 Wagner vitreoretinal degeneration. (A) Marked chorioretinal atrophy with pigment migration into the retina and sparing of the macular area. Visual acuity was 20/25. (B) Fluorescein angiogram of the same eye showing early venous phase. There is extensive atrophy of choriocapillaris, sparing only the macular area. (Reproduced with permission from Graemiger RA, Niemeyer G, Schneeberger SA, et al. Wagner vitreoretinal degeneration. Follow-up of the original pedigree. Ophthalmology 1995;102:1830–1839. Copyright © 1995 American Academy of Ophthalmology.)

dot-like cortical cataracts, foveal ectopia, abnormal retinal vessels (inverted papilla), perivascular pigmentation and sheathing, retinal thinning, as well as slowly progressive chorioretinal atrophy. Patients with Wagner syndrome have pseudostrabismus from congenital temporal displacement of the fovea. They also have nyctalopia early in life and final dark adaptation thresholds are elevated in some patients.[32] Most patients under the age of 20 have normal vision; however, cataract, retinal detachment, optic atrophy, and chorioretinal atrophy may be progressive and cause visual loss with advancing age[20,23,25–27] (Fig. 41.1). In addition to the clinical features of Wagner syndrome, ERVR reveals progressive nyctalopia and visual field constriction. A conspicuous loss of retinal pigment epithelium and choriocapillaries is observed by fluorescein angiography.[19] The vitreous findings are marked syneresis with prominent membranes. Rhegmatogenous retinal detachment is usually described as a feature of ERVR, and is less frequent in the original description of Wagner syndrome.[33]

Visual psychophysics

Nyctalopia can be present early in life in some patients. Vision is usually normal as the pathologic process initially involves the retinal periphery, but severe loss of vision will occur in patients when diffuse cone–rod loss ensues as there is progressive chorioretinal atrophy.[1,25]

Electrophysiology

Both the ERG and dark adaptation of patients with the chromosome 5q retinopathies appear to be normal early in life but become progressively abnormal throughout the patient's life. The rod and cone systems are affected to varying degrees but in a family-specific manner. While both a-wave and b-wave amplitudes are reduced, b-wave amplitudes are generally better preserved. Visual field findings can be variable and may include diffuse peripheral loss or partial/complete midperipheral ring scotomas as the chorioretinal atrophy progresses.[34]

Differential diagnosis

Ophthalmologic examination, an autosomal dominant inheritance pattern of family history, visual field examination, ERG, and orthoptic assessment are critical for definitive diagnosis and timely management. The differential diagnosis includes both autosomal dominant and recessive vitreoretinopathies.

Autosomal dominant vitreoretinopathies

Snowflake vitreoretinal degeneration

SVD is a progressive hereditary eye disorder caused by mutations in *KCNJ13*. Diagnostic features of SVD consist of fibrillar vitreous degeneration, early-onset cataract, minute crystalline deposits in the neurosensory retina, and retinal detachment.[4] However, membranous degeneration of the vitreous with avascular strands and veils is not observed in SVD. Retinal defects typically start in the superficial retinal layers and retinal detachment is uncommon.[4,27]

Stickler syndrome

Stickler syndrome is genetically distinguished from Wagner syndrome and other chromosome 5q retinopathies. Type I Stickler syndrome is due to *COL2A1* mutation and is associated with retrolental membranous vitreous, while type II Stickler syndrome is due to mutations in *COL11A1* and is associated with a fibrillar or beaded vitreous phenotype. Both type I and II Stickler syndrome have ocular and systemic manifestations, while type III Stickler syndrome, associated with *COL11A2* mutations, has systemic manifestations only. Most, but not all, patients with Stickler syndrome have congenital, nonprogressive, and high-degree myopia. The cataracts may be congenital and nonprogressive, and have an unusual characteristic curved cortical distribution.[35] Retinal detachment is much more common in Stickler syndrome (50%) than in chromosome 5q vitreoretinopathies (15%). Systemic abnormalities are present in Stickler syndrome, such as midface hypoplasia, midline cleft of the palate, bifid uvula, sensorineural hearing loss, and skeletal abnormalities.[24,27–29] Abnormal dark adaptation associated with alterations in the ERG that is common in chromosome 5q retinopathies has not been described in Stickler syndrome.[1,27]

Autosomal dominant vitreoretinochoroidopathy

ADVIRC is caused by mutations in *VMD2* and also has characteristic retinal and vitreous findings, in particular a peripheral retinal circumferential hyperpigmented band, vitreous fibrillar condensation, punctate white opacities in the retina, breakdown of the blood–retinal barrier, and retinal neovascularization.[36]

Autosomal recessive vitreoretinopathies

Goldmann–Favre syndrome (GFS) and enhanced S-cone syndrome

GFS and ESCS share common mutations in the *NR2E3* gene and are usually associated with night blindness and visual field abnormalities. ERG typically reveals a severe reduction in rod function and a relatively enhanced function of the short-wavelength-sensitive cones.[27,37] GFS manifests with progressive vitreous changes, hemeralopia, chorioretinal atrophy, and pigmentary retinal degeneration, later resulting in marked visual field loss, retinoschisis in the periphery and/or macula, presenile cataract, and hyperopia rather than myopia.[27,38,39] ESCS lacks the typical marked vitreous changes of GFS.

Knobloch syndrome

Knobloch syndrome is an autosomal recessive disorder characterized by pathogenic mutations in the *COL18A1* gene.[40] Characteristic features of Knobloch syndrome are high myopia, vitreoretinal degeneration with retinal detachment, and congenital encephalocele.

Management

Genetic counseling

Chromosome 5q retinopathies are inherited in an autosomal dominant manner, so prenatal testing is very important. Each child with these diseases has a 50% chance of inheriting the mutation.

Treatments

Refractive error is corrected by spectacles or contact lenses. Cataract is managed by the phacoemulsification and implantation of an intraocular lens. Retinal breaks without retinal detachment are treated with laser photocoagulation. Vitreoretinal surgery is needed for retinal detachment, vitreoretinal traction involving the macula, or epiretinal membranes involving the macula. Prophylactic cryotherapy has been recently reported to reduce the risk of retinal detachment markedly.[1]

CHONDRODYSPLASIAS ASSOCIATED WITH VITREORETINAL DEGENERATION: THE STICKLER SYNDROMES, MARSHALL SYNDROME, KNIEST DYSPLASIA, KNOBLOCH SYNDROME, AND WEISSENBACHER–ZWEYMULLER SYNDROME

General features

Chondrodysplasias refer to a group of hereditary and systematic disorders that affect skeletal development and growth. These conditions may also feature ocular, central nervous system, or renal abnormalities. The genes involved in these syndromes affect types II, III, V, X, or XI, collagen molecules that are found mainly in cartilage and vitreous and are essential for the normal development of bones and other connective tissue, thus accounting for the symptoms observed clinically. Antenatal diagnosis, including fetal magnetic resonance imaging, computed tomography, ultrasonography, and genetic testing of fetal DNA obtained from aminocentesis or chorionic villus sampling, is important for the proper management of children and counseling of parents.[41–43]

According to the various "chondrodysplasia genes" and clinical presentations, five syndromes with distinct ocular dysfunctions – Stickler syndrome, Marshall syndrome, Kniest dysplasia, Knobloch syndrome, and Weissenbacher–Zweymuller syndrome – belong to the family of chondrodysplasias associated with vitreoretinal degeneration.

Stickler syndrome, also known as hereditary progressive arthro-ophthalmopathy, is considered to be the most common chondrodysplasia associated with vitreoretinal degeneration. Types I, II, and III are the three subgroups of Stickler syndrome classified by genetic heterogeneity. Types I and II Stickler syndrome, respectively caused by mutations in the *COL2A1* gene encoding type II collagen[44] and in the *COL11A1* gene encoding type XI collagen,[45] can be differentiated successfully by vitreous phenotypes. Mutations in *COL2A1* usually result in a congenital membranous vitreous anomaly, while mutations in *COL11A1* result in an irregular and beaded vitreous.[46,47] Recently, a new subgroup of *COL2A1* mutations was found that lead to a hypoplastic vitreous which is either optically empty or contains sparse irregular lamellae.[13] Due to the differential splicing, *COL2A1* gene transcription products can be divided into two types: collagen IIA with an exon2-encoded length of 69 (rich in amino acid homocysteine) and collagen IIB without the exon2-encoded peptide. Whereas both collagen IIA and IIB loss results in systemic connective tissues disease, collagen IIA loss also leads to ocular abnormalities. It is because collagen IIA primarily exists in the vitreous.[48,49] Recent studies have indicated that mutations in any collagen IX genes, like *COL9A1*, *COL9A2*, or *COL9A3*, can cause autosomal recessive Stickler syndrome.[50–52] Thus far, the diagnosis of Stickler syndrome has been based on clinical manifestations without consensus on the minimal clinical diagnostic criteria. The anomalous formation of the vitreous gel structure and its corresponding characteristic abnormalities are essential for the diagnosis of types I and II Stickler syndrome. In additional to these clinical manifestations, a detailed family history should be obtained and the diagnosis can be confirmed by genetic analysis. Recently, the *COL2A1* mutation in peripheral white blood cells has been used to identify patients with type I Stickler syndrome.[51]

Marshall syndrome, an autosomal dominant chondrodysplasia, is caused by a splicing mutation of 54-bp exons in the c-terminal region of the *COL11A1* gene which is located on the short arm of chromosome 1. Although Marshall syndrome and Stickler syndrome are now considered two distinct diseases, a case of a patient with overlapping phenotypes has been described.[53]

Kniest dysplasia, inherited in an autosomal dominant pattern, is a moderately severe collagenopathy. Like type I Stickler syndrome, Kniest dysplasia is caused by mutations in *COL2A1* gene which encodes type II collagen, so cartilage and vitreous are mainly involved. It is reported that small deletions or splice site alterations between *COL2A1* gene exons 12 and 24 may cause the inframe deletions of type II collagen.

Knobloch syndrome is a rare and clinically heterogeneous autosomal recessive disorder. Collagen XVIII, which is a basement membrane proteoglycan, distributes in multiple organs of the body and plays an important role in the function and development of the eye, kidney, and nervous system. In most patients with this symptom, null mutations in the *COL18A1* gene mapped to the long arm of chromosome 21 are supposed to induce the changes in collagen XVIII.[54] There are also case reports of Knobloch syndrome without *COL18A1* gene mutations, and thus immunofluorescent histochemistry of skin biopsy samples has proved to be a useful preliminary and complementary test for the diagnosis of Knobloch syndrome.[55]

Weissenbacher–Zweymuller syndrome, also called Pierre Robin syndrome with fetal chondrodysplasia, is an autosomal recessive disorder characterized by a single-base mutation in the *COL11A2* gene, which substitutes glutamate for glycine.[56] In the past, it was often misdiagnosed as Stickler syndrome. Recently, investigators have differentiated these two syndromes successfully by prenatal ultrasonography.[57]

Clinical findings

Extraocular features

Stickler syndrome features a highly variable systemic phenotype, including conductive and sensorineural hearing loss, immunoglobulin deficiency,[20] cleft palate, mid facial underdevelopment, mild spondyloepiphyseal dysplasia, and precocious arthritis[58] (Fig. 41.2).

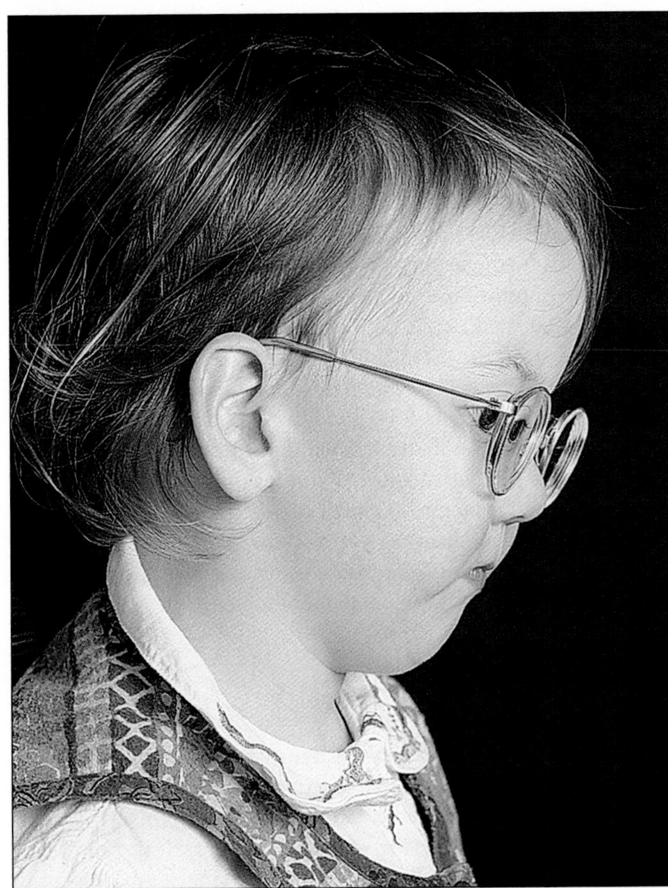

Fig. 41.2 Stickler syndrome. Child with facial features including mid facial hypoplasia and Pierre Robin sequence.

Like Stickler syndrome, Marshall syndrome is also characterized by mid facial hypoplasia, sensorineural deafness, and ocular defects (cataract and high myopia). More importantly, it also includes ectodermal dysplasia, absence of frontal sinuses, calcifications of falx and tentorial meninges, as well as distal femoral and proximal tibial epiphyses, and wide tufts of the distal phalanges. Thus neural system, limb, and trunk abnormalities are important features.

Kniest dysplasia has the typical manifestations of short-trunk dwarfism with kyphoscoliosis, enlarged joints with decreased motion, flat midface, cleft palate, and hearing loss.[59]

Extraocular features of Knobloch syndrome are mainly characterized by the occipital encephalocele caused by a midline defect in the occipital bone. Due to its rarity, the spectrum of clinical variability is not fully understood.

Weissenbacher–Zweymuller syndrome is characteristic of midface hypoplasia with a flat nasal bridge, small upturned nasal tip, micrognathia, sensorineural hearing loss, and rhizomelic limb shortening. Radiographic examination may detect dumbbell-shaped femora and humeri, and vertebral coronal clefts in these patients.[53] However, some congenital abnormalities, such as dwarfism, developmental delays, and radiological abnormalities, may return to normality at school age, so it is hypothesized to be dysmaturational other than syndromic.[60]

Ocular features

Types I and II Stickler syndrome have a high risk of ocular complications, including congenital high myopia, cataract, and retinal problems,[46] such as vitreous changes, radial perivascular retinal degeneration, and rhegmatogenous retinal detachment[61] (Fig. 41.3). These findings may manifest at any age and produce vision loss. Unlike Stickler syndrome, rhegmatogenous retinal detachment is unusual in Marshall syndrome and cataracts may be spontaneously absorbed.

The ocular manifestations of Kniest dysplasia mainly consist of high myopia, optically empty vitreous with retrolental and peripheral vitreous membranes, lattice degeneration, and retinal detachment. Ocular manifestations involved in Knobloch syndrome include high myopia, cataract, vitreoretinal degeneration, and retinal detachment which lead to progressive and

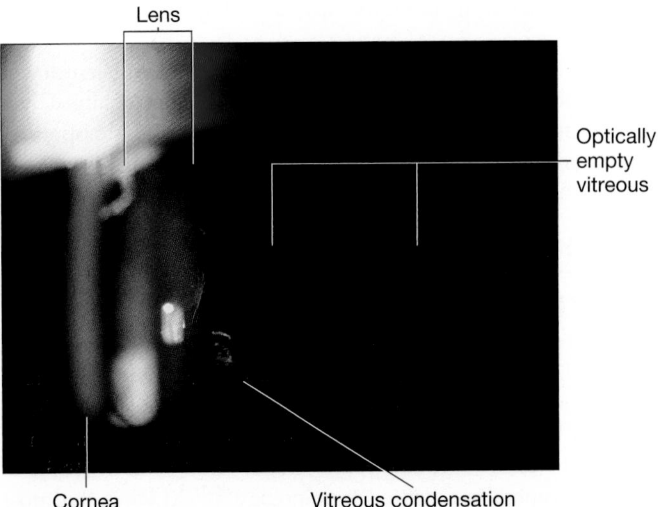

Fig. 41.3 Stickler syndrome. Slit-lamp photograph of the child shown in Figure 41.2 showing congenital vitreous abnormality.

irreversible vision loss. Weissenbacher–Zweymuller syndrome mainly shows strabismus and various refractive errors, which should be treated at an early age to prevent amblyopia.[62]

Differential diagnosis

Marfan syndrome

Marfan syndrome is an autosomal dominant disorder characterized by ocular, skeletal, and cardiovascular abnormalities. The ocular manifestations include flat cornea, high myopia, lens subluxation lens, and retinal detachment. It is believed that mutations in the gene *FBN1*, which encodes a component of the extracellular matrix-connective tissue protein fibrillin-1, may result in the pathological changes of Marfan syndrome.

Wagner syndrome

As noted above, Wagner syndrome is often confused with Stickler syndrome. Key differentiating features are the typical vitreous abnormalities, higher risk of retinal detachment, and systemic findings of Stickler syndrome versus the characteristic nyctalopia, retinal pigmentary changes, and dark adaption problems of Wagner syndrome.[20,23]

Erosive vitroeretinopathy

ERVR, as described above, is characterized by an "optically empty vitreous" and avascular vitreous strands and veils, mild or occasionally moderate to severe myopia, presenile cataract, night blindness of variable degree associated with progressive chorioretinal atrophy, retinal detachment at advanced stages, and reduced visual acuity. Systemic abnormalities are not observed. Rhegmatogenous retinal detachment occurs more frequently in ERVR than in Wagner syndrome.[63]

Management

The most common management strategy is symptomatic treatment for complications such as mandibular distraction osteogenesis for pediatric airway management,[64] mandibular advancement for malocclusion and micrognathia, correction of refractive errors with spectacles, vitrectomy with silicone oil injection for retinal detachment, and symptomatic treatment for arthropathy.

Prevention of secondary complications and surveillance are essential.[65] The rate of retinal detachment has been reported to be as high as 60%,[24] so frequent follow-up and potential interventions, including laser therapy, are of great importance in prevention.

Recently, several transgenic mouse models have been developed with mutations in the pro-alpha collagen chain. These animals may serve as useful models for arthro-ophthalmopathies and eventually provide a basis for gene-directed therapy for these conditions.[43,48]

X-LINKED RETINOSCHISIS

General features

X-linked retinoschisis (XLRS) is a human inherited retinal degenerative disease caused by mutations of the *RS1* gene on Xp22.1. Haas[66] first described the disease that is now known as retinoschisis in 1898. XLRS was first documented as being X-linked in 1913.[67] The term "X-linked retinoschisis," first used in 1953,[68] is now the generally accepted terminology.[69–71] XLRS is the most common form of juvenile-onset retinal degeneration in males, with a prevalence of between 1 in 15000 and 1 in 30000, and causes vision loss.[72,73] XLRS is characterized by schisis of the neural retina, including cystic maculopathy, peripheral schisis, and reduced amplitude of the b-wave on the ERG.[74] The common sight-threatening complications of XLRS include retinal detachment, vitreous hemorrhage, and foveal schisis.[75] Females who are heterozygous for the *RS1* mutation commonly have no clinical symptoms of XLRS.[76] To date, no treatment is available to halt the development of schisis in patients with XLRS. Surgical interventions are required for XLRS patients with severe complications, such as retinal detachment and nonclearing vitreous hemorrhage.[77]

Since the causative gene *RS1* was identified in 1997,[78] approximately 177 mutations of the *RS1* gene responsible for XLRS have been found (http://www.dmd.nl/rs/index.html). *RS1* is exclusively expressed in the photoreceptors and retinal bipolar cells,[79,80] and encodes a 224-amino-acid homo-oligomeric secretory protein complex – retinoschisin. Retinoschisin can be detected throughout the neural retina layers despite its restricted pattern of gene expression.[79–81] A mutant *RS1* gene appears to interfere with the secretion and/or octamerization and function of retinoschisin.[82–84] Wu et al.[82] found that *RS1* exists as a novel octamer in which the eight subunits are joined together by Cys59-Cys223 intermolecular disulfide bonds. Each subunit consists of a 157-amino-acid discoidin domain. Within the discoidin domain, one cysteine (Cys83) exists in its reduced state, and two cysteine pairs (Cys63-Cys219 and Cys110-Cys142) form intramolecular disulfide bonds that are important in protein folding. Mutations of *RS1* disrupt subunit assembly and then cause XLRS. Although insertions, deletions, and splice site mutations have been described, the mutations that encode the discoidin domain are predominantly missense and clustered in exons 4–6.

Many studies have been focused on understanding the function and role of retinoschisin in retinal cell adhesion. Recently, retinoschisin has been reported to interact with β2 laminin within the extracellular space and αB crystallin intracellularly as it moves through the secretory pathway.[73,85,86] Molday et al.[87] have confirmed the co-localization of retinoschisin with Na/K-ATPase and SARM1 in photoreceptors and retinal bipolar cells. Gehrig et al.[88] suggested that activation of microglia/glia may trigger the photoreceptor degeneration in retinoschisin-deficient mice and that the Erk1/2-Egr1 pathway may be activated in the pathogenesis of RS. Also, *RS1* efficiently and reversely binds galactose-agarose and lactose-agarose, indicating the possibility of interaction between RS1 and glycosylation sites on Na/K ATPase, providing a method for the purification of RS1, which may facilitate further functional studies of RS1.[89] There may be other influencing factors such as genetic modifiers or environmental influences, since no correlations are between mutation type and disease severity or progression exists.[90,91] Certainly, the roles of these potential molecular interactions in XLRS require further investigation.

Clinical findings

Ocular features

XLRS has variable disease severity, even when caused by the same *RS1* mutation.[90] Each eye of a patient may have asymmetric progression, but both eyes are invariably involved. Foveal schisis is the characteristic sign of XLRS and is present in 98–100% of cases.[92,93] Although macular changes are present in almost all XLRS patients, the typical foveal schisis, seen as a spokewheel pattern of folds radiating out from the fovea

(Fig. 41.4), has been found to appear in only about 70% of XLRS patients. Peripheral retinoschisis is often noted in the inferotemporal region and is present in around 50% of patients[94] (Fig. 41.5). The splitting occurs in the superficial retinal layers, and so retinal vessels may lie in either the outer or inner leaf or cross from one to the other through the schisis cavity. Breaks occur within the inner layer, varying from small holes to large tears,[92] and the fragmentation of the inner leaf can lead to membranous remnants referred to vitreous veils. Other changes, including subretinal linear fibrosis, pigmentation, white retinal flecks, and vascular attenuation or sheathing, often appear in peripheral retina. The common sight-threatening complications of XLRS include traction or rhegmatogenous retinal detachment, dense vitreous hemorrhage, hemorrhage within a large schisis cavity, and intraretinal splitting involving the macula. Other less common complications include neovascular glaucoma,[95] vitreoretinal traction with secondary macular dragging,[96,97] and optic atrophy.[98] For most retinal detachments associated with XLRS, fluid usually accesses the subretinal space through either outer leaf/layer breaks in the areas of peripheral retinoschisis with inner leaf holes, or full-thickness retinal tears following vitreous detachment. Vitreous hemorrhage and retinal detachment are the most serious complications of XLRS. About 5–20% of XLRS patients may progress to retinal detachment,[92,93] and up to a third of patients develop vitreous hemorrhage,[73,99] which causes severe vision loss.

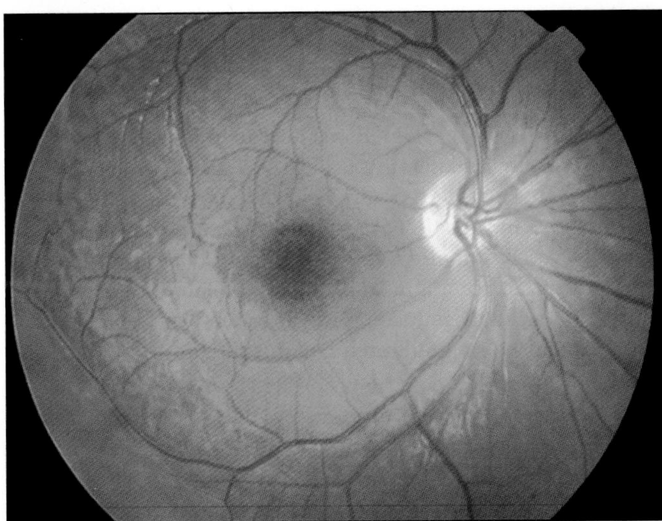

Fig. 41.4 Fundus photograph of X-linked retinoschisis with foveal cysts in a spokewheel pattern.

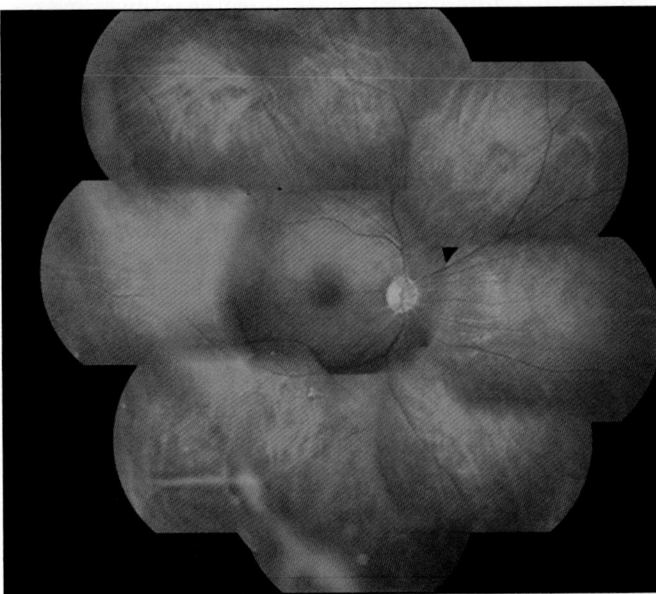

Fig. 41.5 Mosaic fundus photograph of X-linked retinoschisis with peripheral retinoschisis. The retinal vessels can be seen to be elevated from the retina into the vitreous cavity.

Less commonly, the disorder may present in early infancy with strabismus, nystagmus, axial hyperopia, foveal ectopia, or bilateral very large bullous retinoschisis, often with hemorrhage within the schisis cavity or into the vitreous.[99–101]

Visual psychophysics

Vision loss is the most common clinical presentation in XLRS patients. Visual acuity may deteriorate during the first and second decades of life, presenting as young as 3 months,[77] then remain relatively stable with very slow progression of macular atrophy until the fifth or sixth decade,[102] with eventual progression to legal blindness (acuity <20/200) by the sixth or seventh decade. XLRS patients are often detected when having reading difficulties and poor vision at school age. Visual acuity ranges from 20/20 to less than 20/200. The average visual acuity in young adults is around 20/70. Retinal detachment and vitreous hemorrhage may be the cause of a precipitous drop in visual acuity. Defective color vision (red–green dyschromatopsia) can also be present in XLRS patients.[103] The visual field shows an absolute scotoma in the field corresponding to the location of the peripheral retinal schisis.

Optical coherence tomography

Optical coherence tomography (OCT) helps to enhance the visualization of macular pathologic features in XLRS (Fig. 41.6).[104] The schisis can occur in different layers of the neural retina.[75] OCT findings may vary depending on the disease stage.[105]

Electrophysiology

ERG is helpful in the diagnosis of XLRS. There is typically reduced b-wave amplitude with a relatively preserved a-wave amplitude, although a few patients may have a relatively preserved b-wave amplitude.[94] The alteration of the b:a ratio ("negative" waveform, with a-wave amplitude exceeding the b-wave amplitude) is considered to be an important diagnostic parameter.[106] However, not all individuals with XLRS show

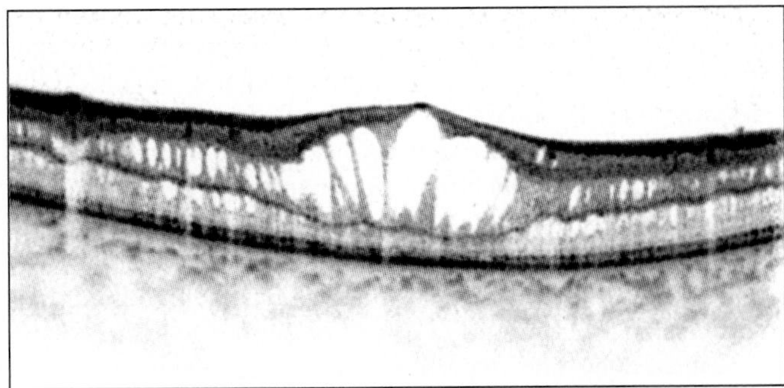

Fig. 41.6 Optical coherence tomography of X-linked retinoschisis demonstrating the splitting of the inner and outer retinal layers.

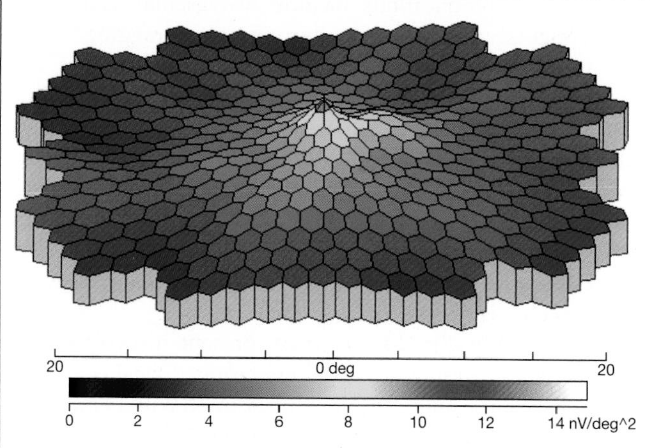

Fig. 41.7 Trace array and three-dimensional response density plot of multifocal electroretinography in X-linked retinoschisis showing reduced response amplitude in the macula.

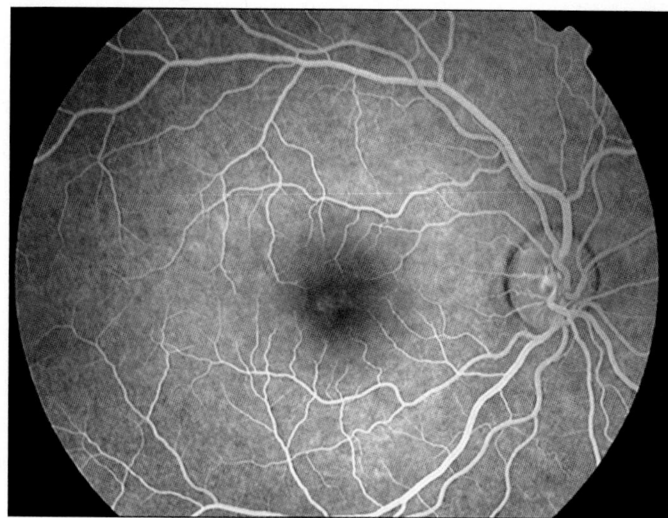

Fig. 41.8 Fluorescein angiogram demonstrating the foveal schisis cavity of X-linked retinoschisis and absence of leakage.

the classic electronegative ERG, and b-wave amplitudes may not be significantly different from normal. The a-wave can be normal or near-normal in an XLRS patient, whereas it may also be reduced due to the progressive atrophy of the retinal pigment epithelium.[107] The severity of ERG abnormalities does not appear to correlate with the mutation type.[108] Multifocal ERG can also demonstrate the reduced amplitudes and longer implicit times in the central macula (Fig. 41.7).

Differential diagnosis

The typical foveal schisis in a male with a reduced b-wave on ERG and a family history consistent with X-linked inheritance makes the diagnosis of XLRS very likely.[73] A domelike or slight elevation of a very thin layer of retinal tissue containing blood vessels can be visualized by ophthalmoscopy. Ancillary studies, including OCT and fluorescein angiography, may be useful in supporting the clinical diagnosis when minute foveal schisis is difficult to find by ophthalmoscopy. XLRS patients can be further confirmed with gene diagnosis of the *RS1* gene mutation.

Unlike many full-thickness neurosensory retinal detachments, the very thin and transparent layers of the neural retina in the setting of schsis do not undulate or shift when the position of the eye is changed. Moreover, the retinal abnormalities are always noted in both eyes of patients with XLRS.

In addition to retinal detachment, other disorders, such as cystoid macular edema, degenerative retinoschisis, acquired retinoschisis, amblyopia, Goldmann–Favre vitreoretinal degeneration, ESCS, Eales disease, and *VCAN*-related vitreoretinopathy, should be considered in the differential diagnosis of XLRS.

Cystoid macular edema is often observed in association with disorders such as retinal vein occlusion, diabetic retinopathy, uveitis, retinitis pigmentosa, dominantly inherited cystoid macular edema, or intraocular surgery (Irvine–Gass syndrome).[109] Although angiography is not required for diagnosis of XLRS, the absence of leakage in XLRS may aid in differentiating foveal schisis from other causes of cystoid macular edema characterized by late hyperfluorescence in a petaloid pattern (Fig. 41.8).

Degenerative retinoschisis is an idiopathic, degenerative splitting of the outer layers of the peripheral retina without ERG abnormalities or *RS1* mutations, occurring in an older age group, typically unilaterally.[73,110]

Goldmann–Favre vitreoretinal degeneration and ESCS caused by mutations in the *NR2E3* gene can also lead to foveal schisis, but the severely impaired vision, including marked visual field loss and nyctalopia, pigmentary clumping, absence of vitreous veils, and markedly reduced a-waves and b-waves with altered timing, should help to differentiate this disease from XLRS.[39]

Management

Genetic counseling

X-linked inheritance should be explained to XLRS patients. Carrier women have a 50% chance of transmitting the retinoschisis mutation in each pregnancy: males with the mutation will be affected and females with the mutation will be carriers and nearly always have normal visual function. Affected males pass the disease-causing mutation to all of their daughters and none of their sons. Carrier testing for at-risk female relatives and prenatal testing for pregnancy at increased risk are possible if the retinoschisis mutation in the family is known.

Treatment

Pharmacological treatment

The successful treatment of schisis cavities with carbonic anhydrase inhibitor has been previously reported.[111] Genead et al.[112] treated 29 eyes of 15 XLRS patients with topical dorzolamide for 4–41 months and noted some positive effects on visual acuity, cystoid macular lesions, and central foveal thickness. Further studies are required to elucidate the true frequency and completeness of the response to dorzolamide, as well as to evaluate for possible recurrence of foveal cystic change.[113] More specific pharmacotherapies may become possible as the pathogenetic mechanisms of XLRS are better understood.

Laser

Laser photocoagulation is often considered as an adjuvant or preventive treatment for XLRS.[114,115] However, scatter laser photocoagulation performed in order to flatten peripheral schisis cavities and reduce the likelihood of retinal detachment resulted in retinal detachment in many cases.[116] So the administration time and effectiveness of laser treatment for XLRS should be carefully considered.

Surgery

Surgical intervention may be required for XLRS patients with severe complications, such as retinal detachment and vitreous hemorrhage. Currently, the main surgeries include scleral buckle,[115] vitrectomy, and perfluorocarbon liquid, perfluorodecalin or sulfur hexafluoride gas tamponade. Vitreous surgery includes core vitrectomy, surgical induction of posterior vitreous detachment, removal of the internal limiting membrane, and gas tamponade.[117]In addition, Wu et al.[118] used autologous plasmin enzyme-assisted vitreoretinal surgery to treat XLRS patients and achieved retinal reattachment in 91% (20/21) of eyes and postoperative visual improvement in 53% (8/15).

Gene therapy

Gene therapy also holds great promise for the treatment of inherited retinal degenerations.[119] Gene therapy might be an effective treatment for XLRS patients.[120] The *RS1* gene delivered intraocularly in *RS1*-knockout mice was found to restore b-wave amplitude of the treated mice.[121,122] XLRS patients may benefit from the replacement of *RS1* gene, even at advanced stages, and gene replacement may be a promising treatment for XLRS patients in the near future.[123]

Retina and/or progenitor cell transplantation

Retinal transplantation or replacement also holds promise as a potential future therapy for XLRS disease in conjunction with the development of new surgical techniques and instrumentation. However, due to the limited source of human tissue and ethical considerations, it is important to find an alternative cell source for retinal replacement therapy. Transplantation of stem cells and/or progenitor cells, including retinal progenitor cells, bone marrow-derived cells, and induced pluripotent cells, may eventually provide an alternative approach to restore vision.[124] Compared to human embryonic stem cells, the use of human bone marrow-derived cells and induced pluripotent cells does not have significant ethical issues and may eliminate the risk of immunorejection.

RETINAL NUCLEAR RECEPTOR (NR2E3)-RELATED DISEASES: ENHANCED S-CONE SYNDROME AND GOLDMANN–FAVRE VITREOTAPETORETINAL DEGENERATION

General features

NR2E3 (retinal nuclear receptor subfamily 2, group E, member 3), formerly called photoreceptor-specific nuclear receptor (PNR), is a transcription factor of the nuclear hormone receptor superfamily whose expression is uniquely restricted to photoreceptors. Its physiological activity is essential for proper rod and cone development and maintenance. Mutations in NR2E3 may suppress cone proliferation during retinal development[125] and lead to an autosomal recessive retinal degeneration of variable severity, encompassing GFS,[126,127] ESCS,[128] and clumped pigmentary retinal degeneration.[39,129]

Goldmann–Favre vitreotapetoretinal degeneration (also called Favre microfibrillar vitreoretinal degeneration), a rare condition that affects the retina, vitreous body, and crystalline lens, was first described in 1958.[130,131] The characteristic features are early-onset nyctalopia, fibrillar vitreous degeneration, foveal cysts, peripheral retinoschisis, and retinal degeneration with clumped pigment, and an unusual ERG.[132] An estimated 0.5% of patients with retinitis pigmentosa have clumps of pigment in the mid-peripheral fundus, referred to as "clumped pigmentation." To et al. reviewed the clinical and pathological findings in patients with clumped pigmentation and found that they had signs and symptoms of NR2E3 disease. Histopathologic study showed that the clinically distinct areas of clumped pigment are due to excessive accumulation of melanin granules in retinal pigment epithelial cells.[129]

ESCS was described in 1990 and named after the enhanced sensitivity of the S-cone system[128,133] due to an increase in the blue cone population with associated variable degeneration of the rod and red and green cone photoreceptors. Clinical features include early-onset night blindness, cystic maculopathy, and peripheral retinal degeneration characterized by mild visual field loss. The enhanced S-cone ERG shows no response to dim light in the dark-adapted state, but a large, slow response to bright light which persists with light adaptation.[128]

Many psychophysical,[134] histological,[129,135,136] and animal studies[137,138] have demonstrated that mutations in NR2E3 lead to an absolute increase in S cones at the expense of M and L cones, decreased rod development, and retinal disorganization and degeneration. Severe loss of rod sensitivity is evident throughout the retina, along with the characteristic enhanced S-cone ERG.

Clinical findings

Ocular features

Patients with GFS have progressive loss of vision similar to retinitis pigmentosa, which is caused by retinoschisis, cataract, and pigmentary chorioretinal degeneration. It is the macular retinoschisis that most often accounts for the poor central vision and central scotoma in this disorder (Fig. 41.9). The presenting symptom is frequently night blindness, which is often detected in the first decade of life.[132,139] The intraretinal pigmentation is

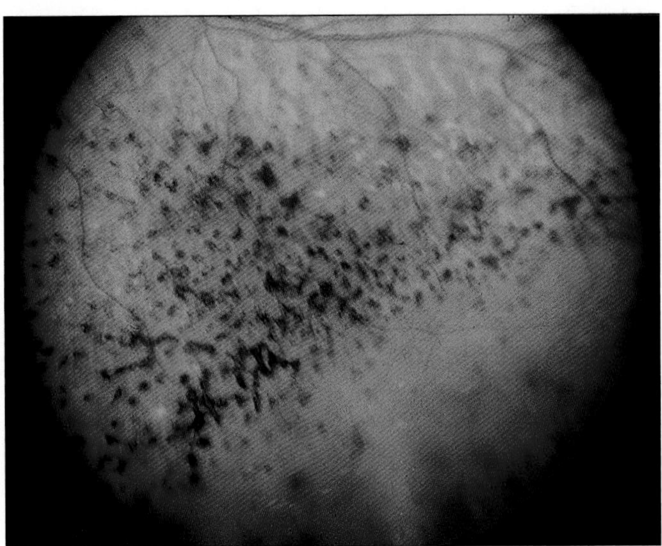

Fig. 41.9 Goldmann–Favre vitreotapetoretinal degeneration, illustrating pigment spots and retinoschisis. (Courtesy of Gerald A. Fishman, MD.)

described as spots of pigment, rather than the bone spicule pattern seen in typical retinitis pigmentosa. The retinoschisis in some patients affects both the central and peripheral retina, and resembles juvenile XLRS. Macular lesions may be isolated from or continuous with the peripheral area of schisis. The peripheral retinoschisis frequently shows oval holes in the inner layer and causes absolute field defects in the peripheral visual field.

The most striking vitreous change is liquefaction, which converts a large portion of the vitreous body into an optically empty space, somewhat similar to that found in Wagner syndrome.[139] The space may contain fine fibrous strands and is surrounded by semiliquefied gel containing loose, plated membranes. These membranes have no visible edge and vary in density from one part of the vitreous body to another. The outer layer of the posterior cortex is condensed, resembling a preretinal membrane. When the posterior cortex is detached, it shows depressions that appear to be molded to retinal vessels. The cortex usually adheres to the retinoschisis and to areas with chorioretinal pigmentary proliferation.

Visual psychophysics

Results of visual field and dark adaptation studies are similar to those from patients with retinitis pigmentosa. The areas of visual field loss correspond to the areas of schisis and pigmentary retinal degeneration. The degree of abnormality of color vision appears to be related to foveal dysfunction.

Electrophysiology

The characteristic ERG shows an undetectable rod-specific response, similar photopic and scotopic responses to a standard single flash, and a 30-Hz lower-amplitude photopic a-wave response. High variability is common and at least partially related to the severity of retinal degeneration.[132] As discussed earlier, the response from the S-cone system accounts for much of the waveform under both scotopic and photopic conditions. The ERG may become undetectable over time.

In addition, ERGs of patients with either ESCS or GFS have greater amplitudes to short-wavelength (e.g., blue) light flashes than to intensity-matched, long-wavelength (e.g., orange) light flashes.[135,140,141] Although rods and S cones are both maximally sensitive to blue light and either might hypothetically mediate this hypersensitivity, the similar ERG amplitudes under scotopic and photopic conditions to single flashes of bright white light indicate that it is mediated predominantly by S cones.[141–143] Evidence from the shape of the ERG a-wave and from psychophysical studies of color sensitivity indicates that the affected retinas have an overabundance of S-cone photoreceptors at birth, a reduced number of L and M cones, and few, if any, functional rod photoreceptors.[143] The relative abundance of S-cone photoreceptors persists even late in the disease, when visual function is severely reduced, as shown by histopathological examination at autopsy of the eyes of a patient with ESCS.[135]

Differential diagnosis

Goldmann–Favre vitreotapetoretinal degeneration and ESCS share features with other vitreoretinal degenerations and retinitis pigmentosa.

X-linked retinoschisis

Goldmann–Favre vitreotapetoretinal degeneration and ESCS are distinguished from XLRS by autosomal inheritance, presence of severe nyctalopia, and ERG findings. The presence of clumped pigment suggests NR2E3-related disease whereas vascular attenuation is suggestive of retinitis pigmentosa.

Cystoid macular edema

The microcystic changes at the posterior pole have sometimes been confused with those of cystoid macular edema and fluorescein angiography has been helpful in making this differentiation, showing a characteristic late leakage that is absent in NR2E3-related disease.

Management

There is no satisfactory treatment for this condition. Standard vitreoretinal approaches are used for rhegmatogenous retinal detachment and prophylactic treatment of retinal tears using laser photocoagulation should be performed. As discussed in the section on congenital XLRS, prophylactic treatment of breaks in the outer layer of the retinoschisis is generally not recommended. Laser photocoagulation has been used to treat elevated macular retinoschisis.[144]

OTHER VITREORETINAL DEGENERATIONS AND VITREORETINOPATHIES

Autosomal dominant vitreoretinochoroidopathy

Kaufman and colleagues described a unique condition with 360° of peripheral chorioretinal atrophy between the ora serrata and a very distinct posterior border near the equator.[145] This feature is not seen in any other disorder to our knowledge. Cataract, moderate fibrillar vitreous degeneration with pigmented cells, cystoid macular edema, neovascularization of the disc, punctate white opacities on the surface of the retina, and retinal detachment may be observed.[146–148] The electro-oculogram may be abnormal,[149] but the ERG is typically normal and nyctalopia is absent.

Autosomal recessive inherited vitreoretinal dystrophy

Sarra and colleagues reported a family with 4 of 8 siblings affected with early-onset high myopia, vitreous liquefaction, macular staphyloma with chorioretinal atrophy, diffuse peripheral atrophy of the retinal pigment epithelium, and early cataract. There was also a peripheral veil in one subject, but no extraocular manifestations.[150] Monophasic dark adaptation was observed and the ERG showed a severe rod–cone retinal degeneration.[150] Linkage analysis identified chromosome 22q13 with a 2-point lod score of 2.18 as the likely locus.

HEREDITARY NEOVASCULAR VITREORETINOPATHIES

These conditions are characterized by hereditary peripheral retinal neovascularization with vitreoretinal traction. We discuss here hereditary conditions without primary vitreal degeneration, unaccompanied by systemic clinical manifestations, and incontinentia pigmenti, sickle-cell retinopathy, and other peripheral proliferative retinopathies that have been reviewed previously.[151]

Autosomal dominant neovascular inflammatory vitreoretinopathy

ADNIV is an apparently rare condition characterized by cataract, cystoid macular edema, peripheral retinal scarring and pigmentation, peripheral arteriolar closure, and neovascularization of the peripheral retina at the ora serrata.[152] Young adults are asymptomatic, but have vitreous cell and selective b-wave loss on the ERG. Neovascularization may result in tractional retinal detachment. About half of patients will develop rubeosis or neovascular glaucoma by age 60 or older. The gene was localized to chromosome 11q13.[153] Vitreous bands and sheets are not observed and the vitreous was not optically empty, enabling differentiation from classical vitreoretinal degenerations such as Stickler, Wagner, and SVD. The peripheral retinal vessels are initially normal in ADNIV, and dragging of the macular vessels as seen in familial exudative vitreoretinopathy is absent.

Dominantly inherited peripheral retinal neovascularization

Gitter and colleagues described a family with 7 of 15 members affected with early cataract, uveitis, prominence of the vitreous base, lattice degeneration, and severe peripheral retinal neovascularization leading to vitreous hemorrhage and retinal detachment. The syndrome appears similar to ADNIV, but after reviewing photographs of the ADNIV family, the condition was deemed to be distinct.[154]

REFERENCES

1. Edwards AO. Clinical features of the congenital vitreoretinopathies. Eye (Lond) 2008;22:1233–42.
2. Hirose T, Lee KY, Schepens CL. Snowflake degeneration in hereditary vitreoretinal degeneration. Am J Ophthalmol 1974;77:143–53.
3. Lee MM, Ritter R, 3rd, Hirose T, et al. Snowflake vitreoretinal degeneration: follow-up of the original family. Ophthalmology 2003;110:2418–26.
4. Hejtmancik JF, Jiao X, Li A, et al. Mutations in KCNJ13 cause autosomal-dominant snowflake vitreoretinal degeneration. Am J Hum Genet 2008;82:174–80.
5. Gheiler M, Pollack A, Uchenik D, et al. Hereditary snowflake vitreoretinal degeneration. Birth Defects Orig Artic Ser 1982;18:577–80.
6. Pollack A, Uchenik D, Chemke J, et al. Prophylactic laser photocoagulation in hereditary snowflake vitreoretinal degeneration. A family report. Arch Ophthalmol 1983;101:1536–9.
7. Robertson DM, Link TP, Rostvold JA. Snowflake degeneration of the retina. Ophthalmology 1982;89:1513–7.
8. Chen CJ, Everett TK, Marascalco D. Snowflake degeneration: an independent entity or a variant of retinitis pigmentosa? South Med J 1986;79:1216–23.
9. Jiao X, Ritter R, 3rd, Hejtmancik JF, et al. Genetic linkage of snowflake vitreoretinal degeneration to chromosome 2q36. Invest Ophthalmol Vis Sci 2004;45:4498–503.
10. Hirose T, Wolf E, Schepens CL. Retinal functions in snowflake degeneration. Ann Ophthalmol 1980;12:1135–46.
11. Aylward B, daCruz L, Ezra E, et al. Stickler syndrome. Ophthalmology 2008;115:1636–7; author reply 7–8.
12. Ang A, Ung T, Puvanachandra N, et al. Vitreous phenotype: a key diagnostic sign in Stickler syndrome types 1 and 2 complicated by double heterozygosity. Am J Med Genet A 2007;143:604–7.
13. Richards AJ, McNinch A, Martin H, et al. Stickler syndrome and the vitreous phenotype: mutations in COL2A1 and COL11A1. Hum Mutat 2010;31:E1461–71.
14. Richards AJ, Yates JR, Williams R, et al. A family with Stickler syndrome type 2 has a mutation in the COL11A1 gene resulting in the substitution of glycine 97 by valine in alpha 1 (XI) collagen. Hum Mol Genet 1996;5:1339–43.
15. Annunen S, Korkko J, Czarny M, et al. Splicing mutations of 54-bp exons in the COL11A1 gene cause Marshall syndrome, but other mutations cause overlapping Marshall/Stickler phenotypes. Am J Hum Genet 1999;65:974–83.
16. Shanske AL, Bogdanow A, Shprintzen RJ, et al. The Marshall syndrome: report of a new family and review of the literature. Am J Med Genet 1997;70:52–7.
17. Brubaker JW, Mohney BG, Pulido JS, et al. Vitreous veils and radial lattice in Marshall syndrome. Ophthalmic Genet 2008;29:184–5.
18. Kloeckener-Gruissem B, Bartholdi D, Abdou MT, et al. Identification of the genetic defect in the original Wagner syndrome family. Mol Vis 2006;12:350–5.
19. Mukhopadhyay A, Nikopoulos K, Maugeri A, et al. Erosive vitreoretinopathy and Wagner disease are caused by intronic mutations in CSPG2/Versican that result in an imbalance of splice variants. Invest Ophthalmol Vis Sci 2006;47:3565–72.
20. Meredith SP, Richards AJ, Flanagan DW, et al. Clinical characterisation and molecular analysis of Wagner syndrome. Br J Ophthalmol 2007;91:655–9.
21. Batioglu F. Goldmann–Favre vitreoretinal degeneration. Eur J Ophthalmol 2003;13:307–10.
22. Ang A, Poulson AV, Goodburn SF, et al. Retinal detachment and prophylaxis in type 1 Stickler syndrome. Ophthalmology 2008;115:164–8.
23. Ronan SM, Tran-Viet KN, Burner EL, et al. Mutational hot spot potential of a novel base pair mutation of the CSPG2 gene in a family with Wagner syndrome. Arch Ophthalmol 2009;127:1511–9.
24. Carroll C, Papaioannou D, Rees A, et al. The clinical effectiveness and safety of prophylactic retinal interventions to reduce the risk of retinal detachment and subsequent vision loss in adults and children with Stickler syndrome: a systematic review. Health Technol Assess 2011;15:iii–xiv, 1–62.
25. Brown DM, Graemiger RA, Hergersberg M, et al. Genetic linkage of Wagner disease and erosive vitreoretinopathy to chromosome 5q13–14. Arch Ophthalmol 1995;113:671–5.
26. Black GC, Perveen R, Wiszniewski W, et al. A novel hereditary developmental vitreoretinopathy with multiple ocular abnormalities localizing to a 5-cM region of chromosome 5q13-q14. Ophthalmology 1999;106:2074–81.
27. Kloeckener-Gruissem B, Amstutz C. VCAN-related vitreoretinopathy. In: Pagon RA, Bird TD, Dolan CR, et al, editors. GeneReviews (internet). Seattle, WA: University of Washington; 2009.
28. Fryer AE, Upadhyaya M, Littler M, et al. Exclusion of COL2A1 as a candidate gene in a family with Wagner–Stickler syndrome. J Med Genet 1990;27:91–3.
29. Snead MP, Yates JR. Clinical and Molecular genetics of Stickler syndrome. J Med Genet 1999;36:353–9.
30. McLeod D, Black GC, Bishop PN. Vitreous phenotype: genotype correlation in Stickler syndrome. Graefes Arch Clin Exp Ophthalmol 2002;240:63–5; author reply 6.
31. Perveen R, Hart-Holden N, Dixon MJ, et al. Refined genetic and physical localization of the Wagner disease (WGN1) locus and the genes CRTL1 and CSPG2 to a 2- to 2.5-cM region of chromosome 5q14.3. Genomics 1999;57:219–26.
32. Maumenee IH, Stoll HU, Mets MB. The Wagner syndrome versus hereditary arthroophthalmopathy. Trans Am Ophthalmol Soc 1982;80:349–65.
33. Go SL, Maugeri A, Mulder JJ, et al. Autosomal dominant rhegmatogenous retinal detachment associated with an Arg453Ter mutation in the COL2A1 gene. Invest Ophthalmol Vis Sci 2003;44:4035–43.
34. Graemiger RA, Niemeyer G, Schneeberger SA, et al. Wagner vitreoretinal degeneration. Follow-up of the original pedigree. Ophthalmology 1995;102:1830–9.
35. Seery CM, Pruett RC, Liberfarb RM, et al. Distinctive cataract in the Stickler syndrome. Am J Ophthalmol 1990;110:143–8.
36. Yardley J, Leroy BP, Hart-Holden N, et al. Mutations of VMD2 splicing regulators cause nanophthalmos and autosomal dominant vitreoretinochoroidopathy (ADVIRC). Invest Ophthalmol Vis Sci 2004;45:3683–9.
37. Audo I, Michaelides M, Robson AG, et al. Phenotypic variation in enhanced S-cone syndrome. Invest Ophthalmol Vis Sci 2008;49:2082–93.
38. Chavala SH, Sari A, Lewis H, et al. An Arg311Gln NR2E3 mutation in a family with classic Goldmann–Favre syndrome. Br J Ophthalmol 2005;89:1065–6.
39. Sharon D, Sandberg MA, Caruso RC, et al. Shared mutations in NR2E3 in enhanced S-cone syndrome, Goldmann–Favre syndrome, and many cases of clumped pigmentary retinal degeneration. Arch Ophthalmol 2003;121:1316–23.
40. Menzel O, Bekkeheien RC, Reymond A, et al. Knobloch syndrome: novel mutations in COL18A1, evidence for genetic heterogeneity, and a functionally impaired polymorphism in endostatin. Hum Mutat 2004;23:77–84.
41. Cui YX, Xia XY, Bu Y, et al. Rapid molecular prenatal diagnosis of spondyloepiphyseal dysplasia congenita by PCR-SSP assay. Genet Test 2008;12:533–6.
42. Wada R, Sawai H, Nishimura G, et al. Prenatal diagnosis of Kniest dysplasia with three-dimensional helical computed tomography. J Matern Fetal Neonatal Med 2011;24:1181–4.
43. Yazici Z, Kline-Fath BM, Laor T, et al. Fetal MR imaging of Kniest dysplasia. Pediatr Radiol 2010;40:348–52.
44. Hoornaert KP, Vereecke I, Dewinter C, et al. Stickler syndrome caused by COL2A1 mutations: genotype–phenotype correlation in a series of 100 patients. Eur J Hum Genet 2010;18:872–80.
45. Majava M, Hoornaert KP, Bartholdi D, et al. A report on 10 new patients with heterozygous mutations in the COL11A1 gene and a review of genotype-phenotype correlations in type XI collagenopathies. Am J Med Genet A 2007;143:258–64.
46. Vu CD, Brown Jr J., Korkko J, et al. Posterior chorioretinal atrophy and vitreous phenotype in a family with Stickler syndrome from a mutation in the COL2A1 gene. Ophthalmology 2003;110:70–7.
47. Donoso LA, Edwards AO, Frost AT, et al. Identification of a stop codon mutation in exon 2 of the collagen 2A1 gene in a large stickler syndrome family. Am J Ophthalmol 2002;134:720–7.
48. Donoso LA, Edwards AO, Frost AT, et al. Clinical variability of Stickler syndrome: role of exon 2 of the collagen COL2A1 gene. Surv Ophthalmol 2003;48:191–203.
49. McAlinden A, Majava M, Bishop PN, et al. Missense and nonsense mutations in the alternatively-spliced exon 2 of COL2A1 cause the ocular variant of Stickler syndrome. Hum Mutat 2008;29:83–90.
50. Baker S, Booth C, Fillman C, et al. A loss of function mutation in the COL9A2 gene causes autosomal recessive Stickler syndrome. Am J Med Genet A 2011;155:1668–72.
51. Nikopoulos K, Schrauwen I, Simon M, et al. Autosomal recessive Stickler syndrome in two families caused by mutations in the COL9A1 gene. Invest Ophthalmol Vis Sci 2011;52:4774–9.
52. Yaguchi H, Ikeda T, Osada H, et al. Identification of the COL2A1 mutation in patients with type I Stickler syndrome using RNA from freshly isolated peripheral white blood cells. Genet Test Mol Biomarkers 2011;15:231–7.

53. Al Kaissi A, Ganger R, Klaushofer K, et al. Significant ophthalmoarthropathy associated with ectodermal dysplasia in a child with Marshall–Stickler overlap: a case report. Cases J 2008;1:270.
54. Passos-Bueno MR, Suzuki OT, Armelin-Correa LM, et al. Mutations in collagen 18A1 and their relevance to the human phenotype. An Acad Bras Cienc 2006;78:123–31.
55. Suzuki O, Kague E, Bagatini K, et al. Novel pathogenic mutations and skin biopsy analysis in Knobloch syndrome. Mol Vis 2009;15:801–9.
56. Pihlajamaa T, Prockop DJ, Faber J, et al. Heterozygous glycine substitution in the COL11A2 gene in the original patient with the Weissenbacher–Zweymuller syndrome demonstrates its identity with heterozygous OSMED (nonocular Stickler syndrome). Am J Med Genet 1998;80:115–20.
57. Pacella E, Malvasi A, Tinelli A, et al. Stickler syndrome in Pierre-Robin sequence prenatal ultrasonographic diagnosis and postnatal therapy: two cases report. Eur Rev Med Pharmacol Sci 2010;14:1051–4.
58. Couchouron T, Masson C. Early-onset progressive osteoarthritis with hereditary progressive ophthalmopathy or Stickler syndrome. Joint Bone Spine 2011;78:45–9.
59. Spranger J, Winterpacht A, Zabel B. Kniest dysplasia: Dr. W. Kniest, his patient, the molecular defect. Am J Med Genet 1997;69:79–84.
60. Galil A, Carmi R, Goldstein E, et al. Weissenbacher–Zweymuller syndrome: long-term follow-up of growth and psychomotor development. Dev Med Child Neurol 1991;33:1104–9.
61. Watanabe H, Kohzaki K, Kubo H, et al. [Stickler syndrome with rhegmatogenous retinal detachment.] Nippon Ganka Gakkai Zasshi 2010;114:454–8.
62. Rabinowitz R, Gradstein L, Galil A, et al. The ocular manifestations of Weissenbacher–Zweymuller syndrome. Eye (Lond) 2004;18:1258–63.
63. Parma ES, Korkko J, Hagler WS, et al. Radial perivascular retinal degeneration: a key to the clinical diagnosis of an ocular variant of Stickler syndrome with minimal or no systemic manifestations. Am J Ophthalmol 2002;134: 728–34.
64. Miloro M. Mandibular distraction osteogenesis for pediatric airway management. J Oral Maxillofac Surg 2010;68:1512–23.
65. Ihanamäki T, Metsäranta M, Rintala M, et al. Ocular abnormalities in transgenic mice harboring mutations in the type II collagen gene. Eur J Ophthalmol 1996;6:427–35.
66. Haas J. Ueber das Zusammenvorkommen von Veranderungen der Retina und Choroidea. Arch Augenheilkd 1898;37:343–8.
67. Pagenstecher H. Uebereine unter dem Bildeder Natzhauterblosung verlaufende, erbiche Erkankung der Retina. Graefes Arch Clin Exp Ophthalmol 1913;86:457–62.
68. Jager G. A hereditary retinal disease. Trans Ophthalmol Soc UK 1953;73: 617–9.
69. Kim SY, Ko HS, Yu YS, et al. Molecular genetic characteristics of X-linked retinoschisis in Koreans. Mol Vis 2009;15:833–43.
70. Lamey T, Laurin S, Chelva E, et al. Genotypic analysis of X-linked retinoschisis in Western Australia. Adv Exp Med Biol 2010;664:283–91.
71. Teixeira C, Rocha-Sousa A, Trump D, et al. Identification of XLRS1 gene mutation (608C > T) in a Portuguese family with juvenile retinoschisis. Eur J Ophthalmol 2005;15:638–40.
72. Biswas S, Funnell CL, Gray J, et al. Nidek MP-1 microperimetry and Fourier domain optical coherence tomography (FD-OCT) in X linked retinoschisis. Br J Ophthalmol 2010;94:949–50.
73. Sikkink SK, Biswas S, Parry NR, et al. X-linked retinoschisis: an update. J Med Genet 2007;44:225–32.
74. Garcia-Arumi J, Corcostegui IA, Navarro R, et al. Vitreoretinal surgery without schisis cavity excision for the management of juvenile X linked retinoschisis. Br J Ophthalmol 2008;92:1558–60.
75. Lesch B, Szabo V, Kanya M, et al. Clinical and genetic findings in Hungarian patients with X-linked juvenile retinoschisis. Mol Vis 2008;14:2321–32.
76. Vainio-Mattila B, Eriksson AW, Forsius H. X-chromosomal recessive retinoschisis in the region of Pori. An ophthalmo-genetical analysis of 103 cases. Acta Ophthalmol (Copenh) 1969;47:1135–48.
77. Riveiro-Alvarez R, Trujillo-Tiebas MJ, Gimenez-Pardo A, et al. Correlation of genetic and clinical findings in Spanish patients with X-linked juvenile retinoschisis. Invest Ophthalmol Vis Sci 2009;50:4342–50.
78. Sauer CG, Gehrig A, Warneke-Wittstock R, et al. Positional cloning of the gene associated with X-linked juvenile retinoschisis. Nat Genet 1997;17: 164–70.
79. Grayson C, Reid SN, Ellis JA, et al. Retinoschisin, the X-linked retinoschisis protein, is a secreted photoreceptor protein, and is expressed and released by Weri-Rb1 cells. Hum Mol Genet 2000;9:1873–9.
80. Molday LL, Hicks D, Sauer CG, et al. Expression of X-linked retinoschisis protein RS1 in photoreceptor and bipolar cells. Invest Ophthalmol Vis Sci 2001;42:816–25.
81. Reid SN, Yamashita C, Farber DB. Retinoschisin, a photoreceptor-secreted protein, and its interaction with bipolar and Müller cells. J Neurosci 2003;23:6030–40.
82. Wu WW, Wong JP, Kast J, et al. RS1, a discoidin domain-containing retinal cell adhesion protein associated with X-linked retinoschisis, exists as a novel disulfide-linked octamer. J Biol Chem 2005;280:10721–30.
83. Wang T, Zhou A, Waters CT, et al. Molecular pathology of X linked retinoschisis: mutations interfere with retinoschisin secretion and oligomerisation. Br J Ophthalmol 2006;90:81–6.
84. Fraternali F, Cavallo L, Musco G. Effects of pathological mutations on the stability of a conserved amino acid triad in retinoschisin. FEBS Lett 2003;544: 21–6.
85. Steiner-Champliaud MF, Sahel J, Hicks D. Retinoschisin forms a multimolecular complex with extracellular matrix and cytoplasmic proteins: interactions with beta2 laminin and alphaB-crystallin. Mol Vis 2006;12:892–901.
86. Horwitz J. Alpha-crystallin can function as a molecular chaperone. Proc Natl Acad Sci U S A 1992;89:10449–53.
87. Molday LL, Wu WW, Molday RS. Retinoschisin (RS1), the protein encoded by the X-linked retinoschisis gene, is anchored to the surface of retinal photoreceptor and bipolar cells through its interactions with a Na/K ATPase-SARM1 complex. J Biol Chem 2007;282:32792–801.
88. Gehrig A, Langmann T, Horling F, et al. Genome-wide expression profiling of the retinoschisin-deficient retina in early postnatal mouse development. Invest Ophthalmol Vis Sci 2007;48:891–900.
89. Dyka FM, Wu WW, Pfeifer TA, et al. Characterization and purification of the discoidin domain-containing protein retinoschisin and its interaction with galactose. Biochemistry 2008;47:9098–106.
90. Pimenides D, George ND, Yates JR, et al. X-linked retinoschisis: clinical phenotype and RS1 genotype in 86 UK patients. J Med Genet 2005;42:e35.
91. Iannaccone A, Mura M, Dyka FM, et al. An unusual X-linked retinoschisis phenotype and biochemical characterization of the W112C RS1 mutation. Vision Res 2006;46:3845–52.
92. Kellner U, Brummer S, Foerster MH, et al. X-linked congenital retinoschisis. Graefes Arch Clin Exp Ophthalmol 1990;228:432–7.
93. Mitamura Y, Miyanishi K, Shizukawa N, et al. A case of X-linked retinoschisis diagnosed in an infant. Retina 2003;23:731–2.
94. Peachey NS, Fishman GA, Derlacki DJ, et al. Psychophysical and electroretinographic findings in X-linked juvenile retinoschisis. Arch Ophthalmol 1987;105:513–6.
95. Ando A, Takahashi K, Sho K, Matsushima M, et al. Histopathological findings of X-linked retinoschisis with neovascular glaucoma. Graefes Arch Clin Exp Ophthalmol 2000;238:1–7.
96. Greven CM, Moreno RJ, Tasman W. Unusual manifestations of X-linked retinoschisis. Trans Am Ophthalmol Soc 1990;88:211–25; discussion 26–8.
97. Tasman W, Greven C, Moreno R. Nasal retinal dragging in X-linked retinoschisis. Graefes Arch Clin Exp Ophthalmol 1991;229:319–22.
98. Sorsby A, Klein M, Gann JH, et al. Unusual retinal detachment possibly sex-linked. Br J Ophthalmol 1951;35:1–10.
99. George ND, Yates JR, Moore AT. Clinical features in affected males with X-linked retinoschisis. Arch Ophthalmol 1996;114:274–80.
100. George ND, Yates JR, Bradshaw K, et al. Infantile presentation of X linked retinoschisis. Br J Ophthalmol 1995;79:653–7.
101. Garg SJ, Lee HC, Grand MG. Bilateral macular detachments in X-linked retinoschisis. Arch Ophthalmol 2006;124:1053–5.
102. Apushkin MA, Fishman GA, Rajagopalan AS. Fundus findings and longitudinal study of visual acuity loss in patients with X-linked retinoschisis. Retina 2005;25:612–8.
103. McKibbin M, Booth AP, George ND. Foveal ectopia in X-linked retinoschisis. Retina 2001;21:361–6.
104. Muscat S, Fahad B, Parks S, et al. Optical coherence tomography and multifocal electroretinography of X-linked juvenile retinoschisis. Eye (Lond) 2001;15: 796–9.
105. Yu J, Ni Y, Keane PA, et al. Foveomacular schisis in juvenile X-linked retinoschisis: an optical coherence tomography study. Am J Ophthalmol 2010;149:973–8 e2.
106. Tanimoto N, Usui T, Takagi M, et al. Electroretinographic findings in three family members with X-linked juvenile retinoschisis associated with a novel Pro192Thr mutation of the XLRS1 gene. Jpn J Ophthalmol 2002;46: 568–76.
107. Miyake Y, Shiroyama N, Ota I, et al. Focal macular electroretinogram in X-linked congenital retinoschisis. Invest Ophthalmol Vis Sci 1993;34:512–5.
108. Bradshaw K, George N, Moore A, et al. Mutations of the XLRS1 gene cause abnormalities of photoreceptor as well as inner retinal responses of the ERG. Doc Ophthalmol 1999;98:153–73.
109. Deutman AF, Pinckers AJ, Aan de Kerk AL. Dominantly inherited cystoid macular edema. Am J Ophthalmol 1976;82:540–8.
110. Gehrig A, White K, Lorenz B, et al. Assessment of RS1 in X-linked juvenile retinoschisis and sporadic senile retinoschisis. Clin Genet 1999;55:461–5.
111. Iannaccone A, Fung KH, Eyestone ME, et al. Treatment of adult-onset acute macular retinoschisis in enhanced s-cone syndrome with oral acetazolamide. Am J Ophthalmol 2009;147:307–12 e2.
112. Genead MA, Fishman GA, Walia S. Efficacy of sustained topical dorzolamide therapy for cystic macular lesions in patients with X-linked retinoschisis. Arch Ophthalmol 2010;128:190–7.
113. Bastos AL, Freitas Bde P, Villas Boas O, et al. Use of topical dorzolamide for patients with X-linked juvenile retinoschisis: case report. Arq Bras Oftalmol 2008;71:286–90.
114. Gopal L, Shanmugam MP, Battu RR, et al. Congenital retinoschisis: successful collapse with photocoagulation. Ind J Ophthalmol 2001;49:265–6.
115. Avitabile T, Ortisi E, Scott IU, et al. Scleral buckle for progressive symptomatic retinal detachment complicating retinoschisis versus primary rhegmatogenous retinal detachment. Can J Ophthalmol 2010;45:161–5.
116. Tantri A, Vrabec TR, Cu-Unjieng A, et al. X-linked retinoschisis: a clinical and molecular genetic review. Surv Ophthalmol 2004;49:214–30.
117. Ikeda F, Iida T, Kishi S. Resolution of retinoschisis after vitreous surgery in X-linked retinoschisis. Ophthalmology 2008;115:718–22 e1.
118. Wu WC, Drenser KA, Capone A, et al. Plasmin enzyme-assisted vitreoretinal surgery in congenital X-linked retinoschisis: surgical techniques based on a new classification system. Retina 2007;27:1079–85.

119. Simonelli F, Maguire AM, Testa F, et al. Gene therapy for Leber's congenital amaurosis is safe and effective through 1.5 years after vector administration. Mol Ther 2010 Mar;18(3):643–50.
120. Dyka FM, Molday RS. Coexpression and interaction of wild-type and missense RS1 mutants associated with X-linked retinoschisis: its relevance to gene therapy. Invest Ophthalmol Vis Sci 2007;48:2491–7.
121. Zeng Y, Takada Y, Kjellstrom S, et al. RS-1 gene delivery to an adult Rs1h knockout mouse model restores ERG b-wave with reversal of the electronegative waveform of X-linked retinoschisis. Invest Ophthalmol Vis Sci 2004;45: 3279–85.
122. Min SH, Molday LL, Seeliger MW, et al. Prolonged recovery of retinal structure/function after gene therapy in an Rs1h-deficient mouse model of x-linked juvenile retinoschisis. Mol Ther 2005;12:644–51.
123. Janssen A, Min SH, Molday LL, et al. Effect of late-stage therapy on disease progression in AAV-mediated rescue of photoreceptor cells in the retinoschisin-deficient mouse. Mol Ther 2008;16:1010–7.
124. Ballios BG, Cooke MJ, van der Kooy D, et al. A hydrogel-based stem cell delivery system to treat retinal degenerative diseases. Biomaterials 2010;31: 2555–64.
125. Yanagi Y, Takezawa S, Kato S. Distinct functions of photoreceptor cell-specific nuclear receptor, thyroid hormone receptor beta2 and CRX in one photoreceptor development. Invest Ophthalmol Vis Sci 2002;43:3489–94.
126. Schorderet DF, Escher P. NR2E3 mutations in enhanced S-cone sensitivity syndrome (ESCS), Goldmann–Favre syndrome (GFS), clumped pigmentary retinal degeneration (CPRD), and retinitis pigmentosa (RP). Hum Mutat 2009;30:1475–85.
127. Brydak-Godowska J, Makowiec-Tabernacka M. [Goldmann–Favre syndrome – case report.] Klin Oczna. 2009;111:346–7.
128. Marmor MF, Jacobson SG, Foerster MH, et al. Diagnostic clinical findings of a new syndrome with night blindness, maculopathy, and enhanced S cone sensitivity. Am J Ophthalmol 1990;110:124–34.
129. To KW, Adamian M, Jakobiec FA, et al. Clinical and histopathologic findings in clumped pigmentary retinal degeneration. Arch Ophthalmol 1996;114: 950–5.
130. Favre M. [Two cases of hyaloid-retinal degeneration.] Ophthalmologica 1958;135:604–9.
131. Francois J, de Rouck A, Cambie E. [Goldmann–Favre vitreo-tapeto-retinal degeneration.] Ophthalmologica 1974;168:81–96.
132. Fishman GA, Jampol LM, Goldberg MF. Diagnostic features of the Favre–Goldmann syndrome. Br J Ophthalmol 1976;60:345–53.
133. Marmor MF. A teenager with nightblindness and cystic maculopathy: enhanced S cone syndrome (Goldmann–Favre syndrome). Doc Ophthalmol 2006;113:213–5.
134. Hood DC, Cideciyan AV, Roman AJ, et al. Enhanced S cone syndrome: evidence for an abnormally large number of S cones. Vision Res 1995;35: 1473–81.
135. Milam AH, Rose L, Cideciyan AV, et al. The nuclear receptor NR2E3 plays a role in human retinal photoreceptor differentiation and degeneration. Proc Natl Acad Sci U S A 2002;99:473–8.
136. Peyman GA, Fishman GA, Sanders DR, et al. Histopathology of Goldmann–Favre syndrome obtained by full-thickness eye-wall biopsy. Ann Ophthalmol 1977;9:479–84.
137. Haider NB, Naggert JK, Nishina PM. Excess cone cell proliferation due to lack of a functional NR2E3 causes retinal dysplasia and degeneration in rd7/rd7 mice. Hum Mol Genet 2001;10:1619–26.
138. Mitton KP, Swain PK, Khanna H, et al. Interaction of retinal bZIP transcription factor NRL with Flt3-interacting zinc-finger protein Fiz1: possible role of Fiz1 as a transcriptional repressor. Hum Mol Genet 2003;12:365–73.
139. Feiler-Ofry V, Adam A, Regenbogen L, et al. Hereditary vitreoretinal degeneration and night blindness. Am J Ophthalmol 1969;67:553–8.
140. Jacobson SG, Marmor MF, Kemp CM, et al. SWS (blue) cone hypersensitivity in a newly identified retinal degeneration. Invest Ophthalmol Vis Sci 1990;31: 827–38.
141. Jacobson SG, Roman AJ, Roman MI, et al. Relatively enhanced S cone function in the Goldmann–Favre syndrome. Am J Ophthalmol 1991;111:446–53.
142. Fishman GA, Peachey NS. Rod–cone dystrophy associated with a rod system electroretinogram obtained under photopic conditions. Ophthalmology 1989;96:913–8.
143. Greenstein VC, Zaidi Q, Hood DC, et al. The enhanced S cone syndrome: an analysis of receptoral and post-receptoral changes. Vision Res 1996;36:3711–22.
144. Khairallah M, Ladjimi A, Ben Yahia S, et al. Elevated macular retinoschisis associated with Goldmann–Favre syndrome successfully treated with grid laser photocoagulation. Retina 2002;22:234–7.
145. Kaufman SJ, Goldberg MF, Orth DH, et al. Autosomal dominant vitreoretinochoroidopathy. Arch Ophthalmol 1982;100:272–8.
146. Lafaut BA, Loeys B, Leroy BP, et al. Clinical and electrophysiological findings in autosomal dominant vitreoretinochoroidopathy: report of a new pedigree. Graefes Arch Clin Exp Ophthalmol 2001;239:575–82.
147. Roider J, Fritsch E, Hoerauf H, et al. Autosomal dominant vitreoretinochoroidopathy. Retina 1997;17:294–9.
148. Blair NP, Goldberg MF, Fishman GA, et al. Autosomal dominant vitreoretinochoroidopathy (ADVIRC). Br J Ophthalmol 1984;68:2–9.
149. Han DP, Lewandowski MF. Electro-oculography in autosomal dominant vitreoretinochoroidopathy. Arch Ophthalmol 1992;110:1563–7.
150. Sarra GM, Weigell-Weber M, Kotzot D, et al. Clinical description and exclusion of candidate genes in a novel autosomal recessively inherited vitreoretinal dystrophy. Arch Ophthalmol 2003;121:1109–16.
151. Jampol LM, Ebroon DA, Goldbaum MH. Peripheral proliferative retinopathies: an update on angiogenesis, etiologies and management. Surv Ophthalmol 1994;38:519–40.
152. Bennett SR, Folk JC, Kimura AE, et al. Autosomal dominant neovascular inflammatory vitreoretinopathy. Ophthalmology 1990;97:1125–35; discussion 35–6.
153. Stone EM, Kimura AE, Folk JC, et al. Genetic linkage of autosomal dominant neovascular inflammatory vitreoretinopathy to chromosome 11q13. Hum Mol Genet 1992;1:685–9.
154. Gitter KA, Rothschild H, Waltman DD, et al. Dominantly inherited peripheral retinal neovascularization. Arch Ophthalmol 1978;96:1601–5.

For additional online content visit http://www.expertconsult.com

Chapter 42

Macular Dystrophies

Elliott H. Sohn, Robert F. Mullins, Edwin M. Stone

INTRODUCTION

Historically, the term "macular dystrophy" has been used to refer to a group of heritable disorders that cause ophthalmoscopically visible abnormalities in the portion of the retina bounded by the temporal vascular arcades. Most medical terms tend to suffer over time because evolving scientific knowledge reveals inconsistencies with their conventional use, and "macular dystrophy" is no exception. For example, age-related macular degeneration (AMD) affects the macula and has a significant genetic component. However, the genes that cause AMD interact with each other and with the environment in a sufficiently non-Mendelian fashion that it is not typically considered one of the macular dystrophies. Achromatopsia, foveal hypoplasia, and albinism are also Mendelian disorders that cause ophthalmoscopically visible abnormalities of the macula, but these, too, are not typically grouped among the macular dystrophies. In the first case, it is probably because the visible macular lesions first appear decades after the visual dysfunction is evident, while in the latter cases, it is probably because the macular abnormalities are developmental, completely stationary, and do not cause any discoloration of the macular structures. The unifying features of the conditions presented in this chapter are: they are inherited in a Mendelian fashion; the associated pathology is limited to the eye; and lesions are biomicroscopically visible in the macula when symptoms first occur (and in some cases, before symptoms occur). For most of the disorders, the mechanism underlying their macular predilection is unclear but may be related to the anatomical differences in density, structure, and composition of the choriocapillaris, Bruch's membrane, retinal pigment epithelium (RPE), and photoreceptor cells; differences in light exposure; regional gene expression patterns; blood flow; or other factors. A better understanding of the development and cell biology of the macular region, and how it differs from the extramacular retina, will be crucial in developing a deeper understanding of macular dystrophies and devising improved therapies for them.

The genes that cause most of the disorders in this chapter have been identified and it is tempting to try to eliminate the inconsistencies in the historical clinical nomenclature by abandoning it in favor of a scheme that is solely based on the causative genes. However, there are several serious disadvantages to such an approach. First, patients present with symptoms and signs – not with genetic test results. In addition, the near-term disease course in a given patient is usually more tightly correlated to their current clinical appearance and visual function than it is to their genotype. Thus, even in the molecular era, clinicians need to think first in terms of clinical patterns and second about the molecular mechanisms underlying these patterns. Prior to 1985 the clinical diagnosis was for all practical purposes the final diagnosis. Today the initial clinical diagnosis is really a hypothesis that has some prognostic weight by itself, and also serves to focus the search for a more precise and definitive molecular understanding of the patient's disease through genetic testing. Clinicians are often bothered by the fact that there is an imperfect correlation between mutations in specific genes and the resulting clinical outcomes. That is, mutations in a single gene (e.g., *PRPH2* and *ABCA4*) can cause quite different clinical appearances in different patients (e.g., retinitis pigmentosa and macular dystrophy) while a single clinical appearance (e.g., retinitis pigmentosa) can be caused by mutations in many different genes. The best way to cope with this imperfect correlation is to simply accept that the clinical diagnosis has greater validity in certain contexts while the molecular diagnosis has greater validity in others – and that the one can often strengthen the other. For example, prior to the discovery of the causative genes, characteristic clinical features were used to select genetically similar patients from heterogeneous clinic populations for the purpose of gene discovery. Now that many of the disease genes are known, genetic testing can be used to select genetically similar cohorts from clinically heterogeneous populations for the purpose of identifying the range of clinical features that can be associated with mutations in each gene. In this chapter we have taken advantage of molecular diagnosis in our patients to illustrate some unusual clinical presentations of these macular dystrophies that would have been difficult to include in such a chapter in the pre-molecular era. For the most part, we have retained the historical names associated with specific phenotypes and have grouped these whenever they are known to be caused by mutations in a single gene. We have also organized the disorders in the approximate order of their prevalence in the population with the more common diseases first. Table 42.1 summarizes the genetic characterization for all of the macular dystrophies discussed in this chapter.

THE INITIAL APPROACH TO A PATIENT WITH MACULAR DYSTROPHY

Perhaps the most important step in managing a patient with a macular dystrophy is to convince oneself that the patient truly has a Mendelian condition and not one of the many toxic, infectious, autoimmune, and multigenic disorders that can mimic them. Except in extraordinary circumstances, macular dystrophies are bilateral, and in the early years of the disease are usually extremely symmetrical in their fundus appearance.

Autoimmune disorders like the presumed ocular histoplasmosis syndrome and multifocal choroiditis are often bilateral but much less symmetrical in their appearance (Fig. 42.1). Most of the macular dystrophies are inherited in an autosomal dominant fashion and thus one or more living affected relatives often exist. Identification of such a relative is one of the most powerful and most underutilized diagnostic maneuvers the clinician has at his or her disposal. One should always take a careful family history from patients suspected to have a macular dystrophy, realizing that affected individuals over the age of 50 will often carry the diagnosis of age-related macular degeneration (AMD). One should also remember that dominant macular dystrophies often exhibit variable expressivity and incomplete penetrance, such that a patient's parents can be normal by history while more distant relatives can exhibit macular disease. Thus, when taking the history one should be very suspicious of any relative reported to have a macular disease of any kind. One should also examine any first-degree relatives who accompany the patient to the clinic and request fundus photographs and other ophthalmic records from all relatives with a history of macular disease. Not infrequently an affected relative will exhibit the "classic" features of a specific macular dystrophy but carry the diagnosis of

Table 42.1 Macular dystrophies

Disease name	Gene	Chromosome	Inheritance
Best macular dystrophy	*BEST1*	11	AD/AR
Stargardt disease	*ABCA4*	1	AR
Stargardt-like dominant macular dystrophy	*ELOVL4*	6	AD
Pattern dystrophy	*PRPH2*	6	AD
Sorsby fundus dystrophy	*TIMP3*	22	AD
Autosomal dominant radial drusen	*EFEMP1*	2	AD
North Carolina macular dystrophy	Unknown	5 and 6	AD
Spotted cystic dystrophy	Unknown	Unknown	AD
Dominant cystoid macular edema	Unknown	7	AD
Fenestrated sheen macular dystrophy	Unknown	Unknown	AD
Glomerulonephritis type II	*CFH*	1	AR

AD, autosomal dominant; AR, autosomal recessive.

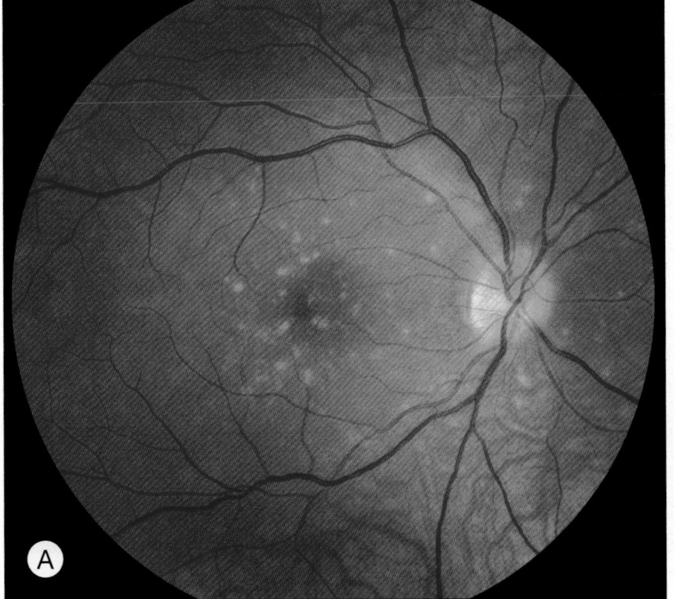

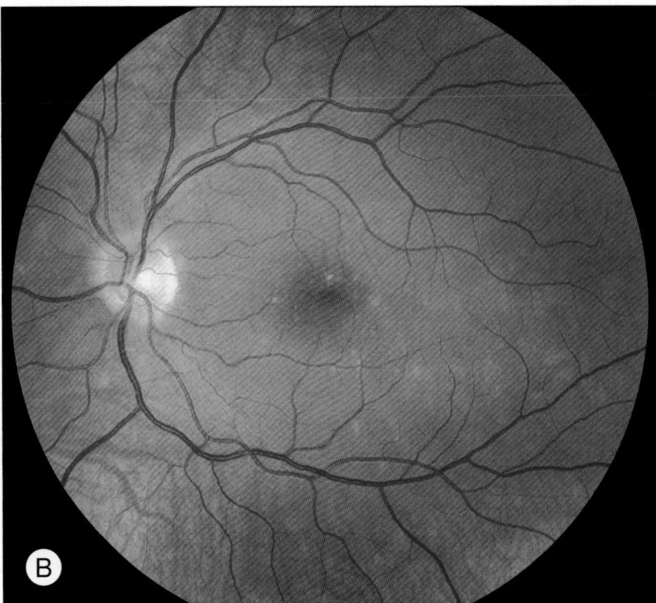

Fig. 42.1 A 33-year-old female with 20/20 visual acuity in both eyes and ovoid-circular fleck-like changes in the macula and around the disc. Although the appearance of either eye could be mistaken for disease due to *ABCA4* or *RDS* mutations, the asymmetry is more suggestive of inflammatory disease. This patient has multifocal choroiditis.

AMD while the patient before you will exhibit a more puzzling fundus appearance and/or set of symptoms.

There are two classes of disease one should be especially careful to think about when initially considering a diagnosis of macular dystrophy: neuronal ceroid lipofuscinosis (NCL) and drug toxicity. In children between the ages of six and eight years, NCL (a fatal systemic disease) can present with a Stargardt-like appearance and no systemic features of any kind (Fig. 42.2). The electroretinogram is usually markedly abnormal in visually symptomatic patients with NCL but is much less likely to be abnormal in a Stargardt patient of that age. The visual dysfunction associated with NCL (both visual field and visual acuity) also tends to progress much more rapidly than Stargardt disease – over months instead of years. The other class of disease to explicitly consider and exclude in every patient suspected to have a macular dystrophy is drug toxicity. One should ask patients whether they are taking or have ever taken any medications over an extended period of time, especially medications for arthritis or skin disease (Fig. 42.3). Table 42.2 provides a list of medications that can cause macular lesions that mimic a macular dystrophy.

Most macular dystrophies are inherited in an autosomal dominant fashion and the identification of affected individuals in multiple generations make ABCA4-associated disease less likely. As a general rule, patients with any of the autosomal dominant macular dystrophies often have visual acuities that are better than one might expect given the striking nature of their fundus findings (e.g., Fig. 42.59) while patients with autosomal recessive Stargardt disease caused by mutations in *ABCA4* often have acuities that are poorer than one might expect given the relatively mild abnormality of their fundus (e.g., Fig. 42.29).

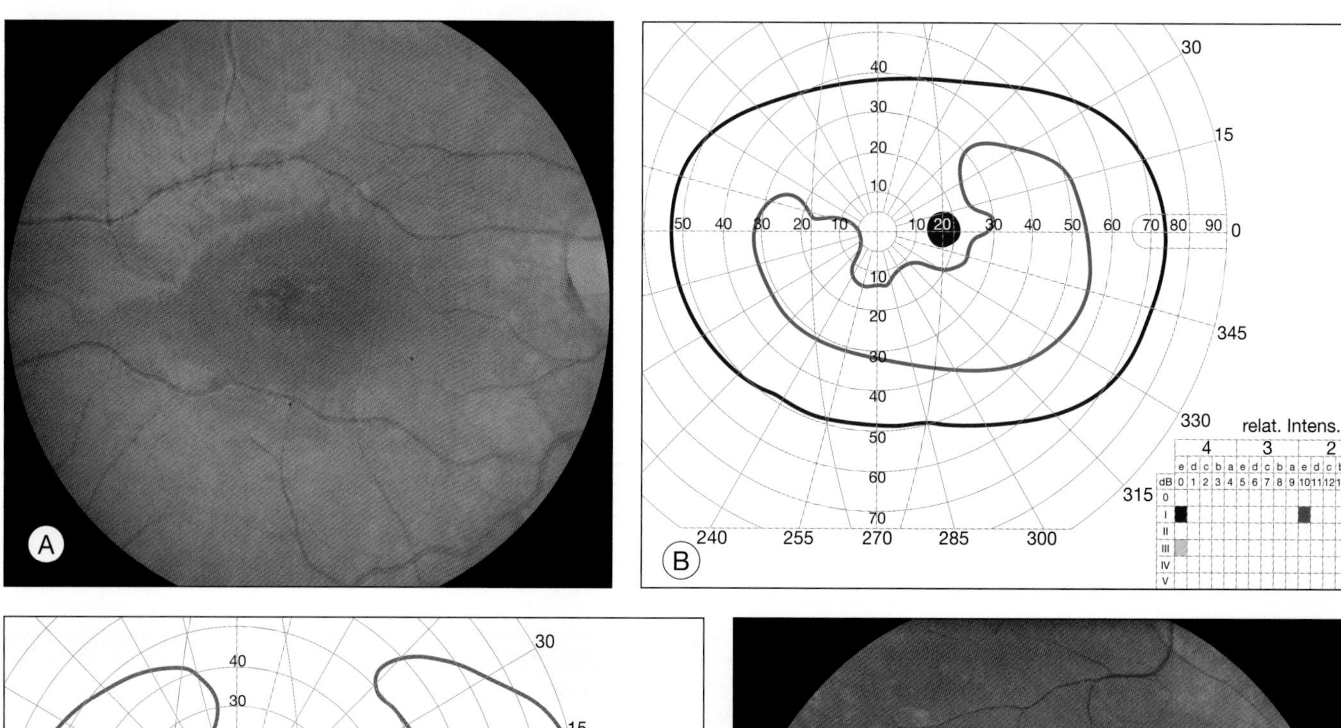

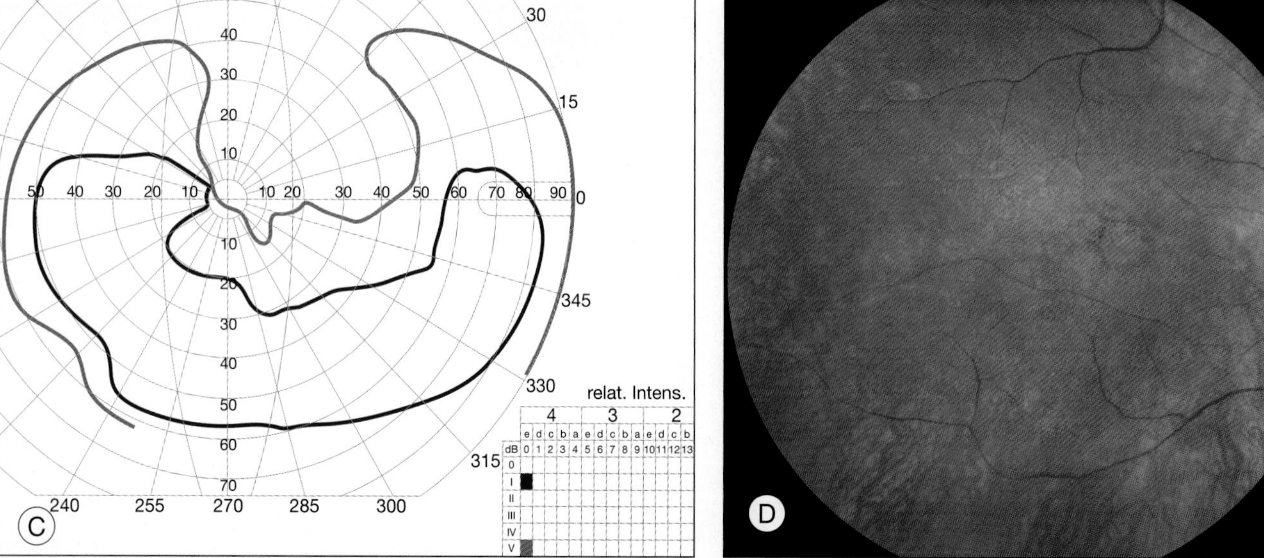

Fig. 42.2 A 5-year-old male with mutations in PPT1 (Thr75Pro/Arg122Trp) causing neuronal ceroid lipofuscinosis. (A) When first seen he had 20/125 visual acuity and an ovoid area of macular thinning. (B) On Goldmann perimetry, the I4e isopter is full and the I2e is still detectable. (C) By age 7 years the visual acuity had fallen to counting fingers, and the I2e isopter has been lost and there is a central and superior scotoma to the V4e target. (D) This was accompanied by progressive thinning of the retinal pigment epithelium and narrowing of the retinal vessels throughout the posterior pole.

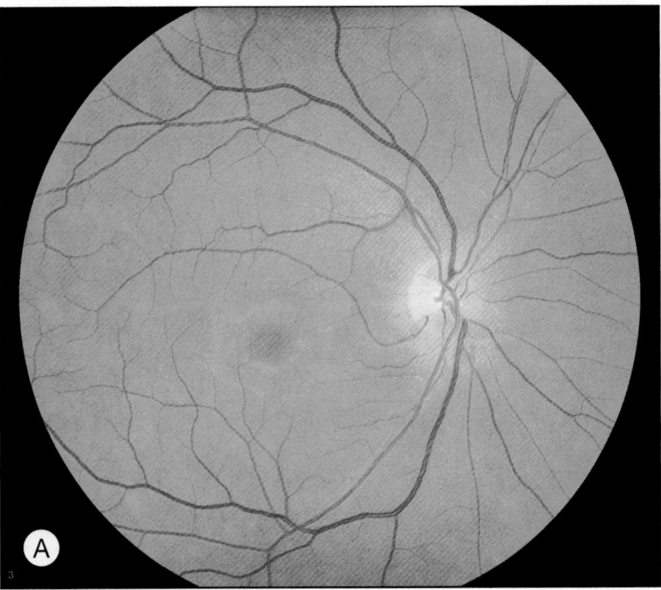

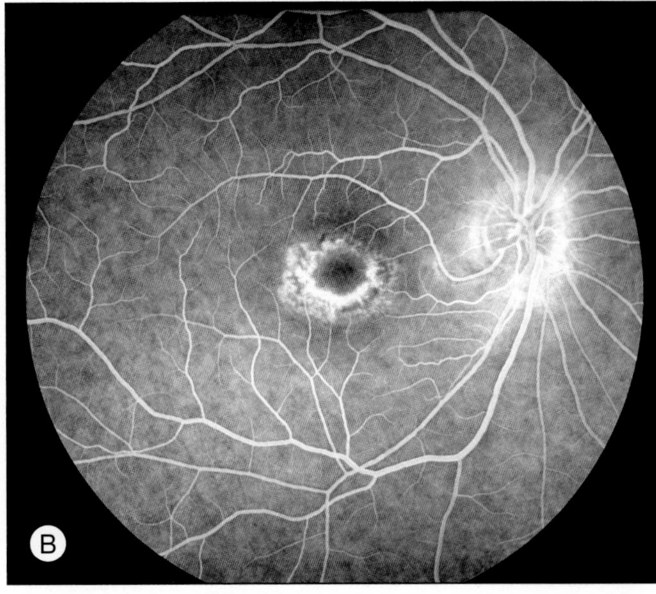

Fig. 42.3 Panels (A) and (B) depict the right eye of a 50-year-old female with plaquenil toxicity and a bull's-eye fundus appearance that could easily be mistaken for Stargardt disease without flecks (compare with Fig. 42.30). Her visual acuity was 20/30.

BEST MACULAR DYSTROPHY

Best macular dystrophy (BMD), or Best disease, is an autosomal dominant condition caused by mutations in the *BEST1* gene (OMIM #607854, formerly known as *VMD2*).[1,2] The first family with this dystrophy was described by Friedrich Best in 1905.[3] Other designations for this disease have since been used, including vitelline dystrophy,[4] vitelliruptive degeneration,[5] and vitelliform dystrophy.[6] It is one of the most common Mendelian macular dystrophies, occurring in about 1 in 10000 individuals. BMD refers to the "classic" form of a single, symmetric egg-yolk-like lesion centered on the fovea of each eye (Figs 42.4–42.7). However it is important to realize that *BEST1* mutations are also associated with multiple other phenotypes (multifocal Best dystrophy (Fig. 42.8), autosomal dominant vitreoretinochoroidopathy (Fig. 42.9), and autosomal recessive bestrophinopathy (Fig. 42.10), which share only a few clinical features, detailed below.

Clinical features of BMD

The fundus findings associated with BMD are quite varied. The macular lesions that are most characteristic of the disease are known as "vitelliform" because of their egg-yolk-like appearance (Figs 42.4–42.7). These lesions are typically solitary, round or horizontally oval, yellow, slightly elevated, and are centered on the fovea. Vitelliform lesions in patients with BMD can range in size from a few hundred microns (Fig. 42.5) to a few millimeters in diameter (Fig. 42.4). The larger lesions can be seen within the first few years of life, while the smaller lesions typically develop after age 20 and sometimes as late as age 60. As a result, the smaller lesions are sometimes referred to as "adult vitelliform" lesions (Fig. 42.5, Fig. 42.11), a phenotype that also occurs in patients with mutations in the *PRPH2* gene (discussed more fully below). Some individuals who harbor disease-causing mutations in *BEST1* never develop significant macular lesions.

Over time, many vitelliform lesions develop a "pseudohypopyon" appearance in which the yellow material gravitates inferiorly in the subretinal space (Figs 42.12, 42.13). Other lesions develop varying amounts of subretinal and sub-RPE fibrosis, RPE atrophy in addition to hyperpigmentation, and atrophy of the RPE. This is sometimes known as a "scrambled-egg lesion" (Fig. 42.14). Many patients develop a single nodule of sub-RPE fibrosis centered very near the fovea (Fig. 42.15). Geographic atrophy is also fairly common after age 60 (Figs 42.16, 42.17), but can occur earlier in some patients. As with all diseases that disturb the RPE, true choroidal neovascularization can develop in a few percent of cases (Fig. 42.18).[7] In addition, a few patients with vitelliform lesions develop subretinal hemorrhage following fairly modest blunt trauma to the head or eye (Fig. 42.19). Fortunately, these hemorrhages usually resolve and good vision returns without treatment. While these many clinical patterns have been described as "stages" by some authors, there is not always a predictable progression of these fundus changes from one to the other in a given patient. Although the maculas of patients with BMD are usually quite symmetric in the early years of the disease, the two eyes can become quite strikingly different in function and appearance as the disease progresses.

Although most patients with Best disease exhibit a single lesion centered on the fovea, there have also been numerous reports of patients with multiple vitelliform lesions who also manifest abnormalities on electro-oculography (EOG)[8,9] and mutations in the *BEST1* gene.[10–14] In the most striking form of this multifocal phenotype, sometimes called multifocal Best dystrophy, there are multiple vitelliform lesions scattered throughout the posterior pole of both eyes (see Fig. 42.8). As with typical Best disease, these patients are asymptomatic unless the vitelliform lesions develop fibrotic scarring affecting the center of the macula. Autofluorescence and optical coherence tomography (OCT) imaging of multifocal lesions demonstrate characteristics similar to the solitary lesions seen in typical Best disease. This condition is distinguished from acute exudative polymorphous vitelliform maculopathy[15,16] as patients with the latter disorder have a normal EOG and lack variations in *BEST1*.

Table 42.2 Drug toxicities mimicking dystrophies

Agent	Reference(s)
Chloroquine	Hobbs et al., 1959; Marmor et al., 2011
Hydroxychloroquine	Shearer et al., 1965; Marmor et al., 2011;
Thioridazine (mellaril)	Weekley et al., 1960
Chloropromazine (thorazine)	Delong et al., 1965
Clofazimine	Craythorn et al., 1986
Tamoxifen	Kaiser-Kupfer and Lippman, 1978
Oxalosis/methoxyfluorane	Bullock and Albert, 1975; Albert et al., 1975
Canthaxanthine	Boudreault et al., 1983; Ros et al., 1985
Nitrofurantoin	Ibanez et al., 1994
Talc	AtLee, 1972
Deferoxamine	Haimovici et al., 2002; Gonzales et al., 2004

Albert DM, Bullock JD, Lahav M, et al. Flecked retina secondary to oxalate crystals from methoxyflurane anesthesia: clinical and experimental studies. Trans Sect Ophthalmol Am Acad Ophthalmol Otolaryngol 1975;79(6): OP817–26.

AtLee WE, Jr. Talc and cornstarch emboli in eyes of drug abusers. JAMA 1972;219(1):49–51.

Boudreault G, Cortin P, Corriveau LA, et al. [Canthaxanthine retinopathy: 1. Clinical study in 51 consumers.] Can J Ophthalmol 1983;18(7):325–8.

Bullock JD, Albert DM. Flecked retina. Appearance secondary to oxalate crystals from methoxyflurane anesthesia. Arch Ophthalmol 1975;93(1):26–31.

Craythorn JM, Swartz M, Creel DJ. Clofazimine-induced bull's-eye retinopathy. Retina 1986;6(1):50–2.

Delong SL, Poley BJ, McFarlane JR, Jr. Ocular changes associated with long-term chlorpromazine therapy. Arch Ophthalmol 1965;73:611–17.

Gonzales CR, Lin AP, Engstrom RE, et al. Bilateral vitelliform maculopathy and deferoxamine toxicity. Retina 2004;24(3):464–7.

Haimovici R, D'Amico DJ, Gragoudas ES, et al. The expanded clinical spectrum of deferoxamine retinopathy. Ophthalmology 2002;109(1):164–71.

Hobbs HE, Sorsby A, Freedman A. Retinopathy following chloroquine therapy. Lancet 1959;2(7101):478–80.

Ibanez HE, Williams DF, Boniuk I. Crystalline retinopathy associated with long-term nitrofurantoin therapy. Arch Ophthalmol 1994;112(3):304–5.

Kaiser-Kupfer MI, Lippman ME. Tamoxifen retinopathy. Cancer Treat Rep 1978;62(3):315–20.

Marmor MF, Kellner U, Lai TY, et al. Revised recommendations on screening for chloroquine and hydroxychloroquine retinopathy. Ophthalmology 2011;118(2):415–22.

Ros AM, Leyon H, Wennersten G. Crystalline retinopathy in patients taking an oral drug containing canthaxanthine. Photodermatol 1985;2(3):183–5.

Shearer RV, Dubois EL. Ocular changes induced by long-term hydroxychloroquine (plaquenil) therapy. Am J Ophthalmol 1967;64(2):245–52.

Weekley RD, Potts AM, Reboton J, et al.. Pigmentary retinopathy in patients receiving high doses of a new phenothiazine. Arch Ophthalmol 1960;64:65–76.

Notably, the canine model for BMD, which is due to a recessive mutation in the canine *BEST1* gene, is associated with multifocal vitelliform lesions[17,18] and some human patients with mutations in both alleles of *BEST1* also exhibit multifocal vitelliform lesions.[10,11,13] However, a few individuals with dominantly inherited disease and solitary lesions as children or young adults will also develop additional extramacular lesions later in life (Figs 42.20, 42.21).

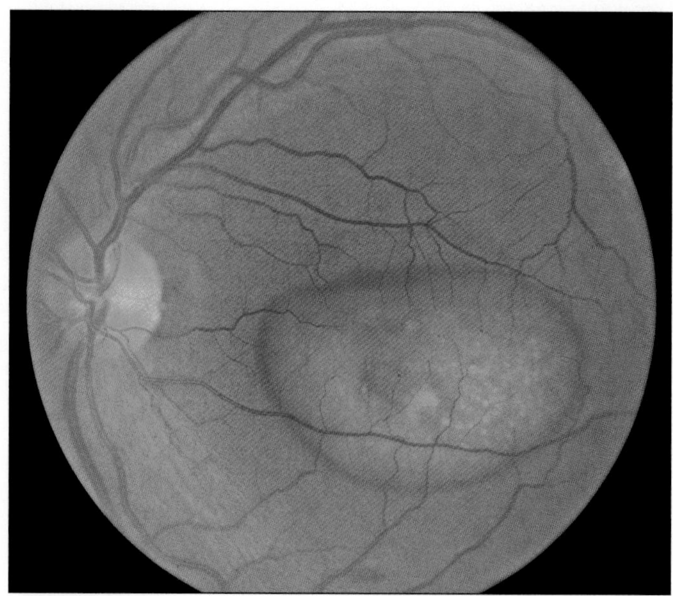

Fig. 42.4 Fundus photograph of the left eye of a 56-year-old male with a Lys30Arg mutation in *BEST1*. This eye has 20/20 visual acuity despite a very large vitelliform lesion centered on the fovea.

Visual function

Visual acuity sufficient to drive is usually preserved in at least one eye throughout the first six decades of life, with more substantial visual loss occurring when BMD is complicated by nodular fibrosis, choroidal neovascularization[19–21] or central geographic atrophy.[22] Visual acuity is often 20/20 or better in eyes with undisturbed vitelliform lesions, which is surprising considering the substantial physical separation of the photoreceptor outer segments and the RPE (see Fig. 42.6) that exists for decades in some individuals (see Fig. 42.7). This suggests that the fluid within vitelliform lesions has an ionic composition relatively similar to that of the normal interphotoreceptor matrix and quite distinct from the composition of the subretinal fluid associated with rhegmatogenous retinal detachments. Some vitelliform lesions gradually flatten over time with persistence of good acuity, while others develop nodular sub-RPE scars or RPE atrophy which are associated with poorer visual acuities that are somewhat proportional to the size of the scar. Peripheral visual fields are usually completely normal in BMD, although patients with other *BEST1* phenotypes do exhibit abnormal visual fields in some cases (see below).

Refractive error

It is not uncommon for patients with BMD to have hyperopia,[22,23] which is likely due to shortened axial length.[24] These findings are sometimes associated with narrow angles and/or angle closure glaucoma[22,24,25] requiring peripheral iridotomy. Hyperopia and angle closure have also been demonstrated in other *BEST1* phenotypes, including autosomal dominant vitreoretinochoroidopathy (ADVIRC)[26,27] and autosomal recessive bestrophinopathy (ARB).[13] Examination of the anterior segment with particular attention to the intraocular pressure and angle is warranted in patients with BMD and other phenotypes associated with *BEST1* mutations.

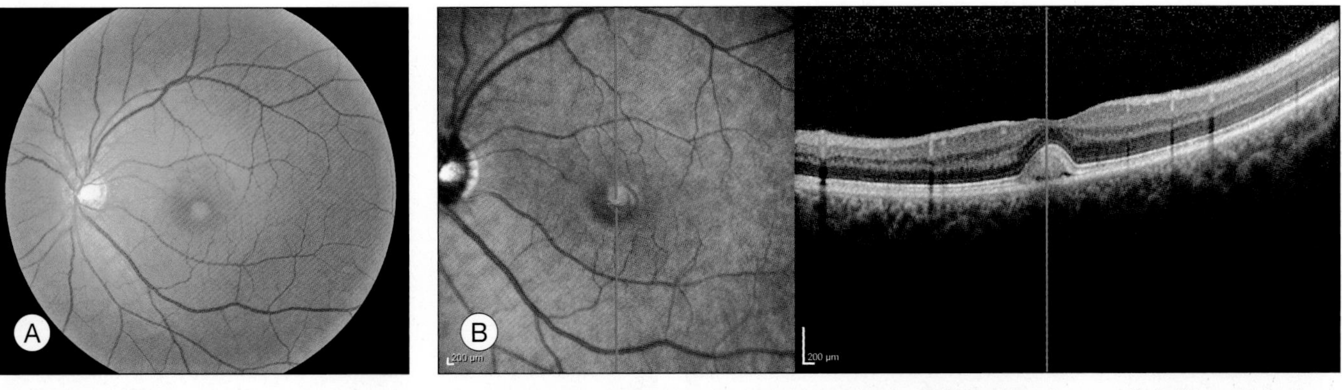

Fig. 42.5 (A) Fundus photograph of the left eye of a 40-year-old male with a Lys30Arg mutation in *BEST1.* There is a small vitelliform lesion in this eye and 20/20 visual acuity. (B) SD-OCT demonstrates hyperreflectivity of the vitelliform material in the subretinal space.

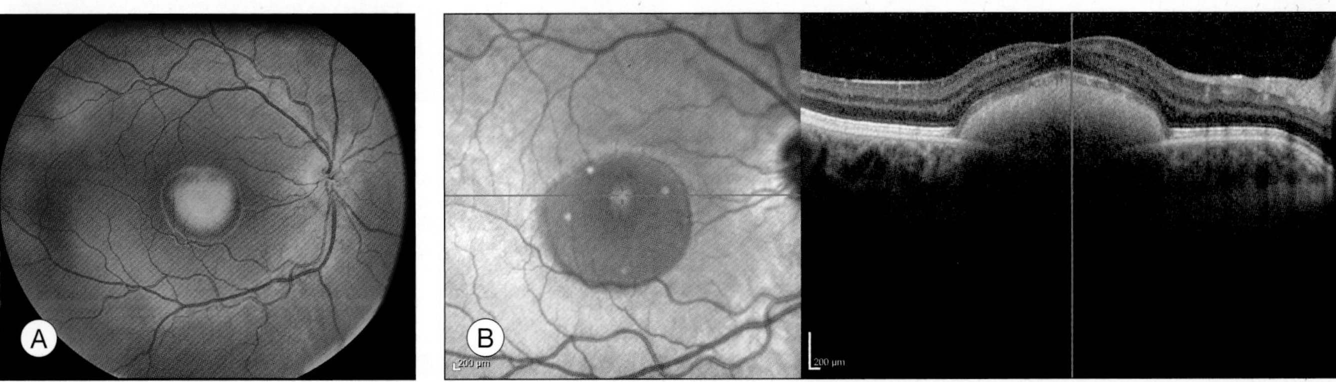

Fig. 42.6 (A) Fundus photograph of the right eye of a 15-year-old male with a Tyr227Asn mutation in *BEST1.* There is a classic vitelliform lesion in this eye and 20/40 visual acuity. (B) SD-OCT demonstrates hyperreflectivity of the vitelliform material in the subretinal space.

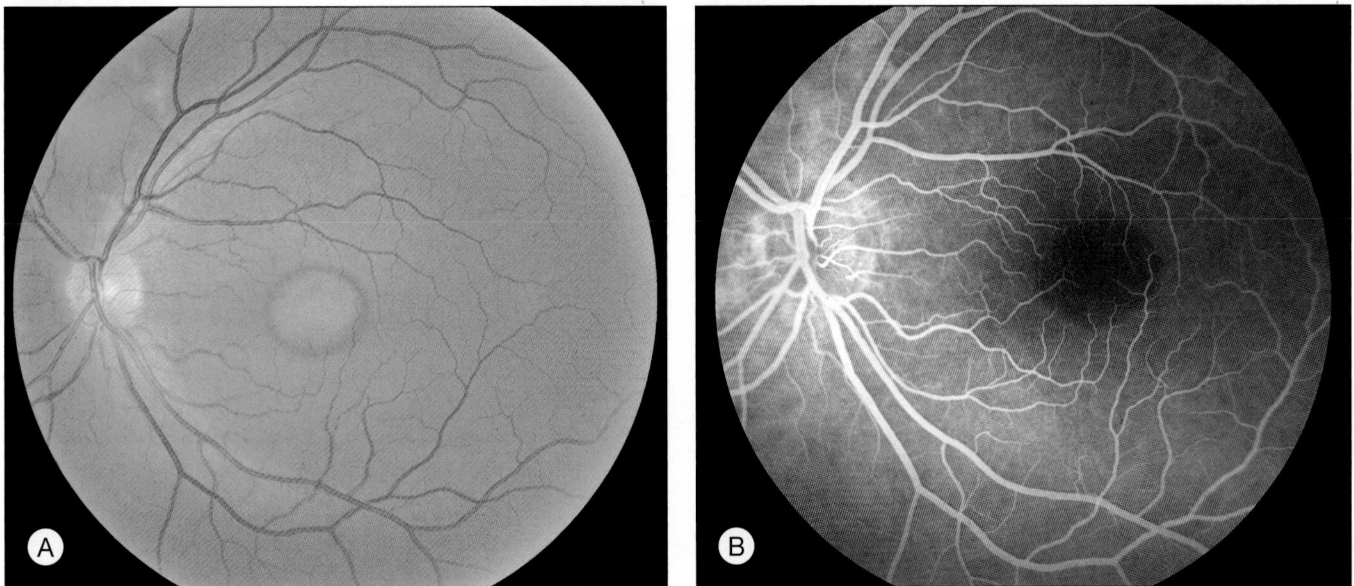

Fig. 42.7 (A) Fundus photograph of the left eye of a 51-year-old male with a 3 nucleotide deletion in *BEST1* (Leu294 del3cTCA). The visual acuity is 20/30 in this eye. The classic vitelliform lesion remains completely homogeneous after more than five decades of life. (B) Fluorescein angiography of this eye reveals almost complete masking of the normal choroidal circulation underlying the lesion.

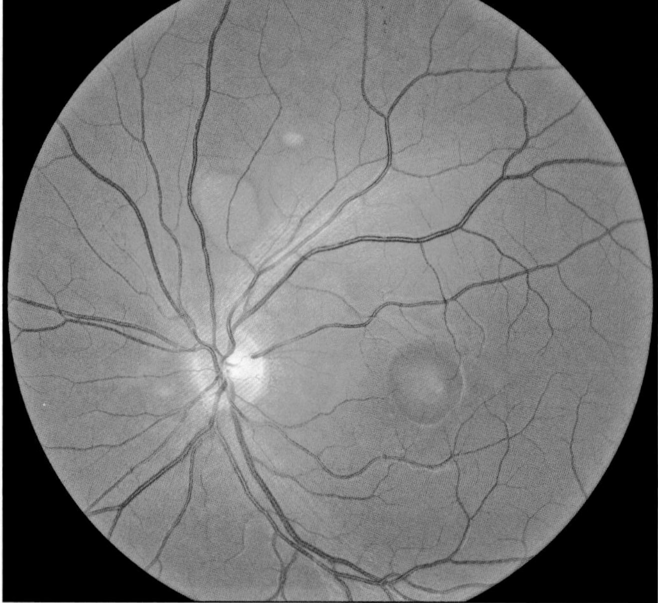

Fig. 42.8 Fundus photograph of the left eye of a 24-year-old male with a Lys30Arg mutation in *BEST1*. There is a vitelliform lesion centered on fixation and a similar lesion superior to the disc. The acuity in this eye is 20/20.

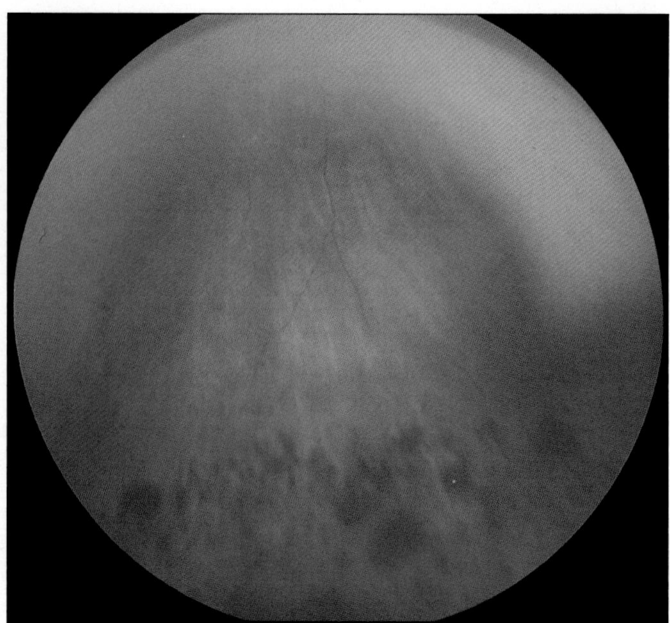

Fig. 42.9 Fundus photograph of the peripheral retina of a 70-year-old woman with ADVIRC caused by an Val239Met mutation in *BEST1*. The visual acuity is 20/100. There is a well-defined border between the normal retinal pigment epithelium and an anterior zone of retinal pigment epithelium clumping and atrophy. (Courtesy of Dr Kean Oh, Associated Retinal Consultants, Petoskey, Michigan.)

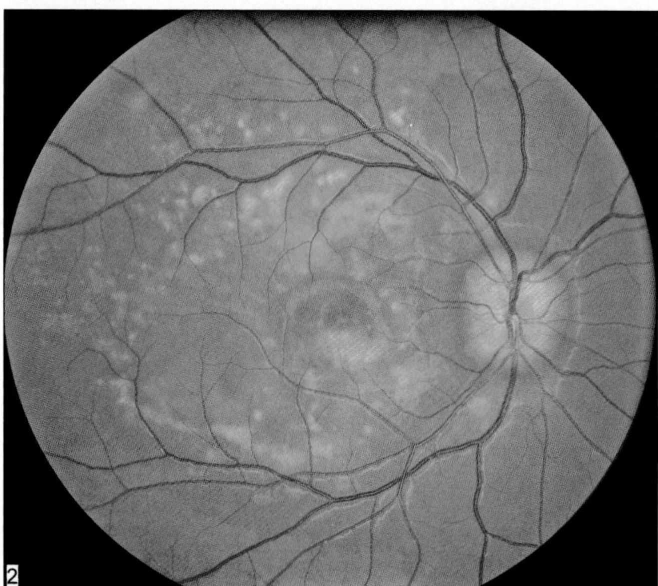

Fig. 42.10 Fundus photograph of an 11-year-old male with two mutations in *BEST1* (Arg141His/Pro152Ala) causing autosomal recessive bestrophinopathy. The visual acuity in this eye is 20/20. There are numerous yellow deposits scattered throughout the posterior pole and a patch of subretinal fibrosis just inferior to the fovea. (Reproduced with permission from Kinnick TR, Mullins RF, Dev S, et al. Autosomal recessive vitelliform macular dystrophy in a large cohort of vitelliform macular dystrophy patients. Retina 2011;31(3): 581–95.)

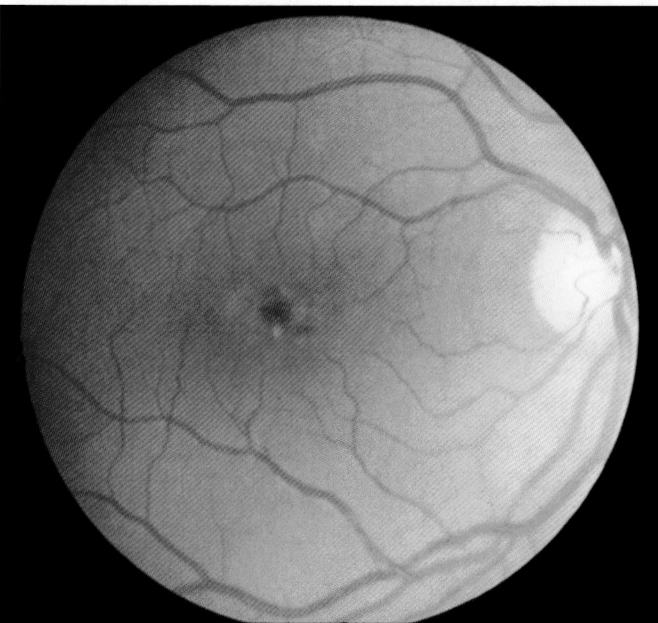

Fig. 42.11 Fundus photograph of the right eye of a 36-year-old female with an Ala243Thr mutation in *BEST1*. The visual acuity in this eye is 20/50. There is a small, oval "dot and halo" lesion centered on the fovea that is reminiscent of pattern dystrophy.

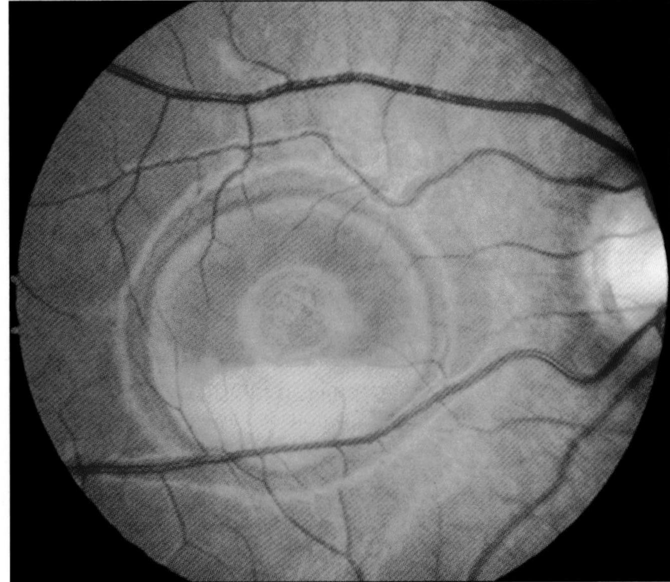

Fig. 42.12 Fundus photograph of the right eye of a 9-year-old male with a Tyr227Asn mutation in *BEST1*. This eye has 20/25 visual acuity. There is a large vitelliform lesion with a pseudohypopyon appearance characterized by layering of the lipofuscin pigment in the inferior aspect of the lesion. Some lipofuscin remains at the very margin of the lesion for its entire circumference.

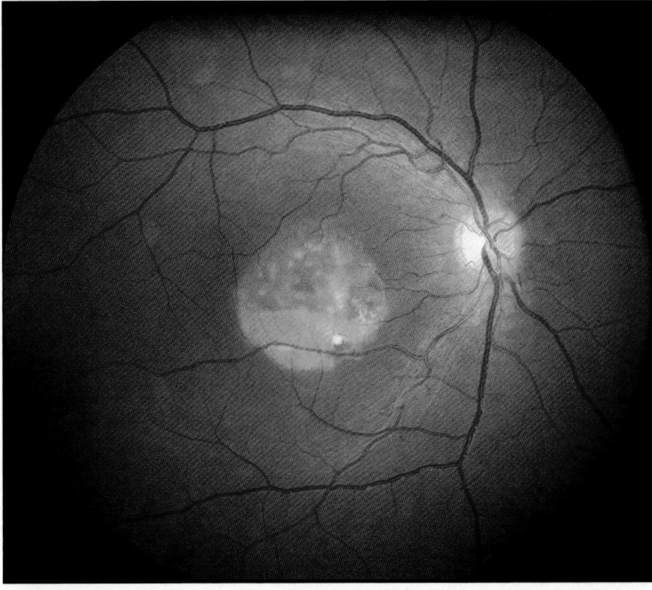

Fig. 42.13 Fundus photograph of the right eye of a 14-year-old male with a Asp302Ala mutation in *BEST1*. This eye has 20/20 visual acuity. The vitelliform lesion has a pseudohypopyon appearance.

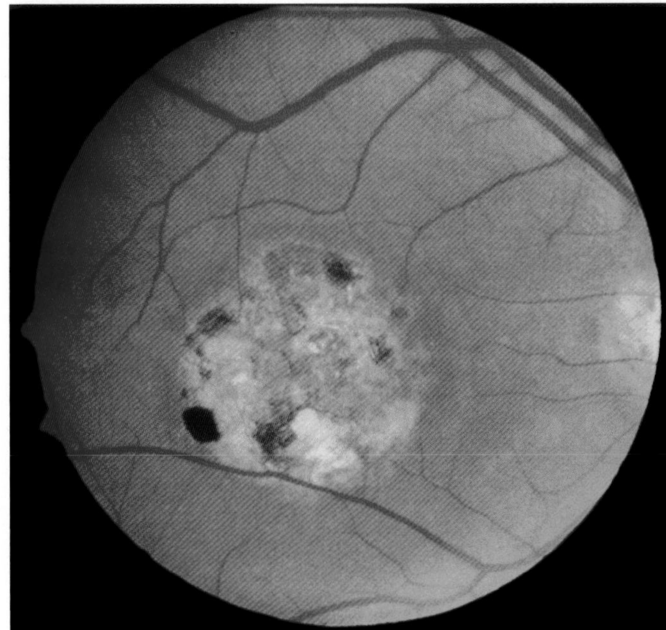

Fig. 42.14 Fundus photograph of the right eye of a 47-year-old male with a Tyr227Asn mutation in *BEST1*. The acuity in this eye is 20/200. There is a sharply circumscribed area of RPE atrophy and RPE pigment disruption at the site of a previous vitelliform lesion.

Optical coherence tomography (OCT)

Although there have been no histopathologic studies of eyes with undisturbed vitelliform lesions, spectral domain OCT allows *in vivo* determination of the anatomy of macular lesions at near histopathologic resolution. The yellow material of a classic vitelliform lesion lies in the subretinal space and appears fairly homogeneous on OCT (see Figs 42.5B, 42.6B).[28–32] In some patients, over time, some of the yellow pigment disappears and is replaced by clear fluid. The yellow pigment is denser than the clear fluid and settles gravitationally to the bottom of the vitelliform lesion with a fairly sharp horizontal line demarcating the pigment–fluid interface (see Figs 42.12, 42.13). This configuration is known as a "pseudohypopyon" and on OCT the yellow pigment appears hyperreflective while the clear subretinal fluid appears hyporeflective (black). Another lesion that is quite common in patients with Best disease and that has a very dramatic appearance on OCT is a fibrotic pillar that develops in the sub-RPE space, usually within 100 μm of the foveal center. These lesions appear hyperreflective on spectral domain OCT and seem to elevate the retina like a circus tent such that they are usually flanked by clear (hyporeflective on OCT) subretinal fluid (see Fig. 42.15B).

The origin of these fibrotic pillars remains obscure. Their sub-RPE location suggests a neovascular origin, but they rarely exhibit a classic neovascular pattern on fluorescein angiography and they tend to become stably fibrotic more rapidly than self-involuting choroidal neovascular membranes (CNVMs) associated with other macular diseases like the presumed ocular histoplasmosis syndrome. Although their height is exaggerated by the normal presentation of SD-OCT data, they do exhibit an unusual height-to-base ratio compared to involuted CNVMs of other disorders. The development of a fibrotic pillar is associated with a relatively rapid loss of yellow pigment from the vitelliform lesion and a drop in visual acuity, although the acuity typically remains much better than it would if a lesion of similar size and configuration developed in a patient with a different macular disease such as age-related macular degeneration.

Fluorescein angiography and autofluorescence

The primary clinical use of fluorescein angiography (FA) in patients with Best disease is to help differentiate

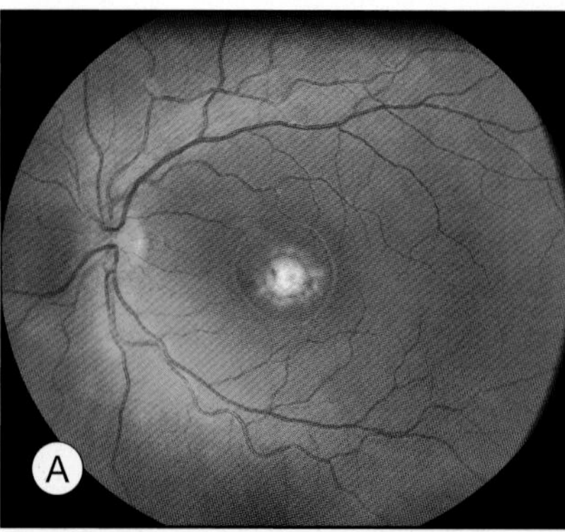

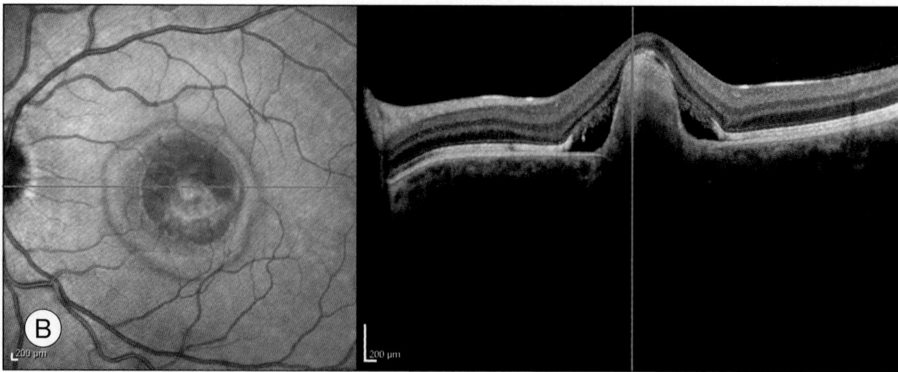

Fig. 42.15 (A) Fundus photograph of the left eye of a 15-year-old male with a Tyr227Asn mutation in *BEST1* and 20/40 visual acuity. There is a fibrotic pillar centered on fixation. (B) SD-OCT of this eye reveals the fibrotic pillar to lie beneath the RPE, surrounded by small amounts of subretinal fluid. Long outer segments can be seen extending from the retina into the subretinal fluid.

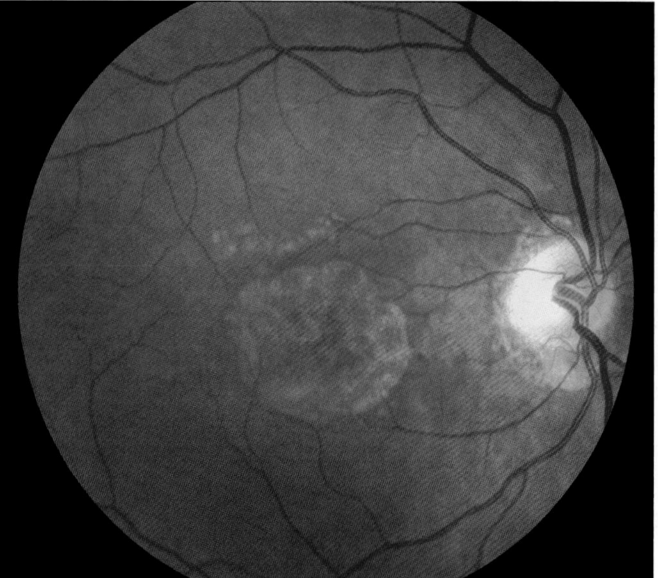

Fig. 42.16 Fundus photograph of the right eye of a 72-year-old female with a Thr307Ile mutation in *BEST1*. She has 20/80 visual acuity in this eye. There is a circular zone of geographic atrophy centered on fixation, flanked superiorly by a few drusen-like deposits.

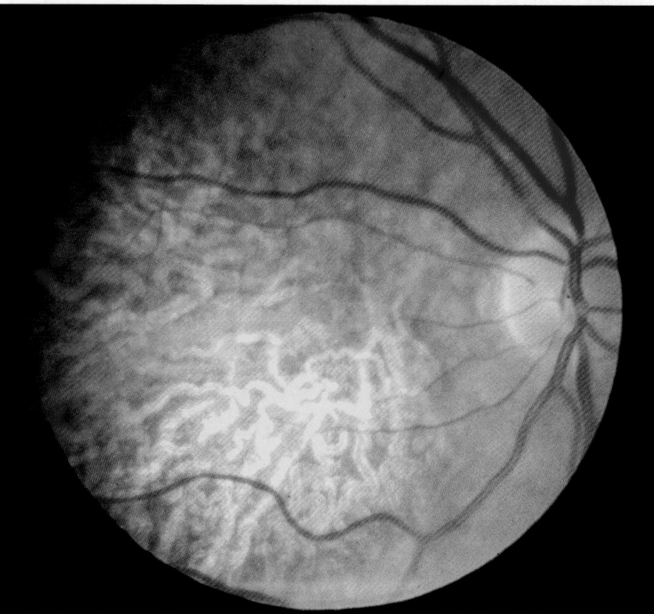

Fig. 42.17 Fundus photograph of the right eye of a 73-year-old female with an Ala243Thr mutation in *BEST1*. She has counting fingers visual acuity in this eye associated with extensive RPE atrophy and depigmentation of the choroidal vessels of the macula.

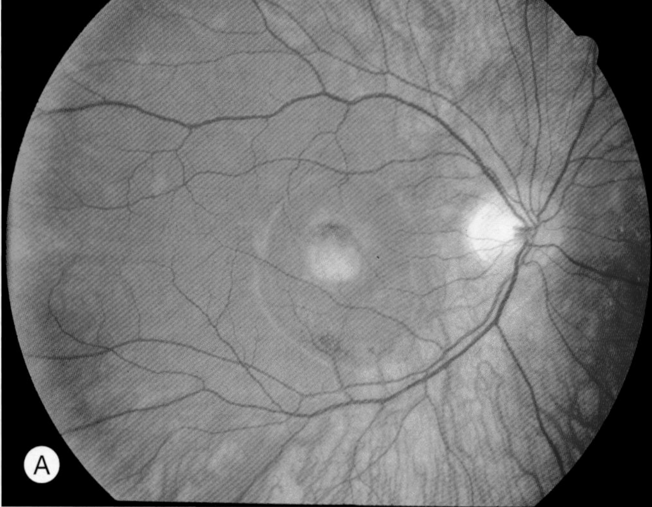

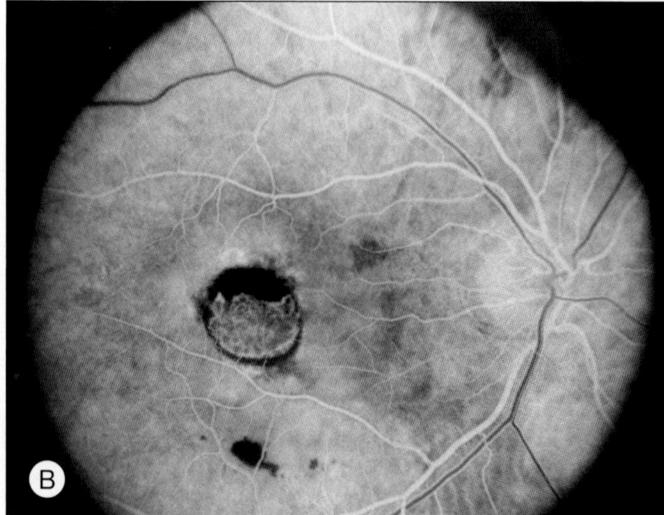

Fig. 42.18 (A) Fundus photograph of the right eye of a 23-year-old female with Best disease and an evolving subretinal fibrotic nodule. A small amount of subretinal blood can be seen at the inferior margin of the associated serous macular detachment. The acuity in this eye is 20/100. (B) The early phase of the fluorescein angiogram of this eye shows a classic choroidal neovascular membrane centered on the fibrotic nodule.

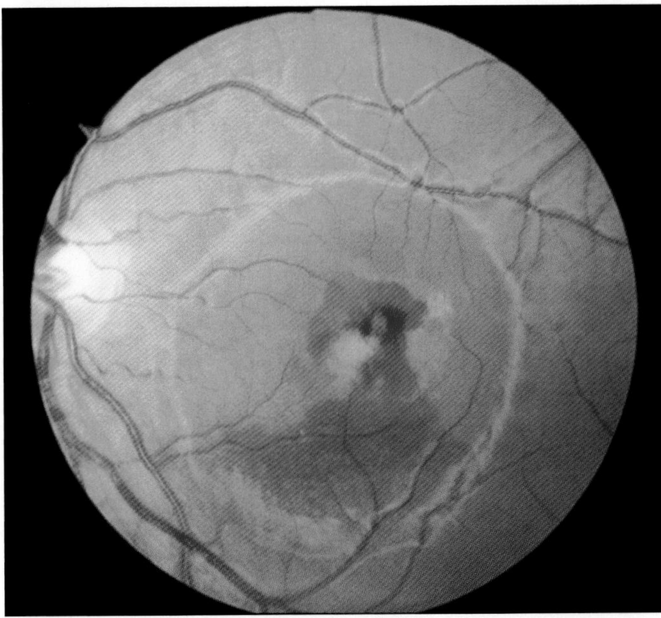

Fig. 42.19 Fundus photograph of the left eye of an 8-year-old male with an Arg218His mutation in *BEST1* and 20/70 visual acuity. The subretinal hemorrhage in the macula was first noted following a moderate blow to the head not involving the eye. Six months later the acuity in this eye improved to 20/40 and the hemorrhage resolved without treatment.

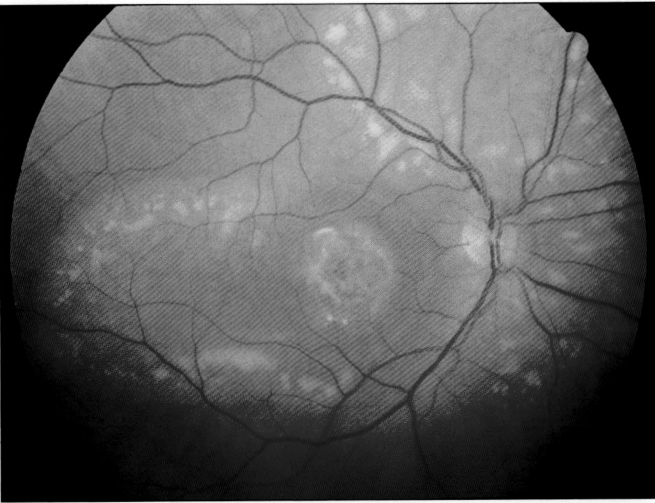

Fig. 42.20 Fundus photograph of the right eye of a 42-year-old male with a Tyr227Asn mutation in *BEST1*. This eye has 20/100 visual acuity and two large areas of subretinal fluid, one involving the entire macula and the other situated superior to the disc There are subretinal deposits of lipofuscin along the edges of both lesions.

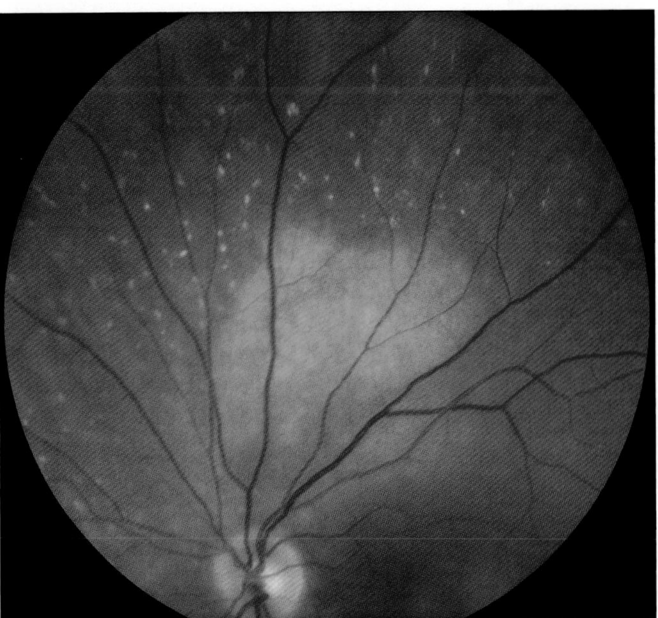

Fig. 42.21 Fundus photograph of the left eye of an 83-year-old female with a Tyr227Asn mutation in *BEST1*. This eye has 20/80 visual acuity. There is a large vitelliform lesion superior to the disc in addition to a number of more peripheral fleck-like deposits.

non-neovascular alterations in lesion anatomy (e.g., irregular resorption of yellow pigment) from active choroidal neovascularization in patients with a recent decrease in visual acuity. Although the vitelliform lesions of Best disease resemble the pigment epithelial detachments that occur in AMD, their anatomy and composition, however, are quite different and this causes some difficulty when interpreting fluorescein angiograms in patients with Best disease. For example, the yellow pigment filling some vitelliform lesions, especially in very young patients, is extremely hydrophobic and completely excludes fluorescein from the lesion. In such patients the vitelliform lesion blocks the underlying choroidal fluorescence almost as completely as blood would in a patient with AMD (see Fig. 42.7). Over time, the contents of the subretinal vitelliform cavities in some patients become more hydrophilic and in such cases the lesions briskly and completely fill with dye during an angiogram, much as a serous pigment epithelial detachment would in a patient with AMD (Fig. 42.22). In patients with the pseudohypopyon configuration the serous component of the lesion will fill with dye while the yellow pigment in the inferior portion of the lesion will both exclude the fluorescein from the vitelliform cavity and block the underlying choroidal fluorescence. This results in an angiogram that closely resembles a "notched" pigment epithelial detachment, which in AMD patients would suggest the presence of a choroidal neovascular membrane. In patients with Best disease this appearance is much less ominous. Autofluorescence imaging is not typically needed to make the diagnosis of Best disease or to make treatment decisions. From a research perspective, however, it is interesting that undisturbed vitelliform lesions usually exhibit uniform hyperfluorescence while those that have some amount of sub-RPE fibrosis or atrophy usually exhibit hypofluorescence.[22,33,34] The increased autofluorescence in the undisturbed vitelliform lesions is likely a reflection of the increased amounts of lipofuscin in eyes with Best disease.[35–38]

Electrophysiology

Before the discovery of the gene responsible for Best disease, electrophysiologic testing played a very prominent role in the diagnosis. The electro-oculogram is usually markedly abnormal in molecularly affected individuals, even when macular lesions

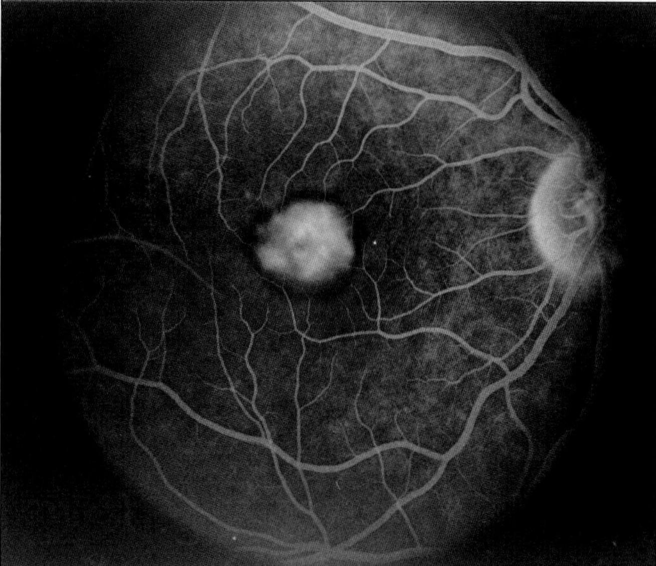

Fig. 42.22 Mid-phase fluorescein angiogram of the right eye of a 31-year-old female with an Ala243Thr mutation in *BEST1*. The acuity in this eye is 20/20. The vitelliform lesion briskly fills with dye simulating a serous pigment epithelial detachment.

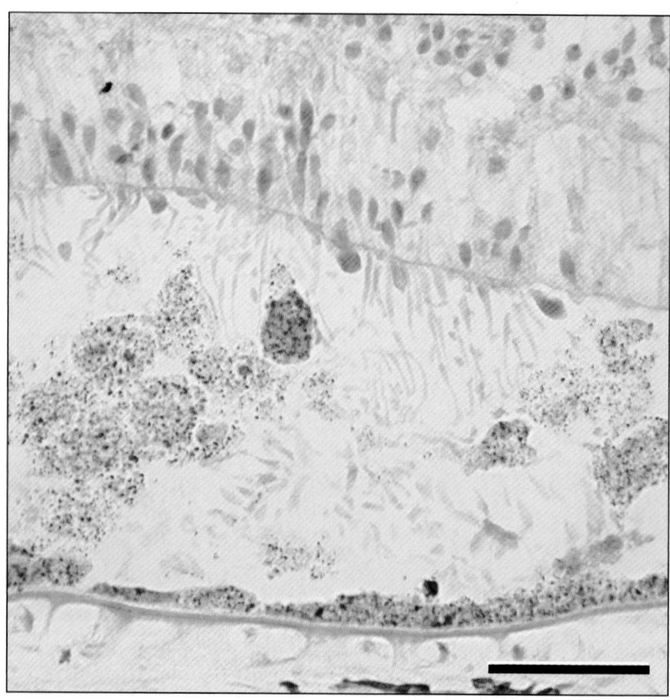

Fig. 42.23 Histological section of the left eye of an 86-year-old donor with Best disease due to a Thr6Arg mutation in *BEST1*. Note the presence of pigment-laden cells and outer-segment debris in the subretinal space. Scale bar indicates 50 μm.

are not evident. In normal individuals the cornea positive standing potential of the eye is nearly twofold higher in bright light than it is in darkness, while in patients with Best disease the ratio of the light peak to dark trough (the Arden ratio) is typically less than 1.5. Full-field electroretinography (ERG) cone and rod a- and b-wave amplitudes are usually normal. The advantage of EOG over genetic testing is that diagnostic information can be obtained within an hour or two, while the patient is in the clinic. The disadvantage is that it is usually more expensive and less sensitive than molecular testing. That is, a normal EOG does not exclude the possibility of Best disease,[39–43] as 37.5% of patients in one series had a *BEST1* mutation despite normal a EOG.[39]

Genetics

Best disease was mapped to chromosome 11q13 in 1992[44] and the causative gene was identified six years later.[1,45,46] Now known as *BEST1*, this gene encodes a 585 amino acid protein known as bestrophin that localizes to the basolateral membrane of the RPE.[47] To date, more than 100 different mutations in *BEST1* have been associated with Best disease.[1,2,22,23,34,41,42,48–62] Most disease-causing mutations are missense variants, and a substantial fraction (about 25%) occur in exon 8, suggesting that the portion of the protein encoded by this exon may be critical to its function.[22] More than 90% of families that have two or more individuals with the clinical diagnosis of Best disease will have a detectable mutation in the coding sequence of *BEST1*. As a result, a negative molecular result is clinically meaningful and suggests that the patient's disease is caused by another gene or that it is a non-Mendelian phenocopy. The gene that most commonly causes macular lesions that are clinically similar to those of Best disease is *PRPH2* (formerly *RDS*), while the most common non-Mendelian phenocopy is a pigment epithelial detachment associated with age-related macular degeneration.

Pathophysiology and histopathology

Although Best disease is rare, there have been a number of histopathologic reports describing the structural changes that accompany this condition. Histopathologic findings include increased RPE lipofuscin,[37,38,63] loss of photoreceptors[38] (often seen over a relatively intact RPE layer[35,58]), sub-RPE drusenoid material,[35,36] and accumulation of cells and material in the subretinal space (Fig. 42.23). Following the discovery of the Best disease gene, efforts have also been made to identify the relationship between anatomical findings and specific genotypes. For example, eyes have been characterized from patients with Tyr227Asn,[58] Thr6Arg,[63] and a homozygous Trp93Cys donor.[38] From these studies it has been suggested that the eyes of patients with Tyr227Asn mutations are notable for extramacular flecks.[58] A donor eye with this mutation was also found to mislocalize bestrophin.[58]

The molecular pathophysiology of Best disease is somewhat controversial – owing in part to the difficulty of comparing the behavior of different types of cultured cells with the RPE in vivo – and a thorough discussion of the evidence for the possible functions of the bestrophin-1 protein is beyond the scope of this chapter; it has been well reviewed elsewhere.[64–66] Briefly, the normal function of bestrophin-1 appears to include the regulation of the ionic milieu in the RPE and/or the subretinal space. When overexpressed in some cell types, bestrophin-1 appears to function as a calcium-sensitive chloride channel,[67,68] whereas mice lacking bestrophin-1[69] or harboring a mutant allele (Tryp93Cys)[70] show altered uptake of calcium by the RPE. It has been suggested that impaired ionic flow across the RPE could result in alterations in the adhesiveness between the interphotoreceptor matrix and the RPE or a diminution of outer

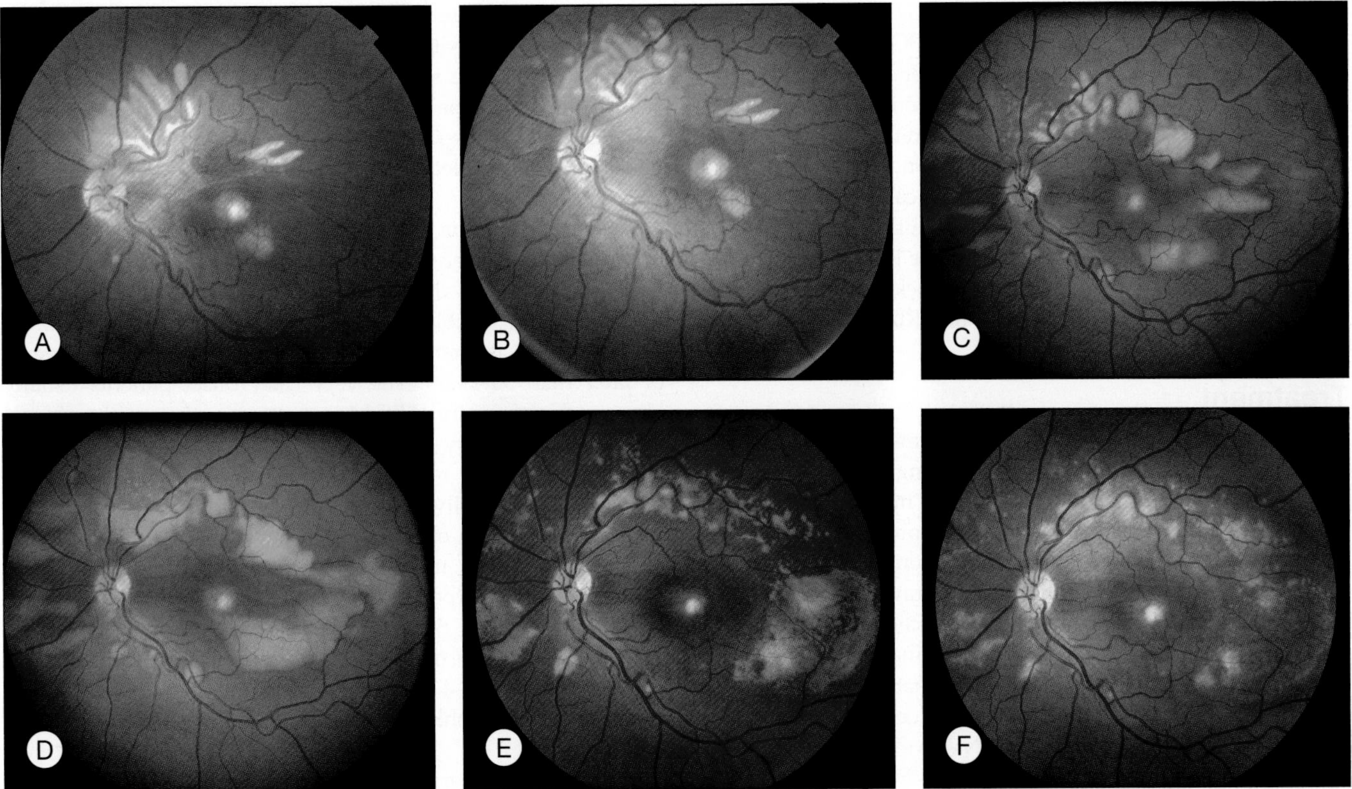

Fig. 42.24 (A) Fundus photograph of the left eye of an 18-year-old female with an Asp302Ala mutation in *BEST1*. This eye has 20/200 visual acuity and a thick epiretinal membrane that has thrown the neurosensory retina into folds. Yellow vitelliform material has formed beneath several of these folds. (B) One week after successful membrane peeling, the visual acuity remains 20/200 but there is little change in the subretinal deposits. (C) Two months after surgery, the acuity has improved to 20/160, the distortion is much less, and the vitelliform deposits have actually increased in number and extent. (D) Ten months after surgery, at age 19, the acuity has improved to 20/125 and the vitelliform material has coalesced. (E) Four years after surgery, at age 22, the acuity has improved to 20/100 and the vitelliform material has started to disappear. (F) Four and a half years after surgery, the acuity remains 20/100 and the resolution of the vitelliform material is more complete. (A,B, Courtesy of Dr Richard Spaide.)

segment phagocytosis, both of which are sensitive to levels of calcium.[71,72]

Bestrophin-1 is expressed in all RPE cells, not just those underlying the macula. Moreover, the large response of the EOG to changes in light (the Arden ratio) suggests that the entire retina participates in this response, not just the macula. Why then are the most typical Best lesions found in the macula, centered on fixation? The answer may be in part due to differences in bestrophin-1 expression in different regions of the retina.[63] However, it also seems likely that there are regional differences in the adhesion of the photoreceptors to the retinal pigment epithelium. The patient shown in Fig. 42.24 is supportive of this hypothesis. She developed an aggressive epiretinal membrane that created localized traction detachments in her left eye and she developed yellow vitelliform material in each of these locations. After successful surgery to remove the membrane and relieve the traction, the extramacular vitelliform deposits persisted for years.

Additional phenotypes associated with mutations in *BEST1*

Autosomal dominant vitreoretinochoroidopathy (ADVIRC)

ADVIRC was first described by Kaufman et al. in 1982[73] as a condition with: (1) an autosomal dominant inheritance pattern; (2) peripheral pigmentary retinopathy for 360 degrees, with a discrete posterior boundary near the equator (see Fig. 42.9); (3) punctate whitish opacities in the retina; (4) vitreous cells and fibrillar condensation; (5) blood–retinal barrier breakdown; (6) retinal arteriolar narrowing and occlusion; (7) retinal neovascularization; (8) choroidal atrophy; and (9) presenile cataracts (see Fig. 42.9).[74] The EOG is usually abnormal with a relatively normal ERG,[75] but the first electrophysiologic studies of ADVIRC patients[27,75,76] occurred in the pre-molecular era when genetic testing was not available. It has since been discovered that ADVIRC is caused by splice-altering mutations in *BEST1* and that these patients can also have concomitant developmental abnormalities, including microcornea, hyperopia, and shortened axial length.[26,77,78] Some patients have a severe form of ADVIRC in which both the ERG and EOG are abnormal, thus resembling retinitis pigmentosa.[79,80]

Autosomal recessive bestrophinopathy (ARB)

The first description of compound heterozygous *BEST1* mutations causing multifocal yellowish changes in the macula and cystoid macular edema was published in 2006.[11] Subsequent descriptions of patients with mutation in both *BEST1* alleles have included both compound heterozygous and homozygous mutations and demonstrate a wide spectrum of fundus findings that are not present in their carrier parents.[10,13,81–83] Burgess et al.[13] coined the term autosomal recessive bestrophinopathy (ARB) to refer to this unusual presentation of *BEST1*-associated retinal disease. Hyperopia and an abnormal EOG are common. The visual acuity in ARB can be normal but tends to be worse than in autosomal dominant Best disease. Some patients exhibit cystoid macular edema or shallow subretinal fluid that can extend throughout the macula and beyond the arcades. Both solitary and mutifocal vitelliform lesions can occur, sometimes associated with flecks within and outside the macula (see Fig. 42.10). OCT can be helpful in detecting the low-lying subretinal fluid, especially in young patients who lack vitelliform lesions. Subretinal fibrosis is more common in ARB than in autosomal dominant disease.

Treatment

Treatment for *BEST1* disease consists primarily of recognizing choroidal neovascularization and hastening its regression with anti-VEGF therapy. Though the natural history of subretinal hemorrhage in BMD is relatively good,[19] preservation of visual function for choroidal neovascularization (CNV) has been reported in retrospective studies using intravitreal bevacizumab and ranibizumab.[81,84–88] In our experience, it is not usually possible to completely eradicate subretinal fluid that exists adjacent to the nodular fibrotic pillars that occur beneath the RPE (see Fig. 42.15B). Thus, when this configuration is seen following treatment of suspected CNV, we would recommend elongating the intervals between anti-VEGF injections, and then discontinuing them altogether, once the visual acuity is stabilized and all subretinal blood has been resorbed. Even in the absence of CNV, subretinal hemorrhage can occur in patients with Best disease following relatively modest head or eye trauma (see Fig. 42.19).[19,89,90] As a result, we usually caution patients against playing sports in which frequent blows to the head are to be expected. Protective eyewear is recommended for all sports. Many patients with Best disease have poor vision in one eye but retain vision sufficient in the fellow eye to drive for many years. In such individuals we recommend wearing spectacles with safety plastic lenses at all times.

STARGARDT DISEASE

Variations in *ABCA4* (OMIM #601691) are the most common cause of autosomal recessive retinal disease in humans. *ABCA4* mutations were first found in patients with autosomal recessive Stargardt disease[91] and were later shown to also cause cone dystrophy, cone–rod dystrophy, and retinitis pigmentosa.[92–97] As discussed more fully below, a patient's position within this disease spectrum is determined largely by the total amount of residual ABCA4 function.[97] First described in 1909,[98] Stargardt disease is the mildest of the ABCA4 phenotypes while a form of retinitis pigmentosa is the most severe.

Clinical features of Stargardt disease

The clinical presentation of Stargardt disease is quite variable in age of onset, presenting symptoms, and fundus appearance, and this variability is often daunting to ophthalmologists who see the condition infrequently. Most of the differences in clinical findings in patients with *ABCA4* disease can be explained by the interplay of three factors that vary among patients: (1) the severity of their *ABCA4* genotype (and hence the rate at which toxic bisretinoids form in the photoreceptors); (2) the relative sensitivity of the foveal cones to the genotype; and (3) the relative sensitivity of the retinal pigment epithelium to the genotype (Fig. 42.25).[97] The first of these variables can be directly assessed by molecular testing of the *ABCA4* gene while the molecular nature of the latter two remains to be determined.

The most common presenting complaint is a loss of visual acuity, which can be as mild as 20/30 or as severe as 20/200 depending on the degree to which this drop in acuity is noticeable and troubling to the patient. The age at which the loss of acuity is first recognized can be as early as 5 years or later than 50 years. The very early onset patients usually have a fairly severe *ABCA4* genotype and sensitive foveal cones while the very late onset patients have a milder *ABCA4* genotype and fairly resistant foveal cones. That is, the younger onset patients usually have less observable extrafoveal disease while the very late onset patients have foveal photoreceptors and RPE that are more preserved anatomically than their extrafoveal counterparts. The second most common reason for a patient with Stargardt disease to present to a retina specialist is an abnormal fundus appearance that is incidentally discovered during a routine eye examination. Patients who present in this fashion almost always have fairly resistant foveal cones.

The most characteristic fundus findings in Stargardt disease are light-colored flecks at the level of the retinal pigment epithelium (Fig. 42.26). These flecks differ from drusen in that they are usually more elongated than round and they often contact each other at angles that create a branching or net-like appearance. Occasionally, two adjacent flecks form an obtuse angle that Franceschetti called "pisciform" because of its resemblance to a fish tail.[99] In some patients a cluster of flecks is entirely contained within a one-by-two disc diameter horizontal ellipse centered on fixation (Fig. 42.27), while in other patients the flecks extend well beyond the temporal vascular arcades (Fig. 42.28), almost reaching the equator.

In addition to the difference in distribution, Stargardt flecks also differ widely in number, size, color, aspect ratio, and edge definition among different patients. Some patients have no flecks at all (Fig. 42.29) while others have hundreds (see Fig. 42.28). Flecks are most commonly yellow but can range from dirty-white to orange. Some flecks have pigmented edges and in a few cases this RPE hyperpigmentation can be quite dramatic. Some patients have very small deposits near the fovea that have a crystalline character on biomicroscopy (Fig. 42.30). Flecks outside the central 2 mm of the macula tend to be a bit larger than those nearer the fovea. Some patients have flecks that are almost round while others have flecks that are several times longer than they are wide. In some individuals with severe *ABCA4* genotypes, the flecks are small and white and are admixed with small patches of subretinal fibrosis that resemble confetti (Fig. 42.31). This is presumably because the widespread photoreceptor injury associated with such genotypes reduces the production of bisretinoids. Some flecks are stable in position, size and number for many years, while others grow in number and/or progress to RPE atrophy (Fig. 42.32).

In addition to the many different fleck configurations, the RPE itself responds to *ABCA4* mutations quite differently in different patients depending in part on the severity of the *ABCA4*

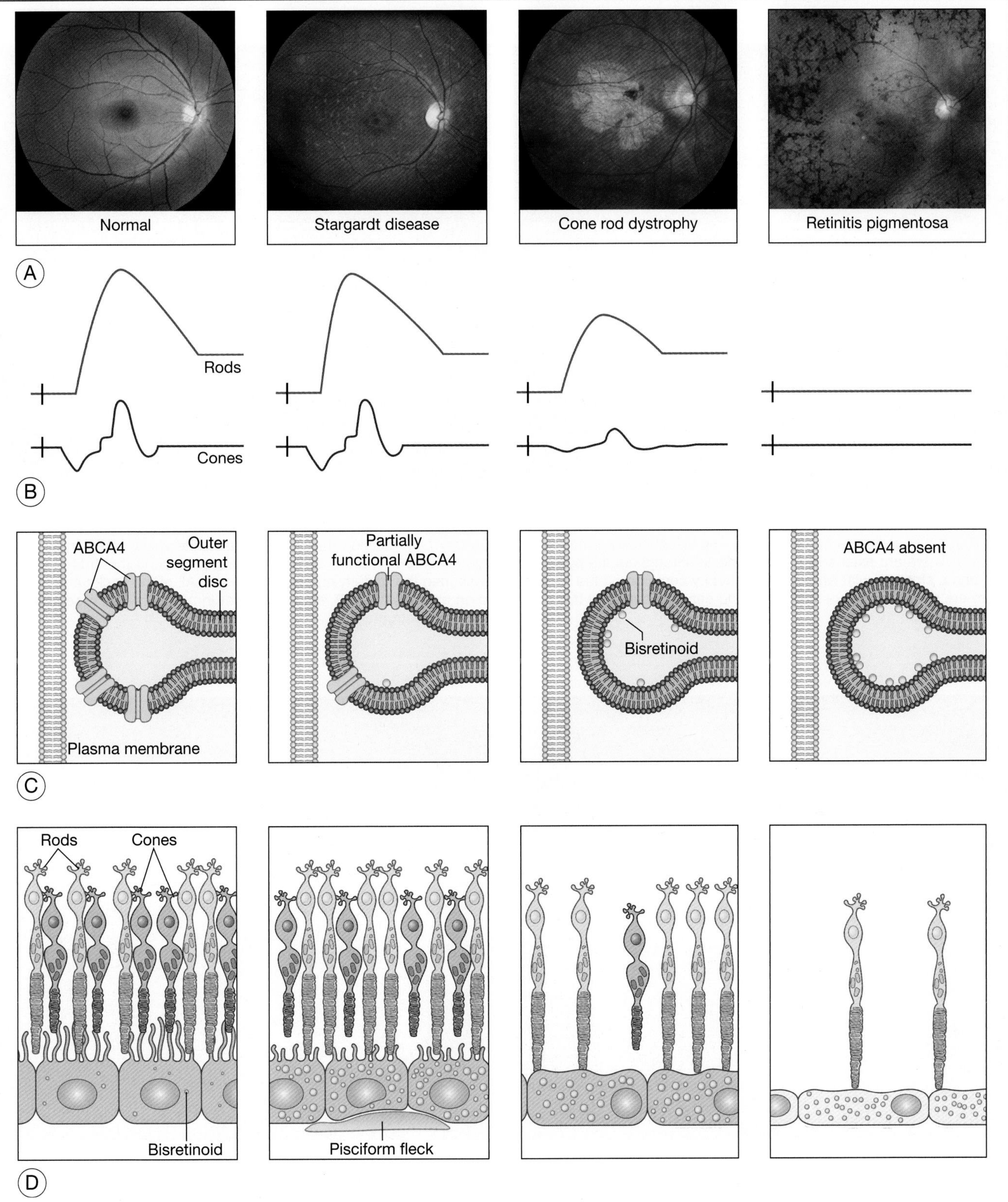

Fig. 42.25 Panel A shows a series of retinal photographs from patients with progressively decreasing amounts of ABCA4 function (from left to right), ranging from a normal retina to those of patients with Stargardt disease, cone–rod dystrophy, and retinitis pigmentosa. Panel B shows the effects of reduced ABCA4 function on full-field electroretinograms. The relatively mild reduction in ABCA4 activity in patients with Stargardt disease has little effect on global photoreceptor function. Moderate loss of ABCA4 function in patients with cone–rod dystrophy has a greater effect on cone photoreceptors than it does on rods. Complete loss of ABCA4 function in some patients with retinitis pigmentosa is associated with extensive loss of both cones and rods and a nonrecordable electroretinogram. Panel C shows the effects of reduced ABCA4 function on the accumulation of bisretinoid (yellow symbols) on the inner leaflet of the photoreceptor outer-segment disc membranes. Mild reduction in ABCA4 activity in Stargardt disease is associated with some bisretinoid formation; moderate loss of function in cone–rod dystrophy is associated with intermediate amounts of accumulation; and complete loss of function in retinitis pigmentosa results in maximal accumulation. Panel D shows the histopathological effects of reduced ABCA4 activity. In patients with Stargardt disease, the rate of bisretinoid formation in the outer segments is relatively slow and the photoreceptors are not directly injured. Bisretinoids are delivered to the secondary lysosomes of the RPE during the normal phagocytosis of photoreceptor outer segments. Some of this material accumulates beneath the RPE causing pisciform flecks that are visible on ophthalmoscopy. In patients with cone–rod dystrophy, moderate loss of ABCA4 function results in sufficient accumulation of bisretinoids in photoreceptor outer segments to cause some apoptosis of photoreceptors (in cones more than rods). In patients with retinitis pigmentosa, complete loss of ABCA4 function causes extensive accumulation of bisretinoids in photoreceptor outer segments, apoptosis of both rod and cone photoreceptors, and associated RPE thinning. (Reproduced with permission from Sheffield VC, Stone EM. Genomics and the eye. *N Engl J Med* 2011;364(20):1932–42.)

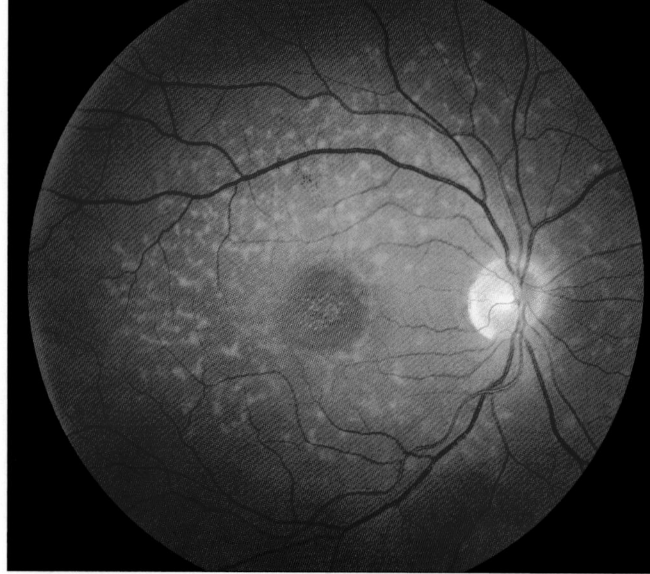

Fig. 42.26 Fundus photograph of the right eye of a 26-year-old female with compound heterozygous mutations in *ABCA4* (IVS40+5 G>A/Val1793Met) causing Stargardt disease. The visual acuity in this eye is 20/60. There are extensive pisciform flecks throughout the posterior pole and a small circular area of RPE atrophy centered on the fovea. There are numerous very small crystalline deposits overlying this atrophy.

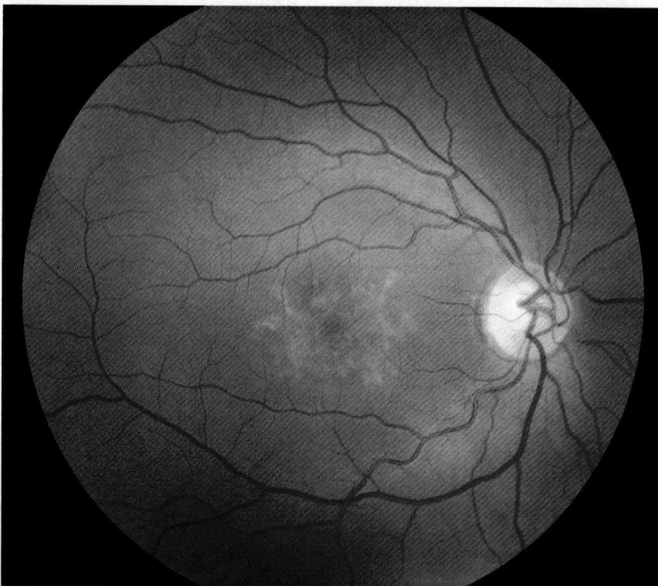

Fig. 42.27 Fundus photograph of the right eye of a 33-year-old female with compound heterozygous mutations in *ABCA4* (Tyr362Stop/Gly1961Glu) causing Stargardt disease. The visual acuity in this eye is 20/125. There is a vermillion appearance to the entire fundus obscuring the underlying choroidal detail. All of the flecks are confined to an area less than 3 mm in diameter in a pattern that resembles butterfly dystrophy.

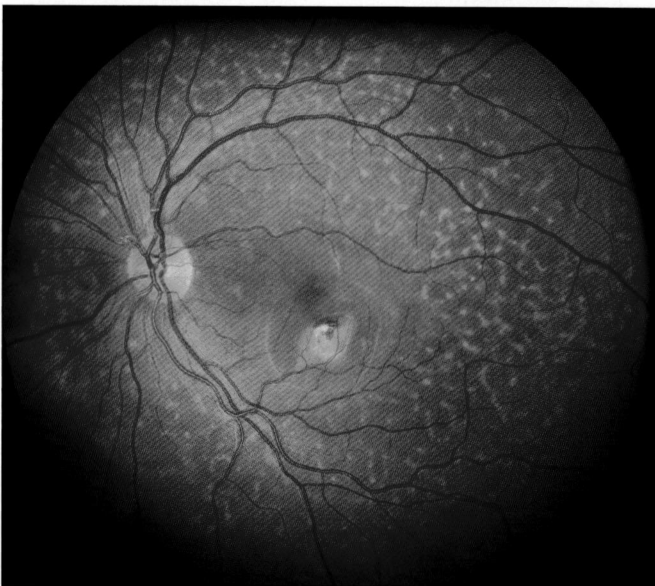

Fig. 42.28 Fundus photograph of the left eye of a 17-year-old male with compound heterozygous mutations in *ABCA4* (IVS40+5 G>A/Val256Val) causing the fundus flavimaculatus variant of Stargardt disease. The visual acuity in this eye is 20/20. There are extensive flecks throughout the posterior pole and a small fibrotic nodule just inferior to the fovea.

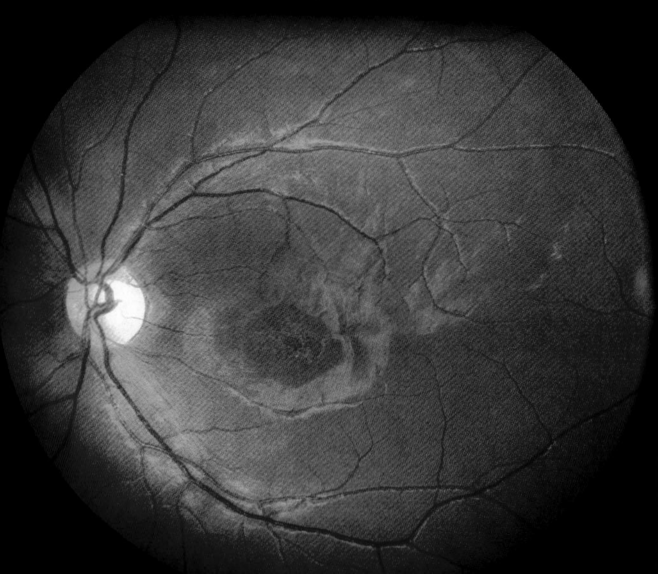

Fig. 42.29 Fundus photograph of the left eye of a 6-year-old male with compound heterozygous mutations in *ABCA4* (IVS9+1 G>A/IVS37+1 G>(A) causing cone–rod dystrophy. The visual acuity is 20/200. The arterioles are slightly narrow for a child of this age and are a clinical sign of a relatively severe *ABCA4* genotype.

genotype and in part on the sensitivity of the RPE to the accumulation of bisretinoids. In some patients with relatively mild genotypes, there is little photoreceptor injury and thus there is a steady supply of bisretinoid to the RPE. In some patients the RPE retains this material intracellularly and as a result becomes somewhat opaque to visible light. On ophthalmoscopy this is recognized as a very uniform vermillion or light-brown color to the fundus with complete obscuration of the underlying choroidal details (see Fig. 42.27, Figs 42.33, 42.34). On fluorescein angiography, this is seen as a complete masking of the choroidal circulation. As a result, the dye-filled retinal vessels lie upon a completely hypofluorescent background (see Fig. 42.43). In other patients with a very similar bisretinoid load emanating from the photoreceptors, the RPE gradually thins, presumably from apoptotic death of some RPE cells and compensatory stretching of those that survive (Fig. 42.35). Frank RPE atrophy is commonly seen in the center of the macula and the bases of these atrophic lesions have a metallic sheen to them (Fig. 42.32) that is distinctly different from the geographic atrophy that occurs in age-related macular degeneration. In some patients these atrophic lesions become dusted with dark pigment over time (Fig. 42.35). In the later stages of disease patients with severe genotypes can develop nummular atrophy of the extramacular RPE and choriocapillaris that somewhat resembles choroideremia (Fig. 42.36).

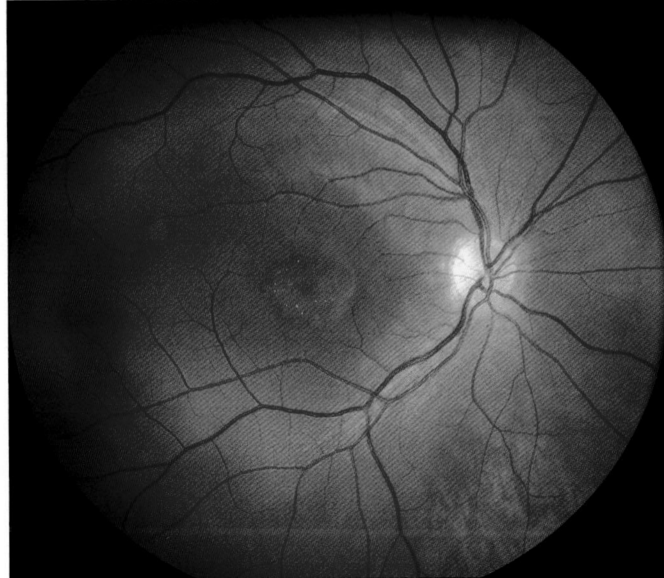

Fig. 42.30 Fundus photograph of the right eye of a 26-year-old male with compound heterozygous mutations in *ABCA4* (Cys2150Tyr/Gly863Ala) causing Stargardt disease. The visual acuity in this eye is 20/80. There is a vermillion appearance to the fundus obscuring the underlying choroidal detail. There are no typical flecks. However, there are tiny intraretinal crystals overlying a circular region of RPE atrophy centered on the fovea.

A fairly reliable diagnostic sign of *ABCA4*-associated retinal disease is a relative sparing of the peripapillary RPE. This sign is often more visible on fluorescein angiography[100] (see Fig. 42.31) or autofluorescence;[101,102] however, it can also be easily observed on ophthalmoscopy alone (Fig. 42.37). The mechanism of this sparing is currently unknown. Patients with *ABCA4*-associated retinal disease are not immune to inflammatory or traumatic retinal injuries and the coexistence of these disorders can make it difficult to establish the correct diagnoses. Although the frequency with which epiretinal membranes (Fig. 42.38A-D), subretinal fibrosis (Figs 42.39, 42.40) and inflammatory nodules (see Fig. 42.38A) occur in Stargardt patients may not be greater than would be expected by chance, the exuberant nature of some of these lesions suggests an adjuvant effect of either the bisretinoids themselves or the

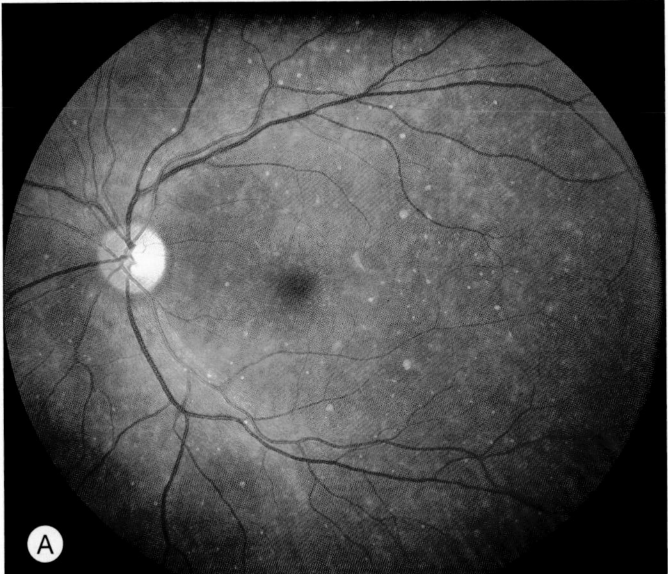

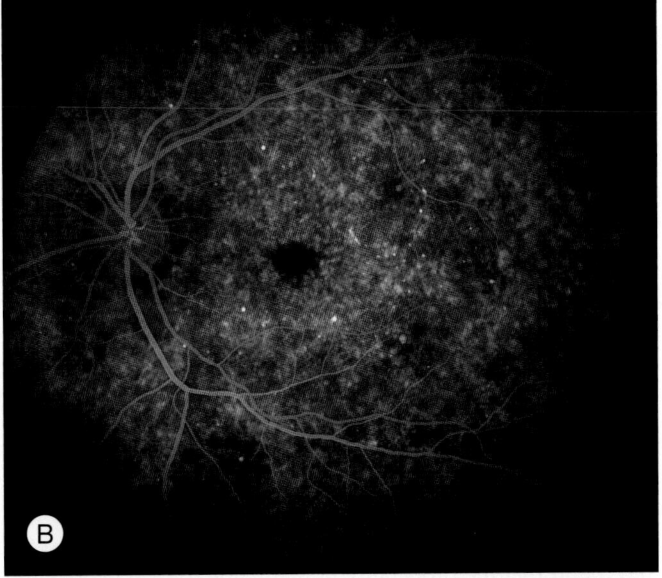

Fig. 42.31 (A) Fundus photograph of the left eye of a 25-year-old female with compound heterozygous mutations in *ABCA4* (Thr1019Met/Lys583Asn) causing Stargardt disease. The photoreceptors and RPE of the fovea are relatively spared in this patient and the visual acuity remains 20/80 despite extensive injury to the RPE throughout the remainder of the posterior pole. There are numerous superficial confetti-like flecks that seem to represent tiny foci of subretinal fibrosis. (B) Fluorescein angiography of this eye reveals the relative preservation of the foveal and peripapillary retina and RPE. The confetti-like flecks are intensely hyperfluorescent.

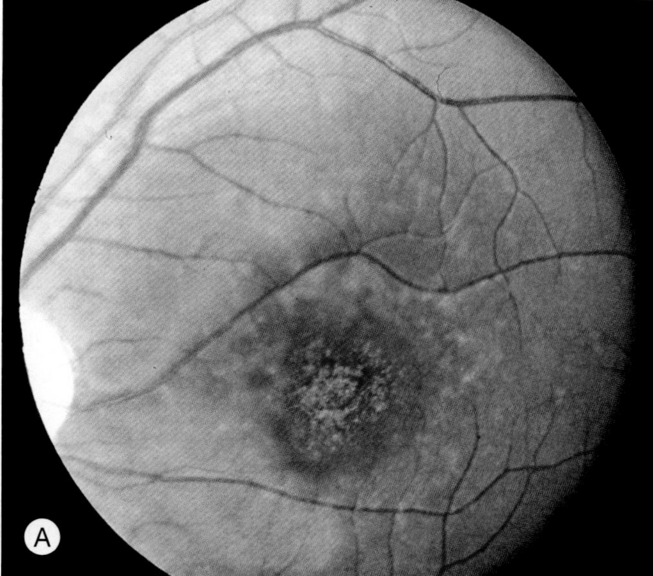

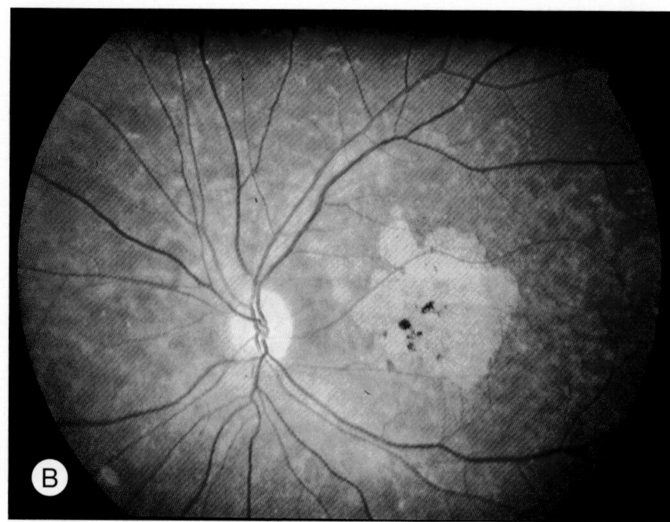

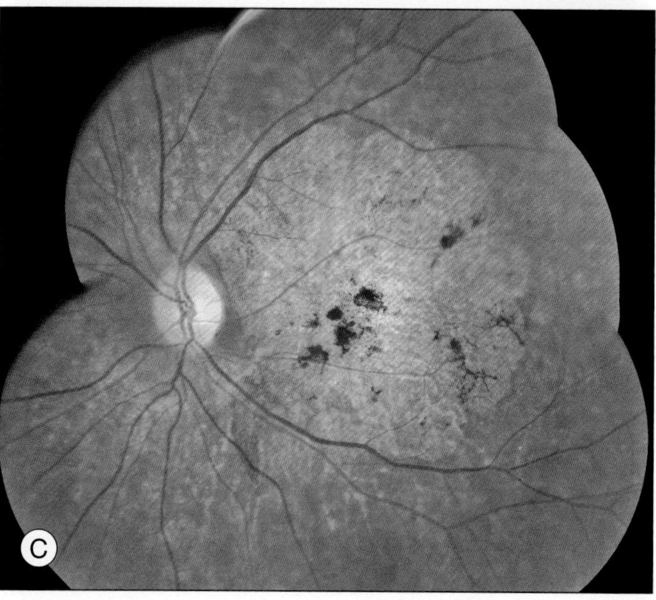

Fig. 42.32 (A) Fundus photograph of the left eye of a 27-year-old female with compound heterozygous mutations in *ABCA4* (Ala1038Val-Ala854Thr/Arg1108Cys) causing Stargardt disease. The visual acuity is 20/200. The small patch of geographic atrophy has a shiny base that glistens in this photograph. A few small flecks can also be seen ringing the atrophy. (B) At age 30, there has been a modest enlargement of the central atrophy and an increase in the number of peripheral flecks but the acuity remains 20/200. (C) At age 42, the area of central atrophy has continued to enlarge but the acuity has fallen to only 20/250. Some clumps of dark pigment have developed within the atrophic lesion. The peripapillary retina is noticeably spared.

low-grade inflammation that is commonly present in degenerative retinal disease.

Visual function

It is important to recognize that the effect of *ABCA4* mutations on visual acuity (VA) is frequently at odds with their effect on the visual field. As a result, many patients will have quite full visual fields for many years after their acuity has fallen below the threshold of legal blindness (Fig. 42.41), while a few patients will retain acuity of better than 20/40 despite extensive field loss (Fig. 42.42). Fishman studied 95 patients with Stargardt disease and found that the probability of maintaining a VA of 20/40 in at least one eye was 52% by age 19, 32% by age 29, and 22% by age 39.[103] In a larger cohort of Stargardt disease patients, cross-sectional analysis showed that almost a quarter had VA of 20/40 or better, whereas 4% had VA worse than 20/400.[104] In general, patients with extensive extramacular flecks have a poorer long-term visual prognosis than patients with flecks and/or atrophy that are limited to the macula.[105,106] Similarly, patients with significant loss of the I2e isopter on Goldmann perimetry have more severe genotypes than those with a more normal I2e response.[97]

Fluorescein angiography and autofluorescence

The accumulation of A2E within the retinal pigment epithelium results in a detectable abnormality on both fluorescein angiography and autofluorescence imaging. With angiography, the A2E blocks the exciting blue light from reaching the dye in the choroidal circulation, resulting in a finding that is variously known as a dark, silent, or masked choroid.[107,108] In these angiograms, the retinal vessels stand out in sharp contrast to the dark background (Fig. 42.43). Flecks and any

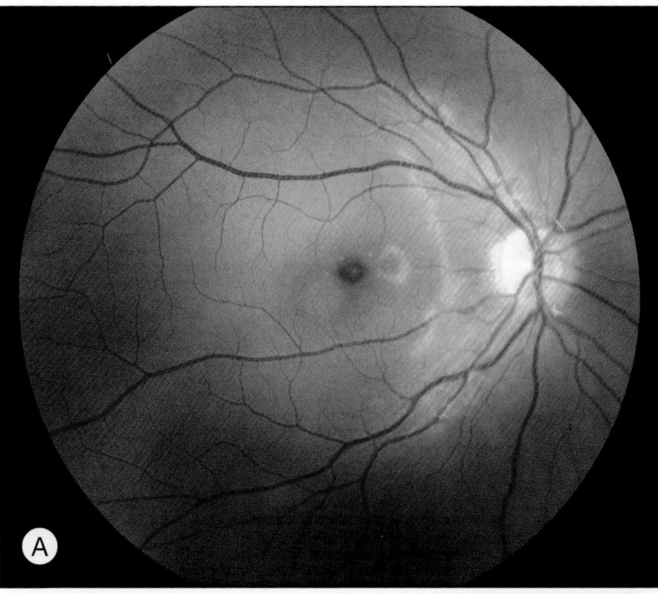

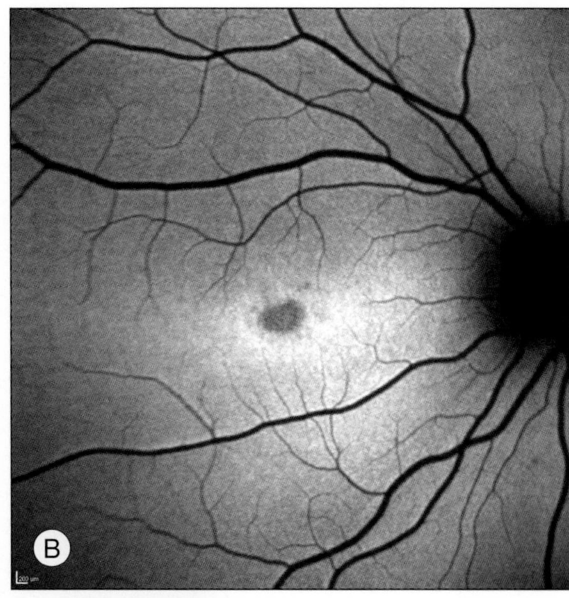

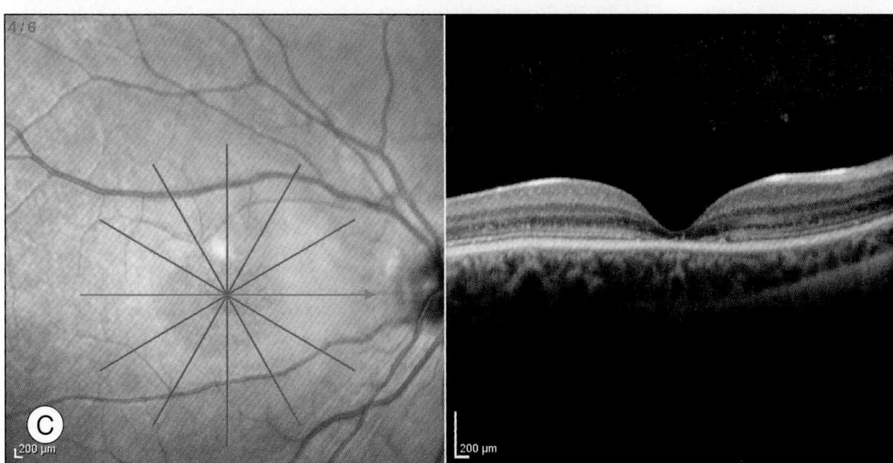

Fig. 42.33 (A) Fundus photograph of the right eye of a 13-year-old female with compound heterozygous mutations in *ABCA4* (IVS38–10 T>C/Gly1961Glu) causing Stargardt disease. The visual acuity in this eye is 20/40. There is a uniform light brown color to the fundus that completely obscures the underlying choroidal detail. This is the ophthalmoscopic equivalent to the "masked choroid" evident by fluorescein angiography. A few small flecks are visible ringing the atrophic fovea. (B) Autofluorescence imaging reveals a loss of autofluorescence in the atrophic fovea and slightly increased autofluorescence elsewhere. (C) SD-OCT reveals selective loss of foveal photoreceptors.

areas of atrophy are hyperfluorescent, although an annulus of a few hundred microns around the optic disc usually remains hypofluorescent even in the presence of very extensive disease.[100] Although quite helpful in the past, we do not routinely employ fluorescein angiography in the workup of patients suspected of *ABCA4* disease for several reasons. First, there is some evidence that exposure to visible light is a cofactor in the disease (knockout mice reared in darkness do not accumulate A2E[109] and there is certainly a lot of light exposure associated with a fluorescein angiogram). Second, molecular testing is becoming more sensitive and more widely available (https://www.carverlab.org/; cited February 2012) and has the added utility of providing some prognostic information when well-characterized mutations are present.[97] Third, many patients with molecularly proven *ABCA4* disease have a readily visible choroidal circulation on angiography (Fig. 42.44). Thus, as with current molecular tests, the absence of a positive result is not helpful. Fourth, there is a small risk of serious complications from the intravenous dye, and finally, the dynamic range of digital cameras is noticeably less than film, tending to accentuate the contrast between the retinal circulation and the normal choroidal circulation, resulting in a false-positive interpretation of the test in some cases. In patients with Stargardt disease, autofluorescence (AF) imaging can also show areas of RPE atrophy, bull's-eye changes in the macula (see Fig. 42.33B), flecks and peripapillary sparing.[42,101,102,110–123] However, AF uses high-intensity illumination at the low end of the visible light spectrum and thus we do not routinely employ this testing modality in patients with suspected *ABCA4* disease.

Optical coherence tomography

OCT can reveal the extent of outer retinal loss and RPE atrophy (see Fig. 42.33C), and it can also distinguish the anatomic level of flecks with accuracy.[112,116,124–126] The test is very sensitive to early changes; one study revealed three patients with photoreceptor abnormalities on OCT without an equivalent abnormality on AF.[116] Peripapillary nerve fiber layer thickness can also be altered on OCT but the significance of this is not yet known.[127]

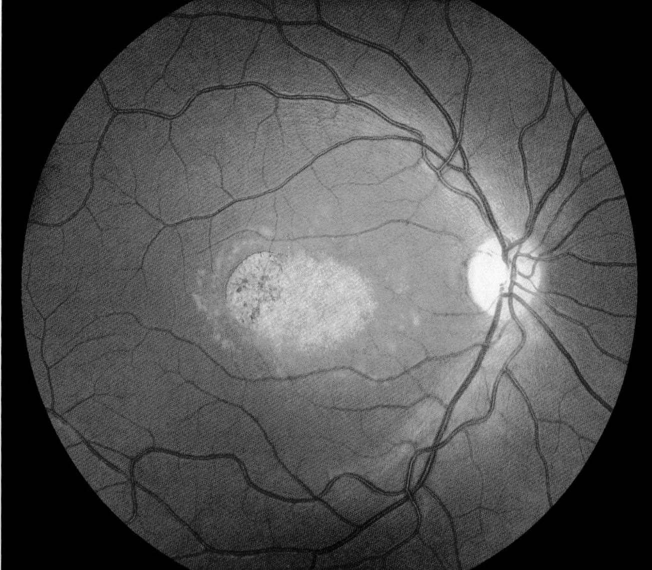

Fig. 42.34 Fundus photograph of the right eye of a 36-year-old female with compound heterozygous mutations in *ABCA4* (Phe608Ile/Gly1961Glu) causing Stargardt disease. The visual acuity in this eye is 20/100. There is a vermillion appearance to the entire fundus obscuring the underlying choroidal detail. The central macular lesion has two distinct components. The temporal third is atrophic with a sharply defined edge and some dark pigment dusting over the atrophy. The nasal two-thirds is more crystalline in appearance. Coarse pisciform flecks ring the central lesion.

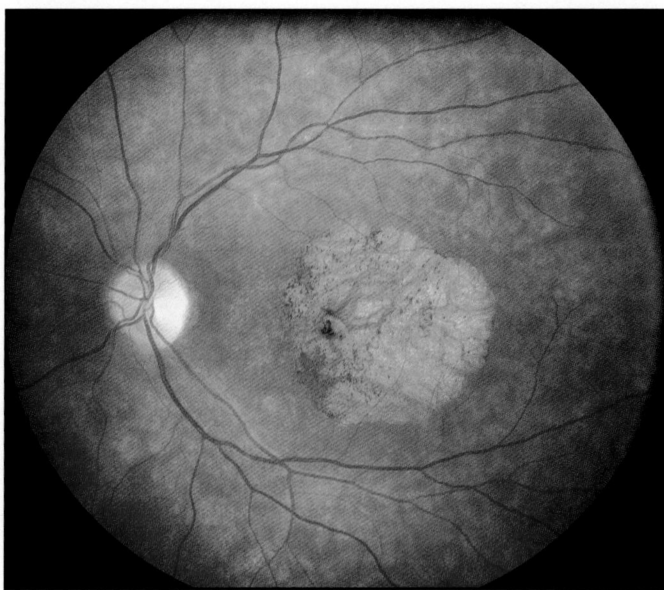

Fig. 42.35 Fundus photograph of the left eye of a 38-year-old female with compound heterozygous mutations in *ABCA4* (Gly863Ala/Leu2109Pro) causing Stargardt disease. The visual acuity in this eye is 5/300. There is a dusting of dark pigment over a sharply demarcated circular area of RPE atrophy centered over the fovea. In addition, there is a reticular network of RPE atrophy throughout the posterior pole. Peripapillary sparing is subtle but present.

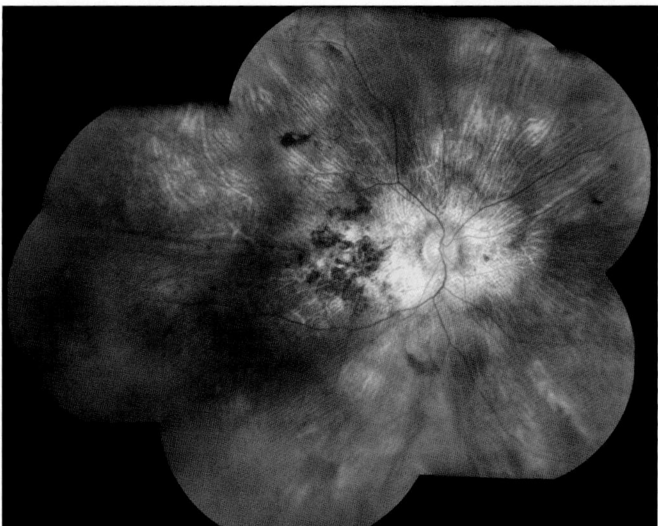

Fig. 42.36 Fundus photograph of the right eye of a 47-year-old male with compound heterozygous mutations in *ABCA4* (Leu2109Pro/IVS38–10 T>C) causing retinitis pigmentosa. The visual acuity is counting fingers at 3 feet. There are nummular areas of RPE and choroidal atrophy admixed with intraretinal pigmentation, some of which is perivascular. The two clinical features that would suggest mutations in *ABCA4* as the cause of this patient's disease are the extensive macular involvement and the noticeable peripapillary sparing.

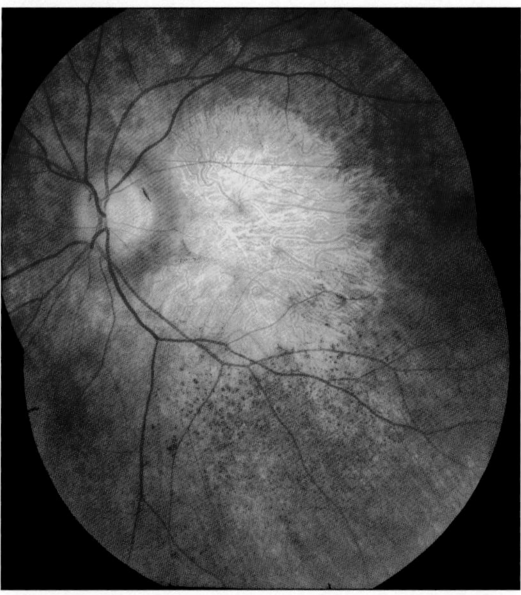

Fig. 42.37 Fundus photograph of the right eye of a 52-year-old male with compound heterozygous mutations in *ABCA4* (Ala1038Val-Leu541Pro/IVS40+5 G>(A) causing cone–rod dystrophy. The visual acuity is 20/50. There is a large area of RPE and choroidal atrophy in the macula and some fine intraretinal pigmentation inferiorly. The two clinical features that would suggest mutations in *ABCA4* as the cause of this patient's disease are extensive macular involvement and the noticeable peripapillary sparing.

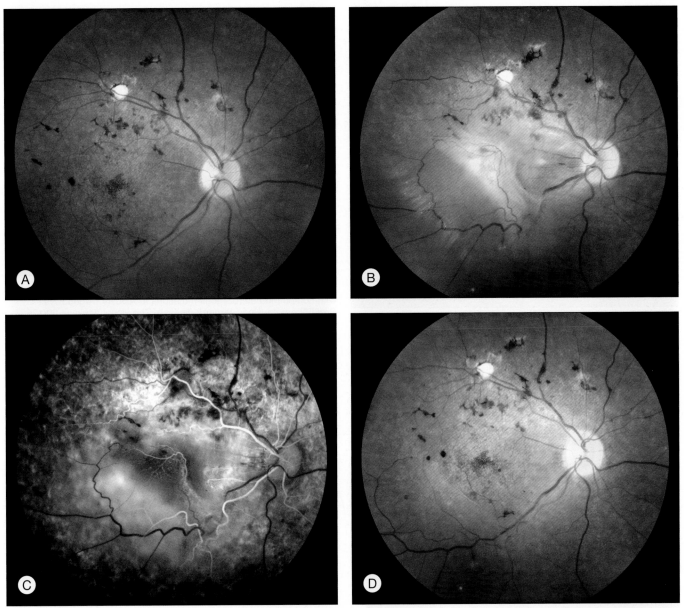

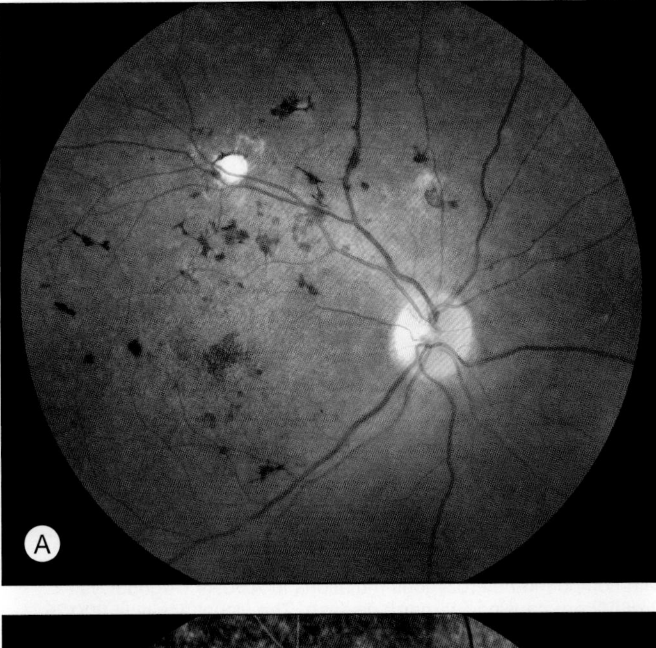

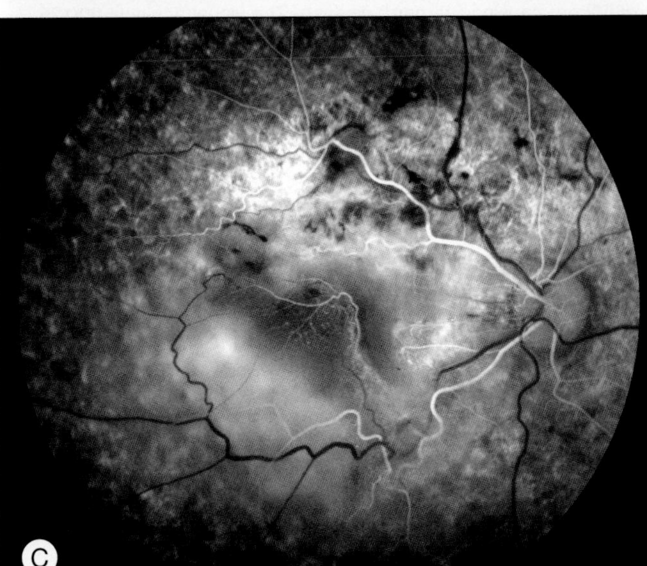

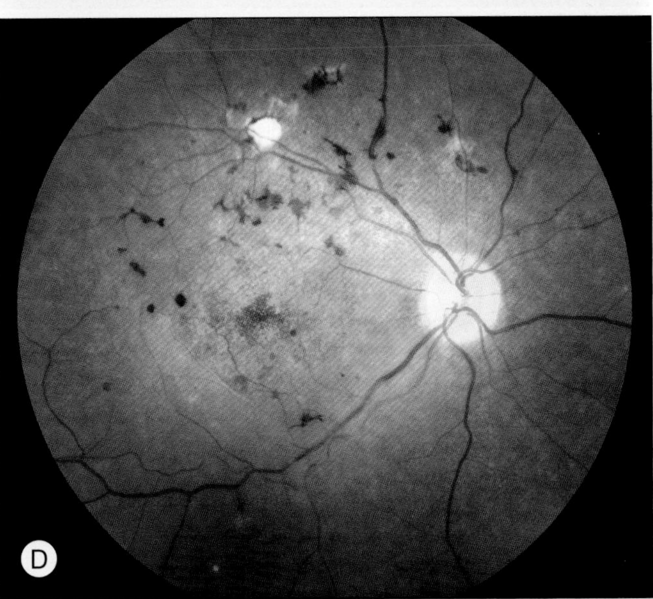

Fig. 42.38 (A) Fundus photograph of the right eye of a 26-year-old female with compound heterozygous mutations in *ABCA4* (Glu1087Lys/IVS38-10 T>C) causing cone-rod dystrophy. The visual acuity on this visit is 20/400. Narrowed arterioles and bone-spicule like pigmentation are signs of moderate photoreceptor cell loss. The normal xanthophyll pigment gives a golden appearance to the thinned macular RPE. There is an inflammatory nodule along the superotemporal arcade. Five months later, the patient returns, reporting a sudden decrease in vision in the right eye. The acuity is counting fingers and ophthalmoscopy reveals an aggressive epiretinal membrane (B) Fluorescein angiography (C) reveals the retina to be folded on itself with no evidence of a significant choroidal neovascular component despite the small hemorrhages at the superior margin of the lesion. (Photographs B, C, and D courtesy of Dr H. Culver Boldt, The University of Iowa.) (D) Following vitrectomy and membrane peeling, only a small remnant of the epiretinal membrane persists temporally. The visual acuity has returned to 20/400.

Electrophysiology

Somewhat by definition, the full-field ERG is typically normal in patients with Stargardt disease while cone and cone–rod dysfunction are seen in more severe forms of *ABCA4* disease.[111,128–133] With mild *ABCA4* genotypes, bisretinoids do not seem to accumulate rapidly enough to injure the photoreceptors directly, except for cones in and near the fovea, which seem to be the most sensitive to *ABCA4* dysfunction in most patients. Loss of the latter cells can cause quite a bit of acuity loss without any detectable effect on the full-field ERG. With moderate *ABCA4* genotypes cones throughout the fundus are directly affected, leading to cone-selective abnormalities in the ERG. With the most severe *ABCA4* genotypes even rods experience direct injury from A2E accumulation, resulting in effects on all components of the ERG and a fundus appearance that can reasonably be called retinitis pigmentosa (Fig. 42.39).[97,134] It is important to realize that patients with the more severe *ABCA4* genotypes can progress from a clinical pattern consistent with the label "Stargardt disease" to one consistent with "retinitis pigmentosa" over the course of their disease and it can be very distressing to patients to have their diagnosis change from one doctor to the next. A few minutes spent explaining that these descriptive labels are used to describe different aspects (e.g., ophthalmoscopic and

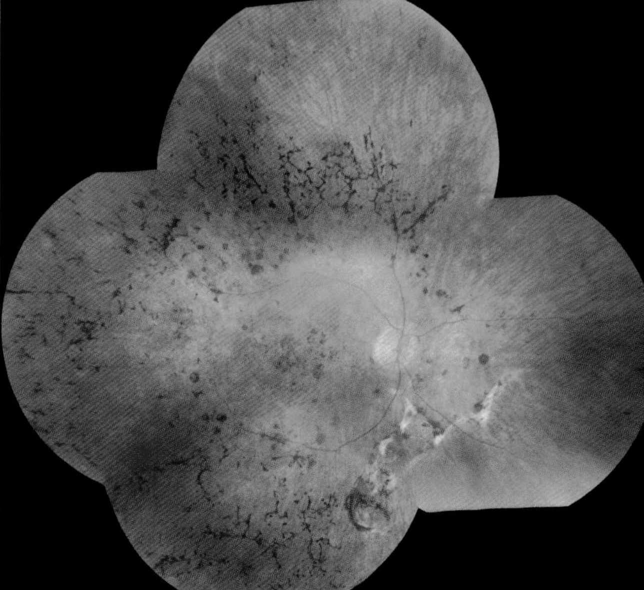

Fig. 42.39 Fundus photograph of the right eye of a 39-year-old female with compound heterozygous mutations in *ABCA4* (Ala1038Val-Leu541Pro/Arg2149Stop) causing retinitis pigmentosa. The visual acuity is 5/300. The two clinical features that would suggest mutations in *ABCA4* as the cause of this patient's disease are the early macular involvement and the extensive subretinal fibrosis inferior to the disc.

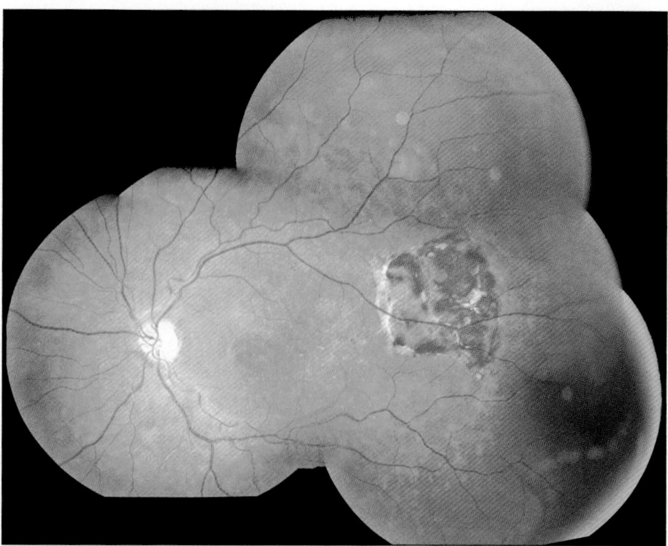

Fig. 42.40 Fundus photograph of the left eye of a 13-year-old female with compound heterozygous mutations in *ABCA4* (Arg653Cys / Pro656Leu) causing Stargardt disease. The visual acuity is 20/125. There is a large plaque of pigmented subretinal fibrosis temporally, possibly related to mild blunt trauma to the eye 5 years earlier. There is some atrophy in the center of the macula and typical flecks are visible along the arcades.

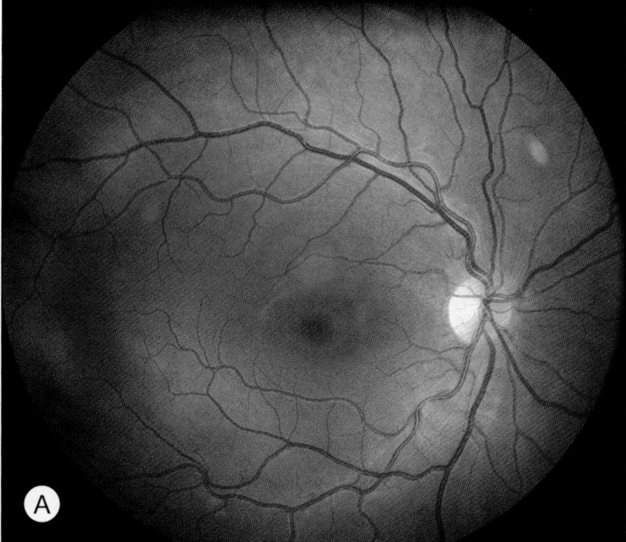

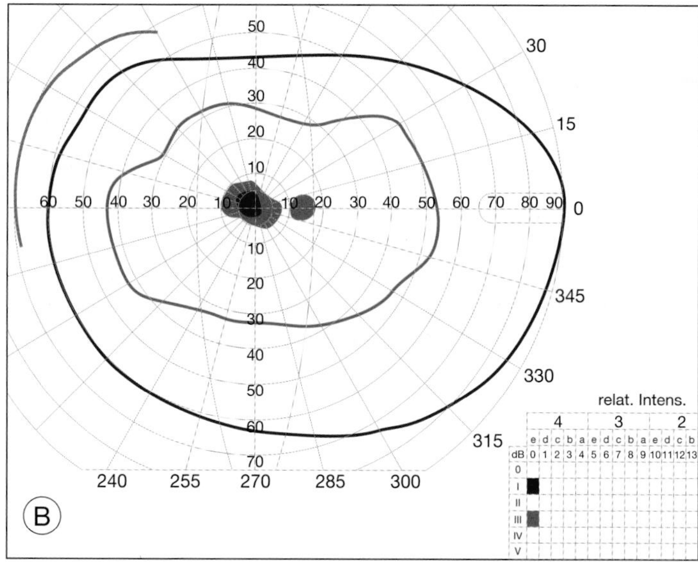

Fig. 42.41 (A) Fundus photograph of the right eye of a 16-year-old female with compound heterozygous mutations in *ABCA4* (Gly1961Glu/Pro1511Arg) causing Stargardt disease. The visual acuity in this eye is 20/70. The fundus is normal except for a very subtle oval area of RPE granularity beneath the fovea a few hundred microns in diameter. (B) Goldmann perimetry is normal except for a small scotoma to the I4e stimulus centered on fixation.

electrophysiologic) and stages (early and late) of a single disease, and that these descriptions can change over time in an individual patient, can reduce this distress significantly. One of the most valuable uses of the full-field ERG in patients suspected to have *ABCA4*-related retinal disease is in differentiating the earliest onset forms of this condition from juvenile NCL (see Fig. 42.2). In patients with NCL, the ERG is usually severely reduced or extinguished before the age of 10 years. If it is recordable at all, the rod ERG is more severely affected than the cone ERG, and the maximum stimulus intensity scotopic response typically shows an electronegative configuration (greater loss of b-wave than a-wave).[135] In contrast, profound reduction in the full-field scotopic ERG response to the standard maximum stimulus intensity is rare in the first decade of life in patients with *ABCA4* disease, and any reductions that do occur are noticeably cone-selective. Finally, electronegative waveforms have not been

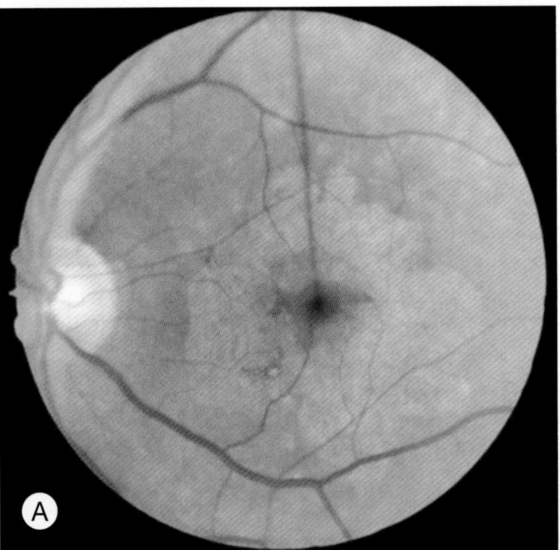

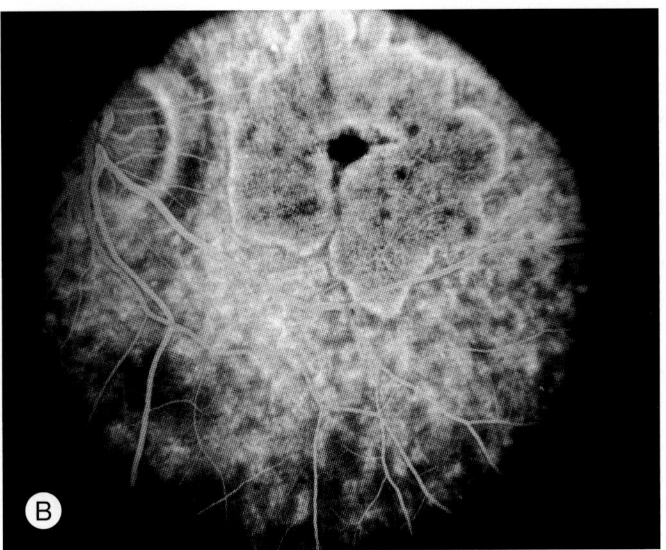

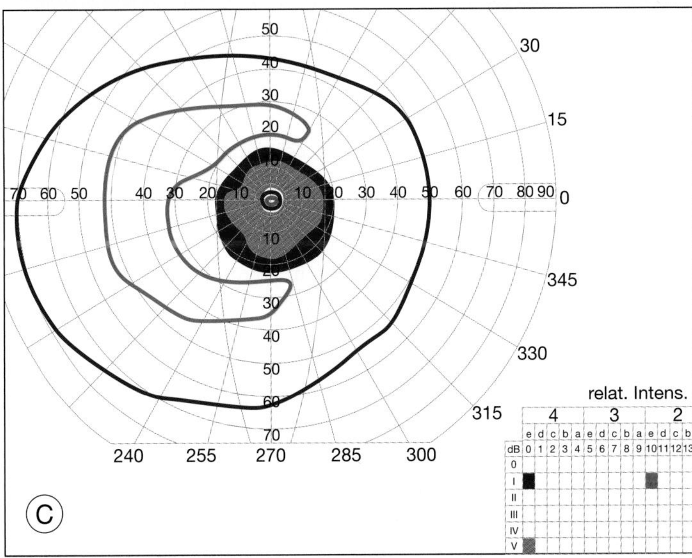

Fig. 42.42 (A) Fundus photograph of the left eye of a 32-year-old male with compound heterozygous mutations in *ABCA4* (Cys1488Arg/Leu2027Phe) causing cone–rod dystrophy. The visual acuity is 20/20. There is an irregular area of complete sparing centered on the fovea, which is surrounded by a large annulus of RPE atrophy. The nasal edge of the atrophic lesion is concave, paralleling the edge of the optic disc. (B) Fluorescein angiography of this eye reveals the completely spared fovea surrounded by RPE atrophy. Relative sparing of the peripapillary retina is also evident. Flecks appear as hyperfluorescent window defects in the otherwise hypofluorescent RPE. (C) Goldmann perimetry of this eye reveals an absolute scotoma corresponding to the perifoveal atrophy. There is a window within this scotoma corresponding to the preserved fovea.

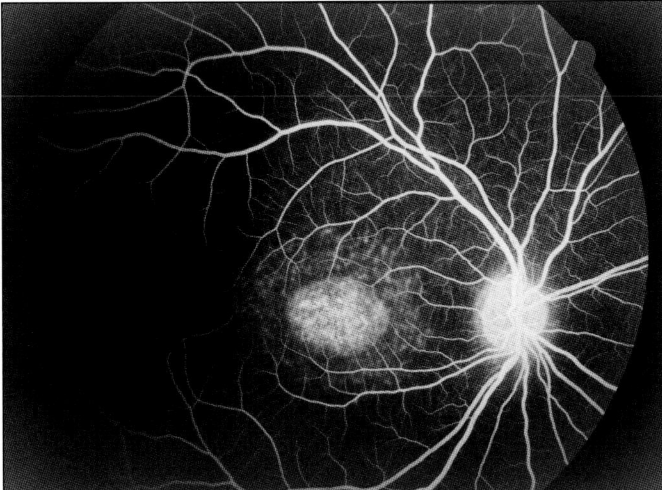

Fig. 42.43 Fluorescein angiogram of the right eye of a 9-year-old female with compound heterozygous mutations in *ABCA4* (Cys54Tyr/Gly550Arg) causing Stargardt disease. The visual acuity in this eye is 20/200. The fluorescence of the choroidal circulation is completely masked by the bisretinoid-containing RPE except in the center of the macula where flecks and atrophy have created window defects. As a result, the fluorescent retinal vasculature stands out in sharp contrast against the unusually hypofluorescent background.

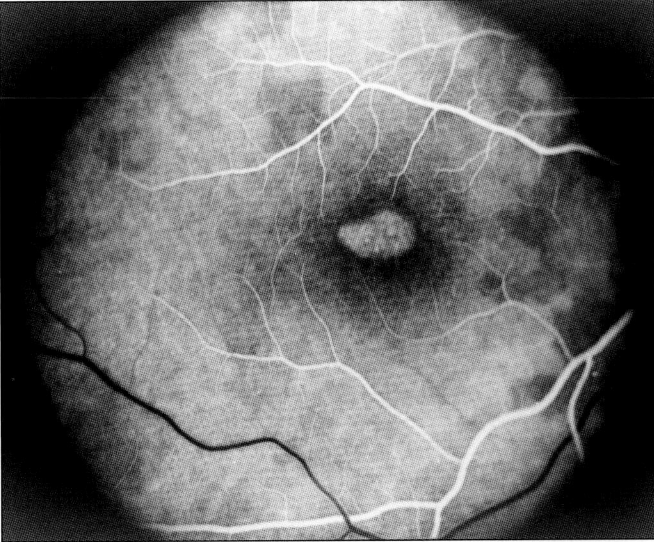

Fig. 42.44 Fluorescein angiogram of the right eye of a 14-year-old male with compound heterozygous mutations in *ABCA4* (Gly1961Glu/Pro1380Leu) causing Stargardt disease. The visual acuity in this eye is 20/250. In this very early frame of the angiogram the choroid is not yet completely filled, making it readily apparent that the choroidal circulation is incompletely masked in this individual.

reported in ABCA4-associated retinal disease. The pattern ERG can be abnormal in patients with Stargardt disease even when the fundus looks relatively normal.[111,126] This led to the proposal of three groups of SD based on electrophysiology: in group 1 there is a severe pattern ERG abnormality with normal scotopic and full-field ERGs; in group 2 there is additional loss of photopic function; and in group 3 there is loss of both photopic and scotopic function.[111] The multifocal ERG is less useful in Stargardt patients than the full-field ERG. Its test–retest reliability and interocular symmetry in SD is significantly lower than in controls.[136]

Genetics

Since the discovery in 1997 that a recessively inherited *ABCA4* mutation causes Stargardt disease,[91] there have been more than 250 different disease-causing alleles identified in *ABCA4* and many non-disease-causing polymorphisms as well. Individuals who counsel patients about their *ABCA4* genotype need to have a thorough understanding of the differences between these two classes of genetic variation. Some laboratories provide a pathogenicity score for the mutations they identify that can be helpful in this regard.[137,138] Another challenge in counseling patients with *ABCA4*-associated retinal disease is that a significant number of disease-causing mutations lie outside the coding and promoter sequences of the gene, making them difficult to identify. Thus, many patients will have only one of their two disease alleles identified by current testing methods. Mutations in *ABCA4* are thought to be responsible for more than 95% of cases of clinical Stargardt disease, 30–50% of cases of cone–rod dystrophy[96] and 8% of autosomal recessive retinitis pigmentosa.[97] Most of the remaining 5% of cases with a Stargardt disease phenotype are caused by mutations in *ELOVL4*, *PRPH2*, or *BEST1*.

The wide range of phenotypes seen in *ABCA4*-associated disease can be attributed to: (1) the variable severity of the many disease alleles in the population; (2) the interaction of these alleles with genetic and environmental modifiers (e.g. light exposure, smoking, and diet); and (3) the complex interaction between rods, cones, and RPE cells. Systematic investigation of the clinical findings of large cohorts of patients with known *ABCA4* genotypes has the potential to deduce the specific pathogenic contribution of individual alleles. For example, multiple regression analysis based on an additive model of *ABCA4* function recently enabled the quantification of specific disease-causing power of some of the more common disease-causing *ABCA4* alleles.[97] As additional studies of this kind are performed and combined, it will allow clinicians to better inform patients of their prognosis, help balance enrollment in clinical trials of novel treatments, and facilitate the identification of disease-modifying factors that may form the basis of such treatments.

Pathophysiology and histopathology

Histological studies of eyes with Stargardt disease reveal remarkable lipofuscin accumulation in the RPE. For example, an eye from a 9-year-old child with Stargardt, enucleated for retinoblastoma at 16 months of age, showed striking RPE autofluorescence when compared to normal aging.[139] Another unusual finding observed in autopsy tissue from a 62-year-old donor is the presence of significant lipofuscin accumulation within photoreceptor cell inner segments, suggesting significantly altered processing of retinoids in the outer retina.[140] Attenuation of photoreceptor inner and outer segments over areas of still-organized RPE cells was also noted, consistent with a primary photoreceptor cell defect. In addition, end-stage central atrophy of the outer retina, gliosis, and RPE hypertrophy or loss have been seen.[140,141]

The pathophysiology of *ABCA4*-associated disease has been recently reviewed[134,142,143] and was elucidated in large part through elegant biochemical studies of the *Abca4*$^{-/-}$ mouse.[144] The normal role of ABCA4 is the clearance of a retinoid intermediate of the visual cycle (N-retinylidene phosphatidylethanolamine) from the intradiscal lumen of the outer segments of rods and cones. Condensation of this retinoid with a second vitamin A moiety, which may occur in the photoreceptor cell or in the RPE following outer segment phagocytosis, results in the formation of A2E, a toxic detergent-like compound that can trigger death of RPE cells[145,146], complement activation,[147] and both direct and indirect loss of photoreceptors (see Fig. 42.25).

Treatment

There is currently no proven treatment for *ABCA4* disease. However, there is extensive ongoing research in genetics, disease mechanisms, gene therapy, and cell replacement, and these studies have already identified a number of promising therapeutic strategies that have been tested in animal models and are just entering human trials.

Since a primary defect in *ABCA4*-associated retinal disease is an accumulation of toxic bisretinoids in the RPE and photoreceptors, drugs that modulate the visual cycle (e.g. isoretinoin and fenretinide), have been investigated for their potential to slow the formation of these toxic products in *Abca4* knockout mice.[148–150] Similarly, gene replacement therapy has been proposed for *ABCA4* disease and efficacy has been demonstrated in the mouse model.[151–153] Proof of concept, safety, and efficacy for ocular gene therapy in humans has already been shown for *RPE65*-associated Leber congenital amaurosis[154,155] and thus gene therapy for *ABCA4*-associated disease seems promising for patients who still have substantial visual function. Patients who have already experienced extensive loss of RPE and photoreceptors will likely need some type of cell replacement therapy, and one human clinical trial of RPE cell replacement is already underway (http://clinicaltrials.gov/ct2/show/NCT01345006?term=advanced+cell+technology&rank=2; cited February 2012).

Pending the successful demonstration of safety and efficacy of one or more of these interventions, we recommend that our patients wear dark glasses and a hat whenever they are exposed to prolonged bright light (to reduce the rate of formation of all-*trans* retinol in the photoreceptors). We also recommend avoidance of cigarette smoking as our Stargardt patients have anecdotally reported dimming of their vision while smoking. Finally, we recommend avoidance of high-dose vitamin A supplements, including AREDS vitamins, because of their potential to increase the formation of bisretinoids in the retina.

STARGARDT-LIKE DOMINANT MACULAR DYSTROPHY (SLDMD)

In 1994 Stone and coworkers described a large family with a Stargardt-like phenotype and mapped the gene to chromosome 6.[156] In contrast to typical Stargardt disease, this family displayed a clear autosomal dominant pattern of inheritance with high penetrance. Zhang et al. later identified a 5 base pair deletion in the gene *ELOVL4* in the affected members of five families affected with this disease.[157] Although additional disease-causing

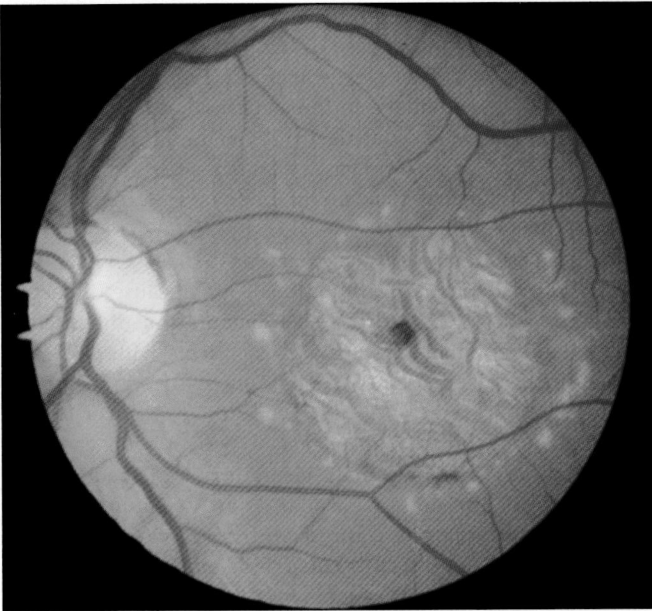

Fig. 42.45 Fundus photograph of the left eye of a 61-year-old male with the common Leu263 del5tttCTTAA mutation in *ELOVL4* causing Stargardt-like dominant macular dystrophy. The visual acuity in this eye is 20/100. All of the most-characteristic features of this disease are present in this patient, including a circular zone of RPE atrophy, a pigmented spot beneath the fovea, and a ring of flecks just beyond the margin of the atrophy.

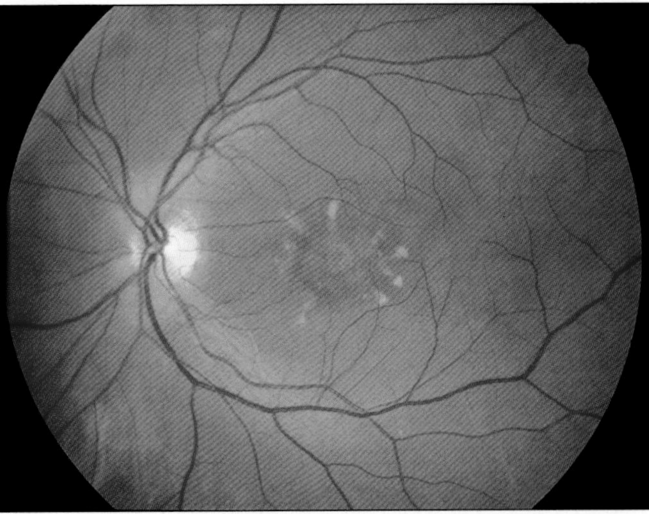

Fig. 42.46 Fundus photograph of the left eye of a 53-year-old male with the common Leu263 del5tttCTTAA mutation in *ELOVL4* causing Stargardt-like dominant macular dystrophy. The visual acuity in this eye is 20/100. There are several branching arms of yellow material at the level of the RPE that extend from a circular area of geographic atrophy centered on fixation. This fundus appearance could easily be confused with *PRPH2*-assocated pattern dystrophy.

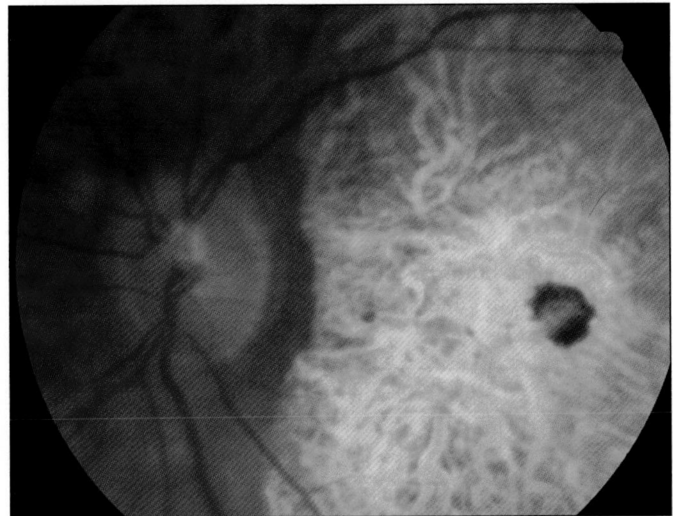

Fig. 42.47 Fundus photograph of the left eye of a 77-year-old female with the common Leu263 del5tttCTTAA mutation in *ELOVL4* causing Stargardt-like dominant macular dystrophy. The visual acuity in this eye is 20/400. At the nasal margin of the large macular lesion there is clear peripapillary sparing.

mutations in *ELOVL4* have been identified,[158,159] the 5 bp deletion is responsible for more than 90% of cases in North America. This condition is characterized by progressive central vision loss; some patients develop symptoms in the first decade of life and the majority have a visual acuity of 20/200 or worse by 30 years of age.[156] The range of fundus findings is almost identical to that of autosomal recessive Stargardt disease and includes pisciform flecks (Figs 42.45, 42.46), peripapillary sparing (Fig. 42.47) and macular atrophy. The bases of the atrophic macular lesions are less likely to have a distinct reflective sheen than those of autosomal recessive Stargardt disease and some patients display a round or cuneiform clump of dark pigment very near fixation (Fig. 42.47). As in *ABCA4*-associated Stargardt disease, a few patients have a severe loss of foveal cones with an otherwise normal fundus (Fig. 42.48). The lipofuscin deposits in SLDMD tend to be a bit larger than those of recessive Stargardt disease and often take on a "butterfly" appearance at some point in the evolution of the macular lesions (Fig. 42.46). For a given degree of fundus abnormality, however, the acuity is usually much more affected in patients with SLDMD than it is in patients with *PRPH2*-associated pattern dystrophy. The ERG is usually normal. These patients are less likely than patients with autosomal recessive Stargardt disease to have a dark choroid on fluorescein angiography but the flecks are similarly hyperfluorescent in both conditions.

Pathophysiology

The *ELOVL4* gene encodes the protein "elongation of very long chain fatty acids-4," a biosynthetic enzyme in the endoplasmic reticulum responsible for the synthesis of fatty acids with more than 26 carbons.[160,161] This gene is expressed in brain and retina, where expression is restricted to photoreceptor cells.[157] Mutations associated with Stargardt-like macular degeneration cause mistrafficking of the mutant protein in vitro,[162] which results in cell death.[163] Mice harboring a single mutant allele of *Elovl4* display mistrafficking of the ELOVL4 protein, show increased lipofuscin formation, and develop peripheral photoreceptor loss.[164,165]

PATTERN DYSTROPHY

Pattern dystrophy (PD) refers to a group of inherited retinal dystrophies characterized by pigment changes at the level of the RPE.[166–168] PD encompasses a broad spectrum of clinical appearances that were originally given names based on the pattern of pigment distribution; such as, butterfly-shaped pigment dystrophy (Fig. 42.49),[166] adult-onset vitelliform pattern dystrophy[169,170] (Fig. 42.50) peculiar foveomacular dystrophy[171] (Fig. 42.51A, B), Sjögren reticular dystrophy of the RPE,[172–174] (Figs 42.51C, 42.52), and fundus pulverulentus.[175,176] The most common causes of all of these different patterns have proven to be mutations in a single gene, *PRPH2* (originally *RDS* – OMIM #179605). Mutations in this gene also cause some cases of central areolar choroidal dystrophy (Fig. 42.53),[177] retinitis pigmentosa,[178–181] and some cases that are nearly identical to the fundus flavimaculatus variant of Stargardt disease (Fig. 42.54). Patients with extensive RPE atrophy will sometimes exhibit peripapillary sparing very similar to that seen in *ABCA4* disease (Fig. 42.55). *PRPH2* mutations usually cause disease in the heterozygous state and the disorders are thus inherited in an autosomal dominant fashion. Most patients with a *PRPH2*-associated PD will experience macular photostress in their daily life; that is, their central acuity will be slow to recover following exposure to bright light. Thus, a patient who can read 20/30 in a dim clinic lane may be incapable of reading their mail for tens of minutes after walking down a sunlit driveway to retrieve it. Similarly, a waitress with excellent acuity under optimal circumstances may be unable to make change for her customers after walking through a bright kitchen and returning to a dark restaurant. All of the *PRPH2*-associated pattern dystrophies also share an 18% lifetime risk of choroidal neovascularization.[182]

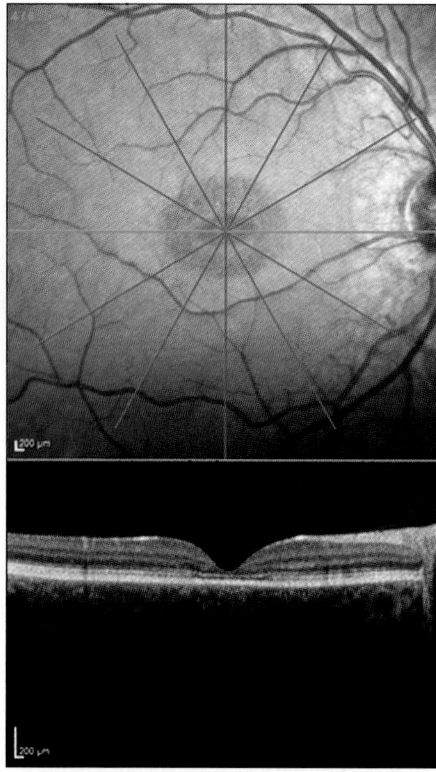

Fig. 42.48 Infrared fundus photograph and spectral domain optical coherence tomogram of the right eye of a 14-year-old male with the common Leu263 del5tttCTTAA mutation in *ELOVL4* causing Stargardt-like dominant macular dystrophy. The visual acuity in this eye is 20/125. Ophthalmoscopically, the fundus is near normal, but SD-OCT reveals loss of foveal photoreceptors. This selective loss of foveal cones is also seen in a subset of patients with *ABCA4*-associated recessive Stargardt disease (see for example Fig. 42.33).

Like most autosomal dominant disorders, the genetic background plays an important role in the specific clinical manifestations that result from *PRPH2* mutations and the same point mutation can cause vitelliform lesions in one patient, peculiar foveomacular dystrophy in another, and butterfly-shaped pigment dystrophy in others.[179,183] Gutman described a patient with a vitelliform lesion in one eye and a butterfly-shaped lesion in the other.[184]

Clinical features and history of specific pattern dystrophies

Butterfly-shaped pigment dystrophy

Deutman described a family with autosomal dominant inheritance that had butterfly-shaped pigmentation located in the RPE.[166] The pigmentation can be yellow, white, or black and

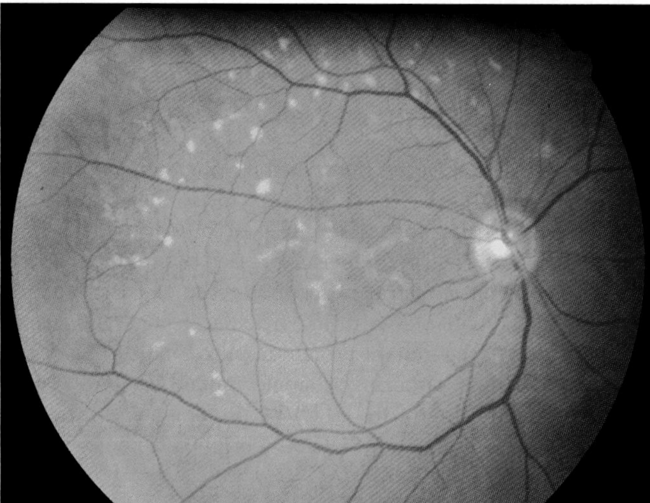

Fig. 42.49 Fundus photograph of the right eye of a 42-year-old female with a Gly167Asp mutation in *PRPH2* causing a butterfly pattern dystrophy. The visual acuity in this eye is 20/20. Although the flecks in the periphery are somewhat reminiscent of Stargardt disease, their globular nature is more consistent with *PRPH2*-associated disease.

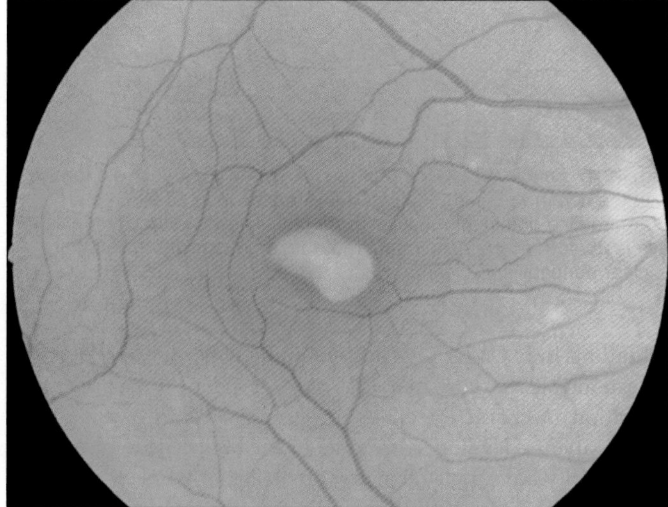

Fig. 42.50 Fundus photograph of the right eye of a 47-year-old male with a Gly167Asp mutation in *PRPH2* causing an adult vitelliform pattern dystrophy. The visual acuity in this eye is 20/70. Although this lesion is very similar to those caused by *BEST1* mutations, its slightly polygonal shape is more consistent with *PRPH2*-associated disease.

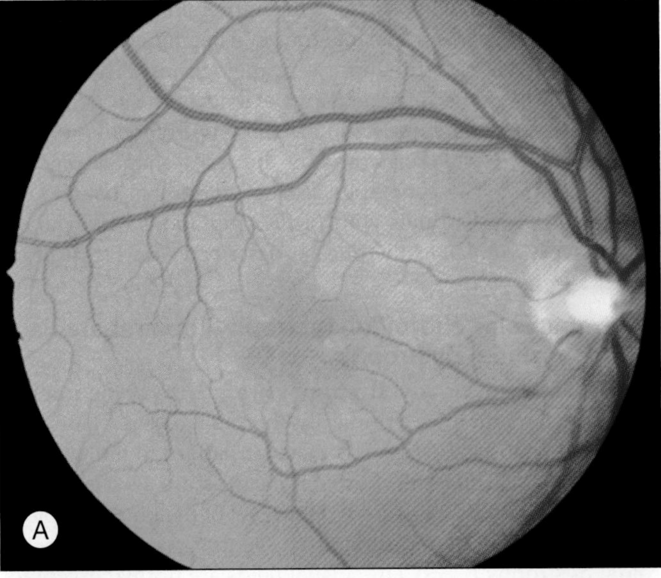

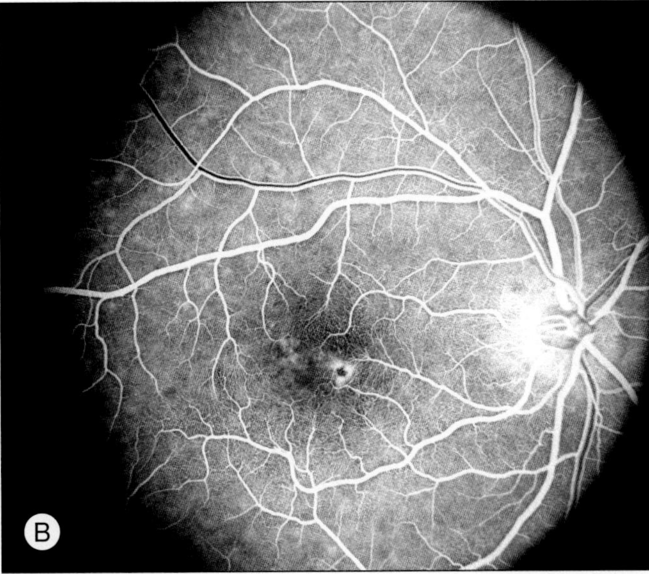

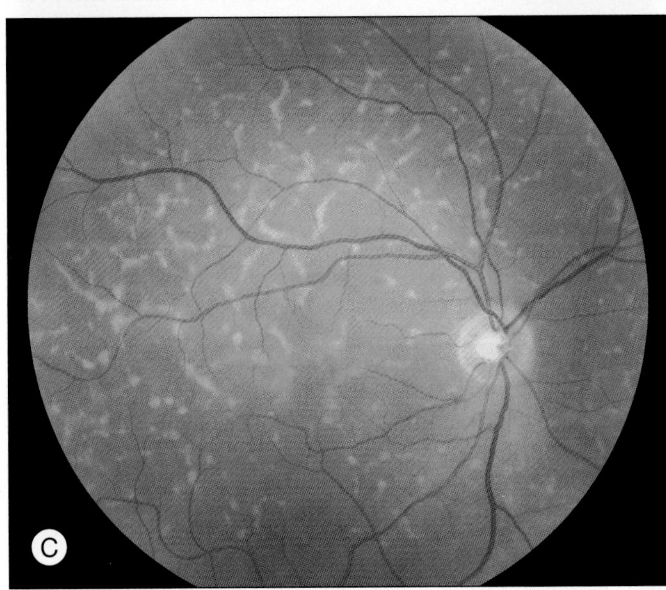

Fig. 42.51 (A) Fundus photograph of the right eye of a 42-year-old female with a Gly167Asp mutation in *PRPH2* causing pattern dystrophy. The visual acuity in this eye is 20/20. With ophthalmoscopy alone there is very little evidence of disease. (B) An early phase fluoroscein angiogram of this eye reveals a small dot and halo lesion and a hint of extramacular disease along the superotemporal arcades. (C) This same eye at age 61 exhibits an extensive reticular network of yellow deposits throughout the posterior pole.

accumulate in an unusual configuration of three to five "arms" or "wings" that resemble the wings of a butterfly (see Fig. 42.49). An area of depigmentation often occurs around the pigment. Additional pigment deposits that look like drusen or flecks can be seen peripheral to the central lesion. These changes can occasionally be seen in the teens but symptoms usually do not occur until patients are in their 20s–30s. Several mutations in *PRPH2* have been shown to be causative of this macular pattern.[183,185–188]

Adult-onset foveomacular vitelliform pattern dystrophy

Patients with adult-onset foveomacular vitelliform dystrophy (described by Gass as a "peculiar foveomacular dystrophy"[171]) present asymptomatically or with mild blurring. Fundus examination reveals symmetric, solitary, autofluorescent vitelliform lesions in the macula (usually centered on or just adjacent to the fovea) that are much smaller in size (less than one-third disc diameter) than the vitelliform lesions of Best disease. These lesions often have a central pigmented spot (see Fig. 42.51B) that is best seen when a narrow beam of a slit lamp is placed just adjacent to the lesion. Partial or complete resorption of the vitelliform material is common and is usually accompanied by outer retinal loss and decreased visual acuity.[189]

Arnold et al. performed histopathologic evaluation of eyes from patients with adult vitelliform lesions. Although genotypes were not determined, the phenotype was consistent with a mutation in *PRPH2* or *BEST1*. These authors noted significant material in the subretinal space beneath the fovea, consisting of outer-segment material and pigment-laden cells. Atrophic changes appeared to be secondary to the accumulation of subretinal material.[190]

Sjögren reticular dystrophy of the RPE

In reticular dystrophy of the RPE, first reported by Sjögren,[172] the fundus is characterized by a clearly defined network of black-pigmented lines at the level of the RPE that resemble a fishnet with knots or chicken wire. Early cases may have only pigment

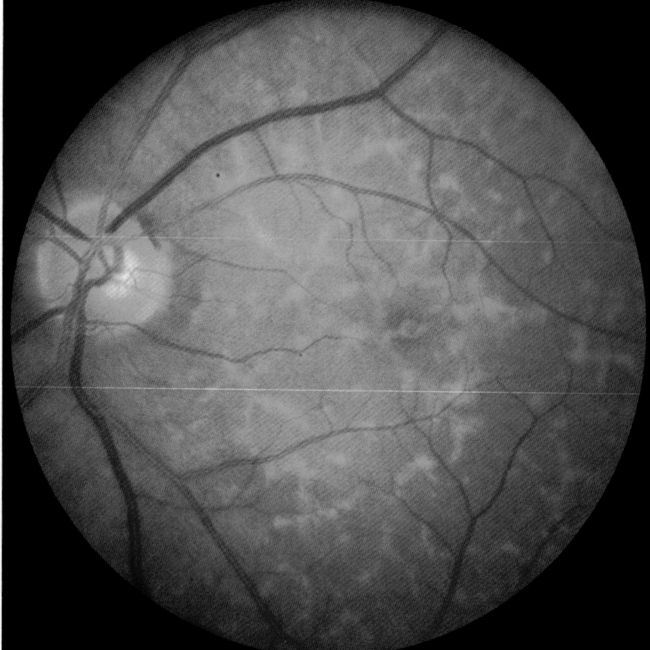

Fig. 42.52 Fundus photograph of the left eye of a 47-year-old male with a Cys82Stop mutation in *PRPH2* causing a reticular pattern dystrophy. The visual acuity in this eye is 20/20. The "knots in the fishnet" described by Sjögren are particularly evident in this patient.

granules in the fovea but still give the impression of a pigmented network in the process of disintegration. The pigment alterations may be more visible with fluorescein angiography. The network usually starts in the fovea and can extend into the periphery. Some patients in the same family as those with reticular dystrophy also have vitelliform and/or butterfly-shaped pigment changes.[174,191–195] The genotypes of Sjögren original patients are unknown but individuals with *PRPH2* mutations can exhibit a pattern very similar to the one he described (see Figs 42.51C, 42.52).

Central areolar choroidal dystrophy (central areolar retinochoroidal dystrophy)

Central areolar choroidal dystrophy was, as its name implies, originally thought to be a primarily choroidal disease. However, numerous reports also link this macular pattern to mutations in *PRPH2*.[177,196–204] Thus, the choroidal changes are secondary to a genetic abnormality expressed at the level of the photoreceptors, and a more accurate term might be "central areolar retinochoroidal dystrophy (CARCD)." Visual fields are normal except for central scotomas corresponding to the macular lesions. The earliest change is a fine, mottled depigmentation in the macula of both eyes that appears between the second and fourth decades and gradually evolves into symmetric, sharply outlined, bull's-eye oval or round areas of geographic atrophy of the RPE (see Fig. 42.53). Within the area of RPE atrophy, the reddish-orange

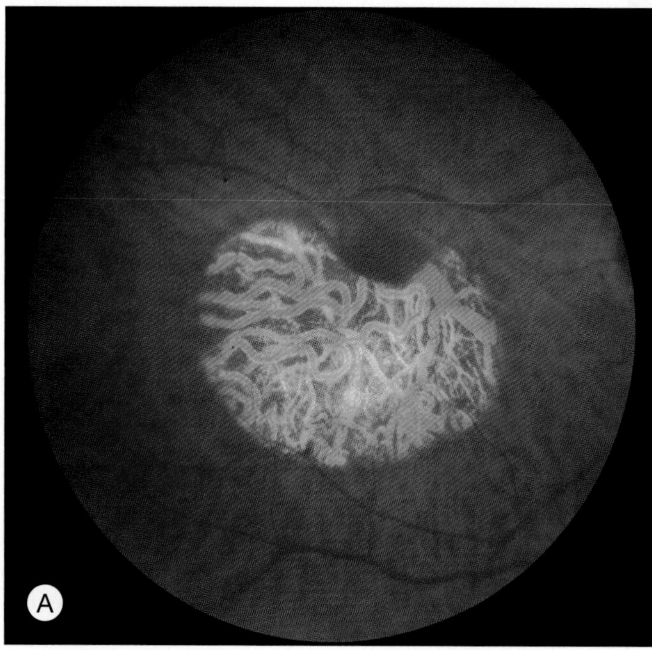

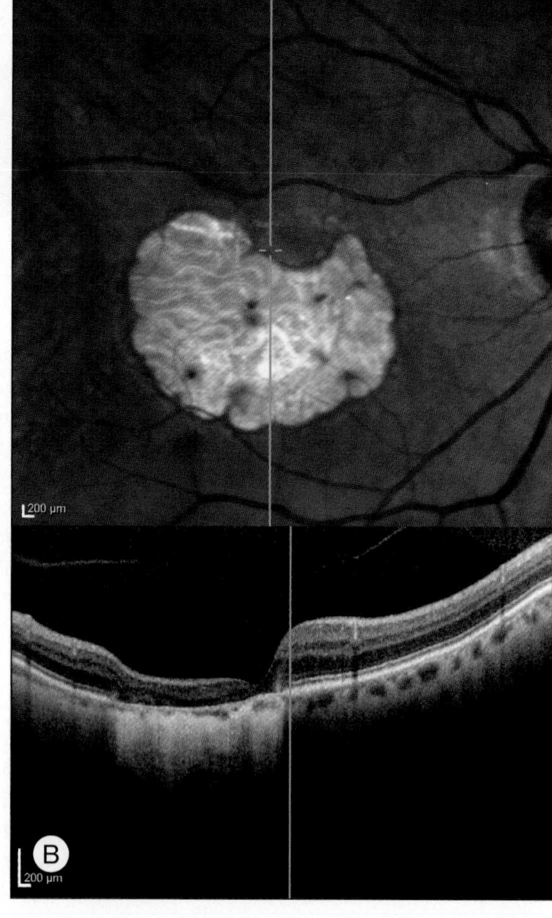

Fig. 42.53 (A) Fundus photograph of the right eye of a 74-year-old male with a Gly108Asp mutation in *PRPH2* causing a central areolar form of pattern dystrophy. The visual acuity in this eye is 20/25. (B) SD-OCT reveals a remarkable preservation of photoreceptors and RPE on the superior edge of the fovea.

color of the large choroidal vessels is replaced by a yellow–white color, sometimes called "choroidal sclerosis" in older literature. Visual acuity deteriorates somewhat in the fourth and fifth decades but can remain as good as 20/100 to 20/200 into the seventh and eighth decades.[205–210]

Electrophysiology

Most patients with pattern dystrophy show normal cone and rod amplitudes and implicit times on the full-field ERG[211] but some reduction can be seen when there are more extensive changes. EOG light-peak to dark-trough ratios are most frequently normal or only modestly subnormal.[211] Genetic testing for variations in *PRPH2* is less expensive than electrophysiology in most institutions and thus we reserve electrophysiologic testing for patients who lack mutations in *PRPH2* and/or who have ophthalmoscopic or perimetric findings suggestive of more widespread photoreceptor disease.

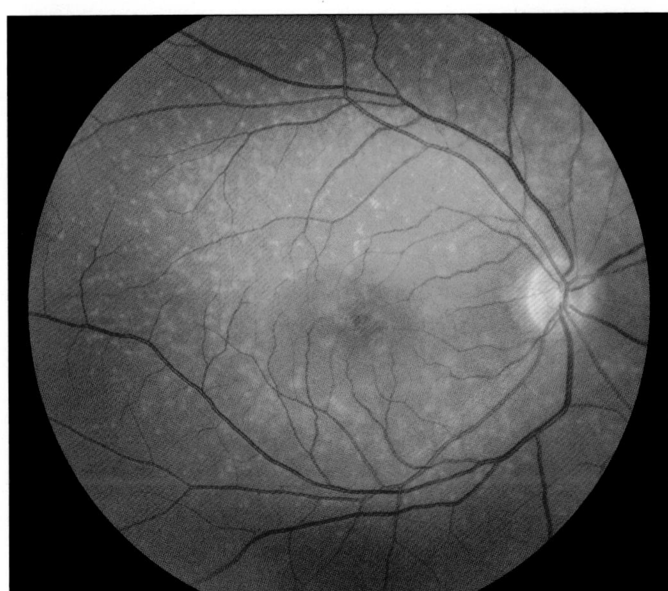

Fig. 42.54 Fundus photograph of the right eye of a 38-year-old female with a IVS2+3 A>T mutation in *PRPH2* causing pattern dystrophy. The visual acuity in this eye is 20/25. The fundus findings are very similar to the fundus flavimaculatus phenotype of *ABCA4*-associated Stargardt disease. However, the dark pigment within the flecks adjacent to the fovea is more characteristic of *PRPH2*-associated disease.

Pathophysiology

PRPH2 encodes a structural protein (peripherin) that plays a critical role in establishing and maintaining the morphology of photoreceptor outer-segment discs.[212,213] Zhang et al.[187] studied eyes from a donor with butterfly dystrophy due to a Cys213Tyr mutation in *PRPH2* and noted an abrupt transition between healthy and degenerated retina and RPE, with massively lipofuscin-laden RPE cells at the transitions. In another report, surgical samples of retina were collected from a living patient with an Arg172Trp mutation in *PRPH2* and manifested abnormal localization of mutant peripherin protein, as well as ultrastructural alterations in outer-segment disc structure.[214] resembling the whorls observed in mice heterozygous for the *rds* mutation.[215] Thus, the primary defect is both genetically and structurally present in photoreceptor cells, with presumed subsequent injury to the RPE and choriocapillaris. The pathophysiologic interplay between the photoreceptors, the RPE, and the choriocapillaris plays a very important role in *PRPH2*-associated diseases, just as it does in the diseases caused by mutations in *ABCA4*. The most severe mutations in both genes cause direct photoreceptor death and this in turn leads to bone-spicule-like pigmentation, narrowed arterioles, and clinical symptoms and signs characteristic of retinitis pigmentosa. In such patients, there is very little yellow pigment deposition because the source of the pigment (the photoreceptor outer segments) is lost. In contrast, the milder mutations of both genes, although expressed in the photoreceptors, have their most visible pathologic effects at the level of the retinal pigment epithelium because the normal

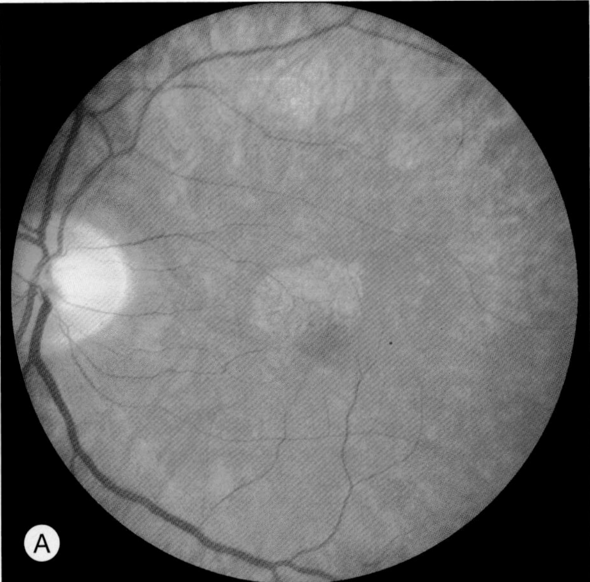

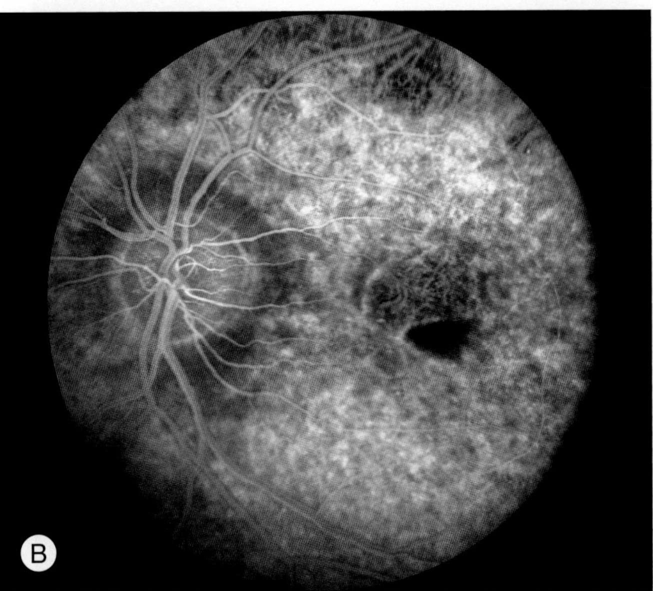

Fig. 42.55 (A) Fundus photograph of the left eye of a 54-year-old male with a Thr146 ins1aC mutation in *PRPH2* causing pattern dystrophy. The visual acuity in this eye is 20/40. There is nummular atrophy in the macula but relative sparing of the inferior edge of the fovea and the peripapillary retina. (B) On fluorescein angiography, the spared areas of RPE block the fluorescence from the underlying choroidal vessels.

phagocytic activity of the latter tissue imports the toxic bisretinoid (in the case of ABCA4) or misshaped discs (in the case of PRPH2). Apoptotic death of the RPE in response to this long-term stress causes death of the underlying choriocapillaris just as it does in age-related macular degeneration.

Treatment

A significant risk for vision loss exists for patients with PD; Francis et al. reported 50% eventually developed poor central acuity due to either geographic atrophy or subretinal neovascularization.[182] However, as in Best disease, many patients can retain driving vision in at least one eye well into their seventh decade of life. Although CNV is slightly less frequent than in age-related macular degeneration, it can be just as devastating to vision and anti-VEGF injections may result in regression and limitation of vision loss.[216] It is also helpful to discuss the practical aspects of delayed recovery from exposure to bright light with PD patients because wearing dark glasses and a hat when outside can allow them to adapt more readily when coming inside. Similarly, adjusting the lighting in the patient's home or office to minimize large changes in illumination from one room to the next (e.g., bright kitchen, dim family room) can make a big difference in their activities of daily living.

SORSBY FUNDUS DYSTROPHY

In 1949 Sorsby described five families with an autosomal dominantly inherited "fundus dystrophy with unusual features" characterized by macular hemorrhages that usually begin early in the fifth decade of life and pigmentary changes in both maculae.[217] Progressive atrophy of the peripheral choroid and RPE is common and can severely limit ambulatory vision later in life. Now known as Sorsby fundus dystrophy (SFD), this disease is caused by mutations in *TIMP-3* (OMIM #188826).[218]

Clinical features of SFD

One of the earliest symptoms of the disease is night blindness,[219,220] although this is not typically severe enough to bring a patient to medical attention. When individuals are seen at this early stage, it is often because they are concerned about the severe macular disease in one of their parents. At this point in the disease course ophthalmoscopically visible yellow-to-gray material is present at the level of Bruch's membrane. In some parts of the fundus this material can take the form of drusen (Fig. 42.56) while in other areas the material coalesces into a fairly uniform yellowish-gray sheet that becomes more prominent with increasing age (Fig. 42.57A). Patients most commonly present to an ophthalmologist in the fourth or fifth decade of life,[217] when they develop bilateral subfoveal neovascular

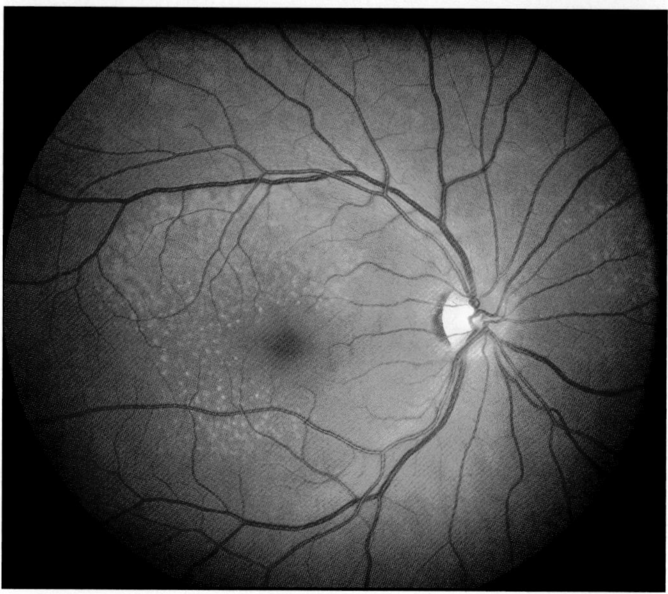

Fig. 42.56 Fundus photograph of the right eye of a 36-year-old female with Ser181Cys mutation in *TIMP-3* causing Sorsby fundus dystrophy. The visual acuity in this eye is 20/15. There are numerous small to medium-sized drusen incompletely ringing the fovea. Superiorly, these drusen merge into a confluent yellow sheet.

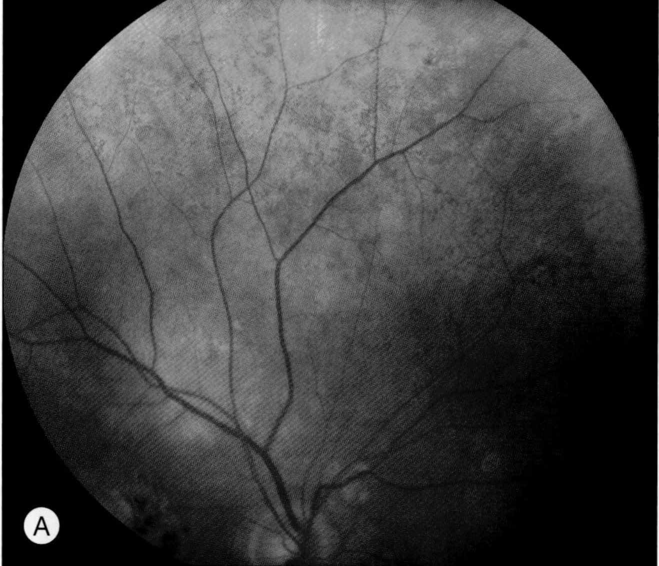

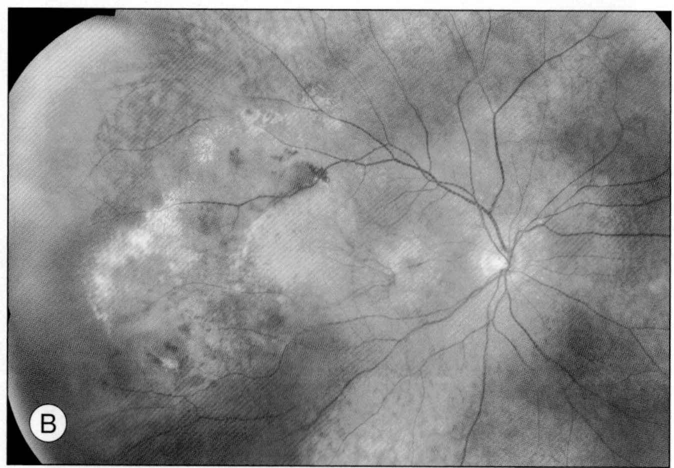

Fig. 42.57 (A) Fundus photograph montage of the right eye of a 55-year-old female with a Ser15Cys mutation in *TIMP-3* causing Sorsby fundus dystrophy. The visual acuity in this eye is 20/125. There is geographic atrophy in the macula and subretinal hemorrhage and exudate temporally indicative of an active choroidal neovascular membrane. (B) A higher magnification view of the retina superior to the disc shows a yellow-gray sheet-like discoloration that corresponds to thickening of Bruch's membrane.

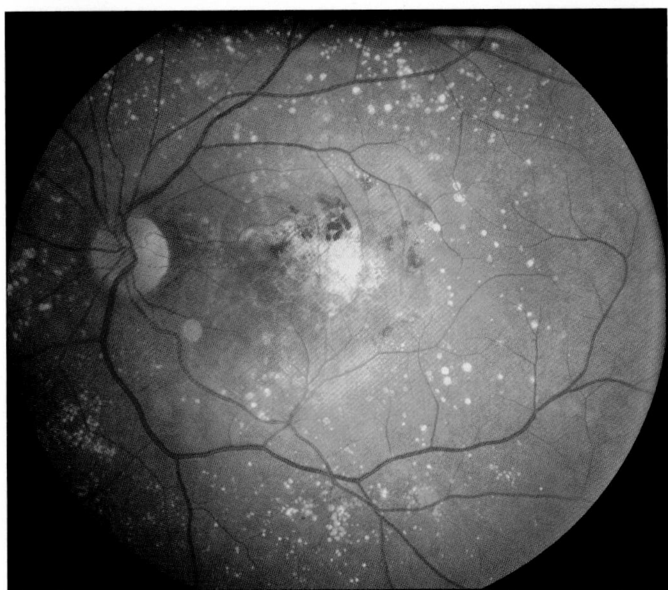

Fig. 42.58 Fundus photograph of the left eye of a 61-year-old female with Trp175Cys mutation in *TIMP-3* causing Sorsby fundus dystrophy. The visual acuity in this eye is 20/125. There is a central disciform scar and temporal subretinal hemorrhage consistent with an active choroidal neovascular membrane. There are numerous drusen of varying sizes in the periphery.

membranes (Figs 42.57A, 42.58) and their visual acuity worsens suddenly. Untreated CNV often results in extensive disciform scarring that severely reduces visual acuity.[221] Marked pigment alterations consisting of atrophy admixed with angular pigment proliferation commonly develop in the macula with or without CNV. Unlike age-related macular degeneration, which rarely extends beyond the temporal vascular arcades, SFD relentlessly extends peripherally and commonly reduces a patient's acuity to hand motions late in life.

Genetics

Since its discovery in 1994, at least 14 mutations in *TIMP3* have been identified.[218,222-229] Most people with SFD in the United Kingdom share a common ancestor and thus harbor the same mutation, Ser181Cys.[230,231] A very unusual feature of SFD is that almost all of the reported mutations create a new cysteine residue in the mutant protein, suggesting that a perturbation of tertiary structure through altered disulfide bonding is required for the development of the disease.

Pathophysiology

The *TIMP3* gene encodes a protein, tissue inhibitor of metalloproteinases-3 (TIMP3), which belongs to a family of negative regulators of matrix metalloproteinase activity. TIMP3 physically interacts with several metalloproteinases[232] and regulates their activity in normal tissue homeostasis. Mutations in this gene are likely to cause altered turnover of extracellular matrix. Given that pathologic angiogenesis is a major clinical feature of SFD, it is notable that TIMP3 suppresses angiogenesis by blocking the interaction of VEGF with its receptor KDR.[233]

The most striking characteristic of eyes with SD is the accumulation of lipidic and proteinaceous material between Bruch's membrane and the RPE up to 30 μm in thickness.[234] Histopathologic analyses of eyes from a donor with SFD due to a Ser181Cys mutation in *TIMP3* revealed CNV and thick deposits beneath the RPE that contained TIMP3 and other extracellular matrix components. The presence of basement membrane proteins in the SFD lesions is consistent with the notion that TIMP3 gain-of-function mutations are pathogenic by their dysregulation of matrix turnover. Ultrastructurally, this material contains banded proteinaceous aggregates with a periodicity suggestive of type VI collagen.[235] Type VI collagen has also been shown to be present at the margins of the lesions by immunohistochemistry.[236]

The TIMP3 protein is a normal component of Bruch's membrane[237] as well as a component of drusen[238] and the abnormal deposits in SFD.[236,239] The accumulation of TIMP3 in SFD may result from the relatively poor turnover of the mutant protein caused by missense mutations.[240]

Dominant mutations in TIMP3 have been recapitulated in mice. Mice harboring a mutant allele of TIMP3 (Ser156Cys) show abnormalities in the RPE basal infoldings and increased extracellular material between the RPE plasma membrane and its basal lamina.[241] Thus, animal studies and biochemical findings strongly suggest that SFD-causing mutations in TIMP3 cause impaired regulation of metalloproteinases and reduced remodeling of the matrix. Normal synthesis, reduced remodeling of extracellular matrix, and impaired control of angiogenesis would appear sufficient to describe the pathology of SFD. However, when Fogarasi et al. assayed the proteinase inhibitory activity of a TIMP3 protein carrying a common SFD mutation, they found no impairment of proteinase inhibition.[242] Thus, some significant questions about the molecular basis of SFD remain to be answered.

Treatment

Treatment of patients with SFD is aimed at CNV control. Argon laser therapy and PDT are not effective in treating SFD-associated CNVs, possibly due to the thickening of Bruch's membrane.[221,243] However, intravenous bevacizumab has been used in one patient and resulted in CNV regression and improvement in visual acuity.[244]

AUTOSOMAL DOMINANT RADIAL DRUSEN (DOYNE HONEYCOMB RETINAL DYSTROPHY, MALATTIA LEVENTINESE)

A familial macular condition with a honeycomb appearance was described by Doyne in the UK in 1899[245] and a similar condition (malattia leventinese, ML) was recognized by Vogt in patients residing in the Leventine Valley of Switzerland in 1925.[246] Surprisingly, it was not until the late 1980s that Gass drew specific attention to one of the most striking clinical features of the condition, the radial distribution of drusen at the temporal periphery of the macular lesions (Fig. 42.59),[247] although at that time he did not explicitly connect this observation to the entities described by Doyne and Vogt. In 1996 Héon and colleagues mapped the disease-causing gene for malattia leventinese to chromosome 2,[248] and in 1999 Stone and coworkers showed that Doyne's honeycomb retinal dystrophy and ML were in fact one disorder caused by a single point mutation (Arg345Trp) in the *EFEMP1* gene.[249] In this chapter, we will use the descriptive term "autosomal dominant radial drusen" (ADRD) to refer to this disease.

Clinical features of ADRD

As with most autosomal dominant conditions, ADRD has a wide range of clinical appearances, presumably due to the variable effect of other genes and environmental factors in different affected individuals. Drusen can be seen in the second decade in some patients while others have barely detectable drusen in the seventh decade. The drusen in the center of the macula and on the nasal edge of the optic disc tend to be large and round (Fig. 42.60), while those at the temporal margin of the macula tend to be smaller, elongated, and radial (see Fig. 42.59). In some patients the small radial drusen can be nearly invisible and reticular pigment changes in the macula can simulate a pattern dystrophy (Fig. 42.61). Most eyes have a group of drusen abutting the nasal aspect of the nerve, even when macular drusen are few or absent.[250] Over time, many eyes develop central atrophy, scarring, and pigment proliferation that can look similar to SFD (Fig. 42.62). However, for a given degree of macular abnormality, the visual acuity in ADRD is typically much better than SFD. Choroidal neovascularization can also complicate ADRD but this occurs much less frequently than it does in SFD.

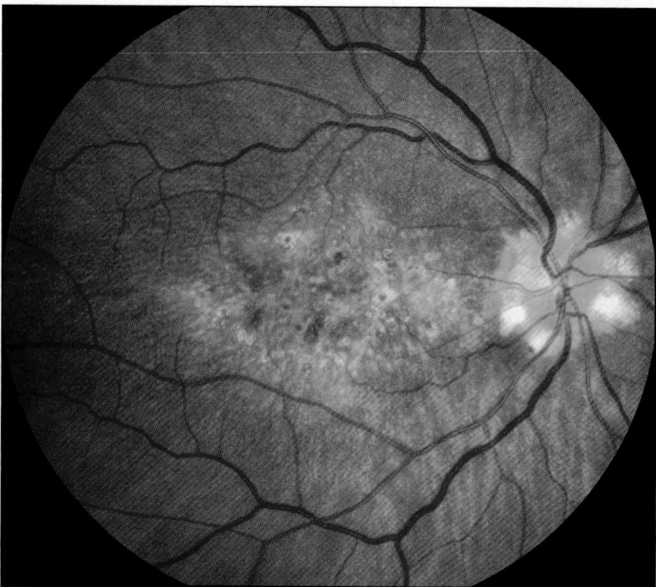

Fig. 42.59 Fundus photograph of the right eye of a 46-year-old female with an Arg345Trp mutation in *EFEMP1* causing ADRD. The visual acuity in this eye is 20/40. The large drusen abutting the optic disc are characteristic of this disease as are the delicate radially oriented drusen that are visible along the temporal edge of the macular lesion. A few of the medium-to-large drusen in the central lesion have fused into a honeycomb configuration.

Visual function and electrophysiology

Even in the presence of extensive drusen, the visual acuity is usually excellent until central atrophy, pigment proliferation, or CNV develop later in life.[250,251] Scotopic sensitivity is reduced and dark-adaptation kinetics are prolonged over confluent macular deposits but are normal elsewhere. The full-field ERG is usually normal but the pattern ERG is abnormal in most eyes.[252]

Imaging

In contrast to drusen in AMD that tend to be hypoautofluorescent, the drusen in ADRD are hyperautofluorescent.[250,253] Autofluorescence can also be useful to distinguish areas of atrophy that can be challenging to see on clinical examination when there is extensive pathology present. Fluorescein angiography is useful for the detection of active choroidal neovascularization, while OCT can demonstrate retinal edema, loss of foveal contour, pigment epithelial detachments, and intense sub-RPE reflectivity.[251]

Pathophysiology and histopathology

The *EFEMP1* gene encodes an extracellular matrix protein known as fibulin-3. Marmorstein et al. studied eyes from an 86-year-old donor with ADRD and found large sub-RPE deposits containing fibulin-3, localized along the apical (i.e., sub-RPE) surface of the deposit, but generally not throughout the druse.[254] Ultrastructural studies have also shown deposition of membranous material in Bruch's membrane.[255] Histologically, drusen in ADRD have a layered appearance that is distinct from

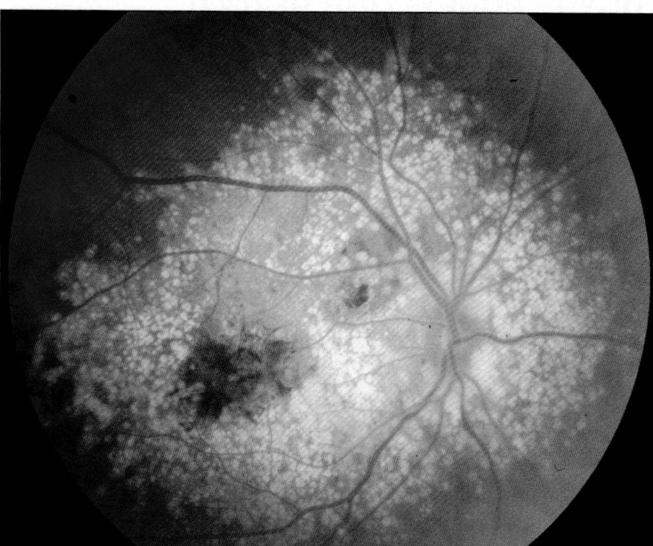

Fig. 42.60 Fundus photograph of the right eye of a 34-year-old male with an Arg345Trp mutation in *EFEMP1* causing ADRD. The visual acuity in this eye is 20/80. There is a dense honeycomb of large drusen occupying most of the posterior pole, with dark pigment and RPE atrophy near the center of the macula.

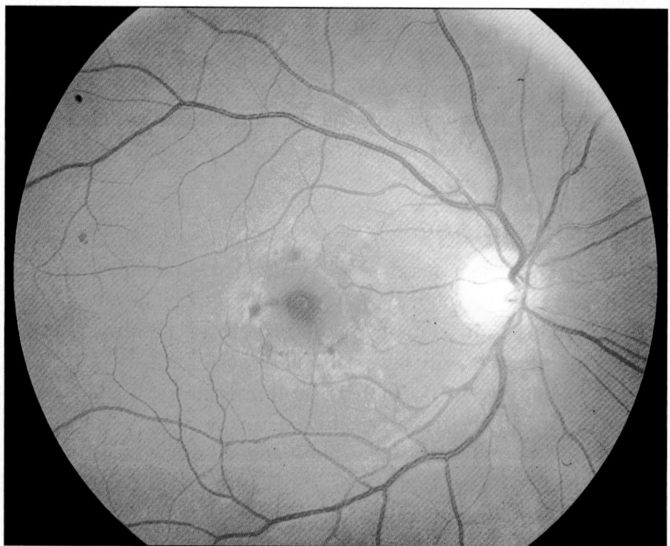

Fig. 42.61 Fundus photograph of the right eye of a 29-year-old female with an Arg345Trp mutation in *EFEMP1* causing ADRD. The visual acuity in this eye is 20/20. Reticular pigment changes outline the large central drusen. Fine radial drusen along the temporal and inferior aspects of the macular lesion are nearly invisible.

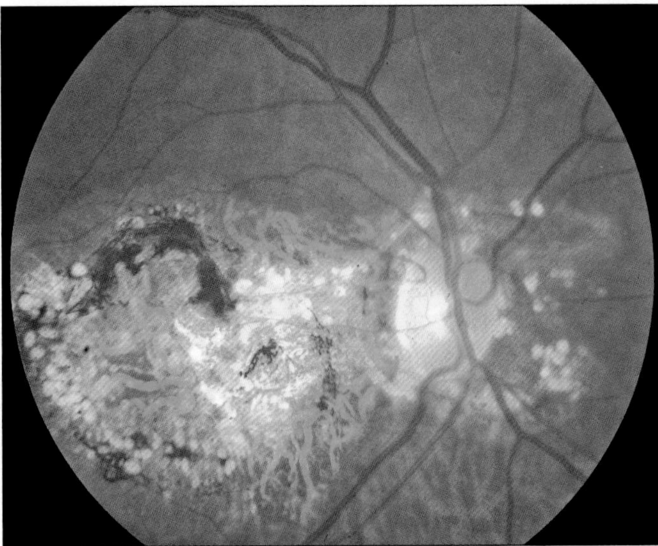

Fig. 42.62 Fundus photograph of the right eye of a 57-year-old female with an Arg345Trp mutation in *EFEMP1* causing ADRD. The visual acuity in this eye is counting fingers. There are extensive atrophic changes in the central macula, papillomacular bundle, and peripapillary regions. A few large drusen are present nasal to the nerve head. This eye had a choroidal neovascular membrane treated with photocoagulation 17 years earlier.

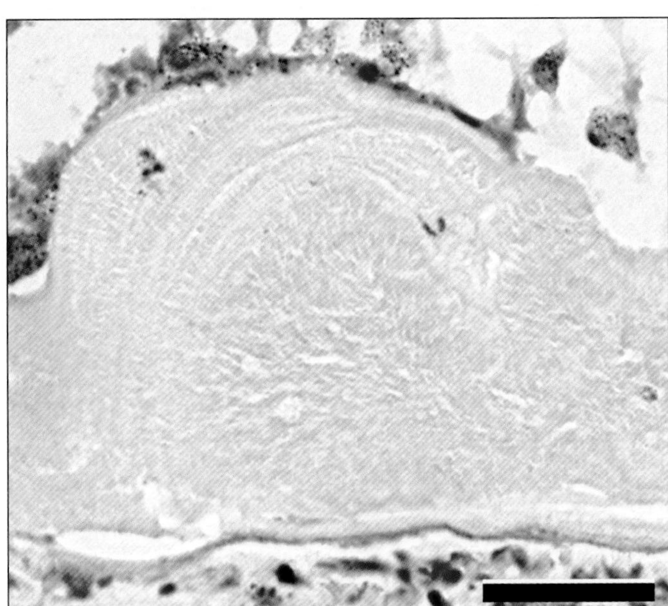

Fig. 42.63 Histological section of a 66-year-old donor eye with ADRD due to an Arg345Trp mutation in the *EFEMP1* gene. The drusen are notable for their size and their unusual tree-ring-like lamination. Scale bar indicates 50 μm.

age-related drusen (see Fig. 42.63). The drusen tend to be large and are often fused together. Cellular infiltration may be present.

Physiological studies have provided some insight into the pathogenesis of ADRD. Fibulin-3 bearing the Arg345Trp mutation is poorly secreted by RPE cells in vitro and its accumulation in the endoplasmic reticulum activates the unfolded protein response.[256] Knockin mice harboring one or more Arg345Trp alleles develop sub-RPE deposits that, while modest in size compared to the drusen observed in ADRD, share molecular components such as fibulin-3 and TIMP3.[257,258] *EFEMP1* is expressed in both neural retina and RPE/choroid layers[259] and fibulin-3 has been detected in photoreceptor cells, inner retinal neurons, and Bruch's membrane.[254]

Treatment

There is currently no treatment for the underlying disease process of ADRD but intravitreal anti-VEGF therapy can cause regression of choroidal neovascularization and restore visual function as long as atrophic changes are minimal.[251]

NORTH CAROLINA MACULAR DYSTROPHY

North Carolina Macular Dystrophy (NCMD) was first described as "dominant macular degeneration and aminoaciduria" by Lefler, Wadsworth, and Sidbury,[260] who studied a kindred originating from two Irish brothers who settled in North Carolina in the 1830s.[261] The original North Carolina pedigree now consists of more than 5000 individuals,[262] but families with similar phenotypes have been identified throughout the world.[263–267] It has also been called central areolar pigment epithelial dystrophy[268] and dominant progressive foveal dystrophy.[261] The latter term is a particularly unfortunate misnomer because Small and colleagues clearly demonstrated that NCMD is a developmental abnormality that is almost completely stationary in most individuals.[269] Large lesions are large at birth and do not progress from smaller ones. This complete lack of progression is one of the most reliable diagnostic features of the disease, and accounts to some degree for the amazingly good visual acuity in some patients with very large lesions. That is, because the lesions are present well before maturation of the visual system, patients learn to fixate on the edges of the lesions and develop their visual pathways accordingly. The fundus findings in NCMD tend to be bilateral and quite symmetric. The most characteristic lesion is a circular coloboma centered on fixation with a shiny concave base surrounded by a thick, white fibrotic rim (Fig. 42.64A). Much more difficult to diagnose correctly in the absence of other family members is the milder manifestation of the disease that can appear as nothing more than a patch of drusen in a young adult with excellent acuity (Fig. 42.64B,C). The visual acuity in NCMD correlates fairly well with the size of the fundus lesions as follows: 20/20 to 20/30 for small (less than 50 μm) lesions; 20/25 to 20/60 for confluent yellow specks in the central macula; and 20/40 to 20/200 when large (500–1000 μm) colobomatous lesions are present (Fig. 42.64A,D).[269,270]

NCMD was mapped by Small and coworkers to chromosome 6[271–273] but the causative gene has not yet been identified. Another dominant macular dystrophy with clinical features very similar to that of NCMD has recently been mapped to chromosome 5[274,275] but the causative gene at this locus has also not yet been identified. In a histopathologic study of one eye from a donor with NCMD, lipofuscin and choriocapillaris atrophy were noted.[276] Currently little is known about the pathophysiology of this disorder or the site of expression of the mutant gene.

SPOTTED CYSTIC DYSTROPHY

Mahajan et al.[277] recently described seven members of a three-generation family with autosomal dominant inheritance of a new dystrophy limited to the macula and characterized by round, flat pigmented spots with or without surrounding hypopigmentation (Fig. 42.65A), cysts in multiple retinal layers

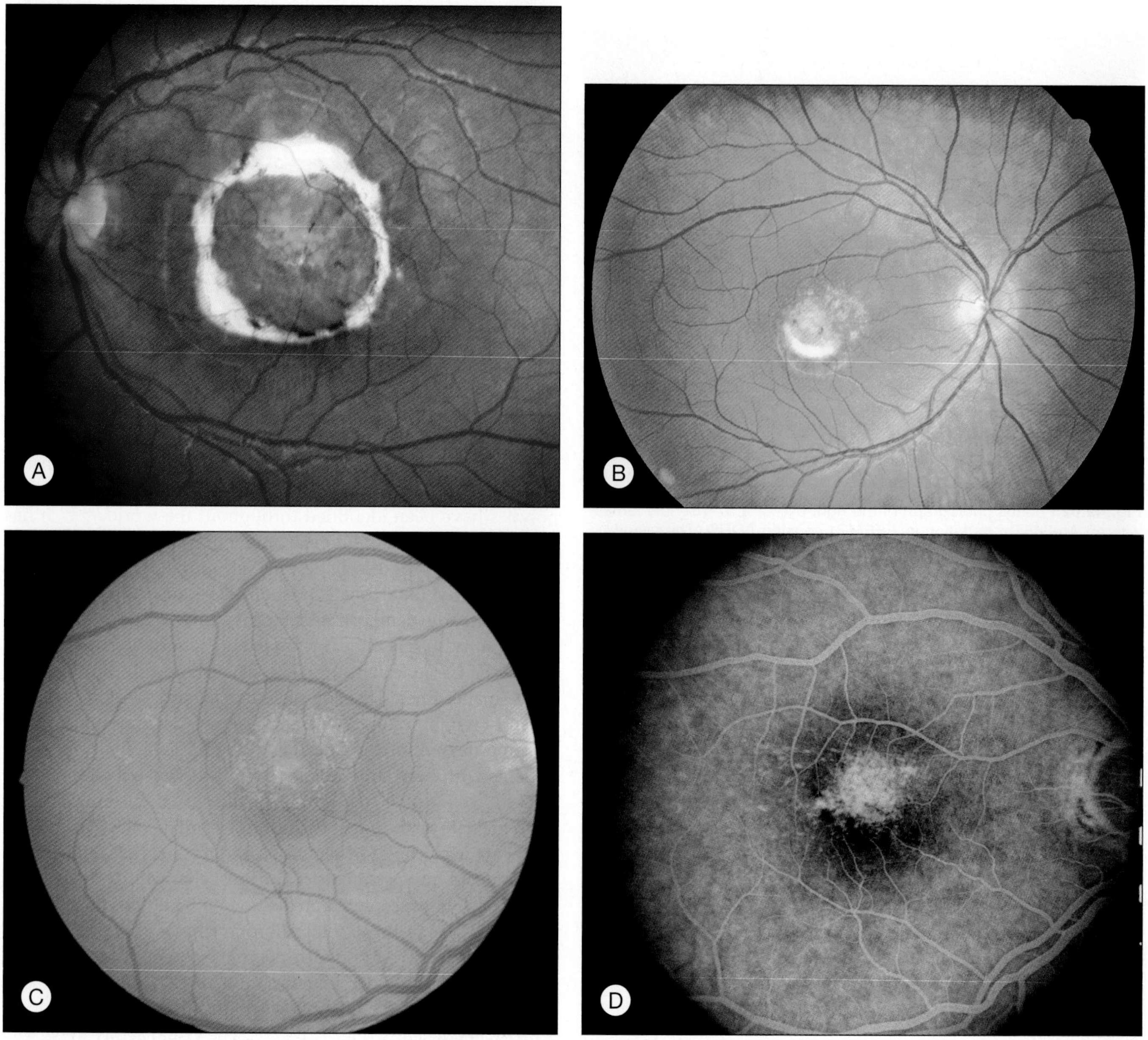

Fig. 42.64 (A) Fundus photograph of the left eye of a 12-year-old female with North Carolina macular dystrophy. The visual acuity in this eye is 20/400 (when fixating on the edge of the lesion). The characteristic fundus findings include a staphylomatous lesion centered in the macula, with a shiny concave base and a thick white fibrotic rim. The disc, vessels, and periphery are all completely normal. (B) The right eye of the 14-year-old sister of the patient shown in (A). The visual acuity is 20/40. The central concavity is smaller than that of her sister and the fibrotic rim is incomplete. The retina opposite the fibrotic rim exhibits drusen-like changes. (C) Fundus photograph of the right eye of the 31-year-old mother of the individuals shown in (A) and (B). The visual acuity is 20/20 and the fundus findings are limited to a patch of small drusen-like deposits centered just above the fovea. (D) The extent of these drusen-like deposits is more easily seen in a fluorescein angiogram of the same eye.

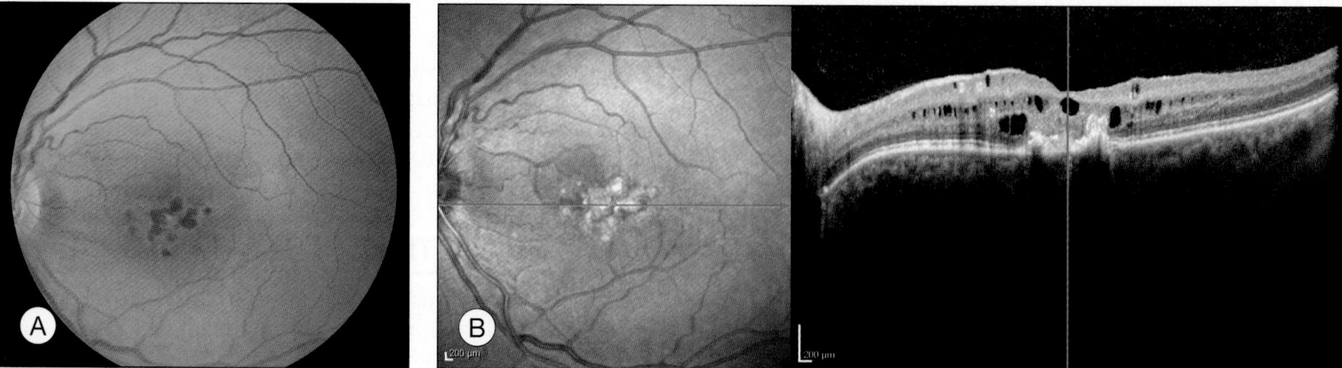

Fig. 42.65 (A) Fundus photograph of the left eye of a 25-year-old female with spotted cystic dystrophy. The visual acuity is 20/70. There are deeply pigmented spots with hypopigmented halos clustered around the fovea. (B) SD-OCT reveals intraretinal cysts and hyperreflective lesions that project from the RPE into the outer retina.

on OCT (Fig. 42.65B), and neovascularization. Amblyopia and strabismus were frequently present in affected individuals. Visual acuity ranged from 20/20 to 20/200. The pathophysiology and genetic mutation responsible for this condition have not been identified. When active macular neovascularization occurs in affected individuals, it has been responsive to either focal laser or a single injection of bevacizumab.[277]

DOMINANT CYSTOID MACULAR DYSTROPHY

Dominant cystoid macular dystrophy (DCMD) was described in 1976 by Deutman[278] as an autosomal dominant condition characterized by leaking perimacular capillaries, whitish punctate deposits in the vitreous, a normal ERG, a subnormal EOG, and hyperopia (Fig. 42.66). In the late stages of the disease, an atrophic central "beaten-bronze" macula was common. A second family was identified a few years later[279] and linkage analysis mapped the chromosomal location of the disease-causing gene to the short arm of chromosome 7.[280] The disease-causing gene for DCMD has not yet been identified. Hogewind and coworkers evaluated intramuscular injections of a somatostatin analog (octreotide acetate) in four patients with DCMD and seven of the eight eyes showed improvement on fluorescein angiography, with stabilization of visual acuity.[281]

FENESTRATED SHEEN MACULAR DYSTROPHY (FSMD)

Several families have been described with an autosomal dominant macular disorder characterized by central macular sheen with small red fenestrations, occurring as early as the first decade of life and seen as late as the fifth decade (Fig. 42.67). Some middle-aged family members develop a bull's-eye pattern of stippled hypopigmentation in the central macula. Mild functional abnormalities roughly correlate with more advanced age but patients with the red fenestrations have 20/20 visual acuity. Normal or mildly abnormal ERG findings have been reported.[282-285] The chromosomal location of the disease-causing gene is currently unknown.

GLOMERULONEPHRITIS TYPE II AND DRUSEN

The majority of patients with membranproliferative glomerulonephritis (MPGN) type II (also known as dense-deposit disease) develop subretinal deposits with the clinical appearance of basal laminar drusen (Fig. 42.68)[286] D'Souza and coworkers followed four MPGN patients with such drusen for 10 years and observed no progression and no vision loss during this interval.[287] In

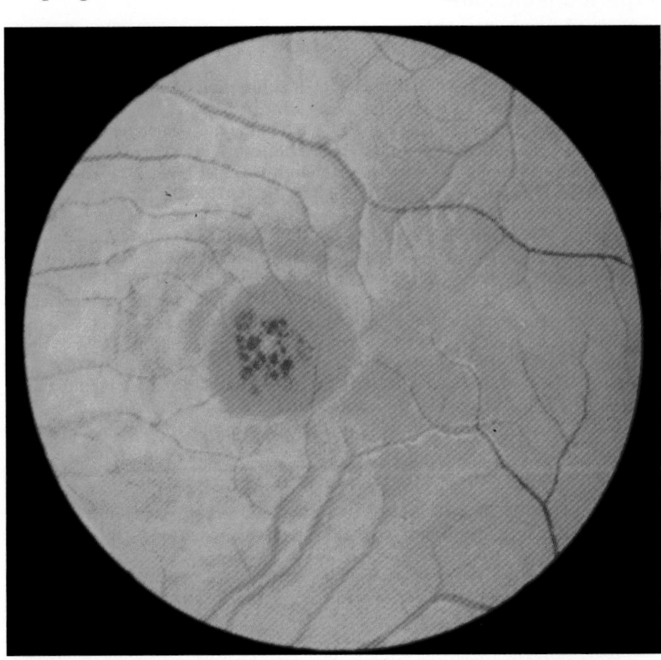

Fig. 42.67 Fundus photograph of the left eye of a 7-year-old patient with fenestrated sheen macular dystrophy. The visual acuity is 20/20. The characteristic lesions are flat red spots clustered about the fovea. (Reproduced with permission from Sneed SR, Sieving PA. Fenestrated sheen macular dystrophy. Am J Ophthalmol 1991;112(1):1–7.)

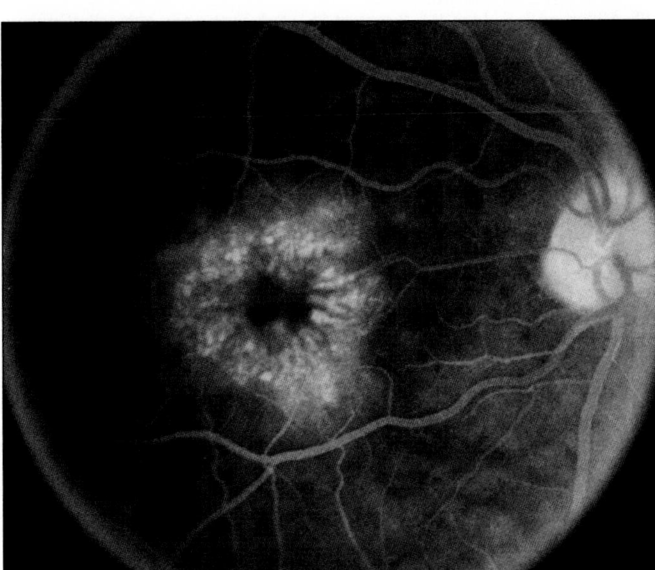

Fig. 42.66 Fluorescein angiogram of the right eye of a patient with dominant cystoid macular edema showing leakage from perifoveal capillaries. (Courtesy of Dr Gerald Fishman, University of Illinois at Chicago.)

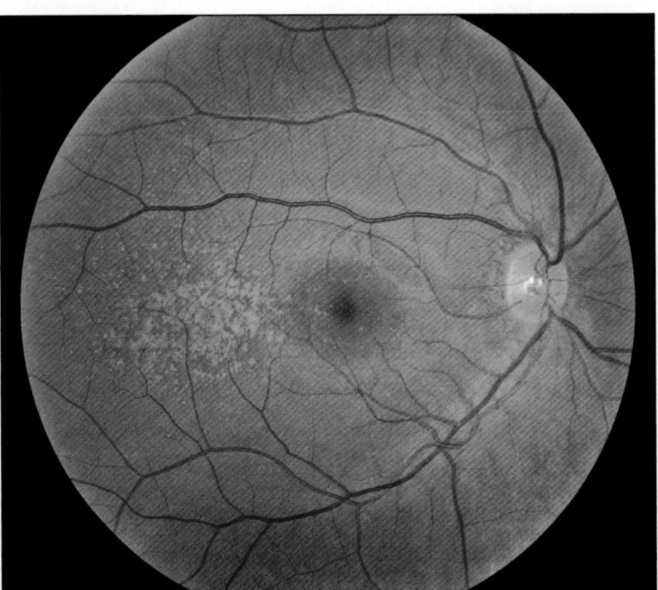

Fig. 42.68 Fundus photograph of the right eye of a 25-year-old female with biopsy-confirmed membranoproliferative glomerulonephritis type II. The visual acuity is 20/20. There are numerous small drusen in the posterior pole, almost all of which are temporal to the fovea.

general, visual acuity tends to be preserved unless CNV, exudative drusen, or serous detachment complicate the disease.[288–290] An abnormal EOG with a relatively normal ERG can be seen in some patients, suggesting a more global retinal dysfunction than the visible drusen would suggest.[291,292] Histopathologic studies of the Bruch's membrane deposits found in MPGN II demonstrate that they are morphologically[293] and compositionally[294] similar to the drusen found in AMD.[295] Abnormal urinalysis with this phenotype in young adults should prompt a referral for work-up of kidney disease.

For online acknowledgments visit **http://www.expertconsult.com**

REFERENCES

1. Petrukhin K, Koisti MJ, Bakall B, et al. Identification of the gene responsible for Best macular dystrophy. Nat Genet 1998;19(3):241–7.
2. Marquardt A, Stohr H, Passmore LA, et al. Mutations in a novel gene, VMD2, encoding a protein of unknown properties cause juvenile-onset vitelliform macular dystrophy (Best's disease). Hum Mol Genet 1998;7(9):1517–25.
3. Best F. Ueber eine hereditaere Makulaaffection. Zschr Augenheilk 1905: 199–212.
4. Braley AE, Spivey BE. Hereditary Vitelline macular degeneration: a clinical and functional evaluation of a new pedigree with variable expressivity and dominant inheritance. Trans Am Ophthalmol Soc 1963;61:339–71.
5. Krill AE, Morse PA, Potts AM, et al. Hereditary vitelliruptive macular degeneration. Am J Ophthalmol 1966;61(6):1405–15.
6. Zanen J, Rausin G. Kyste vitelliforme congenital de la macula. Bull Soc Belge Ophtalmol 1950;96:544.
7. Miller SA, Bresnick GH, Chandra SR. Choroidal neovascular membrane in Best's vitelliform macular dystrophy. Am J Ophthalmol 1976;82(2):252–5.
8. Miller SA. Multifocal Best's vitelliform dystrophy. Arch Ophthalmol 1977;95(6):984–90.
9. Ciulla TA, Frederick AR, Jr. Acute progressive multifocal Best's disease in a 61-year-old man. Am J Ophthalmol 1997;123(1):129–31.
10. Kinnick TR, Mullins RF, Dev S, et al. Autosomal recessive vitelliform macular dystrophy in a large cohort of vitelliform macular dystrophy patients. Retina 2011;31(3):581–95.
11. Schatz P, Klar J, Andreasson S, et al. Variant phenotype of Best vitelliform macular dystrophy associated with compound heterozygous mutations in VMD2. Ophthalmic Genet 2006;27(2):51–6.
12. Wittstrom E, Ekvall S, Schatz P, et al. Morphological and functional changes in multifocal vitelliform retinopathy and biallelic mutations in BEST1. Ophthalmic Genet 2011;32(2):83–96.
13. Burgess R, Millar ID, Leroy BP, et al. Biallelic mutation of BEST1 causes a distinct retinopathy in humans. Am J Hum Genet 2008;82(1):19–31.
14. Querques G, Zerbib J, Santacroce R, et al. Functional and clinical data of Best vitelliform macular dystrophy patients with mutations in the BEST1 gene. Mol Vis 2009;15:2960–72.
15. Chan CK, Gass JD, Lin SG. Acute exudative polymorphous vitelliform maculopathy syndrome. Retina 2003;23(4):453–62.
16. Gass JD, Chuang EL, Granek H. Acute exudative polymorphous vitelliform maculopathy. Trans Am Ophthalmol Soc 1988;86:354–66.
17. Guziewicz KE, Zangerl B, Lindauer SJ, et al. Bestrophin gene mutations cause canine multifocal retinopathy: a novel animal model for best disease. Invest Ophthalmol Vis Sci 2007;48(5):1959–67.
18. Guziewicz KE, Slavik J, Lindauer SJ, et al. Molecular consequences of BEST1 gene mutations in canine multifocal retinopathy predict functional implications for human bestrophinopathies. Invest Ophthalmol Vis Sci 2011.
19. Chung MM, Oh KT, Streb LM, et al. Visual outcome following subretinal hemorrhage in Best disease. Retina 2001;21(6):575–80.
20. Mohler CW, Fine SL. Long-term evaluation of patients with Best's vitelliform dystrophy. Ophthalmology 1981;88(7):688–92.
21. Fishman GA, Baca W, Alexander KR, et al. Visual acuity in patients with best vitelliform macular dystrophy. Ophthalmology 1993;100(11):1665–70.
22. Sohn EH, Francis PJ, Duncan JL, et al. Phenotypic variability due to a novel Glu292Lys variation in exon 8 of the BEST1 gene causing best macular dystrophy. Arch Ophthalmol 2009;127(7):913–20.
23. Renner AB, Tillack H, Kraus H, et al. Late onset is common in Best macular dystrophy associated with VMD2 gene mutations. Ophthalmology 2005;112(4): 586–92.
24. Wittstrom E, Ponjavic V, Bondeson ML, et al. Anterior Segment abnormalities and angle-closure glaucoma in a family with a mutation in the Best1 gene and Best vitelliform macular dystrophy. Ophthalmic Genet 2011;32(4):217–27.
25. Wabbels B, Preising MN, Kretschmann U, et al. Genotype-phenotype correlation and longitudinal course in ten families with Best vitelliform macular dystrophy. Graefes Arch Clin Exp Ophthalmol 2006;244(11):1453–66.
26. Burgess R, MacLaren RE, Davidson AE, et al. ADVIRC is caused by distinct mutations in BEST1 that alter pre-mRNA splicing. J Med Genet 2009;46(9): 620–5.
27. Lafaut BA, Loeys B, Leroy BP, et al. Clinical and electrophysiological findings in autosomal dominant vitreoretinochoroidopathy: report of a new pedigree. Graefes Arch Clin Exp Ophthalmol 2001;239(8):575–82.
28. Kay CN, Abramoff MD, Mullins RF, , et al. Three dimensional distribution of the vitelliform lesion, photoreceptors, and retinal pigment epithelium in the macula of patients with Best vitelliform macular dystrophy. Retina (submitted).
29. Querques G, Regenbogen M, Quijano C, et al. High-definition optical coherence tomography features in vitelliform macular dystrophy. Am J Ophthalmol 2008;146(4):501–7.
30. Ferrara DC, Costa RA, Tsang S, et al. Multimodal fundus imaging in Best vitelliform macular dystrophy. Graefes Arch Clin Exp Ophthalmol 2010; 248(10):1377–86.
31. Spaide RF, Noble K, Morgan A, et al. Vitelliform macular dystrophy. Ophthalmology 2006;113(8):1392–400.
32. Pianta MJ, Aleman TS, Cideciyan AV, et al. In vivo micropathology of Best macular dystrophy with optical coherence tomography. Exp Eye Res 2003;76(2):203–11.
33. von Ruckmann A, Fitzke FW, Bird AC. In vivo fundus autofluorescence in macular dystrophies. Arch Ophthalmol 1997;115(5):609–15.
34. Boon CJ, Theelen T, Hoefsloot EH, et al. Clinical and molecular genetic analysis of best vitelliform macular dystrophy. Retina 2009;29(6):835–47.
35. Frangieh GT, Green WR, Fine SL. A histopathologic study of Best's macular dystrophy. Arch Ophthalmol 1982;100(7):1115–21.
36. O'Gorman S, Flaherty WA, Fishman GA, et al. Histopathologic findings in Best's vitelliform macular dystrophy. Arch Ophthalmol 1988;106(9):1261–8.
37. Weingeist TA, Kobrin JL, Watzke RC. Histopathology of Best's macular dystrophy. Arch Ophthalmol 1982;100(7):1108–14.
38. Bakall B, Radu RA, Stanton JB, et al. Enhanced accumulation of A2E in individuals homozygous or heterozygous for mutations in BEST1 (VMD2). Exp Eye Res 2007;85(1):34–43.
39. Meunier I, Senechal A, Dhaenens CM, et al. Systematic screening of BEST1 and PRPH2 in juvenile and adult vitelliform macular dystrophies: a rationale for molecular analysis. Ophthalmology 2011;118(6):1130–6.
40. Pollack K, Kreuz FR, Pillunat LE. [Best's disease with normal EOG. Case report of familial macular dystrophy.] Ophthalmologe 2005;102(9):891–4.
41. Testa F, Rossi S, Passerini I, et al. A normal electro-oculography in a family affected by Best disease with a novel spontaneous mutation of the BEST1 gene. Br J Ophthalmol 2008;92(11):1467–70.
42. Wabbels B, Demmler A, Paunescu K, et al. Fundus autofluorescence in children and teenagers with hereditary retinal diseases. Graefes Arch Clin Exp Ophthalmol 2006;244(1):36–45.
43. Yu K, Qu Z, Cui Y, et al. Chloride channel activity of bestrophin mutants associated with mild or late-onset macular degeneration. Invest Ophthalmol Vis Sci 2007;48(10):4694–705.
44. Stone EM, Nichols BE, Streb LM, et al. Genetic linkage of vitelliform macular degeneration (Best's disease) to chromosome 11q13. Nat Genet 1992;1(4): 246–50.
45. Graff C, Forsman K, Larsson C, et al. Fine mapping of Best's macular dystrophy localizes the gene in close proximity to but distinct from the D11S480/ROM1 loci. Genomics 1994;24(3):425–34.
46. Nichols BE, Bascom R, Litt M, et al. Refining the locus for Best vitelliform macular dystrophy and mutation analysis of the candidate gene ROM1. Am J Hum Genet 1994;54(1):95–103.
47. Marmorstein AD, Marmorstein LY, Rayborn M, et al. Bestrophin, the product of the Best vitelliform macular dystrophy gene (VMD2), localizes to the basolateral plasma membrane of the retinal pigment epithelium. Proc Natl Acad Sci U S A 2000;97(23):12758–63.
48. Allikmets R, Seddon JM, Bernstein PS, et al. Evaluation of the Best disease gene in patients with age-related macular degeneration and other maculopathies. Hum Genet 1999;104(6):449–53.
49. Bakall B, Marknell T, Ingvast S, et al. The mutation spectrum of the bestrophin protein – functional implications. Hum Genet 1999;104(5):383–9.
50. Ponjavic V, Eksandh L, Andreasson S, et al. Clinical expression of Best's vitelliform macular dystrophy in Swedish families with mutations in the bestrophin gene. Ophthalmic Genet 1999;20(4):251–7.
51. Lotery AJ, Munier FL, Fishman GA, et al. Allelic variation in the VMD2 gene in Best disease and age-related macular degeneration. Invest Ophthalmol Vis Sci 2000;41(6):1291–6.
52. White K, Marquardt A, Weber BH. VMD2 mutations in vitelliform macular dystrophy (Best disease) and other maculopathies. Hum Mutat 2000;15(4): 301–8.
53. Kramer F, White K, Pauleikhoff D, et al. Mutations in the VMD2 gene are associated with juvenile-onset vitelliform macular dystrophy (Best disease) and adult vitelliform macular dystrophy but not age-related macular degeneration. Eur J Hum Genet 2000;8(4):286–92.
54. Eksandh L, Bakall B, Bauer B, et al. Best's vitelliform macular dystrophy caused by a new mutation (Val89Ala) in the VMD2 gene. Ophthalmic Genet 2001;22(2):107–15.
55. Seddon JM, Afshari MA, Sharma S, et al. Assessment of mutations in the Best macular dystrophy (VMD2) gene in patients with adult-onset foveomacular vitelliform dystrophy, age-related maculopathy, and bull's-eye maculopathy. Ophthalmology 2001;108(11):2060–7.
56. Stohr H, Marquardt A, Nanda I, et al. Three novel human VMD2-like genes are members of the evolutionary highly conserved RFP-TM family. Eur J Hum Genet 2002;10(4):281–4.
57. Seddon JM, Sharma S, Chong S, et al. Phenotype and genotype correlations in two Best families. Ophthalmology 2003;110(9):1724–31.
58. Mullins RF, Oh KT, Heffron E, et al. Late development of vitelliform lesions and flecks in a patient with Best disease: clinicopathologic correlation. Arch Ophthalmol 2005;123(11):1588–94.

59. Apushkin MA, Fishman GA, Taylor CM, et al. Novel de novo mutation in a patient with Best macular dystrophy. Arch Ophthalmol 2006;124(6): 887–9.
60. Marchant D, Yu K, Bigot K, et al. New VMD2 gene mutations identified in patients affected by Best vitelliform macular dystrophy. J Med Genet 2007;44(3):e70.
61. Boon CJ, Klevering BJ, Leroy BP, et al. The spectrum of ocular phenotypes caused by mutations in the BEST1 gene. Prog Retin Eye Res 2009;28(3): 187–205.
62. Schatz P, Bitner H, Sander B, et al. Evaluation of macular structure and function by OCT and electrophysiology in patients with vitelliform macular dystrophy due to mutations in BEST1. Invest Ophthalmol Vis Sci 2010;51(9): 4754–65.
63. Mullins RF, Kuehn MH, Faidley EA, et al. Differential macular and peripheral expression of bestrophin in human eyes and its implication for Best disease. Invest Ophthalmol Vis Sci 2007;48(7):3372–80.
64. Marmorstein AD, Cross HE, Peachey NS. Functional roles of bestrophins in ocular epithelia. Prog Retin Eye Res 2009;28(3):206–26.
65. Xiao Q, Hartzell HC, Yu K. Bestrophins and retinopathies. Pflugers Arch 2010;460(2):559–69.
66. Hartzell C, Qu Z, Putzier I, et al. Looking chloride channels straight in the eye: bestrophins, lipofuscinosis, and retinal degeneration. Physiology (Bethesda) 2005;20:292–302.
67. Sun H, Tsunenari T, Yau KW, et al. The vitelliform macular dystrophy protein defines a new family of chloride channels. Proc Natl Acad Sci U S A 2002;99(6):4008–13.
68. Fischmeister R, Hartzell HC. Volume sensitivity of the bestrophin family of chloride channels. J Physiol 2005;562(Pt 2):477–91.
69. Marmorstein LY, Wu J, McLaughlin P, et al. The light peak of the electroretinogram is dependent on voltage-gated calcium channels and antagonized by bestrophin (best-1). J Gen Physiol 2006;127(5):577–89.
70. Zhang Y, Stanton JB, Wu J, et al. Suppression of Ca^{2+} signaling in a mouse model of Best disease. Hum Mol Genet 2010;19(6):1108–18.
71. Marmor MF, Yao XY, Hageman GS. Retinal adhesiveness in surgically enucleated human eyes. Retina 1994;14(2):181–6.
72. Hall MO, Abrams TA, Mittag TW. ROS ingestion by RPE cells is turned off by increased protein kinase C activity and by increased calcium. Exp Eye Res 1991;52(5):591–8.
73. Kaufman SJ, Goldberg MF, Orth DH, et al. Autosomal dominant vitreoretinochoroidopathy. Arch Ophthalmol 1982;100(2):272–8.
74. Blair NP, Goldberg MF, Fishman GA, et al. Autosomal dominant vitreoretinochoroidopathy (ADVIRC). Br J Ophthalmol 1984;68(1):2–9.
75. Han DP, Lewandowski MF. Electro-oculography in autosomal dominant vitreoretinochoroidopathy. Arch Ophthalmol 1992;110(11):1563–7.
76. Kellner U, Jandeck C, Kraus H, et al. Autosomal dominant vitreoretinochoroidopathy with normal electrooculogram in a German family. Graefes Arch Clin Exp Ophthalmol 1998;236(2):109–14.
77. Vincent A, McAlister C, Vandenhoven C, et al. BEST1-related autosomal dominant vitreoretinochoroidopathy: a degenerative disease with a range of developmental ocular anomalies. Eye (Lond) 2011;25(1):113–8.
78. Yardley J, Leroy BP, Hart-Holden N, et al. Mutations of VMD2 splicing regulators cause nanophthalmos and autosomal dominant vitreoretinochoroidopathy (ADVIRC). Invest Ophthalmol Vis Sci 2004;45(10):3683–9.
79. Oh KT, Vallar C. Central cone dysfunction in autosomal dominant vitreoretinochoroidopathy (ADVIRC). Am J Ophthalmol 2006;141(5):940–3.
80. Davidson AE, Millar ID, Urquhart JE, et al. Missense mutations in a retinal pigment epithelium protein, bestrophin-1, cause retinitis pigmentosa. Am J Hum Genet 2009;85(5):581–92.
81. Iannaccone A, Kerr NC, Kinnick TR, et al. Autosomal recessive best vitelliform macular dystrophy: report of a family and management of early-onset neovascular complications. Arch Ophthalmol 2011;129(2):211–17.
82. Davidson AE, Sergouniotis PI, Burgess-Mullan R, et al. A synonymous codon variant in two patients with autosomal recessive bestrophinopathy alters in vitro splicing of BEST1. Mol Vis 2010;16:2916–22.
83. Gerth C, Zawadzki RJ, Werner JS, et al. Detailed analysis of retinal function and morphology in a patient with autosomal recessive bestrophinopathy (AR(B). Doc Ophthalmol 2009;118(3):239–46.
84. Leu J, Schrage NF, Degenring RF. Choroidal neovascularisation secondary to Best's disease in a 13-year-old boy treated by intravitreal bevacizumab. Graefes Arch Clin Exp Ophthalmol 2007;245(11):1723–5.
85. Montero JA, Ruiz-Moreno JM, De La Vega C. Intravitreal bevacizumab for adult-onset vitelliform dystrophy: a case report. Eur J Ophthalmol 2007;17(6): 983–6.
86. Querques G, Bocco MC, Soubrane G, et al. Intravitreal ranibizumab (Lucentis) for choroidal neovascularization associated with vitelliform macular dystrophy. Acta Ophthalmol 2008;86(6):694–5.
87. Rishi E, Rishi P, Mahajan S. Intravitreal bevacizumab for choroidal neovascular membrane associated with Best's vitelliform dystrophy. Indian J Ophthalmol 2010;58(2):160–2.
88. Heidary F, Hitam WH, Ngah NF, et al. Intravitreal ranibizumab for choroidal novascularization in Best's vitelliform macular dystrophy in a 6-year-old boy. J Pediatr Ophthalmol Strabismus 2011;48 Online:e19–22.
89. Boon CJ, den Hollander AI, Hoyng CB, et al. The spectrum of retinal dystrophies caused by mutations in the peripherin/RDS gene. Prog Retin Eye Res 2008;27(2):213–35.
90. Chowers I, Zamir E, Banin E, et al. Blunt trauma in Best's vitelliform macular dystrophy. Br J Ophthalmol 2000;84(11):1330–1.
91. Allikmets R. A photoreceptor cell-specific ATP-binding transporter gene (ABCR) is mutated in recessive Stargardt macular dystrophy. Nat Genet 1997;17(1):122.
92. Cremers FP, van de Pol DJ, van Driel M, et al. Autosomal recessive retinitis pigmentosa and cone-rod dystrophy caused by splice site mutations in the Stargardt's disease gene ABCR. Hum Mol Genet 1998;7(3):355–62.
93. Martinez-Mir A, Paloma E, Allikmets R, et al. Retinitis pigmentosa caused by a homozygous mutation in the Stargardt disease gene ABCR. Nat Genet 1998;18(1):11–2.
94. Fishman GA, Stone EM, Grover S, et al. Variation of clinical expression in patients with Stargardt dystrophy and sequence variations in the ABCR gene. Arch Ophthalmol 1999;117(4):504–10.
95. Maugeri A, Klevering BJ, Rohrschneider K, et al. Mutations in the ABCA4 (ABCR) gene are the major cause of autosomal recessive cone-rod dystrophy. Am J Hum Genet 2000;67(4):960–6.
96. Fishman GA, Stone EM, Eliason DA, et al. ABCA4 gene sequence variations in patients with autosomal recessive cone-rod dystrophy. Arch Ophthalmol 2003;121(6):851–5.
97. Schindler EI, Nylen EL, Ko AC, et al. Deducing the pathogenic contribution of recessive ABCA4 alleles in an outbred population. Hum Mol Genet 2010;19(19):3693–701.
98. Stargardt K. Uber familiare, progressive degeneration in der maculagegend des auges. Albrecht von Graefes Arch Ophthalmol 1909;71:534–50.
99. Franceschetti A. La Retinopathie ponctuée albescente. In: Bulletins et memoires de la Société Française d'Ophthalmologie. Paris: Masson&Cie; 1963. p. 14–9.
100. Jayasundera T, Rhoades W, Branham K, et al. Peripapillary dark choroid ring as a helpful diagnostic sign in advanced Stargardt disease. Am J Ophthalmol 2010;149(4):656–60 e2.
101. Cideciyan AV, Swider M, Aleman TS, et al. ABCA4-associated retinal degenerations spare structure and function of the human parapapillary retina. Invest Ophthalmol Vis Sci 2005;46(12):4739–46.
102. Lois N, Halfyard AS, Bird AC, et al. Fundus autofluorescence in Stargardt macular dystrophy-fundus flavimaculatus. Am J Ophthalmol 2004;138(1): 55–63.
103. Fishman GA, Farber M, Patel BS, et al. Visual acuity loss in patients with Stargardt's macular dystrophy. Ophthalmology 1987;94(7):809–14.
104. Rotenstreich Y, Fishman GA, Anderson RJ. Visual acuity loss and clinical observations in a large series of patients with Stargardt disease. Ophthalmology 2003;110(6):1151–8.
105. Oh KT, Weleber RG, Oh DM, et al. Clinical phenotype as a prognostic factor in Stargardt disease. Retina 2004;24(2):254–62.
106. Hadden OB, Gass JD. Fundus flavimaculatus and Stargardt's disease. Am J Ophthalmol 1976;82(4):527–39.
107. Anmarkrud N. Fundus fluorescein angiography in fundus flavimaculatus and Stargardt's disease. Acta Ophthalmol (Copenh) 1979;57(2):172–82.
108. Ernest JT, Krill AE. Fluorescein studies in fundus flavimaculatus and drusen. Am J Ophthalmol 1966;62(1):1–6.
109. Radu RA, Mata NL, Bagla A, et al. Light exposure stimulates formation of A2E oxiranes in a mouse model of Stargardt's macular degeneration. Proc Natl Acad Sci U S A 2004;101(16):5928–33.
110. Lois N, Holder GE, Fitzke FW, et al. Intrafamilial variation of phenotype in Stargardt macular dystrophy-fundus flavimaculatus. Invest Ophthalmol Vis Sci 1999;40(11):2668–75.
111. Lois N, Holder GE, Bunce C, et al. Phenotypic subtypes of Stargardt macular dystrophy-fundus flavimaculatus. Arch Ophthalmol 2001;119(3): 359–69.
112. Ergun E, Hermann B, Wirtitsch M, et al. Assessment of central visual function in Stargardt's disease/fundus flavimaculatus with ultrahigh-resolution optical coherence tomography. Invest Ophthalmol Vis Sci 2005;46(1): 310–16.
113. Sunness JS, Ziegler MD, Applegate CA. Issues in quantifying atrophic macular disease using retinal autofluorescence. Retina 2006;26(6):666–72.
114. Boon CJ, Jeroen Klevering B, Keunen JE, et al. Fundus autofluorescence imaging of retinal dystrophies. Vision Res 2008;48(26):2569–77.
115. Sunness JS, Steiner JN. Retinal function and loss of autofluorescence in stargardt disease. Retina 2008;28(6):794–800.
116. Gomes NL, Greenstein VC, Carlson JN, et al. A comparison of fundus autofluorescence and retinal structure in patients with Stargardt disease. Invest Ophthalmol Vis Sci 2009;50(8):3953–9.
117. Smith RT, Gomes NL, Barile G, et al. Lipofuscin and autofluorescence metrics in progressive STGD. Invest Ophthalmol Vis Sci 2009;50(8):3907–14.
118. Shah SN, Koozekanani DD, Kim JE. Phenotypic heterogeneity and lesion size measurements in Stargardt macular dystrophy. Ophthalmic Surg Lasers Imaging 2009;40(5):506–12.
119. Sodi A, Bini A, Passerini I, et al. Different patterns of fundus autofluorescence related to ABCA4 gene mutations in Stargardt disease. Ophthalmic Surg Lasers Imaging 2010;41(1):48–53.
120. Burke TR, Allikmets R, Smith RT, et al. Loss of peripapillary sparing in non-group I Stargardt disease. Exp Eye Res 2010;91(5):592–600.
121. Anastasakis A, Fishman GA, Lindeman M, et al. Infrared scanning laser ophthalmoscope imaging of the macula and its correlation with functional loss and structural changes in patients with Stargardt disease. Retina 2011;31(5):949–58.
122. Chen Y, Ratnam K, Sundquist SM, et al. Cone photoreceptor abnormalities correlate with vision loss in patients with Stargardt disease. Invest Ophthalmol Vis Sci 2011;52(6):3281–92.

123. Chen B, Tosha C, Gorin MB, et al. Analysis of autofluorescent retinal images and measurement of atrophic lesion growth in Stargardt disease. Exp Eye Res 2010;91(2):143–52.
124. Cella W, Greenstein VC, Zernant-Rajang J, et al. G1961E mutant allele in the Stargardt disease gene ABCA4 causes bull's eye maculopathy. Exp Eye Res 2009;89(1):16–24.
125. Lim JI, Tan O, Fawzi AA, et al. A pilot study of Fourier-domain optical coherence tomography of retinal dystrophy patients. Am J Ophthalmol 2008;146(3):417–26.
126. Lenassi E, Jarc-Vidmar M, Glavac D, et al. Pattern electroretinography of larger stimulus field size and spectral-domain optical coherence tomography in patients with Stargardt disease. Br J Ophthalmol 2009;93(12):1600–5.
127. Genead MA, Fishman GA, Anastasakis A. Spectral-domain OCT peripapillary retinal nerve fibre layer thickness measurements in patients with Stargardt disease. Br J Ophthalmol 2011;95(5):689–93.
128. Klevering BJ, Deutman AF, Maugeri A, et al. The spectrum of retinal phenotypes caused by mutations in the ABCA4 gene. Graefes Arch Clin Exp Ophthalmol 2005;243(2):90–100.
129. Oh KT, Weleber RG, Stone EM, et al. Electroretinographic findings in patients with Stargardt disease and fundus flavimaculatus. Retina 2004;24(6):920–8.
130. Fukui T, Yamamoto S, Nakano K, et al. ABCA4 gene mutations in Japanese patients with Stargardt disease and retinitis pigmentosa. Invest Ophthalmol Vis Sci 2002;43(9):2819–24.
131. Gerth C, Andrassi-Darida M, Bock M, et al. Phenotypes of 16 Stargardt macular dystrophy/fundus flavimaculatus patients with known ABCA4 mutations and evaluation of genotype-phenotype correlation. Graefes Arch Clin Exp Ophthalmol 2002;240(8):628–38.
132. Scholl HP, Besch D, Vonthein R, et al. Alterations of slow and fast rod ERG signals in patients with molecularly confirmed Stargardt disease type 1. Invest Ophthalmol Vis Sci 2002;43(4):1248–56.
133. Birch DG, Peters AY, Locke KL, et al. Visual function in patients with cone-rod dystrophy (CRD) associated with mutations in the ABCA4(ABCR) gene. Exp Eye Res 2001;73(6):877–86.
134. Sheffield VC, Stone EM. Genomics and the eye. N Engl J Med 2011;364(20):1932–42.
135. Weleber RG. The dystrophic retina in multisystem disorders: the electroretinogram in neuronal ceroid lipofuscinoses. Eye (Lond) 1998;12(Pt 3b):580–90.
136. Tosha C, Gorin MB, Nusinowitz S. Test-retest reliability and inter-ocular symmetry of multi-focal electroretinography in Stargardt disease. Curr Eye Res 2010;35(1):63–72.
137. Stone EM. Finding and interpreting genetic variations that are important to ophthalmologists. Trans Am Ophthalmol Soc 2003;101:437–84.
138. Philp AR, Jin M, Li S, et al. Predicting the pathogenicity of RPE65 mutations. Hum Mutat 2009;30(8):1183–8.
139. Steinmetz RL, Garner A, Maguire JI, et al. Histopathology of incipient fundus flavimaculatus. Ophthalmology 1991;98(6):953–6.
140. Birnbach CD, Jarvelainen M, Possin DE, et al. Histopathology and immunocytochemistry of the neurosensory retina in fundus flavimaculatus. Ophthalmology 1994;101(7):1211–9.
141. Klien BA, Krill AE. Fundus flavimaculatus. Clinical, functional and histopathologic observations. Am J Ophthalmol 1967;64(1):3–23.
142. Tsybovsky Y, Molday RS, Palczewski K. The ATP-binding cassette transporter ABCA4: structural and functional properties and role in retinal disease. Adv Exp Med Biol 2010;703:105–25.
143. Molday RS, Zhang K. Defective lipid transport and biosynthesis in recessive and dominant Stargardt macular degeneration. Prog Lipid Res 2010;49(4):476–92.
144. Weng J, Mata NL, Azarian SM, et al. Insights into the function of Rim protein in photoreceptors and etiology of Stargardt's disease from the phenotype in abcr knockout mice. Cell 1999;98(1):13–23.
145. Sparrow JR, Nakanishi K, Parish CA. The lipofuscin fluorophore A2E mediates blue light-induced damage to retinal pigmented epithelial cells. Invest Ophthalmol Vis Sci 2000;41(7):1981–9.
146. Suter M, Remé C, Grimm C, et al. Age-related macular degeneration. The lipofusion component N-retinyl-N-retinylidene ethanolamine detaches proapoptotic proteins from mitochondria and induces apoptosis in mammalian retinal pigment epithelial cells. J Biol Chem 2000;275: 39625–30.
147. Zhou J, Kim SR, Westlund BS, et al. Complement activation by bisretinoid constituents of RPE lipofuscin. Invest Ophthalmol Vis Sci 2009;50(3):1392–9.
148. Radu RA, Mata NL, Nusinowitz S, et al. Treatment with isotretinoin inhibits lipofuscin accumulation in a mouse model of recessive Stargardt's macular degeneration. Proc Natl Acad Sci U S A 2003;100(8):4742–7.
149. Radu RA, Han Y, Bui TV, et al. Reductions in serum vitamin A arrest accumulation of toxic retinal fluorophores: a potential therapy for treatment of lipofuscin-based retinal diseases. Invest Ophthalmol Vis Sci 2005;46(12):4393–401.
150. Ma L, Kaufman Y, Zhang J, et al. C20-D3-vitamin A slows lipofuscin accumulation and electrophysiological retinal degeneration in a mouse model of Stargardt disease. J Biol Chem 2011;286(10):7966–74.
151. Allocca M, Doria M, Petrillo M, et al. Serotype-dependent packaging of large genes in adeno-associated viral vectors results in effective gene delivery in mice. J Clin Invest 2008;118(5):1955–64.
152. Cideciyan AV, Swider M, Aleman TS, et al. ABCA4 disease progression and a proposed strategy for gene therapy. Hum Mol Genet 2009;18(5):931–41.
153. Kong J, Kim SR, Binley K, et al. Correction of the disease phenotype in the mouse model of Stargardt disease by lentiviral gene therapy. Gene Ther 2008;15(19):1311–20.
154. Bainbridge JW, Smith AJ, Barker SS, et al. Effect of gene therapy on visual function in Leber's congenital amaurosis. N Engl J Med 2008;358(21):2231–9.
155. Maguire AM, Simonelli F, Pierce EA, et al. Safety and efficacy of gene transfer for Leber's congenital amaurosis. N Engl J Med 2008;358(21):2240–8.
156. Stone EM, Nichols BE, Kimura AE, et al. Clinical features of a Stargardt-like dominant progressive macular dystrophy with genetic linkage to chromosome 6q. Arch Ophthalmol 1994;112(6):765–72.
157. Zhang K, Kniazeva M, Han M, et al. A 5-bp deletion in ELOVL4 is associated with two related forms of autosomal dominant macular dystrophy. Nat Genet 2001;27(1):89–93.
158. Bernstein PS, Tammur J, Singh N, et al. Diverse macular dystrophy phenotype caused by a novel complex mutation in the ELOVL4 gene. Invest Ophthalmol Vis Sci 2001;42(13):3331–6.
159. Maugeri A, Meire F, Hoyng CB, et al. A novel mutation in the ELOVL4 gene causes autosomal dominant Stargardt-like macular dystrophy. Invest Ophthalmol Vis Sci 2004;45(12):4263–7.
160. Vasireddy V, Wong P, Ayyagari R. Genetics and molecular pathology of Stargardt-like macular degeneration. Prog Retin Eye Res 2010;29(3):191–207.
161. Agbaga MP, Brush RS, Mandal MN, et al. Role of Stargardt-3 macular dystrophy protein (ELOVL4) in the biosynthesis of very long chain fatty acids. Proc Natl Acad Sci U S A 2008;105:12843–8.
162. Ambasudhan R, Wang X, Jablonski MM, et al. Atrophic macular degeneration mutations in ELOVL4 result in the intracellular misrouting of the protein. Genomics 2004;83(4):615–25.
163. Karan G, Yang Z, Zhang K. Expression of wild type and mutant ELOVL4 in cell culture: subcellular localization and cell viability. Mol Vis 200431;10:248–53.
164. Vasireddy V, Jablonski MM, Khan NW, et al. Elovl4 5-bp deletion knock-in mouse model for Stargardt-like macular degeneration demonstrates accumulation of ELOVL4 and lipofuscin. Exp Eye Res 2009;89(6):905–12.
165. Vasireddy V, Jablonski MM, Mandal MN, et al. Elovl4 5-bp-deletion knock-in mice develop progressive photoreceptor degeneration. Invest Ophthalmol Vis Sci 2006;47(10):4558–68.
166. Deutman AF, van Blommestein JD, Henkes HE, et al. Butterfly-shaped pigment dystrophy of the fovea. Arch Ophthalmol 1970;83(5):558–69.
167. Hsieh RC, Fine BS, Lyons JS. Patterned dystrophies of the retinal pigment epithelium. Arch Ophthalmol 1977;95(3):429–35.
168. Marmor MF, Byers B. Pattern dystrophy of the pigment epithelium. Am J Ophthalmol 1977;84(1):32–44.
169. Epstein GA, Rabb MF. Adult vitelliform macular degeneration: diagnosis and natural history. Br J Ophthalmol 1980;64(10):733–40.
170. Bloom LH, Swanson DE, Bird AC. Adult vitelliform macular degeneration. Br J Ophthalmol 1981;65(11):800–1.
171. Gass JD. A clinicopathologic study of a peculiar foveomacular dystrophy. Trans Am Ophthalmol Soc 1974;72:139–56.
172. Sjogren H. Dystrophia reticularis laminae pigmentosae retinae, an earlier not described hereditary eye disease. Acta Ophthalmol (Copenh) 1950;28(3):279–95.
173. Kingham JD, Fenzl RE, Willerson D, et al. Reticular dystrophy of the retinal pigment epithelium. A clinical and electrophysiologic study of three generations. Arch Ophthalmol 1978;96(7):1177–84.
174. Deutman AF, Rumke AM. Reticular dystrophy of the retinal pigment epithelium. Dystrophia reticularis laminae pigmentosa retinae of H. Sjogren. Arch Ophthalmol 1969;82(1):4–9.
175. Slezak H, Hommer K. [Fundus pulverulentus.] Albrecht Von Graefes Arch Klin Exp Ophthalmol. 1969;178(2):176–82.
176. de Jong PT, Delleman JW. Pigment epithelial pattern dystrophy. Four different manifestations in a family. Arch Ophthalmol 1982;100(9):1416–21.
177. Hoyng CB, Heutink P, Testers L, et al. Autosomal dominant central areolar choroidal dystrophy caused by a mutation in codon 142 in the peripherin/RDS gene. Am J Ophthalmol 1996;121(6):623–9.
178. Kajiwara K, Hahn LB, Mukai S, et al. Mutations in the human retinal degeneration slow gene in autosomal dominant retinitis pigmentosa. Nature 1991;354(6353):480–3.
179. Weleber RG, Carr RE, Murphey WH, et al. Phenotypic variation including retinitis pigmentosa, pattern dystrophy, and fundus flavimaculatus in a single family with a deletion of codon 153 or 154 of the peripherin/RDS gene. Arch Ophthalmol 1993;111(11):1531–42.
180. Farrar GJ, Kenna P, Jordan SA, et al. A three-base-pair deletion in the peripherin-RDS gene in one form of retinitis pigmentosa. Nature 1991; 354(6353):478–80.
181. Farrar GJ, Jordan SA, Kenna P, et al. Autosomal dominant retinitis pigmentosa: localization of a disease gene (RP6) to the short arm of chromosome 6. Genomics 1991;11(4):870–4.
182. Francis PJ, Schultz DW, Gregory AM, et al. Genetic and phenotypic heterogeneity in pattern dystrophy. Br J Ophthalmol 2005;89(9):1115–9.
183. Nichols BE, Sheffield VC, Vandenburgh K, et al. Butterfly-shaped pigment dystrophy of the fovea caused by a point mutation in codon 167 of the RDS gene. Nat Genet 1993;3(3):202–7.
184. Gutman I, Walsh JB, Henkind P. Vitelliform macular dystrophy and butterfly-shaped epithelial dystrophy: a continuum? Br J Ophthalmol 1982;66(3):170–3.
185. Nichols BE, Drack AV, Vandenburgh K, et al. A 2 base pair deletion in the RDS gene associated with butterfly-shaped pigment dystrophy of the fovea. Hum Mol Genet 1993;2(8):1347.

186. Fossarello M, Bertini C, Galantuomo M, et al. Deletion in the peripherin/RDS gene in two unrelated Sardinian families with autosomal dominant butterfly-shaped macular dystrophy. Arch Ophthalmol 1996;114:448–56.
187. Zhang K, Garibaldi DC, Li Y, et al. Butterfly-shaped pattern dystrophy: a genetic, clinical, and histopathological report. Arch Ophthalmol 2002;120(4):485–90.
188. Yang Z, Li Y, Jiang L, et al. A novel RDS/peripherin gene mutation associated with diverse macular phenotypes. Ophthalmic Genet 2004;25(2):133–45.
189. Querques G, Forte R, Querques L, et al. Natural course of adult-onset foveomacular vitelliform dystrophy: a spectral-domain optical coherence tomography analysis. Am J Ophthalmol 2011;152(2);304–13.
190. Arnold JJ, Sarks JP, Killingsworth MC, et al. Adult vitelliform macular degeneration: a clinicopathological study. Eye (Lond) 2003;17(6):717–26.
191. Fishman GA, Woolf MB, Goldberg MF, et al. Reticular tapeto-retinal dystrophy. As a possible late stage of Sjogren's reticular dystrophy. Br J Ophthalmol 1976;60(1):35–40.
192. Chopdar A. Reticular dystrophy of retina. Br J Ophthalmol 1976;60(5):342–4.
193. Kempeneers HP, Dewachter A, Kempeneers GM. Pattern dystrophies of the retinal pigment epithelium. The study of three generations in a family. Doc Ophthalmol 1990;76(3):261–72.
194. Cardillo Piccolino F, Zingirian M. Pattern dystrophy of the retinal pigment epithelium with vitelliform macular lesion: evolution in ten years. Int Ophthalmol 1988;11(4):207–17.
195. Giuffre G, Lodato G. Vitelliform dystrophy and pattern dystrophy of the retinal pigment epithelium: concomitant presence in a family. Br J Ophthalmol 1986;70(7):526–32.
196. Boon CJ, Klevering BJ, Cremers FP, et al. Central areolar choroidal dystrophy. Ophthalmology 2009;116(4):771–82, 82 e1.
197. Yanagihashi S, Nakazawa M, Kurotaki J, et al. Autosomal dominant central areolar choroidal dystrophy and a novel Arg195Leu mutation in the peripherin/RDS gene. Arch Ophthalmol 2003;121(10):1458–61.
198. Reig C, Serra A, Gean E, Vidal M, et al. A point mutation in the RDS-peripherin gene in a Spanish family with central areolar choroidal dystrophy. Ophthalmic Genet 1995;16(2):39–44.
199. Klevering BJ, van Driel M, van Hogerwou AJ, et al. Central areolar choroidal dystrophy associated with dominantly inherited drusen. Br J Ophthalmol 2002;86(1):91–6.
200. Keilhauer CN, Meigen T, Weber BH. Clinical findings in a multigeneration family with autosomal dominant central areolar choroidal dystrophy associated with an Arg195Leu mutation in the peripherin/RDS gene. Arch Ophthalmol 2006;124(7):1020–7.
201. Keilhauer CN, Meigen T, Stohr H, et al. Late-onset central areolar choroidal dystrophy caused by a heterozygous frame-shift mutation affecting codon 307 of the peripherin/RDS gene. Ophthalmic Genet 2006;27(4):139–44.
202. Hoyng CB, van Rijn PM, Deutman AF. Central areolar choroidal dystrophy and slowly progressive sensorineural hearing loss. Acta Ophthalmol Scand 1996;74(6):639–41.
203. Renner AB, Fiebig BS, Weber BH, et al. Phenotypic variability and long-term follow-up of patients with known and novel PRPH2/RDS gene mutations. Am J Ophthalmol 2009;147(3):518–30 e1.
204. Coco RM, Telleria JJ, Sanabria MR, et al. PRPH2 (Peripherin/RDS) mutations associated with different macular dystrophies in a Spanish population: a new mutation. Eur J Ophthalmol 2010;20(4):724–32.
205. Nettleship E. Central senile areolar choroidal atrophy. Trans Ophthalmol Soc UK 1884;4:165–6.
206. Hoyng CB, Pinckers AJ, Deutman AF. Early findings in central areolar choroidal dystrophy. Acta Ophthalmol (Copenh) 1990;68(3):356–60.
207. Carr RE. Central areolar choroidal dystrophy. Arch Ophthalmol 1965;73:32–5.
208. Mansour AM. Central areolar choroidal dystrophy in a family with pseudoachondroplastic spondyloepiphyseal dysplasia. Ophthalmic Paediatr Genet 1988;9(1):57–65.
209. Noble KG. Central areolar choroidal dystrophy. Am J Ophthalmol 1977;84(3):310–8.
210. Gass J. Stereoscopic atlas of macular diseases. 4th ed. St Louis: Mosby; 2001.
211. Fishman GA, Birch DG, Holder GE, et al. Electrophysiologic testing in disorders of the retina, optic nerve, and visual pathway. 2nd ed. (Ophthalmology Monograph 2.) San Francisco: Foundation of the American Academy of Ophthalmology; 2001.
212. Farjo R, Naash MI. The role of Rds in outer segment morphogenesis and human retinal disease. Ophthalmic Genet 2006;27(4):117–22.
213. Bok D. Cellular mechanisms of retinal degenerations: RPE65, ABCA4, RDS, and bicarbonate transporter genes as examples. Retina 2005;(8 Suppl):S18–20.
214. Wickham L, Chen FK, Lewis GP, et al. Clinicopathological case series of four patients with inherited macular disease. Invest Ophthalmol Vis Sci 2009;50(8):3553–61.
215. Kedzierski W, Lloyd M, Birch DG, et al. Generation and analysis of transgenic mice expressing P216L-substituted rds/peripherin in rod photoreceptors. Invest Ophthalmol Vis Sci 1997;38(2):498–509.
216. Parodi MB, Iacono P, Cascavilla M, et al. Intravitreal bevacizumab for subfoveal choroidal neovascularization associated with pattern dystrophy. Invest Ophthalmol Vis Sci 2010;51(9):4358–61.
217. Sorsby A, Mason ME. A fundus dystrophy with unusual features. Br J Ophthalmol 1949;33(2):67–97.
218. Weber BH, Vogt G, Pruett RC, et al. Mutations in the tissue inhibitor of metalloproteinases-3 (TIMP3) in patients with Sorsby's fundus dystrophy. Nat Genet 1994;8(4):352–6.
219. Lin RJ, Blumenkranz MS, Binkley J, et al. A novel His158Arg mutation in TIMP3 causes a late-onset form of Sorsby fundus dystrophy. Am J Ophthalmol 2006;142(5):839–48.
220. Lip PL, Good PA, Gibson JM. Sorsby's fundus dystrophy: a case report of 24 years follow-up with electrodiagnostic tests and indocyanine green angiography. Eye (Lond) 1999;13 (Pt 1):16–25.
221. Sivaprasad S, Webster AR, Egan CA, et al. Clinical course and treatment outcomes of Sorsby fundus dystrophy. Am J Ophthalmol 2008;146(2):228–34.
222. Tabata Y, Isashiki Y, Kamimura K, et al. A novel splice site mutation in the tissue inhibitor of the metalloproteinases-3 gene in Sorsby's fundus dystrophy with unusual clinical features. Hum Genet 1998;103(2):179–82.
223. Langton KP, McKie N, Curtis A, et al. A novel tissue inhibitor of metalloproteinases-3 mutation reveals a common molecular phenotype in Sorsby's fundus dystrophy. J Biol Chem 2000;275(35):27027–31.
224. Barbazetto IA, Hayashi M, Klais CM, et al. A novel TIMP3 mutation associated with Sorsby fundus dystrophy. Arch Ophthalmol 2005;123(4):542–3.
225. Jacobson SG, Cideciyan AV, Bennett J, et al. Novel mutation in the TIMP3 gene causes Sorsby fundus dystrophy. Arch Ophthalmol 2002;120(3):376–9.
226. Jacobson SG, Cideciyan AV, Regunath G, et al. Night blindness in Sorsby's fundus dystrophy reversed by vitamin A. Nat Genet 1995;11(1):27–32.
227. Felbor U, Stohr H, Amann T, et al. A novel Ser156Cys mutation in the tissue inhibitor of metalloproteinases-3 (TIMP3) in Sorsby's fundus dystrophy with unusual clinical features. Hum Mol Genet 1995;4(12):2415–6.
228. Felbor U, Benkwitz C, Klein ML, et al. Sorsby fundus dystrophy: reevaluation of variable expressivity in patients carrying a TIMP3 founder mutation. Arch Ophthalmol 1997;115(12):1569–71.
229. Saihan Z, Li Z, Rice J, et al. Clinical and biochemical effects of the E139K missense mutation in the TIMP3 gene, associated with Sorsby fundus dystrophy. Mol Vis 2009;15:1218–30.
230. Wijesuriya SD, Evans K, Jay MR, et al. Sorsby's fundus dystrophy in the British Isles: demonstration of a striking founder effect by microsatellite-generated haplotypes. Genome Res 1996;6(2):92–101.
231. Gregory-Evans K. What is Sorsby's fundus dystrophy? Br J Ophthalmol 2000;84(7):679–80.
232. Apte SS, Olsen BR, Murphy G. The gene structure of tissue inhibitor of metalloproteinases (TIMP)-3 and its inhibitory activities define the distinct TIMP gene family. J Biol Chem 1995;270(24):14313–8.
233. Qi JH, Ebrahem Q, Moore N, et al. A novel function for tissue inhibitor of metalloproteinases-3 (TIMP3): inhibition of angiogenesis by blockage of VEGF binding to VEGF receptor-2. Nat Med 2003;9(4):407–15.
234. Capon MR, Marshall J, Krafft JI, et al. Sorsby's fundus dystrophy. A light and electron microscopic study. Ophthalmology 1989;96(12):1769–77.
235. Knupp C, Chong NH, Munro PM, et al. Analysis of the collagen VI assemblies associated with Sorsby's fundus dystrophy. J Struct Biol 2002;137(1–2):31–40.
236. Chong NH, Alexander RA, Gin T, et al. TIMP-3, collagen, and elastin immunohistochemistry and histopathology of Sorsby's fundus dystrophy. Invest Ophthalmol Vis Sci 2000;41(3):898–902.
237. Fariss RN, Apte SS, Olsen BR, et al. Tissue inhibitor of metalloproteinases-3 is a component of Bruch's membrane of the eye. Am J Pathol 1997;150(1):323–8.
238. Kamei M, Apte SS, Rayborn ME, et al. TIMP-3 accumulation in Bruch's membrane and drusen in eyes from normal and age-related macular degeneration donors. In: LaVail MM, Anderson RE, Hollyfield JG, editors. Degenerative retinal diseases. New York: Plenum Press; 1997. p. 11–5.
239. Fariss RN, Apte SS, Luthert PJ, et al. Accumulation of tissue inhibitor of metalloproteinases-3 in human eyes with Sorsby's fundus dystrophy or retinitis pigmentosa. Br J Ophthalmol 1998;82(11):1329–34.
240. Langton KP, McKie N, Smith BM, et al. Sorsby's fundus dystrophy mutations impair turnover of TIMP-3 by retinal pigment epithelial cells. Hum Mol Genet 2005;14(23):3579–86.
241. Weber BH, Lin B, White K, et al. A mouse model for Sorsby fundus dystrophy. Invest Ophthalmol Vis Sci 2002;43(8):2732–40.
242. Fogarasi M, Janssen A, Weber BH, et al. Molecular dissection of TIMP3 mutation S156C associated with Sorsby fundus dystrophy. Matrix Biol 2008;27(5):381–92.
243. Holz FG, Haimovici R, Wagner DG, et al. Recurrent choroidal neovascularization after laser photocoagulation in Sorsby's fundus dystrophy. Retina 1994;14(4):329–34.
244. Prager F, Michels S, Geitzenauer W, et al. Choroidal neovascularization secondary to Sorsby fundus dystrophy treated with systemic bevacizumab (Avastin). Acta Ophthalmol Scand 2007;85(8):904–6.
245. Doyne R. A peculiar condition of choroiditis occurring in several members of the same family. Trans Ophthalmol Soc UK 1899;19:71.
246. Vogt A. Handbuch der gesammten Augenheilkunde. Untersuchungsmethoden. 3rd ed. Berlin: Springer Verlag; 1925.
247. Gass J. Diseases causing choroidal exudative and hemorrhagic localized (disciform) detachment of the retina and pigment epithelium. In: Stereoscopic atlas of macular diseases. St Louis: Mosby; 1987. p. 96–7.
248. Heon E, Piguet B, Munier F, et al. Linkage of autosomal dominant radial drusen (malattia leventinese) to chromosome 2p16–21. Arch Ophthalmol 1996;114(2):193–8.
249. Stone EM, Lotery AJ, Munier FL, et al. A single EFEMP1 mutation associated with both Malattia Leventinese and Doyne honeycomb retinal dystrophy. Nat Genet 1999;22(2):199–202.

250. Michaelides M, Jenkins SA, Brantley MA, Jr., et al. Maculopathy due to the R345W substitution in fibulin-3: distinct clinical features, disease variability, and extent of retinal dysfunction. Invest Ophthalmol Vis Sci 2006;47(7): 3085–97.
251. Sohn EH Patel PJ, MacLaren RE, et al. Responsiveness of choroidal neovascular membranes in patients with R345W mutation in fibulin-3 (Doyne honeycomb retinal dystrophy) to anti-VEGF therapy. Arch Ophthalmol 2011;129(12):1626–8.
252. Haimovici R, Wroblewski J, Piguet B, et al. Symptomatic abnormalities of dark adaptation in patients with EFEMP1 retinal dystrophy (Malattia Leventinese/ Doyne honeycomb retinal dystrophy). Eye (Lond) 2002;16(1):7–15.
253. Evans K, Gregory CY, Wijesuriya SD, et al. Assessment of the phenotypic range seen in Doyne honeycomb retinal dystrophy. Arch Ophthalmol 1997;115(7):904–10.
254. Marmorstein LY, Munier FL, Arsenijevic Y, et al. Aberrant accumulation of EFEMP1 underlies drusen formation in Malattia Leventinese and age-related macular degeneration. Proc Natl Acad Sci U S A 2002;99(20):13067–72.
255. Holz FG, Owens SL, Marks J, et al. Ultrastructural findings in autosomal dominant drusen. Arch Ophthalmol 1997;115(6):788–92.
256. Roybal CN, Marmorstein LY, Vander Jagt DL, et al. Aberrant accumulation of fibulin-3 in the endoplasmic reticulum leads to activation of the unfolded protein response and VEGF expression. Invest Ophthalmol Vis Sci 2005; 46(11):3973–9.
257. Fu L, Garland D, Yang Z, et al. The R345W mutation in EFEMP1 is pathogenic and causes AMD-like deposits in mice. Hum Mol Genet 2007;16(20): 2411–22.
258. Marmorstein LY, McLaughlin PJ, Peachey NS, et al. Formation and progression of sub-retinal pigment epithelium deposits in Efemp1 mutation knock-in mice: a model for the early pathogenic course of macular degeneration. Hum Mol Genet 2007;16(20):2423–32.
259. Blackburn J, Tarttelin EE, Gregory-Evans CY, et al. Transcriptional regulation and expression of the dominant drusen gene FBLN3 (EFEMP1) in mammalian retina. Invest Ophthalmol Vis Sci 2003;44(11):4613–21.
260. Lefler WH, Wadsworth JA, Sidbury JB, Jr. Hereditary macular degeneration and amino-aciduria. Am J Ophthalmol 1971;71(1 Pt 2):224–30.
261. Frank HR, Landers MB, 3rd, Williams RJ, et al. A new dominant progressive foveal dystrophy. Am J Ophthalmol 1974;78(6):903–16.
262. Small KW. North Carolina macular dystrophy: clinical features, genealogy, and genetic linkage analysis. Trans Am Ophthalmol Soc 1998;96:925–61.
263. Reichel MB, Kelsell RE, Fan J, et al. Phenotype of a British North Carolina macular dystrophy family linked to chromosome 6q. Br J Ophthalmol 1998;82(10):1162–8.
264. Pauleikhoff D, Sauer CG, Muller CR, et al. Clinical and genetic evidence for autosomal dominant North Carolina macular dystrophy in a German family. Am J Ophthalmol 1997;124(3):412–5.
265. Small KW, Puech B, Mullen L, et al. North Carolina macular dystrophy phenotype in France maps to the MCDR1 locus. Mol Vis 1997;3:1.
266. Rabb MF, Mullen L, Yelchits S, et al. A North Carolina macular dystrophy phenotype in a Belizean family maps to the MCDR1 locus. Am J Ophthalmol 1998;125(4):502–8.
267. Kim SJ, Woo SJ, Yu HG. A Korean family with an early-onset autosomal dominant macular dystrophy resembling North Carolina macular dystrophy. Korean J Ophthalmol 2006;20(4):220–4.
268. Fetkenhour CL, Gurney N, Dobbie JG, et al. Central areolar pigment epithelial dystrophy. Am J Ophthalmol 1976;81(6):745–53.
269. Small KW, Killian J, McLean WC. North Carolina's dominant progressive foveal dystrophy: how progressive is it? Br J Ophthalmol 1991;75(7):401–6.
270. Small KW. North Carolina macular dystrophy, revisited. Ophthalmology 1989;96(12):1747–54.
271. Small KW, Weber JL, Hung WY, et al. North Carolina macular dystrophy: exclusion map using RFLPs and microsatellites. Genomics 1991;11(3):763–6.
272. Small KW, Weber JL, Roses A, et al. North Carolina macular dystrophy is assigned to chromosome 6. Genomics 1992;13(3):681–5.
273. Small KW, Udar N, Yelchits S, et al. North Carolina macular dystrophy (MCDR1) locus: a fine resolution genetic map and haplotype analysis. Mol Vis 1999;5:38.
274. Michaelides M, Johnson S, Tekriwal AK, et al. An early-onset autosomal dominant macular dystrophy (MCDR3) resembling North Carolina macular dystrophy maps to chromosome 5. Invest Ophthalmol Vis Sci 2003;44(5): 2178–83.
275. Rosenberg T, Roos B, Johnsen T, et al. Clinical and genetic characterization of a Danish family with North Carolina macular dystrophy. Mol Vis 2010; 16:2659–68.
276. Small KW, Voo I, Flannery J, et al. North Carolina macular dystrophy: clinicopathologic correlation. Trans Am Ophthalmol Soc 2001;99:233–7; discussion 7–8.
277. Mahajan VB, Russell SR, Stone EM. A new macular dystrophy with anomalous vascular development, pigment spots, cystic spaces, and neovascularization. Arch Ophthalmol 2009;127(11):1449–57.
278. Deutman AF, Pinckers AJ, Aan de Kerk AL. Dominantly inherited cystoid macular edema. Am J Ophthalmol 1976;82(4):540–8.
279. Fishman GA, Goldberg MF, Trautmann JC. Dominantly inherited cystoid macular edema. Ann Ophthalmol 1979;11(1):21–7.
280. Kremer H, Pinckers A, van den Helm B, et al. Localization of the gene for dominant cystoid macular dystrophy on chromosome 7p. Hum Mol Genet 1994;3(2):299–302.
281. Hogewind BF, Pieters G, Hoyng CB. Octreotide acetate in dominant cystoid macular dystrophy. Eur J Ophthalmol 2008;18(1):99–103.
282. Sneed SR, Sieving PA. Fenestrated sheen macular dystrophy. Am J Ophthalmol 1991;112(1):1–7.
283. Daily MJ, Mets MB. Fenestrated sheen macular dystrophy. Arch Ophthalmol 1984;102(6):855–6.
284. Slagsvold JE. Fenestrated sheen macular dystrophy. A new autosomal dominant maculopathy. Acta Ophthalmol (Copenh) 1981;59(5):683–8.
285. O'Donnell FE, Jr., Welch RB. Fenestrated sheen macular dystrophy. A new autosomal dominant maculopathy. Arch Ophthalmol 1979;97(7):1292–6.
286. McAvoy CE, Silvestri G. Retinal changes associated with type 2 glomerulonephritis. Eye (Lond) 2005;19(9):985–9.
287. D'Souza Y, Short CD, McLeod D, et al. Long-term follow-up of drusen-like lesions in patients with type II mesangiocapillary glomerulonephritis. Br J Ophthalmol 2008;92(7):950–3.
288. Leys A, Vanrenterghem Y, Van Damme B, et al. Sequential observation of fundus changes in patients with long standing membranoproliferative glomerulonephritis type II (MPGN type II). Eur J Ophthalmol 1991;1(1):17–22.
289. Leys A, Vanrenterghem Y, Van Damme B, et al. Fundus changes in membranoproliferative glomerulonephritis type II. A fluorescein angiographic study of 23 patients. Graefes Arch Clin Exp Ophthalmol 1991;229(5):406–10.
290. Ulbig MR, Riordan-Eva P, Holz FG, et al. Membranoproliferative glomerulonephritis type II associated with central serous retinopathy. Am J Ophthalmol 1993;116(4):410–3.
291. Kim RY, Faktorovich EG, Kuo CY, et al. Retinal function abnormalities in membranoproliferative glomerulonephritis type II. Am J Ophthalmol 1997; 123(5):619–28.
292. O'Brien C, Duvall-Young J, Brown M, et al. Electrophysiology of type II mesangiocapillary glomerulonephritis with associated fundus abnormalities. Br J Ophthalmol 1993;77(12):778–80.
293. Duvall-Young J, MacDonald MK, McKechnie NM. Fundus changes in (type II) mesangiocapillary glomerulonephritis simulating drusen: a histopathological report. Br J Ophthalmol 1989;73(4):297–302.
294. Mullins RF, Aptsiauri N, Hageman GS. Structure and composition of drusen associated with glomerulonephritis: implications for the role of complement activation in drusen biogenesis. Eye (Lond) 2001;15(Pt 3):390–5.
295. Mullins RF, Russell SR, Anderson DH, et al. Drusen associated with aging and age-related macular degeneration contain proteins common to extracellular deposits associated with atherosclerosis, elastosis, amyloidosis, and dense deposit disease. FASEB J 2000;14(7):835–46.

For additional online content visit http://www.expertconsult.com

Chapter 43

Hereditary Choroidal Diseases

Mohamed A. Genead, Gerald A. Fishman, Sandeep Grover

INTRODUCTION

The term "choroidal dystrophy" is likely a misnomer as it implies a primary degenerative process involving the choroidal circulation. However, the current evidence focuses on the retinal pigment epithelium (RPE) as playing an important, if not pivotal, role in the disorders categorized under the rubric of choroidal dystrophy since genetic mutations that affect the RPE can lead to atrophic changes of both the RPE and choriocapillaris.

Nonetheless, the hereditary choroidal dystrophies can be classified in the following manner: (1) choroidal atrophy phenotypes, which can be further subdivided into: (a) central areolar choroidal dystrophy (CACD); (b) peripapillary choroidal dystrophy; and (c) diffuse choroidal dystrophy; (2) gyrate atrophy of the choroid and retina; and (3) choroideremia (CHM). While each of the choroidal dystrophies has characteristic fundus features, in certain instances at advanced stages of disease an overlap in fundus appearance may be observed (Table 43.1).

The common feature of these disorders is degenerative changes of the RPE in the early stages that progress to involve the choriocapillaris, photoreceptor cell layer, and in later stages, the larger choroidal vessels. Whether an abnormality in the choriocapillaris or even photoreceptor cells occurs concurrently with degenerative changes in the RPE has not been conclusively determined. Certain of these dystrophies are generalized and progressive (CHM, gyrate atrophy, and diffuse choroidal dystrophy) whereas others are more localized, either remaining geographically confined (CACD) or progressively expanding (peripapillary choroidal dystrophy) to involve more extensive regions of the fundus. In the advanced stages of certain choroidal dystrophies, the loss of RPE cells, retinal and choroidal tissue, as well as pigment accumulation, may not be easily differentiated from the fundus changes observed in certain other hereditary degenerative or inflammatory retinal disorders.

Table 43.1 Brief outline of chapter layout

1. Choroidal atrophy phenotypes
   A. Central areolar choroidal dystrophy
   B. Peripapillary choroidal dystrophy
   C. Diffuse choroidal dystrophy
2. Gyrate atrophy of the choroid and retina
3. Choroideremia
4. Clinical phenotypes resembling hereditary choroidal diseases
   A. Advanced stage of X-linked retinitis pigmentosa
   B. Advanced stage of Kearns–Sayre syndrome
   C. Bietti's crystalline dystrophy
   D. Thioridazine (Mellaril) retinal toxicity
   E. Advanced stage of Stargardt disease
   F. Advanced stage of pattern dystrophy

CHOROIDAL ATROPHY PHENOTYPES

According to Sorsby,[1] this group of disorders can be subdivided into three clinical phenotypes based on their geographical distribution. They include: central areolar, peripapillary, and more diffuse or generalized choroidal dystrophy. All can be inherited as either autosomal dominant or autosomal recessive traits.

Central areolar choroidal dystrophy

CACD was first described by Nettleship in 1884. It is inherited primarily as an autosomal dominant trait,[2,3] although autosomal recessive cases have been occasionally reported.[4,5] Yanagihashi and colleagues[6] identified a novel mutation in the peripherin/RDS (retinal degeneration slow) gene in a Japanese family with an autosomal dominant form of CACD.

The initial symptoms of diminished central vision generally begin in the latter part of the second to the early part of the fourth decade. Characteristic bilateral macular lesions are solitary with well-defined margins, and circular or ovoid in shape (Fig. 43.1). Although they may increase in size and become irregular in shape, they do not involve the peripapillary region or extend beyond the vascular arcades.

The early fundus changes include a mottling of the RPE in the macula. At this stage, the underlying choroid may appear ophthalmoscopically normal. With the subsequent loss of RPE and choriocapillaris, the underlying choroidal vessels are more readily visualized. With continued loss of RPE and choriocapillaris, the larger choroidal vessels may undergo degeneration. In

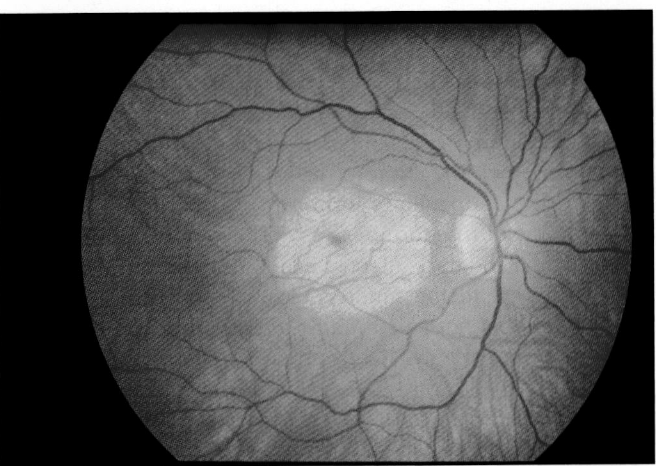

Fig. 43.1 Color fundus photograph from the right eye of a patient with central areolar choroidal dystrophy shows a well-defined, oval-shaped hypopigmented atrophic macular lesion.

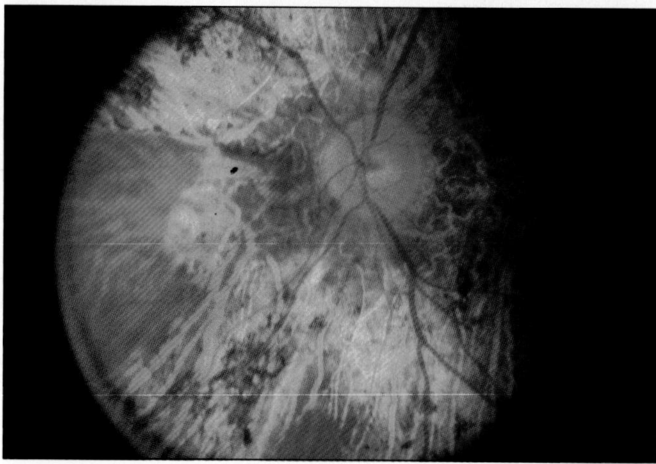

Fig. 43.2 Color fundus photograph from the left eye of a patient with peripapillary choroidal dystrophy shows both retinal pigment epithelium and choroidal atrophy in a region predominantly around the optic disc.

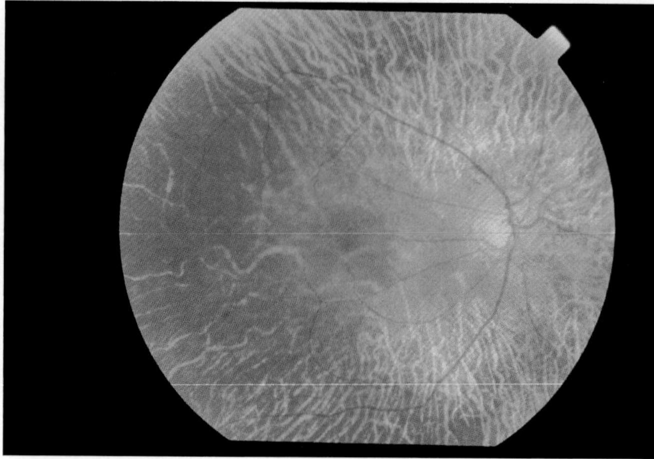

Fig. 43.3 Color fundus photograph from the right eye of a patient with an advanced stage of diffuse choroidal dystrophy shows diffuse retinal pigment epithelium and choroidal atrophy. Both the posterior pole and the retinal periphery are involved to varying degrees.

advanced stages of disease, the sclera is visible as a consequence of choroidal atrophy. Fluorescein angiography at the early stages of the disease shows hyperfluorescence (window defect) due to increased transmission from the underlying normal choriocapillaris. The optic disc and retinal vessels remain normal. Traditionally, full-field electroretinographic (ERG) amplitudes are normal. In some cases, patients may show reduced cone function. In these instances, consideration should be given to the diagnosis of cone dystrophy.

A few other inherited retinal disorders may show a CACD macular phenotype in their more advanced stages. These, in part, include Stargardt disease, cone dystrophy, North Carolina macular dystrophy, and pattern dystrophy as well as the geographic atrophic macular lesion that can be observed in age-related macular degeneration.

Peripapillary choroidal dystrophy

The peripapillary form of choroidal dystrophy is usually inherited as an autosomal recessive trait,[7] although in some instances autosomal dominant transmission may be encountered.

The fundus findings in this form of choroidal dystrophy initially include changes seen in the RPE and later an ophthalmoscopically apparent loss of RPE and choroidal tissue. The important distinction between CACD and the peripapillary phenotype is their location. The peripapillary form begins in the region surrounding the optic disc and slowly enlarges, in finger-like projections, nasally, temporally, and into the macula, eventually occupying the entire posterior pole (Fig. 43.2). In some instances the peripapillary form can progress to a phenotype similar to the diffuse form.

Visual field and dark-adapted final thresholds testing indicate that peripheral to the fundoscopically involved area, retinal function is either normal or mildly impaired. The full-field ERG is either normal or only slightly reduced, reflecting the extent of the disease.[7,8]

The differential diagnosis includes peripapillary pigment epithelial dystrophy in which there are well-defined areas of RPE loss, with direct visualization of the underlying choroidal vasculature. Fluorescein angiography shows an intact choriocapillaris that differentiates it from those with choriocapillaris loss.[7] Another disorder that mimics peripapillary choroidal dystrophy is serpiginous choroiditis, which usually begins in the peripapillary region and then extends into the retina in pseudopod-like extensions, sometimes involving the macula.

Diffuse choroidal dystrophy

This diffuse disorder of the RPE and choriocapillaris is most often inherited as an autosomal dominant trait;[9] however, autosomal recessive transmission may occur. The onset of symptoms occurs most often in the fourth and fifth decade and is usually manifested by poor central vision, impairment of night vision, or both.

The early fundus changes include retinal pigment mottling and hypopigmentation. The disease may initially show a predilection for the posterior pole of the retina before progressing to a more diffuse phenotype. Later there is diffuse atrophy of both the RPE and choriocapillaris while the larger choroid vessels appear sclerotic as yellowish-white bands. Both the posterior pole and the periphery are involved to varying degrees. Even with diffuse involvement in the more advanced stages, the retinal vessels usually remain normal[10] (Fig. 43.3). In the end stages, diffuse choroidal dystrophy cannot be easily differentiated from other diffuse chorioretinal diseases such as thioridazine (Mellaril) retinal toxicity, advanced stages of both pattern dystrophy and Stargardt disease, in addition to the advanced retinopathy seen in the Kearns–Sayre syndrome.

Psychophysical and electrophysiological studies reflect the diffuse involvement. Visual fields show a concentric peripheral constriction, while ERG recordings are either subnormal[10] or undetectable.[7] Fluorescein angiography shows a loss of the choriocapillaris and visualization of the larger choroidal vessels beneath atrophic-appearing RPE.[7,11] A few scattered areas show a patchy choroidal flush pattern indicative of some remnants of the choriocapillaris.

GYRATE ATROPHY OF THE CHOROID AND RETINA

The first case of this disease was described in 1888 by Jacobsohn[12] as an example of "atypical retinitis pigmentosa"; however,

Cutler[13] in 1895 and Fuchs[14] in 1896 were the first to recognize the disease as a distinct clinical entity. Gyrate atrophy is a rare choroidal disease with a prevalence of about 1 in 50 000 in Finland.[15] It is inherited as an autosomal recessive trait, although dominant pedigrees have also been reported.[10] The biochemical abnormalities observed in this disorder were initially described by Simell and Takki[16] in 1973; these included a deficiency of the enzyme ornithine-delta-aminotransferase (OAT), which results in an increase in the plasma ornithine concentration (10–15 times the normal levels). The enzyme OAT is a mitochondrial-encoded enzyme with pyridoxal phosphate (vitamin B_6) enzyme as a cofactor that catalyzes the interconversion of ornithine, glutamate, and proline. This results in systemic biochemical abnormalities, including hyperornithinemia, and reductions in plasma lysine, glutamine, glutamate, and creatine.[17–19] Either an absence or a marked reduction of OAT in cultured skin fibroblasts and in lymphocytes has been observed.[20] A number of different mutations have been identified within the OAT gene on chromosome 10.[21–23] Kellner and colleagues[24] previously described a gyrate atrophy-like phenotype in 6 male patients, 3 of whom were patients of the same family, with normal serum ornithine levels.

The onset of visual symptoms, including poor night vision and constricted peripheral vision, usually begins in the second and third decades. Since both structural and visual functional changes spread from more peripheral to a central location, loss of visual acuity is a later complaint in the disease. Myopia and posterior subcapsular cataracts are frequently observed and vitreous opacities may also be present.[15]

The fundus changes begin in the midperipheral and peripheral retina with a thinning and atrophic appearance of the RPE in which the underlying choroidal vessels may appear either normal or sclerotic. These areas are typically scalloped in shape and are initially separate but tend to become confluent as they slowly progress both centrally and peripherally (Fig. 43.4). Progression of the disease leads to pigment clumping, RPE and choriocapillaris atrophy, and eventual total atrophy of the choroid exposing the white sclera. In the late stages, an annular ring of choroidal atrophy may be seen from the periphery to the posterior pole, usually sparing the macula. The retinal vessels may appear normal initially or attenuated in later stages of the disease when the optic nerve may appear pale.[7,10]

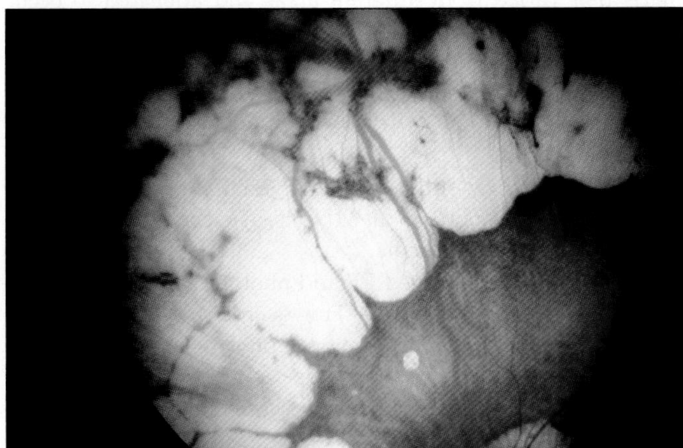

Fig. 43.4 Color fundus photograph from the left eye of a patient with gyrate atrophy of the choroid and retina shows the typical scalloped areas of retinal pigment epithelium and choroidal atrophy.

There are reports on the presence of cystoid macular edema in patients with gyrate atrophy.[25–27] A study by Vasconcelos-Santos et al.[27] showed a short-term therapeutic effect with the use of a 4-mg intravitreal triamcinolone acetonide injection for gyrate atrophy-related macular edema. After drug clearance, the edema recurred, with return of visual acuity to the pretreatment level.

Visual function varies considerably from case to case and seems to be related to the extent of fundus involvement. Visual field testing shows a concentric peripheral constriction of the visual field as the most often observed abnormality. However, an annular ring and paracentral scotomas may develop as the disease progresses. Eventually, if the fovea becomes involved, a central scotoma will be seen.[7,28]

Early in the disease, dark adaptation testing shows only mild threshold elevations while significant elevation of the final rod thresholds is eventually noted in most patients. In the early stage, full-field ERG recordings may show only a mild abnormality in rod and cone amplitudes, while, as the disease progress, the ERG responses deteriorate and may eventually become undetectable. The rod responses are affected more severely in the early stages, but later both cone as well as rod function is severely impaired.[29,30] The electro-oculogram (EOG) is normal or only mildly reduced at very early stages. The EOG light peak to dark trough ratio becomes markedly reduced in the later stages. Electromyograms are often abnormal, although only a few patients complain of mild muscle weakness. Muscle biopsy shows atrophic type 2 muscle fibers with tubular aggregates visible on electron microscopy.[31,32] Both electrocardiographic and electroencephalographic abnormalities may be observed in some patients.[33,34] Histopathologic studies show early changes in RPE cells, with subsequent loss of photoreceptors and choriocapillaris, suggesting that these latter changes may be secondary to the loss of RPE cell integrity.[35] A report of a histologic study in the ornithine-deficient mouse model of gyrate atrophy[36] is available online.

An arginine-restricted diet has been pursued as a form of therapy in patients with gyrate atrophy of the choroid and retina.[17,37–39] Since ornithine is produced from other amino acids, mainly arginine, some investigators advocate that patients be restricted to a rigid low-protein diet, including near-total elimination of arginine with supplementation of essential amino acids. Orally administered pyridoxal phosphate (vitamin B_6), can result in a reduction in plasma ornithine levels in some patients, while others are nonresponsive to B_6.[29] Overall, ERG responses are better maintained by B_6-responsive patients compared to those who are nonresponders.[29,37] While Kaiser-Kupfer et al.[38] concluded that a dietary approach to reducing plasma ornithine was effective, this was not similarly observed to occur in patients with gyrate atrophy in studies by Vannas-Sulonen et al.[39] or Berson et al.[37]

CHOROIDEREMIA

Mauthner in 1872[40] was the first to describe the clinical features of CHM, which is a generalized degeneration of the retina, inherited as an X-linked recessive trait,[41] with an estimated prevalence of 1 in 50 000.[42] The onset of symptoms occurs in the first and second decades with impairment of night vision and peripheral visual field loss. Central vision is most often preserved until later in life. Males in their 40s generally have useful visual acuity, but typically only a small residual visual field. Later (ages 50–70 years), central vision is more substantially reduced. In a study of 115 males with CHM (mean age 39 years), a slow rate of visual acuity loss with the retention of central visual acuity until the seventh decade was found.[43]

Fundus changes are readily apparent by the second decade of life or earlier. A 22-month-old infant with fundus changes has been described.[41] The clinical diagnosis of affected males is characterized by the following:[43]

- A history of defective dark adaptation, manifesting as poor visual function in dim illumination is commonly the first symptom. Males may not show this impairment until their early teens.
- The fundus changes in affected males undergo a characteristic progression. The initial appearance is a fine, peppery-like retinal pigment mottling at the midperipheral retina and posterior pole. At this stage, the ERG is abnormal, showing reduced or absent scotopic responses.[10] Focal disturbances in the RPE consisting of pigmentary loss or a metallic sheen follow the "salt and pepper" mottling while the underlying choroid may appear normal or show choriocapillaris atrophy. Occasionally, these areas of focal disturbances assume a shape similar to gyrate atrophy, and the distinction between the two diseases may be difficult on the basis of the fundus appearance (Fig. 43.5). Atrophy of the choroid follows with eventual loss of the entire layer and exposure of bare sclera. The rate of progression will vary from individual to individual and from family to family. These changes are initially most apparent in the midperipheral retina and progress centrally, the macula being the last affected, with central vision preserved until later in the disease. In the final stage, the fundus shows an extensive yellowish-white reflex from the sclera (Fig. 43.6). Cystoid macular edema has recently been described by Genead and Fishman[44] to be present in 63% of patients in a small ($n = 16$) cohort.

1. Peripheral visual field loss manifests as a ring scotoma that corresponds to areas of chorioretinal degeneration.
2. Even in the early stages of the disease, the ERG is most often abnormal under both light- and dark-adapted conditions. The ERG may be normal early in the course of the disease when only a few focal lesions are present,[45] but eventually becomes undetectable in most.[45] Nonetheless, a wide intrafamilial and interfamilial variability in ERG amplitudes with age has been observed.[46] EOG recordings show an abnormally low light peak to dark trough ratio.

Visual field testing in affected males is generally normal when only minor pigmentary changes are present at the early stages of the disease. With the occurrence of equatorial and peripapillary choroidal vascular atrophy, there is not infrequently the development of corresponding equatorial diminished retinal sensitivity or ring scotomas and an enlarged blind spot. Gradual deterioration of visual field occurs and ultimately, by the fifth and sixth decades, the patient may show a field of less than 10°. Occasionally, a few peripheral islets of vision remain.

Dark adaptation testing is normal if the patient is seen at an early stage. In general, there is initially an abnormality of the rod portion of the dark adaptation curve. There is progressive deterioration of rod dark adaptation, and eventually the cone portion of the curve becomes involved as well.

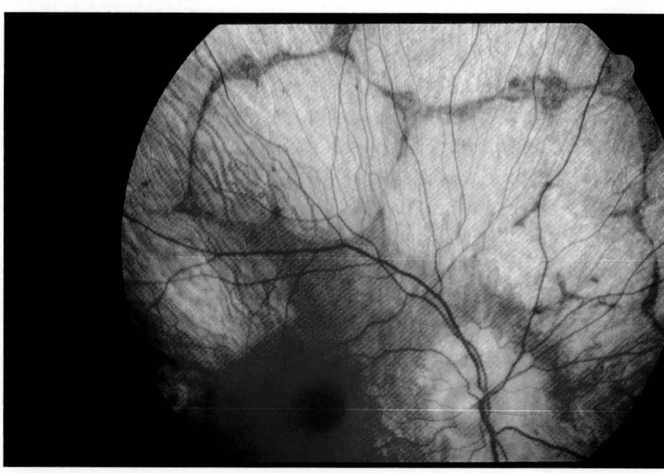

Fig. 43.5 Color fundus photograph from the right eye of a patient with choroideremia shows scalloped areas of retinal pigment epithelium and choroidal atrophy that shows a similarity to lesions observed in patients with gyrate atrophy of the choroid and retina.

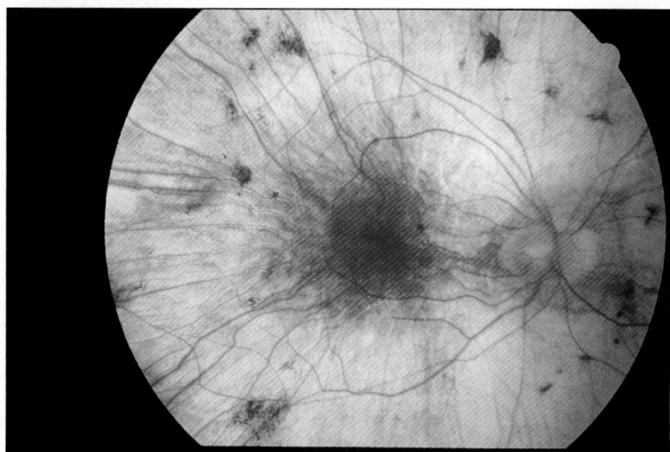

Fig. 43.6 Color fundus photograph from the right eye of a patient with an advanced stage of choroideremia shows a yellowish-white reflex from the sclera due to the extensive atrophy of the retinal pigment epithelium and choroid in the midperipheral retina and posterior pole with scattered pigment clumps. The macula shows relative sparing.

Histopathologic examination of a 30-year-old man with CHM showed diffuse abnormalities of the retina, RPE, and choriocapillaris that varied from different areas and appeared to occur independently of each other. In addition, mild T-lymphocyte infiltration was found within the choroid.[47] Prior pathological specimens[41,48–50] from patients afflicted with CHM showed the following:

1. Extensive atrophy of the choroidal vasculature and Bruch's membrane was found in all subjects. The choroid was most recognizable at the macula.
2. Extensive atrophy of the RPE and photoreceptors was common even in the macula. However, in the eye from the youngest patient, distinct photoreceptor nuclei were seen in the macula.
3. In general, the retinal bipolar, ganglion, and nerve fiber layers were normal.
4. The optic nerve showed an increase in glial tissue within the septa and mild cystoid degeneration among the axons in the neural channels.

The CHM gene was localized to the long arm of the X chromosome (Xq21).[51,52] The gene encodes the Rab escort protein-1 (REP-1) that is involved in the prenylation of Rabs. The REP-1 protein facilitates posttranslational modification of Rab proteins, which regulate intracellular trafficking in the RPE and photoreceptors and is likely involved in the removal of outer-segment disc membranes by the RPE.[53] All currently described mutations in *REP-1/CHM*, including deletions, translocations, and mutations, result in protein truncation due to replacement of an arginine residue with a stop codon.[54] In 1998, MacDonald et al.[55] observed the absence of *REP-1* in peripheral lymphocytes of affected individuals that led to the development of an immunoblot assay using anti-REP-1 antibodies to diagnose patients with CHM.

The carrier females of X-linked CHM show the following:

1. With few exceptions, fundus changes are considerably milder than those observed in affected males. Typically there is pigment mottling, best seen in the midperipheral retina, which may also be apparent in the macula. This finding becomes more readily evident after the second decade and has been described as showing a "moth-eaten appearance." Some of the pigmentary changes in carriers consist of radial bands that course from the midperipheral retina toward the ora serrata (Fig. 43.7). There is no apparent relation between the degree of fundus pigmentary changes and the age of a carrier. The pigmentary changes observed in carriers are due to a skewed X-chromosome inactivation or the presence of an X-chromosome translocation involving Xq21.[56]
2. In most instances, carrier females do not experience significant visual impairment and in general are asymptomatic. However, carrier females may show changes on ERG, dark adaptation, visual field, and macular microperimetry testing.[57] The ERG may be normal, even in carriers with pigmentary fundus changes. EOG recordings characteristically show no abnormality in the light peak to dark trough ratio.[58] Measurement of fundus autofluorescence may demonstrate patchy areas of autofluorescence loss.[59]
3. There are occasional case reports[60,61] in which the carrier female may have retinal and functional changes similar to affected male patients, but such findings are a rarity.

A histopathologic study[62] of an eye from an 88-year-old carrier of CHM showed a patchy degeneration of photoreceptors and RPE cells that were not strictly concordant. The choriocapillaris was described as normal, except in regions of severe retinal degeneration. Immunofluorescence analysis, with a mouse monoclonal antibody, localized the CHM gene product, *REP-1*, to the rod cytoplasm and amacrine cells but not in cone cells.[62] This observation suggests the possibility that the primary site of this disease may reside in the rods rather than in the RPE or choroid. Labeling observed within small vesicles in the rod cytoplasm is consistent with the association of *REP-1* with intracellular vesicular transport.

CLINICAL PHENOTYPES RESEMBLING HEREDITARY CHOROIDAL DISEASES

X-linked retinitis pigmentosa (XLRP)

RP is a group of inherited disorders in which abnormalities of the RPE and photoreceptors lead to progressive visual loss. The initial symptoms of RP include night vision impairment and restriction of the peripheral visual field. A diagnosis of RP includes abnormalities on ERG testing. RP can be inherited in an autosomal dominant, autosomal recessive, or X-linked manner. Mutations in *RPGR* (also called *RP3*) and *RP2* genes are the most common causes of XLRP. Linkage studies suggest that they account for 70–90% and 10–20%, respectively, of XLRP. In the later stages of particularly CHM, when the loss of choroid and retina is significant, the fundus appearance may be confused with end-stage XLRP; however, the degree and appearance of pigment migration into the retina that typifies RP are not characteriscally seen in individuals with CHM (Figs 43.8 and 43.9).

Kearns–Sayre syndrome (KSS)

This disease represents a multisystem mitochondrial DNA deletion syndrome that is observed before 20 years of age and consists of a pigmentary retinopathy (Figs 43.10 and 43.11),

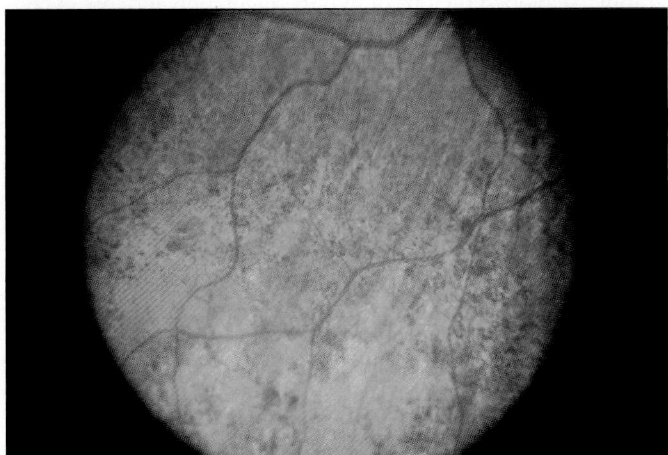

Fig. 43.7 Color fundus photograph from the right eye of a carrier for X-linked choroideremia shows the typical pigment granularity or mottling in the midperipheral retina referred to as a "moth-eaten appearance."

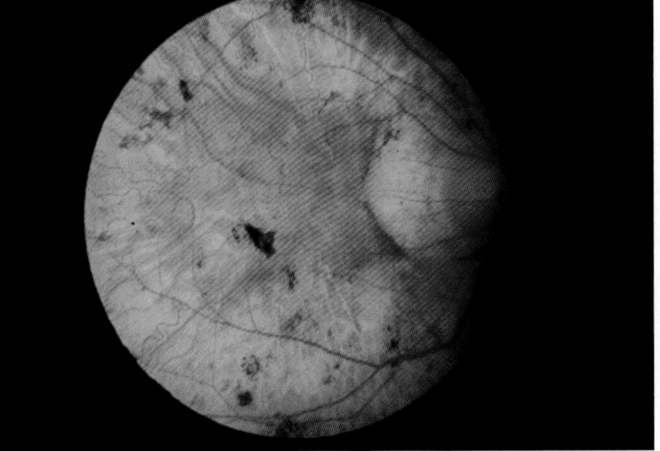

Fig. 43.8 Color fundus photograph from the right eye of a patient with an advanced stage of X-linked retinitis pigmentosa shows extensive atrophy of retinal pigment epithelium and choroid in the posterior pole and midperipheral retina with scattered pigment clumps. The retinal vessels are attenuated.

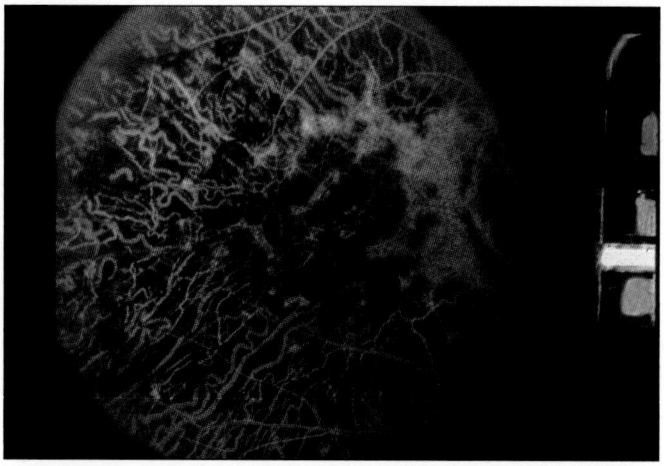

Fig. 43.9 Fluorescein angiogram from the right eye from the same patient depicted in Figure 43.8 with X-linked retinitis pigmentosa shows extensive atrophy of the retinal pigment epithelium and choriocapillaris corresponding to the pigmentary changes seen ophthalmoscopically.

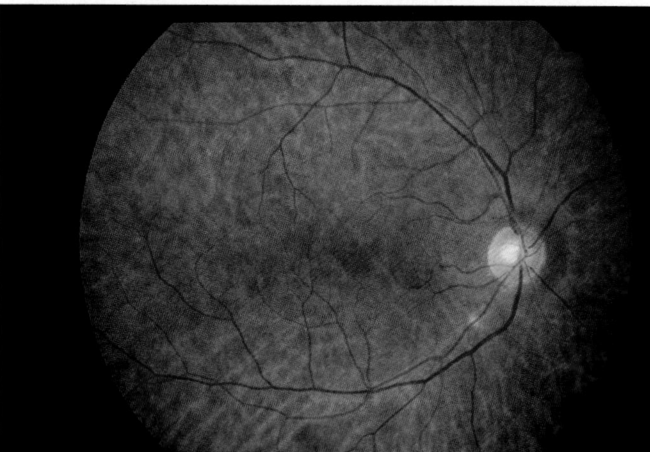

Fig. 43.10 Color fundus photograph from the right eye of a patient with Kearns–Sayre syndrome shows diffuse hypopigmentary changes in the posterior pole and midperipheral retina.

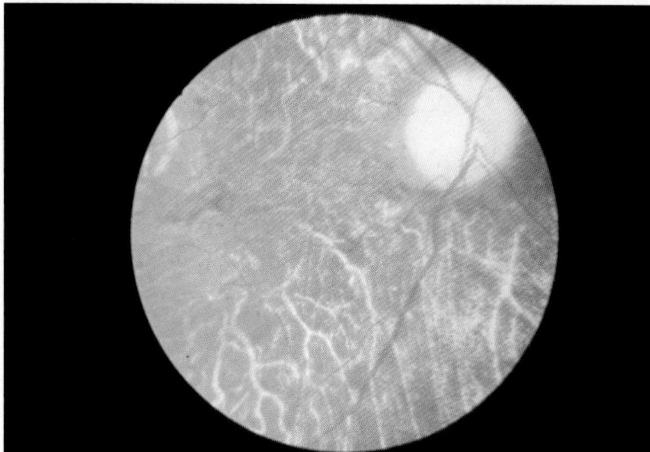

Fig. 43.11 Color fundus photograph from the right eye of a patient with Kearns–Sayre syndrome shows generalized atrophy of the retinal pigment epithelium and choroid that resembles diffuse choroidal dystrophy.

progressive external ophthalmoplegia, as well as ptosis. In addition, patients may have at least one of the following: cardiac conduction block, cerebellar ataxia, or cerebrospinal fluid protein concentration greater than 100 mg/dL. Muscle biopsy in such patients shows ragged red fibers by light microscopy and mitochondrial abnormalities by high-resolution microscopy. Three phenotypes were described by Bastiaensen et al.,[63] including infantile, juvenile, and adult-onset forms. In some patients with advanced disease, a generalized atrophy of the RPE and choriocapillaris can be encountered (Fig. 43.11). Subnormal cone and rod a- and b-wave amplitudes are most frequently observed in patients with Kearns–Sayre syndrome.

Bietti's crystalline dystrophy

Patients affected with Bietti's crystalline dystrophy most often present within the third decade of life with visual impairment and glistening crystalline-like changes in the posterior pole of the retina. Approximately one-third will also show crystals in the superficial stromal layer of the paralimbal region of the cornea. These cholesterol or cholesterol esters can also be found in fibroblasts as well as circulating lymphocytes, suggesting that this disorder may be a systemic abnormality of lipid metabolism. Both diffuse and more localized forms of retinal degenerative changes may be encountered. These changes involve both RPE and choriocapillaris atrophy and in this sense represent an overlap with the changes observed in choroidal dystrophies. ERG amplitude reduction often parallels the degree of fundus pigmentary changes. The disease is most often transmitted as an autosomal recessive trait. Gekka and colleagues[64] identified a mutation in the *CYP4V2* gene in two Japanese patients with Bietti's crystalline dystrophy.

Thioridazine (Mellaril) retinal toxicity

Thioridazine was initially introduced in 1959 for the treatment of psychosis. Patients who receive relatively high doses of the drug can experience a decrease in their visual acuity as well as night blindness. Both central and ring scotomas have been observed. In earlier stages, a pigmentary granularity or mottling occurs in the macular or paramacular regions. Subsequently, extensive degenerative changes of the RPE, choriocapillaris, and photoreceptors are seen (Fig. 43.12). A phenotype with geographic, scalloped regions of hypopigmentation and loss of choriocapillaris vessels may become evident. Both this intermediate and a more advanced and more diffuse disease stage can mimic fundus changes seen in CHM, gyrate atrophy and diffuse choroidal dystrophy phenotypes. ERG recordings show various degrees of diminished photopic and scotopic a- and b-wave responses that parallel in severity the clinically evident fundus changes.

Stargardt disease

This disease is typically characterized by impairment of central vision within the first 10–20 years of life that often progresses to the level of legal blindness. The peripheral vision is most often preserved. There is a characteristic "beaten bronze" appearance of the macula, with small pisciform yellow-white flecks scattered within the posterior pole and, to a lesser extent, in the midperipheral retina. In the majority of affected patients, fluorescein angiography shows a masking of the fluorescence from the choroidal circulation (dark choroid).[65–68] Although the inheritance is usually autosomal recessive,[69] rare families have been reported

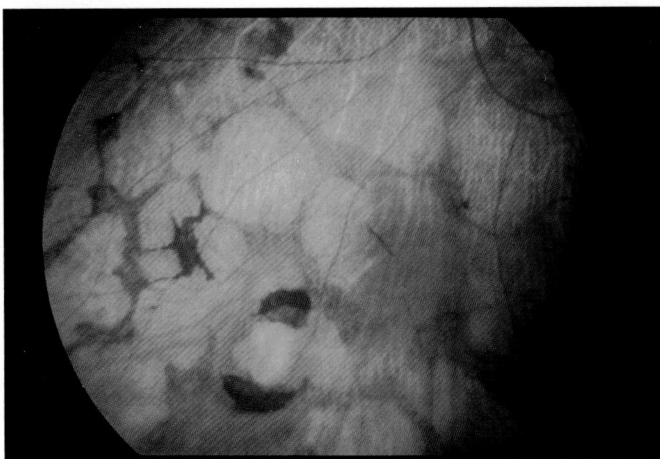

Fig. 43.12 Color fundus photograph from the left eye of a patient with thioridazine (Mellaril) retinal toxicity shows geographic, scalloped regions of hypopigmentation and loss of the retinal pigment epithelium and choroid that are similar to the fundus changes observed in patients with choroideremia and gyrate atrophy of the choroid and retina.

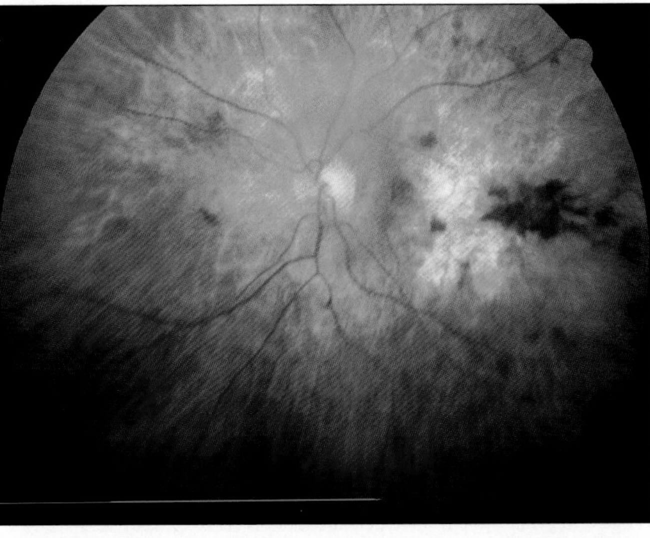

Fig. 43.13 Color fundus photograph from the left eye of a patient with an advanced stage of Stargardt disease shows the extensive atrophy of the retinal pigment epithelium and choroid in the posterior pole and anterior to vascular arcades phenotypically similar to the changes in diffuse choroidal dystrophy.

with autosomal dominant inheritance.[70-72] The autosomal dominant form has been attributed to mutations in the gene *ELOVL4* (chromosome 6q),[73] whereas the recessive form has been linked to mutations in *ABCA4* (chromosome 1p).[69,74] More information is available online.

The advanced stages of Stargardt disease[75] may appear as extensive atrophy of the RPE and choroid in the posterior pole and anterior to the vascular arcades (Fig. 43.13). Although the ERG is most often normal to modestly subnormal in the early to middle course of typical autosomal recessive Stargardt disease, it is often more notably abnormal by the advanced stage of disease.

Pattern macular dystrophy

This disease is an autosomal dominant, fundoscopically variable disorder that involves the accumulation of lipofuscin within RPE cells with subsequent cell degeneration and secondary choriocapillaris loss.[76] The lesions often begin in midlife and can be associated with mild to moderate visual acuity loss.[77,78] Pattern dystrophy can, in late stages, occasionally produce diffusely atrophic changes of the RPE and choroid that resembles CHM or localized RPE and choroidal atrophy resembling CACD.[79]

CONCLUSION

Currently there is no defined treatment for hereditary choroidal dystrophies; however, periodic ophthalmic examination to monitor progression of these diseases is recommended as affected individuals need counsel regarding their level of visual function loss and prognosis. Ultraviolet and short-wavelength (blue)-blocking sunglasses may have a protective role when an affected individual is outdoors. Low-vision services are designed to benefit those whose ability to function is compromised by clinically significant visual impairment. A low-vision examination may be useful to help optimize the use of remaining visual function. Cataract surgery may be required for individuals with clinically significant lens opacity. Genetic counseling is warranted that can provide patients and families with information on the genetic implications of these disorders which, in turn, can help them make informed personal decisions.

Gene therapy for individuals with hereditary choroidal dystrophies is likely to be a treatment strategy that is available in the future. Introduction of recombinant adenovirus containing the full-length *REP-1* CHM coding region can restore protein levels and *REP-1* activity in enzyme-deficient lymphocytes and fibroblasts in vitro.[80] A recent report by Genead et al.[81] showed that treatment of cystoid macular edema in CHM patients with a topical dorzolamide 2% ophthalmic formulation can reduce central macular thickness associated with cystoid macular edema on spectral-domain optical coherence tomography testing with a potential improvement for visual acuity, while the study by Vasconcelos-Santos et al.[27] showed a short-term beneficial effect on cystoid macular edema in patients with gyrate atrophy and the use of intravitreal triamcinolone acetonide.

With treatment strategies for various inherited retinal diseases emerging, the future looks promising for potentially improving or delaying loss of visual function in patients with inherited choroidal diseases.

Bonus material for this chapter is available online at **http://www.expertconsult.com**

REFERENCES

1. Sorsby A. Choroidal angiosclerosis with special reference to its hereditary character. Br J Ophthalmol 1939;23:433–44.
2. Carr RE. Central areolar choroidal dystrophy. Arch Ophthalmol 1965;73:32–5.
3. Sandvig K. Familial, central, areolar, choroidal atrophy of autosomal dominant inheritance. Acta Ophthalmol (Copenh) 1955;33:71–8.
4. Waardenburg PJ. Familial angiosclerosis of the choroid. J Genet Hum 1952;1:83–90.
5. Sorsby A, Crick RP. Central areolar choroidal sclerosis. Br J Ophthalmol 1953;37:129–39.
6. Yanagihashi S, Nakazawa M, Kurotaki J, et al. Autosomal dominant central areolar choroidal dystrophy and a novel Arg195Leu mutation in the peripherin/RDS gene. Arch Ophthalmol 2003;121:1458–61.
7. Krill AE, Archer D. Classification of the choroidal atrophies. Am J Ophthalmol 1971;72:562–85.
8. Carr RE, Mittl RN, Noble KG. Choroidal abiotrophies. Trans Sect Ophthalmol Am Acad Ophthalmol Otolaryngol 1975;79:OP796–816.
9. Sorsby A, Davey JB. Generalized choroidal sclerosis; course and mode of inheritance. Br J Ophthalmol 1955;39:257–76.
10. Franceschetti A, Francois J, Babel J. Chorioretinal heredodegenerations. Springfield, Ill: Charles C Thomas; 1974.
11. Curry Jr HF, Schonberg SS. Fluorescein photography in choroidal sclerosis. Arch Ophthalmol 1969;81:177–83.

12. Jacobsohn E. Ein fall von Retinitis pigmentosa atypica. Klin Monatsbl Augenheilkd 1888;26:202-6.
13. Cutler C. Dri ungewohnliche Falle von retino-choroideak Degeneration. Arch Augenheilkd 1895;30:117.
14. Fuchs E. Ueber awei der Retinitis pigmentosa verwandte Krankheiten (retinitis punctate albescens und atrophia gyrate chorioideae et retinae). Arch Augenheilkd 1896;32:111.
15. Takki KK, Milton RC. The natural history of gyrate atrophy of the choroid and retina. Ophthalmology 1981;88:292-301.
16. Simell O, Takki K. Raised plasma-ornithine and gyrate atrophy of the choroid and retina. Lancet 1973;1:1031-3.
17. Valle D, Walser M, Brusilow SW, et al. Gyrate atrophy of the choroid and retina: amino acid metabolism and correction of hyperornithinemia with an arginine-deficient diet. J Clin Invest 1980;65:371-8.
18. Valle D, Walser M, Brusilow S, et al. Gyrate atrophy of the choroid and retina. Biochemical considerations and experience with an arginine-restricted diet. Ophthalmology 1981;88:325-30.
19. Kaiser-Kupfer MI, de Monasterio FM, Valle D, et al. Gyrate atrophy of the choroid and retina: improved visual function following reduction of plasma ornithine by diet. Science 1980;210:1128-31.
20. Heinänen K, Näntö-Salonen K, Leino L, et al. Gyrate atrophy of the choroid and retina: lymphocyte ornithine-delta-aminotransferase activity in different mutations and carriers. Pediatr Res 1998;44:381-5.
21. Inana G, Hotta Y, Zintz C, et al. Expression defect of ornithine aminotransferase gene in gyrate atrophy. Invest Ophthalmol Vis Sci 1988;7:1001-5.
22. Mitchell GA, Brody LC, Siplia I, et al. At least two mutant alleles of ornithine delta-aminotransferase cause gyrate atrophy of the choroid and retina in Finns. Proc Natl Acad Sci USA 1989;86:197-201.
23. McClatchey AI, Kaufman DL, Berson EL, et al. Splicing defect at the ornithine amino-transferase (OAT) locus in gyrate atrophy. Am J Hum Genet 1990;47: 790-4
24. Kellner U, Weleber RG, Kennaway NG, et al. Gyrate atrophy-like phenotype with normal plasma ornithine. Retina 1997;17:403-13.
25. Feldman RB, Mayo SS, Robertson DM, et al. Epiretinal membranes and cystoid macular edema in gyrate atrophy of the choroid and retina. Retina 1989;9: 139-42.
26. Oliveira TL, Andrade RE, Muccioli C, et al. Cystoid macular edema in gyrate atrophy of the choroid and retina: a fluorescein angiography and optical coherence tomography evaluation. Am J Ophthalmol 2005;140:147-9.
27. Vasconcelos-Santos DV, Magalhães EP, Nehemy MB. Macular edema associated with gyrate atrophy managed with intravitreal triamcinolone: a case report. Arq Bras Oftalmol 2007;70:858-61.
28. Kurstjens JH. Choroideremia and gyrate atrophy of the choroid and retina. Docum. Ophtal 1965;19:1.
29. Weleber RG, Kennaway NG. Clinical trial of vitamin B_6 for gyrate atrophy of the choroid and retina. Ophthalmology 1981;88:316-24.
30. Raitta C, Carlson S, Vannas-Sulonen K. Gyrate atrophy of the choroid and retina: ERG of the neural retina and the pigment epithelium. Br J Ophthalmol 1990;74:363-7.
31. Sipilä I, Simell O, Rapola J, et al. Gyrate atrophy of the choroid and retina with hyperornithinemia: tubular aggregates and type 2 fiber atrophy in muscle. Neurology 1979;29:996-1005.
32. Kaiser-Kupfer MI, Kuwabara T, Askanas V, et al. Systemic manifestations of gyrate atrophy of the choroid and retina. Ophthalmology 1981;88:302-6.
33. McCulloch JC, Arshinoff SA, Marliss EB, et al. Hyperornithinemia and gyrate atrophy of the choroid and retina. Ophthalmology 1978;85:918-28.
34. Takki K. Gyrate atrophy of the choroid and retina associated with hyperornithinaemia. Br J Ophthalmol 1974;58:3-23.
35. Wilson DJ, Weleber RG, Green WR. Ocular clinicopathologic study of gyrate atrophy. Am J Ophthalmol 1991;111:24-33.
36. Wang T, Milam AH, Steel G, et al. A mouse model of gyrate atrophy of the choroid and retina. Early retinal pigment epithelium damage and progressive retinal degeneration. J Clin Invest 1996;97:2753-62.
37. Berson EL, Hanson 3rd AH, Rosner B, et al. A two year trial of low protein, low arginine diets or vitamin B_6 for patients with gyrate atrophy. Birth Defects Orig Artic Ser 1982;18:209-18.
38. Kaiser-Kupfer MI, Caruso RC, Valle D. Gyrate atrophy of the choroid and retina. Long-term reduction of ornithine slows retinal degeneration. Arch Ophthalmol 1991;109:1539-48.
39. Vannas-Sulonen K, Simell O, Sipilä I. Gyrate atrophy of the choroid and retina. The ocular disease progresses in juvenile patients despite normal or near normal plasma ornithine concentration. Ophthalmology 1987;94: 1428-33.
40 Mauthner L. Ein Fall von Chorioideremie. Berl Natur-med. Ver Innsbruck 1872;2:191.
41. McCulloch C, McCulloch RJP. A hereditary and clinical study of choroideremia. Trans. Am. Acad. Ophthal. Otolaryngol 1948;52:160.
42. MacDonald IM, Sereda C, McTaggart K, et al. Choroideremia gene testing. Expert Rev Mol Diagn 2004;4:478-84.
43. Roberts MF, Fishman GA, Roberts DK, et al. Retrospective, longitudinal, and cross sectional study of visual acuity impairment in choroideraemia. Br J Ophthalmol 2002;86:658-62.
44. Genead MA, Fishman GA. Cystic macular oedema on spectral-domain optical coherence tomography in choroideremia patients without cystic changes on fundus examination. Eye (Lond) 2011;25:84-90.
45. Francis PJ, Fishman GA, Trzupek KM, et al. Stop mutations in exon 6 of the choroideremia gene, CHM, associated with preservation of the electroretinogram. Arch Ophthalmol 2005;123:1146-9.
46. Ponjavic V, Abrahamson M, Andréasson S, et al. Phenotype variations within a choroideremia family lacking the entire CHM gene. Ophthalmic Genet 1995;16:143-50.
47. MacDonald IM, Russell L, Chan CC. Choroideremia: new findings from ocular pathology and review of recent literature. Surv Ophthalmol 2009;54:401-7.
48. Rafuse EV, McCulloch C. Choroideremia. A pathological report. Can J Ophthalmol 1968;3:347-52.
49. McCulloch C. Choroideremia: a clinical and pathological review. Trans Am Ophthalmol Soc 1969;67:142-95.
50. McCulloch JC. The pathologic findings in two cases of choroideremia. Trans Am Acad Ophthalmol Otolaryngol 1950;54:565-72.
51. Lewis RA, Nussbaum RL, Ferrell R. Mapping X-linked ophthalmic diseases. Provisional assignment of the locus for choroideremia to Xq13-q24. Ophthalmology 1985;92:800-6.
52. Nussbaum RL, Lewis RA, Lesko JG, et al. Choroideremia is linked to the restriction fragment length polymorphism DXYS1 at XQ13-21. Am J Hum Genet 1985;37:473-81.
53. Seabra MC, Brown MS, Slaughter CA, et al. Purification of component A of Rab geranylgeranyl transferase: possible identity with the choroideremia gene product. Cell 1992;70:1049-57.
54. van den Hurk JA, Schwartz M, van Bokhoven H, et al. Molecular basis of choroideremia (CHM): mutations involving the Rab escort protein-1 (REP-1) gene. Hum Mutat 1997;9:110-7.
55. MacDonald IM, Mah DY, Ho YK, et al. A practical diagnostic test for choroideremia. Ophthalmology 1998;105:1637-40.
56. Lorda-Sanchez IJ, Ibañez AJ, Sanz RJ, et al. Choroideremia, sensorineural deafness, and primary ovarian failure in a woman with a balanced X-4 translocation. Ophthalm Genet 2000;21:185-9.
57. Thobani A, Anastasakis A, Fishman GA. Microperimetry and OCT findings in female carriers of choroideremia. Ophthalmic Genet 2010;31:235-9.
58. Yau RJ, Sereda CA, McTaggart KE, et al. Choroideremia carriers maintain a normal electro-oculogram (EOG). Doc Ophthalmol 2007;114:147-51.
59. Preising MN, Wegscheider E, Friedburg C, et al. Fundus autofluorescence in carriers of choroideremia and correlation with electrophysiologic and psychophysical data. Ophthalmology 2009;116:1201-9.
60 Fraser GR, Friedmann AI. Choroideremia in a female. Br Med J 1968;2: 732-4.
61. Harris GS, Miller JR. Choroideremia. Visual defects in a heterozygote. Arch Ophthalmol 1968;80:423-9.
62. Syed N, Smith JE, John SK, et al. Evaluation of retinal photoreceptors and pigment epithelium in a female carrier of choroideremia. Ophthalmology 2001;108:711-20.
63. Bastiaensen LA, Notermans SL, Ramaekers CH, et al. Kearns syndrome or Kearns disease: further evidence of a genuine entity in a case with uncommon features. Ophthalmologica 1982;184:40-50.
64. Gekka T, Hayashi T, Takeuchi T, et al. CYP4V2 mutations in two Japanese patients with Bietti's crystalline dystrophy. Ophthalm Res 2005;37:262-9.
65. Fishman GA, Farber M, Patel BS, et al. Visual acuity loss in patients with Stargardt's macular dystrophy. Ophthalmology 1987;94:809-14.
66. Rotenstreich Y, Fishman GA, Anderson RJ. Visual acuity loss and clinical observations in a large series of patients with Stargardt disease. Ophthalmology 2003;110:1151-8.
67. Armstrong JD, Meyer D, Xu S, et al. Long-term follow-up of Stargardt's disease and fundus flavimaculatus. Ophthalmology 1998;105:448-57.
68. Aaberg TM. Stargardt's disease and fundus flavimaculatus: evaluation of morphologic progression and intrafamilial co-existence. Trans Am Ophthalmol Soc 1986;84:453-87.
69. Allikmets R, Singh N, Sun H, et al. A photoreceptor cell-specific ATP-binding transporter gene (ABCR) is mutated in recessive Stargardt macular dystrophy. Nat Genet 1997;15:236-46.
70. Cibis GW, Morey M, Harris DJ. Dominantly inherited macular dystrophy with flecks (Stargardt). Arch Ophthalmol 1980;98:1785-9.
71. Zhang K, Bither PP, Park R, et al. A dominant Stargardt's macular dystrophy locus maps to chromosome 13q34. Arch Ophthalmol 1994;112:759-64.
72. Stone EM, Nichols BE, Kimura AE, et al. Clinical features of a Stargardt-like dominant progressive macular dystrophy with genetic linkage to chromosome 6q. Arch Ophthalmol 1994;112:765-72.
73. Zhang K, Kniazeva M, Han M, et al. A 5-bp deletion in ELOVL4 is associated with two related forms of autosomal dominant macular dystrophy. Nat Genet 2001;27:89-93.
74. Kaplan J, Gerber S, Larget-Piet D, et al. A gene for Stargardt's disease (fundus flavimaculatus) maps to the short arm of chromosome 1. Nat Genet 1993;5: 308-11.
75. Fishman GA. Fundus flavimaculatus: a clinical classification. Arch Ophthalmol 1976;94:2061-7.
76. Zhang K, Garibaldi DC, Li Y, et al. Butterfly-shaped pattern dystrophy: a genetic, clinical, and histopathological report. Arch Ophthalmol 2002;120:485-90.
77. Marmor MF, Byers B. Pattern dystrophy of the pigment epithelium. Am J Ophthalmol 1977;84:32-44.
78. de PTVM, Delleman JW. Pigment epithelial pattern dystrophy: four different manifestations in a family. Arch Ophthalmol 1982;100:1416-21.
79. Watzke RC, Folk JC, Lang RM. Pattern dystrophy of the retinal pigment epithelium. Ophthalmology 1982;89:1400-6.
80. Anand V, Barral DC, Zeng Y, et al. Gene therapy for choroideremia: in vitro rescue mediated by recombinant adenovirus. Vision Res 2003;43:919-26.
81. Genead MA, McAnany JJ, Fishman GA. Topical dorzolamide for treatment of cystoid macular edema in patients with choroideremia. Retina 2012;32: 826-33.

For additional online content visit http://www.expertconsult.com

Chapter 44

Abnormalities of Cone and Rod Function

David M. Wu, Amani A. Fawzi

This chapter will review a genetically heterogeneous group of retinal disorders, which often have subtle clinical findings in the face of distinct visual symptoms. Clinical suspicion paired with the appropriate psychophysical and electrophysiological testing can lead to a correct diagnosis. Research toward identifying molecular causes for these diseases continues at a rapid pace. As the underlying genetic mutations responsible for each entity are identified, phenotype/genotype correlations may lead to improved understanding of disease pathophysiology and pave the way for new classifications based on molecular mechanisms. Also, as new therapies emerge for a subset of these previously untreatable disorders, identifying the causative mutation will be of utmost importance to patients.

Congenital color vision deficits as well as retinitis pigmentosa and its related disorders are covered in separate chapters (respectively, Chapter 10, Color vision and night vision, and Chapter 40, Retinitis pigmentosa and related disorders).

DISORDERS OF THE CONE SYSTEM

Cone disorders can be divided into congenital defects that have early onset and are usually stationary, or those with later onset that tend to be progressive. The stationary disorders include complete and incomplete achromatopsia and blue cone monochromatism. Progressive dystrophies include those that involve only the cones (cone dystrophies) and those that have a component of rod degeneration (cone–rod dystrophies).

Achromatopsia

Congenital achromatopsia is a rare disorder, with an incidence of roughly 1 in 30 000.[1] Individuals with this disorder have poor vision from birth and complain of poor color discrimination and photosensitivity, which relates to their visual acuity decreasing in bright light rather than actual discomfort. Patients with complete achromatopsia, also known as rod monochromatism, are generally considered to lack cones and have vision worse than 20/200. On the other hand, patients with incomplete achromatopsia, also known as atypical achromatopsia, may have slightly better visual acuity in the range of 20/80–20/200. Complete achromats have no color vision whereas incomplete achromats may have some residual color vision. Interestingly, because their color vision loss is congenital, even complete achromats may be able to identify colors. They generally perceive colors as lighter or darker shades of gray and may have learned that red is a darker shade of gray and yellow is a lighter shade of gray and so forth. Consequently, specific color vision tests (discussed below and in Chapter 10,) are designed to uncover this characteristic. Pendular nystagmus may be present, which can improve with age. Family history can be useful as achromatopsia displays an autosomal recessive inheritance pattern.

Diagnosis

On clinical examination, patients may have a normal fundus, or have subtle granularity or atrophy of the macula. The nerve may be normal or show some temporal pallor. Electrophysiologial testing is crucial to making the diagnosis in achromatopsia. Photopic and 30 Hz-flicker electroretinograms will show nearly or completely nonrecordable cone responses in the face of normal or near-normal rod responses (Fig. 44.1). Multifocal electroretinograms will be severely diminished. Full-field electroretinography (ERG) is critical to diagnosis as it helps differentiate achromatopsia from other entities that share a normal fundus exam and associated symptoms. For instance, an infant with Leber congenital amaurosis will also have nystagmus, extremely poor vision, and photosensitivity but will have extinguished photopic and scotopic ERGs. A blue cone monochromat will have poor vision, but will have recordable cone responses when stimulated with blue light on a yellow background. A patient with optic neuropathy would have optic nerve pallor with otherwise unremarkable fundus findings as well as decreased vision and color perception, but would show normal photopic and scotopic ERGs.

Other ancillary tests are also helpful in the diagnosis. Congenital achromats may be able to identify several of the pseudochromatic (Ishihara) color plates because they may have learned to distinguish colors as different shades of gray. Farnsworth D-15 testing may reveal a scotopic axis between the deutan and tritan axes. The Sloan achromatopsia test uses an achromat's correlation of different shades of gray to various colors in order to distinguish them from normal individuals.[2] Dark-adaptation curves will show a lack of a cone–rod break, reflecting the lack of cone function (Fig. 44.2). Visual field testing may reveal a small central scotoma but the peripheral visual fields should be either mildly constricted or normal, and, most importantly, they remain stable over time. Progression on serial visual field testing should raise suspicion for other disorders such as a cone–rod dystrophy or retinitis pigmentosa with a cone–rod pattern.

The ERG changes precede the less specific and sometimes more subtle findings seen on optical coherence tomography (OCT) (Fig. 44.1). A recent report calculated the frequency of these findings in a large series of 77 eyes of achromatopsia patients.[3] Among the most obvious and common is disruption of the inner/outer-segment (IS–OS) junction occurring in 70% of these eyes. A hyporeflective, optically empty cavity may be seen in the cone layer of the foveola (60%), preferentially weighted to the nasal side of the foveal center, where there is higher density

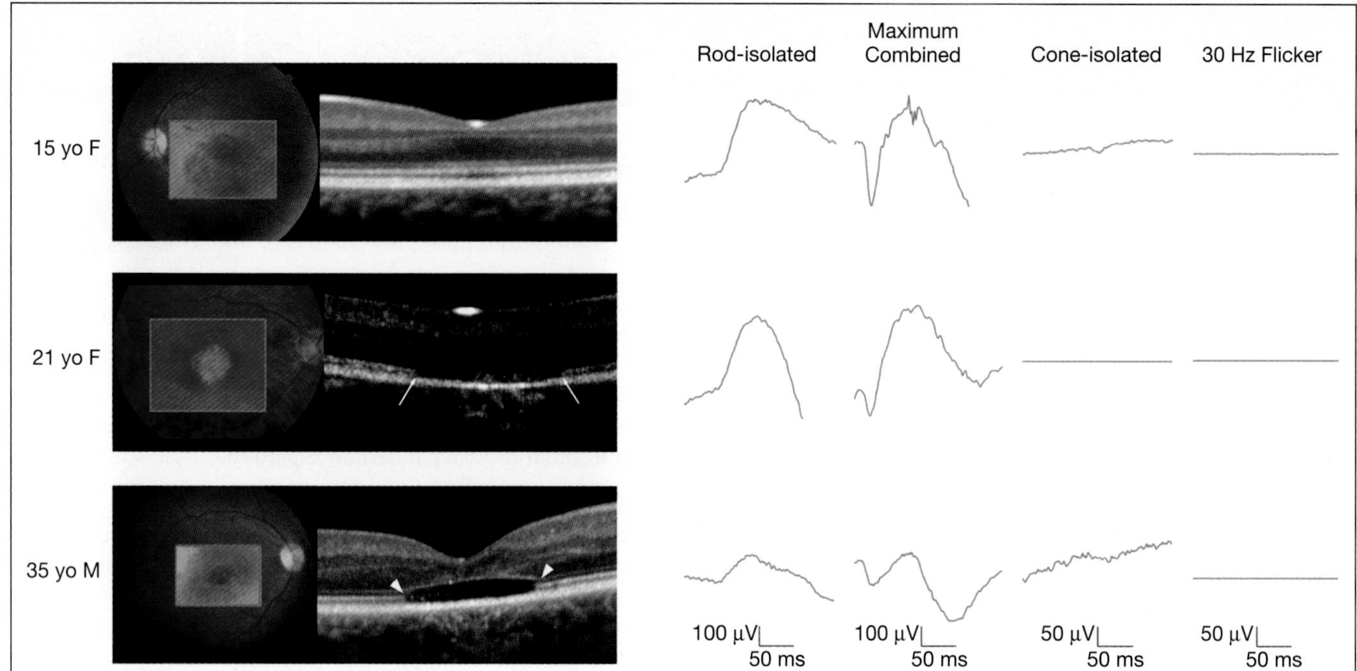

Fig. 44.1 Color fundus photographs, optical coherence tomography (OCT), and electroretinography (ERG) of a series of patients with achromatopsia (yo = years old). The OCTs display a range of the most common features seen in achromatopsia. These findings include foveal hypoplasia, illustrated by preservation of the inner retinal layers through the fovea, most prominent in the top and middle OCTs. The middle OCT demonstrates, in addition, disruption of the IS–OS junction and thinning of the retinal pigment epithelium within the fovea (arrows), which is manifesting as increased signal transmission and increased visibility of the vasculature in the underlying choroid. The bottom OCT demonstrates an optically empty hyporeflective zone involving the outer fovea (arrowheads) with loss of the IS–OS junction and relative preservation of the external limiting membrane and the bare retinal pigment epithelium. To the right of each panel, the corresponding ERG shows normal to near-normal rod-isolated and maximum-combined ERG but unrecordable cone-isolated and 30 Hz flicker ERGs. (Courtesy of Dr Stephen Tsang, Columbia University.)

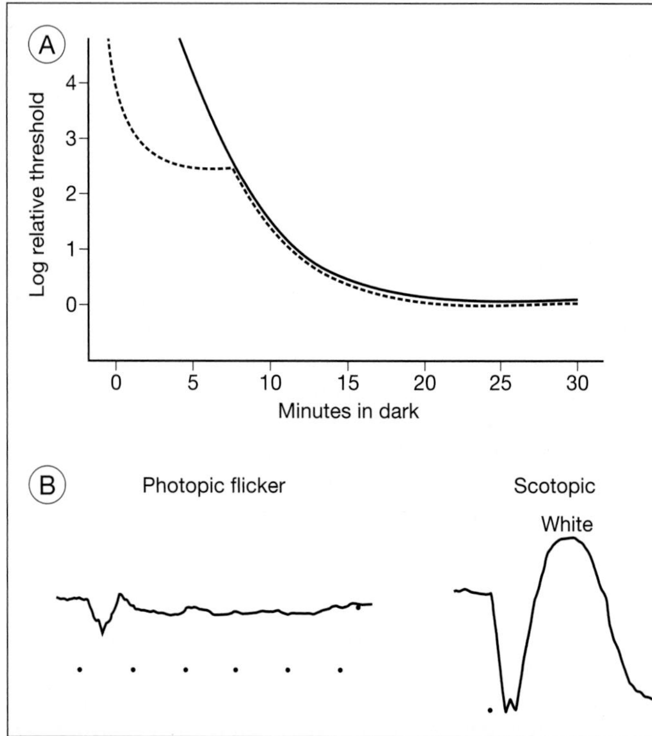

Fig. 44.2 Rod monochromatism. The dark-adaptation curve (A) shows an absence of the initial (cone) segment with a normal rod segment.

of cone photoreceptors. Also present in the majority of patients is foveal hypoplasia (83%). Disruption of the RPE and outer retinal atrophy can be seen in a minority of patients (18%). Although achromatopsia has traditionally been thought to be stationary, the imaging studies suggest that this view should be reconsidered.[4] Progressive cone death may occur in achromatopsia patients with age as suggested by comparing the patient's OCT to age-matched controls as well as a preferential age-dependence of features such as the hyporeflective zone, thinning of the outer nuclear layer, and RPE atrophy.[3,5] Given the overlap in genetic and clinical findings, it is also plausible that some patients diagnosed with complete achromatopsia were incomplete achromats who later progressed.

Although the technique is not readily available in most clinics, adaptive optics scanning laser ophthalmoscopic imaging of the macular photoreceptor mosaic in a patient with complete achromatopsia has helped shed light on the pathophysiology.[6] This case has revealed that the macular area has significant gaps within the photoreceptor mosaic, with a total absence of photoreceptors bearing the characteristics of normal healthy cones. These remaining photoreceptors appeared to have morphologic characteristics typical of rods.

Clinical molecular genetic testing for the four known genes responsible for the majority of achromatopsia cases is available from multiple laboratories (http://www.ncbi.nlm.nih.gov/sites/GeneTests/lab/clinical_disease_id/211350?db=genetests;

accessed February 2012). A brief discussion of our molecular understanding of achromatopsia is available online.

Treatment

There is currently no treatment for the underlying defects in achromatopsia. Photophobia can be reduced with tinted lenses, particularly orange or red lenses since rod photoreceptors are less sensitive to orange and red lights. Red-tinted soft contact lenses that transmit between 400 and 480 nm can reduce the stigma of having to wear dark glasses even indoors.[14] Low vision aids may help to enhance visual acuity. Great strides have been made in research whereby adenoviral-mediated gene transfer has been used to correct the defect in all three genetic forms of human achromatopsia in corresponding animal models.[15–17] As these gene-based therapies eventually move to human trials, identification of mutations in patients with achromatopsia will become crucial.

Cone monochromatism and blue cone monochromatism

Cone monochromatism is a congenital disorder in which two of the three cone systems (long- [L], middle- [M], and short-wavelength [S]) are absent or nearly absent. Monochromatism involving preservation of either the red or the green cone system is extremely rare, with an incidence estimated at 1 in 100 million.[18] These patients have a normal visual acuity, no nystagmus and a normal ERG, residual red and green sensitive pigments by fundus densitometry, and spectral sensitivity curves similar to normal patients.[19–21] Given its rarity, the mechanism remains poorly understood and is mentioned here mainly for completeness.

The remainder of this subsection will concentrate on the relatively more common entity of congenital blue cone monochromatism, which affects approximately 1 in 100,000 people. In blue cone monochromatism, there is preservation of normal S-cone function with absent L- and M-cone function. The signs and symptoms resemble congenital achromatopsia, where those affected have poor vision in the range of 20/80–20/200 from birth. They may also have a pendular nystagmus and photosensitivity. Family history is a useful clue to distinguish the two entities, since patients with blue cone monochromatism have an X-linked recessive, compared to an autosomal recessive inheritance pattern in congenital achromatopsia.

Diagnosis

Fundus examination may be normal, or may reveal progressive pigment irregularities and macular atrophy on ophthalmoscopy and autofluorescence.[22–24] By history, symptoms, and visual acuity, these individuals resemble achromatopsia and thus there are several tests that may help the clinician distinguish between the two. Because they have functional S cones, these patients will have rudimentary dichromatic color discrimination and they can be distinguished from achromats based on the presence of residual tritan discrimination on color testing. One can also use Berson plates that have been specifically developed for this purpose.[25–27] Although the photopic and 30 Hz cone flicker will be absent under normal testing conditions, an S-cone signal can be recorded with a blue light-flash on a yellow background.[28] Scotopic and bright-flash ERGs can be normal or attenuated.[22,28,29] The disorder has been reported to be either stable or progressive, and it is unclear whether this variability is due to the specific mutation, epigenetic influences, and/or environmental factors. Clinical molecular genetic testing is currently available for some of the mutations involved with blue cone monochromatism (see online for a discussion of molecular mechanisms).

Treatment

There is currently no treatment for blue cone monochromatism, but visual acuity and contrast may be improved by blue cutoff filters.[35] Patients should be counseled regarding the X-linked inheritance mechanism of the disorder.

Progressive cone dystrophies

These are inherited retinal dystrophies that usually present within the first three decades of life, although there are rare reports of patients presenting after the fifth decade.[36–38] Decreased visual acuity and central scotomas, some degree of color vision loss, and photophobia are the usual symptoms. The visual defects become worse over time. Some are purely cone dystrophies in which rod function remains normal. In these individuals, night blindness is not a major complaint, nor is peripheral field loss. However, there are many patients who, sooner or later, will have diminished rod function and will manifest the accompanying symptoms at that time. Cone–rod dystrophies are primarily nonsyndromic, but can also be associated with syndromes including Bardet–Biedl and spinocerebellar ataxia, so attention must be paid to a review of systems and the medical history. All mechanisms of inheritance are possible with cone–rod dystrophies, and a careful collection of family history will assist with narrowing down the myriad of mutations responsible for this phenotype, as well as with genetic counseling.

Diagnosis

When confronted with a patient with a relatively normal-appearing fundus and the complaint of uncorrectable bilateral decreased acuity and photosensitivity, the diagnosis of a cone disorder should be entertained. When macular atrophy appears in cone dystrophies it is usually symmetric between the two eyes. Peripheral pigmentary deposits are a rare occurrence. The progressive history rules out stationary disorders of cone photoreceptors (achromatopsia or blue cone monochromatism) discussed earlier in this chapter, and Leber congenital amaurosis. Although the symptoms may be consistent with Stargardt disease, the absence of the characteristic Stargardt findings (fundus flavimaculatus, bull's eye, and dark choroid on fluorescein angiography) can help distinguish between the two. Later in the course of cone and cone–rod dystrophies there may be changes in fundus appearance ranging from pigment deposition, macular atrophy, vessel attenuation, and optic disc pallor. At that time, it may be more difficult to use fundus appearance alone to distinguish from entities such as retinitis pigmentosa.

Electrophysiology continues to be the mainstay diagnostic test to confirm the diagnosis and differentiate between cone or cone–rod dystrophies. Patients are expected to have significantly decreased photopic and 30 Hz flicker ERGs with delays in the implicit times. Multifocal ERGs will be diminished. Early in the course of the disease, when the clinical examination may be normal, this is the most definitive way to confirm the diagnosis. Scotopic ERGs may be reduced as well, especially in later stages depending on the degree of rod involvement in cone–rod dystrophies. However, significant reduction in scotopic amplitudes of the ERG in the early stages would argue strongly in favor of retinitis pigmentosa.

Visual field examinations are useful adjuncts to the diagnostic workup and follow-up evaluations. Early in the course of the disease the fields can show central scotomas with sparing of the periphery. This will remain stable in those with cone dystrophies, whereas patients with cone–rod dystrophies will show progressive peripheral loss over time.

OCT may show thinning of the outer retinal layers, limited mostly to the central retina.[39] Fundus autofluorescence can show central or parafoveal areas of increased or decreased autofluorescence with variable involvement of the periphery. However, the OCT and autofluorescence changes are nonspecific and may be similar in a number of other retinal degenerations as well. It is therefore important to remember that it is the electrophysiological evaluation coupled with these imaging studies which will help make the definitive diagnosis.[40]

Although not readily available in most clinics, adaptive optics imaging has been used to investigate eyes with cone dystrophy. With this technique the photoreceptor mosaic shows increased cone spacing in cone dystrophy compared to normal subjects or retinitis pigmentosa patients.[41]

The diversity of mutations responsible for cone and cone–rod dystrophies currently precludes widespread screening for mutations. However, this may change as more efficient screening mechanisms such as microarrays become more readily available.[42] A brief discussion of the molecular mechanisms of cone–rod dystrophies is given online.

Treatment

There are currently no therapies available to reverse the retinal degeneration process in cone dystrophies. Low vision aids, lenses that reduce photosensitivity, and occupational and psychosocial support remain the primary treatment modalities.

CONGENITAL STATIONARY NIGHT BLINDNESS

Congenital stationary night blindness (CSNB) is generally associated with nonprogressive defects in scotopic vision and/or dark adaptation with otherwise normal visual function. The initial description of the Nougaret family by Belgian ophthalmologist Cunier,[50] which was later expanded by Nettleship,[51] ultimately encompassed nine generations and 2121 patients, and established that this was indeed a nonprogressive "stationary" night blindness. In fact, this classic description still bears the name Nougaret and represents one of the largest pedigrees in ophthalmology and one of the first documentations of a dominantly inherited disorder.[52]

Since these initial reports, CSNB is now recognized to have many variants, which are associated with various inheritance patterns (autosomal dominant, recessive, or X-linked). Although most are truly stationary, some mutations lead to progressive visual loss. Myopia is linked to some forms, but not all. Finally, while the original family had a normal fundus, CSNB variants with fundus abnormalities are well characterized. We now know that the heterogeneity of CSNB is secondary to the variety of mutations that cause this condition. Clinical testing of some of the CSNB genes is currently available (for a list of genes and laboratories offering testing, see the GeneReviews website http://www.ncbi.nlm.nih.gov/sites/GeneTests/?db=GeneTests; accessed February 2012). At the time of publication, a new gene array is being developed in order to facilitate rapid and economical screening of all known mutations for CSNB.[53] As emerging therapies become available, there is a continued need for clinicians to recognize the clinical characteristics to determine whether their patients may benefit from emerging treatments.[54]

Clinical suspicion, careful clinical examination and testing, in conjunction with appropriate genetic testing will ultimately help clinicians make the diagnosis of the particular variant of CSNB. A molecular classification that parallels and supplements the conventional clinical classification was elegantly laid out by Dryja in his Jackson Memorial Lecture from 2000.[55]

CSNB with normal fundi

CSNB patients with normal fundus examination may have normal visual acuity and may not complain of night blindness. Only some forms (X-linked variants) are associated with myopia and generally have subnormal vision (~20/50). On electrophysiologic testing, patients with CSNB and normal fundi generally have severely abnormal rod-mediated ERGs, and some forms have modestly reduced cone amplitudes. Even when reduced in amplitude, cone responses are expected to have a normal implicit time in these patients. A delay in the rod or cone peak implicit time with relatively high amplitudes is more likely a harbinger of progressive retinal degeneration.[56] Other ancillary tests are of less value in these patients, who have normal visual fields. Color vision as measured by conventional psychophysical testing is also typically normal.

In the approach to a patient with suspected CSNB with normal fundi, one must consider the differential diagnosis for those with poor night vision for other reasons. This may include vitamin A deficiency from dietary deficiency or malabsorption, paraneoplastic syndromes, retinitis pigmentosa, and other retinal degenerations, such as choroideremia. A careful history will help elucidate additional symptoms and identify some of these entities. During the examination, most of these other causes will reveal additional fundus findings, such as gray white spots (vitamin A deficiency), peripheral pigmentation (retinitis pigmentosa), or choroidal changes (choroideremia), that exclude them from further consideration.

Diagnosis

In a CSNB patient with a normal fundus, the ERG and dark-adaptation curve are very helpful in characterizing the disorder and determining the specific variant. These patients may broadly be divided into two groups depending on the presence or absence of an a-wave on ERG (Fig. 44.3). Riggs type (also known as type I) patients lack a scotopic ERG, lack both an a- and b-wave on maximum bright-field stimulation ERG, and lack a rod–cone break on their dark-adaptation curve. Without a scotopic ERG and a rod–cone break on the dark-adaptation curve, the molecular defect is predictably located at the rod photoreceptor level (Fig. 44.4).

Schubert–Bornschein (also known as type II) patients possess an a-wave on maximum bright-field stimulation ERG but no b-wave, hence exhibiting a negative waveform. They are further classified into those who possess a scotopic ERG (incomplete form) and those who do not (complete form). In the incomplete form there is a rod–cone break on the dark-adaptation curve whereas in the complete form there is not.[57] Because there is an intact a-wave (originating in the photoreceptors) but diminished b-wave (originating in the inner retina) the defect is expected to originate not in the photoreceptors but within the inner retina.

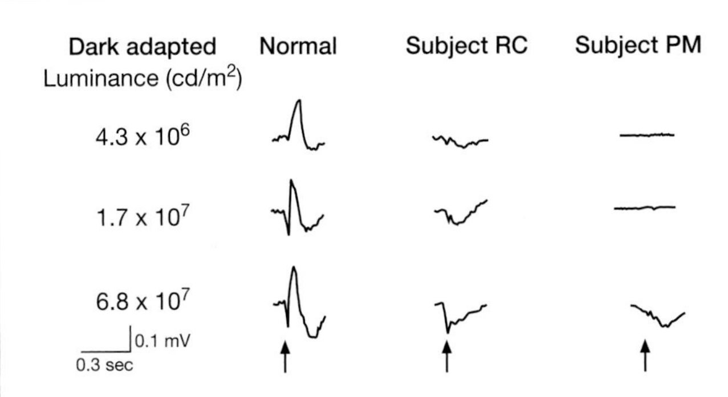

Fig. 44.3 Congenital stationary night blindness (CSNB), normal fundi. Schematics of dark-adapted ERGs at varying stimulus intensities. Subject RC has type II (Schubert–Bornschein), and subject PM has type I (Nougaret).

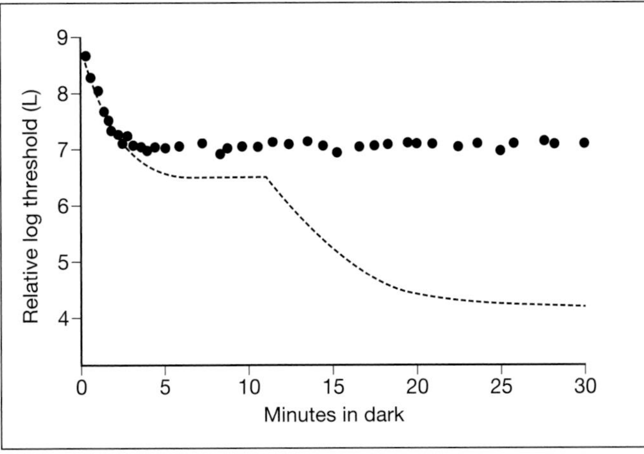

Fig. 44.4 CSNB, normal fundus, showing dark-adaptation curve of subject PM in Fig. 44.3. There is no evidence of a rod–cone break.

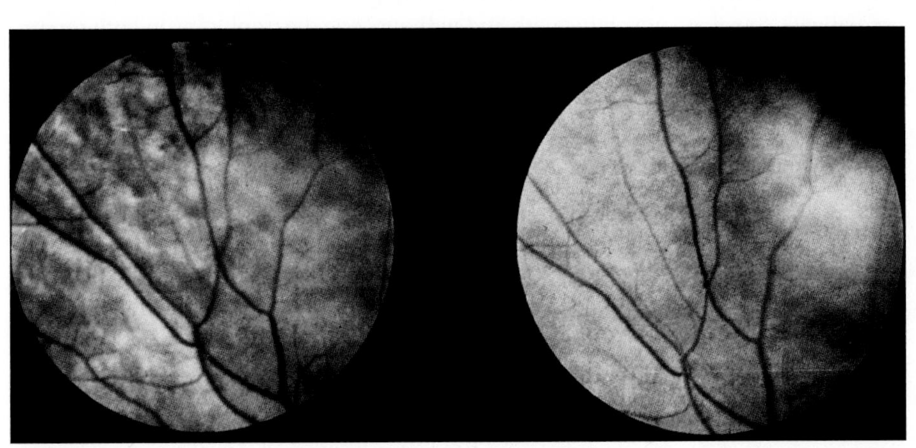

Fig. 44.5 Oguchi disease. (Left) Fundus appearance showing a metallic reflex with vessels standing out in bold relief against this background. (Right) After 3 hours of dark adaptation the retina reverts to normal color.

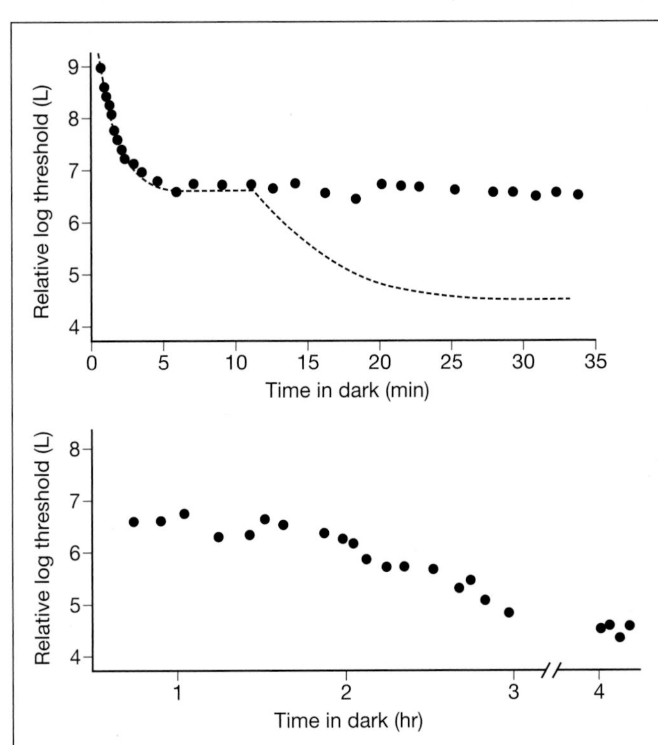

Fig. 44.6 Dark-adaptation curve in Oguchi disease. Normal cone adaptation is obtained, but there is marked delay in obtaining a normal rod threshold.

Our molecular understanding of CSNB correlates with these clinical findings. More detail is available online.

CSNB with abnormal fundi

CSNB with abnormal fundi includes two entities: Oguchi disease and fundus albipunctatus.

Oguchi disease

Oguchi disease refers to cases of CSNB in which there is a particular fundus finding known as the Mizuo-Nakamura phenomenon.[69] In this variant, the retina appears normal following prolonged dark adaptation, but on exposure to light the retina displays a golden sheen with an unusually dark macula[70] (Fig. 44.5).

Diagnosis

Visual acuity and color vision are typically normal in this disorder. On clinical testing, in addition to the abnormal fundus appearance, patients have a dark-adaptation curve with a cone component (Fig. 44.6) but no rod–cone break, and exhibit gradual recovery of full rod sensitivity after prolonged dark adaptation of 1–2 hours. There is no scotopic ERG under normal testing conditions.[71] A single-flash ERG following prolonged dark adaptation will be normal, but then subsequent flashes will not generate a response until the patient undergoes another prolonged period of dark adaptation.[72]

The mechanism underlying the Mizuo-Nakamura phenomenon and fundus sheen seen in Oguchi disease remains a subject of speculation. Histopathological study suggests the presence of an abnormal layer between photoreceptor outer segments and the retinal pigment epithelium (RPE).[73] Recent OCT studies showed that the outer segments appeared shortened in areas with the golden sheen reflex seen in light and suggested that the sheen is related to accumulation of photoactivated rhodopsin in shortened rod outer segments.[74] Other authors have shown that the IS–OS junction was better visualized on OCT following prolonged dark adaptation (and disappearance of the golden sheen), suggesting that reversible changes in the rod photoreceptors related to this mutation may explain the golden sheen reflex.[75] More detail on the molecular basis is available online.

Fundus albipunctatus

Fundus albipunctatus describes a subgroup of CSNB in which white or yellow dots can be seen scattered through the fundus (Fig. 44.7). Individuals may complain of night blindness early in childhood without progression, though most patients remain asymptomatic until the characteristic flecks are detected incidentally on routine fundoscopy.

Diagnosis

As with other forms of CSNB, visual acuity and color vision are typically normal in this disorder. A scotopic ERG can be recorded but only after unusually long dark adaptation, whereas the cone ERG is usually normal. The dark-adaptation curve of fundus albipunctatus features prolongation of both rod and cone sensitivities (Fig. 44.8). Consistent with this, rod and cone visual pigment regeneration is significantly slower in patients with fundus albipunctatus (Fig. 44.9).[79] Of note, there is also a form of fundus albipunctatus associated with cone dystrophy, in which there is progressive decrease in visual acuity and color vision with bull's-eye maculopathy and significantly reduced cone ERGs.[80]

Optical coherence tomography and autofluorescence imaging have recently been used to investigate the flecks in fundus albipunctatus with and without cone dystrophy.[81,82] In both reports,

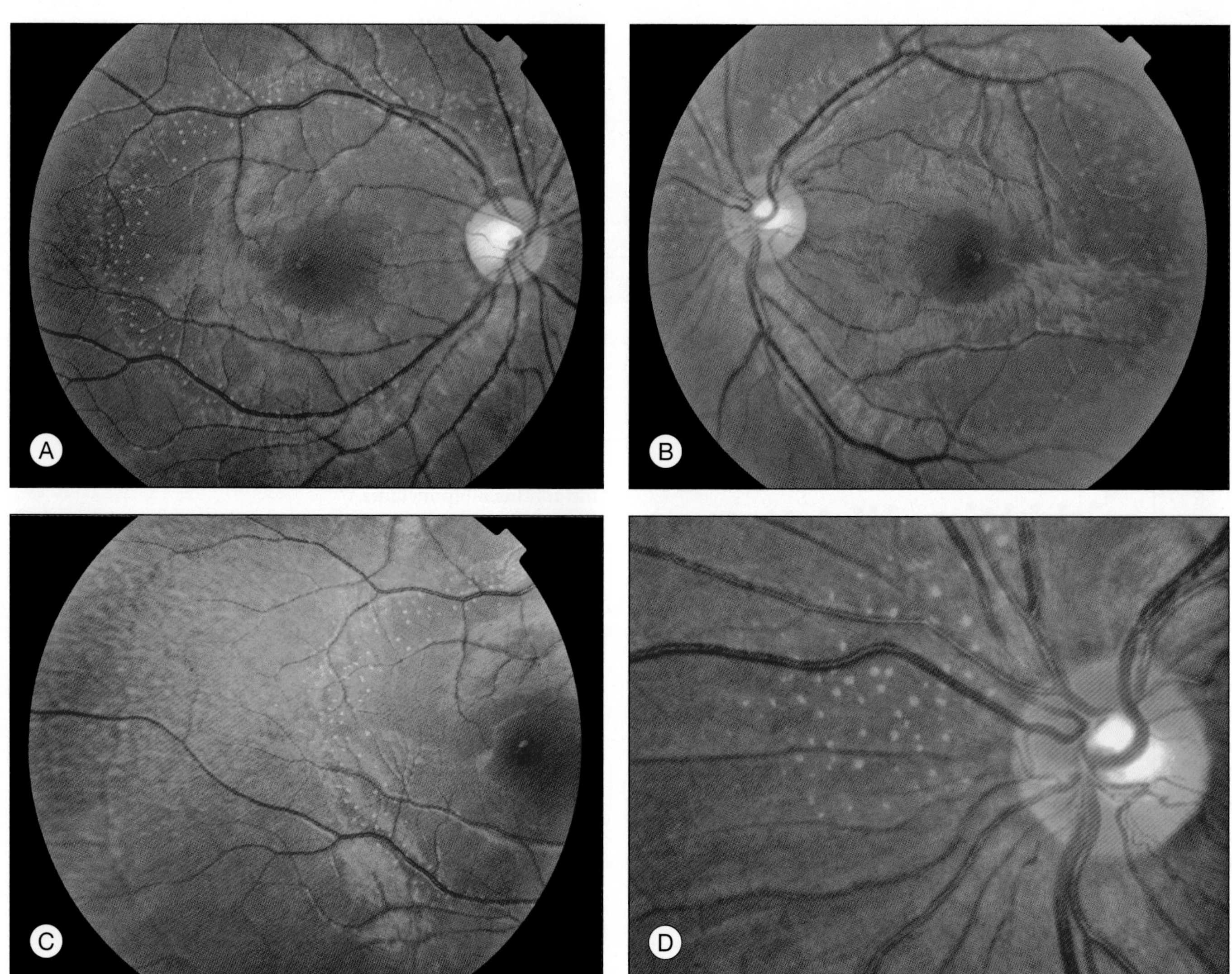

Fig. 44.7 Color fundus photographs of a 10-year-old girl with fundus albipunctatus. By history, she has had poor vision under scotopic conditions since a very young age. The scotopic ERG was borderline abnormal, while the final dark-adapted thresholds were elevated 2.0 log units above normal. (A) and (B) Fundus photographs showing the typical yellowish-white spots in the paramacular region of the right and left eyes. (C) Peripheral temporal view of the right eye illustrating the tendency of the deposits to become larger in the peripheral fundus compared to the paramacular region. (D) Higher magnification of the deposits nasal to the optic nerve. (Courtesy of Dr Thomas O' Hearn.)

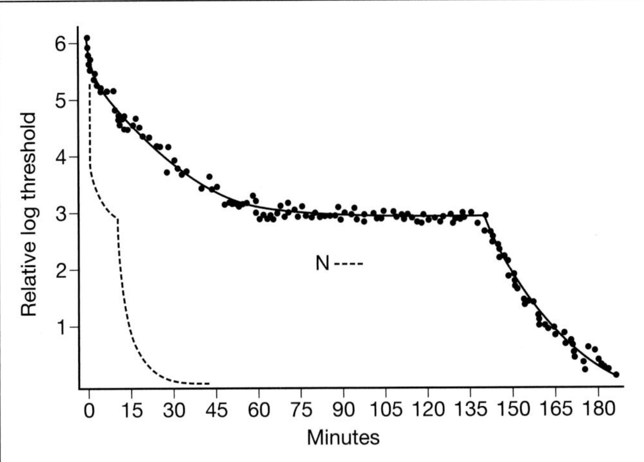

Fig. 44.8 Dark adaptation in fundus albipunctatus compared with normal (N). There is marked prolongation of both cone and rod segments until normal thresholds are reached.

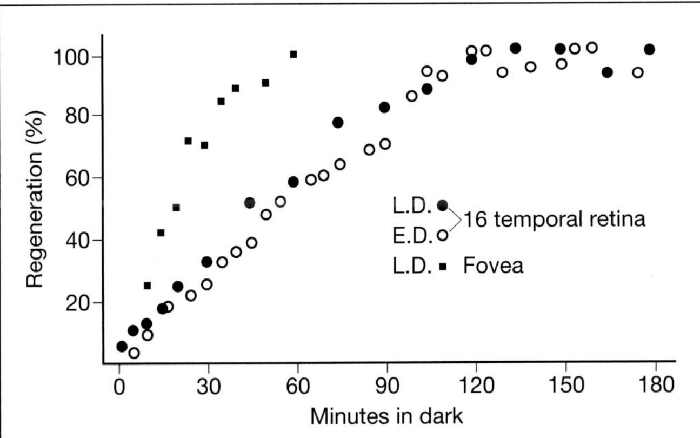

Fig. 44.9 Regeneration times of visual pigments in fundus albipunctatus. Sixteen degrees temporal retina (circles) shows the very prolonged regeneration times of rhodopsin (half-time = 6 minutes). The prolonged regeneration time of the cone pigments (squares) is shown in such patients (normal half-time of regeneration = 55 seconds).

OCT demonstrated homogeneous dome-shaped hyperreflective deposits originating from the inner RPE that correlated with the white fundus spots and were noted to project into the outer retina, disrupting the IS–OS junction, the external limiting membrane, and the outer nuclear layer. Autofluorescence revealed areas of hyperautofluorescence corresponding to the elevated lesions on OCT. It is hypothesized that these lesions represent accumulations of retinoids secondary to the disruption of production of 11-*cis* retinal. The patient with cone dystrophy in conjunction with fundus albipunctatus also had a bull's-eye lesion with corresponding loss of the IS–OS junction on OCT and abnormal circular hypoautofluoresence. More detail on the molecular basis is available online.

Treatment for CSNB

There is currently no treatment available for most forms of CSNB. However, because the defect in fundus albipunctatus affects regeneration of 11-*cis* retinal, supplementation has been explored as a potential avenue for therapy. A recent nonrandomized study in which 9-*cis* retinal was given to such patients showed significant improvement in Humphrey visual field mean deviation, rod dark-adaptation recovery rates, and rod ERG.[54] It is believed that the 9-*cis* retinal is transported from the liver to the retina, where it combines with opsin to generate isorhodopsin, a visual pigment with light absorption peak very close to rhodopsin. The 9-*cis* retinal may also reduce the activity of the retinoid cycle and decrease mislocation of opsin, all of which may potentially stabilize photoreceptors.[88]

For additional online content visit **http://www.expertconsult.com**

REFERENCES

1. Sharpe LT, Stockman A, Jagle H, et al. Opsin genes, cone photopigments, and colour blindness. In: Gegenfurtner KS, Sharpe LT, editors. Color vision: From genes to perception. Cambridge: Cambridge University Press; 1999. p. 3–52.
2. O'Connor PS, Tredici TJ, Ivan DJ, et al. Achromatopsia. Clinical diagnosis and treatment. J Clin Neuroophthalmol 1982;2(4):219–26.
3. Thiadens AA, Somervuo V, van den Born LI, et al. Progressive loss of cones in achromatopsia: an imaging study using spectral-domain optical coherence tomography. Invest Ophthalmol Vis Sci 2010;51(11):5952–7.
4. Thiadens AA, Slingerland NW, Roosing S, et al. Genetic etiology and clinical consequences of complete and incomplete achromatopsia. Ophthalmology 2009;116(10):1984–9 e1981.
5. Thomas MG, Kumar A, Kohl S, et al. High-resolution in vivo imaging in achromatopsia. Ophthalmology 2011;118(5):882–7.
6. Carroll J, Choi SS, Williams DR. In vivo imaging of the photoreceptor mosaic of a rod monochromat. Vision Res 2008;48(26):2564–8.
7. Sundin OH, Yang JM, Li Y, et al. Genetic basis of total colourblindness among the Pingelapese islanders. Nat Genet 2000;25(3):289–93.
8. Kohl S, Marx T, Giddings I, et al. Total colourblindness is caused by mutations in the gene encoding the alpha-subunit of the cone photoreceptor cGMP-gated cation channel. Nat Genet 1998;19(3):257–9.
9. Wissinger B, Gamer D, Jagle H, et al. CNGA3 mutations in hereditary cone photoreceptor disorders. Am J Hum Genet 2001;69(4):722–37.
10. Aligianis IA, Forshew T, Johnson S, et al. Mapping of a novel locus for achromatopsia (ACHM4) to 1p and identification of a germline mutation in the alpha subunit of cone transducin (GNAT2). J Med Genet 2002;39(9):656–60.
11. Kohl S, Baumann B, Rosenberg T, et al. Mutations in the cone photoreceptor G-protein alpha-subunit gene GNAT2 in patients with achromatopsia. Am J Hum Genet 2002;71(2):422–5.
12. Chang B, Grau T, Dangel S, et al. A homologous genetic basis of the murine cpfl1 mutant and human achromatopsia linked to mutations in the PDE6C gene. Proc Natl Acad Sci U S A 2009;106(46):19581–6.
13. Michaelides M, Aligianis IA, Holder GE, et al. Cone dystrophy phenotype associated with a frameshift mutation (M280fsX291) in the alpha-subunit of cone specific transducin (GNAT2). Br J Ophthalmol 2003;87(11):1317–20.
14. Park WL, Sunness JS. Red contact lenses for alleviation of photophobia in patients with cone disorders. Am J Ophthalmol 2004;137(4):774–5.
15. Alexander JJ, Umino Y, Everhart D, et al. Restoration of cone vision in a mouse model of achromatopsia. Nat Med 2007;13(6):685–7.
16. Michalakis S, Muhlfriedel R, Tanimoto N, et al. Restoration of cone vision in the CNGA3-/- mouse model of congenital complete lack of cone photoreceptor function. Mol Ther Dec 2010;18(12):2057–63.
17. Komaromy AM, Alexander JJ, Rowlan JS, et al. Gene therapy rescues cone function in congenital achromatopsia. Hum Mol Genet Jul 1 2010;19(13): 2581–93.
18. Pitt FHG. Monochromatism. Nature 1944;154:466–8.
19. Weale RA. Cone-monochromatism. J Physiol 1953;121(3):548–69.
20. Weale RA. Photosensitive reactions in foveae of normal and cone-monochromatic observers. Opt Acta 1959;6:158–74.
21. Gibson IM. Visual mechanisms in a cone-monochromat. J Physiol 1962;161: 10P–11P.
22. Kellner U, Wissinger B, Tippmann S, et al. Blue cone monochromatism: clinical findings in patients with mutations in the red/green opsin gene cluster. Graefes Arch Clin Exp Ophthalmol 2004;242(9):729–35.
23. Ayyagari R, Kakuk LE, Bingham EL, et al. Spectrum of color gene deletions and phenotype in patients with blue cone monochromacy. Hum Genet 2000;107(1):75–82.
24. Ayyagari R, Kakuk LE, Coats CL, et al. Bilateral macular atrophy in blue cone monochromacy (BCM) with loss of the locus control region (LCR) and part of the red pigment gene. Mol Vis 28 1999;5:13.
25. Berson EL, Sandberg MA, Rosner B, et al. Color plates to help identify patients with blue cone monochromatism. Am J Ophthalmol 1983;95(6):741–7.
26. Weiss AH, Biersdorf WR. Blue cone monochromatism. J Pediatr Ophthalmol Strabismus 1989;26(5):218–23.
27. Alpern M, Lee GB, Maaseidvaag F, Miller SS. Colour vision in blue-cone 'monochromacy'. J Physiol 1971;212(1):211–33.
28. Gouras P, MacKay CJ. Electroretinographic responses of the short-wavelength-sensitive cones. Invest Ophthalmol Vis Sci 1990;31(7):1203–9.
29. Moskowitz A, Hansen RM, Akula JD, et al. Rod and rod-driven function in achromatopsia and blue cone monochromatism. Invest Ophthalmol Vis Sci 2009;50(2):950–8.
30. Nathans J, Davenport CM, Maumenee IH, et al. Molecular genetics of human blue cone monochromacy. Science 1989;245(4920):831–8.

31. Nathans J, Thomas D, Hogness DS. Molecular genetics of human color vision: the genes encoding blue, green, and red pigments. Science 1986;232(4747): 193–202.
32. Nathans J, Maumenee IH, Zrenner E, et al. Genetic heterogeneity among blue-cone monochromats. Am J Hum Genet 1993;53(5):987–1000.
33. Gardner JC, Michaelides M, Holder GE, et al. Blue cone monochromacy: causative mutations and associated phenotypes. Mol Vis 2009;15:876–84.
34. Michaelides M, Johnson S, Simunovic MP, et al. Blue cone monochromatism: a phenotype and genotype assessment with evidence of progressive loss of cone function in older individuals. Eye (Lond) 2005;19(1):2–10.
35. Zrenner E, Magnussen S, Lorenz B. [Blue cone monochromasia: diagnosis, genetic counseling and optical aids]. Klin Monbl Augenheilkd 1988;193(5): 510–7.
36. Krill AE, Deutman AF, Fishman M. The cone degenerations. Doc Ophthalmol 1973;35(1):1–80.
37. Rowe SE, Trobe JD, Sieving PA. Idiopathic photoreceptor dysfunction causes unexplained visual acuity loss in later adulthood. Ophthalmology 1990;97(12): 1632–7.
38. Ladewig M, Kraus H, Foerster MH, Kellner U. Cone dysfunction in patients with late-onset cone dystrophy and age-related macular degeneration. Arch Ophthalmol 2003;121(11):1557–61.
39. Sergouniotis PI, Holder GE, Robson AG, et al. High-resolution optical coherence tomography imaging in KCNV2 retinopathy. Br J Ophthalmol May 10, 2011. E-pub ahead of print, PMID21558291.
40. Wang NK, Chou CL, Lima LH, et al. Fundus autofluorescence in cone dystrophy. Doc Ophthalmol 2009;119(2):141–4.
41. Duncan JL, Zhang Y, Gandhi J, et al. High-resolution imaging with adaptive optics in patients with inherited retinal degeneration. Invest Ophthalmol Vis Sci 2007;48(7):3283–91.
42. Kitiratschky VB, Grau T, Bernd A, et al. *ABCA4* gene analysis in patients with autosomal recessive cone and cone rod dystrophies. Eur J Hum Genet 2008;16(7):812–9.
43. Hamel CP. Cone rod dystrophies. Orphanet J Rare Dis 2007;2:7.
44. Rivolta C, Berson EL, Dryja TP. Dominant Leber congenital amaurosis, cone-rod degeneration, and retinitis pigmentosa caused by mutant versions of the transcription factor CRX. Hum Mutat 2001;18(6):488–98.
45. Kitiratschky VB, Nagy D, Zabel T, et al. Cone and cone-rod dystrophy segregating in the same pedigree due to the same novel CRX gene mutation. Br J Ophthalmol 2008;92(8):1086–91.
46. Maugeri A, Klevering BJ, Rohrschneider K, et al. Mutations in the *ABCA4* (ABCR) gene are the major cause of autosomal recessive cone-rod dystrophy. Am J Hum Genet 2000;67(4):960–6.
47. Nakazawa M, Kikawa E, Chida Y, et al. Autosomal dominant cone–rod dystrophy associated with mutations in codon 244 (Asn244His) and codon 184 (Tyr184Ser) of the peripherin/RDS gene. Arch Ophthalmol 1996;114(1):72–8.
48. Demirci FY, Rigatti BW, Wen G, et al. X-linked cone–rod dystrophy (locus COD1): identification of mutations in RPGR exon ORF15. Am J Hum Genet 2002;70(4):1049–53.
49. Perrault I, Rozet JM, Gerber S, et al. A retGC-1 mutation in autosomal dominant cone–rod dystrophy. Am J Hum Genet 1998;63(2):651–4.
50. Cunier R. Historie d'une hemerolopie, hereditaire depuis siecles dans' un famille de la commune de Vendemian, pres Montpellier. Ann Soc Med de Gand 1838;4:385.
51. Nettleship E. A history of congenital stationary nightblindness in nine consecutive generations. Trans Ophthalmol Soc UK 1907;27:269–93.
52. Carr RE. Congenital stationary nightblindness. Trans Am Ophthalmol Soc 1974;72:448–87.
53. Zeitz C, Labs S, Lorenz B, et al. Genotyping microarray for CSNB-associated genes. Invest Ophthalmol Vis Sci 2009;50(12):5919–26.
54. Rotenstreich Y, Harats D, Shaish A, et al. Treatment of a retinal dystrophy, fundus albipunctatus, with oral 9-cis-{beta}-carotene. Br J Ophthalmol 2010;94(5):616–21.
55. Dryja TP. Molecular genetics of Oguchi disease, fundus albipunctatus, and other forms of stationary night blindness: LVII Edward Jackson Memorial Lecture. Am J Ophthalmol 2000;130(5):547–63.
56. Berson EL. Retinitis pigmentosa. The Friedenwald Lecture. Invest Ophthalmol Vis Sci 1993;34(5):1659–76.
57. Miyake Y. [Establishment of the concept of new clinical entities - complete and incomplete form of congenital stationary night blindness]. Nippon Ganka Gakkai Zasshi 2002;106(12):737–55; discussion 756.
58. Strom TM, Nyakatura G, Apfelstedt-Sylla E, et al. An L-type calcium-channel gene mutated in incomplete X-linked congenital stationary night blindness. Nat Genet 1998;19(3):260–3.
59. Sieving PA. Photopic ON- and OFF-pathway abnormalities in retinal dystrophies. Trans Am Ophthalmol Soc 1993;91:701–73.
60. Nakamura M, Ito S, Terasaki H, Miyake Y. Novel CACNA1F mutations in Japanese patients with incomplete congenital stationary night blindness. Invest Ophthalmol Vis Sci 2001;42(7):1610–6.
61. Bech-Hansen NT, Naylor MJ, Maybaum TA, et al. Mutations in NYX, encoding the leucine-rich proteoglycan nyctalopin, cause X-linked complete congenital stationary night blindness. Nat Genet 2000;26(3):319–23.
62. Zeitz C, Kloeckener-Gruissem B, Forster U, et al. Mutations in CABP4, the gene encoding the Ca^{2+}-binding protein 4, cause autosomal recessive night blindness. Am J Hum Genet 2006;79(4):657–67.
63. Dryja TP, McGee TL, Berson EL, et al. Night blindness and abnormal cone electroretinogram ON responses in patients with mutations in the GRM6 gene encoding mGluR6. Proc Natl Acad Sci U S A Mar 29 2005;102(13):4884–9.
64. Zeitz C, van Genderen M, Neidhardt J, et al. Mutations in GRM6 cause autosomal recessive congenital stationary night blindness with a distinctive scotopic 15-Hz flicker electroretinogram. Invest Ophthalmol Vis Sci 2005;46(11): 4328–35.
65. Audo I, Kohl S, Leroy BP, et al. TRPM1 is mutated in patients with autosomal-recessive complete congenital stationary night blindness. Am J Hum Genet 2009;85(5):720–9.
66. Li Z, Sergouniotis PI, Michaelides M, et al. Recessive mutations of the gene TRPM1 abrogate ON bipolar cell function and cause complete congenital stationary night blindness in humans. Am J Hum Genet 2009;85(5):711–9.
67. Nakamura M, Sanuki R, Yasuma TR, et al. TRPM1 mutations are associated with the complete form of congenital stationary night blindness. Mol Vis 2010;16:425–37.
68. van Genderen MM, Bijveld MM, Claassen YB, et al. Mutations in TRPM1 are a common cause of complete congenital stationary night blindness. Am J Hum Genet 2009;85(5):730–6.
69. Oguchi C. Ueber einen Fall von eigenartiger Hemeralopie. Nippon Ganka Gakkai Zasshi 1907;11:123.
70. Mizuo G. On a new discovery in the dark adaptation on Oguchi's dsease. Acta Soc Ophthalmol 1913;17:1148.
71. Carr RE, Gouras P. Oguchi's disease. Arch Ophthalmol 1965;73:646–56.
72. Gouras P. Electroretinography: Some basic principles. Invest Ophthalmol 1970;9(8):557–69.
73. Kuwakara Y, Ishihara K, Akiya S. Histopathological and electron microscopic studies of the reitna of Oguchi's disease. Acta Soc Ophthalmol Jpn 1963; 67:1323.
74. Hashimoto H, Kishi S. Shortening of the rod outer segment in Oguchi disease. Graefes Arch Clin Exp Ophthalmol 2009;247(11):1561–3.
75. Yamada K, Motomura Y, Matsumoto CS, et al. Optical coherence tomographic evaluation of the outer retinal architecture in Oguchi disease. Jpn J Ophthalmol 2009;53(5):449–51.
76. Fuchs S, Nakazawa M, Maw M, et al. A homozygous 1-base pair deletion in the arrestin gene is a frequent cause of Oguchi disease in Japanese. Nat Genet 1995;10(3):360–2.
77. Yamamoto S, Sippel KC, Berson EL, et al. Defects in the rhodopsin kinase gene in the Oguchi form of stationary night blindness. Nat Genet 1997;15(2):175–8.
78. Carr RE, Ripps, H. Rhodopsin kinetics and rod adaptation in Oguchi's disease. Invest Ophthalmol Vis Sci 1967;6:426–36.
79. Carr RE, Ripps, H, Siegel, IM. Visual pigment kinetics and adaptation in fundus albipunctatus. Doc Ophthalmol 1974:193–204.
80. Nakamura M, Lin J, Miyake Y. Young monozygotic twin sisters with fundus albipunctatus and cone dystrophy. Arch Ophthalmol 2004;122(8): 1203–7.
81. Querques G, Carrillo P, Querques L, et al. High-definition optical coherence tomographic visualization of photoreceptor layer and retinal flecks in fundus albipunctatus associated with cone dystrophy. Arch Ophthalmol 2009;127(5): 703–6.
82. Genead MA, Fishman GA, Lindeman M. Spectral-domain optical coherence tomography and fundus autofluorescence characteristics in patients with fundus albipunctatus and retinitis punctata albescens. Ophthalmic Genet 2010;31(2):66–72.
83. Gonzalez-Fernandez F, Kurz D, Bao Y, et al. 11-cis retinol dehydrogenase mutations as a major cause of the congenital night-blindness disorder known as fundus albipunctatus. Mol Vis 30 1999;5:41.
84. Yamamoto H, Simon A, Eriksson U, et al. Mutations in the gene encoding 11-cis retinol dehydrogenase cause delayed dark adaptation and fundus albipunctatus. Nat Genet 1999;22(2):188–91.
85. Schatz P, Preising M, Lorenz B, et al. Fundus albipunctatus associated with compound heterozygous mutations in RPE65. Ophthalmology 2011;118(5): 888–94.
86. Voigt M, Querques G, Atmani K, et al. Analysis of retinal flecks in fundus flavimaculatus using high-definition spectral-domain optical coherence tomography. Am J Ophthalmol 2010;150(3):330–7.
87. Niwa Y, Kondo M, Ueno S, et al. Cone and rod dysfunction in fundus albipunctatus with RDH5 mutation: an electrophysiological study. Invest Ophthalmol Vis Sci 2005;46(4):1480–5.
88. Maeda A, Maeda T, Palczewski K. Improvement in rod and cone function in mouse model of fundus albipunctatus after pharmacologic treatment with 9-cis-retinal. Invest Ophthalmol Vis Sci 2006;47(10):4540–6.

The Epidemiology of Diabetic Retinopathy

Ronald Klein, Barbara E.K. Klein

INTRODUCTION

Despite the efficacy of glycemic and blood pressure control and photocoagulation, diabetic retinopathy remains an important cause of visual loss in working-age people. With the growing number of people expected to develop diabetes due to changes in diet and physical activity, the number of people at risk for visual impairment due to retinopathy has the potential to increase further. Recent evidence suggests, however, that the incidence of visual impairment due to diabetic retinopathy may be decreasing owing to changes in the management of diabetes over the past 25 years. The purpose of this chapter is to provide an overview of the epidemiology of diabetic retinopathy using data from large population-based epidemiological cohort studies and clinical trials.

PREVALENCE OF DIABETIC RETINOPATHY

Population-based studies such as the Wisconsin Epidemiologic Study of Diabetic Retinopathy (WESDR)[1–3] that use stereoscopic fundus photographs of seven standard photographic fields and objective grading by standard protocols have provided precise estimates of the prevalence and severity of diabetic retinopathy. In 1980–82, the WESDR showed that 71%, 23%, and 11% of those with type 1 diabetes (insulin-dependent diabetes mellitus, IDDM) and 47%, 6%, and 8% of those with type 2 diabetes (noninsulin-dependent diabetes mellitus, NIDDM) had retinopathy, proliferative retinopathy, and macular edema, respectively.[3,4] These prevalence estimates, derived from data collected approximately 30 years ago in an 11-county area of southern Wisconsin (99% white), are higher than more recent prevalence data reported in other population-based studies (Table 45.1, Figs 45.1, 45.2).

A recent effort to provide more up-to-date estimates of prevalence using pooled data from eight studies including the WESDR[5] included 615 individuals who were black and 1415 who were Hispanic. The prevalence estimates were limited to persons 40 years of age and older. The estimates of retinopathy were higher in the WESDR group compared to the seven other studies, all of which were performed at least 10 years after the WESDR (Figs 45.1, 45.2). Based on pooled analyses from these studies, it was estimated that among persons with diabetes, the crude prevalence of diabetic retinopathy was 40% and the crude prevalence of severe vision-threatening retinopathy (pre-proliferative and proliferative retinopathy or macular edema) was 8%. Projection

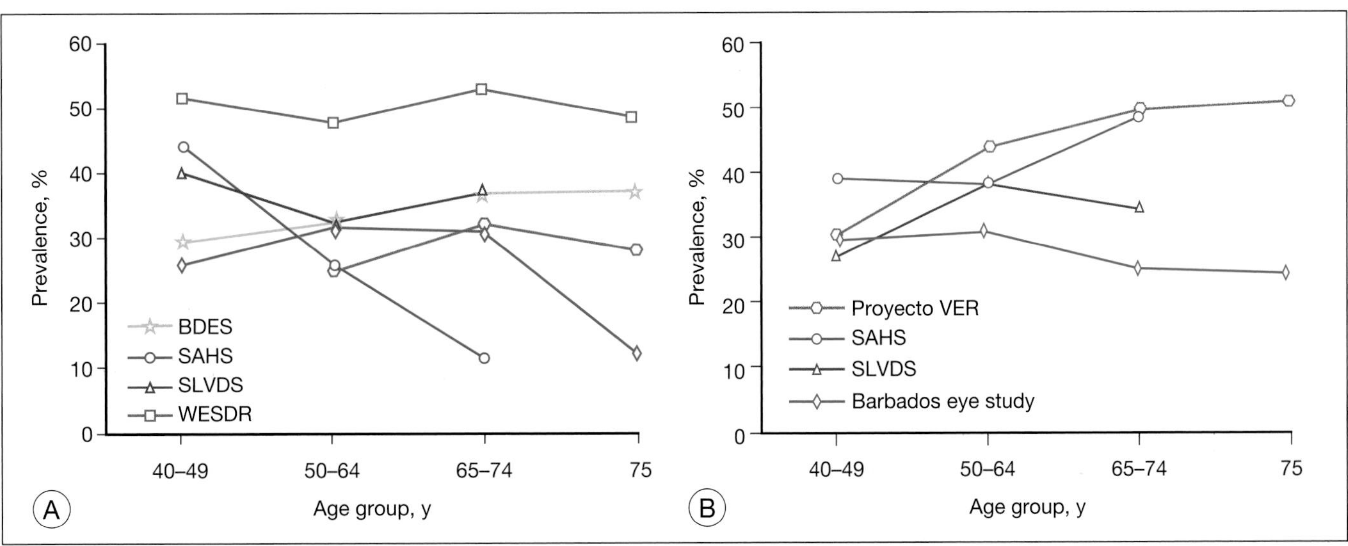

Fig. 45.1 (A) Prevalence of diabetic retinopathy among white subjects who have diabetes mellitus. (B) Prevalence of diabetic retinopathy among Hispanic and black subjects who have diabetes mellitus. BDES, Beaver Dam Eye Study, Beaver Dam, Wisconsin; SAHS, San Antonio Heart Study, San Antonio, Texas; SLVDS, San Luis Valley Diabetes Study, San Luis Valley, Colorado; VER, Vision Evaluation Research, Nogales and Tucson, Arizona; WESDR, Wisconsin Epidemiologic Study of Diabetic Retinopathy, southern Wisconsin. The Barbados Eye Study was conducted in Barbados, West Indies; all participants were black. (Reproduced with permission from The Eye Diseases Prevalence Research Group. The prevalence of diabetic retinopathy among adults in the United States. Arch Ophthalmol 2004;122:552–63. Copyright © 2004 American Medical Association. All rights reserved.)

Table 45.1 Studies included in estimates of the prevalence of diabetic retinopathy*

Variable	Barbados Eye Study, Barbados, West Indies	BDES, Beaver Dam, Wis.	BMES, Blue Mountain, Australia	Melbourne VIP, Melbourne, Australia	Proyecto VER, Nogales and Tucson, Ariz.	SAHS, San Antonio, Tex.†	SLVDS, San Luis Valley, Colo.	WESDR, Southern Wis.
Years study conducted	1988–1992	1988–1990	1992–1994	1991–1998	1999–2000	1985–1987	1984–1988	1980–1982
No. of participants with DM‡	615	410	252	233	899	351	360	1313
Photographic fields taken§	1 and 2	1–7	1–5	1 and 2	1, 2, and 4	1–7	1, 2, and 4	1–7
Age (yr)								
40–49	19.2	6.6	0.0	9.9	17.8	31.2	22.9	7.4
50–64	47.2	36.3	38.9	40.8	44.6	66.7	55.8	35.9
65–74	26.3	34.9	36.5	31.7	25.4	12.5	31.4	33.8
≥75	7.3	22.2	24.6	17.6	12.2	NA	NA	22.8
Gender								
Women	63.4	56.8	47.2	43.8	63.0	58.7	56.4	53.2
Men	36.6	43.2	52.8	56.2	37.0	41.3	33.6	46.8
Race/ethnicity								
Black	100.0	NA	NA	NA	NA	NA	NA	NA
Hispanic	NA	NA	NA	NA	100.0	80.6	64.7	NA
White	NA	100.0	100.0	100.0	NA	19.4	35.3	100.0
Crude prevalence								
Mild NPDR	19.8	22.9	21.0	16.3	36.6	18.2	20.6	36.6
Moderate NPDR	8.0	10.0	4.4	6.9	1.7	13.7	10.3	6.8
Severe NPDR and/or PDR	1.0	2.2	3.6	4.3	6.0	4.3	4.4	6.9
Macular edema	8.6	1.2	4.8	2.2	8.9	2.6	3.3	5.1
DR of any type	28.8	35.1	29.0	27.5	44.3	36.2	35.3	50.3
VTDR	9.1	3.2	6.4	4.3	8.9	5.3	6.4	10.0

Abbreviations: BDES, Beaver Dam Eye Study; BMES, Blue Mountains Eye Study; VIP, Visual Impairment Project; VER, Vision Evaluation Research; SAHS, San Antonio Heart Study; SLVDS, San Luis Valley Diabetes Study; WESDR, Wisconsin Epidemiologic Study of Diabetic Retinopathy; DM, diabetes mellitus; NA, not applicable; NPDR, nonproliferative diabetic retinopathy; PDR, proliferative diabetic retinopathy; DR, diabetic retinopathy; VTDR, vision-threatening diabetic retinopathy.
**Data are given as percentage of persons unless otherwise indicated.*
†Persons with adult-onset diabetes mellitus only.
‡The number of persons reported for each study in this table reflects the number contributing to our estimates in the current article [in the published source] and not necessarily the total number of participants in the original study as published.
§The photographic fields are described in reference 8 [in the published source; the reference is Early Treatment Diabetic Retinopathy Study Research Group. Grading diabetic retinopathy from stereoscopic color fundus photographs – an extension of the modified Airlie House classification. ETDRS report number 10. Ophthalmology 1991;98(5 Suppl):786–806.]
(Reproduced with permission from The Eye Diseases Prevalence Research Group. The prevalence of diabetic retinopathy among adults in the United States. Arch Ophthalmol 2004;122:552–63. Copyright © 2004 American Medical Association. All rights reserved.)

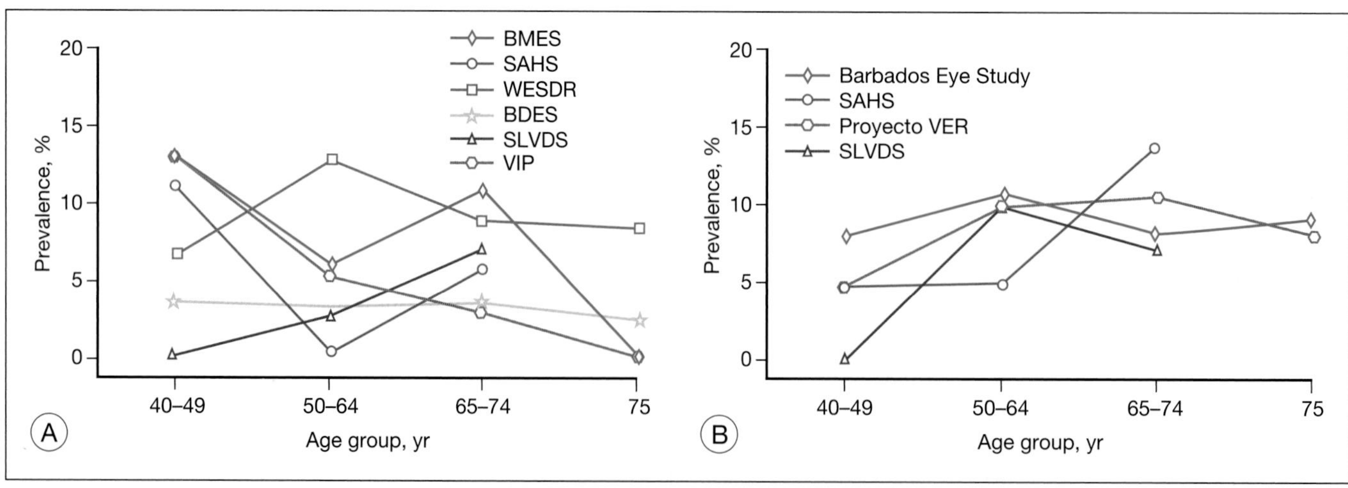

Fig. 45.2 (A) Prevalence of vision-threatening diabetic retinopathy among white subjects who have diabetes mellitus. (B) Prevalence of vision-threatening diabetic retinopathy among Hispanic and black subjects who have diabetes mellitus. BDES, Beaver Dam Eye Study, Beaver Dam, Wisconsin; SAHS, San Antonio Heart Study, San Antonio, Texas; SLVDS, San Luis Valley Diabetes Study, San Luis Valley, Colorado; VIP, Melbourne VIP Study; VER, Vision Evaluation Research, Nogales and Tucson, Arizona; WESDR, Wisconsin Epidemiologic Study of Diabetic Retinopathy, southern Wisconsin. The Barbados Eye Study was conducted in Barbados, West Indies; all participants were black. (Reproduced with permission from The Eye Diseases Prevalence Research Group. The prevalence of diabetic retinopathy among adults in the United States. Arch Ophthalmol 2004;122:552–63. Copyright © 2004 American Medical Association. All rights reserved.)

of these rates to the diabetic population 40 years of age or older in the United States resulted in an estimate of 4 million persons with retinopathy, of whom 900000 have signs of vision-threatening retinopathy. Based on grading of fundus images in the 2005–8 National Health and Nutrition Examination Survey (NHANES), 4.2 million people 40 years of age or older with diabetes were estimated to have diabetic retinopathy, of whom 650000 had signs of vision-threatening retinopathy. With expectations that diabetes will continue to become more prevalent, without a significant decline in the incidence of diabetic retinopathy, the actual number of persons with vision-threatening retinopathy is likely to continue to increase.

The lower prevalence of diabetic retinopathy in more recent studies is thought to be due, in part, to changes in the management of diabetes.[6–46] In persons with type 1 diabetes in the WESDR, there have been dramatic changes in management that include an increase in the use of blood glucose self-monitoring (from 72% in 1984–6 to 91% in 2005–7) and a greater frequency of using three or more injections of insulin per day (from 4% in 1980–2 to 85% in 2005–7). In the WESDR, this was associated with a 25% drop in the mean glycosylated hemoglobin A1c (A1c) from 10.1% to 7.6% and a 29% increase in those achieving American Diabetes Association (ADA) guidelines of A1c of <7% from 4% to 33% over the same period.[47]

There have also been changes in the management of glycemia in people with type 2 diabetes. In 1988–94, the use of only one oral hypoglycemic agent was the primary treatment to manage hyperglycemia in people with type 2 diabetes. After the findings from the United Kingdom Prospective Diabetes Study (UKPDS), there was an increase in the use of more than one oral hypoglycemic agent over a 5-year period (1999–2004).[48,49] This was associated with a decrease in the mean A1c levels from 7.8% to 7.2%, with a 41% increase (from 41% to 58%) in persons achieving A1c levels of <7.0% in the periods 1999–2000 and 2005–6.

INCIDENCE AND PROGRESSION OF DIABETIC RETINOPATHY AND INCIDENCE OF CLINICALLY SIGNIFICANT MACULAR EDEMA

There are fewer reports of incidence of retinopathy in population-based studies.[8,21,50–63] The incidence of retinopathy in a 4-year interval in the entire WESDR population was 40.3%.[50,51] The 4-year incidence and rates of progression of diabetic retinopathy and macular edema in the WESDR are presented in Table 45.2. Those with type 1 diabetes had a higher incidence of any retinopathy, progression, and progression to proliferative retinopathy than those with type 2 diabetes (Table 45.2).[52] The highest 4-year incidence of clinically significant macular edema was in those with type 2 diabetes taking insulin, while the lowest was in those with type 2 diabetes not taking insulin. While the incidence of proliferative retinopathy was higher in those with type 1 diabetes, the estimates of the number of incident cases in the 4-year period were higher in the group with type 2 diabetes than in the group with type 1 diabetes (120 vs 83 persons) due to the higher frequency of people with type 2 diabetes.

There is also evidence that the prevalence and incidence of diabetic retinopathy may be decreasing in subjects more recently diagnosed with type 1 diabetes. Hovind et al.[64] first showed a declining incidence of proliferative diabetic retinopathy and macular edema in a study of 600 patients with type 1 diabetes diagnosed between 1965 and 1984 in Denmark. In that study, the cumulative incidence of proliferative diabetic retinopathy and macular edema after 20 years of diabetes declined from 31% and 19%, respectively, in those diagnosed from 1965 to 1969, to 13% and 7%, respectively, in those diagnosed from 1979 to 1984. There was also significant improvement in visual acuity and lower prevalence of severe visual impairment in those diagnosed with type 1 diabetes more recently than those

Table 45.2 Four-year incidences of any retinopathy, improvement or progression of retinopathy, progression to proliferative diabetic retinopathy (PDR) and incidence of clinically significant macular edema (CSME) in younger-onset type 1 diabetes and older-onset type 2 diabetes in the Wisconsin Epidemiologic Study of Diabetic Retinopathy, 1980–1986

	Younger-onset		Older-onset Taking insulin		Older-onset Not taking insulin	
Retinopathy	No. at risk	%	No. at risk	%	No. at risk	%
Any retinopathy	271	59.0	154	47.4	320	34.4
Improvement	376	6.9	215	15.3	101	19.8
No change	713	55.1	418	58.1	486	71.0
Progression	713	41.2	418	34.0	486	24.9
Progression to PDR	713	10.5	418	7.4	486	2.3
Incidence of CSME	610	4.3	273	5.1	379	1.3

Note: Number at risk for incidence of any retinopathy refers to group that had no retinopathy (level 10/10) at baseline exam and who were at risk of developing retinopathy at follow-up exam. Number at risk for improvement in retinopathy refers to those with retinopathy levels of 21/21 to 51/51 at baseline exam who could have a decrease in their retinopathy severity by at least two steps or more at follow-up exam. Number at risk for no change, progression or progression to PDR refers to those with retinopathy levels of 10/10 to 51/51 who either did not change by two or more steps or progressed by two or more steps.

(Modified from Klein R, Klein BEK, Moss SE, et al: The Wisconsin Epidemiologic Study of Diabetic Retinopathy, IX: four-year incidence and progression of diabetic retinopathy when age at diagnosis is less than 30 years. Arch Ophthalmol 1989;107:237–243; Klein R, Klein BEK, Moss SE et al: [Table 2 page 240] The Wisconsin Epidemiologic Study of Diabetic Retinopathy, X: four-year incidence and progression of diabetic retinopathy when age at diagnosis is 30 years or more. Arch Ophthalmol 1989;107:244–249. Source for the last line comes in part from: Klein R, Moss SE, Klein BEK, et al: The Wisconsin Epidemiologic Study of Diabetic Retinopathy, XI: the incidence of macular edema. Ophthalmology 1989;96:1501–1510.)

diagnosed in earlier periods. These changes were attributed by the authors to improved glycemic control, more aggressive treatment of blood pressure sooner after diagnosis of diabetes, and reduced smoking rates in the more recently diagnosed type 1 diabetic group than in previous years. There was also a decline in the cumulative proportion with severe laser-treated diabetic retinopathy after 25 years of type 1 diabetes from 47% in subjects diagnosed in 1961–5 to 24% in subjects diagnosed in 1971–5 in the Swedish Linköping Diabetes Complications Study.[65,66] However, the Pittsburgh Epidemiology of Diabetic Complications Study did not show a significant decrease in proliferative diabetic retinopathy in those diagnosed more recently.[67] In the WESDR, the annualized estimates for the progression of diabetic retinopathy (4.5 vs 2.5%) and the incidence of proliferative diabetic retinopathy (3.4 vs 1.5%), clinically significant macular edema (1.0 vs 0.4%), and visual impairment (0.7 vs 0.3%) were higher in the first 12 years of the study (1980–92) than in the latest 13 years of the study (1994–2007).[68–71] While controlling for duration of diabetes, there was also evidence in the WESDR of lower prevalence of proliferative diabetic retinopathy (4% lower per more recent time period) and visual impairment (9% lower per more recent time period) but not of macular edema in those diagnosed with type 1 diabetes more recently than those diagnosed longer ago. The relationships remained when adjusting for hypertension and A1c levels over time.

THE RELATIONSHIP OF RACE/ETHNICITY TO DIABETIC RETINOPATHY

In contrast to whites, there are fewer epidemiological studies regarding the prevalence and incidence of diabetic retinopathy in other racial/ethnic groups in the United States, especially in persons with type 1 diabetes. Data from the New Jersey 725 study cohort, which used similar methods to detect and classify retinopathy severity as in the WESDR cohort, showed a similar frequency and severity of retinopathy in African Americans with type 1 diabetes as found in whites with type 1 diabetes in the WESDR.[45,46] At the 6-year follow-up of the same cohort, 56% showed progression of diabetic retinopathy, 15% showed progression to proliferative diabetic retinopathy, and 16% developed macular edema.[62] These findings were similar to those in whites in the WESDR (52).

In four population-based studies, the NHANES 1988–94 and 2005–8,[36] the Atherosclerosis Risk in Communities (ARIC) study,[72] the Cardiovascular Health Study,[73] and the Multi-Ethnic Study of Atherosclerosis (MESA),[74] retinopathy was more prevalent in African Americans with type 2 diabetes than in whites. In the NHANES III in 1988–94, compared to whites, African Americans had a higher frequency of people with poor glycemic control (A1c greater than 8.3%, 37% vs 30%), high systolic blood pressure (>142 mmHg, 42% vs 32%), longer duration of diabetes (>14 years, 29% vs 23%), and on insulin therapy (43% vs 24%). There was no difference (odds ratio [OR] 0.94; 95% confidence interval [CI] 0.54–1.66) in the prevalence of retinopathy between African Americans and whites while controlling for these factors (36). In addition, there were no statistically significant interactions of race with diabetes severity variables or systolic blood pressure, suggesting that the effect of risk factors was similar in both racial/ethnic groups. Similarly, the higher prevalence of retinopathy in the ARIC study (28% vs 17%) and in the MESA (37% vs 25%) in blacks as compared to whites was no longer statistically significant after controlling for differences in glycemic and blood pressure control between the races. Higher prevalence of retinopathy in African Americans with type 2 diabetes appears to be partially due to poorer glycemic and blood pressure control. These data suggest that programs designed to better control blood sugar and blood pressure in diabetic African Americans might be beneficial.

In most population-based studies, Mexican Americans have been shown to have higher frequencies and more severe diabetic retinopathy than non-Hispanic whites.[5,22,31,36,40,74–76] Haffner et al.[22] found that after controlling for all measured risk factors, the frequency of retinopathy in Mexican Americans in San Antonio was 2.4 times as high as the frequency of retinopathy in non-Hispanic whites studied in the WESDR. Similarly, in the NHANES 1988–94 and 2005–8, the MESA, Proyecto VER, and the Los Angeles Latino Eye Study (LALES), retinopathy was more frequent in Mexican Americans compared to non-Hispanic whites 40 years of age or older.[31,36,74,76] In the NHANES 1988–94, retinopathy was more prevalent in Mexican Americans (OR 2.15; 95% CI 1.15–4.04) compared to non-Hispanic whites, even while controlling for duration of diabetes, A1c level, blood pressure, and type of antihyperglycemic medication used.[5] In the NHANES 2005–8, vision-threatening retinopathy was approximately 3.5 times (95% CI 1.05–12.56) as frequent in Mexican Americans compared to non-Hispanic whites.[75] These variations in prevalence among ethnic groups may be a result of differences in how long it takes to diagnose diabetes after its onset, how it was defined, and levels of glycemia and blood pressure. Differences among Hispanic whites may be due to the degree of gene-sharing with Native Americans, a group with a high prevalence of retinopathy (see below).

Among population-based studies, only the LALES has provided data on the incidence and progression of diabetic retinopathy in Mexican Americans with type 2 diabetes.[63] The 4-year incidence of diabetic retinopathy and clinically significant macular edema was 34% and 7%, respectively, and progression of retinopathy and progression from nonproliferative diabetic retinopathy to proliferative diabetic retinopathy was 39% and 5%, respectively, over the 4-year period. While these rates are comparable to those found in the WESDR, they are higher than in most other contemporaneous studies of whites with type 2 diabetes.

The prevalence and severity of retinopathy appears to vary among different Native American groups.[41,77–80] In studies done in the 1970s, Native Americans were reported to have higher rates of severe retinopathy for a given duration of type 2 diabetes compared to whites.[9,10] However, data from more recent studies on the incidence and progression of diabetic retinopathy in Pima Indians show a lower 4-year cumulative incidence and progression of diabetic retinopathy (17% and 18%, respectively) than reported in whites with type 2 diabetes, reflecting possible improvements in glycemic and blood pressure control.[81]

There are few data on the prevalence of retinopathy in Asian Americans and other racial/ethnic groups.[27,37,43,74] The prevalence of retinopathy in second generation (Nisei) Japanese American men, 12%, was significantly lower than that reported in the diabetes clinic at Tokyo University Hospital (49% among patients with onset of diabetes at 20–59 years of age and 47% among those with onset after 59 years of age) and in whites reported in the WESDR (36%).[3,27] In the MESA, the prevalence of any retinopathy (26% vs 25%) in Chinese Americans was similar to whites.[74] However, clinically significant macular edema and proliferative diabetic retinopathy was higher (13% vs 2%) in Chinese than in whites. More data on the prevalence and incidence of retinopathy in Chinese and other Asian American groups are needed.

GENETIC FACTORS

Data from a number of studies that examined familial clustering suggested that genetic factors may be involved more strongly in the susceptibility to diabetic retinopathy than previously thought.[82,83] In addition, data showing that the time of appearance of retinopathy and its severity are more likely to be similar among diabetic identical twins than dizygotic twins suggested that the tendency to develop diabetic retinopathy, and possibly its progression, are influenced by genetic factors. However, unlike the strong associations of complement factor H and other single nucleotide polymorphisms (SNPs) that have been found to be related to age-related macular degeneration, the putative genes and genetic variants have not been found to be as strongly or consistently associated with diabetic retinopathy (see Chapter 46, Diabetic retinopathy: Genetics and etiologic mechanisms). This may be a result of the stronger environmental influence of glycemic and blood pressure control than found for age-related macular degeneration. The fact that retinopathy is not specific to diabetes in its earliest stages may also contribute to inability to find and replicate genes associated with diabetic retinopathy.

Study of specific genetic factors associated with the hypothesized pathogenetic factors for retinopathy, such as aldose reductase activity, collagen formation, inflammatory processes, protein kinase activity, glycation, oxidative stress and platelet adhesiveness and aggregation may yield a better understanding of the possible causal relationships between genetic factors and diabetic retinopathy. There are already a number of studies that have reported associations between retinopathy and mitochondrial DNA mutations[84] and polymorphisms of the aldose reductase gene,[85,86] TNF-beta NcoI gene,[87] epsilon4 allele of apolipoprotein E gene,[88] paraoxonase (an enzyme that prevents oxidation of low-density lipoprotein cholesterol) gene,[89] endothelial nitric oxide synthase gene,[90] intercellular adhesion molecule-1 (ICAM-1),[91] alpha2beta1 integrin gene (involved with platelet function),[92] cytokine vascular endothelial growth factor (VEGF) gene, and many others.[93,94] The reader is referred to a more comprehensive, in-depth discussion of the rapidly evolving field of genetic epidemiology of diabetic retinopathy in Chapter 46.

SEX

In the WESDR, higher frequencies of proliferative retinopathy were present in younger-onset men compared to women.[2] However, there were no significant differences in the 4-, 10-, or 14-year incidence or progression of diabetic retinopathy between the sexes.[50,53,58] There were no significant differences in the prevalence or 10-year incidence of retinopathy or rates of progression to proliferative retinopathy between the sexes in people with type 2 diabetes in the WESDR.[3,51,53]

AGE AND PUBERTY

The prevalence and severity of diabetic retinopathy increased with increasing age in persons with type 1 diabetes in the WESDR.[2] In persons under 13 years of age, diabetic retinopathy was infrequent, irrespective of the duration of diabetes. The 4-year incidence of retinopathy increased with increasing age, with the sharpest increase occurring in persons who were 10–12 years of age at baseline.[50] Four-year rates of progression of retinopathy in younger-onset persons rose steadily with increasing age until 15–19 years of age, after which there was a gradual decline. No child younger than 13 years of age at baseline in the WESDR was found to have proliferative retinopathy at the 4-year follow-up. These findings have formed the rationale for guidelines for not screening for retinopathy in children with type 1 diabetes.[95]

In the WESDR, menarchal status, a crude marker of puberty, at the time of the baseline examination was related to the prevalence and severity of retinopathy.[96] While controlling for other risk factors, those who were postmenarchal were three times as likely to have retinopathy as those who were premenarchal. In a follow-up study of 60 children with type 1 diabetes, Frost-Larsen and Starup[97] found the incidence of retinopathy to be higher after puberty than before, independent of duration or metabolic control of diabetes or type of treatment. These findings have been observed in other studies.[98,99] Increases in growth hormone, insulin-like growth factor I, sex hormones, and blood pressure as well as poorer glycemic control (due to increased insulin resistance, poorer compliance, and/or inadequate insulin dosage) have been hypothesized to explain the higher risk of developing retinopathy after puberty.

In older-onset persons taking insulin in the WESDR, the 4-year incidence of retinopathy and progression of retinopathy had a tendency to decrease with age.[51] The 4-year incidence of improvement tended to increase with age. For those not taking insulin, the 4-year rate of progression to proliferative retinopathy decreased with age. Few persons 75 years of age or older with type 2 diabetes developed proliferative retinopathy over the 10 years of follow-up. These findings are consistent with data from other population-based studies.[8,21] In one such study of people with type 2 diabetes in Rochester, Minnesota, Ballard et al.[14] reported a lower incidence of retinopathy with increasing age in persons with diabetes older than 60 years of age. These findings might reflect a less severe disease in those with older-onset or selective survival, that is, older persons who develop severe retinopathy are at higher risk of dying and not being seen at follow-up in these studies.

DURATION OF DIABETES

Perhaps the most consistent relationship found in persons with diabetes is the increase in the frequency and severity of diabetic retinopathy and macular edema with increasing duration of diabetes.[2] The prevalence of retinopathy 3–4 years after diagnosis of diabetes in the WESDR younger-onset group with type 1 diabetes was 14% in men and 24% in women. However, in persons who had had diabetes for 19–20 years, 50% of men and 33% of women had proliferative retinopathy. Shortly after diagnosis of diabetes, retinopathy was more frequent in persons with type 2 diabetes compared with those with type 1 diabetes (Figs 45.3, 45.4).[3] In the first 3 years after diagnosis of diabetes, 23% of the type 2 diabetic group not taking insulin had retinopathy, and 2% had proliferative retinopathy (PDR).

Based on recent follow-up of the WESDR cohort, the prevalence estimates for a given duration likely overestimate the

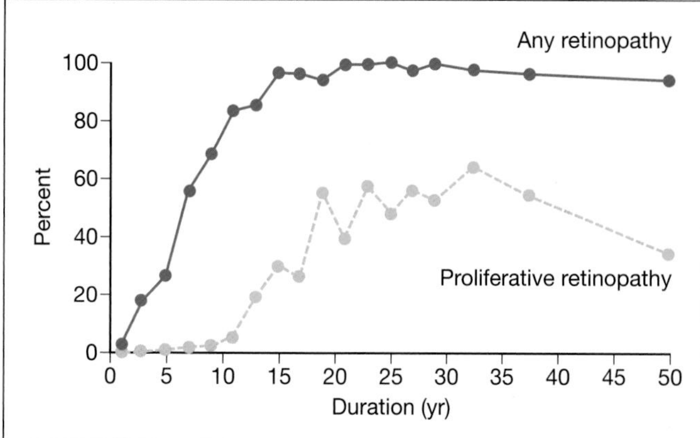

Fig. 45.3 Prevalence of any retinopathy and of PDR in insulin-taking patients diagnosed with diabetes at age <30 years, by duration of diabetes. Data are from WESDR 1980-2. (Reproduced with permission from Klein R, Klein BE, Moss SE. Risk factors for retinopathy. In: Feman SS, editor. Ocular problems in diabetes mellitus. Boston, MA: Blackwell Scientific Publications; 1992. p. 39.)

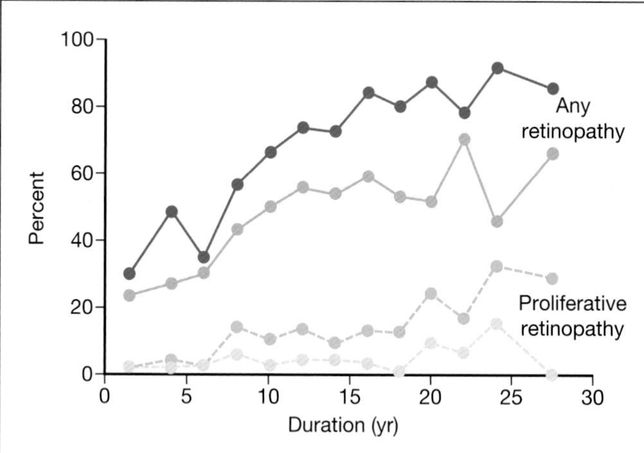

Fig. 45.4 Prevalence of any retinopathy and of PDR in patients diagnosed with diabetes at age ≥30 years, by duration of diabetes. Closed circles = on insulin; open circles = not on insulin. Data are from WESDR 1980–2. (Reproduced with permission from Klein R, Klein BE, Moss SE. Risk factors for retinopathy. In: Feman SS, editor. Ocular problems in diabetes mellitus. Boston, MA: Blackwell Scientific Publications; 1992. p. 39.)

actual prevalence now found in the population.[68] For a specific duration of type 1 diabetes, people diagnosed between 1975 and 1980 had a statistically significantly lower prevalence than persons diagnosed in earlier periods ($P < 0.001$). This difference remained while controlling for A1c, systolic and diastolic blood pressure, and presence of proteinuria. Similarly, for specific duration of type 2 diabetes, those diagnosed more recently had a lower prevalence of diabetic retinopathy than those diagnosed in earlier periods.

Harris et al.,[100] using retinopathy prevalence data at different durations of diabetes from persons with type 2 diabetes in the WESDR and from a study in Australia, extrapolated to the time when retinopathy prevalence was estimated to be zero. They estimated that the onset of detectable retinopathy occurred approximately 4–7 years after diagnosis of type 2 diabetes in these populations.

In the WESDR, the 4- and 10-year incidence of diabetic retinopathy increased with increasing duration of diabetes at baseline.[50,51,53] The risk of developing retinopathy in the younger-onset group was high (74%) after 10 years of diabetes. The 4-year incidence of proliferative retinopathy varied from 0% during the first 3 years after diagnosis of diabetes to 28% in those with 13–14 years of diabetes. Thereafter, the incidence remained stable.[50] A similar trend was found in a cohort of patients with type 1 diabetes followed at the Joslin Clinic.[101] In the older-onset WESDR group, 2% of those with less than 5 years and 5% of those with 15 or more years of diabetes who were not taking insulin at baseline developed signs of proliferative retinopathy at the 4-year follow-up.[51]

AGE AT DIAGNOSIS

Age at diagnosis was not related to incidence or progression of diabetic retinopathy in any of the diabetes groups followed in the WESDR.[50,51] In contrast, while controlling for other risk factors, in a cohort with type 2 diabetes in Rochester, Minnesota, the development of retinopathy was significantly associated with younger age at diagnosis.[14]

GLYCEMIA

In 1978, in his textbook on the epidemiology of diabetes and its complications, Kelly West wrote: "The extent to which hyperglycemia determines the risk of retinopathy is not at all clear. This is the most important issue at hand and deserves high priority in epidemiologic research."[102] Thirty years later, this issue has largely been resolved by epidemiologic studies and clinical trials.

The Diabetes Control and Complications Trial (DCCT) was "designed to compare intensive with conventional diabetes therapy with regard to their effects on the development and progression of the early vascular and neurologic complications of IDDM."[103] Two of the main questions asked in the study were: "Will intensive therapy prevent the development of diabetic retinopathy in patients with no retinopathy (primary prevention)?" and "Will intensive therapy affect the progression of early retinopathy (secondary intervention)?" In addition, the DCCT examined the magnitude of the effect of intensive insulin treatment on progression of retinopathy, the degree to which this effect changes over time, and the relation of the effect to the level of severity of the retinopathy at baseline.[104–106]

Subjects included persons with type 1 diabetes who were C-peptide-deficient, 13–39 years of age, who were in general good health except for the presence of type 1 diabetes, and did not have hypertension, hypercholesterolemia, or other severe medical conditions. There were two groups. In the primary prevention group, subjects were required to have had type 1 diabetes for 1–5 years, have no retinopathy as detected by stereoscopic fundus photography of seven fields of both eyes, a best-corrected visual acuity of 20/25 or better in each eye, and a urinary excretion rate of <40 mg of albumin in 24 hours. In the secondary prevention group, subjects were required to have had type 1 diabetes for 1–15 years, minimal to moderate nonproliferative retinopathy in at least one eye, best corrected visual acuity of 20/32 or better in each eye, and a urinary excretion rate of <200 mg of albumin per 24 hours.

Randomization was used to assign conventional or intensive insulin therapy.[103] Conventional therapy consisted of one or two daily injections of insulin per day, daily self-monitoring of urine or blood glucose, and education about exercise and diet. No attempts were made to adjust the insulin dosage on a daily basis. Intensive therapy consisted of administration of insulin three or more times daily by injections or an external pump. In addition, there was adjustment of the insulin dosage under the direction of an expert team, taking into account self-monitoring of blood glucose performed four times per day, dietary intake, and anticipated exercise.[104]

From 1983 through 1989, 1441 patients were randomized. The primary outcome measure was a sustained (at two consecutive 6-month visits) three-step progression of diabetic retinopathy. This was based on an ordinal severity scale based on retinopathy scores in both eyes, determined by grading of stereoscopic color fundus photographs of the seven standard fields. Nonocular outcomes measured in the study were development of urinary albumin excretion of >40 mg per 24 hours (microalbuminuria) or >300 mg per 24 hours (gross proteinuria), and the incidence of clinical neuropathy. Adverse events included mortality, incidence of severe hypoglycemia, weight gain, myocardial infarction, and stroke.

The average follow-up in the study was 6.5 years (range 3–9 years) after randomization. The average difference in A1c between the intensive and conventional treatment groups for both the primary and secondary prevention was nearly 2%. Less than 5% of the cohort in the intensively treated group were able to maintain their A1c level at 6.0% or less over the course of the study.

An important finding of the trial was the statistically significant reduction in risk of sustained progression of retinopathy by three or more steps by 76% (Table 45.3, Fig. 45.5). In the secondary-intervention cohort, the intensive therapy group had a reduction of average risk of progression by 54% during the entire study period compared to the patients assigned to the conventional-therapy group. In addition, when both cohorts were combined, the intensive therapy group also had a reduction in risk for development of severe nonproliferative retinopathy or proliferative retinopathy by 47% and of treatment with photocoagulation by 51% (Table 45.3). There was a decrease in the incidence of clinically significant macular edema in the group assigned to intensive therapy compared to those assigned to conventional therapy. However, this difference did not reach statistical significance.

Early worsening of retinopathy in the first year of treatment of the intensive therapy group in the secondary-intervention cohort was observed, as had been reported previously.[107–109] On average, it took about 3 years to demonstrate the beneficial effect of intensive treatment. After 3 years, the beneficial effect of intensive insulin treatment increased over time.

The DCCT investigators also examined whether there was an association of A1c values <8% versus those of ≥8% for progression of retinopathy. When they combined the two groups (conventional and intensive treatment), they found no evidence to support the concept of a glycemic threshold regarding progression of retinopathy, as had been described by others.[110]

Intensive insulin treatment reduced but did not prevent the incidence and progression of retinopathy in persons without signs of retinopathy at the baseline examination. The 9-year cumulative incidence of one microaneurysm or more severe retinopathy in eyes with no retinopathy present at baseline was 70% in persons with <2.5 years of type 1 diabetes and 62% in persons with >2.5 years of type 1 diabetes at baseline. Approximately 40% of these individuals developed a three-step progression of their retinopathy.[105]

The DCCT examined whether intensive therapy was more beneficial when started earlier in the course of type 1 diabetes. They found that the 9-year cumulative incidence of sustained three-step progression in persons without retinopathy with <2.5

Table 45.3 Development and progression of long-term complications of diabetes in the study cohorts and reduction in risk with intensive as compared with conventional therapy*

	Primary prevention			Secondary intervention			Both cohorts**
	Conventional therapy	Intensive therapy	Risk reduction	Conventional therapy	Intensive therapy	Risk reduction	Risk reduction
Complications	Rate/100 patient yr		% (95% CI)	Rate/100 patient yr		% (95% CI)	% (95% CI)
≥3-step sustained retinopathy	4.7	1.2	76 (62–85)†	7.8	3.7	54 (39–66)†	63 (52–71)†
Macular edema‡	–	–	–	3.0	2.0	23 (–13–48)	26 (–8–50)
Severe nonproliferative or proliferative retinopathy‡	–	–	–	2.4	1.1	47 (14–67)§	47 (15–67)§
Laser treatment§§	–	–	–	2.3	0.9	56 (26–74)†	51 (21–70)§

*Rates shown are absolute rates of the development and progression of complications per 100 patient-years. Risk reductions represent the comparison of intensive with conventional treatment, expressed as a percentage and calculated from the proportional-hazards model with adjustment for baseline values as noted, except in the case of neuropathy. CI denotes confidence interval.
**Stratified according to the primary-prevention and secondary-prevention cohorts.
†$P \leq 0.002$ by the two-tailed rank-sum test.
‡Too few events occurred in the primary-prevention cohort to allow meaningful analysis of this variable.
§$P < 0.04$ by the two-tailed rank-sum test.
§§Denotes the first episode of laser therapy for macular edema or proliferative retinopathy.
(Reprinted with permission from The Diabetes Control and Complications Trial Research Group (DCCT). The effect of intensive treatment of diabetes on the development and progression of long-term complications in insulin-dependent diabetes mellitus. N Engl J Med 1993;329:977–86. Copyright © 1993 Massachusetts Medical Society.)

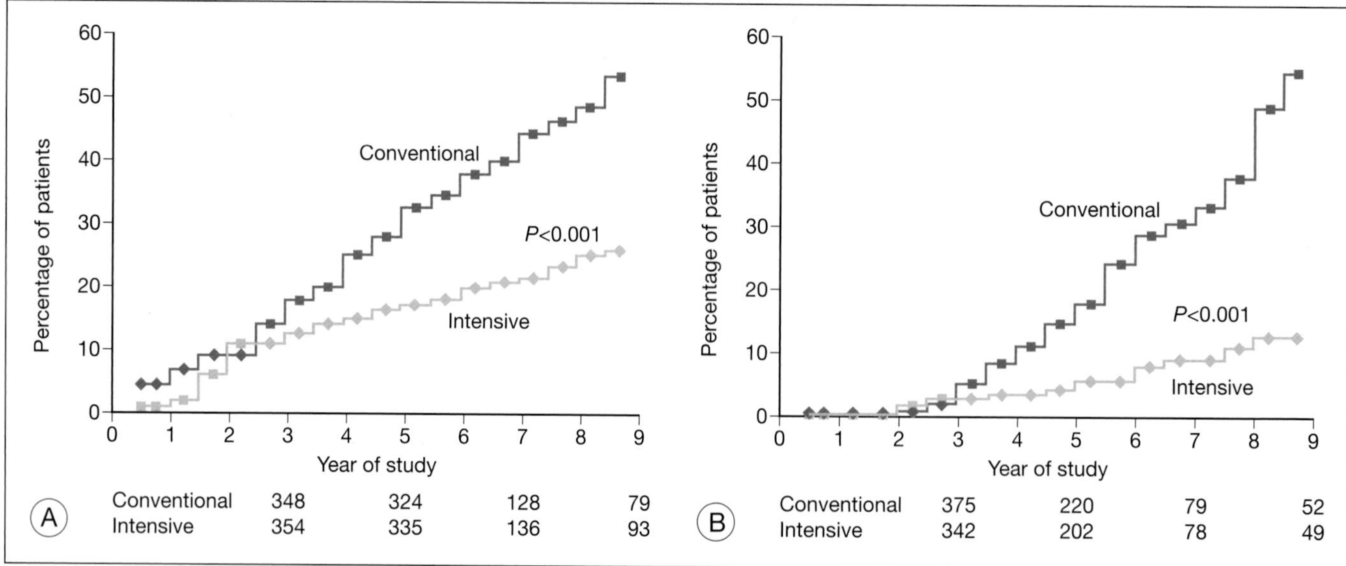

Fig. 45.5 Cumulative incidence of a sustained change in retinopathy in patients with type 1 diabetes mellitus receiving intensive or conventional therapy in (A) the primary prevention and (B) the secondary intervention arms of the Diabetes Control and Complications Trial. (Reproduced with permission from The Diabetes Control and Complications Trial Research Group (DCCT). The effect of intensive treatment of diabetes on the development and progression of long-term complications in insulin-dependent diabetes mellitus. N Engl J Med 1993; 329:977–86. Copyright © 1993 Massachusetts Medical Society.)

years of type 1 diabetes in the intensive therapy group was 7% compared to 20% in those with >2.5 years. The 9-year cumulative incidence of sustained three-step progression in the intensive therapy group was lower in eyes with minimal to early nonproliferative retinopathy at baseline compared to eyes with more severe nonproliferative retinopathy at baseline (11.5–18.2% vs 43.8%). These data suggested a benefit of beginning intensive treatment earlier in the course of diabetes, prior to the onset of diabetic retinopathy.[105]

The most important adverse event was a two- to threefold increase in severe hypoglycemia in the intensive insulin-treatment group compared to the conventional group. There was a 33% increase in the mean adjusted risk of becoming overweight (body weight more than 120% above the ideal) in persons in the intensive compared to the conventional insulin-treatment group, also considered an adverse outcome.

From the trial, it was estimated that intensive therapy would result in a "gain of 920,000 years of sight, 691,000 years free from end-stage renal disease, 678,000 years free from lower extremity amputation, and 611,000 years of life at an additional cost of $4.0 billion over the lifetime" of the 120000 persons with IDDM in the United States who meet DCCT eligibility criteria.[111] The incremental cost per year of life gained was $28661, and when adjusted for quality of life, intensive therapy costs $19987 per quality-of-life year gained. These findings were similar to cost-effectiveness ratios for other medical interventions in the United States.

Fourteen years of additional follow-up of the DCCT cohort after the study was stopped revealed that despite convergence of A1c levels in the intensive and conventional groups, the protective effect of glycemic control was maintained in the intensive group.[112–114] This has been labeled "metabolic memory" and has been found also in persons with type 2 diabetes in the UKPDS (see below).[115] The reason for this finding remains speculative. Recent data suggest that biochemical pathways involving advanced glycation endproducts and oxidative stress may affect genes and proteins involved in the pathogenesis of diabetic microvascular and macrovascular complications.[114]

The UK Prospective Diabetes Study (UKPDS) was a randomized controlled clinical trial involving 3867 patients newly diagnosed with type 2 diabetes.[116–118] After 3 months of diet treatment, patients with a mean of two fasting plasma glucose concentrations of 6.1–15.0 mmol/L were randomly assigned to intensive glycemic control with either a sulfonylurea or insulin or conventional glycemic control. The latter group was further divided into those who were overweight or not. Metformin was included as one of the treatment arms for 1704 overweight patients, and analyses included comparison of the effect of metformin against conventional therapy in overweight patients. After 12 years of follow-up, there was a reduction in rate of progression of diabetic retinopathy of 21% and reduction in need for laser photocoagulation of 29% in the intensive versus the conventional treatment group. In addition, there were no differences in reduction in the incidence of the retinopathy endpoints among the three agents used in the intensive treatment group (chlorpropamide, glibenclamide, and insulin) but the chlorpropamide treatment group failed to show a reduced rate of retinopathy requiring photocoagulation. Furthermore, there was no difference in vision outcomes between conventional and intensive treatments. It was concluded that metformin was preferred as the first-line pharmacological therapy in newly diagnosed type 2 diabetic patients who were overweight, based on their finding of a significant (39%) reduction in myocardial infarction compared to the conventional treatment group. When metformin was added to sulfonlyureas (in both obese and nonobese patients), however, it was associated with increased diabetes-related (96%) and all-cause mortality (60%) when compared to conventional therapy. The intensive treatment group suffered significantly more major hypoglycemic episodes and weight gain than patients in the conventional group. Economic analyses of the clinical trial data suggested that intensive glucose control increased treatment costs but substantially reduced complication costs and increased the time free of such complications.[118]

The development of new treatment modalities for achieving glycemic control has resulted in two recently completed randomized clinical trials that permitted evaluation of near normalization of glycemic level on the incidence of cardiovascular disease and retinopathy. The first trial involved 1791 military veterans with an average age of 60 years and an average duration of 11 years of type 2 diabetes, who had a suboptimal response to therapy for their diabetes. They were randomly assigned to receive either intensive or standard glucose control, with an aim in the intensive therapy group of achieving an absolute reduction of 1.5 percentage points in the A1c level as compared with the standard therapy group. The primary outcome was the time to the first occurrence of a major cardiovascular disease event, and a secondary objective was to evaluate the effect of glycemic control on the incidence and progression of diabetic retinopathy and other microvascular complications.[119,120] The subjects were followed for up to 7.5 years (median: 5.6 years). Despite reaching their glycemic goal (median A1c level at 6 months: 8.4% in the group receiving standard therapy and 6.9% in the intensive therapy group), there were no statistically significant differences in any of the retinopathy outcomes between groups receiving intensive and standard therapy (incidence of retinopathy 42% vs 49%, P = 0.27; progression of retinopathy by two or more steps on the Early Treatment Diabetic Retinopathy Study [ETDRS] severity scale 17% vs 22%, P = 0.07; progression to proliferative diabetic retinopathy 4% vs 5%, P = 0.27) or in progression to clinically significant macular edema (3% vs 5%, P = 0.31). While it is possible that a benefit might have been seen if the study was continued, these data lead to the conclusion that decreasing the A1c level from 8.4% to 6.9% in persons with relatively long-standing type 2 diabetes has little benefit in preventing the incidence and progression of retinopathy.

Another recently concluded large randomized controlled clinical trial is Action to Control Cardiovascular Risk in Diabetes (ACCORD), which examined whether intensive treatment with an even lower targeted A1c level (<6.0%) than in the military veteran study versus standard treatment (targeted A1c level 7.0–7.9%) would reduce the risk of morbidity and mortality from cardiovascular disease (primary endpoint) and microvascular events, such as the incidence of photocoagulation treatment for diabetic retinopathy and incidence of microalbuminuria and macroalbuminuria over a 5-year period (secondary endpoints) in persons with a mean age of 60 years with an average duration of 10 years of type 2 diabetes.[121,122] They reported findings on the same composite microvascular endpoints measured in the UKPDS. They also reported the incidence and progression of diabetic retinopathy on the basis of the grading of fundus photographs in a sample of 4065 of the 10 251 participants. They did not find a statistically significant difference in their composite microvascular endpoints (one combining a history of advanced kidney and eye disease, and the other adding peripheral neuropathy to that outcome) or for some of the other specified ocular or renal outcomes. In the eye study, using the grading of fundus photographs to assess intensive glycemic control, they reported a 33% reduction in the relative risk of progression from 7.3% with intensive glycemia treatment, versus 10.4% with standard therapy (adjusted OR 0.67; 95% CI 0.51–0.87; P = 0.003) in a relatively short period (4 years). The ACCORD intensive glycemic strategy was prematurely discontinued because of a statistically significant 22% increase in overall mortality in the intensive glycemic group of the study. Median A1c was 6.3% compared with 7.6% in the standard glycemic group. The study closure of the glycemic phase of the trial made it too short and the power too low to observe a protective effect for the severe microvascular endpoints, which usually evolve over a longer period.[53]

An additional clinical trial that was recently concluded, the Action in Diabetes and Vascular Disease: Preterax and Diamicron Modified Release Controlled Evaluation (ADVANCE) study of patients with type 2 diabetes, showed no statistically significant effect of glycemic control on severe diabetes related to ocular endpoints.[123]

Based on the results of these studies, it appears that intensive therapy should be the primary public healthcare strategy aimed at reducing the risk of visual loss from diabetic retinopathy in persons with both type 1 and 2 diabetes. The data from the DCCT and UKPDS provided further support for the ADA guidelines of a target goal of A1c level of 7.0% for persons with diabetes, and suggest that this level of control, when achieved earlier after diagnosis of diabetes, may have greater long-term benefit in terms of reducing the incidence and progression of retinopathy.[124] However, data from the NHANES III[125] and the WESDR[126] suggest that few persons with diabetes reach this targeted level of glycemic control. The data from the military veterans study, the ACCORD, and the ADVANCE suggest that further lowering the level of glycemia does not support applying intensive glycemic control with the current technology to achieve such control in patients with long-standing type 2 diabetes who have or who are at risk of cardiovascular disease.[127,128]

C-PEPTIDE STATUS

The relationship of endogenous insulin secretion to diabetic retinopathy independent of glycemic control is uncertain.[129–132] In the WESDR, the highest prevalence and most severe retinopathy were found in individuals with undetectable or low plasma C-peptide (<0.3 nM), whereas the lowest frequencies and least severe retinopathy were found in older-onset individuals not using insulin who were overweight.[133] Older- and younger-onset individuals who were using insulin and who had no detectable C-peptide had similar frequencies of proliferative retinopathy. While controlling for other risk factors associated with the incidence and progression of diabetic retinopathy, there was no relationship of C-peptide level to incident or progressed retinopathy in persons with type 1 diabetes in the WESDR.[134] In the DCCT, however, higher C-peptide levels at entry were associated with reduced incidence of retinopathy and lower incidence of hypoglycemic episodes.[135] In the WESDR, while controlling for characteristics associated with retinopathy in older-onset people who were not taking insulin (type 2 diabetes), there was no protection associated with higher levels of C-peptide.[133,134] These findings suggest that the level of glycemia, and not the level of endogenous insulin secretion as indicated by C-peptide level, is more important in determining the presence and severity of retinopathy in individuals with type 2 diabetes.

EXOGENOUS INSULIN

It has been suggested that exogenous insulin may be a possible cause of atherosclerosis and retinopathy in people with type 2 diabetes.[136] In the WESDR, there was no association between the amount or type of exogenous insulin used and the presence, severity, incidence or progression of retinopathy in the older-onset group using insulin whose C-peptide was 0.3 nM or greater.[133,134] These data suggest that exogenous insulin in itself is unlikely to be causally related to retinopathy in diabetic people with normal C-peptide levels.

BLOOD PRESSURE

In the WESDR, blood pressure was a significant predictor of the 14-year incidence of diabetic retinopathy in people with type 1 diabetes.[58] While controlling for other risk factors such as retinopathy severity, A1c, and duration of diabetes at baseline, the relationships between blood pressure and the incidence or progression of retinopathy remained in the younger-onset group. However, in the WESDR, neither the systolic nor the diastolic blood pressure was found to be related to the 10-year incidence and progression of retinopathy in those with type 2 diabetes.[137] The UKPDS did find that the incidence of retinopathy was associated with systolic blood pressure. For each 10 mmHg decrease in mean systolic blood pressure, a 13% reduction was found for microvascular complications. No threshold was found for any retinopathy endpoint.[138] In the WESDR, a 10 mmHg rise in diastolic blood pressure was found to be associated with a 330% increased 4-year risk of developing macular edema in those with type 1 diabetes and a 210% increased risk in those with type 2 diabetes.[139]

The UKPDS sought to determine whether lowering blood pressure was beneficial in reducing macrovascular and microvascular complications associated with type 2 diabetes.[140] A series of 1048 patients with hypertension (mean blood pressure 160/94 mmHg) were randomized to a regimen of tight control with either captopril (an angiotensin-converting enzyme [ACE] inhibitor) or atenolol (a beta-blocker) and another 390 patients to less tight control of their blood pressure. The aim in the group randomized to tight control of blood pressure (by the standards at the beginning of the clinical trial) was to achieve blood pressure values <150/<85 mmHg. If these goals were not met with maximal doses of a beta-blocker or ACE inhibitor, additional medications were prescribed, including a loop diuretic, a calcium-channel blocker, and a vasodilator. The aim in the group randomized to less tight control was to achieve blood pressure values <180/<105 mmHg. Tight blood pressure control resulted in a 35% reduction in retinal photocoagulation compared to conventional control, presumably due to a lower incidence of macular edema. After 7.5 years of follow-up, there was a 34% reduction in the rate of progression of retinopathy by two or more steps using the modified ETDRS severity scale and a 47% reduction in the deterioration of visual acuity by 3 lines or more using the ETDRS charts (for example, a reduction in vision from 20/30 to 20/60 or worse on a Snellen chart). Atenolol and captopril were equally effective in reducing the risk of developing these microvascular complications, suggesting that blood pressure reduction itself was more important than the type of medication used to reduce it. The effects of blood pressure control were independent of those of glycemic control. These findings support the recommendations for blood pressure control in patients with type 2 diabetes as a means of preventing visual loss from diabetic retinopathy.

The ACCORD also examined whether in the context of good glycemic control, a "therapeutic strategy that targets a systolic blood pressure of <120 mmHg would reduce cardiovascular disease events compared to a strategy that targets a systolic blood pressure of <140 mmHg in persons with type 2 diabetes."[121] There were 1263 ACCORD-Eye study participants enrolled in the ACCORD blood pressure study. After 1 year, the baseline median systolic blood pressure lowered significantly (from 133 to 117 mmHg) in the intensive blood pressure therapy group compared to the standard blood pressure therapy group and remained stable throughout the remainder of the trial. The rates of progression of diabetic retinopathy were 10% in the group undergoing intensive blood pressure control compared to 9% in the group undergoing standard blood pressure control (adjusted OR 1.23; 95% CI 0.84–1.79; $P = 0.29$).

The ADVANCE study also found no beneficial effect of intensive blood pressure control on progression of diabetic retinopathy.[141] These findings from the ACCORD, ADVANCE, and UKPDS suggest that the benefit in preventing the progression of diabetic retinopathy may be limited to those with type 2 diabetes with uncontrolled high blood pressure.

A number of randomized controlled clinical trials have examined whether specific antihypertensive agents had a protective effect in preventing the progression of retinopathy independent of its effect on blood pressure.[142–148] The Epidemiology and Prevention of Diabetes (EURODIAB) Controlled Trial of Lisinopril in Insulin-Dependent Diabetes Mellitus (EUCLID) study sought to examine the role of an ACE inhibitor in reducing the incidence and progression of retinopathy in a group of largely normotensive type 1 diabetic patients, of whom 85% did not have microalbuminuria at baseline.[142] This study showed a statistically significant 50% reduction in the progression of retinopathy in those taking lisinopril over a two-year period after adjustment for glycemic control. Progression to proliferative retinopathy was also reduced, although the relation was not statistically significant. There was no significant interaction with blood glucose control. It was postulated that ACE inhibitors might have an effect independent of lowering of blood pressure.[143]

The Diabetic Retinopathy Candesartan Trials (DIRECT) comprised of three randomized double-masked, parallel, placebo-controlled studies, involving 5231 patients with type 1 or type 2 diabetes. The aim of the trials was to determine the impact of treatment with 32 mg of candesartan, an angiotensin II type 1 receptor blockade, on the incidence and progression of diabetic retinopathy over a 4-year period.[144,145,148] The DIRECT-Prevent 1 ($n = 1421$) involved prevention of incident diabetic retinopathy while the DIRECT-Protect 1 ($n = 1905$) involved protection against progression of diabetic retinopathy in normoalbuminuric normotensive individuals with type 1 diabetes, respectively, while the DIRECT-Protect 2 ($n = 1905$) involved protection against progression of diabetic retinopathy in persons with type 2 diabetes who were normoalbuminuric, and either normotensive or only mildly hypertensive.[147,148] In the DIRECT-Prevent 1, candesartan had a borderline effect ($P = 0.0508$) on the primary endpoint, reducing the incidence of retinopathy by two or more steps on the ETDRS severity scale by 18%. In post-hoc analyses, candesartan reduced the incidence of retinopathy by three or more steps by 35% (hazard ratio 0.65; 95% CI 0.48–0.87) in the DIRECT-Prevent 1. In the DIRECT-Protect 1 and 2, candesartan had no statistically significant effect on the progression of retinopathy (defined as three or more steps on the ETDRS severity scale in persons with minimal to moderately severe nonproliferative diabetic retinopathy at baseline). However, in the

DIRECT-Protect 2, treatment with candesartan significantly increased a secondary outcome, regression of retinopathy, by 34% (hazard ratio 1.34; 95% CI 1.08–1.68). The effects were limited to those participants with early retinopathy. Thus, the DIRECT, while suggestive of a beneficial effect of candesartan in reducing the incidence of retinopathy, did not achieve the prespecified primary endpoint in any of the three trials.

The ADVANCE study involved more than 11 000 participants and examined whether lowering of blood pressure via a perindopril–indapamide combination provided additional benefit in preventing diabetic macrovascular and microvascular complications.[141] Although mean systolic and diastolic blood pressure reduction by 5.6 mmHg and 2.2 mmHg, respectively, was achieved, there was no reduction in the 4-year incidence or progression of diabetic retinopathy (5.2% in both treatment and placebo groups).

The Renin-Angiotensin System Study (RASS) was a multicenter controlled trial involving 285 normotensive patients with type 1 diabetes and normoalbuminuria and who were randomly assigned to receive losartan (100 mg daily), enalapril (20 mg daily), or placebo and followed for 5 years.[146] It showed that, as compared with placebo, the odds of retinopathy progression by two or more steps was reduced by 65% with enalapril (OR 0.35; 95% CI 0.14–0.85) and by 70% with losartan (OR 0.30; 95% CI 0.12–0.73), independently of changes in blood pressure.

These clinical trial data show a protective effect on incidence of retinopathy by angiotensin inhibitors or receptor blockers in normotensive, normoalbuminuric persons with no retinopathy, and an inconsistent effect on progression in those with early to moderately severe nonproliferative retinopathy. The reasons for the differences in findings in the RASS, DIRECT, and ADVANCE are not known. Any decision to use these agents to prevent diabetic retinopathy must be tempered by the findings in the RASS and DIRECT of an increase in the albumin excretion rate in those receiving losartan or candesartan compared to those in the placebo group.

PROTEINURIA AND DIABETIC NEPHROPATHY

Data from most studies show an association between the prevalence of diabetic nephropathy, as manifest by microalbuminuria or gross proteinuria, and diabetic retinopathy.[2,3,17,22,23,26,53,77,149,150] There are anecdotal reports of patients with renal failure having more severe macular edema that improves after dialysis or renal transplantation. Lipid, rheological, and platelet abnormalities associated with nephropathy may be involved in the pathogenesis of retinopathy. In the WESDR, in those with type 1 diabetes, the relative risk of proliferative retinopathy developing over four years in those with gross proteinuria at baseline was 2.32 (95% CI 1.40–3.83) compared with those without gross proteinuria.[149] However, after controlling for other relevant risk factors, the relationship was of borderline significance. For the older-onset group with type 2 diabetes in the WESDR taking insulin, the relative risk was 2.02 (95% CI 0.91–4.44), and for those not taking insulin it was 1.13 (95% CI 0.15–8.50).

A greater proportion of those with type 1 diabetes participating in a cohort study in Pittsburgh who had microalbuminuria or overt nephropathy at entry to the study progressed to proliferative disease over a 2-year follow-up.[151] However, in the same study nephropathy at baseline was not associated with overall progression of retinopathy. Data from these studies suggest that in those with type 1 diabetes, gross proteinuria is a risk indicator for proliferative retinopathy. These patients may benefit from having regular ophthalmologic evaluation. There have been no clinical trial data to suggest that interventions that prevent or slow diabetic nephropathy will reduce the incidence and progression of retinopathy.

SERUM LIPIDS AND LIPID LOWERING

Macular edema is an important cause of loss of vision in people with diabetes.[152] Hard exudate, a lipoprotein deposit, is often associated with macular edema. Data from early clinical studies showed an association of elevated plasma triglycerides and lipids with hard exudate.[153]

In the WESDR, higher serum total cholesterol was associated with higher prevalence of retinal hard exudates in both the younger- and the older-onset groups taking insulin but not in those with type 2 diabetes using oral hypoglycemic agents.[154] In the ETDRS, higher levels of serum lipids (triglycerides, low-density lipoproteins, and very-low-density lipoproteins) at baseline were associated with increased risk of developing hard exudates in the macula and decreased visual acuity.[155] In a study of Mexican patients with type 2 diabetes, Santos et al.[88] showed the frequency of severe retinal hard exudates was higher in those with the epsilon4 allele polymorphism of the apolipoprotein E gene.

While small pilot studies suggest possible efficacy of statin therapy in preventing or reducing the severity of macular edema there are few large clinical trials showing the efficacy of statins of other lipid-lowering agents in reducing the progression of retinopathy, the incidence of macular edema or the loss of vision.[121,156–158] One is the ACCORD Lipid study, which enrolled a total of 1593 persons with type 2 diabetes and examined whether a "therapeutic strategy of treatment with fenofibrate and statins that raises the serum high-density lipoprotein cholesterol and lowers triglyceride levels in the context of desirable levels of serum LDL cholesterol and good glycemic control reduces the incidence of macular edema and progression of retinopathy compared to a strategy that only achieves desirable levels of LDL cholesterol and glycemic control using statins alone." Serum triglycerides fell from 162 mg/dL at baseline to 120 mg/dL in the fenofibrate treatment group as compared with a decrease to 147 mg/dL in the placebo group after 1 year ($P < 0.001$). The rate of progression of diabetic retinopathy at 4 years was 6.5% in the fenofibrate treatment group compared to 10.2% in the placebo group (adjusted OR 0.60; 95% CI 0.42–0.87; $P = 0.006$). These findings are consistent with the findings from the Fenofibrate Intervention and Event Lowering in Diabetes (FIELD) study, a randomized trial of monotherapy with fenofibrate, which showed a significant reduction in the need for laser therapy for either macular edema or proliferative retinopathy in the fenofibrate treatment group as compared with the placebo group (3.4% vs 4.9%, $P < 0.001$).[159] These findings suggest a beneficial effect of the use of fenofibrate therapy in diabetic patients with elevated triglycerides at risk of progression of diabetic retinopathy and macular edema.

SMOKING

Smoking would be expected to be associated with retinopathy because it is known to cause tissue hypoxia by increasing blood carbon monoxide levels, which causes vasoconstriction of the small blood vessels.[160] Additionally, smoking may lead to increased platelet aggregation and adhesiveness.[161] However, most epidemiologic data show no relationship between cigarette smoking and the incidence or progression of diabetic retinopathy.[14,23,26,77,79,162–164] In the WESDR, cigarette smoking was not associated with the 4- or 10-year incidence or progression of diabetic retinopathy nor of macular edema.[163,164] Despite this, diabetic patients should be advised not to smoke because of an increased risk of cardiovascular and respiratory disease, to which persons with diabetes are already prone, as well as cancer. In the WESDR, after controlling for other risk factors, younger-onset people who smoked were 2.4 times as likely and older-onset people were 1.6 times as likely to die as those who did not smoke.[165]

ALCOHOL

Because moderate alcohol consumption is associated with decreased platelet aggregation and adhesiveness, improved glycemic control, and reduction of inflammation, one might anticipate a possible protective effect in reducing the incidence and progression of retinopathy.[166–168] Data from one study suggested such a beneficial effect, while that from another study suggested an increased risk of proliferative retinopathy.[169,170] No relation between alcohol consumption and diabetic retinopathy was found in a population-based study in Australia.[32] In the UKPDS, a relation of increased alcohol consumption to increased severity of retinopathy was found only in men with newly diagnosed type 2 diabetes.[38] In the EURODIAB Prospective Study of Complications in persons with type 1 diabetes, alcohol consumption was associated with a reduction in progression of diabetic retinopathy.[171] In the ADVANCE Retinopathy Measurements (ADREM), a clinical trial of persons with type 2 diabetes, there was no relation of alcohol consumption to progression of diabetic retinopathy, but for unknown reasons, a decline in the visual acuity at follow-up was seen in those who consumed alcohol when compared with those who abstained from alcohol.[172] In the WESDR, alcohol consumption was associated with a lower frequency of proliferative retinopathy in persons with type 1 diabetes.[173] There was no relationship, however, between alcohol consumption at the 4-year examination and the incidence and progression of retinopathy in either the younger- or older-onset groups at the 10-year follow-up,[174] nor was there a relation to a change in visual acuity. Of interest in the WESDR was an association of reduction in cardiovascular disease mortality in persons with type 1 diabetes who consumed an average of one drink of alcohol per day.[175]

BODY MASS INDEX (BMI)

The relationship between diabetic retinopathy and BMI is inconsistent among various studies.[2,14,77,80,176–179] In the WESDR, body mass was inversely related to the presence or severity of diabetic retinopathy only in persons with type 2 diabetes not using insulin.[179] While controlling for other risk factors, older-onset persons in the WESDR who were underweight at baseline (BMI <20 kg/m^2 for both men and women) were three times as likely to develop retinopathy as those who were of normal weight (BMI of 20–27.7 kg/m^2 for men and 20–27.2 kg/m^2 for women). It has been speculated that underweight older-onset subjects are more likely to be in a "severe" phase of their type 2 diabetes or have late-onset type 1 diabetes. Persons obese at baseline (BMI >31.0 kg/m^2 for men and >32.1 kg/m^2 for women) were 35% more likely to have progression of retinopathy and 41% more likely to develop proliferative retinopathy than those who were of normal weight at baseline. However, these associations were not statistically significant.

PHYSICAL ACTIVITY

Physical activity, through its beneficial effect on glycemic control, would be expected to be associated with decreased prevalence and incidence of diabetic retinopathy.[180] However, few epidemiologic data are available describing the relationship between diabetic retinopathy and physical activity.[177,181–183] One study found no relationship between participating in team sports in high school or college and a history of laser treatment or blindness in people with type 1 diabetes.[177] The same group reported that physical activity in youth did not relate to complications of diabetes.[181,182] In the WESDR, women diagnosed with diabetes before 14 years of age who participated in team sports were less likely to have proliferative diabetic retinopathy than those who did not.[183] There was no association between physical activity or leisure time energy expenditure and the presence and severity of diabetic retinopathy in men. In addition, physical activity was associated with either an increased or decreased risk of progression of retinopathy or the development of proliferative retinopathy over a 6-year interval in people with type 1 diabetes in this study.[184]

SOCIOECONOMIC STATUS

Inconsistent relationships between socioeconomic status and retinopathy severity have been reported.[31,77,185,186] Hanna et al.[185] reported a significant correlation between proliferative retinopathy and occupational status (working class) or lower income in a case–control study of 49 people with type 1 diabetes. Haffner et al.[186] did not find a relationship between socioeconomic status, measured using a combination of the Duncan Index, educational attainment or income, and severe retinopathy in 343 Mexican Americans and 79 non-Hispanic whites with type 2 diabetes in San Antonio. West et al.[77] also did not observe a relationship between retinopathy severity and education level in a population of Oklahoma Indians with type 2 diabetes. In the Proyecto VER cohort of Mexican Americans, low income, once adjusted for other factors, was related to proliferative retinopathy (OR 3.93; 95% CI 1.31–11.80).[31]

There are few studies that have examined the relation of socioeconomic factors to incidence and progression of diabetic retinopathy.[62,187] In the New Jersey 725 study, low socioeconomic status was significantly associated with the 6-year incidence of macular edema but not incidence or progression of diabetic retinopathy. In that study, education, income, medical or eye care, and health insurance at baseline were not significantly different between patients with and without macular edema at follow-up. In the WESDR, except for an association of lower incidence of proliferative retinopathy in women with type 1 diabetes of 25 years of age or older with more education, socioeconomic status (education level and Duncan Socioeconomic Index score) was not associated with risk of developing proliferative retinopathy.[187] It may be that the absence of a relationship of socioeconomic status and retinopathy severity in the WESDR and San Antonio Study is related to the lack of an association of glycemia to socioeconomic status in these populations.

HORMONE AND REPRODUCTIVE EXPOSURES IN WOMEN

In the WESDR, menarchal status at the baseline examination was related to the prevalence and severity of retinopathy[96] as noted previously in the section on puberty. Sex hormones have been hypothesized to explain the higher risk of developing retinopathy after puberty as well.[96] However, it seems unlikely that increased estrogen associated with the onset of puberty is responsible for the increase in retinopathy. Use of oral contraceptives, which contain estrogens as well as progestins, does not appear to increase the risk of retinopathy[188] nor does use of hormone replacement therapy.[189]

Pregnancy, a condition associated with high levels of estrogens, is associated with more rapid progression of retinopathy. When pregnant women were compared with nonpregnant diabetic women of similar age and duration of diabetes, the pregnant women were more likely to develop retinopathy if they had not had it before or to have greater likelihood of progression of their retinopathy when the groups were followed for a time interval roughly equal to the length of the pregnancy.[190] This remained true after controlling for level of glycemia and blood pressure. Similar findings have been reported by others.[191,192] This may occur in those with type 2 as well as type 1 diabetes.[193] A complementary finding was reported by Lovestam-Adrian et al.[194] who found that progression of retinopathy was more likely to occur in pre-eclamptic diabetic women than in those without pre-eclampsia. Similarly, Rosenn et al.[195] found that glycemia and blood pressure were important determinants of progression of retinopathy during pregnancy. While these are important factors in nonpregnant women, pregnancy in all likelihood accelerates the process. Other investigators have found that progression of retinopathy was related to prior duration of diabetes.[196,197] Because duration of diabetes is a risk factor for progression of retinopathy irrespective of pregnancy status, this is also not a novel finding. However, it may be useful information in tailoring a follow-up plan for eye care during pregnancy. It has been suggested that laser treatment before pregnancy for women with moderate to severe retinopathy be considered to protect against progression during pregnancy,[198] although a clinical trial of the efficacy of such an approach is lacking. Aside from diabetic retinopathy, diabetic macular edema that occurs during pregnancy poses a threat to vision and this may benefit from laser treatment,[199] although it is unclear how many women with this sight-threatening complication will have remission after parturition.

There are limited data to suggest that serum IGF-1 levels are associated with progression of retinopathy during pregnancy.[200,201] A small study was performed to determine whether the vasoconstrictor endothelin-1 (ET-1), which is elevated in hypertension and diabetes, was associated with severity of retinopathy in pregnancy. While diabetic women had higher levels of ET-1 in pregnancy than nondiabetic women in the same trimester, there was no relationship to severity of diabetic retinopathy.[202] The study was hampered by its small number of patients and so must be regarded as inconclusive.

Despite the apparent deleterious effect of pregnancy on retinopathy, however, the number of past pregnancies was unrelated to the severity of diabetic retinopathy in younger-onset women in the WESDR.[189] Similarly, in a study in Oulu, Finland, there appeared to be little influence of second and subsequent pregnancies on retinopathy.[203] These data may be interpreted to suggest that pregnancy imparts a transient increased risk for incidence or progression of retinopathy. However, since there may be decreased fertility that results from more severe or more complicated diabetes, it may be that those who sustain repeated pregnancies are more robust, and this is reflected in relative protection against more severe or more progressive retinopathy.

Another source of exposure to estrogens is hormone replacement therapy. Although this treatment has come under intense scrutiny, there is no evidence to suggest that exposure to these medicines increases the risk of diabetic retinopathy.[189]

COMORBIDITY AND MORTALITY

In the WESDR, the risk of developing a heart attack, stroke, diabetic nephropathy, and amputation was higher in those with proliferative diabetic retinopathy compared to those with no or minimal nonproliferative retinopathy at baseline (Table 45.4).[204] In persons with type 1 diabetes, while controlling for age and sex, retinopathy severity was associated with all-cause and ischemic heart disease mortality and in persons with type 2 diabetes with all-cause, ischemic heart disease mortality, and stroke.[205] After controlling for systemic factors, the relations remained only for all-cause and stroke mortality in persons with type 2 diabetes. These data suggest that the presence of more severe retinopathy in diabetic patients is an indicator for increased risk of ischemic heart disease death, and may identify individuals who should be under care for cardiovascular disease. This had been reported by others.[206-208] The higher risk of cardiovascular disease in persons with more severe retinopathy may be partially due to the association of severe retinopathy with cardiovascular disease risk factors such as increased fibrinogen, increased platelet aggregation, hyperglycemia, and hypertension.

NEW MEDICAL INTERVENTIONS

Aside from glycemic, blood pressure, and lipid control, no other medical intervention has been demonstrated to reduce the incidence and progression of diabetic retinopathy. Randomized controlled clinical trials of inhibitors of aldose reductase, protein kinase C, and metalloproteinases have not shown efficacy of the intervention in preventing the incidence and progression of retinopathy in people with diabetes.[209] Controlled clinical trials of intravitreally administered vascular endothelial growth factor (VEGF) inhibitors and steroid in the treatment of diabetic macular edema are presented elsewhere.[210]

PUBLIC HEALTH APPLICATIONS OF EPIDEMIOLOGICAL DATA

Based on the observation that many diabetic patients with severe retinopathy were not receiving dilated eye examinations, guidelines for these examinations were developed and implemented using epidemiological data.[95,211,212] The guidelines recommended that after the initial screening examination, "subsequent examinations for both type 1 and type 2 diabetic patients should be repeated annually by an ophthalmologist or optometrist who is knowledgeable and experienced in diagnosing the presence of diabetic retinopathy, and is aware of its management."[95]

Table 45.4 The relative risk for the prevalence and four-year incidence of myocardial infarction, stroke, and amputation of lower extremities associated with presence of proliferative retinopathy, corrected for age in the Wisconsin Epidemiologic Study of Diabetic Retinopathy

	Myocardial infarction		Stroke		Amputation of lower extremity	
	RR	95% CI	RR	95% CI	RR	95% CI
Younger-onset group						
Prevalence	3.5	1.5–7.9	2.6	0.7–9.7	7.1	2.6–19.7
Incidence	4.5	1.3–15.4	1.6	0.4–5.7	6.0	2.1–16.9
Older-onset group taking insulin						
Prevalence	0.8	0.4–1.4	1.2	0.6–2.4	4.2	2.3–7.9
Incidence	1.2	0.5–3.4	2.9	1.2–6.8	3.4	0.9–13.2
Older-onset group not taking insulin						
Prevalence	0.3	0–2.4	2.9	0.9–9.4	5.2	0.6–45.0
Incidence	1.5	0.2–12.5	6.0	1.1–32.6	7.0	0.8–64.4

CI, confidence interval; RR, relative risk.
(Reproduced with permission from The American Diabetes Association. Klein R, Klein BEK, Moss SE. The epidemiology of proliferative diabetic retinopathy. Diabetes Care 1992;15:1875–91. Copyright © 1992 American Diabetes Association.)

However, a number of reports have demonstrated poor compliance with these guidelines.[213–215] In one study, only 16% of diabetic patients who received primary care in upstate New York received an annual ophthalmic examination using funduscopy by an optometrist or ophthalmologist in two consecutive years.[216] Reasons for poor compliance with the recommended ADA guidelines have been provided by others.[213,217,218] Physician factors may explain the reasons that patients may not be receiving optimal care. In one study, 52% of primary care physicians reported that they performed in-office ophthalmoscopic examinations, 90% of which were through undilated pupils, an approach shown to have limited sensitivity to detecting vision-threatening retinopathy in other studies.[217] Moss et al.[218] studied persons with type 1 and type 2 diabetes for 10 or more years who were participating in the WESDR. In those not having a dilated eye examination in the previous year, 31% and 35% of those with type 1 diabetes and type 2 diabetes, respectively, reported not having been told by their primary care doctors that they needed one.

Patient factors also explain some of the reasons why guidelines for dilated eye examinations are not being followed. In the WESDR, among those not having a dilated eye examination in the previous year, 79% and 71% of those with type 1 diabetes and type 2 diabetes, respectively, reported not having had one because they had no problems with their eyes, and 32% and 11% said they were too busy. These data suggest the importance of educating patients with diabetes about the asymptomatic nature of diabetic retinopathy, and the benefits of a dilated eye examination. This has become an important priority of the National Eye Institute (National Eye Health Education Program) and other specialty organizations.[219] Of course, patients may elect not to follow the advice given or deny its importance. Another reason is that of cost. Moss et al.[218] found that the ability to afford eye care was also a reason patients gave for not having such care. In that study, 30% of persons with type 1 diabetes and 12% of those with type 2 diabetes said they could not afford an examination.

Reexamination of WESDR data by Batchelder and Barricks[220] led them to conclude that based on the "remarkably low incidence of treatable conditions over 4 years for patients with retinopathy levels 21 or less and over 10 years for patients with no retinopathy at their baseline examination" that "these data do not suggest any difference in effectiveness for screening intervals of 1, 2, 3 or even 4 years for this group of low-risk patients." Others, also using models, have suggested in those with type 2 diabetes without retinopathy, that examinations every 2 years rather than yearly would be adequate to detect vision threatening retinopathy.[221] The National Committee for Quality Assurance[222] released the Health Plan Employer Data and Information Set (HEDIS) 1999 draft which suggested examinations for retinopathy every other year if there was no evidence of retinopathy in the previous year's eye exam, persons were not taking insulin, and if the A1c was less than 8% (unpublished data). However, the WESDR data showed that in individuals with type 2 diabetes with no retinopathy present at baseline, 4 per 1000 developed proliferative retinopathy and 10 per 1000 developed clinically significant macular edema over a 4-year period.[50–52]

There is a need to examine the issue of the sensitivity of the screens in detecting the presence of retinopathy. The epidemiologic data are based on detection of retinopathy by skilled graders using standardized protocols under study conditions to grade stereoscopic color fundus photographs of the Diabetic Retinopathy Study seven standard fields. Studies have demonstrated a variable sensitivity, in practice as low as 33%, in the detection of retinopathy by ophthalmoscopy in people with diabetes.[223] Newer screening approaches, including digital cameras with central reading centers, are being used for the screening of diabetic patients not under the care of an ophthalmologist.

However, a recent meta-analysis showed that retinal photography by a photographer with no specialist medical or eye qualifications (i.e., a health worker or nurse), without using pupil-dilating eye drops (the outreach model), appears unlikely to miss cases of diabetic retinopathy that screening methods using mydriasis or a photographer with specialist medical or eye qualifications would detect.[224] There is a need to conduct further epidemiological studies and controlled clinical trials to evaluate the interval and type of ophthalmic screening in persons with diabetes and no retinopathy in various healthcare settings to provide better evidence of efficacy of specific approaches to validate new guidelines and screening approaches.

CONCLUSION

Prevention of diabetes remains an important goal in reducing the complications and costs of this disease. Until approaches for primary prevention of diabetes itself become available, clinical trial data have shown that secondary prevention through medical interventions designed to control blood glycemia, blood pressure, and lipids will reduce the incidence and progression of retinopathy and loss of vision. However, success of these interventions has been limited, in part, due to inability to achieve normalization of blood sugar with current drug delivery systems. While new secondary medical interventions may be of further benefit, tertiary prevention of visual loss (screening examination through a dilated pupil by skilled eye care providers on a regular basis for early detection and subsequent treatment, when indicated, of vision-threatening retinopathy with photocoagulation) remains an important approach to care for diabetic patients.

REFERENCES

1. Klein R, Klein BE, Moss SE, et al. Prevalence of diabetes mellitus in southern Wisconsin. Am J Epidemiol 1984;119:54–61.
2. Klein R, Klein BE, Moss SE, et al. The Wisconsin Epidemiologic Study of Diabetic Retinopathy. II. Prevalence and risk of diabetic retinopathy when age at diagnosis is less than 30 years. Arch Ophthalmol 1984;102:520–6.
3. Klein R, Klein BE, Moss SE, et al. The Wisconsin Epidemiologic Study of Diabetic Retinopathy. III. Prevalence and risk of diabetic retinopathy when age at diagnosis is 30 or more years. Arch Ophthalmol 1984;102:527–32.
4. Klein R, Klein BE, Moss SE, et al. The Wisconsin Epidemiologic Study of Diabetic Retinopathy. IV. Diabetic macular edema. Ophthalmology 1984;91:1464–74.
5. Kempen JH, O'Colmain BJ, Leske MC, et al. The prevalence of diabetic retinopathy among adults in the United States. Arch Ophthalmol 2004;122:552–63.
6. Klein R, Klein BE. Vision disorders in diabetes. In: Harris MI, Cowie CC, Stern MP, et al, editors. Diabetes in America. 2nd ed. Bethesda, MD: National Diabetes Data Group; 1995. p. 293–338. (NIH Publication No. 95-1468.)
7. Houston A. Retinopathy in the Poole area: An epidemiological inquiry. In: Eschwege E, editor. Advances in diabetes epidemiology. Amsterdam: Elsevier; 1982.
8. Dwyer MS, Melton III LJ, Ballard DJ, et al. Incidence of diabetic retinopathy and blindness: a population-based study in Rochester, Minnesota. Diabetes Care 1985;8:316–22.
9. Dorf A, Ballintine EJ, Bennett PH, et al. Retinopathy in Pima Indians. Relationships to glucose level, duration of diabetes, age at diagnosis of diabetes, and age at examination in a population with a high prevalence of diabetes mellitus. Diabetes 1976;25:554–60.
10. Bennett PH, Rushforth NB, Miller M, et al. Epidemiologic studies of diabetes in the Pima Indians. Recent Prog Horm Res 1976;32:333–76.
11. West KM, Erdreich LJ, Stober JA. A detailed study of risk factors for retinopathy and nephropathy in diabetes. Diabetes 1980;29:501–8.
12. Kahn HA, Leibowitz HM, Ganley JP, et al. The Framingham Eye Study. I. Outline and major prevalence findings. Am J Epidemiol 1977;106:17–32.
13. King H, Balkau B, Zimmet P, et al. Diabetic retinopathy in Nauruans. Am J Epidemiol 1983;117:659–67.
14. Ballard DJ, Melton III LJ, Dwyer MS, et al. Risk factors for diabetic retinopathy: a population-based study in Rochester, Minnesota. Diabetes Care 1986;9:334–42.
15. Danielsen R, Jonasson F, Helgason T. Prevalence of retinopathy and proteinuria in type 1 diabetics in Iceland. Acta Med Scand 1982;212:277–80.
16. Constable IJ, Knuiman MW, Welborn TA, et al. Assessing the risk of diabetic retinopathy. Am J Ophthalmol 1984;97:53–61.
17. Knuiman MW, Welborn TA, McCann VJ, et al. Prevalence of diabetic complications in relation to risk factors. Diabetes 1986;35:1332–9.
18. Sjolie AK. Ocular complications in insulin treated diabetes mellitus. An epidemiological study. Acta Ophthalmol Suppl 1985;172:1–77.
19. Nielsen NV. Diabetic retinopathy II. The course of retinopathy in diabetics treated with oral hypoglycaemic agents and diet regime alone. A one year epidemiological cohort study of diabetes mellitus. The Island of Falster, Denmark. Acta Ophthalmol (Copenh) 1984;62:266–73.
20. Nielsen NV. Diabetic retinopathy I. The course of retinopathy in insulin-treated diabetics. A one year epidemiological cohort study of diabetes mellitus. The Island of Falster, Denmark. Acta Ophthalmol (Copenh) 1984;62:256–65.
21. Teuscher A, Schnell H, Wilson PW. Incidence of diabetic retinopathy and relationship to baseline plasma glucose and blood pressure. Diabetes Care 1988;11:246–51.
22. Haffner SM, Fong D, Stern MP, et al. Diabetic retinopathy in Mexican Americans and non-Hispanic whites. Diabetes 1988;37:878–84.
23. Jerneld B. Prevalence of diabetic retinopathy. A population study from the Swedish island of Gotland. Acta Ophthalmol Suppl 1988;188:3–32.
24. Hamman RF, Mayer EJ, Moo-Young GA, et al. Prevalence and risk factors of diabetic retinopathy in non-Hispanic whites and Hispanics with NIDDM. San Luis Valley Diabetes Study. Diabetes 1989;38:1231–7.
25. McLeod BK, Thompson JR, Rosenthal AR. The prevalence of retinopathy in the insulin-requiring diabetic patients of an English country town. Eye (Lond) 1988;2 (Pt 4):424–30.
26. Kostraba JN, Klein R, Dorman JS, et al. The epidemiology of diabetes complications study. IV. Correlates of diabetic background and proliferative retinopathy. Am J Epidemiol 1991;133:381–91.
27. Fujimoto W, Fukuda M. Natural history of diabetic retinopathy and its treatment in Japan. In: Baba S, Goto Y, Fukui I, editors. Diabetes mellitus in Asia. Amsterdam: Excerpta Medica; 1976. p. 225–31.
28. Kullberg CE, Abrahamsson M, Arnqvist HJ, et al. Prevalence of retinopathy differs with age at onset of diabetes in a population of patients with Type 1 diabetes. Diabet Med 2002;19:924–31.
29. Lopez IM, Diez A, Velilla S, et al. Prevalence of diabetic retinopathy and eye care in a rural area of Spain. Ophthalmic Epidemiol 2002;9:205–14.
30. Broadbent DM, Scott JA, Vora JP, et al. Prevalence of diabetic eye disease in an inner city population: the Liverpool Diabetic Eye Study. Eye (Lond) 1999;13(Pt 2):160–5.
31. West SK, Klein R, Rodriguez J, et al. Diabetes and diabetic retinopathy in a Mexican-American population: Proyecto VER. Diabetes Care 2001;24:1204–9.
32. McKay R, McCarty CA, Taylor HR. Diabetic retinopathy in Victoria, Australia: the Visual Impairment Project. Br J Ophthalmol 2000;84:865–70.
33. Toeller M, Buyken AE, Heitkamp G, et al. Prevalence of chronic complications, metabolic control and nutritional intake in type 1 diabetes: comparison between different European regions. EURODIAB Complications Study group. Horm Metab Res 1999;31:680–5.
34. Leske MC, Wu SY, Hyman L, et al. Diabetic retinopathy in a black population: the Barbados Eye Study. Ophthalmology 1999;106:1893–9.
35. Rajala U, Laakso M, Qiao Q, et al. Prevalence of retinopathy in people with diabetes, impaired glucose tolerance, and normal glucose tolerance. Diabetes Care 1998;21:1664–9.
36. Harris MI, Klein R, Cowie CC, et al. Is the risk of diabetic retinopathy greater in non-Hispanic blacks and Mexican Americans than in non-Hispanic whites with type 2 diabetes? A U.S. population study. Diabetes Care 1998;21:1230–5.
37. Dowse GK, Humphrey AR, Collins VR, et al. Prevalence and risk factors for diabetic retinopathy in the multiethnic population of Mauritius. Am J Epidemiol 1998;147:448–57.
38. Kohner EM, Aldington SJ, Stratton IM, et al. United Kingdom Prospective Diabetes Study, 30: diabetic retinopathy at diagnosis of non-insulin-dependent diabetes mellitus and associated risk factors. Arch Ophthalmol 1998;116:297–303.
39. Mitchell P, Smith W, Wang JJ, et al. Prevalence of diabetic retinopathy in an older community. The Blue Mountains Eye Study. Ophthalmology 1998;105:406–11.
40. Gonzalez Villalpando ME, Gonzalez VC, Arredondo PB, et al. Moderate-to-severe diabetic retinopathy is more prevalent in Mexico City than in San Antonio, Texas. Diabetes Care 1997;20:773–7.
41. Berinstein DM, Stahn RM, Welty TK, et al. The prevalence of diabetic retinopathy and associated risk factors among Sioux Indians. Diabetes Care 1997;20:757–9.
42. Kernell A, Dedorsson I, Johansson B, et al. Prevalence of diabetic retinopathy in children and adolescents with IDDM. A population-based multicentre study. Diabetologia 1997;40:307–10.
43. Collins VR, Dowse GK, Plehwe WE, et al. High prevalence of diabetic retinopathy and nephropathy in Polynesians of Western Samoa. Diabetes Care 1995;18:1140–9.
44. Klein R, Klein BE, Moss SE, et al. The Beaver Dam Eye Study. Retinopathy in adults with newly discovered and previously diagnosed diabetes mellitus. Ophthalmology 1992;99:58–62.
45. Roy MS. Diabetic retinopathy in African Americans with type 1 diabetes: The New Jersey 725: I. Methodology, population, frequency of retinopathy, and visual impairment. Arch Ophthalmol 2000;118:97–104.

46. Roy MS, Klein R. Macular edema and retinal hard exudates in African Americans with type 1 diabetes: the New Jersey 725. Arch Ophthalmol 2001;119:251–9.
47. Klein R, Klein BE. Are individuals with diabetes seeing better? A long-term epidemiological perspective. Diabetes 2010;59:1853–60.
48. Suh DC, Choi IS, Plauschinat C, et al. Impact of comorbid conditions and race/ethnicity on glycemic control among the US population with type 2 diabetes, 1988–1994 to 1999–2004. J Diabetes Complications 2010;24:382–91.
49. Ong KL, Cheung BM, Wong LY, et al. Prevalence, treatment, and control of diagnosed diabetes in the U.S. National Health and Nutrition Examination Survey 1999–2004. Ann Epidemiol 2008;18:222–9.
50. Klein R, Klein BE, Moss SE, et al. The Wisconsin Epidemiologic Study of Diabetic Retinopathy. IX. Four-year incidence and progression of diabetic retinopathy when age at diagnosis is less than 30 years. Arch Ophthalmol 1989;107:237–43.
51. Klein R, Klein BE, Moss SE, et al. The Wisconsin Epidemiologic Study of Diabetic Retinopathy. X. Four-year incidence and progression of diabetic retinopathy when age at diagnosis is 30 years or more. Arch Ophthalmol 1989;107:244–9.
52. Klein R, Moss SE, Klein BE, et al. The Wisconsin epidemiologic study of diabetic retinopathy. XI. The incidence of macular edema. Ophthalmology 1989;96:1501–10.
53. Klein R, Klein BE, Moss SE, et al. The Wisconsin Epidemiologic Study of Diabetic Retinopathy. XIV. Ten-year incidence and progression of diabetic retinopathy. Arch Ophthalmol 1994;112:1217–28.
54. Henricsson M, Nystrom L, Blohme G, et al. The incidence of retinopathy 10 years after diagnosis in young adult people with diabetes: results from the nationwide population-based Diabetes Incidence Study in Sweden (DISS). Diabetes Care 2003;26:349–54.
55. Lloyd CE, Becker D, Ellis D, et al. Incidence of complications in insulin-dependent diabetes mellitus: a survival analysis. Am J Epidemiol 1996;143:431–41.
56. Klein R, Palta M, Allen C, et al. Incidence of retinopathy and associated risk factors from time of diagnosis of insulin-dependent diabetes. Arch Ophthalmol 1997;115:351–6.
57. Tudor SM, Hamman RF, Baron A, et al. Incidence and progression of diabetic retinopathy in Hispanics and non-Hispanic whites with type 2 diabetes. San Luis Valley Diabetes Study, Colorado. Diabetes Care 1998;21:53–61.
58. Klein R, Klein BE, Moss SE, et al. The Wisconsin Epidemiologic Study of Diabetic Retinopathy. XVII. The 14-year incidence and progression of diabetic retinopathy and associated risk factors in type 1 diabetes. Ophthalmology 1998;105:1801–15.
59. Porta M, Sjoelie AK, Chaturvedi N, et al. Risk factors for progression to proliferative diabetic retinopathy in the EURODIAB Prospective Complications Study. Diabetologia 2001;44:2203–9.
60. Ling R, Ramsewak V, Taylor D, et al. Longitudinal study of a cohort of people with diabetes screened by the Exeter Diabetic Retinopathy Screening Programme. Eye (Lond) 2002;16:140–5.
61. Younis N, Broadbent DM, Vora JP, et al. Incidence of sight-threatening retinopathy in patients with type 2 diabetes in the Liverpool Diabetic Eye Study: a cohort study. Lancet 2003;361:195–200.
62. Roy MS, Affouf M. Six-year progression of retinopathy and associated risk factors in African American patients with type 1 diabetes mellitus: the New Jersey 725. Arch Ophthalmol 2006;124:1297–306.
63. Varma R, Choudhury F, Klein R, et al. Four-year incidence and progression of diabetic retinopathy and macular edema: the Los Angeles Latino Eye Study. Am J Ophthalmol 2010;149:752–61.
64. Hovind P, Tarnow L, Rossing K, et al. Decreasing incidence of severe diabetic microangiopathy in type 1 diabetes. Diabetes Care 2003;26:1258–64.
65. Bojestig M, Arnqvist HJ, Karlberg BE, et al. Unchanged incidence of severe retinopathy in a population of Type 1 diabetic patients with marked reduction of nephropathy. Diabet Med 1998;15:863–9.
66. Nordwall M, Bojestig M, Arnqvist HJ, et al. Declining incidence of severe retinopathy and persisting decrease of nephropathy in an unselected population of Type 1 diabetes: the Linköping Diabetes Complications Study. Diabetologia 2004;47:1266–72.
67. Pambianco G, Costacou T, Ellis D, et al. The 30-year natural history of type 1 diabetes complications: the Pittsburgh Epidemiology of Diabetes Complications Study experience. Diabetes 2006;55:1463–9.
68. Klein R, Knudtson MD, Lee KE, et al. The Wisconsin Epidemiologic Study of Diabetic Retinopathy. XXII. The twenty-five-year progression of retinopathy in persons with type 1 diabetes. Ophthalmology 2008;115:1859–68.
69. Klein R, Knudtson MD, Lee KE, et al. The Wisconsin Epidemiologic Study of Diabetic Retinopathy. XXIII. The twenty-five-year incidence of macular edema in persons with type 1 diabetes. Ophthalmology 2009;116:497–503.
70. Klein R, Lee KE, Knudtson MD, et al. Changes in visual impairment prevalence by period of diagnosis of diabetes: the Wisconsin Epidemiologic Study of Diabetic Retinopathy. Ophthalmology 2009;116:1937–42.
71. Klein R, Lee KE, Gangnon RE, et al. The 25-year incidence of visual impairment in type 1 diabetes mellitus. The Wisconsin Epidemiologic Study of Diabetic Retinopathy. Ophthalmology 2010;117:63–70.
72. Klein R, Sharrett AR, Klein BE, et al. The association of atherosclerosis, vascular risk factors, and retinopathy in adults with diabetes : the atherosclerosis risk in communities study. Ophthalmology 2002;109:1225–34.
73. Klein R, Marino EK, Kuller LH, et al. The relation of atherosclerotic cardiovascular disease to retinopathy in people with diabetes in the Cardiovascular Health Study. Br J Ophthalmol 2002;86:84–90.
74. Wong TY, Klein R, Islam FM, et al. Diabetic retinopathy in a multi-ethnic cohort in the United States. Am J Ophthalmol 2006;141:446–55.
75. Zhang X, Saaddine JB, Chou CF, et al. Prevalence of diabetic retinopathy in the United States, 2005–2008. JAMA 2010;304:649–56.
76. Varma R, Torres M, Pena F, et al. Prevalence of diabetic retinopathy in adult Latinos: the Los Angeles Latino eye study. Ophthalmology 2004;111:1298–306.
77. West KM, Erdreich LJ, Stober JA. A detailed study of risk factors for retinopathy and nephropathy in diabetes. Diabetes 1980;29:501–8.
78. Lee ET, Lee VS, Lu M, et al. Development of proliferative retinopathy in NIDDM. A follow-up study of American Indians in Oklahoma. Diabetes 1992;41:359–67.
79. Lee ET, Lee VS, Kingsley RM, et al. Diabetic retinopathy in Oklahoma Indians with NIDDM. Incidence and risk factors. Diabetes Care 1992;15:1620–7.
80. Nelson RG, Newman JM, Knowler WC, et al. Incidence of end-stage renal disease in type 2 (non-insulin-dependent) diabetes mellitus in Pima Indians. Diabetologia 1988;31:730–6.
81. Looker HC, Krakoff J, Knowler WC, et al. Longitudinal studies of incidence and progression of diabetic retinopathy assessed by retinal photography in pima indians. Diabetes Care 2003;26:320–6.
82. The Diabetes Control and Complications Trial Research Group. Clustering of long-term complications in families with diabetes in the diabetes control and complications trial. The Diabetes Control and Complications Trial Research Group. Diabetes 1997;46:1829–39.
83. Rema M, Saravanan G, Deepa R, et al. Familial clustering of diabetic retinopathy in South Indian Type 2 diabetic patients. Diabet Med 2002;19:910–6.
84. Fukuda M, Nakano S, Imaizumi N, et al. Mitochondrial DNA mutations are associated with both decreased insulin secretion and advanced microvascular complications in Japanese diabetic subjects. J Diabetes Complications 1999;13:277–83.
85. Demaine A, Cross D, Millward A. Polymorphisms of the aldose reductase gene and susceptibility to retinopathy in type 1 diabetes mellitus. Invest Ophthalmol Vis Sci 2000;41:4064–8.
86. Yamamoto T, Sato T, Hosoi M, et al. Aldose reductase gene polymorphism is associated with progression of diabetic nephropathy in Japanese patients with type 1 diabetes mellitus. Diabetes Obes Metab 2003;5:51–7.
87. Kankova K, Muzik J, Karaskova J, et al. Duration of non-Insulin-dependent diabetes mellitus and the TNF-beta NcoI genotype as predictive factors in proliferative diabetic retinopathy. Ophthalmologica 2001;215:294–8.
88. Santos A, Salguero ML, Gurrola C, et al. The epsilon4 allele of apolipoprotein E gene is a potential risk factor for the severity of macular edema in type 2 diabetic Mexican patients. Ophthalmic Genet 2002;23:13–9.
89. Kao Y, Donaghue KC, Chan A, et al. Paraoxonase gene cluster is a genetic marker for early microvascular complications in type 1 diabetes. Diabet Med 2002;19:212–5.
90. Taverna MJ, Sola A, Guyot-Argenton C, et al. eNOS4 polymorphism of the endothelial nitric oxide synthase predicts risk for severe diabetic retinopathy. Diabet Med 2002;19:240–5.
91. Kamiuchi K, Hasegawa G, Obayashi H, et al. Intercellular adhesion molecule-1 (ICAM-1) polymorphism is associated with diabetic retinopathy in type 2 diabetes mellitus. Diabet Med 2002;19:371–6.
92. Matsubara Y, Murata M, Maruyama T, et al. Association between diabetic retinopathy and genetic variations in alpha2beta1 integrin, a platelet receptor for collagen. Blood 2000;95:1560–4.
93. Yang B, Cross DF, Ollerenshaw M, et al. Polymorphisms of the vascular endothelial growth factor and susceptibility to diabetic microvascular complications in patients with type 1 diabetes mellitus. J Diabetes Complications 2003;17:1–6.
94. Liew G, Klein R, Wong TY. The role of genetics in susceptibility to diabetic retinopathy. Int Ophthalmol Clin 2009;49:35–52.
95. Fong DS, Aiello L, Gardner TW, et al. Diabetic retinopathy. Diabetes Care 2003;26(Suppl 1):S99–S102.
96. Klein BE, Moss SE, Klein R. Is menarche associated with diabetic retinopathy? Diabetes Care 1990;13:1034–8.
97. Frost-Larsen K, Starup K. Fluorescein angiography in diabetic children. A follow-up. Acta Ophthalmol (Copenh) 1980;58:355–60.
98. Murphy RP, Nanda M, Plotnick L, et al. The relationship of puberty to diabetic retinopathy. Arch Ophthalmol 1990;108:215–8.
99. Kostraba JN, Dorman JS, Orchard TJ, et al. Contribution of diabetes duration before puberty to development of microvascular complications in IDDM subjects. Diabetes Care 1989;12:686–93.
100. Harris MI, Klein R, Welborn TA, et al. Onset of NIDDM occurs at least 4–7 yr before clinical diagnosis. Diabetes Care 1992;15:815–9.
101. Aiello LM, Rand LI, Briones JC, et al. Diabetic retinopathy in Joslin Clinic patients with adult-onset diabetes. Ophthalmology 1981;88:619–23.
102. West KM. Epidemiology of diabetes and its vascular lesions. New York: Elsevier; 1978.
103. The Diabetes Control and Complications Trial Research Group. The effect of intensive treatment of diabetes on the development and progression of long-term complications in insulin-dependent diabetes mellitus. N Engl J Med 1993;329:977–86.
104. Diabetes Control and Complications Trial Research Group. The effect of intensive diabetes treatment on the progression of diabetic retinopathy in insulin-dependent diabetes mellitus. Arch Ophthalmol 1995;113:36–51.
105. Diabetes Control and Complications Trial Research Group. Progression of retinopathy with intensive versus conventional treatment in the Diabetes Control and Complications Trial. Ophthalmology 1995;102:647–61.

106. Diabetes Control and Complications Trial Research Group. The absence of a glycemic threshold for the development of long-term complications: the perspective of the Diabetes Control and Complications Trial. Diabetes 1996;45:1289–98.
107. The Kroc Collaborative Study Group. Diabetic retinopathy after two years of intensified insulin treatment. Follow-up of the Kroc Collaborative Study. JAMA 1988;260:37–41.
108. Lauritzen T, Frost-Larsen K, Larsen HW, et al. Two-year experience with continuous subcutaneous insulin infusion in relation to retinopathy and neuropathy. Diabetes 1985;34(Suppl. 3):74–9.
109. Dahl-Jørgensen K, Brinchmann-Hansen O, Hanssen KF, et al. Rapid tightening of blood glucose control leads to transient deterioration of retinopathy in insulin dependent diabetes mellitus: the Oslo study. Br Med J (Clin Res Ed) 1985;290:811–5.
110. Warram JH, Manson JE, Krolewski AS. Glycosylated hemoglobin and the risk of retinopathy in insulin-dependent diabetes mellitus. N Engl J Med 1995;332:1305–6.
111. The Diabetes Control and Complications Trial Research Group. Lifetime benefits and costs of intensive therapy as practiced in the diabetes control and complications trial. JAMA 1996;276:1409–15.
112. The Diabetes Control and Complications Trial/Epidemiology of Diabetes Interventions and Complications Research Group. Retinopathy and nephropathy in patients with type 1 diabetes four years after a trial of intensive therapy. N Engl J Med 2000;342:381–9.
113. The Epidemiology of Diabetes Interventions and Complications (EDIC) Study Group. Sustained effect of intensive treatment of type 1 diabetes mellitus on development and progression of diabetic nephropathy. JAMA 2003;290:2159–67.
114. Cooper ME. Metabolic memory: implications for diabetic vascular complications. Pediatr Diabetes 2009;10:343–6.
115. Holman RR, Paul SK, Bethel MA, et al. 10-year follow-up of intensive glucose control in type 2 diabetes. N Engl J Med 2008;359:1577–89.
116. United Kingdom Prospective Diabetes Study (UKPDS) Group. Intensive blood-glucose control with sulphonylureas or insulin compared with conventional treatment and risk of complications in patients with type 2 diabetes (UKPDS 33). Lancet 1998;352:837–53.
117. United Kingdom Prospective Diabetes Study (UKPDS) Group. Effect of intensive blood-glucose control with metformin on complications in overweight patients with type 2 diabetes (UKPDS 34). Lancet 1998;352:854–65.
118. Gray A, Raikou M, McGuire A, et al. Cost effectiveness of an intensive blood glucose control policy in patients with type 2 diabetes: economic analysis alongside randomised controlled trial (UKPDS 41). United Kingdom Prospective Diabetes Study Group. BMJ 2000;320:1373–8.
119. Duckworth WC, McCarren M, Abraira C. Glucose control and cardiovascular complications: the VA Diabetes Trial. Diabetes Care 2001;24:942–5.
120. Duckworth WC, Abraira C, Moritz T, et al. Glucose control and vascular complications in veterans with type 2 diabetes. N Engl J Med 2009;360:129–39.
121. Chew EY, Ambrosius WT, Davis MD, et al. Effects of medical therapies on retinopathy progression in type 2 diabetes. N Engl J Med 2010;363:233–44.
122. Ismail-Beigi F, Craven T, Banerji MA, et al. Effect of intensive treatment of hyperglycaemia on microvascular outcomes in type 2 diabetes: an analysis of the ACCORD randomised trial. Lancet 2010;376:419–30.
123. Patel A, MacMahon S, Chalmers J, et al. Intensive blood glucose control and vascular outcomes in patients with type 2 diabetes. N Engl J Med 2008;358:2560–72.
124. American Diabetes Association. Standards of medical care for patients with diabetes mellitus. Diabetes Care 1994;17:616–23.
125. Harris MI. Health care and health status and outcomes for patients with type 2 diabetes. Diabetes Care 2000;23:754–8.
126. Klein R, Klein BE, Moss SE, et al. The medical management of hyperglycemia over a 10-year period in people with diabetes. Diabetes Care 1996;19:744–50.
127. Klein BE. Reduction in risk of progression of diabetic retinopathy. N Engl J Med 2010;363:287–8.
128. Klein R. Intensive treatment of hyperglycaemia: ACCORD. Lancet 2010;376:391–2.
129. Smith RB, Pyke DA, Watkins PJ, et al. C-peptide response to glucagon in diabetics with and without complications. N Z Med J 1979;89:304–6.
130. Sjoberg S, Gunnarsson R, Gjotterberg M, et al. Residual insulin production, glycaemic control and prevalence of microvascular lesions and polyneuropathy in long-term type 1 (insulin-dependent) diabetes mellitus. Diabetologia 1987;30:208–13.
131. Sjoberg S, Gjotterberg M, Lefvert AK, et al. Significance of residual insulin production in long-term type I diabetes mellitus. Transplant Proc 1986;18:1498–9.
132. Madsbad S, Lauritzen E, Faber OK, et al. The effect of residual beta-cell function on the development of diabetic retinopathy. Diabet Med 1986;3:42–5.
133. Klein R, Moss SE, Klein BE, et al. Wisconsin Epidemiologic Study of Diabetic Retinopathy. XII. Relationship of C-peptide and diabetic retinopathy. Diabetes 1990;39:1445–50.
134. Klein R, Klein BE, Moss SE. The Wisconsin Epidemiologic Study of Diabetic Retinopathy. XVI. The relationship of C-peptide to the incidence and progression of diabetic retinopathy. Diabetes 1995;44:796–801.
135. Steffes MW, Sibley S, Jackson M, et al. Beta-cell function and the development of diabetes-related complications in the diabetes control and complications trial. Diabetes Care 2003;26:832–6.
136. Serghieri G, Bartolomei G, Pettenello C, et al. Raised retinopathy prevalence rate in insulin-treated patients: a feature of obese type II diabetes. Transplant Proc 1986;18:1576–7.
137. Klein R, Klein BE, Moss SE, et al. Is blood pressure a predictor of the incidence or progression of diabetic retinopathy? Arch Intern Med 1989;149:2427–32.
138. Adler AI, Stratton IM, Neil HA, et al. Association of systolic blood pressure with macrovascular and microvascular complications of type 2 diabetes (UKPDS 36): prospective observational study. BMJ 2000;321:412–9.
139. Klein R, Klein BE, Moss SE, et al. The Wisconsin Epidemiologic Study of Diabetic Retinopathy. XV. The long-term incidence of macular edema. Ophthalmology 1995;102:7–16.
140. United Kingdom Prospective Diabetes Study (UKPDS) Group. Tight blood pressure control and risk of macrovascular and microvascular complications in type 2 diabetes: UKPDS 38. BMJ 1998;317:703–13.
141. Patel A, MacMahon S, Chalmers J, et al. Effects of a fixed combination of perindopril and indapamide on macrovascular and microvascular outcomes in patients with type 2 diabetes mellitus (the ADVANCE trial): a randomised controlled trial. Lancet 2007;370:829–40.
142. Chaturvedi N, Sjolie AK, Stephenson JM, et al. Effect of lisinopril on progression of retinopathy in normotensive people with type 1 diabetes. The EUCLID Study Group. EURODIAB Controlled Trial of Lisinopril in Insulin-Dependent Diabetes Mellitus. Lancet 1998;351:28–31.
143. Chaturvedi N. Modulation of the renin-angiotensin system and retinopathy. Heart 2000;84(Suppl. 1):i29–31.
144. Chaturvedi N, Sjoelie AK, Svensson A. The Diabetic Retinopathy Candesartan Trials (DIRECT) Programme, rationale and study design. J Renin Angiotensin Aldosterone Syst 2002;3:255–61.
145. Chaturvedi N, Porta M, Klein R, et al. Effect of candesartan on prevention (DIRECT-Prevent 1) and progression (DIRECT-Protect 1) of retinopathy in type 1 diabetes: randomised, placebo-controlled trials. Lancet 2008;372:1394–402.
146. Mauer M, Zinman B, Gardiner R, et al. Renal and retinal effects of enalapril and losartan in type 1 diabetes. N Engl J Med 2009;361:40–51.
147. Mitchell P, Wong TY. DIRECT new treatments for diabetic retinopathy. Lancet 2008;372:1361–3.
148. Sjølie AK, Klein R, Porta M, et al. Effect of candesartan on progression and regression of retinopathy in type 2 diabetes (DIRECT-Protect 2): a randomised placebo-controlled trial. Lancet 2008;372:1385–93.
149. Klein R, Moss SE, Klein BE. Is gross proteinuria a risk factor for the incidence of proliferative diabetic retinopathy? Ophthalmology 1993;100:1140–6.
150. Cruickshanks KJ, Ritter LL, Klein R, et al. The association of microalbuminuria with diabetic retinopathy. The Wisconsin Epidemiologic Study of Diabetic Retinopathy. Ophthalmology 1993;100:862–7.
151. Lloyd CE, Klein R, Maser RE, et al. The progression of retinopathy over 2 years: the Pittsburgh Epidemiology of Diabetes Complications (EDC) Study. J Diabetes Complications 1995;9:140–8.
152. Moss SE, Klein R, Klein BE. The incidence of vision loss in a diabetic population. Ophthalmology 1988;95:1340–8.
153. Duncan LJ, Cullen JF, Ireland JT, et al. A three-year trial of atromid therapy in exudative diabetic retinopathy. Diabetes 1968;17:458–67.
154. Klein BE, Moss SE, Klein R, et al. The Wisconsin Epidemiologic Study of Diabetic Retinopathy. XIII. Relationship of serum cholesterol to retinopathy and hard exudate. Ophthalmology 1991;98:1261–5.
155. Chew EY, Klein ML, Ferris III FL, et al. Association of elevated serum lipid levels with retinal hard exudate in diabetic retinopathy. Early Treatment Diabetic Retinopathy Study (ETDRS) Report 22. Arch Ophthalmol 1996;114:1079–84.
156. Gordon B, Chang S, Kavanagh M, et al. The effects of lipid lowering on diabetic retinopathy. Am J Ophthalmol 1991;112:385–91.
157. Freyberger H, Schifferdecker E, Schatz H. [Regression of hard exudates in diabetic background retinopathy in therapy with etofibrate antilipemic agent.] Med Klin (Munich) 1994;89:594–7, 633.
158. Dale J, Farmer J, Jones AF, et al. Diabetic ischaemic and exudative maculopathy: are their risk factors different? Diab Med 2000;17:47.
159. Keech AC, Mitchell P, Summanen PA, et al. Effect of fenofibrate on the need for laser treatment for diabetic retinopathy (FIELD study): a randomised controlled trial. Lancet 2007;370:1687–97.
160. Goldsmith JR, Landaw SA. Carbon monoxide and human health. Science 1968;162:1352–9.
161. Hawkins RI. Smoking, platelets and thrombosis. Nature 1972;236:450–2.
162. Klein R, Klein BE, Davis MD. Is cigarette smoking associated with diabetic retinopathy? Am J Epidemiol 1983;118:228–38.
163. Moss SE, Klein R, Klein BE. Association of cigarette smoking with diabetic retinopathy. Diabetes Care 1991;14:119–26.
164. Moss SE, Klein R, Klein BE. Cigarette smoking and ten-year progression of diabetic retinopathy. Ophthalmology 1996;103:1438–42.
165. Klein R, Moss SE, Klein BE, et al. Relation of ocular and systemic factors to survival in diabetes. Arch Intern Med 1989;149:266–72.
166. Jakubowski JA, Vaillancourt R, Deykin D. Interaction of ethanol, prostacyclin, and aspirin in determining human platelet reactivity in vitro. Arteriosclerosis 1988;8:436–41.
167. Albert MA, Glynn RJ, Ridker PM. Alcohol consumption and plasma concentration of C-reactive protein. Circulation 2003;107:443–7.
168. Greenfield JR, Samaras K, Jenkins AB, et al. Moderate alcohol consumption, estrogen replacement therapy, and physical activity are associated with increased insulin sensitivity: is abdominal adiposity the mediator? Diabetes Care 2003;26:2734–40.

169. Kingsley LA, Dorman JS, Doft BH, et al. An epidemiologic approach to the study of retinopathy: the Pittsburgh diabetic morbidity and retinopathy studies. Diabetes Res Clin Pract 1988;4:99–109.
170. Young RJ, McCulloch DK, Prescott RJ, et al. Alcohol: another risk factor for diabetic retinopathy? Br Med J (Clin Res Ed) 1984;288:1035–7.
171. Beulens JW, Kruidhof JS, Grobbee DE, et al. Alcohol consumption and risk of microvascular complications in type 1 diabetes patients: the EURODIAB Prospective Complications Study. Diabetologia 2008;51:1631–8.
172. Lee CC, Stolk RP, Adler AI, et al. Association between alcohol consumption and diabetic retinopathy and visual acuity - the AdRem Study. Diabet Med 2010;27:1130–7.
173. Moss SE, Klein R, Klein BE. Alcohol consumption and the prevalence of diabetic retinopathy. Ophthalmology 1992;99:926–32.
174. Moss SE, Klein R, Klein BE. The association of alcohol consumption with the incidence and progression of diabetic retinopathy. Ophthalmology 1994;101:1962–8.
175. Valmadrid CT, Klein R, Moss SE, et al. Alcohol intake and the risk of coronary heart disease mortality in persons with older-onset diabetes mellitus. JAMA 1999;282:239–46.
176. Diabetes Drafting Group. Prevalence of small vessel and large vessel disease in diabetic patients from 14 centres. The World Health Organisation Multinational Study of Vascular Disease in Diabetics. Diabetologia 1985;28(Suppl.): 615–40.
177. LaPorte RE, Dorman JS, Tajima N, et al. Pittsburgh Insulin-Dependent Diabetes Mellitus Morbidity and Mortality Study: physical activity and diabetic complications. Pediatrics 1986;78:1027–33.
178. van Leiden HA, Dekker JM, Moll AC, et al. Risk factors for incident retinopathy in a diabetic and nondiabetic population: the Hoorn study. Arch Ophthalmol 2003;121:245–51.
179. Klein R, Klein BE, Moss SE. Is obesity related to microvascular and macrovascular complications in diabetes? The Wisconsin Epidemiologic Study of Diabetic Retinopathy. Arch Intern Med 1997;157:650–6.
180. Wadén J, Tikkanen H, Forsblom C, et al. Leisure time physical activity is associated with poor glycemic control in type 1 diabetic women: the FinnDiane study. Diabetes Care 2005;28:777–82.
181. Orchard TJ, Dorman JS, Maser RE, et al. Factors associated with avoidance of severe complications after 25 yr of IDDM. Pittsburgh Epidemiology of Diabetes Complications Study I. Diabetes Care 1990;13:741–7.
182. Kriska AM, LaPorte RE, Patrick SL, et al. The association of physical activity and diabetic complications in individuals with insulin-dependent diabetes mellitus: the Epidemiology of Diabetes Complications Study - VII. J Clin Epidemiol 1991;44:1207–14.
183. Cruickshanks KJ, Moss SE, Klein R, et al. Physical activity and proliferative retinopathy in people diagnosed with diabetes before age 30 yr. Diabetes Care 1992;15:1267–72.
184. Cruickshanks KJ, Moss SE, Klein R, et al. Physical activity and the risk of progression of retinopathy or the development of proliferative retinopathy. Ophthalmology 1995;102:1177–82.
185. Hanna AK, Roy M, Zinman B, et al. An evaluation of factors associated with proliferative diabetic retinopathy. Clin Invest Med 1985;8:109–16.
186. Haffner SM, Hazuda HP, Stern MP, et al. Effects of socioeconomic status on hyperglycemia and retinopathy levels in Mexican Americans with NIDDM. Diabetes Care 1989;12:128–34.
187. Klein R, Klein BE, Jensen SC, et al. The relation of socioeconomic factors to the incidence of proliferative diabetic retinopathy and loss of vision. Ophthalmology 1994;101:68–76.
188. Klein BE, Moss SE, Klein R. Oral contraceptives in women with diabetes. Diabetes Care 1990;13:895–8.
189. Klein BE, Klein R, Moss SE. Exogenous estrogen exposures and changes in diabetic retinopathy. The Wisconsin Epidemiologic Study of Diabetic Retinopathy. Diabetes Care 1999;22:1984–7.
190. Klein BE, Moss SE, Klein R. Effect of pregnancy on progression of diabetic retinopathy. Diabetes Care 1990;13:34–40.
191. Chew EY, Mills JL, Metzger BE, et al. Metabolic control and progression of retinopathy. The Diabetes in Early Pregnancy Study. National Institute of Child Health and Human Development Diabetes in Early Pregnancy Study. Diabetes Care 1995;18:631–7.
192. Hemachandra A, Ellis D, Lloyd CE, et al. The influence of pregnancy on IDDM complications. Diabetes Care 1995;18:950–4.
193. Rasmussen KL, Laugesen CS, Ringholm L, et al. Progression of diabetic retinopathy during pregnancy in women with type 2 diabetes. Diabetologia 2010;53:1076–83.
194. Lovestam-Adrian M, Agardh CD, Aberg A, et al. Pre-eclampsia is a potent risk factor for deterioration of retinopathy during pregnancy in Type 1 diabetic patients. Diabet Med 1997;14:1059–65.
195. Rosenn B, Miodovnik M, Kranias G, et al. Progression of diabetic retinopathy in pregnancy: association with hypertension in pregnancy. Am J Obstet Gynecol 1992;166:1214–8.
196. Temple RC, Aldridge VA, Sampson MJ, et al. Impact of pregnancy on the progression of diabetic retinopathy in Type 1 diabetes. Diabet Med 2001;18: 573–7.
197. Lauszus F, Klebe JG, Bek T. Diabetic retinopathy in pregnancy during tight metabolic control. Acta Obstet Gynecol Scand 2000;79:367–70.
198. Rahman W, Rahman FZ, Yassin S, et al. Progression of retinopathy during pregnancy in type 1 diabetes mellitus. Clin Experiment Ophthalmol 2007;35: 231–6.
199. Vestgaard M, Ringholm L, Laugesen CS, et al. Pregnancy-induced sight-threatening diabetic retinopathy in women with Type 1 diabetes. Diabet Med 2010;27:431–5.
200. Lauszus FF, Klebe JG, Bek T, et al. Increased serum IGF-I during pregnancy is associated with progression of diabetic retinopathy. Diabetes 2003;52: 852–6.
201. Ringholm L, Vestgaard M, Laugesen CS, et al. Pregnancy-induced increase in circulating IGF-I is associated with progression of diabetic retinopathy in women with type 1 diabetes. Growth Horm IGF Res 2011;21:25–30.
202. Best RM, Hayes R, Hadden DR, et al. Plasma levels of endothelin-1 in diabetic retinopathy in pregnancy. Eye (Lond) 1999;13 (Pt 2):179–82.
203. Vääräsmäki M, Anttila M, Pirttiaho H, et al. Are recurrent pregnancies a risk in Type 1 diabetes? Acta Obstet Gynecol Scand 2002;81:1110–15.
204. Klein R, Klein BE, Moss SE. Epidemiology of proliferative diabetic retinopathy. Diabetes Care 1992;15:1875–91.
205. Klein R, Klein BE, Moss SE, et al. Association of ocular disease and mortality in a diabetic population. Arch Ophthalmol 1999;117:1487–95.
206. Davis MD, Hiller R, Magli YL, et al. Prognosis for life in patients with diabetes: relation to severity of retinopathy. Trans Am Ophthalmol Soc 1979;77: 144–70.
207. Hanis CL, Chu HH, Lawson K, et al. Mortality of Mexican Americans with NIDDM. Retinopathy and other predictors in Starr County, Texas. Diabetes Care 1993;16:82–9.
208. Neil A, Hawkins M, Potok M, et al. A prospective population-based study of microalbuminuria as a predictor of mortality in NIDDM. Diabetes Care 1993;16:996–1003.
209. Sorbinil Retinopathy Trial Research Group. A randomized trial of sorbinil, an aldose reductase inhibitor, in diabetic retinopathy. Arch Ophthalmol 1990;108:1234–44.
210. Elman MJ, Aiello LP, Beck RW, et al. Randomized trial evaluating ranibizumab plus prompt or deferred laser or triamcinolone plus prompt laser for diabetic macular edema. Ophthalmology 2010;117:1064–77.
211. Witkin SR, Klein R. Ophthalmologic care for persons with diabetes. JAMA 1984;251:2534–7.
212. Singer DE, Nathan DM, Fogel HA, et al. Screening for diabetic retinopathy. Ann Intern Med 1992;116:660–71.
213. Sprafka JM, Fritsche TL, Baker R, et al. Prevalence of undiagnosed eye disease in high-risk diabetic individuals. Arch Intern Med 1990;150:857–61.
214. Brechner RJ, Cowie CC, Howie LJ, et al. Ophthalmic examination among adults with diagnosed diabetes mellitus. JAMA 1993;270:1714–18.
215. Weiner JP, Parente ST, Garnick DW, et al. Variation in office-based quality. A claims-based profile of care provided to Medicare patients with diabetes. JAMA 1995;273:1503–8.
216. Kraft SK, Marrero DG, Lazaridis EN, et al. Primary care physicians' practice patterns and diabetic retinopathy. Current levels of care. Arch Fam Med 1997;6:29–37.
217. Bresnick GH, Mukamel DB, Dickinson JC, et al. A screening approach to the surveillance of patients with diabetes for the presence of vision-threatening retinopathy. Ophthalmology 2000;107:19–24.
218. Moss SE, Klein R, Klein BE. Factors associated with having eye examinations in persons with diabetes. Arch Fam Med 1995;4:529–34.
219. National Institutes of Health. The National Eye Health Education Program. From Vision to Research to Health Educations: Planning the Partnership. Bethesda, MD: National Institutes of Health; 1990.
220. Batchelder T, Barricks M. The Wisconsin Epidemiologic Study of Diabetic Retinopathy. Arch Ophthalmol 1995;113:702–3.
221. Vijan S, Hofer TP, Hayward RA. Cost-utility analysis of screening intervals for diabetic retinopathy in patients with type 2 diabetes mellitus. JAMA 2000;283:889–96.
222. National Committee for Quality Assurance. Health Plan Employers Data and Information Set (HEDIS(r)), Version 2.5. Washington, DC: National Committee for Quality Assurance; 1996.
223. Velez R, Haffner SM, Stern MP, et al. Ophthalmologist versus retinal photographs in screening for diabetic retinopathy [abstract]. Clin Res 1987;35: 363A.
224. Bragge P, Gruen RL, Chau M, et al. Screening for presence or absence of diabetic retinopathy: a meta-analysis. Arch Ophthalmol 2011;129(4):435–44.

For additional online content visit http://www.expertconsult.com

Chapter 46

Diabetic Retinopathy: Genetics and Etiologic Mechanisms

Kang Zhang, Henry A. Ferreyra, Seanna Grob, Matthew Bedell, Jun Jun Zhang

This chapter will review our current understanding of the pathogenic mechanisms leading to the development of diabetic retinopathy, with an emphasis on the molecular and genetic pathways. Epidemiology, clinical manifestations, and management of diabetic retinopathy and its complications are discussed in detail elsewhere.

INTRODUCTION

Diabetic retinopathy is the leading cause of blindness among individuals between 25 and 74 years of age in the industrialized world. It affects three out of four diabetic patients after 15 years of disease duration. Chronic hyperglycemia is the primary factor leading to the development of diabetic retinopathy and other complications of the disease. The importance of long-term glycemic control has been conclusively established in the landmark clinical trials including the Diabetes Control and Complications Trial (DCCT),[1] and the UK Prospective Diabetes Study (UKPDS).[2,3] However, the mechanisms by which elevated blood sugar levels lead to the development of diabetic retinopathy and the anatomic changes visible histopathologically remain to be fully elucidated. This chapter will review the biochemical and molecular pathways believed to be responsible for the development of diabetic retinopathy and will highlight recent developments in genetics that provide insight into the influential role of genetic susceptibility.

ANATOMIC LESIONS

Loss of pericytes

Loss of pericytes is one of the earliest and most specific signs of diabetic retinopathy. This finding was first described by Cogan, Kuwabara and coworkers after examining trypsin-digested retinal vasculature flat mounts from diabetic human subjects.[4–6] Since their initial report, their findings have been confirmed by various investigators.[2,7,8] In humans and canines, trypsin digestion of retinal vasculature flat mounts reveals the loss of pericytes as evidenced by the development of pericyte ghosts, empty aneurysmal spaces bulging from the capillary walls that lack the darkly staining nucleus of a viable pericyte (Fig. 46.1A). Pericytes are normally identifiable in these spaces by their nuclei which stain darkly and are spaced regularly along the capillary wall, producing the appearance of "bumps on a log" (Fig. 46.1B).

Pericytes are contractile cells that play an important role in microvascular autoregulation.[9] Loss of pericytes leads to alterations of vascular intercellular contacts and impairment of the inner blood–retina barrier. These effects result in the venous dilation and beading that is visible clinically. Loss of intercellular contacts also appears to promote endothelial cell proliferation resulting in the development of microaneurysms.[10] Loss of pericytes appears to be especially significant in the development of diabetic retinopathy, although pericyte loss has also been

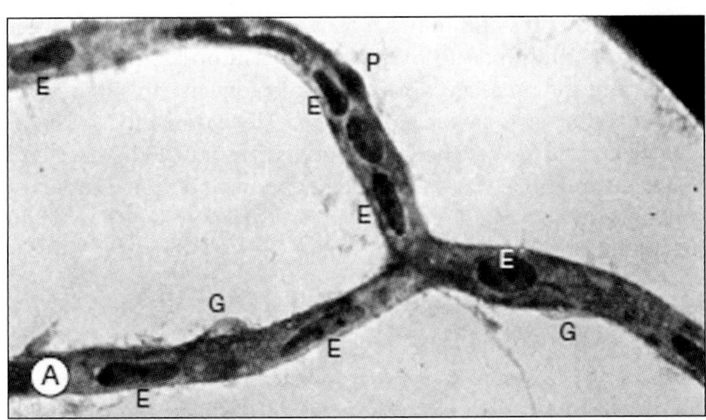

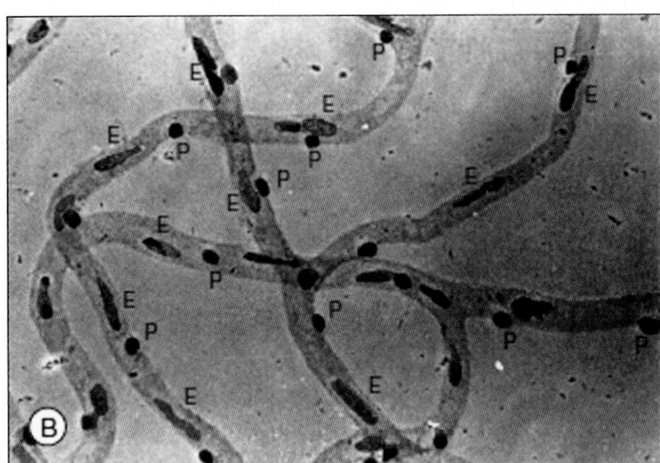

Fig. 46.1 (A) Pericyte ghosts (G) in a trypsin digest preparation from a 42-year-old woman with background diabetic retinopathy who died of a dissecting aneurysm of the aorta. The ghost represents the vacant space in the capillary basement membrane, formerly occupied by an intramural pericyte nucleus that has degenerated. Normal pericyte (P) and endothelial cell (E) nuclei are also shown. The preparation was stained with periodic acid–Schiff (PAS) reagent and hematoxylin. Magnification ×575. (B) A trypsin digest preparation from the retina of a nondiabetic, 55-year-old man who died of a myocardial infarction. Note the regular array of pericyte (P) and endothelial cell (E) nuclei. The preparation was stained with PAS reagent and hematoxylin. Magnification ×450.

reported in diabetic peripheral neuropathy leading to neuronal ischemia.[11] The mechanism by which hyperglycemia leads to pericyte degeneration remains largely unknown. The two leading hypotheses implicate the aldose reductase pathway and platelet-derived growth factor-beta (PDGF-β).

Akagi et al. reported the localization of the enzyme aldose reductase in retinal capillary pericytes but not in endothelial cells in human specimens using immunohistochemistry techniques.[12] These findings would be consistent with the specific loss of capillary pericytes observed in diabetic retinopathy and other microvascular complications of diabetes.[13] Two other groups, however, were unable to identify the presence of aldose reductase in rodent and canine retinal capillaries using immunohistochemistry techniques.[14,15] In addition, a third group reported the presence of aldose reductase activity in cultured bovine retinal capillary pericytes as well as retinal capillary endothelial cells. They also found aldose reductase activity in cultured monkey retinal pericytes.[16] These conflicting reports probably result from species-specific differences in aldose reductase expression and highlight the need to use caution when interpreting animal models of disease.

PDGF-β has been found to be critical in the recruitment of pericytes in the vasculature of various tissues and organs.[17] It is well documented that endothelial cells express PDGF-β,[18–21] and in vitro pericytes are known to express PDGF-β receptors and respond to PDGF-β.[22,23] Lindahl et al. reported that in the PDGF-β-deficient mouse model, pericytes fail to develop in developing capillaries during angiogenesis.[24] Subsequent studies using PDGF-β- and PDGF receptor-β (PDGFR-β)-deficient mice found that while PDGF-β/PDGFR-β-independent induction of pericyte precursors may occur, the expansion of pericytes is dependent on an intact PDGF-β/PDGFR-β paracrine signaling pathway.[25] Ablation of either PDGF-β or PDGFR-β led to identical phenotypes in these mice.[26] These studies suggest that endothelial cell-derived PDGF-β promotes the co-migration of PDGFR-β-expressing pericytes along sprouting new vessels, and the interruption of the PDGF-β/PDGFR-β results in the observed deficiency of pericytes in capillaries. Since PDGF-β has been found to be critical in the recruitment of pericytes during angiogenesis, it has been suggested that PDGF-β may play an important role in maintaining pericyte viability in mature vasculature, although no studies have confirmed this hypothesis.

Capillary basement membrane thickening

Thickening of capillary basement membranes is a well-documented lesion of diabetic retinopathy, visible on electron microscopy. Additional electron microscopic findings include deposition of fibrillar collagen and "Swiss cheese" vacuolization of the otherwise homogenous pattern of basement membrane collagen. The biochemical mechanism leading to basement membrane thickening remains unknown but studies suggest a role for the aldose reductase and the sorbitol pathway.[27–30] Nondiabetic rats fed a galactose-rich diet for prolonged periods of time develop retinal capillary basement membrane thickening, fibrillar collagen deposition, and Swiss cheese vacuolization. By contrast, rats fed a control diet or a galactose-rich diet along with the aldose reductase inhibitor sorbinil do not develop basement membrane thickening.[27,30] However, the observation that basement membrane thickening of renal glomeruli in diabetic and galactosemic rats is not inhibited by aldose reductase inhibitors casts doubt that the aldose reductase pathway is the primary pathway and suggests that basement membrane thickening may be a secondary nonspecific response.[31]

Glycation of basement membrane collagen by enzymatic[32] and nonenzymatic processes[33] may be another mechanism that plays a role in basement membrane thickening. Besides type IV collagen, the predominant type of collagen present in the basement membrane, other collagen types, and noncollagen macromolecules, such as laminin,[34] entactin, heparan sulfate proteoglycan,[35,36] and basement membrane-bound growth factors are also present.[35] Glycation appears to alter the structure of the basement membrane by changing the chemical composition and relative amounts of these components. For example, Shimomura/Spiro and Spiro/Spiro reported decreased heparan sulfate proteoglycan in renal glomeruli from diabetic human subjects.[37,38] Quantitative electron microscopic immunocytochemical studies have found that retinal and renal glomeruli basement membrane thickening in galactosemic rats is associated with a relative increase in the levels of type IV collagen and laminin, while the relative levels of heparan sulfate proteoglycan remain unchanged.[29,31]

Microaneurysms

Although pericyte loss is the earliest sign of diabetic retinopathy, it is only observable histologically. The earliest clinically visible sign of diabetic retinopathy is the microaneurysm.[39] Microaneurysms appear as grape-like or spindle-shaped dilations of retinal capillaries on light microscopy.[4] They can be either hypercellular or acellular. By ophthalmoscopic examination, microaneurysms appear as tiny, intraretinal red dots located in the inner retina. By fluorescein angiography, they appear as punctate hyperfluorescent dots with variable amounts of fluorescein leakage.

Pericyte cell death and loss of vascular intercellular contacts may lead to endothelial cell proliferation and microaneurysm development.[24,40,41] Pericytes appear to exert an antiproliferative effect and pericyte loss may explain the development of hypercellular microaneurysms. However, this mechanism does not account for acellular microaneurysms. Acellular microaneurysms may develop from hypercellular microaneurysms that become acellular from endothelial cell and pericyte apoptosis.[42]

Pericyte loss may also result in weakening of the capillary wall, promoting the development of microaneurysms at the structural weak points. Pericytes contain myofibrils with contractile properties and may act as smooth muscle cells of larger vessels, exerting tone to the vessel wall in order to counteract the transmural pressure. Loss of pericyte tone may result in focal dilation of the vessel wall leading to the development of a microaneurysm. However, the transmural pressure of the capillary bed is low relative to the arterial circulation, and retinal capillary microaneurysms can develop in other diseases in which pericyte loss is not observed.[43,44]

Capillary acellularity

Complete loss of the cellular elements of the retinal capillary network can be seen as a more advanced microvascular lesion in diabetic retinopathy and other microvascular retinopathies. In clinicopathological correlations with fluorescein angiograms performed shortly before the eye was enucleated for therapeutic purposes or because the patient died and the eye was removed during autopsy, the retinal vascular digests of the enucleated eye showed that acellular capillaries are nonfunctional since they appeared as regions of nonperfusion on angiography.[45] The mechanism by which capillaries become acellular is unknown and can be seen in diabetes, other retinal microvascular diseases, or in experimental diabetes or galactosemia in animal models. Since capillary acellularity is not unique to diabetes, a variety of pathogenic mechanisms may result in this nonspecific finding.

Breakdown of blood–retina barrier

Breakdown of the blood–retina barrier is an important pathophysiologic feature of diabetic retinopathy that leads to the development of macular edema, the leading cause of vision loss in diabetic patients. One mechanism by which the function of this barrier becomes altered involves opening of the tight junctions between vascular endothelial cell processes.[46,47] These tight junctions, also known as zonula occludens, appear as a pentalaminar structure on electron microscopy, consisting of two outer and one central electron-dense layer sandwiching two electron-lucent layers, giving the appearance of two "fused" plasma membranes. Using tracers such as lanthanum chloride or horseradish peroxidase, electron microscopy can be used to demonstrate that these molecules cannot pass in the presence of an intact tight junction. However, when the tight junctions are open, they become permeable to these tracer molecules.[47] Several important proteins are involved with the formation and function of tight junctions, with ZO-1 (zonula occludens) and occludin being the best characterized. In the presence of histamine, the expression of ZO-1 in cultured retinal endothelial cells is reduced in a dose-dependent manner.[48] Culturing in astrocyte-conditioned medium increases expression of ZO-1 while high glucose decreases expression of ZO-1.[49] These in vitro results have also been supported by in vivo studies. Reduced expression and anatomic distribution of occludin was found in experimental diabetes.[50] Likewise, in experimentally diabetic rats and in diabetic humans, antihistamines reduce leakage of fluorescein into the vitreous.[51,52]

Vascular endothelial growth factor (VEGF) has been found to be an important mediator leading to the breakdown of the inner blood–retina barrier. Before the discovery of its well-documented role in promoting neovascularization, VEGF was found to increase the permeability of vessels, leading to its alternative name "vascular permeability factor".[53] The mechanism by which VEGF leads to the breakdown of the inner blood–retina barrier appears to involve alteration of endothelial cell tight junctions. Intravitreal injection of VEGF in rats increased the production of the free radical nitric oxide and led to phosphorylation of ZO-1[54,55]

Another important factor promoting retinal vascular permeability involves the kallikrein–kinin system. Proteonomic studies of the vitreous from patients with advanced diabetic retinopathy have identified components of the kallikrein kinin system, including plasma kallikrein, factor XII, and kininogen.[56,57] In rodent models, activation of plasma kallikrein in the vitreous has been found to increase retinal vascular permeability.[58] Likewise, inhibition of the kallikrein kinin system reduces retinal vascular leakage caused by diabetes and hypertension.[58,59] The mechanism by which the kallikrein kinin system promotes vascular permeability probably involves bradykinin. Bradykinin, via nitric oxide, induces vasorelaxation of retinal arterioles.[60] Intravenous infusion of bradykinin results in dilation of retinal arterioles and venules, an effect that is reduced by indomethacin and the cyclooxygenase-2 selective inhibitor nimesulide.[61] Bradykinin is also a neuropeptide with a direct effect on glia and neurons, which can release vasoactive factors that affect blood flow and vascular permeability.[62]

BIOCHEMICAL MECHANISMS IN THE PATHOGENESIS OF DIABETIC RETINOPATHY

Chronic hyperglycemia is known to be the major etiologic factor leading to all of the microvascular complications of diabetes, including diabetic retinopathy. However, the biochemical mechanisms by which hyperglycemia acts currently remain unclear. Proposed theories will be discussed in detail in the subsequent sections of this chapter.

Although diabetic retinopathy does not manifest the classic "rubor, tumor, calor, and dolor" features of an inflammatory disease and lacks a prominent infiltration of inflammatory cells, there are characteristics that imply a chronic low-grade inflammatory component. In the retinas of diabetic rats, increased activation of leukocytes with increased amounts of inflammatory cytokines and adhesion molecules have been observed. The upregulation of these molecules enhances leukocyte adhesion to retinal capillary walls, leading to increased capillary stasis, occlusion, and ultimately hypoxia as seen in diabetic retinopathy.[63–65] Clinically, it has been observed that intravitreal corticosteroid injections decrease diabetic macular edema, often with improvement of visual acuity.[66,67] The mechanism by which intravitreal corticosteroids reduce macular edema in diabetes and other etiologies, like retinal vein occlusions, is unclear, but the anti-inflammatory effects of corticosteroids support an inflammatory component to the development of at least diabetic macular edema as well as macular edema from retinal vein occlusions. Likewise, there is growing evidence that the kinin-kallikrein system, which plays an important role in the inflammatory cascade by acting on phospholipase and promoting the release of arachidonic acid and the production of prostaglandins, contributes to the development of diabetic macular edema.[68]

The aldose reductase theory

Elevation of intracellular glucose levels can cause increased activation of the aldose reductase pathway. Also known as the polyol pathway or the sorbitol pathway, the aldose reductase pathway is a series of intracellular reactions that involves the enzymes aldose reductase and sorbitol dehydrogenase.[69,70] Aldose reductase uses the reduced form of nicotinamide adenine dinucleotide phosphate (NADPH) as a cofactor to reduce many aldose sugars into their respective sugar alcohols. Glucose is reduced to sorbitol, which is then oxidized into fructose by sorbitol dehydrogenase. However, sorbitol may build up to high intracellular levels because the sorbitol dehydrogenase reaction is slow and the accumulating sorbitol does not easily cross the plasma membrane into the extracellular space. In normoglycemic conditions, the aldose reductase pathway is nonoperative because glucose is a poor substrate for aldose reductase due to its high binding constant (kM). However, in the setting of hyperglycemia as seen with uncontrolled diabetes, the aldose reductase pathway becomes activated once the other enzymatic pathways of glucose metabolism become saturated. Lens epithelium expresses high levels of aldose reductase and accumulation of sorbitol is believed to lead to the development of a cataract in diabetes.[71] Osmotic stress has been proposed as the mechanism by which elevated intracellular sorbitol leads to the pathologic changes seen in diabetes.[72] However, the levels of sorbitol in vascular cells are in the nanomolar range, which is orders of magnitude less than other glucose metabolites, which have ranges in the micromolar and millimolar range.[73]

A different mechanism that may account for the role of aldose reductase involves the cellular redox balance. Increases in the utilization of aldose reductase in the hyperglycemic state of diabetes will result in a decline in intracellular NADPH that alters the cellular redox balance. Reduction of intracellular NADPH may also decrease the production of nitric oxide in endothelial cells.[74] Similarly, the increased use of sorbitol dehydrogenase can lead to an increase in the NADH/NAD^+ ratio that alters the cellular redox balance and may lead to oxidative stress and cellular damage.[75]

Of interest to animal models of diabetes, galactose is reduced by aldose reductase into galactilol. However, sorbitol dehydrogenase cannot oxidize galactilol, resulting in the rapid intracellular accumulation of galactilol. In the setting of chronic galactosemia, diabetic-like vascular basement membrane changes,[27,28] and pericyte loss, development of microaneurysms, and capillary acellularity[76] have been reported. When these experiments were repeated and the animals were also treated with aldose reductase inhibitors, it was reported that the development of diabetic-like retinopathy changes was slowed, although most animals developed some degree of changes.[30,77–79] While aldose reductase inhibitors were reported to slow or prevent some of the pathologic changes in animal models of diabetes, the aldose reductase inhibitor sorbinil was found not to be effective in humans in the Sorbinil Retinopathy trial.[80] The lack of efficacy of aldose reductase inhibitors in human trials may, however, reflect dose-limiting side-effects of the drug that may have precluded it from achieving therapeutic levels in the tissues of interest.

Advanced glycation endproduct (AGE) theory

Accelerated aging by nonenzymatic glycation and crosslinking of proteins has been proposed as a mechanism to explain the complications of diabetes.[81] Advanced glycation endproducts (AGEs) is the collective name given to proteins, lipids, and nucleic acids that undergo irreversible modification by reducing sugars or sugar-derived products. The series of chemical reactions that lead to the formation of AGEs is called the Maillard reaction. The Maillard reaction is responsible for the "browning" of tissue seen with aging as well as the "browning" of food during cooking. The initial chemical reaction is known as early glycation and involves reversible nonenzymatic binding of a sugar to amino acid groups on proteins, lipids, or nucleic acids. They form Schiff bases which can undergo rearrangement to form more stable Amadori products. Glycosylated hemoglobin (HbA1c) and fructosamine are well-known examples of Amadori products used clinically as markers of glycemic control. Although they are not AGEs, they can undergo further reactions to eventually lead to the formation of AGEs. Formation of AGEs may directly damage cells by impairing the function of a variety of proteins,[82] including both extracellular proteins like collagen[83] and intracellular proteins.[84,85]

The cellular effect of AGEs is also mediated by its binding to receptors, namely receptor for AGE (RAGE). RAGE is a multiligand transmembrane receptor that is part of the immunoglobulin superfamily of proteins.[86,87] When bound to AGEs, it initiates a cascade of signal transduction involving at least $p21^{ras}$, p44/p42 mitogen-activated protein kinase (MAPK), nuclear factor-kappa B (NF-κB), and protein kinase C (PKC).[88–93] Activation of these intracellular kinases can subsequently lead to cell dysfunction.[94] Other receptors have also been reported to bind to AGEs, such as the macrophage scavenger receptor, P60, P90, and galectin-3.[94–96] Aminoguanidine is an inhibitor of AGE formation and has been reported to block the development of many of the microvascular complications of diabetes in animal models.[97–100] The effects of aminoguanidine cannot be automatically attributed to the blockade of the AGE pathway, however, since aminoguanidine also has parallel action as an inhibitor of inducible nitric oxide synthase and oxidants.[101] Owing to limits secondary to toxicity, clinical trials in humans have been inconclusive; in animal models, however, the use of soluble RAGE to block binding of AGEs to RAGE has been found to prevent many of the effects of hyperglycemia.[102]

Reactive oxygen intermediates (ROI) theory

One of the oldest theories proposes that chronic hyperglycemia leads to the complications of diabetes by increasing oxidative stress. The usual metabolic pathway of glucose is through glycolysis and the tricarboxylic acid cycle, which takes place in the mitochondria and yields reducing equivalents used to drive the synthesis of adenosine triphosphate via oxidative phosphorylation. However, byproducts of oxidative phosphorylation include free radicals, such as superoxide anion, whose production is increased by high levels of glucose.[103] Free radicals can damage mitochondrial DNA[104] as well as cellular proteins[105] and are also produced by the autoxidation of glucose. Elevated oxidative stress also reduces nitric oxide levels,[106,107] promotes leukocyte adhesion to the endothelium and decreases the barrier function of endothelial cells,[108] and damages cellular proteins.[109] In diabetic mice that overexpress Cu^{2+}/Zn^{2+} superoxide dismutase, they develop less mesangial expansion compared to wild-type diabetic mice, suggesting that oxidative stress promotes at least some complications of diabetes.[110] Oxidative stress can also activate PKC by increasing the formation of diacylglycerol (DAG).[111]

There is some evidence of increased oxidative stress in diabetic patients. It has been reported that diabetic patients have lower levels of antioxidants, such as vitamin C, vitamin E, and glutathione,[112–114] although these results have not been unequivocally reproduced by other researchers.[115] However, other markers of oxidative stress, such as oxidized low-density lipoprotein[116] and urinary isoprostanes, are elevated in diabetic patients.[117] In animal models of diabetes, the use of antioxidants has blocked the development of some of the microvascular complications of diabetes.[118–122] One clinical trial reported that high doses of vitamin E (>1000 IU/day) and lipoic acid improved retinal blood flow and creatinine clearance in diabetic patients.[123] However, most studies evaluating antioxidants to prevent the complications of diabetes in people have been unsuccessful.[124]

Protein kinase C (PKC) theory

PKC is a ubiquitous enzyme that appears to promote the development of many of the complications of diabetes without the involvement of the aldose reductase pathway. It has been observed that diabetes and galactosemia can produce elevation of DAG within cells of the retina and aorta in dogs despite treatment with the aldose reductase inhibitor sorbinil.[125,126] Activation of PKC occurs through the activation of phospholipase C, which leads to an increase in intracellular Ca^{2+} and DAG, which in turn results in the activation of PKC.[127] Hyperglycemia can result in pathological activation of PKC. Elevated glucose levels result in activation of the glycolytic pathway and lead to increased levels of intracellular glyceraldehyde-3-phosphate. Glyceraldehyde-3-phosphate can promote the de novo synthesis of DAG through glycerol-3-phosphate, which in turn activates PKC.[128] Activation of PKC can also be mediated by AGE[92] and ROI.[111]

Elevated levels of DAG and PKC activity has been detected in the tissues of animals with diabetes.[129] The pathologic effects of PKC activation that cause vascular damage are mediated through increased vascular permeability,[130] disruption of nitric oxide regulation,[131,132] increased leukocyte adhesion to vessel walls,[133] and changes in blood flow.[134] In fact, the effects of PKC on retinal blood flow as measured by fluorescein video angiography, as well as glomerular filtration rate and albumin excretion rate, were improved in a dose-dependent fashion with ruboxistaurin (LY333531), a PKC-β inhibitor.[135] VEGF[136] and endothelin[137] can also activate PKC, which in turn can promote the expression of growth factors like VEGF[138] and transforming growth factor-beta (TGF-β).[139] PKC activation can influence other signally pathways, such as MAPK or NF-κB.[140]

PKC inhibition by ruboxistaurin has been reported to block many of the vascular abnormalities in endothelial cells and contractile cells from the retina, arteries, and renal glomeruli.[141] In animal models of diabetes, ruboxistaurin protected against or reversed many of the early vascular changes seen with retinopathy, nephropathy, and neuropathy.[135,136,142,143] However, a prospective clinical trial of ruboxistaurin did not meet its primary outcome (progression to sight-threatening diabetic macular edema or application of focal/grid photocoagulation for diabetic macular edema) at 30 months although there was a significant reduction of progression to sight-threatening diabetic macular edema when considered alone.[144] An open-label extension of the Protein Kinase C Diabetic Retinopathy Study 2 (PKCDRS-2) reported that over a 6-year study period patients with the greatest ruboxistaurin exposure (~5 years) had less sustained moderate vision loss (>15-letter decline) compared to those in the original placebo group (~2 years of ruboxistaurin use).[145]

Insulin receptors and glucose transporters

In certain types of cells, such as adipocytes and skeletal muscle cells, insulin is required to transport glucose from the extracellular fluid across the plasma membrane into the cytoplasm. This action requires a specific receptor for insulin on the plasma membrane. Although it has been commonly stated that the microvascular complications of diabetes do not occur in tissues in which insulin is required for the transport of glucose into cells, insulin receptors have been reported on the pericytes and endothelial cells of the retinal microvessels.[146] There is no evidence, however, that the retinal microvascular insulin receptors are required for glucose transport, although insulin does enhance glycogen synthesis from radiolabeled glucose in retinal microvascular pericytes and endothelial cells and aortic smooth-muscle cells, but not in aortic endothelial cells.[146] Insulin in physiologic concentrations (as low as 10 ng/ml) stimulated [3H]-thymidine incorporation into retinal microvascular pericytes and endothelial cells and aortic smooth-muscle cells but not aortic endothelial cells.[146] It is noteworthy that, in these experiments, such low concentrations of insulin produced an effect, because unphysiologically high (e.g., 1 mg/ml) concentrations of insulin will stimulate proliferation of many types of cultured cells. However, since microvascular endothelial cells and pericytes do not normally proliferate in the mature retina,[147] the importance of these results for normal retinal vascular physiology is unclear. Additionally, these results indicate that there are metabolic differences between microvascular endothelial cells and the endothelial cells of larger vessels, so that translation of results from one type of vascular endothelial cell to another must be done with great caution.

There are at least five different types of facilitated cell membrane glucose transporters, designated GLUT1, GLUT2, GLUT3, GLUT4, and GLUT5, that appear to be most important for the intracellular transport of glucose in tissues like the retina that do not require insulin. Of these, GLUT1 appears to be the most prevalent in the retina,[148–150] occurring in microvascular and macrovascular endothelial cells and on RPE cells, as well as in the Müller cells. GLUT2 localization has been reported by immunocytochemistry at the apical ends of the Müller cells of the rat retina, facing the interphotoreceptor matrix,[151] while GLUT3 has been reported by similar techniques to be localized to the plexiform layers of the rat[152] and human[150] retina. An initial report using light microscopic immunocytochemistry in human eyes[148] also reported GLUT1 in the nerve fiber layer of the retina and in photoreceptor cell bodies, but GLUT1 was absent from retinal neovascular proliferations in the eyes of diabetic subjects. Subsequently, these investigators used quantitative immunogold electron microscopic immunocytochemistry to examine GLUT1 localization in the eyes of two nondiabetic subjects and three diabetic subjects with little or no retinopathy.[149] In approximately half of the retinal microvessels from the diabetic subjects there was no quantitative difference in GLUT1 immunoreactivity by comparison with microvessels from the two normal individuals. However, in the other half of the retinal microvessels studied from diabetic individuals, these investigators reported an increase of GLUT1 immunoreactivity of about 18-fold over normal on the luminal plasma membranes. If these findings can be confirmed in a much larger number of eyes, such upregulation could be a mechanism that initiates glucose-mediated cellular damage by permitting a much greater influx of glucose into cells.

Whether galactose also enters cells by one or more of these facilitated glucose transporters has not been directly tested. However, the fact that rats fed a 50% galactose diet – which also contains the normal amount of glucose – double their food intake by comparison with normal rats, but nevertheless gain weight at only 60–70% of the rate of the normal animals,[153] suggests that the excessive amount of galactose competes with glucose for the transport sites, thereby limiting the entry of glucose into cells and diminishing glucose-requiring cellular energy metabolism. However, galactose can participate in other cellular pathways along with glucose, including protein glycation/advanced glycation endproduct formation and synthesis of DAG to activate PKC.[126] Whether glucose or galactose can upregulate the mRNAs governing synthesis of any of the GLUT proteins in a fashion such that this upregulation persists long after cessation of the hyperglycemic or galactosemic state has not yet been explored.

GENETIC FACTORS IN THE PATHOGENESIS OF DIABETIC RETINOPATHY

There is good evidence that diabetic retinopathy has a genetic predisposition.[154] Diabetic Retinopathy Study (DRS) data indicated that only 50% of nonproliferative diabetic retinopathy (NPDR) patients developed PDR, and many diabetic patients never developed diabetic retinopathy (DR). Twin studies of DR also lend support to this notion.[155] Some investigators have also suggested that aldose reductase gene polymorphisms may be associated with risk of DR.[156–162] There appears to be considerable value in further investigation of genetic factors related to the pathogenesis of the more severe forms of diabetic retinopathy: severe nonproliferative and proliferative retinopathy, as well as macular edema. Nearly all individuals with type 1 diabetes, and most with type 2 disease, will demonstrate some of the lesions of early retinopathy with sufficient disease duration, but only 50% or less will develop proliferative disease.[163,164] Like clinically evident diabetic nephropathy, which similarly affects fewer than 50% of all diabetic subjects regardless of the duration of their diabetes, this suggests genetic factors, in addition to chronic hyperglycemia, are likely involved in the development of these severe forms of retinopathy.

Several studies have explored the relationship between human leukocyte antigen (HLA) antigens, expressed on cell surfaces (and customarily tested with leukocytes withdrawn by venipuncture), and the presence, or severity, of diabetic retinopathy. Rand et al.,[165] used a case–control design and found a strong association (relative risk, 3.74) between proliferative retinopathy and the presence of HLA-DR phenotypes 4/0, 3/0, and X/X (neither 3 nor 4). Subjects who had HLA-DR phenotypes 3/4, 3/X, and 4/X had no increased risk of proliferative retinopathy as compared with "control" diabetic subjects, matched for age, sex, and diabetes duration, but without retinopathy. This question was also investigated in a group of 425 subjects with insulin-dependent diabetes who were randomly selected from a much larger population-based study.[166] After adjustments were made for duration of diabetes, glycemic control, hypertension, and nephropathy, these authors also found a significantly increased risk of proliferative diabetic retinopathy in subjects with the HLA DR4^{+} DR3 phenotype.

More recent studies have investigated other aspects of the genetics of diabetic retinopathy. Of particular note is a report from the DCCT research group,[167] which examined familial clustering of severe diabetic retinopathy (Early Treatment Diabetic Retinopathy Study (ETDRS) score >47, i.e., severe preproliferative disease) among families of DCCT subjects with multiple diabetic members. Significant associations were found when the correlation of retinopathy severity among family members was investigated in several different ways. However, a less strong familial clustering of diabetic nephropathy was found. This is surprising since evidence from other studies has demonstrated considerable familial clustering of diabetic nephropathy, a complication of diabetes that is now considered to have a strong genetic component.[168–171] With increased sophistication in molecular biology, a number of investigators have examined several genetic loci for abnormalities that might be related to a hereditary susceptibility to complications of diabetes. Although these studies are not definitive, one of these claimed that a mutation in the aldose reductase gene conferred increased susceptibility to early-onset diabetic retinopathy in patients with type 2 diabetes.[172]

Although many genes and proteins of vascular growth have been studied in association with PDR, few if any definitive predisposing genes for PDR have been identified. Below is a brief summary of several studies performed on candidate genes. One of the best known and most well-studied genes is the *VEGF* gene.[173–175] VEGF refers to 2 families of proteins created by alternate splicing of exon 8 in the *VEGF* gene[176] and is an important mediator of ischemia-induced vascularization and neovascularization. Current research of VEGF has focused on the role that certain single nucleotide polymorphisms (SNP) may play in contributing either a risk or protective effect in patients.[176–178] Recently, three SNPs in the promoter and 5′UTR regions of the gene (C(-7)T, C(-634)G, T(-1498), and G(-1190)A) were studied for frequency differences between patients with and without PDR.[177] These studies have looked at different genetic populations, focusing on Japanese and Indian patients. The results of these genetic studies are at times confusing, as a disease-associated SNP in one population may not confer a risk in another population. For example, in the Japanese population, the CC genotype at the C(-634)G region was significantly associated with PDR, whereas CG genotype at the same site was found to be risk-associated in the Indian population. In addition, disease duration, age, and sex must also be taken into account.

Ramprasad and coworkers in 2007 described work evaluating the role of SNPs within the receptor for advanced glycation end products (RAGE) in PDR.[179] At least 20 different polymorphisms have been studied within the *RAGE* gene. Interaction between the receptor RAGE and its associated glycation ligands plays a role in initiating a proinflammatory cascade, and this interaction has been studied in many disorders of chronic inflammation, including peripheral vascular disease and PDR. Research in these SNPs has shown disease association with the NPDR disease phenotype, yet this association needs to be replicated in other independent cohorts. More recently, Balasubbu et al.[180] analyzed the association of nine candidate genes (*RAGE, PEDF, AKR1B1, EPO, HTRA1, ICAM, HFE, CFH*, and *ARMS2*) but only found a significant association with diabetic retinopathy in one locus (rs2070600 in *RAGE* → reduces risk).

Proliferative diabetic retinopathy (PDR) and endstage renal disease (ESRD) are two of the most common and severe microvascular complications of diabetes. There is a high concordance in the development of PDR and ESRD in diabetic patients, as well as strong familial aggregation of these complications, suggesting a common underlying genetic mechanism. However, the precise gene(s) and genetic variant(s) involved remain largely unknown. Erythropoietin (EPO) is a potent angiogenic factor observed in the diabetic human and mouse eye. By a combination of case–control association and functional studies, Tong et al.[181] demonstrated that the T allele of SNP rs1617640 in the promoter of the *EPO* gene is significantly associated with PDR and ESRD. The study was performed in three European-American cohorts (Utah: $P = 1.91\times10^{-3}$; GoKinD: $P = 2.66\times10^{-8}$; Boston: $P = 2.1\times10^{-2}$). The EPO concentration in human vitreous was 7.5-fold higher in normal subjects with the TT risk genotype than in those with the GG genotype. Computational analysis suggests that the risk allele (T) of rs1617640 creates a matrix match with the EVI1/MEL1 or AP1 binding site, accounting for an observed 25-fold enhancement of luciferase reporter expression as compared to the G allele. These results suggest that rs1617640 in the *EPO* promoter is significantly associated with PDR and ESRD and suggest EPO as a potential pathway mediating severe diabetic microvascular complications.[181]

Genome-wide association studies (GWAS) of diabetic retinopathy have also been pursued. In a Taiwanese population, Huang et al. found genetic associations for susceptibility for development of diabetic retinopathy in five loci, including *PLXDC2* and *ARHGAP22*, which are genes implicated in endothelial cell proliferation and capillary permeability.[182] In addition, one group recently published their preliminary results of a GWAS on a small (286 total) Mexican-American diabetic cohort. They identified 32 SNPs (in 11 regions) with a nominal association for severe diabetic retinopathy, though none was located in traditional candidate genes for diabetes or diabetic retinopathy.[183] These findings have yet to be replicated, and as noted above, the cohort was small. In two large type I diabetes cohorts, several novel genetic loci associated with sight-threatening complications due to diabetic retinopathy, were identified, including rs10521145 in the intron of CCDC101, a histone acetyltransferase.[184]

Catalyzed by the rapid advances in whole-genome SNP genotyping technologies and the construction of reference haplotype maps, genetic variants associated with ~300 traits have successfully been mapped by GWAS in the past few years, using a *P*-value threshold of 10^{-5}. GWAS is based on the hypothesis that common diseases are mainly caused by common genetic variants in the population (Common Disease Common Variants, CD-CV), each having relatively weak effects.[185] This assumption appears to be generally true for many genetic traits such as age-related macular degeneration.[186–188] Another hypothesis is Common Disease Rare Variants (CD-RV), or that common diseases are due to the presence of many rare variants in the same genes or pathways, each having relative strong effects. There is mounting evidence suggesting that CD-RV is also true for many diseases.[189–192] In diseases such as cancer, coronary atherosclerosis, and Parkinson disease, nonsynonymous variants in the disease genes were found more frequently in the disease samples compared to the controls. In addition, a higher proportion of these are predicted to be damaging.[189,193,194] For example, Cohen et al. sequenced genes in individuals at risk for coronary disease.[189] They found that 16% of the individuals in the disease group had novel nonsynonymous variants in candidate genes, in contrast to only 2% for individuals not at risk. Causal variants under the CD-RV hypothesis are difficult to detect in GWAS, because they are in very weak linkage disequilibrium with the tagging SNPs included in genotyping assays. Deep resequencing in the case and control population is required to uncover such variants.[195] Due to the high cost of large-scale resequencing, only a very limited number of candidate genes have been screened.

OTHER OCULAR FACTORS

Becker[196] reported in 1967 that glaucoma was associated with a decreased prevalence and severity of diabetic retinopathy in affected eyes. Other studies have reported similar results. This has never been confirmed in a methodologically precise epidemiologic study, although Becker's claim seems to be correct based on other clinical observations (Fig. 46.2). This is an important point that should be evaluated in a proper case–control study. If it is true, the explanation is unclear. If the effect is observable only in true glaucoma and not in ocular hypertension, in which the intraocular pressure is chronically elevated without damage to the retinal ganglion cell or optic nerve fiber layers, then it may be related in some way to loss of metabolic activity in the retina with degeneration of ganglion cells. If the effect is related simply to elevated intraocular pressure, the explanation for this observation would be less obvious.

It has also been reported that myopia is associated with a decreased prevalence and severity of diabetic retinopathy.[197] This effect of myopia on the prevalence of proliferative diabetic retinopathy has been confirmed by Rand et al.[165] who found an interesting interaction between myopia of greater than 2 diopters and HLA-D-group antigens. Fewer subjects in their "case" group with proliferative retinopathy had myopia of this degree than did subjects in the control group, who had diabetes of 15 years' or more duration and minimal or no retinopathy. Subjects with 2 D or more of myopia and HLA-D group phenotypes 3/0,

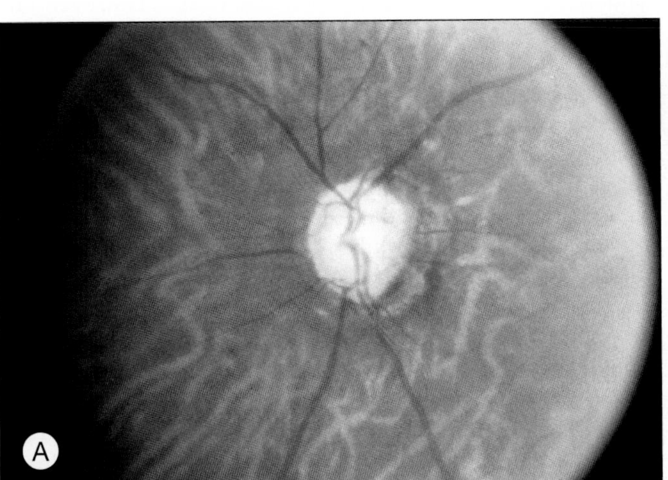

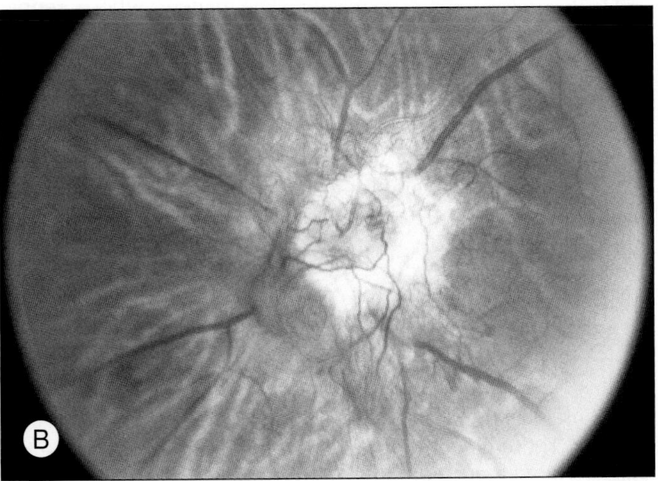

Fig. 46.2 This 64-year-old man presented with asymmetric, chronic open angle glaucoma and markedly asymmetric diabetic retinopathy. Intraocular pressure in the right eye was 32 mmHg, visual acuity was 20/80, and there was a glaucomatous visual field defect and pronounced glaucomatous cupping of the optic nerve head. In the left eye, the pressure was 16 mmHg, visual acuity was 20/20, and there was only physiologic cupping. The patient had had diabetes mellitus for 15 years. (A) Photograph of the right optic nerve head shows extensive cupping of the optic nerve, though without nasal displacement of the vessels. (B) Photograph of the left optic nerve shows extensive neovascularization.

4/0, or X/X had a relative risk for proliferative disease of 1.0 as compared with the control group (i.e., their risk was no different from that of the controls), while the overall risk for all subjects, regardless of refractive error, with these HLA-D group phenotypes was 3.74.

The initial observations leading to the development of panretinal photocoagulation (or scatter) treatment for proliferative diabetic retinopathy were made by Aiello and colleagues at the Symposium on the Treatment of Diabetic Retinopathy,[198] who noted that eyes with a great deal of retinochoroidal scarring from trauma, inflammatory disease, etc. had markedly reduced prevalence and severity of diabetic retinopathy. The effect is unexplained, but the most widespread current hypothesis is that it results from decreased retinal metabolism - in particular, a decreased need for oxygen, with a resultant diminished production of a vasoproliferative (angiogenic) factor.[199,200] The immediate practical application of this observation was the attempt, through extensive photocoagulation of the mid-peripheral retina (panretinal or scatter photocoagulation), to produce the same effect iatrogenically, a technique that significantly reduces the rate of progression to severe visual loss in PDR.[201]

RETINOPATHY IN DIFFERENT FORMS OF DIABETES

There is no evidence that retinopathy differs in different forms of diabetes. Proliferative retinopathy is more prevalent at any given duration of the systemic disease in type 1 than in type 2 diabetes,[163,164] but, as noted earlier, it is not clear whether this is due to different metabolic factors in the two types of diabetes, to differences in the ages of the patients (type 1 patients are, on average, much younger), or to the higher mean blood glucose levels in type 1 patients. Macular edema probably occurs with equal prevalence as a function of disease duration in both type 1 and type 2 diabetes.[202] Type 2 diabetes is more common after the age of 30[164] (although "type 2 diabetes of youth" is becoming increasingly frequently recognized[203]), but, despite the apparently mild metabolic defect, proliferative retinopathy can occur as well in this form of the disease (Fig. 46.3). Similarly, vision-threatening retinopathy can occur in patients with "secondary" diabetes - that which occurs, for example, following pancreatitis, hemochromatosis, or acromegaly. The patient whose retinal photographs are shown in Fig. 46.4A and B had acromegaly secondary to a pituitary adenoma and also developed background diabetic retinopathy with macular edema. Since the acromegaly had been treated and the patient had normal levels of circulating growth hormone, the retinopathy may have been related to diabetes secondary to the acromegaly, or to a type 2 diabetes that would have developed regardless of the presence of acromegaly.

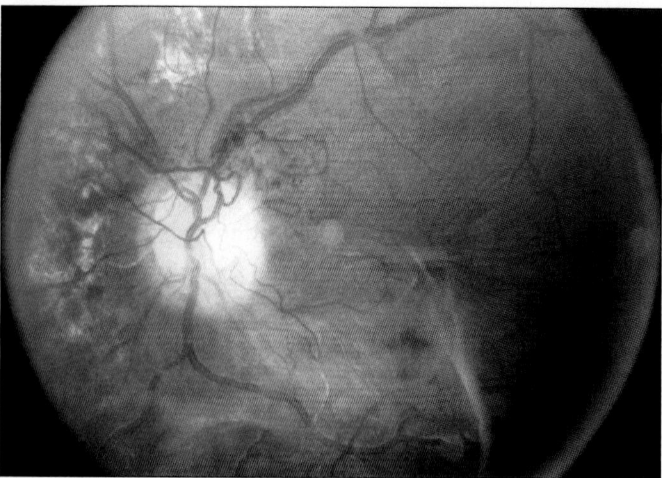

Fig. 46.3 Photograph showing the fundus of the left eye of a 32-year-old woman who had had diabetes mellitus since the age of 12 but had never required insulin. At the time of this photograph she was being maintained on dietary management and sulfonylurea medication. She therefore has the diagnosis of "type 2 diabetes of youth." As the photograph demonstrates, she has developed substantial proliferative diabetic retinopathy with extensive optic nerve head neovascularization and fibroglial proliferation producing traction on the macula. The right eye had been lost because of proliferative diabetic retinopathy with neovascular glaucoma.

ANIMAL MODELS IN THE STUDY OF DIABETIC RETINOPATHY

Studies of the pathogenesis and treatment of human disease can be facilitated by the development of models of the disease in animals. There have been numerous attempts to reproduce the lesions of diabetic retinopathy in animals. Although several authors have claimed positive results, there are only a few animal models in which one or more of the lesions of diabetic retinopathy have been produced with unquestioned validity. Foremost among these are dogs, with spontaneous[204] or induced[205] diabetes of 3–5 years' duration. These animals develop loss of capillary pericytes and ultimately also of endothelial cells with nonfunctional, acellular capillaries; capillary basement membrane thickening, and microaneurysm formation. Early intraretinal neovascularization has also been observed. However, more advanced lesions, including retinal edema (dogs do not have a macula, so true macular edema cannot develop) and neovascularization into the vitreous, have not been reported.

Because of the ease of working with small animals, there have been many attempts to develop diabetic retinopathy in rodents, including mice and, in particular, rats. Claims of producing lesions such as microaneurysms[97] and pericyte dropout[97] in rats with experimental diabetes of less than 1 year have not been validated by Engerman et al.[205] or Tilton et al.[206] However, rats with diabetes or galactosemia[27,28] develop retinal capillary basement membrane thickening, a lesion that has been widely observed in many microvascular systems in the body in human and animal diabetes.[207] In addition, rats that have been galactosemic for 18 months or more develop pericyte loss and, eventually, capillary acellularity,[79,153,208,209] and some rats that have been fed a 30–50% galactose diet for up to 24 months develop a halo of dilated, hypercellular vessels surrounding the optic nerve.[79,153,208,209] Whether these represent intraretinal neovascularization or simply dilated pre-existing vascular channels is uncertain. Of particular interest is a report that pericyte and endothelial cell nuclei in short-term diabetic or galactosemic rats, and in retinal capillaries from donor eyes of humans with diabetes, undergo apoptosis as demonstrated by appropriate nuclear labeling techniques.[42] It is unknown what stimulus is induced by prolonged hyperglycemia, or galactosemia, that causes programmed death of retinal capillary cells to a greater extent than capillary cells elsewhere in the body.

Because of the similarity of their retinal anatomy to that of humans, one might expect that nonhuman primates with

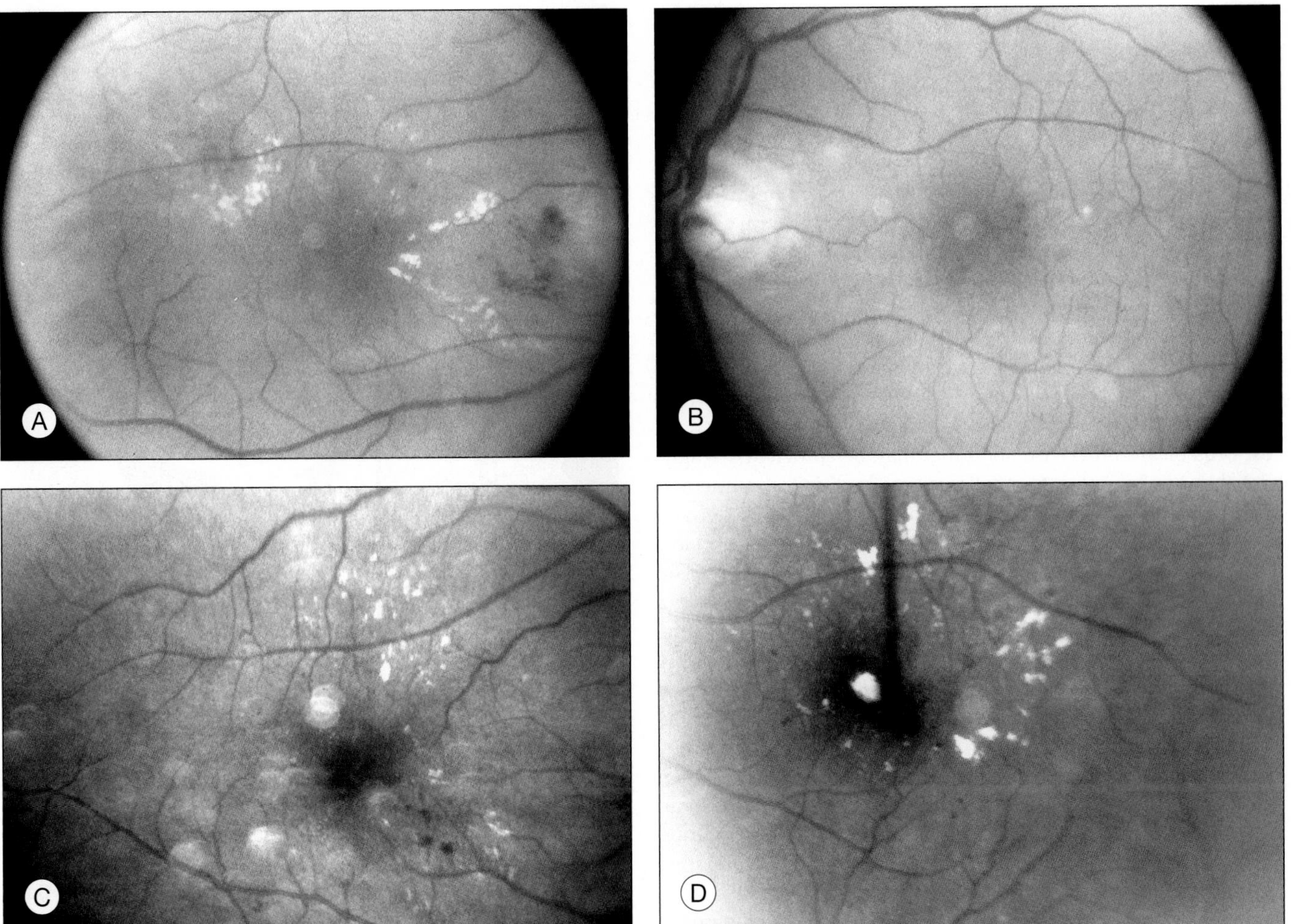

Fig. 46.4 (A) Photograph of the macular region of the right eye of an 84-year-old man who had developed acromegaly 12 years previously. Treatment with bromocriptine has maintained serum growth hormone levels in the normal range. Subsequent to his development of acromegaly, he was found to have type 2 diabetes mellitus, and he developed background diabetic retinopathy with macular edema, for which he received focal argon laser photocoagulation. Subsequently, he developed a central retinal vein occlusion in his right eye, for which he received panretinal argon laser photocoagulation. Nevertheless, neovascular glaucoma ensued, requiring cyclocryotherapy and medical therapy to manage the intraocular pressure and maintain at least some visual acuity. (B) The left eye of the same patient shows a few microaneurysms and minimal lipid deposition. (C) Photograph of the right eye of a 52-year-old man with acromegaly and type 2 diabetes mellitus. Bromocriptine treatment brought serum growth hormone levels to the normal range. Background diabetic retinopathy and macular edema are present. (D) The left macular region of the same patient, also showing background diabetic retinopathy with macular edema.

diabetes of sufficient duration would be good models for human diabetic retinopathy. However, studies of rhesus monkeys with diabetes for as long as 10 years have revealed occasional microaneurysms but no other lesions.[205,210]

Doubtless a major reason for the difficulty in producing lesions of diabetic retinopathy in animals with diabetes is the factor of disease duration. In diabetic dogs a minimum disease duration of 3–5 years is necessary for the development of the earliest lesions of retinopathy, and this is identical to the duration required for retinopathy to develop in humans with type 1 diabetes.[164,211,212] Rats and mice normally have a lifespan of under 3 years, and after the onset of diabetes it is difficult to maintain these animals for much more than 1 year. Several investigators have reported the development of lesions resembling diabetic retinopathy in rats fed a 50% galactose diet for 28 months.[79,153,208] These lesions include pericyte "ghosts," acellular capillaries, and vascular dilation and tortuosity. Whether microaneurysms occur in galactosemic rats is controversial.[42,79,153,208–210] The use of a high-galactose diet to produce a model of diabetic retinopathy originated from the hypothesis that the enzyme sequence known as the "sorbitol pathway" is responsible for the earliest lesions of diabetic retinopathy. Since galactose, along with glucose, is a substrate for this pathway, its use in producing models of retinopathy is a good test of the hypothesis. Previously, Kern and Engerman,[100] as well as Kador and associates,[77,78] have produced a diabetic-like retinopathy in dogs fed a 50% galactose diet for 3–4 years. Kern and Engerman have also reported a diabetic-like retinopathy in mice fed a 30% galactose diet for 21–26 months.[213] They reported that, unlike galactosemic rats, galactosemic mice developed true microaneurysms. These findings raise two important questions. First, why might mice, dogs, and humans develop microaneurysms after chronic diabetes, or galactosemia, and rats do not? Second, how might the presence of retinopathy in chronically galactosemic mice be relevant to the hypothesis that the "sorbitol pathway" is an important causal mechanism for diabetic retinopathy? Both these questions will be considered in more detail in later sections of this chapter.

Species- and organ-specific variations in anatomy and in metabolic pathways may be important considerations in the development of microvascular lesions in the retina or other organs. Pericyte dropout and microaneurysm formation have not been found either in the brains of diabetic human subjects,[214] or in those of diabetic or galactosemic dogs,[215] even though these lesions are common in the retina and were present in the retinas of the same human or animal subjects in whose cerebral cortexes they could not be found. It might be argued that, in these studies, retinas were examined by the trypsin digest procedure in which the entire, intact retinal vasculature can be spread on a microscope slide and examined in detail. This cannot be done with cerebral cortical vasculature, which must be examined histologically following homogenization and sieving through a nylon mesh that retains only vascular fragments. Capillaries that have lost cells or are otherwise abnormal may be sufficiently fragile that they are broken into smaller pieces by this technique and are lost in the sieving process. Although the retina is derived embryologically from the brain, and both retina and brain have a microvasculature featuring thick endothelial cell cytoplasm and tight junctions between endothelial cells that produce a blood–tissue barrier to many molecules, pericyte coverage of the endothelial cell tube of capillaries of the retina is substantially greater in the two species that have been studied (rat and monkey) than it is in the brains of these species.[216,217] The same is probably true in humans, where the data from retina closely resemble data from the retinas of monkeys, but it has not been possible to obtain retinal and brain tissue from the same human donors adequate to perform these morphometric studies. Although galactosemic rats develop a diabetic-like retinopathy, rats have a much smaller ratio of pericytes to endothelial cells in their retinal microcirculations than do humans.[206,216,218] Comparisons of the retinal and cerebral pericyte: endothelial cell ratios in retinas and brains of rats with those of dogs, mice, and humans have not been carried out, but would be of interest because dogs, humans, and (at least according to one group of investigators) mice develop true capillary microaneurysms with long-term diabetes (dogs and humans) and galactosemia (dogs and mice), while rats do not.

Two useful animal models of neovascularization exist, both in nondiabetic animals. The first, originally described by Ashton[196] and by Patz,[219] is produced by exposing neonatal kittens or puppies to an atmosphere high in oxygen for up to a few days just after birth. This produces at least a peripheral, or in more severe cases a generalized,[220] vasoconstriction, followed by the development of retinal new vessels. These vessels are transient, however, and regress spontaneously after a few weeks. This model was initially developed to simulate retinopathy of prematurity, a condition that may develop following exposure of premature human infants to a high-oxygen atmosphere. The development of the new vessels, according to the hypothesis that has been favored for a number of years,[200] presumably resulted from production by the hypoxic retina cells (hypoxic because of the profound vasoconstriction that followed the hyperoxia) of an "angiogenesis factor."[221] More recently, hyperoxygenation during the neonatal period has been applied to mice and rats, producing a model of peripheral retinal neovascularization similar to that of retinopathy of prematurity in human infants (Fig. 46.5), that has been exploited for studies of the production, and inhibition, of angiogenesis factors.[222-224] A second model of intraretinal and subretinal (beneath the neural retina, but arising from the retinal and not the choroidal circulation) neovascularization has recently been described, using transgenic mice that overexpress the gene for VEGF.[225] This model is additional evidence that VEGF is capable of producing retinal neovascularization, although in a quite artificial situation that may not be relevant to human ocular diseases associated with neovascularization. The new vessels in these transgenic mice extend from the retinal circulation to beneath the photoreceptor layer of the neural retina but do not enter the RPE. The reason for this outward growth, rather than inward into the vitreous, is that the promoter used to carry the VEGF gene into the retina is the rhodopsin gene, which is localized to the photoreceptor cells.

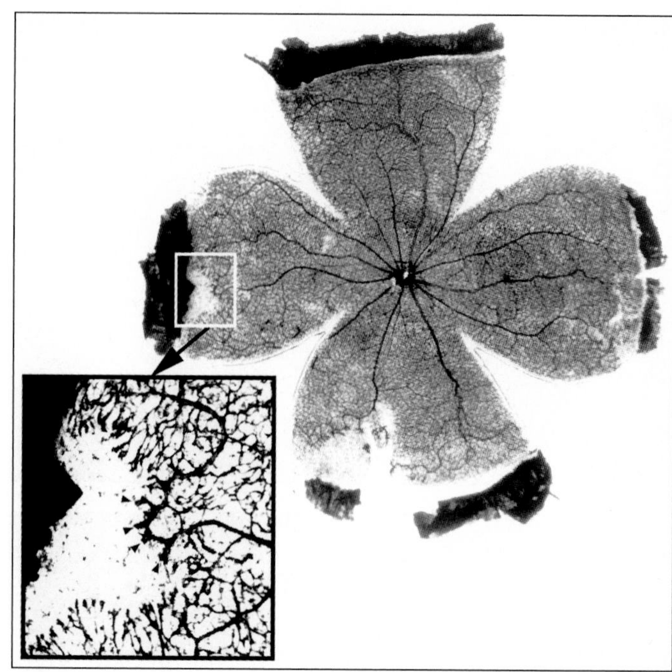

Fig. 46.5 Flat mount of the retinal vessels from an eye of a neonatal albino rat that had been exposed with its mother to an atmosphere in which the oxygen level was varied in stepwise fashion between 50% and 10% every 24 h over the first 14 days after birth. The animal was then returned to room air for the next 6 days and then euthanized, the eyes enucleated, and the retinal vessels visualized using a histochemical technique that demonstrates ADPase activity. The inset demonstrates a tuft of new vessels (arrowheads) in the peripheral retinal vasculature, similar to those that develop in human infants with retinopathy of prematurity. Magnifications: main figure, ×15; inset, ×75. (Courtesy of Bruce Berkowitz, PhD, Department of Anatomy and Cell Biology, Wayne State University School of Medicine.)

CELL CULTURE STUDIES

The intact human, or experimental, animal is a complex organism, in which the study of the intricate metabolic pathways that ultimately lead to diabetic retinopathy may be difficult.

Since the mid-1970s, techniques have been developed to isolate and grow in culture the component cells of both large and small blood vessels, including those from the retina. In 1975, Buzney et al. described the culture of retinal microvascular pericytes from bovine and monkey eyes.[226] Subsequently Frank et al.[227] and several others[228-230] described the culture of retinal microvascular endothelial cells. More recent evidence indicates that glial cells of the retina and optic nerve may also be important in the development, at least in the later stages of diabetic retinopathy, of neovascularization and, perhaps, macular edema. Methods are available for retinal glial cell culture. These techniques add an extra tool for research in diabetic retinopathy, but one that must be used with caution. One can use cell culture studies to investigate certain biochemical processes, but with great caution that the processes being studied have not been greatly modified in culture from those that occur in vivo. The same can be said for the investigation of physiologic function, e.g., phagocytosis, cell contraction, or cell motility. Diabetic retinopathy requires years to develop in the intact human or experimental animal. It has not yet been possible to maintain cultures of retinal cells for that duration, and there is no way of ascertaining that alterations produced in cells by exposure to high glucose or galactose over a short time in culture are truly related to the development of the anatomic and functional lesions of diabetic retinopathy over a very long time in the intact retina. Finally, although capillary tube-like structures composed of micro- and macrovascular endothelial cells have been produced under certain conditions in culture,[231–233] these may not be truly analogous either to normal vessels or to abnormal new vessels in the intact retina.

Despite these caveats, there are several results using cultured retinal microvascular cells that appear to be relevant to the physiology of the intact retinal microcirculation. These include the elegant studies of D'Amore and associates,[40,41] in which microvascular endothelial cells were co-cultured with a variety of other cell types that had been growth-arrested with an antibiotic and were then plated together with endothelial cells in different proportions. Most of the cells used for the co-cultures, including bovine RPE cells, human skin fibroblasts, mouse 3T3 fibroblasts, and Madin–Darby canine kidney cells, greatly stimulated endothelial cell proliferation. By contrast, pericytes and vascular smooth-muscle cells dramatically inhibited endothelial cell proliferation, even when the pericytes or smooth-muscle cells were added in ratios as low as 1:10 with the endothelial cells.[40] For the co-culture to be effective in retarding endothelial cell proliferation, pericyte or smooth-muscle cell processes had to make contact with the endothelial cells. Transfer of "conditioned media" from pericyte or smooth-muscle cell cultures was ineffective in producing growth inhibition. In studying the mechanism of the inhibition, these authors found that it was produced by the release, and activation, of transforming growth factor-beta (TGF-β).[41] Pericytes or smooth-muscle cells alone produce this polypeptide in an inactive form. The co-cultured cells, in physical contact with one another, both produce and activate TGF-beta. This finding suggests that one function of pericytes in the retina is to inhibit the proliferation of endothelial cells. Thus, the loss of pericytes that occurs early in the course of diabetic retinopathy may facilitate the later development of microaneurysms (clusters of newly formed endothelial cells) and of frank neovascularization. In fact, just this result has been reported in an experiment using mice with a targeted disruption ("knock-out") of the gene for the B-chain of platelet-derived growth factor (PDGF-β).[24] This genetic defect is lethal, but histopathologic examination of the fetal PDGF-β-deficient animals shows an absence of capillary pericytes – whose antenatal development is evidently controlled by this growth factor – and the frequent appearance of microaneurysms throughout the microcirculation of the retina and brain.

Pericytes are considered to be contractile cells, regulating flow through the capillaries analogous to the function of the smooth-muscle cells of the larger vessels. Cultured pericytes are immunocytochemically positive for smooth-muscle actin,[234] and in culture they contract either spontaneously[235] or in response to a variety of agents.[236–238] Thus, loss of pericytes from the retinal microcirculation may produce alterations in retinal blood flow. However, direct evidence for pericyte contraction in the circulation of the intact retina has never been obtained. Tilton et al.[239] performed a morphometric study of capillaries in rats following infusion of various vasoconstrictor agents and found evidence of contraction of pericytes in skeletal muscle capillaries but not of those in cardiac muscle. Butryn and coworkers conducted a similar study in the retinal vessels of rats following intravitreal infusion of ET-1, an extremely powerful vasoconstrictor.[240] Although they found evidence of contraction of arteriolar smooth muscle, they could not demonstrate contraction of retinal capillary pericytes.

CONCLUSION

Considerable progress has been made in our understanding of the genetic susceptibility factors and etiologic mechanisms underlying the development of diabetic retinopathy. Considerable additional work is necessary, however, to fully elucidate the sequence of events that lead to this increasingly common blinding disorder.

For online acknowledgments visit **http://www.expertconsult.com**

REFERENCES

1. The Diabetes Control and Complications Trial Research Group. The effect of intensive treatment of diabetes on the development and progression of long-term complications in insulin-dependent diabetes mellitus. N Engl J Med 1993;329:977–86.
2. UK Prospective Diabetes Study (UKPDS) Group. Intensive blood-glucose control with sulphonylureas or insulin compared with conventional treatment and risk of complications in patients with type 2 diabetes (UKPDS 33). Lancet 1998;352:837–53.
3. UK Prospective Diabetes Study Group. Tight blood pressure control and risk of macrovascular and microvascular complications in type 2 diabetes (UKPDS 38). BMJ 1998;317:703–13.
4. Cogan DG, Toussaint D, Kuwabara T. Retinal vascular patterns. IV. Diabetic retinopathy. Arch Ophthalmol 1961;66:366–78.
5. Kuwabara T, Cogan DG. Studies of retinal vascular patterns. I. Normal architecture, Arch Ophthalmol 1960;64:904–11.
6. Kuwabara T, Cogan DG. Retinal vascular patterns. VI. Mural cells of the retinal capillaries. Arch Ophthalmol 1963;69:492–502.
7. Speiser P, Gittelsohn AM, Patz A. Studies on diabetic retinopathy. 3. Influence of diabetes on intramural pericytes. Arch Ophthalmol 1968;80:332–7.
8. Yanoff M. Diabetic retinopathy. N Engl J Med 1966;274:1344–9.
9. Shepro D, Morel NM. Pericyte physiology. FASEB J 1993;7:1031–8.
10. Aiello LP, Cavallerano J, Bursell SE. Diabetic eye disease. Endocrinol Metab Clin North Am 1996;25:271–91.
11. Cameron NE, Eaton SE, Cotter MA, et al. Vascular factors and metabolic interactions in the pathogenesis of diabetic neuropathy. Diabetologia 2001;44:1973–88.
12. Akagi Y, Kador PF, Kuwabara T, et al. Aldose reductase localization in human retinal mural cells. Invest Ophthalmol Vis Sci 1983;24:1516–9.
13. Tilton RG, Hoffmann PL, Kilo C, et al. Pericyte degeneration and basement membrane thickening in skeletal muscle capillaries of human diabetics. Diabetes 1981;30:326–34.
14. Kern TS, Engerman RL. Distribution of aldose reductase in ocular tissues. Exp Eye Res 1981;33:175–82.
15. Ludvigson MA, Sorenson RL. Immunohistochemical localization of aldose reductase. II. Rat eye and kidney. Diabetes 1980;29:450–9.
16. Buzney SM, Frank RN, Varma SD, et al. Aldose reductase in retinal mural cells. Invest Ophthalmol Vis Sci 1977;16:392–6.
17. Brownlee M. Biochemistry and molecular cell biology of diabetic complications. Nature 2001;414:813–20.
18. Barrett TB, Gajdusek CM, Schwartz SM, et al. Expression of the sis gene by endothelial cells in culture and in vivo. Proc Natl Acad Sci U S A 1984;81:6772–4.
19. Collins T, Ginsburg D, Boss JM, et al. Cultured human endothelial cells express platelet-derived growth factor B chain: cDNA cloning and structural analysis. Nature 1985;316:748–50.
20. Collins T, Pober JS, Gimbrone Jr MA, et al. Cultured human endothelial cells express platelet-derived growth factor A chain. Am J Pathol 1987;126:7–12.
21. DiCorleto PE, Bowen-Pope DF. Cultured endothelial cells produce a platelet-derived growth factor-like protein. Proc Natl Acad Sci U S A 1983;80:1919–23.

22. Bernstein LR, Antoniades H, Zetter BR. Migration of cultured vascular cells in response to plasma and platelet-derived factors. J Cell Sci 1982;56: 71–82.
23. D'Amore PA, Smith SR. Growth factor effects on cells of the vascular wall: a survey. Growth Factors 1993;8:61–75.
24. Lindahl P, Johansson BR, Leveen P, et al. Pericyte loss and microaneurysm formation in PDGF-B-deficient mice. Science 1997;277:242–5.
25. Hellstrom M, Kalen M, Lindahl P, et al. Role of PDGF-B and PDGFR-beta in recruitment of vascular smooth muscle cells and pericytes during embryonic blood vessel formation in the mouse. Development 1999;126:3047–55.
26. Leveen P, Pekny M, Gebre-Medhin S, et al. Mice deficient for PDGF B show renal, cardiovascular, hematological abnormalities. Genes Dev 1994;8: 1875–87.
27. Robison Jr WG, Kador PF, Kinoshita JH. Retinal capillaries: basement membrane thickening by galactosemia prevented with aldose reductase inhibitor. Science 1983;221:1177–9.
28. Frank RN, Keirn RJ, Kennedy A, et al. Galactose-induced retinal capillary basement membrane thickening: prevention by Sorbinil. Invest Ophthalmol Vis Sci 1983;24:1519–24.
29. Das A, Frank RN, Zhang NL, et al. Increases in collagen type IV and laminin in galactose-induced retinal capillary basement membrane thickening – prevention by an aldose reductase inhibitor. Exp Eye Res 1990;50:269–80.
30. Robison Jr, WG, Kador PF, Akagi Y, et al. Prevention of basement membrane thickening in retinal capillaries by a novel inhibitor of aldose reductase, tolrestat. Diabetes 1986;35:295–9.
31. Das A, Frank RN, Zhang NL. Sorbinil does not prevent galactose-induced glomerular capillary basement membrane thickening in the rat. Diabetologia 1990;33:515–21.
32. Nishio Y, Warren CE, Buczek-Thomas JA, et al. Identification and characterization of a gene regulating enzymatic glycosylation which is induced by diabetes and hyperglycemia specifically in rat cardiac tissue. J Clin Invest 1995;96:1759–67.
33. Brownlee M, Cerami A. The biochemistry of the complications of diabetes mellitus. Annu Rev Biochem 1981;50:385–432.
34. Timpl R, Rohde H, Robey PG, et al. Laminin – a glycoprotein from basement membranes. J Biol Chem 1979;254:9933–7.
35. Grant DS, Kleinman HK. Regulation of capillary formation by laminin and other components of the extracellular matrix. EXS 1997;79:317–33.
36. Kennedy A, Frank RN, Mancini MA. In vitro production of glycosaminoglycans by retinal microvessel cells and lens epithelium. Invest Ophthalmol Vis Sci 1986;27:746–54.
37. Shimomura H, Spiro RG. Studies on macromolecular components of human glomerular basement membrane and alterations in diabetes. Decreased levels of heparan sulfate proteoglycan and laminin. Diabetes 1987;36: 374–81.
38. Spiro RG, Spiro MJ. Effect of diabetes on the biosynthesis of the renal glomerular basement membrane. Studies on the glucosyltransferase. Diabetes 1971;20:641–8.
39. Friedenwald JS. Diabetic retinopathy. Am J Ophthalmol 1950;33:1187–99.
40. Orlidge A, D'Amore PA. Inhibition of capillary endothelial cell growth by pericytes and smooth muscle cells. J Cell Biol 1987;105:1455–62.
41. Antonelli-Orlidge A, Saunders KB, Smith SR, et al. An activated form of transforming growth factor beta is produced by cocultures of endothelial cells and pericytes. Proc Natl Acad Sci U S A 1989;86:4544–8.
42. Mizutani M, Kern TS, Lorenzi M. Accelerated death of retinal microvascular cells in human and experimental diabetic retinopathy. J Clin Invest 1996;97: 2883–90.
43. Ashton N, Kok DA, Foulds WS. Ocular pathology in macroglobulinaemia. J Pathol Bacteriol 1963;86:453–61.
44. Duke JR, Wilkinson CP, Sigelman S. Retinal microaneurysms in leukaemia. Br J Ophthalmol 1968;52:368–74.
45. Kohner EM, Henkind P. Correlation of fluorescein angiogram and retinal digest in diabetic retinopathy. Am J Ophthalmol 1970;69:403–14.
46. Daneman D, Drash AL, Lobes LA, et al. Progressive retinopathy with improved control in diabetic dwarfism (Mauriac's syndrome). Diabetes Care 1981;4:360–5.
47. Wallow IH, Engerman RL. Permeability and patency of retinal blood vessels in experimental diabetes. Invest Ophthalmol Vis Sci 1977;16:447–61.
48. Gardner TW, Lesher T, Khin S, et al. Histamine reduces ZO-1 tight-junction protein expression in cultured retinal microvascular endothelial cells. Biochem J 1996;320(Pt 3):717–21.
49. Gardner TW. Histamine, ZO-1 and increased blood-retinal barrier permeability in diabetic retinopathy. Trans Am Ophthalmol Soc 1995;93:583–621.
50. Barber AJ, Antonetti DA, Gardner TW. Altered expression of retinal occludin and glial fibrillary acidic protein in experimental diabetes. The Penn State Retina Research Group. Invest Ophthalmol Vis Sci 2000;41:3561–8.
51. Enea NA, Hollis TM, Kern JA, et al. Histamine H1 receptors mediate increased blood–retinal barrier permeability in experimental diabetes. Arch Ophthalmol 1989;107:270–4.
52. Gardner TW, Eller AW, Friberg TR, et al. Antihistamines reduce blood–retinal barrier permeability in type I (insulin-dependent) diabetic patients with nonproliferative retinopathy. A pilot study. Retina 1995;15:134–40.
53. Keck PJ, Hauser SD, Krivi G, et al. Vascular permeability factor, an endothelial cell mitogen related to PDGF. Science 1989;246:1309–12.
54. Antonetti DA, Barber AJ, Hollinger LA, et al. Vascular endothelial growth factor induces rapid phosphorylation of tight junction proteins occludin and zonula occluden 1. A potential mechanism for vascular permeability in diabetic retinopathy and tumors. J Biol Chem 1999;274:23463–7.
55. Lakshminarayanan S, Antonetti DA, Gardner TW, et al. Effect of VEGF on retinal microvascular endothelial hydraulic conductivity: the role of NO. Invest Ophthalmol Vis Sci 2000;41:4256–61.
56. Gao BB, Clermont A, Rook S, et al. Extracellular carbonic anhydrase mediates hemorrhagic retinal and cerebral vascular permeability through prekallikrein activation. Nat Med 2007;13:181–8.
57. Gao BB, Chen X, Timothy N, et al. Characterization of the vitreous proteome in diabetes without diabetic retinopathy and diabetes with proliferative diabetic retinopathy. J Proteome Res 2008;7:2516–25.
58. Phipps JA, Clermont AC, Sinha S, et al. Plasma kallikrein mediates angiotensin II type 1 receptor-stimulated retinal vascular permeability. Hypertension 2009;53:175–81.
59. Abdouh M, Talbot S, Couture R, et al. Retinal plasma extravasation in streptozotocin-diabetic rats mediated by kinin B(1) and B(2) receptors. Br J Pharmacol 2008;154:136–43.
60. Jeppesen P, Aalkjaer C, Bek T. Bradykinin relaxation in small porcine retinal arterioles. Invest Ophthalmol Vis Sci 2002;43:1891–6.
61. Kojima N, Saito M, Mori A, et al. Role of cyclooxygenase in vasodilation of retinal blood vessels induced by bradykinin in Brown Norway rats. Vascul Pharmacol 2009;51:119–24.
62. Parpura V, Basarsky TA, Liu F, et al. Glutamate-mediated astrocyte-neuron signalling. Nature 1994;369:744–7.
63. Adamis AP. Is diabetic retinopathy an inflammatory disease? Br J Ophthalmol 2002;86:363–5.
64. Joussen AM, Murata T, Tsujikawa A, et al. Leukocyte-mediated endothelial cell injury and death in the diabetic retina. Am J Pathol 2001;158:147–52.
65. Joussen AM, Poulaki V, Mitsiades N, et al. Nonsteroidal anti-inflammatory drugs prevent early diabetic retinopathy via TNF-alpha suppression. FASEB J 2002;16:438–40.
66. Martidis A, Duker JS, Greenberg PB, et al. Intravitreal triamcinolone for refractory diabetic macular edema. Ophthalmology 2002;109:920–7.
67. Yilmaz T, Weaver CD, Gallagher MJ, et al. Intravitreal triamcinolone acetonide injection for treatment of refractory diabetic macular edema: a systematic review. Ophthalmology 2009;116:902–11; quiz 912–903.
68. Feener EP. Plasma kallikrein and diabetic macular edema. Curr Diab Rep 2010;10:270–5.
69. Gabbay KH. The sorbitol pathway and the complications of diabetes. N Engl J Med 1973;288:831–6.
70. Kinoshita JH. Cataracts in galactosemia. The Jonas S. Friedenwald Memorial Lecture. Invest Ophthalmol 1965;4:786–99.
71. Kinoshita JH. Mechanisms initiating cataract formation. Proctor Lecture. Invest Ophthalmol 1974;13:713–24.
72. Gabbay KH. Hyperglycemia, polyol metabolism, complications of diabetes mellitus. Annu Rev Med 1975;26:521–36.
73. Van den Enden MK, Nyengaard JR, Ostrow E, et al. Elevated glucose levels increase retinal glycolysis and sorbitol pathway metabolism. Implications for diabetic retinopathy. Invest Ophthalmol Vis Sci 1995;36:1675–85.
74. Tesfamariam B. Free radicals in diabetic endothelial cell dysfunction. Free Radic Biol Med 1994;16:383–91.
75. Williamson JR, Chang K, Frangos M, et al. Hyperglycemic pseudohypoxia and diabetic complications. Diabetes 1993;42:801–13.
76. Engerman RL, Kern TS. Experimental galactosemia produces diabetic-like retinopathy. Diabetes 1984;33:97–100.
77. Kador PF, Akagi Y, Takahashi Y, et al. Prevention of retinal vessel changes associated with diabetic retinopathy in galactose-fed dogs by aldose reductase inhibitors. Arch Ophthalmol 1990;108:1301–9.
78. Kador PF, Akagi Y, Terubayashi H, et al. Prevention of pericyte ghost formation in retinal capillaries of galactose-fed dogs by aldose reductase inhibitors. Arch Ophthalmol 1988;106:1099–102.
79. Robinson Jr, WG, Laver NM, Jacot JL, et al. Diabetic-like retinopathy ameliorated with the aldose reductase inhibitor WAY-121,509. Invest Ophthalmol Vis Sci 1996;37:1149–56.
80. Sorbinil Retinopathy Trial Research Group. A randomized trial of sorbinil, an aldose reductase inhibitor, in diabetic retinopathy. Arch Ophthalmol 1990; 108:1234–44.
81. Monnier VM, Kohn RR, Cerami A. Accelerated age-related browning of human collagen in diabetes mellitus. Proc Natl Acad Sci U S A 1984;81: 583–7.
82. Brownlee M, Vlassara H, Cerami A. Nonenzymatic glycosylation and the pathogenesis of diabetic complications. Ann Intern Med 1984;101:527–37.
83. Brownlee M. Advanced protein glycosylation in diabetes and aging. Annu Rev Med 1995;46:223–34.
84. Chibber R, Molinatti PA, Kohner EM. Intracellular protein glycation in cultured retinal capillary pericytes and endothelial cells exposed to high-glucose concentration. Cell Mol Biol (Noisy-le-grand) 1999;45:47–57.
85. Giardino I, Edelstein D, Brownlee M. Nonenzymatic glycosylation in vitro and in bovine endothelial cells alters basic fibroblast growth factor activity. A model for intracellular glycosylation in diabetes. J Clin Invest 1994;94: 110–7.
86. Neeper M, Schmidt AM, Brett J, et al. Cloning and expression of a cell surface receptor for advanced glycosylation end products of proteins. J Biol Chem 1992;267:14998–5004.
87. Schmidt AM, Vianna M, Gerlach M, et al. Isolation and characterization of two binding proteins for advanced glycosylation end products from bovine lung which are present on the endothelial cell surface. J Biol Chem 1992;267:14987–97.
88. Lander HM, Tauras JM, Ogiste JS, et al. Activation of the receptor for advanced glycation end products triggers a p21(ras)-dependent mitogen-activated

protein kinase pathway regulated by oxidant stress. J Biol Chem 1997;272: 17810–4.
89. Hofmann MA, Drury S, Fu C, et al. RAGE mediates a novel proinflammatory axis: a central cell surface receptor for S100/calgranulin polypeptides. Cell 1999;97:889–901.
90. Huttunen HJ, Fages C, Rauvala H. Receptor for advanced glycation end products (RAGE)-mediated neurite outgrowth and activation of NF-kappaB require the cytoplasmic domain of the receptor but different downstream signaling pathways. J Biol Chem 1999;274:19919–24.
91. Taguchi A, Blood DC, del Toro G, et al. Blockade of RAGE-amphotericin signalling suppresses tumour growth and metastases. Nature 2000;405: 354–60.
92. Beauchamp MC, Michaud SE, Li L, et al. Advanced glycation end products potentiate the stimulatory effect of glucose on macrophage lipoprotein lipase expression. J Lipid Res 2004;45:1749–57.
93. Yan SD, Schmidt AM, Anderson GM, et al. Enhanced cellular oxidant stress by the interaction of advanced glycation end products with their receptors/ binding proteins. J Biol Chem 1994;269:9889–97.
94. Schmidt AM, Stern DM. RAGE: a new target for the prevention and treatment of the vascular and inflammatory complications of diabetes. Trends Endocrinol Metab 2000;11:368–75.
95. el Khoury J, Thomas CA, Loike JD, et al. Macrophages adhere to glucose-modified basement membrane collagen IV via their scavenger receptors. J Biol Chem 1994;269:10197–200.
96. Vlassara H, Li YM, Imani F, et al. Identification of galectin-3 as a high-affinity binding protein for advanced glycation end products (AGE): a new member of the AGE-receptor complex. Mol Med 1995;1:634–46.
97. Hammes HP, Martin S, Federlin K, et al. Aminoguanidine treatment inhibits the development of experimental diabetic retinopathy. Proc Natl Acad Sci U S A 1991;88:11555–8.
98. Brownlee M, Vlassara H, Kooney A, et al. Aminoguanidine prevents diabetes-induced arterial wall protein cross-linking. Science 1986;232:1629–32.
99. Friedman EA. Advanced glycosylated end products and hyperglycemia in the pathogenesis of diabetic complications. Diabetes Care 1999;22(Suppl 2): B65–71.
100. Kern TS, Engerman RL. Pharmacological inhibition of diabetic retinopathy: aminoguanidine and aspirin. Diabetes 2001;50:1636–42.
101. Nilsson BO. Biological effects of aminoguanidine: an update. Inflamm Res 1999;48:509–15.
102. Wautier JL, Zoukourian C, Chappey O, et al. Receptor-mediated endothelial cell dysfunction in diabetic vasculopathy. Soluble receptor for advanced glycation end products blocks hyperpermeability in diabetic rats. J Clin Invest 1996;97:238–43.
103. Nishikawa T, Edelstein D, Du XL, et al. Normalizing mitochondrial superoxide production blocks three pathways of hyperglycaemic damage. Nature 2000;404:787–90.
104. Suzuki S, Hinokio Y, Komatu K, et al. Oxidative damage to mitochondrial DNA and its relationship to diabetic complications. Diabetes Res Clin Pract 1999;45:161–8.
105. Hunt JV, Dean RT, Wolff SP. Hydroxyl radical production and autoxidative glycosylation. Glucose autoxidation as the cause of protein damage in the experimental glycation model of diabetes mellitus and ageing. Biochem J 1988;256:205–12.
106. Giugliano D, Ceriello A, Paolisso G. Oxidative stress and diabetic vascular complications. Diabetes Care 1996;19:257–67.
107. Tesfamariam B. Selective impairment of endothelium-dependent relaxations by prostaglandin endoperoxide. J Hypertens 1994;12:41–7.
108. Lum H, Roebuck KA. Oxidant stress and endothelial cell dysfunction. Am J Physiol Cell Physiol 2001;280:C719–741.
109. Baynes JW. Role of oxidative stress in development of complications in diabetes. Diabetes 1991;40:405–12.
110. Craven PA, Melhem MF, Phillips SL, et al. Overexpression of Cu^{2+}/Zn^{2+} superoxide dismutase protects against early diabetic glomerular injury in transgenic mice. Diabetes 2001;50:2114–25.
111. Taher MM, Garcia JG, Natarajan V. Hydroperoxide-induced diacylglycerol formation and protein kinase C activation in vascular endothelial cells. Arch Biochem Biophys 1993;303:260–6.
112. Jain SK, McVie R. Effect of glycemic control, race (white versus black), duration of diabetes on reduced glutathione content in erythrocytes of diabetic patients. Metabolism 1994;43:306–9.
113. Jennings PE, Chirico S, Jones AF, et al. Vitamin C metabolites and microangiopathy in diabetes mellitus. Diabetes Res 1987;6:151–4.
114. Karpen CW, Cataland S, O'Dorisio TM, et al. Production of 12-hydroxyeicosatetraenoic acid and vitamin E status in platelets from type I human diabetic subjects. Diabetes 1985;34:526–31.
115. Oberley LW. Free radicals and diabetes. Free Radic Biol Med 1988;5: 113–24.
116. Hayden JM, Reaven PD. Cardiovascular disease in diabetes mellitus type 2: a potential role for novel cardiovascular risk factors. Curr Opin Lipidol 2000;11:519–28.
117. Devaraj S, Hirany SV, Burk RF, et al. Divergence between LDL oxidative susceptibility and urinary F(2)-isoprostanes as measures of oxidative stress in type 2 diabetes. Clin Chem 2001;47:1974–9.
118. Cameron NE, Cotter MA. Neurovascular dysfunction in diabetic rats. Potential contribution of autoxidation and free radicals examined using transition metal chelating agents. J Clin Invest 1995;96:1159–63.
119. Cameron NE, Cotter MA, Archibald V, et al. Anti-oxidant and pro-oxidant effects on nerve conduction velocity, endoneurial blood flow and oxygen tension in non-diabetic and streptozotocin-diabetic rats. Diabetologia 1994;37:449–59.
120. Nagamatsu M, Nickander KK, Schmelzer JD, et al. Lipoic acid improves nerve blood flow, reduces oxidative stress, improves distal nerve conduction in experimental diabetic neuropathy. Diabetes Care 1995;18:1160–7.
121. Lal MA, Korner A, Matsuo Y, et al. Combined antioxidant and COMT inhibitor treatment reverses renal abnormalities in diabetic rats. Diabetes 2000;49: 1381–9.
122. Kowluru RA, Tang J, Kern TS. Abnormalities of retinal metabolism in diabetes and experimental galactosemia. VII. Effect of long-term administration of antioxidants on the development of retinopathy. Diabetes 2001;50:1938–42.
123. Bursell SE, Clermont AC, Aiello LP, et al. High-dose vitamin E supplementation normalizes retinal blood flow and creatinine clearance in patients with type 1 diabetes. Diabetes Care 1999;22:1245–51.
124. Yusuf S, Dagenais G, Pogue J, et al. Vitamin E supplementation and cardiovascular events in high-risk patients. The Heart Outcomes Prevention Evaluation Study Investigators. N Engl J Med 2000;342:154–60.
125. Xia P, Aiello LP, Ishii H, et al. Characterization of vascular endothelial growth factor's effect on the activation of protein kinase C, its isoforms, endothelial cell growth. J Clin Invest 1996;98:2018–26.
126. Xia P, Inoguchi T, Kern TS, et al. Characterization of the mechanism for the chronic activation of diacylglycerol-protein kinase C pathway in diabetes and hypergalactosemia. Diabetes 1994;43:1122–9.
127. Nishizuka Y. Intracellular signaling by hydrolysis of phospholipids and activation of protein kinase C. Science 1992;258:607–14.
128. Inoguchi T, Battan R, Handler E, et al. Preferential elevation of protein kinase C isoform beta II and diacylglycerol levels in the aorta and heart of diabetic rats: differential reversibility to glycemic control by islet cell transplantation. Proc Natl Acad Sci U S A 1992;89:11059–63.
129. Ishii H, Koya D, King GL. Protein kinase C activation and its role in the development of vascular complications in diabetes mellitus. J Mol Med 1998;76:21–31.
130. Nagpala PG, Malik AB, Vuong PT, et al. Protein kinase C beta 1 overexpression augments phorbol ester-induced increase in endothelial permeability. J Cell Physiol 1996;166:249–55.
131. Kuboki K, Jiang ZY, Takahara N, et al. Regulation of endothelial constitutive nitric oxide synthase gene expression in endothelial cells and in vivo: a specific vascular action of insulin. Circulation 2000;101:676–81.
132. Bohlen HG, Nase GP. Arteriolar nitric oxide concentration is decreased during hyperglycemia-induced betaII PKC activation. Am J Physiol Heart Circ Physiol 2001;280:H621–627.
133. Nonaka A, Kiryu J, Tsujikawa A, et al. PKC-beta inhibitor (LY333531) attenuates leukocyte entrapment in retinal microcirculation of diabetic rats. Invest Ophthalmol Vis Sci 2000;41:2702–6.
134. Shiba T, Inoguchi T, Sportsman JR, et al. Correlation of diacylglycerol level and protein kinase C activity in rat retina to retinal circulation. Am J Physiol 1993;265:E783–793.
135. Ishii H, Jirousek MR, Koya D, et al. Amelioration of vascular dysfunctions in diabetic rats by an oral PKC beta inhibitor. Science 1996;272:728–31.
136. Aiello LP, Bursell SE, Clermont A, et al. Vascular endothelial growth factor-induced retinal permeability is mediated by protein kinase C in vivo and suppressed by an orally effective beta-isoform-selective inhibitor. Diabetes 1997;46:1473–80.
137. Schiffrin EL, Touyz RM. Vascular biology of endothelin. J Cardiovasc Pharmacol 1998;32(Suppl 3):S2–13.
138. Williams B, Gallacher B, Patel H, et al. Glucose-induced protein kinase C activation regulates vascular permeability factor mRNA expression and peptide production by human vascular smooth muscle cells in vitro. Diabetes 1997;46:1497–503.
139. Koya D, Jirousek MR, Lin YW, et al. Characterization of protein kinase C beta isoform activation on the gene expression of transforming growth factor-beta, extracellular matrix components, prostanoids in the glomeruli of diabetic rats. J Clin Invest 1997;100:115–26.
140. Tomlinson DR. Mitogen-activated protein kinases as glucose transducers for diabetic complications. Diabetologia 1999;42:1271–81.
141. Meier M, King GL. Protein kinase C activation and its pharmacological inhibition in vascular disease. Vasc Med 2000;5:173–85.
142. Danis RP, Bingaman DP, Jirousek M, et al. Inhibition of intraocular neovascularization caused by retinal ischemia in pigs by PKCbeta inhibition with LY333531. Invest Ophthalmol Vis Sci 1998;39:171–9.
143. Nakamura J, Kato K, Hamada Y, et al. A protein kinase C-beta-selective inhibitor ameliorates neural dysfunction in streptozotocin-induced diabetic rats. Diabetes 1999;48:2090–5.
144. Effect of ruboxistaurin in patients with diabetic macular edema: thirty-month results of the randomized PKC-DMES clinical trial. Arch Ophthalmol 2007; 125:318–24.
145. Sheetz MJ, Aiello LP, Shahri N. Effect of ruboxistaurin (RBX) on visual acuity decline over a 6-year period with cessation and reinstitution of therapy: results of an open-label extension of the Protein Kinase C Diabetic Retinopathy Study 2 (PKC-DRS2). Retina 2011;31:1053–9.
146. King GL, Buzney SM, Kahn CR, et al. Differential responsiveness to insulin of endothelial and support cells from micro- and macrovessels. J Clin Invest 1983;71:974–9.
147. Engerman RL, Pfaffenb D, Davis MD. Cell turnover of capillaries. Lab Invest 1967;17:738–43.
148. Kumagai AK, Glasgow BJ, Pardridge WM. GLUT1 glucose transporter expression in the diabetic and nondiabetic human eye. Invest Ophthalmol Vis Sci 1994;35:2887–94.

149. Kumagai AK, Vinores SA, Pardridge WM. Pathological upregulation of inner blood-retinal barrier Glut1 glucose transporter expression in diabetes mellitus. Brain Res 1996;706:313–7.
150. Mantych GJ, Hageman GS, Devaskar SU. Characterization of glucose transporter isoforms in the adult and developing human eye. Endocrinology 1993;133:600–7.
151. Watanabe T, Mio Y, Hoshino FB, et al. GLUT2 expression in the rat retina: localization at the apical ends of Muller cells. Brain Res 1994;655:128–34.
152. Watanabe T, Matsushima S, Okazaki M, et al. Localization and ontogeny of GLUT3 expression in the rat retina. Brain Res Dev Brain Res 1996;94:60–6.
153. Frank RN, Amin R, Kennedy A, et al. An aldose reductase inhibitor and aminoguanidine prevent vascular endothelial growth factor expression in rats with long-term galactosemia. Arch Ophthalmol 1997;115:1036–47.
154. Warpeha KM, Chakravarthy U. Molecular genetics of microvascular disease in diabetic retinopathy. Eye (Lond) 2003;17:305–11.
155. Field LL. Genetic linkage and association studies of Type I diabetes: challenges and rewards. Diabetologia 2002;45:21–35.
156. Kao YL, Donaghue K, Chan A, et al. An aldose reductase intragenic polymorphism associated with diabetic retinopathy. Diabetes Res Clin Pract 1999;46:155–60.
157. Demaine A, Cross D, Millward A. Polymorphisms of the aldose reductase gene and susceptibility to retinopathy in type 1 diabetes mellitus. Invest Ophthalmol Vis Sci 2000;41:4064–8.
158. Demaine AG. Polymorphisms of the aldose reductase gene and susceptibility to diabetic microvascular complications. Curr Med Chem 2003;10:1389–98.
159. Wang Y, Ng MC, Lee SC, et al. Phenotypic heterogeneity and associations of two aldose reductase gene polymorphisms with nephropathy and retinopathy in type 2 diabetes. Diabetes Care 2003;26:2410–5.
160. Sivenius K, Niskanen L, Voutilainen-Kaunisto R, et al. Aldose reductase gene polymorphisms and susceptibility to microvascular complications in Type 2 diabetes. Diabet Med 2004;21:1325–33.
161. Petrovic MG, Peterlin B, Hawlina M, et al. Aldose reductase (AC)n gene polymorphism and susceptibility to diabetic retinopathy in Type 2 diabetes in Caucasians. J Diabetes Complications 2005;19:70–3.
162. Richeti F, Noronha RM, Waetge RT, et al. Evaluation of AC(n) and C(-106)T polymorphisms of the aldose reductase gene in Brazilian patients with DM1 and susceptibility to diabetic retinopathy. Mol Vis 2007;13:740–5.
163. Klein R, Klein BE, Moss SE, et al. The Wisconsin epidemiologic study of diabetic retinopathy. III. Prevalence and risk of diabetic retinopathy when age at diagnosis is 30 or more years. Arch Ophthalmol 1984;102:527–32.
164. Klein R, Klein BE, Moss SE, et al. The Wisconsin epidemiologic study of diabetic retinopathy. II. Prevalence and risk of diabetic retinopathy when age at diagnosis is less than 30 years. Arch Ophthalmol 1984;102:520–6.
165. Rand LI, Krolewski AS, Aiello LM, et al. Multiple factors in the prediction of risk of proliferative diabetic retinopathy. N Engl J Med 1985;313:1433–8.
166. Cruickshanks KJ, Vadheim CM, Moss SE, et al. Genetic marker associations with proliferative retinopathy in persons diagnosed with diabetes before 30 yr of age. Diabetes 1992;41:879–85.
167. The Diabetes Control and Complications Trial Research Group. Clustering of long-term complications in families with diabetes in the diabetes control and complications trial. Diabetes 1997;46:1829–1839.
168. Krolewski AS, Canessa M, Warram JH, et al. Predisposition to hypertension and susceptibility to renal disease in insulin-dependent diabetes mellitus. N Engl J Med 1988;318:140–5.
169. Krolewski AS, Doria A, Magre J, et al. Molecular genetic approaches to the identification of genes involved in the development of nephropathy in insulin-dependent diabetes mellitus. J Am Soc Nephrol 1992;3:S9–17.
170. Pettitt DJ, Saad MF, Bennett PH, et al. Familial predisposition to renal disease in two generations of Pima Indians with type 2 (non-insulin-dependent) diabetes mellitus. Diabetologia 1990;33:438–43.
171. Seaquist ER, Goetz FC, Rich S, et al. Familial clustering of diabetic kidney disease. Evidence for genetic susceptibility to diabetic nephropathy. N Engl J Med 1989;320:1161–5.
172. Ko BC, Lam KS, Wat NM, et al. An (A-C)n dinucleotide repeat polymorphic marker at the 5′ end of the aldose reductase gene is associated with early-onset diabetic retinopathy in NIDDM patients. Diabetes 1995;44:727–32.
173. Aiello LP, Avery RL, Arrigg PG, et al. Vascular endothelial growth factor in ocular fluid of patients with diabetic retinopathy and other retinal disorders. N Engl J Med 1994;331:1480–7.
174. Aiello LP. Angiogenic pathways in diabetic retinopathy. N Engl J Med 2005;353:839–41.
175. Miller JW, Adamis AP, Aiello LP. Vascular endothelial growth factor in ocular neovascularization and proliferative diabetic retinopathy. Diabetes Metab Rev 1997;13:37–50.
176. Robinson CJ, Stringer SE. The splice variants of vascular endothelial growth factor (VEGF) and their receptors. J Cell Sci 2001;114:853–65.
177. Suganthalakshmi B, Anand R, Kim R, et al. Association of VEGF and eNOS gene polymorphisms in type 2 diabetic retinopathy. Mol Vis 2006;12: 336–41.
178. Buraczynska M, Ksiazek P, Baranowicz-Gaszczyk I, et al. Association of the VEGF gene polymorphism with diabetic retinopathy in type 2 diabetes patients. Nephrol Dial Transplant 2007;22:827–32.
179. Ramprasad S, Radha V, Mathias RA, et al. Rage gene promoter polymorphisms and diabetic retinopathy in a clinic-based population from South India. Eye (Lond) 2007;21:395–401.
180. Balasubbu S, Sundaresan P, Rajendran A, et al. Association analysis of nine candidate gene polymorphisms in Indian patients with type 2 diabetic retinopathy. BMC Med Genet 2010;11:158.
181. Tong Z, Yang Z, Patel S, et al. Promoter polymorphism of the erythropoietin gene in severe diabetic eye and kidney complications. Proc Natl Acad Sci U S A 2008;105:6998–7003.
182. Huang YC, Lin JM, Lin HJ, et al. Genome-wide association study of diabetic retinopathy in a Taiwanese population. Ophthalmology 2011;118:642–8.
183. Fu YP, Hallman DM, Gonzalez VH, et al. Identification of Diabetic Retinopathy Genes through a Genome-Wide Association Study among Mexican-Americans from Starr County, Texas. J Ophthalmol 2010 2010.
184. Grassi MA, Tikhomirov A, Ramalingam S, et al. Genome-wide meta-analysis for severe diabetic retinopathy. Hum Mol Genet 2011;20:2472–81.
185. Reich DE, Lander ES. On the allelic spectrum of human disease. Trends Genet 2001;17:502–10.
186. Klein RJ, Zeiss C, Chew EY, et al. Complement factor H polymorphism in age-related macular degeneration. Science 2005;308:385–9.
187. Dewan A, Liu M, Hartman S, et al. HTRA1 promoter polymorphism in wet age-related macular degeneration. Science 2006;314:989–92.
188. Yang Z, Camp NJ, Sun H, et al. A variant of the HTRA1 gene increases susceptibility to age-related macular degeneration. Science 2006;314:992–3.
189. Cohen JC, Kiss RS, Pertsemlidis A, et al. Multiple rare alleles contribute to low plasma levels of HDL cholesterol. Science 2004;305:869–72.
190. Kotowski IK, Pertsemlidis A, Luke A, et al. A spectrum of PCSK9 alleles contributes to plasma levels of low-density lipoprotein cholesterol. Am J Hum Genet 2006;78:410–22.
191. Ahituv N, Kavaslar N, Schackwitz W, et al. Medical sequencing at the extremes of human body mass. Am J Hum Genet 2007;80:779–91.
192. Romeo S, Pennacchio LA, Fu Y, et al. Population-based resequencing of ANGPTL4 uncovers variations that reduce triglycerides and increase HDL. Nat Genet 2007;39:513–6.
193. Smigrodzki R, Parks J, Parker WD. High frequency of mitochondrial complex I mutations in Parkinson's disease and aging. Neurobiol Aging 2004;25: 1273–81.
194. Bielas JH, Loeb KR, Rubin BP, et al. Human cancers express a mutator phenotype. Proc Natl Acad Sci U S A 2006;103:18238–42.
195. Altshuler D, Daly MJ, Lander ES. Genetic mapping in human disease. Science 2008;322:881–8.
196. Becker B. Diabetes and glaucoma; and Ashton N. Oxygen and the growth and development of retinal vessels: in vivo and in vitro studies. In: Kimura SJ, Caygill WM, editors. Vascular complications of diabetes mellitus, with special emphasis on microangiopathy of the eye. St Louis: Mosby; 1967.
197. Jain IS, Luthra CL, Das T. Diabetic retinopathy and its relation to errors of refraction. Arch Ophthalmol 1967;77:59–60.
198. Goldberg MF, Fine SL, United States Public Health Service. Symposium on the Treatment of Diabetic Retinopathy. Arlington, VA: US Neurological and Sensory Disease Control Program; for sale by the Superintendent of Documents, US Government Printing Office, Washington, DC; 1969.
199. Patz A. Studies on retinal neovascularization. Friedenwald Lecture. Invest Ophthalmol Vis Sci 1980;19:1133–8.
200. Weiter JJ, Zuckerman R. The influence of the photoreceptor-RPE complex on the inner retina. An explanation for the beneficial effects of photocoagulation. Ophthalmology 1980;87:1133–9.
201. The Diabetic Retinopathy Study Research Group. Photocoagulation treatment of proliferative diabetic retinopathy. Clinical application of Diabetic Retinopathy Study (DRS) findings, DRS Report number 8. Ophthalmology 1981;88: 583–600.
202. Klein R, Klein BE, Moss SE, et al. The Wisconsin epidemiologic study of diabetic retinopathy. IV. Diabetic macular edema. Ophthalmology 1984;91: 1464–74.
203. Tattersall RB, Fajans SS. A difference between the inheritance of classical juvenile-onset and maturity-onset type diabetes of young people. Diabetes 1975;24:44–53.
204. Patz A, Maumenee AE. Studies on diabetic retinopathy. I. Retinopathy in a dog with spontaneous diabetes mellitus. Am J Ophthalmol 1962;54: 532–41.
205. Engerman R, Finkelstein D, Aguirre G, et al. Ocular complications. Diabetes 1982;31:82–8.
206. Tilton RG, LaRose LS, Kilo C, et al. Absence of degenerative changes in retinal and uveal capillary pericytes in diabetic rats. Invest Ophthalmol Vis Sci 1986;27:716–21.
207. Engerman RL, Colquhoun PJ. Epithelial and mesothelial basement membranes in diabetic patients and dogs. Diabetologia 1982;23:521–4.
208. Kern TS, Engerman RL. Galactose-induced retinal microangiopathy in rats. Invest Ophthalmol Vis Sci 1995;36:490–6.
209. Robison Jr WG, McCaleb ML, Feld LG, et al. Degenerated intramural pericytes ('ghost cells') in the retinal capillaries of diabetic rats. Curr Eye Res 1991;10: 339–50.
210. Bloodworth Jr, JM, Engerman RL, Anderson PJ. Microangiopathy in the experimentally diabetic animal. Adv Metab Disord 1973;2(Suppl 2):245–50.
211. Frank RN, Hoffman WH, Podgor MJ, et al. Retinopathy in juvenile-onset diabetes of short duration. Ophthalmology 1980;87:1–9.
212. Palmberg P, Smith M, Waltman S, et al. The natural history of retinopathy in insulin-dependent juvenile-onset diabetes. Ophthalmology 1981;88:613–8.
213. Kern TS, Engerman RL. A mouse model of diabetic retinopathy. Arch Ophthalmol 1996;114:986–90.
214. de Oliveira F. Pericytes in diabetic retinopathy. Br J Ophthalmol 1966;50: 134–43.
215. Kern TS, Engerman RL. Capillary lesions develop in retina rather than cerebral cortex in diabetes and experimental galactosemia. Arch Ophthalmol 1996;114:306–10.

216. Frank RN, Dutta S, Mancini MA. Pericyte coverage is greater in the retinal than in the cerebral capillaries of the rat. Invest Ophthalmol Vis Sci 1987;28:1086–91.
217. Frank RN, Turczyn TJ, Das A. Pericyte coverage of retinal and cerebral capillaries. Invest Ophthalmol Vis Sci 1990;31:999–1007.
218. Tilton RG, Miller EJ, Kilo C, et al. Pericyte form and distribution in rat retinal and uveal capillaries. Invest Ophthalmol Vis Sci 1985;26:68–73.
219. Patz A. The role of oxygen in retrolental fibroplasia. Trans Am Ophthalmol Soc 1968;66:940–85.
220. Kremer I, Kissun R, Nissenkorn I, et al. Oxygen-induced retinopathy in newborn kittens. A model for ischemic vasoproliferative retinopathy. Invest Ophthalmol Vis Sci 1987;28:126–30.
221. Wise GN, Dollery CT, Henkind P. The retinal circulation. New York: Harper & Row; 1971.
222. Smith LE, Kopchick JJ, Chen W, et al. Essential role of growth hormone in ischemia-induced retinal neovascularization. Science 1997;276: 1706–9.
223. Aiello LP, Pierce EA, Foley ED, et al. Suppression of retinal neovascularization in vivo by inhibition of vascular endothelial growth factor (VEGF) using soluble VEGF-receptor chimeric proteins. Proc Natl Acad Sci U S A 1995;92:10457–61.
224. Penn JS, Rajaratnam VS, Collier RJ, et al. The effect of an angiostatic steroid on neovascularization in a rat model of retinopathy of prematurity. Invest Ophthalmol Vis Sci 2001;42:283–90.
225. Okamoto N, Tobe T, Hackett SF, et al. Transgenic mice with increased expression of vascular endothelial growth factor in the retina: a new model of intraretinal and subretinal neovascularization. Am J Pathol 1997;151: 281–91.
226. Buzney SM, Frank RN, Robison Jr WG. Retinal capillaries: proliferation of mural cells in vitro. Science 1975;190:985–6.
227. Frank RN, Kinsey VE, Frank KW, et al. In vitro proliferation of endothelial cells from kitten retinal capillaries. Invest Ophthalmol Vis Sci 1979;18: 1195–200.
228. Bowman PD, Betz AL, Goldstein GW. Primary culture of microvascular endothelial cells from bovine retina: selective growth using fibronectin coated substrate and plasma derived serum. In Vitro 1982;18:626–32.
229. Buzney SM, Massicotte SJ. Retinal vessels: proliferation of endothelium in vitro, Invest Ophthalmol Vis Sci 1979;18:1191–5.
230. Gitlin JD, D'Amore PA. Culture of retinal capillary cells using selective growth media. Microvasc Res 1983;26:74–80.
231. Madri JA, Williams SK. Capillary endothelial cell cultures: phenotypic modulation by matrix components. J Cell Biol 1983;97:153–65.
232. Montesano R, Orci L, Vassalli P. In vitro rapid organization of endothelial cells into capillary-like networks is promoted by collagen matrices. J Cell Biol 1983;97:1648–52.
233. Goto F, Goto K, Weindel K, et al. Synergistic effects of vascular endothelial growth factor and basic fibroblast growth factor on the proliferation and cord formation of bovine capillary endothelial cells within collagen gels. Lab Invest 1993;69:508–17.
234. Herman IM, D'Amore PA. Microvascular pericytes contain muscle and nonmuscle actins. J Cell Biol 1985;101:43–52.
235. Kelley C, D'Amore P, Hechtman HB, et al. Microvascular pericyte contractility in vitro: comparison with other cells of the vascular wall. J Cell Biol 1987;104:483–90.
236. Das A, Frank RN, Weber ML, et al. ATP causes retinal pericytes to contract in vitro. Exp Eye Res 1988;46:349–62.
237. Kelley C, D'Amore P, Hechtman HB, et al. Vasoactive hormones and cAMP affect pericyte contraction and stress fibres in vitro. J Muscle Res Cell Motil 1988;9:184–94.
238. Chakravarthy U, Gardiner TA, Anderson P, et al. The effect of endothelin 1 on the retinal microvascular pericyte. Microvasc Res 1992;43:241–54.
239. Tilton RG, Kilo C, Williamson JR, et al. Differences in pericyte contractile function in rat cardiac and skeletal muscle microvasculatures. Microvasc Res 1979;18:336–52.
240. Butryn RK, Ruan H, Hull CM, et al. Vasoactive agonists do not change the caliber of retinal capillaries of the rat. Microvasc Res 1995;50:80–93.

Chapter 47

Nonproliferative Diabetic Retinopathy and Diabetic Macular Edema

Henry E. Wiley, Frederick L. Ferris III

Diabetes mellitus (DM) comprises a heterogeneous group of disorders of carbohydrate, protein, and fat metabolism manifesting hyperglycemia. Diabetic retinopathy is a microangiopathy resulting from the chronic effects of the disease, and shares similarities with the microvascular alterations that occur in other tissues vulnerable to DM such as the kidneys and the peripheral nerves. Although the metabolic derangement has direct effects on the neurons and support cells of the retina, the retinal vascular changes dominate the clinical manifestations of disease and are directly implicated in the macular edema and neovascularization that represent the principal causes of vision loss. Diabetic retinopathy is classified into nonproliferative and proliferative stages. Nonproliferative diabetic retinopathy (NPDR) involves progressive intraretinal microvascular alterations that can lead to a more advanced proliferative stage defined by extraretinal neovascularization.

This chapter discusses the clinical manifestations and management of NPDR and diabetic macular edema (DME). Chapter 48 reviews proliferative diabetic retinopathy (PDR).

NATURAL COURSE OF NONPROLIFERATIVE DIABETIC RETINOPATHY

Diabetes mellitus without retinopathy

Retinal microvascular alterations visible on ophthalmoscopy typically develop years following the onset of DM. Chapter 46 (Diabetic retinopathy: Genetics and etiologic mechanisms) reviews what we know about the early biochemical and cellular alterations leading to diabetic retinopathy, while Chapter 45 (The epidemiology of diabetic retinopathy) discusses the incidence and prevalence of retinopathy among diabetics. Experimental models of diabetic retinopathy in dogs and rats, and studies of human autopsy eyes, indicate that early alterations in retinal blood vessels include the loss of capillary pericytes (Fig. 47.1) and thickening of the capillary basement membrane.[1-21]

There is preliminary evidence that parenchymal cells of the retina exhibit changes in the early stages of disease, including glial cell reactivity, alterations in glutamate metabolism, and neuron cell death.[22-28] Several studies have documented subtle changes in contrast sensitivity and color perception in diabetics in the absence of visible retinopathy,[29-34] but it remains unclear whether these effects result from deficits in retinal function, or from other diabetic alterations such as cataractogenesis. Central vision (measured by visual acuity) and peripheral vision (measured by common perimetric tests) typically remain normal in DM prior to onset of clinically evident retinopathy, in the absence of other factors such as cataract.

Microaneurysms

Microaneurysms, identified clinically by ophthalmoscopy as deep-red dots varying from 25 to 100 μm in diameter, are usually the first visible sign of diabetic retinopathy. Although microaneurysms are occasionally seen in normal aging adults and also occur in other retinal vascular diseases, such as retinal vein occlusion and radiation retinopathy, they are a hallmark of NPDR.

Microaneurysms arise as hypercellular saccular outpouchings of the capillary wall that can be well visualized in trypsin-digest retinal mounts (see Fig. 47.1D).[1] Their lumina are sometimes occluded by agglutinated erythrocytes or thrombus. Over time they sometimes become acellular, just as damaged retinal capillaries can evolve into "ghost" vessels devoid of endothelial cells and pericytes. The mechanism for microaneurysm formation is unknown. Possible contributing factors may include alterations in the retinal microenvironment from metabolic effects on neurons, glial cells, and endothelial cells; endothelial cell injury secondary to leukostasis from altered interaction between endothelial cells and leukocytes; response of endothelial cells to altered balance between proliferative and antiproliferative factors; structural changes in the capillary wall (such as from loss of pericytes); or increase in intraluminal pressure.

Microaneurysms visualized by ophthalmoscopy or angiography commonly appear and disappear over time, though some retain a stable appearance for years. The presence of microaneurysms alone, in the absence of other features of diabetic retinopathy, remains compatible with normal vision. However, as the number of microaneurysms increases, there is a greater risk of retinopathy progression.[35-37]

Retinal vascular hyperpermeability

Subtle compromise of the blood–retinal barrier may begin at an early stage of disease, even preceding the appearance of retinopathy, but clinically appreciable retinal vascular hyperpermeability typically follows the appearance of microaneurysms. Visualized clinically by angiography, leakage may arise from microaneurysms, retinal capillaries, or other microvascular abnormalities, and can be highly variable in magnitude and extent. Retinal vascular incompetence may or may not result in localized areas of thickening of the retina. Hard exudates, extravascular deposits of lipid-rich material that result from spillage and incomplete resorption of plasma lipoproteins, may accumulate. Intraretinal hemorrhages appear in the posterior pole and

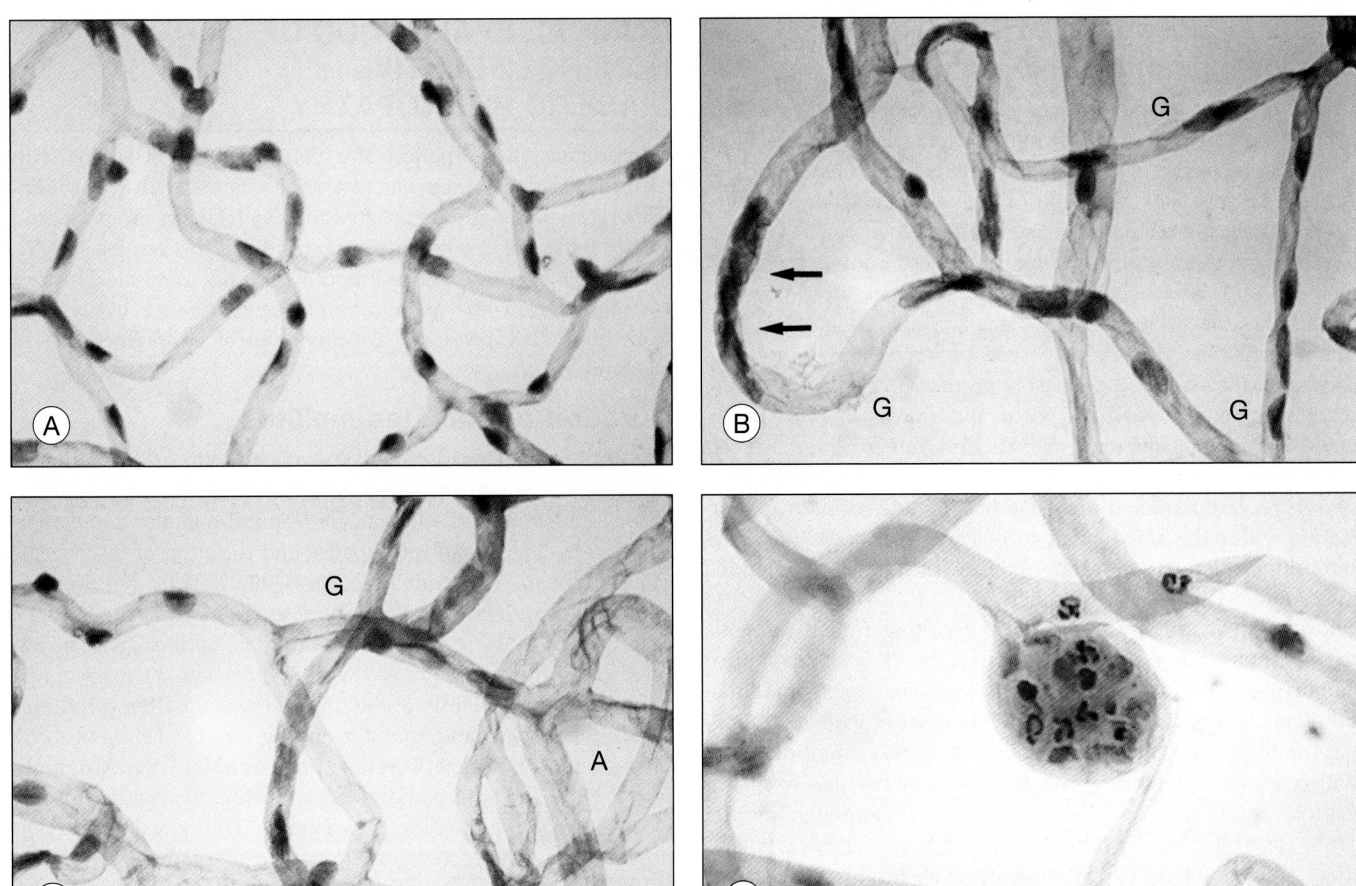

Fig. 47.1 Photomicrographs of mounted retinal capillaries following trypsin digestion and staining with periodic acid-Schiff-hematoxylin, demonstrating retinal capillary alterations in a canine model for diabetic retinopathy. (A) Normal capillaries showing a typical distribution of endothelial cells and pericytes from a control dog fed normal chow (original magnification, ×825). (B,C) Pericyte ghosts (G), focal proliferation of endothelial cells (arrows), and acellular capillaries (A) are visible in a dog fed a galactose diet for 24 months (original magnification, ×825 and ×925, respectively). (D) A microaneurysm is present in a dog fed a galactose diet for 27 months (original magnification, ×570). (Courtesy of Dr Peter Kador.)

in the retinal periphery. The vascular alterations responsible for hyperpermeability in NPDR remain incompletely understood, but may involve dysfunction of the tight junctions between retinal capillary endothelial cells. Possible mechanisms for breakdown of the blood–retinal barrier are discussed in Chapter 27 (Blood–retinal barrier, immune privilege, and autoimmunity).

Diabetic macular edema

Diabetic macular edema (DME), defined as retinal thickening in the posterior pole, results from retinal vascular hyperpermeability and other alterations in the retinal microenvironment, and represents a common cause of vision loss among diabetics. DME can occur in eyes with a wide spectrum of underlying retinopathy, from mild NPDR to PDR. It can occur in areas of demonstrable retinal vascular incompetence, as visualized by angiography, and also in regions of retinal ischemia. In areas of vascular incompetence, DME may result from leakage of microaneurysms, or it may evolve from diffuse leakage of hyperpermeable capillaries. In areas of capillary nonperfusion on angiography, retinal thickening may result from ischemia in the absence of prominent vascular leakage, though hyperpermeable microvascular abnormalities at the borders of such regions may contribute to swelling. Macular edema may or may not be characterized by intraretinal cyst formation. In some cases, usually in the setting of severe cystic thickening involving the fovea, subretinal fluid may also be present.

The pathogenesis of DME remains poorly understood, partly because of the absence of a good animal model. Chapter 46 (Diabetic retinopathy: Genetics and etiologic mechanisms) reviews what we know about the early biochemical and cellular alterations leading to DME, while Chapter 28 (Mechanism of macular edema) discusses factors involved in the pathogenesis of macular edema of different causes.

Extrafoveal foci of retinal thickening and hard exudates may not cause symptoms or affect visual acuity, but DME that involves or threatens the center of the macula carries a significant risk of vision loss. In the Early Treatment of Diabetic Retinopathy Study (ETDRS), the 3-year risk of moderate visual loss (a decrease of three lines or more on a logarithmic visual acuity chart, corresponding to a doubling of the initial visual angle) among untreated eyes with DME involving or threatening the center of the macula was 32%.[38] The natural history of DME is variable. In some eyes, it can persist for years, while in others it may spontaneously resolve. Chapter 45 (The epidemiology of diabetic retinopathy) discusses the incidence and prevalence of DME and consequent vision loss.

Capillary closure, microvascular remodeling, and retinal ischemia

One of the most serious consequences of diabetic retinopathy is progressive loss of functional retinal capillaries. Trypsin-digest preparations of the retina show areas of acellular capillaries, or "ghost" vessels, which have lost the endothelial cells and pericytes that once lined them (see Fig. 47.1C). When patches of such acellular capillaries, first seen early in the course of NPDR, increase and become confluent, the terminal arterioles that supply these capillaries often become occluded. Regions of acellular capillaries in histologic sections have been shown to correspond to areas of capillary nonperfusion visualized by fluorescein angiography.[39] Adjacent to these areas of retinal ischemia, clusters of microaneurysms and hypercellular vessels often develop. It has been difficult to determine whether such vessels represent altered pre-existing capillaries or neovascularization within the retina. Such vessels are described clinically as intraretinal microvascular abnormalities (IRMA), a term intended to accommodate both possibilities.

Progressive capillary closure and resulting retinal ischemia are commonly associated with increasing IRMA, intraretinal hemorrhages, and venous abnormalities such as segmental dilation (venous beading). Occasionally, in cases of extensive capillary nonperfusion, the retina acquires a featureless appearance with a relative dearth of visible vessels, hemorrhages, or microvascular abnormalities. Retinal ischemia represents another cause for vision loss in NPDR, and also plays a central role in the pathogenesis of PDR by stimulating elaboration of vascular endothelial growth factor A (VEGF-A) and other factors promoting the growth of extraretinal neovascularization.[40–47] Chapter 48 (Proliferative diabetic retinopathy) discusses the natural course of PDR.

Alterations of the vitreous gel and vitreoretinal interface

The vitreous gel plays a key role in the fibrovascular proliferation of PDR, but it may also exert important effects at earlier stages of retinopathy. Epiretinal membrane formation, arising from liquefaction of the vitreous gel and consequent effects at the vitreoretinal interface, can occur with advancing age in otherwise healthy eyes but is more common in diabetic eyes.[48–52] It has been hypothesized that liquefaction of the vitreous gel out of proportion to diminution of posterior vitreoretinal adhesion may underlie the pathophysiology of many vitreoretinal diseases,[53] and observations at vitrectomy suggest that the posterior cortical vitreous is frequently more adherent to the retina in the setting of diabetic retinopathy. Studies have documented a number of biochemical changes to the vitreous gel in the setting of DM, including increased collagen fibril cross-linking, accumulation of advanced glycation end products that may augment vitreoretinal adhesion and incite retinal glial cell reactivity, and alterations in the concentration of various soluble proteins.[54–58]

The role of the vitreous gel in the pathophysiology of diabetic retinopathy may extend beyond its capacity to exert mechanical effects on the retina. For example, there is recent evidence that the vitreous may function as an important regulator of intraocular oxygen tension, a finding that could have important implications for diabetic retinopathy and other diseases involving retinal hypoxia.[59,60]

CLINICAL EVALUATION OF NONPROLIFERATIVE DIABETIC RETINOPATHY

Comprehensive evaluation of a patient with DM begins with identification of extraocular factors associated with risk of diabetic retinopathy and its progression. Such factors are presented briefly here and discussed in greater detail in Chapter 45 (The epidemiology of diabetic retinopathy). Pertinent medical history is sought from the patient, and supplemented by records from his or her primary care physician or endocrinologist as warranted.

Duration of diabetes mellitus

The duration of DM is strongly associated with risk of retinopathy. Cross-sectional and longitudinal analyses from population-based epidemiologic studies have established the association between prevalence of retinopathy and duration of disease.[61–70] The Wisconsin Epidemiologic Study of Diabetic Retinopathy (WESDR) examined prevalence and severity of diabetic retinopathy among diabetics categorized into a younger-onset group consisting of those diagnosed with DM prior to 30 years of age who were taking insulin at the time of the evaluation (predominantly type 1 DM) and an older-onset group consisting of those diagnosed with DM at 30 years of age or older (predominantly type 2 DM), the latter subdivided according to whether insulin was being used at the time of evaluation. The prevalence of retinopathy may have changed somewhat since the 1980s when WESDR data was collected, given interim advances and evolving standards of care in management of DM, but the WESDR remains one of our most definitive sources of information about the epidemiology of diabetic retinopathy in the United States. In the younger-onset group, retinopathy (consisting of NPDR or PDR) was seen in 13% of those with less than a 5-year duration of DM and in 90% of those with a duration of 10–15 years.[65] In the older-onset group using insulin, retinopathy was seen in 40% of those with less than a 5-year duration of disease and in 84% of those with a duration of 15–19 years, while the corresponding rates in the older-onset group not taking insulin were 24% and 53%, respectively.[64]

Among those with type 2 DM, in which disease onset is often more insidious than in type 1 DM and in which hyperglycemia can remain asymptomatic for years, age at diagnosis may not always accurately reflect disease duration. The Centers for Disease Control and Prevention estimate that 25.8 million people in the United States have DM, of whom 7.0 million do not know they have it.[71] The prevalence of undiagnosed type 2 DM is felt to be the key factor explaining the higher rates of retinopathy noted soon after diagnosis among type 2 diabetics (24% in the older-onset group not taking insulin with less than a 5-year duration of disease in the WESDR) compared with type 1 diabetics (13% in the younger-onset group with less than a 5-year duration of disease).

Hyperglycemia

The relationship between the degree of hyperglycemia and the presence and severity of diabetic retinopathy has been extensively studied in observational studies and clinical trials. The observational studies have demonstrated that greater hyperglycemia is associated with increased prevalence and severity of diabetic retinopathy.[62,64–67,69,70] Several key randomized controlled clinical trials have demonstrated that better glycemic control is associated with a decreased risk of secondary complications of DM, including diabetic retinopathy.[72–79]

In the Diabetes Control and Complications Trial (DCCT), 1441 participants with type 1 DM were randomly assigned to either conventional or more intensive insulin treatment and followed for a period of 4–9 years.[72,73,76,79] The average difference in glycosylated hemoglobin (hemoglobin A1C [HbA1C]) between the two groups was almost 2%. Intensive insulin treatment as defined by the DCCT was associated with a decreased risk of both the development and progression of diabetic retinopathy. In patients without retinopathy at enrollment, the 3-year risk of developing retinopathy was reduced by 75% in the intensive insulin treatment group compared with the conventional treatment group. The benefit of better glycemic control was also evident in patients with existing retinopathy at baseline, as shown by a 50% reduction in the rate of progression of retinopathy compared with controls. At the 6- and 12-month visits, more intensive insulin treatment exerted a small adverse effect on retinopathy progression, similar to that described in other trials of glycemic control. However, among eyes with little or no retinopathy at the time of initiating better control of hyperglycemia, it was found that such "early worsening" of retinopathy was unlikely to threaten vision. When the DCCT results were stratified by levels of glycosylated hemoglobin, there was a 35–40% reduction in the risk of retinopathy progression for every 10% decrease in HbA1C (e.g., from 8% to 7.2%). This represented a fivefold increase in risk of progression for patients with HbA1C around 10% compared with those with HbA1C around 7%. Notably, there was also a statistically significant reduction in other microvascular complications of DM, including nephropathy and peripheral neuropathy, with more intensive glycemic control in the DCCT.

When the randomized controlled clinical trial was completed, DCCT participants were informed of the results and enrolled in a follow-up phase of the study, known as the Epidemiology of Diabetes Intervention and Complications (EDIC) study.[76] After an additional 7 years of follow-up, during which the HbA1C values in both treatment groups did not differ significantly (8.1% vs 8.2%, P = 0.09), the rate of retinopathy progression remained significantly lower in those who had received more intensive treatment in the DCCT than in those who had received conventional therapy. Thus, more intensive glycemic control over a period of 6.5 years conferred benefits well beyond the period of treatment.

In the United Kingdom Prospective Diabetes Study (UKPDS), 3867 patients with newly diagnosed type 2 DM were randomly assigned to conventional therapy or to more intensive glycemic control with either insulin or a sulfonylurea.[74,75] Among participants treated with conventional therapy, those who were overweight were given metformin and those who were not overweight did not receive this medication. After 12 years, the rate of retinopathy progression was reduced by 21% and the use of laser photocoagulation was reduced by 29% in those getting intensive glycemic control compared with those getting conventional treatment. For every percentage point decrease in HbA1C (e.g., 9% to 8%), there was a 35% reduction in the risk of microvascular complications of disease.

The results of the UKPDS have recently been corroborated by those of another large randomized controlled clinical trial, the Action to Control Cardiovascular Risk in Diabetes (ACCORD) study. The ACCORD study randomly assigned 10251 patients with type 2 DM to very intensive glycemic control (targeting HbA1C less than 6%), or to standard treatment (targeting HbA1C between 7 and 7.9%). A subset of 2856 participants was evaluated for progression of retinopathy by comparison of fundus photographs taken at baseline and at 4 years.[78] In this subset at one year, median HbA1C in the intensive treatment cohort was 6.4% compared with 7.5% in the cohort getting conventional therapy. In the intensive treatment group, the rate of retinopathy progression was 7.3%, compared with 10.4% in the standard therapy group (adjusted odds ratio, 0.67; 95% confidence interval [CI] 0.51–0.87; P = 0.003). The glycemia trial, performed alongside other studies evaluating control of blood pressure and plasma lipids, was halted early at a median of 3.7 years because of an increased rate of death from all causes in participants treated with intensive control compared with those managed with standard control (5% vs 4%, respectively), and the very intensive control approach was abandoned.

Hypertension

In addition to assessing the effects of differential glycemic control, the UKPDS provided a randomized comparison between more intensive blood pressure control (targeting a systolic blood pressure less than 150 mmHg) and less intensive blood pressure control (targeting a systolic blood pressure less than 180 mmHg) in a large cohort of participants with newly diagnosed type 2 DM.[80] Study results demonstrated that intensive blood pressure control was associated with a decreased risk of retinopathy progression. Of 1148 hypertensive participants in the UKPDS, 758 were allocated to more intensive control of blood pressure and 390 to less intensive control with a median follow-up of 8.4 years. More intensive blood pressure control resulted in a 37% reduction in microvascular complications of DM, predominantly a reduced risk of retinal photocoagulation, compared with less intensive control. An earlier report assessing the effects of various blood pressure medications on diabetic retinopathy had suggested that there might be a specific benefit of angiotensin-converting enzyme (ACE) inhibition, even in normotensive persons. The UKPDS included a randomized comparison of beta-blockers and ACE inhibitors within the more intensive blood pressure control arm. Benefit from more intensive blood pressure control was noted in both the beta-blocker and ACE inhibitor treatment groups, with no statistically significant difference between them, suggesting that the treatment effect was probably attributable to blood pressure reduction and not to a specific effect of ACE inhibition.

The ACCORD study attempted to extend the results of the UKPDS by assessing the effect of very tight blood pressure control on retinopathy. In this study, 4733 of the 10251 participants with type 2 DM were randomly assigned to very intensive control of blood pressure (targeting a systolic blood pressure less than 120 mmHg) or standard blood pressure control (targeting a systolic blood pressure less than 140 mmHg). A subset of 1263 participants in the blood pressure trial was evaluated for progression of retinopathy just as in the glycemia arm of the study, with comparison of fundus photographs at baseline and 4 years.[78] Rate of progression of retinopathy was not significantly different in the two groups (10.4% of those treated intensively compared with 8.8% of those treated with standard care, with an adjusted odds ratio of 1.23; 95% CI 0.84–1.79; P = 0.29). The results of the UKPDS and ACCORD study are not necessarily contradictory in this regard, given the very different targets used for more and less intensive control of blood pressure between the two trials.

Dyslipidemia

Elevated levels of plasma cholesterol were associated with greater severity of retinal hard exudates in the WESDR and in the ETRDS.[81,82] Independent of coincident retinal thickening, the severity of retinal hard exudates at baseline was associated with decreased visual acuity in the ETDRS. The severity of retinal hard exudates was also a significant risk factor for moderate visual loss during the course of the study. Elevated levels of plasma triglycerides were associated with a greater risk of developing high-risk PDR in the ETDRS patients.[83] Two recent randomized controlled clinical trials evaluating the plasma lipid-modulatory agent fenofibrate in combination with statins in individuals with elevated plasma lipids have demonstrated that fenofibrate reduces the risk of diabetic retinopathy progression while only providing modest alterations in the plasma lipid profile.[78,84] It is presently uncertain whether the effects of fenofibrate on diabetic retinopathy are secondary to its plasma lipid-modulatory activity or to some other mechanism.

Other extraocular factors

Diabetic retinopathy can worsen precipitously in the setting of pregnancy. Chapter 92 (Pregnancy-related diseases) reviews the natural history of retinopathy in pregnancy. Diabetic nephropathy, as measured by albuminuria, proteinuria, or manifestations of renal failure, has been inconsistently associated with progression of retinopathy.[83,85,86] Anemia has been associated with progression of diabetic retinopathy in two small case series and two epidemiologic studies.[83,87–89] The ETDRS found association between decrease in hematocrit and increase in the incidence of high-risk PDR in an adjusted multivariate model. A few reports have suggested an association between diabetic neuropathy or cardiovascular autonomic neuropathy and progression of retinopathy.[83,90,91] Significant progress has been made in understanding the heritable contributions to the development of DM, particularly the type 1 form and certain familial and syndromic variants of the disease, but the identification of genetic risk factors for development and progression of diabetic retinopathy has been challenging. Chapter 46 (Diabetic retinopathy: Genetics and etiologic mechanisms) reviews our present knowledge about the genetics of diabetic retinopathy.

Ophthalmic evaluation

Ophthalmic evaluation of a patient with DM begins with identification of pertinent features of ocular history, including previous diagnosis of diabetic retinopathy or DME, comorbid ophthalmic conditions, and previous medical or surgical treatment. The severity of existing retinopathy is a powerful predictor of risk of retinopathy progression and vision loss, as discussed below in the section "Classification of diabetic retinopathy." Knowledge of any previous treatment has recently become more relevant for management of NPDR and DME. A proliferating array of therapeutic options and the variability of treatment efficacy among individuals have made management algorithms more complex and clinical decision-making more contingent on assessment of the success of previous treatment strategies. Most pharmacologic therapies leave no lasting marks like the telltale scars of laser photocoagulation, making clinicians more reliant on history-taking and review of records for evidence of prior treatment.

A comprehensive eye examination in a person with DM includes: measurement of visual acuity and intraocular pressure; evaluation of the anterior segment by slit-lamp biomicroscopy; gonioscopy when warranted (such as in the setting of elevated intraocular pressure, neovascularization of the iris, or glaucoma); and dilated funduscopic examination.[92] Evaluation of the anterior segment prior to dilation of the pupil may allow visualization of neovascularization of the iris or anterior chamber angle not visible following mydriasis. Dilation of the pupil is important for adequate assessment of the posterior segment. In the absence of pupil dilation, only 50% of eyes are correctly diagnosed for the presence and severity of retinopathy.[93]

Ophthalmoscopy, including stereoscopic evaluation of the posterior pole and visualization of the vitreous gel and peripheral retina, remains the standard for clinical diagnosis and characterization of NPDR and DME. Examination of the posterior pole is best achieved using slit-lamp biomicroscopy with accessory lenses. A hand-held accessory lens may provide sufficient visualization of the posterior pole and midperipheral retina, but in cases where superior stereopsis and discrimination are desired, an examination contact lens coupled to the eye surface after application of topical anesthetic drops can be used. The peripheral retina is typically surveyed using indirect ophthalmoscopy, but slit-lamp biomicroscopy with an accessory lens may serve as a supplement or substitute when visualization with high magnification is warranted. A three- or four-mirror contact lens coupled to the eye surface can also be used to examine peripheral lesions under high magnification. Red-free illumination can be useful at highlighting retinal vessels and associated lesions of NPDR such as microaneurysms, hemorrhages, and IRMA.

Ancillary ocular imaging

Imaging modalities in common clinical use for management of NPDR and DME include fundus photography, fluorescein angiography (FA), and optical coherence tomography (OCT).

Fundus photography

Fundus photography is a valuable clinical tool for evaluating progression of retinopathy in individual patients and in participants in clinical trials. Photography is used in clinical practice to document the status of retinopathy and effects of treatment. Though not always as sensitive as ophthalmoscopy at detecting subtle features of diabetic retinopathy such as IRMA and early extraretinal neovascularization, photography can be useful in documenting certain findings in select patients. For example, it can be used to record the extent and distribution of hard exudates in DME, the extent of retinal alterations in severe NPDR, and the appearance of laser photocoagulation burns. Chapter 48 (Proliferative diabetic retinopathy) discusses its role in documenting the extent and characteristics of neovascularization, fibrous proliferation, and retinal traction. The development of digital systems capable of high-resolution images immediately accessible to the clinician has expanded the role of fundus photography in clinical practice, facilitating record-keeping, information-sharing among providers, and use of images as a teaching tool with patients.

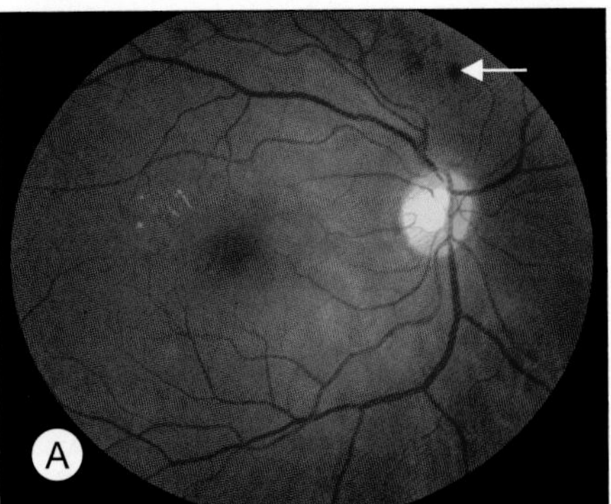

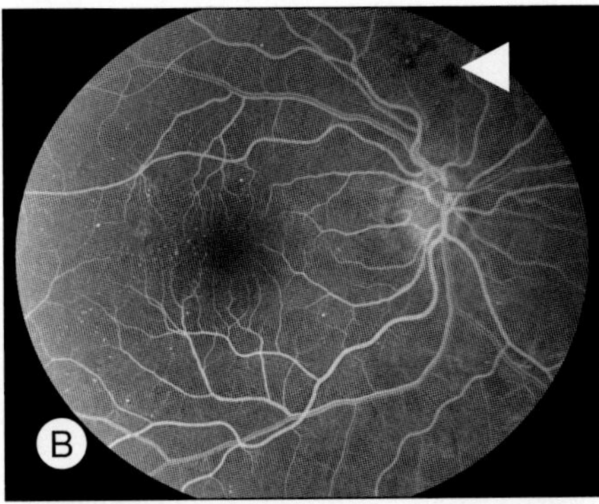

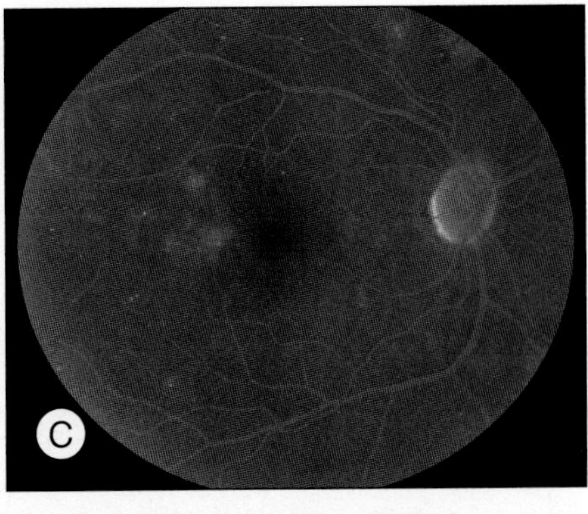

Fig. 47.2 Moderate NPDR and DME. (A) Photograph illustrating microaneurysms, intraretinal hemorrhages, and hard exudates. Retinal thickening visible with stereoscopic viewing on biomicroscopy is present temporal to the foveal center. Microaneurysms appear as variably-sized small red dots most prominent temporal to the fovea. Hemorrhages (arrow) can sometimes be distinguished from microaneurysms because of their size and less sharply demarcated borders. Mild hard exudates appear as small yellow-white intraretinal deposits with sharply demarcated borders. (B) Early frame of the FA. Microaneurysms are visible as variably sized hyperfluorescent dots. Note that angiography allows visualization of microaneurysms not readily seen in the color photograph. Hemorrhages (arrowhead) and hard exudates are hypofluorescent. Microvascular abnormalities not visible in the color photograph are present temporal to the fovea. Degree of capillary nonperfusion is minimal. (C) Late frame of the FA. Mild late leakage is visible as poorly demarcated hyperfluorescence surrounding clusters of microaneurysms temporal to the fovea. (National Eye Institute, Bethesda, MD.)

Fluorescein angiography

Fluorescein angiography (FA), consisting of photography or videography of the fundus using cameras equipped with appropriate filters following intravenous injection of the hydrocarbon dye fluorescein sodium, has been used clinically in ophthalmology for over 40 years and is described in detail in Chapter 1 (Fluorescein angiography). FA has multiple uses in the clinical evaluation of diabetic retinopathy. Because intravenous injection of fluorescein sodium can be associated with life-threatening adverse reactions (with risk of death estimated at approximately 1/200 000),[94] FA for evaluation of diabetic retinopathy is largely confined to settings in which important aspects of management hinge on the results of the test. FA has been used extensively for evaluation of diabetic retinopathy, and is not known to pose any special hazards in DM. Nephropathy or renal failure is not a contraindication to testing.[95] In NPDR, FA is most commonly indicated for further characterization of DME diagnosed on ophthalmoscopy (Fig. 47.2), and its utility in this setting is discussed below in the section "Clinical evaluation of diabetic macular edema."

FA can also be used to investigate vision loss incompletely explained by ophthalmoscopy and other less-invasive testing. In some cases, significant capillary nonperfusion involving the fovea and parafovea, best visualized during the arteriovenous transit phase of the angiogram, implicates macular ischemia as a cause for vision loss. In other cases, FA may suggest other causes for vision loss unrelated to diabetic retinopathy.

FA is occasionally used in eyes with presumed NPDR to search for early lesions of extraretinal neovascularization not detected by ophthalmoscopy or fundus photography, such as in cases where preretinal or vitreous hemorrhage suggests PDR but no cause for bleeding is seen by ophthalmoscopy. The technique in this setting requires a view of the fundus not overly obscured by hemorrhage, and use of either wide-angle lenses or "sweep" fields to image as much of the retina as possible. Its success depends on the prominent leakage of fluorescein dye characteristic of extraretinal neovascularization, typically readily visible against the background of other vascular alterations, but it is important to note that intraretinal alterations such as IRMA can exhibit similar leakage. Sometimes stereoscopic images or further ophthalmoscopy may clarify the extraretinal nature of neovascularization and associated leakage.

Commonly used grading systems for severity of diabetic retinopathy do not consider findings on FA, and FA is not indicated for classification of disease. While FA is a sensitive means for detection of early features of NPDR such as microaneurysms and retinal capillary hyperpermeability, it is not clinically indicated to screen for mild retinopathy.[92]

Optical coherence tomography

Optical coherence tomography (OCT), which utilizes low-coherence interferometry involving near-infrared light for cross-sectional imaging of intraocular structures, has emerged over the last decade as a fast, noninvasive means of imaging the retina, vitreoretinal interface, and the retinal pigment epithelium (RPE) in NPDR and other macular diseases. The basic principles of OCT and the applications of this technology to evaluation of the retina are discussed in Chapter 3 (Optical coherence tomography). In NPDR, OCT is commonly used to characterize DME (Fig. 47.3) and abnormalities of the vitreoretinal interface.

Investigators of the Diabetic Retinopathy Clinical Research Network (DRCR.net),[96] a collaborative network of over 100 sites in the United States dedicated to multicenter clinical research of diabetic retinopathy, have rigorously evaluated OCT as a test yielding measures of macular thickness in diabetic eyes. The standardization required for DRCR.net clinical trials has necessitated use of a common OCT platform and scanning technique. OCT scanning in DRCR.net studies to date involves acquisition of images of the macula by certified operators after pupil dilation, with use of a time-domain system called the Stratus OCT (Carl Zeiss Meditec, Inc., Dublin, CA) and a scanning algorithm known as the fast macular thickness map, which obtains 128 axial scans (A scans) along each of six radial lines (each 6 mm in length) intersecting at a common center, with a total scan time of 1.9 seconds. Stratus processing software includes an automated segmentation algorithm that identifies an inner and outer retinal border on line scans and calculates retinal thickness. A retinal thickness map is generated using data from all line scans

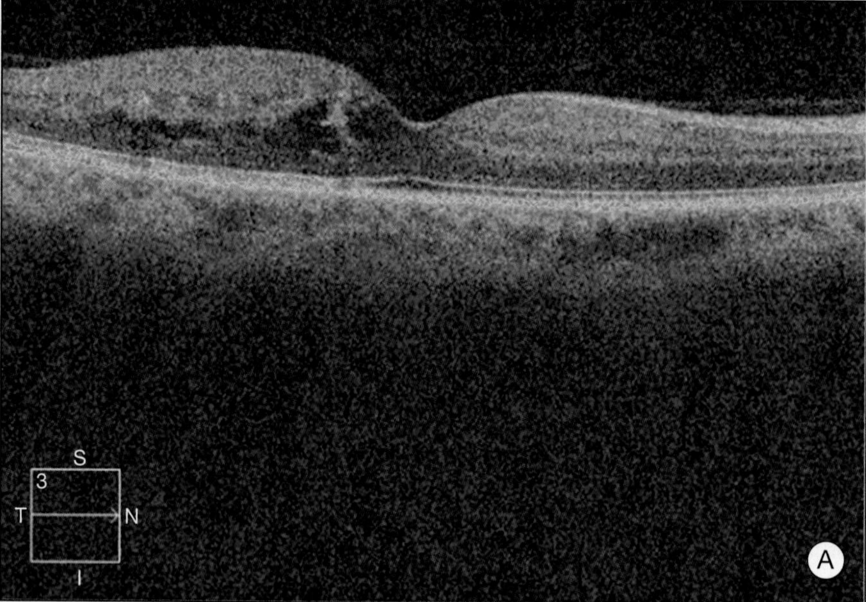

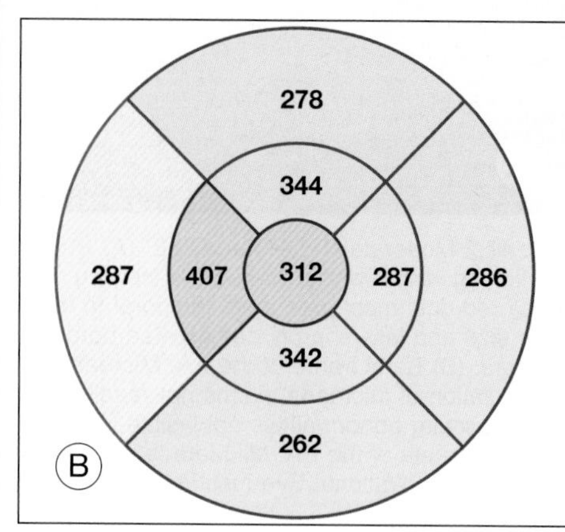

Fig. 47.3 OCT characterization of macular thickening in NPDR and DME. (A) A 6 mm horizontal line scan obtained with a spectral domain OCT system (Cirrus, Carl Zeiss Meditec, Dublin, CA) imaging the macula of the eye illustrated in Fig. 47.2 shows mild retinal thickening temporally, corresponding to the area of microaneurysms leaking on FA. (B) The retinal thickness map generated by automated segmentation of a 6×6 mm 512×128 Macular Cube scan shows mean thickness values for nine standard subfields. Mean thickness is greater than in 99% of normals in the central and inner temporal subfields (shaded purple) and greater than in 95% of normals in the outer temporal subfield (shaded red), based on a comparison to data in the Cirrus normative database. (National Eye Institute, Bethesda, MD.)

obtained by the scanning algorithm. Output includes center-point thickness, total macular volume, and mean values for retinal thickness in a grid comprised of a central subfield, four inner subfields, and four outer subfields. Assessment of the quality of output depends on assessment of other parameters such as signal strength and standard deviation of center-point thickness. Software offers a comparison of thickness values to those from a normative database of measurements obtained from normal individuals.

DRCR.net investigators compared central subfield mean thickness (CSMT) values in 97 diabetics with minimal or no retinopathy and no central macular thickening on examination to normal values for nondiabetics in the Stratus OCT database.[97] Results showed no significant difference between CSMT of diabetic eyes with minimal or no retinopathy and normal values imputed from nondiabetic individuals in the database, suggesting that the presence of DM is not associated with clinically important changes in CSMT in the absence of retinopathy. The study noted a statistically significant difference between CSMT in men and women, similar to findings in other reports.

DRCR.net investigators evaluated the reproducibility of OCT in eyes with DME, and established thresholds indicative of meaningful change in retinal thickness. In a prospective multicenter one-day study evaluating diurnal variation of DME, 212 eyes of 107 participants with DME involving the foveal center on biomicroscopy and CSMT of 225 microns or greater were imaged multiple times on Stratus OCT and the scans were evaluated by a reading center.[98] Both eyes were imaged six times during the day, and at each of these six sittings a pair of scans was generated, with repeat imaging done for scans of suboptimal quality. Of a possible 1284 pairs, 1223 were analyzed. Reproducibility was better for CSMT than for center-point thickness, not surprising considering that CSMT incorporates more data points. The median absolute difference between replicate measurements of CSMT was 7 µm. Expressed as a percentage difference between the two measurements, the half-width of the 95% CI for a change in retinal thickness for CSMT was 10% for eyes with CSMT less than 400 µm, and 13% for eyes with CSMT equal to or greater than 400µm. The authors concluded that a change in CSMT greater than 11% using the Stratus OCT for DME is likely to be real.

The rapid pace of technological progress, resulting in recent improvements such as spectral domain imaging and image-registration capability in some systems, makes for substantial variability in image acquisition, processing, and output metrics among presently available OCT platforms. For example, the spectral domain Cirrus OCT (Carl Zeiss Meditec, Dublin, CA), though its output is similar in many ways to that of the time domain Stratus OCT, uses a distinct automated segmentation algorithm that results in retinal thickness values that are approximately 30–55µm greater than those reported by the Stratus OCT in eyes with DME.[99] Meaningful interpretation of an OCT scan requires familiarity with the system utilized, including understanding of scan acquisition, indicators of scan quality, processing of raw data, algorithms for automated segmentation, and format of output metrics, as well as knowledge of any normative database used by system software to compare a given set of measurements to a normal range. Caution is warranted in comparing OCT scans obtained using different systems, and clinical researchers using OCT must grapple with such issues in planning studies that require standardization of procedures among clinical sites. The DRCR.net is presently evaluating issues related to integrating new OCT systems into future research studies.

Funduscopic lesions of nonproliferative diabetic retinopathy

Small or nonperfused microaneurysms may not be discernible on ophthalmoscopy, but those that are visible appear as small deep-red dots between 25 and 100μm in diameter within the retina (see Figs 47.2A, 47.4). Microaneurysms in NPDR typically arise in the posterior pole, but they can also be present in the midperipheral and peripheral retina, particularly in more severe retinopathy. They may be solitary or may appear in clusters. They may remain stable across months or even years, but many appear and eventually disappear. On FA, microaneurysms are visible during arteriovenous transit as hyperfluorescent dots within the retina (see Fig. 47.2B). This hyperfluorescence typically persists in later phases of the angiogram, and may or may not be associated with leakage in mid- and late frames (see Fig. 47.2C). FA is a sensitive means of detecting microaneurysms, and may reveal lesions that were poorly visible or not visible on ophthalmoscopy.

Intraretinal hemorrhages in NPDR are variable in appearance, just as in other retinal diseases (Figs 47.2A, 47.4). Dot-blot hemorrhages are typically small with sharply demarcated borders, and are sometimes indistinguishable from microaneurysms on ophthalmoscopy. Flame hemorrhages can be larger, and manifest wispy margins as a consequence of their location in the nerve fiber layer. Intraretinal hemorrhages appear hypofluorescent on FA, blocking normal fluorescence from the underlying choroid, and consequently FA offers ready distinction between microaneurysms and hemorrhages (Fig. 47.2B). Intraretinal hemorrhages can be present in the posterior pole and in more peripheral retina, and frequently appear and disappear over weeks or months. Hemorrhages on the optic disc are not typical for diabetic retinopathy, and should raise suspicion for neovascularization or a comorbid condition affecting the optic nerve head. Variability in the density of hemorrhages between one sector of the retina and another is common, but striking asymmetry sometimes suggests a superimposed process such as a branch retinal vein occlusion.

Hard exudates are visible on ophthalmoscopy as sharply demarcated yellow-white deposits within the retina (Figs 47.2A, 47.5). They are visible on OCT line scans as hyperreflective foci within the retina. With stereoscopic viewing they are readily distinguishable from drusen, which reside external to the retina. Hard exudates are often distributed at the border between edematous and nonedematous retina. They may form a circinate ring around areas of prominent vascular hyperpermeability such as a cluster of microaneurysms. They tend to form in the posterior pole in association with macular thickening, but small collections are sometimes present in more peripheral retina. They are hypofluorescent on FA, blocking underlying choroidal fluorescence (see Fig. 47.2B). Hard exudates may appear and disappear over months or years. When severe, they may undergo organization and may cause subretinal fibrosis.

Cotton-wool spots, patches of relative ischemia affecting the nerve fiber layer of the retina, are visible on ophthalmoscopy as small white patches with wispy borders situated in the inner retina (Fig. 47.6). They are hypofluorescent on FA, blocking underlying choroidal fluorescence. They commonly appear and disappear over weeks or months.

The major retinal vessels can exhibit changes in appearance in the setting of advanced retinopathy. Arterioles may appear thin or white. Venules may appear dilated and tortuous. Venous loops are occasionally present. Venous beading consists of localized areas of change in vessel caliber, visible as alternating regions of relative dilation and constriction (Fig. 47.7).

Intraretinal microvascular abnormalities (IRMA) appear as segments of dilated and tortuous retinal vasculature amidst retinal vessels that are normally too small to be visible on ophthalmoscopy (see Fig. 47.6). They are usually readily distinguishable from extraretinal neovascularization on careful biomicroscopy. On FA they appear hyperfluorescent during the arteriovenous transit phase, may leak in later phases, and are often situated at the borders of areas of capillary nonperfusion. They may persist for months or years.

In occasional cases, typical lesions of severe NPDR such as intraretinal hemorrhages, venous abnormalities, and IRMA,

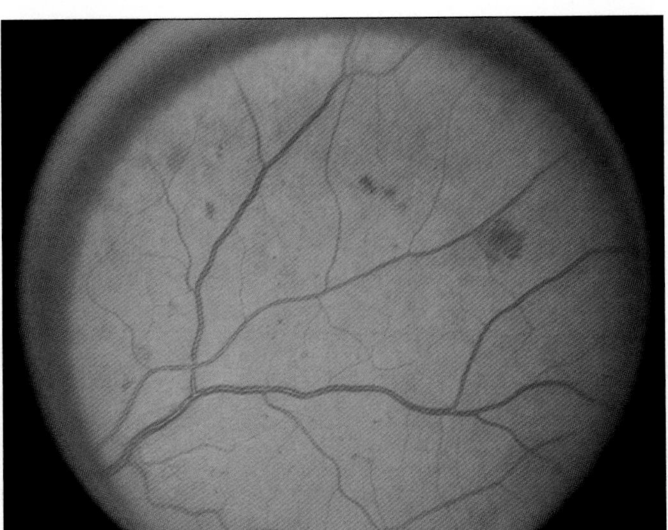

Fig. 47.4 Standard photograph 2A, intermediate standard for hemorrhages/microaneurysms. ETDRS extension of the Modified Airlie House classification of diabetic retinopathy. (Courtesy of the Diabetic Retinopathy Study Research Group.)

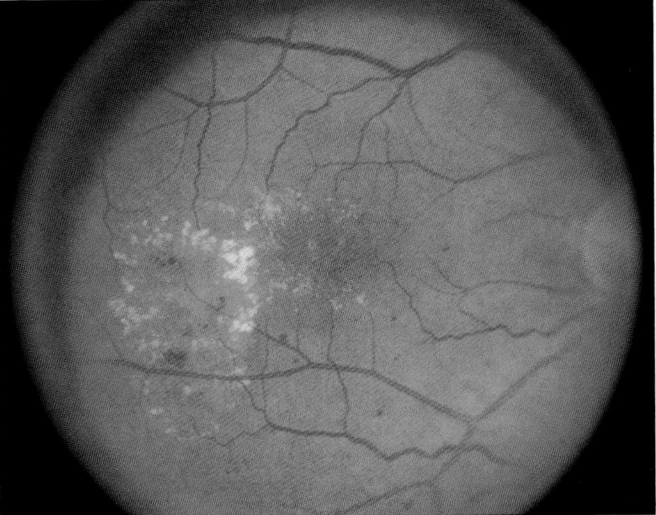

Fig. 47.5 Standard photograph 4, severe standard for hard exudates. ETDRS extension of the Modified Airlie House classification of diabetic retinopathy. Hard exudates in the temporal macula form a circinate ring. (Courtesy of the Diabetic Retinopathy Study Research Group.)

may be sparse or absent in regions of the retina despite profound underlying microvascular alterations poorly visible on ophthalmoscopy. When such areas of "featureless" retina are widespread, the bland appearance may belie the severity of disease. Careful ophthalmoscopy usually reveals manifestations of severe retinal ischemia such as arteriolar narrowing and sheathing, absence of normal vessel markings, and retinal thinning in the setting of an eye at high risk for advanced retinopathy. FA can be used to confirm clinical suspicion when necessary, characteristically revealing widespread capillary nonperfusion in areas of featureless retina.

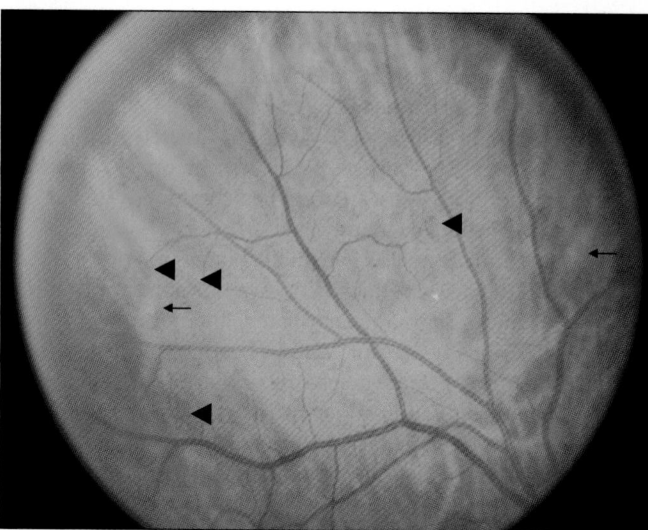

Fig. 47.6 Standard photograph 8A, less severe of two standards for cotton-wool spots and IRMA. ETDRS extension of the Modified Airlie House classification of diabetic retinopathy. Cotton-wool spots are visible in two areas as subtle white patches with wispy borders (arrows). Several areas of IRMA are visible as abnormal, tortuous, dilated retinal vessels (arrowheads). (Courtesy of the Diabetic Retinopathy Study Research Group.)

Classification of diabetic retinopathy

The Diabetic Retinopathy Study, a landmark clinical trial that established the efficacy of scatter laser photocoagulation for reduction of severe vision loss secondary to PDR, used an adaptation of the Airlie House classification of diabetic retinopathy originally developed in 1968.[100] This modified Airlie House system was extended for grading severity of retinopathy in the ETDRS.[101] Grading of retinopathy in the ETDRS involved evaluation of seven-field 30-degree nonsimultaneous stereo color fundus photographs by trained readers. Over 30 characteristics were separately graded, using standard photographs to define thresholds for scoring (see Figs 47.4, 47.5, 47.6, 47.7 for some of the standard photographs utilized in the system), and a summary grade was assigned. The ETDRS diabetic retinopathy severity scale was evaluated for its reproducibility as part of the study and was validated as a grading system with prognostic power.[101–103] ETDRS investigators assigned thresholds to define mild NPDR, moderate NPDR, severe NPDR, early PDR, and high-risk PDR (Box 47.1). The 5-year rates of development of high-risk PDR in eyes randomly assigned to deferral of photocoagulation (no laser treatment unless features of high-risk PDR developed) for eyes with mild, moderate, and severe NPDR at baseline were 15.5%, 26.5%, and 56%, respectively.

The prognostic utility of a 1-step or a 2-or-greater-step progression in the ETDRS diabetic retinopathy severity scale has been evaluated using data from the WESDR.[104] Findings indicated that 1-step or 2-or-greater-step worsening in level of retinopathy over 4 years strongly predicted the development of PDR during the subsequent 6 years. The ETDRS diabetic retinopathy severity scale remains the standard for photographic grading of retinopathy in clinical trials. The schema is impractical for routine clinical use because of its complexity and its basis in photographic – not ophthalmoscopic – assessment of the fundus, but the ETDRS definitions for mild, moderate, and severe NPDR and early and high-risk PDR were incorporated

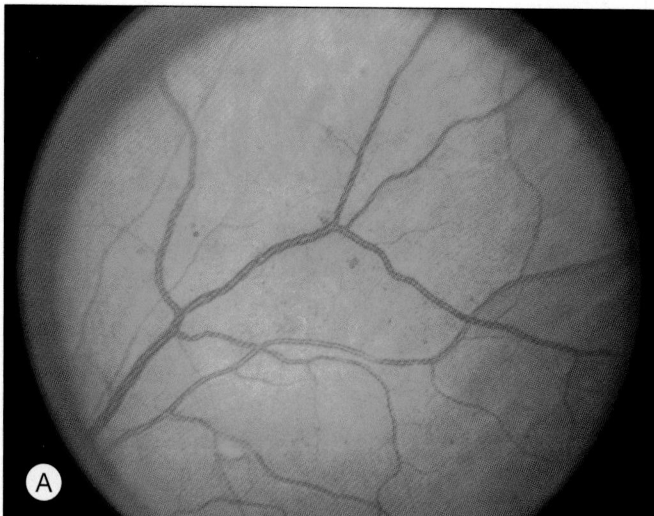

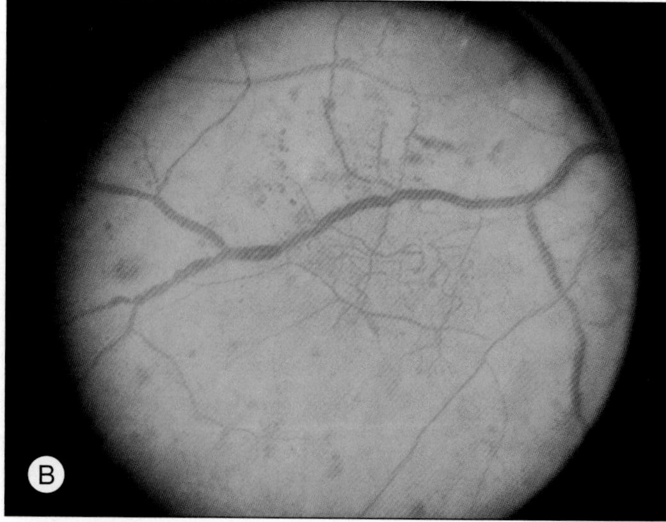

Fig. 47.7 Standard photographs 6A and 6B, less and more severe standards for venous beading. ETDRS extension of the Modified Airlie House classification of diabetic retinopathy. (A) Less severe standard (6A). Two branches of the superior temporal venule show beading that is definite but not severe. (B) More severe standard (6B). Most large and small venule branches show severe beading. (Courtesy of the Diabetic Retinopathy Study Research Group.)

Box 47.1 Classification of diabetic retinopathy in the ETDRS

Mild NPDR
At least one microaneurysm, AND criteria not met for more severe retinopathy.

Moderate NPDR
Hemorrhages/microaneurysms ≥ standard photograph 2A (Fig. 47.4); AND/OR cotton-wool spots, venous beading, or IRMA definitely present; AND criteria not met for more severe retinopathy

Severe NPDR
Cotton-wool spots, venous beading, and IRMA definitely present in at least two of photographic fields 4 to 7; OR two of the three preceding features present in at least two of fields 4 to 7 and hemorrhages/microaneurysms present in fields 4 to 7 ≥ standard photograph 2A (Fig. 47.4) in at least one of them; OR IRMA present in each of fields 4 to 7 and ≥ standard photograph 8A (Fig. 47.6) in at least two of them; AND criteria not met for more severe retinopathy.

Early PDR
New vessels; AND criteria not met for high-risk PDR.

High-risk PDR
New vessels on or within one disc diameter of the optic disc (neovascularization of the disc [NVD]) ≥ standard photograph 10A (approximately 1/4 to 1/3 disc area) with or without vitreous or preretinal hemorrhage; OR vitreous and/or preretinal hemorrhage accompanied by new vessels, either NVD < standard photograph 10A or new vessels elsewhere (NVE) ≥ 1/4 disc area.

Grading and classification of retinopathy in the ETDRS involved evaluation of modified Airlie House seven-field 30-degree non-simultaneous stereo color fundus photographs by trained readers. Photographic fields 4 and 6 image superior retina and are tangential to both a vertical line through the center of the optic disc and a horizontal line crossing its superior border. Photographic fields 5 and 7 image inferior retina and are tangential to both a vertical line through the center of the optic disc and a horizontal line crossing its inferior border. A set of standard photographs was used to define thresholds for grading and classification (see Figs 47.3, 47.4, 47.5, 47.6 for some of the standard photographs utilized in the system).

into clinical practice. A 4–2–1 rule was popularized to simplify the definition of severe NPDR.[105] Upon examination of the four midperipheral quadrants of the retina, the presence of any one of the following features was considered sufficient for diagnosis of severe NPDR (in the absence of evidence for PDR): (1) severe intraretinal hemorrhages and microaneurysms in all *four* quadrants (≥ standard photograph 2A [see Fig. 47.4]); (2) venous beading in *two* or more quadrants; or (3) moderate IRMA in at least *one* quadrant (≥ standard photograph 8A [see Fig. 47.6]). If any two of these features were present, the retinopathy was considered very severe. It is worth pointing out that the 4–2–1 rule uses a threshold for definition of severe NPDR inclusive of milder retinopathy than the definition of severe NPDR used in the ETDRS.

In answer to the need for a simplified classification of diabetic retinopathy to facilitate communication among clinicians worldwide, the Global Diabetic Retinopathy Project Group published proposed International Clinical Diabetic Retinopathy and Diabetic Macular Edema Severity Scales in 2003 (Table 47.1).[106] The classification was developed using evidence from studies such as the ETDRS and WESDR to draw distinctions in retinopathy severity most important for prognosis and management, and approximates the definitions used in the ETDRS.

CLINICAL EVALUATION OF DIABETIC MACULAR EDEMA

Clinical evaluation of DME involves consideration of a number of features relevant to prognosis and treatment. Careful

Table 47.1 Disease severity scales for diabetic retinopathy and diabetic macular edema

Proposed disease severity level	Findings observable on dilated ophthalmoscopy
No apparent retinopathy	No abnormalities
Mild NPDR	Microaneurysms only
Moderate NPDR	More than just microaneurysms but less than severe NPDR
Severe NPDR	One or more of the following, in the absence of PDR: More than 20 intraretinal hemorrhages in each of four quadrants Definite venous beading in two or more quadrants Prominent intraretinal microvascular abnormalities (IRMA) in one or more quadrants
PDR	One or more of the following: Extraretinal neovascularization Vitreous or preretinal hemorrhage
No apparent DME	No retinal thickening or hard exudates in the posterior pole
Mild DME	Some retinal thickening or hard exudates in the posterior pole, distant from the center of the macula
Moderate DME	Retinal thickening or hard exudates near the center of the macula but not involving the center
Severe DME	Retinal thickening or hard exudates involving the center of the macula

DME is defined as retinal thickening, assessed by stereoscopic evaluation of the fundus by slit-lamp biomicroscopy or assessment of photographs. Hard exudates are a sign of present or past retinal thickening.
(Adapted with permission from Wilkinson CP, Ferris FL 3rd, Klein RE, et al. Proposed international clinical diabetic retinopathy and diabetic macular edema disease severity scales. Ophthalmology 2003;110:1677–82.)

assessment of relevant systemic factors, underlying retinopathy severity, and coexisting ocular conditions (cataract, glaucoma, history of intraocular surgery, etc.), as previously outlined above, supplements the characterization of DME discussed below.

Distribution of retinal thickening and hard exudates

The ETDRS defined clinically significant macular edema (CSME) as any of the following noted on biomicroscopy: (1) thickening of the retina at or within 500 µm of the center of the macula; (2) hard exudates at or within 500 µm of the center of the macula, if associated with thickening of the adjacent retina (not residual hard exudates remaining after the disappearance of retinal thickening); or (3) a zone or zones of retinal thickening one disc area or larger, any part of which is within one disc diameter of the center of the macula.[38]

The definition for CSME was based on observation that retinal thickening or hard exudation involving or threatening

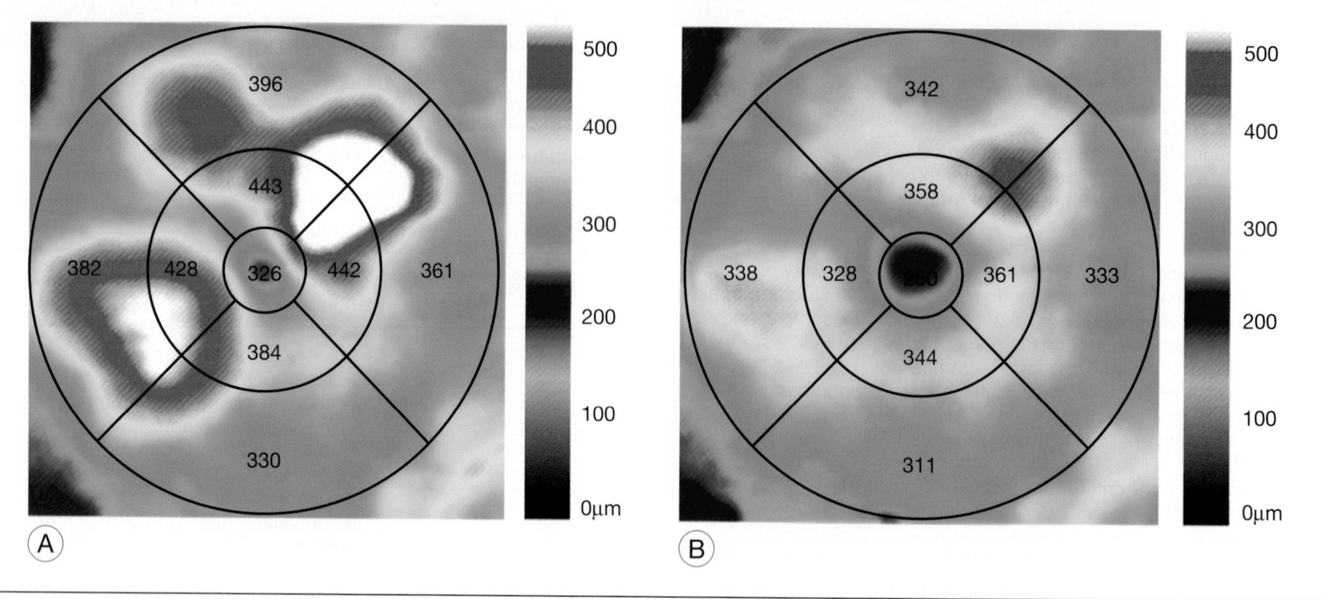

Fig. 47.8 OCT quantification of change in retinal thickness in DME. (A) A retinal thickness map generated using a spectral domain OCT system (Cirrus, Carl Zeiss Meditec, Dublin, CA) shows areas of severe macular edema juxtafoveally in an eye responsive to previous focal/grid laser photocoagulation and serial intravitreous bevacizumab injections. Another intravitreous bevacizumab (1.25 mg) injection was given at this time. (B) The retinal thickness map 5 weeks following injection shows near-resolution of macular edema, with only subtle areas of residual retinal thickening (areas shaded red and yellow) still present. (National Eye Institute, Bethesda, MD.)

the fovea frequently leads to vision loss. Careful assessment of the distribution of retinal thickening and hard exudates and their relation to the center of the macula remains paramount to management of DME. Severity of DME in the International Clinical Diabetic Macular Edema Disease Severity Scale is based solely on whether retinal thickening and hard exudates involve or threaten the center of the macula, reflecting the importance of foveal involvement for prognosis and management.[106]

While diagnosis on biomicroscopic examination remains the clinical standard for detection of DME, OCT is increasingly used as a fast and noninvasive tool to quantitatively map areas of macular thickening (see Fig. 47.3). Subtle changes in distribution of thickening over time and relationship to the fovea can be documented with good-quality scans that serially image the same region of the macula (Fig. 47.8). The standardization afforded by OCT has proven valuable in clinical practice and in research. Hard exudates can be visualized on OCT as hyperreflective foci within the retina, but biomicroscopic examination and fundus photography remain important to document their extent and proximity to the fovea.

Magnitude of retinal thickening

The degree of thickening at any given point in the retina has traditionally been estimated on biomicroscopy and stereoscopic photographs, but OCT has recently emerged as a superior means of quantifying retinal thickness. The sensitivity of OCT for retinal thickening exceeds that of contact lens-assisted biomicroscopy performed by experienced examiners.[107] Correlation between the estimated degree of retinal thickening at the center of the macula on stereoscopic photographs and the center-point thickness measured on time domain OCT is modest, reflecting the limitations of grading retinal thickness on photographs.[108]

OCT processing yields several metrics useful in characterizing the thickness of the retina in DME. For example, the Stratus OCT used by DRCR.net sites calculates a center-point thickness, CSMT, inner and outer subfield mean thicknesses, and macular volume for commonly used scanning algorithms. A DRCR.net study concluded that CSMT is well suited as a metric for central macular thickness in clinical research, with high reproducibility and good correlation to other metrics in the setting of DME.[109] Mean thickness in other subfields and total macular volume are useful in assessing extrafoveal macular edema.

OCT is capable of detecting areas of subtle macular edema that are sometimes not suspected on ophthalmoscopy (Fig. 47.8B). Easy detection of such "subclinical" thickening has added a new and provocative facet to management of DME, challenging clinicians to incorporate knowledge of more mild pathology into clinical decision-making. Conversely, OCT can illustrate areas of retinal thinning that sometimes result from advanced retinopathy. Occasionally, the presence of mild macular edema in retina that would be thinner than normal in the absence of such edema can result in a retinal thickness that appears "normal" relative to typical thickness in diabetics without retinopathy. Such abnormal thickening of retina that would otherwise be abnormally thin can make it challenging to define what constitutes complete resolution of macular edema in some eyes.

Retinal microvascular alterations and vascular hyperpermeability

Findings on ophthalmoscopy may suggest areas of vascular incompetence or retinal ischemia responsible for macular edema.

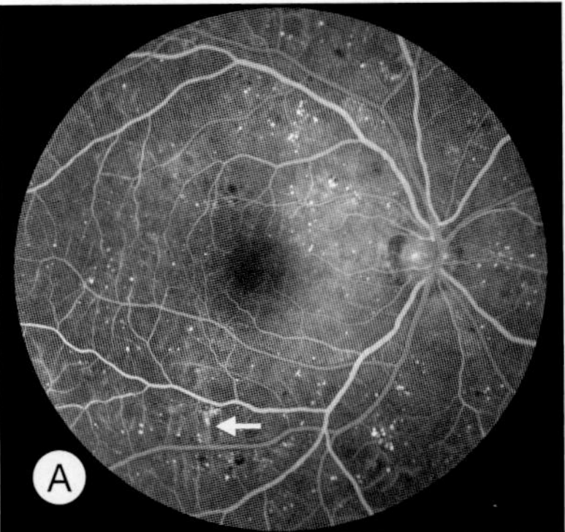

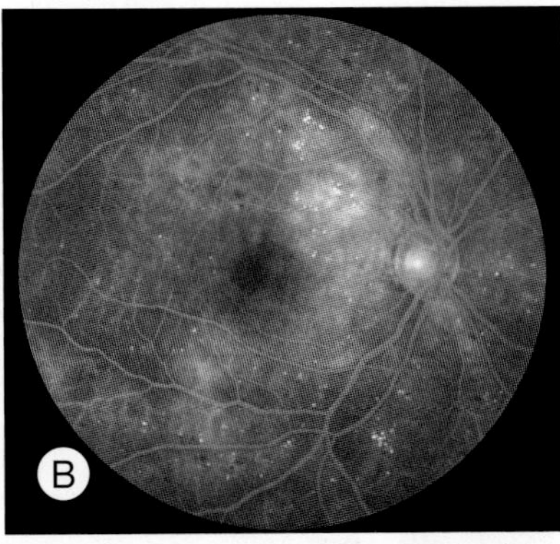

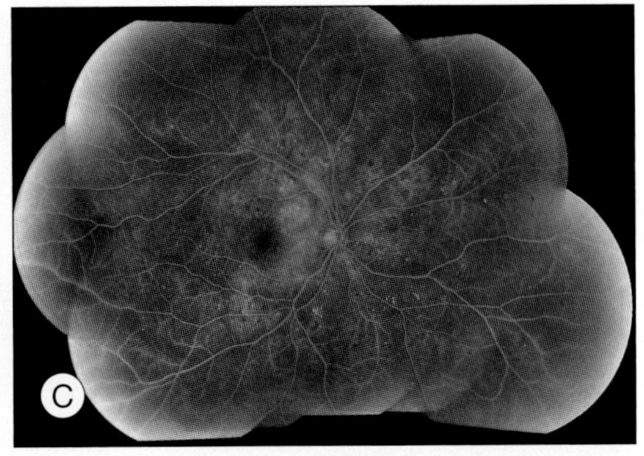

Fig. 47.9 Visualization of capillary nonperfusion and microvascular hyperpermeability by FA. (A) An early frame during arteriovenous transit highlights areas of capillary nonperfusion (visualized as a patchy absence of normal faint diffuse hyperfluorescence from capillaries, sometimes bordered by hyperfluorescent microvascular abnormalities [arrow]), microaneurysms, and microvascular abnormalities. (B) A late frame (5 minutes) illustrates focal fluorescein leakage from microaneurysms and patchy diffuse leakage from retinal capillaries. (C) A montage image created with frames from the mid-phase of the angiogram demonstrates widespread peripheral capillary nonperfusion and leakage of fluorescein from venules. Note that despite significant microvascular alterations and fluorescein leakage, visual acuity measured 20/16 and no macular thickening was present. Also note hyperfluorescence on the temporal aspect of the disc from early neovascularization. (National Eye Institute, Bethesda, MD.)

For example, a circinate lipid ring may imply leakage from a particular cluster of microaneurysms, or intraretinal microvascular abnormalities may highlight the borders of a region of capillary closure. But more definitive information about the extent of microvascular alterations and any associated vascular hyperpermeability can be gained using FA. Stereoscopic images are sometimes helpful, allowing visualization of areas of retinal thickening and localization of angiographic features to various depths within or external to the retina.

The retinal microvasculature and any areas of capillary nonperfusion are best imaged in the arteriovenous transit phase of the angiogram. Microaneurysms and microvascular abnormalities, sometimes unsuspected on ophthalmoscopy, are readily visualized (Fig. 47.2). The absence of normal hyperfluorescence from capillaries in a region where they should usually exist indicates capillary nonperfusion (Fig. 47.9). Areas of foveal capillary nonperfusion manifest as an abnormally large foveal avascular zone (FAZ) or as irregularity in the borders of the FAZ. Unfortunately, visualization of capillary nonperfusion requires resolution near the limit of present camera systems, and even slight decreases in image quality (such as from poor focus or cataract) can impair assessment. The retina in areas of capillary nonperfusion may be edematous, normal thickness, or thin.

FA is useful in evaluating retinal vascular competence, illustrating areas of hyperpermeability where dye leaks into the extravascular space (Fig. 47.9). Fluorescein leakage may emanate from discrete microaneurysms or microvascular abonormalities visible on the angiogram, or it may accumulate in areas of diffuse retinal capillary incompetence. Microaneurysms, microvascular abnormalities, and capillary telangiectasis visualized in the early phase of the angiogram can exhibit progressive leakage best appreciated in later phases, between 5 and 10 minutes after injection of dye. Fluorescein leakage may be present in a region of the retina that is edematous, normal thickness, or thin, and is therefore not synonymous with macular edema. However, ETDRS investigators and others have demonstrated correlation between area of fluorescein leakage and extent of retinal thickening on stereoscopic photographs and OCT.[110–112]

Traction by vitreous gel and epiretinal proliferation

Macular edema can occur secondary to traction exerted by cortical vitreous gel and epiretinal membranes at points of attachment to the retina. In some cases retinal thickening may result solely from the mechanical forces transmitted to the retina, without significant secondary alterations in vascular permeability. Macular edema in such cases can result from traction even in the absence of retinal vascular leakage demonstrable by FA. In other cases, mechanical traction may exert an effect on the competence of retinal capillaries. Macular edema in these cases results from the combined effects of mechanical distortion and retinal microvascular leakage. Complicating clinical assessment of the role of mechanical traction in diabetic eyes is the backdrop of microvascular alterations present as a consequence of the metabolic disease. The clinician is faced with presence of macular edema, a visible hyaloid or epiretinal membrane with attachment to the retina, and a pattern of retinal vascular leakage on FA, and must judge how significant a role the membrane plays in the retinal thickening and vascular leakage.

In some cases, findings on biomicroscopy, OCT, and FA strongly suggest a tractional component to DME (Fig. 47.10). A thickened posterior hyaloid membrane or epiretinal membrane with attachment in the area of macular edema, with or without retinal striae, may be visible on biomicroscopic examination. OCT may show a hyaloid or epiretinal membrane stretched taut over an area of retinal thickening. This membrane may appear uniformly attached to the retina, or may show multiple points of focal attachment, the latter frequently associated with focal tentings of the inner aspect of the retina. The region of macular edema may correspond closely with the area in which the membrane has attachment to the retina, and retina outside this area of attachment may be uninvolved, with an appreciable step-off in thickness at the borders of membrane attachment. Fluorescein leakage, if present, may arise diffusely from telangiectatic retinal capillaries in the region of macular edema. These features are similar to those seen in vitreomacular traction in the setting of incomplete posterior vitreous separation or epiretinal membrane formation with macular edema in nondiabetic eyes.

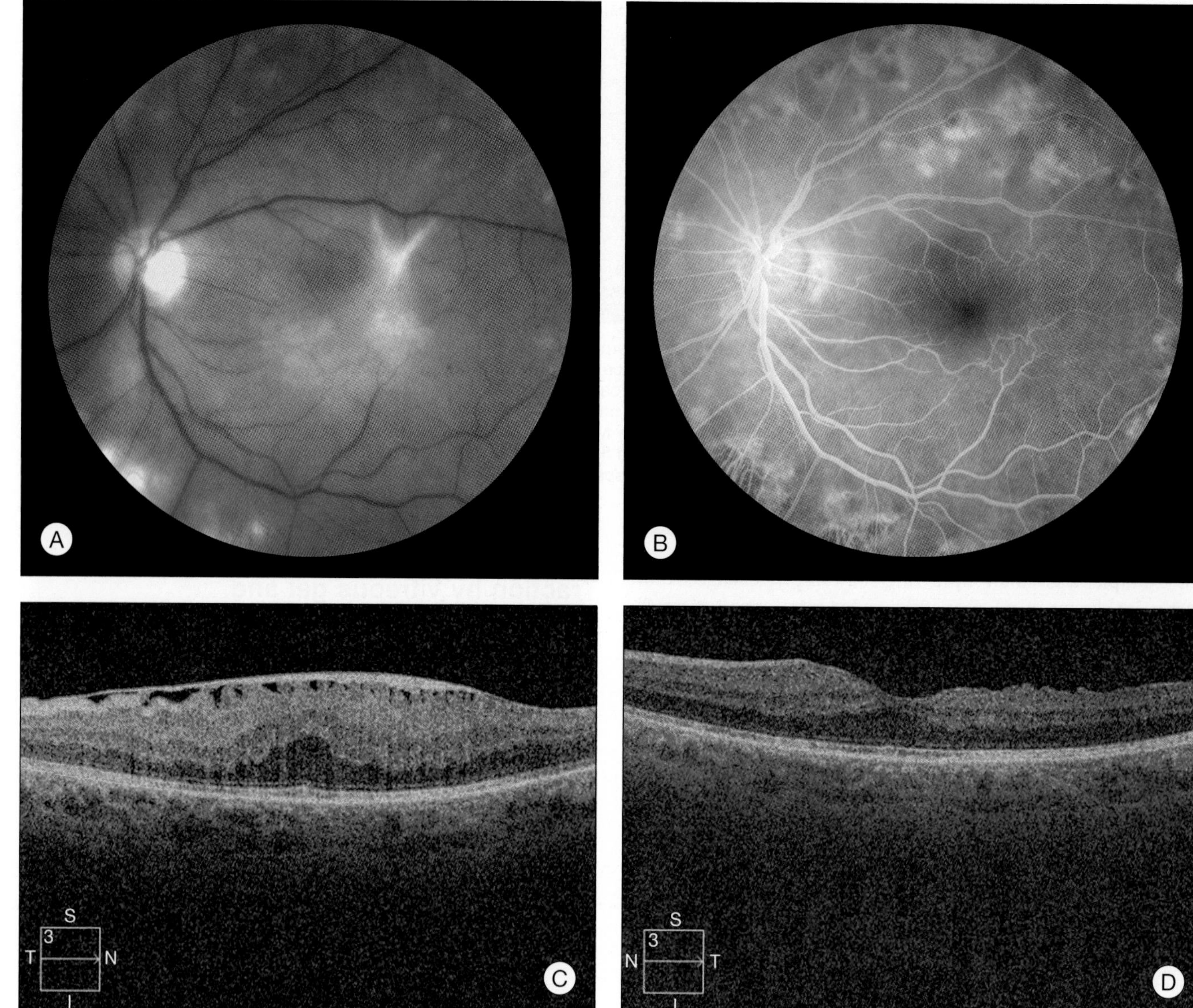

Fig. 47.10 Macular edema predominantly secondary to vitreomacular traction and epiretinal proliferation. (A) A photograph of the left macula shows a thick epiretinal membrane in a 61-year-old woman with history of PDR treated with scatter laser photocoagulation. Retinal striae are visible in the nasal macula. There was no visible separation of the posterior hyaloid on biomicroscopy. Visual acuity measured 20/80. (B) An early frame of the FA shows relatively mild microvascular alterations with only occasional microaneurysms. Later frames (not pictured) showed only very mild diffuse leakage from capillaries. (C) An OCT 6 mm horizontal line scan through the foveal center shows presence of a thick epiretinal membrane with multiple focal attachments to the retina, resulting in a serrated appearance to the inner retinal surface. Severe central thickening is present. (D) A corresponding OCT line scan following vitrectomy with membrane peeling shows relief of traction and near-resolution of retinal thickening. Intraoperative medications included subconjunctival dexamethasone and cefazolin and postoperative medications included topical prednisolone acetate 1% and moxifloxacin. No laser photocoagulation was performed. Visual acuity improved to 20/40. (National Eye Institute, Bethesda, MD.)

In other cases, a posterior hyaloid or epiretinal membrane visible on ophthalmoscopy or OCT may not appear to exert a predominant mechanical effect on the retina, and findings may suggest that retinal microvascular alterations from the metabolic disease are responsible for DME (Fig. 47.11). A subtle glistening of the vitreoretinal interface on biomicroscopy may belie the presence of the membrane, or the membrane may only be visible on OCT. A membrane visible on OCT may parallel the contour of the inner aspect of the retina with areas of attachment, but without any serrated distortion of the inner retina or retinal striae visible on biomicroscopy. The area of macular edema may exhibit a gradually tapering convexity, with or without presence of cysts, without any abrupt step-off to noninvolved areas at its borders. Biomicroscopy may show discrete microaneurysms in the area of macular edema, and FA may show areas of focal leakage from such microaneurysms or other microvascular abnormalities. Incomplete posterior vitreous separation or epiretinal membrane formation in the absence of retinal distortion or thickening in nondiabetic eyes is often compatible with normal vision. Such membranes, when present in eyes with DME, may be incidental to the macular edema associated with the retinopathy.

In many eyes with a visible membrane and at least some evidence for mechanical distortion of the retina, DME may result

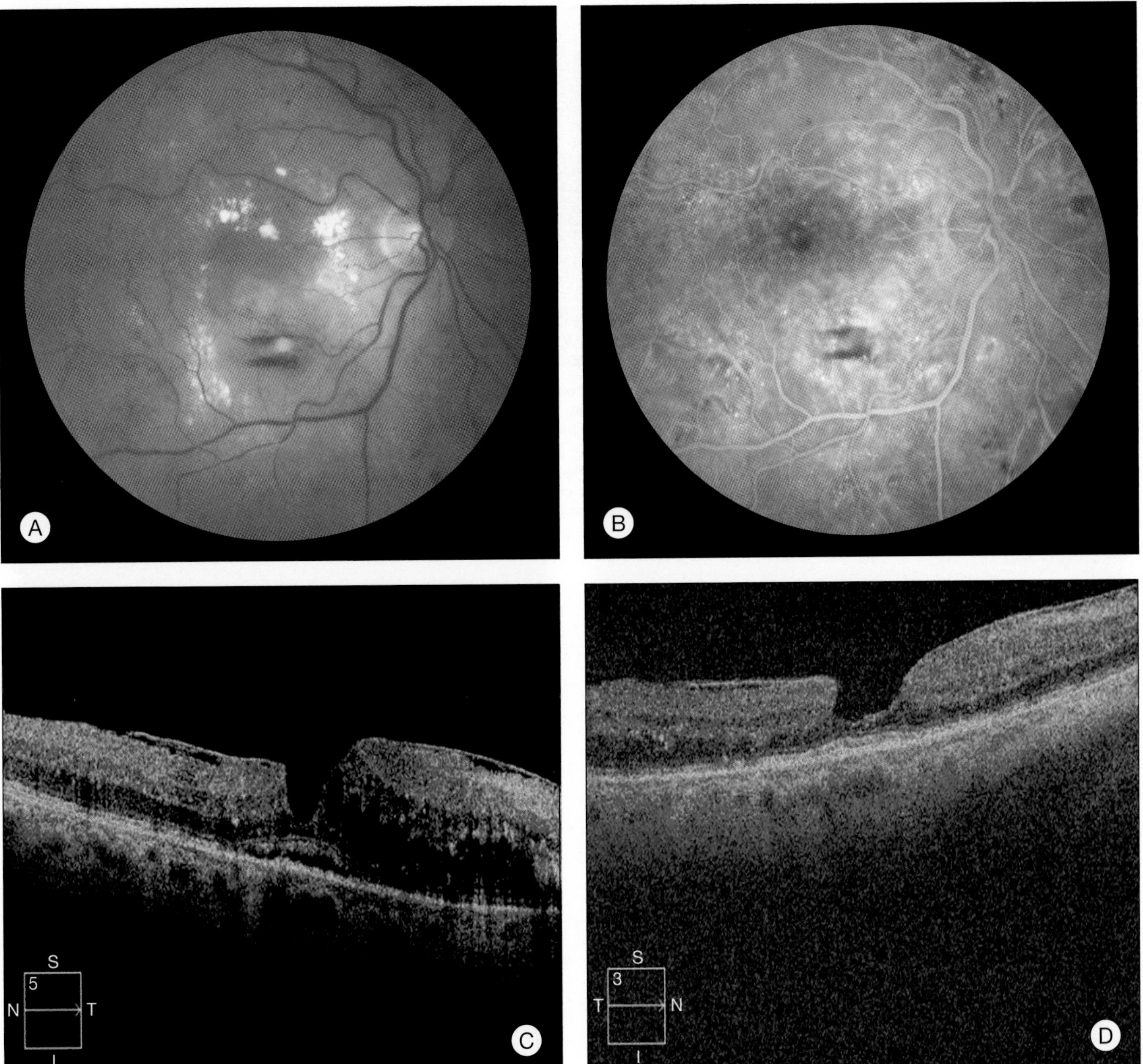

Fig. 47.11 Macular edema predominantly secondary to retinal vascular alterations from DM, with presence of an epiretinal or posterior hyaloid membrane exerting only mild mechanical effects. (A) A photograph of the right macula shows microaneurysms, intraretinal hemorrhages, cotton-wool spots, and hard exudates in a 74-year-old woman with severe NPDR. There is no visible epiretinal membrane or retinal striae formation. The pseudo-hole appearance at the foveal center is likely secondary to presence of shallow subfoveal fluid (see panel C). Visual acuity measured 20/50. (B) An early frame of the FA shows extensive vascular alterations, including presence of microaneurysms, patches of capillary nonperfusion, and microvascular abnormalities. Later frames (not pictured) showed severe leakage, most prominent in the areas of greatest retinal thickening inferonasal to the fovea. (C) An OCT 6 mm horizontal line scan through the foveal center shows presence of severe retinal thickening nasal to the fovea and mild retinal thickening temporal to the fovea, with presence of intraretinal cysts and scant subfoveal fluid. A thin epiretinal or posterior hyaloid membrane is present nasal and temporal to the foveal center. There is minimal distortion of the inner retinal surface, except at the temporal margin of the foveal depression, where an abrupt step-off in thickness suggests a local mechanical effect. (D) A corresponding OCT line scan 2 years later following treatment with multiple sessions of focal/grid laser photocoagulation, one bevacizumab injection, and one subtenon triamcinolone acetonide injection shows significant improvement in retinal thickening, with resolution of intraretinal cysts and subretinal fluid. Persistence of an abrupt step-off of the inner retinal surface at the temporal margin of the foveal depression suggests a mild local mechanical effect. No vitrectomy was performed. (National Eye Institute, Bethesda, MD.)

from a combination of tractional effects and microvascular alterations associated with the diabetic retinopathy. It may be unclear which factor predominates, and in such cases, evaluation across time can be helpful. In clinical practice, this often involves treatment of DME, starting with less-invasive nonsurgical approaches, with careful assessment of the response to treatment.

Alterations in the retinal pigment epithelium

In most eyes with untreated DME, the RPE appears normal on ophthalmoscopy, OCT, and FA. Longstanding macular edema is occasionally accompanied by pigmentary alterations or atrophy of RPE. More commonly, RPE changes reflect stigmata

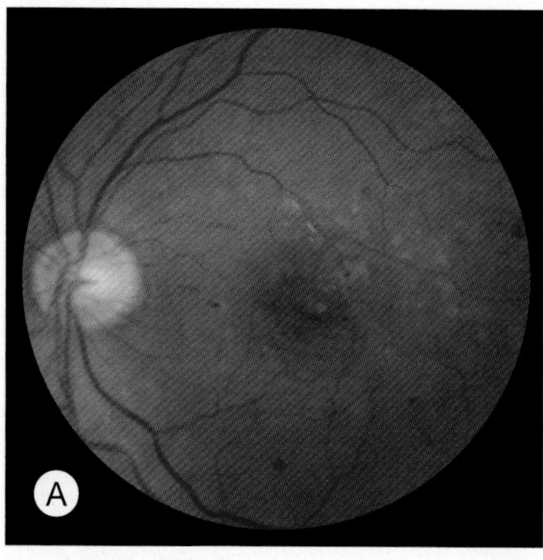

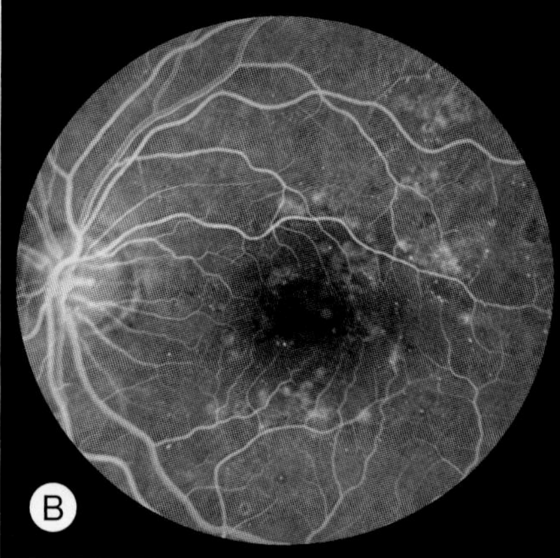

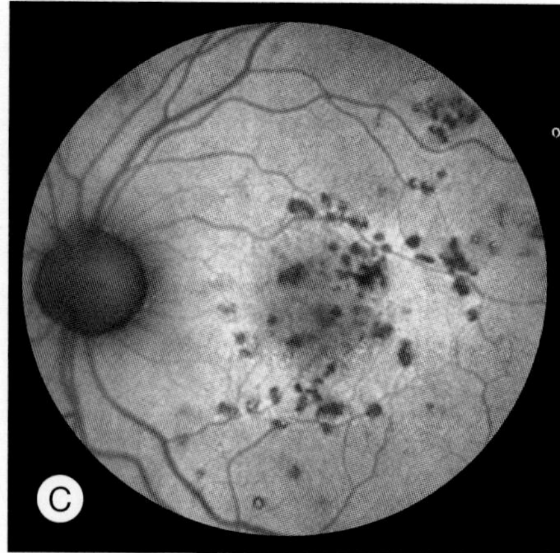

Fig. 47.12 Pigmentary alterations of the RPE secondary to laser photocoagulation. (A) Color photograph showing scattered microaneurysms and intraretinal hemorrhages in the setting of NPDR and DME previously treated with focal/grid laser photocoagulation, with focal hypo- and hyperpigmented alterations of the RPE most prominent temporal to the foveal center. (B) An early frame of the FA shows multiple circular spots of hyperfluorescence, some with hypofluorescent centers, corresponding to laser scars. Note that more laser scars are visible on the FA than on the color photograph. (C) A fundus autofluorescence photograph (modified fundus camera, single-flash, 580/700 nanometers) demonstrates circular spots of hypofluorescence, some with hyperfluorescent centers, corresponding to the same laser scars visualized by FA. Intraretinal hemorrhages also appear hypofluorescent. (National Eye Institute, Bethesda, MD.)

of previous laser photocoagulation in eyes previously treated for DME (Fig. 47.12A). Visualization of discrete laser scars on FA, not always visible on ophthalmoscopy, allows assessment of the adequacy and extent of past treatment and can be helpful in planning further therapy (Fig. 47.12B). Autofluorescence photography has recently emerged as a less invasive means of evaluating such RPE alterations, and may largely supplant angiography for this application in DME (Fig. 47.12C).[113,114]

Subretinal fibrosis

Subretinal fibrosis is an uncommon feature of DME associated with severe hard exudates or disruption of the RPE by overaggressive laser treatment. In the ETDRS, investigators identified 109 eyes with subretinal fibrosis, defined as a mound or sheet of gray-to-white tissue beneath the retina at or near the center of the macula.[115] Very severe hard exudates were present in the macula of 74% of these eyes prior to appearance of subretinal fibrosis; by comparison, exudates this severe were seen only in 2.5% of eyes with CSME that did not develop subretinal fibrosis (P <0.001). Among 264 eyes with very severe hard exudates in the macula at any time during the ETDRS, subretinal fibrosis developed in 31%, while among 5498 eyes with CSME and lesser levels of hard exudation, such fibrosis developed in only 0.05%. In the 4823 eyes that underwent laser photocoagulation for treatment of DME, only 9 eyes developed subretinal fibrosis adjacent to a laser photocoagulation scar, making this at worst a rare complication of such treatment.

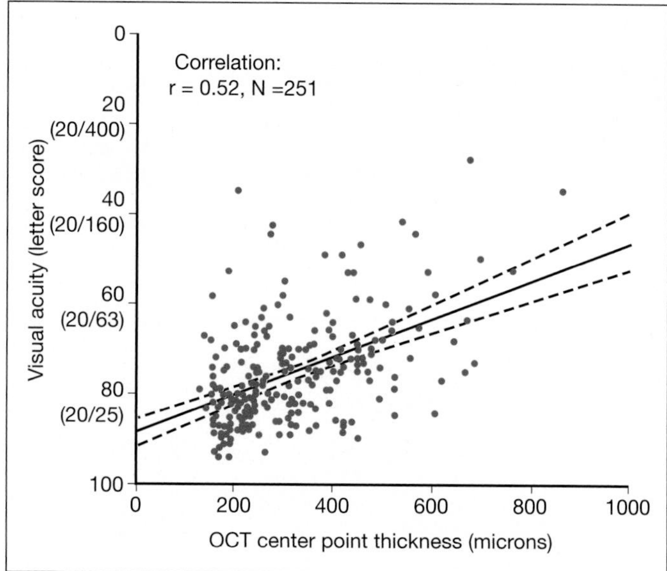

Fig. 47.13 Scatterplot comparing concurrently measured OCT center-point thickness and visual acuity at a single timepoint (baseline) in 251 eyes (210 participants) with DME in a randomized clinical trial evaluating laser techniques. The solid line represents the regression line and the dotted lines represent the 95% CI for the mean. (Adapted with permission from Diabetic Retinopathy Clinical Research Network. Relationship between optical coherence tomography-measured central retinal thickness and visual acuity in diabetic macular edema. Ophthalmology 2007;114:525–36.)

Visual acuity and its correlation to retinal thickening and fluorescein leakage

Retinal thickening that involves or threatens the fovea frequently leads to vision loss. In the ETDRS, the 3-year risk of moderate vision loss was 32% among eyes observed with CSME.[38] However, studies have shown variable but generally modest correlation between central retinal thickness and concurrently measured visual acuity.[116–124] In one study of 251 eyes of 210 participants in a randomized clinical trial evaluating laser techniques, in which vision was tested with an electronic ETDRS protocol following standardized refraction and central retinal thickening was measured using time domain OCT and evaluated by a reading center, the correlation between visual acuity and center-point thickness was 0.52 at the baseline time point (Fig. 47.13).[125] The slope of the corresponding best-fit line was 4.4 letters (95% CI 3.5–5.3) of better visual acuity for every 100 µm decrease in center-point thickness.

Fluorescein leakage on FA has low correlation with concurrently measured visual acuity. Among 422 eyes (a mix of study and nonstudy eyes) of participants in the randomized clinical trial evaluating laser techniques mentioned previously, the area of fluorescein leakage within an ETDRS macular grid was graded at baseline and correlated to several other baseline measures.[111] Correlation of the area of fluorescein leakage with visual acuity was 0.33, compared with a value of 0.38 for OCT CSMT and 0.58 for OCT total macular volume.

Diurnal variation of DME

On average, retinal thickness in DME decreases slightly during the day, but the proportion of eyes with DME exhibiting clinically meaningful changes is small. In the largest study to date, 156 eyes of 96 participants with center-involved DME on ophthalmoscopy and CSMT of 225 microns or greater were evaluated at six time points between 8am and 4pm using the Stratus OCT.[126] Two scans of adequate quality were obtained at each time point and sent to a reading center. The mean change in relative central subfield thickening, defined to represent the change in excess retinal thickness, was a decrease of 6% (95% CI −9% to −3%) between the 8am and 4pm time points. The mean absolute change was a decrease in 13 µm (95% CI −17 to −8 µm). Three percent (5 of 156) of eyes met a composite endpoint of 25% or greater decrease in relative central subfield thickening and 50 µm or greater decrease in CSMT at two consecutive time points, and 1% (2 of 156) of eyes exhibited increases in both measures by at least these amounts.

MANAGEMENT OF NONPROLIFERATIVE DIABETIC RETINOPATHY AND DIABETIC MACULAR EDEMA

Modification of systemic risk factors

Control of hyperglycemia is critical to minimizing risk of onset and progression of diabetic retinopathy. The benefits of better glycemic control in reducing risk for retinopathy progression have been demonstrated in multiple randomized controlled clinical trials, including the DCCT, EDIC study, UKPDS, and ACCORD study mentioned previously and further discussed in Chapter 45 (The epidemiology of diabetic retinopathy).[72,73,75,76,78,79] The American Diabetes Association recommends glycemic control targeting a hemoglobin A1C of 7.0% or lower for most diabetics.[127] Not only does such a target lower risk of retinopathy onset and progression, it also lowers risk of other microvascular complications of disease, such as neuropathy and nephropathy. The ACCORD study has provoked recent controversy about whether more aggressive targeting of near-normal hemoglobin A1C values is desirable.[128,129] As discussed earlier, the ACCORD study included a trial that randomly assigned 10 251 patients with type 2 DM to intensive glycemic control targeting HbA1C of less than 6% or to standard treatment targeting HbA1C between 7 and 7.9%. The glycemia trial was stopped after a median of 3.7 years because of an increase in all-cause mortality in the intensive treatment group (5% in the intensive treatment group versus 4% in the standard treatment group; hazard ratio 1.21; 95% CI 1.02–1.44).[130] Rates of hypoglycemia requiring assistance were significantly higher in the intensive treatment group than in the standard treatment group (10.5% vs 3.5%; P = 0.001), corroborating similar findings among intensively treated participants in other clinical trials of glycemic control, but the higher mortality rate noted in participants in the ACCORD study could not be readily attributed to complications of hypoglycemia. Despite evidence that aggressive targeting of near-normal glycosylated hemoglobin levels may offer benefit in reducing microvascular complications of DM, there is consensus that such an approach should be pursued cautiously based on the mortality findings of the ACCORD study.[127]

Control of hypertension is also beneficial in lowering risk of progression of diabetic retinopathy, as demonstrated in the UKPDS.[74,80] Hypertensive participants with newly diagnosed type 2 DM in the UKPDS were randomly assigned to more intensive blood pressure control (targeting a systolic blood pressure less than 150 mmHg) and less intensive blood pressure control (targeting a systolic blood pressure less than 180 mmHg) and also randomly assigned to treatment with beta-blockers or ACE inhibitors. The UKPDS showed benefit of better control of blood pressure, as discussed previously. The ACCORD study, which included a blood pressure trial that randomly assigned participants to more or less intensive control of blood pressure (targeting a systolic blood pressure less than 120 mmHg or less than 140 mmHg, respectively), did not show benefit in reducing risk of retinopathy progression in a subset of participants evaluated for eye disease.[78] While provocative, the results of the ACCORD study do not necessarily contradict the findings of the UKPDS, given the very different targets used for more and less intensive control of blood pressure between the two trials. It is possible that modest control of severe hypertension (as done in the UKPDS) lowers retinopathy progression, while very aggressive lowering of blood pressure below present standard of care (as done in the ACCORD study) lends no additional benefit. Alternatively, the disparity in findings could be attributable to differences in the study populations.

Treatment of dyslipidemia may be beneficial to retinopathy, based on consideration of observational data from studies like the WESDR and the ETDRS.[81,82] However, there is no evidence from randomized controlled clinical trials that plasma lipid-lowering reduces risk of retinopathy onset or progression, largely because persons with dyslipidemia need to lower their lipid levels to reduce the risk of cardiovascular disease, making such trials difficult or impossible. The ACCORD study, together with another randomized controlled clinical trial called the Fenofibrate Intervention and Event Lowering in Diabetes (FIELD) study, suggests a possible role for fenofibrate in reducing risk of retinopathy progression, but it is unclear whether the mechanism of action involves alteration of the plasma lipid profile.[78,84] Fenofibrate is discussed further below as a potential systemic treatment for diabetic retinopathy.

Retinopathy screening and surveillance

Sight-threatening retinopathy may not cause symptoms prompting evaluation until disease is advanced. Treatment to reduce risk of vision loss in eyes with sight-threatening complications of diabetic retinopathy is most effective when initiated before severe vision loss has occurred. These facts underpin the importance of screening and surveillance for retinopathy, but reports suggest that many diabetics do not receive eye examination on the schedule recommended by organizations such as the American Diabetes Association and the American Academy of Ophthalmology.[92,131–135] For example, an analysis of Medicare claims data for beneficiaries 65 years of age and older revealed that only between 50 and 60% of diabetics received annual eye examinations over a 15-month period.[133] In many less-developed countries the situation is much worse, with only a small fraction of diabetics receiving any eye evaluation at all.

The recommended schedule for screening and surveillance for NPDR reflects knowledge about the epidemiology and natural history of disease. Initial eye examination is recommended 3–5 years following diagnosis of type 1 DM, and at time of diagnosis for those with type 2 DM.[92] Recommended follow-up examination for type 1 and type 2 diabetics with no retinopathy is yearly. In the absence of DME, those with mild to moderate NPDR should be evaluated every 6–12 months, and those with severe NPDR should be seen every 2–4 months. Diabetics with DME merit frequent follow-up, generally at least every 2–4 months, and sometimes monthly depending on treatment. Any new ocular symptoms should prompt timely evaluation tailored to the circumstances.

In the setting of pregnancy, eye examinations are recommended prior to conception and early during the first trimester.[92] Follow-up for pregnant patients with no retinopathy, mild NPDR, or moderate NPDR should be individualized based on the severity and recent changes in retinopathy. Pregnant patients with severe NPDR should be evaluated every 1–3 months. Specific circumstances, such as presence of DME, may dictate need for more frequent follow-up.

A comprehensive eye evaluation including dilated funduscopic examination by an ophthalmologist experienced in management of diabetic eye disease remains the standard of care for retinopathy screening in areas with adequate access to ophthalmic care. However, as imaging and information-sharing technologies continue to improve, remote screening for diabetic retinopathy, such as review of digital fundus photographs acquired outside the ophthalmologist's office, may offer a cost-effective alternative. In such a model, patients manifesting findings indicative of a certain level of retinopathy and patients for whom adequate images cannot be obtained are referred to an ophthalmologist for full evaluation.[136] Such an approach has particular promise in settings where access to ophthalmic care is limited. A number of studies have demonstrated reasonable sensitivity and specificity of various remote screening platforms compared with the standard of dilated funduscopic examination by an ophthalmologist or expert evaluation of seven-field fundus photographs obtained by an ophthalmic photographer.[137–143]

Ocular treatment for diabetic macular edema

For years following the ETDRS, the standard of care for treatment of clinically significant diabetic macular edema has been focal/grid laser photocoagulation, with consideration of other measures such as vitrectomy in select circumstances. Recent studies and clinical experience with intravitreous injection of agents inhibiting the activity of vascular endothelial growth factor A (VEGF-A) isoforms, often done in combination with focal/grid laser photocoagulation, have demonstrated short-term efficacy superior to laser photocoagulation alone in certain circumstances. An expanding array of corticosteroid formulations and delivery systems has also been evaluated in recent clinical trials, adding to our knowledge about the efficacy and hazards of these medications.

Recent success of certain pharmacologic agents for treatment of DME has been exciting, but even the most informative studies raise important unsettled questions. Management algorithms for DME have been made more complex by the availability of alternatives to laser photocoagulation, resulting in decision-making individualized to a variety of factors. The value of information gained from high-quality randomized controlled clinical trials and the importance of long-term outcomes in evaluating new therapies cannot be overstated. Recent experience with use of intravitreous injection of triamcinolone acetonide for treatment of DME illustrates both points. Early clinical experience, case series, and small trials with short-term follow-up suggested significant and occasionally dramatic improvement in macular edema following intravitreous administration of triamcinolone, and the treatment gained popularity, particularly in diabetics refractory to laser photocoagulation therapy.[121,144–150] A randomized controlled clinical trial was carried out comparing focal/grid laser photocoagulation and intravitreous injections of triamcinolone acetonide (1 mg or 4 mg) for treatment of DME involving the center of the macula.[151,152] At 4 months, mean visual acuity was significantly better in eyes treated with triamcinolone (4 mg) than in eyes treated with laser photocoagulation. However, at evaluation of the primary outcome at 2 years, mean visual acuity was significantly better in eyes treated with focal laser than in eyes from either of the triamcinolone groups, a difference that could not be attributed solely to cataract progression in eyes receiving triamcinolone. The results of this trial offered critical clarification of the benefits and limitations of intravitreous triamcinolone not discernible from short-term studies and anecdotal experience.

Despite important progress in treatment, DME remains a significant cause of vision loss. This reflects shortcomings in diagnosis and treatment of DM, inadequacies in screening and surveillance of diabetic retinopathy, and limitations of present treatment for DME. Ocular therapy for DME reduces risk of future vision loss, and may improve vision, but often does not restore normal macular function or structure. In a recent randomized controlled clinical trial demonstrating some of the most significant benefits seen to date for any treatment of DME, groups gaining most vision (those treated with intravitreous injections of the VEGF antagonist ranibizumab plus prompt or deferred focal/grid laser photocoagulation) demonstrated an 8- or 9-letter mean gain in visual acuity at the 2-year visit compared with a baseline mean visual acuity of 63 letters.[153] Such results indicate that on average vision in these eyes improved from approximately 20/50– to 20/40+. At 2 years, the percentage of eyes with CSMT equal to or greater than 250 μm (using a time domain system for which normal CSMT measures approximately 200μm) was 43% in the ranibizumab plus prompt laser group and 42% in the ranibizumab plus deferred laser group, reflecting a significant number of eyes with residual macular edema despite treatment.

The ETDRS concept of clinically significant macular edema (CSME), discussed earlier in this chapter, remains relevant to management of DME. The ETDRS demonstrated that eyes with DME involving or threatening the center of vision are at high risk of vision loss,[38] and there is consensus that such eyes merit treatment to reduce the chance of further vision loss. However, eyes with clinically significant macular edema that threatens but does not involve the macular center have often been excluded from recent clinical trials, making for greater uncertainty about the best treatment options in this subset of eyes. Such eyes received focal/grid laser photocoagulation in the ETDRS, but it is not known how laser treatment compares to other therapeutic options. Likewise, recent trials have frequently excluded eyes with very good and very poor visual acuity, making evidence-based decision-making more difficult in these cases as well. Finally, as mentioned previously, the sensitivity of OCT for retinal thickening allows identification of very mild disease, often termed "subclinical" macular edema because it is not easily visible on biomicroscopy. OCT thickness parameters designated in eligibility criteria and retreatment algorithms from clinical trials indicate what threshold of thickening was considered significant enough to treat and retreat in a given study; however, such information provides no guidance on whether outcomes would have differed if other thickness thresholds had been used instead. Areas of macular thickening and hard exudate not meeting criteria for CSME can usually be observed vigilantly, with institution of treatment if CSME evolves.[38]

Attention to the context of DME is important for management. The principles of treatment of DME remain the same regardless of the underlying severity of diabetic retinopathy, but management may differ depending on the circumstances. There are special considerations for treatment of DME in the context of PDR, given the imperative to administer any necessary treatment to lower risk of vision loss from the complications of proliferative disease. Chapter 48 (Proliferative diabetic retinopathy) discusses considerations for management of DME in the setting of PDR. Other ocular conditions may impact DME or the choice of treatment. For example, postoperative cystoid macular edema may complicate DME following intraocular surgery and may warrant different treatment. Presence of glaucoma may contraindicate use of local corticosteroids. Some such considerations are included in the following discussion, but an exhaustive review is beyond the scope of this chapter.

Focal/grid laser photocoagulation

The efficacy of focal/grid laser photocoagulation for treatment of DME was established in the ETDRS,[38] though its mechanisms of action remain uncertain even two decades later. Chapter 39 (Retinal laser therapy: Biophysical basis and applications) describes the principles of ophthalmic laser therapy and discusses hypotheses about its mechanisms. The ETDRS was a landmark randomized controlled trial with a complex study design enrolling 3711 participants to test the effect of different strategies of focal/grid and scatter laser photocoagulation and the use of daily aspirin on retinopathy progression and vision loss in eyes with disease ranging from mild NPDR to early (non-high-risk) PDR.[154] At 3 years, eyes with mild or moderate NPDR plus macular edema at baseline treated with immediate focal/grid laser photocoagulation showed an approximately 50% decrease in the rate of moderate vision loss (defined as a decrease of three lines or more on a logarithmic visual acuity chart, corresponding to a doubling of the initial visual angle) compared with similar eyes randomly assigned to deferral of photocoagulation (11.2% vs 21.1%; $P < 0.001$). Eyes with severe NPDR or early PDR and macular edema at baseline treated with immediate focal/grid laser photocoagulation were concomitantly treated with immediate full or mild scatter laser, and showed reduction in moderate vision loss apparent at time points later than 3 years, reflecting an early detrimental effect of immediate scatter photocoagulation.

Treatment of eyes assigned to immediate focal/grid laser photocoagulation in the ETDRS involved argon laser application to areas of retinal thickening identified on biomicroscopy and characterized by FA.[155] Study treatment involved "direct" treatment of all microaneurysms exhibiting leakage of fluorescein dye in regions of retinal thickening between 500 and 3000 μm from the foveal center. Burn characteristics for direct treatment included size 50–100 μm, exposure 0.05–0.10 seconds, and intensity sufficient to whiten or darken large microaneurysms. The study treatment technique also included "grid" treatment applied to areas of diffuse leakage of fluorescein dye and areas of capillary nonperfusion in regions of retinal thickening between 500 and 3000 μm from the foveal center, with spacing between spots of at least one burn-width. Burn characteristics for grid treatment included size less than 200 μm, exposure 0.05–0.10 seconds, and intensity described as "mild." Eyes were assessed every 4 months, and retreatment was performed for CSME exhibiting any treatable areas. Minor effects on visual field were attributed to focal/grid laser photocoagulation, but at 4 months the occurrence of scotomata within 20 degrees of fixation identified by kinetic perimetry among eyes with mild or moderate NPDR and macular edema was similar between eyes assigned to immediate focal/grid laser photocoagulation and eyes assigned to deferral of photocoagulation.[103] More significant effects on visual field were attributed to full and mild scatter laser. Additional adverse effects of laser treatment included choroidal neovascularization and subsequent fibrosis that can occur in areas of disruption of the RPE caused by laser photocoagulation, sometimes years following the procedure, but this complication is infrequent and is often self-limited. Subretinal fibrosis was noted in proximity to a laser scar in only 9 of 4823 eyes treated with focal/grid laser photocoagulation in the ETDRS.[115]

The technique for focal/grid laser photocoagulation has evolved since the ETDRS, trending toward application of smaller, less intense burns, and less frequently making use of a fluorescein angiogram to guide treatment. Present standard technique is well summarized by parameters for "modified-ETDRS" focal/grid laser photocoagulation specified by the DRCR.net for use in its protocols (Table 47.2).[156] The development and availability of novel ophthalmic laser systems has led to extrapolation of the argon green laser parameters to other platforms. One randomized prospective study treating 171 eyes (91 participants) with modified grid laser for treatment of DME found no significant difference in visual acuity or other measures comparing the argon green laser to the diode (810 nm) laser.[157] Some uncertainty persists regarding whether other systems and techniques vary in clinically important ways from focal/grid laser photocoagulation using the argon laser.[120,158-167] The value of applying laser photocoagulation in ETDRS-style to areas of retinal thickening and fluorescein leakage was tested in a randomized DRCR.net study comparing standard modified-ETDRS technique to a novel procedure consisting of milder but more extensive burns applied throughout the macula in 323 eyes with DME involving the foveal center.[168] Standard modified-ETDRS laser resulted in significantly greater reduction in retinal thickening in CSMT on OCT compared with the modified grid treatment (adjusted mean difference, 33 μm; 95% CI 5–61 μm; $P = 0.02$). Mean change in visual acuity was similar (0 and −2 letters, respectively, 95% CI −0.5 to 5 letters; $P = 0.10$) at 12 months.

The benefits of focal/grid laser photocoagulation have been highlighted by more recent clinical trials following the ETDRS. Many of the eyes treated in the ETDRS had good visual acuity at baseline, limiting the amount of potential vision gain from any intervention; accordingly, the efficacy of laser in the treated ETDRS cohort as a whole consisted chiefly of a reduction of

Table 47.2 Modified-ETDRS focal/grid laser photocoagulation technique used by the Diabetic Retinopathy Clinical Research Network (DRCR.net)

Treatment parameter	DRCR.net technique for modified-ETDRS focal/grid laser photocoagulation
Direct treatment	Directly treat all leaking microaneurysms in areas of retinal thickening between 500 and 3000 µm from the center of the macula (although may treat between 300 and 500 µm microns of center if center-involved edema persists after initial focal photocoagulation, but generally not if the visual acuity is better than 20/40)
Change in microaneurysm color with direct treatment	Not required, but at least a mild gray-white burn should be evident beneath all microaneurysms
Spot size for direct treatment	50 µm
Burn duration for direct treatment	0.05 to 0.1 seconds
Grid treatment	Apply to all areas with edema not associated with microaneurysms; if fluorescein angiography is obtained, grid is applied to areas of edema with angiographic non-perfusion when judged indicated by the investigator
Area considered for grid treatment	500–3000 µm superiorly, nasally, and inferiorly from center of macula; 500–3500 µm temporally from macular center; no burns placed within 500 µm of disc
Burn size for grid treatment	50 µm
Burn duration for grid treatment	0.05 to 0.1 sec
Burn intensity for grid treatment	Barely visible (light gray)
Burn separation for grid treatment	Two visible burn widths apart
Wavelength (grid and direct treatment)	Green to yellow wavelengths

Use of fluorescein angiography to direct the treatment is at the discretion of the physician. Laser treatment following an injection, if needed, is based on the preinjection macular appearance. Any laser wavelength for photocoagulation within the green to yellow spectrum may be chosen. Lenses used for treatment cannot increase or reduce the burn size by more than 10%.*
**The DRCR.net provides separate guidelines for the PASCAL photocoagulation system.*
(Adapted with permission. Modified-ETDRS Focal Photocoagulation Technique accessed at http://publicfiles.jaeb.org/drcrnet/Misc/FocalGridProcedure42711.pdf.)

vision loss. However, in an ETDRS subgroup of 114 eyes with thickening of the foveal center, visual acuity worse than 20/32, and mild or moderate NPDR treated with immediate focal/grid laser photocoagulation in the ETDRS, change in mean visual acuity from baseline at two years was +4 letters, with 29% of eyes improving 10 letters or more. By comparison, in a subset of 235 eyes meeting the same baseline criteria for which laser was deferred, change in mean visual acuity from baseline at two years was –6 letters, with 12% improving 10 letters or more (Ferris FL, unpublished data, 2008). Recent trials enrolling eyes with more advanced disease corroborate the suggestion that the benefits of focal/grid laser photocoagulation may exceed those demonstrated in the treated ETRS cohort as a whole. In the previously mentioned study comparing focal/grid laser photocoagulation to injection of intravitreous triamcinolone, which enrolled 840 eyes with visual acuity of 20/40 to 20/320 with retinal thickening involving the center of the fovea and a range of underlying diabetic retinopathy, the 330 eyes randomly assigned to laser treatment showed a change in mean visual acuity of +1 letter (standard deviation, ±17 letters) at 2 years, with improvement of 15 letters or more in 18% of laser-treated eyes.[151] In another recent study comparing focal/grid laser photocoagulation alone to intravitreous injection of ranibizumab or triamcinolone acetonide combined with laser treatment in eyes with center-involved DME and baseline visual acuity of 20/32 to 20/320, the change in mean visual acuity at 2 years was +3 letters (standard deviation, ±15 letters) in 211 eyes treated with focal/grid laser photocoagulation alone.[169]

Although focal/grid laser photocoagulation mitigates the morbidity of DME, it is often insufficient to restore normal vision or completely resolve macular edema. Requirement for multiple treatments is common. Even with retreatment, a significant proportion of eyes continue to manifest residual DME. In the aforementioned DRCR.net trial testing focal/grid laser photocoagulation alone versus intravitreous injection of ranibizumab or triamcinolone acetonide plus laser, eyes treated with laser alone manifested a median CSMT of 266 µm at 2 years, representing a median improvement of 113 µm.[169] However, this represents an appreciable amount of residual thickening compared with normal CSMT (approximately 200 µm). Only 39% of eyes in the laser group achieved a CSMT of less than 250 µm with at least a 25 µm decrease in thickness from baseline. Ten percent of eyes treated with laser alone lost 15 or more letters of visual acuity at 2 years from baseline.

Pharmacotherapy with vascular endothelial growth factor (VEGF) antagonists

VEGF-A has been demonstrated to exert potent effects on retinal vascular permeability, and concentrations of certain VEGF-A isoforms in the retina and vitreous are elevated in diabetic retinopathy.[40,41,170] Various VEGF antagonists have been developed for ophthalmic and nonophthalmic uses, including bevacizumab, a humanized murine monoclonal antibody binding VEGF-A; ranibizumab, a humanized murine monoclonal antibody fragment, also binding VEGF-A; pegaptanib sodium, an aptamer specifically inhibiting the VEGF-A 165 isoform; and aflibercept, a human fusion protein incorporating ligand-binding elements from VEGF receptors and the Fc region of an IgG1 molecule. Intravenous administration for ophthalmic disease has been studied for some agents,[171–173] but intravitreous injection has rapidly become the most common mode of delivery to the eye following seminal clinical trials in neovascular age-related macular degeneration and recent clinical experience demonstrating a reasonable safety profile. Following demonstration of efficacy in neovascular age-related macular degeneration, choroidal neovascularization from other causes, and macular edema following retinal vein occlusion, various VEGF antagonists have been evaluated for treatment of DME in a number of small studies with short-term follow-up.[174–180] Encouraging results have led to several larger clinical trials.

The first major clinical trial to report results was designed by DRCR.net investigators to compare four strategies for treatment of DME including focal/grid laser photocoagulation alone, intravitreous injection of ranibizumab (0.5 mg) with deferral of early laser, intravitreous injection of ranibizumab (0.5 mg) with early laser, and intravitreous injection of triamcinolone acetonide (4 mg) with early laser.[153,169] A total of 854 eyes of 691 participants with DME involving the center of the fovea and visual acuity of 20/32 to 20/320 were randomly assigned to one of four treatments. The main outcome measure, best-corrected visual acuity, was evaluated at one year, with follow-up planned for 3 years. Eyes in a prompt laser plus sham injection group received modified-ETDRS focal/grid laser photocoagulation within 3–10 days following sham injection. Those in a ranibizumab plus prompt laser group were given an intravitreous injection of ranibizumab followed by focal/grid laser photocoagulation within 3–10 days. Those in a ranibizumab and deferred laser group received intravitreous injection of ranibizumab as required by protocol without any laser treatment for at least 24 weeks. Finally, those in a triamcinolone plus prompt laser were given an intravitreous injection of a preservative-free formulation of triamcinolone acetonide followed by focal/grid laser photocoagulation within 3–10 days. Retreatment algorithms were complex, but were generally intended to require further therapy in eyes with residual disease in order to maximize treatment effects in the first year. Focal/grid laser photocoagulation was repeated as often as every 13 weeks, ranibizumab was readministered as frequently as every 4 weeks, and triamcinolone acetonide was reinjected as often as every 16 weeks. At one year, mean change in visual acuity was significantly better in the ranibizumab plus prompt laser (+9 letters) and ranibizumab and deferred laser (+9 letters) groups compared with the prompt laser plus sham injection group (+3 letters; both P <0.001). Mean change in visual acuity was not significantly different from the prompt laser plus sham injection group in the triamcinolone plus prompt laser group (+4 letters; P = 0.31). Results at 2 years were similar (Fig. 47.14). Median number of injections in the first year was 8 in the ranibizumab plus prompt laser group, 9 in the ranibizumab and deferred laser group, and 3 in the triamcinolone plus prompt laser group. Median number of laser treatments in the first year in these groups was 2, 0, and 2, respectively, compared with 3 in the prompt laser plus sham injection group. Median number of injections in the second year in these groups decreased to 2, 3, and 1, respectively. There were 3 cases of postinjection endophthalmitis among 3973 ranibizumab injections (0.08%; 95% CI 0.02–0.22%), and 1 case of progression of pre-existing tractional retinal detachment in the ranibizumab and deferred laser group. There were no significant differences in rates of systemic adverse events between groups, and specifically no increase in cardiovascular or cerebrovascular events in the ranibizumab groups.

The results of this study have established a role for ranibizumab in treatment of DME, and have already been supplemented by findings from other trials, including one-year results of a small randomized controlled trial evaluating use of intravitreous bevacizumab.[181–183] The RESTORE study randomly assigned 345 participants with DME and visual acuity of 20/32 to 20/160 to intravitreous injection of ranibizumab (0.5 mg) and sham laser, injection of ranibizumab (0.5 mg) and focal/grid laser photocoagulation, or sham injection and focal/grid laser photocoagulation.[182] Participants received ranibizumab or sham injections monthly for 3 months, then as needed according to retreatment criteria; participants received laser photocoagulation at baseline and then as needed as often as every 3 months at the discretion of investigators. At 12 months, the mean change in visual acuity in the group getting ranibizumab alone (+6.1 letters) and in the group getting ranibizumab plus laser (+5.9 letters) was significantly better compared with the group getting laser alone (+0.8 letters; both P <0.0001). The BOLT study randomly assigned 80 eyes of 80 participants with DME involving the foveal center and visual acuity of 20/40 to 20/200 to intravitreous injection of bevacizumab (1.25 mg) or modified-ETDRS focal/grid laser photocoagulation.[183] Participants getting bevacizumab received three injections spaced apart by 6 weeks each, followed by repeat injections every 6 weeks as needed according to retreatment criteria. Participants getting laser treatment received focal/grid laser photocoagulation at baseline and as often as every 4 months thereafter as needed based on ETDRS guidelines. At 12 months, the mean change in visual acuity was significantly better in bevacizumab group (+5.6 letters) than in the laser group (–4.6 letters; P = 0.0006). The results from these studies should soon be supplemented by longer-term follow-up data and findings from other large clinical trials presently underway.

A host of new questions heralds the beginning of what will probably be a period of rapid evolution in treatment paradigms involving VEGF antagonists for DME. What will long-term follow-up of eyes receiving ranibizumab injections reveal? Can we identify factors that reliably predict which eyes stand to benefit most or least from treatment? What retreatment criteria are sensible in different circumstances? What should be the role of focal/grid laser photocoagulation relative to pharmacotherapy in a variety of circumstances? Does treatment with bevacizumab or other VEGF antagonists yield results appreciably different from those of ranibizumab? Can we devise methods superior to frequent intravitreous injection for drug delivery to the retina? Can we identify other pharmacotherapies that complement anti-VEGF treatment and allow better treatment of residual macular edema?

Pharmacotherapy with corticosteroids

Corticosteroids have immune modulatory and antiangiogenic properties and have been utilized for treatment of ophthalmic disease since the 1950s.[184–189] Common adverse effects, including hyperglycemia and other metabolic alterations difficult to manage in the setting of DM, limit their long-term systemic use, but a number of formulations allowing local delivery to the eye have been developed. The poor intraocular penetration of existing topical preparations makes them unsuitable for treatment of most retinal diseases, but injectable corticosteroids and sustained-release formulations for intraocular use have been evaluated for efficacy in DME.

Our most definitive knowledge about intravitreous injection of triamcinolone acetonide for treatment of DME comes from two randomized controlled clinical trials conducted by the DRCR.net.[151,152,153,169] The first study enrolled 840 eyes of 693 participants with DME involving the foveal center and visual acuity of 20/32 to 20/320, with a primary outcome measure of mean change in best-corrected visual acuity at two years.[151,152]

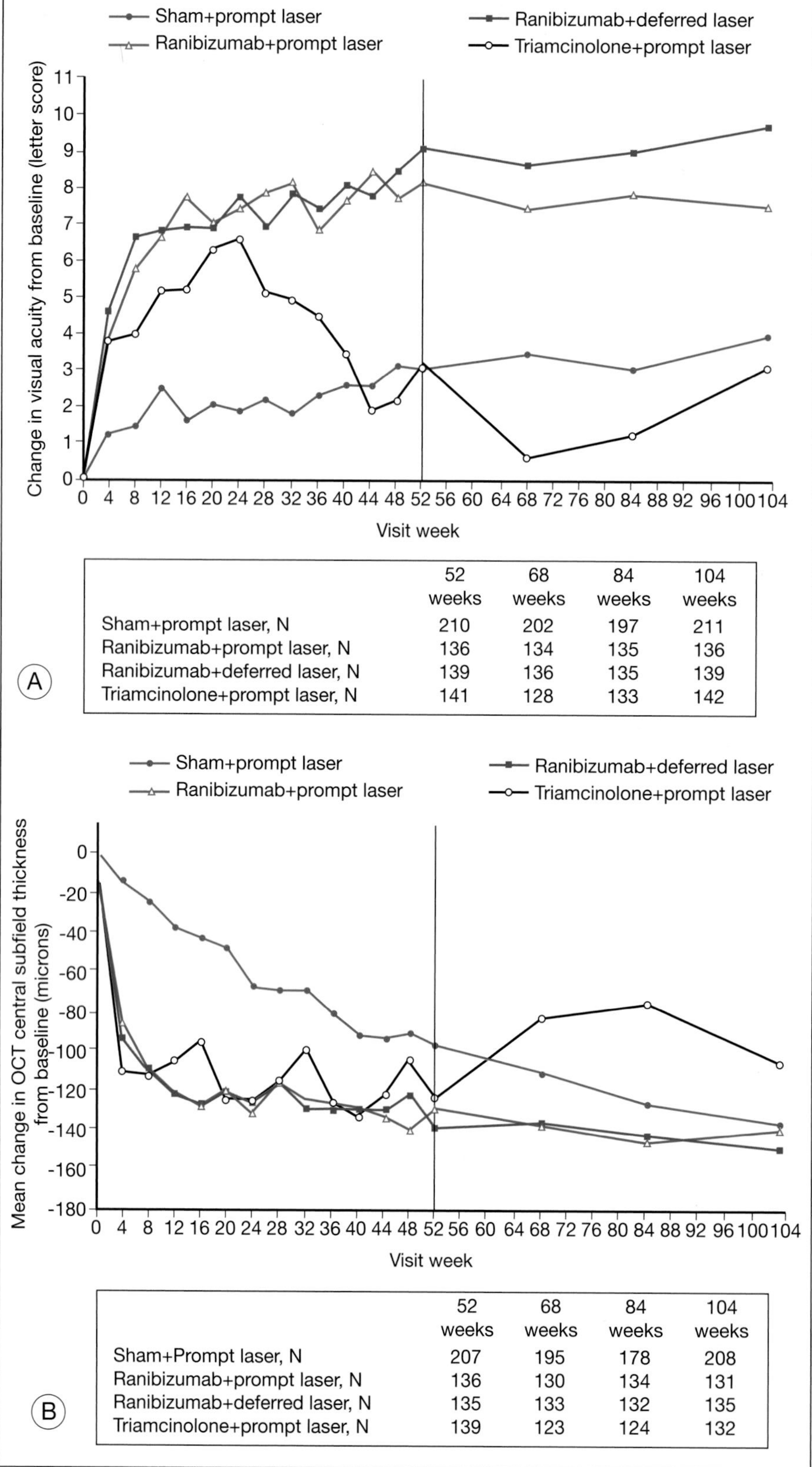

	52 weeks	68 weeks	84 weeks	104 weeks
Sham+prompt laser, N	210	202	197	211
Ranibizumab+prompt laser, N	136	134	135	136
Ranibizumab+deferred laser, N	139	136	135	139
Triamcinolone+prompt laser, N	141	128	133	142

	52 weeks	68 weeks	84 weeks	104 weeks
Sham+Prompt laser, N	207	195	178	208
Ranibizumab+prompt laser, N	136	130	134	131
Ranibizumab+deferred laser, N	135	133	132	135
Triamcinolone+prompt laser, N	139	123	124	132

Fig. 47.14 Two-year results of a randomized clinical trial of 854 eyes (691 participants) evaluating intravitreous injection of ranibizumab (0.5 mg) or triamcinolone acetonide (4 mg) combined with focal/grid laser photocoagulation compared to focal/grid laser photocoagulation alone for treatment of DME. The primary outcome was measured at 52 weeks (corresponding to vertical line on graphs). (A) Mean change in visual acuity at follow-up visits for cohort that completed 2-year visit. Values that were ±30 or more letters were assigned a value of 30. P values for difference in mean change in visual acuity from sham+prompt laser at the 104-week study visit: ranibizumab+prompt laser = 0.03, ranibizumab+deferred laser <0.001, and triamcinolone+prompt laser = 0.35. (B) Mean change in OCT mean central subfield thickness at follow-up visits for cohort that completed 2-year visit. P values for difference in mean change in OCT mean central subfield thickness from sham+prompt laser at the 104-week visit: ranibizumab+prompt laser = 0.003, ranibizumab+deferred laser = 0.01, and triamcinolone+prompt laser = 0.37. (Adapted with permission from Elman MJ, Bressler NM, Qin H, et al. Expanded 2-year follow-up of ranibizumab plus prompt or deferred laser or triamcinolone plus prompt laser for diabetic macular edema. Ophthalmology 2011;118:609–14.)

Eyes were randomly assigned to receive modified-ETDRS focal/grid laser photocoagulation, intravitreous injection of triamcinolone acetonide (1 mg), or intravitreous injection of triamcinolone acetonide (4 mg), both corticosteroid arms utilizing a preservative-free formulation of the drug. Persistent or new macular edema was retreated every 4 months. Mean change in visual acuity at two years was significantly better in laser-treated eyes (+1 letter) than in eyes receiving 1 mg triamcinolone (–2 letters; P = 0.02) and likewise significantly better than in eyes receiving 4 mg triamcinolone (–3 letters; P = 0.002). The mean number of treatments over two years was 2.9 in the laser group, 3.5 in the 1 mg triamcinolone group, and 3.1 in the 4 mg triamcinolone group. Corticosteroids are well-known to promote cataract and to elevate intraocular pressure in some eyes, and such effects were carefully documented in this study. Cataract surgery was performed in 13% of eyes in the laser group, 23% of eyes in the 1 mg triamcinolone group, and 51% of eyes in the 4 mg triamcinolone group by two years. Intraocular pressure elevation of 10 mmHg or more from baseline at any study visit was noted in 4, 16, and 33% of eyes in the three groups, respectively, by two years. There were no cases of endophthalmitis or inflammatory pseudoendophthalmitis among 1649 intravitreous injections. Addressing whether cataract formation obscured benefit of treatment of DME in eyes treated with corticosteroids, subgroup analysis of 145 eyes pseudophakic at baseline was performed and at two years showed mean change in visual acuity of +2 letters in the laser group, +2 letters in the 1 mg triamcinolone group, and –1 in the 4 mg triamcinolone group. Investigators judged that the superiority of focal/grid laser photocoagulation could not be explained solely by cataract progression in triamcinolone-injected groups. This conclusion was supported by data on change in retinal thickness. At 2 years, mean improvement in CSMT was significantly greater in the laser group (139 µm) compared with the 1 mg triamcinolone group (86 µm; P <0.001) and the 4 mg triamcinolone group (77 µm; P <0.001).

The other study, already discussed above in the section "Pharmacotherapy with VEGF antagonists," compared a combination of intravitreous injection of preservative-free triamcinolone (4 mg) and focal/grid laser photocoagulation to three other strategies, including focal/grid laser photocoagulation alone, intravitreous injection of ranibizumab plus early focal/grid laser photocoagulation, and intravitreous injection of ranibizumab and deferral of early laser.[153,169] At the primary endpoint of one year, mean change in visual acuity was not significantly different in the triamcinolone plus laser group (+4 letters) compared with the prompt laser plus sham injection group (+3 letters; P = 0.31). However, subgroup analysis of eyes pseudophakic at baseline showed a trend toward benefit in the triamcinolone plus laser group comparable to that seen in ranibizumab groups and superior to that seen in the laser group (Fig. 47.15). Investigators judged that cataract formation, cataract surgery, or both may have adversely impacted benefit of combination therapy with intravitreous injection of triamcinolone and focal/grid laser photocoagulation in phakic eyes. Taken together, the results of these two trials suggest that while monotherapy with intravitreous injection of triamcinolone acetonide is inferior to monotherapy with focal/grid laser photocoagulation, the combination of the two treatments in pseudophakic eyes might possibly be superior to laser alone.

Sustained-release devices designed for intraocular delivery of fluocinolone acetonide and dexamethasone have been developed and tested for various ophthalmic applications, including treatment of DME. The first to achieve wide clinical use was the fluocinolone acetonide intravitreal implant (Retisert, Bausch & Lomb, Rochester, NY), consisting of a 0.59 mg pellet embedded in a nonbiodegradable scaffold designed to be implanted in the vitreous cavity via a sclerotomy and anchored by a suture to the eye wall. The Retisert, which releases drug at steady state between 0.3 and 0.4µg/day for approximately 30 months, has been used most commonly for treatment of chronic non-infectious posterior uveitis.[190–193] Though small studies were initiated for treatment of DME, the requirement for incisional surgery and the high rates of cataract progression and intraocular pressure

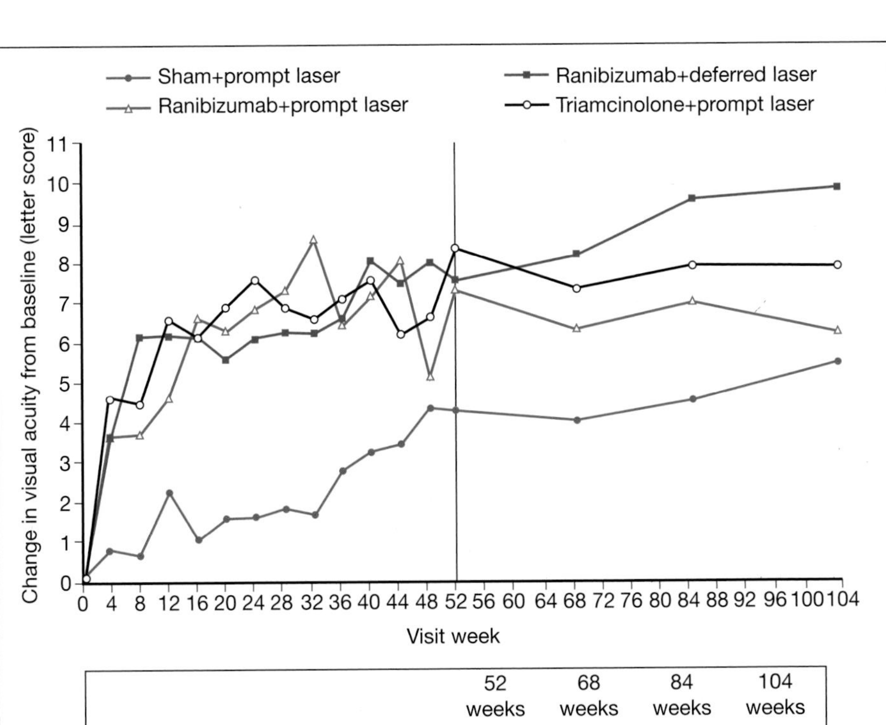

	52 weeks	68 weeks	84 weeks	104 weeks
Sham+Prompt laser, N	78	75	73	78
Ranibizumab+Prompt laser, N	41	41	41	41
Ranibizumab+deferred laser, N	40	40	40	40
Triamcinolone+Prompt laser, N	46	43	42	47

Fig. 47.15 Two-year mean change in visual acuity for eyes pseudophakic at baseline in a randomized clinical trial evaluating intravitreous injection of ranibizumab (0.5 mg) or triamcinolone acetonide (4 mg) combined with focal/grid laser photocoagulation compared to focal/grid laser photocoagulation alone for treatment of DME. The primary outcome was measured at 52 weeks (corresponding to vertical line on graph). Values that were ±30 or more letters were assigned a value of 30. P values for difference in mean change in visual acuity from sham+prompt laser at the 104-week study visit: ranibizumab+prompt laser = 0.83, ranibizumab+deferred laser = 0.15, and triamcinolone+prompt laser groups = 0.53. (Adapted with permission from Elman MJ, Bressler NM, Qin H, et al. Expanded 2-year follow-up of ranibizumab plus prompt or deferred laser or triamcinolone plus prompt laser for diabetic macular edema. Ophthalmology 2011;118:609–14.)

elevation associated with the device have limited its use for this indication.[194]

An intravitreous insert (Iluvien, Alimera Sciences, Alpharetta, GA) releasing stable quantities of fluocinolone acetonide for at least a year, consisting of a non-biodegradable cylinder (3.5×0.37 mm) containing the same polymer matrix as the Retisert implant and introduced into the vitreous cavity via injection by 25-gauge needle, was recently evaluated for treatment of DME in a large randomized controlled clinical trial.[195] Statistically significant benefit was demonstrated at 2 years for inserts releasing 0.2 and 0.5µg/day compared with sham injection in a study design that involved use of "rescue" focal/grid laser photocoagulation for persistent macular edema in all three groups. Progression of cataract and elevation of intraocular pressure were common in eyes receiving steroid inserts. Visual gain in eyes receiving inserts was greater in those that were pseudophakic at baseline and similar in magnitude to benefit seen in eyes treated with intravitreous triamcinolone and prompt focal/grid laser photocoagulation in the DRCR.net trial.

A dexamethasone intravitreous implant (Ozurdex, Allergan, Irvine, CA) consisting of a biodegradable pellet releasing high levels of drug for approximately 60 days and delivered via surgical sclerotomy or 22-gauge needle-injector system has been evaluated in a randomized clinical trial for macular edema.[196] Two versions, a 350 µg and 700 µg version, were tested for efficacy in 171 eyes with DME comprising a subgroup of a short-term larger study also enrolling eyes with macular edema secondary to branch and central retinal vein occlusion, uveitis, and cataract surgery. At the primary endpoint at 90 days, the percentage of eyes gaining 10 or more letters was significantly higher in the dexamethasone 700 µg microgram implant group than in the observation group (33% vs 12%; $P = 0.007$).

Although there is ample evidence for benefit of various corticosteroids in treatment of DME, none has shown superiority to focal/grid laser photocoagulation or intravitreous injection of VEGF antagonists when used as monotherapy. However, these medications show promise as components of combination therapy, particularly in the setting of DME refractory to other therapies and in the setting of pseudophakia. The need for less frequent administration is a present advantage over monthly intravitreous injection of ranibizumab or bevacizumab, but frequent follow-up is still necessary to monitor for intraocular pressure elevation and glaucoma.

Vitrectomy

A number of small case series have reported benefit of vitrectomy in the setting of demonstrable vitreomacular traction and epiretinal proliferation in DME.[197-200] Differences in patient populations, definition of clinically significant vitreoretinal traction, surgical approach, use of laser and medications as adjunct treatment, outcome measures, and follow-up, alongside the customary limitations and biases of retrospective studies, make it difficult to assess the efficacy of surgery. A noncontrolled prospective study representing one of the largest series published to date evaluated vitrectomy for 87 eyes with DME and evidence for vitreomacular traction as judged by the investigator.[201] Intervention was nonstandardized, with vitrectomy variably accompanied by epiretinal membrane peeling, internal limiting membrane peeling, use of scatter laser, and injection of corticosteroids. At the primary endpoint at 6 months, visual acuity improved by 10 letters or more in 38% (95% CI 28–49%) and worsened by 10 letters or more in 22% (95% CI 13–31%). Adverse events included endophthalmitis in one eye, retinal detachment in 3 eyes, vitreous hemorrhage in 5 eyes, and elevated intraocular pressure necessitating treatment in 7 eyes.

Results of case series evaluating vitrectomy for DME even in the absence of any visible vitreoretinal traction have been mixed, with some reports suggesting efficacy and others not.[202-210] Two very small randomized trials showed no evidence for significant benefit.[211,212] In the absence of any data from large, well-designed clinical trials, efficacy remains uncertain at best, and, weighed against well-known risks of surgery, does not typically warrant vitrectomy for this indication alone. The possibility of benefit is presently most relevant to surgical decision-making in PDR, in which treatment of DME is undertaken simultaneously with surgical management of fibrovascular proliferation, vitreous hemorrhage, and retinal detachment. The role for surgery in management of PDR is discussed in Chapter 111 (Surgery for proliferative diabetic retinopathy).

Ocular treatment for nonproliferative diabetic retinopathy

Various local therapies have been evaluated for their effects on altering the course of NPDR. The efficacy of scatter laser photocoagulation for reduction of severe vision loss among eyes with advanced retinopathy (severe NPDR and PDR) was established in the Diabetic Retinopathy Study.[213] The ETDRS was designed partly to clarify the optimal point during the course of retinopathy for administration of scatter laser photocoagulation. In the ETDRS, eyes were randomly assigned to early laser photocoagulation or deferral of laser treatment. Eyes were categorized according to presence or absence of macular edema and according to severity of retinopathy, and further randomly assigned to various laser strategies in a complex study design. In addition to testing the effects of focal/grid laser photocoagulation for macular edema, the ETDRS also evaluated the effects of immediate "mild" and "full" scatter photocoagulation in eyes with more severe retinopathy (severe NPDR and non-high-risk PDR) with and without macular edema and delayed mild and full scatter photocoagulation in eyes with less severe retinopathy and macular edema. At 5 years, the rate of severe vision loss (defined as visual acuity less than 5/200 at two consecutive visits) was low in eyes receiving early laser treatment (2.6%) and in those with deferral of laser (3.7%) (Fig. 47.16).[103] Rates of severe vision loss in the subset of eyes with mild or moderate NPDR were even lower. On the basis of these findings, ETDRS investigators recommended against scatter laser photocoagulation for mild and moderate NPDR, provided that adequate follow-up could be anticipated. They suggested consideration of scatter laser photocoagulation for severe NPDR and non-high risk PDR, with potential benefit balanced against adverse effects of laser on visual acuity and visual fields. The use of scatter laser photocoagulation in diabetic retinopathy is further discussed in Chapter 48 (Proliferative diabetic retinopathy).

There is preliminary evidence suggesting that local administration of VEGF antagonists or corticosteroids for treatment of DME may also benefit the course of NPDR. In the aforementioned DRCR.net study comparing various strategies of focal/grid laser photocoagulation and intravitreous administration of ranibizumab or triamcinolone acetonide combined with laser for treatment of DME, ranibizumab- and triamcinolone-treated eyes

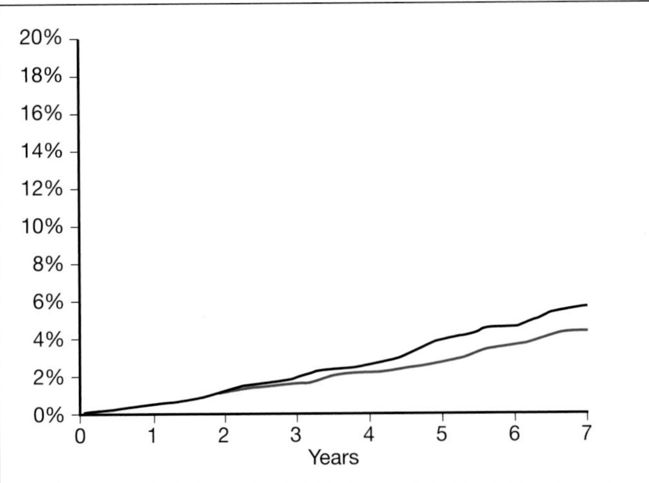

Fig. 47.16 Life table cumulative event rates of severe vision loss in all eyes assigned to immediate laser photocoagulation (blue) or deferral of laser photocoagulation (black) in the ETDRS. (Adapted with permission from Early Treatment Diabetic Retinopathy Study Research Group. ETDRS report number 9. Early photocoagulation for diabetic retinopathy. Ophthalmology 1991;98(5 Suppl):766–85.)

appeared less likely to exhibit progression of retinopathy and more likely to exhibit improvement of retinopathy than eyes treated with focal/grid laser photocoagulation alone, as assessed by reading-center evaluation of fundus photographs taken at baseline and one year.[153,169] The trend in most subgroups was not statistically significant. Ranibizumab- and triamcinolone-treated eyes were significantly less likely to manifest vitreous hemorrhage or receive scatter laser photocoagulation during the first year than eyes treated with focal/grid laser photocoagulation alone. A similar exploratory analysis was performed on data from the DRCR.net study comparing focal/grid laser photocoagulation to intravitreous injection of triamcinolone acetonide (1 mg or 4 mg), with worsening of retinopathy defined as a composite measure including evidence of progression on fundus photographs evaluated by a reading center, any documentation of vitreous hemorrhage, or receipt of scatter laser photocoagulation.[214] At 2 years, the cumulative probability of retinopathy progression was significantly lower in the 4 mg triamcinolone group (21%) but not in the 1 mg triamcinolone group (29%) compared with the laser group (31%; P = 0.005 and P = 0.64, respectively). Such preliminary findings are intriguing, but merit more definitive investigation to characterize any benefit and its clinical significance.

Other systemic treatment for nonproliferative diabetic retinopathy

Antiplatelet agents have been evaluated for treatment of diabetic retinopathy in a few randomized controlled clinical trials. In a 3-year study, 475 participants with early retinopathy were randomly assigned to daily aspirin, aspirin plus dipyridamole, or placebo, and progression of retinopathy was measured as the change in the number of microaneurysms visualized on FA.[215] The annual increase in macroaneurysms was significantly greater in the placebo group than in the treatment groups, but the growth rate was low (less than two microaneurysm per year) in all groups. In an analogous 3-year study involving 435 participants randomly assigned to daily ticlopidine or placebo, the annual increase in microaneurysms was greater in the placebo group than in the treatment group in an analysis that showed low appearance rates and borderline statistical significance.[216] Neither study showed a change in severity level of retinopathy, and the clinical significance of differences in microaneurysm counts remains uncertain.

The most definitive evidence for effects of antiplatelet therapy comes from the ETDRS, in which 3711 participants were randomly assigned to aspirin (650 mg per day) or placebo. Eyes assigned to deferral of laser photocoagulation were assessed for the effects of aspirin on progression of diabetic retinopathy. Aspirin use did not affect the severity of retinopathy or the risk of visual loss over 7 years.[217] Aspirin use did not increase the incidence, severity, or duration of preretinal or vitreous hemorrhage in eyes with deferral of photocoagulation or in eyes randomly assigned to early laser treatment.[217,218] Participants randomly assigned to aspirin exhibited a 17% reduction in morbidity and mortality from cardiovascular disease compared with participants receiving placebo, corroborating benefits seen in other studies. Aspirin remains an important therapy for control of cardiovascular risk in many diabetics, and no level of retinopathy severity, including PDR, should contraindicate its use. The ETDRS results apply to persons with significant diabetic retinopathy, and some uncertainty remains about any effects of antiplatelet agents in very mild NPDR.

Sorbinil, an inhibitor of the enzyme aldose reductase, which catalyzes the conversion of glucose to sorbitol, was evaluated in a randomized controlled clinical trial following animal studies, suggesting that these drugs might slow the development of diabetic retinopathy.[7,11,12] The Sorbinil Retinopathy Trial randomized 497 participants with type 1 DM and mild or no retinopathy to sorbinil or placebo.[219] The percentage of participants showing significant progression of diabetic retinopathy, defined as a two-step or greater change in the ETDRS diabetic retinopathy severity scale on fundus photographs, was not significantly different between the two groups after 3–4 years of follow-up.

Inhibitors targeting the protein kinase C family, which is implicated in VEGF-mediated vasopermeability and endothelin-mediated vasoconstriction in animal models of diabetic retinopathy,[220-223] have been developed and evaluated for effects on diabetic retinopathy. Ruboxistaurin, an inhibitor of beta-isoforms of protein kinase C, has been evaluated in two randomized controlled clinical trials. In the first, which randomly assigned 252 participants with moderate to very severe NPDR to receive ruboxistaurin or placebo for 36–46 months, rates of retinopathy progression were not significantly different between groups, but participants taking ruboxistaurin (32 mg/day) showed a significant delay in time to moderate vision loss (doubling of the visual angle) compared with those taking placebo (P = 0.038).[224] In a second larger study, 685 participants with moderate to very severe NPDR were randomly assigned to ruboxistaurin or placebo and evaluated at 3 years for rates of sustained moderate vision loss, defined as decrease in ETDRS visual acuity score of 15 letters or more (doubling of the visual angle) for 6 months or longer.[225] The rate of sustained moderate vision loss was significantly lower in the ruboxistaurin group (5.5%) than in the placebo group (9.1%), representing a 40% risk reduction (P = 0.034). Focal/grid laser photocoagulation was initiated 26% less frequently among those treated with ruboxistaurin than among those receiving placebo (P = 0.008). There was no significant difference between rates of retinopathy progression between the two groups. Despite intriguing results, further clinical testing necessary for regulatory approval in the United States and in Europe has not been pursued and the drug remains unavailable.

Fenofibrate, a peroxisome proliferator-activated receptor (PPAR) alpha agonist, has been evaluated for efficacy in treatment of diabetic retinopathy in combination with statin therapy as a plasma lipid-modulating agent capable of lowering triglyceride levels and raising high-density lipoprotein (HDL) cholesterol levels. Two randomized controlled clinical trials have suggested benefit of fenofibrate for diabetic retinopathy. The Fenofibrate Intervention and Event Lowering in Diabetes (FIELD) study was a large trial randomizing 9795 participants with type 2 DM to fenofibrate (200 mg/day) or placebo.[84] The cumulative percentage of participants receiving initiation of laser treatment for retinopathy (including focal/grid and scatter laser photocoagulation), a prespecified tertiary endpoint in the main study, was significantly lower in the fenofibrate group (3.4%) than in the placebo group (4.9%; hazard ratio, 0.69; 95% CI 0.56–0.84; P = 0.0002) over six years. Progression by two steps or greater on an adapted ETDRS diabetic retinopathy severity scale, the primary endpoint of a substudy involving analysis of two-field 45-degree fundus photographs for 1012 participants, did not differ significantly between fenofibrate and placebo groups. Investigators commented on a significantly higher rate of retinopathy progression in the placebo group compared with the fenofibrate group among participants with retinopathy at baseline, but the number of incident cases was small in both groups. The ACCORD study, discussed above, was a complex trial that included a lipid study randomizing 5518 participants with type 2 DM and dyslipidemia to receive simvastatin plus fenofibrate (160 mg/day) or simvastatin plus placebo. In the lipid study 1593 participants were evaluated for effects of fenofibrate on retinopathy.[78] At 4 years, the rate of progression of retinopathy, defined as a composite measure of three-step or greater progression on the ETDRS diabetic retinopathy severity scale or worsening requiring laser photocoagulation or vitrectomy, was significantly lower in the fenofibrate group (6.5%) compared with the placebo group (10.2%; adjusted odds ratio 0.60; 95% CI 0.42–0.87; P = 0.006).

The results of the FIELD and ACCORD studies are intriguing, particularly in the setting of some uncertainty about whether the benefit of fenofibrate on retinopathy is secondary to its effects on plasma lipid alterations or not given relatively modest effects on plasma HDL cholesterol and triglyceride levels among fenofibrate-treated participants in both trials.

A number of other agents have been evaluated for benefit in treatment of diabetic retinopathy, including ACE inhibitors, inhibitors of advanced glycation endproduct formation, growth hormone antagonists, antioxidants, and others. At the present time, the systemic strategies with a definite role in the management of diabetic retinopathy involve those interventions effective in controlling underlying hyperglycemia, hypertension, and dyslipidemia.

CONCLUSION

Diabetic retinopathy is a leading cause of vision loss in working-age Americans and a significant cause of blindness worldwide.[226,227] Its impact is expected to grow in the setting of profound increases in prevalence of DM projected in coming decades. At the present time, one in 10 American adults has DM. The Centers for Disease Control and Prevention predict prevalence among Americans will increase to between one in 5 and one in 3 by 2050.[71,228] The International Diabetes Federation estimates that as many as 438 million people worldwide will have DM in 2030, an increase from the approximately 285 million people estimated to have the disease in 2010.[228]

We have made tremendous progress in managing diabetic retinopathy. Large well-designed clinical trials have provided important information about the benefits of controlling hyperglycemia and hypertension to lower risk of retinopathy and its complications. Landmark trials in the 1970s and 1980s established the efficacy of laser photocoagulation, which reduces risk of moderate vision loss from DME by 50% and risk of blindness from PDR by 90%. Recent studies suggest efficacy of local administration of certain VEGF antagonists and corticosteroids used alone or in combination with laser photocoagulation for DME. Present treatment strategies offer vision gain in a significant proportion of patients.

Significant challenges remain, however. To combat the increasing burden of disease, we must develop better preventive strategies. To realize the benefits of existing treatments, we must greatly improve our success at screening and surveillance for diabetic retinopathy and facilitate access to timely therapy. To develop more effective treatments, we must better understand the biochemical and cellular basis for disease and rationally target key pathways. The recent success of intravitreous pharmacotherapy for treatment of DME represents a significant milestone in rational design of therapy, and will hopefully galvanize development of better methods for sustained drug delivery to the retina. If the achievements of the last several decades are predictive of further progress, we stand to make significant further strides in eliminating vision loss secondary to diabetic retinopathy in the near future.

REFERENCES

1. Cogan DG, Toussaint D, Kuwabara T. Retinal vascular patterns. IV. Diabetic retinopathy. Arch Ophthalmol 1961;66:366–78.
2. Cogan DG, Kuwabara T. Capillary shunts in the pathogenesis of diabetic retinopathy. Diabetes 1963;12:293–300.
3. Kuwabara T, Cogan DG. Retinal vascular patterns. VI. Mural cells of the retinal capillaries. Arch Ophthalmol 1963;69:492–502.
4. Toussaint D, Dustin P. Electron microscopy of normal and diabetic retinal capillaries. Arch Ophthalmol 1963;70:96–108.
5. Speiser P, Gittelsohn AM, Patz A. Studies on diabetic retinopathy. 3. Influence of diabetes on intramural pericytes. Arch Ophthalmol 1968;80:332–7.
6. Babel J, Leuenberger P. A long term study on the ocular lesions in streptozotocin diabetic rats. Albrecht Von Graefes Arch Klin Exp Ophthalmol 1974;189:191–209.
7. Robison Jr WG, Kador PF, Kinoshita JH. Retinal capillaries: basement membrane thickening by galactosemia prevented with aldose reductase inhibitor. Science 1983;221:1177–9.
8. Sima AA, Garcia-Salinas R, Basu PK. The BB Wistar rat: an experimental model for the study of diabetic retinopathy. Metabolism 1983;32:136–40.
9. Engerman RL, Kern TS. Experimental galactosemia produces diabetic-like retinopathy. Diabetes 1984;33:97–100.
10. Kozak WM, Marker NA, Elmer KK. Effects of aldose reductase inhibition on the retina and health indices of streptozotocin-diabetic rats. Doc Ophthalmol 1986;64:355–77.
11. Kador PF, Akagi Y, Terubayashi H, et al. Prevention of pericyte ghost formation in retinal capillaries of galactose-fed dogs by aldose reductase inhibitors. Arch Ophthalmol 1988;106:1099–102.
12. Kador PF, Akagi Y, Takahashi Y, et al. Prevention of retinal vessel changes associated with diabetic retinopathy in galactose-fed dogs by aldose reductase inhibitors. Arch Ophthalmol 1990;108:1301–9.
13. Takahashi Y, Wyman M, Ferris 3rd F, et al. Diabeteslike preproliferative retinal changes in galactose-fed dogs. Arch Ophthalmol 1992;110:1295–302.
14. Kern TS, Engerman RL. Comparison of retinal lesions in alloxan-diabetic rats and galactose-fed rats. Curr Eye Res 1994;13:863–7.
15. Engerman RL, Kern TS. Retinopathy in animal models of diabetes. Diabetes Metab Rev 1995;11:109–20.
16. Kador PF, Takahashi Y, Wyman M, et al. Diabeteslike proliferative retinal changes in galactose-fed dogs. Arch Ophthalmol 1995;113:352–4.

17. Kern TS, Engerman RL. Galactose-induced retinal microangiopathy in rats. Invest Ophthalmol Vis Sci 1995;36:490–6.
18. Robison Jr WG. Diabetic retinopathy: galactose-fed rat model. Invest Ophthalmol Vis Sci 1995;36:4A, 1743–4.
19. Kobayashi T, Kubo E, Takahashi Y, et al. Retinal vessel changes in galactose-fed dogs. Arch Ophthalmol 1998;116:785–9.
20. Kador PF, Takahashi Y, Akagi Y, et al. Age-dependent retinal capillary pericyte degeneration in galactose-fed dogs. J Ocul Pharmacol Ther 2007;23: 63–9.
21. Roy S, Ha J, Trudeau K, et al. Vascular basement membrane thickening in diabetic retinopathy. Curr Eye Res 2010;35:1045–56.
22. Barber AJ. A new view of diabetic retinopathy: a neurodegenerative disease of the eye. Prog Neuropsychopharmacol Biol Psychiatry 2003;27:283–90.
23. Barber AJ, Lieth E, Khin SA, et al. Neural apoptosis in the retina during experimental and human diabetes. Early onset and effect of insulin. J Clin Invest 1998;102:783–91.
24. Lieth E, Barber AJ, Xu B, et al. Glial reactivity and impaired glutamate metabolism in short-term experimental diabetic retinopathy. Penn State Retina Research Group. Diabetes 1998;47:815–20.
25. Lieth E, Gardner TW, Barber AJ, et al.Retinal neurodegeneration: early pathology in diabetes. Clin Experiment Ophthalmol 2000;28:3–8.
26. Martin PM, Roon P, Van Ells TK, et al. Death of retinal neurons in streptozotocin-induced diabetic mice. Invest Ophthalmol Vis Sci 2004;45: 3330–6.
27. Mizutani M, Gerhardinger C, Lorenzi M. Muller cell changes in human diabetic retinopathy. Diabetes 1998;47:445–9.
28. Whitmire W, Al-Gayyar MM, Abdelsaid M, et al. Alteration of growth factors and neuronal death in diabetic retinopathy: what we have learned so far. Mol Vis 2011;17:300–8.
29. Della Sala S, Bertoni G, Somazzi L, et al. Impaired contrast sensitivity in diabetic patients with and without retinopathy: a new technique for rapid assessment. Br J Ophthalmol 1985;69:136–42.
30. Greenstein V, Sarter B, Hood D, et al. Hue discrimination and S cone pathway sensitivity in early diabetic retinopathy. Invest Ophthalmol Vis Sci 1990;31: 1008–14.
31. Kurtenbach A, Wagner U, Neu A, et al. Brightness matching and colour discrimination in young diabetics without retinopathy. Vision Res 1994;34: 115–22.
32. Sokol S, Moskowitz A, Skarf B, et al. Contrast sensitivity in diabetics with and without background retinopathy. Arch Ophthalmol 1985;103:51–4.
33. Tregear SJ, Knowles PJ, Ripley LG, et al. Chromatic-contrast threshold impairment in diabetes. Eye (Lond) 1997;11(Pt 4):537–46.
34. Trick GL, Burde RM, Gordon MO, et al. The relationship between hue discrimination and contrast sensitivity deficits in patients with diabetes mellitus. Ophthalmology 1988;95:693–8.
35. Klein R, Meuer SM, Moss SE, et al. The relationship of retinal microaneurysm counts to the 4-year progression of diabetic retinopathy. Arch Ophthalmol 1989;107:1780–5.
36. Klein R, Meuer SM, Moss SE, et al. Retinal microaneurysm counts and 10-year progression of diabetic retinopathy. Arch Ophthalmol 1995;113:1386–91.
37. Kohner EM, Sleightholm M. Does microaneurysm count reflect severity of early diabetic retinopathy? Ophthalmology 1986;93:586–9.
38. Early Treatment Diabetic Retinopathy Study Research Group. Photocoagulation for diabetic macular edema. Early Treatment Diabetic Retinopathy Study report number 1. Arch Ophthalmol 1985;103:1796–806.
39. Kohner EM, Henkind P. Correlation of fluorescein angiogram and retinal digest in diabetic retinopathy. Am J Ophthalmol 1970;69:403–14.
40. Adamis AP, Miller JW, Bernal MT, et al. Increased vascular endothelial growth factor levels in the vitreous of eyes with proliferative diabetic retinopathy. Am J Ophthalmol 1994;118:445–50.
41. Aiello LP, Avery RL, Arrigg PG, et al. Vascular endothelial growth factor in ocular fluid of patients with diabetic retinopathy and other retinal disorders. N Engl J Med 1994;331:1480–7.
42. Aiello LP, Northrup JM, Keyt BA, et al. Hypoxic regulation of vascular endothelial growth factor in retinal cells. Arch Ophthalmol 1995;113:1538–44.
43. Miller JW, Adamis AP, Shima DT, et al. Vascular endothelial growth factor/vascular permeability factor is temporally and spatially correlated with ocular angiogenesis in a primate model. Am J Pathol 1994;145:574–84.
44. Pe'er J, Shweiki D, Itin A, et al. Hypoxia-induced expression of vascular endothelial growth factor by retinal cells is a common factor in neovascularizing ocular diseases. Lab Invest 1995;72:638–45.
45. Shweiki D, Itin A, Soffer D, et al. Vascular endothelial growth factor induced by hypoxia may mediate hypoxia-initiated angiogenesis. Nature 1992;359: 843–5.
46. Adamis AP, Shima DT, Tolentino MJ, et al. Inhibition of vascular endothelial growth factor prevents retinal ischemia-associated iris neovascularization in a nonhuman primate. Arch Ophthalmol 1996;114:66–71.
47. Robinson GS, Pierce EA, Rook SL, et al. Oligodeoxynucleotides inhibit retinal neovascularization in a murine model of proliferative retinopathy. Proc Natl Acad Sci U S A 1996;93:4851–6.
48. Fraser-Bell S, Ying-Lai M, Klein R, et al. Prevalence and associations of epiretinal membranes in Latinos: the Los Angeles Latino Eye Study. Invest Ophthalmol Vis Sci 2004;45:1732–6.
49. Kawasaki R, Wang JJ, Sato H, et al. Prevalence and associations of epiretinal membranes in an adult Japanese population: the Funagata study. Eye (Lond) 2009;23:1045–51.
50. Klein R, Klein BE, Wang Q, et al. The epidemiology of epiretinal membranes. Trans Am Ophthalmol Soc 1994;92:403–25; discussion 25–30.
51. Mitchell P, Smith W, Chey T, et al. Prevalence and associations of epiretinal membranes. The Blue Mountains Eye Study, Australia. Ophthalmology 1997;104:1033–40.
52. Ng CH, Cheung N, Wang JJ, et al. Prevalence and risk factors for epiretinal membranes in a multi-ethnic United States population. Ophthalmology 2011;118:694–9.
53. Sebag J. Anomalous posterior vitreous detachment: a unifying concept in vitreo-retinal disease. Graefes Arch Clin Exp Ophthalmol 2004;242:690–8.
54. Barile GR, Pachydaki SI, Tari SR, et al. The RAGE axis in early diabetic retinopathy. Invest Ophthalmol Vis Sci 2005;46:2916–24.
55. Gao BB, Chen X, Timothy N, et al. Characterization of the vitreous proteome in diabetes without diabetic retinopathy and diabetes with proliferative diabetic retinopathy. J Proteome Res 2008;7:2516–25.
56. Kim T, Kim SJ, Kim K, et al. Profiling of vitreous proteomes from proliferative diabetic retinopathy and nondiabetic patients. Proteomics 2007;7:4203–15.
57. Sebag J, Buckingham B, Charles MA, et al. Biochemical abnormalities in vitreous of humans with proliferative diabetic retinopathy. Arch Ophthalmol 1992;110:1472–6.
58. Shitama T, Hayashi H, Noge S, et al. Proteome profiling of vitreoretinal diseases by cluster analysis. Proteomics Clin Appl 2008;2:1265–80.
59. Holekamp NM. The vitreous gel: more than meets the eye. Am J Ophthalmol 2010;149:32–6.
60. Shui YB, Holekamp NM, Kramer BC, et al. The gel state of the vitreous and ascorbate-dependent oxygen consumption: relationship to the etiology of nuclear cataracts. Arch Ophthalmol 2009;127:475–82.
61. Chen MS, Kao CS, Chang CJ, et al. Prevalence and risk factors of diabetic retinopathy among noninsulin-dependent diabetic subjects. Am J Ophthalmol 1992;114:723–30.
62. Cikamatana L, Mitchell P, Rochtchina E, et al. Five-year incidence and progression of diabetic retinopathy in a defined older population: the Blue Mountains Eye Study. Eye (Lond) 2007;21:465–71.
63. Klein R, Klein BE, Moss SE, et al. The Wisconsin Epidemiologic Study of diabetic retinopathy. XIV. Ten-year incidence and progression of diabetic retinopathy. Arch Ophthalmol 1994;112:1217–28.
64. Klein R, Klein BE, Moss SE, et al. The Wisconsin Epidemiologic Study of diabetic retinopathy. III. Prevalence and risk of diabetic retinopathy when age at diagnosis is 30 or more years. Arch Ophthalmol 1984;102:527–32.
65. Klein R, Klein BE, Moss SE, et al. The Wisconsin Epidemiologic Sstudy of diabetic retinopathy. II. Prevalence and risk of diabetic retinopathy when age at diagnosis is less than 30 years. Arch Ophthalmol 1984;102:520–6.
66. Leske MC, Wu SY, Hennis A, et al. Hyperglycemia, blood pressure, and the 9-year incidence of diabetic retinopathy: the Barbados Eye Studies. Ophthalmology 2005;112:799–805.
67. Svensson M, Eriksson JW, Dahlquist G. Early glycemic control, age at onset, and development of microvascular complications in childhood-onset type 1 diabetes: a population-based study in northern Sweden. Diabetes Care 2004;27:955–62.
68. Varma R, Choudhury F, Klein R, et al. Four-year incidence and progression of diabetic retinopathy and macular edema: the Los Angeles Latino Eye Study. Am J Ophthalmol 2010;149:752–61 e1–3.
69. Wong TY, Cheung N, Tay WT, et al. Prevalence and risk factors for diabetic retinopathy: the Singapore Malay Eye Study. Ophthalmology 2008;115: 1869–75.
70. Zhang X, Saaddine JB, Chou CF, et al. Prevalence of diabetic retinopathy in the United States, 2005–2008. JAMA 2010;304:649–56.
71. Centers for Disease Control and Prevention. [Internet]. Atlanta, GA: CDC [update 2011 May 23; cited 2012 Feb 2]. National Diabetes Fact Sheet: Diagnosed and undiagnosed diabetes in the United States, all ages, 2010. Available from: http://www.cdc.gov/diabetes/pubs/estimates11.htm#1.
72. The Diabetes Control and Complications Trial Research Group. The effect of intensive treatment of diabetes on the development and progression of long-term complications in insulin-dependent diabetes mellitus. N Engl J Med 1993;329:977–86.
73. Diabetes Control and Complications Trial Research Group. The relationship of glycemic exposure (HbA1c) to the risk of development and progression of retinopathy in the diabetes control and complications trial. Diabetes 1995;44:968–83.
74. UK Prospective Diabetes Study (UKPDS) Group. Intensive blood-glucose control with sulphonylureas or insulin compared with conventional treatment and risk of complications in patients with type 2 diabetes (UKPDS 33). Lancet 1998;352:837–53.
75. UK Prospective Diabetes Study (UKPDS) Group. Effect of intensive blood-glucose control with metformin on complications in overweight patients with type 2 diabetes (UKPDS 34). Lancet 1998;352:854–65.
76. The Diabetes Control and Complications Trial/Epidemiology of Diabetes Intervention and Complications Study Research Group. Effect of intensive therapy on the microvascular complications of type 1 diabetes mellitus. JAMA 2002;287:2563–9.
77. Holman RR, Paul SK, Bethel MA, et al. 10-year follow-up of intensive glucose control in type 2 diabetes. N Engl J Med 2008;359:1577–89.
78. Chew EY, Ambrosius WT, Davis MD, et al. Effects of medical therapies on retinopathy progression in type 2 diabetes. N Engl J Med 2010;363:233–44.
79. The effect of intensive diabetes treatment on the progression of diabetic retinopathy in insulin-dependent diabetes mellitus. The Diabetes Control and Complications Trial. Arch Ophthalmol 1995;113:36–51.
80. UK Prospective Diabetes Study Group. Tight blood pressure control and risk of macrovascular and microvascular complications in type 2 diabetes: UKPDS 38. BMJ 1998;317:703–13.

81. Klein BE, Moss SE, Klein R, et al. The Wisconsin Epidemiologic Study of Diabetic Retinopathy. XIII. Relationship of serum cholesterol to retinopathy and hard exudate. Ophthalmology 1991;98:1261–5.
82. Chew EY, Klein ML, Ferris 3rd FL, et al. Association of elevated serum lipid levels with retinal hard exudate in diabetic retinopathy. Early Treatment Diabetic Retinopathy Study (ETDRS) Report 22. Arch Ophthalmol 1996;114: 1079–84.
83. Davis MD, Fisher MR, Gangnon RE, et al. Risk factors for high-risk proliferative diabetic retinopathy and severe visual loss: Early Treatment Diabetic Retinopathy Study Report #18. Invest Ophthalmol Vis Sci 1998;39:233–52.
84. Keech AC, Mitchell P, Summanen PA, et al. Effect of fenofibrate on the need for laser treatment for diabetic retinopathy (FIELD study): a randomised controlled trial. Lancet 2007;370:1687–97.
85. Janka HU, Warram JH, Rand LI, et al. Risk factors for progression of background retinopathy in long-standing IDDM. Diabetes 1989;38:460–4.
86. Rand LI, Prud'homme GJ, Ederer F, et al. Factors influencing the development of visual loss in advanced diabetic retinopathy. Diabetic Retinopathy Study (DRS) Report No. 10. Invest Ophthalmol Vis Sci 1985;26:983–91.
87. Berman DH, Friedman EA. Partial absorption of hard exudates in patients with diabetic end-stage renal disease and severe anemia after treatment with erythropoietin. Retina 1994;14:1–5.
88. Qiao Q, Keinanen-Kiukaanniemi S, Laara E. The relationship between hemoglobin levels and diabetic retinopathy. J Clin Epidemiol 1997;50:153–8.
89. Shorb SR. Anemia and diabetic retinopathy. Am J Ophthalmol 1985;100: 434–6.
90. Krolewski AS, Barzilay J, Warram JH, et al. Risk of early-onset proliferative retinopathy in IDDM is closely related to cardiovascular autonomic neuropathy. Diabetes 1992;41:430–7.
91. Tesfaye S, Stevens LK, Stephenson JM, et al. Prevalence of diabetic peripheral neuropathy and its relation to glycaemic control and potential risk factors: the EURODIAB IDDM Complications Study. Diabetologia 1996;39:1377–84.
92. American Academy of Ophthalmology [homepage on the Internet]. San Francisco, CA: AAO; 2008 [cited 2012 Feb 2]. American Academy of Ophthalmology Retina Panel. Preferred Practice Pattern® guidelines. Diabetic retinopathy. Available from: http://www.aao.org/ppp.
93. Klein R, Klein BE, Neider MW, et al. Diabetic retinopathy as detected using ophthalmoscopy, a nonmydriatic camera and a standard fundus camera. Ophthalmology 1985;92:485–91.
94. Yannuzzi LA, Rohrer KT, Tindel LJ, et al. Fluorescein angiography complication survey. Ophthalmology 1986;93:611–7.
95. AK-FLUOR (fluorescein sodium) injection for intravenous use. Full prescribing information. Package insert. Revised 7/2008.
96. Diabetic Retinopathy Clinical Research Network [homepage on the Internet]. 2007–12 [cited 2012 Feb 2]. Available from: http://drcrnet.jaeb.org/.
97. Bressler NM, Edwards AR, Antoszyk AN, et al. Retinal thickness on Stratus optical coherence tomography in people with diabetes and minimal or no diabetic retinopathy. Am J Ophthalmol 2008;145:894–901.
98. Krzystolik MG, Strauber SF, Aiello LP, et al. Reproducibility of macular thickness and volume using Zeiss optical coherence tomography in patients with diabetic macular edema. Ophthalmology 2007;114:1520–5.
99. Forooghian F, Cukras C, Meyerle CB, et al. Evaluation of time domain and spectral domain optical coherence tomography in the measurement of diabetic macular edema. Invest Ophthalmol Vis Sci 2008;49:4290–6.
100. Diabetic Retinopathy Study Research Group. A modification of the Airlie House classification of diabetic retinopathy. Report Number 7. Invest Ophthalmol Vis Sci 1981;21:210–26.
101. Grading diabetic retinopathy from stereoscopic color fundus photographs – an extension of the modified Airlie House classification. ETDRS report number 10. Early Treatment Diabetic Retinopathy Study Research Group. Ophthalmology 1991;98:786–806.
102. Fundus photographic risk factors for progression of diabetic retinopathy. ETDRS report number 12. Early Treatment Diabetic Retinopathy Study Research Group. Ophthalmology 1991;98:823–33.
103. Early photocoagulation for diabetic retinopathy. ETDRS report number 9. Early Treatment Diabetic Retinopathy Study Research Group. Ophthalmology 1991;98:766–85.
104. Klein R, Klein BE, Moss SE. How many steps of progression of diabetic retinopathy are meaningful? The Wisconsin Epidemiologic Study of diabetic retinopathy. Arch Ophthalmol 2001;119:547–53.
105. Murphy RP. Management of diabetic retinopathy. Am Fam Physician 1995;51:785–96.
106. Wilkinson CP, Ferris 3rd FL, Klein RE, et al. Proposed international clinical diabetic retinopathy and diabetic macular edema disease severity scales. Ophthalmology 2003;110:1677–82.
107. Brown JC, Solomon SD, Bressler SB, et al. Detection of diabetic foveal edema: contact lens biomicroscopy compared with optical coherence tomography. Arch Ophthalmol 2004;122:330–5.
108. Davis MD, Bressler SB, Aiello LP, et al. Comparison of time-domain OCT and fundus photographic assessments of retinal thickening in eyes with diabetic macular edema. Invest Ophthalmol Vis Sci 2008;49:1745–52.
109. Browning DJ, Glassman AR, Aiello LP, et al. Optical coherence tomography measurements and analysis methods in optical coherence tomography studies of diabetic macular edema. Ophthalmology 2008;115:1366–71, 71 e1.
110. Fluorescein angiographic risk factors for progression of diabetic retinopathy. ETDRS report number 13. Early Treatment Diabetic Retinopathy Study Research Group. Ophthalmology 1991;98:834–40.
111. Danis RP, Scott IU, Qin H, et al. Association of fluorescein angiographic features with visual acuity and with optical coherence tomographic and stereoscopic color fundus photographic features of diabetic macular edema in a randomized clinical trial. Retina 2010;30:1627–37.
112. Neubauer AS, Chryssafis C, Priglinger SG, et al. Topography of diabetic macular oedema compared with fluorescein angiography. Acta Ophthalmol Scand 2007;85:32–9.
113. Framme C, Roider J. Immediate and long-term changes of fundus autofluorescence in continuous wave laser lesions of the retina. Ophthalmic Surg Lasers Imaging 2004;35:131–8.
114. Muqit MM, Gray JC, Marcellino GR, et al. Fundus autofluorescence and Fourier-domain optical coherence tomography imaging of 10 and 20 millisecond Pascal retinal photocoagulation treatment. Br J Ophthalmol 2009;93: 518–25.
115. Fong DS, Segal PP, Myers F, et al. Subretinal fibrosis in diabetic macular edema. ETDRS report 23. Early Treatment Diabetic Retinopathy Study Research Group. Arch Ophthalmol 1997;115:873–7.
116. Bandello F, Polito A, Del Borrello M, et al. "Light" versus "classic" laser treatment for clinically significant diabetic macular oedema. Br J Ophthalmol 2005;89:864–70.
117. Catier A, Tadayoni R, Paques M, et al. Characterization of macular edema from various etiologies by optical coherence tomography. Am J Ophthalmol 2005;140:200–6.
118. Goebel W, Kretzchmar-Gross T. Retinal thickness in diabetic retinopathy: a study using optical coherence tomography (OCT). Retina 2002;22:759–67.
119. Hee MR, Puliafito CA, Wong C, et al. Quantitative assessment of macular edema with optical coherence tomography. Arch Ophthalmol 1995;113: 1019–29.
120. Laursen ML, Moeller F, Sander B, et al. Subthreshold micropulse diode laser treatment in diabetic macular oedema. Br J Ophthalmol 2004;88:1173–9.
121. Martidis A, Duker JS, Greenberg PB, et al. Intravitreal triamcinolone for refractory diabetic macular edema. Ophthalmology 2002;109:920–7.
122. Massin P, Duguid G, Erginay A, et al. Optical coherence tomography for evaluating diabetic macular edema before and after vitrectomy. Am J Ophthalmol 2003;135:169–77.
123. Otani T, Kishi S. Tomographic findings of foveal hard exudates in diabetic macular edema. Am J Ophthalmol 2001;131:50–4.
124. Ozdemir H, Karacorlu M, Karacorlu SA. Regression of serous macular detachment after intravitreal triamcinolone acetonide in patients with diabetic macular edema. Am J Ophthalmol 2005;140:251–5.
125. Browning DJ, Glassman AR, Aiello LP, et al. Relationship between optical coherence tomography-measured central retinal thickness and visual acuity in diabetic macular edema. Ophthalmology 2007;114:525–36.
126. Danis RP, Glassman AR, Aiello LP, et al. Diurnal variation in retinal thickening measurement by optical coherence tomography in center-involved diabetic macular edema. Arch Ophthalmol 2006;124:1701–7.
127. American Diabetes Association. Standards of medical care in diabetes – 2011. Diabetes Care 2011;34(Suppl 1):S11–61.
128. Lachin JM. Point: Intensive glycemic control and mortality in ACCORD – a chance finding? Diabetes Care 2010;33:2719–21.
129. Riddle MC. Counterpoint: Intensive glucose control and mortality in ACCORD – still looking for clues. Diabetes Care 2010;33:2722–4.
130. Gerstein HC, Miller ME, Genuth S, et al. Long-term effects of intensive glucose lowering on cardiovascular outcomes. N Engl J Med 2011;364:818–28.
131. Fong DS, Sharza M, Chen W, et al. Vision loss among diabetics in a group model Health Maintenance Organization (HMO). Am J Ophthalmol 2002;133:236–41.
132. Kraft SK, Marrero DG, Lazaridis EN, et al. Primary care physicians' practice patterns and diabetic retinopathy. Current levels of care. Arch Fam Med 1997;6:29–37.
133. Lee PP, Feldman ZW, Ostermann J, et al. Longitudinal rates of annual eye examinations of persons with diabetes and chronic eye diseases. Ophthalmology 2003;110:1952–9.
134. Paz SH, Varma R, Klein R, et al. Noncompliance with vision care guidelines in Latinos with type 2 diabetes mellitus: the Los Angeles Latino Eye Study. Ophthalmology 2006;113:1372–7.
135. Schoenfeld ER, Greene JM, Wu SY, et al. Patterns of adherence to diabetes vision care guidelines: baseline findings from the Diabetic Retinopathy Awareness Program. Ophthalmology 2001;108:563–71.
136. Zimmer-Galler IE, Zeimer R. Telemedicine in diabetic retinopathy screening. Int Ophthalmol Clin 2009;49:75–86.
137. Ahmed J, Ward TP, Bursell SE, et al. The sensitivity and specificity of nonmydriatic digital stereoscopic retinal imaging in detecting diabetic retinopathy. Diabetes Care 2006;29:2205–9.
138. Bursell SE, Cavallerano JD, Cavallerano AA, et al. Stereo nonmydriatic digital-video color retinal imaging compared with Early Treatment Diabetic Retinopathy Study seven standard field 35-mm stereo color photos for determining level of diabetic retinopathy. Ophthalmology 2001;108:572–85.
139. Fransen SR, Leonard-Martin TC, Feuer WJ, et al. Clinical evaluation of patients with diabetic retinopathy: accuracy of the Inoveon diabetic retinopathy-3DT system. Ophthalmology 2002;109:595–601.
140. Lin DY, Blumenkranz MS, Brothers RJ, et al. The sensitivity and specificity of single-field nonmydriatic monochromatic digital fundus photography with remote image interpretation for diabetic retinopathy screening: a comparison with ophthalmoscopy and standardized mydriatic color photography. Am J Ophthalmol 2002;134:204–13.
141. Schiffman RM, Jacobsen G, Nussbaum JJ, et al. Comparison of a digital retinal imaging system and seven-field stereo color fundus photography to detect diabetic retinopathy in the primary care environment. Ophthalmic Surg Lasers Imaging 2005;36:46–56.

142. Tennant MT, Greve MD, Rudnisky CJ, et al. Identification of diabetic retinopathy by stereoscopic digital imaging via teleophthalmology: a comparison to slide film. Can J Ophthalmol 2001;36:187–96.
143. Whited JD. Accuracy and reliability of teleophthalmology for diagnosing diabetic retinopathy and macular edema: a review of the literature. Diabetes Technol Ther 2006;8:102–11.
144. Jonas JB, Sofker A. Intraocular injection of crystalline cortisone as adjunctive treatment of diabetic macular edema. Am J Ophthalmol 2001;132:425–7.
145. Chan CK, Chan WM, Cheung BT, et al. Intravitreal injection of triamcinolone for diffuse diabetic macular edema. Arch Ophthalmol 2004;122:1083–5; author reply 6–8.
146. Ip MS. Intravitreal injection of triamcinolone: an emerging treatment for diabetic macular edema. Diabetes Care 2004;27:1794–7.
147. Kuhn F, Barker D. Intravitreal injection of triamcinolone acetonide for diabetic macular edema. Arch Ophthalmol 2004;122:1082–3; author reply 6–8.
148. Massin P, Audren F, Haouchine B, et al. Intravitreal triamcinolone acetonide for diabetic diffuse macular edema: preliminary results of a prospective controlled trial. Ophthalmology 2004;111:218–24; discussion 24–5.
149. Rodriguez-Coleman H, Yuan P, Kim H, et al. Intravitreal injection of triamcinolone for diffuse macular edema. Arch Ophthalmol 2004;122:1085–6; author reply 6–8.
150. Wong R, Sherefat H, Bartholomew D, et al. Intravitreal injection of triamcinolone for diffuse diabetic macular edema. Arch Ophthalmol 2004;122:1082; author reply 6–8.
151. Diabetic Retinopathy Clinical Research Network. A randomized trial comparing intravitreal triamcinolone acetonide and focal/grid photocoagulation for diabetic macular edema. Ophthalmology 2008;115:1447–9, 9 e1–10.
152. Beck RW, Edwards AR, Aiello LP, et al. Three-year follow-up of a randomized trial comparing focal/grid photocoagulation and intravitreal triamcinolone for diabetic macular edema. Arch Ophthalmol 2009;127:245–51.
153. Elman MJ, Aiello LP, Beck RW, et al. Randomized trial evaluating ranibizumab plus prompt or deferred laser or triamcinolone plus prompt laser for diabetic macular edema. Ophthalmology 2010;117:1064–77 e35.
154. Early Treatment Diabetic Retinopathy Study design and baseline patient characteristics. ETDRS report number 7. Ophthalmology 1991;98:741–56.
155. Treatment techniques and clinical guidelines for photocoagulation of diabetic macular edema. Early Treatment Diabetic Retinopathy Study Report Number 2. Early Treatment Diabetic Retinopathy Study Research Group. Ophthalmology 1987;94:761–74.
156. Diabetic Retinopathy Clinical Research Network [Internet]. 2011 [cited 2012 Feb 20. Modified-ETDRS focal photocoagulation technique. Available from: http://publicfiles.jaeb.org/drcrnet/Misc/FocalGridProcedure42711.pdf.
157. Akduman L, Olk RJ. Diode laser (810 nm) versus argon green (514 nm) modified grid photocoagulation for diffuse diabetic macular edema. Ophthalmology 1997;104:1433–41.
158. Bolz M, Kriechbaum K, Simader C, et al. In vivo retinal morphology after grid laser treatment in diabetic macular edema. Ophthalmology 2010;117:538–44.
159. Kumar V, Ghosh B, Mehta DK, et al. Functional outcome of subthreshold versus threshold diode laser photocoagulation in diabetic macular oedema. Eye (Lond) 2010;24:1459–65.
160. Lavinsky D, Cardillo JA, Melo Jr LA, et al. Randomized clinical trial evaluating mETDRS versus normal or high-density micropulse photocoagulation for diabetic macular edema. Invest Ophthalmol Vis Sci 2011;52:4314–23.
161. Muqit MM, Gray JC, Marcellino GR, et al. Barely visible 10-millisecond pascal laser photocoagulation for diabetic macular edema: observations of clinical effect and burn localization. Am J Ophthalmol 2010;149:979–86 e2.
162. Nakamura Y, Mitamura Y, Ogata K, et al. Functional and morphological changes of macula after subthreshold micropulse diode laser photocoagulation for diabetic macular oedema. Eye (Lond) 2010;24:784–8.
163. Ohkoshi K, Yamaguchi T. Subthreshold micropulse diode laser photocoagulation for diabetic macular edema in Japanese patients. Am J Ophthalmol 2010;149:133–9.
164. Venkatesh P, Ramanjulu R, Azad R, et al. Subthreshold micropulse diode laser and double frequency neodymium: YAG laser in treatment of diabetic macular edema: a prospective, randomized study using multifocal electroretinography. Photomed Laser Surg 2011.
165. Figueira J, Khan J, Nunes S, et al. Prospective randomised controlled trial comparing sub-threshold micropulse diode laser photocoagulation and conventional green laser for clinically significant diabetic macular oedema. Br J Ophthalmol 2009;93:1341–4.
166. Jain A, Collen J, Kaines A, et al. Short-duration focal pattern grid macular photocoagulation for diabetic macular edema: four-month outcomes. Retina 2010;30:1622–6.
167. Luttrull JK, Musch DC, Mainster MA. Subthreshold diode micropulse photocoagulation for the treatment of clinically significant diabetic macular oedema. Br J Ophthalmol 2005;89:74–80.
168. Fong DS, Strauber SF, Aiello LP, et al. Comparison of the modified Early Treatment Diabetic Retinopathy Study and mild macular grid laser photocoagulation strategies for diabetic macular edema. Arch Ophthalmol 2007;125: 469–80.
169. Elman MJ, Bressler NM, Qin H, et al. Expanded 2-year follow-up of ranibizumab plus prompt or deferred laser or triamcinolone plus prompt laser for diabetic macular edema. Ophthalmology 2011;118:609–14.
170. Hofman P, Blaauwgeers HG, Tolentino MJ, et al. VEGF-A induced hyperpermeability of blood–retinal barrier endothelium in vivo is predominantly associated with pinocytotic vesicular transport and not with formation of fenestrations. Vascular endothelial growth factor-A. Curr Eye Res 2000;21: 637–45.
171. Michels S, Rosenfeld PJ, Puliafito CA, et al. Systemic bevacizumab (Avastin) therapy for neovascular age-related macular degeneration twelve-week results of an uncontrolled open-label clinical study. Ophthalmology 2005;112: 1035–47.
172. Moshfeghi AA, Rosenfeld PJ, Puliafito CA, et al. Systemic bevacizumab (Avastin) therapy for neovascular age-related macular degeneration: twenty-four-week results of an uncontrolled open-label clinical study. Ophthalmology 2006;113:2002 e1–12.
173. Nguyen QD, Shah SM, Hafiz G, et al. A phase I trial of an IV-administered vascular endothelial growth factor trap for treatment in patients with choroidal neovascularization due to age-related macular degeneration. Ophthalmology 2006;113:1522 e1–e14.
174. Cunningham Jr ET, Adamis AP, Altaweel M, et al. A phase II randomized double-masked trial of pegaptanib, an anti-vascular endothelial growth factor aptamer, for diabetic macular edema. Ophthalmology 2005;112:1747–57.
175. Faghihi H, Roohipoor R, Mohammadi SF, et al. Intravitreal bevacizumab versus combined bevacizumab-triamcinolone versus macular laser photocoagulation in diabetic macular edema. Eur J Ophthalmol 2008;18:941–8.
176. Lam DS, Lai TY, Lee VY, et al. Efficacy of 1.25 MG versus 2.5 MG intravitreal bevacizumab for diabetic macular edema: six-month results of a randomized controlled trial. Retina 2009;29:292–9.
177. Nguyen QD, Shah SM, Heier JS, et al. Primary end point (six months) results of the Ranibizumab for Edema of the mAcula in diabetes (READ-2) study. Ophthalmology 2009;116:2175–81 e1.
178. Paccola L, Costa RA, Folgosa MS, et al. Intravitreal triamcinolone versus bevacizumab for treatment of refractory diabetic macular oedema (IBEME study). Br J Ophthalmol 2008;92:76–80.
179. Scott IU, Edwards AR, Beck RW, et al. A phase II randomized clinical trial of intravitreal bevacizumab for diabetic macular edema. Ophthalmology 2007;114:1860–7.
180. Soheilian M, Ramezani A, Obudi A, et al. Randomized trial of intravitreal bevacizumab alone or combined with triamcinolone versus macular photocoagulation in diabetic macular edema. Ophthalmology 2009;116:1142–50.
181. Massin P, Bandello F, Garweg JG, et al. Safety and efficacy of ranibizumab in diabetic macular edema (RESOLVE Study): a 12-month, randomized, controlled, double-masked, multicenter phase II study. Diabetes Care 2010;33: 2399–405.
182. Mitchell P, Bandello F, Schmidt-Erfurth U, et al. The RESTORE study: ranibizumab monotherapy or combined with laser versus laser monotherapy for diabetic macular edema. Ophthalmology 2011;118:615–25.
183. Michaelides M, Kaines A, Hamilton RD, et al. A prospective randomized trial of intravitreal bevacizumab or laser therapy in the management of diabetic macular edema (BOLT study) 12-month data: report 2. Ophthalmology 2010;117:1078–86 e2.
184. Crum R, Szabo S, Folkman J. A new class of steroids inhibits angiogenesis in the presence of heparin or a heparin fragment. Science 1985;230:1375–8.
185. Folkman J, Ingber DE. Angiostatic steroids. Method of discovery and mechanism of action. Ann Surg 1987;206:374–83.
186. Gordon DM. Prednisone and prednisolone in ocular disease. Am J Ophthalmol 1956;41:593–600.
187. Ingber DE, Madri JA, Folkman J. A possible mechanism for inhibition of angiogenesis by angiostatic steroids: induction of capillary basement membrane dissolution. Endocrinology 1986;119:1768–75.
188. Fauci A. Clinical aspects of immunosuppression: use of cytotoxic agents and corticosteroids. In: Bellanti JA, editor. Immunology II. Philadelphia: WB Saunders; 1978.
189. Nussenblatt R, Whitcup S, Palestine A. Uveitis: fundamentals and clinical practice. St Louis: Mosby; 1996.
190. Callanan DG, Jaffe GJ, Martin DF, et al. Treatment of posterior uveitis with a fluocinolone acetonide implant: three-year clinical trial results. Arch Ophthalmol 2008;126:1191–201.
191. Pavesio C, Zierhut M, Bairi K, et al. Evaluation of an intravitreal fluocinolone acetonide implant versus standard systemic therapy in noninfectious posterior uveitis. Ophthalmology 2010;117:567–75, 75 e1.
192. The effect of ruboxistaurin on visual loss in patients with moderately severe to very severe nonproliferative diabetic retinopathy: initial results of the Protein Kinase C beta Inhibitor Diabetic Retinopathy Study (PKC-DRS) multicenter randomized clinical trial. Diabetes 2005;54:2188–97.
193. Jaffe GJ, Martin D, Callanan D, et al. Fluocinolone acetonide implant (Retisert) for noninfectious posterior uveitis: thirty-four-week results of a multicenter randomized clinical study. Ophthalmology 2006;113:1020–7.
194. Schwartz SG, Flynn Jr HW. Fluocinolone acetonide implantable device for diabetic retinopathy. Curr Pharm Biotechnol 2011;12:347–51.
195. Campochiaro PA, Brown DM, Pearson A, et al. Long-term benefit of sustained-delivery fluocinolone acetonide vitreous inserts for diabetic macular edema. Ophthalmology 2011;118:626–35 e2.
196. Haller JA, Kuppermann BD, Blumenkranz MS, et al. Randomized controlled trial of an intravitreous dexamethasone drug delivery system in patients with diabetic macular edema. Arch Ophthalmol 2010;128:289–96.
197. Harbour JW, Smiddy WE, Flynn Jr HW, et al. Vitrectomy for diabetic macular edema associated with a thickened and taut posterior hyaloid membrane. Am J Ophthalmol 1996;121:405–13.
198. Kaiser PK, Riemann CD, Sears JE, et al. Macular traction detachment and diabetic macular edema associated with posterior hyaloidal traction. Am J Ophthalmol 2001;131:44–9.
199. Lewis H, Abrams GW, Blumenkranz MS, et al. Vitrectomy for diabetic macular traction and edema associated with posterior hyaloidal traction. Ophthalmology 1992;99:753–9.

200. Pendergast SD, Hassan TS, Williams GA, et al. Vitrectomy for diffuse diabetic macular edema associated with a taut premacular posterior hyaloid. Am J Ophthalmol 2000;130:178–86.
201. Haller JA, Qin H, Apte RS, et al. Vitrectomy outcomes in eyes with diabetic macular edema and vitreomacular traction. Ophthalmology 2010;117: 1087–93 e3.
202. Dillinger P, Mester U. Vitrectomy with removal of the internal limiting membrane in chronic diabetic macular oedema. Graefes Arch Clin Exp Ophthalmol 2004;242:630–7.
203. Figueroa MS, Contreras I, Noval S. Surgical and anatomical outcomes of pars plana vitrectomy for diffuse nontractional diabetic macular edema. Retina 2008;28:420–6.
204. Hartley KL, Smiddy WE, Flynn Jr HW, et al. Pars plana vitrectomy with internal limiting membrane peeling for diabetic macular edema. Retina 2008;28:410–9.
205. Higuchi A, Ogata N, Jo N, et al. Pars plana vitrectomy with removal of posterior hyaloid face in treatment of refractory diabetic macular edema resistant to triamcinolone acetonide. Jpn J Ophthalmol 2006;50:529–31.
206. Ikeda T, Sato K, Katano T, et al. Vitrectomy for cystoid macular oedema with attached posterior hyaloid membrane in patients with diabetes. Br J Ophthalmol 1999;83:12–4.
207. La Heij EC, Hendrikse F, Kessels AG, et al. Vitrectomy results in diabetic macular oedema without evident vitreomacular traction. Graefes Arch Clin Exp Ophthalmol 2001;239:264–70.
208. Recchia FM, Ruby AJ, Carvalho Recchia CA. Pars plana vitrectomy with removal of the internal limiting membrane in the treatment of persistent diabetic macular edema. Am J Ophthalmol 2005;139:447–54.
209. Rosenblatt BJ, Shah GK, Sharma S, et al. Pars plana vitrectomy with internal limiting membranectomy for refractory diabetic macular edema without a taut posterior hyaloid. Graefes Arch Clin Exp Ophthalmol 2005;243:20–5.
210. Yanyali A, Horozoglu F, Celik E, et al. Long-term outcomes of pars plana vitrectomy with internal limiting membrane removal in diabetic macular edema. Retina 2007;27:557–66.
211. Patel JI, Hykin PG, Schadt M, et al. Diabetic macular oedema: pilot randomised trial of pars plana vitrectomy vs macular argon photocoagulation. Eye (Lond) 2006;20:873–81.
212. Thomas D, Bunce C, Moorman C, et al. A randomised controlled feasibility trial of vitrectomy versus laser for diabetic macular oedema. Br J Ophthalmol 2005;89:81–6.
213. The Diabetic Retinopathy Study Research Group. Photocoagulation treatment of proliferative diabetic retinopathy. Clinical application of Diabetic Retinopathy Study (DRS) findings, DRS Report Number 8 Ophthalmology 1981;88: 583–600.
214. Bressler NM, Edwards AR, Beck RW, et al. Exploratory analysis of diabetic retinopathy progression through 3 years in a randomized clinical trial that compares intravitreal triamcinolone acetonide with focal/grid photocoagulation. Arch Ophthalmol 2009;127:1566–71.
215. The DAMAD Study Group. Effect of aspirin alone and aspirin plus dipyridamole in early diabetic retinopathy. A multicenter randomized controlled clinical trial. Diabetes 1989;38:491–8.
216. The TIMAD Study Group. Ticlopidine treatment reduces the progression of nonproliferative diabetic retinopathy. Arch Ophthalmol 1990;108: 1577–83.
217. Effects of aspirin treatment on diabetic retinopathy. ETDRS report number 8. Early Treatment Diabetic Retinopathy Study Research Group. Ophthalmology 1991;98:757–65.
218. Chew EY, Klein ML, Murphy RP, et al. Effects of aspirin on vitreous/preretinal hemorrhage in patients with diabetes mellitus. Early Treatment Diabetic Retinopathy Study report no. 20. Arch Ophthalmol 1995;113: 52–5.
219. Sorbinil Retinopathy Trial Research Group. A randomized trial of sorbinil, an aldose reductase inhibitor, in diabetic retinopathy. Arch Ophthalmol 1990; 108:1234–44.
220. Aiello LP, Bursell SE, Clermont A, et al. Vascular endothelial growth factor-induced retinal permeability is mediated by protein kinase C in vivo and suppressed by an orally effective beta-isoform-selective inhibitor. Diabetes 1997;46:1473–80.
221. Xu X, Zhu Q, Xia X, et al. Blood–retinal barrier breakdown induced by activation of protein kinase C via vascular endothelial growth factor in streptozotocin-induced diabetic rats. Curr Eye Res 2004;28:251–6.
222. Yokota T, Ma RC, Park JY, et al. Role of protein kinase C on the expression of platelet-derived growth factor and endothelin-1 in the retina of diabetic rats and cultured retinal capillary pericytes. Diabetes 2003;52:838–45.
223. Zhu Q, Xu X, Xia X, et al. Role of protein kinase C on the alteration of retinal endothelin-1 in streptozotocin-induced diabetic rats. Exp Eye Res 2005;81: 200–6.
224. PKC-DRS Study Group. The effect of ruboxistaurin on visual loss in patients with moderately severe to very severe nonproliferative diabetic retinopathy: initial results of the Protein Kinase C beta Inhibitor Diabetic Retinopathy Study (PKC-DRS) multicenter randomized clinical trial. Diabetes 2005;54: 2188–97.
225. Aiello LP, Davis MD, Girach A, et al. Effect of ruboxistaurin on visual loss in patients with diabetic retinopathy. Ophthalmology 2006;113:2221–30.
226. Congdon N, O'Colmain B, Klaver CC, et al. Causes and prevalence of visual impairment among adults in the United States. Arch Ophthalmol 2004;122: 477–85.
227. World Health Organization [Internet]. Geneva: WHO; 2011 August [cited 2012 2 Feb]. Fact sheet no. 312: Diabetes. Available from: http://www.who.int/mediacentre/factsheets/fs312/en/.
228. Centers for Disease Control and Prevention [Press release on the Internet]. CDC: Atlanta, GA; 2010 Oct [cited 2012 Feb 2]. Number of Americans with diabetes projected to double or triple by 2050. Available from: http://www.cdc.gov/media/pressrel/2010/r101022.html.

Proliferative Diabetic Retinopathy

Paolo A.S. Silva, Jerry D. Cavallerano, Jennifer K. Sun, Barbara A. Blodi, Matthew D. Davis, Lloyd M. Aiello, Lloyd Paul Aiello

"Since we are not yet able to prevent retinal changes in diabetic patients we must be content to accept, lessen, or slow the progress of these degenerative retinal vascular changes."

(William Parkes Beetham, Visual prognosis of proliferating diabetic retinopathy. British Journal of Ophthalmology, 1963)

The earliest diabetes-induced changes in the retina are biochemical, hemodynamic, and cellular in nature. Often these are initially imperceptible clinically and may have no or minimal effect on vision. In contrast, proliferative diabetic retinopathy (PDR) represents an advanced stage of diabetic eye disease characterized by the growth of newly formed retinal vessels on the retina or optic disc that extend along the retinal surface or into the vitreous cavity, significantly increasing the risk for vision loss.[1,2] Among patients with diabetes, nearly 25% with type 1 and 16% with type 2 will develop PDR after 15 years of diabetes.[3,4] The rate of progression to PDR is highest among type 1 patients, with a 42% cumulative risk over 25 years.[5] Furthermore, there is a strong association between PDR and uncontrolled systemic disease.[6,7] The publication of landmark clinical trials establishing the importance of intensive glycemic control in preventing the onset and progression of retinopathy and other diabetic complications in both type 1 and type 2 diabetes has led to marked improvement in the medical care of patients with diabetes over the past two decades. With these improvements there has been a corresponding decline in the incidence of PDR.[8–11] Nevertheless, the ocular complications arising from development of PDR remain a leading cause of severe vision loss in developed countries worldwide.[10]

This section begins with a brief discussion of the pathogenesis of PDR and the circumstances under which preretinal new vessels appear and are recognized clinically. A detailed description of the natural course of PDR follows, emphasizing four fundamental processes: (1) the cycle of proliferation and regression typical of new vessels; (2) proliferation of fibrous tissue accompanying new vessels; (3) formation of adhesions between the fibrovascular proliferations and the posterior vitreous surface; and (4) contraction of the posterior vitreous surface and associated proliferations. Other sections of this chapter consider the relationship of PDR to duration and type of diabetes, glycemic control, and other factors. The treatment of PDR is reviewed with emphasis on findings of clinical trials and guidelines for management. Finally, evolving novel treatment strategies are presented that hold promise as less invasive interventions or adjunctive therapy when photocoagulation response is inadequate.

PATHOGENESIS OF PROLIFERATIVE DIABETIC RETINOPATHY

Hyperglycemia and metabolic changes from diabetes lead to alterations in the retinal vasculature that result in reduced perfusion of the retinal tissue.[12] This state of relative retinal ischemia is thought to be the primary angiogenic stimulus that plays a central role in the pathogenesis of PDR. Various angiogenic factors such as angiopoietin, erythropoietin, basic fibroblast growth factor (bFGF), insulin-like growth factor (IGF), protein kinase C (PKC), tumor growth factor (TGF), and platelet-derived growth factor (PDGF) have stimulatory or modulating activities during the development of PDR. However, based on *in vivo* and *in vitro* studies, the protein called vascular endothelial growth factor (VEGF) appears to be primarily responsible for the ischemia-driven angiogenic pathology in PDR.[13–15] The role of VEGF in PDR is well supported by studies demonstrating high concentrations of VEGF in the vitreous of patients with PDR which are closely correlated with extent of disease activity.[13,16] Following successful laser treatment and in patients with naturally quiescent PDR, VEGF vitreous concentrations were low or undetectable.[13] Furthermore, the direct role for VEGF mediation of the neovascular response in PDR was demonstrated by showing that vitreous fluids from patients with active PDR were angiogenic in vitro, and this angiogenic stimulus could be blocked using a VEGF-specific inhibitor. Intraocular vessels from PDR and diabetes-induced iris neovascularization are exquisitely sensitive to VEGF inhibitors, often showing initial regression within one day.[17]

Although VEGF appears to be the primary direct causative angiogenic factor in PDR, the complex mechanisms regulating in vivo angiogenesis likely involve factors other than VEGF as well. Angiogenic pathways such as the angiopoietin/Tie-2 system modulate the effect of VEGF and directly affect retinal pericytes and endothelial cells, which are the principal cell types thought to be involved in the pathological processes of PDR.[18,19] In addition, hyperglycemia reduces PDGF survival-promoting activity, thus leading to pericyte apoptosis and diabetic vasculopathy. This mechanism is driven by hyperglycemia-induced activation of protein kinase C-δ (PKC-δ) which leads to increased expression of a protein tyrosine phosphatase called Src homology-2 domain–containing phosphatase-1 (SHP-1). SHP-1 activation in turn mediates resistance to PDGF, resulting in loss of cellular survival mechanisms and increased pericyte apoptosis.[20] Inhibition of SHP-1 is being investigated as a possible protective mechanism against initial retinal changes that underlie subsequent development of PDR.[20] VEGF independent pathways such as that mediated by erythropoietin (EPO) have also been implicated in the development of PDR.[21] Single nucleotide polymorphisms (SNPs) that increase EPO expression have been associated with development of PDR and severe renal disease in a small genetic study of three independent patient populations.[22,23] Antiangiogenic mediators such as pigment epithelium-derived factor (PEDF) are reportedly lower in patients with diabetes and in patients with active PDR compared to other retinopathies.[24] An interplay between both angiogenic and antiangiogenic pathways may be important in the eye at various stages of retinopathy.[25] A more detailed discussion regarding the pathological angiogenesis of PDR is presented in Chapter 26.

ORIGIN AND EARLY RECOGNITION OF PRERETINAL NEW VESSELS

The risk of PDR is greatest in eyes with severe nonproliferative diabetic retinopathy (NPDR), characterized by the presence and severity of soft exudates (cotton-wool spots), intraretinal microvascular abnormalities (IRMA, a term chosen so as to be neutral about whether these abnormal vessels represent intraretinal new vessels or dilated pre-existing vessels), venous beading, and extensive retinal hemorrhages or microaneurysms (H/MA) (Fig. 48.1). In the Diabetic Retinopathy Study (DRS), severe NPDR was defined as the presence of at least three of the above four characteristics, each generally involving at least two quadrants of the fundus. Approximately 50% of such eyes assigned to the untreated control group developed PDR within 15 months.[26] Today, a quick assessment of severe or very severe NPDR can be derived from determining the extent and severity of H/MA (moderately severe in 4 quadrants), VB (definitely present in 2 or more quadrants), and IRMA (obvious in 1 or more quadrant) – the 4–2–1 rule (see Box 48.1). Any one of these findings indicates severe NPDR and two or more represent very severe NPDR. As noted above, these levels of NPDR are associated with a high likelihood of developing PDR.

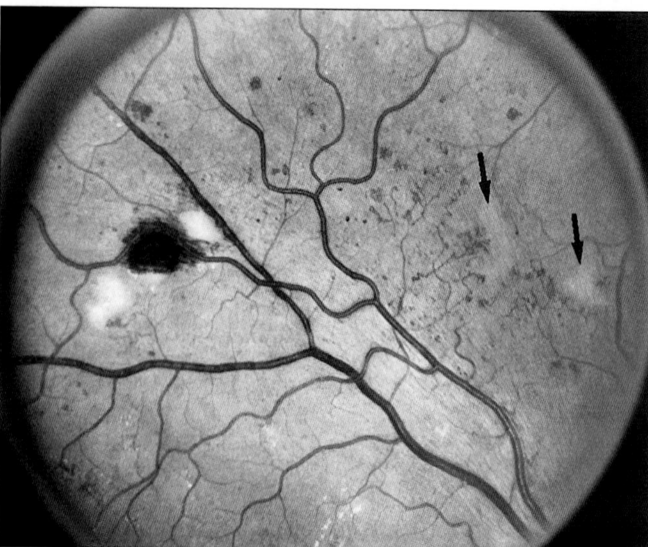

Fig. 48.1 Severe nonproliferative diabetic retinopathy (NPDR). On the left are two prominent soft exudates with a large blot hemorrhage between them. Venous beading is present where the superior branch of the superotemporal vein passes by the upper exudate. On the right are two faint soft exudates (arrows) and many intraretinal microvascular abnormalities. (Courtesy of Early Treatment Diabetic Retinopathy Study Research Group.)

The lesions characterizing severe NPDR are related to retinal capillary closure, and their frequent presence in eyes that are about to develop preretinal new vessels is one important observation linking these processes. Further evidence has been provided by the fluorescein angiographic montages of Shimizu and coworkers,[27] who found that the extent of capillary closure observed using angiography increased as the severity of new vessels increased on the following four-step scale: (1) none, (2) new vessels involving the retina but sparing the disc, (3) new vessels involving the disc, and (4) neovascularization of the anterior chamber angle with neovascular glaucoma. Muraoka and Shimizu[28] have provided serial fluorescein angiographic observations supporting the view that some lesions designated as IRMA or reduplication of small venules are in fact intraretinal new vessels revascularizing areas of capillary loss.

Although there is little doubt that the presence of severe NPDR is predictive of subsequent neovascularization, the characteristic intraretinal lesions are not always present when preretinal new vessels are first recognized. A possible explanation for this absence is the relatively transient nature of some of these lesions. Soft exudates usually disappear within 6–12 months.[29] H/MA have a half-life of approximately 3 months.[30] Blot hemorrhages and IRMA tend to disappear after extensive capillary closure, when the number of small vascular branches decreases and some small arterioles become sclerosed with a white thread-like appearance. This condition is sometimes described as "featureless retina" (Fig. 48.2B). However, in some eyes intraretinal lesions are mild, and signs of extensive capillary closure are absent when new vessels are first recognized.

New vessels may arise anywhere in the retina; however, they are most frequently seen posteriorly, within about 45 degrees of the optic disc. They are particularly common on the disc itself (Davis reported 69% of 155 eyes with PDR[31]; Taylor and Dobree, 73% of 86 eyes[32]). In the DRS, among 1377 control-group eyes with new vessels present in baseline photographs 15% had new vessels only on or within 1 disc diameter (DD) of the disc or in the vitreous cavity anterior to this area (new vessels on disc, or NVD), 40% had new vessels only outside this zone (new vessels elsewhere, or NVEs), and 45% had new vessels in both zones.[33] Also from the DRS, NVE had been shown to occur most frequently in the superotemporal quadrant (field 4, 27%), followed in frequency by the inferonasal (field 7, 21%) quadrant.[34] Although rare, the appearance of neovascularization arising from the perifoveal capillaries has been reported,[35] and possibly may provide insight on the association of DR and perifoveal telangiectasia.[36]

NVD (defined as NV at or within 1 disc diameter of the diskc[37]) begins as fine loops or networks of vessels lying on the surface

Box 48.1 The 4–2–1 rule

Severe NPDR (any one of the following)
- H/MA ≥ Standard photograph 2A (Fig. 48.20) in four quadrants
- VB definitely present in two or more quadrants
- IRMA ≥ Standard photograph 8A (Fig. 48.21) in one or more quadrants

Very severe NPDR (two or more of the above)

H/MA, hemorrhage/microaneurysms; VB, venous bleeding; IRMA, intraretinal microvascular abnormalities.

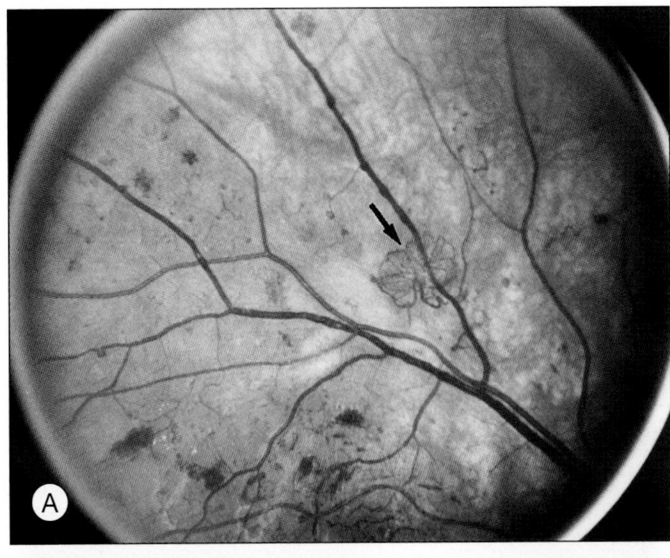

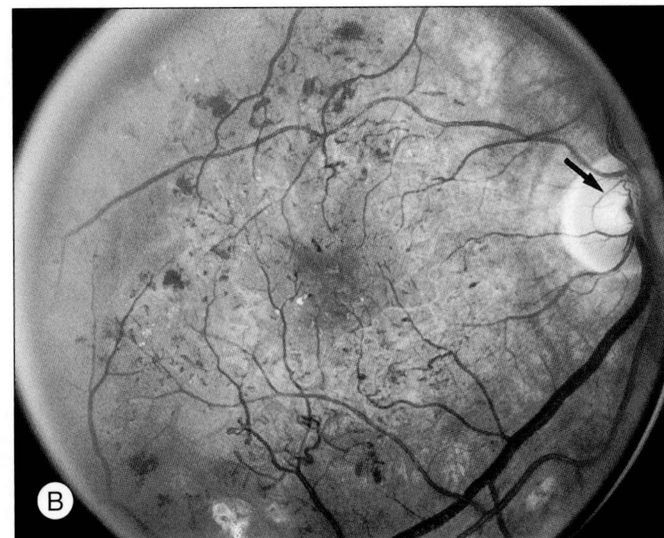

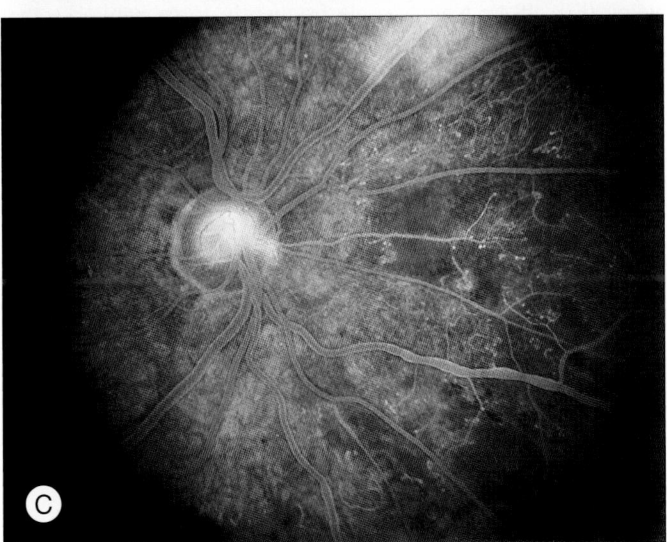

Fig. 48.2 Early proliferative diabetic retinopathy (PDR). (A) New vessels form a small wheel-like network (arrow) in the superotemporal quadrant of an eye with venous beading, soft exudates, intraretinal microvascular abnormalities (IRMA), and blot hemorrhages. (B) Posterior pole of the same eye, showing IRMA and retinal hemorrhages centrally and a featureless retina near the left edge of the figure. With stereoscopic examination, the vascular loop on the disc (arrow) can be seen to bridge the physiologic cup and is clearly a new vessel. (C) In the late-stage angiogram, new vessels on the disc are no longer filled with fluorescent blood; they stand out in contrast to the pool of fluorescein that has leaked from them. Prominent fluorescein leakage along the superonasal vein at the upper edge of the figure is from new vessels there. An area of capillary dropout is located nasal to the disc. (Courtesy of Early Treatment Diabetic Retinopathy Study Research Group.)

of the disc or bridging across the physiologic cup. They are usually easily identified once established, but in their earliest stages they may be overlooked, especially with the low magnification of binocular indirect ophthalmoscopy. They also may be difficult to distinguish from normal vessels in nonstereoscopic photographs or with monocular direct ophthalmoscopy. The most satisfactory examination methods are those that provide a magnified stereoscopic view, either biomicroscopy with contact or precorneal lens or stereoscopic 30-degree photography. If necessary, new vessels can be identified using fluorescein angiography where they will leak profusely, unlike normal physiologic vasculature (Fig. 48.2).

Evaluation of early NVE requires identification of the lesion and differentiation from IRMA. Binocular indirect ophthalmoscopy of the retina combined with a biomicroscopic or direct ophthalmoscopic examination of any suspicious lesions and careful review within 5 or 6 DD of the disc is a useful approach. Indirect ophthalmoscopy alone is not adequate. When new vessels or fibrous proliferation are extensive, wide-angle (45-degree or, preferably, 60-degree) photographs have the advantage of providing in one or two fields an integrated view of all or most of these lesions. For detection of early NVE, stereophotographs with a 30-degree camera are superior, and in most patients an adequate stereoscopic effect can be obtained in all the seven standard fields of the modified Airlie House classification[33,37] (Fig. 48.3), even with a maximum pupillary dilation of only 4 or 5 mm. The fundus should be scanned for definite or questionable NVE outside the standard fields, particularly between and above fields 4 and 6, between and below fields 5 and 7, and temporal to fields 4 and 5. Subsequent follow-up visits are greatly facilitated by a set of 30-degree stereophotographs from the baseline examination.

Ultrawide field imaging is a newer modality allowing visualization of retinal areas previously difficult or impossible to image. A single 200-degree field taken with ultrawide field scanning laser ophthalmoscopes resulted in detection of lesions that were beyond the field of routine standard 30- and 45-degree photography.[38] This capability of ultrawide field retinal imaging may enhance the detection of areas of peripheral vessel leakage and non-perfusion by flourescein angiography.[39] Potentially, when validated in a broader patient population, imaging of the retinal periphery may provide prognostic and early risk stratification for visual loss in patients with diabetic retinopathy.

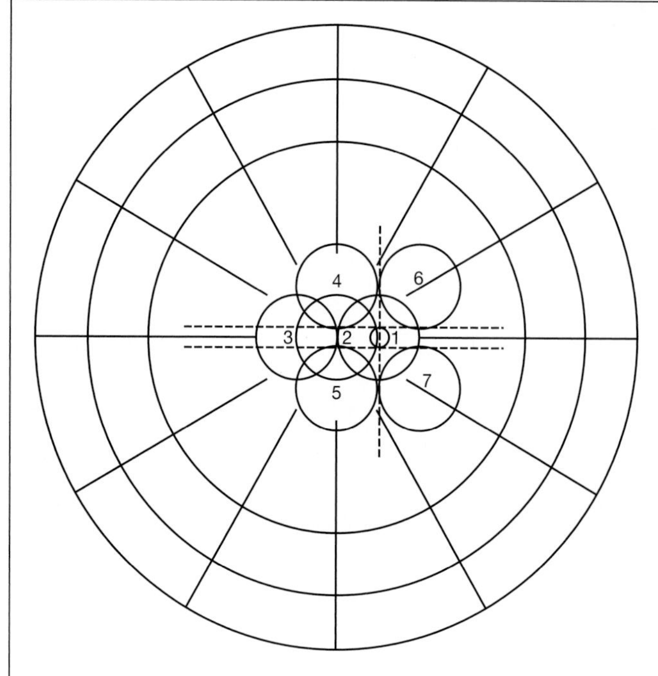

Fig. 48.3 Modified Airlie House classification. Seven standard photographic fields are shown for the right eye. Field 1 is centered on the disc, field 2 on the macula, and field 3 temporal to the macula so that its nasal edge passes through the center of the macula. Fields 4 to 7 are tangential to a vertical line passing through the center of the disc and to horizontal lines passing through its upper and lower poles, as shown. (Reproduced with permission from Diabetic Retinopathy Study Research Group. A modification of the Airlie House classification of diabetic retinopathy. DRS report number 7. Invest Ophthalmol Vis Sci 1981;21:210–26.)

When new vessels are not discovered by any of these techniques but are strongly suspected because of recent vitreous hemorrhage, examination of the more peripheral retina with biomicroscopy and a Goldmann three-mirror lens may be helpful. In this situation fluorescein angioscopy using the binocular indirect ophthalmoscope with a dark-blue filter over the light source can also be used effectively. The possibility that the vitreous hemorrhage may come from a peripheral retinal tear, unrelated to DR, should be kept in mind, and a careful examination of the peripheral fundus with scleral depression should be performed.

More difficult than finding NVE may be distinguishing between NVE and IRMA. This differentiation is particularly difficult if IRMA are extensive and NVE do not yet show any of their unique features – more superficial location, formation of wheel-like networks, extension across both arterial and venous branches of the underlying retinal vascular network, and accompanying fibrous proliferation. In unusual borderline cases, fluorescein angiography can distinguish between the profuse leakiness of preretinal new vessels and the more competent IRMA.

NATURAL COURSE OF PROLIFERATIVE DIABETIC RETINOPATHY

The natural course of PDR involves the development of new vessels on the retina and optic disc that extend along the retinal surface and the vitreous. These new vascular growths are commonly accompanied by progressively increasing fibrous proliferation. The subsequent contraction of the fibrous tissue can lead to traction retinal detachment and vitreous hemorrhage – the two most common complications associated with visual loss in PDR. Invariably, treated or untreated, PDR will eventually reach an involutional quiescent stage which may remain stable for decades. Visual outcome is dependent on the degree of damage to critical visual structures that has occurred by that point. Laser photocoagulation induces this quiescent state earlier, usually with less associated retinal damage and visual loss.

Development and proliferation of new vessels

Initially, new vessels may be barely visible. Later, their caliber is commonly one-eighth to one-quarter that of a major retinal vein at the disc margin, and occasionally they are as large as such veins (Fig. 48.4). New vessels frequently form networks that often resemble part or all of a carriage wheel. The vessels radiate like spokes from the center of the complex to a circumferential vessel bounding its periphery (see Figs 48.2A and 48.4). New vessel networks may also be irregular in shape, without a distinct radial pattern. New vessel patches often lie over retinal veins and appear to drain into them. The superotemporal vein is involved somewhat more frequently than others.[31,32] In the 1158 DRS control-group eyes that had NVE in at least one of the five photographic fields in which they were graded (fields 3 to 7 in Fig. 48.3), the number of times each field was involved was assessed. In each eye a count of one was divided equally among all fields containing NVE, and the counts for each field were totaled for all eyes. Field 4, which usually includes a major portion of the superotemporal vein, had a score of 308 (27% of 1158), whereas other scores ranged from 194 (17%) for field 5 to 242 (21%) for field 7.[2]

At times new vessels grow for several DD across the retina without forming prominent networks. The new vessels appear much like normal retinal vessels but are easily recognized as new vessels because of their unique capability of crossing both arterioles and veins in the underlying retina (Figs 48.5. 48.6). New vessels of this type commonly arise on the disc and are often accompanied during their actively growing phase by mild-to-moderate thickening (presumably edema) of the disc and surrounding retina (Fig. 48.7). This appearance is similar to typical cases of diabetic papillopathy,[40] in which all or most of the dilated small vessels on and adjacent to the disc are intraretinal and characteristically do not leak on fluorescein angiography.

The growth rate of new vessels is extremely variable. In some patients a patch of vessels may show little change over many months, whereas in others a definite increase may be seen in 1–2 weeks. Early in their evolution new vessels appear bare, but later, delicate white fibrous tissue usually becomes visible adjacent to them. The common clinical convention of referring to such tissue as "fibrous" is adhered to in this chapter, even though it has been shown to contain both fibrocytes and glial cells.[41,42] New vessels characteristically follow a cycle of proliferation followed by partial or complete regression.[31,43] Regression of a wheel-shaped net of new vessels typically begins with a decrease in the number and caliber of the vessels at the center of the patch, followed by their partial replacement with fibrous tissue. Simultaneously, the peripheral vessels tend to become

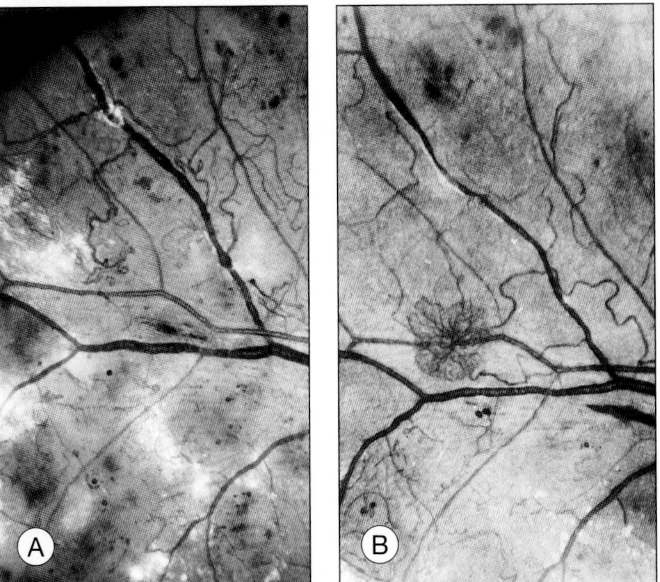
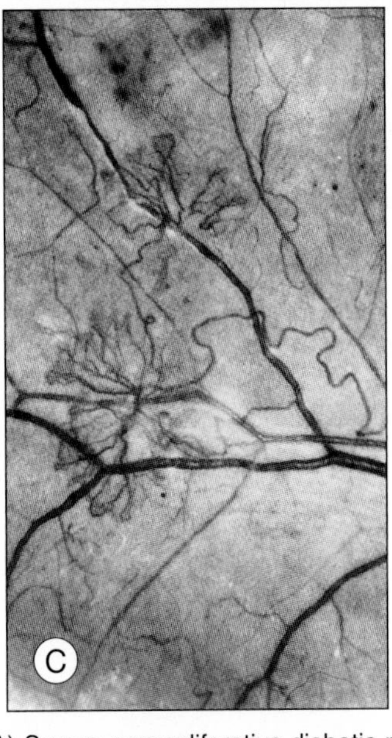
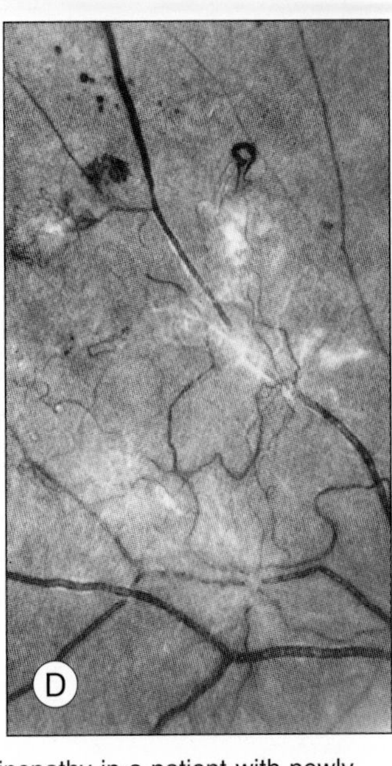

Fig. 48.4 Proliferation and regression of new vessels elsewhere (NVE). (A) Severe nonproliferative diabetic retinopathy in a patient with newly diagnosed type 2 diabetes (superotemporal quadrant of the right eye). Present were many microaneurysms, hemorrhages, and hard exudates, as well as extensive retinal edema and venous beading. Most of the tortuous small vessels appeared to be within the retina (large intraretinal microvascular abnormalities), but some may have been on its surface (NVE). (B) Eight months later, marked improvement in the intraretinal abnormalities was noted, but a wheel-like network of new vessels had appeared on the surface of the retina. Venous beading had decreased, and venous sheathing had increased. (C) Three months later, the new vessel patch had enlarged, and a second patch had developed above it. During the next 2 years, the new vessels continued to grow slowly at the edges of the patches, while regressing at their centers. (D) Three years after they had appeared, most of the new vessels had regressed, although there was still one dilated loop at the upper edge of the upper patch. No contraction of fibrous proliferation or vitreous had occurred, no vitreous hemorrhage was present, and vision remained good.

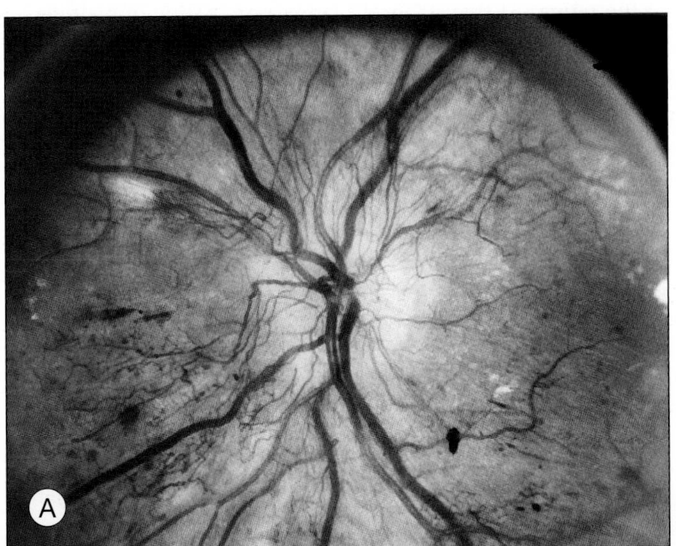
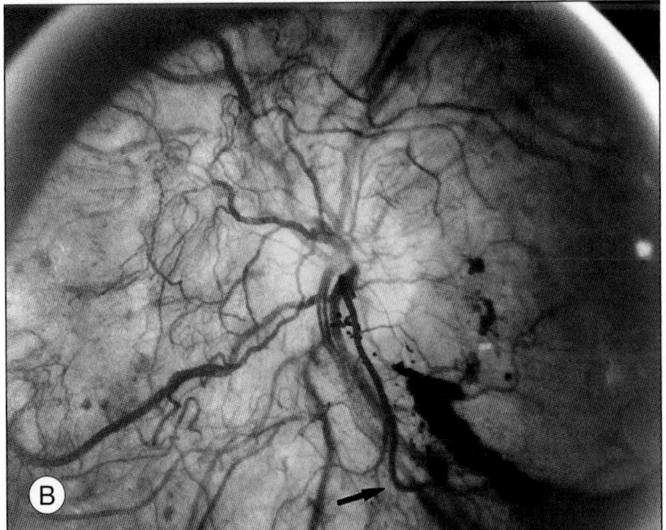
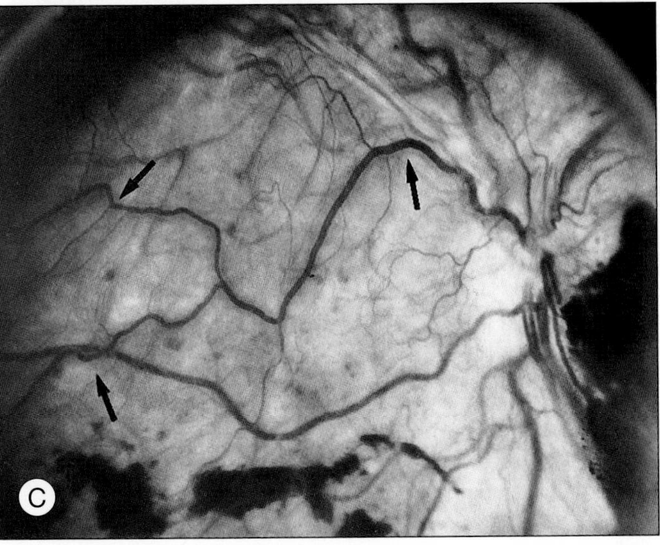

Fig. 48.5 Rapid development of large-caliber new vessels from the disc. (A) In the left eye of this 21-year-old white woman, whose age at diagnosis of diabetes was 7 years, new vessels arose on the disc and extended across its margins in all quadrants. The disc margins were blurred. There were soft and hard exudates, intraretinal microvascular abnormalities, and hemorrhages in the retina and on its surface. Blood pressure was 126/96 mmHg. (B) Two months later, new vessels had grown remarkably, and preretinal hemorrhage had increased. Arrow indicates large new vessel that crosses the inferotemporal artery and vein. (C) Three months later, one of the new vessels (arrows) had become as large as a major retinal vein and extended nasally beyond the edge of the figure. The new vessels on and adjacent to the disc had regressed partially. Two months later, the patient died suddenly of a myocardial infarction.

more narrow, although they may still be growing in length and the patch may still be enlarging (Fig. 48.4). At times, regressing new vessels appear to become sheathed. The width of the sheath, which presumably represents opacification and thickening of the vessel wall, increases until only a network of white lines without visible blood columns remains (Fig. 48.8). At times certain new vessels seem to become preferential channels, enlarging while adjacent vessels regress and disappear. Fresh, active new vessels are commonly seen emerging from the edges of partially regressed patches, and new vessels are frequently seen at different stages of development in different areas of the same eye. Early in their evolution, the fibrous components of fibrovascular proliferations tend to be translucent and are easily underestimated. Subsequently, with increasing growth, contraction, or separation from the retina, they become more prominent. If contraction of the vitreous and fibrovascular proliferations does not occur, new vessels may pass through all the stages described here without causing any visual symptoms. Concurrently, a decrease in intraretinal lesions and in the caliber of major retinal vessels may occur as retinopathy enters the quiescent stage. Occasionally, new vessels appear to regress completely, leaving no trace of their previous presence.[44]

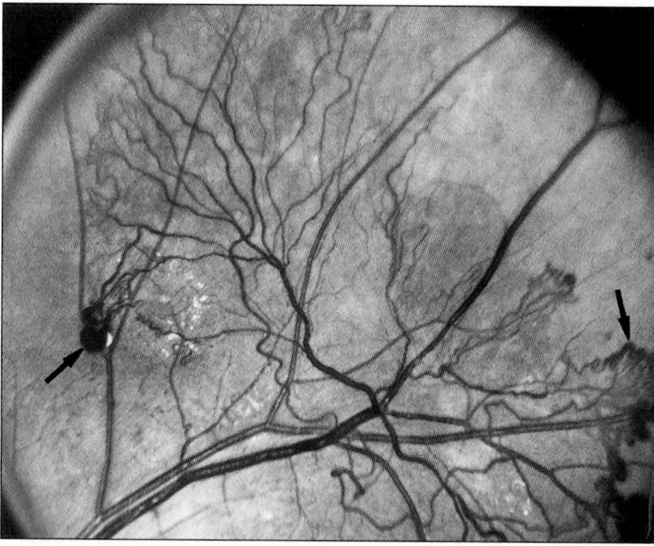

Fig. 48.6 New vessels elsewhere (NVE) without prominent network formation. Over much of their course, these new vessels did not form networks. Large aneurysmal dilations were present at the end of a long new-vessel loop (left arrow) and at the circumference of a partial wheel-like network (right arrow). (Courtesy of Diabetic Retinopathy Study Research Group.)

Based on the findings of the DRS, the development of PDR with high-risk characteristics places the patient at an increased risk for visual loss and generally requires prompt laser treatment. PDR with high-risk characteristics is defined by one or more of the following lesions: (1) NVD that is approximately one-quarter to one-third disc area or more in size (i.e., greater than or equal to NVD in standard photograph 10A); (2) any amount of NVD if fresh vitreous or preretinal hemorrhage is present; or (3) NVE greater than or equal to one-half disc area in size if fresh vitreous or preretinal hemorrhage is present Therefore, attention must be paid to the presence, location, and severity of new vessels, as well as the presence or absence of preretinal or vitreous hemorrhages.[2]

Contraction of the vitreous and fibrovascular proliferation

Before the onset of posterior vitreous detachment, neovascular networks appear to propagate primarily on or slightly anterior to the retina. At this stage, slit-lamp examination of new vessel patches that appear to be slightly elevated shows no change in the vitreous adjacent to them nor any separation between them and the retina. This finding suggests that mild thickening of the retina may be responsible for the slightly elevated appearance of the new vessels. Typically, the edges of such a new vessel patch are tightly apposed to the retina, and its center appears slightly elevated, giving the patch as a whole a mildly convex curvature. Nearly all new vessel patches are adherent to the posterior vitreous surface. This adhesion becomes apparent when posterior vitreous detachment occurs adjacent to the patch, pulling its edge forward. If vitreous detachment surrounds the patch, all its edges become more elevated than its center, giving its anterior surface a concave appearance.

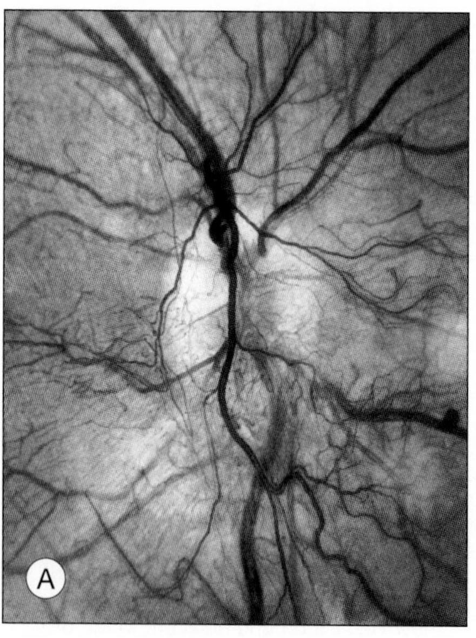

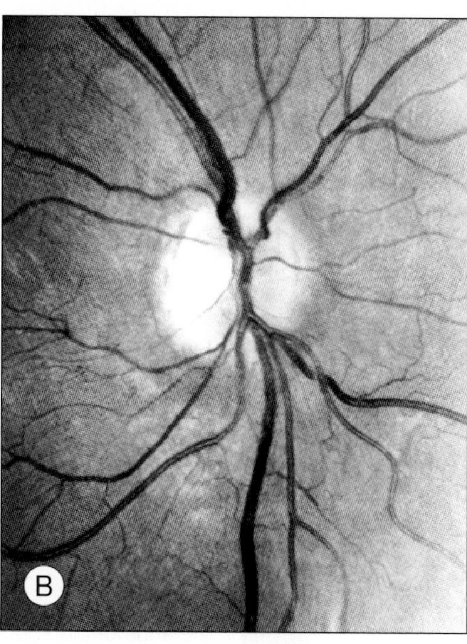

Fig. 48.7 Optic disc swelling. This 20-year-old man, whose diabetes had been diagnosed at age 14, sought ophthalmologic attention because of the sudden onset of floaters, first in the left eye and several days later in the right eye. (A) The disc was swollen, had blurred margins, and was partially obscured by extensive new vessels arising on it and extending on to the retina in all quadrants. (B) Five months later, disc swelling had resolved, and all new vessels had regressed spontaneously. Vision remained 20/15. (Courtesy of Diabetic Retinopathy Study Research Group.)

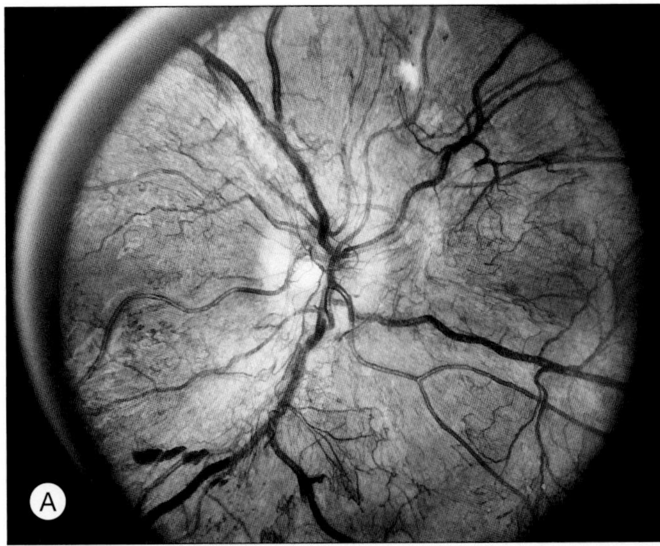

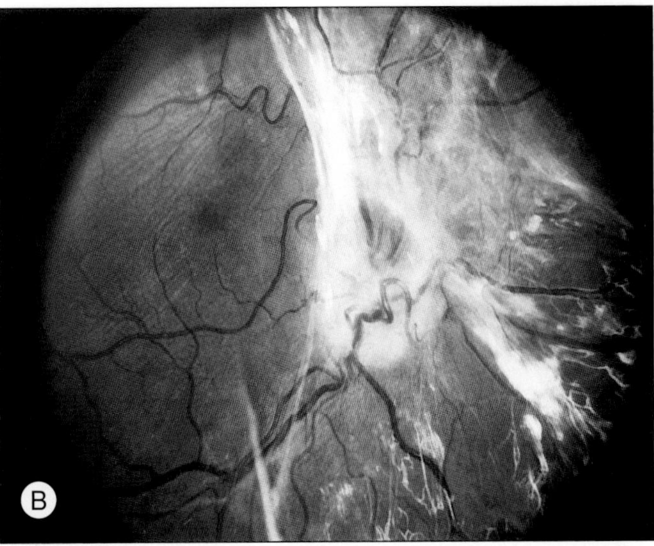

Fig. 48.8 Dragging of the macula by contraction of fibrovascular proliferations; regression of new vessels. (A) In the right eye of this 21-year-old woman, whose age at diagnosis of diabetes was 10 years, extensive new vessels were present on the surface of the disc and retina, as well as many dilated intraretinal vessels (intraretinal microvascular abnormalities). A soft exudate was noted about 1 disc diameter (DD) superonasally to the disc, and several small preretinal hemorrhages were found (near bottom left). The macula was in its normal position, centered at or just temporal to the left edge of the figure. Fibrous tissue accompanying the new vessels was visible adjacent to the temporal vascular arcades and nasal to the disc. Fibrous proliferations were actually much more extensive but were transparent and difficult to detect. Visual acuity was 20/20. Contraction of the proliferations occurred within the next several months, dragging the retina nasally and superiorly, and new vessels regressed. (B) Four years later, the center of the macula was above the disc and about 1 DD temporal to it. The central dark retinal pigment epithelial pigmentation appeared to coincide with the neurosensory macula. The first major bifurcation of the inferotemporal vein had been pulled upward to the disc margin from its previous position. New vessels had regressed completely, some of them now appearing as networks of white lines. Visual acuity was 20/30. (Courtesy of Diabetic Retinopathy Vitrectomy Study Research Group.)

Before the beginning of posterior vitreous detachment, new vessels are usually asymptomatic.[31,43] Small hemorrhages in the posterior vitreous are occasionally seen near the growing ends of the new vessels, but they usually remain subhyaloid or hang suspended in the most posterior portion of the vitreous without becoming apparent to the patient. When symptomatic vitreous hemorrhages occur, some evidence of localized posterior vitreous detachment can usually be found. When only a small area of the posterior vitreous surface is detached, it appears flat and very close to the retina, but as detachment becomes more extensive, this surface moves forward and assumes a curved contour more or less parallel to the retina and about 0.5–2 DD anterior to it. This otherwise smoothly curved surface is held posteriorly by vitreoretinal adhesions at the sites of new vessels. The new vessels in turn tend to be pulled forward in these same areas. Vitreous strands and opacities can usually be seen anterior to the posterior vitreous surface, whereas posteriorly the vitreous cavity is optically empty or contains red blood cells.[31,45] The principal force pulling the posterior vitreous surface forward usually appears to be the forward vector resulting from contraction of this surface and the fibrovascular proliferation growing along it. In explaining this process to students and patients, it helps to use the analogy of a bowl lined with a piece of cloth attached to the rim of the bowl: if the cloth shrinks, it eventually becomes tightly stretched across the top of the bowl.

The thickness of the posterior vitreous surface varies, as indicated by three different appearances. Immediately adjacent to the site of new vessels, the surface is often thick enough to be seen easily with the ophthalmoscope. Presumably this increased opacity is due to proliferation of fibrous tissue along the posterior vitreous surface. In other areas some distance from any visible new vessels, the surface is also sometimes thick enough to be detected ophthalmoscopically or in stereoscopic fundus photographs. In these areas the surface is usually somewhat shiny, with thinner and thicker areas alternating to give a "Swiss cheese" effect but without actual holes; presumably a thin layer of fibrous tissue is also present here. In still other areas the posterior vitreous surface is so thin that it can be appreciated only by mentally integrating many separate slit-lamp sections. Only the portion directly illuminated by the slit beam is visible, and the impression of a continuous surface is gained by watching the slit beam glide along smoothly over the surface as the slit lamp is moved. Frequently in the same eye all these various appearances can be seen in different areas of the same surface, the general course of the surface continuing without change as its thickness varies (Fig. 48.9).

Posterior vitreous detachment usually begins near the posterior pole, the most common locations being the region of the superotemporal vessels, temporal to the macula, and above or below the disc.[31] Detachment often spreads fairly rapidly (within hours, days, or weeks) to the periphery of the quadrant in which it begins, unless such spread is impeded by vitreoretinal adhesions associated with patches of new vessels. Extension circumferentially into other quadrants of the fundus tends to be slower, sometimes requiring months or years to reach completion. Detachment of the vitreous from the disc is usually prevented by adhesions between the vitreous and fibrovascular proliferations arising there. Vitreous detachment is not a smoothly progressive process. It occurs in abrupt steps, usually halting whenever its advancing edge meets a patch of active or regressed new vessels. If contraction continues, the patch is pulled forward,

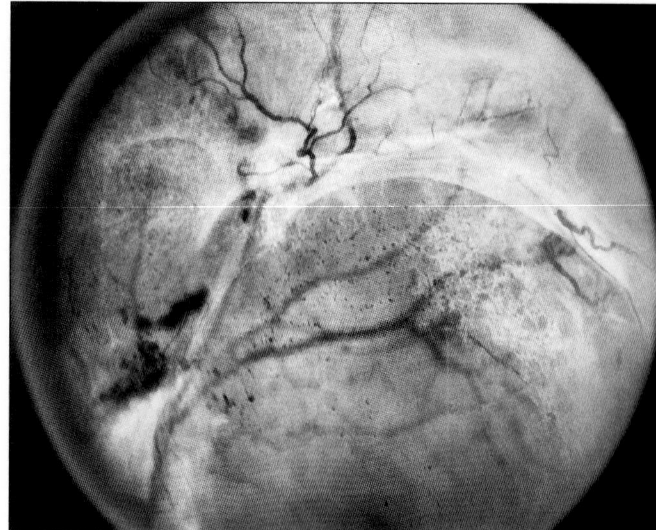

Fig. 48.9 The posterior vitreous surface. In this left eye fibrovascular proliferations were present at the disc and above the superotemporal vascular arcade. The posterior vitreous surface was adherent to these proliferations but was detached elsewhere. In the center of the figure the posterior vitreous surface was thin (visible only with slit illumination), but its position is marked by fine dots of hemorrhage deposited on it. Temporal to this area, the posterior vitreous surface has the typical "Swiss cheese" appearance; that is, the surface can be seen as a semiopaque sheet in which there are round and oval clear areas. This same appearance is present 1 to 2 disc diameters above the disc, near the left edge of the figure. The retina was attached but is blurred, in part because the camera was focused on the elevated proliferations and also because of blood present in the posterior fluid vitreous. (Courtesy of Diabetic Retinopathy Vitrectomy Study Research Group.)

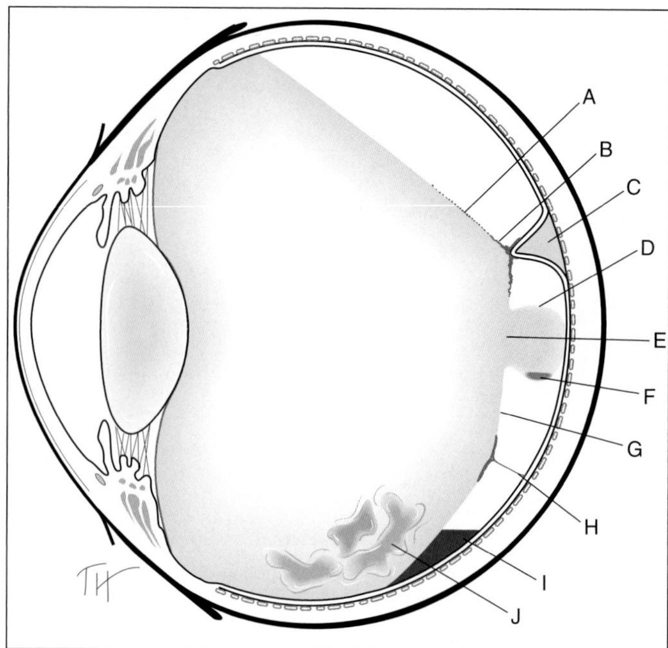

Fig. 48.10 Vitreous detachment in proliferative diabetic retinopathy. (A) Blood deposited on the detached posterior surface of the formed vitreous after hemorrhage into the posterior fluid vitreous. (B) Neovascular and fibrous proliferations creating a tight vitreoretinal adhesion, which pulls the retina forward and holds the formed vitreous posteriorly. (C) Localized collection of subretinal fluid. (D) Curved upper surface of a "mushroom" of formed vitreous extending posteriorly to reach the retina through a "hole" in the posterior vitreous surface. (E) Hole in the posterior vitreous surface. (F) Blood collected in the dependent portion of the mushroom of vitreous after hemorrhage into the formed vitreous. (G) Posterior vitreous surface. (H) A single new vessel stretching between the retina and proliferations on the detached posterior vitreous surface without traction retinal detachment. (I) Blood with fluid level pooling between the retina and the posterior vitreous surface above the inferior limit of vitreous detachment after hemorrhage into the posterior fluid vitreous. (J) Blood settled out in the inferior part of the formed vitreous.

with or without the underlying retina, and vitreous detachment spreads beyond it. At times the peripheral spread of posterior vitreous detachment is halted temporarily by invisible adhesions to the retina in areas where no new vessels are present. These adhesions are indicated by a subtle linear elevation of the inner surface of the retina at the junction of posteriorly detached and anteriorly attached vitreous. After several weeks or months, vitreous detachment usually spreads farther peripherally, and the subtle retinal fold flattens.

Traction exerted on the new vessels appears to be a factor contributing to the recurrent vitreous hemorrhages that often coincide with extension of vitreous detachment. Hemorrhages also occur independently, sometimes apparently in relation to bouts of severe coughing or vomiting and occasionally at the time of insulin reactions. More often they occur during sleep and are unrelated to any obvious factor.[46,47] Blood in the fluid vitreous posterior to the detached vitreous framework usually absorbs within weeks or several months, retaining its red color until absorbed. Hemorrhage in the formed vitreous tends to lose its red color and become white before absorption is complete. Absorption of a large hemorrhage from the formed vitreous is usually slow, requiring many months.

The arrangement and movement of blood in the posterior fluid vitreous often make it possible to define the limits of posterior vitreous detachment ophthalmoscopically.[31,48] In areas of vitreous detachment, the presence of fresh blood in the posterior fluid vitreous obscures fundus details, distinguishing these areas from adjacent areas in which the vitreous remains attached and details of the retina are clear. In the upper quadrants of the fundus, blood tends to become deposited in thin meridional streaks on the detached posterior vitreous surface, identifying its position. Inferiorly, blood pools between the detached vitreous and attached retina, outlining the inferior extent of vitreous detachment and often forming a fluid-level or "boat-shaped" hemorrhage. At times, even when posterior vitreous detachment cannot definitely be identified with slit lamp and contact lens, a thin, curving line of subhyaloid hemorrhage parallel to and behind the inferior equator can be seen, presumably marking the lower edge of an area of vitreous detachment. Occasionally the posterior vitreous surface can be traced across the macula on slit-lamp examination, but usually its continuity is lost in this region. In some of these cases a round or oval hole with sharp edges can be detected in the posterior vitreous surface, occupying an area 2–4 DD wide in the posterior pole. The posterior vitreous surface in this area appears broken, with solid vitreous protruding back through the hole and coming into contact with the retina. At times the surface of a bulging mushroom of vitreous can be seen extending posteriorly through such a hole, occasionally with hemorrhage suspended within its lower part (Fig. 48.10).

Retinal distortion and tractional detachment

With contraction of an extensive sheet of fibrovascular proliferations, distortion or displacement ("dragging") of the macula may occur.[49] In some cases the central, more intensely pigmented area of the retinal pigment epithelium (RPE) appears to be dragged with the neurosensory macula toward the major focus of contracted tissue, whereas in other cases only the neurosensory macula appears displaced. Since the most common site of extensive fibrovascular proliferations is on and near the disc, the macula is usually dragged nasally and often also somewhat vertically (Figs 48.11, 48.12).

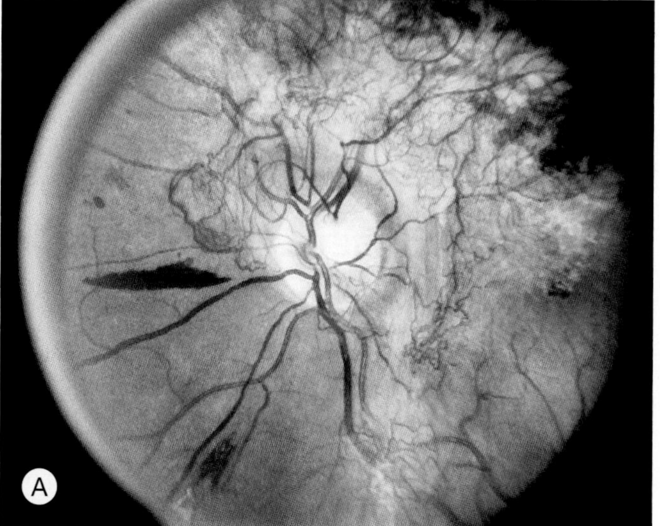

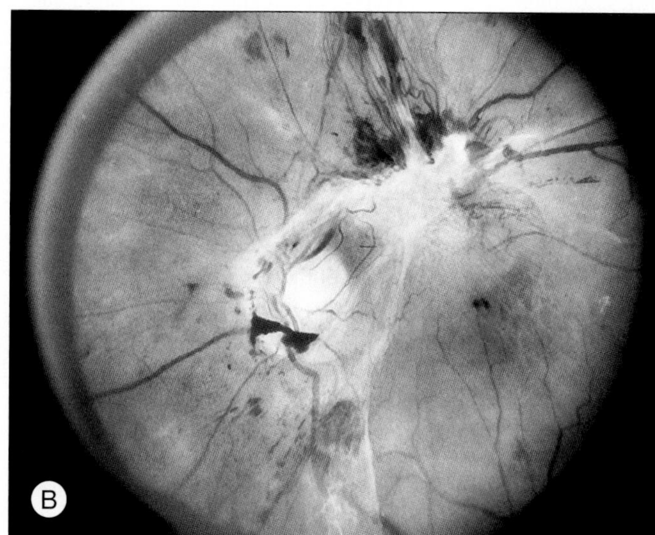

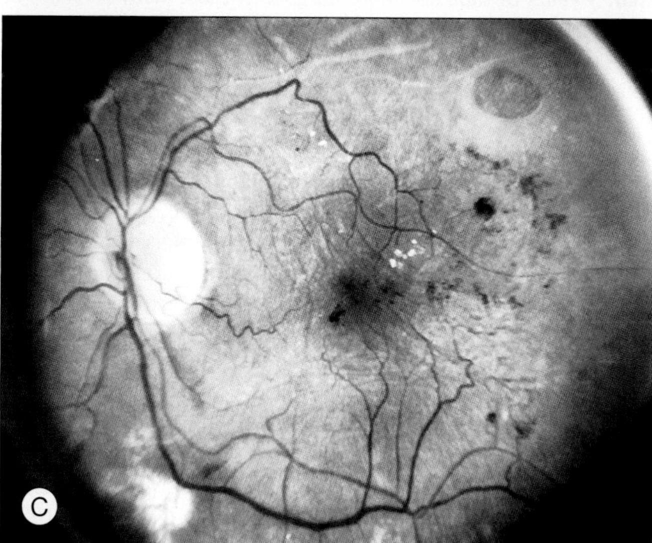

Fig. 48.11 Dragging of the macula. (A) In the left eye of this 39-year-old white woman, whose age at diagnosis of diabetes was 10 years, extensive fibrovascular proliferations were present on and adjacent to the disc, centered superotemporally. The temporal edge of the patch of proliferations was tightly apposed to the retina, and the nasal edge was elevated about one-third of a disc diameter by localized posterior vitreous detachment, the lower edge of which was marked by a preretinal hemorrhage. Visual acuity was 20/60. Scatter photocoagulation was initiated. (B) Three weeks after photocoagulation, the patient noted a marked decrease in visual acuity and returned for examination. There had been marked regression of the new vessels. Contraction of the proliferations had pulled the neurosensory macula (but not the corresponding, more deeply pigmented retinal pigment epithelium) up and nasally. Vitrectomy was carried out. (C) Two months later, visual acuity had improved to 20/30, and the neurosensory macula had returned to near-normal position. There appeared to be a rather large, full-thickness retinal break (near upper right corner), but this did not lead to retinal detachment during the remaining 3 years of follow-up. At 4-year follow-up, vision had improved to 20/20. (Courtesy of Diabetic Retinopathy Vitrectomy Study Research Group.)

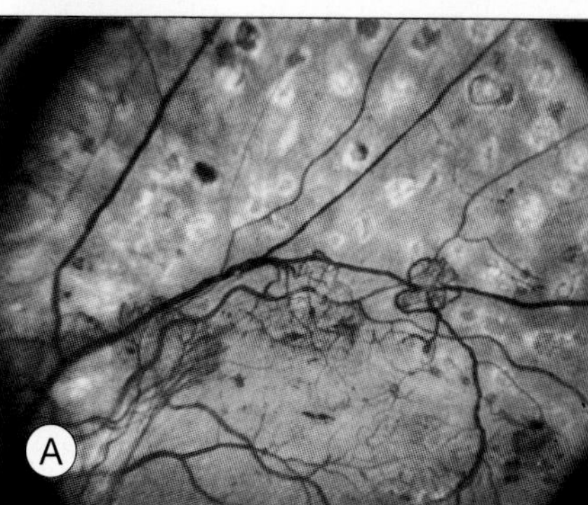

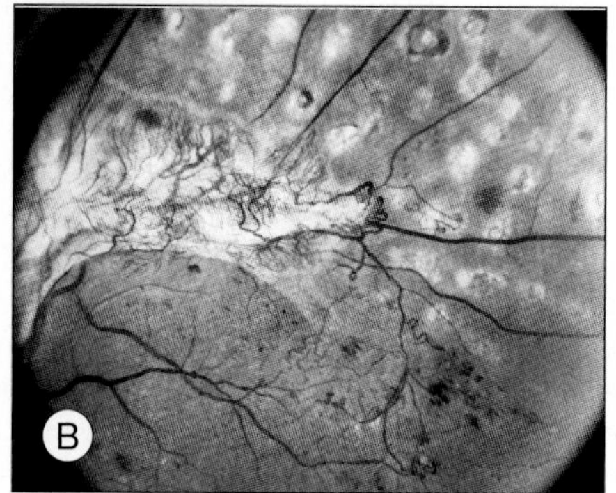

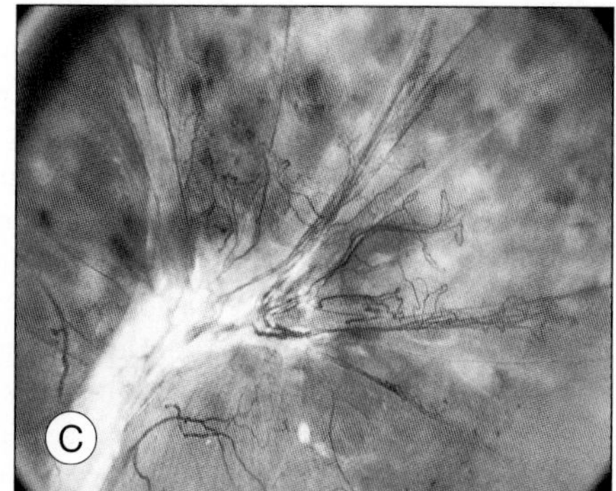

Fig. 48.12 Contraction of fibrovascular proliferations leading to extensive retinal detachment. (A) In the left eye of this 35-year-old man, whose age at diagnosis of diabetes was 14 years, networks of new vessels extended over the surface of the retina along the superotemporal vein. Scars were typical of initial scatter photocoagulation, with space between scars available for additional treatment. (B) Four months later, new vessels had increased, and dense fibrous tissue had appeared. (C) Seven months later, fibrous proliferations had contracted. Broad adhesions prevented them from pulling away from the retina. Instead, the retina was pulled forward (detached) throughout the area shown in the figure. The photocoagulation scars were blurred by the overlying detached retina (and are out of focus). (Courtesy of Diabetic Retinopathy Vitrectomy Study Research Group.)

Contraction of vitreous or areas of fibrovascular proliferation may also lead to retinal detachment. This retinal detachment may be limited to avulsion of a retinal vessel, usually a vein, sometimes accompanied by vitreous hemorrhage. Alternatively, a relatively thin fold of retina may become elevated, with only a narrow zone of retinal detachment adjacent to its base, sometimes outlined by a pigmented demarcation line. In other cases retinal detachment may be more extensive, but the concave shape that is typical of traction detachment is generally maintained. At times, small, apparently full-thickness retinal holes may be seen near the proliferation; these sometimes, but not always, lead to rhegmatogenous detachment. When such detachment does occur, it tends to have a flat or convex anterior surface and be more extensive, often reaching the ora serrata. The occurrence and severity of retinal detachment are influenced by the timing and degree of shrinkage of the vitreous and fibrovascular proliferations and by the type, extent, and location of the new vessels responsible for vitreoretinal adhesions. Extensive nets of large-caliber new vessels accompanied by heavy fibrous tissue produce broad, tight vitreoretinal adhesions. Contraction of such proliferations is often followed by extensive retinal detachment (Fig. 48.12). New vessels with little accompanying fibrous tissue tend to produce less extensive vitreoretinal adhesions and less risk of retinal detachment, particularly when posterior vitreous detachment begins soon after the onset of neovascularization (Fig. 48.13). At times, new vessels that extend for a considerable distance along the surface of the retina appear to be adherent to the retina only at their sites of origin and to the vitreous only near their distal ends. In this case, the posterior vitreous surface can pull away from the retina by a distance equal to the length of the vessels before exerting traction on the retina. When new vessels are confined to the surface of the disc, vitreous detachment can reach completion without producing traction on the retina, since there are no vitreoretinal adhesions. Retinal detachment does not occur in such eyes, but recurrent vitreous hemorrhage from the new vessels is common.

Involutional or "Quiescent" Proliferative Diabetic Retinopathy

DR ultimately reaches an involutional stage wherein the retinopathy has "burned-out" and is termed "quiescent." At this stage vitreous contraction has reached completion and the vitreous is detached from all areas of the retina except where vitreoretinal adhesions associated with new vessels prevent such detachment.[31,43,50,51] Vitreous hemorrhages decrease in frequency and severity and may stop entirely, although many months may elapse before substantial vitreous clearing occurs. Some degree of retinal detachment may be present at this stage. If the detachment is localized and the macula remains intact, visual acuity may be good. However, dragging or distortion of the macula or long-standing macular edema can lead to substantial reduction in vision. In some cases, retinal detachment involves the entire posterior pole, with resultant severe loss of vision. Although spontaneous partial reattachment occasionally occurs, if the macula has been detached for months or years, usually little significant return of vision occurs.

A marked reduction in the caliber of retinal vessels is characteristic of this stage. Previously dilated or beaded veins return to normal caliber or become narrower and often appear sheathed. Fewer small venous branches are visible. Changes in the arterioles are often even more striking, with decreased caliber and reduction of the number of visible branches. Some small arterioles can appear to be white threads without visible blood columns. Characteristically, only occasional retinal hemorrhages and microaneurysms are present. New vessels are usually reduced in caliber and number and at times no patent new vessels can be seen. Fibrous tissue may become thinner and more transparent, allowing the retina to be observed more clearly. Vision loss at this stage is related to macular detachment, macular ischemia, chronic macular edema, optic nerve disease or media opacity. Marked vision loss is likely due to severe retinal ischemia.

RELATIONSHIP OF PROLIFERATIVE DIABETIC RETINOPATHY TO TYPE AND DURATION OF DIABETES

In a population-based stereophotographic study carried out by Klein and coworkers,[52] the prevalence of PDR in insulin-taking patients younger than 30 at diagnosis (exclusively or mainly type 1) was near zero when duration of diabetes was less than 10 years and then rose rapidly to about 50% in persons with 20 years or more of diabetes. In an older-onset (30 years or more) insulin-taking group, which included both diabetes types, prevalence of PDR rose fairly steadily, from 2% in persons with less than 5 years of diabetes to about 25% in those with 20 years or more. In the older-onset, noninsulin-taking (type 2) group, prevalence of PDR increased only slightly with duration, from less than 5% before 20 years to about 5% thereafter (Fig. 48.14).[53] Among patients with PDR, its severity did not appear to differ between the younger-onset and the combined older-onset groups. In each case, in the worse eye about 25% of patients had DRS high-risk characteristics and 15% had retinopathy severity ungradable because of extensive vitreous hemorrhage, phthisis bulbi, or enucleation secondary to complications of DR.[7] In patients with PDR, macular edema was more common in the combined older-onset group with retinal thickening or scars of previous focal photocoagulation present in at least one eye in about 45% (versus 30% in the younger-onset group).[54]

The Diabetic Retinopathy Vitrectomy Study (DRVS) found a substantial variation in severity of PDR by diabetes type among persons with vitreous hemorrhage severe enough to reduce visual acuity to 5/200 or less for a period of at least 1 month.[55–58] In this study the severity of new vessels, fibrous proliferation, and vitreoretinal adhesions decreased significantly as diabetes type shifted from type 1 to type 2 (Table 48.1).

Diabetes with onset after age 30 is more common than the younger-onset type, and in clinical practice PDR is seen with about equal frequency in the younger- and older-onset groups. Klein et al.[52,53] estimated that in the population they surveyed, 43% of patients with PDR were in the younger-onset group, 42% were in the older-onset insulin-taking group, and 15% were in the noninsulin-taking group. In the DRS, in which more than 90% of the 1742 patients examined had PDR in at least one eye, 44% were classified as juvenile-onset (younger than 20 years at diagnosis and taking insulin at entry into the study); 28% as adult-onset, possibly insulin-dependent (age 20 years or older at diagnosis, not overweight, and taking insulin); and 26% as classic adult-onset (mild symptomatic or asymptomatic onset at age 20 years or older and either overweight or not taking insulin at study entry). The remaining 2% were not classifiable.[33] Aiello and coworkers[59] described the distribution of age at diabetes

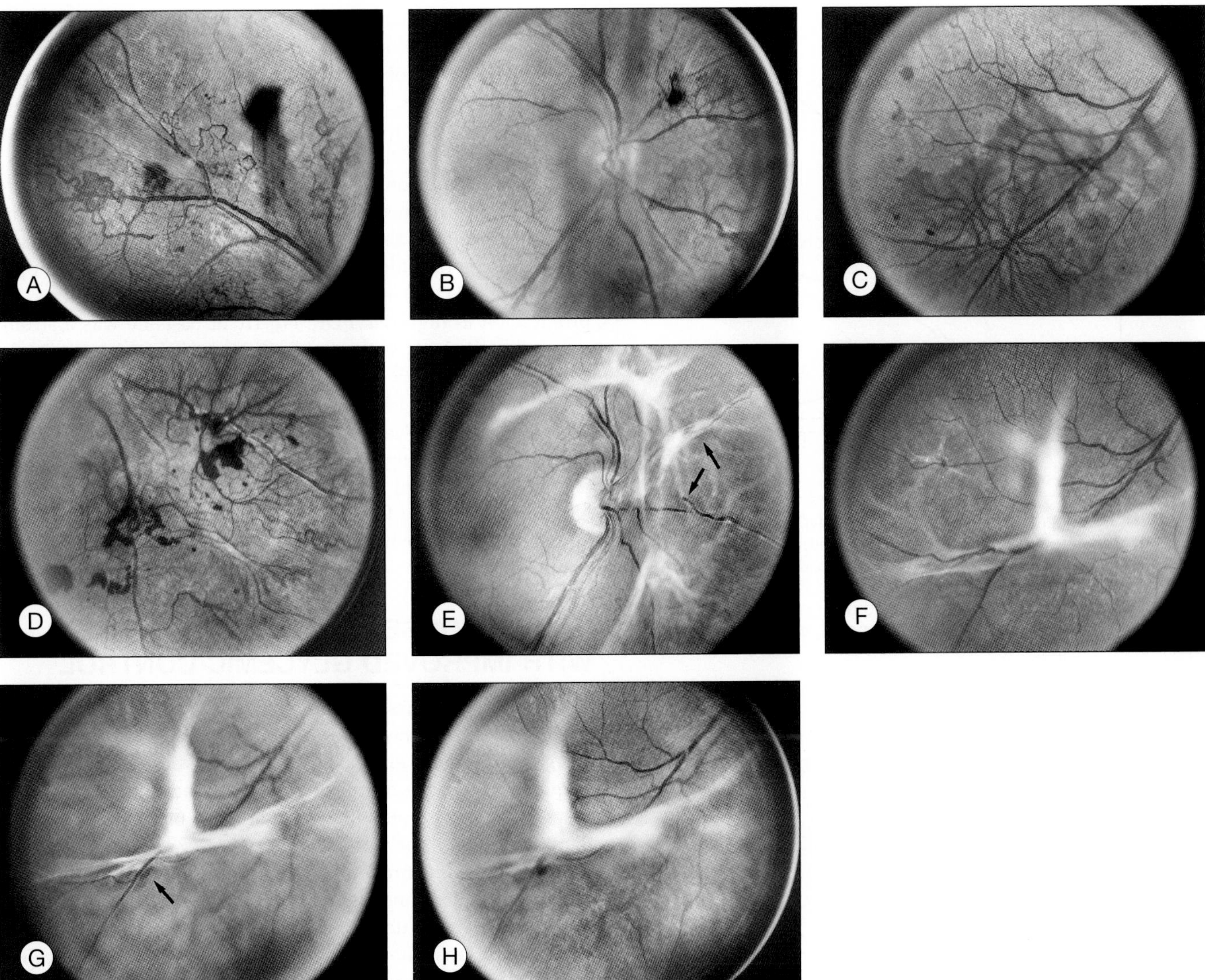

Fig. 48.13 Contraction of fibrovascular proliferations with limited vitreoretinal adhesions, leading to pulled-up retinal vessels and localized retinal detachment, and spontaneous regression of new vessels. (A) In the superotemporal quadrant of the right eye of this 25-year-old man, whose age at diagnosis of diabetes was 8 years, several small, wheel-shaped networks of new vessels on the surface of the retina, venous beading, intraretinal microvascular abnormalities, and localized hemorrhage far anterior to the retina in the formed vitreous were noted. Several small, white, threadlike arterioles were present superiorly, where the retina appeared featureless, indicating loss of much of the retinal capillary bed. (B) The disc and new vessels nasal to it are blurred by vitreous hemorrhage. The macula is visible in its normal position at the left edge of the figure. (C) New vessels along the inferior temporal vein were in focus inferiorly, where they were on the surface of the retina, but were out of focus above the vein, where they were about a half-disc diameter (DD) anterior to the retina, growing along the detached posterior vitreous surface. (D) New vessels and thin fibrous proliferations inferonasal to the disc. Inferiorly, the new vessels were flat on the surface of the retina; superiorly, they were elevated about a half-DD in front of the retina, on the detached posterior vitreous surface. Preretinal hemorrhages marked the inferior extent of posterior vitreous detachment. Visual acuity was 20/20. (E) One year later, following spontaneous regression of the new vessels and completion of posterior vitreous detachment, most of the proliferations were far anterior to the retina and out of focus. The inferonasal vein had been pulled upward to the horizontal meridian, and a loop of it had been pulled forward (lower arrow) without adjacent retinal detachment. The superonasal vein was also pulled forward, together with a narrow fold of retina (upper arrow). Tension lines ran through the macula, which had been displaced somewhat downward. (F) The inferotemporal vein had been pulled forward, together with a narrow fold of retina, but the adjacent retina was flat. Visual acuity was 20/30. (G) (focused on the elevated inferotemporal vein) Three years later, a small oval retinal hole (arrow) could be seen just below the point where the inferotemporal vein was most highly elevated. Retinal detachment extended inferotemporally past the edge of the figure. (H) (focused on the attached posterior retina) The retina above the superotemporal vein remained flat, and visual acuity had improved to 20/20. Panels (G) and (H) may be viewed stereoscopically by relaxing convergence (or using a base-out prism). (Courtesy of Diabetic Retinopathy Vitrectomy Study Research Group.)

diagnosis among 244 patients with PDR at the Joslin Clinic during a 5-month period: diagnosis age less than 20 years, 53%; 20–39 years, 25%; and 40 years or older, 22%.

In a comprehensive meta-analysis including 28 prospective interventional or observational studies comprising 27120 diabetic patients with at least 10 years of follow-up, lower rates of progression to PDR and severe visual loss were observed in those more recently diagnosed with diabetes.[10] The 4-year risk of progression to PDR and severe visual loss was substantially lower among participants in 1986–2008 (2.6% and 3.2%) than in 1975–1985 (19.5% and 9.7%). At 10 years, similar patterns were observed with participants in 1986–2008 studies having lower

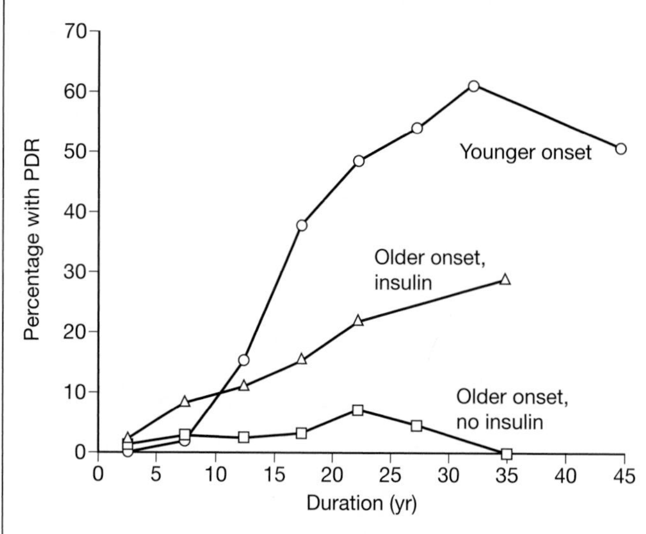

Fig. 48.14 Percentage of people with proliferative diabetic retinopathy (PDR) by duration of diabetes in each of the three groups. (Reproduced with permission from Klein R, Davis M, Moss S, et al. The Wisconsin Epidemiologic Study of Diabetic Retinopathy: a comparison of retinopathy in younger and older onset diabetic persons. In: Vranic M, Hollenberg C, Steiner G, editors. Comparison of type I and II diabetes. New York: Plenum Press; 1985.)

Table 48.1 Percentage of Diabetic Retinopathy Vitrectomy Study (DRVS) group H eyes assigned to early vitrectomy with specified severity level of new vessels, fibrous proliferations, and vitreoretinal adhesions, by diabetes type

	Diabetes type*		
Fundus abnormality	Type 1	Mixed	Type 2
New vessels ≥ 1 disc area	81.1%	58.2%	42.2%
Fibrous proliferations ≥ 2 disc areas	68.2%	47.7%	44.5%
Vitreoretinal adhesions ≥ 4 disc areas	47.8%	34.5%	23.6%

**Type I, age at diagnosis 20 years or younger and taking insulin at study entry; mixed, age at diagnosis 21–39 years and taking insulin at study entry; type II, age at diagnosis 40 years or older, or not taking insulin at study entry.*
(Reproduced with permission from Diabetic Retinopathy Vitrectomy Study (DRVS) Research Group: report number 2. Arch Ophthalmol 1985;103:1644–52.

proportions of PDR and NPDR at all time points than participants in 1975–1985 studies. National population-based estimates have reflected this trend of a reduction in the prevalence of PDR, presumably reflecting improved glycemic and systemic control as well as earlier detection of retinal complications.[60] These trends in the reduction of PDR and visual loss are discussed in greater detail in Chapter 45 (The epidemiology of diabetic retinopathy).

PROLIFERATIVE DIABETIC RETINOPATHY AND BLOOD GLUCOSE CONTROL

The results from the Diabetes Control and Complications Trial (DCCT)/Epidemiology of Diabetes Interventions and Complications (EDIC) and the United Kingdom Prospective Diabetes Study (UKPDS) have established the benefit of intensive blood glucose control in reducing the risk for DR in both type 1 and type 2 patients.[61–70] These large multicenter trials demonstrated conclusively that the long-term risks for the development and progression of DR can be reduced dramatically by improving blood glucose control with intensive treatment.[61–70]

Additional evidence that better glycemic control in patients with severe NPDR or early PDR reduces their risk of further progression is provided by Early Treatment Diabetic Retinopathy Study (ETDRS) multivariable analyses of risk factors for progression to high-risk PDR. HbA1c at baseline was a strong risk factor. Patients with HbA1c >12% had the highest risk of progression and patients with HbA1c <8.3% had the lowest risk of progression (OR 1.59 vs 1.00, P <0.0001).[71] Even in the lowest A1c category, the 5-year rate of developing high-risk PDR from severe NPDR was high (50%). These data suggest that the benefits of better control continue to be manifest even once severe NPDR or PDR has developed; however, they do address the effects, beneficial or harmful (see below), of improving control at this stage.

EARLY WORSENING OF RETINOPATHY WITH IMPROVED GLYCEMIC CONTROL

Soon after HbA1c assays, home blood glucose monitoring and continuous subcutaneous insulin infusion became widely available, several small clinical trials and case series reported the frequent occurrence of unexpected worsening of DR[72–75] in the first 3–12 months following the initiation of intensive insulin therapy (termed "early worsening").[73,76–78] In most of these early trials the patients enrolled had no more than mild-to-moderate NPDR at baseline and the early worsening, when it occurred, was usually mild (development of cotton-wool spots and/or IRMA) and transient. In some reports, however, when glycemic control was very poor and/or retinopathy more severe at baseline, some eyes developed severe PDR and/or macular edema and substantial visual loss.[63,72–75]

In the DCCT, cotton-wool spots or IRMA, or both, developed in only 1% of 348 patients entering the trial with no retinopathy. This proportion increased to 48% in the 60 patients with mild nonproliferative retinopathy, defined as the presence of microaneurysms plus mild retinal hemorrhages and/or hard exudates. Recovery was frequent and at the 4-year follow-up visit progression from baseline on the ETDRS scale was about the same in intensive treatment group eyes that had experienced early worsening as in conventional treatment group eyes that had not (1.3 vs 1.0 steps). Clinically important early worsening (defined as development of PDR, severe NPDR, or clinically significant macular edema) was not observed in patients with no retinopathy or with microaneurysms involving only one eye, but it occurred in 6 of the 32 patients with moderate NPDR. DCCT patients were followed closely, and early worsening did not lead to serious visual loss, but DCCT findings support the conclusion that early worsening may be more common and more sight-threatening in patients with more severe retinopathy and/or very poor glycemic control. For this reason, patients with advanced nonproliferative or active proliferative DR should be monitored closely before and for several months after initiation of intensive insulin treatment.[70,72,75,79] Panretinal photocoagulation prior to initiation of such treatment may be considered when factors suggest a particular need to protect against advancing severe retinopathy. Such considerations include very severe NPDR or active PDR, long-standing very poor glycemic control and high likelihood of suboptimal follow-up.[72] The most important risk factors for early worsening were higher baseline HbA1c and greater reduction of HbA1c after enrollment. Possible mechanisms include[72,75] alterations in retinal blood flow, decreased autoregulation of the retinal circulation, transient ischemia owing to a decrease in nutrient substrate, and insulin-induced changes in retinal homeostasis that lead to an increase in growth factors such as VEGF.[80–82] Because the short- and long-term benefits of improved glycemic control in reducing the risk of retinopathy progression are remarkable[67] and because treatments for sight-threatening retinopathy are highly effective in preventing visual loss, intensive glycemic control should not be discouraged for fear of retinopathy progression.[69]

ABSENCE OF PROLIFERATIVE DIABETIC RETINOPATHY IN INDIVIDUALS WITH DIABETES OF EXTREME DURATION

Despite the nearly universal development of some degree of retinopathy in people with diabetes given sufficient time, the development of PDR plateaus at approximately 60%. This observation has generated significant research interest, as it suggests that there may be protective mechanisms that may delay or prevent the progression to PDR. There are published reports on two unique cohorts of type 1 patients with more than 50 years of type 1 diabetes. The Golden Years cohort from the United Kingdom was noted to have characteristic normal body mass, low insulin dose, a favorable lipid profile, and a positive family history of longevity consistent with possibly genetically determined favorable outcomes.[83] The Joslin 50-year Medalist cohort has been characterized for all four major diabetic vascular complications of retinopathy, nephropathy, neuropathy, and cardiovascular disease. The 50-Year Medalist Study[84,85] has demonstrated that substantial proportions of individuals may survive diabetes duration of 50 years or more and remain free of advanced diabetic vasculopathy including PDR (49.4%). Longitudinal data from a subgroup of 97 Medalists followed for an average of 20.6 years and 39.4 visits suggests that retinopathy worsening occurs almost entirely within the first two decades of follow-up and eyes that do not develop PDR have a slower rate of retinopathy progression. These findings strongly suggest the existence of a subgroup of individuals who develop early protection against the long-term adverse effects of hyperglycemia. Furthermore, despite multiple studies that have strongly associated worse glycemic control, hypertension, and hyperlipidemia with more severe diabetic retinopathy or diabetic macular edema in patients with shorter duration diabetes, no relationship has been found between these factors and PDR status in the Medalists. Instead, initial findings suggest that specific combinations of advanced glycation endproducts may be associated with increased risk for (carboxyethyl-lysine and pentosidine) or protection from (carboxymethyl-lysine and fructose-lysine) PDR in this unique cohort. Ongoing studies in the Medalists and other populations with extremely long duration of diabetes may yield additional insights into protective mechanisms against PDR development, including novel genetic, biochemical, and physiologic factors.

SYSTEMIC MEDICATIONS AND PROLIFERATIVE DIABETIC RETINOPATHY

Systemic medications are often used in the setting of diabetes mellitus to attain optimal glycemic control and treat coexisting conditions. These drugs can have beneficial or deleterious effects on the onset or progression of diabetic eye disease. There is mounting evidence that oral systemic medications can reduce microvascular complications possibly though mechanisms other than their effect on glycemic control, blood pressure and lipid lowering. The results of clinical trials on glycemic control (DCCT,[61,65] EDIC,[69,70] UKPDS,[62,67,68] ACCORD,[86] ADVANCE[87]), lipid-lowering medications (ACCORD-EYE,[88] FIELD[89]) and angiotensin-converting enzyme inhibitors (EURODIAB,[90] EUCLID,[90] ADVANCE[86]) angiotensin II type 1-receptor blockers (DIRECT[91,92], RASS[93]) on retinopathy progression are discussed in detail in Chapter 45 (The epidemiology of diabetic retinopathy) and Chapter 47 (Nonproliferative diabetic retinopathy and diabetic macular edema).

Evidence to support the rationale of using systemically active therapeutic agents to prevent or limit local microvascular complications such as PDR is also growing. Thiazolidinediones are a class of oral hypoglycemic agents used in the treatment of type 2 diabetes that activate the peroxisome proliferator-activated receptor (PPAR) γ - a transcription factor known to regulate the expression of genes primarily located in adipose tissue, but also present in other tissues such as the retina.[94] The thiazolidinedione rosiglitazone has been reported to delay the onset of PDR, possibly because of antiangiogenic effects mediated by PPARγ agonist activity.[95,96] Shen and colleagues[95] performed a longitudinal medical record review of 124 patients treated with rosiglitazone and 158 patients not receiving rosiglitazone as controls, who were matched by baseline characteristics including level of HbA1c. Among patients with severe NPDR receiving rosiglitazone, the relative risk of progression to PDR at 3 years was reduced by 59% ($P = 0.045$), and this effect continued over 5 years of follow-up. Furthermore, at 5 years of follow-up, a significantly smaller proportion of patients in the rosiglitazone group experienced a decline of 3 or more lines in visual acuity (0.5% vs 38.0%; $P = 0.03$). No difference was found in the incidence of DME or CSME between the groups ($P = 0.28$). Initial case series and a prospective cohort-based electronic medical record-based review have reported the association of thiazolidinedione use and diabetic macular edema (OR 2.6; 95% CI 2.4–3.0). However, data from the largest clinical trial study to date to evaluate an association between thiazolidinedione exposure and DME in patients with type 2 diabetes demonstrated no such association. Thus, it appears that DME can occur at least sporadically with thiazolidinedione use, although this is relatively rare.

OTHER RISK FACTORS FOR PROLIFERATIVE DIABETIC RETINOPATHY

Most studies seeking to identify risk factors for the development of PDR begin with patients who have various levels of NPDR or no visible retinopathy at all, and make comparisons of baseline factors between those who do and do not develop PDR. As expected, the significant risk factors for the development of PDR include increasing NPDR severity, decreased visual acuity, and elevated HbAlc. Additional risk factors included the presence of diabetic neuropathy, decreased hematocrit, increased serum triglyceride, and decreased plasma albumin.[71] However, it should be noted that if the risk factors for progression from severe NPDR to PDR differ substantially from those mediating onset or progression of earlier NPDR previous studies may not have readily identified these differences.

The association of elevated serum lipids with increased risk of progression to high-risk PDR, as well as their association with increased hard exudates and decreased visual acuity,[97] provide additional motivation for lowering the frequently elevated lipid levels observed in diabetic patients. Data from the ACCORD-EYE study show that DR progression rates were reduced from 10.2% with placebo to 6.5% with fenofibrate therapy for dyslipidemia (adjusted OR 0.60; 95% CI 0.42–0.87; P = 0.006).[88] Severe anemia is a less frequently encountered problem in diabetic patients, but its association with increased risk of severe retinopathy has been suggested by ETDRS analyses and three other reports.[71] Hypertension was not identified as a risk factor for development of high-risk PDR in the ETDRS, while findings in previous studies have been variable.[7,71] In the UKPDS, patients with hypertension were randomized between more- and less-intensive regimens of blood pressure control, and retinopathy progression was significantly less common in the former, as was the incidence of photocoagulation and of a 3 or more line decrease in visual acuity. Risk reductions after 7.5 years ranged from 35% to 45% for these outcomes. Progression to PDR was too infrequent for meaningful analysis. A more detailed discussion of the epidemiology and risk factors for DR is presented in Chapter 45.

MANAGEMENT OF PROLIFERATIVE DIABETIC RETINOPATHY

Familiarity with the natural course of PDR suggests two principal therapeutic approaches: first, to discourage the proliferation of new vessels, and, second, to prevent or relieve the effects of contraction of the posterior vitreous surface and fibrovascular proliferation. This section deals mainly with the first aim as the second is discussed in Chapter 111 (Surgery for proliferative diabetic retinopathy). The cornerstone of diabetes eye care is the maintenance of intensive glycemic control which is remarkably effective in reducing the risk of onset and progression of DR and the development of PDR.[61–70] Once active proliferative changes have begun, glycemic control alone is usually insufficient. A variety of other approaches have been attempted including pituitary ablation, which was supplanted by laser photocoagulation as the treatment of choice for more than four decades now. In addition, new therapeutic interventions are now on the horizon. The following section discusses these past, present, and future approaches.

Pituitary ablation

Building on the fundamental discovery of Biasotti and Houssay[98] and that hypophysectomy reduced the severity of diabetes in pancreatectomized dogs, Luft and coworkers[99] carried out hypophysectomy in the hope of ameliorating the vascular complications of diabetes. Further impetus was provided by Poulsen's report[100,101] of remission of DR in a woman with post-partum anterior pituitary insufficiency (Sheehan syndrome). Over the next 25 years, various types of pituitary suppression were used, ranging from external irradiation to transfrontal hypophysectomy, and consensus developed among advocates of these procedures that complete or nearly complete suppression of anterior pituitary function (pituitary ablation) produced rapid improvement in eyes with the intraretinal lesions characteristic of severe NPDR and actively growing new vessels not yet accompanied by extensive fibrous proliferations. Although only two randomized trials have been reported,[102] both small and neither in itself compelling, the weight of evidence supports the strongly held opinion of those most experienced with this procedure that it was beneficial. Particularly persuasive are comparisons between patients in whom transsphenoidal implantation of radioactive yttrium was followed by complete or nearly complete anterior pituitary suppression and similar patients in whom little or no suppression was achieved. Substantially better outcome was observed in the former group.[103] Additional support is provided by a nonrandomized comparison of eyes with very extensive new vessels and IRMA, in which outcome was better in the eyes of patients undergoing pituitary ablation than in similar eyes receiving photocoagulation or no treatment.[104] Pituitary ablation is now primarily of historical interest because photocoagulation is more effective and is free of the many substantial disadvantages of inducing and living in the hypopituitary state with concomitant diabetes (e.g., operative and immediate postoperative risks, increased susceptibility to severe insulin reactions, need for continuing replacement of adrenal corticosteroids, sterility).

The favorable effect of pituitary ablation on retinopathy is thought to be mediated by suppression of growth hormone activity and effects on insulin-like growth factor 1 (IGF-1).[105] Daily subcutaneous injections of a genetically engineered growth hormone receptor antagonist, pegvisomant, have been given for 3 months in 25 patients with non-high-risk PDR. Regression of new vessels did not occur in any patient, although the serum level of insulin-like growth factor 1 (IGF-1), a growth factor whose secretion is stimulated by growth hormone, did decrease an average of 55% compared to baseline levels.[106] In a small randomized clinical trial, multiple daily subcutaneous injections of octreotide, a somatostatin analog that inhibits both growth hormone and insulin-like growth factor, were given to 11 patients with severe NPDR or non-high-risk PDR. During 15 months' follow-up, 1 out of 22 of these patients' eyes required scatter laser photocoagulation compared to 9 out of 24 eyes of 12 patients randomly assigned to an untreated control group.[107] Unfortunately, larger clinical trials of somatostatin analogs were not found to be effective.

Early laser trials

Early observations noted that certain ocular conditions seemed to prevent severe diabetic retinopathy. In addition, as many as 10% of patients experienced spontaneous resolution of PDR.[51] In these eyes the retinopathy becomes stable, the hemorrhages resolve, the retinal vasculature becomes quiescent, the proliferating tissue thins, the retinal veins lose their distended appearance, the retinal arteries become small and attenuated and many obliterated vessel branches are observed. This appearance of the retina is strikingly similar to eyes that have undergone chorioretinal scarring, optic atrophy, high myopia, retinitis pigmentosa, and the end stage of the desired outcome following pituitary ablation.[108,109] The initial use of the xenon arc photocoagulator developed by Meyer-Schwickerath[110] in the treatment of PDR involved direct treatment of new vessels on the surface of the retina, particularly those that appeared to be the source of vitreous hemorrhage.[111–113] Large, slow, moderately intense burns were used, turning the retina white adjacent to the new vessels and sometimes causing them to narrow and the flow within them to slow. These effects were the result of heat generated when light was absorbed by the retinal pigment epithelium (RPE) or by hemorrhage within the retina or on its surface. Direct destruction of new vessels required heavy burns, which usually involved the full thickness of the retina and often led to nerve fiber bundle field defects, particularly if hemorrhages were present in or on the retina. When new vessels were located some distance from the RPE, either in the vitreous or on the optic disc, they could not be treated directly with the xenon arc photocoagulator because it was not possible to concentrate enough energy in a short enough time to coagulate the rapidly flowing blood within them. The hope that this effect would be possible with the narrow, intense, blue–green beam of the argon laser was part of the rationale for its development.

Before the argon laser became widely available, and before recognition of the tendency for NVD and elevated NVE to regrow after apparently successful direct treatment, the novel concept of panretinal treatment described above began to evolve. Based on observations of remarkable asymmetry of retinopathy favoring the involved eye in diabetic patients who had unilateral disseminated chorioretinal scarring, high myopia, or optic atrophy, Beetham and Aiello began a study in which ruby laser burns were scattered across the retina from the posterior pole to the midperiphery.[109,114,115] The hope was that the induced scarring might have a distant effect across the retina and promote regression of new vessels and diminution of retinal edema and vascular congestion.[109,116,117] The long wavelength and very brief exposure time of the ruby laser limited burns mainly to the outer layers of the retina, without immediately visible effects in new vessels on its surface.

The mechanisms by which panretinal photocoagulation mediates its remarkable benefit are not fully understood. Several mechanisms have been proposed and all may contribute toward the beneficial effect. Ischemic retina, which produces growth factors, is destroyed, thus reducing the angiogenic stimulus. Another possibility is that retinal cells may produce growth-inhibiting factors or reduce production of growth-promoting factors in response to photocoagulation injury. Such factors have not been shown to be of importance in vivo to date.[118,119] It is thought that the primary mediating factor is an increase in oxygenation from the choroid to the inner retina that occurs through the laser scars due to the thinning of the retina in the treated area.[120–124] Indeed, retinal blood flow decreases and the autoregulatory response to breathing pure oxygen improves following scatter photocoagulation, as might be expected if more oxygen reached the inner retina from the choroid.[125,126] Furthermore, direct measurements of increased vitreous oxygen have been made using intraocular microelectrodes.[127]The oxygen concentration of the vitreous is much higher overlying the areas of laser burns than over the untreated retina. Regardless of the relative contributions of these mechanisms, the remarkable efficacy of panretinal photocoagulation in the treatment of PDR has been thoroughly documented in multiple randomized clinical trials.

Panretinal photocoagulation

The initial reports concerning photocoagulation suffered from small numbers of patients, brief periods of follow-up, or lack of a randomly selected control group.[119] Randomized clinical trials were needed to evaluate the possible benefits and risks of this treatment objectively. Two collaborative studies were initiated in the early 1970s: the British multicenter trial using xenon arc photocoagulation[128] and the National Eye Institute's Diabetic Retinopathy Study (DRS), which compared xenon arc and argon laser photocoagulation to no photocoagulation in patients with PDR.[129] The DRS provided the initial evidence to establish the safety and efficacy of modern panretinal (scatter) photocoagulation (PRP).

The DRS conclusively demonstrated that PRP significantly reduces the risk of severe visual loss (SVL) from PDR, particularly when high-risk PDR is present.[1,26,130] Patients entering the DRS had PDR in at least one eye or severe NPDR in both eyes. Visual acuity of 20/100 or better was present in each eye. Each patient was randomly assigned to either the argon or xenon treatment group. One eye was randomly assigned to photocoagulation treatment and the other to indefinite deferral of treatment (i.e., no treatment ever), unless evidence that treatment was beneficial resulted in a change of study protocol. Patients were followed at 4-month intervals according to a protocol that provided for measurement of best-corrected visual acuity under standard lighting conditions, with separate charts for each eye. The visual acuity examiners did not know the identity of the treated eye or type of treatment and attempted to reduce patient bias by urging the patient to read as far down the chart as possible with each eye, guessing at letters until more than one in a line was missed.[1]

DRS treatment techniques are summarized in Table 48.2. Both techniques included scatter treatment with burns spaced about

Table 48.2 Diabetic retinopathy study photocoagulation techniques

	Argon laser	Xenon arc
Scatter treatment		
No. of burns	800–1600 (500 μm)	400–800 (3 degrees)
	or 500–1000	or 200–400
	(1000 μm)	(4.5 degrees)
Exposure time	0.1 s	Not specified
Direct treatment*		
Surface NVE	+	+
Elevated NVE	+	–
NVD	+	–
Macular edema	+	+
Follow-up treatment	+	+

NVE, new vessels elsewhere (more than 1 disc diameter [DD] from the disc); NVD, new vessels on or within 1 DD of the disc.
(Reproduced with permission from Diabetic Retinopathy Study Research Group. Photocoagulation treatment of proliferative diabetic retinopathy: clinical application of Diabetic Retinopathy Study (DRS) findings. DRS report number 8. Ophthalmology 1981; 88:583–600. Copyright © 1981 American Academy of Ophthalmology.)

one-half to one burn-width apart, extending from the posterior pole to the equator and often completed in a single sitting. The argon treatment technique specified 800–1600 500 μm scatter burns of 0.1 second duration and direct treatment of new vessels on the disc and elsewhere, whether flat or elevated. Direct treatment was also applied to microaneurysms or other lesions thought to be causing macular edema. Follow-up treatment was applied as needed at 4-month intervals. The xenon technique was similar, but burns were fewer, of longer duration, and stronger. Direct treatment was not applied to elevated new vessels or those on the surface of the disc in the xenon treated group.

The principal outcome of the DRS was visual acuity of <5/200 at each of two consecutively completed follow-up visits, scheduled at least 4-months apart (termed severe visual loss). Visual acuity of <5/200 was chosen as the level at which vision becomes too poor to be useful for walking about or for other self-care activities. The requirement of two consecutive visits was included because the rate of recovery to better visual acuity after a single visit at the <5/200 level was 29% in the control group and 49% in the treated group whereas after two visits it was 12% and 29%, respectively, and after three visits, 8% and 21%.[1] Because recovery was somewhat more common in treated eyes, the chosen endpoint tends to underestimate the treatment benefit.

Table 48.3 presents 2-year cumulative rates of severe visual loss in eyes grouped by baseline retinopathy severity and treatment assignment.[2] For severe visual loss to be present at the 2-year visit, visual acuity had to be <5/200 no later than the 20-month visit. For all eyes in the untreated control group, the risk of severe visual loss within 2 years was 15.9%, and this risk was reduced to 6.4% by treatment. The risk was greatest in group J (36.9% in the control group). These eyes had preretinal or vitreous hemorrhage and NVD exceeding those in standard photograph 10A of the modified Airlie House classification (Fig. 48.15). The risk appeared somewhat lower for eyes with NVD of

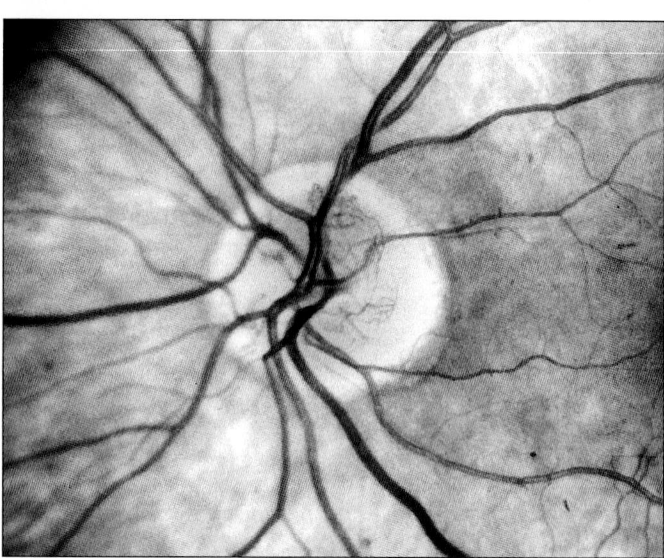

Fig. 48.15 Standard photograph 10A of the modified Airlie House classification, defining the lower limit of moderate new vessels on or within 1 disc diameter of the disc. (Reproduced with permission from Diabetic Retinopathy Study Research Group. A modification of the Airlie House classification of diabetic retinopathy. DRS report number 7. Invest Ophthalmol Vis Sci 1981;21:210–26.)

Table 48.3 Cumulative 2-year rates of severe visual loss in eyes grouped by baseline retinopathy severity and treatment assignment

Retinopathy severity group	NVE	NVD	VH/PRH	No. of NV-VH risk factors	Control		Treated		Z-value
					SVL (%)	No. at risk*	SVL (%)	No. at risk*	
A	0	0	0	0	3.6	195	3.0	182	0.4
B	0	0	+	1	4.2	11	0.0	16	1.0
C	<1/2DA	0	0	1	6.8	120	2.0	96	1.8
D	<1/2DA	0	+	2	6.4	18	0.0	19	1.1
E	≥1/2DA	0	0	2	6.9	125	4.3	141	1.0
F	≥1/2DA	0	+	3	29.7	40	7.2	41	3.0
G	+ or 0	<10A	0	2	10.5	114	3.1	126	2.4
H	+ or 0	<10A	+	3	25.6	39	4.3	35	2.9
I	+ or 0	≥10A	0	3	26.2	150	8.5	174	4.7
J	+ or 0	≥10A	+	4	36.9	76	20.1	107	3.2
All eyes					15.9	897	6.4	946	7.2

NVD, new vessels on or within 1 disc diameter of the optic disc; NVE, new vessels elsewhere (i.e., outside the area defined as NVD); VH/PRH, vitreous/preretinal hemorrhage; NV-VH risk factors, new vessel–vitreous hemorrhage risk factors (see text); SVL, severe visual loss (visual acuity < 5/200 at two or more consecutively completed follow-up visits scheduled at 4-month intervals); DA, disc area (NVE < 1/2 DA indicates that NVE do not equal or exceed one-half the area of the disc in any of the standard photographic fields, NVE ≥ 1/2 DA indicates that NVE equal or exceed this area in at least one of these fields); 10A, standard photograph 10A of the modified Airlie House classification (Fig. 48.15).

*In the 20- to 24-month interval.

(Reproduced with permission from the Diabetic Retinopathy Study Research Group. Indications for photocoagulation treatment of diabetic retinopathy. DRS report number 14. Int Ophthalmol Clin 1987;27:239–53.)

this severity without hemorrhage (group I, 26.2% in the control group). Similar risks (25.6 and 29.7%, respectively) were observed for untreated eyes in groups H and F, eyes with vitreous or preretinal hemorrhage, and less severe new vessels. Eyes in these four groups were referred to in the DRS as eyes with high-risk characteristics or, alternatively, eyes with three or four new vessel-vitreous hemorrhage (NV-VH) risk factors, these factors being: (1) new vessels present; (2) new vessels located on or within 1 DD of the disc (NVD); (3) new vessels moderate to severe (NVD equaling or exceeding those in standard photograph 10A or, for eyes without NVD, NVE equaling or exceeding one-half disc area in at least one photographic field); and (4) vitreous or preretinal hemorrhage (or both) present. In counting risk factors, the presence and severity of NVE were considered only in eyes without NVD because a subgroup analysis indicated that in eyes with NVD the presence of moderate or severe NVE did not further increase the risk of severe visual loss.[2] In the remaining groups (A through E and G), the risk without treatment varied from 3.6 to 10.5%. Treatment reduced the rate of severe visual loss in each group, most impressively in groups F through J. Since it appeared that a small permanent reduction in visual acuity might occur in 10–20% of treated eyes, the DRS investigators concluded in 1976 that prompt photocoagulation treatment was usually desirable for eyes with high-risk characteristics. The protocol was therefore modified to allow treatment of eyes originally assigned to the untreated control group, if they had high-risk characteristics at the time or developed them subsequently.[1]

In Table 48.4 the retinopathy severity groups presented in Table 48.3 have been combined, and observations from follow-up visits completed after the 1976 protocol change have been included.[1] Forty-three percent of the 2-year visits and all the 4-year visits included in this analysis were carried out after the 1976 protocol change. At the 2-year visit, 12% of control-group eyes had been treated, and by the 4-year visit 35% had been treated. All eyes were classified in the group to which they were originally randomly assigned, without reference to treatment of control-group eyes. In the control group the 2-year risk of severe visual loss increased from 3.2% in eyes with NPDR to 7% in eyes with PDR without high-risk characteristics, and to 26.2% in eyes with high-risk characteristics. The 4-year rates in these groups were, respectively, 12.8, 20.9, and 44.0%. Treatment reduced the risk of severe visual loss by 50% to 65% in all three groups at both 2 and 4 years, except for the NPDR group at 2 years.

Figure 48.16 depicts cumulative rates of severe visual loss by treatment assignment (argon and xenon groups combined) for up to 6 years. Two separate analyses are summarized, one excluding and the other including visits made after the 1976 protocol change. The curves for control-group eyes are very similar over the first 20 months of follow-up, and those for treated eyes are similar over at least the first 28 months. The difference between the two control-group curves is probably due, at least in part, to the beneficial effect of treatment experienced by some of these eyes after the protocol change, and the long-term analysis probably underestimates treatment effect. In each of these analyses, treatment reduced the risk of severe visual loss by 50% or more at and after the 16-month visit.[130] In Fig. 48.17, the plots from Fig. 48.16, including all visits, are presented separately for the argon and xenon groups. The treatment effect (i.e., the difference between treatment and control groups) appeared somewhat greater in the xenon group, but this difference was small, its statistical significance was borderline, and its clinical importance was outweighed by the greater harmful effects of DRS xenon treatment.

A temporary decrease in visual acuity is frequently noted after extensive scatter photocoagulation, with recovery to the pretreatment level in most cases within several weeks. In the DRS,

Table 48.4 Cumulative 2- and 4-year rates of severe visual loss in eyes grouped by baseline retinopathy severity and treatment assignment*

Retinopathy severity	Groups†	No. of NV–VH risk factors	Follow-up	Control		Treated		
				SVL (%)	No. at risk‡	SVL (%)	No. at risk‡	Z-value
NPDR	A	0	2-year	3.2	297	2.8	303	0.3
			4-year	12.8	183	4.3	188	3.6
PDR without HRC	B–E, G	1 or 2	2-year	7.0	603	3.2	615	3.1
			4-year	20.9	332	7.4	390	6.5
PDR with HRC	F, H–J	3 or 4	2-year	26.2	473	10.9	570	7.1
			4-year	44.0	238	20.4	324	8.5
All eyes			2-year	14.0	1278	6.2	1489	7.4
			4-year	28.5	754	12.0	903	11.0

*As in Table 48.3.
NPDR, nonproliferative diabetic retinopathy; PDR, proliferative diabetic retinopathy; HRC, high-risk characteristics.
†NV–VH risk factors, new vessel–vitreous hemorrhage risk factors (see text); SVL, severe visual loss (visual acuity < 5/200 at two or more consecutively completed follow-up visits scheduled at 4-month intervals).
‡In the 20- to 24-month interval for the 2-year rates at the 44- to 48-month interval for the 4-year rates.
(Reproduced with permission from Diabetic Retinopathy Study Research Group. Indications for photocoagulation treatment of diabetic retinopathy. DRS report number 14. Int Ophthalmol Clin 1987;27:239–53. Copyright © 1981 American Academy of Ophthalmology.)

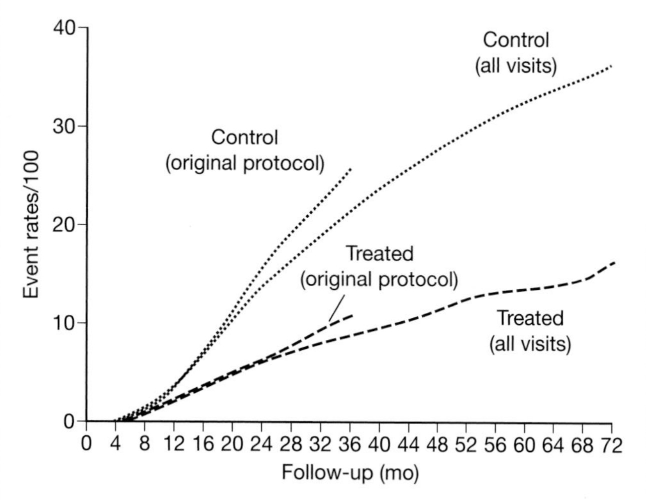

Fig. 48.16 Cumulative rates of severe visual loss, including and excluding observations made after the 1976 protocol change, for argon and xenon groups combined. (Reproduced with permission from Diabetic Retinopathy Study Research Group. Photocoagulation treatment of proliferative diabetic retinopathy: clinical application of Diabetic Retinopathy Study (DRS) findings. DRS report number 8. Ophthalmology 1981;88:583–600. Copyright © 1981 American Academy of Ophthalmology.)

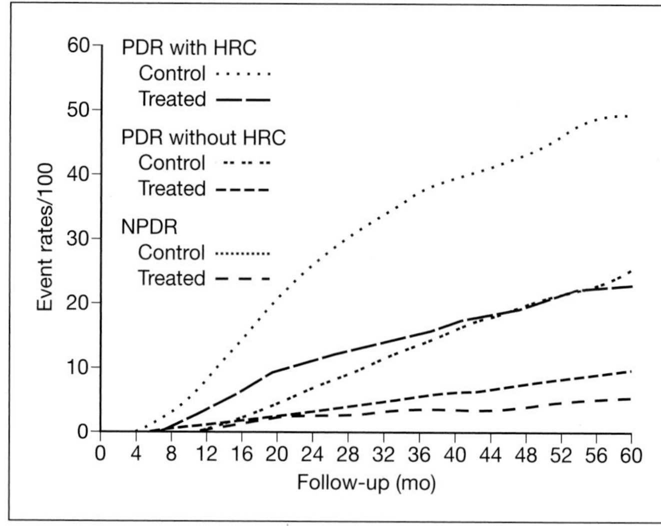

Fig. 48.18 Cumulative rates of severe visual loss for eyes classified by the presence of proliferative retinopathy (PDR) and high-risk characteristics (HRC) in baseline fundus photographs, argon, and xenon groups combined. NPDR, Nonproliferative diabetic retinopathy. (Reproduced with permission from Diabetic Retinopathy Study Research Group. Photocoagulation treatment of proliferative diabetic retinopathy: clinical application of Diabetic Retinopathy Study (DRS) findings. DRS report number 8. Ophthalmology 1981;88:583–600. Copyright © 1981 American Academy of Ophthalmology.)

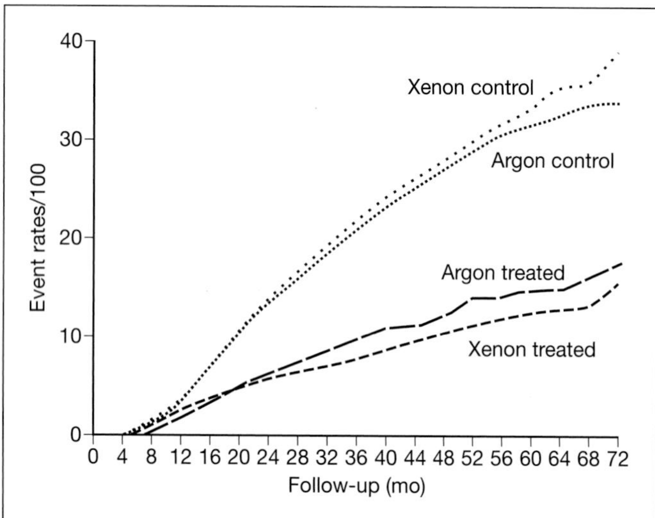

Fig. 48.17 Cumulative rates of severe visual loss by treatment group. (Reproduced with permission from Diabetic Retinopathy Study Research Group. Photocoagulation treatment of proliferative diabetic retinopathy: clinical application of Diabetic Retinopathy Study (DRS) findings. DRS report number 8. Ophthalmology 1981;88:583–600. Copyright © 1981 American Academy of Ophthalmology.)

Table 48.5 Estimated percentages of eyes with harmful effects attributable to diabetic retinopathy study treatment

	Argon (%)	Xenon (%)
Constriction of visual field		
(Goldmann IVe4 test object)		
to an average of		
≤ 45 degree, > 30 degree per meridian	5	25
≤ 30 degree per meridian	0	25
Decrease in visual acuity		
1 line	11	19
≥ 2 lines	3	11

(Reproduced with permission from Diabetic Retinopathy Study Research Group. Photocoagulation treatment of proliferative diabetic retinopathy: clinical application of Diabetic Retinopathy Study (DRS) findings. DRS report number 8. Ophthalmology 1981;88:583–600. Copyright © 1981 American Academy of Ophthalmology.)

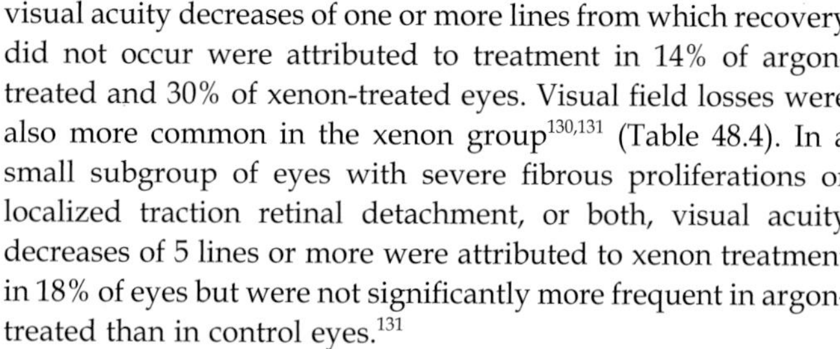

visual acuity decreases of one or more lines from which recovery did not occur were attributed to treatment in 14% of argon-treated and 30% of xenon-treated eyes. Visual field losses were also more common in the xenon group[130,131] (Table 48.4). In a small subgroup of eyes with severe fibrous proliferations or localized traction retinal detachment, or both, visual acuity decreases of 5 lines or more were attributed to xenon treatment in 18% of eyes but were not significantly more frequent in argon-treated than in control eyes.[131]

In Fig. 48.18, the Fig. 48.16 plots including all visits are presented separately for the three subgroups shown in Table 48.4. In each subgroup treatment reduced the risk of severe visual loss to about one-half of that observed in control-group eyes, but this effect became apparent later, and the percentage of eyes treated that benefited (the arithmetic difference between treated and control groups) was smaller as retinopathy severity decreased. On the basis of this analysis and the estimates of the harmful effects of treatment summarized in Table 48.5, the DRS confirmed its previous conclusion that, for eyes with high-risk characteristics, the chance of benefit from treatment clearly outweighed its risk and recommended prompt photocoagulation for most such eyes.[130]

For eyes with severe NPDR or PDR without high-risk characteristics, the DRS concluded that either prompt treatment or careful follow-up with prompt treatment if high-risk characteristics developed was satisfactory and that DRS results were not helpful in choosing between these strategies. In unadjusted analyses of DRS control-group eyes that had PDR without high-risk characteristics, the severity of each of three retinopathy characteristics was associated with risk of visual loss: retinal hemorrhages or microaneurysms, arteriolar abnormalities, and venous caliber abnormalities. These lesions – and soft exudates and IRMA – were also risk factors for visual loss in control-group eyes with NPDR.[33] A multivariable analysis that included all DRS control-group eyes found baseline visual acuity, extent of NVD, elevation of NVD (a measure of contraction of vitreous and fibrous proliferations), and severity of hemorrhages or microaneurysms, arteriolar abnormalities, venous caliber abnormalities, and vitreous or preretinal hemorrhage all to be risk factors for visual loss. Neither in this analysis, nor in a similar one confined to DRS control-group eyes that were free of NVD, was the extent of NVE found to be a risk factor.[132] These findings support clinical impressions that NVE on the surface of the retina often proliferate and regress over a period of years, remaining asymptomatic unless contraction of vitreous and fibrous proliferations begins, and that the severity of intraretinal lesions may be of greater prognostic importance than the extent of NVE.

When the DRS first reported evidence of a beneficial treatment effect and modified its protocol to encourage treatment of control-group eyes with high-risk characteristics, it also modified its treatment protocol. Because the harmful effects of the DRS argon treatment were less than those observed with the xenon treatment used in the DRS, argon was given preference and, in the hope of further reducing harmful side-effects, scatter treatment was more often divided between two or more episodes several days apart. However, because the beneficial treatment effect in the xenon group, in which no focal treatment had been applied to NVD or elevated NVE, had been at least as great as that in the argon group, these technically difficult parts of the argon protocol were dropped. Two large case series[133,134] and two smaller randomized trials reported beneficial treatment effects similar to those found in the DRS.[135,136]

Early treatment diabetic retinopathy study and the timing of treatment

As mentioned previously for eyes with severe NPDR or early (not high-risk) PDR, DRS results were not helpful in determining which of two treatment strategies would be attended by a more favorable visual outcome: (1) immediate photocoagulation or (2) frequent follow-up and prompt initiation of photocoagulation only if high-risk PDR developed. One of the goals of the Early Treatment Diabetic Retinopathy Study (ETDRS), a randomized clinical trial sponsored by the National Eye Institute, was to compare these alternatives (designated "early photocoagulation" and "deferral of photocoagulation," respectively) in patients with mild to severe NPDR or early PDR, with or without macular edema.[137] Other goals were to evaluate photocoagulation for diabetic macular edema[138] and to determine the possible effects of aspirin on DR.[139] Between 1980 and 1985, 3711 patients were enrolled and assigned randomly to aspirin 650 mg/day or placebo. One eye of each patient was randomly assigned to early photocoagulation and the other to deferral. Follow-up ranged from 3 to 8 years. Eyes assigned to early photocoagulation were randomly assigned to either of two scatter treatment protocols, full or mild. The full scatter protocol called for 500 μm, 0.1 sec argon blue–green or green laser burns of moderate intensity, placed one-half burn apart, extending from the posterior pole to the equator. Between 1200 and 1600 burns were applied, divided between two or more sittings. The mild scatter protocol was the same, except that 400–650 more widely spaced burns were applied to the same area in a single sitting. Direct (local) treatment was specified for patches of flat surface NVE that were two disc areas or less in extent (the area of a circle about 1.4 times the diameter of the disc), using confluent, moderately intense burns that extended 500 μm beyond the edges of the patch. For larger patches or several small ones close together, full scatter alone to this area was an acceptable alternative. No direct treatment was carried out for NVD.[140]

One important outcome measure used in the ETDRS was the first occurrence of either severe visual loss, as defined in the DRS, or vitrectomy.[137] These events were combined because progression to a stage requiring vitrectomy may rightly be considered an undesirable outcome for ETDRS-eligible eyes and since presumably most eyes selected for vitrectomy before the occurrence of severe visual loss (68% of the 243 ETDRS eyes undergoing vitrectomy) would have developed severe visual loss within several months if vitrectomy had not been performed. Five-year life-table rates of severe visual loss or vitrectomy, and relative risks for early photocoagulation compared to deferral over the entire follow-up period, are shown in Table 48.6. The first two rows include eyes with macular edema, subdivided by retinopathy severity. As anticipated, the poor outcome was more frequent in eyes with more severe retinopathy (in the deferral group, 10% in eyes with severe NPDR or early PDR versus 4% in eyes with mild to moderate NPDR). In both of these retinopathy subgroups, early treatment reduced the event rate to about one-half that of the deferral group, but the percentage of eyes treated that benefited was only 2–4%. The third row of the table includes all eyes without macular edema regardless of retinopathy severity (eyes with mild NPDR were not eligible unless macular edema was present), and outcome here was intermediate between that in rows 1 and 2. Some harmful effects of scatter photocoagulation were also observed in the ETDRS, including an early decrease in visual acuity (a doubling or more of the visual angle at the 4-month visit in about 10% of eyes assigned to early full scatter, compared to about 5% of eyes assigned to deferral) and some decrease in visual field. Both beneficial and harmful effects were somewhat greater with full than with mild scatter.

Figure 48.19 presents cumulative incidence rates of high-risk PDR in ETDRS eyes assigned to deferral of photocoagulation, by severity of retinopathy at baseline. It is of interest that high-risk PDR developed at about equal rates in eyes with moderate PDR or very severe NPDR, with rates of about 50% after 18 months. Figures 48.15, 48.20, and 48.21 present the standard photographs used in the definitions of high-risk PDR and very severe NPDR, the most important severity levels for application to clinical practice. It is convenient to express the approximate definitions of severe and very severe NPDR with the 4–2–1 rule described earlier (see Box 48.1).

The ETDRS recommended that scatter treatment not be used in eyes with mild to moderate NPDR but that it be considered for eyes approaching the high-risk stage (i.e., eyes with very

Table 48.6 Cumulative 5-year rates of severe visual loss or vitrectomy, and relative risks for the entire period of follow-up, by baseline retinopathy status and treatment group*

	Treatment group				
	Early photocoagulation		Deferral		
Baseline retinopathy	No. at baseline	5-year rate (%)	No. at baseline	5-year rate (%)	Relative risk (99% CI)
Mild to moderate NPDR with macular edema (0.33–0.94)	1448	2	1429	4	0.55
Severe NPDR or early PDR with macular edema (0.47–0.99)	1090	6	1103	10	0.68
Moderate to severe NPDR or early PDR without macular edema	1173	4	1179	5	0.78 (0.47–1.29)

**CI, confidence interval; NPDR, nonproliferative diabetic retinopathy; PDR, proliferative diabetic retinopathy.*
(Reproduced with permission from Early Treatment of Diabetic Retinopathy Study report number 9. Early Treatment of Diabetic Retinopathy Study Group. Ophthalmology 1991;98:766–85. Copyright © 1991 American Academy of Ophthalmology.)

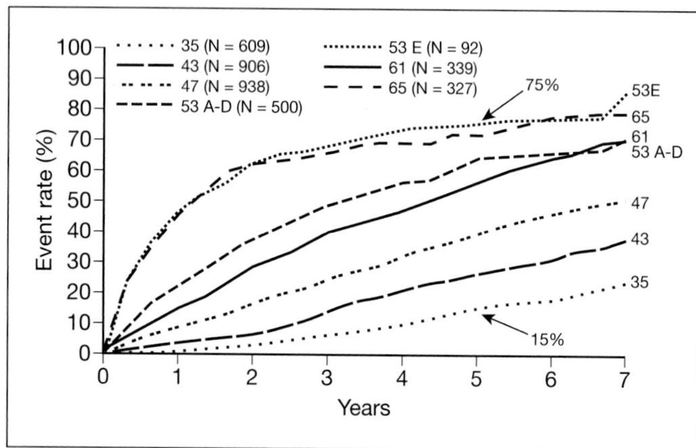

Fig. 48.19 Cumulative incidence of high-risk proliferative diabetic retinopathy in the eyes of Early Treatment Diabetic Retinopathy Study (ETDRS) patients assigned to deferral of photocoagulation. The 5-year rate for eyes with mild nonproliferative diabetic retinopathy (NPDR: level 35) was 15%. For eyes with very severe NPDR (level 53E) or moderate PDR (level 65), the 5-year rate was about 75% and the 1-year rate was almost 50%. Levels 43 and 47 represent moderate NPDR; level 53A–D, severe NPDR; and level 61, mild PDR (nVE less than half disc area or fibrous proliferation only). (Reproduced with permission from Early Treatment of Diabetic Retinopathy Study Group. Early photocoagulation for diabetic retinopathy. ETDRS report no. 9. Ophthalmology 1991;98:766–85. Copyright © 1991 American Academy of Ophthalmology.)

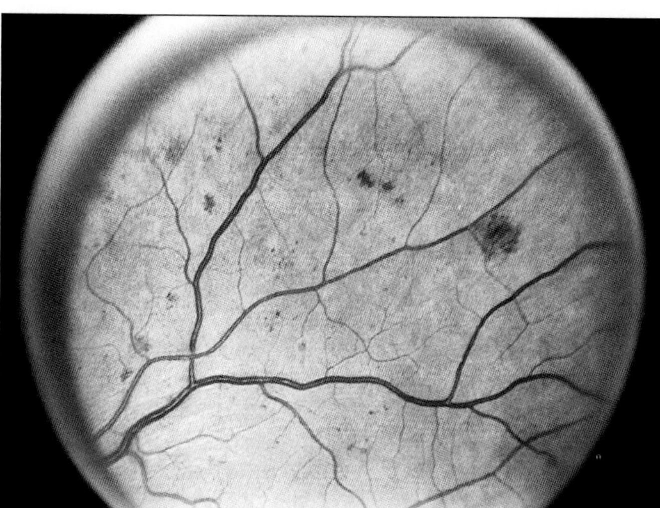

Fig. 48.20 Standard photograph 2A of the modified Airlie House classification, defining lower margin of the "severe" category for retinal hemorrhages and microaneurysms. (Reproduced with permission from Diabetic Retinopathy Study Research Group. A modification of the Airlie House classification of diabetic retinopathy. DRS report number 7. Invest Ophthalmol Vis Sci 1981;21:210–26. Copyright © 1981 American Academy of Ophthalmology.)

severe NPDR or moderate PDR) and that it usually should not be delayed when the high-risk stage is present. The recommendation to consider photocoagulation for eyes approaching the high-risk stage was made because, although both the benefits and risks of treatment were small and roughly in balance, the risk–benefit ratio was approaching a clearly favorable range. A policy of continued observation would be expected to spare only a minority of eyes from the risks of treatment, while increasing the risk that rapid progression might occur between follow-up visits and that entry into the high-risk stage might be marked by occurrence of a large vitreous hemorrhage, making satisfactory treatment difficult. In choosing between prompt treatment and deferral, the commitment of the patient to careful follow-up and the state of the fellow eye were important factors. If visual function decreased in the fellow eye after scatter photocoagulation, deferral of treatment in the second eye may be desirable. On the other hand, in a patient whose first eye had an unfortunate outcome without photocoagulation or one with photocoagulation only after PDR was advanced, prompt treatment may be preferable, particularly if close follow-up will be difficult.

These initial ETDRS recommendations were made without regard to patient age or type of diabetes. Subsequent analyses of ETDRS data suggest that, among patients whose retinopathy is in the severe NPDR to non-high-risk PDR range, the benefit of prompt treatment is greater in those who have type 2 diabetes or are older than 40 years of age (these characteristics are highly correlated, and analyses using either gave almost identical results)[141] (Fig. 48.22). In the type 2 group, the 5-year rate of severe visual loss or vitrectomy was about 5% in eyes assigned

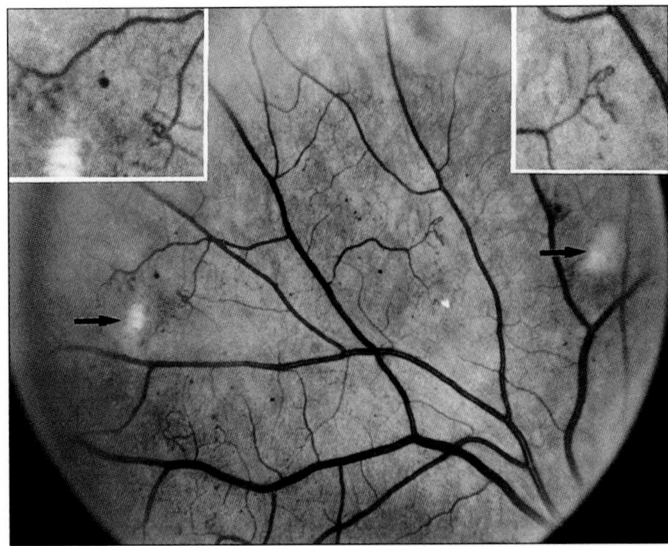

Fig. 48.21 Standard photograph 8A of the modified Airlie House classification, defining the lower margin of the "moderate" category for intraretinal microvascular abnormalities (IRMA) (and for soft exudates, indicated by arrows). IRMA are prominent in three areas, two of which are shown in insets. Additional IRMA can be seen when the color transparencies used in grading are viewed stereoscopically with ∞5 magnification. (Reproduced with permission from Diabetic Retinopathy Study Research Group. A modification of the Airlie House classification of diabetic retinopathy. DRS report number 7. Invest Ophthalmol Vis Sci 1981;21:210–26. Copyright © 1981 American Academy of Ophthalmology.)

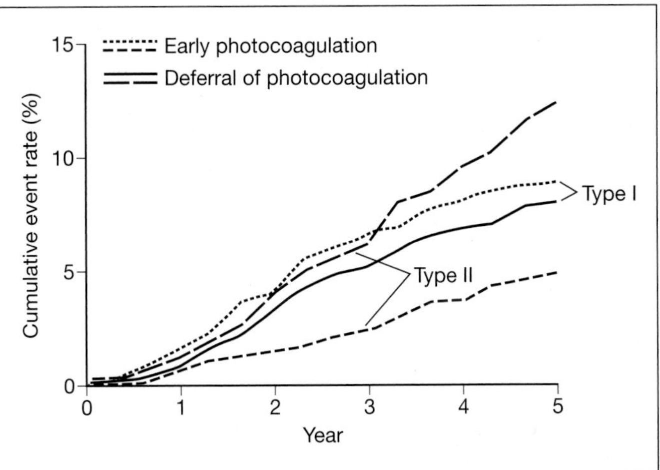

Fig. 48.22 Development of severe visual loss or vitrectomy in eyes with severe nonproliferative or early proliferative retinopathy at baseline. Early treated eyes compared with deferred eyes, for those with type 1 (P = 0.43) and type 2 (P = 0.0001) diabetes. Test for interaction of treatment and type (P = 0.0002). (Reproduced with permission from Ferris F. Early photocoagulation in patients with either type 1 or type 2 diabetes. Trans Am Ophthalmol Soc 1996;94:505–37.)

to early photocoagulation versus 13% in eyes assigned to deferral, whereas in the type 1 group the rates were about 8% in both treatment groups (Fig. 48.19). In eyes assigned to deferral, severe visual loss or vitrectomy developed over the first 3 years at about the same rate in both diabetes types; apparently the greater treatment effect in type 2 diabetes resulted mainly from greater responsiveness to early treatment. The DRS also found greater photocoagulation treatment benefit in patients with type 2 diabetes.[141] Greater responsiveness to photocoagulation in older versus younger patients has also been observed in other studies.[142,143] These studies are consistent with the clinical impression that, in patients with type 2 diabetes, high-risk PDR is often first detected on the basis of a symptomatic vitreous hemorrhage in an eye in which new vessels had not been observed on previous visits, whereas in patients with type 1 diabetes, NVD is more often the first sign of high-risk PDR, an occurrence more easily managed with photocoagulation.

Thus, in older patients with type 2 diabetes who have very severe NPDR or early PDR, ETDRS results and clinical impression suggest that prompt photocoagulation is probably safer than deferral. In younger patients with type 1 diabetes, ETDRS results suggest that there is little to lose from deferring scatter photocoagulation until high-risk PDR develops assuming appropriate compliance with follow-up. However, even in younger patients, when early NVD (less than shown in Fig. 48.15) is accompanied by the intraretinal signs of severe or very severe NPDR (see Fig. 48.2), prompt treatment is generally recommended. On the other hand, when younger patients have only mild intraretinal lesions and NVE (only) that appear stable, an initial period of observation is generally recommended. If new vessels are demonstrated to be growing, photocoagulation is usually recommended. However, these eyes often remain asymptomatic for many years, with little new vessel growth and often demonstrate spontaneous regression of the new vessels. In such eyes vitreoretinal adhesions tend to be delicate, and when posterior vitreous detachment occurs, there is less tendency for traction retinal detachment. When the process of posterior vitreous detachment has reached completion in such an eye, new vessels are likely to be few, narrow, elevated, and partially replaced by fibrous proliferations, and there may be little to be gained from photocoagulation at this stage unless vitreous hemorrhages are occurring. Presumably the reduced aggressiveness of new vessels in the setting of posterior vitreous detachment results from the lack of the posterior vitreous face scaffold for proliferation and less possibility for retinal traction. These findings support studies regarding the therapeutic usefulness of pharmacologic vitreolysis described later in this chapter.

Systemic factors should also be considered when deciding whether to initiate treatment in patients with very severe NPDR or moderate PDR. The progression of retinopathy may accelerate during pregnancy,[144,145] development of renal failure,[146] extreme illness, and poor glycemic control. If photocoagulation is deferred until high-risk characteristics develop in these situations, these more pressing problems may make it difficult to provide prompt and complete photocoagulation.

Scatter photocoagulation and macular edema

Macular edema sometimes increases, at least temporarily, after scatter photocoagulation, and this edema may be followed by transient or persistent reduction of visual acuity.[147–149] In the ETDRS, 18% of eyes had center-involved DME and less severe retinopathy without center involvement at baseline at 4 months.[137] The DRS also found early harmful effects, which were greater in the xenon group.[131] At the 6-week post-treatment visit, 21% of argon-treated and 46% of xenon-treated eyes that had DME and were free of high-risk characteristics at baseline had a decrease in visual acuity of two or more lines, compared with 9% of untreated eyes. Comparable percentages for eyes with neither DME nor high-risk characteristics were 9% argon, 18% xenon, and 3% untreated. After one year of follow-up in the group with DME at baseline, the greater progression of retinopathy in untreated eyes had led them to catch up with treated eyes; the percentages with a decrease in visual acuity of 2 or more lines were 32% argon, 33% xenon, and 34% untreated.[130,150] Both the ETDRS and the DRS support the clinical impression that eyes with DME requiring scatter treatment are at less risk of visual acuity loss when focal or grid treatment to reduce the DME precedes scatter photocoagulation. If a delay of scatter treatment seems undesirable, the ETDRS protocol can be used, combining focal/grid treatment for macular edema with scatter treatment during the first photocoagulation sitting.[140,151] VEGF inhibitors combined with either immediate or deferred macular laser have been shown to be more effective at reducing visual loss than laser alone.[152–154] In eyes with DME and PDR, VEGF inhibitors used to treat the edema may have a temporary beneficial effect on the retinal neovascularization until PRP can be performed. Certainly, scatter treatment should not be delayed when the risks of vitreous hemorrhage or neovascular glaucoma seem high, regardless of the status of the macula.

The Diabetic Retinopathy Clinical Research Network (DRCR.net) evaluated 364 eyes with center-involved ME to evaluate the short-term effects of intravitreal ranibizumab or intravitreal triamcinolone on preexisting ME in eyes receiving both PRP for severe NPDR (or non-high risk PDR) and focal/grid laser for concurrent ME.[155] Mean change in visual acuity from baseline was significantly better in the ranibizumab (+1 letters; $P < 0.001$) and triamcinolone (+2 letters; $P < 0.001$) groups compared with the sham group (–4 letters) at the 14-week visit. The effect on retinal thickness mirrored these results. These differences were not maintained when study participants were followed for 56 weeks for safety outcomes. These data suggested that at least in the short term, exacerbation of DME and visual acuity loss following PRP in eyes also receiving focal/grid laser for ME can be reduced by intravitreal triamcinolone or ranibizumab. Whether continued long-term intravitreal treatment is beneficial cannot be determined from this study.

As noted above, the ETDRS divided PRP into two or more sittings in an effort to reduce side effects, including exacerbation of ME. Utilizing optical coherence tomography (OCT), studies have evaluated the effect of PRP on macular thickness. Alterations in OCT measured macular thickening during and after PRP in patients with severe DR and good vision were evaluated in a study comparing weekly versus biweekly spacing between episodes of PRP.[156] Thirty-six patients with severe nonproliferative or early proliferative retinopathy and 20/20 vision in each eye at baseline received scatter photocoagulation in the following manner: in one eye, one quadrant was treated every week for 4 weeks and in the other eye, one quadrant was treated every other week for 8 weeks. OCT assessment of macular thickness was performed at baseline, before each session of photocoagulation, and at 16 weeks, the end of the follow-up period. Four of 36 eyes in the weekly treatment group and 3 of 36 in the biweekly group developed center-involved DME with decreased visual acuity (from 20/40 to 20/200), which was treated with photocoagulation. Additional photocoagulation for residual neovascularization was carried out in 35–40% of eyes in each group. The response of the remaining eyes is shown in Fig. 48.23. At baseline, mean retinal thickness was 191 μm in the central zone of the macular grid (1000 μm in diameter) in both groups.

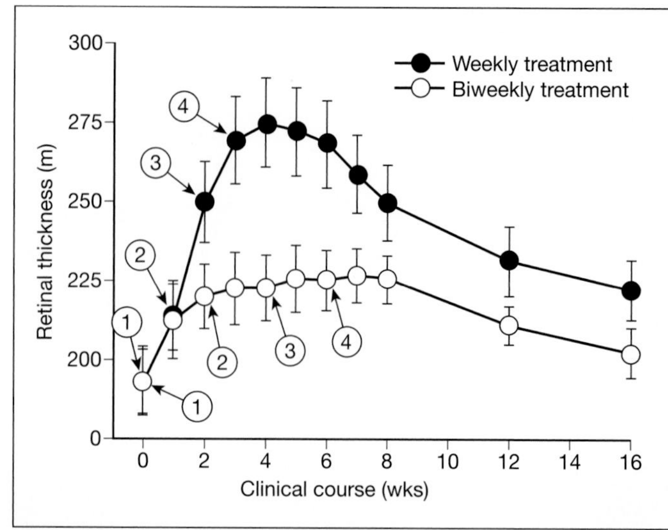

Fig. 48.23 Comparison of retinal thickness in the central zone between the weekly treated eyes and biweekly treated eyes. Each point and vertical bar indicates mean retinal thickness ± standard error of the mean. Arrows indicate each session of weekly treatment at 0-, 1-, 2-, and 3-week time points and biweekly treatment at 0-, 2-, 4-, and 6-week time points. (Reproduced with permission from Shimura M, Yasuda K, Nakazawa T, et al. Quantifying alterations of macular thickness before and after panretinal photocoagulation in patients with severe diabetic retinopathy and good vision. Ophthalmology 2003;110:2386–94. Copyright © 2003 American Academy of Ophthalmology.)

Thickness increased progressively after each weekly treatment to a maximum of 275 μm at week 4 and then decreased to 225 μm at 16 weeks. The increase was less after the biweekly treatments and at 16 weeks was closer to, but had not reached, the baseline value. There was little change in retinal thickness outside the central zone with either treatment technique.

The DRCR.net conducted an observational study to compare the effects of 1-sitting vs 4-sitting PRP on DME in subjects with severe nonproliferative or early proliferative diabetic retinopathy with relatively good visual acuity and no or mild center-involved macular edema.[157] Patients enrolled in the study were treated with 1 sitting or 4 sittings of PRP in a nonrandomized, prospective, multicenter clinical trial. The median change in central subfield thickness was slightly greater in the 1-sitting group ($n = 84$) than in the 4-sitting group ($n = 71$) at the 3-day (+9 μm vs +5 μm, $P = 0.01$) and 4-week visits (+ 13 μm vs +5 μm, $P = 0.003$). At the 34-week primary outcome visit, the slight differences had reversed, with the thickness being slightly greater in the 4-sitting group than in the 1-sitting group (+14 μm vs +22 μm, $P = 0.06$). Visual acuity changes paralleled OCT changes: 1 vs 4 sittings at 3 days (–3 vs –1 letters, $P = 0.005$), 4 weeks (–1 vs –1 letters, $P = 0.37$) and 34 weeks (0 vs –2 letters, $P = 0.006$). The results of the study suggest that clinically meaningful differences are unlikely in OCT thickness or visual acuity following application of PRP in a single sitting compared with 4 sittings in patients without center-involved macular edema and good vision.

Panretinal photocoagulation and advanced proliferative diabetic retinopathy

There is widespread agreement that PRP should be performed promptly in most eyes with PDR and high-risk characteristics. However, progressive contraction of fibrous proliferations leading to displacement or detachment of the macula sometimes follows PRP in eyes with extensive fibrous proliferations (see Fig. 48.11). Such cases have led to some reluctance to advise photocoagulation in this situation. Few such eyes were included in the DRS, but analyses of such cases indicated that outcome was better with photocoagulation than without it and suggested that it is only excessively heavy treatment that should be avoided. The adverse treatment effect was only evident in the xenon group, and even there the benefit of treatment outweighed its risks.[131] When high-risk characteristics are definitely present, PRP should usually be carried out, despite the presence of fibrous proliferation or localized traction retinal detachment. Treatment directly over areas of fibrous proliferation and retinal detachment should be avoided, and treatment strength should be mild to moderate.

Extensive neovascularization in the anterior chamber angle is a strong indication for PRP regardless of the presence of high-risk characteristics as regression of these new vessels before extensive closure of the angle has occurred can prevent neovascular glaucoma.[133,158]

CURRENT TECHNIQUES OF PANRETINAL PHOTOCOAGULATION

The DRS and ETDRS validated the effectiveness of PRP and established the indications and parameters for the treatment of PDR several decades ago.[130,140] These concepts persist mostly unchanged to this day as a result of their remarkable efficacy. A summary of the current protocol for PRP is presented in Table 48.7.

Direct (local) treatment of NVE

In the ETDRS, investigators had the option of applying direct photocoagulation (referred to as "local treatment") to flat new vessels on the retina. Confluent argon laser burns of 200–1000 μm spot size and a 0.1–0.5 second duration were specified with a resulting appearance (Fig. 48.24A) very similar to that obtained with mild xenon arc photocoagulation. Local treatment was limited to patches of NVE <2 disc areas in size in order to avoid large scotomas or nerve fiber bundle field defects. Although most retina specialists today do not perform local treatment, the efficacy of PRP without it, although clearly good, is not precisely known.

Distribution and strength of panretinal photocoagulation

A common feature of most scatter laser treatment protocols is the location of burns beginning about 2–3 DD from the center of the macula and extending peripherally to the equator. It is important to realize that the size of the burn produced depends not only on the spot-size setting used, but also on power and

Table 48.7 Current treatment protocol for panretinal (PRP) laser photocoagulation

Burn characteristic	Recommendations
Conventional slit-lamp laser delivery systems	
Size (on retina)	500 μm (e.g., argon laser using 200 μm spot size with Rodenstock lens (or equivalent), 400 μm (e.g., 200 μm spot size with Mainster 165, Volk Quadraspheric or SuperQuad 160) or 500 μm spot size with 3-mirror contact lens)
Exposure	0.1 seconds recommended, 0.05–0.2 allowed
Intensity	Mild white retinal burns
Distribution	Edges 1 burn width apart
No. of Sessions/Sittings	Unrestricted (generally should be completed in <6)
Nasal proximity to disk	No closer than 500 μm
Temp. proximity to center	No closer than 3000 μm
Superior/inferior limit	No further posterior than 1 burn within the temporal arcades
Extent	Arcades (~3000 μm from the macular center) to at least the equator
Number of Final Burns:	1200 to 1600
Wavelength	Green or yellow (red can be used if vitreous hemorrhage is present precluding use of green or yellow)
Automated pattern scanning laser delivery systems	
Size (on retina)	400 μm (e.g. 200 μm spot size with Mainster 165, Volk Quadraspheric or SuperQuad 160)
Exposure	0.020 seconds
Intensity	Mild white retinal burns
Distribution	0.5 spot diameter spacing

Continued

Table 48.7 Current treatment protocol for panretinal (PRP) laser photocoagulation—Cont'd

Burn characteristic	Recommendations
No. of sessions/sittings	1 to 3
Nasal proximity to disc	No closer than 500 μm
Temp. proximity to center	No closer than 3000 μm
Superior/inferior limit	No further posterior than 1 burn within the temporal arcades
Extent	Arcades (~3000 μm from the macular center) to at least the equator
Number of final burns	1800 to 2400
Wavelength	Green (532 nm) only
Patterns	2×2, 3×3, 4×4, 5×5 as needed for uniform focus/uptake
Indirect laser delivery systems	
Size (on retina)	400 to 500 μm spot size with 20D, 28D, or 30D indirect lens (depending on diopter of Indirect lens)
Exposure	0.050–0.10 seconds
Intensity	Mild white retinal burns
Distribution	500 μm spot diameter spacing
No. of Sessions/Sittings	1 to 3
Nasal proximity to disk	No closer than 500 μm
Temp. proximity to center	No closer than 3000 μm
Superior/inferior limit	No further posterior than 1 burn within the temporal arcades
Extent	Arcades (~3000 μm from the macular center) to at least the equator
Number of final burns:	1200 to 2000
Wavelength	Green (532 nm) only

(Adapted from the Diabetic Clinical Research Network Procedure Manuals.)

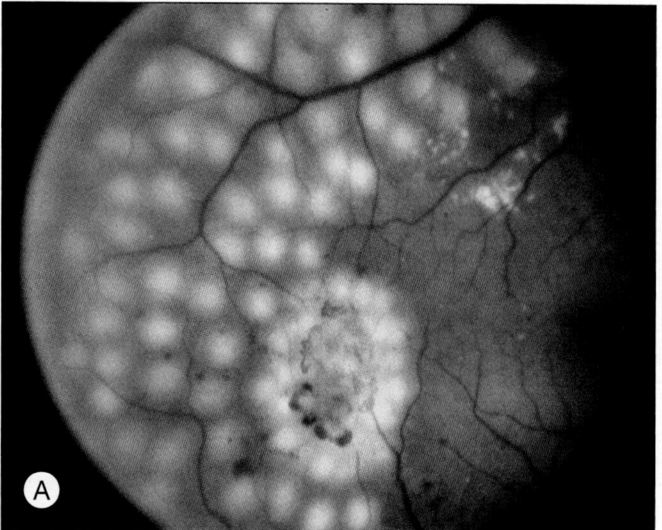

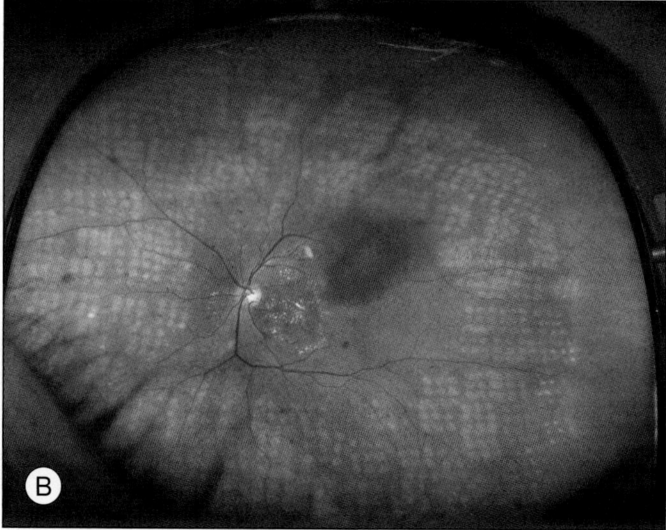

Fig. 48.24 (A) Immediate post-treatment photograph illustrating Early Treatment Diabetic Retinopathy Study full-scatter treatment and local confluent treatment of a patch of new vessels everywhere (NVE). (B) Appearance of pattern scanning laser burns 1 week after treatment. (Panel (A) reproduced with permission from Early Treatment of Diabetic Retinopathy Study Research Group. Techniques for scatter and local photocoagulation treatment of diabetic retinopathy: the ETDRS report no. 3. Int Ophthalmol Clin 1987;27:254–64; panel (B) Courtesy of the Beetham Eye Institute Library.)

duration, so it is difficult to compare techniques precisely, even those using the same wavelength and spot-size setting, on the basis of number and theoretical size of burns. It is also difficult to describe burn strength. Reporting power level is not particularly helpful, since the required power for a burn of given strength, even if spot-size setting and duration are kept constant, depends on the clarity of the media and the pigmentation of the fundus. The ETDRS protocol for full scatter treatment provides useful guidelines for initial treatment,[140] calling for a total of 1200–1600 500 µm 0.1 s argon laser burns of moderate intensity placed one-half to one burn apart and divided between two or more sittings (at least 2 weeks apart if two sittings and at least 4 days apart if three or more sittings). Burns appear to enlarge slightly within several minutes after their application, resulting in the closer spacing of the scatter burns shown in Fig. 48.24A.

Pattern scanning laser delivery systems

The development of scanning laser delivery systems (PASCAL®, OptiMedica, Inc., Santa Clara, CA and Zeiss VITE, Carl Zeiss Meditec, Dublin, CA) has given ophthalmologists the ability to deliver various semi-automated operator-selected burn patterns. These systems utilize a 532 nm frequency-doubled neodymium-doped yttrium aluminum garnet (Nd:YAG) solid-state laser and typically have a 20 ms pulse duration for each laser burn that is 5–10 times shorter as compared with conventional lasers. This allows defined multispot patterns to be delivered nearly simultaneously with a single application of the foot pedal. The shorter duration results in less thermal damage, less burn spread, and potentially improves patient comfort and safety without apparently compromising efficacy.

Preclinical animal experiments on the effects of various pulse durations demonstrated that laser burns of pulse durations greater than 20 ms resulted in significant diffusion of heat with a less homogeneous lesion on histological examination.[159] Pulse durations of approximately 20 ms have been shown to represent an optimal compromise between the favorable impact of speed, spatial localization, and reduced collateral damage with a sufficient therapeutic window.[160] The 10–30 ms pulse of the pattern laser systems is associated clinically with a more uniform and predictable burn dimension with minimal thermal spread compared with conventional photocoagulation.[159,161,162] Clinically, pattern scanning laser burns are typically lighter in intensity and more uniform, as confirmed by clinical retinal morphologic studies that demonstrated pattern scanning laser burns to be nearly identical in size and sharply delineated from the surrounding untreated retina.[163] Furthermore, the area of tissue destruction was confined to the outer retinal layers, from the outer nuclear layer to the RPE, reflecting less energy spread and less damage to the inner retinal layers and choriod[163] (Fig. 48.24).

Number of episodes used for scatter treatment

The effect of single and multiple laser sittings on DME has been discussed earlier in this chapter, noting that complete application within a single sitting did not appear to be detrimental as compared with dividing treatment over multiple sittings. Among the techniques in use for PDR alone, the number of sittings in which initial scatter treatment is carried out varies from one to four or more. Those techniques using a smaller number of larger burns tend toward a single sitting, sometimes with retrobulbar anesthesia, whereas those using a larger number of smaller burns have generally been divided into two or more sittings. In general, multiple sittings may reduce discomfort, but may cause delays and inconvenience for patients. Angle-closure glaucoma secondary to serous detachment of the peripheral choroid and ciliary body is reportedly less common when treatment is carried out in two or more sessions over a period of 1 or 2 weeks.[164]

Doft and Blankenship[165] addressed this question in a small randomized trial. They randomly assigned one eye from each of 50 patients with DRS high-risk characteristics to scatter photocoagulation with 1200, 500 µm, 0.1 s argon laser burns of moderate intensity applied in either of two ways: (1) at a single sitting or (2) in three sittings at 1-week intervals. Retrobulbar anesthesia was used in the single-sitting group and for the first of the multiple-sitting group. In this latter group at the first episode, several rows of burns were placed surrounding the posterior pole, and treatment was extended temporally and nasally to the periphery, leaving the remainder of the upper quadrants (from the 10 o'clock to the 2 o'clock position) for the second episode and the remainder of the lower quadrants (from the 4 o'clock to the 8 o'clock position) for the third. Surrounding the posterior pole with treatment at the initial sitting is different from most protocols, where posterior burns are usually divided between multiple sittings.

Patients were examined 3, 7, 14, 21, 60, and 180 days after completion of the initial treatment episode. Peripheral choroidal detachment was noted more frequently at the 3-day visit in the single than in the multiple-sitting group (17 of 25 and 10 of 25 eyes, respectively), and three eyes in the single-sitting group developed angle closure which resolved spontaneously without any adverse effect. Transient (present at the 3-day and 7-day visit but not at the 14-day visit) exudative retinal detachment involving the macula was noted in 7 of 25 (28%) eyes treated in a single sitting and in 2 of 25 (8%) eyes treated in three sittings. Eyes with exudative macular detachment had, on average, a visual acuity decrease of about 5 lines at the 3-day visit, but at the 6-month visit they had recovered to approximately the same level as eyes without transient detachments. At the 6-month visit the numbers of eyes with a decrease in visual acuity of 1 line, 2–4 lines, and 5 or more lines from the baseline visit were 3, 6, and 1 in the single-sitting group, compared with 4, 4, and 1 in the multiple-sitting group. These differences were not statistically significant in this small low-power study.

Wavelength

The Krypton-Argon Regression of Neovascularization Study (KARNS) randomly assigned 907 eyes (of 696 patients) that had NVD equaling or exceeding those in Fig. 48.15 to scatter photocoagulation (1600–2000 moderate-intensity 500 mm burns) with either blue-green argon or red krypton wavelengths.[142] If, after the initial treatment, NVD increased by more than 0.5 disc area, retreatment was recommended (and could also be applied for other reasons, such as increasing NVE or vitreous hemorrhage). Retreatment was carried out in 36% and 33%, respectively, of the argon and krypton groups. Worsening NVD was the reason for the retreatment in ~40% of retreated eyes in each group. Regression of NVD to less than that shown in Fig. 48.15 was observed in almost identical proportions of the two groups (41.4% and 41.8%, respectively, at 3 months and 55.0% and 52.8%, respectively, at 1 year). No differences were found in the effectiveness of argon versus krypton treatment, although retrobulbar anesthesia was used more frequently with krypton treatment. In two small randomized trials, diode (810 nm) and double-frequency Nd:YAG (532 nm) lasers gave results similar to those of the argon green laser.[166,167]

REGRESSION OF NEW VESSELS AFTER INITIAL PHOTOCOAGULATION AND INDICATIONS FOR RETREATMENT

There is general agreement that substantial regression of new vessels usually occurs within days or weeks after the initial application of scatter photocoagulation and that eyes in which new vessels continue to grow despite initial treatment or recur after partial or complete regression may respond well to additional treatment. However, data documenting the rapidity and completeness of regression are sparse, and many reports do not clearly separate results after initial treatment and results after initial treatment plus retreatment as needed. Table 48.8 summarizes much of the available information. Doft and Blankenship[168] combined the single- and multiple-treatment groups previously discussed and described the course of new-vessel regression over a 6-month period without retreatment. At the 3-day post-treatment visit 10 (20%) of the 50 eyes had regressed from the high-risk stage; at 2 weeks, 25 (50%); at 3 weeks, 36 (72%); and at 6 months, 31 (62%). About one-third of the eyes that were still in the high-risk stage after 3 weeks were no longer high-risk at 6 months. Conversely, approximately one-third of those with regression at 3 weeks had progressed to the high-risk stage again at 6 months. Blankenship[169] reported similar findings in his study comparing peripheral and posterior laser treatment. In both groups combined there were 31 eyes with NVD greater than or equal to one-quarter disc area at baseline. In all but one of these 31 eyes, NVD were less than one-quarter disc area at the 1-month follow-up visit while at the 6-month visit, 24 of the 31 (77%) met this criterion. Vander and coworkers [170] reported that 59% of 59 eyes with high-risk PDR had a satisfactory response (retinopathy no longer in the high-risk category) 3 months after initial full-scatter photocoagulation. In the KARNS, 3 months after the initial treatment (with or without retreatment), NVD had decreased to less than 50% of the baseline area in 54% of eyes and had decreased by a lesser amount in an additional 19%.[142] Among DRS eyes with NVD equaling or exceeding those in Fig. 48.15 at baseline (with or without NVE), all new vessels had regressed completely 1 year after the initial treatment in 20% of argon-treated eyes, and regression of NVD to less than those in Fig. 48.15 had occurred in an additional 34%. Results after xenon arc photocoagulation were similar.[26] Because the DRS

Table 48.8 Regression of neovascularization after scatter photocoagulation

	Initial photocoagulation				
Author (publication year)	No. of eyes	Pretreatment retinopathy severity (no. of burns)	Response criterion	Time to evaluation	No. (%) with favorable response
Doft and Blankenship, 1984[163]	50	High-risk PDR (1200 one episode)	Absence of high-risk PDR	3 days	10 (20%)
				2 weeks	25 (50%)
				3 weeks	36 (72%)
				6 month	31 (62%)
Blankenship. 1988[158]	31	NVD ≥ 1/4 disc area	NVD < 1/4 disc area	1 month	30 (97%)
				6 months	24 (77%)
Vander et al., 1991[164]	59	High-risk PDR ("full-scatter")	Absence of high-risk PDR	3 months	35 (59%)
KARNS, 1993[150]	907	NVD ≥ standard 10A (1600–2	NVD < 50% of baseline	3 months	490 (54%)
		NVD ≥ standard 10A (1600–2000)	NVD 50–99% of baseline	3 months	172 (19%)
DRS, 1978[13]	188	NVD ≥ standard 10A	No NVD or NVE	1 year	38 (20%)
		Argon (800–1000)	NVD < standard 10A	1 year	64 (34%)
	163	Xenon arc (200–800)	No NVD or NVE	1 year	36 (22%)
			NVD < standard 10A	1 year	62 (38%)
Rogell, 1983[165]	55	PDR (1100–1500 total in two episodes)	"Substantial regression"	1 month	21 (38%)
	34	Retreatment (300–400)	"Substantial regression"	1 month	30 (88%)

PDR, proliferative diabetic retinopathy; NVD, neovascularization of disc; NVE, neovascularization elsewhere.

protocol did not provide mandated guidelines for retreatment, and because treatment was being compared with no treatment, these results probably reflect outcomes to be expected after initial treatment.

Efficacy of retreatment can be difficult to compare between studies. After applying 1100–1500 500 μm moderately intense argon laser burns, divided between two sittings about 1 week apart, Rogell[171] followed patients at monthly intervals, applying 300–400 additional burns at each visit until "substantial regression" of new vessels had occurred. In 21 of 55 eyes (38%) with PDR, the initial treatment was sufficient. Additional photocoagulation was carried out once or twice in 29 eyes (53%), three to five times in 5 eyes (1%), and peripheral retinal cryotherapy was added in 2 eyes (4%). Response to retreatment was considered satisfactory in 30 of 34 eyes (88%). In a retrospective case review of 182 patients (294 eyes), Reddy and coworkers[172] assessed the need for retreatment after initial full-scatter photocoagulation in patients with two or more NV-VH risk factors. In 177 of 294 eyes (60%) the response to initial treatment was considered satisfactory. The remaining 117 eyes were retreated, 71 with photocoagulation alone and 46 with a combination of photocoagulation and anterior retinal cryotherapy. Retreatment was successful in 98 of 117 eyes (84%). Among an unspecified number of eyes with high-risk PDR treated initially with extensive argon laser scatter photocoagulation during a 2-year period, 23 eyes remained in the high-risk stage 8 weeks after completion of the initial treatment and were given follow-up treatment by Vine.[173] Eyes were observed at 6- to 8-week intervals, and follow-up treatment (1000–2000 low-intensity burns placed between scars) was applied until regression from the high-risk stage occurred or further treatment was not feasible. Retreatment was successful in 12 of 23 eyes (52%).

From these studies it appears that, on average, about two-thirds of eyes have a satisfactory response to initial scatter treatment. As mentioned earlier, this ratio tends to be more favorable in patients with type 2 diabetes. Patients with severe intraretinal lesions and actively growing new vessels, who typically have type 1 diabetes, often need multiple treatments.[174]

The ETDRS protocol contains guidelines for follow-up treatment that seem suitable for general use. Six factors are considered: (1) change in new vessels since the last visit or last photocoagulation treatment; (2) appearance of the new vessels (caliber, degree of network formation, extent of accompanying fibrous tissue); (3) frequency and extent of vitreous hemorrhage since the last visit or last photocoagulation treatment; (4) status of vitreous detachment; (5) extent of photocoagulation scars; and (6) extent of traction retinal detachment and fibrous proliferations.[140] If new vessels appear to be active, as suggested by formation of tight networks, paucity of accompanying fibrous tissue, and increase in extent in comparison to the previous visit, additional photocoagulation is considered. The case for additional treatment is stronger if the extent of new vessels is substantially greater than it was at the time of initial treatment for high-risk characteristics or if vitreous or preretinal hemorrhages are occurring repeatedly (Fig. 48.6). Decreased caliber of new vessels and fibrous proliferation development suggest that retinopathy is entering a quiescent stage in which additional treatment may not be needed. A single episode of vitreous hemorrhage coincident with the occurrence of extensive posterior vitreous detachment, particularly if the only vitreoretinal adhesion remaining is at the disc, argues less for additional photocoagulation than do recurrent hemorrhages unrelated to such an occurrence. Additional photocoagulation may be needed less frequently in the setting of extensive posterior vitreous detachment because additional growth of new vessels is limited as is the extent of vitreoretinal adhesions. The extent and location of photocoagulation scars may also influence the decision regarding additional photocoagulation treatment. If the scars are widely spaced, or if there are areas where treatment was omitted, benefit from additional photocoagulation is more likely. In the presence of extensive scars where additional treatment would be placed over old scars, additional treatment may be less beneficial and be associated with increased risk of side-effects such as loss of visual field or nyctalopia. In such cases indefinite deferral of photocoagulation may sometimes be the best alternative, even though there are extensive new vessels on the detached posterior vitreous surface and/or small vitreous hemorrhages are occurring occasionally. If severe vitreous hemorrhage or vision threatening proliferation occurs, vitrectomy may be the best treatment option.

COMPLICATIONS OF PRP

Although remarkably effective, visually threatening complications from PRP may arise (Box 48.2). It is important that such complications are identified and treated promptly to prevent further vision loss. Diabetes affects most ocular structures and may increase risks of potential complications following PRP. Diabetes-related corneal neuropathy may predispose eyes to corneal epithelial trauma possibly leading to secondary infection or recurrent corneal erosions if undetected.[175] The use of the appropriate coupling solution, proper placement and minimal manipulation of the contact lens during laser treatment may minimize shearing and friction of the corneal surface. Iritis or iris burns and lenticular burns may occur with poorly dilated pupils, cataractous lenses or improper laser focus.[176] Careful

Box 48.2 Complications of scatter (PRP) photocoagulation

- Loss of visual function
  - Moderate visual loss
  - Diminished or loss of visual field
  - Diminished contrast sensitivity
  - Diminished color vision
  - Reduced or loss of dark adaptation
- Damage to posterior ocular structures
  - Inadvertent foveal or optic disc damage
  - Retinal nerve fiber thinning
  - Retinal tear
  - Choriodal hemorrhage
  - Choriodal neovascularization
  - Vitreous, preretinal or subhyaloid hemorrhage
- Complications related to blood retinal barrier breakdown
  - Macular edema
  - Choriodal detachment/effusion and secondary angle closure
  - Iritis and increased intraocular pressure
  - Exudative retinal detachment
- Complications related to the destructive nature of the procedure
  - Pain during treatment and shortly after treatment
  - Corneal epithelial defects and recurrent erosions
  - Mydriasis and paresis of accommodation
  - Iris burns and damage
  - Lenticular burns or opacification
- Complications related to contraction of fibrovascular tissue
  - Progressive traction retinal detachment
  - Vitreous, preretinal or subhyaloid hemorrhage

focusing and optimizing papillary dilation can help avoid these complications, particularly when high-power, long-duration laser treatment is used. Some degree of discomfort is reported in most patients undergoing PRP. Carefully titrating burn intensity, shortening exposure time, and avoiding the ciliary nerves at the horizontal meridian will minimize patient discomfort. Judicious use of retrobulbar, peribulbar, subtenon or subconjunctival anesthesia may be used to increase patient comfort and effectively complete treatment in some patients. Such procedures are usually not required, however, in the vast majority of individuals.

The inherent destructive nature of PRP may also lead to adverse effects on the retina, including macular edema, serous macular/retinal detachment, contraction of preretinal membranes, choroidal detachment and angle closure glaucoma.[177] Choroidal effusion is commonly observed after PRP within the first week. These effusions are usually asymptomatic but may cause angle closure, especially in predisposed hyperopic eyes with shallow chambers. Inadvertent direct photocoagulation of the central macula is a potential and obviously detrimental complication that can result in permanent scotoma and substantial visual loss. Careful attention of anatomic landmarks and adherence to a strict standardized treatment regimen for each patient can reduce this risk. Intense, small spot-size burns, especially in the red light spectrum, may predispose to the rupture of Bruch's membrane. Clinically, Bruch's membrane rupture is associated with risk of hemorrhage and secondary choroidal neovascularization. Intermittent direct pressure on the globe with the contact lens often stops any associated hemorrhaging and low intensity, confluent large laser burns may be applied to the bleeding area to help control hemorrhaging. Inadvertent photocoagulation of the long posterior ciliary nerve may result in permanent mydriasis and loss of accommodation.[178] Substantial visual field loss may be caused by high-density, high-intensity PRP and a sudden decrease in central vision may occur with occlusion of limited remaining arterioles supplying the macula.[132] Even with uncomplicated PRP, some decline in visual function has been reported, including moderate visual loss, impaired night vision, diminished visual field, reduced color vision, and reduced contrast sensitivity.[179]

Despite these complications, the long-term safety and efficacy of PRP in reducing the risk for severe visual loss has been confirmed by numerous large multicenter clinical trials and PRP is the only proven long-term therapy for PDR. However, our understanding of the molecular and biochemical pathways underlying the onset and regression of retinal neovascularization has increased dramatically. With this knowledge, new therapeutic targets and novel potential treatment methods have been identified and are under extensive investigation. It is likely that additional treatment options for PDR may become available within the next several years.

ANTIANGIOGENIC THERAPIES FOR PROLIFERATIVE DIABETIC RETINOPATHY

Intravitreal antiangiogenic agents can induce rapid initial regression of ischemia-related ocular neovascularization. Although the neovascular regression effect can be remarkable in terms of its speed and extent, the effect generally appears to be temporary, requiring either additional definitive treatment (such as laser photocoagulation) or repeated dosing. Generalized use of VEGF inhibitors for PDR will likely be limited until there is development of tolerable continuous delivery mechanisms or identification of anti-VEGF agents with long duration of action. Various VEGF inhibitors have shown at least transient beneficial activity in PDR. Mendrinos and coworkers published a case report demonstrating rapid regression of neovascularization after a single injection of pegaptanib which was sustained for more than 15 months.[180] Bevacizumab has been shown by Avery et al. to induce regression of new vessels in PDR as early as 24 hours after injection, but with a variable sustained effect ranging between 2 and 11 weeks.[181] Jorge et al. demonstrated short-term resolution of leakage from retinal neovascularization at 6 weeks after a single intravitreal injection of bevacizumab in 15 patients with persistent new vessels despite panretinal laser photocoagulation. At 12 weeks, 14 out of 15 patients had recurrent leakage but to a lesser extent than at baseline.[182] Other studies have reported similar short-term efficacy of bevacizumab in inducing regression of retinal neovascularization.[183–185] The Diabetic Retinopathy Clinical Research Network (DRCR.net) is conducting two trials: one to study the efficacy of ranibizumab in cases of vitreous hemorrhage due to PDR, and another to assess the efficacy of adjunctive use of ranibizumab compared to triamcinolone with laser treatment in PDR. The results of these trials will help further define the role of VEGF inhibitors in the management of diabetic ocular neovascular complications and provide additional safety data for long-term exposure that is presently unknown.

It has been postulated that VEGF inhibition for PDR would require extended treatment durations since the underlying ischemia leading to VEGF expression would not be ameliorated. Some initial data suggest, however, that this may not be the case. The natural history of PDR is to become quiescent eventually with or without laser treatment (although of course visual outcomes are improved with laser photocoagulation). Intraocular VEGF concentrations have been shown to be lower in quiescent PDR, whether following laser photocoagulation or spontaneously.[13]A similar argument regarding the need for prolonged treatment might be made for DME; however, studies from DRCR.net and others have shown a reduced need for VEGF inhibitors over time.[152] The mean number of intravitreal ranibizumab injections was 8–9 of 13 possible the first year but fell to 2–3 the second year without a loss of visual acuity or an increase in retinal thickness. Together, these data suggest that after a period of VEGF inhibitor treatment, it may be possible to reduce such treatment without reactivation of disease. Whether this holds true, and to what extent, remains to be demonstrated by ongoing and upcoming clinical trials.

PHARMACEUTICAL VITREOLYSIS FOR TREATMENT OF PDR

As discussed earlier in this chapter, the vitreous plays a key role in the pathology and natural course of PDR. The presence of a complete posterior vitreous detachment (PVD) has been observed in diabetic eyes to be associated with lower risk for developing PDR.[186,187] The widespread utilization of the intravitreal injections has led to research into pharmacologic agents such as plasmin, tissue plasminogen activator, microplasmin, hyaluronidase, chondroitinase, collagenase, dispase, and nattokinase.[188] These agents may be used to facilitate the cleavage of the cortical hyaloid at the vitreoretinal junction, thereby inducing complete PVD and liquefaction of the vitreous gel.[189] In a pooled analysis of the initial clinical trials with hyalonidase involving 1125 patients with persistent vitreous hemorrhage who were randomized to receive one of two doses of intravitreal hyaluronidase (55 or 75 IU) or saline,[190] only patients receiving 55 IU reached the primary efficacy endpoint, defined as (3 months after baseline) clearance of hemorrhage sufficient to see the underlying pathology or allow completion of treatment when indicated. Acute self-limited iritis was the most common adverse event, occurring in a dose-dependent fashion.[184]

Microplasmin, a recombinant protein that contains only the catalytic domain of human plasmin, has shown ability to induce vitreolysis in patients with vitreomacular adhesion. A phase II randomized double-masked clinical trial with control sham injection enrolled 60 patients. Patients in each of the four cohorts were randomized (4:1) to active treatment or sham injection. In the first three cohorts, increasing doses of microplasmin (75, 125, and 175 µg) were administered. In the fourth cohort, an initial injection of 125 µg microplasmin or sham was administered followed 1 month later by an injection of 125 µg microplasmin if no release of vitreoretinal adhesion occurred. A third dose was injected 4 weeks later if there was still no release of adhesion. Within 28 days of sham, 75, 125, and 175 µg microplasmin resulted in nonsurgical resolution of vitreomacular adhesion in 8%, 25%, 44%, and 27% of the patients, respectively. When the 125 µg dose was repeated up to two times, adhesion release was observed in 58% of patients 28 days after the final injection.[191] These data suggest that nonsurgical enzymatic release of vitreoretinal adhesions may potentially provide a less invasive means to achieve a more nearly complete cleavage of the vitreous as compared to conventional vitrectomy. In addition to the mechanical removal of vitreoretinal adhesions, complete vitreolysis changes the molecular flux across the vitreoretinal interface and improves oxygen supply to the retina.[12,192] This action could potentially delay the onset or progression of PDR. Further studies are underway to better define the role of pharmacologic vitreolysis in the treatment of PDR.

INDICATIONS FOR VITRECTOMY

When vitrectomy was initially introduced in 1970 by Machemer et al.,[193] the major indications in eyes with PDR were severe vitreous hemorrhage that had failed to clear spontaneously after a year and traction retinal detachment involving the center of the macula. As this procedure came into widespread use, it was recognized that it can be of value earlier in the course of severe PDR and its indications have broadened[56,57] (Box 48.3). A more extensive discussion of vitrectomy and surgical interventions for the proliferative complications of diabetic retinopathy is presented in Chapter 111 (Surgery for proliferative diabetic retinopathy).

Box 48.3 Indications for vitrectomy

1. To permit visualization of the retinal and adequate photocoagulation of active retinopathy
   a. Severe nonclearing vitreous hemorrhage
   b. Dense subhyaloid or premacular hemorrhage
   c. Anterior segment neovascularization with an associated media opacity
2. To relieve traction of the retina that is threatening or causing visual impairment
   a. Traction retinal detachment involving or threatening the fovea
   b. Vitreomacular traction , macular striae or distortion causing visual loss
   c. Combined traction-rhegmatogeous retinal detachment
   d. Epiretinal membranes or opacified posterior vitreous face causing visual loss
3. To control progressive retinopathy or complications despite adequate retinal photocoagulation
   a. Progressive fibrovascular proliferation
   b. Anterior hyloidal fibrovascular proliferation
   c. Ghost cell/hemolytic glaucoma

CONCLUSION

Proliferative diabetic retinopathy is a severe sight-threatening complication of diabetes. While PDR cannot be prevented, scatter (panretinal) laser photocoagulation is very effective in preserving vision and preventing vision loss. Increased understanding of the biochemical mechanisms underlying PDR are providing new therapeutic approaches with the promise to be both effective and less destructive than current photocoagulation techniques. Furthermore, it is important to keep in mind that a comprehensive approach to diabetes care is particularly critical for patients with advanced retinopathy. Only with the coordinated care between eye care providers and the many other members of the diabetic patient's medical care team can optimal ophthalmic outcomes be achieved. The development of PDR is strongly associated with the presence of significant systemic disease. Progressive retinal ischemia and the release of local growth factors are the main pathogenic mechanisms underlying the development of PDR. The natural course of PDR involves highly active phases of retinal neovascularization and fibrous proliferation, potentially leading to visual loss if left untreated. Timely panretinal laser photocoagulation can reduce the risk of severe visual loss by 96%, with long-term preservation of vision. Multiple studies have suggested that systemic and intravitreal pharmacologic therapies may induce regression of retinal neovascularization and prevent the onset or slow the progression to PDR. These approaches, if adequately sustained and proven safe and efficacious in rigorous clinical trials, will represent a major treatment advance. Fortunately, the vast majority of severe visual loss from PDR can already be prevented, albeit necessitating access to specialized care and with attendant side-effects and complications. Given the advances underway in the systemic and ocular management of diabetes, it is likely that the future of PDR therapy will be marked by even greater benefit and reduced risk.

REFERENCES

1. Diabetic Retinopathy Study Research Group. Preliminary report on effects of photocoagulation therapy. Am J Ophthalmol 1976;81:383–96.
2. Diabetic Retinopathy Study Research Group. Four risk factors for severe visual loss in diabetic retinopathy. The third report from the Diabetic Retinopathy Study. Arch Ophthalmol 1979;97:654–5.
3. Klein R, Klein BE, Moss SE, et al. The Wisconsin Epidemiologic Study of Diabetic Retinopathy. IX. Four-year incidence and progression of diabetic retinopathy when age at diagnosis is less than 30 years. Arch Ophthalmol 1989;107:237–43.
4. Klein R, Klein BE, Moss SE, et al. The Wisconsin Epidemiologic Study of Diabetic Retinopathy. X. Four-year incidence and progression of diabetic retinopathy when age at diagnosis is 30 years or more. Arch Ophthalmol 1989;107:244–9.
5. Klein R, Knudtson MD, Lee KE, et al. The Wisconsin Epidemiologic Study of Diabetic Retinopathy. XXII. The twenty-five-year progression of retinopathy in persons with type 1 diabetes. Ophthalmology 2008;115(11):1859–68.
6. Aiello LP, Cahill MT, Wong JS. Systemic considerations in the management of diabetic retinopathy. Am J Ophthalmol 2001;132:760–6.
7. Klein R, Klein BE, Moss SE. Epidemiology of proliferative diabetic retinopathy. Diabetes Care 1992;15:1875–91.

8. Hovind P, Tarnow L, Rossing K, et al. Decreasing incidence of severe diabetic microangiopathy in type 1 diabetes. Diabetes Care 2003;26:1258–64.
9. Klein R, Klein BE, Moss SE, et al. The medical management of hyperglycemia over a 10-year period in people with diabetes. Diabetes Care 1996;19:744–50.
10. Wong TY, Mwamburi M, Klein R, et al. Rates of progression in diabetic retinopathy during different time periods: a systematic review and meta-analysis. Diabetes Care 2009;32:2307–13.
11. Klein R, Klein BE. Are individuals with diabetes seeing better? A long-term epidemiological perspective. Diabetes 2010;59:1853–60.
12. Stefansson E. Ocular oxygenation and the treatment of diabetic retinopathy. Surv Ophthalmol 2006;51:364–80.
13. Aiello LP, Avery RL, Arrigg PG, et al. Vascular endothelial growth factor in ocular fluid of patients with diabetic retinopathy and other retinal disorders. N Engl J Med 1994;331:1480–7.
14. Miller JW, Adamis AP, Shima DT, et al. Vascular endothelial growth factor/vascular permeability factor is temporally and spatially correlated with ocular angiogenesis in a primate model. Am J Pathol 1994;145:574–84.
15. Pierce EA, Avery RL, Foley ED, et al. Vascular endothelial growth factor/vascular permeability factor expression in a mouse model of retinal neovascularization. Proc Natl Acad Sci U S A 1995;92:905–9.
16. Adamis AP, Miller JW, Bernal MT, et al. Increased vascular endothelial growth factor levels in the vitreous of eyes with proliferative diabetic retinopathy. Am J Ophthalmol 1994;118:445–50.
17. Avery RL. Regression of retinal and iris neovascularization after intravitreal bevacizumab (Avastin) treatment. Retina 2006;26:352–4.
18. Cai J, Kehoe O, Smith GM, et al. The angiopoietin/Tie-2 system regulates pericyte survival and recruitment in diabetic retinopathy. Invest Ophthalmol Vis Sci 2008;49:2163–71.
19. Takagi H, Koyama S, Seike H, et al. Potential role of the angiopoietin/tie2 system in ischemia-induced retinal neovascularization. Invest Ophthalmol Vis Sci 2003;44:393–402.
20. Geraldes P, Hiraoka-Yamamoto J, Matsumoto M, et al. Activation of PKC-delta and SHP-1 by hyperglycemia causes vascular cell apoptosis and diabetic retinopathy. Nat Med 2009;15:1298–306.
21. Watanabe D, Suzuma K, Matsui S, et al. Erythropoietin as a retinal angiogenic factor in proliferative diabetic retinopathy. N Engl J Med 2005;353:782–92.
22. Tong Z, Yang Z, Patel S, et al. Promoter polymorphism of the erythropoietin gene in severe diabetic eye and kidney complications. Proc Natl Acad Sci U S A 2008;105:6998–7003.
23. Abhary S, Burdon KP, Casson RJ, et al. Association between erythropoietin gene polymorphisms and diabetic retinopathy. Arch Ophthalmol 2010;128: 102–6.
24. Ogata N, Tombran-Tink J, Nishikawa M, et al. Pigment epithelium-derived factor in the vitreous is low in diabetic retinopathy and high in rhegmatogenous retinal detachment. Am J Ophthalmol 2001;132:378–82.
25. Praidou A, Androudi S, Brazitikos P, et al. Angiogenic growth factors and their inhibitors in diabetic retinopathy. Curr Diabetes Rev 2010;6:304–12.
26. Diabetic Retinopathy Study Research Group. Photocoagulation treatment of proliferative diabetic retinopathy: the second report of diabetic retinopathy study findings. Ophthalmology 1978;85:82–106.
27. Shimizu K, Kobayashi Y, Muraoka K. Midperipheral fundus involvement in diabetic retinopathy. Ophthalmology 1981;88:601–12.
28. Muraoka K, Shimizu K. Intraretinal neovascularization in diabetic retinopathy. Ophthalmology 1984;91:1440–6.
29. Kohner EM, Dollery CT, Bulpitt CJ. Cotton-wool spots in diabetic retinopathy. Diabetes 1969;18:691–704.
30. Kohner EM, Dollery CT. The rate of formation and disappearance of microaneurysms in diabetic retinopathy. Trans Ophthalmol Soc U K 1970;90: 369–74.
31. Davis MD. Vitreous contraction in proliferative diabetic retinopathy. Arch Ophthalmol 1965;74:741–51.
32. Taylor E, Dobree JH. Proliferative diabetic retinopathy. Site and size of initial lesions. Br J Ophthalmol 1970;54:11–8.
33. Diabetic Retinopathy Study. Report number 6. Design, methods, and baseline results. Report number 7. A modification of the Airlie House classification of diabetic retinopathy. Prepared by the Diabetic Retinopathy Study Research Group. Invest Ophthalmol Vis Sci 1981;21:1–226.
34. Prud'homme G, Rand L. The Diabetic Retinopathy Study Research Group: distribution of maximum grade of lesion in proliferative diabetic retinopathy. Invest Ophthalm Vis Sci 1981;20(Suppl):59.
35. Joondeph BC, Joondeph HC, Flood TP. Foveal neovascularization in diabetic retinopathy. Arch Ophthalmol 1987;105:1672–5.
36. Chew EY, Murphy RP, Newsome DA, et al. Parafoveal telangiectasis and diabetic retinopathy. Arch Ophthalmol 1986;104:71–5.
37. Early Treatment Diabetic Retinopathy Study Research Group. Grading diabetic retinopathy from stereoscopic color fundus photographs – an extension of the modified Airlie House classification. ETDRS report no. 10. Ophthalmology 1991;98:786–806.
38. Wilson PJ, Ellis JD, MacEwen CJ, et al. Screening for diabetic retinopathy: a comparative trial of photography and scanning laser ophthalmoscopy. Ophthalmologica 2010;224:251–7.
39. Oliver SC, Schwartz SD. Peripheral vessel leakage (PVL): a new angiographic finding in diabetic retinopathy identified with ultra wide-field fluorescein angiography. Semin Ophthalmol 2010;25:27–33.
40. Schwartz JS, Pavan PR. Optic disc edema. Int Ophthalmol Clin 1984;24: 83–91.
41. Kampik A, Kenyon KR, Michels RG, et al. Epiretinal and vitreous membranes. Comparative study of 56 cases. Arch Ophthalmol 1981;99:1445–54.
42. Nork TM, Wallow IH, Sramek SJ, et al. Muller's cell involvement in proliferative diabetic retinopathy. Arch Ophthalmol 1987;105:1424–9.
43. Dobree JH. Proliferative diabetic retinopathy: evolution of the retinal lesions. Br J Ophthalmol 1964;48:637–49.
44. Bandello F, Gass JD, Lattanzio R, et al. Spontaneous regression of neovascularization at the disk and elsewhere in diabetic retinopathy. Am J Ophthalmol 1996;122:494–501.
45. Tolentino FI, Lee PF, Schepens CL. Biomicroscopic study of vitreous cavity in diabetic retinopathy. Arch Ophthalmol 1966;75:238–46.
46. Anderson Jr B. Activity and diabetic vitreous hemorrhages. Ophthalmology 1980;87:173–5.
47. Tasman W. Diabetic vitreous hemorrhage and its relationship to hypoglycemia. Mod Probl Ophthalmol 1979;20:413–4.
48. Larsen HW. Diabetic retinopathy. An ophthalmoscopic study with a discussion of the morphologic changes and the pathogenetic factors in this disease. Acta Ophthalmol 1960;(Suppl 60):1–89.
49. Bresnick GH, Haight B, De Venecia G. Retinal wrinkling and macular heterotopia in diabetic retinopathy. Arch Ophthalmol 1979;97:1890–5.
50. Ramsay WJ, Ramsay RC, Purple RL, et al. Involutional diabetic retinopathy. Am J Ophthalmol 1977;84:851–8.
51. Beetham WP. Visual prognosis of proliferating diabetic retinopathy. Br J Ophthalmol 1963;47:611–9.
52. Klein R, Klein BE, Moss SE, et al. The Wisconsin epidemiologic study of diabetic retinopathy. II. Prevalence and risk of diabetic retinopathy when age at diagnosis is less than 30 years. Arch Ophthalmol 1984;102:520–6.
53. Klein R, Klein BE, Moss SE, et al. The Wisconsin epidemiologic study of diabetic retinopathy. III. Prevalence and risk of diabetic retinopathy when age at diagnosis is 30 or more years. Arch Ophthalmol 1984;102:527–32.
54. Klein R, Klein BE, Moss SE, et al. The Wisconsin Epidemiologic Study of Diabetic Retinopathy. XV. The long-term incidence of macular edema. Ophthalmology 1995;102:7–16.
55. Diabetic Retinopathy Vitrectomy Study Research Group. Early vitrectomy for severe vitreous hemorrhage in diabetic retinopathy. Two-year results of a randomized trial. Diabetic Retinopathy Vitrectomy Study report 2. Arch Ophthalmol 1985;103:1644–52.
56. Diabetic Retinopathy Vitrectomy Study Research Group. Early vitrectomy for severe proliferative diabetic retinopathy in eyes with useful vision. Clinical application of results of a randomized trial – Diabetic Retinopathy Vitrectomy Study report 4. Ophthalmology 1988;95:1321–34.
57. Diabetic Retinopathy Vitrectomy Study Research Group. Early vitrectomy for severe proliferative diabetic retinopathy in eyes with useful vision. Results of a randomized trial. Diabetic Retinopathy Vitrectomy Study report 3. Ophthalmology 1988;95:1307–20.
58. Diabetic Retinopathy Vitrectomy Study Research Group. Early vitrectomy for severe vitreous hemorrhage in diabetic retinopathy. Four-year results of a randomized trial. Diabetic Retinopathy Vitrectomy Study report 5. Arch Ophthalmol 1990;108:958–64.
59. Aiello LM, Rand LI, Briones JC, et al. Diabetic retinopathy in Joslin Clinic patients with adult-onset diabetes. Ophthalmology 1981;88:619–23.
60. Zhang X, Saaddine JB, Chou CF, et al. Prevalence of diabetic retinopathy in the United States, 2005–2008. JAMA 2010;304:649–56.
61. The effect of intensive treatment of diabetes on the development and progression of long-term complications in insulin-dependent diabetes mellitus. The Diabetes Control and Complications Trial Research Group. N Engl J Med 1993;329:977–86.
62. UK Prospective Diabetes Study (UKPDS) Group. Intensive blood-glucose control with sulphonylureas or insulin compared with conventional treatment and risk of complications in patients with type 2 diabetes (UKPDS 33). Lancet 1998;352:837–53.
63. Diabetes Control and Complications Trial Research Group. Progression of retinopathy with intensive versus conventional treatment in the Diabetes Control and Complications Trial. Ophthalmology 1995;102:647–61.
64. The effect of intensive diabetes treatment on the progression of diabetic retinopathy in insulin-dependent diabetes mellitus. The Diabetes Control and Complications Trial. Arch Ophthalmol 1995;113:36–51.
65. Effect of intensive therapy on the microvascular complications of type 1 diabetes mellitus. JAMA 2002;287:2563–9.
66. Sustained effect of intensive treatment of type 1 diabetes mellitus on development and progression of diabetic nephropathy: the Epidemiology of Diabetes Interventions and Complications (EDIC) study. JAMA 2003;290: 2159–67.
67. Gerstein HC, Miller ME, Byington RP, et al. Effects of intensive glucose lowering in type 2 diabetes. N Engl J Med 2008;358:2545–59.
68. Holman RR, Paul SK, Bethel MA, et al. 10-year follow-up of intensive glucose control in type 2 diabetes. N Engl J Med 2008;359:1577–89.
69. White NH, Sun W, Cleary PA, et al. Prolonged effect of intensive therapy on the risk of retinopathy complications in patients with type 1 diabetes mellitus: 10 years after the Diabetes Control and Complications Trial. Arch Ophthalmol 2008;126:1707–15.
70. White NH, Cleary PA, Dahms W, et al. Beneficial effects of intensive therapy of diabetes during adolescence: outcomes after the conclusion of the Diabetes Control and Complications Trial (DCCT). J Pediatr 2001;139:804–12.
71. Davis MD, Fisher MR, Gangnon RE, et al. Risk factors for high-risk proliferative diabetic retinopathy and severe visual loss: Early Treatment Diabetic Retinopathy Study (ETDRS) report no. 18. Invest Ophthalmol Vis Sci 1998;39: 233–52.
72. Early worsening of diabetic retinopathy in the Diabetes Control and Complications Trial. Arch Ophthalmol 1998;116:874–86.

73. Dahl-Jorgensen K, Brinchmann-Hansen O, Hanssen KF, et al. Rapid tightening of blood glucose control leads to transient deterioration of retinopathy in insulin dependent diabetes mellitus: the Oslo study. Br Med J (Clin Res Ed) 1985;290:811–5.
74. Dandona P, Bolger JP, Boag F, et al. Rapid development and progression of proliferative retinopathy after strict diabetic control. Br Med J (Clin Res Ed) 1985;290:895–6.
75. Funatsu H, Yamashita H, Ohashi Y, et al. Effect of rapid glycemic control on progression of diabetic retinopathy. Jpn J Ophthalmol 1992;36:356–67.
76. Lauritzen T, Frost-Larsen K, Larsen HW, et al. Two-year experience with continuous subcutaneous insulin infusion in relation to retinopathy and neuropathy. Diabetes 1985;34(Suppl 3):74–9.
77. Brinchmann-Hansen O, Dahl-Jorgensen K, Hanssen KF, et al. The response of diabetic retinopathy to 41 months of multiple insulin injections, insulin pumps, and conventional insulin therapy. Arch Ophthalmol 1988;106: 1242–6.
78. Blood glucose control and the evolution of diabetic retinopathy and albuminuria. A preliminary multicenter trial. The Kroc Collaborative Study Group. N Engl J Med 1984;311:365–72.
79. Agardh CD, Eckert B, Agardh E. Irreversible progression of severe retinopathy in young type I insulin-dependent diabetes mellitus patients after improved metabolic control. J Diabetes Complications 1992;6:96–100.
80. Ernest JT, Goldstick TK, Engerman RL. Hyperglycemia impairs retinal oxygen autoregulation in normal and diabetic dogs. Invest Ophthalmol Vis Sci 1983;24:985–9.
81. Grunwald JE, Brucker AJ, Braunstein SN, et al. Strict metabolic control and retinal blood flow in diabetes mellitus. Br J Ophthalmol 1994;78:598–604.
82. Grunwald JE, Brucker AJ, Schwartz SS, et al. Diabetic glycemic control and retinal blood flow. Diabetes 1990;39:602–7.
83. Bain SC, Gill GV, Dyer PH, et al. Characteristics of type 1 diabetes of over 50 years duration (the Golden Years Cohort). Diabet Med 2003;20:808–11.
84. Keenan HA, Costacou T, Sun JK, et al. Clinical factors associated with resistance to microvascular complications in diabetic patients of extreme disease duration: the 50-year medalist study. Diabetes Care 2007;30:1995–7.
85. Sun JK, Keenan HA, Cavallerano JD, et al. Protection from retinopathy and other complications in patients with type 1 diabetes of extreme duration: the Joslin 50-year medalist study. Diabetes Care. 2011;34(4):968–74.
86. Ismail-Beigi F, Craven T, Banerji MA, et al. Effect of intensive treatment of hyperglycaemia on microvascular outcomes in type 2 diabetes: an analysis of the ACCORD randomised trial. Lancet 2010;376:419–30.
87. Patel A, MacMahon S, Chalmers J, et al. Effects of a fixed combination of perindopril and indapamide on macrovascular and microvascular outcomes in patients with type 2 diabetes mellitus (the ADVANCE trial): a randomised controlled trial. Lancet 2007;370:829–40.
88. Chew EY, Ambrosius WT, Davis MD, et al. Effects of medical therapies on retinopathy progression in type 2 diabetes. N Engl J Med 2010;363:233–44.
89. Keech AC, Mitchell P, Summanen PA, et al. Effect of fenofibrate on the need for laser treatment for diabetic retinopathy (FIELD study): a randomised controlled trial. Lancet 2007;370:1687–97.
90. Chaturvedi N, Sjolie AK, Stephenson JM, et al. Effect of lisinopril on progression of retinopathy in normotensive people with type 1 diabetes. The EUCLID Study Group. EURODIAB controlled trial of lisinopril in insulin-dependent diabetes mellitus. Lancet 1998;351:28–31.
91. Chaturvedi N, Porta M, Klein R, et al. Effect of candesartan on prevention (DIRECT-Prevent 1) and progression (DIRECT-Protect 1) of retinopathy in type 1 diabetes: randomised, placebo-controlled trials. Lancet 2008;372: 1394–402.
92. Sjolie AK, Klein R, Porta M, et al. Effect of candesartan on progression and regression of retinopathy in type 2 diabetes (DIRECT-Protect 2): a randomised placebo-controlled trial. Lancet 2008;372:1385–93.
93. Mauer M, Zinman B, Gardiner R, et al. Renal and retinal effects of enalapril and losartan in type 1 diabetes. N Engl J Med 2009;361:40–51.
94. Pershadsingh HA, Moore DM. PPARgamma agonists: potential as therapeutics for neovascular retinopathies. PPAR Res 2008;2008:164273.
95. Shen LQ, Child A, Weber GM, et al. Rosiglitazone and delayed onset of proliferative diabetic retinopathy. Arch Ophthalmol 2008;126:793–9.
96. Panigrahy D, Singer S, Shen LQ, et al. PPARgamma ligands inhibit primary tumor growth and metastasis by inhibiting angiogenesis. J Clin Invest 2002;110:923–32.
97. Chew EY, Klein ML, Ferris III FL, et al. Association of elevated serum lipid levels with retinal hard exudate in diabetic retinopathy. Early Treatment Diabetic Retinopathy Study (ETDRS) report no. 22. Arch Ophthalmol 1996;114:1079–84.
98. Biasotti A, Houssay BA. Phlorrhizin diabetes in fasting or fed hypophysectomized dogs. J Physiol 1932;77:81–91.
99. Luft R, Olivecrona H, Sjogren B. [Hypophysectomy in man.] Nord Med 1952;47:351–4.
100. Poulsen JE. Recovery from retinopathy in a case of diabetes with Simmonds' disease. Diabetes 1953;2:7–12.
101. Poulsen JE. Diabetes and anterior pituitary insufficiency. Final course and postmortem study of a diabetic patient with Sheehan's syndrome. Diabetes 1966;15:73–7.
102. Kohner EM, Joplin GF, Blach RK, et al. Pituitary ablation in the treatment of diabetic retinopathy. (A randomized trial). Trans Ophthalmol Soc U K 1972; 92:79–90.
103. Panisset A, Kohner EM, Cheng H, et al. Diabetic retinopathy: new vessels arising from the optic disc. II. Response to pituitary ablation by yttrium 90 implant. Diabetes 1971;20:824–33.
104. Kohner EM, Hamilton AM, Joplin GF, et al. Florid diabetic retinopathy and its response to treatment by photocoagulation or pituitary ablation. Diabetes 1976;25:104–10.
105. Smith LE, Shen W, Perruzzi C, et al. Regulation of vascular endothelial growth factor-dependent retinal neovascularization by insulin-like growth factor-1 receptor. Nat Med 1999;5:1390–5.
106. Growth Hormone Antagonist for Proliferative Diabetic Retinopathy Study Group (2001). The effect of a growth hormone receptor antagonist drug on proliferative diabetic retinopathy. Ophthalmology 2001;108:2266–72.
107. Boehm BO, Lang GK, Jehle PM, et al. Octreotide reduces vitreous hemorrhage and loss of visual acuity risk in patients with high-risk proliferative diabetic retinopathy. Horm Metab Res 2001;33:300–6.
108. Beetham WP. Visual prognosis of proliferating diabetic retinopathy. Br J Ophthalmol 1963;47:611–19.
109. Aiello LM, Beetham WP, Balodimos MC, et al. Ruby laser photocoagulation in treatment of diabetic proliferating retinopathy: Preliminary report. In: Goldberg MF, Fine SL, editors. Symposium on the treatment of diabetic retinopathy. Arlington, VA: U S Department of Health, Education, and Welfare, 1968. pp. 437–63.
110. Meyer-Schwickerath G. [Light coagulation; a method for treatment and prevention of the retinal detachment.] Albrecht Von Graefes Arch Ophthalmol 1954;156:2–34.
111. Okun E, Cibis PA. The role of photocoagulation in the therapy of proliferative diabetic retinopathy. Arch Ophthalmol 1966;75:337–52.
112. Wetzig PC, Jepson CN. Treatment of diabetic retinopathy by light coagulation. Am J Ophthalmol 1966;62:459–65.
113. Wetzig PC, Worlton JT. Treatment of diabetic retinopathy by light-coagulation: a preliminary study. Br J Ophthalmol 1963;47:539–41.
114. Beetham WP, Aiello LM, Balodimos MC, et al. Ruby-laser photocoagulation of early diabetic neovascular retinopathy: preliminary report of a long-term controlled study. Trans Am Ophthalmol Soc 1969;67:39–67.
115. Beetham WP, Aiello LM, Balodimos MC, et al. Ruby laser photocoagulation of early diabetic neovascular retinopathy. Preliminary report of a long-term controlled study. Arch Ophthalmol 1970;83:261–72.
116. Meyer-Schwickerath RE, Schott K. Diabetic retinopathy and photocoagulation. Am J Ophthalmol 1968;66:597–603.
117. Okun E. The effectiveness of photocoagulation in the therapy of proliferative diabetic retinopathy (PDR). (A controlled study in 50 patients.) Trans Am Acad Ophthalmol Otolaryngol 1968;72:246–52.
118. Glaser BM, Campochiaro PA, Davis Jr JL, et al. Retinal pigment epithelial cells release an inhibitor of neovascularization. Arch Ophthalmol 1985;103: 1870–5.
119. Ederer F, Hiller R. Clinical trials, diabetic retinopathy and photocoagulation. A reanalysis of five studies. Surv Ophthalmol 1975;19:267–86.
120. Stefansson E, Hatchell DL, Fisher BL, et al. Panretinal photocoagulation and retinal oxygenation in normal and diabetic cats. Am J Ophthalmol 1986;101: 657–64.
121. Gerstein DD, Dantzker DR. Retinal vascular changes in hereditary visual cell degeneration. Arch Ophthalmol 1969;81:99–105.
122. Molnar I, Poitry S, Tsacopoulos M, et al. Effect of laser photocoagulation on oxygenation of the retina in miniature pigs. Invest Ophthalmol Vis Sci 1985;26:1410–4.
123. Weiter JJ, Zuckerman R. The influence of the photoreceptor-RPE complex on the inner retina. An explanation for the beneficial effects of photocoagulation. Ophthalmology 1980;87:1133–9.
124. Wolbarsht ML, Landers III MB. The rationale of photocoagulation therapy for proliferative diabetic retinopathy: a review and a model. Ophthalmic Surg 1980;11:235–45.
125. Grunwald JE, Riva CE, Brucker AJ, et al. Altered retinal vascular response to 100% oxygen breathing in diabetes mellitus. Ophthalmology 1984;91: 1447–52.
126. Patel V, Rassam S, Newsom R, et al. Retinal blood flow in diabetic retinopathy. BMJ 1992;305:678–83.
127. Stefansson E, Machemer R, de Juan Jr E, et al. Retinal oxygenation and laser treatment in patients with diabetic retinopathy. Am J Ophthalmol 1992;113: 36–8.
128. Cheng H. Multicentre trial of xenon-arc photocoagulation in the treatment of diabetic retinopathy. A Randomized controlled study. Interim report. Trans Ophthalmol Soc U K 1975;95:351–7.
129. Editorial: The diabetic retinopathy study. Arch Ophthalmol 1973;90: 347–8.
130. Diabetic Retinopathy Study Research Group. Photocoagulation treatment of proliferative diabetic retinopathy. Clinical application of Diabetic Retinopathy Study (DRS) findings. Diabetic Retinopathy Study report 8. Ophthalmology 1981;88:583–600.
131. Diabetic Retinopathy Study Research Group. Photocoagulation treatment of proliferative diabetic retinopathy: relationship of adverse treatment effects to retinopathy severity. Diabetic Retinopathy Study report 5. Dev Ophthalmol 1981;2:248–61.
132. Rand LI, Prud'homme GJ, Ederer F, et al. Factors influencing the development of visual loss in advanced diabetic retinopathy. Diabetic Retinopathy Study (DRS) report 10. Invest Ophthalmol Vis Sci 1985;26:983–91.
133. Little HL, Rosenthal AR, Dellaporta A, et al. The effect of pan-retinal photocoagulation on rubeosis iridis. Am J Ophthalmol 1976;81:804–9.
134. Okun E, Johnston GP, Boniuk I, et al. Xenon arc photocoagulation of proliferative diabetic retinopathy. A review of 2688 consecutive eyes in the format of the Diabetic Retinopathy Study. Ophthalmology 1984;91: 1458–63.

135. British Multicentre Study Group. Photocoagulation for proliferative diabetic retinopathy: a randomised controlled clinical trial using the xenon-arc. Diabetologia 1984;26:109–15.
136. Hercules BL, Gayed II, Lucas SB, et al. Peripheral retinal ablation in the treatment of proliferative diabetic retinopathy: a three-year interim report of a randomised, controlled study using the argon laser. Br J Ophthalmol 1977;61:555–63.
137. Early Treatment Diabetic Retinopathy Study Research Group. Early photocoagulation for diabetic retinopathy. ETDRS report no. 9. Ophthalmology 1991;98:766–85.
138. Early Treatment Diabetic Retinopathy Study Research Group. Photocoagulation for diabetic macular edema. ETDRS report no. 1. Arch Ophthalmol 1985;103:1796–806.
139. Early Treatment Diabetic Retinopathy Study Research Group. Effects of aspirin treatment on diabetic retinopathy. ETDRS report no. 8. Ophthalmology 1991;98:757–65.
140. Early Treatment Diabetic Retinopathy Study Research Group. Techniques for scatter and local photocoagulation treatment of diabetic retinopathy. ETDRS report no. 3. Int Ophthalmol Clin 1987;27:254–64.
141. Ferris F. Early photocoagulation in patients with either type I or type II diabetes. Trans Am Ophthalmol Soc 1996;94:505–37.
142. Chey EY for the Krypton Argon Regression Neovascularization Study Research Group. Randomized comparison of krypton versus argon scatter photocoagulation for diabetic disc neovascularization: KARNS Study report number 1. Ophthalmology 1993;100:1655–64
143. Meyer-Schwickerath G, Gerke E. Bjerrum lecture. Treatment of diabetic retinopathy with photocoagulation. Results of photocoagulation therapy of proliferative retinopathy in childhood-onset and maturity-onset diabetes and an approach to the dosage in photocoagulation. Acta Ophthalmol (Copenh) 1983;61:756–68.
144. Chew EY, Mills JL, Metzger BE, et al. Metabolic control and progression of retinopathy. The Diabetes in Early Pregnancy Study. National Institute of Child Health and Human Development Diabetes in Early Pregnancy Study. Diabetes Care 1995;18:631–7.
145. Klein BE, Moss SE, Klein R. Effect of pregnancy on progression of diabetic retinopathy. Diabetes Care 1990;13:34–40.
146. Mathiesen ER, Ronn B, Storm B, et al. The natural course of microalbuminuria in insulin-dependent diabetes: a 10-year prospective study. Diabet Med 1995;12:482–7.
147. McDonald HR, Schatz H. Macular edema following panretinal photocoagulation. Retina 1985;5:5–10.
148. McDonald HR, Schatz H. Visual loss following panretinal photocoagulation for proliferative diabetic retinopathy. Ophthalmology 1985;92:388–93.
149. Meyers SM. Macular edema after scatter laser photocoagulation for proliferative diabetic retinopathy. Am J Ophthalmol 1980;90:210–6.
150. Ferris III FL, Podgor MJ, Davis MD. Macular edema in diabetic retinopathy study patients. Diabetic Retinopathy Study report number 12. Ophthalmology 1987;94:754–60.
151. Early Treatment Diabetic Retinopathy Study Research Group. Treatment techniques and clinical guidelines for photocoagulation of diabetic macular edema. ETDRS report no. 2. Ophthalmology 1987;94:761–74.
152. Elman MJ, Aiello LP, Beck RW, et al. Randomized trial evaluating ranibizumab plus prompt or deferred laser or triamcinolone plus prompt laser for diabetic macular edema. Ophthalmology 2010;117:1064–77.
153. Sultan MB, Zhou D, Loftus J, et al. A phase 2/3, multicenter, randomized, double-masked, 2-year trial of pegaptanib sodium for the treatment of diabetic macular edema. Ophthalmology 2011;118:1107–18.
154. Arevalo JF, Sanchez JG, Fromow-Guerra J, et al. Comparison of two doses of primary intravitreal bevacizumab (Avastin) for diffuse diabetic macular edema: results from the Pan-American Collaborative Retina Study Group (PACORES) at 12-month follow-up. Graefes Arch Clin Exp Ophthalmol 2009;247:735–43.
155. Googe J, Brucker AJ, Bressler NM, et al. for the Diabetic Retinopathy Clinical Research Network. Randomized trial evaluating short-term effects of intravitreal ranibizumab or triamcinolone acetonide on macular edema after focal/grid laser for diabetic macular edema in eyes also receiving panretinal photocoagulation. Retina 2011;31(6):1009–27.
156. Shimura M, Yasuda K, Nakazawa T, et al. Quantifying alterations of macular thickness before and after panretinal photocoagulation in patients with severe diabetic retinopathy and good vision. Ophthalmology 2003;110:2386–94.
157. Diabetic Retinopathy Clinical Research Network, Brucker AJ, Qin H, Antoszyk AN, et al. Observational study of the development of diabetic macular edema following panretinal (scatter) photocoagulation given in 1 or 4 sittings. Arch Ophthalmol 2009;127:132–40.
158. Pavan PR, Folk JC, Weingeist TA, et al. Diabetic rubeosis and panretinal photocoagulation. Arch Ophthalmol 1983;101:882–4.
159. Blumenkranz MS, Yellachich D, Andersen DE, et al. Semiautomated patterned scanning laser for retinal photocoagulation. Retina 2006;26:370–6.
160. Jain A, Blumenkranz MS, Paulus Y, et al. Effect of pulse duration on size and character of the lesion in retinal photocoagulation. Arch Ophthalmol 2008;126:78–85.
161. Muqit MM, Sanghvi C, McLauchlan R, et al. Study of clinical applications and safety for Pascal((R)) laser photocoagulation in retinal vascular disorders. Acta Ophthalmol 2010. Epub ahead of print February 16, 2010; PMID 20163363
162. Velez-Montoya R, Guerrero-Naranjo JL, Gonzalez-Mijares CC, et al. Pattern scan laser photocoagulation: safety and complications, experience after 1301 consecutive cases. Br J Ophthalmol 2010;94:720–4.
163. Kriechbaum K, Bolz M, Deak GG, et al. High-resolution imaging of the human retina in vivo after scatter photocoagulation treatment using a semiautomated laser system. Ophthalmology 2010;117:545–51.
164. Liang JC, Huamonte FU. Reduction of immediate complications after panretinal photocoagulation. Retina 1984;4:166–70.
165. Doft BH, Blankenship GW. Single versus multiple treatment sessions of argon laser panretinal photocoagulation for proliferative diabetic retinopathy. Ophthalmology 1982;89:772–9.
166. Bandello F, Brancato R, Lattanzio R, et al. Double-frequency Nd:YAG laser vs argon-green laser in the treatment of proliferative diabetic retinopathy: randomized study with long-term follow-up. Lasers Surg Med 1996;19:173–6.
167. Bandello F, Brancato R, Trabucchi G, et al. Diode versus argon-green laser panretinal photocoagulation in proliferative diabetic retinopathy: a randomized study in 44 eyes with a long follow-up time. Graefes Arch Clin Exp Ophthalmol 1993;231:491–4.
168. Doft BH, Blankenship G. Retinopathy risk factor regression after laser panretinal photocoagulation for proliferative diabetic retinopathy. Ophthalmology 1984;91:1453–7.
169. Blankenship GW. A clinical comparison of central and peripheral argon laser panretinal photocoagulation for proliferative diabetic retinopathy. Ophthalmology 1988;95:170–7.
170. Vander JF, Duker JS, Benson WE, et al. Long-term stability and visual outcome after favorable initial response of proliferative diabetic retinopathy to panretinal photocoagulation. Ophthalmology 1991;98:1575–9.
171. Rogell GD. Incremental panretinal photocoagulation. Results in treating proliferative diabetic retinopathy. Retina 1983;3:308–11.
172. Reddy VM, Zamora RL, Olk RJ. Quantitation of retinal ablation in proliferative diabetic retinopathy. Am J Ophthalmol 1995;119:760–6.
173. Vine AK. The efficacy of additional argon laser photocoagulation for persistent, severe proliferative diabetic retinopathy. Ophthalmology 1985;92:1532–7.
174. Early Treatment Diabetic Retinopathy Study Research Group. Case reports to accompany Early Treatment Diabetic Retinopathy Study reports 3 and 4. Int Ophthalmol Clin 1987;27:273–333.
175. Dogru M, Kaderli B, Gelisken O, et al. Ocular surface changes with applanation contact lens and coupling fluid use after argon laser photocoagulation in noninsulin-dependent diabetes mellitus. Am J Ophthalmol 2004;138:381–8.
176. Bloom SM, Mahl CF, Schiller SB. Lenticular burns following argon panretinal photocoagulation. Br J Ophthalmol 1992;76:630–1.
177. Moriarty AP, Spalton DJ, Shilling JS, et al. Breakdown of the blood-aqueous barrier after argon laser panretinal photocoagulation for proliferative diabetic retinopathy. Ophthalmology 1996;103:833–8.
178. Patel JI, Jenkins L, Benjamin L, et al. Dilated pupils and loss of accommodation following diode panretinal photocoagulation with sub-tenon local anaesthetic in four cases. Eye (Lond) 2002;16:628–32.
179. Fong DS, Girach A, Boney A. Visual side effects of successful scatter laser photocoagulation surgery for proliferative diabetic retinopathy: a literature review. Retina 2007;27:816–24.
180. Mendrinos E, Donati G, Pournaras CJ. Rapid and persistent regression of severe new vessels on the disc in proliferative diabetic retinopathy after a single intravitreal injection of pegaptanib. Acta Ophthalmol 2009;87:683–4.
181. Avery RL, Pearlman J, Pieramici DJ, et al. Intravitreal bevacizumab (Avastin) in the treatment of proliferative diabetic retinopathy. Ophthalmology 2006;113:1695–15.
182. Jorge R, Costa RA, Calucci D, et al. Intravitreal bevacizumab (Avastin) for persistent new vessels in diabetic retinopathy (IBEPE study). Retina 2006;26:1006–13.
183. Erdol H, Turk A, Akyol N, et al. The results of intravitreal bevacizumab injections for persistent neovascularizations in proliferative diabetic retinopathy after photocoagulation therapy. Retina 2010;30:570–7.
184. Mirshahi A, Roohipoor R, Lashay A, et al. Bevacizumab-augmented retinal laser photocoagulation in proliferative diabetic retinopathy: a randomized double-masked clinical trial. Eur J Ophthalmol 2008;18:263–9.
185. Tonello M, Costa RA, Almeida FP, et al. Panretinal photocoagulation versus PRP plus intravitreal bevacizumab for high-risk proliferative diabetic retinopathy (IBeHi study). Acta Ophthalmol 2008;86:385–9.
186. Takahashi M, Trempe CL, Maguire K, et al. Vitreoretinal relationship in diabetic retinopathy. A biomicroscopic evaluation. Arch Ophthalmol 1981;99:241–5.
187. Ono R, Kakehashi A, Yamagami H, et al. Prospective assessment of proliferative diabetic retinopathy with observations of posterior vitreous detachment. Int Ophthalmol 2005;26:15–9.
188. Rheaume MA, Vavvas D. Pharmacologic vitreolysis. Semin Ophthalmol 2010;25:295–302.
189. Gandorfer A. Objective of pharmacologic vitreolysis. Dev Ophthalmol 2009;44:1–6.
190. Kuppermann BD, Thomas EL, de Smet MD, et al., Vitrase for Vitreous Hemorrhage Study Groups. Pooled efficacy results from two multinational randomized controlled clinical trials of a single intravitreous injection of highly purified ovine hyaluronidase (Vitrase) for the management of vitreous hemorrhage. Am J Ophthalmol 2005;140:573–84.
191. Stalmans P, Delaey C, de Smet MD, et al. Intravitreal injection of microplasmin for treatment of vitreomacular adhesion: results of a prospective, randomized, sham-controlled phase II trial (the MIVI-IIT trial). Retina 2010;30:1122–7.
192. Goldenberg DT, Trese MT. Pharmacologic vitreodynamics and molecular flux. Dev Ophthalmol 2009;44:31–6.
193. Machemer R, Buettner H, Norton EW, et al. Vitrectomy: a pars plana approach. Trans Am Acad Ophthalmol Otolaryngol 1971;75:813–20.

Hypertension

Chapter 49

Carol Yim Lui Cheung, Tien Yin Wong

INTRODUCTION

Hypertension is the leading risk factor for cardiovascular disease (CVD) and mortality worldwide,[1] with a projected number of 1.56 billion individuals with hypertension by 2025.[2]

Hypertension has profound effects on both the structure and function of the vasculature in the eye. The retinal, choroidal, and optic nerve circulations undergo a range of pathophysiological changes in response to elevated blood pressure resulting in a spectrum of clinical signs known as hypertensive retinopathy, choroidopathy, and optic neuropathy, respectively.[3] Hypertension is also a major risk factor for many other eye diseases, including the development and progression of diabetic retinopathy,[4] retinal vein occlusion,[5] retinal arterial macroaneurysm,[6] and possibly age-related macular degeneration and glaucoma.[3,7]

HYPERTENSIVE RETINOPATHY

Definition and classification

Retinopathy is the most common manifestation of hypertension which develops due to acute and/or chronic elevations in blood pressure. Hypertensive retinopathy is broadly divided into different stages.[8] The initial response to elevated blood pressure is vasospasm and an increase in vasomotor tone, with consequent narrowing of retinal arterioles to control for optimal blood volume ("vasoconstrictive" phase). This stage is seen clinically as generalized or diffuse retinal arteriolar narrowing.

Persistently elevated blood pressure leads to the "sclerotic" phase, which manifests pathologically as intimal thickening, media wall hyperplasia and hyaline degeneration. This stage accords with diffused and localized (focal) retinal arteriolar narrowing, arteriolar wall opacification ("silver" or "copper wiring"), and compression of the venules by structural changes in the arterioles (arteriovenous "nicking" or "nipping").

With chronically sustained blood pressure elevation, the blood–retinal barrier is disrupted. Pathological changes at this stage ("exudative" phase) include necrosis of the smooth muscles and endothelial cells, exudation of blood and lipids and retinal nerve fiber layer ischemia, which results in microaneurysms, retinal hemorrhages, hard exudates, and cotton-wool spots seen in the retina.

Very severe hypertension (i.e. "malignant hypertension" phase) may lead to optic disc swelling which may reflect underlying hypertensive encephalopathy with raised intracranial pressure.[3,7–9]

The above phases of hypertensive retinopathy are not always sequential. For example, in patients with acutely raised blood pressure, signs of retinopathy reflecting the "exudative" stage (e.g. retinal hemorrhage) may be present without features of the "sclerotic" stage (e.g. arteriovenous nicking). Furthermore, elevated blood pressure does not fully explain all the pathophysiological mechanisms of hypertensive retinopathy. Other processes involved in the pathogenesis of hypertensive retinopathy signs include inflammation,[10] endothelial dysfunction,[11] abnormal angiogenesis,[12] and oxidative stress.[13] In fact, hypertensive retinopathy signs are detected frequently in persons without a known history of hypertension.[14]

There have been many different classifications for hypertensive retinopathy. Traditionally, the Keith–Wagener–Baker system classifies patients with hypertension into four groups of increasing severity.[15] However, it is difficult to distinguish early retinopathy grades (e.g. group 1 signs are not easily distinguished from group 2 signs).[9,16] A simplified classification of hypertensive retinopathy based on prognosis of different signs from recent population-based data has been proposed[9]:

1. **None**: no detectable signs.
2. **Mild**: Generalized arteriolar narrowing, focal arteriolar narrowing, arteriovenous nicking, arteriolar wall opacification (silver or copper wiring), or a combination of these signs (Fig. 49.1).
3. **Moderate**: Hemorrhages (blot, dot, or flame-shaped), microaneurysms, cotton-wool spots, hard exudates, or a combination of these signs (Fig. 49.2).
4. **Malignant**: Signs of moderate retinopathy in combination with optic disc swelling, in the presence of severely elevated blood pressure (Fig. 49.3).

Recently, the application of digital retinal photography and imaging software has allowed measurements of retinal vessel widths to quantify generalized arteriolar narrowing objectively.[17,18] Studies using such methods show that generalized retinal arteriolar narrowing is strongly related to blood pressure and risk of hypertension.[19,20] There is also evidence that retinal venular diameter may convey independent prognostic information.[21] However, the measurement of retinal vessel width using these methods require specialized computer software and trained technicians and is thus not yet widely available for clinical use.

It has been argued that the clinical assessment of hypertensive retinopathy signs is of limited additional value in the management of patients with hypertension.[22] Most international hypertension management guidelines, however, including those of the US Joint National Committee on Prevention, Detection,

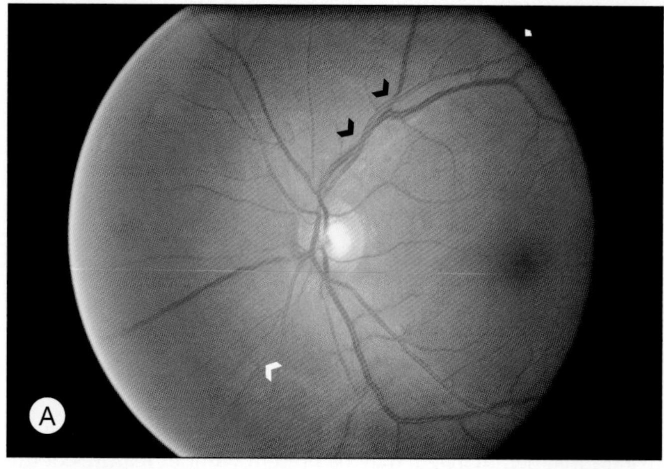

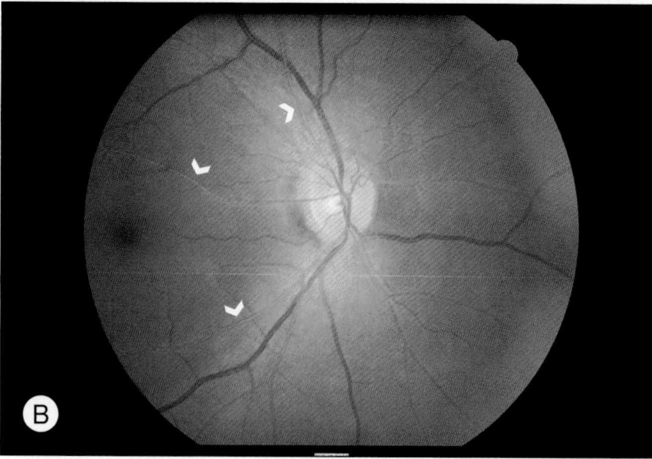

Fig. 49.1 Examples of mild hypertensive retinopathy. Panel A shows arteriovenous nicking (black arrows) and focal narrowing (white arrow). Panel B shows opacification (silver or copper wiring) of arteriolar wall (white arrows).

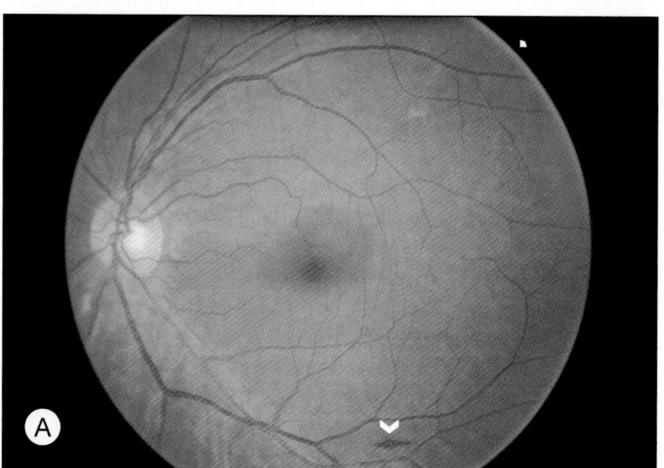

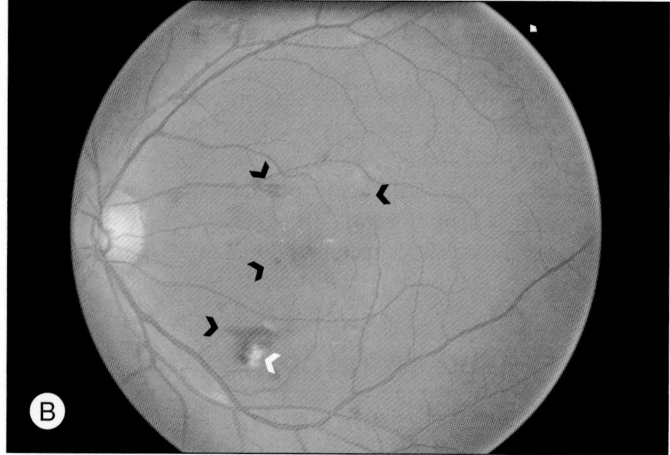

Fig. 49.2 Examples of moderate hypertensive retinopathy. Panel A shows a flame-shaped retinal hemorrhage (white arrow). Panel B shows a cotton-wool spot (white arrow), retinal hemorrhages and microaneurysms (black arrows).

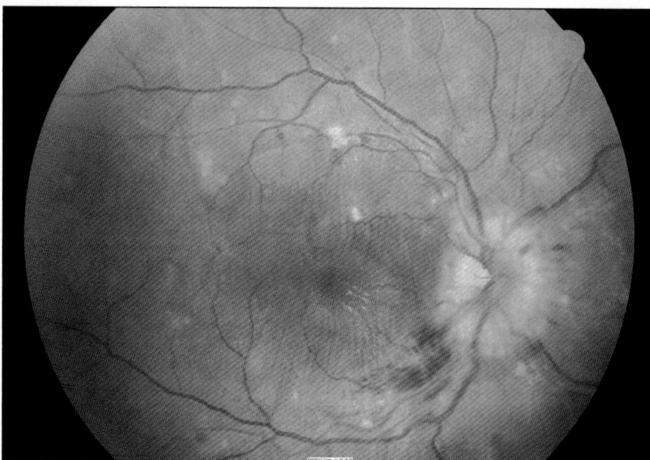

Fig. 49.3 Example of malignant hypertensive retinopathy. Retinal hemorrhages, cotton-wool spots, hard exudates, and swelling of the optic disc are present.

Evaluation, and Treatment of High Blood Pressure (JNC), the British Society of Hypertension and the European Society of Hypertension (ESH), and the European Society of Cardiology (ESC),[23–25] still emphasize that hypertensive retinopathy, with left ventricular hypertrophy and renal impairment, is an indicator of target organ damage, and that its presence should be an indication for a more aggressive approach in managing these hypertensive patients.[24] Whether the retinal examinations should be performed by physicians using the direct ophthalmoscope, by ophthalmologists, or via standardized assessment using digital retinal photography remains unclear.

Epidemiology

In the past 30 years, epidemiological studies that have used retinal photography and standardized assessment methods to document and define hypertensive retinopathy have contributed to a greater understanding of the epidemiology, risk factors, and systemic associations of hypertensive retinopathy signs in the general population with different racial samples.[26]

With the exception of optic disc swelling, hypertensive retinopathy signs are generally common in persons 40 years of age or older, even in the absence of diabetes mellitus, with prevalence ranges from 2 to 17%.[27–33] These studies also demonstrate that hypertensive retinopathy signs increase with age, and may vary by race/ethnicity (Chinese have a higher prevalence of hypertensive retinopathy than Caucasian whites) and possibly gender (men have higher rates than women).

While it is well established that hypertensive retinopathy signs are strongly correlated with blood pressure levels,[26,34,35] new epidemiological studies show three particularly interesting features. First, there is now good evidence that some signs, particularly generalized retinal arteriolar narrowing, may precede the development of hypertension.[19,20,36] In some studies, normotensive persons with this sign were more likely to develop hypertension and, among those with mild hypertension, were more likely to develop the severe stages of hypertension.[37] Thus, generalized retinal arteriolar narrowing, possibly reflecting more widespread systemic peripheral vasoconstriction, may be an early preclinical marker of hypertension.

Second, new studies in children have demonstrated that the association between retinal arteriolar narrowing and elevated blood pressure can be observed even in children as young as 4–5 years of age. These findings suggest that the impact of elevated blood pressure on the retinal microcirculation occurs in early life,[38,39] which may then "track" through to adulthood, even before the onset of overt hypertension.

Third, there is now evidence to show that the patterns of associations of specific retinopathy signs vary with current and past blood pressure levels. Generalized retinal arteriolar narrowing and arteriovenous nicking, for example, are related not only to current blood pressure levels, but also to blood pressure levels measured in the past, suggesting these two retinal signs reflect the cumulative effects of long-standing hypertension and are persistent markers of chronic hypertensive damage. In contrast, focal arteriolar narrowing, retinal hemorrhages, microaneurysms and cotton-wools spots are related only to concurrently measured blood pressure, mirroring the effects of short-term blood pressure changes.[35]

Finally, retinal venular diameter, not traditionally considered part of the spectrum of hypertensive retinopathy signs, may convey additional information regarding the state of the retinal vasculature and systemic health. Studies found that retinal venular widening or dilation is also related to elevated blood pressure levels,[20,21,34,40] suggesting that the venule may exhibit different optimal flow characteristics across the vascular network compared with arterioles in the presence of hypertension.[41] Whether retinal venular dilation should be included as part of the classification of hypertensive retinopathy remains unclear at this time.

Relationship with stroke

Retinal and cerebral small vessels share similar embryological origin, anatomical features, and physiological properties. There are now numerous studies that have reported the strong link between the presence of hypertensive retinopathy and both subclinical and clinical stroke as well as other cerebrovascular conditions.

In one large multicenter US study, middle-aged, generally healthy persons with moderate hypertensive retinopathy signs were more likely to have subclinical MRI-defined cerebral infarction, cerebral white matter lesions, and cerebral atrophy than those without these signs.[42–45] Furthermore, persons with moderate hypertensive signs at baseline were more likely to develop an incident clinical stroke,[46] incident lacunar stroke,[47] cognitive impairment,[48] and cognitive decline[49] than persons without these signs, even controlling for traditional risk factors. Another large cohort study based in Rotterdam, Netherlands, have further reported associations of larger retinal venular diameter with incidence of hemorrhagic stroke and the development of dementia.[50,51]

Some recent studies further demonstrated that hypertensive retinopathy may allow further refinement and subtyping of stroke. In a multicenter study of patients with acute stroke, different hypertensive retinopathy signs were associated with specific stroke subtypes.[52] For example, retinal arteriolar narrowing was associated with lacunar stroke, while retinal hemorrhages were linked with cerebral hemorrhages. These findings suggest that hypertensive signs reflect specific cerebral microvasculopathy and may further help to understand the underlying pathologic mechanisms.[47,52–54]

Relationship with coronary heart disease

The presence of hypertensive retinopathy signs is associated with multiple markers of subclinical atherosclerotic diseases, including coronary artery calcification,[55] aortic stiffness,[56] left ventricular hypertrophy,[57] and carotid intima-media thickness.[58] There is also evidence that hypertensive retinopathy signs are predictive of clinical coronary artery disease events and congestive heart failure; however, the results of these studies show less consistent associations than with stroke.[59–61] In one study, persons with moderate hypertensive retinopathy were three times more likely to develop congestive heart failure than those without retinopathy, while controlling for the presence of other cardiovascular risk factors.[62]

Hypertensive retinopathy has also been associated with increased risk of CVD mortality, stroke mortality, and coronary heart disease mortality.[14,63,64] In one study, persons with moderate hypertensive retinopathy were more likely to die from coronary heart disease than persons without this sign, with an equivalent risk similar to that of diabetes.[63] These data suggest that hypertensive retinopathy may convey additional prognostic information than other risk measures of CVD.

Relationship with other end-organ damage of hypertension

The significance of hypertensive retinopathy signs as risk indicators has long been recognized in patients with renal disease.[65] Retinopathy signs have also been associated with other indicators of hypertensive target organ damage, such as microalbuminuria and renal impairment.[66,67] Such association was independent of blood pressure, diabetes, and other risk factors, and was also seen in persons without diabetes or hypertension. Furthermore, hypertensive retinopathy was correlated with left ventricular hypertrophy, even in patients with mild-to-moderate hypertensive retinopathy, suggesting that its presence is an indicator of other target organ damage.[68–70]

Taken in totality, these data suggest hypertensive retinopathy signs are markers of systemic vascular disease which may mirror preclinical structural changes in the cerebral and coronary microcirculations, and represent a greater burden of cardiovascular risk factors that predispose people to develop CVD. The presence of hypertensive retinopathy may therefore convey additional prognostic information than other risk measures of CVD.

HYPERTENSIVE CHOROIDOPATHY

Hypertensive choroidopathy is less well recognized compared with hypertensive retinopathy. The underlying mechanism of hypertensive choroidopathy is related to choroidal ischemia which has effects on the retinal pigment epithelium and retina.

Like the retinal vessels, the choroidal vessels may also undergo fibrinoid necrosis at the level of the choroidal capillaries in the presence of elevated blood pressure, leading to hypertensive choroidopathy signs that include Elschnig spots (round, deep, and gray-yellow patches at the level of the retinal pigment epithelium) and Siegrist streaks (linear hyperpigmented streaks along choroidal arteries). In severe cases, there may also be serous retinal detachment which can lead to vision loss.[71-73]

HYPERTENSIVE OPTIC NEUROPATHY

Bilateral optic disc swelling or papilloedema is commonly caused by accelerated or malignant hypertension, representing the "malignant hypertensive retinopathy" stage in the above classification. The pathogenesis of optic disc swelling secondary to accelerated hypertension remains controversial. Ischemia, raised intracranial pressure and hypertensive encephalopathy are all possible mechanisms that can result in papilloedema.[73] Bilateral disc swelling is strongly correlated with CVD risk and mortality,[14,15,64] and these patients need urgent antihypertensive management.[9]

FUTURE DIRECTIONS

There are several areas of research in the field of hypertensive retinopathy. First, advances in digital retinal imaging and computer software analysis have provided the opportunity to quantify and monitor hypertensive retinopathy signs in a more objective manner. In addition to the measurement of retinal vascular caliber used in previous studies, new research has identified a number of other retinal vascular features, such as branching angles, bifurcation, fractal dimension, tortuosity, vascular length-to-diameter ratio, and wall-to-lumen ratio, that may also be related to hypertension.[74-78] These newer, quantitatively measured retinal vascular changes may offer increasingly accurate and reliable parameters reflecting early and subtle retinal vascular abnormalities, which potentially provide additional predictive value of CVD risk outcomes.

Furthermore, advanced state-of-the-art cellular-level retinal imaging using adaptive optics retinal cameras, retinal vessel oxygen saturation using the retinal oximeter, retinal blood flow using Doppler optical coherence tomography, and choroidal vasculature imaging using spectral domain optical coherence tomography are recently developed technologies that hold promise for better examining the link between eye and hypertension.

Second, genetic epidemiology studies have provided clues to new vascular pathophysiological processes linked to hypertensive retinopathy signs.[40] For example, a recent population-based genome-wide association study demonstrated four novel loci associated with retinal venular caliber, an endophenotype of the microcirculation associated with clinical CVD.[79] These genetic studies may allow understanding of the contribution and biological mechanisms of microcirculatory changes that underlie CVD.

Retinal vasculature assessment also allows the study of new therapies for hypertension. Studies have demonstrated regression of hypertensive retinopathy signs in response to blood pressure reduction and that regression patterns are different in response to different antihypertensive regimens (e.g., angiotensin-converting enzyme inhibitors appear to have a more favorable effect on the retinal vasculature).[80-82] Further prospective controlled trials are required to clarify whether specific reduction of hypertensive retinopathy also reduces the morbidity and mortality associated with CVD.

CONCLUSION

Hypertension has widespread effects on the ocular vasculature. Hypertensive retinopathy signs are commonly seen in the general adult population and are associated with both subclinical and clinical measures of CVD. Patients with hypertensive retinopathy may therefore benefit from a careful assessment of blood pressure and other vascular factors and appropriate CVD risk management.

REFERENCES

1. Lawes CM, Vander HS, Rodgers A. Global burden of blood-pressure-related disease, 2001. Lancet 2008;371(9623):1513–18.
2. Kearney PM, Whelton M, Reynolds K, et al. Global burden of hypertension: analysis of worldwide data. Lancet 2005;365(9455):217–23.
3. Wong TY, Mitchell P. The eye in hypertension. Lancet 2007;369(9559): 425–35.
4. Cheung N, Mitchell P, Wong TY. Diabetic retinopathy. Lancet 2010;376(9735): 124–36.
5. Wong TY, Scott IU. Clinical practice. Retinal-vein occlusion N Engl J Med 2010;363(22):2135–44.
6. Panton RW, Goldberg MF, Farber MD. Retinal arterial macroaneurysms: risk factors and natural history. Br J Ophthalmol 1990;74:595–600.
7. Bhargava M, Ikram MK, Wong TY. How does hypertension affect your eyes? J Hum Hypertens 2011.
8. Tso MO, Jampol LM. Pathophysiology of hypertensive retinopathy. Ophthalmology 1982;89(10):1132–45.
9. Wong TY, Mitchell P. Hypertensive retinopathy. N Engl J Med 2004;351(22): 2310–7.
10. Klein R, Sharrett AR, Klein BE, et al. Are retinal arteriolar abnormalities related to atherosclerosis?: The Atherosclerosis Risk in Communities Study. Arterioscler Thromb Vasc Biol 2000;20(6):1644–50.
11. Delles C, Michelson G, Harazny J, et al. Impaired endothelial function of the retinal vasculature in hypertensive patients. Stroke 2004;35(6):1289–93.
12. Tsai WC, Li YH, Huang YY, et al. Plasma vascular endothelial growth factor as a marker for early vascular damage in hypertension. Clin Sci (Lond) 2005;109(1):39–43.
13. Coban E, Alkan E, Altuntas S, et al. Serum ferritin levels correlate with hypertensive retinopathy. Med Sci Monit 2010;16(2):CR92–CR95.
14. Wong TY, Klein R, Klein BE, et al. Retinal microvascular abnormalities and their relationship with hypertension, cardiovascular disease, and mortality. Surv Ophthalmol 2001;46(1):59–80.
15. Keith NM, Wagener HP, Barker NW. Some different types of essential hypertension: their course and prognosis. Am J Med Sci 1939;197(3):332–43.
16. Dodson PM, Lip GY, Eames SM, et al. Hypertensive retinopathy: a review of existing classification systems and a suggestion for a simplified grading system. J Hum Hypertens 1996;10(2):93–8.
17. Wong TY, Knudtson MD, Klein R, et al. Computer-assisted measurement of retinal vessel diameters in the Beaver Dam Eye Study: methodology, correlation between eyes, and effect of refractive errors. Ophthalmology 2004;111(6): 1183–90.
18. Cheung CY, Hsu W, Lee ML, et al. A new method to measure peripheral retinal vascular caliber over an extended area. Microcirculation 2010;17(7):495–503.
19. Wong TY, Klein R, Sharrett AR, et al. Retinal arteriolar diameter and risk for hypertension. Ann Intern Med 2004;140(4):248–55.
20. Ikram MK, Witteman JC, Vingerling JR, et al. Retinal vessel diameters and risk of hypertension: the Rotterdam Study. Hypertension 2006;47(2):189–94.
21. Wong TY, Kamineni A, Klein R, et al. Quantitative retinal venular caliber and risk of cardiovascular disease in older persons: the cardiovascular health study. Arch Intern Med 2006;166(21):2388–94.
22. van den Born BJ, Hulsman CA, Hoekstra JB, et al. Value of routine funduscopy in patients with hypertension: systematic review. BMJ 2005;331(7508):73.
23. Williams B, Poulter NR, Brown MJ, et al. British Hypertension Society guidelines for hypertension management 2004 (BHS-IV): summary. BMJ 2004; 328(7440):634–40.
24. Chobanian AV, Bakris GL, Black HR, et al. The Seventh Report of the Joint National Committee on Prevention, Detection, Evaluation, and Treatment of High Blood Pressure: the JNC 7 report. JAMA 2003;289(19):2560–72.
25. Mansia G, De Backer G, Dominiczak A, et al. 2007 ESH-ESC Guidelines for the management of arterial hypertension: the task force for the management of arterial hypertension of the European Society of Hypertension (ESH) and of the European Society of Cardiology (ESC). Blood Press 2007;16(3):135–232.
26. Hubbard LD, Brothers RJ, King WN, et al. Methods for evaluation of retinal microvascular abnormalities associated with hypertension/sclerosis in the Atherosclerosis Risk in Communities Study. Ophthalmology 1999;106(12): 2269–80.
27. Klein R. Retinopathy in a population-based study. Trans Am Ophthalmol Soc 1992;90:561–94.

28. Jeganathan VS, Cheung N, Tay WT, et al. Prevalence and risk factors of retinopathy in an Asian population without diabetes: the Singapore Malay Eye Study. Arch Ophthalmol 2010;128(1):40–5.
29. Peng XY, Wang FH, Liang YB, et al. Retinopathy in persons without diabetes: the Handan Eye Study. Ophthalmology 2010;117(3):531–7, 537.
30. Chao JR, Lai MY, Azen SP, et al. Retinopathy in persons without diabetes: the Los Angeles Latino Eye Study. Invest Ophthalmol Vis Sci 2007;48(9):4019–25.
31. Wong TY, Liew G, Tapp RJ, et al. Relation between fasting glucose and retinopathy for diagnosis of diabetes: three population-based cross-sectional studies. Lancet 2008;371(9614):736–43.
32. Ojaimi E, Nguyen TT, Klein R, et al. Retinopathy signs in people without diabetes: the multi-ethnic study of atherosclerosis. Ophthalmology 2011;118(4):656–62.
33. Wong TY, Klein R, Duncan BB, et al. Racial differences in the prevalence of hypertensive retinopathy. Hypertension 2003;41(5):1086–91.
34. Cheung CY, Tay WT, Mitchell P, et al. Quantitative and qualitative retinal microvascular characteristics and blood pressure. J Hypertens 2011;29(7):1380–91.
35. Wong TY, Hubbard LD, Klein R, et al. Retinal microvascular abnormalities and blood pressure in older people: the Cardiovascular Health Study. Br J Ophthalmol 2002;86(9):1007–13.
36. Klein R, Klein BE, Moss SE, et al. The relationship of retinopathy in persons without diabetes to the 15-year incidence of diabetes and hypertension: Beaver Dam Eye Study. Trans Am Ophthalmol Soc 2006;104:98–107.
37. Smith W, Wang JJ, Wong TY, et al. Retinal arteriolar narrowing is associated with 5-year incident severe hypertension: the Blue Mountains Eye Study. Hypertension 2004;44(4):442–7.
38. Mitchell P, Cheung N, de Haseth K, et al. Blood pressure and retinal arteriolar narrowing in children. Hypertension 2007;49(5):1156–62.
39. Li LJ, Cheung CY, Liu Y, et al. Influence of blood pressure on retinal vascular caliber in young children. Ophthalmology 2011;118(7):1459–65.
40. Sun C, Wang JJ, Mackey DA, et al. Retinal vascular caliber: systemic, environmental, and genetic associations. Surv Ophthalmol 2009;54(1):74–95.
41. Patton N, Aslam T, Macgillivray T, et al. Asymmetry of retinal arteriolar branch widths at junctions affects ability of formulae to predict trunk arteriolar widths. Invest Ophthalmol Vis Sci 2006;47(4):1329–33.
42. Kawasaki R, Cheung N, Mosley T, et al. Retinal microvascular signs and 10-year risk of cerebral atrophy: the Atherosclerosis Risk in Communities (ARIC) Study. Stroke 2010;41(8):1826–8.
43. Wong TY, Klein R, Sharrett AR, et al. Cerebral white matter lesions, retinopathy, and incident clinical stroke. JAMA 2002;288(1):67–74.
44. Cooper LS, Wong TY, Klein R, et al. Retinal microvascular abnormalities and MRI-defined subclinical cerebral infarction: the Atherosclerosis Risk in Communities Study. Stroke 2006;37(1):82–6.
45. Cheung N, Mosley T, Islam A, et al. Retinal microvascular abnormalities and subclinical magnetic resonance imaging brain infarct: a prospective study. Brain 2010;133(Pt 7):1987–93.
46. Wong TY, Klein R, Couper DJ, et al. Retinal microvascular abnormalities and incident stroke: the Atherosclerosis Risk in Communities Study. Lancet 2001;358(9288):1134–40.
47. Yatsuya H, Folsom AR, Wong TY, et al. Retinal microvascular abnormalities and risk of lacunar stroke: Atherosclerosis Risk in Communities Study. Stroke 2010;41(7):1349–55.
48. Wong TY, Klein R, Sharrett AR, et al. Retinal microvascular abnormalities and cognitive impairment in middle-aged persons: the Atherosclerosis Risk in Communities Study. Stroke 2002;33(6):1487–92.
49. Lesage SR, Mosley TH, Wong TY, et al. Retinal microvascular abnormalities and cognitive decline: the ARIC 14-year follow-up study. Neurology 2009;73(11):862–8.
50. de Jong FJ, Schrijvers EM, Ikram MK, et al. Retinal vascular caliber and risk of dementia: the Rotterdam study. Neurology 2011;76(9):816–21.
51. Wieberdink RG, Ikram MK, Koudstaal et al. Retinal vascular calibers and the risk of intracerebral hemorrhage and cerebral infarction: the Rotterdam Study. Stroke 2010;41(12):2757–61.
52. Lindley RI, Wang JJ, Wong MC, et al. Retinal microvasculature in acute lacunar stroke: a cross-sectional study. Lancet Neurol 2009;8(7):628–34.
53. Baker ML, Hand PJ, Wong TY, et al. Retinopathy and lobar intracerebral hemorrhage: insights into pathogenesis. Arch Neurol 2010;67(10):1224–30.
54. Baker ML, Hand PJ, Liew G, et al. Retinal microvascular signs may provide clues to the underlying vasculopathy in patients with deep intracerebral hemorrhage. Stroke 2010;41(4):618–23.
55. Wong TY, Cheung N, Islam FM, et al. Relation of retinopathy to coronary artery calcification: the multi-ethnic study of atherosclerosis. Am J Epidemiol 2008;167(1):51–8.
56. Cheung N, Sharrett AR, Klein R, et al. Aortic distensibility and retinal arteriolar narrowing: the multi-ethnic study of atherosclerosis. Hypertension 2007;50(4):617–22.
57. Cheung N, Bluemke DA, Klein R, et al. Retinal arteriolar narrowing and left ventricular remodeling: the multi-ethnic study of atherosclerosis. J Am Coll Cardiol 2007;50(1):48–55.
58. Kawasaki R, Cheung N, Islam FM, et al. Is diabetic retinopathy related to subclinical cardiovascular disease? Ophthalmology 2011;118(5):860–5.
59. Michelson EL, Morganroth J, Nichols CW, et al. Retinal arteriolar changes as an indicator of coronary artery disease. Arch Intern Med 1979;139(10):1139–41.
60. Wong TY, Klein R, Sharrett AR, et al. Retinal arteriolar narrowing and risk of coronary heart disease in men and women. The Atherosclerosis Risk in Communities Study. JAMA 2002;287(9):1153–9.
61. Duncan BB, Wong TY, Tyroler HA, et al. Hypertensive retinopathy and incident coronary heart disease in high risk men. Br J Ophthalmol 2002;86(9):1002–6.
62. Wong TY, Rosamond W, Chang PP, et al. Retinopathy and risk of congestive heart failure. JAMA 2005;293(1):63–9.
63. Liew G, Wong TY, Mitchell P, et al. Retinopathy predicts coronary heart disease mortality. Heart 2009;95(5):391–4.
64. Wong TY, Klein R, Nieto FJ, et al. Retinal microvascular abnormalities and 10-year cardiovascular mortality: a population-based case-control study. Ophthalmology 2003;110(5):933–40.
65. Gunn RM. Ophthalmoscopic evidence of (1) arterial changes associated with chronic renal diseases and (2) of increased arterial tension. Trans Ophthalmol Soc UK 1982;12:124–5.
66. Saitoh M, Matsuo K, Nomoto S, et al. Relationship between left ventricular hypertrophy and renal and retinal damage in untreated patients with essential hypertension. Intern Med 1998;37(7):576–80.
67. Wong TY, Coresh J, Klein R, et al. Retinal microvascular abnormalities and renal dysfunction: the atherosclerosis risk in communities study. J Am Soc Nephrol 2004;15(9):2469–76.
68. Kim GH, Youn HJ, Kang S, et al. Relation between grade II hypertensive retinopathy and coronary artery disease in treated essential hypertensives. Clin Exp Hypertens 2010;32(7):469–73.
69. Cuspidi C, Meani S, Valerio C, et al. Prevalence and correlates of advanced retinopathy in a large selected hypertensive population. The Evaluation of Target Organ Damage in Hypertension (ETODH) study. Blood Press 2005;14(1):25–31.
70. Tikellis G, Arnett DK, Skelton TN, et al. Retinal arteriolar narrowing and left ventricular hypertrophy in African Americans: the Atherosclerosis Risk in Communities (ARIC) study. Am J Hypertens 2008;21(3):352–9.
71. Luo BP, Brown GC. Update on the ocular manifestations of systemic arterial hypertension. Curr Opin Ophthalmol 2004;15(3):203–10.
72. Bourke K, Patel MR, Prisant LM, et al. Hypertensive choroidopathy. J Clin Hypertens (Greenwich) 2004;6(8):471–2.
73. Chatterjee S, Chattopadhyay S, Hope-Ross M, et al. Hypertension and the eye: changing perspectives. J Hum Hypertens 2002;16(10):667–75.
74. Witt N, Wong TY, Hughes AD, et al. Abnormalities of retinal microvascular structure and risk of mortality from ischemic heart disease and stroke. Hypertension 2006;47(5):975–81.
75. Cheung CY, Zheng Y, Hsu W, et al. Retinal vascular tortuosity, blood pressure, and cardiovascular risk factors. Ophthalmology 2011;118(5):812–18.
76. Liew G, Wang JJ, Cheung N, et al. The retinal vasculature as a fractal: methodology, reliability, and relationship to blood pressure. Ophthalmology 2008;115(11):1951–6.
77. Hughes AD, Martinez-Perez E, Jabbar AS, et al. Quantification of topological changes in retinal vascular architecture in essential and malignant hypertension. J Hypertens 2006;24(5):889–94.
78. Ritt M, Schmieder RE. Wall-to-lumen ratio of retinal arterioles as a tool to assess vascular changes. Hypertension 2009;54(2):384–7.
79. Ikram MK, Sim X, Jensen RA, et al. Four novel Loci (19q13, 6q24, 12q24, and 5q14) influence the microcirculation in vivo. PLoS Genet 2010;6(10):e1001184.
80. Hughes AD, Stanton AV, Jabbar AS, et al. Effect of antihypertensive treatment on retinal microvascular changes in hypertension. J Hypertens 2008;26(8):1703–7.
81. Dahlof B, Stenkula S, Hansson L. Hypertensive retinal vascular changes: relationship to left ventricular hypertrophy and arteriolar changes before and after treatment. Blood Press 1992;1(1):35–44.
82. Thom S, Stettler C, Stanton A, et al. Differential effects of antihypertensive treatment on the retinal microcirculation: an Anglo-Scandinavian cardiac outcomes trial substudy. Hypertension 2009;54(2):405–8.

Chapter 50

Telescreening for Diabetic Retinopathy

Rajiv Raman, Aditi Gupta, Tarun Sharma

INTRODUCTION

The criteria for human diseases amenable to screening approaches were defined by the World Health Organization in 1968[1] and diabetic retinopathy fulfills all of these. Visual impairment due to diabetic retinopathy is a significant health problem; however, it has a recognizable presymptomatic stage.[2] The DCCT and the UKPDS established that intensive diabetes management to obtain near-euglycemic control can prevent and delay the progression of diabetic retinopathy in patients with diabetes.[3,4] Timely laser photocoagulation therapy can also prevent loss of vision in a large proportion of patients with sight-threatening diabetic retinopathy.[5] Screening for diabetic retinopathy saves vision at a relatively low cost, which has been demonstrated in various studies.[6,7] The American Academy of Ophthalmology recommends annual dilated eye examinations beginning at the time of diagnosis for patients with type II diabetes.[2] For those with type I diabetes, the recommendation is retinal examination 3–5 years after diagnosis, with annual exams thereafter.[2] The barriers for successful screening are numerous and include the high cost of care, poor awareness levels, lack of symptoms in the early stages of disease, socioeconomic factors and poor geographical access to care.[8] Current screening programs for diabetic retinopathy are either ophthalmologist-based (with actual presence of the ophthalmologist at the site of screening) or ophthalmologist-led (no ophthalmologist at the site of screening). Table 50.1 summarizes the key differences between the two models. Telemedicine for retinopathy screening is an ophthalmologist-led screening model, which may be a logical potential alternative for patients who have been noncompliant with the traditional face-to-face examination by an ophthalmologist. Telemedicine is the exchange of medical data by electronic telecommunications technology allowing a patient's medical problems to be evaluated, monitored, and possibly treated while the patient and physician are located at sites physically remote from each other.[9] Ophthalmology is uniquely suited for telemedicine as it is a highly visual and image intensive specialty and digital imagery is easily transmitted by electronic means. Remote assessment for diabetic retinopathy provides an ideal model for telehealth screening initiatives and, in fact, has become one of the most common uses for telemedicine in ophthalmology.

Table 50.1 Differences between the ophthalmologist-led and ophthalmologist-based models for screening for diabetic retinopathy

	Ophthalmologist-led model (Telescreening)	Ophthalmologist-based model
Brief description	Paramedical staff acquire data/images, which are then transferred for interpretation by ophthalmologist	Screening is performed by ophthalmologist
Feasibility	Yes, with less human resources	Needs trained expert
Maintenance	Required	Not required
Capital expenditure	More	Less
Revenue expenditure	Less	More
Interobserver bias	Less	More
Digital photo archiving	Yes	No
Acceptance by community	Yes	Yes

GUIDELINES FOR TELESCREENING PROGRAM

American Telemedicine Association telehealth practice recommendations for diabetic retinopathy

American Telemedicine Association (ATA), Ocular Telehealth Special Interest Group, and the National Institutes of Standards and Technology Working Group, established the telescreening guidelines for diabetic retinopathy.[10] The ATA recommends that telehealth programs for diabetic retinopathy should demonstrate an ability to compare favorably with ETDRS film or digital photography. For screening programs with low thresholds for referral, the International Clinical Diabetic Retinopathy Disease Severity Scale may be used in place of ETDRS scales, however, protocols should state the reference standard used for validation and relevant datasets used for comparison.

The ATA recognizes four categories of telescreening programs, of which higher categories (3 and 4) are generally not necessary for screening programs which do not involve actual management of diabetic eye disease:

Category 1: The program allows identification of patients who have no or minimal diabetic retinopathy and distinguishes them from those who have more than minimal diabetic retinopathy.

Category 2: The program allows identification of patients who do not have sight-threatening diabetic retinopathy and distinguishes them from those who have potentially sight-threatening diabetic retinopathy.

STEPS OF TELESCREENING

The flow of steps of the telescreening process is diagrammed in Fig. 50.1. In brief, patient enrollment is performed after defining the data to be collected. Since ocular telescreening services for diabetic retinopathy satisfy the criteria of low risk telehealth procedures and are within commonly accepted standards of practice, signature consent may not be required. However, practitioners should provide patients with information about the telescreening program they would reasonably want to know, including differences between care delivered using ocular telehealth approaches versus traditional face-to-face encounters, and a description of what is to be done at the patient's site and the remote site. The data collected includes fundus images, along with patient examination findings (identification, demographic, and medical information) and some morphological information that is used to make a clinical decision. Fundus images of both eyes of the patient are acquired under a fixed, predetermined imaging protocol. These images are taken by a trained technician using a fundus camera. Due to various factors, the quality of the acquired images may be below the grading standard, thus not providing any meaningful information for examination by the reader. This can be addressed by employing an automatic image quality assessment module. An automatic image quality assessment module will ensure that the images transmitted for diagnosis conform to prescribed gradability standards. During the quality assurance process, the gradable images are selected for compression, whereas the identification of poor quality images can trigger reimaging by the technician. The patient data comprising the clinical data and the fundus images are compressed to make them suitable for low-bandwidth network connectivity. The patient data are transmitted to the servers via the Internet or satellite. At the reading center, the images are graded for presence of retinal lesions and the determination of a diabetic retinopathy level; referred to "next level" graders if necessary; and a retinopathy structured report is generated. Only qualified readers should perform retinal image grading and interpretation. If a reader is not a licensed eye care provider, specific training is required. A licensed, qualified eye care provider with expertise in diabetic retinopathy and familiarity with telescreening program technology should supervise the readers. An adjudicating reader (an ophthalmologist with special qualifications in diabetic retinopathy by training or experience) may resolve discrepant interpretations. Image processing algorithms should undergo rigorous clinical validation. A report comprising the findings, the results and the medical advice given by the expert is made available to the patient and the care team at the remote site through an accessible interface.

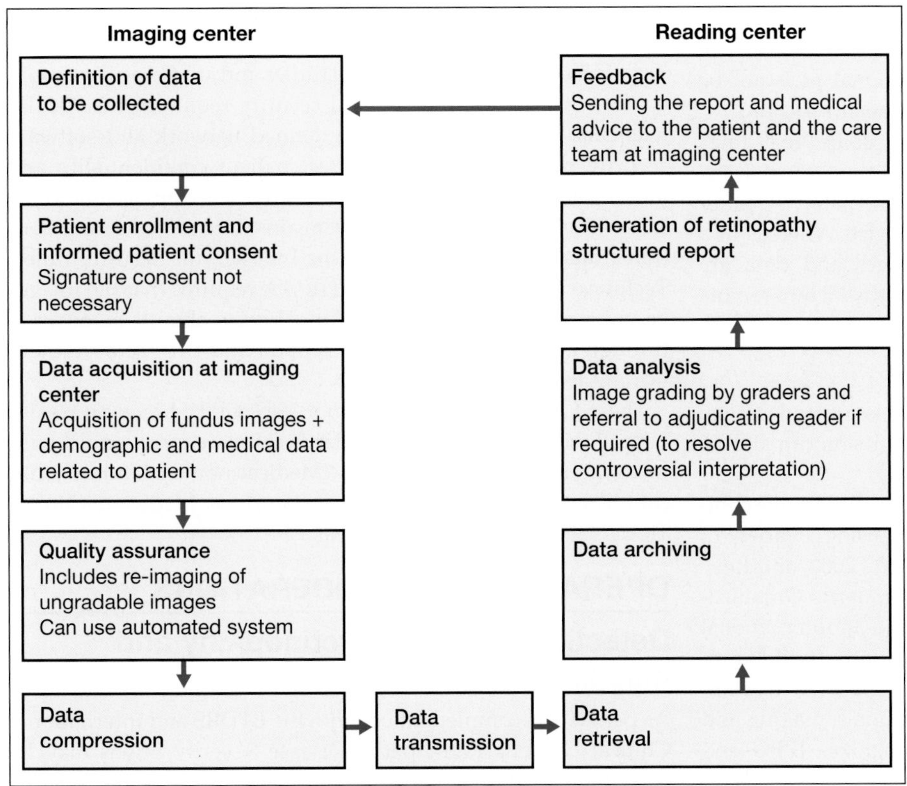

Fig. 50.1 Flowchart representing the steps of telescreening. This figure shows the sequential steps of telescreening carried out at the imaging center and the reading center.

TECHNICAL CONSIDERATIONS

Image acquisition

The gold standard for telescreening is the ETDRS 7 mydriatic standard field 35 mm stereoscopic color fundus photographs.[11] However, more practical alternatives, such as digital fundus photography[12,13] and nonmydriatic fundus photography,[14,15] have been evaluated. Digital imaging has the advantage of faster and easier acquisition, transmission, and storage. Several investigators have reported a high level of correlation between stereoscopic digital imaging and slide film for the identification of most features of diabetic retinopathy.[12,13]

Regarding nonmydriatic fundus photography, a higher rate of unreadable photographs has been reported through undilated versus dilated pupils.[14,15] Diabetic persons often have smaller pupils and a greater incidence of cataracts, which may limit image quality if the procedure is performed through an undilated pupil. Pupil dilation using 0.5% tropicamide is associated with a minimal risk of angle closure glaucoma. Programs using pupil dilation should have a defined protocol to recognize and address this potential complication.

The unsatisfactory performance of nonmydriatic photography has led to the concept of "targeted mydriasis," offering mydriasis only to a preselected group of patients, in whom undilated photography is known to produce dismal results.[15] However, the exact "target" remains to be defined. Based on ROC curve analysis, Raman et al.[16] predetermined the cutoff values for "target mydriasis" groups as vision <6/12 (20/40 Snellen equivalent) and age >59 years. Staged mydriasis is another option.[17] In this model, a nonmydriatic single digital photograph for screening is taken. If an unsatisfactory nonmydriatic photograph is obtained, the patient undergoes immediate pupillary dilation with 1% tropicamide and the photograph is then repeated. Using this protocol, 75–80% of patients do not require mydriasis.

According to ATA recommendations, image acquisition personnel ("imagers") should possess the knowledge and skills for independent imaging or with assistance and consultation by telephone, since a licensed eye care professional may not be physically available at all times during a telehealth session.

After acquisition, the transfer of the images can be "real-time" or by a "store-and-forward" technique. In real-time transfer, the captured images and associated data are immediately ("simultaneously") seen by the remote ophthalmologist. Whereas in a store-and-forward technique, captured images and data are compressed, stored, and then forwarded for retrieval by a remote ophthalmologist later.

Compression

Data and image compression facilitates transmission and storage of retinal images. The time needed for transmission can also be dramatically reduced by image compression.

Compression may be used if algorithms have undergone clinical validation. Image data can be compressed using a variety of standards, including JPEG, JPEG Lossless, JPEG 2000, and Run-length encoding (RLE). The International Standards Organization (ISO/IEC JTC1/SC2/WG10) has prepared an International Standard, ISO/IS-15444-1 (JPEG 2000 Part 1), for the digital compression and coding of continuous-tone still images. This standard is known as the JPEG 2000 Standard. Digital Imaging and Communication in Medicine (DICOM) recognizes JPEG and JPEG 2000 for lossy compression of medical images.[18] ATA recommends that the compression types and ratios should be periodically reviewed to ensure appropriate clinical image quality and diagnostic accuracy. Some studies have attempted to look at the effect of various levels of compression on the quality of the image with both subjective and objective parameters.[19,20] The level of acceptable compression ranges from 1:28 to 1:52.[19,20]

Data transfer, archiving, and retrieval

The described telemedicine models reported earlier used the Internet to transmit images.[21,22] In rural areas and mobile clinics, satellite transmission is a more preferred option because of poor infrastructure. A variety of technologies are available for data communication and transfer. Telescreening programs should determine specifications for transmission technologies best suited to their needs.

The images and reports are transmitted digitally via electronic picture archiving and communication systems (PACS); this eliminates the need for manual file transfer or retrieval. A PACS consists of four major components: the imaging instrumentation, a secured network for the transmission of patient information, workstations for interpreting and reviewing images, and archives for the storage and retrieval of images and reports. The universal format for PACS image storage and transfer is DICOM. To minimize errors, data communications should be compliant with DICOM standards.

Telescreening systems should provide storage capacities in compliance with facility, state, and federal medical record retention regulations. Digital images obtained by telescreening are typically stored locally on a PACS for rapid retrieval. Past images and reports should also be available for retrieval. It is important and is required in the United States by the Security Rule's Administrative Safeguards section of the Health Insurance Portability and Accountability Act (HIPAA) that facilities have a means of recovering images in the event of an error or disaster.

Security and documentation

Transmission of retinal imaging studies and study results should conform to HIPAA privacy and security requirements. Ocular telehealth systems should have defined network and software security protocols so as to protect patient confidentiality and identification of image data. Protective measures should be taken to safeguard data integrity against intentional or unintentional data corruption. If using the Internet, the Security Rule's Technical Safeguards section of HIPAA requires that the images be encrypted during transmission. Privacy should be ensured through a minimum 128-bit encryption and two-factor authentication technology.

The ATA recommends that reports should be based on Health Level 7 (HL7) and DICOM standards software forms and should meet interoperability standards. Medical nomenclature should conform to Systematized Nomenclature of Medicine Clinical Terms (SNOMED CT®) standards.

OPERATIONAL CONSIDERATIONS

Detection of diabetic retinopathy and macular edema

As per ATA recommendation, both the ETDRS and International Clinical Diabetic Retinopathy Disease Severity Scales may be used for classifying diabetic retinopathy and macular edema.

Nonstereo imaging methods can detect diabetic retinopathy quite well but diabetic macular thickening cannot be detected as reliably. Hence, all nonstereo imaging methods need additional information about retinal thickness for an accurate assessment of macular edema. The retinal thickness analyzer (RTA), which combines two imaging modalities – a wide-angle, red-free black-on-white fundus photograph and a detailed map of retinal thickness at the posterior pole – had mean 93% sensitivity for diagnosis of proliferative diabetic retinopathy and 100% for macular edema when compared with clinical examination.[23]

Role of the reading center to grade retinal images

Pathways of grading

At the reading center, the grader examines the retinal images for evidence of diabetic change in the eye and assesses those images for disease against the minimum dataset. There are two possible routes for a grading pathway.

Pathway 1: Disease/no disease grading

This involves three stages of grading prior to any referral to an arbitration-level grader:

Stage 1: The grader assesses patient image sets to classify into disease and no disease without grading the level of disease. Urgent referrals should be passed for immediate assessment by an ophthalmologist.

Stage 2: A random 10% of the patient's no disease image sets, together with all the disease image sets are reviewed for an initial full disease grade by a different grader accredited to carry out that level of grading. That second grader should not see the result of the first grader prior to grading.

Stage 3: This is carried out in all cases where an initial full disease grade indicates evidence of diabetic retinopathy in the eye. All referable image sets are reassessed by a different grader who carries out a second full disease grade on these images masked to the initial grading.

Pathway 2: Full disease grading

This involves two stages of grading prior to any referral to an arbitration grader:

Stage 1: A grader carries out a full disease grade on all image sets. Urgent referrals should be passed to the grading center for immediate assessment by an ophthalmologist.

Stage 2: A different masked grader will assess a random 10% of the images where no diabetic retinopathy is evident and carry out a second full grade on all the disease image sets from the stage 1 grade.

Arbitration grade

An arbitration grading procedure is carried out in both the pathways, if there is a difference of opinion between the first full disease grader and the second full disease grader on the level of disease or whether or not there should be a referral. Usually this will be done by an ophthalmologist or an experienced screener, accredited for this level of work. Most grading centers find it helpful if arbitration grading is carried out on all referable retinopathy diagnoses in advance of a referral to an ophthalmologist for treatment in order to reduce the burden of avoidable referrals to eye clinics.

To make best use of limited resources, it has been proposed that the assessment of image quality and the presence or absence of any diabetic retinopathy could be performed by relatively inexperienced "disease/no disease" graders after a short period of training. Experienced "full disease" graders would then identify patients, deemed to have retinopathy, for referral to an ophthalmologist.[24]

Reading personnel

The gold standard of image reading by ophthalmologists is impractical in rural areas. Ruamviboonsuk et al.[25] evaluated the interobserver differences among the nonphysician personnel (local ophthalmic photographers and certified ophthalmic nurses, who attended an intensive instruction course for this screening program) and ophthalmologists (retina specialists and general ophthalmologists without additional training), in the interpretation of single-field digital fundus images for diabetic retinopathy screening. Retinal specialists had the best agreement among the groups. Photographers were more reliable than the nurses. The authors concluded that the retina specialists should be effective interpreters without additional training, general ophthalmologists may need more training, but nonphysician personnel must have comprehensive training.

Handling of ungradable images

ATA guidelines recommend that the inability to obtain or read images should be considered a positive finding and patients with unobtainable or unreadable images should be promptly re-imaged or referred for evaluation by an eye care specialist. Authors from the Joslin Vision Network (JVN) reported that of those images that were judged ungradable, a large proportion had pathology that required referral for comprehensive examination.[26] In the Gloucestershire Study, 3.7% of patients had unassessable images (including those with cataract), of whom 10.3% had referable retinopathy.[14]

The United Kingdom National Screening Committee (UKNSC) recommends that arrangements should be made for patients with ungradable images to be examined either by an ophthalmologist or by a trained and accredited person supervised by an ophthalmologist (as in the Scottish scheme). It may still not be possible to assess a very small number of patients due to a range of disabilities (for example it may not be possible for a patient to hold still in one position either for assessment or for treatment). It should be noted that some patients with ungradable images may be unsuitable for treatment due to a condition that is not going to be improved with treatment in either eye. Clearly great care must be taken before such a decision is made.

While nonmydriatic photography screening is being successfully used, several factors have been reported to result in ungradable images in nonmydriatic retinal photography. Increasing age is an important factor.[27] Media opacity such as cataract and small pupil are other major factors. Scanlon et al.[27] suggested that a 20% failure rate for nonmydriatic photography might be acceptable. They also supported the use of nonmydriatic photography for the group of individuals <50 years of age who are at the lowest risk of ungradable images, if the screening programs are directed towards the detection of sight-threatening diabetic retinopathy.

QUALITY ASSURANCE

In 2000, the UKNSC stressed the integration of quality assurance as a core feature of telescreening programs for diabetic retinopathy and proposed the criteria and minimal/achievable standards for each quality assurance objective.[28] Since then, other ongoing quality assurance programs have published their methods and outcomes.[29,30] Different screening programs have different criteria for image regrading, resulting in different numbers of retinal photographs that need to be regraded for quality assurance (6% to 46%).[31]

There are two categories of quality assurance:[32]

(a) Internal quality assurance that is integrated as part of the day-to-day workflow in a screening program measured against national standards.
(b) External quality assurance which has three main functions: the monitoring of ongoing program performance against the quality standards, the organization of peer-review visits, and the administration of an external proficiency testing system for all graders.

There is international consensus that screening programs for diabetic retinopathy should achieve at least 80% sensitivity, 95% specificity, and <5% technical failure rates.[33] The quality assurance group of the National Screening Committee has recommended that quality assurance should involve the second examination of all images initially reported to have any diabetic retinopathy, together with 10% of the negative images, independently as part of the internal quality assurance system.[34]

The ATA and UKNSC have established the national standards for quality assurance for a diabetic retinopathy screening program. ATA has specified major categories of performance to be evaluated, as applicable to the program, at the level of the originating site and at the reading center. The UKNSC has provided 19 standards or parameters for quality assurance. Several authors have suggested further measures. Leese et al.[31] recommended the use of automated grading systems running in parallel with manual grading; and concentrating quality assurance in the smaller number of patients with high-risk nonproliferative disease.

EVALUATING TELESCREENING PROGRAMS

Efficacy

Telescreening has been shown to detect diabetic retinopathy and macular edema with a reasonably high sensitivity and specificity.[9,35] Whited et al.[35] reviewed the available literature and noted that the sensitivity and specificity values ranged from 50% to 93% for detection of diabetic retinopathy. Similar high efficacy was reported on comparing teleophthalmology for macular edema detection to both gold standards, i.e. slit-lamp biomicroscopy and stereoscopic photography.[35]

Patient satisfaction

Since telescreening involves remote care without evaluation by the doctor in person, there are concerns regarding lack of satisfaction among patients. Studies have shown, however, that telescreening has equal, if not better, satisfaction than in-person evaluation by a doctor.[36,37] Paul et al. assessed patient satisfaction levels and factors influencing satisfaction during teleophthalmology consultation in India using a patient satisfaction questionnaire. He found that 37.34% of the patients felt that telescreening is more satisfying than an in-person evaluation, and 60% felt that both models are equally satisfying. It was also noted that patients who asked questions during the screening were 2.18 times more likely to be satisfied with teleophthalmology than those who did not.

Cost-effectiveness

Bjorvig et al.,[38] in an economic analysis, concluded that telemedicine was a less costly option for screening in places with higher patient workloads. Telemedicine was also proven to be cost-effective in the prison populations by Aoki et al.,[39] where it may have special utility due to costs and safety issues associated with transporting prisoners.

Gomez-Ulla et al.[6] did a comparative cost analysis of diabetic retinopathy telescreening versus standard ophthalmoscopy, from both Public Healthcare System (PHS) and patient perspectives. The authors concluded that from the PHS perspective, direct fundus examination is less costly than telescreening owing to the higher capital costs required for the purchase of digital imaging equipment. From a global perspective, however, the digital imaging alternative is more convenient because the travel cost and loss of income for the patient are lower.

Recently, Jones et al.[7] reviewed the evidence available on cost-effectiveness. They concluded that telemedicine is cost-effective for retinopathy screening in remote and rural communities and other groups with travel difficulties and the cost-effectiveness increases with an increase in patient workload.

ADVANCES IN TELESCREENING

Recent advances resulting in better and faster telecommunication, miniaturization of diagnostic equipment including digital cameras, and automation of retinal image analysis, offer excellent opportunities to expand telescreening services in more remote areas.

Automated retinal image analysis

The shortage of manpower imposes a limitation on the screening capability of telehealth programs serving a steadily growing diabetic population. Therefore, an automated image analysis system able to detect diabetic retinopathy is a vital necessity, especially in the coming years.

Over the past decade several attempts have been made to either semi-automate or fully-automate retinal image analysis. Tools have been developed for analyzing and enhancing the image quality (correction of illumination, increasing image contrast, histogram equalization, vessel segmentation, edge sharpening, and image deconvolution), and for providing automated identification of pathologic retinal lesions (neural networks, region growing, morphological analysis, and classification algorithms).[40] Automated identification of retinal lesions can identify the absence or presence of diabetic retinopathy based on the detection of microaneurysms and dot hemorrhages (dark lesions),[41] or can detect referable retinopathy based on the detection of exudates (bright lesions) and blot hemorrhages (dark lesions).[42]

Winder et al.[40] conducted a structured survey of algorithms for the automatic detection of retinopathy in digital color retinal images. The authors pointed out the need for clear guidelines and goals in image processing research in order to avoid producing results that are difficult to compare in terms of the success of the algorithms or techniques.

CONCLUSION

Telescreening has the enormous potential to offer remote care to patients with diabetes without compromising the quality of care. However, to maximize the chance for success, it is essential that all telescreening programs should define clear goals, establish appropriate quality control measures, and adhere to regulatory and statutory requirements. Prospective studies demonstrating a reduction in vision loss from diabetic retinopathy as a result of telescreening programs will be of critical importance, before telescreening strategies can be adopted as the standard for routine clinical management of patients with diabetes.

REFERENCES

1. Wilson JMG, Jungner G. Principles and practice of screening for disease. WHO Chronicle 1968;22:473.
2. American Diabetes Association. Standards of medical care in diabetes - 2008. Diabetes Care 2008;31(Suppl 1):S12–54.
3. The DCCT Research Group. The effect of intensive diabetes treatment on the progression of diabetic retinopathy in insulin-dependent diabetes mellitus. Arch Ophthalmol 1995;113:36–51.
4. UK Prospective Diabetes Study (UKPDS) Group. Intensive blood-glucose control with sulphonylureas or insulin compared with conventional treatment and risk of complications in patients with type 2 diabetes (UKPDS 33). Lancet 1998;352:837–53.
5. Early Treatment Diabetic Retinopathy Study Research Group. Early photocoagulation treatment for diabetic retinopathy, ETDRS report number 9. Ophthalmology 1991;98: 766–85.
6. Gomez-Ulla F, Alonso F, Aibar B, et al. A comparative cost analysis of digital fundus imaging and direct fundus examination for assessment of diabetic retinopathy. Telemed J E Health 2008;14:912–8.
7. Jones S, Edwards RT. Diabetic retinopathy screening: a systematic review of the economic evidence. Diabet Med 2010;27:249–56.
8. Hazin R, Barazi MK, Summerfield M. Challenges to establishing nationwide diabetic retinopathy screening programs. Curr Opin Ophthalmol 2011;22: 174–9.
9. Zimmer-Galler IE, Zeimer R. Telemedicine in diabetic retinopathy screening. Ophthalmol Clin 2009(Spring); 49:75–86.
10. Cavallerano J, Lawrence MG, Zimmer-Galler I, et al. American Telemedicine Association, Ocular Telehealth Special Interest Group; National Institute of Standards and Technology Working Group. Telehealth practice recommendations for diabetic retinopathy. Telemed J E Health 2004;10:469–82.
11. Early Treatment Diabetic Retinopathy Study Research Group. Grading diabetic retinopathy from stereoscopic color fundus photographs: an extension of the modified Airlie House classification. ETDRS report number 10. Ophthalmology 1991;98:786–806.
12. Tennant MT, Greve MD, Rudnisky CJ, et al. Identification of diabetic retinopathy by stereoscopic digital imaging via teleophthalmology: a comparison to slide film. Can J Ophthalmology 2001;36:187–96.
13. Liesenfeld B, Kohner E, Piehlmeier W, et al. A telemedical approach to the screening of diabetic retinopathy: digital fundus photography. Diabetes Care 2000;23:345–8.
14. Scanlon PH, Malhotra R, Thomas G, et al. The effectiveness of screening for diabetic retinopathy by digital imaging photography and technician ophthalmoscopy. Diabet Med 2003;20:467–74.
15. Murgatroyd H, Ellingford A, Cox A, et al. Effect of mydriasis and different field strategies on digital image screening of diabetic eye disease. Br J Ophthalmol 2004;88:920–4.
16. Raman R, Rani PK, Mahajan S, et al. The tele-screening model for diabetic retinopathy: evaluating the influence of mydriasis on the gradability of a single-field 45 degrees digital fundus image. Telemed J E Health 2007;13: 597–602.
17. Murgatroyd H, Cox A, Ellingford A, et al. Can we predict which patients are at risk of having an ungradeable digital image for screening for diabetic retinopathy? Eye (Lond) 2008;22:344–8.
18. Digital Imaging and Communications in Medicine (DICOM) Supplement 61:JPEG 2000 Transfer Syntaxes. Available at: ftp://medical.nema.org/medical/dicom/final/sup61_ft.pdf.
19. Eikelboom RH, Yogesan K, Barry CJ, et al. Methods and limits of digital image compression of retinal images for telemedicine. Invest Ophthalmol Vis Sci 2000;41:1916–24.
20. Newsom RSB, Clover A, Costen MTJ, et al. Effect of digital image compression on screening for diabetic retinopathy. Br J Ophthalmol 2001;85:799–802.
21. Luzio S, Hatcher S, Zahlmann G, et al. Feasibility of using the TOSCA telescreening procedures for diabetic retinopathy. Diabet Med 2004;21:1121–8.
22. Aiello LM, Bursell SE, Cavallerano J, et al. Joslin Vision Network Validation Study: pilot image stabilization phase. J Am Optom Assoc 1998;69:699–710.
23. Neubauer AS, Welge-Lüssen UC, Thiel MJ, et al. Tele-screening for diabetic retinopathy with the retinal thickness analyzer. Diabetes Care 2003;26:2890–7.
24. Harding S, Greenwood R, Aldington S, et al. Grading and disease management in national screening for diabetic retinopathy in England and Wales. Diabet Med 2003;20:965–71.
25. Ruamviboonsuk P, Teerasuwanajak K, Tiensuwan M, et al. Thai Screening for Diabetic Retinopathy Study Group. Interobserver agreement in the interpretation of single-field digital fundus images for diabetic retinopathy screening. Ophthalmology 2006;113:826–32.
26. Cavallerano AA, Cavallerano JD, Katalinic P, et al. Use of Joslin Vision Network digital-video nonmydriatic retinal imaging to assess diabetic retinopathy in a clinical program. Retina 2003;23:215–23.
27. Scanlon PH, Foy C, Malhotra R, et al. The influence of age, duration of diabetes, cataract, and pupil size on image quality in digital photographic retinal screening. Diabetes Care 2005;28:2448–53.
28. Garvican L, Clowes J, Gillow T. Preservation of sight in diabetes: developing a national risk reduction programme. Diabet Med 2000;17:627–34.
29. Arun CS, Young D, Batey D, et al. Establishing ongoing quality assurance in a retinal screening programme. Diabet Med 2006;23:629–34.
30. Schneider S, Aldington SJ, Kohner EM, et al. Quality assurance for diabetic retinopathy telescreening. Diabet Med 2005;22:794–802.
31. Leese GP, Ellis JD. Quality assurance for diabetic retinal screening. Diabet Med 2007;24:579–81.
32. UK National Screening Committee [Internet]. Gloucester, UK: NHS Diabetic Eye Screening Programme; January 2012 [cited 2012 4 Feb]. Workbook 4.4. Essential elements in developing a diabetic retinopathy screening programme. Available at http://diabeticeye.screening.nhs.uk/workbook.
33. Taylor R, Broadbent DM, Greenwood R et al. Mobile retinal screening in Britain. Diabet Med 1998;15:344–7.
34. Garvican L, Scanlon PH. A pilot quality assurance scheme for diabetic retinopathy risk reduction programmes. Diabet Med 2004;21:1066–74.
35. Whited JD. Accuracy and reliability of teleophthalmology for diagnosing diabetic retinopathy and macular edema: a review of the literature. Diabetes Technol Ther 2006;8:102–11.
36. Luzio S, Hatcher S, Zahlmann G, et al. Feasibility of using the TOSCA telescreening procedures for diabetic retinopathy. Diabetic Med 2004;21:1121–8.
37. Paul PG, Raman R, Rani PK, et al. Patient satisfaction levels during teleophthalmology consultation in rural South India. Telemed J E Health 2006;12: 571–8.
38. Bjorvig S, Johansen MA, Fossen K. An economic analysis of screening for diabetic retinopathy. J Telemed Telecare 2002;8:32–5.
39. Aoki N, Dunn K, Fukui T, et al. Costeffectiveness analysis of telemedicine to evaluate diabetic retinopathy in a prison population. Diabetes Care 2004;27: 1095–101.
40. Winder RJ, Morrow PJ, McRitchie IN, et al. Algorithms for digital image processing in diabetic retinopathy. Comput Med Imaging Graph 2009;33:608–22.
41. Philip S, Fleming AD, Goatman KA, et al. The efficacy of automated "disease/no disease" grading for diabetic retinopathy in a systematic screening programme. Br J Ophthalmol 2007;91:1512–7.
42. Fleming AD, Goatman KA, Philip S, et al. The role of haemorrhage and exudate detection in automated grading of diabetic retinopathy. Br J Ophthalmol 2010;94:706–11.

Chapter 51

Retinal Artery Obstructions

Purnima S. Patel, SriniVas R. Sadda

CRAO was first described in 1859 in von Graefe's report of multiple systemic emboli in the setting of endocarditis causing obstruction of the central retinal artery.[1] Since then significant literature has been published on retinal arterial occlusions and their classification, epidemiology, presentation, prognosis, and treatment. Here we use an arbitrary classification, as indicated below, to discuss these disorders in sequence:

- Central retinal artery obstruction (CRAO)
- Branch retinal artery obstruction (BRAO)
- Cilioretinal artery obstruction (CLRAO)
- Combined retinal artery and vein obstruction
- Cotton-wool spots.

CENTRAL RETINAL ARTERY OBSTRUCTION

Epidemiology

The true incidence of CRAOs is unknown. The estimated incidence of CRAO is reported to be roughly 1 in 10000 cases at tertiary referral centers.[2,3] The incidence may be even lower for the general population, at approximately 8.5 cases per 100000.[3] Similar to other vascular disorders, this condition is largely seen in older adults but cases in children and young adults have also been reported.[4,5] The average age at presentation is in the early sixties, with greater than 90% of patients presenting at over 40 years of age. Men are affected more frequently than women. No predilection for one eye over the other has been reported; however, 1–2% of cases may manifest bilateral involvement.[6]

Clinical features

Typically, patients with acute CRAO present with monocular, painless, severe loss of vision which occurs acutely, possibly over the span of a few seconds. In some cases, premonitory episodes of amaurosis fugax may be reported. Amaurosis fugax represents transient acute retinal ischemia and typically suggests an embolic source of occlusion; however, it has also been reported in association with giant cell arteritis.[7] Presence of amaurosis fugax also has a higher correlation with stroke compared with retinal emboli alone.[8] The risk of CRAO after amaurosis fugax is estimated to be only 1% per year.[9] Although CRAO rarely presents simultaneously in both eyes, it may occur sequentially.[10]

Visual acuity at the time of initial presentation ranges from counting fingers to light perception in 74–90% of eyes.[6,11] Central visual acuity may be near normal in patients who have a transient CRAO or a cilioretinal artery providing sufficient vascular supply to the fovea. Connolly et al. reported a trend toward better visual acuities in patients with monocular CRAO secondary to giant cell arteritis as compared with those with CRAO due to other, largely embolic causes.[12] The presence of an embolus is usually associated with poorer vision. The absence of light perception is rare; therefore, in such cases, concomitant choroidal circulation deficit (e.g., due to ophthalmic artery occlusion) or optic nerve involvement should be considered.[6] Visual acuity tends only to improve within the first week of onset with minimal chance for appreciable improvement subsequently.[11] Visual recovery after treatment has been shown to correlate with presenting visual acuity and the duration of visual impairment.[13] Although visual acuity may spontaneously improve in up to 22% of patients with nonarteritic CRAO,[11] less than 10% of patients report a meaningful recovery of vision.[14]

Typically an afferent pupillary defect develops within seconds following obstruction of the central retinal artery regardless of macular sparing.[4] Intraocular pressure is often normal at presentation but may become elevated in the setting of rubeosis iridis.

In a majority of cases of acute CRAO, the anterior-segment exam is normal initially. If rubeosis iridis is present acutely, ocular ischemia secondary to the presence of a concomitant carotid artery obstruction should be considered. The incidence of rubeosis in CRAO is 16.6–18.8%.[15–17] As compared to central retinal vein occlusions (CRVO), iris rubeosis tends to occur earlier after CRAO – at a mean of 4–5 weeks after onset compared to 5 months after onset in CRVO. Not surprisingly, rubeosis is more common in more severe and complete obstructions with extensive nonperfusion. The risk of developing iris neovascularization is greater for obstruction lasting greater than 1 week versus those lasting only a few days after onset.[15–17] In the case of carotid obstruction, rubeosis iridis can cause elevated intraocular pressure to the point of exceeding the perfusion pressure in the central retinal artery and lead to an obstruction via this mechanism. Laser panretinal photocoagulation causes successful regression in approximately 65% of cases.[18]

In his 1891 report, Nettleship described in detail the ophthalmoscopic appearance of CRAO. "The classic dense, white haze of the central region in the retina with a well-marked clear patch at the yellow-spot was very well shown (Fig. 51.1); there were no hemorrhages; the arteries and veins were of about normal size, but no pulsation could be produced in any of them by pressure with the finger upon the globe."[19] Hayreh and Zimmerman investigated fundus changes in CRAOs in a large retrospective review in 2007 of 248 eyes of 240 patients. In the acute phase, his group noted a cherry-red spot (90%), posterior pole retinal opacity or whitening (58%), box-carring of retinal arteries and

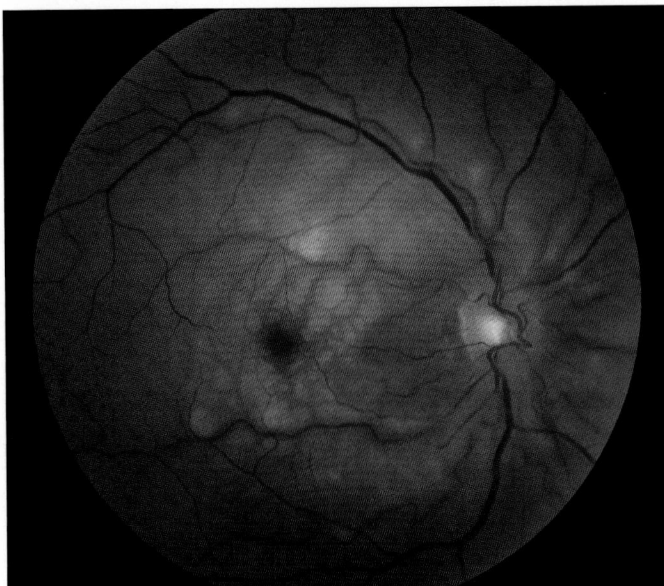

Fig. 51.1 Acute central retinal artery obstruction. Superficial retinal whitening or opacification is noted in the posterior pole with evidence of a central cherry-red spot. The opacification is most prominent in the peripheral fovea. (Courtesy of Dr Steven Yeh, Emory Eye Center, Atlanta.)

veins (19% and 20% respectively), retinal arterial attenuation (32%), optic disc edema (22%), and optic nerve pallor (39%). The retinal findings were predominantly located in the posterior pole with a normal-appearing periphery.[20]

Typically, retinal whitening in the posterior pole and a cherry-red spot are the earliest characteristic changes in CRAO. Both of these findings are clinical signs for which ophthalmologists have a high degree of clinical agreement.[21] The retinal whitening corresponds to ischemic damage to the inner half of the retina and is due to opacification of the retinal nerve fiber and ganglion cell layer as a result of cessation of axoplasmic transport caused by the acute ischemic insult. The opacification is visible ophthalmoscopically where the ganglion cell layer is more than one cell thick, i.e., the macula, except in the foveal region, where a cherry-red spot is seen. The outer nuclear and plexiform layers and photoreceptors remain intact, as demonstrated in histologic studies.[22,23] The size of the cherry-red spot is variable and is dependent on the width of the foveola. The cherry-red spot is actually normal-appearing retina and is observed in high contrast against the surrounding opacified retina because the thin retina in this location is nourished by the underlying choroidal circulation and as a result does not become hypoxic or opacified, permitting continued visualization of the underlying retinal pigment epithelium (RPE) and choroid.[24] Similarly, the retinal periphery in CRAO cases appears normal because the retina is also thinner with a single layer of ganglion cells, such that the nutrition of the inner retinal layers can be maintained by the choroidal circulation alone. In experimental primate models of transiently induced CRAOs, retinal opacification was observed as early as 7 minutes after complete occlusion. The probability of a cherry-red spot still being present decreases with increasing duration from the onset of CRAO: 88% after 1 week, 59% after 2 weeks, 47% after 3 weeks, and 19% after 4 weeks after onset. Typically, the retinal opacification resolves over a period of 4–6 weeks, although at least some retinal whitening is noted in 17% of patients with complete, nontransient CRAO after 1 month.[20] Pathologically, this evolution corresponds to a resolution of initial acute ischemia-induced intracellular edema with subsequent loss of neuronal cells and the development of an acellular scar of the inner retinal cell layers.[25]

A patent cilioretinal artery supplying some or all of the papillomacular bundle is seen in approximately one-third of cases. In cases of cilioretinal sparing, retinal whitening will be clearly demarcated around the area of preserved macula perfused by the cilioretinal circulation (Fig. 51.2A). In these cases, the visual acuity will be dictated by the location and extent of the area of the papillomacular bundle perfused by the patent cilioretinal artery.[11,26–28] Sparing of the fovea may be associated with excellent visual acuity, albeit with a significant visual field deficit corresponding to the topography of the occlusion.

The appearance of the retinal vasculature can be quite variable soon after the onset of CRAO, and the presence of a normal-appearing vasculature should not exclude the diagnosis. In Nettleship's 19th-century description of CRAO, he noted the appearance of the retinal vasculature to have a stagnated arterial blood column without attenuation.[19] In the natural history study by Hayreh and Zimmerman,[20] only 15% of acute CRAO had normal-appearing retinal arteries. Box-carring or segmentation of the blood column of both the arteries and veins can occur secondary to separation of blood serum from erythrocytes in a stacked or rouleaux formation.

Retinal emboli are visible in 20–40% of eyes with CRAO.[4,21] Retinal emboli are the most common cause of nonarteritic CRAO and BRAO.[29] The most common variant is a yellow, refractile cholesterol embolus (Hollenhorst plaque) (Fig. 51.3). According to a study by Arruga and Sanders, retinal emboli consist of cholesterol in 74% of cases, calcified material in 15.5%, and platelet and fibrin in 15.5%.[30] These cholesterol emboli typically originate from the carotid arteries in the setting of atherosclerotic disease, but can also arise from the aortic arch, ophthalmic artery, or proximal central retinal artery. Cholesterol emboli are often small, do not completely obstruct retinal arterial blood flow, and are frequently found at bifurcation sites (Fig. 51.3). Emboli can often be asymptomatic and migration with disappearance of retinal emboli is common.[20] Calcific emboli are less common than cholesterol emboli but are typically larger and cause more severe or complete obstruction. They most commonly originate from the cardiac valves.[24,31]

The optic nerve is acutely edematous in nearly all cases of arteritic CRAO as a result of the associated anterior ischemic optic neuropathy that is typically observed in these patients. In the acute phase of nonarteritic CRAO, the disc may be normal, hyperemic, edematous, and, rarely, pale. Acute-phase optic nerve pallor is due to ischemic opacification of the surface nerve fiber layer since this layer of the optic nerve is supplied by retinal circulation.[32] Neovascularization of the disc in acute CRAO is rare but has been reported, typically in association with a chronically hypoxic retina (e.g., concomitant diabetic retinopathy, ischemic CRVO, or ocular ischemia).[19,20]

The most frequent findings in the chronic stage of eyes with CRAO are optic atrophy (91%), retinal arterial attenuation (58%), cilioretinal collaterals (18%), macular RPE changes (11%), and cotton-wool spots (3%) (Fig. 51.4). In experimental studies in rhesus monkeys, the extent of optic nerve and nerve fiber layer damage has been correlated with the duration of CRAO.[33] Chronic-phase optic nerve pallor is due to optic atrophy and

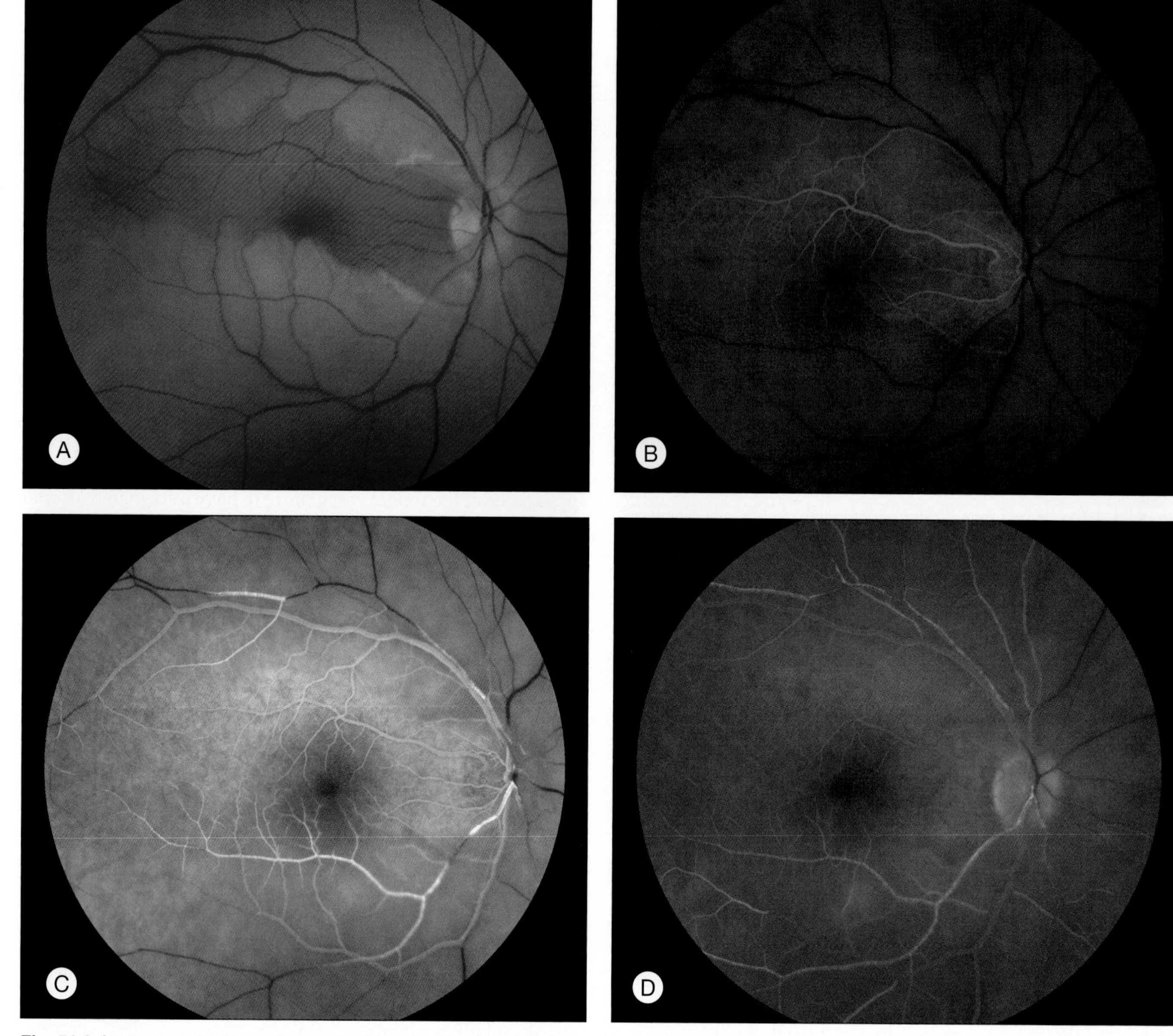

Fig. 51.2 Acute central retinal artery occlusion with cilioretinal artery sparing. (A) Retinal opacification is clearly demarcated around the preserved macula perfused by the patent cilioretinal artery. The perfused area includes the fovea; therefore the patient's presenting visual acuity was good. (B) At 19 seconds, the cilioretinal artery is perfused with retrograde flow into the retinal veins. (C) At 47 seconds, incomplete appearance of fluorescein dye is noted in the retinal arteries. (D) At 9 minutes the arterial circulation is still not completely filled, demonstrating a severely delayed arteriovenous transit time. (Courtesy of Dr John Payne, Emory Eye Center, Atlanta.)

nerve fiber loss (Fig. 51.5). In arteritic CRAO, the associated anterior ischemic optic neuropathy also contributes to the development of pallor.[20] In chronic CRAO, neovascularization of the optic disc rarely occurs, presumably because nonviable tissue is less likely to elaborate angiogenic factors compared with chronically ischemic but viable retinal tissue seen in cases of diabetic retinopathy or retinal vein occlusion.[34] Incidence of neovascularization of the disc in one retrospective study was only 1.8%.[35] Concomitant rubeosis iridis may also occur in the setting of chronic CRAO. Retinal arterial attenuation is more common in the chronic phase of disease than in the acute phase.[20] Months after an acute CRAO, cilioretinal collaterals may develop as a result of a compensatory enlargement of capillary anastomoses between retinal capillaries on the surface of the disc and ciliary capillaries in deeper parts of the optic nerve head. The probability of developing cilioretinal disc collaterals was 4% at 1 month and 18% at 3 months from onset of CRAO in one study.[20] Macular RPE changes are seen with CRAO but are much less common than in ophthalmic artery obstruction, where the choroidal circulation is also involved.

Ancillary studies

Fluorescein angiography in CRAO almost always initially shows some variable residual retinal circulation with delayed and sluggish filling of the retinal vasculature. Complete absence of retinal filling is rare. Appearance of dye in the central retinal artery is typically delayed by 5–20 seconds. However, the delay in retinal arterial branches is even more substantial. The fluorescein dye lines the arterial walls in a pattern similar to the laminar flow filling of normal retinal veins. In cases with visible intra-arterial emboli, the arteriovenous transit time can be even further delayed (Fig. 51.2B–D).[36] The severity of obstruction and retinal ischemia correlates with less favorable initial visual acuities. Staining of the optic disc can be variable; however, staining of the retinal vessels is rare. Areas of delayed choroidal perfusion, characterized by a delay in filling of more than 10 seconds compared to adjacent normal choroid, may be seen in about 11% of eyes with acute CRAO.[6] Leakage of fluorescein dye at the level of the RPE is generally not seen with CRAO unless the choroidal circulation is involved.[37] Typically, the retinal circulation is re-established after an acute CRAO but the inner retinal tissue has generally already infarcted by then. Therefore, although the fluorescein angiogram may return to relatively normal appearance, the vision loss, optic nerve atrophy, and arterial narrowing persist.[24] For patients with a normalized fluorescein angiogram who do not go on to develop optic atrophy, the diagnosis of a true CRAO should be called into question, though it is possible that some individuals may have reperfusion before the irreversible damage has occurred.

In the acute stage, optical coherence tomography (OCT) shows an irregular macular contour with increased reflectivity of the inner retina. This corresponds to intracellular edema and explains the lack of intraretinal, hyporeflective fluid spaces in cases of CRAO or BRAO. The reflectivity of the outer retinal layers and RPE is blocked by the highly reflective inner retinal layer. No retinal thickening secondary to the accumulation of serous fluid escaping from retinal capillaries into the extracellular space is seen (Fig. 51.6). OCT images of chronic CRAO

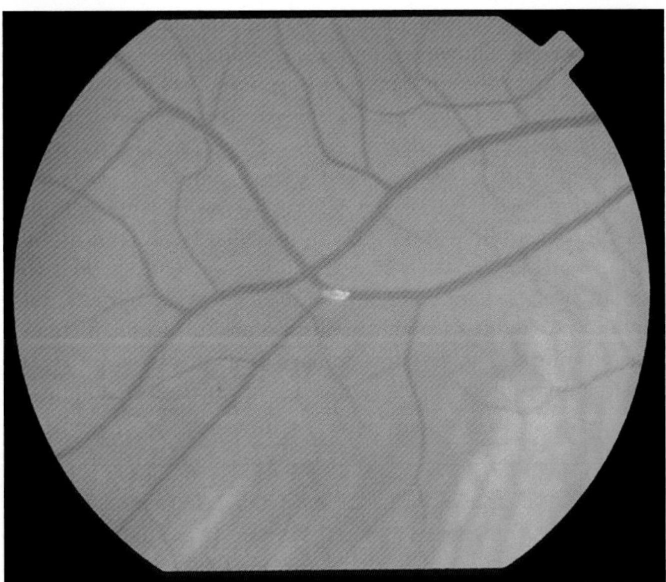

Fig. 51.3 Cholesterol embolus at an arterial bifurcation along the superotemporal arcade.

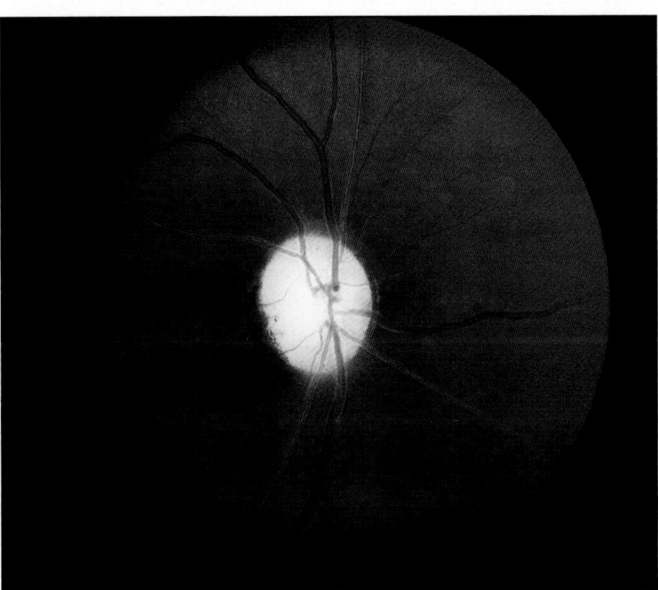

Fig. 51.4 Chronic central retinal artery occlusion. Optic nerve pallor from atrophy and severe arterial attenuation is seen in this patient with a remote central artery occlusion.

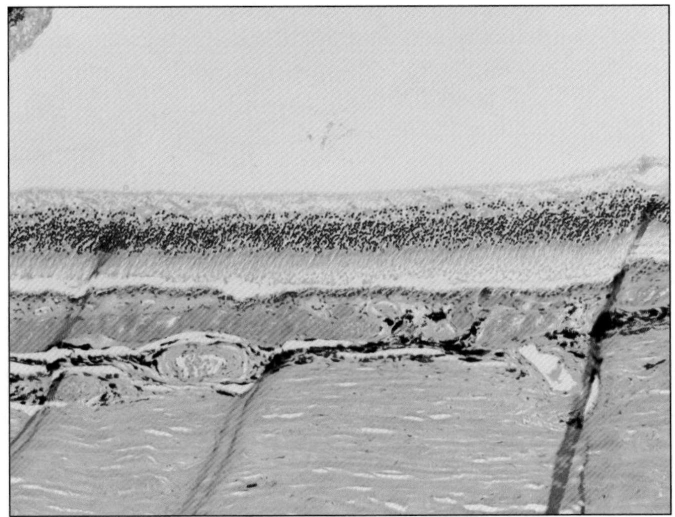

Fig. 51.5 Histopathologic findings in central retinal artery obstruction. In the chronic stage of the disease, the inner retinal layers show significant atrophy. Hematoxylin and eosin ×25. (Courtesy of Dr Hans Grossniklaus, Emory Eye Center, Atlanta.)

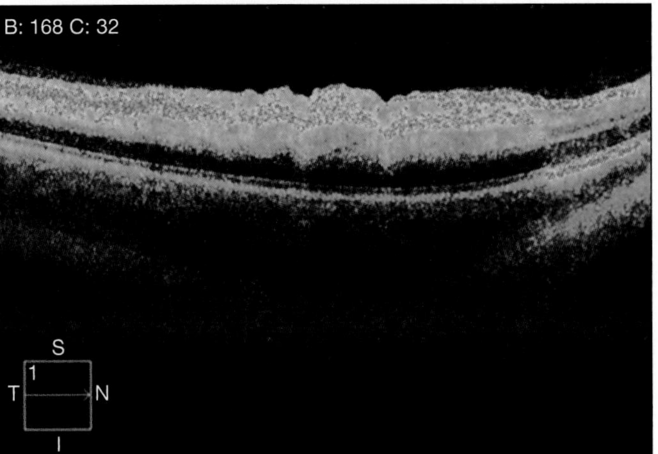

Fig. 51.6 Spectral-domain optical coherence tomography (SD-OCT) of acute central retinal artery occlusion (CRAO). An irregular foveal contour is seen with a highly reflective, thickened inner retina. The outer retina is relatively hyporeflective because of blocking from the thickened inner retina. The inner-segment–outer-segment junction and the external limiting membrane are intact, as would be expected with acute CRAO.

show thinning and atrophy of the inner retina. OCT can be helpful in cases of chronic CRAO where the fundus may appear featureless but the OCT shows inner retinal atrophy with preservation of the outer retina.[38–40]

Central scotoma is the most common defect observed on macular visual field testing followed by paracentral scotoma. Patients with cilioretinal sparing show a preserved central island of vision corresponding to the area perfused by the patent cilioretinal artery. Peripheral constriction is the most common visual field deficit noted in these patients.[11] A preserved temporal island may be seen in some patients, presumably secondary to choroid-derived perfusion of the nasal retina.[26] Visual field defects improve in approximately 28% of patients, remain stable in 57%, and worsen in 7%.[11]

In a CRAO, electroretinography typically demonstrates more severe attenuation of the b-wave than the a-wave since the inner retinal layers are more affected – this produces a characteristic negative waveform with the scotopic white stimulus (Fig. 51.7). Diminution of the a-wave and b-wave may suggest outer retinal damage secondary to choroidal vascular hypoperfusion in the setting of an ophthalmic artery occlusion in addition to a CRAO.[41]

Autofluorescence imaging in the area supplied by the occluded retinal artery acutely shows decreased autofluorescence due to blockage of the normal autofluorescence of the RPE by the thickened inner retina. This blockage resolves over time and may evolve into a window defect with increased autofluorescence in the chronic phase as areas of significant inner retinal thinning develop.[39]

Systemic associations

The distribution of systemic associations for CRAO varies depending on age. Overall, embolism from carotid artery atherosclerosis is the most common etiology for retinal arterial occlusion; however, carotid disease is relatively rare in patients under the age of 40 in whom cardiac embolism is the most common etiology.[4,5,42] The systemic and ocular abnormalities that have been associated with retinal arterial occlusions are summarized in Box 51.1.

The Beaver Dam Eye Study, a large population-based study in Wisconsin, found a 10-year cumulative incidence of retinal emboli of 1.5%. The incidence of retinal emboli varied with age; persons who were 65 years of age or older at baseline were 2.4 times as likely to develop a retinal embolus compared with persons 43–54 years of age at baseline. Retinal emboli were more likely to occur in men than in women. Incidence of bilateral emboli was rare; however, multiple emboli in the same eye may be seen in up to one-third of cases (Fig. 51.8). Persons with retinal emboli in Beaver Dam were 2.4 times as likely to have a diagnosis of stroke on their death certificate over an 11-year period compared with those without retinal emboli.[43] The large population-based studies, the Atherosclerosis Risk in Communities (North Carolina) and the Cardiovascular Health Study (Australia), both looked at a biracial population and showed that retinal arteriolar emboli were associated with hypertension, higher systolic blood pressure, carotid artery plaque, increased plasma fibrinogen levels, coronary heart disease, increased plasma lipoprotein levels, and current cigarette smoking. In

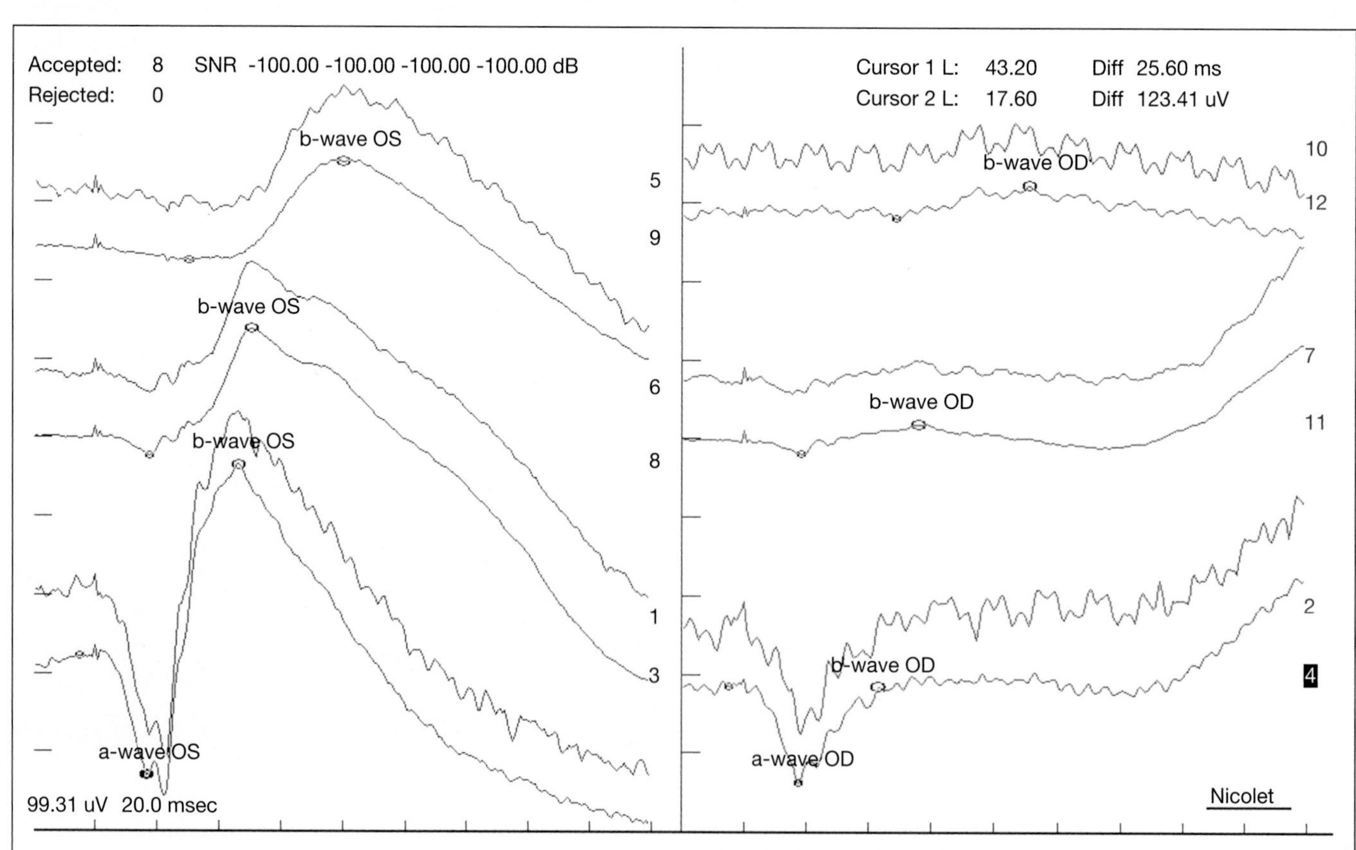

Fig. 51.7 Electroretinogram. The responses from a normal eye are seen on the left. The tracings on the right are from an eye with a central retinal artery occlusion (CRAO). The bottom right tracing shows the maximum response to the scotopic white stimulus. The a-wave is of normal amplitude; however, the b-wave does not reach the baseline, yielding a negative waveform, as is typically seen with a CRAO.

Box 51.1 Systemic and ocular abnormalities associated with retinal arterial occlusion

Embolic sources
- Systemic arterial hypertension (via atherosclerotic plaque formation)[6,24]
- Carotid atherosclerosis[8,99,100]
- Cardiac valvular disease (rheumatic,[49] mitral valve prolapse,[49,50] aortic stenosis,[49] mitral annular calcification[56])
- Left ventricular hypertrophy[56] and segmental wall motion abnormalities[56]
- Thrombus after myocardial infarction
- Cardiac myxoma[45–47]
- Tumors[51,101]
- Carotid artery dissection[102]
- Intravenous drug use[4,103,104]
- Lipid emboli (pancreatitis)[104]
- Purtscher's retinopathy (trauma)[105]
- Loiasis[106,107]
- Radiologic studies (carotid angiography,[102] cerebral angiography,[74] cardiac catheterization,[60] lymphography,[61] hysterosalpingography[64])
- Carotid endarterectomy[108]
- Deep-vein thrombosis (via paradoxical embolus through a cardiac wall defect)[67]
- Nasal oxymethazoline use[68]

Trauma
- Retrobulbar injection[70]
- Orbital floor fracture repair[71]
- Anesthesia[72]
- Penetrating injury[75]
- Nasal surgery[109]

Coagulopathies
- Sickle-cell disease[110]
- Homocystinuria[111]
- Lupus anticoagulant[112]
- Protein C and/or S deficiency[113]
- Antithrombin III deficiency[113]
- Activated protein C resistance[114]
- Factor V Leiden[115]
- Platelet abnormalities[4]
- Oral contraceptives[116]
- Pregnancy[4]
- Leukemia/lymphoma[89,90]

Ocular conditions
- Prepapillary arterial loops[117]
- Optic disc drusen[118]
- Increased intraocular pressure (from intravitreal injection,[91] gas expansion after vitrectomy,[119] prone intraoperative positioning,[120] retrobulbar hemorrhage,[121] orbital emphysema[122])
- Optic neuritis[123]

Collagen vascular disease
- Giant cell arteritis[124]
- Systemic lupus erythematosus[125]
- Polyarteritis nodosa[124]
- Wegener's granulomatosis[126]
- Fibromuscular dysplasia[68]

Other vasculitides and inflammatory conditions
- Orbital mucormycosis[127]
- Toxoplasmosis[128]
- *Toxocara*[129]
- Lyme disease[130]
- Behçet disease[131]
- Cat-scratch disease[132]

Miscellaneous associations
- Susac's syndrome[133] (Fig. 51.10)
- Fabry's disease[134]
- Sydenham's chorea[135]
- Migraine[136]
- Hypotension[24]

(Adapted from Ryan SJ. Retina. 4th edn. Philadelphia: Elsevier/Mosby; 2006.)

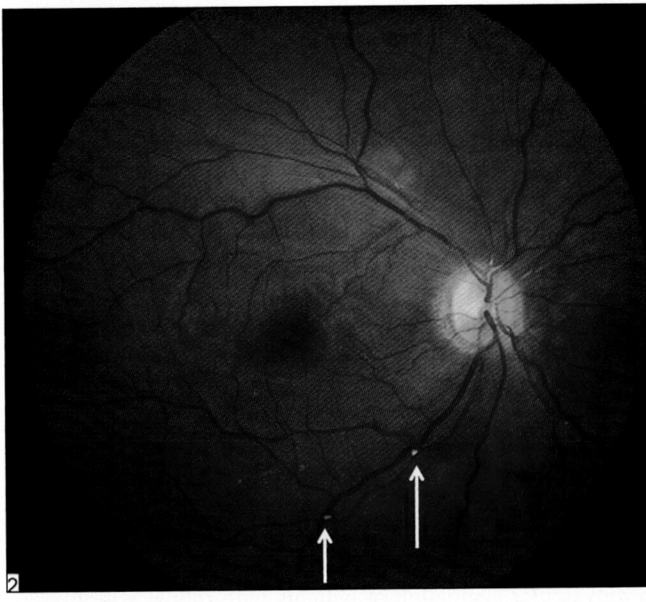

Fig. 51.8 Multiple cholesterol emboli are seen in the same eye (arrows) within the inferotemporal arcade.

multivariable models, significant independent predictors were carotid artery plaque, hypertension status, and current cigarette smoking.[44] In the heart, sources of emboli are aortic or mitral valve lesions, patent foramen ovale, left atrial tumor, and myxoma.[45–47]

The presence of a Hollenhorst plaque or retinal artery occlusion is associated with a low prevalence of carotid atherosclerosis requiring carotid endarterectomy. Furthermore, in contrast to amaurosis fugax, these ocular findings are not associated with a high risk for hemispheric neurological events.[48] However, patients with retinal emboli do have an associated higher mortality rate.[43,45,49,50] Pooled data from the Beaver Dam Eye Study and the Blue Mountain Eye study of two older populations suggests that retinal emboli predict a modest increase in all-cause and stroke-related mortality independent of cardiovascular risk factors.[51] The prevalence of diabetes, hypertension, ischemic heart disease, cerebrovascular accidents, and smoking is significantly higher in patients with retinal arterial occlusions.[6,42–44,48,52–54]

Evaluation

Patients with CRAO typically present to a physician several days after the acute onset; therefore, the etiologic workup is generally recommended on an outpatient basis along with a primary care physician. The only true emergency in such a circumstance would be to rule out giant cell arteritis in patients older than 50 years with a positive review of systems. Evaluation for giant cell arteritis includes compete blood count, including platelets, erythrocyte sedimentation rate, and C-reactive protein. If suspicion is high, the patient should be started on steroid therapy and scheduled for a temporal artery biopsy. Rarely, a patient with acute CRAO may present within the first few hours of visual deficit. These patients should be admitted for observation, treatment, and immediate workup as their risk is higher for cerebral infarction.[14]

The evaluation of embolic source often includes carotid Doppler imaging and echocardiography since the most common sources of retinal emboli are from the carotid artery or the heart. As most retinal emboli are relatively small, from the ophthalmic point of view, when evaluating the results of carotid Doppler ultrasonography, the presence or absence of plaque is more important than whether a hemodynamically significant stenosis is present; the latter is more important in determining the need for carotid endarterectomy. Carotid Doppler also has its limitations, including the lack of imaging of the thoracic and intracranial portion of the carotid artery and poor resolution for detection of microemboli.[55]

Although a cardiogenic cause is less common, identifying this is important as chronic anticoagulation may be indicated to prevent more serious adverse events.

A cardiac evaluation is especially important in young patients and those with calcific emboli. In patients with acute retinal arterial obstruction at low cardioembolic risk, transthoracic echocardiography (TTE) results in anticoagulation or cardiac surgery in only 1.5% of patients.[56] Transesophageal echocardiography (TEE) has a higher yield than the transthoracic approach in the cardiovascular evaluation of patients with retinal artery occlusion. In patients without a cardiac history and a normal TTE examination (including normal size and function of cardiac chambers and normal valves with no calcification, along with the absence of atrial fibrillation), the yield of subsequent TEE for identifying intracardiac pathology is low. However, in patients in whom clinical and TTE findings are suggestive of possible intracardiac or aortic thrombus, TEE should be considered as an adjunct to the systemic workup.[57] A computed tomography (CT) angiogram or magnetic resonance imaging angiogram should be considered in special cases such as suspected carotid or aortic dissection. Since the cardiac morbidity and mortality are significant in patients with retinal artery occlusion, a baseline electrocardiogram is recommended.[10,14]

A hypercoagulability evaluation should be considered for patients less than 50 years of age with a suggestive history (e.g., prior thrombosis, miscarriage, or family history) or unknown embolic source. Workup includes blood tests for factor V Leiden mutation; protein C, protein S, and antithrombin III deficiencies; homocysteine levels; sickle-cell disease; and antiphospholipid antibodies. Other tests for monoclonal gammopathy, cancer, infection, and disseminated intravascular coagulation may be ordered depending on the clinical circumstance.[14]

Treatment

CRAO continues to be a challenging disease entity to treat. Typically treatment is either conservative or invasive. Most reports of treatment outcome are anecdotal as a result of low incidence.[58] Spontaneous resolution can occur in up to 22% of patients[11] and has been reported to occur up to 3 days after initial onset.[59] However, less than 10% of patients report meaningful visual recovery.[60,61] Rarely do patients have complete spontaneous recovery.[62]

Based on experimental models of CRAO in elderly and atherosclerotic rhesus monkeys, the retina suffers no damage up to 97 minutes after an acute CRAO but after 4 hours the retina suffers massive irreversible damage. Therefore, no treatment instituted after about 4 hours from onset can logically restore any vision in the setting of complete obstruction. Additionally, this model showed the longer the ischemia, the longer the time to recovery.[11] However, unlike the animal model, humans rarely have complete obstruction. As a result, treatment for CRAO has been recommended within 24 hours of symptom onset. Given the relative rarity of CRAO and variability in time to presentation, therapeutic trials have been limited in sample size, thus reducing the power to detect small treatment benefits. Thus, for a new therapy to have a major impact on the management of this disease, it will likely need to double or triple the success rate of current conventional therapy yet still maintain a low risk for morbidity and mortality.

Current conventional therapy consists of dislodging emboli, reducing intraocular pressure and increasing retinal blood flow, vasodilating the ocular blood supply, improving retinal circulation, decreasing retinal edema, maintaining retinal oxygenation until spontaneous reperfusion, and acting on the thrombus.[14] None of these treatments have proven effective and their use is largely based on anecdotal reports and small case series. In a small study of 11 patients, Rumelt et al. found that a systematic regimen involving multiple, sequential treatment steps had better visual outcomes than arbitrary treatment with conservative measures. The protocol included ocular massage, sublingual isosorbide dinitrate, intravenous acetazolamide, intravenous mannitol or oral glycerol, anterior-chamber paracentesis, intravenous methylprednisolone, streptokinase, and retrobulbar tolazine. Treatment with one or two conservative modalities was usually insufficient.[3,63,64] In a Cochrane Controlled Trials Register comparing any treatment for CRAO with another treatment, Fraser and Siriwardena found no randomized controlled trials meeting their inclusion criteria. They concluded that insufficient data existed to decide if any beneficial treatments existed for CRAO.[65]

Ocular massage is performed using either a Goldmann contact lens or digital massage to apply ocular pressure with an in-and-out movement to dislodge a possibly obstructing embolus. Repeated massage with 10–15 seconds of pressure followed by a sudden release is recommended.[66] This maneuver can produce retinal arterial vasodilation, thereby improving retinal blood flow.[67,68] A mixture of 95% oxygen and 5% carbon dioxide (carbogen) can be provided to induce vasodilation and improve oxygenation, but efficacy has not been proven.[69] Hyperbaric oxygen provides oxygen at levels of atmospheric pressure. The purpose of hyperbaric oxygen is to preserve the retina in an oxygenated state until recanalization and reperfusion occur, typically at 72 hours. The hyperbaric oxygen increases the arterial oxygen pressure and thereby increases nitric oxide synthesis, leading to vasodilation. Case reports of successful treatment have been published,[70–72] but currently treatment for ocular diseases is an off-label use of hyperbaric oxygen.[73] Anterior-chamber paracentesis causes a sudden decrease in intraocular pressure, possibly causing the arterial perfusion pressure behind the obstruction to force an obstructing embolus downstream. This treatment has shown some success in retrospective analyses;[74,75] however, a study by Atebara et al. compared anterior-chamber paracentesis and carbogen therapy with no intervention and found no significant difference in visual outcome.[69] Vasodilating medications that have been utilized to increase retinal blood flow in retinal arterial occlusion include pentoxifylline, nitroglycerin, and isosorbide dinitrate.[3,76,77] Isovolemic hemodilution is used to increase oxygen supply to the retinal tissue. It includes the replacement of 500 mL of blood with the same volume of hydroxy-ethyl starch. In vascular disease, the limiting factor in tissue oxygenation is blood flow and not oxygen-carrying capacity. In this situation lowering blood viscosity by decreasing the hematocrit and plasma viscosity will improve tissue oxygen levels.[65,78]

Various surgical techniques have also been explored for treatment of CRAO. Neodymium:yttrium aluminum garnet (Nd-YAG) laser arteriotomy in patients with CRAO has been reported to result in extrusion of an embolus, reopening of the central retinal artery, and return of vision. A fundus contact lens is used with the laser in single-burst mode. The laser is focused slightly deep to the vessel wall at the site of the embolus to avoid photodisruption and opacification of the overlying nerve fiber layer. In patients with small emboli, the laser is focused on the center of the plaque. In patients with elongated emboli, the laser is focused slightly on the distal or downstream end to reduce the chance of hemorrhage. Pulses are delivered directly to the emboli, beginning with the lowest power setting and then with increasing energy until either (1) achieving photofragmentation of the embolus within the arteriole without creating an opening in the vessel wall and without vitreous hemorrhage or (2) creating visible removal of the embolus from within arteriole into the vitreous cavity, typically associated with a limited vitreous hemorrhage. Digital pressure can be applied to the globe to help stop bleeding, if it occurs.[79]

Corticosteroids should only be used when arteritic CRAO from giant cell arteritis is suspected.[14] Anticoagulants should be reserved for secondary prevention of cerebral and ocular infarction in those rare patients who have an underlying systemic disease such as atrial fibrillation, acute internal carotid artery dissection, or a hypercoagulable condition.[14]

With the common use of thrombolytics for acute cerebrovascular accidents, their potential application in the setting of acute CRAO has been considered. Intravenously or intra-arterially administered thrombolytics currently in use include streptokinase, urokinase, and tissue plasminogen activator (t-PA). Intravenous administration is relatively easy and workup prior to treatment is minimal, including blood tests and a brain CT; however intravenous thrombolytics do increase the risk of systemic hemorrhage. Because of the increased systemic risks, most thrombolysis strategies currently in use are intra-arterial.[14] A meta-analysis of all published literature pertaining to intra-arterial thrombolysis for treatment of acute CRAO done in 2000 found that this treatment did not improve visual acuity beyond the disease's natural course. No prospective randomized studies were available to be included at that time.[80] In 2010 the European Assessment Group for Lysis in the Eye (EAGLE) study group published the results of the first prospective, randomized clinical trial evaluating the effect of intra-arterial t-PA compared with conservative treatment. Of note, no true placebo arm was included in the study. At 1 month, the mean best-corrected visual acuity improved significantly in both groups but no significant difference was noted between groups. Clinically significant visual improvement (0.3 logMAR) was noted in 60.0% of patients in the conventional therapy group and 57.1% of patients in the thrombolysis group. The trial was stopped early because of the apparent similarity in efficacy between groups and the higher rate of adverse events, namely cerebral hemorrhage, in the intra-arterial t-PA group.[78] The EAGLE study highlights the importance of careful randomized controlled trials, as the rate of visual improvement in the conventional therapy group was higher than one might expect from prior retrospective studies.

BRANCH RETINAL ARTERY OCCLUSION

BRAOs are thought to represent 38% of all acute retinal artery obstructions.[26] Patients generally present with monocular vision loss, which may be restricted to one part of the visual field. Initial visual acuity is better than 20/40 in approximately three-fourths of patients.[81,82] Presenting visual field defects include a central scotoma in 20%, a central altitudinal defect in 13%, and sector defects in 49%.[82]

Fundoscopically, a sectoral pattern of retinal opacification is seen. The whitening is most prominent in the posterior pole along the distribution of the obstructed vessel. Areas of more intense whitening are often seen at the borders of the ischemic area (Fig. 51.9). These probably occur secondary to blocked axoplasmic flow in the nerve fiber layer as it reaches the hypoxic retina. BRAOs typically occur at vessel bifurcations, and 98% of the time the temporal vessels are affected – this may, however, be due to a presentation bias, as nasal occlusions may be asymptomatic and undetected. Emboli are visible 62% of the time.[81]

In the chronic stage of BRAO, sectoral nerve fiber layer loss and arterial attenuation may be seen (Fig. 51.10). Rarely in the chronic phase, posterior-segment and/or iris neovascularization will be seen after BRAO, particularly in patients with diabetes.[83] Artery-to-artery collaterals may also be seen and are pathognomonic for BRAO.[84]

The visual prognosis in eyes with symptomatic BRAO is generally good, and acuity usually improves to 20/40 or better in 80% of eyes.[4] In a retrospective study of 52 eyes, Mason et al. reported visual prognosis after BRAO correlated with the presenting visual acuity;[85] however, Hayreh et al., in their natural history study of 133 eyes, did not find such a correlation.[82] They reported visual acuity to correlate with foveal involvement and the extent of irreversible ischemic damage to the retina.[82] Ros et al. showed an improvement in visual field deficit by Goldmann perimetry in 80% of 201 eyes surveyed.[81]

Risk factors for BRAO are similar to CRAO; therefore a similar evaluation is generally recommended.[81] Giant cell arteritis tends to present much less often with a BRAO than a CRAO. In cases

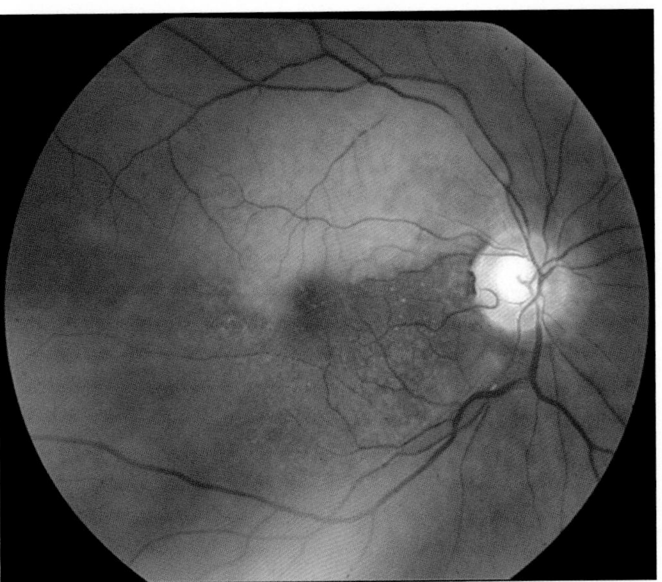

Fig. 51.9 Branch retinal artery occlusion of the superotemporal arcade. Retinal opacification of the superior macula is seen with segmentation within the superior temporal arterioles.

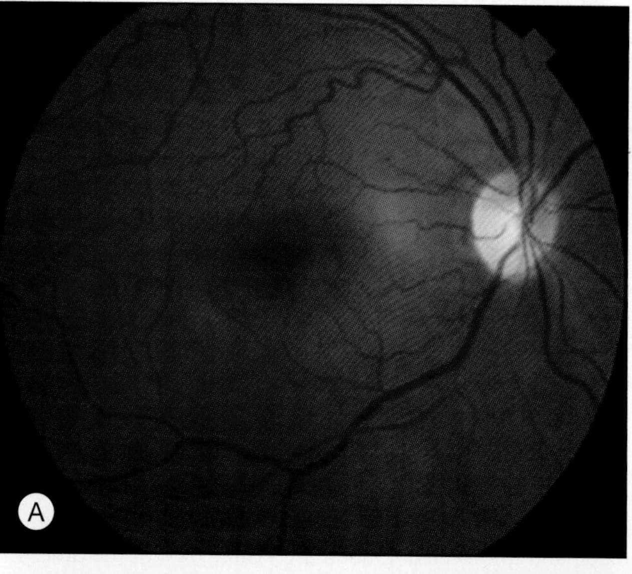

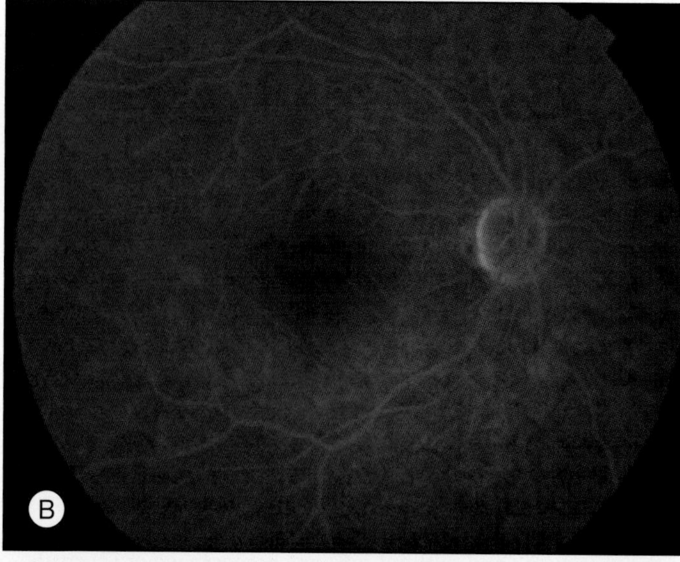

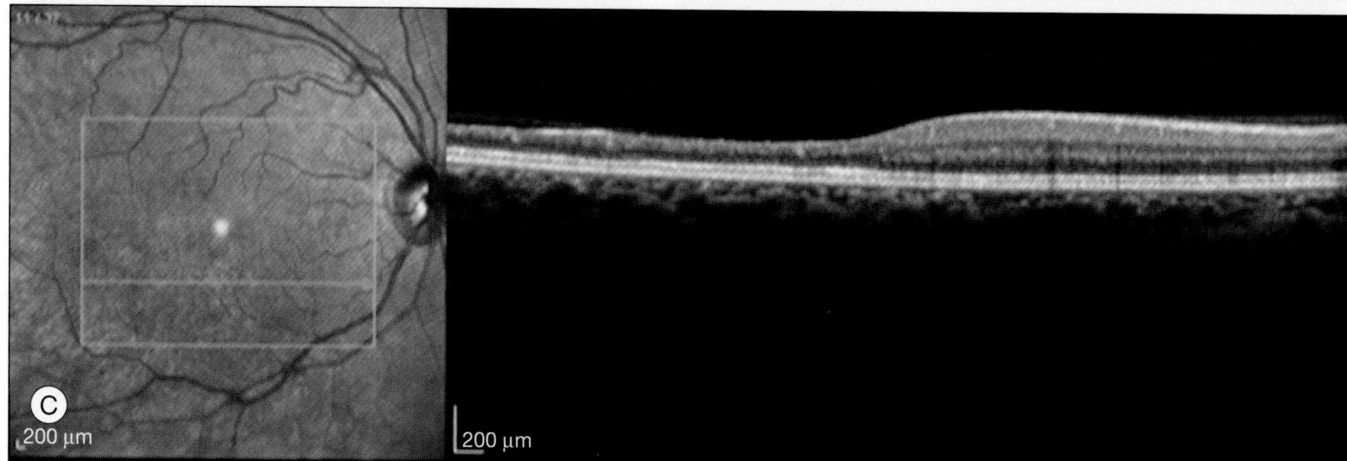

Fig. 51.10 (A) Color fundus photograph of the right eye in a patient with Susac's disease with a history of a remote inferotemporal branch retinal artery occlusion. Inferotemporal nerve fiber layer loss and arterial attenuation can be seen compared to the superotemporal area. (B) Fluorescein angiography shows restoration of arterial blood flow. (C) Spectral-domain optical coherence tomography shows sectoral inner retinal atrophy down to the inner nuclear layer in the inferotemporal macula.

of an obstruction at a bifurcation, the etiology is more often embolic.

Since the visual prognosis is typically good for BRAO, aggressive therapy is generally not pursued unless significant foveal involvement is seen. Additionally, the good prognosis makes the positive effect of treatment more difficult to discern from natural history.

CILIORETINAL ARTERY OCCLUSION

CLRAOs account for 5% of retinal arterial obstructions.[37] Cilioretinal arteries enter the retina from the temporal optic disc, separate from the central retinal artery, and can be seen on exam in 20% of eyes. On fluorescein angiography, they are seen 32% of the time and fill concomitantly with the choroidal circulation.[27] Fundoscopically, an area of superficial retinal whitening is seen along the course of the cilioretinal artery.

When evaluating CLRAO, typically three distinct groups are found: (1) isolated CLRAO; (2) CLRAO associated with CRVO; and (3) CLRAO in conjunction with anterior ischemic optic neuropathy. Brown et al. found 90%, 70%, and 0% of eyes achieved 20/40 or better vision in the first, second, and third group, respectively.[86] Initial visual field defects include cecocentral scotoma, central scotoma, and central superior or inferior altitudinal defect.[82]

Isolated CLRAOs typically have a good prognosis, with nearly 90% achieving 20/40 or better vision and 60% returning to 20/20. Even with severe damage to the papillomacular bundle, potential visual acuity can be quite good, presumably secondary to intact superior and inferior nerve fiber layer bundles supplying the fovea.

CLRAO in conjunction with a CRVO comprises 40% of CLRAO.[86] Approximately 5% of eyes with CRVO also have a CLRAO.[87] Visual acuity correlates with the degree of venous obstruction. The venous obstructions are usually nonischemic and tend not to cause iris neovascularization or neovascular glaucoma.[86] Reduced hydrostatic pressure in the cilioretinal artery may predispose the cilioretinal artery to stasis and thrombosis in the setting of increased hydrostatic pressure within the retinal venous system. Optic disc edema may also contribute by decreasing the area of the cilioretinal artery and thereby the flow.[87]

CLRAO in association with anterior ischemic optic neuropathy is seen in 15% of eyes with CLRAO and has a poor visual prognosis, ranging from 20/400 to no light perception secondary to optic nerve damage. Typically a hyperemic or pale, edematous optic disc is seen with superficial retinal whitening along the course of the cilioretinal artery.[86] Acute pale swelling is more suggestive of giant cell arteritis and is usually associated with more severe vision loss. Giant cell arteritis has a selective tendency to involve the posterior ciliary artery, resulting in its occlusion, which in turn results in simultaneous development of both arteritic anterior ischemic optic neuropathy and CLRAO.[82]

Systemic evaluation is similar to CRAO except investigation for embolic sources is likely not indicated for cases associated with CRVO. Ocular treatment is generally not pursued unless concern for underlying giant cell arteritis exists.

COMBINED RETINAL ARTERY AND VEIN OCCLUSION

CRVO can be seen in association with CRAO,[88] BRAO,[89] and CLRAO.[90,91] Patients with combined CRAO/BRAO and CRVO generally present with sudden decreased vision. The fundus exam shows superficial retinal whitening with a cherry-red spot and signs of venous obstruction, such as dilated, tortuous veins, intraretinal hemorrhages, optic disc edema, cotton-wool spots, and marked thickening of the retina (Figs 51.11 and 51.12).[88]

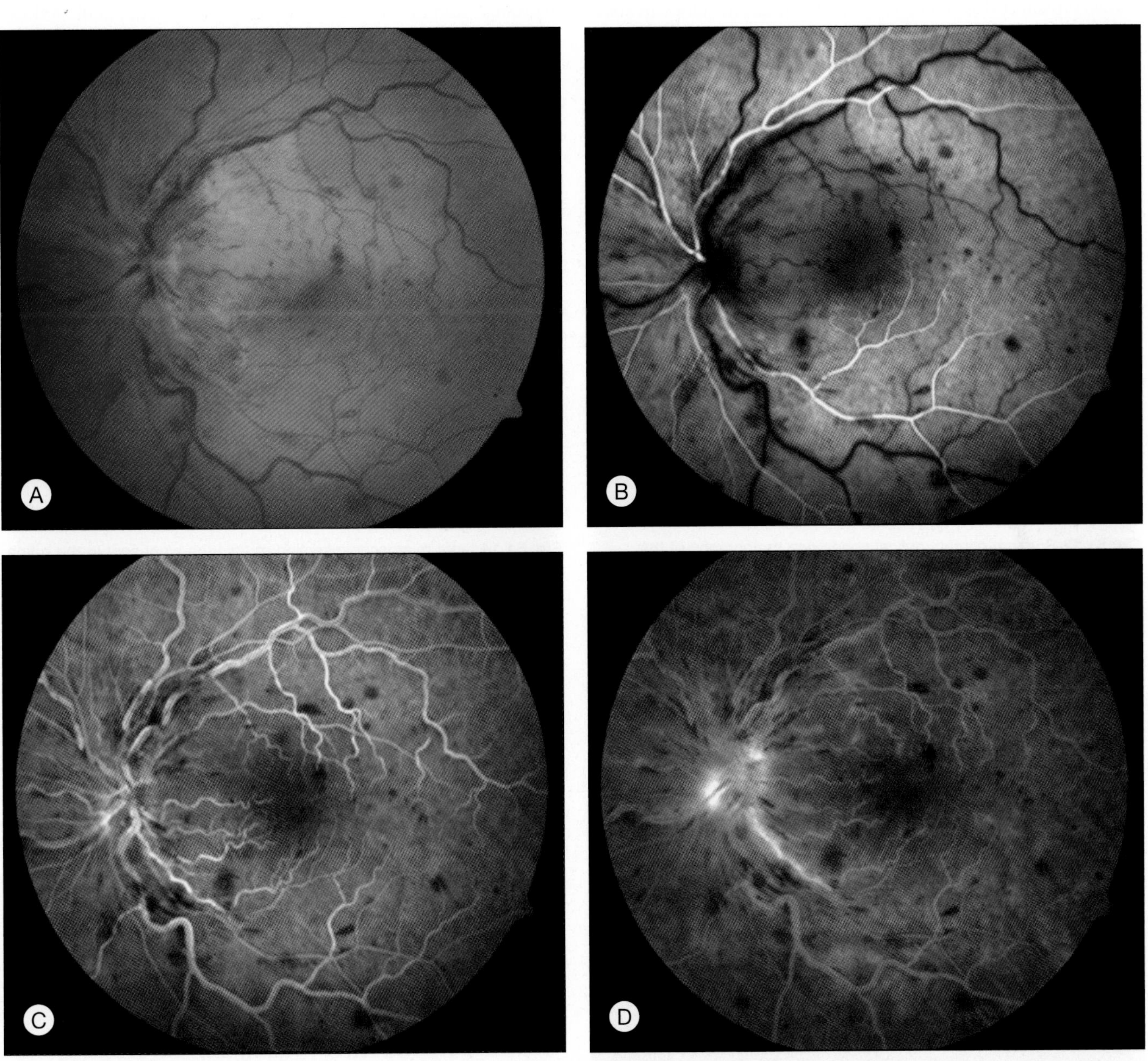

Fig. 51.11 (A) Fundus photograph of an acute central retinal venous occlusion (CRVO) with a branch retinal artery occlusion in a patient with the factor V Leiden mutation. Optic disc hyperemia and edema, dilated and tortuous veins, intraretinal hemorrhages, and cotton-wool spots are seen consistent with a CRVO. Superotemporal to the disc, retinal opacification is seen consistent with a branch retinal artery occlusion. (B) Fluorescein angiography shows initial nonperfusion of the branch retinal artery superior to the fovea. (C) Marked delay in transit consistent with the occlusive process is seen. The arteriole occlusion is not complete as the dye eventually does get into the artery. (D) In the late frames, disc leakage is seen consistent with the CRVO.

The CRAO seen with a CRVO may not be a true CRAO but may be secondary to the occlusion of the central retinal vein in the region of the lamina cribrosa. The blood cannot exit out of the retinal vascular bed as a result of complete blockage of the central retinal vein, and secondarily compromises entry of blood into the eye.[55] Fluorescein angiography shows severe widespread retinal capillary nonperfusion with sudden termination or pruning of the mid-sized retinal vessels. Minimal macular leakage is seen as a result of closure of these vessels despite the clinical appearance.[92]

The visual prognosis is generally poor, with visual acuity in the hand motions range.[92] After 6–8 weeks, optic nerve pallor is seen with severe arterial attenuation. Histopathology of the chronic phase shows hemorrhagic retinal necrosis and inner retinal atrophy consistent with a CRVO and CRAO. The macula shows typical cystoid changes. Rubeosis iridis develops in about 80% of eyes, leading to neovascular glaucoma as the end result.[88] This can be seen as early as 1–2 weeks but is seen on average at about 6 weeks. Aggressive treatment with panretinal photocoagulation is recommended.[92]

Combined CRAO and CRVO has been associated with many diverse entities, including syphilis, optic neuritis, leukemia, lymphoma, temporal arteritis, orbital inflammatory disease, posterior scleritis, systemic lupus erythematosus, trauma, retrobulbar injections, and superior ophthalmic vein thrombosis.[89] Intravitreal gentamicin injection may cause a similar appearance; however, angiography would show normal filling of the choroid, retinal arteries, and veins.[93]

COTTON-WOOL SPOTS

Cotton-wool spots are often referred to using the misnomer "soft exudates" and are described as slightly elevated, small, yellow-white or gray-white, cloud-like, linear or serpentine lesions with

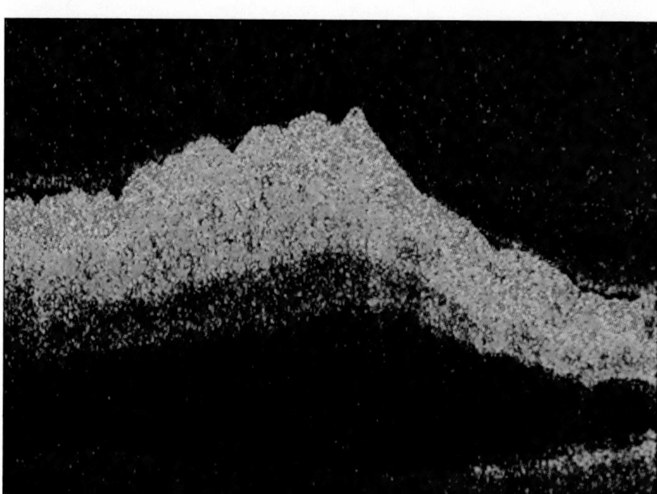

Fig. 51.12 Spectral-domain optical coherence tomography of the patient shown in Figure 51.11. Inner and outer retinal edema can be seen consistent with the combined central retinal venous occlusion and branch retinal artery occlusion.

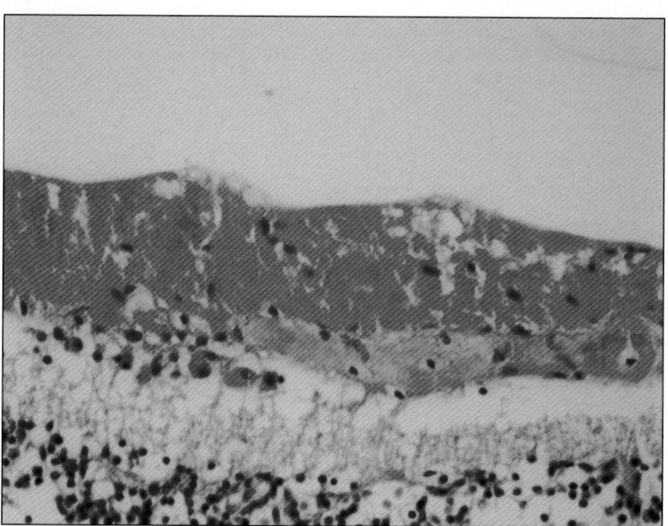

Fig. 51.14 Light microscopic section of a cotton-wool spot in the retina showing swelling of the nerve fiber layer with the presence of cytoid bodies. Hematoxylin and eosin, ×100. (Courtesy of Dr. Hans Grossniklaus, Emory Eye Center, Atlanta.)

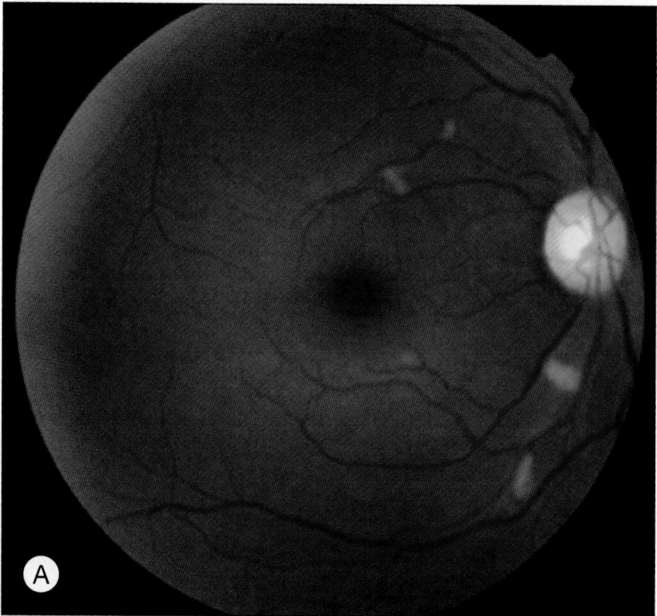

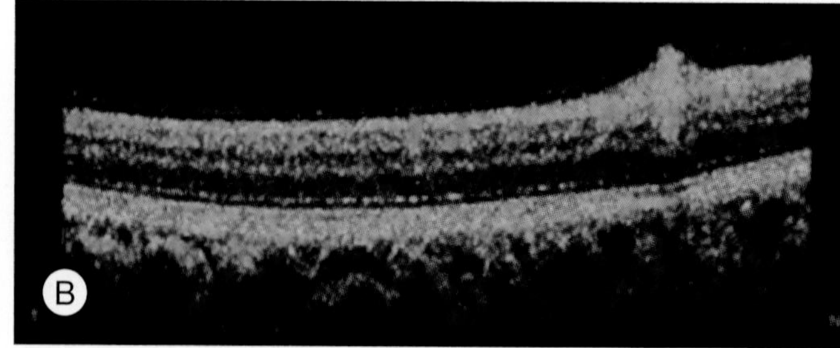

Fig. 51.13 (A) Fundus photo showing multiple cotton-wool spots in a patient with interferon-β1a retinopathy. (B) Spectral-domain optical coherence tomography through one of the cotton-wool spots shows focal thickening and elevation of the nerve fiber layer.

Box 51.2 Etiologies for cotton-wool spots

Ischemic
- Diabetes
- Hypertension
- Retinal vein occlusion
- Ocular ischemic syndrome
- Severe anemia
- Hyperviscosity/hypercoagulable state/dysproteinemia
- Radiation
- Acute blood loss

Embolic
- Carotid emboli
- Cardiac emboli
  - Cardiac valvular disease
  - Endocarditis
  - Rheumatic heart disease
- Deep venous emboli
- White cell emboli/Purtscher and Purtscher-like retinopathy (head trauma, long bone fractures, acute pancreatitis, chest compression injury, amniotic fluid emboli, fat emboli)
- Foreign-body emboli (intravenous drug abuse, talc)

Collagen vascular disease
- Systemic lupus erythematosus
- Dermatomyositis
- Scleroderma
- Polyarteritis nodosa
- Giant cell arteritis

Infectious
- HIV retinopathy
- Fungemia
- Bacteremia
- Rocky Mountain spotted fever (*Rickettsia rickettsii*)
- Cat-scratch disease (*Bartonella henselae*)
- Leptospirosis
- Onchocerciasis (*Onchocerca volvulus*)

Toxic
- Interferon (α_{2a}, β_{1a})

Neoplastic
- Leukemia
- Lymphoma
- Metastatic carcinoma

Miscellaneous
- Traumatic
- Tractional (epiretinal membrane)
- High-altitude retinopathy
- Papilledema/papillitis

Idiopathic

HIV, human immunodeficiency virus.
(Reproduced with permission from Brown GC, Brown MM, Hiller T, et al. Cotton-wool spots. Retina 1985;5:206–14.)

fimbriated borders in the superficial retina (Fig. 51.13). They are usually restricted to the posterior segment of the fundus and they rarely exceed one-third of the area of the optic disc.[94] Cotton-wool spots rarely cause vision loss unless they involve the fovea and typically resolve within 6–12 weeks,[94] though they may last longer in diabetics.[95]

A cotton-wool spot is hypothesized to develop secondary to obstruction of a retinal arteriole with resultant ischemia. The focal hypoxia causes blockage of axoplasmic flow within the nerve fiber layer with subsequent deposition of intra-axonal organelles.[96] Early light microscopy of cotton-wool spots in the retina revealed the presence of a cytoid body, a round, dark-staining "pseudonucleus" within a grossly swollen nerve fiber layer (Fig. 51.14). The application of electron microscopic techniques revealed the composition of cytoid bodies to be an accumulation of intracytoplasmic organelles, largely mitochondria, with a major lipid component.[97]

Diabetes mellitus and systemic hypertension are by far the most common etiologies of cotton-wool spots, followed by undiagnosed diabetes and hypertension. In patients who have a cotton-wool spot and no known history of diabetes, an elevated blood sugar level is identified in 20% of patients and an elevated blood pressure (diastolic blood pressure of 90 mmHg or greater) in 50% of patients. Cotton-wool spots, however, may be observed in association with numerous other diseases (Box 51.2). Fortunately, most patients who present with cotton-wool spots have other systemic or ocular findings that help narrow down their specific etiology. The presence of even one cotton-wool spot in an otherwise normal fundus necessitates an investigation to ascertain systemic etiologic factors. A giant cell arteritis workup is not necessary unless a positive review of systems is noted. In approximately 95% of cases, a systemic underlying condition can be found. Almost any etiology that can cause a CRAO or BRAO can potentially also produce cotton-wool spots.[98]

REFERENCES

1. von Graefe A. Ueber Embolie der arteria centralis retinae als Urscahe plotzlicher Erblingdung. Arch Ophthalmol 1859;5:136–57.
2. Ryan SJ. Retina. 4th ed. Philadelphia: Elsevier/Mosby; 2006.
3. Rumelt S, Dorenboim Y, Rehany U. Aggressive systematic treatment for central retinal artery occlusion. Am J Ophthalmol 1999;128:733–8.
4. Brown GC, Magargal LE, Shields JA, et al. Retinal arterial obstruction in children and young adults. Ophthalmology 1981;88:18–25.
5. Greven CM, Slusher MM, Weaver RG. Retinal arterial occlusions in young adults. Am J Ophthalmol 1995;120:776–83.
6. Brown GC, Magargal LE. Central retinal artery obstruction and visual acuity. Ophthalmology 1982;89:14–9.
7. Alwitry A, Holden R. One hundred transient monocular central retinal artery occlusions secondary to giant cell arteritis. Arch Ophthalmol 2003;121:1802–3.
8. Breen LA. Atherosclerotic carotid disease and the eye. Neurol Clin 1991;9:131–45.
9. Kline L. The natural history of patients with amaurosis fugax. Ophthalmol Clin North Am 1996;9:351–7.
10. Appen RE, Wray SH, Cogan DG. Central retinal artery occlusion. Am J Ophthalmol 1975;79:374–81.
11. Hayreh SS, Zimmerman MB. Central retinal artery occlusion: visual outcome. Am J Ophthalmol 2005;140:376–91.
12. Connolly BP, Krishnan A, Shah GK, et al. Characteristics of patients presenting with central retinal artery occlusion with and without giant cell arteritis. Can J Ophthalmol 2000;35:379–84.
13. Augsburger JJ, Magargal LE. Visual prognosis following treatment of acute central retinal artery obstruction. Br J Ophthalmol 1980;64:913–7.
14. Biousse V, Calvetti O, Bruce BB, et al. Thrombolysis for central retinal artery occlusion. J Neuroophthalmol 2007;27:215–30.
15. Duker JS, Brown GC. Iris neovascularization associated with obstruction of the central retinal artery. Ophthalmology 1988;95:1244–50.
16. Duker JS, Sivalingam A, Brown GC, et al. A prospective study of acute central retinal artery obstruction. The incidence of secondary ocular neovascularization. Arch Ophthalmol 1991;109:339–42.
17. Hayreh SS, Rojas P, Podhajsky P, et al. Ocular neovascularization with retinal vascular occlusion – II. Incidence of ocular neovascularization with retinal vein occlusion. Ophthalmology 1983;90:488–506.
18. Duker JS, Brown GC. The efficacy of panretinal photocoagulation for neovascularization of the iris after central retinal artery obstruction. Ophthalmology 1989;96:92–5.
19. Nettleship E. Unusual appearance in a case of retinal embolism about 30 hours after its occurence. In: Festschrift zur Feier Siebzigsten Geburtstage, vol. 7. Stuttgardt: Hermann von Helmholz; 1891. pp. 7–8.
20. Hayreh SS, Zimmerman MB. Fundus changes in central retinal artery occlusion. Retina 2007;27:276–89.
21. Sharma S, ten Hove MW, Pinkerton RM, et al. Interobserver agreement in the evaluation of acute retinal artery occlusion. Can J Ophthalmol 1997;32:441–4.
22. Hayreh SS, Kolder HE, Weingeist TA. Central retinal artery occlusion and retinal tolerance time. Ophthalmology 1980;87:75–8.
23. Hayreh SS, Zimmerman MB, Kimura A, et al. Central retinal artery occlusion. Retinal survival time. Exp Eye Res 2004;78:723–36.
24. Gold D. Retinal arterial occlusion. Trans Sect Ophthalmol Am Acad Ophthalmol Otolaryngol 1977;83:OP392–408.
25. Yanoff MFB. Retinal ischemia. Ocular pathology – a text and atlas. Philadelphia: J.B. Lippincott; 1989.
26. Brown GC, Shields JA. Cilioretinal arteries and retinal arterial occlusion. Arch Ophthalmol 1979;97:84–92.
27. Justice Jr J, Lehmann RP. Cilioretinal arteries. A study based on review of stereo fundus photographs and fluorescein angiographic findings. Arch Ophthalmol 1976;94:1355–8.

28. Singh S, Dass R. The central artery of the retina. II. A study of its distribution and anastomoses. Br J Ophthalmol 1960;44:280–99.
29. Hayreh SS. Acute retinal arterial occlusive disorders. Prog Retin Eye Res 2011;30:359–94.
30. Arruga J, Sanders MD. Ophthalmologic findings in 70 patients with evidence of retinal embolism. Ophthalmology 1982;89:1336–47.
31. Ramakrishna G, Malouf JF, Younge BR, et al. Calcific retinal embolism as an indicator of severe unrecognised cardiovascular disease. Heart 2005;91: 1154–7.
32. Hayreh SS. Blood supply of the optic nerve head and its role in optic atrophy, glaucoma, and oedema of the optic disc. Br J Ophthalmol 1969;53:721–48.
33. Hayreh SS, Jonas JB. Optic disk and retinal nerve fiber layer damage after transient central retinal artery occlusion: an experimental study in rhesus monkeys. Am J Ophthalmol 2000;129:786–95.
34. Hayreh SS, Podhajsky P. Ocular neovascularization with retinal vascular occlusion. II. Occurrence in central and branch retinal artery occlusion. Arch Ophthalmol 1982;100:1585–96.
35. Duker JS, Brown GC. Neovascularization of the optic disc associated with obstruction of the central retinal artery. Ophthalmology 1989;96: 87–91.
36. David NJ, Norton EW, Gass JD, et al. Fluorescein angiography in central retinal artery occlusion. Arch Ophthalmol 1967;77:619–29.
37. Brown GC, Magargal LE, Sergott R. Acute obstruction of the retinal and choroidal circulations. Ophthalmology 1986;93:1373–82.
38. Chen SN, Hwang JF, Chen YT. Macular thickness measurements in central retinal artery occlusion by optical coherence tomography. Retina 2011;31: 730–7.
39. Mathew R, Papavasileiou E, Sivaprasad S. Autofluorescence and high-definition optical coherence tomography of retinal artery occlusions. Clin Ophthalmol 2010;4:1159–63.
40. Schuman JS, Puliafito CA, Fujimoto JG. Optical coherence tomography of ocular diseases. 2nd ed. Thorofare, NJ: Slack; 2004.
41. Henkes HE. Electroretinography in circulatory disturbances of the retina. II. The electroretinogram in cases of occlusion of the central retinal artery or of its branches. Arch Ophthalmol 1954;51:42–53.
42. Hayreh SS, Podhajsky PA, Zimmerman MB. Retinal artery occlusion: associated systemic and ophthalmic abnormalities. Ophthalmology 2009;116: 1928–36.
43. Klein R, Klein BE, Moss SE, et al Retinal emboli and cardiovascular disease: the Beaver Dam Eye Study. Arch Ophthalmol 2003;121:1446–51.
44. Wong TY, Larsen EK, Klein R, et al. Cardiovascular risk factors for retinal vein occlusion and arteriolar emboli: the Atherosclerosis Risk in Communities & Cardiovascular Health studies. Ophthalmology 2005;112:540–7.
45. Jampol LM, Wong AS, Albert DM. Atrial myxoma and central retinal artery occlusion. Am J Ophthalmol 1973;75:242–9.
46. Campbell JK. Early diagnosis of an atrial myxoma with central retinal artery occlusion. Ann Ophthalmol 1974;6:1207–8, 10–1.
47. Cogan DG, Wray SH. Vascular occlusions in the eye from cardiac myxomas. Am J Ophthalmol 1975;80:396–403.
48. Dunlap AB, Kosmorsky GS, Kashyap VS. The fate of patients with retinal artery occlusion and Hollenhorst plaque. J Vasc Surg 2007;46:1125–9.
49. Wilson LA, Warlow CP, Russell RW. Cardiovascular disease in patients with retinal arterial occlusion. Lancet 1979;1:292–4.
50. Greven CM, Weaver RG, Harris WR, et al. Transesophageal echocardiography for detecting mitral valve prolapse with retinal artery occlusions. Am J Ophthalmol 1991 ;111:103–4.
51. Tarkkanen A, Merenmies L, Makinen J. Embolism of the central retinal artery secondary to metastatic carcinoma. Acta Ophthalmol (Copenh) 1973;51: 25–33.
52. Klein R, Klein BE, Jensen SC, et al. Retinal emboli and stroke: the Beaver Dam Eye Study. Arch Ophthalmol 1999;117:1063–8.
53. Wong TY, Klein R. Retinal arteriolar emboli: epidemiology and risk of stroke. Curr Opin Ophthalmol 2002;13:142–6.
54. Cheung N, Lim L, Wang JJ, et al. Prevalence and risk factors of retinal arteriolar emboli: the Singapore Malay Eye Study. Am J Ophthalmol 2008;146: 620–4.
55. Hayreh SS. Prevalent misconceptions about acute retinal vascular occlusive disorders. Prog Retin Eye Res 2005;24:493–519.
56. Sharma S, Naqvi A, Sharma SM, et al. Transthoracic echocardiographic findings in patients with acute retinal arterial obstruction. A retrospective review. Retinal Emboli of Cardiac Origin Group. Arch Ophthalmol 1996;114: 1189–92.
57. Kramer M, Goldenberg-Cohen N, Shapira Y, et al. Role of transesophageal echocardiography in the evaluation of patients with retinal artery occlusion. Ophthalmology 2001;108:1461–4.
58. Rumelt S, Brown GC. Update on treatment of retinal arterial occlusions. Curr Opin Ophthalmol 2003;14:139–41.
59. Duker JS, Brown GC. Recovery following acute obstruction of the retinal and choroidal circulations. A case history. Retina 1988;8:257–60.
60. Meyer CH, Holz FG. Images in clinical medicine. Blurred vision after cardiac catheterization. N Engl J Med 2009 ;361:2366.
61. Rasmussen KE. Retinal and cerebral fat emboli following lymphography with oily contrast media. Acta Radiol Diagn (Stockh) 1970;10:199–202.
62. Perkins SA, Magargal LE, Augsburger JJ, et al. The idling retina: reversible visual loss in central retinal artery obstruction. Ann Ophthalmol 1987; 19:3–6.
63. Kim RW, Juzych MS, Eliott D. Ocular manifestations of injection drug use. Infect Dis Clin North Am 2002;16:607–22.
64. Charawanamuttu AM, Hughes-Nurse J, Hamlett JD. Retinal embolism after hysterosalpingography. Br J Ophthalmol 1973;57:166–9.
65. Fraser S, Siriwardena D. Interventions for acute non-arteritic central retinal artery occlusion. Cochrane Database Syst Rev 2002;1:CD001989.
66. Ffytche TJ. A rationalization of treatment of central retinal artery occlusion. Trans Ophthalmol Soc U K 1974;94:468–79.
67. Nakagawa T, Hirata A, Inoue N, et al. A case of bilateral central retinal artery obstruction with patent foramen ovale. Acta Ophthalmol Scand 2004;82: 111–2.
68. Sawada T, Harino S, Ikeda T. Central retinal artery occlusion in a patient with fibromuscular dysplasia. Retina 2004;24:461–4.
69. Atebara NH, Brown GC, Cater J. Efficacy of anterior chamber paracentesis and Carbogen in treating acute nonarteritic central retinal artery occlusion. Ophthalmology 1995;102:2029–34; discussion 34–5.
70. Morgan CM, Schatz H, Vine AK, et al. Ocular complications associated with retrobulbar injections. Ophthalmology 1988;95:660–5.
71. Emery JM, Huff JD, Justice J, Jr. Central retinal artery occlusion after blow-out fracture repair. Am J Ophthalmol 1974;78:538–40.
72. Hollenhorst RW, Svien HJ, Benoit CF. Unilateral blindness occurring during anesthesia for neurosurgical operations. AMA Arch Ophthalmol 1954;52: 819–30.
73. Oguz H, Sobaci G. The use of hyperbaric oxygen therapy in ophthalmology. Surv Ophthalmol 2008;53:112–20.
74. Johnson LN, Krohel GB, Hong YK, et al. Central retinal artery occlusion following transfemoral cerebral angiography. Ann Ophthalmol 1985;17:359–62.
75. Brown GC, Magargal LE. Sudden occlusion of the retinal and posterior choroidal circulations in a youth. Am J Ophthalmol 1979;88:690–3.
76. Incandela L, Cesarone MR, Belcaro G, et al. Treatment of vascular retinal disease with pentoxifylline: a controlled, randomized trial. Angiology 2002;53 (Suppl 1):S31–4.
77. Kuritzky S. Nitroglycerin to treat acute loss of vision. N Engl J Med 1990;323:1428.
78. Schumacher M, Schmidt D, Jurklies B, et al. Central retinal artery occlusion: local intra-arterial fibrinolysis versus conservative treatment, a multicenter randomized trial. Ophthalmology 2010;117:1367–75 e1.
79. Opremcak E, Rehmar AJ, Ridenour CD, et al. Restoration of retinal blood flow via translumenal Nd:YAG embolysis/embolectomy (TYL/E) for central and branch retinal artery occlusion. Retina 2008;28:226–35.
80. Beatty S, Au Eong KG. Local intra-arterial fibrinolysis for acute occlusion of the central retinal artery: a meta-analysis of the published data. Br J Ophthalmol 2000;84:914–6.
81. Ros MA, Magargal LE, Uram M. Branch retinal-artery obstruction: a review of 201 eyes. Ann Ophthalmol 1989;21:103–7.
82. Hayreh SS, Podhajsky PA, Zimmerman MB. Branch retinal artery occlusion: natural history of visual outcome. Ophthalmology 2009;116:1188–94 e1–4.
83. Shah GK, Sharma S, Brown GC. Iris neovascularization following branch retinal artery occlusion. Can J Ophthalmol 1998;33:389–90.
84. Sharma MC, Volpe NJ. Collaterals in branch retinal artery occlusion. Ophthalmic Surg Lasers 1999;30:324–5.
85. Mason 3rd JO, Shah AA, Vail RS, et al. Branch retinal artery occlusion: visual prognosis. Am J Ophthalmol 2008;146:455–7.
86. Brown GC, Moffat K, Cruess A, et al. Cilioretinal artery obstruction. Retina 1983;3:182–7.
87. Fong AC, Schatz H, McDonald HR, et al. Central retinal vein occlusion in young adults (papillophlebitis). Retina 1992;12:3–11.
88. Richards R. Simultaneous occlusion of the central retinal artery and vein. Tr Am Ophth Soc 1967;78:191–209.
89. Duker JS, Cohen MS, Brown GC, et al. Combined branch retinal artery and central retinal vein obstruction. Retina 1990;10:105–12.
90. McLeod D. Cilio-retinal arterial circulation in central retinal vein occlusion. Br J Ophthalmol 1975;59:486–92.
91. Hayreh SS, Fraterrigo L, Jonas J. Central retinal vein occlusion associated with cilioretinal artery occlusion. Retina 2008;28:581–94.
92. Brown GC, Duker JS, Lehman R, et al. Combined central retinal artery-central vein obstruction. Int Ophthalmol 1993;17:9–17.
93. Brown GC, Eagle RC, Shakin EP, et al. Retinal toxicity of intravitreal gentamicin. Arch Ophthalmol 1990;108:1740–4.
94. Cotton-wool spots. Br Med J 1966;2:1474.
95. Hodge JV, Dollery CT. Retinal soft exudates. A clinical study by colour and fluorescence photography. Q J Med 1964;33:117–31.
96. McLeod D, Marshall J, Kohner EM, et al. The role of axoplasmic transport in the pathogenesis of retinal cotton-wool spots. Br J Ophthalmol 1977;61: 177–91.
97. Ashton N. Pathophysiology of retinal cotton-wool spots. Br Med Bull 1970;26:143–50.
98. Brown GC, Brown MM, Hiller T, et al. Cotton-wool spots. Retina 1985;5: 206–14.
99. Sharma S, Brown GC, Pater JL, et al. Does a visible retinal embolus increase the likelihood of hemodynamically significant carotid artery stenosis in patients with acute retinal arterial occlusion? Arch Ophthalmol 1998; 116(12):1602–6.
100. Kollarits CR, Lubow M, Hissong SL. Retinal strokes. I. Incidence of carotid atheromata. JAMA 1972;222(10):1273–5.
101. Masuda H, Ohira A, Shibuya Y, et al. Branch retinal artery occlusion caused by an embolus of metastatic gastric adenocarcinoma. Arch Ophthalmol 2002; 120(9):1209–11.
102. Hwang JF, Chen SN, Chiu SL, et al. Embolic cilioretinal artery occlusion due to carotid artery dissection. Am J Ophthalmol 2004;138(3):496–8.

103. AtLee WE, Jr. Talc and cornstarch emboli in eyes of drug abusers. JAMA 1972;219(1):49–51.
104. Inkeles DM, Walsh JB. Retinal fat emboli as sequela to acute pancreatitis. Am J Ophthalmol 1975;80(5):935–8.
105. Madsen PH. Traumatic retinal angiopathy (Purtscher). Ophthalmologica 1972;165(5):453–8.
106. Toussaint D, Danis P. Retinopathy in generalized loa-loa filariasis. A clinicopathological study. Arch Ophthalmol 1965;74(4):470–6.
107. Corrigan MJ, Hill DW. Retinal artery occlusion in loiasis. Br J Ophthalmol 1968;52(6):477–80.
108. Treiman RL, Bloemendal LC, Foran RF, et al. Ipsilateral blindness: a complication of carotid endarterectomy. Arch Surg 1977;112(8):928–32.
109. Lee DH, Yang HN, Kim JC, et al. Sudden unilateral visual loss and brain infarction after autologous fat injection into nasolabial groove. Br J Ophthalmol 1996;80(11):1026–7.
110. Goldberg MF. Retinal vaso-occlusion in sickling hemoglobinopathies. Birth Defects Orig Artic Ser 1976;12(3):475–515.
111. Wilson RS, Ruiz RS. Bilateral central retinal artery occlusion in homocystinuria. A case report. Arch Ophthalmol 1969;82(2):267–8.
112. Kleiner RC, Najarian LV, Schatten S, et al. Vaso-occlusive retinopathy associated with antiphospholipid antibodies (lupus anticoagulant retinopathy). Ophthalmology 1989;96(6):896–904.
113. Bertram B, Remky A, Arend O, et al Protein C, protein S, and antithrombin III in acute ocular occlusive diseases. Ger J Ophthalmol 1995;4(6):332–5.
114. Vignes S, Wechsler B, Elmaleh C, et al. Retinal arterial occlusion associated with resistance to activated protein C. Br J Ophthalmol 1996;80(12):1111.
115. Talmon T, Scharf J, Mayer E, et al. Retinal arterial occlusion in a child with factor V Leiden and thermolabile methylene tetrahydrofolate reductase mutations. Am J Ophthalmol 1997;124(5):689–91.
116. Friedman S, Golan A, Shoenfeld A, et al Acute opthalmologic complications during the use of oral contraceptives. Contraception 1974;10(6):685–92.
117. Brown GC, Magargal L, Augsburger JJ, et al. Preretinal arterial loops and retinal arterial occlusion. Am J Ophthalmol 1979;87(5):646–51.
118. Purcell Jr JJ, Goldberg RE. Hyaline bodies of the optic papilla and bilateral acute vascular occlusions. Ann Ophthalmol 1974;6(10):1069–72, 74.
119. Fang IM, Huang JS. Central retinal artery occlusion caused by expansion of intraocular gas at high altitude. Am J Ophthalmol 2002;134(4):603–5.
120. Stambough JL, Dolan D, Werner R, et al. Ophthalmologic complications associated with prone positioning in spine surgery. J Am Acad Orthop Surg 2007;15(3):156–65.
121. Goldsmith MO. Occlusion of the central retinal artery following retrobulbar hemorrhage. Ophthalmologica 1967;153(3):191–6.
122. Linberg JV. Orbital emphysema complicated by acute central retinal artery occlusion: case report and treatment. Ann Ophthalmol 1982;14(8):747–9.
123. Abrams JD. Papillitis Complicated by Central Retinal Artery Occlusion. Br J Ophthalmol 1963;47:53.
124. Solomon SM, Solomon JH. Bilateral central retinal artery occlusions in polyarteritis nodosa. Ann Ophthalmol 1978;10(5):567–9.
125. Gold DH, Morris DA, Henkind P. Ocular findings in systemic lupus erythematosus. Br J Ophthalmol 1972;56(11):800–4.
126. Haynes BF, Fishman ML, Fauci AS, et al. The ocular manifestations of Wegener's granulomatosis. Fifteen years experience and review of the literature. Am J Med 1977;63(1):131–41.
127. Luo QL, Orcutt JC, Seifter LS. Orbital mucormycosis with retinal and ciliary artery occlusions. Br J Ophthalmol 1989;73(8):680–3.
128. Willerson Jr D, Aaberg TM, Reeser F, et al. Unusual ocular presentation of acute toxoplasmosis. Br J Ophthalmol 1977;61(11):693–8.
129. Brown GC, Tasman WS. Retinal arterial obstruction in association with presumed Toxocara canis neuroretinitis. Ann Ophthalmol 1981;13(12):1385–7.
130. Lightman DA, Brod RD. Branch retinal artery occlusion associated with Lyme disease. Arch Ophthalmol 1991;109(9):1198–9.
131. Colvard DM, Robertson DM, O'Duffy JD. The ocular manifestations of Behcet's disease. Arch Ophthalmol 1977;95(10):1813–7.
132. Solley WA, Martin DF, Newman NJ, et al. Cat scratch disease: posterior segment manifestations. Ophthalmology 1999;106(8):1546–53.
133. Susac JO, Hardman JM, Selhorst JB. Microangiopathy of the brain and retina. Neurology 1979;29(3):313–6.
134. Andersen MV, Dahl H, Fledelius H, et al. Central retinal artery occlusion in a patient with Fabry's disease documented by scanning laser ophthalmoscopy. Acta Ophthalmol (Copenh) 1994;72(5):635–8.
135. Ling W, Oftedal G, Simon T. Central retinal artery occlusion in Sydenham's chorea. Am J Dis Child 1969;118(3):525–7.
136. Beversdorf D, Stommel E, Allen C, et al. Recurrent branch retinal infarcts in association with migraine. Headache 1997;37(6):396–9.

Chapter 52

Acquired Retinal Macroaneurysms

Emily Y. Chew, Robert P. Murphy

CLINICAL DESCRIPTION

Acquired retinal macroaneurysms are fusiform or round dilations of the retinal arterioles that occur in the posterior fundus within the first three orders of arteriolar bifurcation. Often they are located at the site of an arteriolar bifurcation or an arteriovenous crossing (Fig. 52.1). The supratemporal artery is the most commonly reported site of involvement because patients with such involvement are more likely to have visual impairment. Women make up the majority of reported cases. Most cases are unilateral, while 10% may be bilateral. Retinal macroaneurysm was estimated to occur in 1 in 9000 in the Beijing Eye Study.[1]

Most commonly, retinal macroaneurysm affects patients in the sixth and seventh decades of life. Often associated are vascular problems such as hypertension and general arteriosclerotic cardiovascular disease, as noted by Robertson,[2] who first coined the term *retinal macroaneurysm*. Uncontrolled hypertension can present with a retinal artery macroaneurysm and its accompanying vitreous hemorrhage.[3] Other investigators have confirmed this association with hypertension.[4] Serum lipid and lipoprotein abnormalities have also been reported in patients with this condition.[5] Systemic investigations for hypertension and cardiovascular disease should be conducted in patients who have a retinal arteriolar macroaneurysm.

Although a patient with a retinal arteriolar macroaneurysm may be asymptomatic if the macula is not involved (Fig. 52.2), the most common clinical symptom is decline in central visual acuity as a result of retinal edema, exudation, or hemorrhage.[6] Bleeding from macroaneurysms can occur in the subretinal space, into the retina, beneath the internal limiting membrane, or into the vitreous. So-called hourglass hemorrhages are typical. Hemorrhage in the space beneath the retinal pigment epithelium may produce a dark lesion simulating an ocular tumor such as malignant melanoma,[7] or a lesion associated with age-related macular degeneration. A complication of the vitreous hemorrhage also includes the development of angle closure glaucoma.[8]

The hemorrhage may also partially or completely obscure the aneurysm (Fig. 52.3). Occasionally, multiple macroaneurysms occur. Other retinal microvascular changes associated with macroaneurysms include widening of the periarterial capillary-free zone around the area of the aneurysm, capillary dilation and nonperfusion, microaneurysms, and artery-to-artery collaterals.

DIAGNOSIS OF RETINAL MACROANEURYSM

Fluorescein angiography initially may fail to demonstrate the macroaneurysm because of blockage by the surrounding

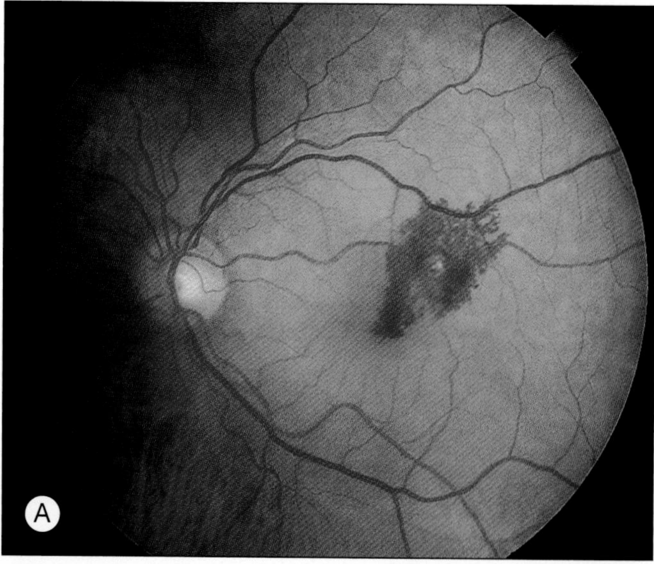

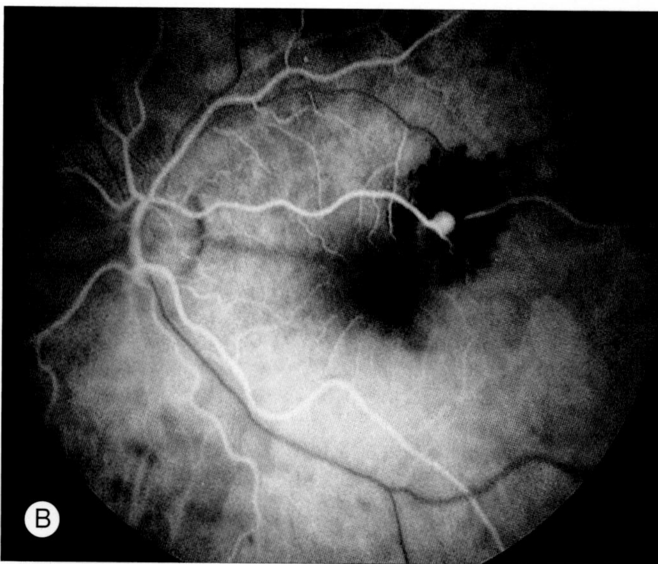

Fig. 52.1 (A) A 62-year-old woman with hypertension had a subretinal hemorrhage associated with a macroaneurysm in her left supratemporal artery. (B) The fluorescein angiogram demonstrated hypofluorescence from blockage from the retinal hemorrhage and hyperfluorescence of the retinal macroaneurysm itself, apparent as a round dilation located at the arteriolar bifurcation.

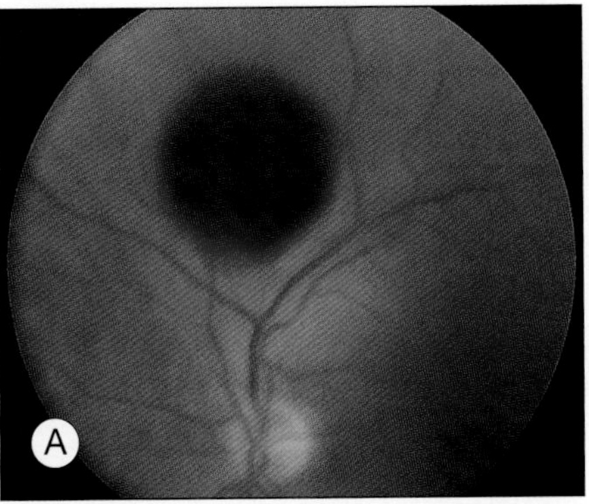

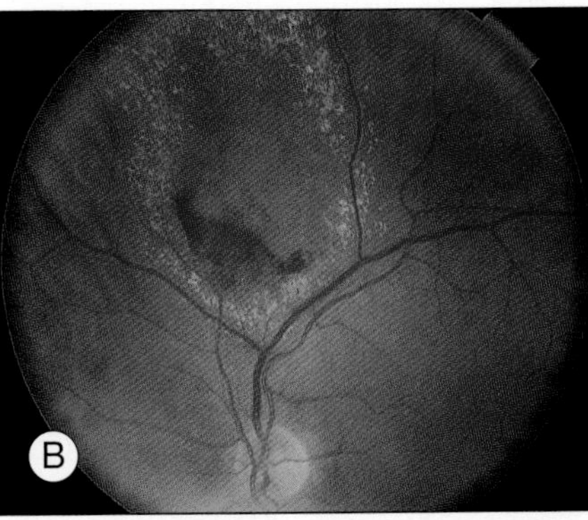

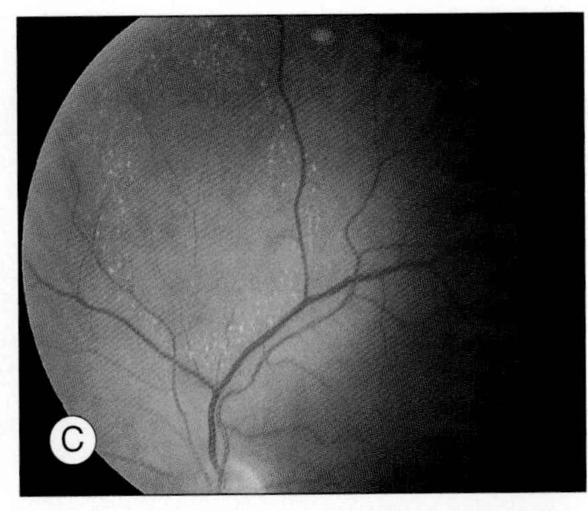

Fig. 52.2 (A) The retinal hemorrhage superior to the optic disc, associated with a retinal macroaneurysm, caused no ocular symptoms. (B) Six months later, the retinal macroaneurysm is partially obstructed by the resolving retinal hemorrhage, with a surrounding ring of lipid. (C) Eight months later, the macroaneurysm has spontaneously involuted, with complete resolution of the hemorrhage and a decrease in the lipid.

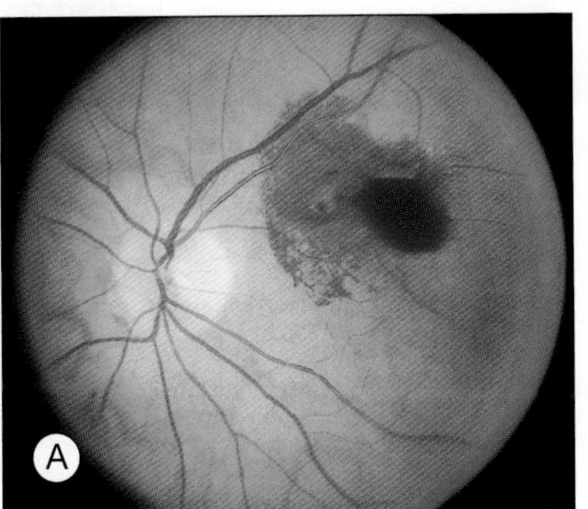

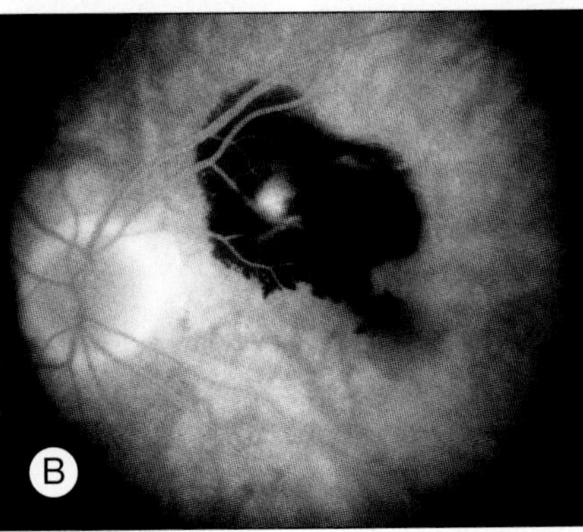

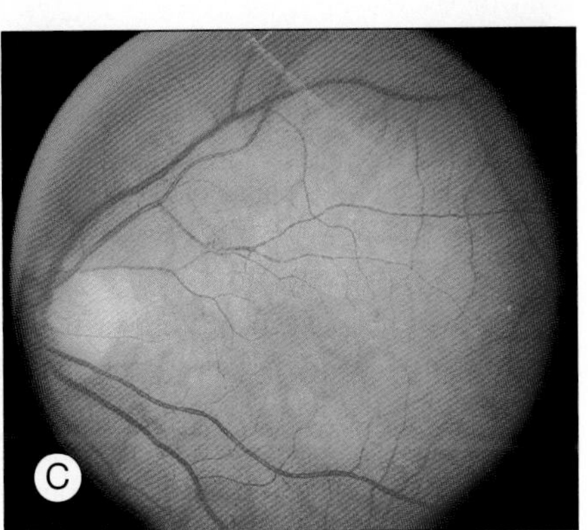

Fig. 52.3 (A) A preretinal hemorrhage partially obscures the retinal macroaneurysm. (B) The fluorescein angiogram shows the hyperfluorescence that corresponds to the hemorrhage and the hyperfluorescence of the retinal macroaneurysm. (C) At 20 months later, there is spontaneous resolution of the hemorrhage and the retinal macroaneurysm.

hemorrhage. Dense hemorrhage in the retina can cause marked hypofluorescence. In such cases of dense hemorrhage, indocyanine green angiography may be useful because its absorption and emission peak in the near-infrared range allow the light to penetrate the hemorrhage to a greater extent than fluorescein angiography.[9] A small case series using indocyanine green angiography has demonstrated these lesions to be pulsatile and contiguous with the arterial wall, pathognomonic of an insolated retinal artery macroaneurysm.[10] The macroaneurysm typically fills in the early arterial phase of the angiogram. The appearance of the late phase of the fluorescein angiogram varies, ranging from little staining of the vessel wall to marked leakage. Leakage of surrounding dilated capillaries also may be seen. The lipid often present in the macular area fails to block fluorescein unless the amount of lipid is massive. Macular hole formation following rupture of a retinal arterial macroaneurysm has been reported.[11,12]

Histopathologic studies of macroaneurysms have shown gross distension of the involved retinal arteriole. Surrounding this are fibroglial proliferation, dilated capillaries, extravasated blood, lipoidal exudates, and hemosiderin deposits.

Evaluation of the retinal structure with optical coherence tomography was conducted in a series of patients with retinal macroaneurysm.[13] Although most of the retinal structure was intact at the initial exam, subretinal hemorrhage or extensive exudative changes from retinal macroaneurysm can cause the deterioration of the foveal outer photoreceptor layer with a poor visual outcome.

NATURAL COURSE AND TREATMENT OF RETINAL MACROANEURYSMS

Several series have reported on the natural history and treatment response of macroaneurysms.[5,14,15] The yellow dye laser has been considered for treatment because of its theoretical advantages.[16] Some investigators believe the visual prognosis is excellent in most patients who have macroaneurysms and do not have treatment because the lesions can thrombose and undergo spontaneous involution with clearing of the macular exudate.[2] However, the exudative process may progress in some patients and cause structural damage to the macula with loss of vision (Fig. 52.4).[17] Moderate visual loss also may occur if bleeding causes secondary morphologic changes in the macula. No clear indication for treatment with laser photocoagulation has been established, and the beneficial effects of such treatments have not been proven.

Vitrectomy was performed for clearing the macular hemorrhage associated with the rupture of a macroaneurysm.[18] The results of vitrectomy are variable depending on the location of the hemorrhage from the retinal macroaneurysms. The vision is particularly poor in those patients who have dense submacular hemorrhage.[19]

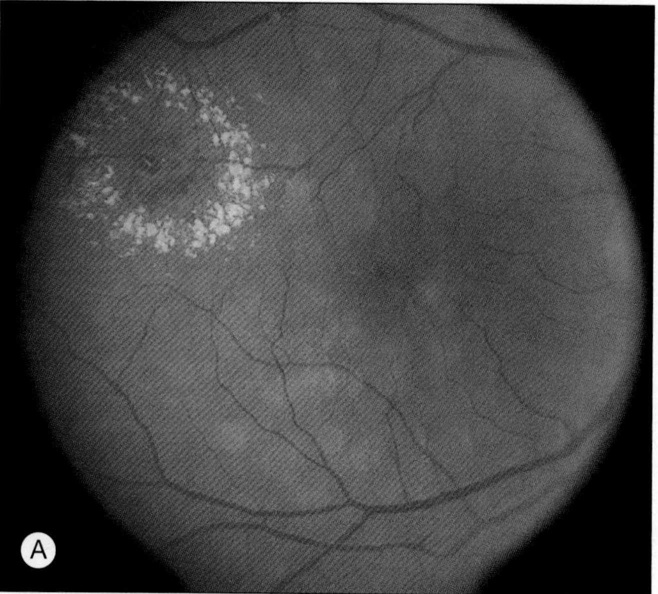

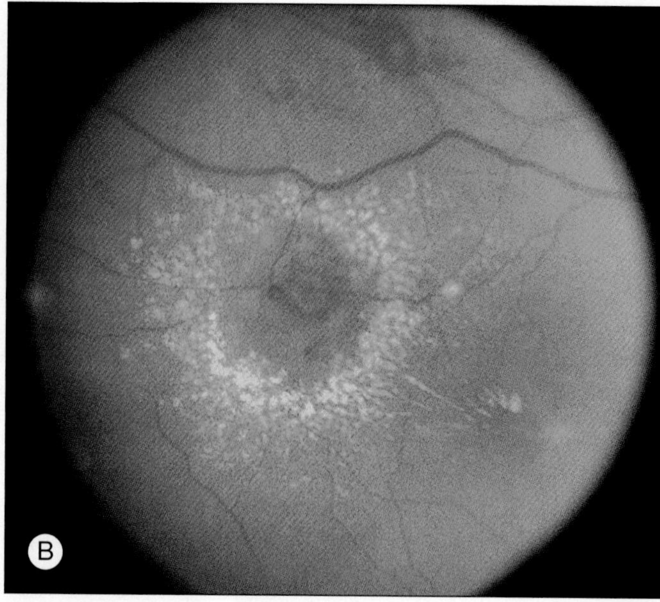

Fig. 52.4 (A) The retinal macroaneurysm caused a progressive increase in the retinal hard exudate, resulting in a visual acuity decrease to 20/25 in the right eye over a period of 22 months. (B) The edema and lipid were threatening the macula. The patient was offered treatment.

Pneumatic displacement with or without tissue plasminogen activator has also been used for the therapy of submacular hemorrhage associated with a macroaneurysms.[20] Yag laser has also been used to treat such premacular hemorrhage.[21] The surgical excision of the retinal macroaneruysm with scissors and diathermy followed by the drainage of the submacular hemorrhage was also explored in 2 cases, with some improvement in vision.[22]

Many investigators consider direct laser photocoagulation of the macroaneurysm if the lipid exudate coming from it threatens the fovea. Treatment when hemorrhage is present is fraught with difficulties. There is also the danger of occluding the retinal arteriole during treatment. This potential complication must always be considered when the distal portion of the arteriole being considered for treatment supplies the macula.

The differential diagnoses of retinal macroaneurysms include other retinal vascular abnormalities, including diabetic retinopathy, retinal telangiectasia, retinal capillary angioma, cavernous hemangioma, malignant melanoma,[7] and the hemorrhagic pigment epithelial detachment of age-related macular degeneration.[23]

REFERENCES

1. Xu L, Wang Y, Jonas JB. Frequency of retinal macroaneurysm in adult Chinese, Beijing Eye Study. Br J Ophthalmol 2007;91:840–1.
2. Robertson DM. Macroaneurysms of the retinal arteries. Trans Am Acad Ophthalmol Otolaryngol 1973;77:55–67.
3. Sekuri C, Kayikcioglu M, Kaykcioglu O. Retinal artery macroaneurysm as initial presentation of hypertension. Int J Cardiol 2004;93:87–8.
4. Moosavi RA, Fong KCS, Chopdar A. Retinal artery macroaneurysms: clinical and fluorescein angiographic features in 34 patients. Eye 2006;20:1011–20.
5. Cleary PE, Kohner EM, Hamilton AM, et al. Retinal macro-aneurysms. Br J Ophthalmol 1975;59:355–61.
6. Rabb MF, Gagliano DA, Teske MP. Retinal arterial macro-aneurysms, Surv Ophthalmol 1988;33:73–96.
7. Fritsche PL, Flipsen E, Polak BC. Subretinal hemorrhage from retinal arterial macroaneurysm simulating malignancy. Arch Ophthalmol 2000;118: 1704–5.
8. Arthur SN, Mason J, Roberts B, et al. CA. Secondary acute angle-closure glaucoma associated with vitreous hemorrhage after ruptured retinal arterial macroaneurysm. Am J Ophthalmol 2004;138:682–3.
9. Townsend-Pico WA, Meyers SM, Lewis H. Indocyanine green angiography in the diagnosis of retinal arterial macroaneurysms associated with submacular and preretinal hemorrhages: a case series. Am J Ophthalmol 2000;129:33–7.
10. Schneider U, Wagner AL, Kreissig I. Indocyanine green videoangiography of hemorrhagic retinal arterial macroaneurysms. Ophthalmologica 1997;211: 115–18.
11. Mitamura Y, Terashima H, Takeuchi S. Macular hole formation following rupture of retinal arterial macroaneurysm. Retina 2002;22:113–15.
12. Sato R, Yasukawa T, Hirano Y, et al. Early-onset macular holes following ruptured retinal arterial macroaneurysms. Graefes Arch Clin Exp Ophthalmol 2008;246:1779–82.
13. Tsujikawa A, Sakamoto A, Ota M, et al. Retinal structural changes associated with retinal arterial macroaneurysm examined with optical coherence tomography. Retina 2009;29:782–92.
14. Abdel-Khalek MN, Richardson J. Retinal macroaneurysm: natural history and guidelines for treatment. Br J Ophthalmol 1986;70:2–11.
15. Lewis RA, Norton EWD, Gass JDM. Acquired arterial macro-aneurysms of the retina. Br J Ophthalmol 1976;60:21–30.
16. Mainster MA, Whitacre MM. Dye yellow photocoagulation of retinal arterial macroaneurysms. Am J Ophthalmol 1988;105:97–8.
17. Yang CS, Tsai DC, Lee FL, et al. Retinal arterial macroaneurysms: risk factors of poor visual outcome. Ophthalmologica 2005;219:366–72.
18. Zhao P, Hayashi H, Oshima K, et al. Vitrectomy for macular hemorrhage associated with retinal arterial macroanerusym. Ophthalmol 2000;107: 613–17.
19. Nakamura H, Hayakawa K, Sawguchi S, et al. Visual outcome after vitreous, sub-internal limiting membrane, and/or submacular hemorrhage removal associated with ruptured retinal arterial macroaneurysms. Graefes Arch Lin Exp Ophthalmol 2008;246:661–9.
20. Mizutani T, Yasukawa T, Ito Y, et al. Pneumatic displacement of submacular hemorrhage with or without tissue plasminogen activator. Graefes Arch Clin Exp Ophthalmol 2011;249:1153–7.
21. Dahreddine M, Eldirani H, Mutsinzi E. Retinal macroaneurysm complicated by premacular hemorrhage: treatment by YAG laser disruption. J Fr Ophthalmol 2011;34:131.
22. Oie Y, Emi K. Surgical excision of retinal macroaneurysms with submacular hemorrhage. Jpn J Ophthalmol 2006;50:550–3.
23. Hochman MA, Seery CM, Zarbin MA. Pathophysiology and management of subretinal hemorrhage. Surv Ophthalmol 1997;42:195–213.

Branch Vein Occlusion

Alex Yuan, Peter K. Kaiser

Chapter 53

INTRODUCTION

Branch retinal vein occlusion (BRVO) is a common cause of retinal vascular disease.[1] The Beaver Dam Study estimated the 15-year cumulative incidence of retinal vein occlusions (RVO) at 2.3% in the population, with a majority of these (78%) being BRVO.[2] BRVO affects males and females equally and occurs most frequently between the ages of 60 and 70. The pathologic interruption of venous flow in these eyes almost always occurs at a retinal arteriovenous intersection, where a retinal artery crosses over a retinal vein.[3–7] Systemic vascular diseases such as hypertension and arteriosclerosis are risk factors for BRVO, probably because they lead to thickening of the retinal artery.[3,7] Other risk factors for BRVO include diabetes, smoking, hyperlipidemia, glaucoma, and ocular inflammatory disease.[8] Antiphospholipid antibodies, elevated plasma homocysteine levels, and low serum folate levels have also been associated with increased risk of vein occlusion.[9–11] A decreased risk is present in those with higher serum levels of high-density lipoprotein and light to moderate alcohol consumption.[8] Other studies have suggested an increased risk of BRVO in eyes with shorter axial lengths.[12–15] This section discusses the pathophysiology, clinical features, evaluation, and treatment of patients with BRVO.

PATHOGENESIS

Because BRVO mostly occurs at arteriovenous crossings,[4,8,16] underlying arterial disease may play a causative role. In 99% of 106 eyes with BRVO, the artery was located anterior to the vein at the obstructed site.[7,8] Histopathologically, the retinal artery and vein share a common adventitial sheath, and in some cases, a common medium.[17] The lumen of the vein may be compressed up to 33% at the crossing site.[7,18] The vitreous may also play a role in compression of susceptible arteriovenous crossing sites, as evidenced by studies demonstrating that eyes with decreased axial length and higher likelihood of vitreomacular attachment at the arteriovenous crossing are at increased risk of BRVO.[13,19]

Some have postulated that turbulent blood flow at the crossing site causes focal swelling of the endothelium and deeper vein wall tissue, leading to venous obstruction.[17,19,20] Other reports have demonstrated actual venous thrombus formation at the point of occlusion.[3,18] The resulting venous obstruction leads to elevation of venous pressure that may overload the collateral drainage capacity[21] and lead to macular edema and ischemia by mechanisms that are still under investigation. Unrelieved venous pressure can also result in rupture of the vein wall with intraretinal hemorrhage.[17] Vision loss from RVOs is typically due to macular ischemia, macular edema, or complications from neovascular disease.

CLINICAL FEATURES

Symptoms

Patients with BRVO present with sudden painless loss of vision or a visual field defect. Subclinical presentations may occur if a tributary distal to the macula or a nasal retinal vein is involved. Rarely, patients with BRVO will present with floaters from a vitreous hemorrhage if the initial vein occlusion was unrecognized and retinal neovascularization has occurred.

Signs

Patients typically present with a wedge-shaped distribution of intraretinal hemorrhage that is less marked if the occlusion is perfused (or nonischemic), and more extensive if the occlusion is nonperfused (or ischemic) and associated with retinal capillary nonperfusion. The Branch Vein Occlusion Study Group defined ischemic BRVO as those with greater than a total of five disc diameters of nonperfusion on fluorescein angiography (FA).[1] The location of the venous blockage determines the distribution of the intraretinal hemorrhage; if the venous obstruction is at the optic nerve head, two quadrants of the fundus may be involved, whereas if the occlusion is peripheral to the disc, one quadrant or less may be involved with the intraretinal hemorrhage. If the venous blockage is peripheral to tributary veins draining the macula, there may be no macular involvement and no decrease in visual acuity. The most common location for BRVOs is in the superotemporal quadrant.[5,6,22] This favored location may be attributed to a larger number of arteriovenous crossings in the superotemporal quadrant.

Figure 53.1 demonstrates the typical acute appearance of a BRVO involving the superotemporal quadrant of the right eye. A narrowed branch retinal vein passing under a retinal artery can sometimes be identified proximal to the hemorrhage. Rarely, a patient may present initially with very little intraretinal hemorrhage, which then becomes more extensive in the succeeding weeks to months. In these instances, it is presumed that an incomplete block at the arteriovenous crossing has progressed to more complete occlusion.

Over time the intraretinal hemorrhage may completely resorb. Without the characteristic segmental distribution of intraretinal hemorrhage, the ophthalmoscopic diagnosis may be more difficult, but the segmental distribution of retinal vascular abnormalities that occurred during the acute phase will persist and be apparent on FA. In many cases, macular edema may also be detected by optical coherence tomography (OCT). Consequently, in the chronic phase of the disease, after intraretinal hemorrhage absorption, the diagnosis may depend on detecting a segmental distribution of retinal vascular abnormalities that may include capillary nonperfusion, dilation of capillaries, microaneurysms, telangectatic vessels, and collateral vessel formation (Fig. 53.2).

Nonocular signs such as systemic hypertension have been associated with BRVOs.[2,8,23] Thus, systemic blood pressure may be elevated. In bilateral cases or cases involving young patients, systemic manifestations of infectious disease, inflammatory or autoimmune conditions, neoplasm, or hypercoagulable states may be present.

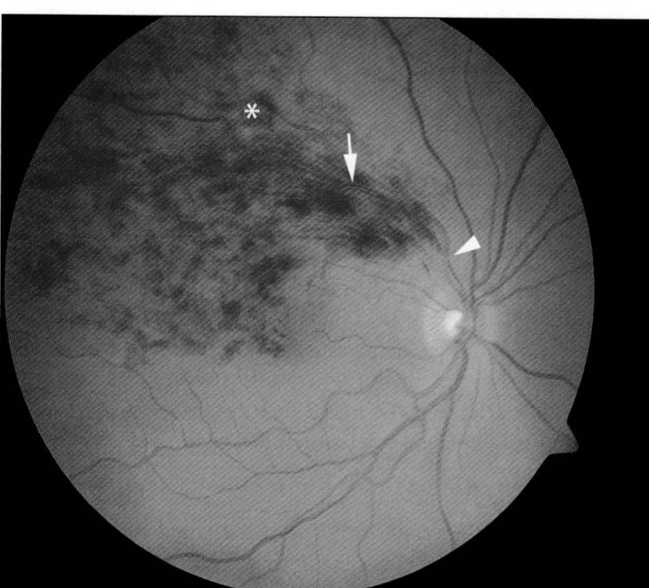

Fig. 53.1 Acute branch retinal vein occlusion. Intraretinal hemorrhages in a wedge-shaped pattern delineating the area drained by the occluded vein. The occluded vessel is often seen passing underneath a retinal artery (arrowhead). Cotton-wool spots (asterisk) are sometimes seen. Note the dilated and tortuous occluded vein (arrow) compared to the normal retinal vein in the inferior arcade.

Complications

There are three common vision-limiting complications of BRVO: (1) macular edema; (2) macular ischemia; and (3) sequelae of neovascularization. It is important to appreciate the variability of these complications before considering the benefits of treatment.[24–26]

During the acute phase, extensive intraretinal hemorrhages may obscure macular ischemia and macular leakage on FA. Under these circumstances it is impossible to evaluate the perfusion status by FA because the hemorrhage itself blocks the view of the vasculature. In addition, the hemorrhage in the foveal center may reduce visual acuity independently of any macular edema or ischemia. Since this reduction in visual acuity may recover completely if there is no other cause for the visual loss, such as macular edema or macular capillary nonperfusion, observation in these cases can be considered. When there is extensive foveal hemorrhage, OCT is an important ancillary test to look for macular edema. Although it may be difficult to provide a prognosis in the acute phase, it is helpful to recognize that about one-third to one-half of patients with BRVO have a return of vision to 20/40 or better without any therapy.

Retinal and iris neovascularization, vitreous hemorrhage, traction retinal detachment, and neovascular glaucoma are complications that manifest late in the course of the disease due to ischemia. With the exception of macular ischemia, these complications can largely be treated or prevented. Thus, it is important that patients with BRVO be closely followed. From the Branch Vein Occlusion Study, 31–41% of patients with ischemic BRVO (defined as >5 disc diameters of nonperfusion on FA) developed neovascularization or vitreous hemorrhage, compared with 11% of patients with nonischemic BRVO.[1]

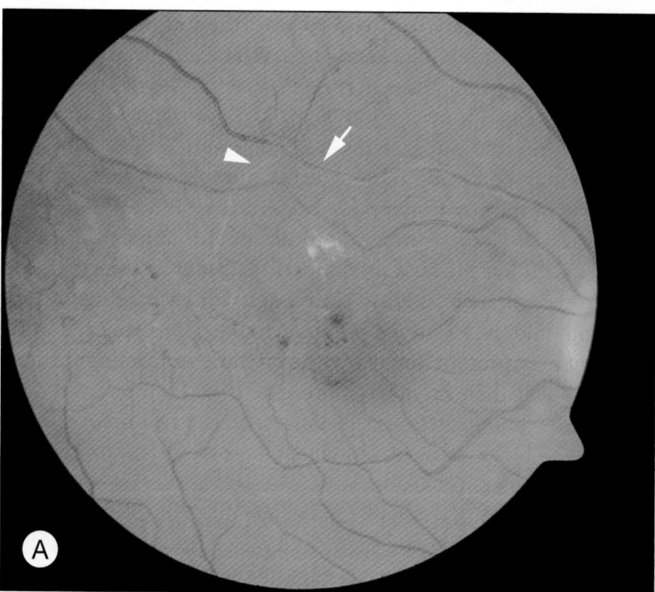

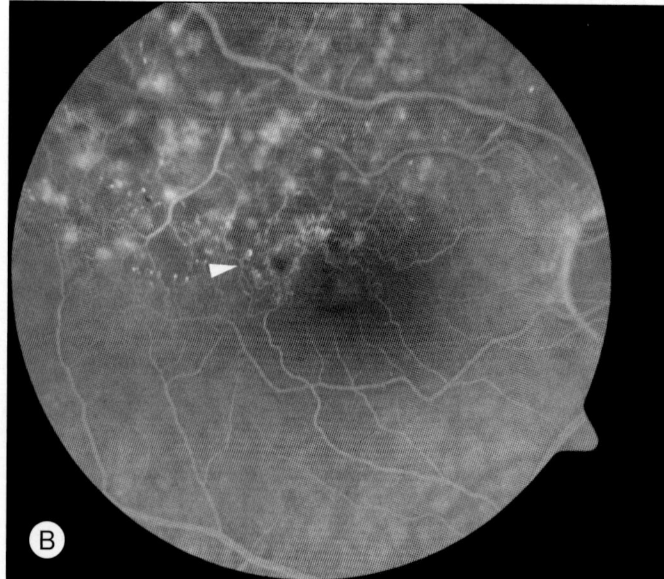

Fig. 53.2 Chronic branch retinal vein occlusion. (A) Color fundus photograph showing microaneurysms, exudates, and a sclerosed retinal vein (arrowhead) draining into a sheathed vessel (arrow). (B) Corresponding mid- to late-phase fluorescein angiogram shows abundant collaterals (arrowhead) and highlights the microvascular abnormalities.

CLINICAL EVALUATION

Clinical examination

A complete ophthalmic examination should be performed, paying particular attention to the history of glaucoma and signs of intraocular inflammation, since these are risk factors for BRVO. Careful examination of the iris and angle should be performed in appropriate cases to monitor for early signs of rubeosis or neovascular glaucoma. Initially, when the risk of macular edema and neovascularization is higher, patients should be followed every month. Once stable, and if visually significant macular edema and other complications are not present, follow-up can be extended.

Fluorescein angiography

To help verify the diagnosis and evaluate for complications, FA should be obtained to delineate the retinal vascular characteristics that may have prognostic significance: macular leakage and edema, macular ischemia, and large segments of capillary nonperfusion that may portend eventual neovascularization. FA is the only technique that will accurately define the capillary abnormalities in BRVO; it is therefore particularly important that high-quality angiography be obtained (Fig. 53.3).

The characteristic finding on FA is delayed filling of the occluded retinal vein. Varying amounts of capillary nonperfusion, blockage from intraretinal hemorrhages, microaneurysms, telangiectatic collateral vessels, and dye extravasation from macular edema or retinal neovascularization are other features encountered. In chronic cases, when the hemorrhages have resolved, microvascular changes on FA may provide the only clues of a previous BRVO.

When FA demonstrates macular leakage and edema with cystoid involvement of the fovea, but no capillary nonperfusion, it is presumed that the macular edema is the cause of vision loss. Under these circumstances, about one-third of patients will spontaneously regain some vision. However, patients who have had decreased vision for over 1 year as a result of macular edema are much less likely to regain vision spontaneously. When macular edema is present ophthalmoscopically within the first 6 months after a BRVO and there is little or no leakage on FA, macular ischemia may be the cause of the macular edema. In such circumstances, the edema almost always spontaneously resorbs in the first year after the occlusion, often with return of vision.[27]

Unfortunately, acute BRVOs with dense intraretinal hemorrhages may make FA interpretation challenging due to blockage of fluorescence by the hemorrhages. Thus, it is advisable to obtain FA only after the intraretinal hemorrhages have cleared significantly from the macula. Other diagnostic tests, such as OCT, can be obtained in the acute phase to aid in the diagnosis of macular edema.

Wide-field angiography

Wide-field angiography is not a commonly used imaging modality for patients with BRVO, but a recent study supports its utility. Ultrawide-field FA using the Optos C200MA revealed a correlation between nonperfusion in the peripheral retina with macular edema and retinal neovascularization.[28] Future studies to determine if laser photocoagulation of the nonperfused peripheral retina decreases macular edema and neovascularization may alter the therapeutic paradigm. In patients with recalcitrant macular edema or retinal neovascularization, wide-field angiography may reveal peripheral areas of nonperfusion helping to guide targeted laser photocoagulation.

Optical coherence tomography

OCT has arguably become the most important imaging modality in the treatment of patients with BRVO and macular edema. OCT offers a noninvasive and rapid method of quantitatively measuring macular edema. OCT is frequently used to monitor the response to treatment of macular edema and has been used in place of FA in some treatment trials for BRVO. Unlike FA,

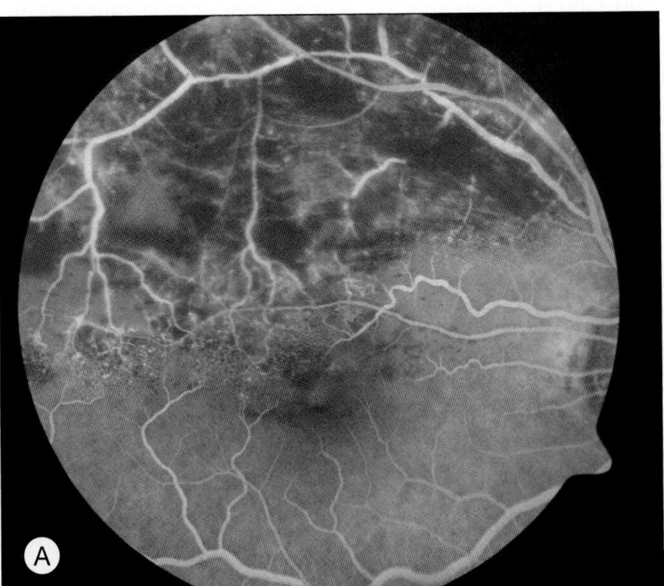

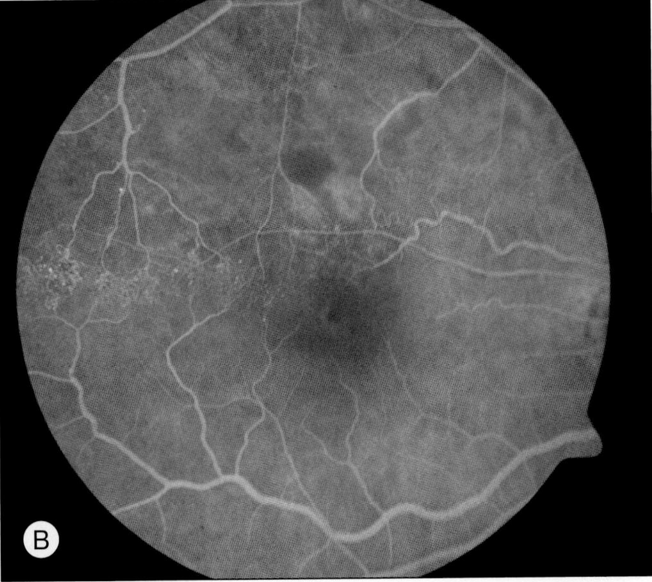

Fig. 53.3 Fluorescein angiogram of branch retinal vein occlusion. (A) Blocked fluorescence from intraretinal hemorrhage is common in acute branch retinal vein occlusion. Note the telangiectatic vessels forming collaterals across the horizontal raphe. The hemorrhages obscure underlying areas of capillary nonperfusion and edema. (B) Six months later, the hemorrhages have cleared, revealing small patches of nonperfusion and macular edema.

intraretinal hemorrhages have a minimal effect on the interpretation of OCT, making this imaging modality helpful, even in the acute setting with foveal hemorrhage. The characteristic findings of BRVO on OCT are cystoid edema, intraretinal hyperreflectivity from hemorrhages, shadowing from edema and hemorrhages, and occasionally subretinal fluid[29,30] (Fig. 53.4A). In chronic cases, photoreceptor inner-segment–outer-segment junction abnormalities from long-standing macular ischemia and macular edema may also be seen (Fig. 53.4B).

Diagnostic workup

Young patient

BRVO typically occurs in patients beyond their sixth decade of life. When they present in younger patients, an underlying predisposing condition may be suspected. In this younger patient population, a detailed history should be taken, including the use of oral contraception in females, or the use of other medications that can promote a hypercoagulable state or thromboembolism. Workup should be performed in consultation with an internist. Systemic blood pressure should be checked and the patient should be screened for diabetes. In suspected cases, infectious causes such as Lyme disease, syphilis, or human immunodeficiency virus should be screened. In young patients with other systemic findings suggestive of inflammatory disease or coagulopathy, workup should include a complete blood count, prothrombin time/partial thromboplastin time/international normalized ratio, lipid panel, serum homocysteine, anticardiolipin antibodies, antinuclear antibodies with lupus anticoagulant, protein C/S, and activated protein C resistance (factor V Leiden).[10,11,31]

In young patients without systemic symptoms suggestive of a coagulopathy, careful consideration should be given in consultation with an internist prior to initiating an exhaustive systemic workup unless a vision-disabling complication has occurred. It is unclear whether the risks involved with lifelong anticoagulation are justified.

Older patient

In patients older than 60, additional workup is not necessary since the majority of these cases are idiopathic or due to hypertension or atherosclerosis.

Bilateral or numerous BRVO patients

In bilateral cases or in cases with a history of multiple BRVOs, searching for an infectious or inflammatory disorder or hypercoagulopathy may be warranted. There are numerous case reports of patients with bilateral vein occlusions and systemic inflammatory disorders or hypercoagulopathies; however the vast majority can be attributed to systemic hypertension.[32–37] The workup should proceed in the manner described for young patients.

TREATMENT OPTIONS

Medical treatment

In cases where a hypercoagulopathy has been identified, anticoagulation may be considered in consultation with an internist. In most cases, however, anticoagulant therapy has not been shown to be beneficial in either the prevention or the management of BRVO. Since the systemic administration of anticoagulants can be associated with systemic complications, and could, in theory, increase the severity of intraretinal hemorrhage occurring in the acute phase, such therapy is not recommended. Treatment of BRVO has focused on the management of vision-limiting complications.

Laser treatment

Branch Vein Occlusion Study for macular edema

The collaborative Branch Vein Occlusion Study (BVOS),[38] a multicenter randomized clinical trial supported by the National Eye Institute, reported that argon laser photocoagulation may reduce visual loss from macular edema for those eyes that meet study eligibility criteria and are treated according to that protocol. Important eligibility criteria included fluorescein-proven perfused macular edema involving the foveal center, absorption of intraretinal hemorrhage from the foveal center, recent BRVO (usually 3–18 months' duration), no diabetic retinopathy, and vision reduced to 20/40 or worse after best refraction.

In the BVOS,[38] argon laser photocoagulation was applied in a grid pattern throughout the leaking area demonstrated by FA (Fig. 53.5). Coagulation extended no closer to the fovea than the edge of the capillary-free zone and no further into the periphery

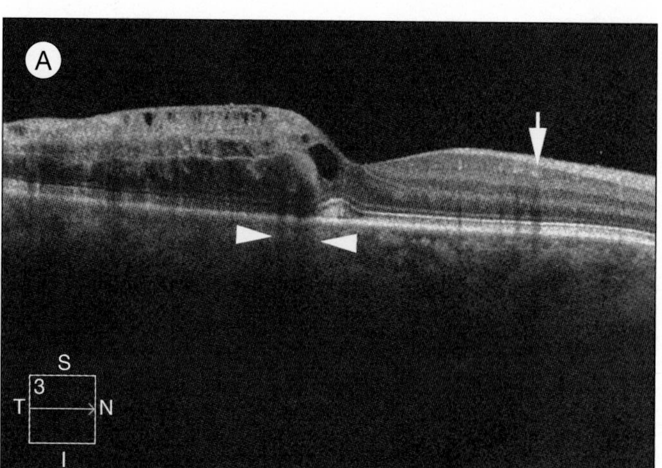

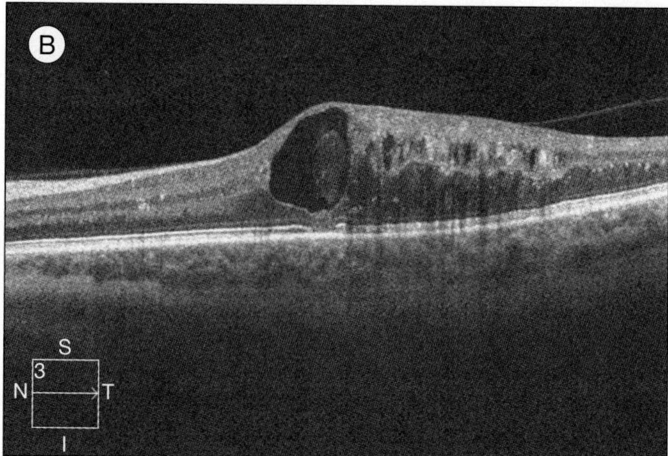

Fig. 53.4 Spectral-domain optical coherence tomography of an eye with a branch retinal vein occlusion (BRVO). (A) Raster scan of the BRVO in Figure 53.1 reveals cystoid macular edema, intraretinal fluid, and shadowing (between the arrowheads). Intraretinal heme (arrow) appears hyperreflective and produces a shadow on optical coherence tomography. (B) Raster scan of a chronic BRVO with inner-segment–outer-segment abnormalities and a large cyst.

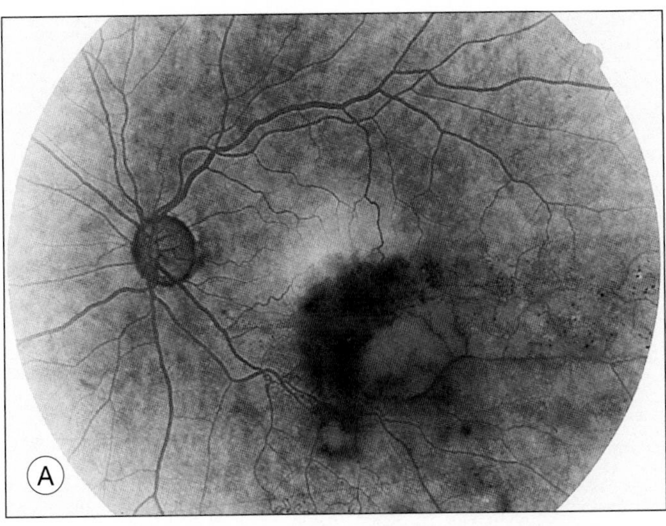

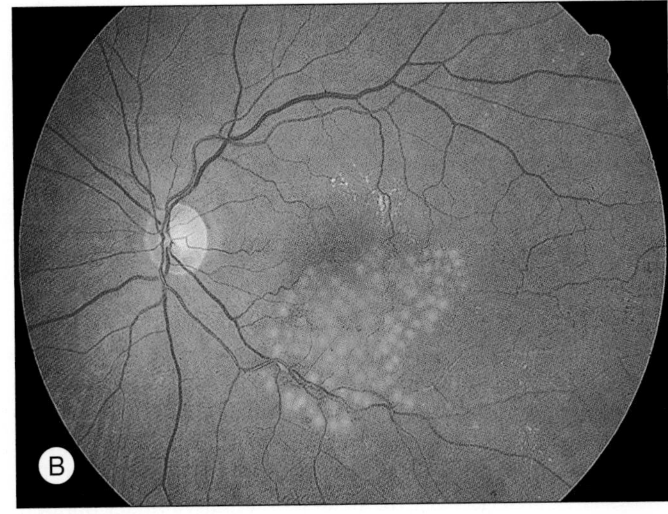

Fig. 53.5 Grid macular laser for macular edema. (A) Fluorescein angiogram, late phase, demonstrating macular edema with foveal involvement. (B) Immediate posttreatment fundus photograph showing grid pattern of laser photocoagulation.

than the major vascular arcade. Recommended treatment parameters included a duration of 0.1 second, a 100-µm diameter spot size, and a power setting sufficient to produce a "medium" white burn. FA was repeated 2–4 months after the treatment, and additional photocoagulation was applied to residual areas of leakage if reduced visual acuity persisted. Improvement in visual acuity was assessed in several ways.[38] When improvement was defined as reading two or more Snellen lines (beyond baseline) at two consecutive visits, treated eyes showed visual improvement more often than untreated eyes. After 3 years of follow-up, 63% of treated eyes gained two or more lines of vision, compared to 36% of untreated eyes. The average gain in visual acuity for treated eyes was one more Snellen line than in untreated eyes.

Before laser photocoagulation is performed, it is important to obtain high-quality FAs of the macula; the FA must demonstrate that the macular edema involves the center of the fovea and that there is not a large amount of capillary nonperfusion adjacent to the capillary-free zone that could explain the visual loss. In addition, it is important to follow patients for a length of time sufficient to ascertain that macular edema is not resolving spontaneously. During this period of follow-up, it should be demonstrated that there is clearing of intraretinal hemorrhage and that there is no hemorrhage in the center of the fovea that could account for a spontaneously reversible cause of visual loss. In the application of the grid photocoagulation, laser absorption occurs at the level of the pigment epithelium; photocoagulation is not applied to close the leaking and dilated capillary vasculature directly and immediately. Although it is not understood how the laser treatment may act in lessening edema, it is interesting to note that preliminary experimental studies in the normal primate have shown a decrease in capillary diameter when this form of therapy is used and when laser absorption occurs at the level of the pigment epithelium.[39] One explanation for the effect of grid pattern photocoagulation is that it results in a thinning of the retina (in particular the outer retina), reducing oxygen consumption and increasing choroidal delivery of oxygen to the inner retina, producing a consequent autoregulatory constriction of the retinal vasculature in the leaking area and thereby decreasing the edema.

In the application of grid pattern laser photocoagulation, it is crucial to obtain good definition of landmarks so that the center of the fovea can be identified and avoided. Since landmarks frequently may be obscured in the macula after BRVO, such cases can be managed more effectively and safely by treating well peripheral to the capillary-free zone in the first sitting. When the patient returns in 2 months for follow-up evaluation, a repeat FA may identify more clearly the amount of further treatment that needs to be applied closer to the edge of the capillary-free zone, because the pigmentation of the previous treatment is then visible. Consequently, treatment in this next sitting may be advanced closer to the edge of the capillary-free zone, if that is deemed necessary because of persistent foveal edema and vision loss. The placement of grid laser treatment in this repetitively staged fashion may be safer and appears to be just as effective as a single treatment. It has never been established that macular edema must be treated quickly or that long-standing edema produces irreversible macular damage in the first 2–3 years.

For the grid treatment used in the BVOS, the argon blue-green wavelength was employed.[38] This is the only wavelength that has been proven effective and it is unknown whether argon green and krypton red photocoagulation are equally effective. In other diseases, when laser treatment is applied inside the capillary-free zone, it is recognized that krypton red and argon green laser photocoagulation are absorbed less than blue-green by the xanthophyll pigment of the inner retina that is present in increasing concentrations close to the foveal center. However, because the grid treatment never comes closer to the fovea than the capillary-free zone, the BVOS did not encounter any problems with the argon blue-green laser in this region; consequently, this laser continues to be recommended.

The summary recommendations for management of acute branch vein occlusion from the BVOS emphasize waiting at least 3–6 months before considering laser therapy. If the vision is reduced to 20/40 or worse, wait 3–6 months for sufficient clearing of retinal hemorrhage to permit high-quality FA and then evaluate for macular edema and macular ischemia. If perfused macular edema accounts for the visual loss, and vision continues to be 20/40 or worse without spontaneous improvement, consider grid macular photocoagulation. However, this conclusion needs to be balanced against the improvements in vision seen with recent anti-vascular endothelial growth factor (VEGF) agents. If macular ischemia accounts for the visual loss, no laser treatment is recommended to improve vision.

Branch Vein Occlusion Study for neovascularization

A separate group of patients in the BVOS were randomized to receive scatter panretinal photocoagulation to prevent neovascular complications. The BVOS demonstrated that prophylactic scatter laser photocoagulation can lessen subsequent neovascularization and, if neovascularization already exists, that peripheral scatter laser photocoagulation can lessen subsequent vitreous hemorrhage.[1] Only eyes with the type of BRVO that shows large areas (>5 disc diameters) of retinal capillary nonperfusion are at risk for developing neovascularization. About 40% of these eyes develop neovascularization, and of this 40%, about 60% will experience periodic vitreous hemorrhage. Retinal or disc neovascularization, or both, may develop at any time within the first 3 years after an occlusion but are most likely to appear within the first 6–12 months after the occlusion. If peripheral scatter laser photocoagulation is applied in eyes with large areas of nonperfusion, the incidence of neovascularization can be reduced from about 40% to 20%. However, if one were to treat prophylactically, many eyes (60%) that would never develop neovascularization would receive peripheral scatter laser photocoagulation. For this reason, it is recommended that laser photocoagulation be applied only after neovascularization is observed.

Iris neovascularization is a rare complication of BRVO; it appears, however, that diabetes (with or without retinopathy) may increase this risk. Retinal neovascularization is particularly difficult to recognize in BRVO because the collaterals that develop frequently may mimic neovascularization. Arising presumably from pre-existing capillaries, these collaterals occur as vein-to-vein channels around the blockage site, across the temporal raphe, and in other locations to bypass the blocked retinal segment. These collaterals frequently become quite tortuous, mimicking the appearance of neovascularization if they are evaluated by ophthalmoscopy alone. When it is unclear whether an abnormal vascular pattern represents collateral formation or true neovascularization, the FA (Fig. 53.6) can be helpful because leakage from neovascularization is more prominent than from collateral vessels.

The BVOS data strongly suggest that photocoagulation after the development of neovascularization is as effective in preventing vitreous hemorrhage as is photocoagulation before the development of neovascularization.[1] When neovascularization is unequivocally confirmed by FA, peripheral scatter laser photocoagulation can reduce the likelihood of vitreous hemorrhage from about 60% to 30%. As demonstrated in Figure 53.7, the scatter laser photocoagulation can be applied with argon blue-green laser to achieve "medium" white burns (200–500 μm in diameter) spaced one burn width apart and covering the entire area of capillary nonperfusion, as defined by FA, but extending no closer than two disc diameters from the center of the fovea and extending peripherally at least to the equator. Retrobulbar anesthesia is used as needed for discomfort associated with the scatter photocoagulation.

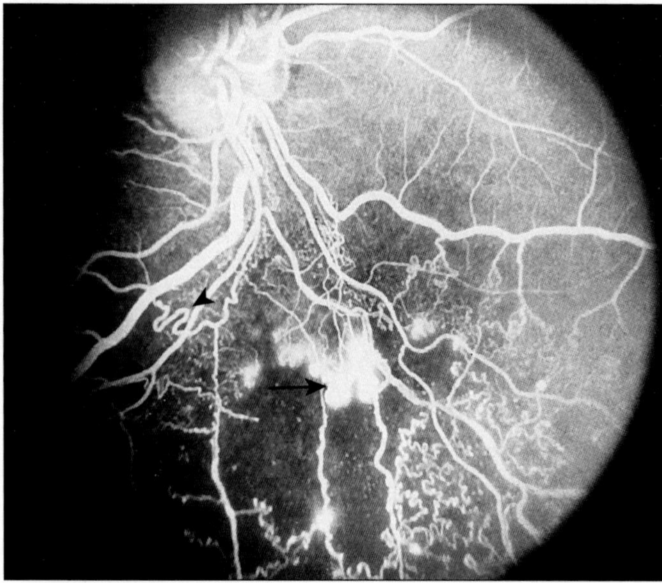

Fig. 53.6 Retinal neovascularization with leakage (arrow) can be differentiated from collaterals that are not leaking (arrowhead).

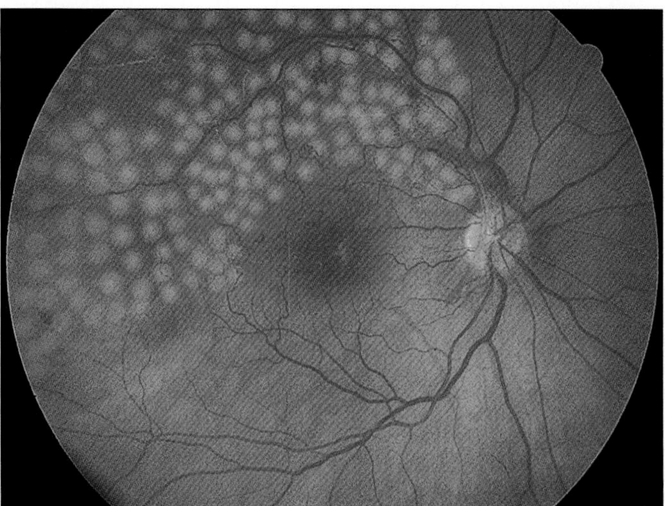

Fig. 53.7 Immediate posttreatment fundus photograph showing pattern of peripheral scatter photocoagulation.

Of patients who develop neovascularization, approximately 60% experience episodes of vitreous hemorrhage if the condition is left untreated. The short- and long-term visual consequences of vitreous hemorrhage in BRVO have not been carefully studied. In some cases, the hemorrhage may be mild or may clear spontaneously without causing permanent visual impairment. However, in some patients, vitreous hemorrhage from neovascularization can lead to prolonged visual disability in the affected eye. When the hemorrhage is dense, B-scan ultrasonography may help rule out an associated traction retinal detachment. Most eyes can be observed. If the vitreous hemorrhage does not spontaneously clear in a few months, a pars plana vitrectomy with sector endolaser photocoagulation should be considered.

Familiarity with the laser treatment technique is required to individualize the treatment. Important variables, such as residual intraretinal hemorrhage, thickness of the retina from edema, location of collaterals, and presence of retinal traction, influence the exact mode of therapy within the above general treatment guidelines for the management of macular edema and neovascularization. There are numerous complications of laser photocoagulation; however, it is generally recognized that with proper attention to detail, complications are infrequent. Side-effects of treatment, including generation of scotoma, merit careful consideration and discussion with the patient before initiation of treatment. It is particularly important to recognize that laser photocoagulation should never be placed over extensive intraretinal hemorrhage in the acute phase of branch vein occlusion because the laser energy will be absorbed by the intraretinal hemorrhage rather than at the level of the pigment epithelium, likely damaging the nerve fiber layer and possibly enhancing the development of preretinal fibrosis.

Steroid treatment

Macular edema results from increased vascular permeability mediated at least in part by an increase in VEGF.[40,41] Corticosteroids have been shown to inhibit the expression of VEGF and therefore reduce macular edema in animal models.[42,43] The anti-inflammatory effects of corticosteroids may further potentiate its anti-VEGF effects and help attenuate macular edema. Intraocular corticosteroids, however, have significant side-effects, including cataract formation and glaucoma. Several trials have evaluated the use of corticosteroids in the treatment of macular edema in BRVO.

SCORE (triamcinolone) study

In the Standard care vs Corticosteroid for Retinal vein occlusion (SCORE) BRVO study, the effectiveness and safety of intravitreal triamcinolone acetate (IVTA) for the treatment of macular edema from BRVO were evaluated.[44] In this multicenter, randomized controlled study, 411 patients were randomized to receive macular grid laser, 1 mg IVTA, or 4 mg IVTA. Retreatment was allowed every 4 months for each group unless the treatment was successful, futile, or contraindicated. There was no significant difference in vision or the reduction of macular edema measured by OCT at the end of 12 months between each group. Respectively, 29%, 26%, and 27% of eyes in the laser, 1 mg IVTA, and 4 mg IVTA groups gained a visual acuity score of ≥15 ETDRS letters. Subgroup analysis of pseudophakic eyes also failed to demonstrate a significant difference in vision. Median (interquartile range) center point thicknesses measured by OCT were 228 (163–364) μm, 354 (183–486) μm, and 274 (180–481) μm in the laser, 1 mg, and 4 mg IVTA groups, respectively. Three-year results from 128 patients suggested that the laser group maintained a significantly greater average increase in vision (12.9 letters) compared with the two IVTA groups (4.4 letters, 1 mg and 8.0 letters, 4 mg). Significant side-effects from IVTA included cataract formation and elevation of intraocular pressure requiring treatment. Both side-effects were dose-dependent.

As a result of this study, IVTA is not recommended as first-line therapy for macular edema in BRVO. However it can be considered in patients where macular grid laser or other therapies are ineffective, as the treatment was found to be relatively safe, especially in pseudophakic eyes.

GENEVA (dexamethasone implant) study

The Global Evaluation of implantable dexamethasone in retinal Vein occlusion with macular edema (GENEVA) study evaluated a sustained-release, biodegradable, dexamethasone intravitreal implant (Ozurdex, Allergan, Irvine, CA) for the treatment of macular edema in central retinal vein occlusion (CRVO) and BRVO patients.[45] Ozurdex is a biodegradable copolymer of poly (D,L-lactide-co-glycolide) acid (PLGA) containing micronized dexamethasone. It is injected intravitreally through a pars plana route using a 23-gauge custom injector, and it gradually releases the total dose of dexamethasone over several months via Krebs cycle breakdown of the PLGA into lactic and glycolic acid, and finally into water and carbon dioxide. In this multicenter, randomized controlled study, an increase in best-corrected visual acuity (BCVA) of ≥15 ETDRS letters was achieved in 30% of the Ozurdex 0.7 mg group ($n = 291$), 26% of the 0.35 mg group ($n = 260$), and 13% of the sham group ($n = 279$) 60 days after injection (peak response) in patients with BRVO ($P < 0.001$ for each group versus sham). A statistically significant difference between both Ozurdex groups and sham was seen up to 90 days after injection. At 90 days after injection, there was a significant improvement ($P < 0.001$) in central retinal thickness measured by OCT in both Ozurdex groups, compared with the sham group. The mean ± SD decrease in central retinal thickness at 90 days was 208 ± 201 μm, 177 ± 197 μm, and 85 ± 173 μm in the 0.7 mg, 0.35 mg, and sham groups, respectively. The OCT results are from pooled data including both BRVO and CRVO patients. The only complications that were significantly greater in the Ozurdex groups compared with sham were elevated intraocular pressure and anterior-chamber cell. Most eyes with elevated intraocular pressures were successfully managed with topical therapy, but five eyes required a procedure to lower the pressure adequately. In the 6 months of this study, there was no difference in the rate of cataract formation, and no endophthalmitis cases were reported. A long-term study of repeated treatments is currently underway and will help determine the safety and optimal interval for retreatment.

A major difference between the GENEVA study and other recent BRVO studies is the absence of a macular grid laser group, or rescue laser treatment for the sham group. The GENEVA study showed that the dexamethasone implant is an alternative treatment to macular grid laser in the appropriate patient population (i.e., no glaucoma, pseudophakic) and is approved by the Food and Drug Administration (FDA) for this indication.

Anti-VEGF treatment

Macular edema results from increased vascular permeability as a response to retinal nonperfusion. In patients with BRVO, retinal ischemia leads to the secretion of VEGF, which leads to increased vascular permeability, vasodilation, migration of endothelial cells, and neovascularization.[40,41,46] Increased vascular permeability and perhaps vasodilation lead to retinal edema. Thus, inhibition of VEGF is an attractive treatment for macular edema from BRVO. There are several anti-VEGF agents currently being investigated for use in treatment of RVOs. We will discuss the use of ranibizumab (Lucentis), bevacizumab (Avastin), pegaptanib (Macugen), and aflibercept (Eylea). Bevacizumab is a full-length, humanized monoclonal antibody that binds all VEGF-A isoforms and is FDA-approved for colorectal cancer, but is used off-label in the eye. Ranibizumab is an affinity-purified, humanized monoclonal antibody fragment (Fab) that binds all VEGF-A isoforms. Pegaptanib is an aptamer targeted against only the VEGF 165 isoform, and no other isoforms. Aflibercept is a fusion protein composed of key binding domains from VEGF receptors 1 and 2 fused to the Fc portion of human immunoglobulin G. Aflibercept binds with high affinity to all VEGF-A isoforms and placental growth factor. At this time, only ranibizumab is FDA-approved for the treatment of RVO.

BRAVO (ranibizumab) study

The Branch Retinal Vein Occlusion (BRAVO) study was a prospective, multicenter, randomized controlled study to evaluate the efficacy and safety of ranibizumab in the treatment of macular edema from BRVO.[47] Patients were randomized into three groups: (1) sham injection ($n = 132$); (2) 0.3 mg ranibizumab ($n = 134$); and (3) 0.5 mg ranibizumab ($n = 131$). In the first 6 months, injections were given monthly. A 28-day screening period excluded patients with spontaneous and rapid improvement in vision of >10 ETDRS letters. At month 3, a patient was eligible for rescue laser if a gain of <5 ETDRS letters, or improvement of <50 µm in central subfield thickness was observed compared with the visit 3 months prior. If rescue laser was not applied at month 3, the same criteria were used to determine eligibility for rescue laser at each subsequent monthly visit. At 6 months, both ranibizumab groups gained +16.6 and +18.3 ETDRS letters (0.3 mg and 0.5 mg groups, respectively) compared with a gain of +7.3 letters in the control group ($P < 0.0001$ for each group versus sham). The percentage of patients who improved greater than 15 ETDRS letters was 55.2% and 61.1% (0.3 mg and 0.5 mg groups, respectively) compared with 28.8% in the control ($P < 0.0001$ for each group versus sham). Concurrent with the improvement in visual acuity, the mean decrease in OCT central retinal thickness was −337.3 µm and −345.2 µm (0.3 mg and 0.5 mg groups, respectively) compared with −157.7 µm in the control ($P < 0.0001$ for each group versus sham). During the first 6 months, 54.5% of the control group required rescue laser therapy compared with 18.7% in the 0.3 mg and 19.8% in the 0.5 mg ranibizumab groups.

After the first 6 months, all three groups were allowed to receive "as needed" (PRN) intravitreal ranibizumab at monthly intervals if they had vision ≤ 20/40 or mean central foveal thickness ≥250 µm. Despite receiving only PRN treatments, patients in both ranibizumab groups maintained their vision gain at 12 months (unpublished results). Although the control group showed a benefit from the PRN treatment regimen, the final vision gained at 12 months was not equivalent in all three groups (unpublished results). Not surprisingly, the mean change in central foveal thickness was maintained in both ranibizumab groups at 12 months while there was a significant improvement observed in the control group after PRN treatment was initiated (unpublished results). At the end of 12 months, the incidence of adverse events in all groups was similar. One patient in the 0.5 mg ranibizumab group suffered from endophthalmitis, which is a known complication of intravitreal injections.

The BRAVO study showed that ranibizumab is superior to traditional laser treatment for macular edema from BRVO with little risk of adverse events. The current recommendation is therefore to treat patients diagnosed with macular edema from BRVO with monthly 0.5 mg ranibizumab. If treatment fails after 3 months (<5 ETDRS letter gain, or improvement of <50 µm in central subfield thickness), then traditional grid macular laser should be performed. The BRAVO study showed that PRN treatment did not adversely affect the visual outcome after five scheduled monthly injections. However, the timing of when to switch to PRN treatment was not evaluated in the BRAVO study and thus the decision to switch to PRN dosing should be based on factors such as improvement in visual acuity, residual macular edema on OCT imaging, success of prior injections, and expectations of the patient.

Other anti-VEGF inhibitors

Bevacizumab

There are numerous case series and small prospective studies evaluating the efficacy of intravitreal bevacizumab in treating macular edema from BRVO.[48–55] All of these studies show that bevacizumab is effective at improving visual acuity and decreasing macular edema, as measured by OCT. One of the larger retrospective studies compared two different doses of bevacizumab, 1.25 and 2.5 mg.[50] Forty-five patients with an average 35.2 weeks of follow-up completed the study. There were no functional or anatomical differences between the two dosages, and both required similar numbers of injections. At 6 months the 1.25 mg group improved by an average +5.1 lines compared with +4.8 lines in the 2.5 mg group. The central macular thickness decreased by −184 µm in the 1.25 mg group and −145 µm in the 2.5 mg group. A second large retrospective review with 1 year of follow-up showed similar results with a mean improvement of +13 letters at 6 months and +15 letters at 1 year with a decrease in central retinal thickness of −161 µm at 6 months and −205 µm at 1 year.[53]

Although there are no studies directly comparing the efficacy of bevacizumab with ranibizumab or macular grid laser, the results reported in the BRAVO study are roughly equivalent to those reported in multiple studies with bevacizumab. It is reasonable to extrapolate that bevacizumab may be effective in treating macular edema from BRVO and may be a viable alternative to macular grid laser, corticosteroids, and other anti-VEGF agents.

Pegaptanib

A phase II study of pegaptanib for the treatment of BRVO showed significant improvements in vision and central macular thickness.[56] However, due to limited enrollment with the increasing use of bevacizumab and ranibizumab, larger trials with pegaptanib have not been conducted. For the most part, with the availability of bevacizumab and ranibizumab, pegaptanib is not used as a primary treatment for macular edema in BRVO patients.

Aflibercept

Currently, there are no trials evaluating intravitreal aflibercept specifically for macular edema from BRVO. However, two multicenter, randomized controlled phase III trials (COPERNICUS and GALILEO) are evaluating its use in patients with macular edema secondary to CRVO. In the COPERNICUS study, patients with macular edema from CRVO were randomized to receive 2 mg aflibercept ($n = 114$) or sham ($n = 74$). Only patients with vision between 20/40 and 20/320 with central retinal thickness of ≥250 µm were included. Patients were retreated every 4 weeks with aflibercept. Preliminary results of the COPERNICUS study[57] showed that, after 24 weeks, 56.1% of the treatment group gained ≥15 ETDRS letters compared with 12.3% of the sham group ($P < 0.0001$). There was an average of +17.3 ETDRS letters gained in the treatment group compared with −4.0 letters lost in the sham

($P < 0.001$). There was a reduction of −457.8 µm in central retinal thickness in the treatment group compared with −144.8 µm in the sham group ($P < 0.001$). A parallel phase III clinical trial (GALILEO) is currently underway with preliminary results that are similar to the COPERNICUS study.

Given the results of ranibizumab in the BRAVO study, and the results of ranibizumab in the phase III study for CRVO (CRUISE), it is likely that the results of aflibercept in COPERNICUS and GALILEO can be extrapolated to BRVO. Currently, aflibercept is not FDA-approved for either indication.

Experimental treatments

FAVOR (iluvien) study

A sustained-release, non-erodable, intravitreal implant of fluocinolone acetonide (Iluvien) is currently under investigation for use in patients with macular edema due to BRVO or CRVO of >3 months' duration in a phase II trial. The implant is introduced through a 25-gauge needle using a special injector during an in-office procedure, and releases 0.2 µg/day of the steroid. The implant is designed to sustain release for 36 months.

Surgical management

Vitrectomy with or without sheathotomy

The majority of the venous lesions in BRVO occur downstream from the arteriovenous crossing site. In a retrospective review of color photographs and FAs of patients with BRVO, Kumar and associates[19] identified venous narrowing at the crossing site, and in the majority of cases, evidence of downstream hemodynamic changes on angiogram, including venous-phase leakage, abnormal flow, and presumed thrombi. The authors also suggested that removal of the compressive factor by sectioning the adventitial sheath (sheathotomy) may be an effective treatment for BRVO.

In the first report of sheathotomy for BRVO, Osterloh and Charles[58] reported significant visual improvement in the one case presented (20/200 to 20/25+ over 8 months). In the second report, Opremcak and Bruce[59] reported equal or improved visual acuity in 12 of 15 patients (80%). Ten of those patients (67%) had improved postoperative visual acuities, with an average gain of four lines of vision. Three patients had a decline in visual acuity, with an average of two lines of vision lost. All patients had marked resolution of the intraretinal hemorrhage and edema. Visual symptoms from BRVO ranged from 1 to 12 months, with an average of 3.3 months. In 2 patients, intraoperative retinal vascular bleeding was controlled with intraocular diathermy. No patient in the series developed worsening edema, ischemia, retinal neovascularization, or secondary vitreous hemorrhage. Mester and Dillinger reported 43 cases of BRVO treated with sheathotomy with similar results. In 16 of the cases, removal of the internal limiting membrane in the area of the arteriovenous crossing was also performed.[60] In contrast, Cahill and colleagues reported 27 cases of BRVO treated with vitrectomy and sheathotomy without a statistically significant improvement in postoperative median visual acuity.[61]

Other authors have experienced difficulty in separating the artery from the vein at the crossing site. Han and colleagues reported 20 cases of vitrectomy and attempted sheathotomy. While the visual outcome results were similar to those reported by Opremcak and Bruce, in 19 of the 20 cases, the authors were unable to separate the artery from the vein.[62] No randomized, controlled study evaluating the benefit of sheathotomy has been published.[63]

There is evidence that vitreomacular attachment itself may contribute to the development of macular edema in BRVO.[64] Saika and coworkers reported reduction in macular edema and restoration of normal foveal contour in 10 of 19 eyes after vitrectomy, posterior hyaloid separation, and intraocular gas tamponade.[65] Possible explanations for the clinical improvements in these studies include removal of vitreous traction, increased oxygenation of the macula, and tamponade of the macula by intraocular gas.

Due to the risk of intraoperative complications and the availability of less invasive alternatives, vitrectomy with or without sheathotomy has limited clinical use as a first-line therapy.

FOLLOW-UP

The major complications that can lead to vision loss in patients with BRVO include macular edema, macular ischemia, and neovascularization. Treatment is available for macular edema and neovascularization and follow-up should be tailored to monitor the development of these complications adequately. Initially, patients should be followed closely every month or 2 months for the development of macular edema and/or neovascularization. Anti-VEGF therapy with or without macular laser should be initiated for patients with macular edema without spontaneous improvement. Once macular edema has stabilized or has resolved, the follow-up interval can be extended to 3–6 months or even longer for stable chronic cases. Patients with previously untreated retinal nonperfusion measuring >5 disc diameters should be followed at closer intervals (3 months) due to the increased risk for neovascular complications. In patients where anti-VEGF therapy and/or laser is not showing sufficient therapeutic efficacy, steroids can be considered, particularly in pseudophakic patients. Only after failure of medical therapy should surgery be considered.

CONCLUSIONS

BRVO is a common cause of vision loss, but many treatment options are available and emerging therapies are under investigation. Current treatments for macular edema include macular grid laser and intravitreal anti-VEGF injections and intraocular corticosteroids. All have side-effects. Anti-VEGF therapy typically lasts 4–6 weeks, necessitating frequent reinjections, and corticosteroids can induce vision-limiting side-effects such as glaucoma and cataract. However, due to its longer duration of action, corticosteroids may play an important role in pseudophakic patients or in patients who do not respond to laser and anti-VEGF agents. Alternate delivery methods, including topical, local depot injections, or perhaps even systemic delivery, will likely emerge. Combination therapy with anti-VEGF agents acting to reduce macular edema rapidly, and therapy aimed at restoring blood flow such as vitrectomy with or without sheathotomy for BRVO may merit future investigation to limit the need for chronic pharmacotherapy.

Disclosure

Peter K. Kaiser is consultant to Genentech, Regeneron, Bayer, Novartis. P.K.K. and the Cole Eye Institute receive research grant support from Research to Prevent Blindness.

REFERENCES

1. Branch Vein Occlusion Study Group. Argon laser scatter photocoagulation for prevention of neovascularization and vitreous hemorrhage in branch vein occlusion. A randomized clinical trial. Arch Ophthalmol 1986;104:34–41.
2. Klein R, Moss SE, Meuer SM, et al. The 15-year cumulative incidence of retinal vein occlusion: the Beaver Dam Eye Study. Arch Ophthalmol 2008;126: 513–8.
3. Bowers DK, Finkelstein D, Wolff SM, et al. Branch retinal vein occlusion. A clinicopathologic case report. Retina 1987;7:252–9.
4. Weinberg D, Dodwell DG, Fern SA. Anatomy of arteriovenous crossings in branch retinal vein occlusion. Am J Ophthalmol 1990;109:298–302.
5. Feist RM, Ticho BH, Shapiro MJ, et al. Branch retinal vein occlusion and quadratic variation in arteriovenous crossings. Am J Ophthalmol 1992;113: 664–8.
6. Zhao J, Sastry SM, Sperduto RD, et al. Arteriovenous crossing patterns in branch retinal vein occlusion. The Eye Disease Case-Control Study Group. Ophthalmology 1993;100:423–8.
7. Frangieh GT, Green WR, Barraquer-Somers E, et al. Histopathologic study of nine branch retinal vein occlusions. Arch Ophthalmol 1982;100:1132–40.
8. Eye Disease Case-control Study Group. Risk factors for branch retinal vein occlusion. Am J Ophthalmol 1993;116:286–96.
9. Lahey JM, Kearney JJ, Tunc M. Hypercoagulable states and central retinal vein occlusion. Curr Opin Pulm Med 2003;9:385–92.
10. Lahey JM, Tunc M, Kearney J, et al. Laboratory evaluation of hypercoagulable states in patients with central retinal vein occlusion who are less than 56 years of age. Ophthalmology 2002;109:126–31.
11. Cahill MT, Stinnett SS, Fekrat S. Meta-analysis of plasma homocysteine, serum folate, serum vitamin B(12), and thermolabile MTHFR genotype as risk factors for retinal vascular occlusive disease. Am J Ophthalmol 2003;136: 1136–50.
12. Ariturk N, Oge Y, Erkan D, et al. Relation between retinal vein occlusions and axial length. Br J Ophthalmol 1996;80:633–6.
13. Majji AB, Janarthanan M, Naduvilath TJ. Significance of refractive status in branch retinal vein occlusion. A case-control study. Retina 1997;17:200–4.
14. Simons BD, Brucker AJ. Branch retinal vein occlusion. Axial length and other risk factors. Retina 1997;17:191–5.
15. Timmerman EA, de Lavalette VW, van den Brom HJ. Axial length as a risk factor to branch retinal vein occlusion. Retina 1997;17:196–9.
16. Duker JS, Brown GC. Anterior location of the crossing artery in branch retinal vein obstruction. Arch Ophthalmol 1989;107:998–1000.
17. Seitz R. The retinal vessels. Saint Louis: CV Mosby; 1964. pp. 20–74.
18. Bandello F, Tavola A, Pierro L, et al. Axial length and refraction in retinal vein occlusions. Ophthalmologica 1998;212:133–5.
19. Kumar B, Yu DY, Morgan WH, et al. The distribution of angioarchitectural changes within the vicinity of the arteriovenous crossing in branch retinal vein occlusion. Ophthalmology 1998;105:424–7.
20. Clemett RS. Retinal branch vein occlusion. Changes at the site of obstruction. Br J Ophthalmol 1974;58:548–54.
21. Christoffersen NL, Larsen M. Pathophysiology and hemodynamics of branch retinal vein occlusion. Ophthalmology 1999;106:2054–62.
22. Klein R, Klein BE, Moss SE, et al. The epidemiology of retinal vein occlusion: the Beaver Dam Eye Study. Trans Am Ophthalmol Soc 2000;98:133–41, discussion 141-3.
23. Mitchell P, Smith W, Chang A. Prevalence and associations of retinal vein occlusion in Australia. The Blue Mountains Eye Study. Arch Ophthalmol 1996;114:1243–7.
24. Gutman FA, Zegarra H. Macular edema secondary to occlusion of the retinal veins. Surv Ophthalmol 1984;28(Suppl):462–70.
25. Hayreh SS, Rojas P, Podhajsky P, et al. Ocular neovascularization with retinal vascular occlusion - III. Incidence of ocular neovascularization with retinal vein occlusion. Ophthalmology 1983;90:488–506.
26. Joffe L, Goldberg RE, Magargal LE, et al. Macular branch vein occlusion. Ophthalmology 1980;87:91–8.
27. Finkelstein D. Ischemic macular edema. Recognition and favorable natural history in branch vein occlusion. Arch Ophthalmol 1992;110:1427–34.
28. Prasad PS, Oliver SC, Coffee RE, et al. Ultra wide-field angiographic characteristics of branch retinal and hemicentral retinal vein occlusion. Ophthalmology 2010;117:780–4.
29. Spaide RF, Lee JK, Klancnik JK, Jr, et al. Optical coherence tomography of branch retinal vein occlusion. Retina 2003;23:343–7.
30. Lerche RC, Schaudig U, Scholz F, et al. Structural changes of the retina in retinal vein occlusion - imaging and quantification with optical coherence tomography. Ophthalmic Surg Lasers 2001;32:272–80.
31. Turello M, Pasca S, Daminato R, et al. Retinal vein occlusion: evaluation of "classic" and "emerging" risk factors and treatment. J Thromb Thrombolysis 2010;29:459–64.
32. Chai SM, Mathur R, Ong SG. Retinal vasculopathy in Fanconi anemia. Ophthalmic Surg Lasers Imaging 2009;40:498–500.
33. Sungur G, Hazirolan D, Hekimoglu E, et al. Late-onset Behcet's disease: demographic, clinical, and ocular features. Graefes Arch Clin Exp Ophthalmol 2010;248:1325–30.
34. De Salvo G, Li Calzi C, Anastasi M, et al. Branch retinal vein occlusion followed by central retinal artery occlusion in Churg–Strauss syndrome: unusual ocular manifestations in allergic granulomatous angiitis. Eur J Ophthalmol 2009;19: 314–7.
35. Mandel ER, Schwartz PL, Rosen DA. Bilateral retinal branch vein occlusion. Ann Ophthalmol 1982;14:387, 390–1.
36. Tseng MY, Chen YC, Lin YY, et al. Simultaneous bilateral central retinal vein occlusion as the initial presentation of acute myeloid leukemia. Am J Med Sci 2010;339:387–9.
37. Yau JW, Lee P, Wong TY, et al. Retinal vein occlusion: an approach to diagnosis, systemic risk factors and management. Intern Med J 2008;38: 904–10.
38. Branch Vein Occlusion Study Group. Argon laser photocoagulation for macular edema in branch vein occlusion. Am J Ophthalmol 1984;98:271–82.
39. Wilson DJ, Finkelstein D, Quigley HA, et al. Macular grid photocoagulation. An experimental study on the primate retina. Arch Ophthalmol 1988;106: 100–5.
40. Aiello LP, Avery RL, Arrigg PG, et al. Vascular endothelial growth factor in ocular fluid of patients with diabetic retinopathy and other retinal disorders. N Engl J Med 1994 ;331:1480–7.
41. Noma H, Minamoto A, Funatsu H, et al. Intravitreal levels of vascular endothelial growth factor and interleukin-6 are correlated with macular edema in branch retinal vein occlusion. Graefes Arch Clin Exp Ophthalmol 2006;244: 309–15.
42. Zhang X, Bao S, Lai D, et al. Intravitreal triamcinolone acetonide inhibits breakdown of the blood–retinal barrier through differential regulation of VEGF-A and its receptors in early diabetic rat retinas. Diabetes 2008;57: 1026–33.
43. McAllister IL, Vijayasekaran S, Chen SD, et al. Effect of triamcinolone acetonide on vascular endothelial growth factor and occludin levels in branch retinal vein occlusion. Am J Ophthalmol 2009;147:838–46, 846.e1–2.
44. Scott IU, Ip MS, VanVeldhuisen PC, et al. A randomized trial comparing the efficacy and safety of intravitreal triamcinolone with standard care to treat vision loss associated with macular edema secondary to branch retinal vein occlusion: the Standard Care vs Corticosteroid for Retinal Vein Occlusion (SCORE) study report 6. Arch Ophthalmol 2009;127:1115–28.
45. Haller JA, Bandello F, Belfort Jr R, et al. Randomized, sham-controlled trial of dexamethasone intravitreal implant in patients with macular edema due to retinal vein occlusion. Ophthalmology 2010;117:1134–46.e3.
46. Bates DO. Vascular endothelial growth factors and vascular permeability. Cardiovasc Res 2010;87:262–71.
47. Campochiaro PA, Heier JS, Feiner L, et al. Ranibizumab for macular edema following branch retinal vein occlusion: six-month primary end point results of a phase III study. Ophthalmology 2010;117:1102–12.e1.
48. Rabena MD, Pieramici DJ, Castellarin AA, et al. Intravitreal bevacizumab (Avastin) in the treatment of macular edema secondary to branch retinal vein occlusion. Retina 2007;27:419–25.
49. Kriechbaum K, Michels S, Prager F, et al. Intravitreal Avastin for macular oedema secondary to retinal vein occlusion: a prospective study. Br J Ophthalmol 2008;92:518–22.
50. Wu L, Arevalo JF, Roca JA, et al. Comparison of two doses of intravitreal bevacizumab (Avastin) for treatment of macular edema secondary to branch retinal vein occlusion: results from the Pan-American Collaborative Retina Study Group at 6 months of follow-up. Retina 2008;28:212–9.
51. Gunduz K, Bakri SJ. Intravitreal bevacizumab for macular oedema secondary to branch retinal vein occlusion. Eye (Lond) 2008;22:1168–71.
52. Jaissle GB, Leitritz M, Gelisken F, et al. One-year results after intravitreal bevacizumab therapy for macular edema secondary to branch retinal vein occlusion. Graefes Arch Clin Exp Ophthalmol 2009;247:27–33.
53. Gregori NZ, Rattan GH, Rosenfeld PJ, et al. Safety and efficacy of intravitreal bevacizumab (avastin) for the management of branch and hemiretinal vein occlusion. Retina 2009;29:913–25.
54. Figueroa MS, Contreras I, Noval S, et al. Results of bevacizumab as the primary treatment for retinal vein occlusions. Br J Ophthalmol 2010;94:1052–6.
55. Pai SA, Shetty R, Vijayan PB, et al. Clinical, anatomic, and electrophysiologic evaluation following intravitreal bevacizumab for macular edema in retinal vein occlusion. Am J Ophthalmol 2007;143:601–6.
56. Wroblewski JJ, Wells 3rd JA, Gonzales CR. Pegaptanib sodium for macular edema secondary to branch retinal vein occlusion. Am J Ophthalmol 2010; 149:147–54.
57. VEGF Trap-Eye In CRVO. Primary endpoint results of the phase 3 COPERNICUS study. ARVO 2011; May 3, 2011; 2011.
58. Osterloh MD, Charles S. Surgical decompression of branch retinal vein occlusions. Arch Ophthalmol 1988;106:1469–71.
59. Opremcak EM, Bruce RA. Surgical decompression of branch retinal vein occlusion via arteriovenous crossing sheathotomy: a prospective review of 15 cases. Retina 1999;19:1–5.
60. Mester U, Dillinger P. Vitrectomy with arteriovenous decompression and internal limiting membrane dissection in branch retinal vein occlusion. Retina 2002;22:740–6.
61. Cahill MT, Kaiser PK, Sears JE, et al. The effect of arteriovenous sheathotomy on cystoid macular oedema secondary to branch retinal vein occlusion. Br J Ophthalmol 2003;87:1329–32.
62. Han DP, Bennett SR, Williams DF, et al. Arteriovenous crossing dissection without separation of the retina vessels for treatment of branch retinal vein occlusion. Retina 2003;23:145–51.
63. Cahill MT, Fekrat S. Arteriovenous sheathotomy for branch retinal vein occlusion. Ophthalmol Clin North Am 2002;15:417–23.
64. Takahashi MK, Hikichi T, Akiba J, et al. Role of the vitreous and macular edema in branch retinal vein occlusion. Ophthalmic Surg Lasers 1997;28:294–9.
65. Saika S, Tanaka T, Miyamoto T, et al. Surgical posterior vitreous detachment combined with gas/air tamponade for treating macular edema associated with branch retinal vein occlusion: retinal tomography and visual outcome. Graefes Arch Clin Exp Ophthalmol 2001;239:729–32.

Central Retinal Vein Occlusion

Paul Hahn, Prithvi Mruthyunjaya, Sharon Fekrat

Central retinal vein occlusion (CRVO) is a retinal vascular condition that may cause significant ocular morbidity. It commonly affects men and women equally and occurs predominantly in persons over the age of 65 years.[1–3] In this population there may be associated systemic vascular disease, including hypertension and diabetes.[4] Younger individuals who present with a clinical picture of CRVO may have an underlying hypercoagulable or inflammatory etiology.[5,6] Population-based studies report the prevalence of CRVO at <0.1 to 0.4%.[2,7,8] CRVO is usually a unilateral disease; however, the annual risk of developing any type of retinal vascular occlusion in the fellow eye is approximately 1% per year, and it is estimated that up to 7% of persons with CRVO may develop CRVO in the fellow eye within 5 years of onset in the first eye.[1,9] Individuals with CRVO demonstrate a significant decrease in vision-related quality of life with increased healthcare costs and resource use as compared to a reference group without ocular disease.[10,11] CRVO may impact a person's ability to perform activities of daily living, especially in cases of bilateral CRVO or when concurrent ocular disease limits vision in the fellow eye.

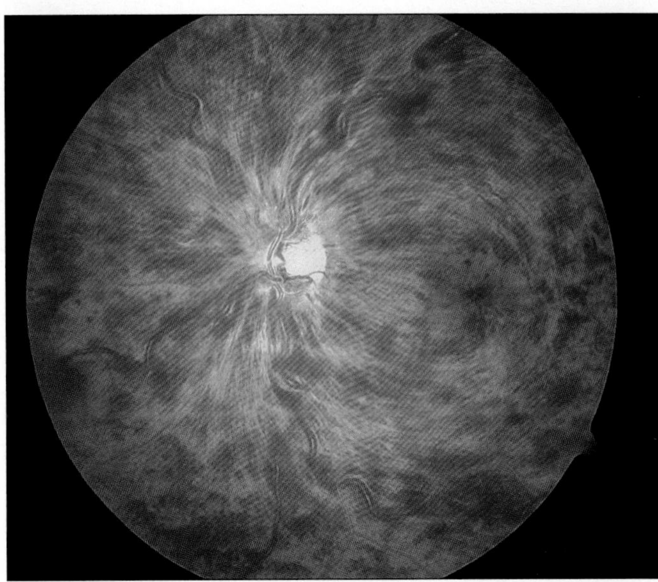

Fig. 54.1 Fundus photograph of a central retinal vein occlusion with extensive intraretinal hemorrhage. Extensive blocking on fluorescein angiography in such an occlusion precludes accurate determination of perfusion status.

CLINICAL FEATURES

CRVO usually presents with sudden painless loss of vision, but it may also present with a history of gradual visual decline that may correlate with a series of less severe occlusions. The typical clinical constellation in CRVO includes retinal hemorrhages (both superficial flame-shaped and deep blot type) in all four quadrants of the fundus with a dilated, tortuous retinal venous system. The hemorrhages radiate from the optic nerve head, are variable in quantity, and may result in the classic "blood and thunder" appearance (Fig. 54.1). Optic nerve head swelling, cotton-wool spots, splinter hemorrhages, and macular edema are present to varying degrees (Figs 54.2 and 54.3). Breakthrough vitreous hemorrhage may also be observed.

A cilioretinal artery occlusion can occur in association with CRVO. Together, these occlusions have been hypothesized to constitute a distinct clinical entity arising from a sudden increase in the intraluminal capillary pressure due to CRVO, inducing relative occlusion of the cilioretinal artery whose perfusion pressure is lower than the central retinal artery.[12,13] Rarely, a central retinal arterial occlusion may also accompany a CRVO.[14]

With time, the extent of retinal hemorrhage may decrease or resolve completely with variable degrees of secondary retinal pigment epithelium alterations. The time course for resolution of the hemorrhages varies and is dependent on the amount of hemorrhage produced by the occlusion. Macular edema often chronically persists despite resolution of retinal hemorrhages (Fig. 54.4). An epiretinal membrane may also form. Optociliary shunt vessels can develop on the optic nerve head, a sign of newly formed collateral channels with the choroidal circulation (Fig. 54.5). Neovascularization of the optic disc (NVD) or retinal neovascularization elsewhere (NVE) may develop as a response to secondary retinal ischemia. The vessels that comprise NVD are typically of smaller caliber than optociliary shunt vessels, branch into a vascular network resembling a net, and will leak on fluorescein angiography. Fibrovascular proliferation from NVD or NVE may result in vitreous hemorrhage or traction retinal detachment.

The natural history of CRVO was examined in the Central Vein Occlusion Study (CVOS), a randomized multicenter clinical trial of 728 eyes with CRVO. In this study, visual acuity at the time of presentation was variable but an important prognostic indicator of final visual outcome. Baseline visual acuity was 20/40 or better in 29% of affected eyes, 20/50–20/200 in 43%, and 20/250 or worse in 28%; median baseline acuity was 20/80.[3,15] Of those with initial visual acuity of 20/40 or better, the majority maintained this acuity. Individuals with intermediate visual acuity (20/50–20/200) had a variable outcome: 21% improved to better than 20/50, 41% stayed in the intermediate group, and 38% were worse than 20/200. Persons with poor visual

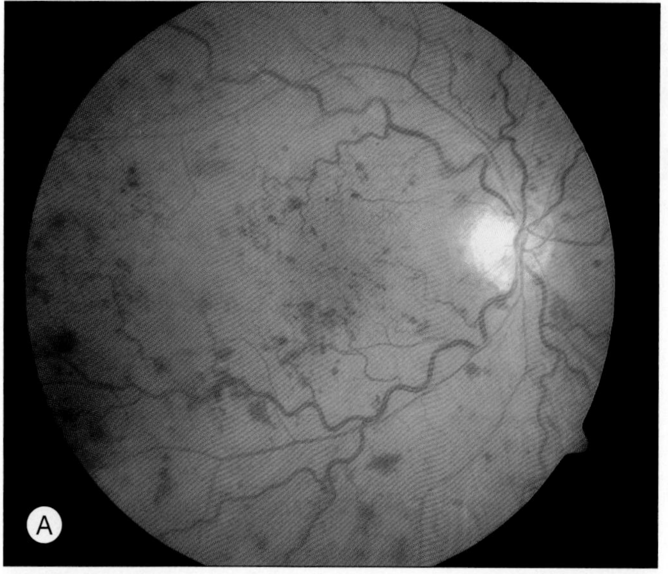

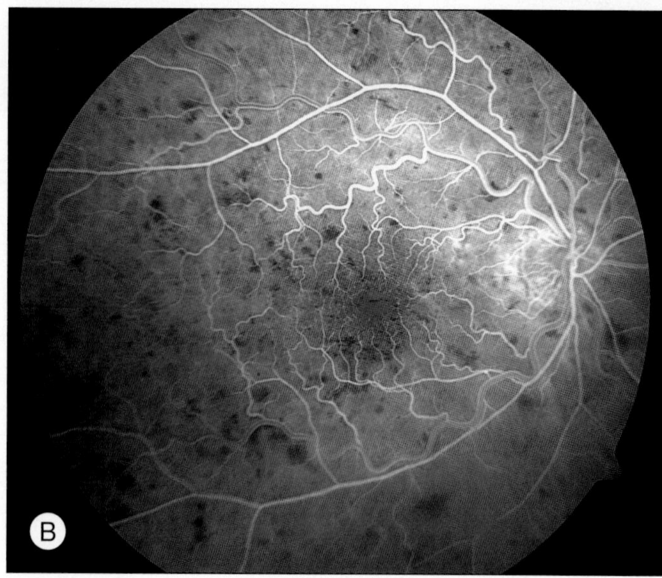

Fig. 54.2 (A) Fundus photograph of a central retinal vein occlusion demonstrating typical features of venous tortuosity, macular thickening, and intraretinal hemorrhage in all four quadrants of the fundus. (B) Early-phase angiogram of the fundus depicted in A, demonstrating an intact parafoveal capillary network in this perfused central retinal vein occlusion.

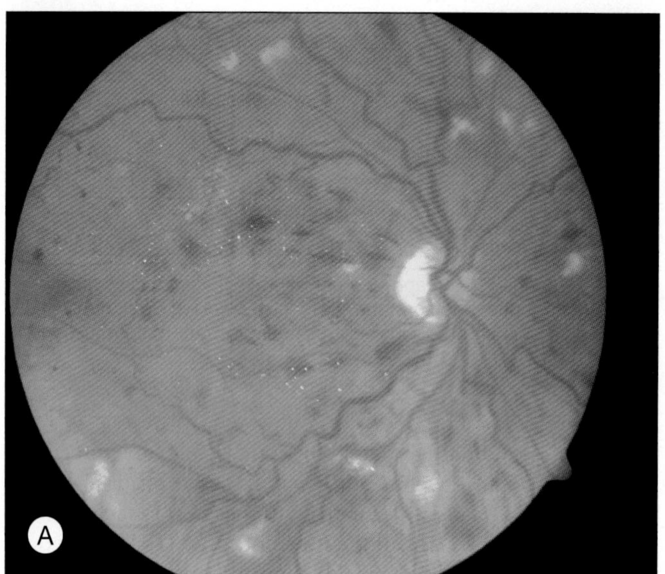

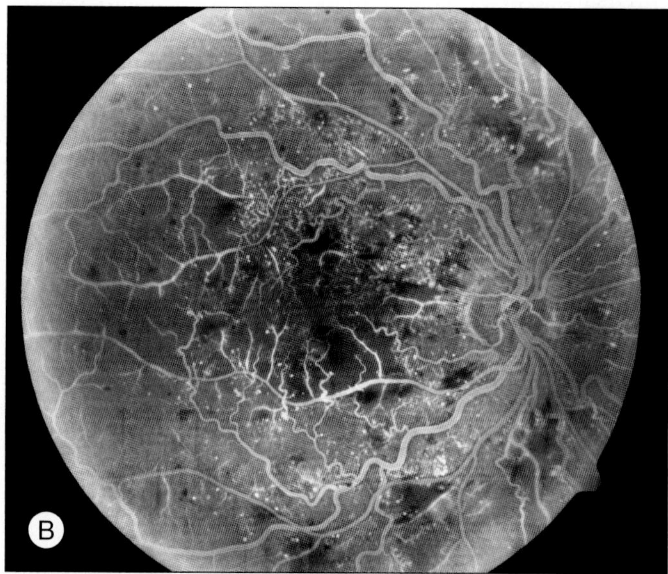

Fig. 54.3 (A) Fundus photograph of an eye with central retinal vein occlusion demonstrating scattered retinal hemorrhages, venous engorgement, and cotton-wool spots. (B) Midphase fluorescein angiogram of the eye shown in A, demonstrating capillary nonperfusion involving the foveal center. This eye also had extensive peripheral nonperfusion and is an example of the nonperfused form of central retinal vein occlusion.

acuity at onset (less than 20/200) had only a 20% chance of improvement.[9]

Anterior-segment findings may include iris and/or angle neovascularization (NVI/NVA). NVI typically begins at the pupillary border but may extend across the iris surface. NVA is detected during undilated gonioscopy as fine branching vessels bridging the scleral spur and may develop without any NVI in 6–12% of eyes with CRVO.[3,9,16] The CVOS used an index of any 2 clock-hours of NVI or any NVA as evidence of significant anterior-segment neovascularization, which was found in 16% of eyes with 10–29 disc areas of angiographic nonperfusion and 52% of eyes with 75 disc areas or more of angiographic nonperfusion.[9] In the CVOS, worse initial visual acuity correlated with the development of NVI/NVA: 5% in eyes with 20/40 or better, 14.8% in eyes with 20/50–20/200, and 30.8% in eyes with worse than 20/200 acuity.[9] Long-standing NVA may lead to secondary angle closure from peripheral anterior synechiae formation. Elevated intraocular pressure associated with NVI/NVA is the hallmark of neovascular glaucoma.

PERFUSION STATUS

The CVOS classified the perfusion status of a CRVO as perfused, nonperfused, or indeterminate based on fluorescein angiographic characteristics. Angiographic assessment of perfusion status in CRVO is based on the photographic protocol from the

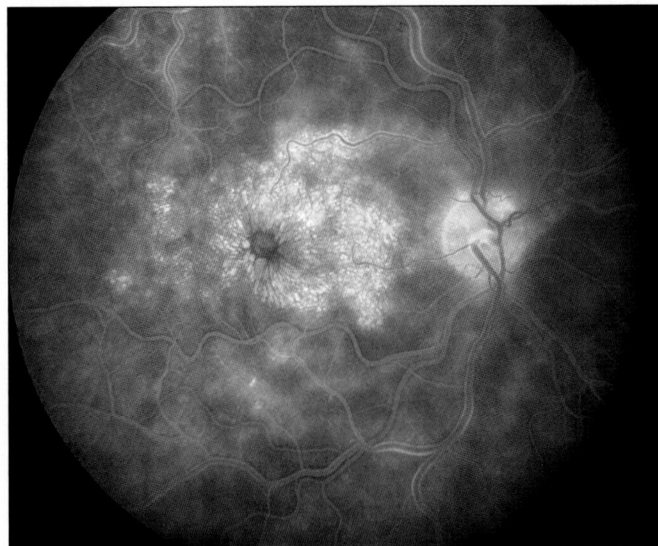

Fig. 54.4 Fluorescein angiogram of a chronic central retinal vein occlusion with resolution of intraretinal hemorrhage but persistence of cystoid macular edema demonstrated by petaloid leakage.

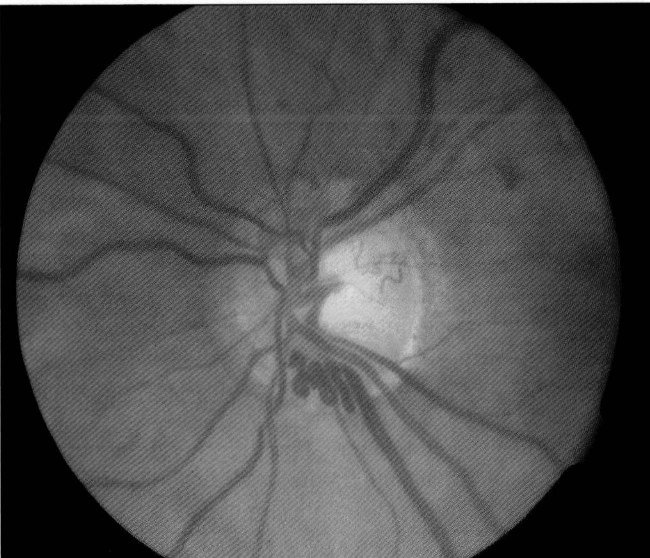

Fig. 54.5 Fundus photograph demonstrating optociliary shunt vessels (better termed collaterals) at the inferior border of the optic nerve head in this patient with a chronic central retinal vein occlusion. These vessels do not leak on fluorescein angiography.

CVOS which used a conventional wide-angle fundus camera with sweeps of the midperiphery 30 seconds after intravenous injection of sodium fluorescein.

A perfused CRVO (also termed nonischemic, incomplete, or partial) demonstrates less than 10 disc areas of retinal capillary nonperfusion on angiography (Fig. 54.2). These eyes typically have a lesser degree of intraretinal hemorrhage on presentation. Generally, eyes with perfused CRVO have better initial and final visual acuity. A nonperfused CRVO (also termed ischemic, hemorrhagic, or complete) demonstrates 10 or more disc areas of retinal capillary nonperfusion on angiography (Fig. 54.3). Acutely, these eyes demonstrate a greater degree of intraretinal hemorrhage, macular and disc edema, and capillary nonperfusion than in perfused CRVO. A CRVO is categorized as indeterminate when there is sufficient intraretinal hemorrhage to prevent angiographic determination of the perfusion status. Other examination features that may help in determining the perfusion status in the acute phase of a CRVO include baseline visual acuity, presence of an afferent pupillary defect, electroretinography (a negative waveform may be seen), and Goldmann perimetry.[5,9,17]

The CVOS classification of initial perfusion status of the CRVO was important for determining the natural history of the disease.[9] Poor visual acuity and large areas of retinal capillary nonperfusion were significant factors associated with an increased risk of developing NVI/NVA. In eyes initially categorized as perfused, 10% (56/538) developed NVI/NVA compared to 35% (61/176) of eyes initially characterized as nonperfused or indeterminate. At 3 years, there was a 45% chance of developing neovascular glaucoma after onset of ischemic CRVO.[1] Overall, 34% of initially perfused eyes converted to nonperfused status after 3 years.[9] In the CVOS, 38 eyes (83%) with an indeterminate CRVO at baseline were ultimately determined to be nonperfused. Initial visual acuity was highly correlated with degree of nonperfusion - eyes with nonperfused CRVO were much more likely than those with perfused CRVO to have poor visual acuity at initial presentation and final visit.[9,18]

Ultrawide-field angiography has enabled mapping of peripheral retinal nonperfusion not easily visualized with a conventional fundus camera. Adjusted protocols for grading extent of nonperfusion are being developed from photographs taken with ultrawide-field angiography, which may prove important in redefining characteristics of perfused versus nonperfused CRVO.[19,20]

PATHOGENESIS

The pathophysiology of CRVO is not clearly understood. Histopathologic studies of eyes enucleated for CRVO demonstrated a thrombus occluding the lumen of the central retinal vein at or just proximal to the lamina cribrosa,[21] suggesting that the anatomic variations at the level of the lamina cribrosa may be important in the development of a CRVO. Within the retrolaminar portion of the optic nerve, the central retinal artery and vein are aligned parallel to each other in a common tissue sheath. The central retinal artery and vein are naturally compressed as they cross through the rigid sieve-like openings in the lamina cribrosa but typically give off branching collateral vessels just before piercing the lamina. These vessels may be subject to compression from mechanical stretching of the lamina, as with increases in intraocular pressure, which may cause a posterior bowing of the lamina and subsequent impingement on the central retinal vein. Furthermore, local factors may predispose to occlusion of the central retinal vein, including compression by an atherosclerotic central retinal artery or primary occlusion of the central retinal vein from inflammation.

Hemodynamic alterations may produce stagnant flow and subsequent thrombus formation in the central retinal vein, including diminished blood flow, increased blood viscosity, and an altered lumen wall (also known as Virchow's triad). Experimentally, occlusion of both the retrolaminar central retinal artery and central retinal vein, posterior to the lamina cribrosa and prior to the branching of collateral channels from the main trunk, was required to produce the clinical appearance of a hemorrhagic (ischemic) CRVO.[18] This implies that concurrent retinal artery insufficiency or occlusion may play a role in an ischemic CRVO. It is hypothesized that a less hemorrhagic, more likely nonischemic, CRVO may be due to occlusion of the central retinal vein at a site further posterior, allowing normal collateral channels to provide alternative routes of venous drainage.

In the largest histopathologic study of eyes with CRVO, 29 eyes enucleated for acute (within 6 hours) and chronic (up to 10 years) occlusions were reviewed,[21] some of which had concurrent neovascular glaucoma. In acute occlusions, a thrombus at the level of the lamina cribrosa was adherent to a portion of the vein wall devoid of an endothelial lining. Subsequently, there was endothelial cell proliferation within the vein and secondary inflammatory cell infiltrates. Recanalization of the thrombus was demonstrated in eyes 1–5 years after the documented occlusion.

Neovascularization of the anterior and posterior segment and severity of macular edema are modulated by growth factors released from the ischemic retina. Green and colleagues demonstrated inner retinal ischemic changes in 25% of eyes enucleated for CRVO.[21] In a study of enucleated eyes with CRVO and neovascular glaucoma, intraretinal vascular endothelial growth factor (VEGF) production from areas of ischemic retina was demonstrated.[22] Analysis of vitreous fluid from patients with CRVO demonstrated increased levels of VEGF along with other cytokines and growth factors, including interleukin-6 (IL-6), IL-8, interferon-induced protein-10, monocyte chemotactic protein-1, and platelet-derived growth factor-AA.[23–25] Intraocular VEGF levels correlate with severity of ocular findings, including neovascularization and vascular permeability,[26] prompting the development of anti-VEGF agents for the treatment of CRVO (see below).

RISK FACTORS AND ASSOCIATIONS

Concurrent systemic vascular disease is a risk factor for CRVO (Box 54.1). The Eye Disease Case-Control Study found an increased risk of any type of CRVO in persons with systemic hypertension and diabetes mellitus.[4] Similar associations with systemic hypertension were found in other studies.[27–31] Diabetes mellitus was more prevalent in individuals with nonperfused CRVO than in matched controls from large population databases.[27,28] Hyperlipidemia, arteriosclerosis, and smoking have also been linked to the development of vein occlusions.[2,30,32]

Box 54.1 Risk factors and associations with central retinal vein occlusion[4,5,39]

- Systemic vascular diseases: diabetes mellitus, hypertension, carotid insufficiency
- Ocular diseases: open angle glaucoma, ischemic optic neuropathy, pseudotumor cerebri, tilted optic nerve heads, optic nerve head drusen
- Hematologic alterations: hyperviscosity syndromes: dysproteinemias (multiple myeloma), blood dyscrasias (polycythemia vera, lymphoma, leukemia, sickle-cell disease or trait), anemia, elevated plasma homocysteine, factor XII deficiency, antiphospholipid antibody syndrome, activated protein C resistance, protein C deficiency, protein S deficiency
- Inflammatory/autoimmune vasculitis: systemic lupus erythematosus
- Medications: oral contraceptives, diuretics, hepatitis B vaccine
- Infectious vasculitis: HIV, syphilis, herpes zoster, sarcoidosis
- Other: after retrobulbar block, dehydration, pregnancy

HIV, human immunodeficiency virus.

Hematologic abnormalities, particularly conditions that predispose to a hypercoagulable state, have been identified in persons with CRVO. Individuals less than 60 years of age may have a greater association with hypercoagulable states and inflammatory conditions compared to older persons with a higher incidence of systemic vascular disease risk factors.[5,6] Lahey and colleagues found one abnormal laboratory value suggesting systemic hypercoagulability in 27% of 55 patients younger than 56 years of age.[33] Studies have demonstrated an increased incidence of coagulation cascade abnormalities, including protein C and S deficiency, activated protein C resistance, presence of factor V Leiden, presence of antiphospholipid antibodies, hyperhomocysteinemia, antithrombin III deficiency, prothrombin gene mutations, and abnormal fibrinogen levels.[34–41] Hyperviscosity from blood dyscrasias, dysproteinemias, and dehydration have also been reported with CRVO.[42–45]

An increased risk of CRVO is present in eyes with open angle glaucoma.[4,46] Other ocular conditions causing deformation or mechanical pressure on the optic nerve head and lamina cribrosa, including ischemic optic neuropathy, tilted optic nerve head, optic nerve head drusen, optic disc traction syndrome, and pseudotumor cerebri,[42,47] have also been associated with CRVO. External compression of the globe and optic nerve from thyroid-related ophthalmopathy, mass lesions, or head trauma with orbital fracture may also result in CRVO.[5]

CLINICAL EVALUATION

At the time of initial presentation, a careful assessment of the CRVO duration and the degree of macular edema and retinal ischemia will determine treatment options and the follow-up schedule. An ocular history may determine the onset of the occlusion, although individuals may not have noted vision loss if the fellow eye has maintained good acuity. A history of systemic diseases, such as hypertension, diabetes, and heart disease, and a personal or family history of thrombosis or hypercoagulable state should be determined.

The ophthalmic examination should be performed on both eyes and include visual acuity, pupillary reaction, and intraocular pressure. Undilated slit-lamp examination is performed to detect NVI or NVA. Undilated gonioscopy is essential to determine the presence of NVA or evidence of angle closure from peripheral anterior synechiae, as NVA may be present without any NVI in up to 12% of eyes.[16] Ophthalmoscopic examination will help differentiate a CRVO from intraretinal hemorrhage associated with carotid occlusive disease.[48] Adjunctive imaging studies, including optical coherence tomography (OCT) and fluorescein angiography, are helpful in evaluating and following the presence of macular edema and perfusion status.

In general, a systemic workup is not indicated in persons older than 60 years of age with known systemic vascular risk factors for CRVO. Younger patients are more likely to have predisposing conditions resulting in thrombotic disease.[6,33] A limited systemic workup may be considered in those with a prior occlusion in the fellow eye, prior systemic thrombotic disease, family history of thrombosis, or other symptoms suggestive of a hematologic or rheumatologic condition. An initial laboratory investigation may include an erythrocyte sedimentation rate, antinuclear antibody, antiphospholipid antibody, and fasting plasma homocysteine levels. An elevated plasma homocysteine level may uncover a correctable etiology of CRVO, which may also influence cardiovascular health.[38] Individuals with bilateral, simultaneous CRVO or mixed-type retinal vascular occlusions should have a detailed evaluation for a hypercoagulable condition, as these persons may be at risk for future, nonocular thrombotic events.[9]

THERAPEUTIC OPTIONS

Treatment for CRVO is directed at treating the sequelae of CRVO, particularly macular edema and neovascularization. The recent development of intravitreal pharmacotherapy has revolutionized the treatment of CRVO-associated macular edema (Fig. 54.6). While these intravitreal agents can also improve secondary neovascularization, panretinal photocoagulation (PRP) remains the definitive treatment. Alternative experimental therapies have sought to modify the anatomic alterations believed to be responsible for CRVO. Of course, appropriate management of blood pressure and other systemic factors is always of paramount importance.

Treatment of macular edema

Observation

The CVOS group M report studied the effect of grid pattern argon laser photocoagulation to improve visual acuity in 155 eyes with perfused CRVO-associated macular edema and 20/50 acuity or worse.[49] Laser treatment involved a grid pattern in the area of leaking capillaries within 2 disc diameters of the foveal center but not within the foveal avascular zone. At 36 months, there was no significant difference in mean visual acuity between treated (20/200) and untreated (20/160) eyes despite reduction of angiographic macular edema. Widespread damage to the perifoveal capillary network has been hypothesized to contribute to the lack of visual recovery. Therefore, the CVOS did not recommend grid laser photocoagulation for CRVO-associated macular edema. In the absence of robust treatment options before the advent of intravitreal pharmacotherapy for retinal diseases,[50] standard of care for CRVO-associated macular edema was observation.

Corticosteroid therapy

The exact mechanism of action of corticosteroids in modulating retinal edema is unknown. It is believed that corticosteroids maintain anti-inflammatory effects with modulation of production of cytokines and growth factors, including VEGF. Corticosteroids are also thought to stabilize the blood–retinal barrier with reduction in vascular permeability.[51,52] There is little evidence for systemic administration of corticosteroids to treat macular edema from CRVO, unless the vein occlusion is associated with underlying systemic inflammatory disease.[53] Intravitreal delivery of corticosteroids provides targeted delivery of the drug to the retinal vessels and macular tissue while limiting potential systemic toxicity.

Following case reports on the use of intravitreal triamcinolone (IVTA) for the treatment of CRVO-associated cystoid macular edema (CME),[54–57] the Standard care vs Corticosteroid for Retinal vein occlusion (SCORE) study compared the efficacy and safety of two doses of preservative-free IVTA (1 mg and 4 mg) versus standard of care (i.e., observation per CVOS) for the treatment of CME in 271 eyes with CRVO.[58] In this randomized, multicenter clinical trial, eyes were retreated with IVTA every 4 months for 1 year unless one of the following reasons was encountered: (1) significant improvement (central subfield OCT

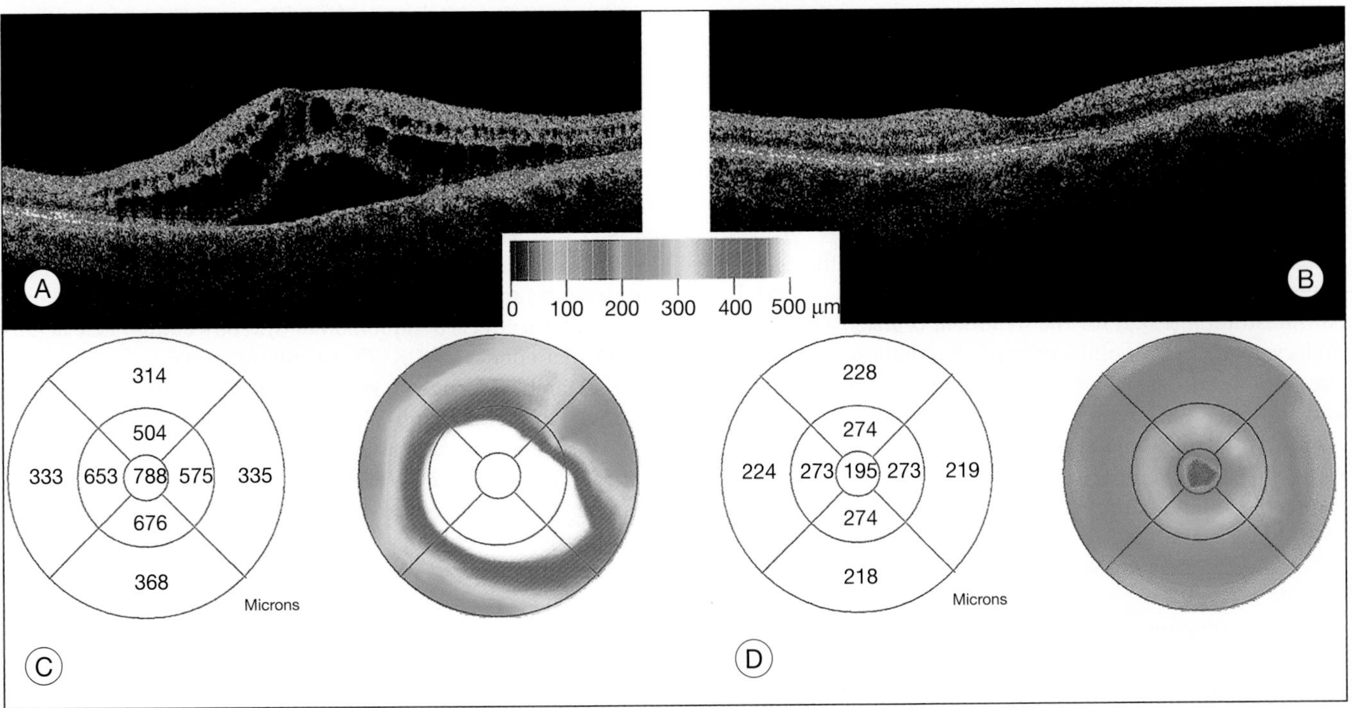

Fig. 54.6 A 67-year-old male with 5-month history of vision loss from a central retinal vein occlusion who received a single intravitreal injection of triamcinolone acetonide (4 mg) to treat persistent cystoid macular edema. (A) Preinjection optical coherence tomography (OCT) demonstrating prominent retinal thickening in the macular region with inner and outer retinal cysts and subretinal fluid accumulation. (B) 4-month postinjection OCT demonstrating dramatic resolution of retinal thickening and return of normal foveal contour. (C) Retinal thickness map and corresponding color map from A with marked macular thickening. (D) Retinal thickness map and corresponding color map from B with normal retinal thickness measurements. Similar resolution of macular edema can be observed with intravitreal injections of antivascular endothelial growth factor agents, including ranibizumab and bevacizumab.

thickness ≤ 225 μm, visual acuity ≥ 20/25, or significant interval improvement with presumed potential for continued improvement without treatment); (2) contraindication due to significant adverse effect (e.g., significant rise in intraocular pressure); or (3) additional treatment considered futile due to no improvement following two consecutive injections.

The SCORE study showed significant improvement in visual acuity with IVTA compared to observation.[58] At 1 year, 26% of eyes in the 4-mg group and 27% of eyes in the 1-mg group gained ≥15 letters at 1 year compared to 7% of untreated eyes. Mean change in visual acuity was a loss of only 1.2 letters in both IVTA groups compared to a loss of 12.1 letters in the observation group. A subgroup analysis of pseudophakic eyes revealed a mean gain in visual acuity of two letters in the 1-mg group and a mean loss of visual acuity of one letter in the 4-mg group compared to a mean loss of 14 letters in the observation group. In these pseudophakic eyes, a gain of three or more lines was achieved in 20% of both IVTA groups compared to 6% in the observation group.

Primary ocular adverse events included cataract formation and elevated intraocular pressure.[58] Cataract formation was observed in 26% and 33% of eyes in the 1-mg and 4-mg IVTA groups, respectively, compared to 18% in the observation group. Over 2 years, 27% of eyes from the 4-mg group and 3% of eyes in the 1-mg group required cataract surgery, but no eyes from the observation group required cataract surgery. Elevated intraocular pressure was observed in 20% and 35% of eyes in the 1-mg and 4-mg IVTA groups, respectively, compared to 8% in the observation group. At 12 months, there were no cases of endophthalmitis or retinal detachment in any group.

The limited duration of the response to IVTA therapy has prompted the development of sustained-release corticosteroids for the treatment of CRVO-associated CME. In a case series of 14 eyes with chronic refractory CME secondary to CRVO, improvements in visual acuity and macular edema after 1 year were observed in eyes surgically implanted with a sustained-release intravitreal fluocinolone acetonide implant (Retisert).[59] In this series, all phakic eyes developed visually significant cataracts, and 92% required medical or surgical intervention for increased intraocular pressure.

In 2009, a sustained-release intravitreal dexamethasone delivery system, Ozurdex, was approved by the Food and Drug Administration (FDA) for the treatment of macular edema secondary to CRVO. A multicentered, international study at 167 sites in 24 countries reported the 6-month outcomes of a 0.35-mg and 0.7-mg Ozurdex dose for CME in eyes with retinal vein occlusion, a group consisting of both branch retinal vein occlusions and CRVO, compared to sham-injected eyes.[60] The Ozurdex implant resulted in improved mean visual acuity, increased rate of ≥15 letter gain, and lower rate of ≤15 letter loss. Subgroup analysis was performed on 136 CRVO eyes injected with Ozurdex. The 0.7-mg group demonstrated significant gains of ≥15 letters compared to sham control at 30 days (28% versus 7%) and at 60 days (29% versus 9%), but not at 90 or 180 days. The 0.35-mg group demonstrated significant gains of ≥15 letters compared to sham at 30 days (20% versus 7%), at 60 days (33% versus 9%), and at 90 days (24% versus 10%), but not at 180 days. No significant difference in cataract formation or cataract surgery was identified between the treated and untreated groups. Ocular hypertension occurred in 4% of eyes receiving the drug delivery system, and most were able to be managed with topical medications. There were no significant differences between the sham and treatment groups in vitreous hemorrhage, vitreous floaters, or retinal hemorrhage. Two retinal detachments occurred in the study, one in the sham group and one in the 0.7-mg group. No cases of endophthalmitis were reported.[60]

Intravitreal anti-VEGF therapy

VEGF plays a key role in the pathophysiology of CRVO and its sequelae. Markedly elevated levels of VEGF have been demonstrated in the vitreous of eyes with ischemic CRVO.[23] It has been hypothesized that VEGF may cause capillary endothelial cell proliferation that leads to progressive vascular closure and nonperfusion in CRVO.[61] Anti-VEGF therapy may result in enhanced blood flow, lowered intravenous pressure, and the normalization of venous diameter and tortuosity.[61] Several intravitreal anti-VEGF treatments have been developed, including ranibizumab (Lucentis), bevacizumab (Avastin), and pegaptanib (Macugen).

The double-masked, multicenter, randomized phase III CRUISE trial prospectively compared monthly intravitreal injections of 0.3 mg or 0.5 mg ranibizumab to sham-injected controls in the treatment of 392 patients with macular edema after CRVO.[62] Eyes treated with 0.3 mg and 0.5 mg ranibizumab gained 12.7 and 14.9 letters, respectively, at 6 months compared to a 0.8 letter gain in the sham group. Additionally 46.2% (0.3 mg) and 47.7% (0.5 mg) of eyes treated with intravitreal ranibizumab gained ≥15 letters from baseline compared to only 16.9% in the sham group. The mean change in central foveal thickness was -434 μm (0.3 mg) and -452 μm (0.5 mg) in the treatment groups compared to -167.7 μm in the sham group. These improvements in visual acuity and foveal thickness were statistically significant at 6 months. There were no cases of retinal detachment or endophthalmitis in any of the groups. Systemic adverse events were also rare. There were no reported strokes in any of the groups. One transient ischemic attack occurred in the 0.5-mg group, and one myocardial infarction occurred in each of the groups. Following the 6-month endpoint, the control group was treated with ranibizumab on an as-needed basis, limiting further information on the natural history of CRVO and any long-term comparison in this study between a true control group and the treatment group.[15] The results of this study prompted FDA approval of ranibizumab for the treatment of CRVO. However, the long-term effects of ranibizumab and other anti-VEGF agents on macular edema for CRVO are still unknown.

Pegaptanib (Macugen) is currently the only other FDA-approved intravitreal anti-VEGF agent which received approval for the treatment of neovascular age-related macular degeneration. Similar to other anti-VEGF agents, the off-label use of pegaptanib for the treatment of retinal diseases has been investigated. In a phase II double-masked, multicenter, randomized trial, patients with CRVO receiving 0.3 mg or 1 mg pegaptanib every 6 weeks for 24 weeks were prospectively compared to sham-injected controls.[63] Patients treated with 0.3 mg and 1 mg pegaptanib had a risk of ≤15 letter loss of 9% and 6%, respectively, which was significantly lower compared to 31% in sham-injected eyes. While there was no significant difference in gain of ≥15 letters among groups, 0.3 mg and 1 mg pegaptanib groups showed 7.1 and 9.9 mean letter improvement, respectively, compared to -3.2 letter loss in sham-injected eyes; only the 1-mg group difference was statistically significant. The 0.3-mg and 1-mg pegaptanib groups also exhibited a significantly greater decrease of -269 µm and -210 µm, respectively, in central retinal thickness compared to -5 µm in the sham group.

Much of our understanding of the role of anti-VEGF agents in the treatment of retinal disease comes from studies with bevacizumab. While bevacizumab is not FDA-approved for intravitreal use, its ophthalmic use quickly grew due to its low cost, reported efficacy, and availability prior to the approval of ranibizumab. Several retrospective and prospective case series have reported decreased retinal thickness and improved visual acuity after intravitreal treatment with bevacizumab in eyes with CRVO-associated macular edema.[61,64–67] In a study using a single injection of bevacizumab, the peak increase in visual acuity was reached between 3 and 6 weeks after the injection, followed by a return of macular edema and secondary decrease in visual acuity.[66] As a result, in most case series, repeated treatment with bevacizumab was given at 4–8-week intervals to avoid recurrence of CME. Improvements in macular edema and visual acuity in CRVO following intravitreal bevacizumab are greater than would be expected by the natural history alone and have been reported in both ischemic and nonischemic CRVO.[67] Additionally, intravitreal bevacizumab has been associated with rapid resolution of anterior-segment neovascularization,[68] indicating that neovascular complications of CRVO, including neovascular glaucoma, may respond well to anti-VEGF agents.

The intravitreal use of bevacizumab is off-label. The lack of large, randomized, controlled clinical trials limits the safety profile data on bevacizumab for rare events, and it is difficult to quantify theoretical systemic risks such as stroke and myocardial infarction. In retrospective studies, the side-effect profile of bevacizumab was similar to that of ranibizumab, with an equivalent rate of endophthalmitis of 0.2%.[69] In another study, the most common adverse events were conjunctival hyperemia and subconjunctival hemorrhage at the injection site.[64] A recent randomized, blinded comparison of bevacizumab and ranibizumab in the treatment of age-related macular degeneration suggests that bevacizumab may be comparable to ranibizumab in efficacy.[70] It is unclear if these results are generalizable to the treatment of CRVO or of other retinal disorders.

Given the efficacy of intravitreal pharmacologic agents in the treatment of CRVO, and given their favorable side-effect profile, the use of intravitreal pharmacotherapy has replaced observation as the previous standard of care established by the CVOS for treatment of CRVO-associated macular edema. The specific indications for anti-VEGF agents compared to corticosteroids are currently being investigated along with the efficacy of combined therapy.[71] In a small study following 32 eyes with CRVO prospectively randomized to either IVTA or intravitreal bevacizumab treatment every 3 months as needed, improvements in visual acuity and central retinal thickness were equivalent at the 9-month endpoint. Significantly fewer injections were required with IVTA (mean 1.31 injections) than with bevacizumab (mean 2.38 injections, $P = 0.004$) over 9 months, but IVTA was associated with significantly more adverse events, particularly increases in intraocular pressure and visually significant premacular membranes.[72] The long-term role of these agents in the treatment of CRVO, the role for early intervention in improving outcome, and their ability to limit progression to the ischemic variant remain unanswered but are currently being investigated.[73,74] Further understanding of duration of effect and frequency of injections required will be important in optimizing dosing of anti-VEGF agents.

Treatment of ocular neovascularization

Laser photocoagulation

The CVOS group N report compared the efficacy of PRP placement at the time of study entry in eyes with nonperfused CRVO that did not have evidence of NVI/NVA (early treatment group, $n = 90$) with delayed, but prompt, PRP application (no early treatment group, $n = 91$) only when NVI/NVA was detected.[75] NVI/NVA developed in 20% of early treatment and 34% of no early treatment eyes. There was greater resolution of NVI/NVA by 1 month after PRP in 56% of no early treatment eyes compared with 22% of early treatment eyes. The CVOS therefore recommended that PRP be delivered promptly after the development of NVI/NVA but not prophylactically in eyes with nonperfused CRVO. In approximately 90% of cases, the regression of NVI/NVA occurs within 1–2 months of PRP. Persistent neovascularization after PRP should be followed closely, and additional PRP may be applied in attempts to halt its progression. Persons presenting with NVD/NVE without NVI/NVA should be treated with PRP, as performed in eyes with proliferative diabetic retinopathy or branch retinal vein occlusion, to prevent anterior-segment neovascularization. Prophylactic placement of PRP may be considered in eyes with nonperfused CRVO and risk factors for developing NVI/NVA (male gender, short duration of CRVO, extensive retinal nonperfusion, and extensive retinal hemorrhage) or in cases where frequent ophthalmologic follow-up is not possible.

Medical therapy

Topical or systemic antiglaucoma agents may be required to reduce elevated intraocular pressure. Topical corticosteroids can reduce anterior-segment inflammation by stabilizing tight junctions in neovascular tissue, thereby reducing vascular exudation. Cycloplegic agents prevent posterior synechiae formation between the iris and lens. Anti-VEGF agents may result in rapid regression of neovascularization, but these agents should be used as a temporizing adjunctive measure with subsequent placement of PRP for definitive treatment.[76] Failure of medical therapy to control intraocular pressure may require surgical intervention (e.g., trabeculectomy or tube placement).

Treatment of systemic medical conditions

Identification and treatment of systemic vascular risk factors, such as systemic hypertension and diabetes mellitus, are of paramount importance in individuals with CRVO. Coordination with the internist is strongly recommended. The role of systemic anticoagulation in CRVO is unclear as there is no evidence that agents, such as aspirin or heparin, can prevent or alter the natural history of CRVO; patients taking warfarin sodium (Coumadin) can still develop CRVO despite maintaining therapeutic levels of anticoagulation.[77] Prophylactic use of these medications, however, may help prevent nonocular thrombotic events, especially in individuals with known systemic vascular disease, and may be considered in coordination with the patient's internist.

Oral pentoxifylline is a potent vasodilator used in systemic vascular diseases to improve perfusion to occluded vessels and enhance the development of collateral circulation. A retrospective series of 11 patients treated with oral pentoxifylline (400 mg three times a day) for an average of 5 months demonstrated a 10% mean reduction in macular thickening by volumetric OCT but did not demonstrate a change in visual acuity or perfusion status.[78]

The reported increased plasma viscosity in persons with CRVO has prompted interest in systemic hemodilution to increase oxygen supply to the retina. A recent prospective, randomized, controlled clinical trial of selected CRVO patients demonstrated significant visual acuity gains and reduced conversion to nonperfusion.[79] Hemodilution is likely not appropriate for patients with anemia, renal insufficiency, or pulmonary insufficiency, which may limit its clinical use.[79,80]

Alternative treatments

Chorioretinal venous anastomosis

In eyes with perfused CRVO, investigators have bypassed the occluded central retinal vein by creating a chorioretinal anastomosis (CRA) between a nasal branch retinal vein and the choroidal circulation. Successful creation of an anastomosis may allow transretinal retrograde flow of venous blood from the eye and prevent the development of retinal ischemia or the reduction of macular edema. CRAs have been created through a surgical transretinal venipuncture technique[81,82] or, more commonly, through argon or neodymium:yttrium aluminum garnet (Nd-YAG) laser delivery directly at a branch retinal vein to rupture the posterior vein wall and Bruch's membrane.[83,84] McAllister and colleagues prospectively randomized 113 patients with nonischemic CRVO to laser-induced CRA or sham treatment.[85] Treated eyes demonstrated a significant 8.3 letter mean improvement compared to sham. Successful anastomosis was created in 76.4% of CRVO patients, and subanalysis of this group revealed 11.7 mean letter improvement compared to sham. Neovascularization developed at the site of anastomosis in 18.2% of treated eyes, and 9.1% of treated eyes required vitrectomy because of macular traction or nonclearing vitreous hemorrhage.

Immediate complications from this technique may include intraretinal, subretinal, or vitreous hemorrhage, while long-term complications include nonclearing vitreous hemorrhage, epiretinal avascular proliferation, fibrovascular proliferation, secondary neovascularization (choroidal, retinal, choroidovitreal, anterior segment), and traction retinal detachment.[81,86,87] Visual recovery may be limited in spite of successful anastomosis creation due to thrombosis of the treated vein with progressive retinal ischemia and development of macular pigment abnormalities following resolution of chronic macular edema.

Tissue plasminogen activator

Thrombolytic agents have been proposed as a treatment against a suspected thrombus in the central retinal vein. Recombinant tissue plasminogen activator (r-tPA) is a synthetic fibrinolytic agent that converts plasminogen to plasmin and destabilizes intravascular thrombi. Reduction in clot size may facilitate dislodging of the entire thrombus or recanalization of the occluded retinal vein. r-tPA, as therapy against CRVO, has been administered by several routes: systemic, intravitreal, and by endovascular cannulation of retinal vessels.

Systemic administration of low-dose (50 mg) front-loaded r-tPA has been attempted in two pilot studies with visual acuity improvement in 30–73% of patients.[88,89] In a prospective, multicentered randomized trial of 41 patients with CRVO, Hattenbach and colleagues demonstrated significant 1-year improvement of three lines of acuity in 45% of patients undergoing low-dose r-tPA compared to 21% of patients undergoing hemodilution.[90] Another study, examining full-dose (≤100 mg) systemic tPA for the treatment of 96 patients with CRVO, reported development of intraocular hemorrhage in 3 patients and a fatal stroke in 1 patient.[91] While Hattenbach et al.[90] did not observe any serious adverse events in their trial of low dose r-tPA, these complications highlight the importance of approaching systemic administration of r-tPA with caution.

Intravitreal delivery of r-tPA has potential advantages, including decreased risk of systemic complications, directed delivery to the vitreous cavity, and subsequent access to the retinal vessels with low risk of ocular morbidity from the procedure. Of 47 persons in three noncontrolled studies of intravitreal r-tPA for both ischemic and nonischemic CRVO of less than 21 days' duration, 28–44% had three lines of visual acuity improvement, with 6-month follow-up.[92–94] Administration of r-tPA did not significantly alter final perfusion status, especially in pretreatment ischemic eyes. Although there were no significant treatment-related complications, differences in inclusion criteria and dosage of r-tPA used (between 66 and 100 mg) limit generalizations from these studies. Ghazi and colleagues reported using a standard dose of 50 mg of intravitreal r-tPA in 12 eyes with acute CRVO of less than 3 days' duration.[95] In all patients, perfusion status remained unchanged at last follow-up, but marked improvement (20/50 or better) was demonstrated in eyes with perfused CRVO. This report did not include a control arm but suggests that prompt use of intravitreal r-tPA in perfused CRVO may provide visual benefit.

Endovascular delivery of r-tPA involves cannulation of retinal vessels, either through a neuroradiologic or a vitreoretinal approach, with delivery of minute quantities of r-tPA directly to the occluded vessels to release the suspected thrombus.[96,97] Weiss and Bynoe reported their technique of pars plana vitrectomy followed by cannulation of a branch vein and infusion of r-tPA towards the optic nerve head.[98] In their report, 50% of 28 eyes with CRVO of greater than 1 month's duration and worse than 20/400 preoperative acuity recovered more than three lines of acuity by a mean follow-up of 12 months. There was a trend towards increased perfusion by fluorescein angiography attributed in part to the resolution of intraretinal hemorrhages after the procedure. This study did not include a control arm. Complications included vitreous hemorrhage in seven eyes and treated retinal detachment in one eye. In another prospective study of 13 patients undergoing endovascular r-tPA delivery, visual recovery did not correspond with successful thrombolysis, and complications including retinal detachment, phthisis, neovascular glaucoma, and cataract were considered unacceptably high.[99]

Surgical treatments

Vitrectomy

Pars plana vitrectomy may be useful to address complications of CRVO and even to attempt to alter the natural course of the disease. Eyes with nonclearing vitreous hemorrhage from secondary retinal neovascularization may benefit from surgical evacuation. At the time of vitrectomy, clearing of the hemorrhage can be combined with removal of epiretinal membranes and removal of fibrovascular proliferations, if present, and the placement of complete endolaser PRP.[100] Although this technique may prevent or aid in regression of anterior-segment neovascularization, visual outcomes may be limited due to the extent of underlying retinal nonperfusion.[101] In eyes with extensive anterior-segment neovascularization and neovascular glaucoma, pars plana vitrectomy and endolaser PRP may be combined with pars plana placement of a glaucoma drainage device to avoid anterior-chamber hemorrhage at the time of tube placement.

The potential role for pars plana vitrectomy with peeling of the internal limiting membrane has also been investigated for treatment of CME secondary to CRVO. Small studies have demonstrated an improvement in CME accompanied by improvement in visual acuity.[102–104] In contrast, one study showed no significant improvement in visual acuity despite improvement of central foveal thickness.[105]

The use of vitrectomy with membrane peel in the treatment of CRVO-associated CME requires further investigation with randomized trials to establish its efficacy, particularly given the development of effective and less invasive intravitreal pharmacologic agents. Vitrectomy alters the pharmacokinetics of these intravitreal agents, resulting in a reduced duration of effect. The use of vitrectomy in the treatment of CRVO may result in decreased efficacy of further intravitreal pharmacotherapy, which should be carefully balanced against the expected benefits of vitrectomy.

Radial optic neurotomy

Opremcak and colleagues first reported combining pars plana vitrectomy with radial optic neurotomy (RON) involving transvitreal incision of the nasal scleral ring to release pressure on the central retinal vein at the level of the scleral outlet. In a nonrandomized study of 117 consecutive eyes undergoing RON, Opremcak et al. reported anatomic resolution of CME in 95% and visual improvement in 71% of eyes.[106] Interpretation of these impressive results must consider the nonrandomized nature of the study and the absence of a control group. While subsequent reports on RON have also demonstrated visual improvement,[107–109] no study has replicated the 71% improvement in Opremcak's study, and some studies have reported that visual improvement following RON is comparable to natural history.[109] In contrast, other studies have not demonstrated improvement in visual acuity[110] or in central retinal hemodynamics,[111,112] questioning the role for RON in CRVO treatment. Importantly, RON has been associated with signficant risks, including postoperative visual field defects, laceration of central retinal vessels, globe perforation, choroidal neovascularization, and retinal detachment.[107,109,110,113] Evidence of the efficacy of RON in management of CRVO is limited by the absence of randomized prospective trials but currently does not clearly demonstrate a beneficial role. With the availability of effective intravitreal pharmacologic agents, the use of RON for patients with CRVO has largely been abandoned.

FOLLOW-UP

Prior to the availability of intravitreal pharmacotherapy for the treatment of CRVO-associated macular edema, follow-up for eyes with CRVO to detect neovascular complications was typically guided by visual acuity at initial presentation. Eyes with initial acuity of 20/40 or better were generally examined every 1–2 months for 6 months, then annually if stable. Eyes with initial acuity worse than 20/200 were seen monthly for the initial 6 months, then bimonthly for the next 6 months, as these eyes have a greater degree of nonperfusion and a higher risk of developing NVI/NVA. Eyes with acuity between 20/50 and 20/200 have an intermediate risk of developing NVI/NVA and were also typically examined monthly for the first 6 months. Eyes that experienced a drop in visual acuity below the 20/200 level during follow-up were re-evaluated with assessment of perfusion status and presence of neovascularization, and monthly follow-up for an additional 6 months was recommended for these eyes.[9] With the development of intravitreal pharmacologic agents, this follow-up paradigm has changed. Follow-up intervals for patients undergoing treatment with intravitreal pharmacotherapy should currently be based on clinical response to treatment.

CONCLUSION

CRVO is a sight-threatening disease with significant ocular morbidity, including macular edema and ocular neovascularization. Before the recent advent of intravitreal pharmacotherapy in the management of CRVO, standard of care was guided by results from the CVOS, which recommended observation of macular edema and retinal ischemia with management of neovascular sequelae using PRP. In the absence of robust treatment options for CRVO,[50] other approaches, including the administration of r-tPA, creation of CRA, and various surgical interventions, had been reported with variable success and often unacceptable adverse effects. More recently, intravitreal corticosteroids and particularly anti-VEGF agents have demonstrated impressive improvements in macular edema, visual acuity, and even neovascular complications with a favorable side-effect profile. The use of ranibizumab (Lucentis) and a sustained-release dexamethasone implant (Ozurdex) have been FDA-approved for the treatment of CRVO. Intravitreal pharmacotherapy has now replaced observation as the standard of care for the management of macular edema associated with CRVO.

REFERENCES

1. Hayreh SS, Zimmerman MB, Podhajsky P. Incidence of various types of retinal vein occlusion and their recurrence and demographic characteristics. Am J Ophthalmol 1994;117:429–41.
2. Mitchell P, Smith W, Chang A. Prevalence and associations of retinal vein occlusion in Australia. The Blue Mountains Eye Study. Arch Ophthalmol 1996;114:1243–7.
3. The Central Vein Occlusion Study. Baseline and early natural history report. Arch Ophthalmol 1993;111:1087–95.
4. The Eye Disease Case-Control Study Group. Risk factors for central retinal vein occlusion. Arch Ophthalmol 1996;114:545–54.
5. Gutman FA. Evaluation of a patient with central retinal vein occlusion. Ophthalmology 1983;90:481–3.
6. Fong AC, Schatz H. Central retinal vein occlusion in young adults. Surv Ophthalmol 1993 ;37:393–417.
7. Klein R, Klein BE, Moss SE, et al. The epidemiology of retinal vein occlusion: the Beaver Dam Eye Study. Trans Am Ophthalmol Soc 2000;98:133–41; discussion 41–3.
8. Rogers S, McIntosh RL, Cheung N, et al. The prevalence of retinal vein occlusion: pooled data from population studies from the United States, Europe, Asia, and Australia. Ophthalmology 2010;117:313–9 e1.
9. The Central Vein Occlusion Study Group. Natural history and clinical management of central retinal vein occlusion. Arch Ophthalmol 1997;115:486–91.
10. Deramo VA, Cox TA, Syed AB, et al. Vision-related quality of life in people with central retinal vein occlusion using the 25-item National Eye Institute Visual Function Questionnaire. Arch Ophthalmol 2003;121:1297–302.
11. Fekrat S, Shea AM, Hammill BG, et al. Resource use and costs of branch and central retinal vein occlusion in the elderly. Curr Med Res Opin 2010;26: 223–30.
12. Schatz H, Fong AC, McDonald HR, et al. Cilioretinal artery occlusion in young adults with central retinal vein occlusion. Ophthalmology 1991;98: 594–601.
13. Hayreh SS, Fraterrigo L, Jonas J. Central retinal vein occlusion associated with cilioretinal artery occlusion. Retina 2008;28:581–94.
14. Brown GC, Duker JS, Lehman R, et al. Combined central retinal artery-central vein obstruction. Int Ophthalmol 1993;17:9–17.
15. Decroos FC, Fekrat S. The natural history of retinal vein occlusion: what do we really know? Am J Ophthalmol 2011;151:739–41 e2.
16. Browning DJ, Scott AQ, Peterson CB, et al. The risk of missing angle neovascularization by omitting screening gonioscopy in acute central retinal vein occlusion. Ophthalmology 1998;105:776–84.

17. Hayreh SS, Klugman MR, Beri M, et al. Differentiation of ischemic from non-ischemic central retinal vein occlusion during the early acute phase. Graefes Arch Clin Exp Ophthalmol 1990;228:201–17.
18. Hayreh SS, Podhajsky PA, Zimmerman MB. Natural history of visual outcome in central retinal vein occlusion. Ophthalmology 2011;118:119–33 e1–2.
19. Tsui I, Kaines A, Havunjian MA, et al. Ischemic index and neovascularization in central retinal vein occlusion. Retina 2011;31:105–10.
20. Spaide RF. Peripheral areas of nonperfusion in treated central retinal vein occlusion as imaged by wide-field fluorescein angiography. Retina 2011;31: 829–37.
21. Green WR, Chan CC, Hutchins GM, et al. Central retinal vein occlusion: a prospective histopathologic study of 29 eyes in 28 cases. Retina 1981;1: 27–55.
22. Pe'er J, Folberg R, Itin A, et al. Vascular endothelial growth factor upregulation in human central retinal vein occlusion. Ophthalmology 1998;105:412–6.
23. Aiello LP, Avery RL, Arrigg PG, et al. Vascular endothelial growth factor in ocular fluid of patients with diabetic retinopathy and other retinal disorders. N Engl J Med 1994;331:1480–7.
24. Funk M, Kriechbaum K, Prager F, et al. Intraocular concentrations of growth factors and cytokines in retinal vein occlusion and the effect of therapy with bevacizumab. Invest Ophthalmol Vis Sci 2009;50:1025–32.
25. Noma H, Funatsu H, Mimura T, et al. Vitreous levels of interleukin-6 and vascular endothelial growth factor in macular edema with central retinal vein occlusion. Ophthalmology 2009;116:87–93.
26. Boyd SR, Zachary I, Chakravarthy U, et al. Correlation of increased vascular endothelial growth factor with neovascularization and permeability in ischemic central vein occlusion. Arch Ophthalmol 2002;120:1644–50.
27. Elman MJ, Bhatt AK, Quinlan PM, et al. The risk for systemic vascular diseases and mortality in patients with central retinal vein occlusion. Ophthalmology 1990;97:1543–8.
28. Hayreh SS, Zimmerman B, McCarthy MJ, et al. Systemic diseases associated with various types of retinal vein occlusion. Am J Ophthalmol 2001;131: 61–77.
29. Koizumi H, Ferrara DC, Brue C, et al. Central retinal vein occlusion case-control study. Am J Ophthalmol 2007;144:858–63.
30. Cheung N, Klein R, Wang JJ, et al. Traditional and novel cardiovascular risk factors for retinal vein occlusion: the multiethnic study of atherosclerosis. Invest Ophthalmol Vis Sci 2008;49:4297–302.
31. Di Capua M, Coppola A, Albisinni R, et al. Cardiovascular risk factors and outcome in patients with retinal vein occlusion. J Thromb Thrombolysis 2010;30:16–22.
32. O'Mahoney PR, Wong DT, Ray JG. Retinal vein occlusion and traditional risk factors for atherosclerosis. Arch Ophthalmol 2008;126:692–9.
33. Lahey JM, Tunc M, Kearney J, et al. Laboratory evaluation of hypercoagulable states in patients with central retinal vein occlusion who are less than 56 years of age. Ophthalmology 2002;109:126–31.
34. Williamson TH, Rumley A, Lowe GD. Blood viscosity, coagulation, and activated protein C resistance in central retinal vein occlusion: a population controlled study. Br J Ophthalmol 1996;80:203–8.
35. Gottlieb JL, Blice JP, Mestichelli B, et al. Activated protein C resistance, factor V Leiden, and central retinal vein occlusion in young adults. Arch Ophthalmol 1998;116:577–9.
36. Hayreh SS, Zimmerman MB, Podhajsky P. Hematologic abnormalities associated with various types of retinal vein occlusion. Graefes Arch Clin Exp Ophthalmol 2002;240:180–96.
37. Hvarfner C, Hillarp A, Larsson J. Influence of factor V Leiden on the development of neovascularisation secondary to central retinal vein occlusion. Br J Ophthalmol 2003;87:305–6.
38. Cahill MT, Stinnett SS, Fekrat S. Meta-analysis of plasma homocysteine, serum folate, serum vitamin B(12), and thermolabile MTHFR genotype as risk factors for retinal vascular occlusive disease. Am J Ophthalmol 2003;136: 1136–50.
39. Yap YC, Barampouti F. Central retinal vein occlusion secondary to protein S deficiency. Ann Ophthalmol (Skokie) 2007;39:343–4.
40. Rehak M, Rehak J, Muller M, et al. The prevalence of activated protein C (APC) resistance and factor V Leiden is significantly higher in patients with retinal vein occlusion without general risk factors. Case–control study and meta-analysis. Thromb Haemost 2008;99:925–9.
41. Incorvaia C, Parmeggiani F, Costagliola C, et al. The heterozygous 20210 G/A genotype prevalence in patients affected by central and branch retinal vein occlusion: a pilot study. Graefes Arch Clin Exp Ophthalmol 2001;239:251–6.
42. Ciardella AP, Clarkson JG, Guyer DR, et al. Central retinal vein occlusion: a primer and review. In: Guyer DR, Yannuzzi LA, Chang S, et al., editors. Retina - vitreous - macula. New York: W.B. Saunders; 1999.
43. Francis PJ, Stanford MR, Graham EM. Dehydration is a risk factor for central retinal vein occlusion in young patients. Acta Ophthalmol Scand 2003;81: 415–6.
44. Alexander P, Flanagan D, Rege K, et al. Bilateral simultaneous central retinal vein occlusion secondary to hyperviscosity in Waldenstrom's macroglobulinaemia. Eye (Lond) 2008;22:1089–92.
45. Al-Abdulla NA, Thompson JT, LaBorwit SE. Simultaneous bilateral central retinal vein occlusion associated with anticardiolipin antibodies in leukemia. Am J Ophthalmol 2001;132:266–8.
46. Dev S, Herndon L, Shields MB. Retinal vein occlusion after trabeculectomy with mitomycin C. Am J Ophthalmol 1996;122:574–5.
47. Rumelt S, Karatas M, Pikkel J, et al. Optic disc traction syndrome associated with central retinal vein occlusion. Arch Ophthalmol 2003;121:1093–7.
48. Kearns TP. Differential diagnosis of central retinal vein obstruction. Ophthalmology 1983;90:475–80.
49. The Central Vein Occlusion Study Group M report. Evaluation of grid pattern photocoagulation for macular edema in central vein occlusion. Ophthalmology 1995;102:1425–33.
50. Hayreh SS. Management of central retinal vein occlusion. Ophthalmologica 2003;217:167–88.
51. Nauck M, Karakiulakis G, Perruchoud AP, et al. Corticosteroids inhibit the expression of the vascular endothelial growth factor gene in human vascular smooth muscle cells. Eur J Pharmacol 1998;341:309–15.
52. Felinski EA, Antonetti DA. Glucocorticoid regulation of endothelial cell tight junction gene expression: novel treatments for diabetic retinopathy. Curr Eye Res 2005;30:949–57.
53. Shaikh S, Blumenkranz MS. Transient improvement in visual acuity and macular edema in central retinal vein occlusion accompanied by inflammatory features after pulse steroid and anti-inflammatory therapy. Retina 2001;21:176–8.
54. Jonas JB, Kreissig I, Degenring RF. Intravitreal triamcinolone acetonide as treatment of macular edema in central retinal vein occlusion. Graefes Arch Clin Exp Ophthalmol 2002;240:782–3.
55. Ip MS, Kumar KS. Intravitreous triamcinolone acetonide as treatment for macular edema from central retinal vein occlusion. Arch Ophthalmol 2002;120:1217–9.
56. Greenberg PB, Martidis A, Rogers AH, et al. Intravitreal triamcinolone acetonide for macular oedema due to central retinal vein occlusion. Br J Ophthalmol 2002;86:247–8.
57. Park CH, Jaffe GJ, Fekrat S. Intravitreal triamcinolone acetonide in eyes with cystoid macular edema associated with central retinal vein occlusion. Am J Ophthalmol 2003;136:419–25.
58. Ip MS, Scott IU, VanVeldhuisen PC, et al. A randomized trial comparing the efficacy and safety of intravitreal triamcinolone with observation to treat vision loss associated with macular edema secondary to central retinal vein occlusion: the Standard Care vs Corticosteroid for Retinal Vein Occlusion (SCORE) study report 5. Arch Ophthalmol 2009;127:1101–14.
59. Ramchandran RS, Fekrat S, Stinnett SS, et al. Fluocinolone acetonide sustained drug delivery device for chronic central retinal vein occlusion: 12-month results. Am J Ophthalmol 2008;146:285–91.
60. Haller JA, Bandello F, Belfort R, Jr., et al. Randomized, sham-controlled trial of dexamethasone intravitreal implant in patients with macular edema due to retinal vein occlusion. Ophthalmology 2010;117:1134–46 e3.
61. Ferrara DC, Koizumi H, Spaide RF. Early bevacizumab treatment of central retinal vein occlusion. Am J Ophthalmol 2007;144:864–71.
62. Brown DM, Campochiaro PA, Singh RP, et al. Ranibizumab for macular edema following central retinal vein occlusion: six-month primary endpoint results of a phase III study. Ophthalmology 2010;117:1124–33 e1.
63. Wroblewski JJ, Wells 3rd JA, Adamis AP, et al. Pegaptanib sodium for macular edema secondary to central retinal vein occlusion. Arch Ophthalmol 2009;127:374–80.
64. Costa RA, Jorge R, Calucci D, et al. Intravitreal bevacizumab (avastin) for central and hemicentral retinal vein occlusions: IBeVO study. Retina 2007; 27:141–9.
65. Pai SA, Shetty R, Vijayan PB, et al. Clinical, anatomic, and electrophysiologic evaluation following intravitreal bevacizumab for macular edema in retinal vein occlusion. Am J Ophthalmol 2007;143:601–6.
66. Stahl A, Agostini H, Hansen LL, et al. Bevacizumab in retinal vein occlusion-results of a prospective case series. Graefes Arch Clin Exp Ophthalmol 2007;245:1429–36.
67. Kriechbaum K, Michels S, Prager F, et al. Intravitreal Avastin for macular oedema secondary to retinal vein occlusion: a prospective study. Br J Ophthalmol 2008;92:518–22.
68. Ehlers JP, Spirn MJ, Lam A, et al. Combination intravitreal bevacizumab/ panretinal photocoagulation versus panretinal photocoagulation alone in the treatment of neovascular glaucoma. Retina 2008;28:696–702.
69. Fintak DR, Shah GK, Blinder KJ, et al. Incidence of endophthalmitis related to intravitreal injection of bevacizumab and ranibizumab. Retina 2008;28: 1395–9.
70. Martin DF, Maguire MG, Ying GS, et al. Ranibizumab and bevacizumab for neovascular age-related macular degeneration. N Engl J Med 2011;364: 1897–908.
71. Ehlers JP, Fekrat S. Differential effects of triamcinolone and bevacizumab in central retinal vein occlusion. Can J Ophthalmol 2011;46:88–9.
72. Ding X, Li J, Hu X, et al. Prospective study of intravitreal triamcinolone acetonide versus bevacizumab for macular edema secondary to central retinal vein occlusion. Retina 2011 ;31:838–45.
73. Chang LK, Spaide RF, Klancnik JM, et al. Longer-term outcomes of a prospective study of intravitreal ranibizumab as a treatment for decreased visual acuity secondary to central retinal vein occlusion. Retina 2011 31: 821–8.
74. DeCroos FC, Ehlers JP, Stinnett S, et al. Intravitreal bevacizumab for macular edema due to central retinal vein occlusion: perfused vs. ischemic and early vs. late treatment. Curr Eye Res 2011;36:1164–70.
75. The Central Vein Occlusion Study Group N report. A randomized clinical trial of early panretinal photocoagulation for ischemic central vein occlusion. Ophthalmology 1995;102:1434–44.
76. Iliev ME, Domig D, Wolf-Schnurrbursch U, et al. Intravitreal bevacizumab (Avastin) in the treatment of neovascular glaucoma. Am J Ophthalmol 2006;142:1054–6.

77. Mruthyunjaya P, Wirostko WJ, Chandrashekhar R, et al. Central retinal vein occlusion in patients treated with long-term warfarin sodium (Coumadin) for anticoagulation. Retina 2006;26:285–91.
78. Park CH, Scott AW, Fekrat S. Effect of oral pentoxifylline on cystoid macular edema associated with central retinal vein occlusion. Retina 2007;27:1020–5.
79. Glacet-Bernard A, Atassi M, Fardeau C, et al. Hemodilution therapy using automated erythrocytapheresis in central retinal vein occlusion: results of a multicenter randomized controlled study. Graefes Arch Clin Exp Ophthalmol 2011;249:505–12.
80. Chen HC, Wiek J, Gupta A, et al. Effect of isovolaemic haemodilution on visual outcome in branch retinal vein occlusion. Br J Ophthalmol 1998;82: 162–7.
81. Fekrat S, de Juan E, Jr. Chorioretinal venous anastomosis for central retinal vein occlusion: transvitreal venipuncture. Ophthalmic Surg Lasers 1999;30: 52–5.
82. Peyman GA, Kishore K, Conway MD. Surgical chorioretinal venous anastomosis for ischemic central retinal vein occlusion. Ophthalmic Surg Lasers 1999;30:605–14.
83. McAllister IL, Constable IJ. Laser-induced chorioretinal venous anastomosis for treatment of nonischemic central retinal vein occlusion. Arch Ophthalmol 1995;113:456–62.
84. Fekrat S, Goldberg MF, Finkelstein D. Laser-induced chorioretinal venous anastomosis for nonischemic central or branch retinal vein occlusion. Arch Ophthalmol 1998;116:43–52.
85. McAllister IL, Gillies ME, Smithies LA, et al. The Central Retinal Vein Bypass Study: a trial of laser-induced chorioretinal venous anastomosis for central retinal vein occlusion. Ophthalmology 2010;117:954–65.
86. McAllister IL, Douglas JP, Constable IJ, et al. Laser-induced chorioretinal venous anastomosis for nonischemic central retinal vein occlusion: evaluation of the complications and their risk factors. Am J Ophthalmol 1998;126:219–29.
87. Bavbek T, Yenice O, Toygar O. Problems with attempted chorioretinal venous anastomosis by laser for nonischemic CRVO and BRVO. Ophthalmologica 2005 ;219:267–71.
88. Hattenbach LO, Steinkamp G, Scharrer I, et al. Fibrinolytic therapy with low-dose recombinant tissue plasminogen activator in retinal vein occlusion. Ophthalmologica 1998;212:394–8.
89. Hattenbach LO, Wellermann G, Steinkamp GW, et al. Visual outcome after treatment with low-dose recombinant tissue plasminogen activator or hemodilution in ischemic central retinal vein occlusion. Ophthalmologica 1999; 213:360–6.
90. Hattenbach LO, Friedrich Arndt C, Lerche R, et al. Retinal vein occlusion and low-dose fibrinolytic therapy (R.O.L.F.): a prospective, randomized, controlled multicenter study of low-dose recombinant tissue plasminogen activator versus hemodilution in retinal vein occlusion. Retina 2009 ;29:932–40.
91. Elman MJ. Thrombolytic therapy for central retinal vein occlusion: results of a pilot study. Trans Am Ophthalmol Soc 1996;94:471–504.
92. Lahey JM, Fong DS, Kearney J. Intravitreal tissue plasminogen activator for acute central retinal vein occlusion. Ophthalmic Surg Lasers 1999;30:427–34.
93. Glacet-Bernard A, Kuhn D, Vine AK, et al. Treatment of recent onset central retinal vein occlusion with intravitreal tissue plasminogen activator: a pilot study. Br J Ophthalmol 2000;84:609–13.
94. Elman MJ, Raden RZ, Carrigan A. Intravitreal injection of tissue plasminogen activator for central retinal vein occlusion. Trans Am Ophthalmol Soc 2001;99:219–21; discussion 22–3.
95. Ghazi NG, Noureddine B, Haddad RS, et al. Intravitreal tissue plasminogen activator in the management of central retinal vein occlusion. Retina 2003;23:780–4.
96. Paques M, Vallee JN, Herbreteau D, et al. Superselective ophthalmic artery fibrinolytic therapy for the treatment of central retinal vein occlusion. Br J Ophthalmol 2000;84:1387–91.
97. Weiss JN. Treatment of central retinal vein occlusion by injection of tissue plasminogen activator into a retinal vein. Am J Ophthalmol 1998;126:142–4.
98. Weiss JN, Bynoe LA. Injection of tissue plasminogen activator into a branch retinal vein in eyes with central retinal vein occlusion. Ophthalmology 2001;108:2249–57.
99. Feltgen N, Junker B, Agostini H, et al. Retinal endovascular lysis in ischemic central retinal vein occlusion: one-year results of a pilot study. Ophthalmology 2007;114:716–23.
100. Lam HD, Blumenkranz MS. Treatment of central retinal vein occlusion by vitrectomy with lysis of vitreopapillary and epipapillary adhesions, subretinal peripapillary tissue plasminogen activator injection, and photocoagulation. Am J Ophthalmol 2002;134:609–11.
101. Yeshaya A, Treister G. Pars plana vitrectomy for vitreous hemorrhage and retinal vein occlusion. Ann Ophthalmol 1983;15:615–7.
102. Liang XL, Chen HY, Huang YS, et al. Pars plana vitrectomy and internal limiting membrane peeling for macular oedema secondary to retinal vein occlusion: a pilot study. Ann Acad Med Singapore 2007;36:293–7.
103. Raszewska-Steglinska M, Gozdek P, Cisiecki S, et al. Pars plana vitrectomy with ILM peeling for macular edema secondary to retinal vein occlusion. Eur J Ophthalmol 2009;19:1055–62.
104. Park DH, Kim IT. Long-term effects of vitrectomy and internal limiting membrane peeling for macular edema secondary to central retinal vein occlusion and hemiretinal vein occlusion. Retina 2010;30:117–24.
105. DeCroos FC, Shuler RK, Jr., Stinnett S, et al. Pars plana vitrectomy, internal limiting membrane peeling, and panretinal endophotocoagulation for macular edema secondary to central retinal vein occlusion. Am J Ophthalmol 2009;147:627–33 e1.
106. Opremcak EM, Rehmar AJ, Ridenour CD, et al. optic neurotomy for central retinal vein occlusion: 117 consecutive cases. Retina 2006;26:297–305.
107. Weizer JS, Stinnett SS, Fekrat S. Radial optic neurotomy as treatment for central retinal vein occlusion. Am J Ophthalmol 2003;136:814–9.
108. Hasselbach HC, Ruefer F, Feltgen N, et al. Treatment of central retinal vein occlusion by radial optic neurotomy in 107 cases. Graefes Arch Clin Exp Ophthalmol 2007;245:1145–56.
109. Arevalo JF, Garcia RA, Wu L, et al. Radial optic neurotomy for central retinal vein occlusion: results of the Pan-American Collaborative Retina Study Group (PACORES). Retina 2008;28:1044–52.
110. Martinez-Jardon CS, Meza-de Regil A, Dalma-Weiszhausz J, et al. Radial optic neurotomy for ischaemic central vein occlusion. Br J Ophthalmol 2005;89: 558–61.
111. Crama N, Gualino V, Restori M, et al. Central retinal vessel blood flow after surgical treatment for central retinal vein occlusion. Retina 2010;30:1692–7.
112. Skevas C, Wagenfeld L, Feucht M, et al. Radial optic neurotomy in central retinal vein occlusion does not influence ocular hemodynamics. Ophthalmologica 2011;225:41–6.
113. Opremcak EM, Bruce RA, Lomeo MD, et al. Radial optic neurotomy for central retinal vein occlusion: a retrospective pilot study of 11 consecutive cases. Retina 2001;21:408–15.

Chapter 55

Macular Telangiectasia

Michael Engelbert, Emily Y. Chew, Lawrence A. Yannuzzi

INTRODUCTION

Macular telangiectasia (mac tel), or idiopathic perifoveal or juxtafoveal telangiectasia, includes several, different vascular diseases affecting the capillaries of the posterior pole. While complex classifications have been used, there are essentially two basic and distinct forms: (1) a developmental or congenital, usually unilateral vascular anomaly, which may be part of the larger spectrum of Coats disease and now often called mac tel type 1; and (2) a presumably acquired bilateral form found in middle-aged and older persons, which has been termed macular, juxtafoveal, or perifoveal telangiectasia and is now known as mac tel type 2. A brief history of the evolving classification of retinal telangiectasis will follow. This chapter will then focus on mac tel type 2, the bilateral, acquired form of perifoveal telangiectasia from unknown cause with characteristic alterations of the macular capillaries and neurosensory degeneration.

HISTORY, NOMENCLATURE, AND CLASSIFICATION OF MACULAR TELANGIECTASIA

The concept of "retinal telangiectasia" has been known for over a century. First alluded to by Graefe in 1808 as "Telangiectasie der Retina" and/or "Aneurismen der Zentralarterie," it was used to describe dilated retinal vessels on all three components of the circulation, arterioles, capillaries, and venules for a variety of abnormalities, mostly cutaneous and cutaneous-ocular in nature.[1] One hundred years later, in 1908, Coats described "exudative retinitis," which was best characterized as vascular abnormalities with massive subretinal exudation.[2] Today, congenital telangiectasia goes by his name, Coats disease, and it consists of dilated retinal capillaries, micro- and macroaneurysms, ischemia, nonperfusion, and retinal vascular leakage, usually unilateral in males. Four years after Coats' original description, Leber described "miliary aneurysms,"[3] which were quite similar clinically to cases seen by Coats. It was not until 1956 that Reese suggested that Coats disease and Leber miliary aneurysms were one and the same, occurring either in child or adulthood.[4] By 1968, Gass acknowledged the contribution by Reese, suggesting that Leber and Coats were indeed manifestations along the spectrum of one disease, but Gass also introduced a new distinct entity, which he called idiopathic juxtafoveolar retinal telangiectasis (IJRT),[5] in order to differentiate it from Coats disease. This resulted in an extensive, detailed classification in 1993.[6] Table 55.1 puts the various diseases and their classifications in context.

Classification

Gass classified what had previously been known as Leber miliary aneurysms into IJRT groups 1A and B; this distinction proved to be useful in terms of prognosis and therapy. IJRT group 2 was to include the common bilateral disease seen in older and elderly patients, but later a group 2B was created to accommodate two brothers, who developed subretinal neovascularization, although these two remain the only cases fitting this category.[6] Another group was introduced and subdivided into IJRT group 3A, which is characterized by telangiectatic changes, vascular occlusion, and minimal exudation in 3 patients, and group 3B, who had similar retinal changes but had additional neurological changes in 3 patients also.

Yannuzzi classification

In 2006, Yannuzzi discussed new diagnostic, adjunctive imaging systems such as optical coherence tomography (OCT) and high-speed stereo angiography in a cohort of 36 patients with mac tel of various types. He introduced the name "idiopathic macular telangiectasia."[7] He proposed to pool together mac tel types 1 A and B and to classify them as "aneurysmal" telangiectasia. Gass group 2A mac tel was preserved but, because of the lack of subjects in the other categories, types 2B, 3A, and 3B were eliminated in this classification.

EPIDEMIOLOGY

Prevalence of disease: estimates from population-based studies

Beaver dam eye study

The Beaver Dam Eye Study[8] regraded the stereoscopic fundus photographs of the eyes of 4926 subjects aged 43–84, 99% of whom were white, for mac tel type 2. Five individuals, one woman and four men, were identified to have mac tel type 2, which translates into a prevalence of 0.1%. The average age was 63 years, with a range from 52 to 68 years. Bilateral manifestations were found in 2 patients.

Melbourne collaborative cohort study

This Australian study[9] analyzed 22415 Caucasians, with regard to the presence of typical features of mac tel type 2 on nonmydriatic color fundus photographs. Twelve patients with "possible" unilateral mac tel type 2 and 5 patients with signs of bilateral mac tel type 2 were identified. The average age amongst bilateral cases was 63 and ranged from 53 to 72 years. Three of the 5 bilateral cases were female. Only one "very convincing case with early gray sheen and telangiectatic vessels temporal to the fovea"

Table 55.1 Various Classifications of Macular Telangiectasia (Types 1 and 2) and the Differential Diagnoses

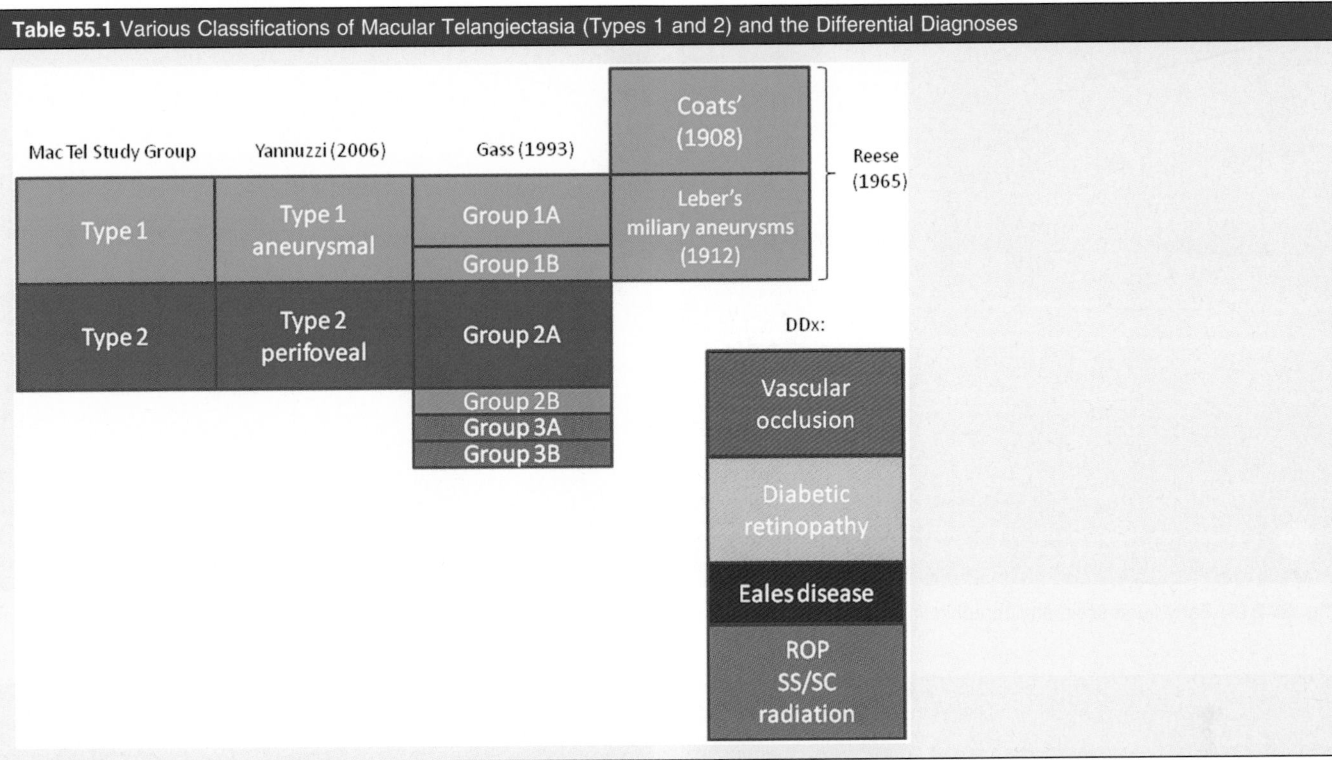

Mac Tel Study Group
Yannuzzi (2006)
Gass (1993)
Coats' (1908)
Leber's miliary aneurysms (1912)
Reese (1965)
Type 1
Type 1 aneurysmal
Group 1A
Group 1B
Type 2
Type 2 perifoveal
Group 2A
Group 2B
Group 3A
Group 3B
DDx:
Vascular occlusion
Diabetic retinopathy
Eales disease
ROP
SS/SC
radiation

DDx, differential diagnosis; ROP, retinopathy of prematurity; SS, sickle cell disease; SC, sickle cell trait.

was reported. The authors concluded that the incidence in their studied population ranged from 0.0045% to 0.022%, a prevalence which is significantly lower than the one found in the Beaver Dam Eye Study.

As noted by Klein et al., this lower prevalence estimate found in the Australian population might be a result of using a screening protocol in which images were only reassessed specifically for mac tel type 2 if a previous grading had suggested at least one feature of the disease[8]. The Beaver Dam Eye Study was conducted by regrading the entire cohort. It is possible that both studies have underestimated the true prevalence because only color fundus images were available. Other imaging technologies such as fluorescein angiography (FA), OCT, or fundus autofluorescence (FAF) have been demonstrated to be sensitive in detecting early and asymptomatic disease stages of mac tel type 2.[10]

These two population-based studies have been mainly in white populations. The Mac Tel Project, which consists of an international consortium of investigators evaluating the natural history of this ocular condition with the goal of conducting clinical trials to assess potential therapies, also enrolled a mostly white population. The involvement of other ethnicities is not well studied.

Although Gass and Blodi did not find gender differences in their cohort of 140 patients (94 with mac tel type 2),[6] the proportions of women reported by the Mac Tel Project ($n = 310$) and by Yannuzzi were about 64% and 58%, respectively.[11] On average, the Mac Tel Project participants (mean age 61 ± 9 years) had their disease diagnosed at age 57 (± 9 years).

CLINICAL PRESENTATION

Fundus appearance

The disease tends to be bilateral, but one eye may be more advanced than the other. All lesions tend to begin temporal to the foveal center but may subsequently involve the entire parafoveolar area. The earliest fundoscopic manifestion of mac tel type 2 is a subtle loss of retinal transparency in the perifoveal region, beginning temporally (Fig. 55.1).[7] This becomes more pronounced over time, and dilation of the parafoveal capillaries in the temporal parafoveal area ensues, and may extend to surround the fovea. These mildly ectatic capillaries were described to affect mainly the deeper capillary network (Fig. 55.2).[6] However, others have identified involvement of both the inner

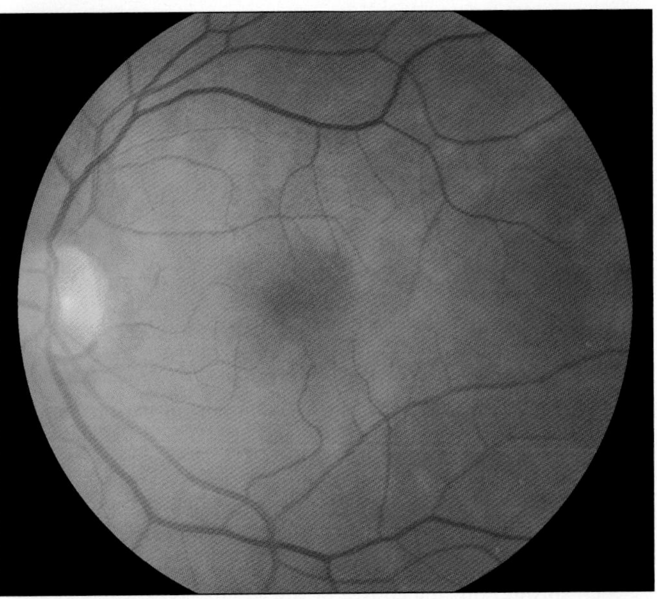

Fig. 55.1 Loss of retinal transparency, resulting in grayish discoloration of the temporal perifovea, may be the earliest fundoscopic sign of macular telangiectasia type 2.

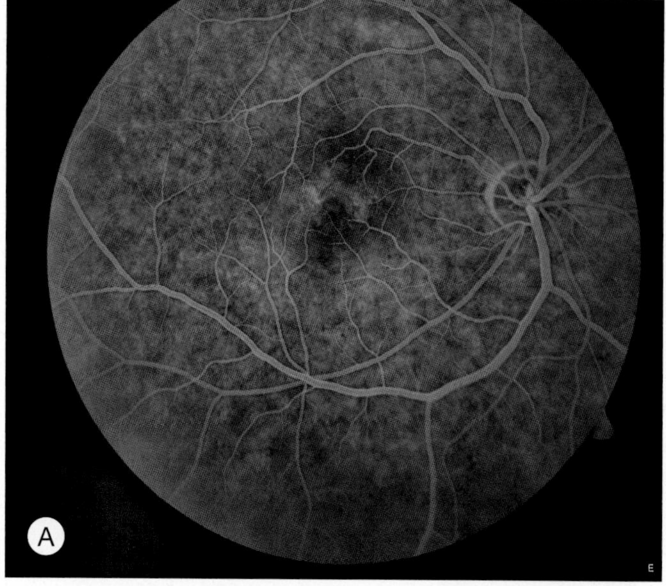

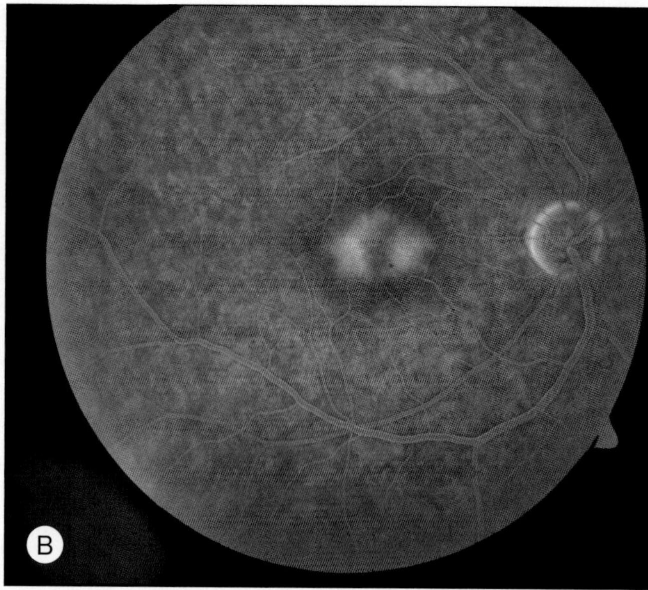

Fig. 55.2 (A) Early fluorescein angiographic findings of macular telangiectasia type 2 and (B) late leakage.

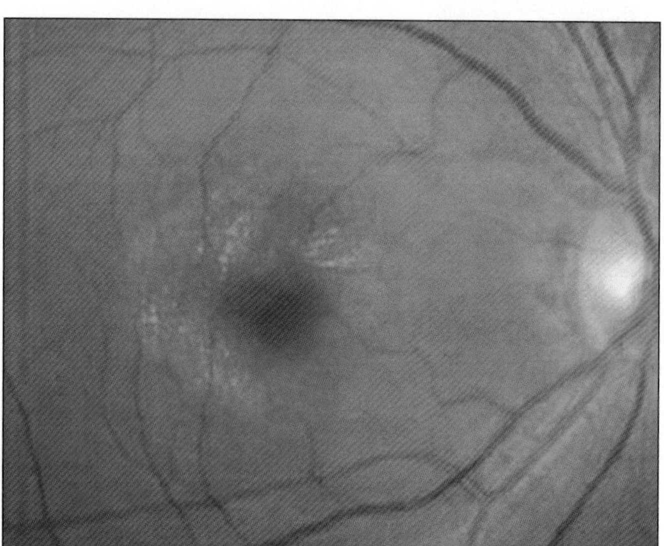

Fig. 55.3 Crystalline dots can be seen at the vitreoretinal interface.

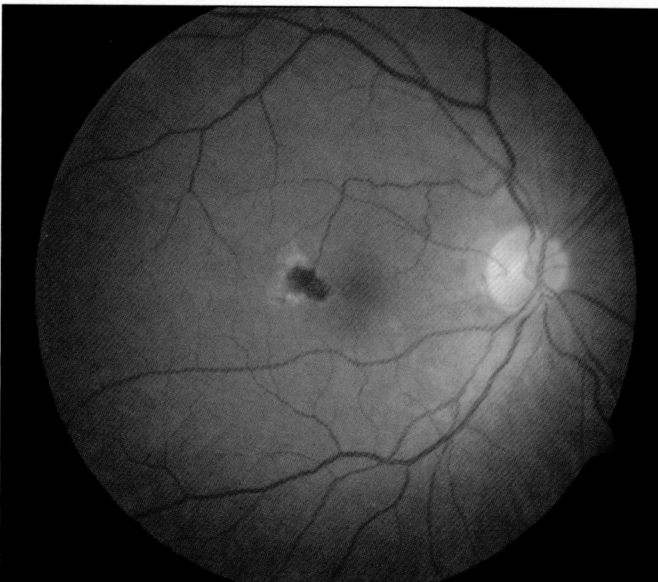

Fig. 55.4 Right-angle retinal vessels, manifest as blunted arterioles or venules that connect the superficial and deeper retinal plexus, are typical fundoscopic features of macular telangiectasia type 2. The right angle vessels may be difficult to appreciate without stereoscopy. A pigment plaque is also seen in this patient's eye.

and outer retinal circulation.[7] In contrast to mac tel type 1, retinal hard exudate is not seen unless there is evidence of neovascularization. Crystalline deposits at the vitreoretinal interface may be seen throughout the course of the disease (Fig. 55.3).[6,12]

Blunted, dilated venules, either as single or multiple vessels, are often associated with ectatic capillaries. As vessels course towards the fovea, they usually decrease in diameter but, in mac tel type 2, they dilate and may make a right-angle turn, diving into the deeper retinal layers (Fig. 55.4). Eventually, intraretinal pigment migration and RPE hyperplasia along these diving dilated venules may occur[7] (Fig. 55.5). In addition to RPE cell migration, atrophic changes in the neurosensory retina are another frequent finding.

A yellow spot, or vitelliform lesion, in the center of the fovea with slight loss of the foveal depression may become apparent in some eyes.[7] Other foveal changes include lamellar or full-thickness macular holes that have been detected on clinical exams and some confirmed by OCT imaging.[7,13–17] The degeneration and atrophy associated with this disease contribute to the formation of such holes. Surgical repair may not necessarily result in either structural or functional improvement.

The development of neovascularization is often, but not always, preceded by the right-angle venule and the intraretinal pigment hyperplasia which is often temporal to the fovea.[6,7] The neovascularization is most commonly seen temporal to the fovea.[18] Retinal hard exudates, intraretinal edema, and subretinal or intraretinal hemorrhage may occur (Fig. 55.6). These neovascular complexes are retinal in origin, as seen by the feeder vessel from the retinal arteries and the drainage into venules (Fig. 55.7). This may be indistinguishable from choroidal neovascularization with chorioretinal anastomosis. A disciform scar may be the advanced stage of this process (Fig. 55.8).

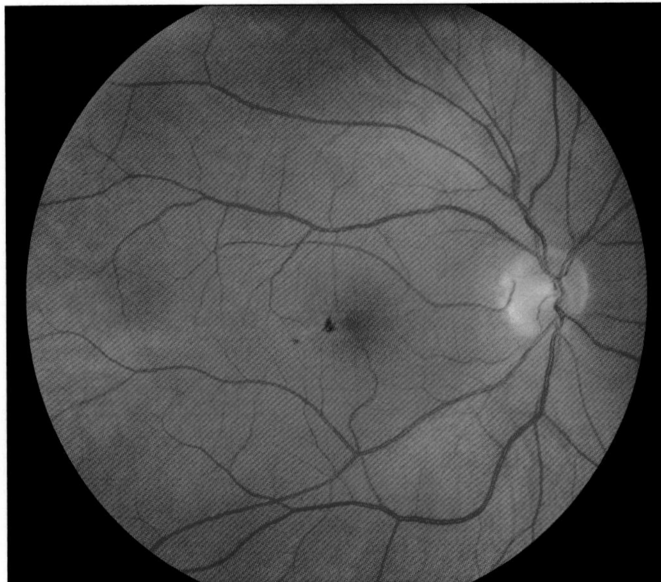

Fig. 55.5 Retinal pigment epithelial hyperplasia surrounds the right-angle venule.

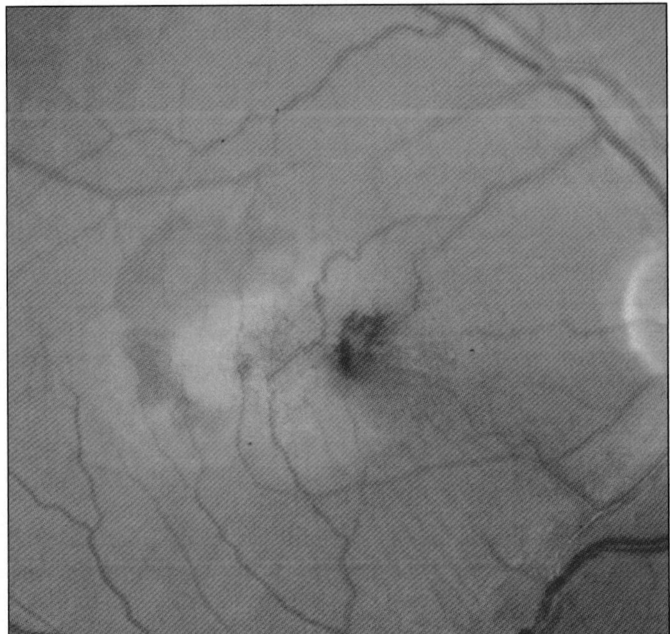

Fig. 55.6 Subretinal neovascularization is a rare complication of macular telangiectasia type 2. Intra- and subretinal hemorrhage, as shown here, are features of neovascular macular telangiectasia type 2.

RETINAL IMAGING

Fundus autofluorescence

One of the earliest signs of mac tel type 2 is the loss of the hypofluorescent center seen normally on blue-light FAF due to the depletion of macular pigment in this condition (Fig. 55.9). Even in the absence of any fluorescein leakage or any other signs, especially in patients with asymmetrical mac tel type 2,[10] this is diagnostic of the ocular condition. The area of retinal pigment hyperplasia will appear hypofluorescent on the FAF (Fig. 55.9).

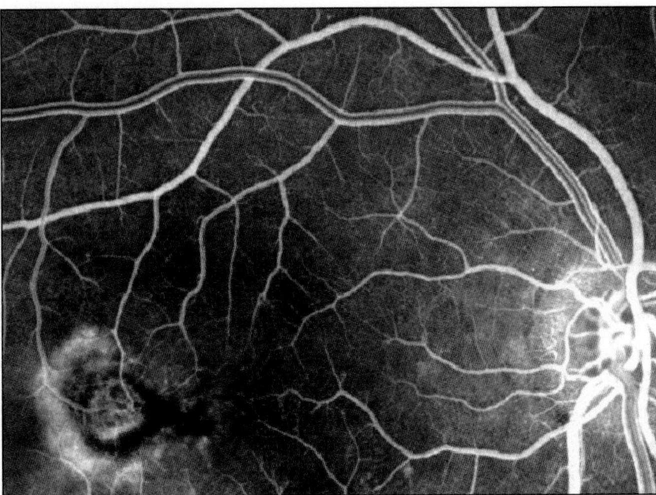

Fig. 55.7 Neovascular macular telangiectasia type 2 shows a subretinal neovascular membrane which is fed by a retinal arteriole, and in turn drained by a retinal venule.

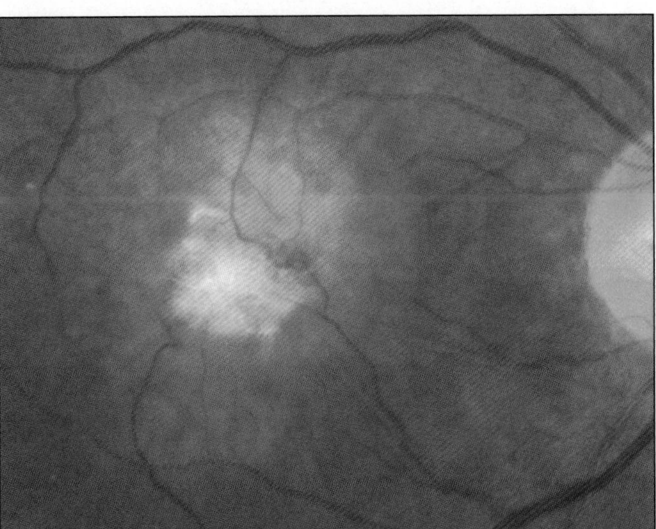

Fig. 55.8 A fibrovascular scar with chorioretinal anastomosis can be the endpoint of the pathogenic process of macular telangiectasia type 2, and is indistinguishable from disciform scarring in wet age-related macular degeneration. However, there is a lack of drusen and usually, the retinal pigment hyperplasia is prominent.

Fluorescein angiography

The hallmark finding in mac tel type 2 has been the characteristic telangiectactic capillaries on FA, again starting predominantly temporal to the fovea (Fig. 55.10). Eventually, the entire parafoveal area is involved (Fig. 5.2). Stereoscopic angiography has demonstrated that the deeper vasculature is involved but more superficial capillaries may also contribute to the fluorescein leakage.[6] Traditionally, the use of FA was essential in the diagnosis of mac tel type 2. However, OCT changes, as described below, may precede the development of any angiographic findings.

Optical coherence tomography

OCT may indeed provide valuable information as to the diagnosis and natural course of mac tel type 2 disease. The most subtle and earliest change may be the temporal enlargement of

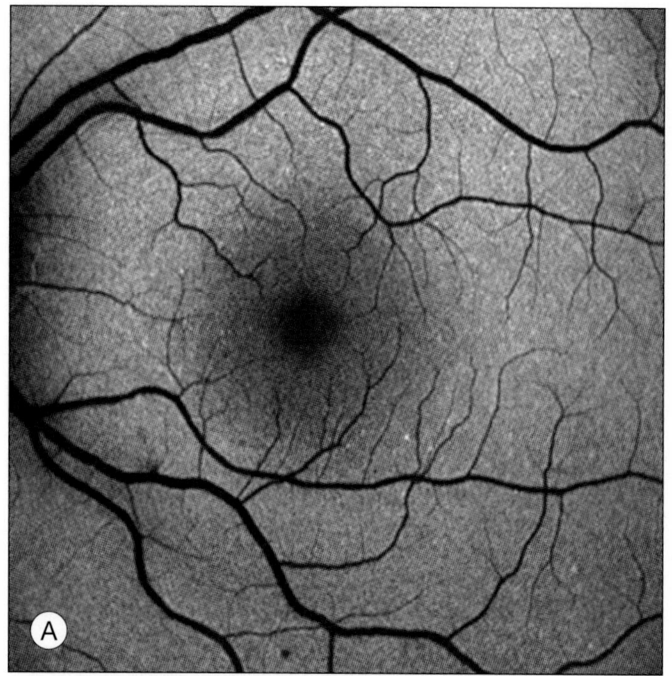

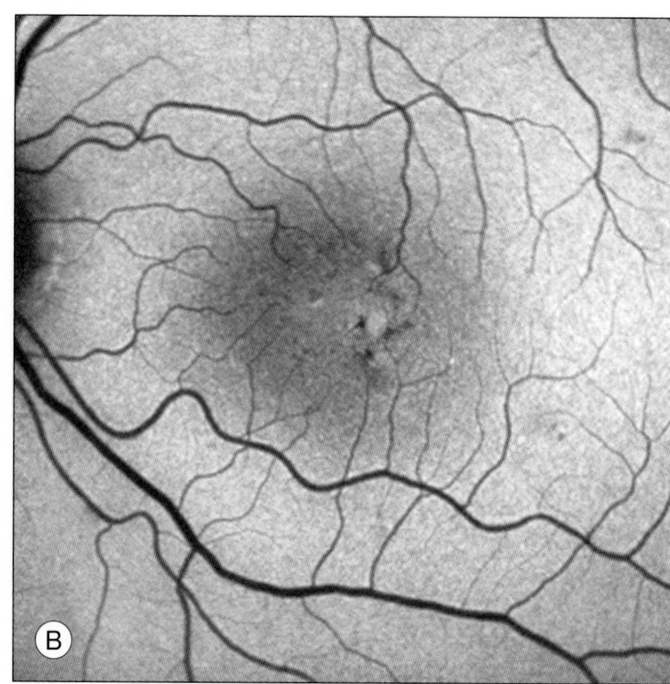

Fig. 55.9 A loss of foveal luteopigment is an early finding in macular telangiectasia type 2. (A) Blocking of autofluorescence in the central macula by healthy luteopigment. (B) Unmasking of hyperautofluorescence as well as spotty blocking from intraretinal pigment.

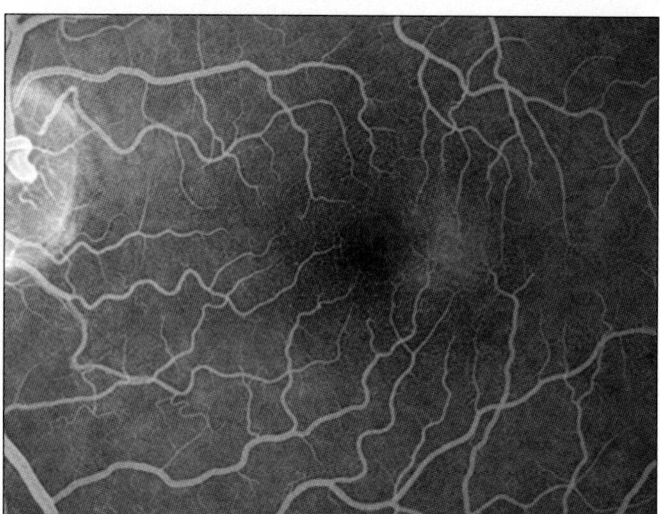

Fig. 55.10 Late staining in the temporal perifoveal area is an early angiographic feature of macular telangiectasia type 2.

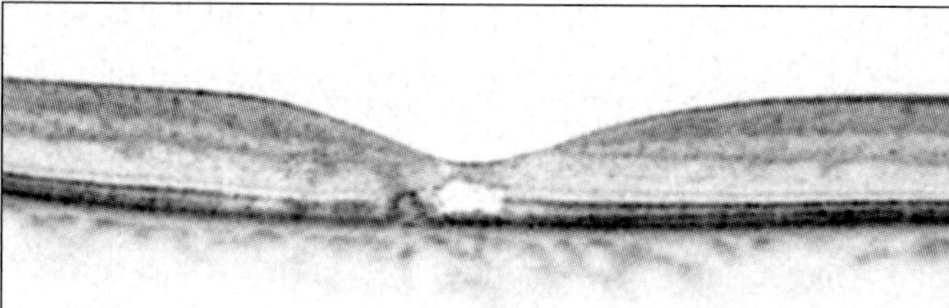

Fig. 55.11 Outer retinal cavity formations from the disruption of the photoreceptor layer and intraretinal pigment migration are associated with decreased central vision.

the foveal pit, resulting in an asymmetric pit with the temporal area being thinner than the nasal.[10] There are corresponding changes to the outer nuclear and/or photoreceptor layer. With time, the disruption of the photoreceptor inner-segment–outer-segment junction is seen, again temporal to the fovea. With progression, there will be hyporeflective cavities in the inner retina and these may clinically be described as "pseudolamellar macular holes." There are no pockets of leakage from the FA that correspond to these hyporeflective cavities. The disease progresses with hyporeflective cavities in the outer neurosensory retina and, eventually, atrophy (Fig. 55.11). The foci of retinal pigment hyperplasia manifest as hyperreflective intraretinal lesions that appear to migrate into the inner retinal layers, with associated posterior shadowing.

Adaptive optics imaging

Adaptive optics imaging, a technique that corrects for the optical aberrations of the eye and utilizes a scanning laser ophthalmoscope, allows evaluation of the cone photoreceptor mosaic.[19] Cone density evaluations in individuals with mac tel have identified areas of paracentral cone loss despite the absence of capillary abnormalities seen on FA.[20]

Visual function

Metamorphopsia or a scotoma may be present in the early stages of the disease.[13] When patients are asked specifically for symptoms of metamorphopsia, a majority will admit to such symptoms, even among those with early disease.[21] Visual impairment may be mild; however, loss of vision in one eye is frequently reported.[6] Vision may decrease gradually with the progression of the disease. Visual acuity less than 20/200 (legal blindness) is rare but may be seen in the advanced stages with marked atrophy of the central photoreceptors or secondary to a large area affected by neovascularization.[6,7,18,22] In the Mac Tel Project, the mean visual acuity at baseline was 20/40 in 522 eyes that had not previously received therapy.[11] Visual acuity was 20/20 or better in 16% and 20/32 or better in approximately 50%. The most common risk factors associated with lower visual acuity in this cohort were characteristics found in more advanced disease, namely retinal pigment hyperplasia and the right-angle venules. Similar visual acuity results were reported by Gass and Blodi.[6] In a retrospective study, 25% of eyes (6/24) remained stable during a follow-up period of 10–17 years.[22]

Despite the mild visual impairment, the vision-related quality of life is impacted markedly. In the Mac Tel Project, the National Eye Institute Visual Functioning Questionnaire (NEI-VFQ-25) was administered to all participants.[23] They reported significantly lower vision-related function in all domains compared to a group of participants in a study of age-related macular degeneration and who had similar visual acuities. A subset of these participants, enrolled in the Mac Tel Project, were tested using the Impact of Vision Impairment questionnaire.[24] Similar results were seen in this second study.

Microperimetry

Another method of evaluating function is the use of microperimetry, which may help to correlate the structural changes with the functional changes.[25–29] Retinal sensitivity defects appear to correlate with the outer retinal atrophy seen on OCT imaging. In areas of retinal pigment hyperplasia, there is often a dense scotoma. The use of microperimetry to correlate with changes seen on OCT may result in a reasonable outcome measurement for measuring changes over time, which may be especially useful for clinical trials that will be designed to test various therapies.

STAGING AND PROGNOSTIC FACTORS

From their extensive clinical experience and review of fundus photographs, Gass and Blodi concluded that various mac tel type 2 lesions appear in an orderly fashion over time.[6] Some lesions, such as retinal opacification, may be easily missed because of image quality. There was no availability of noninvasive tools such as OCT or FAF to assist in their classification of this condition. Nevertheless, the authors had remarkable clinical acumen and developed a scale (shown in Table 55.2) that has been part of this landmark study. However, the present usefulness of this scale is somewhat limited, as it does not incorporate OCT. With further research into the natural history of mac tel type 2, another scale incorporating newer technologies may be of value. A major challenge for studying therapies for mac tel type 2 is the development of reproducible and clinically meaningful outcome measurements. When structural and functional correlations can be made, such outcome measurements may become more evident.

Table 55.2 Clinical Staging of Macular Telangiectasia Type 2 (Gass and Blodi)

	Stages of macular telangiectasia type 2* (idiopathic juxtafoveal retinal telangiectasis of Gass and Blodi)[6]
Stage 1	No biomicroscopic abnormality, no or minimal capillary dilation, mild staining of outer perifoveal retina
Stage 2	Slight graying of perifoveolar retina, no or minimal biomicroscopically visible telangiectatic vessels, but capillary telangiectasis of outer capillary network temporally on fundus autofluorescence
Stage 3	One or several slightly dilated and blunted retinal venules descending into outer perifovea, typically temporally
Stage 4	Pigment hyperplasia, often surrounding right-angle venules
Stage 5	Subretinal neovascularization, often in proximity to intraretinal pigment migration

Based on biomicroscopy and stereoscopic fluorescein angiography.

GENETICS

The occurrence of this condition in monozygotic twins,[10,30–32] siblings, and families[6,10,33–36] suggests a genetic association in mac tel type 2. A vertical transmission pattern would also suggest an autosomal dominant pattern, but there may be variable expressivity or penetrance with monozygotic twins showing different disease severities.[10] Environmental influences or gene-to-gene interaction might account for this variation. The *ataxia telangiectasia mutated* gene, responsible for the ataxia telangiectasia syndrome, has been implicated in the pathogenesis of mac tel type 2.[37,38] A number of candidate genes known to cause other retinal diseases, such as those causing familial exudative vitreoretinopathy and Norrie disease, or those with a role in retinal neovascularization or macular pigment metabolism, have recently been excluded to play a role in the pathogenesis of mac tel type 2.[39] Evaluation of a gene that might be involved with xanthophyll transport also demonstrated no statistically significant association.[40]

ASSOCIATION OF SYSTEMIC DISEASES

Early reports have implicated an increased risk of diabetes in patients with mac tel type 2.[33,41] The Mac Tel Project, the largest population of mac tel type 2 patients to date, found a high prevalence of diabetes mellitus (28%) and also hypertension (52%).[11] Strikingly similar numbers were reported for diabetes and hypertension in another series.[38] These risk factors may further our understanding of the pathogenesis of this condition.

DIFFERENTIAL DIAGNOSIS

Retinal capillary telangiectasia may result from a multitude of retinal vascular inflammatory or occlusive conditions. However, mac tel type 2 is quite distinct from other conditions where retinal telangiectasia is a prominent feature. Branch retinal vein occlusions can give rise to segmental capillary changes, but this can be readily distinguished since it involves an area of distribution distal to an arteriolar-venular crossing, and does not cross the horizontal raphe, unless there is already collateral formation. Radiation retinopathy usually involves a larger retinal area, and is accompanied by cotton-wool spots and preretinal neovascularization, both features that are not characteristic of mac tel type 2. A history of radiation to the eye, orbit, or head can be readily elicited. Neovascular mac tel type 2 may masquerade as neovascular age-related macular degeneration, and vice versa. Since digital angiography (often monoscopic) has largely replaced stereo-film FA, precise localization of the retinal layer displaying the hyperfluorescence may be more difficult. However, in neovascular age-related macular degeneration, drusen and RPE changes are usually present, and retinal capillary disease is uncommon. OCT imaging will help localize the lesion and demonstrate other typical features, either in the same, or in the contralateral eye. Late stages of neovascular mac tel type 2 may, however, be indistinguishable from a disciform scar with chorioretinal anastomosis in age-related macular degeneration.

CLINICOPATHOLOGICAL CORRELATION

It is curious that vascular changes are not prominent features of early mac tel type 2, but blunting of the foveal reflex is typical. Based on the staining of the retina with fluorescein in eyes with minimal edema, Gass has postulated that it is possible that the primary abnormality may be found in the parafoveal retinal neural or Müller cells.[42] This is illustrated in a case where OCT and ERG changes in the form of inner-lamellar holes and reduced cone responses manifested before the development of typical vascular changes.[43] Xanthophyll is probably primarily stored in Müller cells, and this could be a surrogate measure of the health and concentration of Müller cells in that region. Xanthophyll concentration is already diminished in early mac tel.[44] Histopathological examination of the eyes of a 58-year-old woman with mac tel type 2 did not demonstrate telangiectatic capillaries, but did show narrowing of the vessel diameter. Instead, pericyte degeneration and lipid accumulation within the capillary walls, as well as multilaminated basement membrane, were found[45] – all similar to those seen in diabetics and prediabetics. Another histopathological study[46] demonstrated dilation and proliferation of retinal capillaries into the outer retinal, subretinal, and preretinal spaces. Perivascular pigment migration along the telangiectatic vessels was also seen. A sharp demarcation between the edematous and nonedematous retina was present and involved all layers of the retina, including the nerve fiber layer and the ganglion cell layer. The most detailed histopathological study to date examined the eye of a 65-year-old patient with mac tel type 2 and found reduced expression of Müller cell-specific markers in the fovea, which correlated with macroscopically visible pigment depletion in this area.[47]

THERAPEUTIC OPTIONS

There are no generally accepted therapies for lesions of mac tel type 2 not associated with neovascularization. There are anecdotal case reports, but no controlled randomized clinical trials conducted in this ocular condition. Laser photocoagulation[48] or photodynamic therapy[49] does not appear to improve or stabilize visual acuity in nonneovascular mac tel type 2. Anti-angiogenic agents seem to be equally ineffective in most reported series despite angiographic and tomographic effects,[50,51] although individual patients may experience a functional benefit.[52] The same seems to be true for intravitreal injections of triamcinolone acetonide.[53]

For neovascular complications of mac tel type 2, transpupillary therapy[54,55] and photodynamic therapy[56] have been reported to be somewhat efficacious, but have recently been replaced by anti-angiogenic agents, which may be able to stabilize neovascular complications of mac tel type 2.[57] Surgical removal of subretinal neovascularization was associated with a poor visual outcome in 2 patients.[58]

Mac tel type 2 may be complicated by the development of a full-thickness macular hole. The success rate after surgical repair appears to be lower than for idiopathic macular holes, probably depending on the relative contribution of tangential traction versus the neurodegeneration that is part of mac tel type 2.[16,59,60]

Future trials of therapies for mac tel type 2 may include neuroprotective agents to treat the purported neurodegenerative component. Currently, a safety trial is underway for implants of ciliary neurotrophic factor. Other neuroprotective agents may be considered in the future.

SUMMARY AND FUTURE RESEARCH DIRECTIONS

Despite a marked increase in our knowledge of idiopathic mac tel, or mac tel type 2, as it is now commonly called, the pathogenesis remains unknown. It has been well established that it is a bilateral disease that affects patients in the sixth decade of life with a slight predilection for the female sex. Most individuals progress from an asymptomatic, but clinically identifiable state, through a well-characterized pathogenic sequence eventually to develop significant visual disability, despite pharmacological, laser, and surgical attempts at treatment. Future research will hopefully unravel the molecular basis and identify targets for a cure.

REFERENCES

1. Graefe CF. Angiectasie. Ein Beitrag zur rationellen Cur und Erkenntniβ der Gefäβausdehnungen. Leipzig: K.F. Köhler; 1808.
2. Coats G. Forms of retinal disease with massive exudation. R Lond Ophthalmol Hosp Rep 1908;12:440.
3. Leber T. Über eine durch Vorkommen multipler Miliaraneurysmen charakterisierte Form von Retinaldegeneration. Graefes Arch Ophthalmol 1912;81: 1–14.
4. Reese A. Telangiectasis of the retina and Coats' disease. Am J Ophthalmol 1956;42:1.
5. Gass JD. A fluorescein angiographic study of macular dysfunction secondary to retinal vascular disease. V. Retinal telangiectasis. Arch Ophthalmol 1968;80: 592–605.
6. Gass JD, Blodi BA. Idiopathic juxtafoveolar retinal telangiectasis. Update of classification and follow-up study. Ophthalmology 1993;100:1536–46.
7. Yannuzzi LA, Bardal AM, Freund KB, et al. Idiopathic macular telangiectasia. Arch Ophthalmol 2006;124:450–60.
8. Klein R, Blodi BA, Meuer SM, et al. The prevalence of macular telangiectasia type 2 in the Beaver Dam eye study. Am J Ophthalmol 2010;150:55–62.
9. Aung KZ, Wickremasinghe SS, Makeyeva G, et al. The prevalence estimates of macular telangiectasia type 2. Retina 2010;30:473–8.
10. Gillies MC, Zhu M, Chew EY, et al. Familial asymptomatic macular telangiectasia type 2. Ophthalmology 2009;116:2422–9.
11. Clemons TE, Gillies MC, Chew EY, et al. Baseline characteristics of participants in the natural history study of macular telangiectasia (MacTel) MacTel Project Report No. 2. Ophthalmic Epidemiol 2010;17:66–73.
12. Moisseiev J, Lewis H, Bartov E, et al. Superficial retinal refractile deposits in juxtafoveal telangiectasis. Am J Ophthalmol 1990;109:604–5.
13. Gass JD, Oyakawa RT. Idiopathic juxtafoveolar retinal telangiectasis. Arch Ophthalmol 1982;100:769–80.
14. Patel B, Duvall J, Tullo AB. Lamellar macular hole associated with idiopathic juxtafoveolar telangiectasia. Br J Ophthalmol 1988;72:550–1.
15. Koizumi H, Iida T, Maruko I. Morphologic features of group 2A idiopathic juxtafoveolar retinal telangiectasis in three-dimensional optical coherence tomography. Am J Ophthalmol 2006;142:340–3.
16. Charbel Issa P, Scholl HP, Gaudric A, et al. Macular full-thickness and lamellar holes in association with type 2 idiopathic macular telangiectasia. Eye 2009;23: 435–41.
17. Shukla D. Evolution and management of macular hole secondary to type 2 idiopathic macular telangiectasia. Eye (Lond) 2011;25:532–3.
18. Engelbrecht NE, Aaberg Jr TM, Sung J, et al. Neovascular membranes associated with idiopathic juxtafoveolar telangiectasis. Arch.Ophthalmol 2002;120: 320–4.
19. Roorda A, Romero-Borja F, Donnelly Iii W, et al. Adaptive optics scanning laser ophthalmoscopy. Opt Express 2002;10:405–12.
20. Ooto S, Hangai M, Takayama K, et al. High-resolution photoreceptor imaging in idiopathic macular telangiectasia type 2 using adaptive optics scanning laser ophthalmoscopy. Invest Ophthalmol Visual Sci 2011;52:5541–50.
21. Charbel Issa P, Holz FG, Scholl HPN. Metamorphopsia in patients with macular telangiectasia type 2. Doc Ophthalmol 2009b;119:133–40.
22. Watzke RC, Klein ML, Folk JC, et al. Long-term juxtafoveal retinal telangiectasia. Retina 2005;25:727–35.
23. Clemons TE, Gillies MC, Chew EY, et al. The National Eye Institute visual function questionnaire in the Macular Telangiectasia (MacTel) project. Invest Ophthalmol Vis Sci 2008;49:4340–6.
24. Lamoureux EL, Maxwell RM, Marella M, et al. The longitudinal impact of macular telangiectasia (MacTel) type 2 on vision-related quality of life. Invest Ophthalmol Vis Sci 2011;52:2520–4.
25. Charbel Issa P, Helb HM, Rohrschneider K, et al. Microperimetric assessment of patients with type II macular telangiectasia. Invest Ophthalmol Vis Sci 2007;48:3788–95.

26. Charbel Issa P, Helb HM, Holz FG, et al. Correlation of macular function with retinal thickness in nonproliferative type 2 idiopathic macular telangiectasia. Am J Ophthalmol 2008;245:169–75.
27. Maruko I, Iida T, Sekiryu T, et al. Early morphological changes and functional abnormalities in group 2A idiopathic juxtafoveolar retinal telangiectasis using spectral domain optical coherence tomography and microperimetry. Br J Ophthalmol 2008;92:1488–91.
28. Schmitz-Valckenberg S, Ong EE, Rubin GS, et al. Structural and functional changes over time in MacTel patients. Retina 2009;29:1314–20.
29. Wong WT, Forooghian F, Majumdar Z, et al. Fundus autofluorescence in type 2 idiopathic macular telangiectasia: correlation with optical coherence tomography and microperimetry. Am J Ophthalmol 2009;148:573–83.
30. Hannan SR, Madhusudhana KC, Rennie C, et al. Idiopathic juxtafoveolar retinal telangiectasis in monozygotic twins. Br J Ophthalmol 2007;91:1729–30.
31. Menchini U, Virgili G, Bandello F, et al. Bilateral juxtafoveolar telangiectasis in monozygotic twins. Am J Ophthalmol 2000;129:401–3.
32. Siddiqui N, Fekrat S. Group 2A idiopathic juxtafoveolar retinal telangiectasia in monozygotic twins. Am J Ophthalmol 2005;139:568–70.
33. Chew EY, Murphy RP, Newsome DA, et al. Parafoveal telangiectasis and diabetic retinopathy. Arch Ophthalmol 1986;104:71–5.
34. Hutton WL, Snyder WB, Fuller D, et al. Focal parafoveal retinal telangiectasis. Arch Ophthalmol 1978;96:1362–7.
35. Isaacs TW, McAllister IL. Familial idiopathic juxtafoveolar retinal telangiectasis. Eye 1996;10(5):639–42.
36. Oh KT, Park DW. Bilateral juxtafoveal telangiectasis in a family. Retina 1999;19:246–7.
37. Mauget-Faÿsse M, Vuillaume M, Quaranta M, et al. Idiopathic and radiation-induced ocular telangiectasia: the involvement of the ATM gene. Invest Ophthalmol Vis Sci 2003;44:3257–62.
38. Barbazetto IA, Room M, Yannuzzi NA, et al. ATM gene variants in patients with idiopathic perifoveal telangiectasia. Invest Ophthalmol Vis Sci 2008;49:3806–11.
39. Parmalee NL, Schubert C, Merriam JE, et al. Analysis of candidate genes for macular telangiectasia type 2. Mol Vis 2010;16:2718–26.
40. Szental JA, Baird PN, Richardson AJ, et al. Analysis of glutathione S-transferase Pi isoform (GSTP1) single-nucleotide polymorphisms and macular telangiectasia type 2. Int Ophthalmol 2010;30:645–50.
41. Millay RH, Klein ML, Handelman IL, et al. Abnormal glucose metabolism and parafoveal telangiectasia. Am J Ophthalmol 1986;102:363–70.
42. Gass JDM. Histological study of presumed parafoveal telangiectasia. Retina 2000;20:226–7.
43. Barthelmes D, Gillies MC, Fleischhauer JC, et al. A case of idiopathic perifoveal telangiectasia preceded by features of cone dystrophy. Eye (Lond) 2007;21:1534–5.
44. Helb HM, Charbel Issa P, Van der Veen RL, et al. Abnormal macular pigment distribution in type 2 idiopathic macular telangiectasia. Retina 2008;28:808–16.
45. Green WR, Quigley HA, de la Cruz Z et al. Parafoveal retinal telangiectasis: light and electron microscopy studies. Trans Ophthalmol Soc UK 1980;100:162–70.
46. Eliassi-Rad B, Green WR. Histologic study of presumed parafoveal telangiectasis. Retina 1999;19:332–5.
47. Powner MB, Gillies MC, Tretiach M, et al. Perifoveal müller cell depletion in a case of macular telangiectasia type 2. Ophthalmology 2010;117:2407–16.
48. Park DW, Schatz H, McDonald HR, et al. Grid laser photocoagulation for macular edema in bilateral juxtafoveal telangiectasis. Ophthalmology 1997;104:1838–46.
49. De Lahitte GD, Cohen SY, Gaudric A. Lack of apparent short-term benefit of photodynamic therapy in bilateral, acquired, parafoveal telangiectasis without subretinal neovascularization. Am J Ophthalmol 2004;138:892–4.
50. Gamulescu MA, Walter A, Sachs H, et al. Bevacizumab in the treatment of idiopathic macular telangiectasia. Graefes Arch Clin Exp Ophthalmol 2008;246:1189–93.
51. Charbel Issa P, Finger RP, Kruse K, et al. Monthly ranibizumab for nonproliferative macular telangiectasia type 2: a 12-month prospective study. Am J Ophthalmol 2011;151:876–86.
52. Matt G, Sacu S, Ahlers C, et al. Thirty-month follow-up after intravitreal bevacizumab in progressive idiopathic macular telangiectasia type 2. Eye 2010;24:1535–41.
53. Wu L, Evans T, Arévalo JF, et al. Long-term effect of intravitreal triamcinolone in the nonproliferative stage of type II idiopathic parafoveal telangiectasia. Retina 2008;28:314–9.
54. Shukla D, Singh J, Kolluru CM, et al. Transpupillary thermotherapy for subfoveal neovascularization secondary to group 2A idiopathic juxtafoveolar telangiectasis. Am J Ophthalmol 2004;138:147–9.
55. Nachiappan K, Shanmugam MP. Treatment of CNVM secondary to idiopathic juxtafoveal retinal telangiectasis by transpupillary thermotherapy. Am J Ophthalmol 2005;139:577–8.
56. Snyers B, Verougstraete C, Postelmans L, et al. Photodynamic therapy of subfoveal neovascular membrane in type 2A idiopathic juxtafoveolar retinal telangiectasis. Am J Ophthalmol 2004;137:812–9.
57. Kovach JL, Rosenfeld PJ. Bevacizumab (avastin) therapy for idiopathic macular telangiectasia type II. Retina 2009;29:27–32.
58. Berger AS, McCuen II BW, Brown GC, et al. Surgical removal of subfoveal neovascularization in idiopathic juxtafoveolar retinal telangiectasis. Retina 1997;17:94–8.
59. Gregori N, Flynn Jr HW. Surgery for full-thickness macular hole in patients with idiopathic macular telangiectasia type 2. Ophthalmic Surg Lasers Imaging 2010;41:1–4.
60. Shukla D. Evolution and management of macular hole secondary to type 2 idiopathic macular telangiectasia. Eye (Lond) 2011;25:532–3.

Chapter 56

Coats Disease

Nikolas J.S. London, Carol L. Shields, Julia A. Haller

HISTORY

Coats disease is an idiopathic condition characterized by telangiectatic and aneurysmal retinal vessels with intraretinal and subretinal exudation and fluid.[1] Coats disease was first described by Scottish ophthalmologist George Coats in 1908.[2] In his initial classification, Coats separated this new entity into three distinct groups. Group I included eyes with massive subretinal exudation and no demonstrable vascular abnormalities. Group II consisted of eyes with massive subretinal exudation and multiple retinal vascular abnormalities with intraretinal hemorrhage. Group III included eyes with massive subretinal exudation and frank retinal arteriovenous malformations.[2] Eugen von Hippel later demonstrated that group III represented the distinctly separate entity of angiomatosis retinae (later retermed retinal capillary hemangioma or retinal hemangioblastoma), prompting Coats to drop this group from his classification. In 1912, and again in 1915, Theodor von Leber described a disease with similar telangiectatic and aneurysmal retinal vessels that lacked the massive subretinal exudation described by Coats.[3,4] This condition was later named Leber multiple miliary aneurysms. In a 1916 paper, Leber concluded that what he had described was merely an earlier stage of the disease process identified by Coats.[5,6] This conclusion was later reinforced by Reese, who described an eye with Leber miliary aneurysms that progressed into a classic case of Coats disease during long-term follow-up.[7] Although some authors have disagreed, most authorities today classify Leber disease as an early or nonprogressive form of Coats disease.[5,8,9]

HISTOPATHOLOGY, ETIOLOGY, AND PATHOGENESIS

Early descriptions of Coats disease focused primarily on the morphology of the disease and attempted to explain the disease process solely on the basis of fundoscopic and histopathologic changes.[10,11] The first observations published by Coats focused on histopathologic examination of six eyes enucleated for this condition that he received from various colleagues.[2] From these histopathologic specimens, Coats described subretinal masses of fibrous tissue intimately adherent to the outer retina. Most of the eyes had associated retinal thickening, degeneration, and detachment, as well as diffuse vascular abnormalities. Four of the six eyes had associated retinal hemorrhages and most had cholesterol crystals. One eye had evidence of bone formation. Coats believed the vascular changes represented secondary manifestations of the underlying disease and that the exudation was secondary to organization and partial resorption of retinal hemorrhages, as he often found hemorrhages in association with the exudation.[2] Coats also postulated that the primary process might be infectious in light of the mononuclear infiltrate found on histopathologic examination. This infectious theory of Coats disease was supported by a number of other reports, including that of Evens,[12] Straub,[13] and Müller,[13] who suspected toxoplasmosis as the underlying cause. Subsequent investigations and the failure of anti-inflammatory adrenocorticotropic hormone and steroid therapies have refuted early theories of a primary infectious or inflammatory etiology.[13,14]

Pathologic samples of eyes with Coats disease were once abundant owing to enucleations for suspected intraocular tumor.[15] Moreover, most histopathologic reports describe findings in eyes with advanced stages of the disease. Gross examination of enucleated eyes typically reveals bullous retinal detachment.[16] Subretinal fluid has a viscous, lipid-rich, yellow appearance with glistening crystals.[16] Microscopically, the subretinal exudation contains collections of foamy histiocytes and cholesterol clefts.[16] The outer retina is thickened by exudation, with variable penetration of inner retinal layers.[16] Areas of the inner retina also contain numerous, large, dilated, and telangiectatic vessels.[16] Other vascular abnormalities include degenerated and hypocellular walls, narrowed lumen with or without thrombi, capillary dropout, neovascularization, as well as perivascular sheathing and/or pigmentation.[1,9,17–23] Thickened vessel walls show characteristic heavy periodic acid–Schiff-positive deposits.[1] Flat preparations prepared by trypsin digestion reveal vascular aneurysms measuring 50–350 µm, often forming large sausage-like outpouchings and located on shunt vessels.[1] Advanced cases may have intraocular bone formation, with evidence of calcification on echography and computed tomography (CT) scanning that potentially confuses the diagnosis with retinoblastoma.[24,25] Electron microscopy confirms diffuse structural abnormalities of the retinal vasculature. Tripathi and Ashton described prominent structural alterations of retinal vessels in areas of retinal thickening, with thickened walls mostly replaced by a laminated fibrous coating of basement membrane-like material.[18] Most affected vessels were completely devoid of endothelium and pericytes, with red blood cells, plasma, and fibrin filling the lumina. There was patchy thinning or even absence of the vessel wall in some areas, with the vessel lumen extending to the basement membrane of adjacent glial cells.[18] These findings support the widely held view that Coats disease is a disorder of vascular integrity.

Indeed, recent work in molecular genetics suggests that Coats disease may be part of a spectrum of related genetic disorders known as "retinal hypovasculopathies"[26,27] which includes Norrie disease, familial exudative vitreoretinopathy (FEVR), fascioscapulohumeral muscular dystrophy (FSHD), and the osteoporosis pseudoglioma syndrome.[27–35] These diseases share a similar ocular phenotype, characterized by a failure to vascularize fully the retinal periphery and associated telangiectatic, incompetent remnant vasculature. Each of these conditions can be related to abnormalities in the Wnt signalling pathway during retinal angiogenesis.[26,27,36]

Several reports have implicated a deficiency of Norrin, a retinal protein, in the pathogenesis of Coats disease.[37,38] In one case report, a female with unilateral Coats disease gave birth to a son affected by Norrie disease.[37] Both carried a missense mutation within the Norrie disease pseudoglioma (*NDP*) gene on chromosome Xp11.2. Further analysis on archival tissue from nine enucleated eyes from males with unilateral Coats disease revealed a mutation in the *NDP* gene in one subject. Knockout mouse models of Norrie disease model demonstrate abnormalities of the retinal vessels, including telangiectasia, bulb-like dilatations, and underdevelopment of the capillary bed.[39,40] Elevated levels of hypoxia-inducible factor-1α and vascular endothelial growth factor (VEGF), as well as characteristic electroretinogram patterns in these mice, confirmed inner retinal hypoxia.[40] Moreover, ectopic lens expression of Norrin in knockout mice induces the formation of normal deep retinal capillaries, and completely prevents abnormalities in retinal angiogenesis.[41] These observations suggest a genetic basis for Coats disease and that a mutation in the *NDP* gene may be responsible.

Although FEVR and Coats disease share certain clinical features, they likely do not share a common genetic basis. Robataille and associates studied DNA expression of Frizzled-4 (*FZD4*) in 68 cases of FEVR and 16 cases of Coats disease.[42] They found 11 *FZD4* mutations in FEVR cases and no mutations in Coats disease cases. They concluded that germline mutations in *FZD4* do not appear to be a common cause of Coats disease, implying that Coats disease does not likely represent asymmetric FEVR and is a distinct ocular condition.

Other genetic pathways have been explored. Cremers and associates found that 55% of eyes with retinitis pigmentosa and Coats-like secondary exudative vasculopathy contained a mutation in the *CRB1* gene.[43] This suggests that the *CRB1* gene could be involved in primary Coats disease as well as other retinal diseases and dystrophies.

CLINICAL PRESENTATION

Coats disease is classically a painless ophthalmic condition. The disease affects males three times as often as females and has no reported racial or ethnic predilection.[44] Coats disease is unilateral in 80–95% of cases.[5,44,45] Some of the bilateral cases in older reports could represent secondary bilateral Coats-like retinopathy with systemic conditions and not true primary Coats disease. Any patient with bilateral presumed Coats disease should be evaluated for conditions that causes Coats-like exudative retinopathy such as retinitis pigmentosa, pars planitis, FSHD, FEVR, or other diseases.[46] Based on a study of 150 consecutive cases, the mean age at diagnosis is 5 years with a range of 1 month to 63 years.[44] Some speculate that the disease could be present at birth.[13,47]

In an analysis of 150 consecutive cases of Coats disease, presenting symptoms included decreased visual acuity (43%), strabismus (23%: Fig. 56.1), leukocoria/xanthocoria (20%: Fig. 56.1), pain (3%), heterochromia (1%), nystagmus (1%), and no symptom (8%).[44] Visual acuity was 20/20 to 20/50 in 12% of all eyes, 20/60 to 20/100 in 11%, 20/200 to counting fingers in 18%, and hand motions to no light perception in 58%. Nearly 90% of eyes had a normal anterior-segment examination. Those with findings included cataract (8%), iris neovascularization (8%), shallow anterior chamber (4%), corneal edema (3%), cholesterol in the anterior chamber (3%: Fig. 56.1),[48,49] and megalocornea (2%). Retinal findings included telangiectasia (100%), intraretinal exudation (99%), exudative retinal detachment (81% with 42% demonstrating partial retinal detachment and 58% with total retinal detachment), retinal hemorrhage (13%), retinal macrocyst (11%), vasoproliferative tumor (6%), and optic disc neovascularization (1%). No eyes in this cohort presented with vitreous hemorrhage. Other studies have described macular fibrosis in up to 23% of patients, developing in an area of previous dense exudation, and involving the fovea in all cases.[50]

Adult cases of Coats disease are similar in clinical presentation and disease course, but generally have a smaller area of involvement, slower disease progression, more frequent hemorrhage near larger aneurysmal dilated vessels, and typically do not present with strabismus.[51] Although the adult form of the disease has been described as frequently associated with hypercholesterolemia, such an association does not appear to occur in the juvenile form.[14,52]

The typical ophthalmoscopic picture in Coats disease is that of localized, yellow, subretinal exudation associated with adjacent vascular anomalies, including sheathing, telangiectasia, tortuosity, aneurysmal dilation, zones of capillary dropout, and occasionally neovascularization.[13,44] There is variability in this clinical picture.[44] Exudation, hemorrhage, or a combination appears minimal during less active stages of the disease and can progress to massive findings, obscuring the retinal vasculature in more aggressive stages. The vascular abnormalities can be subtle and clinically undetectable or can be obvious as a dominant feature. The clinical course is also variable, but is generally slowly progressive. Spontaneous remission has been observed but is exceptional.[53] Subretinal choroidal neovascularization rarely occurs in areas of lipid deposition. As subretinal fluid and exudation increase, the retinal detachment progresses and can reach a highly elevated state, visible behind the lens (Fig. 56.1). Hemorrhagic and nonhemorrhagic retinal macrocysts can occur as a result of chronic coalescent intraretinal cystoid edema.[54] Secondary complications such as iridocyclitis, cataract, and secondary neovascular glaucoma can lead to phthisis bulbi in severe cases.[2,15,55]

Several staging systems for Coats disease have been proposed.[2,56] The most recent and widely used was introduced by Shields and associates in 2000 (Table 56.1).[57] Stage 1 is characterized by retinal telangiectasia. Stage 2 has telangiectasia and intraretinal exudation, extrafoveal exudation defines stage 2A (Fig. 56.2), whereas foveal involvement defines stage 2B. Stage 3 is defined by exudative retinal detachment, 3A is a subtotal detachment, with 1 and 2 designating extrafoveal and foveal involvement, respectively (Fig. 56.3), and 3B is a total retinal detachment (Fig. 56.4). Stage 4 has total retinal detachment plus elevated intraocular pressure (Fig. 56.3), and stage 5 is endstage disease, occasionally with phthisis bulbi (Fig. 56.1). Using this classification for grouping of 124 cases, Shields and associates found stage 1 in 1%, stage 2 in 14% (2A in 8%, 2B in 6%), stage

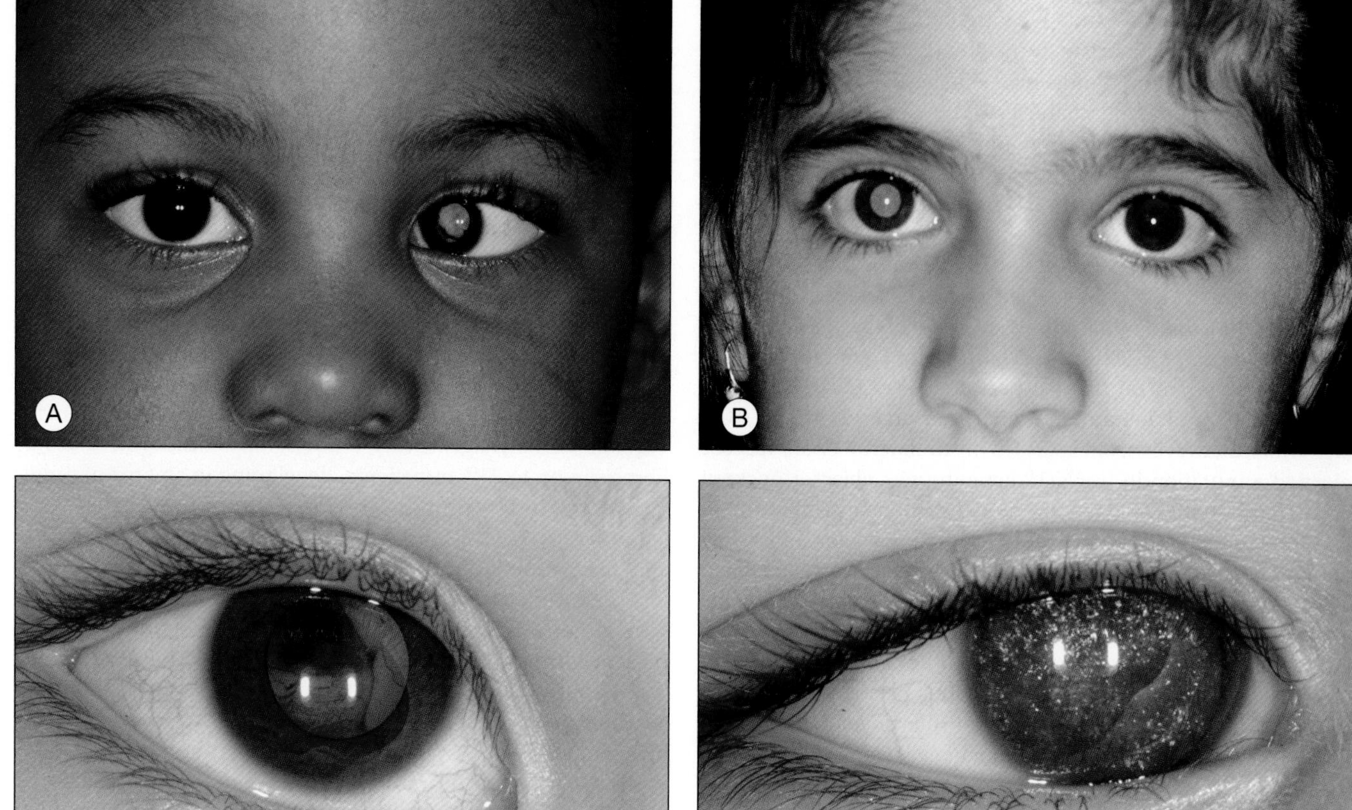

Fig. 56.1 Unique clinical features occasionally seen in Coats disease. (A) Young boy who presented with leukocoria and esotropia of the left eye. He had stage 5 disease, including total retinal detachment, cataract, and prephthisis. The decision was made to observe. (B) Young girl with xanthocoria of the right eye. (C) Young girl who presented with a total retinal detachment abutting the posterior surface of the lens. (D) Young girl with anterior-chamber cholesterolosis of the right eye.

Table 56.1 Staging system for Coats disease with prevalence on presentation

Stage	Simplified format	Criteria	Prevalence[57]
1	T	Retinal telangiectasia (T) only	1%
2	T+E	Telangiectasia and exudation (E)	14%
2A		Extrafoveal	8%
2B		Foveal	6%
3	T+E+D	Exudative retinal detachment (D)	69%
3A		Subtotal	38%
3A1		Extrafoveal	19%
3A2		Foveal	19%
3B		Total	30%
4	T+E+D+G	Total retinal detachment and glaucoma (G)	15%
5	T+E+D+G+P	Advanced endstage disease often with phthisis (P) bulbi	2%

(Adapted from Shields JA, Shields CL, Honavar SG, et al. Classification and management of Coats disease: the 2000 Proctor Lecture. Am J Ophthalmol 2001;131:572–83.)

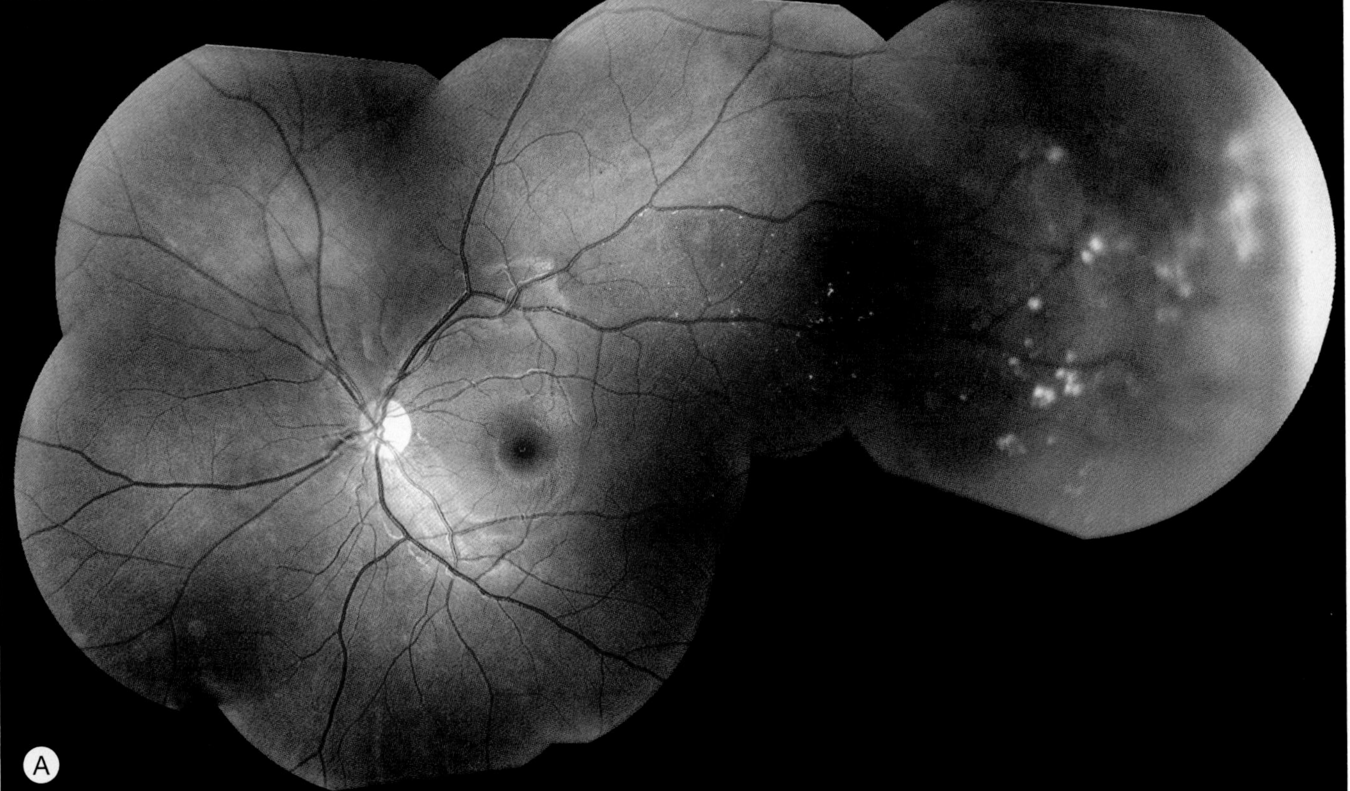

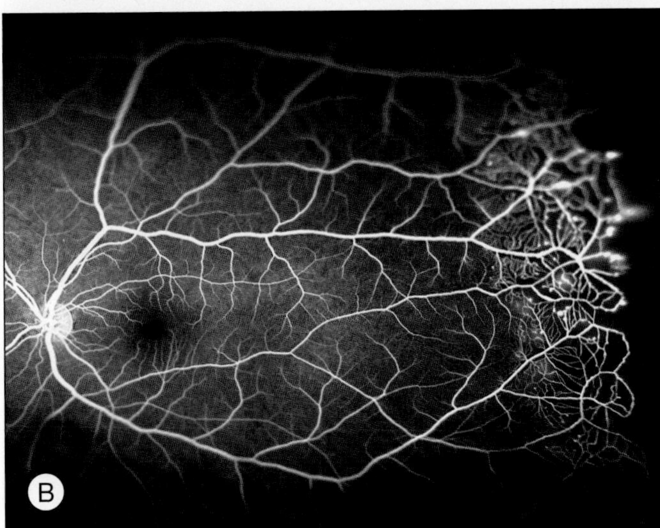

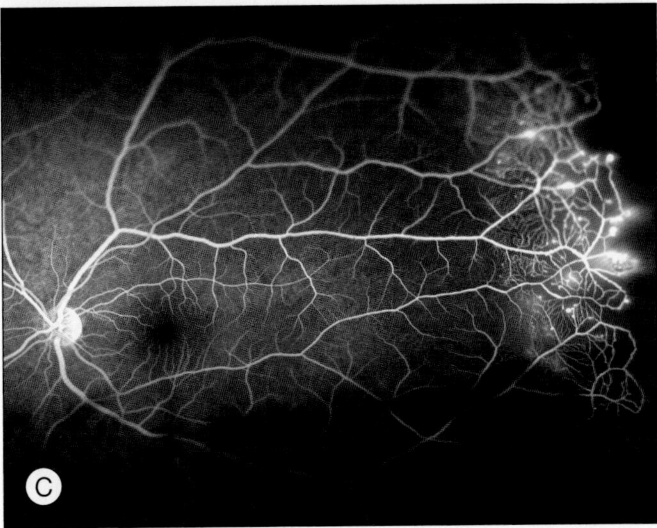

Fig. 56.2 Clinical imaging of a 10-year old Latina girl with stage 2A Coats disease in the left eye. (A) Montage color photograph. Note the exudation and vascular telangiectasia in the far temporal periphery. (B) Midphase wide-field fluorescein angiogram of the same patient. Note the far peripheral avascularity and adjacent telangiectatic vasculature. (C) Late-phase wide-field fluorescein angiogram of the same patient. Note the mild dye leakage from telangiectasia.

3 in 69% (3A1 in 19%, 3A2 in 19%, 3B in 30%), stage 4 in 15%, and stage 5 in 2%.[57] Based on classification and treatment, visual acuity strongly depended on stage at diagnosis.[44,58] At the time of Coats disease control, poor visual acuity (20/200 or worse) was found in 0% of stage 1, 53% of stage 2, 74% of stage 3, and 100% of stage 4 and stage 5.[57]

DIAGNOSTIC TESTING

Ancillary testing may be useful when the diagnosis of Coats disease is suspected, but other clinical entities must be ruled out, most notably retinoblastoma.[59] Particularly when retinal detachment with subretinal exudation and dilated retinal vessels coexist, even an experienced clinician may have difficulty differentiating these entities ophthalmoscopically. Fluorescein angiography is critical to document classic findings to establish the diagnosis. Echography may enable differentiation between Coats disease and retinoblastoma on the basis of features such as the character of the retinal detachment and the presence or absence of subretinal calcifications. Echography is less useful when the retinoblastoma is poorly calcified and also has shortcomings in detecting optic nerve or extraocular extension of retinoblastoma when heavy calcification exists.[60]

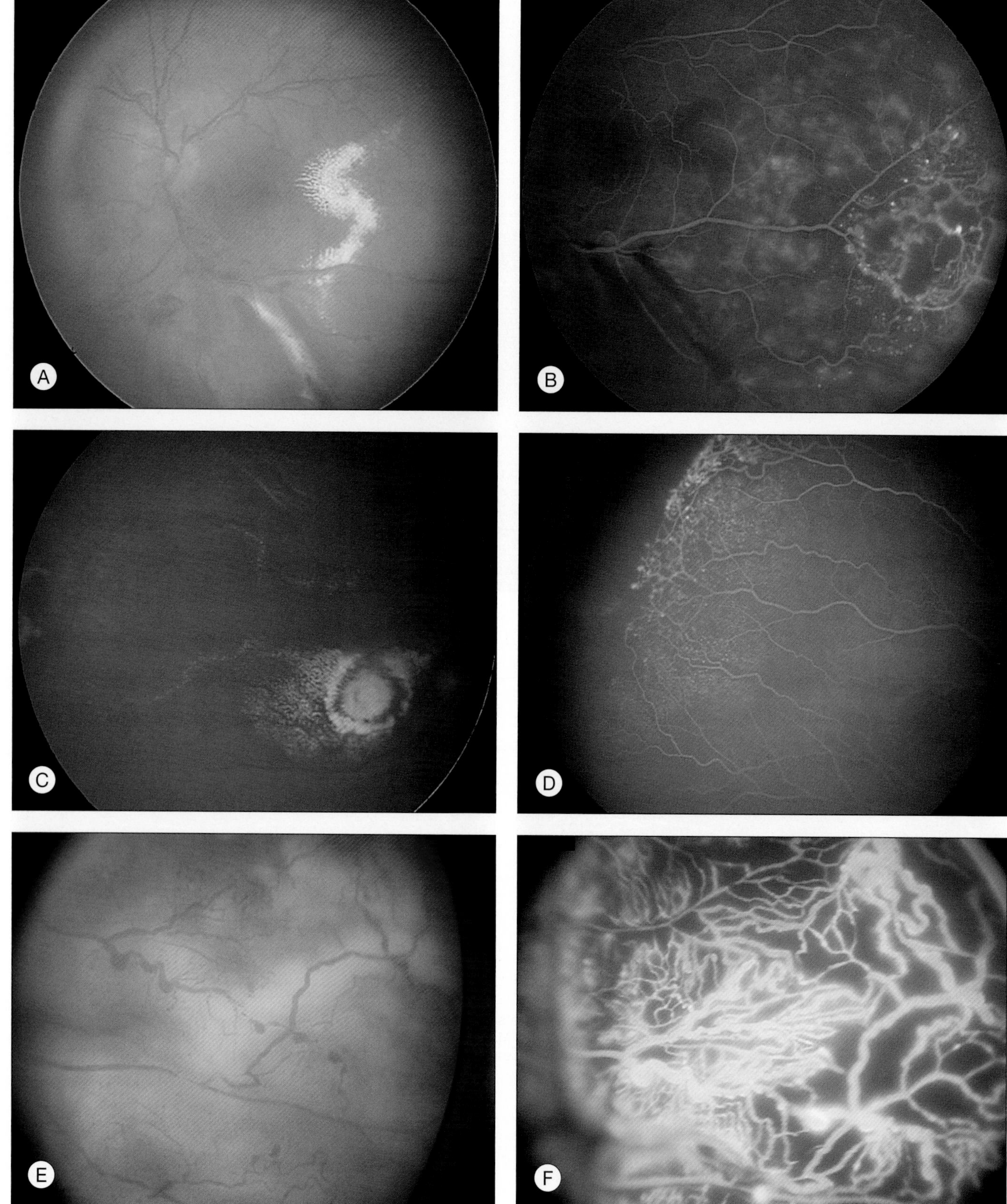

Fig. 56.3 Clinical images of various stages of Coats disease, including 3A1, 3A2, and 4. (A) Color fundus photograph of a patient with stage 3A1 Coats disease. Note the temporal extrafoveal exudation. (B) Recirculation-phase fluorescein angiogram of the same patient as in (A). Note the temporal vascular abnormalities, areas of capillary nonperfusion, and perivascular dye leakage. (C) Color fundus photograph of a patient with stage 3A2 Coats disease with prominent foveal exudation. Also note the subtle temporal vascular telangiectasia and aneurysmal vessels. (D) The extent of vascular abnormalities is more apparent in this midphase fluorescein angiogram. Note the telangiectasia adjacent to a wide zone of peripheral avascularity. (E) Color fundus photograph of a patient with stage 4 disease who presented with a total exudative retinal detachment and elevated intraocular pressure. (F) Fluorescein angiography revealed prominent capillary nonperfusion between dilated, abnormal vasculature.

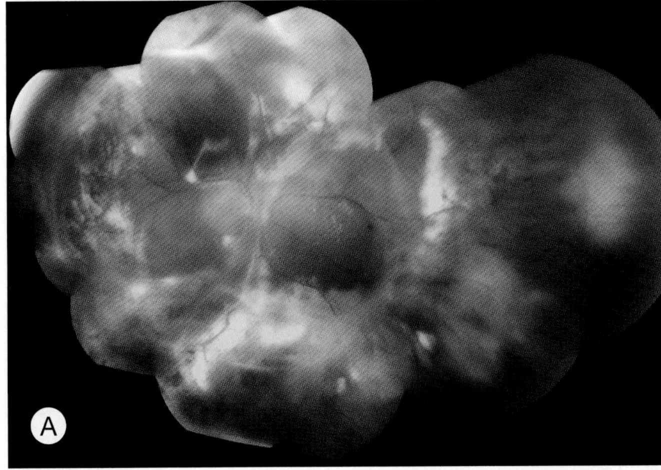

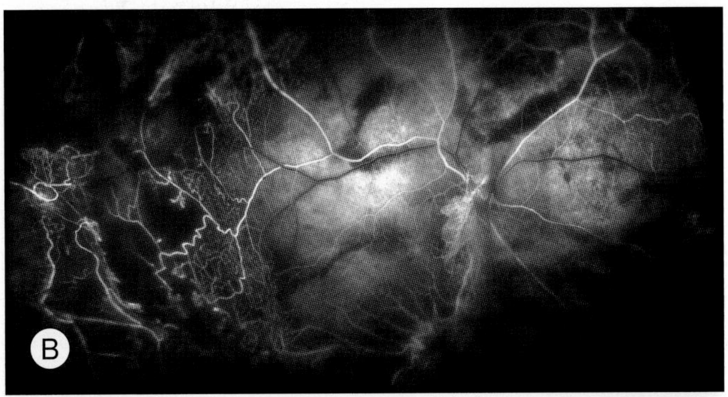

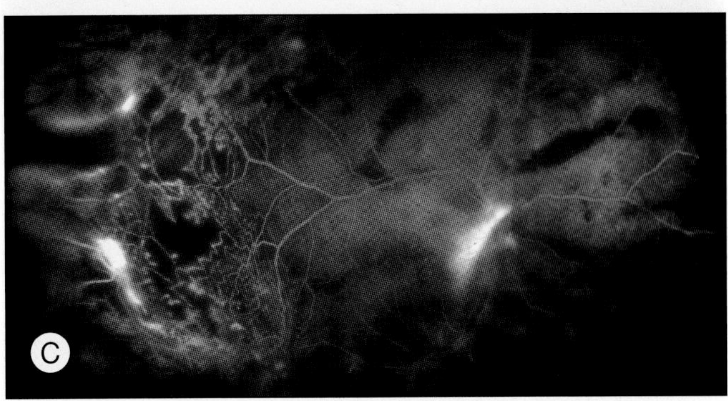

Fig. 56.4 Clinical imaging of a 17-year-old African American man with stage 3B Coats disease in the right eye. (A) Montage color fundus photograph depicting extensive subretinal exudation, a total retinal detachment, diffuse midperipheral vascular abnormalities, and optic nerve head neovascularization. (B) Early-phase fluorescein angiogram, centered more temporally than the color photo, demonstrating filling of telangiectatic and aneurysmal vascular channels, most prominent in the temporal periphery. Adjacent to telangiectatic vessels are large areas of retinal capillary nonperfusion. (C) In the later phase of the angiogram, leakage of dye from telangiectatic vessels and disc neovascularization are seen. (Courtesy of Carl Regillo, MD, Wills Eye Institute.)

Fluorescein angiography

The typical fluorescein angiographic picture of Coats disease is one of numerous localized anomalies of the retinal vasculature with peripheral retinal nonperfusion (Figs 56.2–56.6). Telangiectasia, aneurysms, beading of vessel walls, and various vascular communicating channels are found with larger vessels. These vessels show early and persistent leakage, which verifies their role as the source of exudation and hemorrhage. This leakage represents breakdown of the blood–retinal barrier, which can further be detected by vitreous fluorophotometry.[61] Microvascular involvement is demonstrated with areas of diffuse loss of the capillary bed or areas of complete capillary nonperfusion on angiography. Geographic zones of microvascular involvement are typically surrounded by areas of arteriolar and venular anomalies. Although some early authors described cases of massive exudation or hemorrhage without areas of obvious vascular involvement, fluorescein angiography and histopathologic specimens invariably show unsuspected anomalous vessels. The ability to identify all anomalous vessels, especially those with the greatest degree of leakage, has made adequate treatment of Coats disease a possibility.[5,57,62,63]

Computed tomography

CT is valuable because of its ability to characterize intraocular morphology, quantify subretinal densities, identify vascularities within the subretinal space through the use of contrast enhancement, and detect other abnormalities that may be associated in the orbital or intracranial space. Spiral CT has the advantage of reducing anesthesia risk in small children and also decreases acquisition time and staff and equipment monitoring requirements.[64]

Magnetic resonance imaging

Magnetic resonance imaging (MRI) as an auxiliary test is useful because it permits multiplanar imaging and superior contrast resolution and yields biochemical insight into the structure and composition of tissues.[65,66] It is less useful in detecting calcium than either ultrasound or CT scanning.[60,67] An MRI study of 28 patients with leukocoria or intraocular mass, or both, found that retinoblastomas could be reliably distinguished from Coats disease, toxocariasis, and persistent hyperplastic primary vitreous.[67] Calcification could not be reliably detected on MRI scanning.

Doppler ultrasonography

High-resolution Doppler ultrasound has been suggested as a diagnostic adjunct, providing unique information with real-time imaging and duplex pulse Doppler evaluation.[68] This technique may delineate structural abnormalities not shown by CT or MRI.

Blood testing

Aqueous lactic dehydrogenase and isoenzyme levels have not proved valuable in distinguishing between Coats disease and retinoblastoma. Examination of subretinal fluid, although rarely used, is accurate in confirming the diagnosis of Coats disease on the basis of cholesterol crystal and pigment-laden macrophages in the absence of tumor cells.[60]

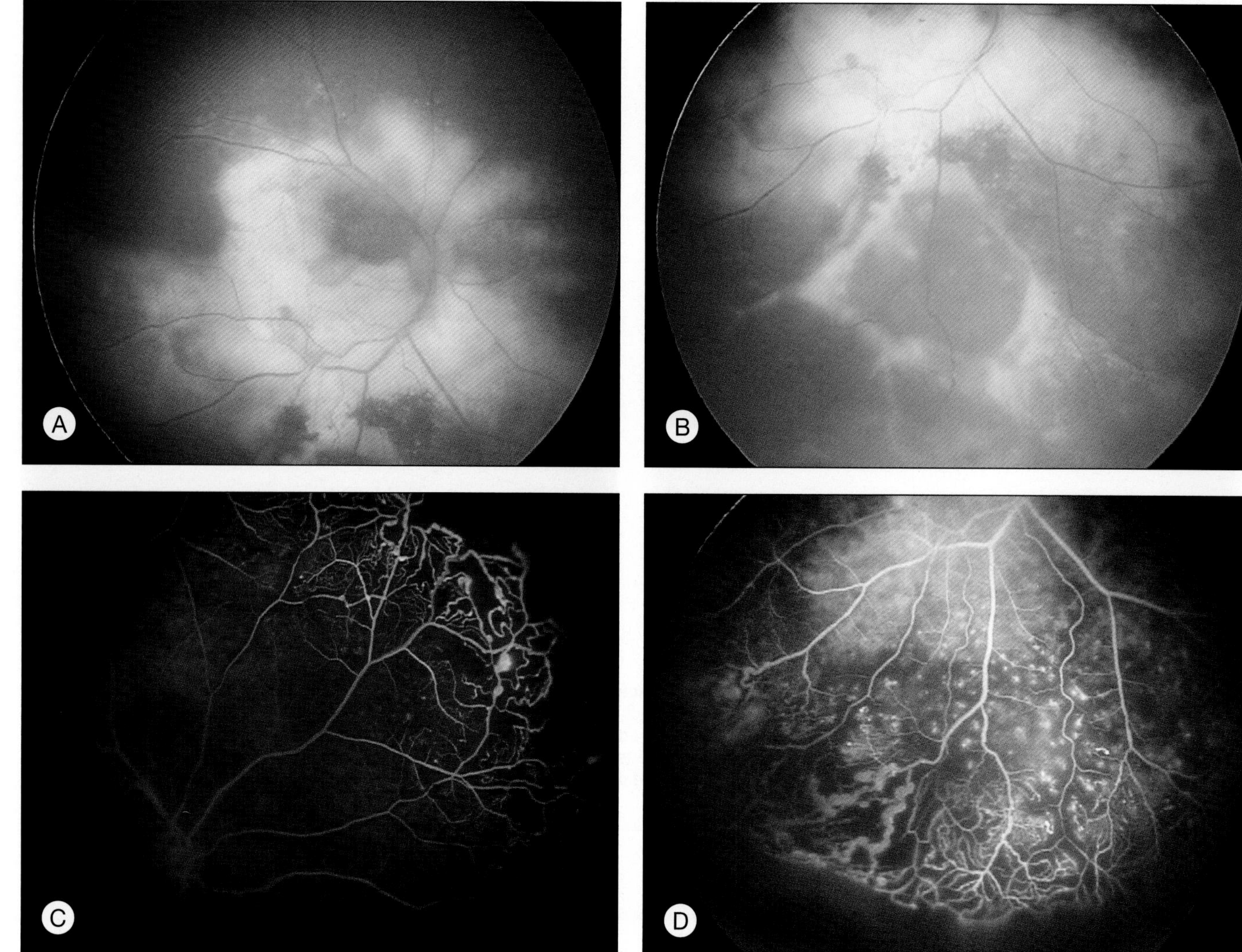

Fig. 56.5 Color fundus photography and fluorescein angiography of a patient with stage 4 Coats disease. Macular (A) and inferior (B) color photographs depicting extensive subretinal exudate. Note the elevated retinal detachment in B. (C) Early-phase fluorescein angiogram of the superonasal retinal periphery. Note the blunted, telangiectatic, and aneurysmal vasculature just posterior to a zone of avascular retina. (D) Midphase fluorescein angiogram of the inferior retina corresponding to (B), depicting similar angiographic findings as well as prominent sausage-like vascular dilations.

DIFFERENTIAL DIAGNOSIS

The differential diagnosis of Coats disease includes other conditions that produce leukocoria or strabismus,[19] including retinoblastoma,[15,69] retinal detachment, persistent hyperplastic primary vitreous, congenital cataract, Norrie disease, and FEVR,[70] among other diagnoses. Shields and associates reviewed 150 cases of Coats disease and found that the diagnosis was correct in 64 cases (41%).[44] The mistaken referring diagnoses included retinoblastoma in 43 cases (27%), retinal detachment in 12 (8%), retinal hemorrhage in 7 (4%), toxocariasis in 4 (3%), choroidal melanoma in 2 (1%), choroidal hemangioma in 2 (1%), coloboma in 2 (1%), endophthalmitis in 2 (1%), and single cases of cytomegalovirus retinitis, retinopathy of prematurity, traumatic retinopathy, and toxoplasmosis. In 18 cases (11%) there was no submitted diagnosis.

Numerous entities have been described as presenting with a Coats-like picture, including several systemic conditions, and Coats disease can also simulate other exudative retinal conditions such as FEVR, peripheral vasculitis, Eales disease, and FSHD (Table 56.2). FEVR is an important consideration and can present with peripheral avascularity with telangiectasia and exudation. FEVR can be differentiated based on the typical presence of retinal dragging, a positive family history, and bilaterality, all of which are rare in Coats disease. A Coats-like picture of bilateral retinal telangiectasia and exudation has been described in patients with deafness and FSHD.[71–73] It is believed that the retinal vascular abnormalities, muscular dystrophy, and deafness in FSHD may all be a consequence of a common mechanism based on abnormal Wnt signaling.[35]

A Coats-like picture associated with varied skeletal defects, cerebellar and extrapyramidal movement disorder, epileptic seizures, leukodystrophic changes, and postnatal growth failure has been referred to as "Coats plus syndrome."[74] In order to avoid confusion, the term "Coats disease" should be reserved for cases of idiopathic retinal telangiectasia associated with intraretinal exudation with or without exudative retinal detachment, without evidence of vitreoretinal traction.[7,44]

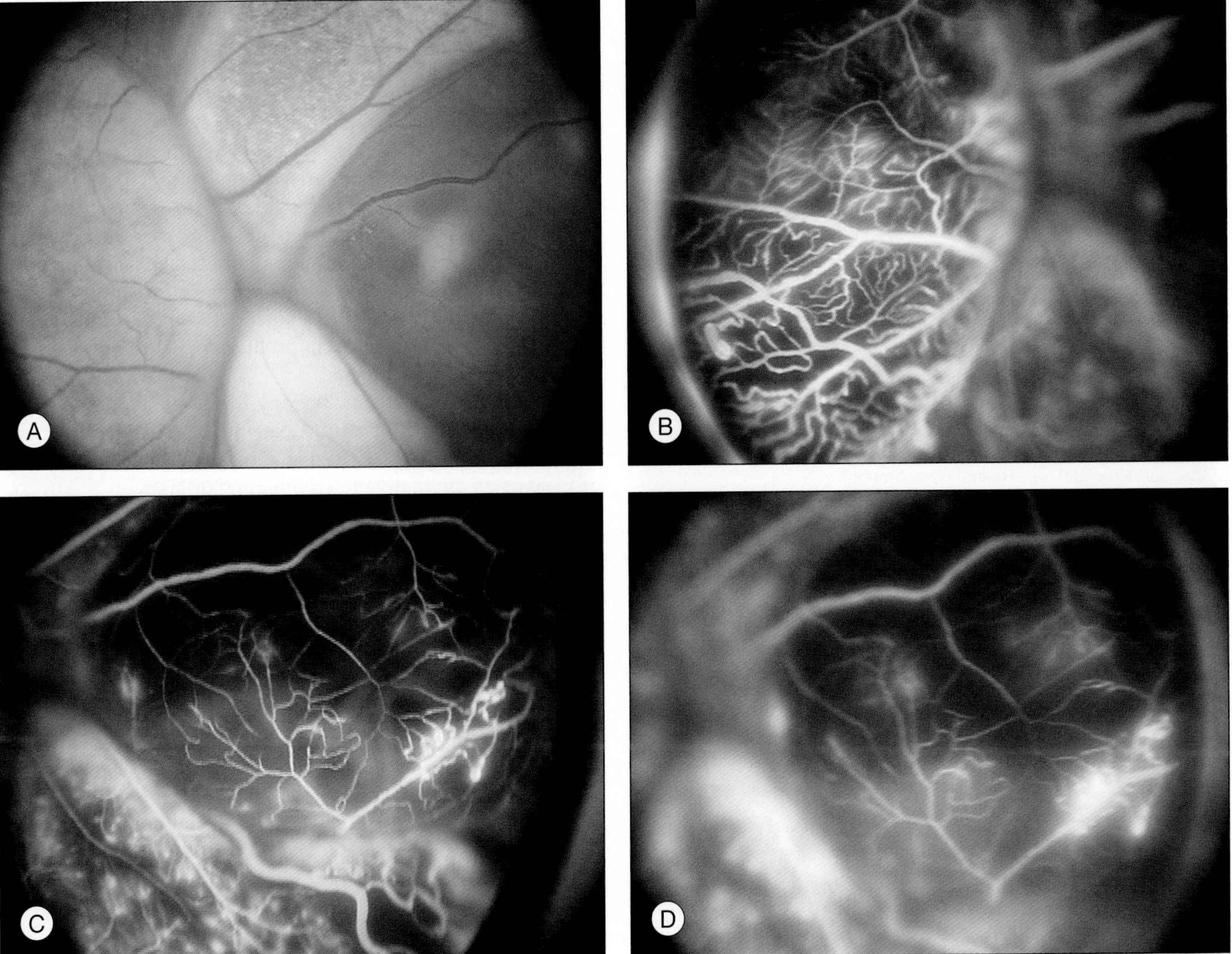

Fig. 56.6 Color fundus photography and fluorescein angiogram of a patient with a total bullous retinal detachment associated with Coats disease. (A) Color fundus photograph depicting the very bullous retinal detachment. (B–D) Fluorescein angiogram images of the same patient depicting typical angiographic features of Coats disease.

Isolated case reports have described a number of other disorders occurring concurrently with Coats disease, including retinitis pigmentosa,[75,76] Senior–Loken syndrome,[77] the ichthyosis hystrix variant of epidermal nevus syndrome,[78] Turner's syndrome,[79] diffuse central nervous system venous abnormality,[80] and Hallermann–Streiff syndrome[81] (Table 56.2). Small, in 1968, reported the combination of mental retardation, muscular dystrophy, and an exudative vasculopathy in four siblings.[71] Egerer and associates noted histologic evidence of rosettes characteristic of retinal dysplasia in a series of nine enucleated eyes carrying the diagnosis of Coats disease.[82] Fogle and colleagues noted an exudative vasculopathy with a clinical picture similar to that of Coats disease arising from abnormal choroidal vessels in both eyes of a patient with retinitis pigmentosa.[83] Despite these reports, no definite connection has been made between other systemic or ocular conditions and Coats disease.

TREATMENT

Treatment for Coats disease depends on the stage of disease. Mild cases with only retinal telangiectasia (stage 1) should be documented with color fundus photography and wide-field fluorescein angiography and followed conservatively. If subretinal fluid or exudation develop, then intervention is necessary. For more advanced stages (2 through 4), treatment involves ablation with photocoagulation or cryotherapy to areas of telangiectatic vasculature and retinal nonperfusion. Surgical intervention to repair traction, hemorrhage, or rhegmatogenous retinal detachment is rarely necessary.

Ablative therapies – laser photocoagulation and cryotherapy

In less severe cases of exudation due to Coats disease, with or without retinal detachment, argon or diode laser photocoagulation is the treatment of choice (Fig. 56.7).[84–86] Fluorescein angiographic guidance assists directed treatment of vascular leakage. Most wavelengths of laser light are adequate for treatment, although those near the yellow portion of the spectrum have better absorption by blood in the target vascular channels and may be particularly useful if the vessels are in detached retina. Leaking lesions are treated directly with moderate to large (100–500 μm, depending on size and location of the target lesions) applications of moderate-intensity light. Scatter

Table 56.2 Clinical conditions that can present with Coats-like retinal findings	
Systemic conditions	Muscular dystrophy[71,120–122] Turner syndrome[123] Epidermal nevus syndrome[78] Cornelia de Lange syndrome[124] Alport syndrome[125] Senior–Loken syndrome (familial renal-retinal dystrophy)[77] 13q deletion syndrome[126] Renal transplantation[127] Ch 3 inversion[128] Hallermann–Streiff syndrome[81] Aplastic anemia[129] Multiple glomus tumors[130] Telangiectasia of the nasal mucosa[131] Osteoporosis pseudoglioma syndrome[132] Focal segmental glomerulosclerosis[133]
Ocular conditions that can simulate juvenile Coats disease	Retinoblastoma[45] Retinal detachment Congenital cataract Norrie disease[37] Persistent hyperplastic primary vitreous Ocular toxocariasis Retinal capillary hemangiomatosis Retinal cavernous hemangiomatosis Vasoproliferative tumor Familial exudative vitreoretinopathy
Ocular conditions that can simulate Coats disease at any age	Branch retinal vein occlusion[134] Eales disease Vasculitis Tumor accompanied by exudation Diabetic vasculopathies with lipid exudation Ocular toxoplasmosis[135] Morning-glory disc anomaly[136] Idiopathic retinal gliosis[137] Retinal dysplasia[82] Type 1 idiopathic juxtafoveolar telangiectasis Retinitis pigmentosa[75,83,138–141] Retinal macroaneurysm Retinal capillary hemangiomatosis Familial exudative vitreoretinopathy Any vasculopathy producing exudation Epiretinal membrane with secondary exudation

photocoagulation to areas of extensive nonperfusion is of unproven value but could decrease the risk of later neovascularization. If lesions are too peripheral to be reached with the slit-lamp delivery system, the indirect ophthalmoscope-mounted laser, transscleral laser, or cryotherapy can be used.[87] These methods may be particularly useful in small children, who usually require general anesthesia for treatment. Of note, extensive laser photocoagulation can result in transient disruption of the blood–retinal barrier, paradoxically increasing retinal exudation. Several sessions of therapy, approximately every 3 months, are often necessary to produce complete resolution of exudation or detachment.[57,84,88] Complications of photocoagulation in Coats disease include inflammation, choroidal detachment, progressive exudation, creation of chorioretinal and vitreochoroidal anastomoses, epiretinal membrane formation, sympathetic ophthalmia, rhegmatogenous retinal detachment, and hemorrhage.

Double freeze–thaw cryotherapy is also useful in ablating affected areas of the retina, and is particularly helpful in cases where laser is ineffective, such as extensive subretinal exudation or retinal detachment. In some cases it may be necessary to drain subretinal fluid to obtain sufficient retinal vascular freezing. As with laser photocoagulation, many more advanced cases require multiple sessions.[57] To minimize side-effects in eyes with extensive vascular abnormalities, selective treatment with cryotherapy to two or fewer quadrants per session may be advised, as well as avoidance of the ciliary body. In some cases with advanced disease and imminent glaucoma, treatment of the entire four quadrants of the retina is necessary. Compared to laser, cryotherapy is associated with more inflammation and patient discomfort as well as potential complications, which include subcapsular cataract, proliferative vitreoretinopathy, and total retinal detachment.[63]

The use of photodynamic therapy in combination with intravitreal bevacizumab for adult Coats disease was reported in a single case report, with apparent success.[89] Diathermy also can be used as an alternative to cryotherapy or laser.

Pharmacologic therapies

Intravitreal triamcinolone acetonide (IVTA) is effective in reducing macular edema and subretinal exudation.[90,91]Othman and colleagues recently described their experience in 15 eyes treated with 4 mg IVTA in combination with traditional treatment modalities and followed for at least 1 year. All patients experienced an improvement in visual acuity, although 40% required cataract surgery and one patient required intraocular pressure-lowering drops.[90]

Intravitreal anti-VEGF agents have been reported to be effective as adjunctive therapy to reduce subretinal fluid and macular exudation in children with Coats if given alone[92–94] or in combination with IVTA,[95,96] laser photocoagulation, or cryotherapy.[94,95,97–99] Intraocular VEGF levels are known to be substantially elevated in eyes with Coats disease, with dramatic decline following intravitreal anti-VEGF injection.[100,101] In a study of four eyes with Coats disease, the intraocular VEGF levels were nearly 2400 pg/mL, compared to 15 pg/mL in five eyes with rhegmatogenous retinal detachment.[101] In one eye with stage 2B disease in that report, the intraocular VEGF level decreased from 1247 pg/mL to 20.4 pg/mL 1 month after a single injection of intravitreal bevacizumab, with a corresponding improvement in visual acuity. VEGF levels may be elevated secondary to retinal ischemia associated with the abnormal vasculature.

Although in most of the available reports anti-VEGF agents appeared to be well tolerated, the case numbers are small, with limited follow-up. In the largest published series to date of eight eyes, Ramasubramanian and Shields noted the development of vitreous fibrosis in four eyes after a mean of 1.75 injections and 5 months of follow-up. In three of these patients, this progressed to tractional retinal detachment.[102] Furthermore, we have no data on the long-term consequences of repeated anti-VEGF injections in children. Larger studies with longer follow-up will be necessary to establish the safety of anti-VEGF in juvenile Coats disease.

In contrast, the safety profile of anti-VEGF injections in adults is well established, and several small studies have shown the efficacy of anti-VEGF agents in adult-onset Coats with macular involvement.[103,104]

Surgery

Less invasive measures are usually effective in treating exudative retinal detachment with Coats disease;[105] however eyes with

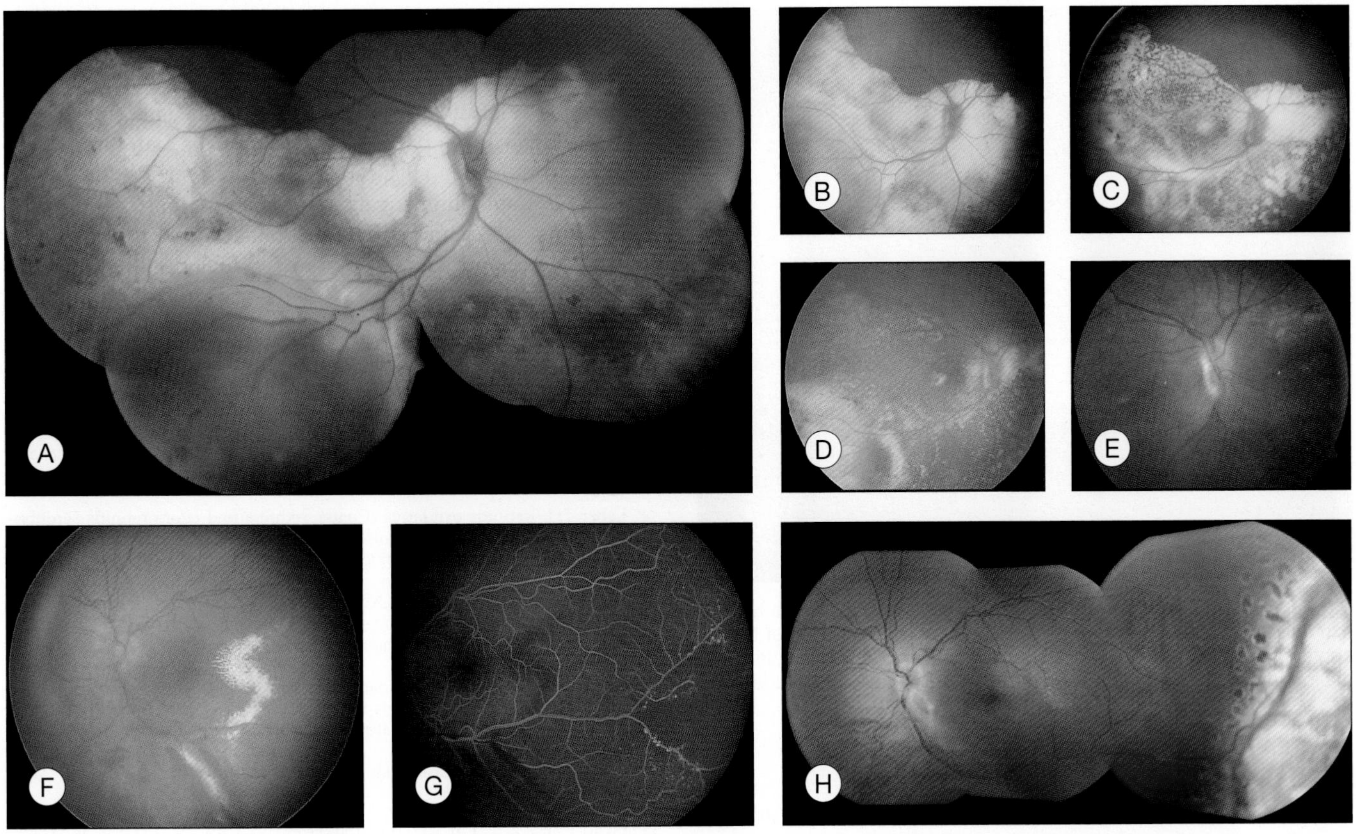

Fig. 56.7 Color fundus photographs from two patients demonstrating the effect of laser photocoagulation. Laser photocoagulation was used to treat focal areas of leakage in the peripheral retina with a modified scatter pattern to zones of capillary nonperfusion. Burns were 100–500 μm and of moderate intensity applied through a fundus contact lens. (A) Montage color fundus photograph of a separate patient with stage 4 Coats disease. Note the extensive exudation. (B–E) Sequential color fundus photographs following treatment with laser photocoagulation; the exudation and retinal detachment were noted to be slowly improving. (F) Color fundus photograph of the left macula in a patient with stage 3A1 Coats disease. (G) Fluorescein angiogram of the same patient delineating areas of retinal nonperfusion and vascular abnormalities that are used to guide laser photocoagulation. (H) Montage color photograph of the same patient following treatment with laser photocoagulation. Note the laser scars in the far temporal periphery as well as the total resolution of retinal exudation. The visual acuity following treatment improved to 20/20.

advanced retinal detachment abutting the crystalline lens or those with a rhegmatogenous component to the detachment may benefit from surgical repair.

Machemer and Williams reported improvement in the clinical course of selected cases of Coats disease with vitreous surgery consisting of removal of vitreal and preretinal membranes to eliminate traction detachment, combined with destruction of leaking vessels.[106] Other authors have advocated the use of vitrectomy with internal drainage of subretinal fluid to flatten the retina, before vasoablative procedures, and intraocular tamponade with gas or silicone oil.[107–109] Silodor and associates have used intraocular infusion, drainage of subretinal fluid, and cryotherapy with success in eyes with advanced bullous retinal detachment.[110] In their series of 13 children with blindness from Coats disease, six that were followed without surgery developed painful neovascular glaucoma necessitating enucleation and seven that were surgically repaired avoided glaucoma and the eyes remained cosmetically acceptable. When transscleral drainage of extensive subretinal fluid is necessary, a pediatric infusion cannula placed in the anterior chamber works well for maintaining the globe (Fig. 56.8).

Endstage cases associated with neovascular or angle closure glaucoma, or a blind painful eye may require enucleation.[57,111] Alternatively, eyes with neovascular glaucoma may respond to transscleral diode laser cyclophotocoagulation.[112]

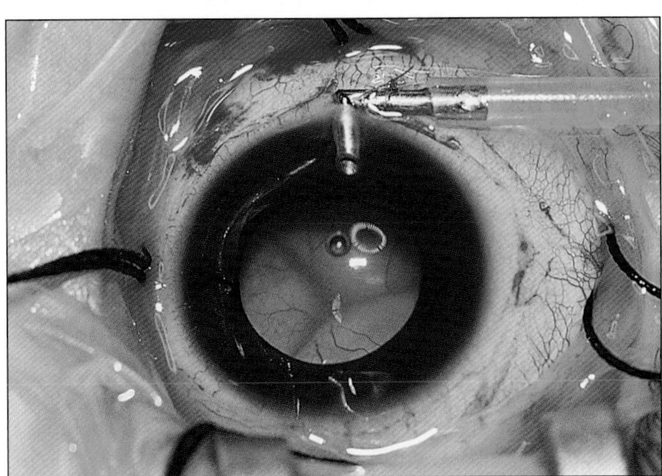

Fig. 56.8 In this eye of an 18-month-old boy with total exudative retinal detachment, anatomic stability was achieved by infusion into the anterior chamber, posterior drainage of subretinal fluid, and cryotherapy to 11 clock-hours of peripheral vascular anomalies. (Reproduced with permission from Haller JA. Coats' disease and retinal telangiectasia. In: Yanoff M, Duker JS, editors. Ophthalmology. London: Mosby; 1999.)

OUTCOMES

In a series of 103 eyes, published by Shields and associates in 2001, telangiectasia resolved completely (47%) or partially (53%) over a mean interval of 15 months following treatment.[57]

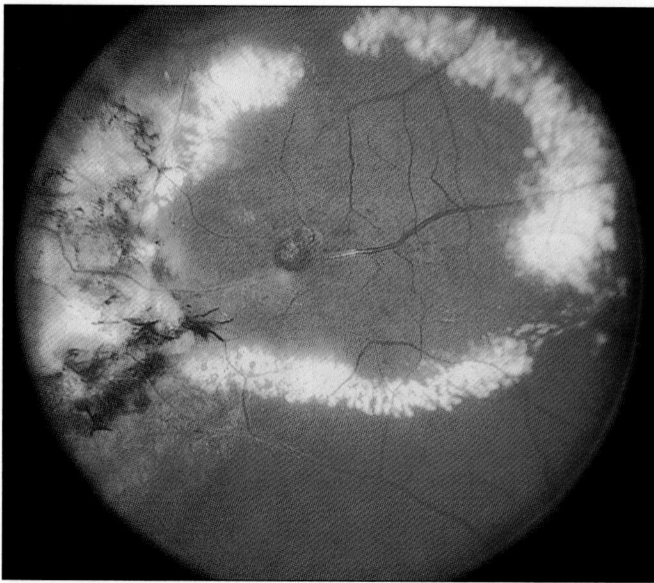

Fig. 56.9 This patient, previously treated successfully for Coats-type exudative retinopathy (see old scarring and fibrosis to the left of the photograph), has now developed a new adjacent area of vascular malformation and aneurysmal dilation, with a circinate lipid exudate.

Following treatment, inactive telangiectasia and old exudation were found in 45% of cases at 17 months.[57] Residual telangiectatic areas are often left untreated, especially if there is no fresh exudation or subretinal fluid. The goal of treatment is to close telangiectasia so that further leakage is halted. In 7% of cases by 10 years, recurrence of leakage from residual or new telangiectasia can occur.[57]

Anatomically, most cases (76%) stabilize or improve following treatment, with the minority (8%) progressively worsening.[57] Approximately 20% require enucleation for neovascular glaucoma or painful phthisis bulbi.[57] In the large series by Shields and colleagues on 150 patients, 117 individuals (124 eyes) were managed and followed for a median of 23 months and outcomes were determined. Management included observation in 22 eyes (18%), photocoagulation in 16 (13%), cryotherapy in 52 (42%), retinal detachment repair with drainage of subretinal fluid and cryotherapy or photocoagulation in 20 (17%), and enucleation in 14 (11%). Often multiple sessions were required. The median interval from initial treatment to complete resolution of telangiectasia was 10 months (range 2–123 months). Exudation resolved completely in 46 cases (45%) over a median of 12 months. Of the 88 eyes with retinal detachment prior to treatment, 50 (57%) had complete resolution of the detachment. Unfortunately, visual outcome with this condition is generally poor as foveal exudation and retinal detachment often destroy macular function. In that series, final visual acuity was 20/50 or better in 16%, 20/60 to 20/100 in 8%, 20/200 to finger counting in 29%, and hand motions to no light perception in 47%.[57] Severe vision loss was due to persistent foveal exudation, retinal detachment, and/or subfoveal fibrosis. Risk factors predictive of poor visual outcome (20/200 or worse) included noncaucasian race, postequatorial ($P = 0.01$), diffuse ($P = 0.01$), or superior ($P = 0.04$) location of telangiectasia and exudation, failed resolution of subretinal fluid after treatment ($P = 0.02$), and presence of retinal macrocysts ($P = 0.02$). Significant risk factors for enucleation included elevated intraocular pressure (greater than 22 mm Hg; $P < 0.001$) and iris neovascularization ($P < 0.001$) at presentation.

Following resolution of exudation, extensive subretinal fibrosis and pigmentation, particularly in the fovea, can limit visual recovery. Intraocular surgical intervention carries the added risks of endophthalmitis, retinal tear formation, rhegmatogenous retinal detachment, and proliferative vitreoretinopathy.[5,79,113–116] Patients should be followed lifelong for recurrence (Fig. 56.9).[57,117–119]

REFERENCES

1. Egbert PR, Chan CC, Winter FC. Flat preparations of the retinal vessels in Coats' disease. J Pediatr Ophthalmol 1976;13:336–9.
2. Coats G. Forms of retinal disease with massive exudation. R Lond Ophthalm Hosp Rep 1908;525:440–525.
3. Leber TH. Über eine durch Vorkommen multipler Miliaraneurysmen charakterisierte Form von Retinaldegeneration. Graefes Arch Ophthalmol 1912;81: 1–14.
4. Leber TH. Retinitis exudativa (Coats), retinitis und chorioretinitis serofibrinosa degenerans. Graefe-Saemisch Augenheilk 1915;7:1267–319.
5. Egerer I, Tasman W, Tomer T. Coats disease. Arch Ophthalmol 1974;92:109–12.
6. Leber T. Die Krankheiten der Netzhaut. In: Handbuch der gesamten Augenheilkunde. Leipzig: Engelmann, Graefe und Saemisch; 1916.
7. Reese AB. Telangiectasis of the retina and Coats' disease. Am J Ophthalmol 1956;42:1–8.
8. Bonnet M. Le syndrome de Coats. J Fr Ophthalmol 1980;3:57–66.
9. Theodossiadis GP, Bairaktaris-Kouris E, Kouris T. Evolution of Leber's miliary aneurysms: a clinicopathological study. J Pediatr Ophthalmol Strabismus 1979;16:364–70.
10. Sugar HS. Coats' disease: telangiectatic or multiple vascular origin. Am J Ophthalmol 1958;45:508–17.
11. Wise GN. Coats' disease. AMA Arch Ophthalmol 1957;58:735–46.
12. Evens L, Francois J, Rabaey M, et al. [Title not available.] Ophthalmologica 1956;132:1–12.
13. Imre G. Coats' disease. Am J Ophthalmol 1962;54:175.
14. Woods AC, Duke JR. Coats's disease. I. Review of the literature, diagnostic criteria, clinical findings, and plasma lipid studies. Br J Ophthalmol 1963;47:385–412.
15. Naumann GD, Portwich E. [Etiology and final clinical cause for 1000 enucleations. (A clinico-pathologic study) (author's transl.).] Klin Monbl Augenheilkd 1976;168:622–30.
16. Eagle Jr RC. Eye pathology. Philadelphia: Lippincott Williams & Wilkins; 2011. pp. 221–2
17. Hogan M, Zimmerman L. Ophthalmic pathology, an atlas and textbook. Philadelphia: WB Saunders; 1962.
18. Tripathi R, Ashton N. Electron microscopical study of Coats' disease. Br J Ophthalmol 1971;55:289–301.
19. Chang MM, McLean IW, Merritt JC. Coats' disease: a study of 62 histologically confirmed cases. J Pediatr Ophthalmol Strabismus 1984;21:163–8.
20. Duke JR, Woods AC. Coats's disease. II. Studies on the identity of the lipids concerned, and the probable role of mucopolysaccharides in its pathogenesis. Br J Ophthalmol 1963;47:413–34.
21. Farkas TG, Potts AM, Boone C. Some pathologic and biochemical aspects of Coats' disease. Am J Ophthalmol 1973; 75:289–301.
22. Takei Y. Origin of ghost cell in Coats' disease. Invest Ophthalmol 1976;15: 677–81.
23. Yannuzzi L, Gitter K, Schatz H. The macula: a comprehensive text and atlas. Baltimore: Williams & Wilkins; 1979.
24. Senft SH, Hidayat AA, Cavender JC. Atypical presentation of Coats disease. Retina 1994;14:36–8.
25. Pe'er J. Calcifications in Coats' disease. Am J Ophthalmol 1988;106: 742–3.
26. Ye X, Wang Y, Cahill H, et al. Norrin, frizzled-4, and Lrp5 signaling in endothelial cells controls a genetic program for retinal vascularization. Cell 2009;139:285–98.
27. Clevers H. Eyeing up new Wnt pathway players. Cell 2009;139:227–9.
28. Lin P, Shankar SP, Duncan J, et al. Retinal vascular abnormalities and dragged maculae in a carrier with a new NDP mutation (c. 268delC) that caused severe Norrie disease in the proband. J AAPOS 2010;14:93–6.
29. Dickinson JL, Sale MM, Passmore A, et al. Mutations in the NDP gene: contribution to Norrie disease, familial exudative vitreoretinopathy and retinopathy of prematurity. Clin Experiment Ophthalmol 2006;34:682–8.
30. Warden SM, Andreoli CM, Mukai S. The Wnt signaling pathway in familial exudative vitreoretinopathy and Norrie disease. Semin Ophthalmol 2007;22: 211–7.
31. Qin M, Hayashi H, Oshima K, et al. Complexity of the genotype–phenotype correlation in familial exudative vitreoretinopathy with mutations in the LRP5 and/or FZD4 genes. Hum Mutat 2005;26:104–12.
32. Jiao X, Ventruto V, Trese MT, et al. Autosomal recessive familial exudative vitreoretinopathy is associated with mutations in LRP5. Am J Hum Genet 2004;75:878–84.

33. Chen ZY, Battinelli EM, Fielder A, et al. A mutation in the Norrie disease gene (NDP) associated with X-linked familial exudative vitreoretinopathy. Nat Genet 1993;5:180–3.
34. Chung BD, Kayserili H, Ai M, et al. A mutation in the signal sequence of LRP5 in a family with an osteoporosis-pseudoglioma syndrome (OPPG)-like phenotype indicates a novel disease mechanism for trinucleotide repeats. Hum Mutat 2009;30:641–8.
35. Fitzsimons RB. Retinal vascular disease and the pathogenesis of facioscapulohumeral muscular dystrophy. A signalling message from Wnt? Neuromuscul Disord 2011;214:263–71.
36. Xu Q, Wang Y, Dabdoub A, et al. Vascular development in the retina and inner ear: control by Norrin and Frizzled-4, a high-affinity ligand-receptor pair. Cell 2004;116:883–95.
37. Black GC, Perveen R, Bonshek R, et al. Coats' disease of the retina (unilateral retinal telangiectasis) caused by somatic mutation in the NDP gene: a role for norrin in retinal angiogenesis. Hum Mol Genet 1999;8:2031–5.
38. Shastry BS, Trese MT. Overproduction and partial purification of the Norrie disease gene product, norrin, from a recombinant baculovirus. Biochem Biophys Res Commun 2003;312:229–34.
39. Berger W, van de Pol D, Bachner D, et al. An animal model for Norrie disease (ND): gene targeting of the mouse ND gene. Hum Mol Genet 1996;5:51–9.
40. Luhmann UF, Lin J, Acar N et al. Role of the Norrie disease pseudoglioma gene in sprouting angiogenesis during development of the retinal vasculature. Invest Ophthalmol Vis Sci 2005;46:3372–82.
41. Ohlmann A, Scholz M, Goldwich A, et al. Ectopic norrin induces growth of ocular capillaries and restores normal retinal angiogenesis in Norrie disease mutant mice. J Neurosci 2005;25:1701–10.
42. Robitaille JM, Zheng B, Wallace K, et al. The role of Frizzled-4 mutations in familial exudative vitreoretinopathy and Coats disease. Br J Ophthalmol 2011;95:574–9.
43. Cremers FP, Maugeri A, den Hollander AI, et al. The expanding roles of ABCA4 and CRB1 in inherited blindness. Novartis Found Symp 2004;255:68–79. discussion 79–84, 177–8.
44. Shields JA, Shields CL, Honavar SG, et al. Clinical variations and complications of Coats disease in 150 cases: the 2000 Sanford Gifford Memorial Lecture. Am J Ophthalmol 2001;131:561–71.
45. Shields JA, Shields CL. Differentiation of coats' disease and retinoblastoma. J Pediatr Ophthalmol Strabismus 2001;38:262–6. quiz 302–263.
46. Vance SK, Wald KJ, Sherman J, et al. Subclinical facioscapulohumeral muscular dystrophy masquerading as bilateral Coats disease in a woman. Arch Ophthalmol 2011;129:807–9.
47. Campbell FP. Coats' disease and congenital vascular retinopathy. Trans Am Ophthalmol Soc 1976;74:365–424.
48. Gupta N, Beri S, D'Souza P. Cholesterolosis bulbi of the anterior chamber in Coats disease. J Pediatr Ophthalmol Strabismus 2009;1–3.
49. Shields JA, Eagle Jr RC, Fammartino J, et al. Coats' disease as a cause of anterior chamber cholesterolosis. Arch Ophthalmol 1995;113:975–7.
50. Jumper JM, Pomerleau D, McDonald HR, et al. Macular fibrosis in Coats disease. Retina 2010;30(Suppl):S9–14.
51. Smithen LM, Brown GC, Brucker AJ, et al. Coats' disease diagnosed in adulthood. Ophthalmology 2005;112:1072–8.
52. Yeung J, Harris GS. Coats' disease: A study of cholesterol transport in the eye. Can J Ophthalmol 1976;11:61–8.
53. Deutsch TA, Rabb MF, Jampol LM. Spontaneous regression of retinal lesions in Coats' disease. Can J Ophthalmol 1982;17:169–72.
54. Goel SD, Augsburger JJ. Hemorrhagic retinal macrocysts in advanced Coats disease. Retina 1991;11:437–40.
55. Friedenwald H, Friedenwald JS. Terminal stage in a case of retinitis with massive exudation. Trans Am Ophthalmol Soc 1929;27:188–94.
56. Cahill M, O'Keefe M, Acheson R, et al. Classification of the spectrum of Coats' disease as subtypes of idiopathic retinal telangiectasis with exudation. Acta Ophthalmol Scand 2001;79:596–602.
57. Shields JA, Shields CL, Honavar SG, et al. Classification and management of Coats disease: the 2000 Proctor Lecture. Am J Ophthalmol 2001;131:572–83.
58. Lai CH, Kuo HK, Wu PC, et al. Manifestation of Coats' disease by age in Taiwan. Clin Experiment Ophthalmol 2007;35:361–5.
59. Smirniotopoulos JG, Bargallo N, Mafee MF. Differential diagnosis of leukokoria: radiologic-pathologic correlation. Radiographics 1994;14:1059–79. quiz 1052–81.
60. Haik BG. Advanced Coats' disease. Trans Am Ophthalmol Soc 1991;89: 371–476.
61. Cunha-Vaz JG. The blood–retinal barriers. Doc Ophthalmol 1976;41:287–327.
62. Ridley ME, Shields JA, Brown GC, et al. Coats' disease. Evaluation of management. Ophthalmology 1982;89:1381–7.
63. Tarkkanen A, Laatikainen L. Coat's disease: clinical, angiographic, histopathological findings and clinical management. Br J Ophthalmol 1983;67:766–76.
64. O'Brien JM, Char DH, Tucker N, et al. Efficacy of unanesthetized spiral computed tomography scanning in initial evaluation of childhood leukocoria. Ophthalmology 1995;102:1345–50.
65. Beets-Tan RG, Hendriks MJ, Ramos LM, et al. Retinoblastoma: CT and MRI. Neuroradiology 1994;36:59–62.
66. Lai WW, Edward DP, Weiss RA, et al. Magnetic resonance imaging findings in a case of advanced Coats' disease. Ophthalmic Surg Lasers 1996;27:234–8.
67. Mafee MF, Goldberg MF, Cohen SB, et al. Magnetic resonance imaging versus computed tomography of leukocoric eyes and use of in vitro proton magnetic resonance spectroscopy of retinoblastoma. Ophthalmology 1989;96:965–75. discussion 966–75.
68. Glasier CM, Brodsky MC, Leithiser RE Jr, et al. High resolution ultrasound with Doppler: a diagnostic adjunct in orbital and ocular lesions in children. Pediatr Radiol 1992;22:174–8.
69. Lam HD, Samuel MA, Rao NA, et al. Retinoblastoma presenting as Coats' disease. Eye (Lond) 2008;22:1196–7.
70. Plager DA, Orgel IK, Ellis FD, et al. X-linked recessive familial exudative vitreoretinopathy. Am J Ophthalmol 1992;114:145–8.
71. Small RG. Coats' disease and muscular dystrophy. Trans Am Acad Ophthalmol Otolaryngol 1968;72:225–31.
72. Padberg GW, Brouwer OF, de Keizer RJ, et al. On the significance of retinal vascular disease and hearing loss in facioscapulohumeral muscular dystrophy. Muscle Nerve 1995;2:S73–80.
73. Shields CL, Zahler J, Falk N, et al. Neovascular glaucoma from advanced Coats disease as the initial manifestation of facioscapulohumeral dystrophy in a 2-year-old child. Arch Ophthalmol 2007;125:840–2.
74. Crow YJ, McMenamin J, Haenggeli CA, et al. Coats' plus: a progressive familial syndrome of bilateral Coats' disease, characteristic cerebral calcification, leukoencephalopathy, slow pre- and post-natal linear growth and defects of bone marrow and integument. Neuropediatrics 2004;35:10–9.
75. Khan JA, Ide CH, Strickland MP. Coats'-type retinitis pigmentosa. Surv Ophthalmol 1988;32:317–32.
76. Pruett RC. Retinitis pigmentosa: clinical observations and correlations. Trans Am Ophthalmol Soc 1983;81:693–735.
77. Schuman JS, Lieberman KV, Friedman AH, et al. Senior-Loken syndrome (familial renal-retinal dystrophy) and Coats' disease. Am J Ophthalmol 1985;100:822–7.
78. Burch JV, Leveille AS, Morse PH. Ichthyosis hystrix (epidermal nevus syndrome) and Coats' disease. Am J Ophthalmol 1980;89:25–30.
79. Asdourian G. Vascular anomalies of the retina. In: Peyman G, Sanders D, Goldberg M, editors. Principles and practices of ophthalmology. Philadelphia: Saunders; 1980.
80. Robitaille JM, Monsein L, Traboulsi EI. Coats' disease and central nervous system venous malformation. Ophthalmic Genet 1996;17:215–8.
81. Newell SW, Hall BD, Anderson CW, et al. Hallermann–Streiff syndrome with Coats disease. J Pediatr Ophthalmol Strabismus 1994;31:123–5.
82. Egerer I, Rodrigues MM, Tasman WS. Retinal dysplasia in Coat's disease. Can J Ophthalmol 1975;10:79–85.
83. Fogle JA, Welch RB, Green WR. Retinitis pigmentosa and exudative vasculopathy. Arch Ophthalmol 1978;96:696–702.
84. Schefler AC, Berrocal AM, Murray TG. Advanced Coats' disease. Management with repetitive aggressive laser ablation therapy. Retina 2008;28(Suppl) :S38–41.
85. Spitznas M, Joussen F, Wessing A. Treatment of Coats' disease with photocoagulation. Graefes Arch Klin Exp Ophthalmol 1976;199:31–7.
86. Shapiro MJ, Chow CC, Karth PA, et al. Effects of green diode laser in the treatment of pediatric Coats disease. Am J Ophthalmol 2011;151:725–31. e722.
87. Sneed SR, Blodi CF, Pulido JS. Treatment of Coats' disease with the binocular indirect argon laser photocoagulator. Arch Ophthalmol 1989;107:789–90.
88. Couvillion SS, Margolis R, Mavrofjides E, et al. Laser treatment of Coats' disease. J Pediatr Ophthalmol Strabismus 2005;42:367–8.
89. Kim J, Park KH, Woo SJ. Combined photodynamic therapy and intravitreal bevacizumab injection for the treatment of adult Coats' disease: a case report. Korean J Ophthalmol 2010;24:374–6.
90. Othman IS, Moussa M, Bouhaimed M. Management of lipid exudates in Coats disease by adjuvant intravitreal triamcinolone: effects and complications. Br J Ophthalmol 2010;94:606–10.
91. Jarin RR, Teoh SC, Lim TH. Resolution of severe macular oedema in adult Coat's syndrome with high-dose intravitreal triamcinolone acetonide. Eye (Lond) 2006;20:163–5.
92. Entezari M, Ramezani A, Safavizadeh L, et al. Resolution of macular edema in Coats' disease with intravitreal bevacizumab. Indian J Ophthalmol 2010;58:80–2.
93. Alvarez-Rivera LG, Abraham-Marin ML, Flores-Orta HJ, et al. [Coat's disease treated with bevacizumab (Avastin).] Arch Soc Esp Oftalmol 2008;83: 329–31.
94. Lin CJ, Hwang JF, Chen YT, et al. The effect of intravitreal bevacizumab in the treatment of Coats disease in children. Retina 2010;30:617–22.
95. Cakir M, Cekic O, Yilmaz OF. Combined intravitreal bevacizumab and triamcinolone injection in a child with Coats disease. J AAPOS 2008;12:309–11.
96. Bergstrom CS, Hubbard GB 3rd. Combination intravitreal triamcinolone injection and cryotherapy for exudative retinal detachments in severe Coats disease. Retina 2008;28(Suppl):S33–7.
97. Venkatesh P, Mandal S, Garg S. Management of Coats disease with bevacizumab in 2 patients. Can J Ophthalmol 2008;43:245–6.
98. Cackett P, Wong D, Cheung CM. Combined intravitreal bevacizumab and argon laser treatment for Coats' disease. Acta Ophthalmol 2010;88: e48–9.
99. Kaul S, Uparkar M, Mody K, et al. Intravitreal anti-vascular endothelial growth factor agents as an adjunct in the management of Coats' disease in children. Indian J Ophthalmol 2010;58:76–8.
100. Sun Y, Jain A, Moshfeghi DM. Elevated vascular endothelial growth factor levels in Coats disease: rapid response to pegaptanib sodium. Graefes Arch Clin Exp Ophthalmol 2007; 45:1387–8.
101. He YG, Wang H, Zhao B, et al. Elevated vascular endothelial growth factor level in Coats' disease and possible therapeutic role of bevacizumab. Graefes Arch Clin Exp Ophthalmol 2010;248:1519–21.

102. Ramasubramanian A, Shields CL. Bevacizumab for Coats' disease with exudative retinal detachment and risk of vitreoretinal traction. Br J Ophthalmol 2012;96:356–9.
103. Goel N, Kumar V, Seth A, et al. Role of intravitreal bevacizumab in adult onset Coats' disease. Int Ophthalmol 2011;31:183–90.
104. Jun JH, Kim YC, Kim KS. Resolution of severe macular edema in adult coats' disease with intravitreal triamcinolone and bevacizumab injection. Korean J Ophthalmol 2008;22:190–3.
105. Zhao T, Wang K, Ma Y, et al. Resolution of total retinal detachment in Coats' disease with intravitreal injection of bevacizumab. Graefes Arch Clin Exp Ophthalmol 2011;249:1745–6.
106. Machemer R, Williams JM Sr. Pathogenesis and therapy of traction detachment in various retinal vascular diseases. Am J Ophthalmol 1988;105:170–81.
107. Yoshizumi MO, Kreiger AE, Lewis H, et al. Vitrectomy techniques in late-stage Coats'-like exudative retinal detachment. Doc Ophthalmol 1995;90: 387–94.
108. Muftuoglu G, Gulkilik G. Pars plana vitrectomy in advanced coats' disease. Case Report Ophthalmol 2011;2:15–22.
109. Peyman GA, Dellacroce JT, Ebrahim SA. Removal of submacular exudates in a patient with coats disease: a case report. Retina 2006;26:836–9.
110. Silodor SW, Augsburger JJ, Shields JA, et al. Natural history and management of advanced Coats' disease. Ophthalmic Surg 1988;19:89–93.
111. Shields JA, Shields CL. Review: coats disease: the 2001 LuEsther T. Mertz lecture. Retina 2002;22:80–91.
112. de Silva DJ, Brookes JL. Cyclodiode treatment of neovascular glaucoma secondary to Coats' disease. Br J Ophthalmol 2007;91:690–1.
113. Harris GS. Coats' disease, diagnosis and treatment. Can J Ophthalmol 1970;5:311–20.
114. Schatz H, Burton T, Yanuzzi L, et al. Abnormal retinal and disc vessels and retinal leak. In: Schatz H, editors. Interpretation of fundus fluorescein angiography. St. Louis: Mosby; 1978.
115. Mondon H, Hamard H, Girard P, et al. [Retinal gliosis associated with Coats' disease.] Bull Soc Ophtalmol Fr 1970;70:881–3.
116. Theodossiadis GP. Some clinical, fluorescein-angiographic, and therapeutic-aspects of Coats' disease. J Pediatr Ophthalmol Strabismus 1979;16:257–62.
117. Shienbaum G, Tasman WS. Coats disease: a lifetime disease. Retina 2006;26:422–4.
118. Tasman W. Coats' disease. Am Fam Physician 1977;15:107.
119. Egerer I, Tasman W, Tomer TT. Coats disease. Arch Ophthalmol 1974; 92:109–12.
120. Matsuzaka T, Sakuragawa N, Terasawa K, et al. Facioscapulohumeral dystrophy associated with mental retardation, hearing loss, and tortuosity of retinal arterioles. J Child Neurol 1986;1:218–23.
121. Desai UR, Sabates FN. Long-term follow-up of facioscapulohumeral muscular dystrophy and Coats' disease. Am J Ophthalmol 1990;110:568–9.
122. Gurwin EB, Fitzsimons RB, Sehmi KS, et al. Retinal telangiectasis in facioscapulohumeral muscular dystrophy with deafness. Arch Ophthalmol 1985;103: 1695–700.
123. Cameron JD, Yanoff M, Frayer WC. Coats' disease and turner's syndrome. Am J Ophthalmol 1974;78:852–4.
124. Folk JC, Genovese FN, Biglan AW. Coats' disease in a patient with Cornelia de Lange syndrome. Am J Ophthalmol 1981;91:607–10.
125. Kondra L, Cangemi FE, Pitta CG. Alport's syndrome and retinal telangiectasia. Ann Ophthalmol 1983;15:550–1.
126. Genkova P, Toncheva D, Tzoneva M, et al. Deletion of 13q12. 1 in a child with Coats disease. Acta Paediatr Hung 1986;27:141–3.
127. Berger M, Lieberman KV, Schoeneman MJ, et al. Coats' disease in a renal transplant recipient. Nephrol Dial Transplant 1987;2:120–3.
128. Skuta GL, France TD, Stevens TS, et al. Apparent Coats' disease and pericentric inversion of chromosome 3. Am J Ophthalmol 1987;104:84–6.
129. Kajtar P, Mehes K. Bilateral coats retinopathy associated with aplastic anaemia and mild dyskeratotic signs. Am J Med Genet 1994;49:374–7.
130. Bhushan M, Kumar S, Griffiths CE. Multiple glomus tumours, Coats' disease and basic fibroblast growth factor. Br J Dermatol 1997;137:454–6.
131. Gärtner J, Draf W. Leber's miliary aneurysms associated with telangiectasia of the nasal mucosa. Am J Ophthalmol 1975;79:56–8.
132. Frontali M, Stomeo C, Dallapiccola B. Osteoporosis-pseudoglioma syndrome: report of three affected sibs and an overview. Am J Med Genet 1985;22: 35–47.
133. Reynolds BC, Lemmers RJ, Tolmie J, et al. Focal segmental glomerulosclerosis, Coats'-like retinopathy, sensorineural deafness and chromosome 4 duplication: a new association. Pediatr Nephrol 2010;25:1551–4.
134. Luckie AP, Hamilton AM. Adult Coats' disease in branch retinal vein occlusion. Aust N Z J Ophthalmol 1994;22:203–6.
135. Frezzotti R, Berengo A, Guerra R, et al. Toxoplasmic Coats' retinitis. A parasitologically proved case. Am J Ophthalmol 1965;59:1099–102.
136. Kremer I, Cohen S, Izhak RB, et al. An unusual case of congenital unilateral Coats's disease associated with morning glory optic disc anomaly. Br J Ophthalmol 1985;69:32–7.
137. Green WR. Bilateral Coats' disease. Massive gliosis of the retina. Arch Ophthalmol 1967;77:378–83.
138. Lanier JD, McCrary 3rd JA, Justice J. Autosomal recessive retinitis pigmentosa and Coats disease: a presumed familial incidence. Arch Ophthalmol 1976;94:1737–42.
139. Spallone A, Carlevaro G, Ridling P. Autosomal dominant retinitis pigmentosa and Coats'-like disease. Int Ophthalmol 1985;8:147–51.
140. Arrigg PG, Lahav M, Hutchins RK, et al. Pigmentary retinal degeneration and Coats' disease: a case study. Ophthalmic Surg 1988;19:432–6.
141. Kim RY, Kearney JJ. Coats-type retinitis pigmentosa in a 4-year-old child. Am J Ophthalmol 1997;124:846–8.

Chapter 57

Hemoglobinopathies

Adrienne W. Scott, Gerard A. Lutty, Morton F. Goldberg

In a landmark 1910 *Archives of Internal Medicine* article,[1] Dr James Herrick noted "peculiar, elongated, sickle-shaped red blood corpuscles" from a peripheral blood smear of a Grenadian dental student with recurring medical illnesses and, thus, penned the first written description of sickle-cell disease (SCD).[1–3] Linus Pauling and colleagues in 1949 were the first to implicate a defective hemoglobin molecule within the erythrocyte as the cause of the disease.[4,5]

The term "sickle-cell disease" encompasses the group of hemoglobinopathies characterized by intravascular hemolysis and by defective oxygen transport. In a normal red blood cell, two α-globin subunits, two β-globin subunits, and a central heme molecule combine to form adult hemoglobin (Hb A). The β-globin gene, an oxygen transport gene, is found on the short arm of chromosome 11.[6,7] Hemoglobin S (Hb S) results from a single amino acid point mutation in which a valine substitutes for a glutamic acid at the sixth position within the β-globin chain. Hemoglobin C (Hb C) is caused by a glutamic acid to lysine mutation in the β-globin molecule.

SCD is transmitted through the autosomal recessive mode of inheritance. Two copies of Hb S may combine with one another (SS disease), or one copy of Hb S and another β-globin variant, such as Hb C, may combine (double heterozygous SC disease).[7] Individuals with one copy of Hb A and one copy of Hb S are described as having the sickle-cell trait, the carrier state for SCD. β-thalassemia occurs when a reduced amount of β-globin is present. This condition is beta-plus (β^+) thalassemia, whereas the absence of β-globin is called beta-zero (β^0). Either of these conditions may combine with Hb S, leading to a compound heterozygous state.[7]

PREVALENCE

To date, SCD remains the most common inherited blood disorder, and affects nearly 80000 people of African American and Hispanic descent.[8] SCD occurs in 1/500 African American births and every 1/36000 Hispanic-American births.[8–10] SCD results in 5% of deaths in children under 5 years in Africa, more than 9% of such deaths in West Africa, and up to 16% of under-5 deaths in individual West African countries.[11] Approximately 8% (or one in 12) of black Americans possess sickle-cell trait, which is not associated with increased mortality or morbidity (except in hyphema), and is thought to confer a genetic protection against malarial infection.[10] Their hemoglobin concentration is typically 35–40% Hb S and 55–60% Hb A.[7] Although sickle-cell trait subjects are generally asymptomatic, they may encounter systemic complications of SCD under conditions of extreme hypoxia.[12]

Populations of African descent possess the highest frequency of Hb S. At-risk genotypes for SCD are also observed in people of Mediterranean, Caribbean, South and Central American, Arab, and East Indian descent.[7] SS disease is displayed in approximately 0.15% of African descendants in North America.[7,13] Those with SS disease do not typically become symptomatic until after 6 months of age, when the fetal hemoglobin (Hb F) is replaced with Hb S. These individuals have a decreased life expectancy, as they are prone to developing severe anemia and are highly susceptible to recurrent infections.[14] Individuals with Hb SC disease, the double heterozygotes, typically exhibit 50% Hb S and 50% Hb C hemoglobin composition and typically display less morbidity from the systemic complications of SCD, and have a normal life expectancy.[7] With a hemoglobin composition of 60–90% Hb S and 10–30% Hb F, sickle β-thalassemia patients are typically encountered in central African and Mediterranean countries. Those with other forms of sickle β-thalassemia may have Hb A as 10–30% of their hemoglobin composition.[7,15]

GENETIC MODIFIERS

The degree of phenotypic expression of SCD is quite variable, even among those with the same genotype. Environmental effects and multiple gene interactions are thought to be at play. Further, the ability of an individual to generate Hb F may lead to reduced disease severity. Different β-globin cluster haplotypes may result in different levels of Hb F.[7,16] Levels of Hb F have been shown to correlate with the clinical manifestations of SCD.[17]

PATHOPHYSIOLOGY

The interplay among abnormal erythrocytes and hypoxic, hyperosmolar, or acidotic conditions leads to the abnormal rheology and hemolysis characteristic of SCD. In Hb S, a strongly hydrophobic polar valine takes the place of a nonpolar strongly hydrophilic glutamic acid residue.[5] Upon deoxygenation in the microcirculation, hydrophobic residues within Hb S are exposed and associate with hydrophobic regions of adjacent molecules. This polymerization results in the generation of rigid fibers of Hb S which damage the red blood cell membrane and cytoskeleton and cause the cell to assume a sickle shape. This polymerization process is reversible as oxygenation increases, and the cell may resume its native discoid shape. However, the repeated cycle of sickling and unsickling of the red blood cell membrane may lead to permanent damage to the erythrocyte membrane, irreversible sickling, and hemolysis. Mean corpuscular hemoglobin concentration (MCHC) may be the most important factor contributing to the rate of Hb S polymerization.[5] The higher the MCHC, the more hemoglobin molecules that are available to participate in polymerization, and the closer these molecules are to one another, further promoting a favorable environment for Hb S polymerization.[18,19]

The erythrocyte's original state of oxygenation also impacts the extent and rate of polymerization.[15,16] An intrinsic property of the normal erythrocyte is the ability to deform easily in order to pass through capillaries with smaller diameters than its own. Decreased erythrocyte deformability and increased rigidity can cause increased capillary transit time.[19] Deoxygenation and sickling promote increased permeability of the cell membrane to potassium, sodium, and calcium cations, which leads to water efflux from the cell, cellular volume contraction, and resultant increase in Hb S concentration.[5,19,20,21]

In addition to mechanical obstruction of blood vessels by dense, sickled erythrocytes, these sickled erythrocytes display increased adhesion to vascular endothelium matrix proteins, such as laminin,[22,23] and thus cause direct damage to the endothelium. Integrin α4β1, integrin-associated protein, sulfated glycolipid, lutheran protein, phosphatidylserine, band 3 protein, and CD36 are adhesion molecules expressed in sickled red blood cells.[24–26] Immature red blood cells called reticulocytes increase in SCD following intravascular hemolysis. These cells also have increased adhesion molecules, such as integrin α4β1,[27–29] which promote pathologic adhesion to the vascular endothelium, specifically to vascular cell adhesion molecule-1 (VCAM-1). Direct activation of endothelial cells occurs in response to elevated circulating cytokines such as tumor necrosis factor-α (TNF-α) and interleukin-1β (IL-1β),[30,31] which upregulate expression of endothelial adhesion molecules like intercellular adhesion molecule-1 (ICAM-1), VCAM-1, E-selectin, and P-selectin.[32,33]

Inflammation likely plays a role in the vaso-occlusive process in SCD. Lutty and colleagues demonstrated retention of SS red cells and adherence of red cells in reticulocyte-rich fractions in retina and choroid of rat eyes in hypoxic conditions or following TNF-α stimulation.[34–36] TNF-α and IL-1 may contribute to vaso-occlusion by accelerating the production of adhesion molecules on the vascular endothelium and by activating polymorphonuclear leukocytes.[30] TNF-α and IL-1 have been shown to be upregulated in the sera of individuals with SCD at baseline.[31,37,38]

Nitric oxide (NO) is a potent vasodilator and regulator of vascular tone; it is derived from the vascular endothelial NO synthase. SCD has been associated with elevated reactive oxygen species, which scavenge NO and metabolize arginine, its precursor.[7] L-arginine as an oral supplement has been given to induce NO production in transgenic sickle-cell mice.[38,39]

Vascular endothelial growth factor (VEGF), which is upregulated by hypoxia, is present in the serum of SCD patients at baseline, and is elevated during vaso-occlusive crises.[40] Elevated VEGF has been demonstrated in eyes with sickle-cell retinopathy.[41,42] VEGF has also been shown to increase levels of cell adhesion molecules, ICAM-1 and VCAM-1.[43,44] Angiopoietin-1 (Ang-1) and angiopoietin-2 (Ang-2) interact with the Tie-2 receptor on endothelial cells, regulating angiogenesis. Ang-1 is responsible for the maintenance and stabilization of mature blood vessels, while Ang-2 leads to vessel destabilization and dissociation of pericytes and is upregulated by hypoxia and VEGF.[45] Interaction among these proteins may be important in the pathogenesis of SCD.

SYSTEMIC MANIFESTATIONS

Over recent years, as the life expectancy of those affected by SCD has increased, so have the number of complications these individuals experience.[12,46] Sickling of the red blood cells, with resultant intravascular hemolysis, thrombosis, tissue necrosis, and ischemia, causes a myriad of systemic complications, including cerebrovascular accident, acute chest syndrome, pulmonary hypertension, splenic sequestration, priapism, osteonecrosis, cholelithiasis, pneumonia, leg ulcers, aplastic crisis, renal disease, need for recurrent transfusions, episodic, painful vaso-occlusive crises, and death.[7]

Severe visual impairment and blindness from complications of proliferative sickle-cell retinopathy (PSR) may also occur. For reasons that are as yet unclear, subjects with Hb SC disease typically display less systemic morbidity from their hemoglobinopathy, but have a higher likelihood of experiencing the ophthalmic complications, than their homozygous Hb SS counterparts.[47] In one study of patients with SCD, retinopathy was detected in 33% of patients with Hb SC disease compared to 3% of patients with Hb SS disease.[37]

Several theories have been proposed to explain this difference. One explanation could be that Hb SS patients typically have a shorter life expectancy than Hb SC patients, and may not live long enough to manifest the ophthalmic disease. Alternatively, the difference in retinopathy among sickle-cell genotypes may be due to the higher hematocrit and cell density, and the lower Hb F, of individuals with Hb SC as compared to Hb SS individuals.[7] The overall lower hematocrit in Hb SS patients, and the resultant lowered viscosity of blood, may confer a relative protection from vaso-occlusion in the retinal circulation.[48] Another theory is that the retinal vaso-occlusions in SS disease may be so complete that no viable tissue remains to produce the growth factors necessary to mount a proliferative response. In Hb SC disease, the vascular occlusions may be less complete, and they occur in the setting of a chronic hypoxic rather than anoxic state. Thus, a steady-state release of angiogenic growth factors from the remaining viable tissue may occur.[49] Finally, Lutty and colleagues showed that irreversibly sickled Hb SS erythrocytes are easily trapped in retinal capillaries and precapillary arterioles in hypoxic conditions in a rat model.[16,35] Hb SC cells, however, regardless of oxygen levels, were less easily trapped in the retinal microvasculature. When the vascular endothelium was stimulated with cytokines, retention of Hb SC cells did occur. The authors suggested that vaso-occlusion in Hb SC disease may be the result of the complex interaction among cytokines, the fibrinolytic cascade, leukocyte interactions, and activation of the vascular endothelium with induction of adhesion molecules.[13,35] This data suggests that retention of sickled cells in the retina is not mechanical (rigid cells retained in a small lumen) but rather due to hypoxia-initiated cytokines and receptors.

OPHTHALMIC CLINICAL FEATURES

Retrobulbar and orbital involvement

Orbital involvement of SCD is uncommon, but has been reported. One study from Oman reported periorbital swelling during vaso-occlusive crises in five patients.[50] The patients ranged in age from 6 to 15 years old. Four of these patients had SS disease, while one had sickle-beta thalassemia. Infarction of orbital bones and orbital hematomas occur, and may lead to the orbital compression syndrome. These patients typically display lid edema, fever, facial pain, proptosis, restriction of motility, and resultant diplopia. The authors concluded that these syndromes usually resolve with conservative management with treatment of the underlying crisis, antibiotics, and steroids. Orbital involvement in SCD may cause sudden permanent unilateral loss of vision without detectable retinal arterial changes due to retrobulbar ischemic optic neuropathy.[7,51] Urgent decompression of the orbit may be required. Recurrent bilateral lacrimal gland swelling has also been reported.[52]

Anterior-segment involvement

Conjunctival and iris findings may be present in SCD. An early reported finding is the saccular and sausage-like dilatations of the tiniest conjunctival vessels.[53] They are most easily seen with the highest power of the slit-lamp biomicroscope. Paton described these comma-shaped capillary segments in the inferior bulbar conjunctival vessels, and coined the term "conjunctival sign."[54] This sign was uncommon in those with high Hb F levels. Local heat from the slit lamp induces vasodilation, and causes reversal of the comma-shaped vessels,[55,56] whereas topical vasoconstricting drops increase the abnormality.[57,58] These conjunctival vascular changes vary with oxygenation status, and are more prevalent in Hb SS disease than in Hb SC disease.[54] Pathophysiology studies show constriction of these conjunctival vessels during painful crises, with normal blood flow returning on recovery.[58] On histopathologic examination, these vessels exhibit endothelial proliferation, dilatation, and thinning of the proximal blood vessel segments, and aggregation of red blood cells in the distal portions of capillaries.[58]

Segmental iris atrophy and pupil abnormalities can be seen in individuals with SCD (Fig. 57.1).[59,60] Iris atrophy is thought to result from sectoral ischemic necrosis involving radial iris vessels. Secondary neovascularization of the iris stroma has also been described and documented with intravenous fluorescein angiography, and in one instance this neovascular frond resembled that classically seen as the "sea fan" in PSR.[13,61] Neovascular glaucoma rarely occurs as a consequence of PSR.[7,62]

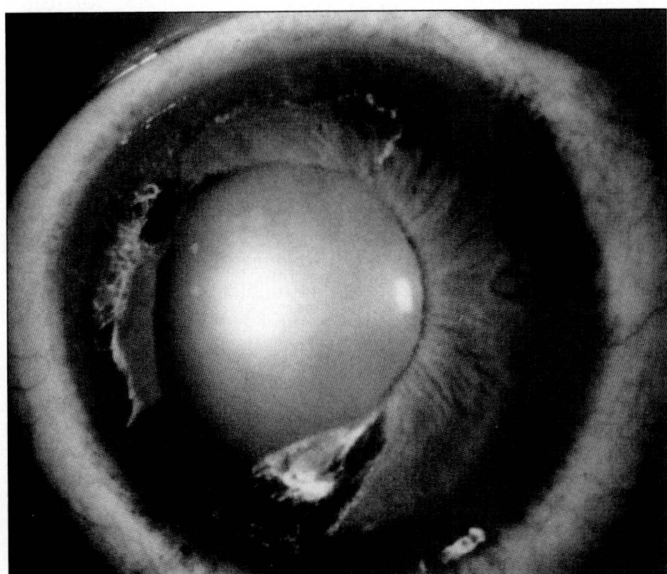

Fig. 57.1 Atrophy and irregularity of the iris at the pupillary border are seen in a patient with sickle-cell disease as a result of sectoral ischemic necrosis.

Hyphema in a patient with SCD and in those with sickle-cell trait represents a sight-threatening emergency, as even modest elevations of intraocular pressure (IOP) have resulted in vision loss from central retinal artery occlusion or macular branch retinal artery occlusion.[62–65] This is likely a mechanical phenomenon, as sickled red blood cells clog the trabecular meshwork,[61] causing elevation in IOP. Although intensive medical management to lower IOP in SCD patients with hyphema is recommended, IOP-lowering medications must be used cautiously. Repetitive use of carbonic anhydrase inhibitors, for example, is contraindicated in SCD patients with hyphema as most of these medications cause intracameral acidotic conditions that may worsen erythrocyte sickling. Early surgical intervention for IOP control should be considered, typically by paracentesis of the anterior chamber.[66] Intracameral tissue plasminogen activator may be a potentially useful agent in the treatment of posttraumatic hyphema in some cases.[67] Hyperoxygenation of the patient may also be helpful.

Posterior-segment involvement

Vitreoretinal interface

The pathologic retinal neovascularization caused by retinal ischemia in SCD can result in vision loss from vitreous hemorrhage.[68,69] Other abnormalities of the vitreoretinal interface have been described, such as peripheral retinal whitening, which may represent abnormal or particularly strong adhesion at the vitreoretinal interface. This has been described in 93% of Hb SS patients,[70] 83% of Hb SC patients,[71] and 82% of Hb S Thal patients.[72] There is no known pathologic significance to this finding. This peripheral whitening is noted in the peripheral retina in the normal population as "white without pressure," and may not be truly unique to those with sickle-cell retinopathy.[13,57]

Correspondingly, flat, brown, ovoid lesions in the retinal periphery have been noted in SCD, and termed "dark without pressure." These lesions can be transient, and may disappear without sequelae. The underlying choroid appears normal on ophthalmoscopy, and the corresponding fluorescein angiogram is also normal.[13,73]

Optic nerve

The optic nerve in patients with SCD may exhibit vascular changes. Dark, dilated capillaries at the optic nerve head appear as small red dots (Fig. 57.2), and represent precapillary arterioles plugged with sickled erythrocytes. These abnormal vessels have a linear or Y-shaped configuration on high-magnification ophthalmoscopy.[13,57,70,74] These changes are not visually significant as the vascular occlusions are transient. Optic disc neovascularization is rare but has been reported in four Hb SC patients[13,75–78] and one Hb SS patient.[13,70]

Macula

Though the hallmark of ocular SCD has been the peripheral retinopathy, the macula is also susceptible to infarction from vaso-occlusive disease. The "macular depression sign" has been described as an oval depression of the bright foveal or parafoveal reflex as a result of macular thinning due to ischemic atrophy.[79] This finding is best detected using red-free illumination. The extent of macular vascular changes has not been shown to correlate with visual acuity. In a study by Sanders and colleagues, an enlarged foveal avascular zone (FAZ) was identified

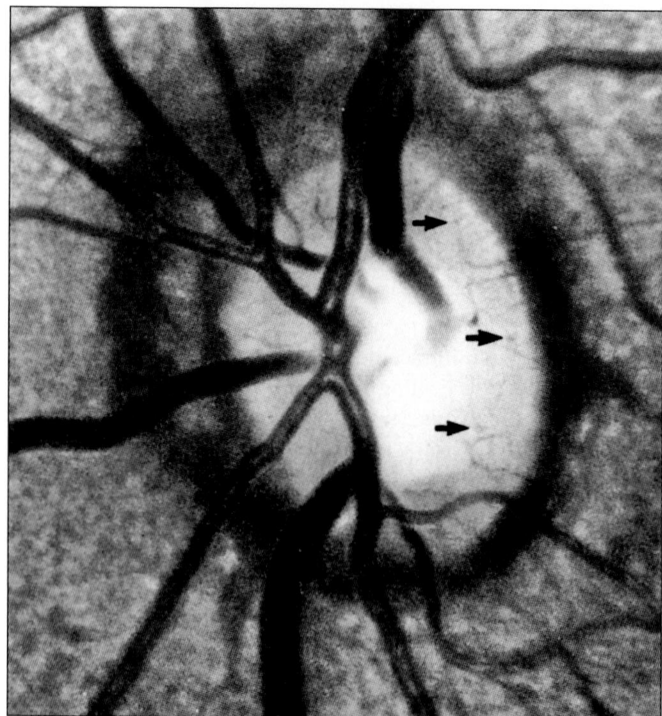

Fig. 57.2 Optic disc sign in sickle-cell disease is shown. The arrows point to occluded precapillary arterioles, seen as small dots on the optic nerve.

in patients with SCD on fluorescein angiography as compared to healthy, age-matched controls.[80] Within the sickle-cell group, visual acuity did not correlate with FAZ size. The authors reported an enlarged FAZ in patients with SCD irrespective of the type of hemoglobinopathy or degree of retinopathy.

Macular infarcts can now be confirmed using optical coherence tomography.[81] In a recent study utilizing spectral-domain optical coherence tomography (SD-OCT), Hoang and coworkers[82] described retinal thinning of the central macula compared to healthy controls, most notably in the outer retinal layers in the central macula and parafoveal retina. Although several previous studies have reported atrophy of inner retinal layers after macular infarction, Hoang *et al.* hypothesize that the outer retinal layers may be thinned due to ischemia and resultant atrophy of the choriocapillaris, as these larger-caliber vessels may possibly be more prone to occlusion than the retinal vessels. Additionally, this study reported "splaying," or blunting of the foveal contour on SD-OCT in asymptomatic patients with SCD with areas of focal parafoveal thinning (Fig. 57.3). A case series by Murthy *et al.* also describes thinning of the temporal macula in patients with PSR on SD-OCT, and suggests that this finding should lead clinicians to perform peripheral wide-field angiography to evaluate the retinal periphery for ischemia.[83] Macular hole,[84] epiretinal membranes,[85] macular schisis,[86] and posterior pole neovascularization[87] have all been reported as rare complications of sickle-cell retinopathy.

Angioid streaks

Angioid streaks, breaks in Bruch's membrane, have a well-documented association with SCD, occurring in 1–2% of patients.[13,70,88] These irregular, reddish subretinal bands are most commonly found in patients with the Hb SS genotype.[70,89] The incidence of angioid streaks in these eyes increases with age, and one Jamaican study found that 22% of 60 patients with Hb SS disease over age 40 had angioid streaks, compared to 2% of 150 patients under 40.[90] Why angioid streaks occur in SCD is unclear. One hypothesis is that elastic tissue injury may occur as the result of oxidative damage due to hypoxia, and inflammatory cells may release cytokines that cause tissue damage.[7,91] Angioid streaks in SCD usually have a benign course and resultant choroidal neovascularization (CNV) is rare.[13]

Retinal vasculature

Vascular tortuosity caused by arteriovenous anastomoses may be more commonly observed in Hb SS patients (Fig. 57.4).[7] One study reported increased retinal vascular tortuosity in 47% of Hb SS patients and 32% of Hb SC patients,[92] while another reported 11% vascular tortuosity in both Hb SS and Hb SC patients.[70,71] This discrepancy could be due to an imprecise definition of vascular tortuosity.[7]

Retinal vascular occlusions frequently occur in the peripheral retina in patients with SCD, and peripheral retinal nonperfusion is a common finding in these eyes. Arteriovenous anastomoses may occur in this setting (Fig. 57.5). Retinal arteriole "silver-wiring" represents permanently occluded arterioles (Fig. 57.6).

Depending on its location, vascular occlusion may cause temporary or permanent vision loss. The precapillary arterioles in eyes with SCD are particularly susceptible to obstruction. The cause of these occlusions may be multifactorial, potentially involving sickled red blood cells attaching to vascular endothelium, or the activation of the coagulation cascade, with secondary intimal injury.[2,93] In the peripheral temporal retina, where vessels become markedly narrow, arterial occlusions are common.

Vaso-occlusion arising from the posterior ciliary arterial circulation may potentially cause choroidal infarction, an event that has been described in numerous reports in the ophthalmic literature in SCD. Histopathologic studies show impacted red blood cells, increased fibrin, and platelet fibrin thrombi in cases of choroidal occlusion.[94,95] As in the retinal circulation, the interaction among adhesion molecules, facilitating adhesion of dense reticulocytes to the endothelium, may play a role.[34] Choroidal neovascularization may rarely occur spontaneously[96] or result after high-energy laser burns.[97]

NONPROLIFERATIVE SICKLE RETINOPATHY

Salmon patch hemorrhages

Salmon patch lesions are pinkish orange hemorrhages located between the retina and its internal limiting membrane (Fig. 57.7). These may arise from areas of bleeding into the retina adjacent to areas of nonperfusion, and have been described as a "blowout" of an occluded arteriole.[98,99] Although the hemorrhage is initially red, it may turn a red-orange or salmon color over time because of progressive hemolysis. The localized collection of blood may remain under the internal limiting membrane, travel into the subretinal space, or spread into the vitreous cavity.[13,98,99]

Iridescent spots

If arteriolar occlusion causes retinal hemorrhage, a small schisis cavity may develop after the intraretinal portion of the hemorrhage resolves.[13] The cavity may contain hemosiderin-laden

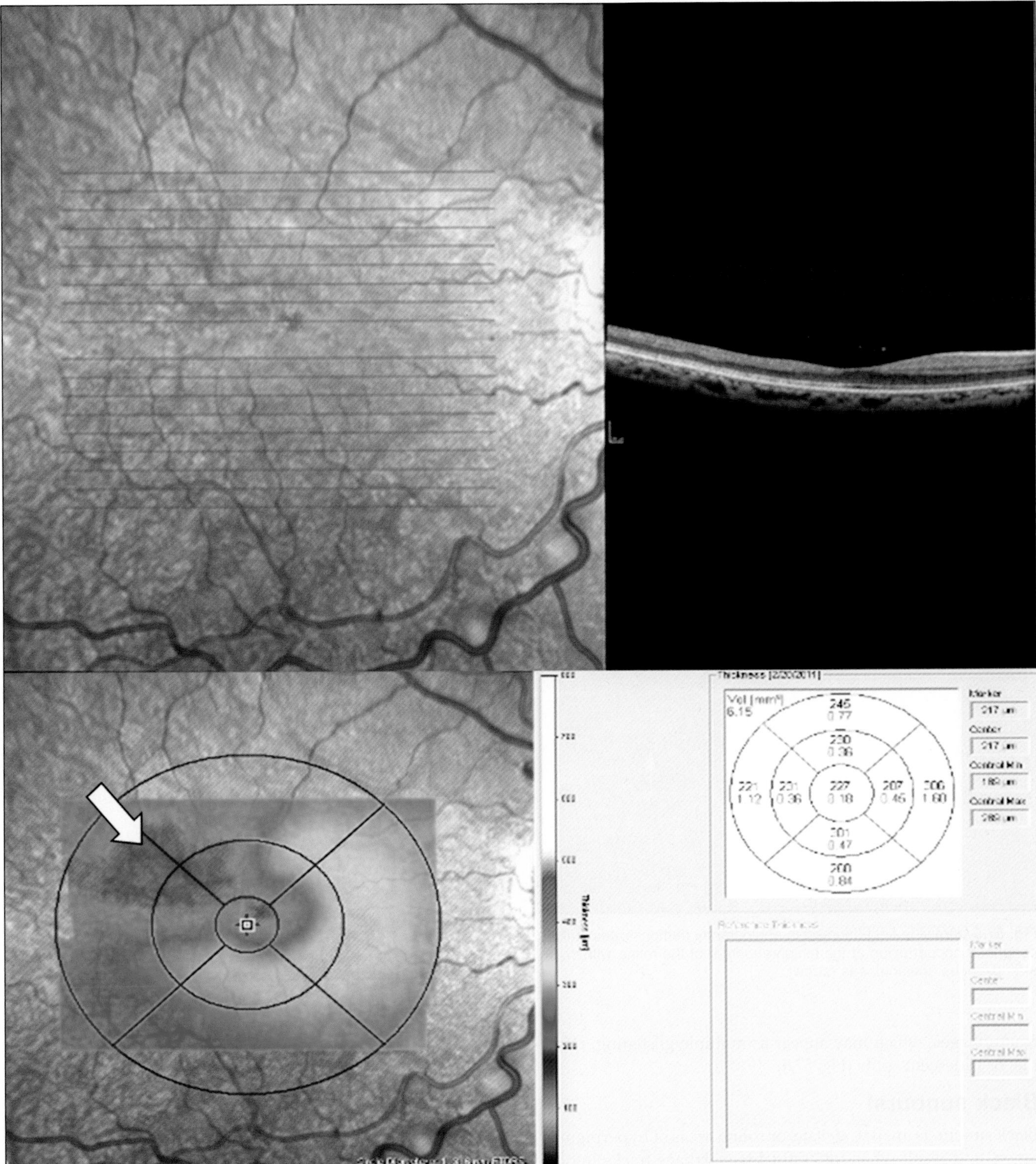

Fig. 57.3 Spectral domain optical coherence tomography demonstrates "foveal splaying" (saucerization of the foveal pit) and focal thinning (arrow) within the temporal foveal region in a patient with Hb SS disease.

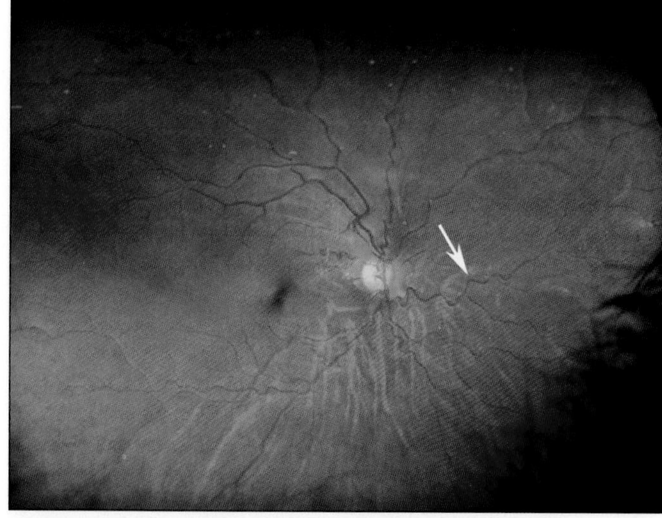
Fig. 57.4 Ultrawide-field fundus photo demonstrates vascular tortuosity (arrow) in a patient with Hb sickle-cell disease and proliferative sickle retinopathy.

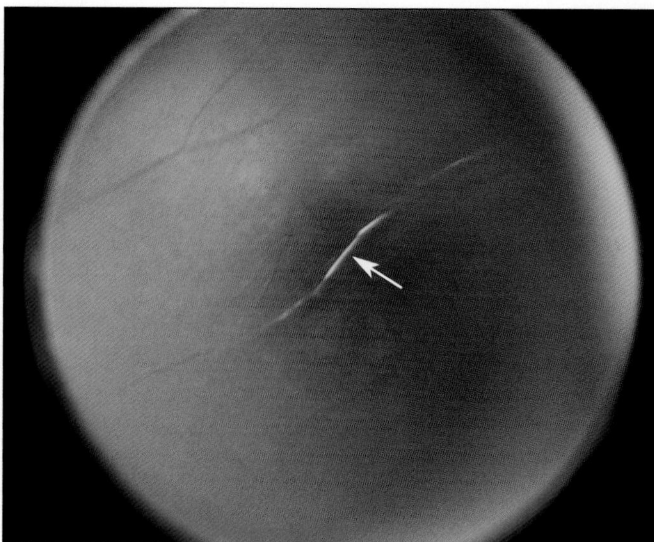
Fig. 57.6 Silver-wiring and occlusion of a peripheral retinal arteriole, is shown (arrow).

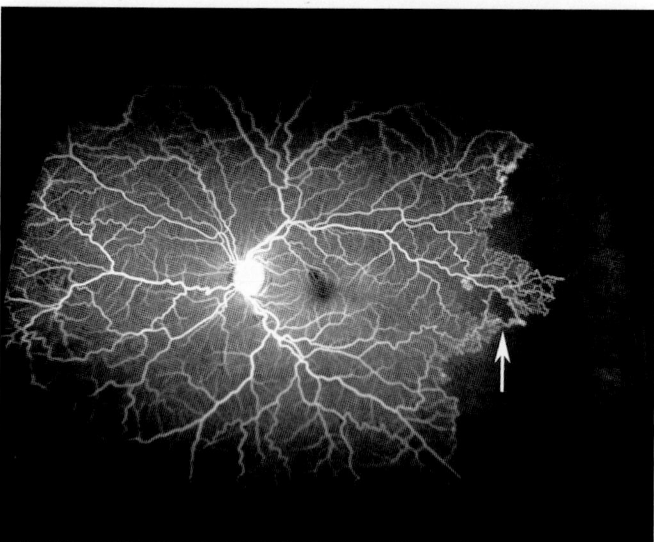
Fig. 57.5 Ultrawide-field fluorescein angiography demonstrates striking peripheral nonperfusion at the temporal border of the retina with arteriovenous anastomoses (arrow).

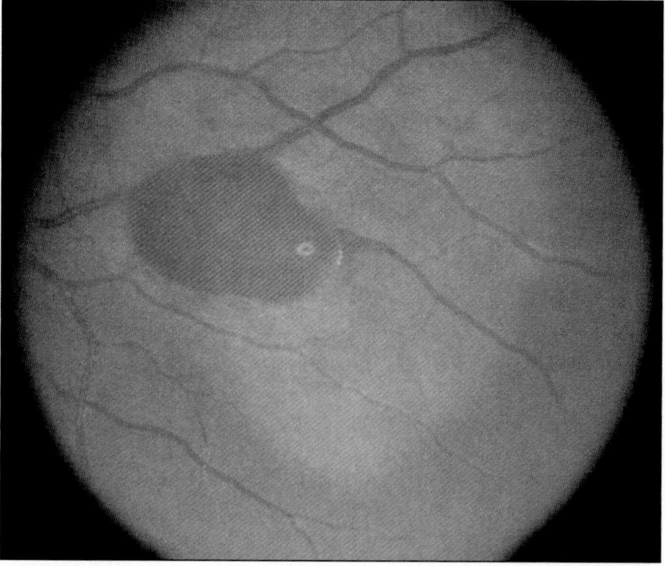
Fig. 57.7 A salmon patch hemorrhage results from "blowout" of blood from an occluded retinal arteriole.

macrophages, which may appear as multiple glistening, refractile, or iridescent spots (Fig. 57.8).

Black sunburst

Black sunbursts are flat, stellate, or round areas of hyperpigmentation, and result when intraretinal hemorrhage tracks into the subretinal space (Fig. 57.9).[98,100] On histopathologic study, black sunbursts appear as focal hypertrophy of the retinal pigment epithelium (RPE).[98] This "sunburst sign" may also represent localized choroidal ischemic damage to the overlying RPE.[101] Another hypothesis is that the black sunburst may be the RPE response to an area of underlying CNV.[96,102]

PROLIFERATIVE SICKLE RETINOPATHY

A critical event in the development of PSR is the formation of the sea fan, the peripheral vascular lesion so named for its close resemblance to the marine invertebrate, *Gorgonia flabellum* (Fig. 57.10). Peripheral retinal arteriolar occlusions are the inciting events in sea-fan formations. Occlusion of the vasculature causes release of growth factors, resulting in formation of these neovascular fronds. PSR complications are the major contributor to vision loss. Sea fans are predisposed to hemorrhage into the vitreous, and to cause vitreous membrane formation, tractional retinoschisis, and tractional or combined rhegmatogenous–tractional retinal detachment.[48] Sea fans often form at arteriovenous crossings and may have multiple feeding arterioles and draining venules (Fig. 57.11).[103]

In 1971, Goldberg devised the widely utilized classification system for PSR (Table 57.1).[104]

Goldberg stages

Stage I

Stage I retinopathy is defined by peripheral vascular occlusion.[57] The peripheral retina may show multiple simultaneous

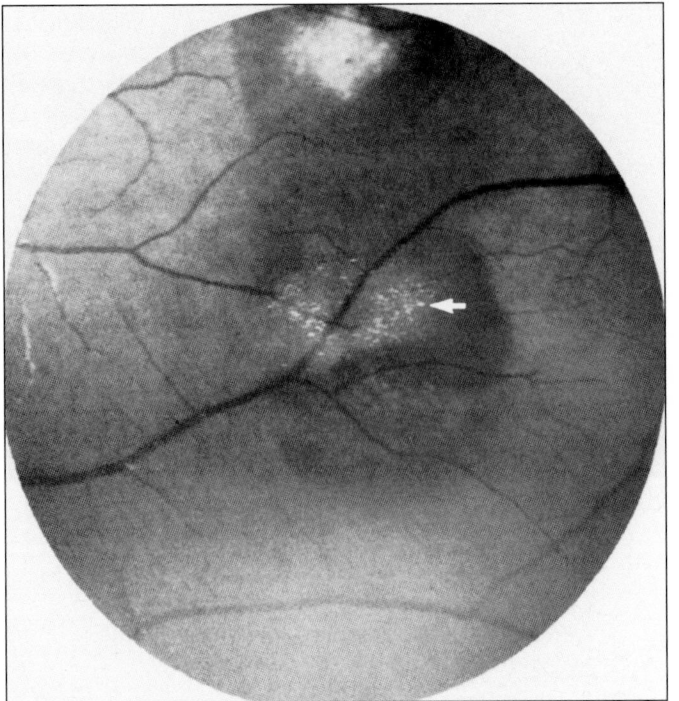

Fig. 57.8 Iridescent spots are shown within a retinal schisis cavity (arrow) and may represent hemosiderin-laden macrophages.

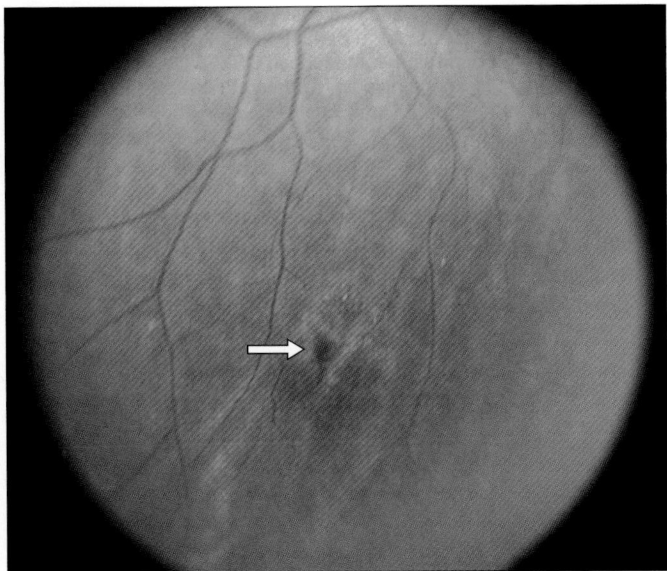

Fig. 57.9 A black sunburst may represent focal hypertrophy or hyperplasia of the retinal pigment epithelium.

arteriolar occlusions, and silver-wiring of the arterioles may be present. Vaso-occlusion occurs primarily in the peripheral temporal retina due to longer arteriovenous transit times (with deoxygenation), an increased number of occludable bifurcation sites, and decreased perfusion.

Stage II

In this stage, vascular remodeling at the border of perfused and nonperfused retina occurs. Arteriovenous anastomoses form connections between occluded arterioles and adjacent terminal venules by way of pre-existing capillaries (Fig. 57.5). The

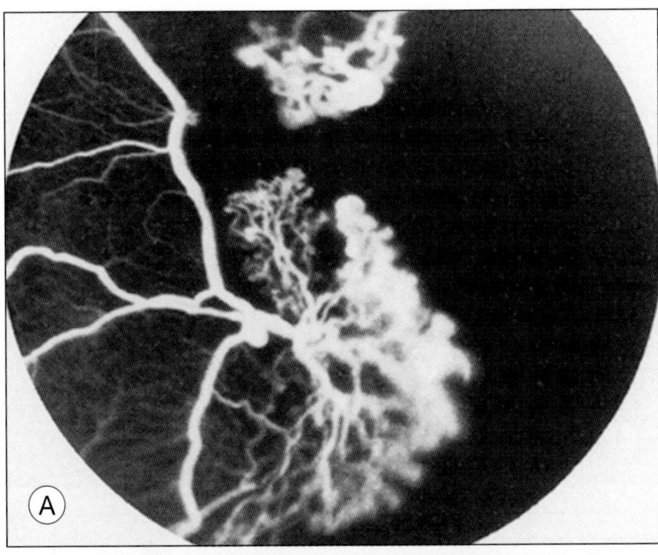

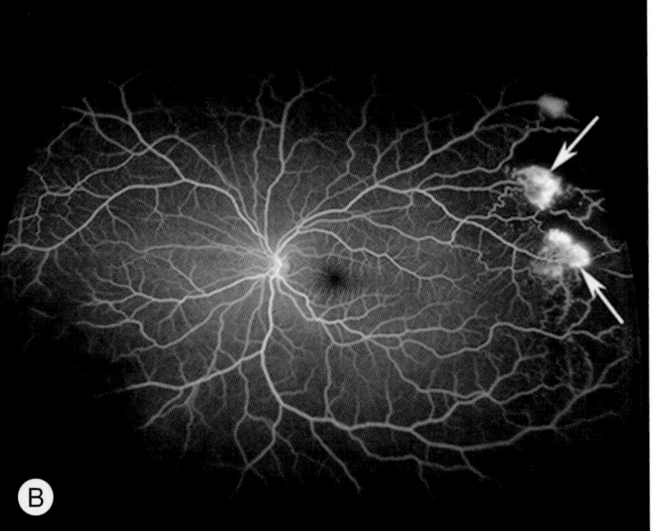

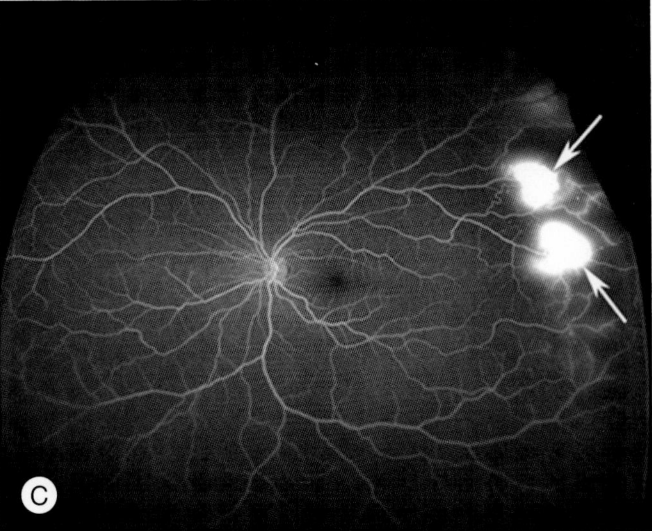

Fig. 57.10 Sea-fan lesions are shown in the peripheral fundus in a patient with Hb SC disease. The frond-like vascular structures (shown in a 30° image in one subject) are typically present at the border of perfused and nonperfused peripheral retina (A). Ultrawide-field fluorescein angiography demonstrates initial bright hyperfluorescence of the sea-fan lesions. In (B) the white arrows point to hyperfluoresence of sea fan neovascularization caused by proliferative sickle retinopathy. The later phase of the angiogram (C) shows diffuse leakage from the neovascular fronds, identified with white arrows.

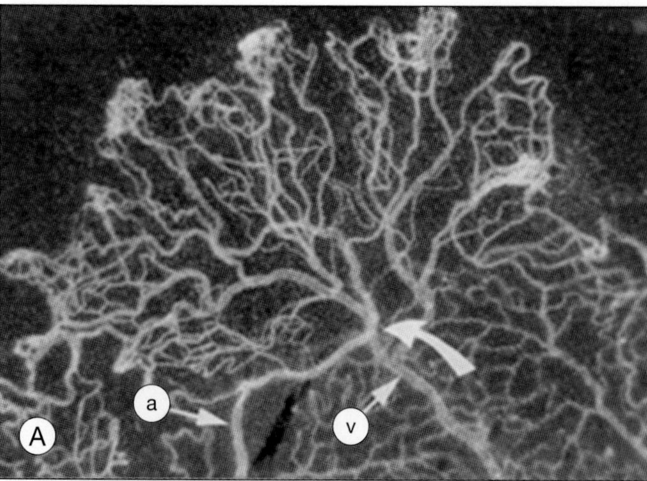

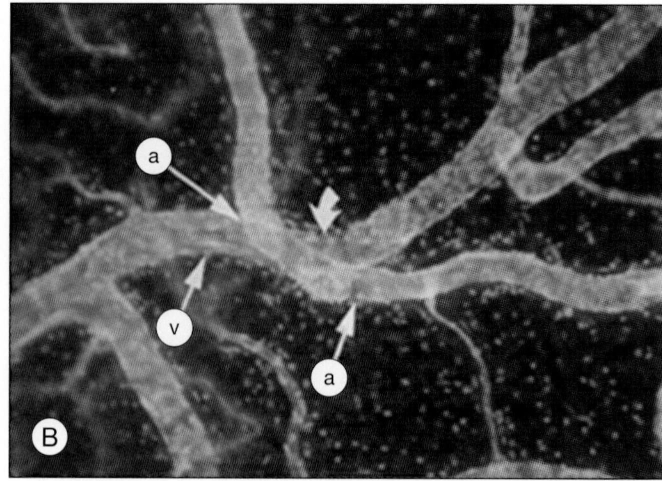

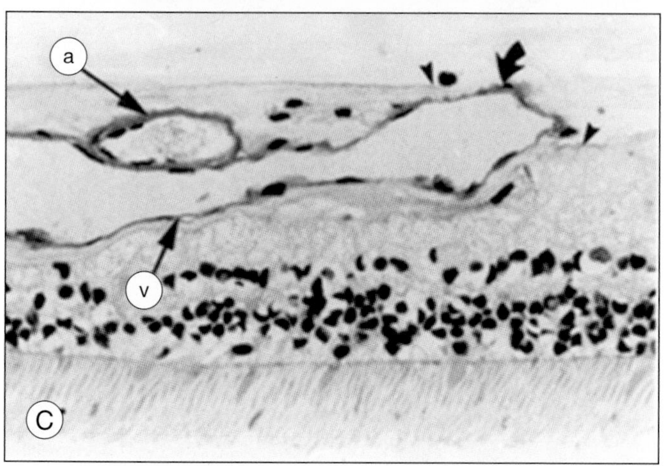

Fig. 57.11 Flat-embedded ADPase retina from a 40-year-old SS subject. (A) A sea-fan formation is shown with dark-field illumination of the retina en bloc before sectioning. This formation occurred at the crossing (curved arrow) of an artery (a) and vein (v) and had five connections to the arterial circulation and four connections to venous channels. (B) Higher magnification of the arteriovenous crossing. (C) Cross-section of the arteriovenous crossing shows the retina is very thin in this region at the border of perfused and nonperfused retina. (Reproduced with permission from McLeod DS, Fukushima A, Goldberg MF, et al. Histopathologic features of neovascularization in sickle-cell retinopathy. Am J Ophthalmol 1997;124:455–72.)

Table 57.1 Goldberg classification of proliferative sickle-cell retinopathy

Stage I	Peripheral arterial occlusions
Stage II	Peripheral arteriovenous anastomoses
Stage III	Neovascular and fibrous proliferations
Stage IV	Vitreous hemorrhage
Stage V	Retinal detachment

anastomoses do not leak, confirming that these early vascular lesions are derived from pre-existing blood vessels with an intact blood–retinal barrier, as opposed to being true neovascular complexes.

Stage III

Sea-fan fronds are the hallmark of stage III PSR, and are perhaps the most recognizable trademark lesion of sickle retinopathy (Fig. 57.10). These lesions are most commonly found in the superotemporal retina, followed by the inferotemporal, superonasal, and inferonasal quadrants. Sea fans represent true neovascularization, and thus, display diffuse leakage on fluorescein angiography (Fig. 57.10). The blood–retinal barrier is not intact. Therefore, sea fans cause chronic transudation into the vitreous from the neovascular lesions, which in turn leads to vitreous degeneration and retinal traction. These may be precursors to vitreous hemorrhage and retinal detachment.[13,48,57]

Most sea fans are found at the border of perfused and nonperfused retina, and they grow toward the ora serrata.[48,78] Sea fan neovascular complexes arise from the venous aspect of the arteriovenous anastomoses, and develop approximately 18 months following the formation of the arteriovenous connections[13,48] (Fig. 57.11). Chronic ischemia within the peripheral retina leads to an increase in angiogenic factors, such as VEGF and basic fibroblastic growth factor.[13,41,94] Pigment epithelial growth factor/VEGF balance may play a role in the angiogenesis of these lesions as well as the subsequent, spontaneous regression of some neovascular complexes.[42]

Another potential mechanism for sea-fan development has been proposed.[95] Occlusive events may create hydrostatic backpressure, causing extrusion of the upstream segment of the blocked vessel into the preretinal space. The rise in intraluminal pressure may cause expansion of the extruded vessel, with resultant stretching of the pericytes and endothelial cells. This process may stimulate endothelial cells, leading to endothelial cell proliferation[105] and subsequent neovascularization.[95,106]

Sea fans typically possess at least one feeding arteriole and one draining venule, and are most commonly found at the sites of arteriovenous anastomoses and arteriovenous crossings.[103,104] A network of these lesions with multiple anastomoses may develop with multiple feeding and draining vessels, and they may form tractional vitreous bands.

Stage IV

Vitreous hemorrhage represents Goldberg stage IV. Sea fans grow or are pulled into the vitreous chamber, and vitreous traction on the delicate neovascular fronds may cause bleeding into the vitreous. Vitreous hemorrhage may be localized over the sea fan, and an individual may remain asymptomatic. However, dramatic, sudden vision loss may occur as the hemorrhage disseminates into the vitreous gel. Vitreous hemorrhage occurs more commonly in the Hb SC than the Hb SS genotype (23% versus 3%).[70,88,92] The risk of recurrent vitreous hemorrhage also increases if an eye has more than 60° of circumferential retinal neovascularization, or if a patient initially presents with vitreous hemorrhage.[107] Chronic vitreous hemorrhage may give rise to fibroglial membranes and vitreous strands, which may produce traction and resultant retinal detachment.[48,57]

Stage V

Presence of traction retinal detachment (TRD) defines Goldberg stage V. TRD develops as the result of chronic vitreous hemorrhage or chronic transudation from neovascular tissue and resultant vitreous membrane formation. Round or horseshoe retinal breaks may also occur, and may be due to localized retinal atrophy and thinning from chronic vaso-occlusion and ischemia.[48] In contrast to the TRD commonly seen in proliferative diabetic retinopathy, the TRD in SCD most commonly involves the peripheral retina as opposed to the posterior pole. Combined TRD and rhegmatogenous retinal detachment may also occur.

ALTERNATIVE CLASSIFICATION SCHEMES

Another classification scheme for PSR was proposed by Penman and colleagues[108] and applies a prognostic significance to varying degrees of PSR. In this angiographic study of eyes of children in a Jamaican sickle cell cohort, two groups were assigned. The type I group showed a normal vascular pattern, and the type 2 group displayed an abnormal vascular pattern. An abnormal vascular pattern was most commonly seen in individuals with Hb SC disease versus individuals with Hb SS disease, and was more likely to develop with age. Over time, the type 2 eyes were more likely to develop proliferative disease. Yet another grading system for PSR has been proposed by Sayag and coworkers[109] to compare clinical outcome of peripheral sea fans in Goldberg stage III lesions treated by laser photocoagulation as compared to the natural course of the disease. The following grades for PSR were described: (A) flat sea fan with leakage <1 Macular Photocoagulation Study (MPS) disc area; (B) elevated sea fan with hemorrhage; (C) elevated sea fan with partial fibrosis; (D) a sea fan with complete fibrosis and without well-demarcated vessels; and (E) a sea fan with complete fibrosis and well-demarcated vessels. In this study, scatter laser photocoagulation is suggested for grade B, grade D, or grade E lesions; however, the authors suggest that grade A or grade C should be observed without laser treatment due to the low rate of progression.[109]

INCIDENCE/PREVALENCE

Among the hemoglobinopathies, the incidence of PSR is higher in those individuals with Hb SC disease and S-β thalassemia than in individuals with Hb SS disease. In the Hb SC genotype, PSR has an earlier onset, with peak prevalence at 15–24 years of age in men and 20–39 years in women. In the SS genotype, peak prevalence of PSR onset falls in the age range of 25–39 years in men and women.[7] In one natural history study of SCD patients followed longitudinally over 20 years, prevalence of PSR was greater in those with Hb SC disease, and by the ages of 24–26 years, PSR had occurred in 43% subjects with Hb SC disease and in 14% subjects with Hb SS disease.[110]

RISK FACTORS

Fox and colleagues described other risk factors that increase an individual's likelihood of developing PSR in addition to genotype, age, and sex.[111] The development of an unstable type IIa border (hairpin loop) conferred an increased risk for PSR. In the Hb SS genotype, high total hemoglobin in males and a low Hb F in both males and females were associated with the development of PSR. In the Hb SC genotype, increased mean cell volume and low Hb F increased the risk in men and women. High total hemoglobin and high MCHC incurred a higher PSR risk in men with Hb SC genotype.[7] In this same study, 70% of patients with Hb SC disease developed bilateral PSR, while 49% of patients with Hb SS disease developed bilateral PSR.[111]

NATURAL HISTORY

Autoinfarction of the proliferative sickle lesions occurs frequently. Spontaneous regression of PSR may occur in 32% of eyes.[110] The mechanism of autoinfarction is not completely understood. This process may be due to chronic and repetitive vaso-occlusion within the vascular channels of the delicate sea-fan neovascular complexes. In a cohort of 120 patients with Hb SS disease and 222 patients with Hb SC disease followed for 10 years, visual acuity loss occurred in 10% of untreated eyes.[112] Vision loss most commonly resulted from PSR, specifically vitreous hemorrhage, TRD, and epiretinal membranes. Patients with nonproliferative disease had a lower incidence of vision loss over the 10-year period than did their counterparts with PSR.[112] Downes and colleagues reported that patients with unilateral PSR had a 16% (11% Hb SS, 17% Hb SC) probability of regressing to no PSR and a 14% (16% Hb SS, 13% Hb SC) probability of progressing to bilateral PSR. Those with bilateral PSR had an 8% (both Hb SC and Hb SS genotypes) probability of regressing to unilateral PSR and a 1% (0 Hb SS, 2% Hb SC) probability of regressing to a PSR-free state.[110]

OPHTHALMIC TREATMENTS

No intervention is indicated for small, asymptomatic peripheral lesions, given the relatively high probability of autoinfarction.[113,114] However, treatment of PSR may be considered in the eye of an individual with significant visual loss from PSR or vision impairment in the contralateral eye. Treatment may also be required in cases of rapid growth of a sea fan, presence of large, elevated sea fans, spontaneous hemorrhage, or bilateral proliferative disease.[13] The goal of intervention in these cases is to prevent the progression of stage III PSR to stages IV or V.

Historically, a goal in PSR treatment had been to occlude the feeder arterioles of the sea-fan lesions.[113] This was accomplished through laser photocoagulation, diathermy, or cryotherapy.[114] This technique was shown to reduce the incidence of vitreous hemorrhage in a small study.[113] Feeder vessel photocoagulation is no longer widely used because of its high rate of complications, which include CNV from breaks in Bruchs membrane and retinal break formation.

Scatter laser photocoagulation is the current mainstay of treatment in PSR. The objective of scatter laser treatment is similar to that employed in the management of proliferative diabetic retinopathy, in which ischemic retina is ablated by laser photocoagulation, thus decreasing the stimulus for pathologic growth factor secretion. Laser photocoagulation of ischemic retina may also help to decrease the overall oxygen requirement of the retina. Through laser destruction of ischemic, damaged peripheral retina, oxygen may be shunted to healthier, more viable retinal tissue (Fig. 57.12).

Anti-VEGF agents have been successful in the treatment of neovascular age-related macular degeneration, retinal venous occlusion, diabetic macular edema, and proliferative diabetic retinopathy. Intravitreal bevacizumab has been reported to cause complete regression of retinal neovascularization and resolution of vitreous hemorrhage following intravitreal injection in eyes with PSR.[115,116] Future study is warranted to assess the role of intravitreal anti-VEGF therapy in PSR.

Vitrectomy may be considered for nonclearing vitreous hemorrhage. Early intervention with vitrectomy may be considered if an individual has an associated retinal detachment or visual impairment in the contralateral eye, or may be indicated to improve visualization of retinal pathology to facilitate treatment. A possible therapeutic approach is combination vitrectomy and scatter laser photocoagulation, with consideration of an anti-VEGF agent in an eye with active PSR. Exchange transfusion, erythropheresis, and hyperbaric oxygen have been attempted to minimize complications from surgically induced anterior-segment ischemia. These methods were without clear benefit and were associated with systemic complications.[117] Vitrectomy in an eye with PSR can be safe with today's modern vitrectomy techniques without these extra measures. The vitreoretinal surgeon should take special care to maximize perfusion in the eye, and work closely with the anesthesiologist to insure the patient is well oxygenated throughout and after the procedure.

Given the propensity for peripheral retinal breaks and other peripheral vitreoretinal pathology to develop, scleral buckling may be considered in SCD to relieve traction from anterior lesions. Though anterior-segment ischemia is a feared complication of scleral buckling in sickle-cell retinopathy eyes, scleral buckles have safely been utilized in sickle-cell retinal detachment surgery.[118] Williamson and colleagues reported their experience with management of vitreoretinal complications of sickle-cell retinopathy.[119] These authors observed flattening of the retina in one patient with rhegmatogenous retinal detachment and one patient with TRD without surgical intervention, though such events are unusual. A high rate of iatrogenic retinal tears was noted by vitreoretinal surgeons while peeling membranes from the atrophic, ischemic peripheral retina with delamination (tangential peeling of preretinal scar tissue from the retinal surface) techniques. Therefore, these authors recommend segmentation (removal of anterior–posterior traction) techniques instead.

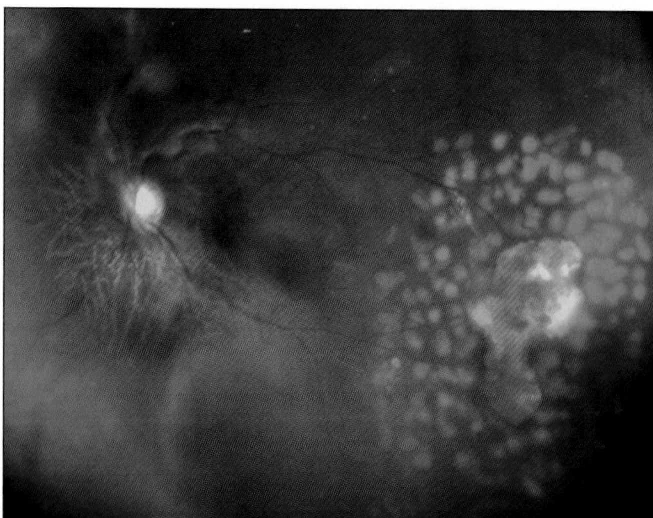

Fig. 57.12 A sea-fan lesion with localized hemorrhage is depicted on ultrawide-field fundus photography immediately after scatter laser treatment in a patient with Hb SC disease.

IMAGING

Selected imaging modalities facilitate diagnosis, monitoring, and assessment of treatment response in sickle-cell retinopathy. As impaired choroidal circulation may be present in eyes with SCD, indocyanine green (ICG) angiography has been studied as a way to assess choroidal perfusion, but the utility of ICG in sickle retinopathy is as yet undetermined.[120] The use of ultrawide-field imaging is particularly helpful to monitor peripheral lesions and to assess treatment response (Fig. 57.12). Fluorescein angiography remains the gold-standard imaging tool for assessment of retinal perfusion status. A potential limitation of conventional fluorescein angiography is the inability to image the pathology of the far peripheral retina in some eyes with sickle retinopathy.[108] Accordingly, ultrawide-field fundus photography and angiography have become useful in the evaluation of the retinal periphery in eyes with sickle-cell retinopathy. As previously mentioned, OCT and especially SD-OCT, with its high resolution, may provide important details about foveal anatomy, which may aid in the diagnosis and management of sickle retinopathy,[79,81–83] even in asymptomatic patients.

POTENTIAL THERAPEUTIC OPTIONS FOR THE FUTURE

Treatment strategies that decrease Hb S and increase Hb F have been shown to decrease the systemic morbidity of SCD. Higher Hb F may interfere with polymerization of Hb S. Agents to increase Hb F include hydroxyurea, omega-3 fatty acids, and erythropoietin. Hydroxyurea may also possess anti-inflammatory properties, and may reduce the load of inflammatory mediators in SCD. The burden of Hb S cells may be reduced through transfusion or hemapheresis. Warfarin, heparin, and ticlopidine all work as antithrombotic agents. Vasodilation of occluded small blood vessels may be improved with NO, or its precursor, arginine. Additional future areas of investigation include hematopoietic stem cell transplantation and gene therapy.[7]

REFERENCES

1. Herrick JB. Peculiar elongated and sickle-shaped red blood corpuscles in a case of severe anemia. Arch Intern Med 1910;6:517–21.
2. Savitt TL. Tracking down the first recorded sickle cell patient in western medicine. J Natl Med Assoc 2010;102:981–92.
3. Savitt TL, Goldberg MF. Herrick's 1910 case report of sickle cell anemia. The rest of the story. JAMA 1989;261:266–71.
4. Pauling L, Itano HA, Singer SJ, et al. Sickle cell anemia, a molecular disease. Science 1949;110:543–48.
5. Barabino GA, Platt NO, Kaul DK. Sickle cell biomechanics. Annu Rev Biomed Eng 2010;12:345–67.

6. Ashley-Koch A, Yang Q, Olney RS. Sickle hemoglobin (HbS) allele and sickle cell disease: a HuGE review. Am J Epidemiol 2000;151:839–45.
7. Elagouz M, Jyothi S, Gupta B, et al. Sickle cell disease and the eye: old and new concepts. Surv Ophthalmol 2010;359–77.
8. Neumayr L, Pringle S, Giles S, et al. Chart card: feasibility of a tool for improving emergency department care in sickle cell disease. J Natl Med Assoc 2010;102:1017–23.
9. Rosenberg JB, Hutcheson K. Pediatric sickle retinopathy: correlation with clinical factors. J AAPOS 2011;15:49–53.
10. National Heart, Lung and Blood Institute. Who is at risk for sickle cell anemia? Available online at: http://www.nhlbi.nih.gov/health/dci/Diseases/Sca/SCA_WhoIsAtRisk.html; 2008 [accessed June 10, 2011].
11. World Health Organization. Sickle-cell anaemia: report by the Secretariat. Available online at: http://www.who.int/gb/ebwha/pdf_files/WHA59/A59_9-en.pdf; 2006 [accessed May 26, 2011].
12. Serjeant G. Sickle cell disease. Oxford: Oxford University Press; 1985.
13. Emerson GG, Harlan JB, Fekrat S, et al. Hemoglobinopathies. In: Ryan SJ, editor. Retina, vol. II. 4th ed. Edinburgh: Elsevier; 2006. p. 1429–45.
14. Gill FM, Sleeper LA, Weiner SJ, et al. Clinical events in the first decade in a cohort of infants with sickle cell disease: Cooperative Study of Sickle Cell Disease. Blood 1995;86:776–83.
15. Bunn HF. Disorders of hemoglobin. In: Braunwald E, Isselbacher KJ, Petersdorf RG, et al, editors. Harrison's principles of internal medicine. 11th ed. New York: McGraw-Hill; 1987. p. 1518–23.
16. Powara D, Hiti A. Sickle cell anemia: beta s gene cluster haplotypes as genetic markers for severe disease expression. Am J Dis Child 1993;147:1197–202.
17. Thomas PW, Higgs DR, Serjeant GR. Benign clinical course in homozygous sickle cell disease: a search for predictors. J Clin Epidemiol 1997;50:121–6.
18. Ferrone FA. Polymerization and sickle cell disease: a molecular review. Microcirculation 2004;11:115–28.
19. Bunn HF. Pathogenesis and treatment of sickle cell disease. N Engl J Med 1997;337:762–9.
20. Mohandas N, Rossi ME, Clark MR. Association between morphologic distortion of sickle cells and deoxygenation-induced cation permeability increase. Blood 1986;68:450–4.
21. Brugnara C, Bunn HF, Tosteson DC. Regulation of erythrocyte cation and water content in sickle cell anemia. Science 1986;232:388–90.
22. Fabry ME, Kaul DK. Sickle cell vasocclusion. Hematol/Oncol Clin North Am 1991;5:375–98.
23. Hebbel RP. Adhesive interactions of sickle erythrocytes with endothelium. J Clin Invest 1997;100:S83–86.
24. Sugihara K, Sugihara T, Mohandas N, et al. Thrombospondin mediates adherence of CD36+ sickle erythrocytes to endothelial cells. Blood 1992;80: 2634–42.
25. Swerlick RA, Eckman JR, Kumar A, et al. Alpha 4 beta 1 expression on sickle reticulocytes; vascular cell adhesion molecule 1 dependent binding to the endothelium. Blood 1993;82:1891–9.
26. Wun T, Paglieroni T, Field CL, et al. Platelet-erythrocyte adhesion in sickle cell disease. J Invest Med 1999;47:121–7.
27. Kaul DK, Fabry ME, Nagel RL. The pathophysiology of vascular obstruction in the sickle syndromes. Blood Rev 1996;10:29–44.
28. Joneckis CC, Ackley RL, Orringer EP, et al. Integrin alpha 4 beta 1 and glycoprotein IV (CD36) are expressed on circulating reticulocytes in sickle cell anemia. Blood 1993;82:3548–55.
29. Setty BN, Stuart MJ. Vascular cell adhesion molecule 1 is involved in mediating hypoxia-induced sickle red blood cell adherence to endothelium; potential role in sickle cell disease. Blood 1996;88:2311–20.
30. Francis Jr RB, Haywood LJ. Elevated immunoreactive tumor necrosis factor and interleukin-1 in sickle cell disease. J Natl Med Assoc 1992;84:611–5.
31. Malave I, Perdomo Y, Escalona E, et al. Levels of tumor necrosis factor α/cachectin (TNFα) in sera from patients with sickle cell disease. Acta Haematol 1993;90:172–6.
32. Solovey A, Lin Y, Browne P, et al. Circulating activated endothelial cells in sickle cell anemia. N Engl J Med 1997;337:1584–90.
33. Kunz Mathews M, McLeod DS, Merges C, et al. Neutrophils and leukocyte adhesion molecules in sickle cell retinopathy. Br J Ophthalmol 2002;86: 684–90.
34. Lutty GA, Otsuji T, Taomoto M, et al. Mechanisms for sickle red blood cell retention in choroid. Curr Eye Res 2002;25:163–71.
35. Lutty GA, Phelan A, Mcleod DS, et al. A rat model for sickle-cell mediated vaso-occlusion in retina. Microvasc Res 1996;52:270–80.
36. Lutty GA, Taomoto M, Cao J, et al. Inhibition of TNF-alpha-induced sickle RBC retention in retina with a VLA-4 antagonist. Invest Ophthalmol Vis Sci 2001;42:1349–55.
37. Lutty GA, Goldberg MF. Ophthalmological complications. In: Embury SH, Hebbel RP, Mohandas N, et al, editors. Sickle cell disease: basic principles and clinical practice. New York: Raven Press; 1992, p. 703–24.
38. Vichinsky E. New therapies in sickle cell disease. Lancet 2002;360:629–31.
39. Wood KC, Hsu LL, Gladwin MT. Sickle cell disease vasculopathy; a state of nitric oxide resistance. Free Radic Biol Med 2008;44:1506–28.
40. Gurkan E, Tanriverdi K, Baslamish F. Clinical relevance of vascular endothelial growth factor levels in sickle cell disease. Ann Hematol 2005;84:71–5.
41 Cao J, Kunz Mathews MK, McLeod DS, et al. Angiogenic factors in human proliferative sickle cell retinopathy. Br J Ophthalmol 1999;83:838–46.
42. Kim DY, Mocanu V, McLeod DS, et al. Expression of pigment epithelium-derived factor (PEDF) and vascular endothelial growth factor (VEGF) in sickle cell retina and choroid. Exp Eye Res 2003;7:433–45.
43. Lu M, Perez VL, Ma N. VEGF increases retinal vascular ICAM-1 expression in vivo. Invest Ophthalmol Vis Sci 1999;40:1808–12.
44 Perlman N, Selvaraj SK, Batra S, et al. Placenta growth factor activates monocytes and correlates with sickle cell disease severity. Blood 2003;102:1506–14.
45. Oh H, Takagi H, Suzuma K, et al. Hypoxia and vascular endothelial growth factor selectively upregulate angiopoietin-2 in bovine microvascular endothelial cells. J Biol Chem 1999;274:15732–9.
46. Fadugbagbe AO, Gurgel RQ, Mendonca CQ, et al. Ocular manifestations of sickle cell disease. Ann Trop Paediatr 2010;30:19–26.
47. Ballas SK, Lewis CN, Noone AM, et al. Clinical, hematological, and biochemical features of Hb SC disease. Am J Hematol 1982;13:37–51.
48. Goldberg MF. Retinal neovascularization in sickle cell retinopathy. Trans Am Acad Ophthalmol Otolaryngol 1977;83:Op409–Op431.
49. Gagliano DA, Jampol L, Rabb M. Sickle cell disease. In: Tasman WS, Jaeger E, editors. Duane's clinical ophthalmology, vol. 3. Philadelphia: Lippincott Raven; 1996. p. 1–40.
50. Ganesh A, William RR, Mitra S, et al. Orbital involvement in sickle cell disease: a report of 5 cases and review literature. Eye 2001;15:774–80.
51. Perlman JI, Forman S, Gonzalez ER. Retrobulbar ischemic optic neuropathy associated with sickle cell disease. J Neuro-Ophthalmol 1994;14:45–8.
52. Adewoye AH, Ramsey J, McMahon L, et al. Lacrimal gland enlargement in sickle cell disease. Am J Hematol 2006;81:888–9.
53. Condon PI, Sergeant GR. Ocular findings in elderly cases of homozygous sickle cell disease in Jamaica. Br J Ophthalmol 1976;60:361–4.
54. Paton D. The conjunctival sign of sickle cell disease. Arch Ophthalmol 1961;66:90–4.
55. Fink AI, Funahashi T, Robinson M, et al. Conjunctival blood flow in sickle cell disease. Preliminary report. Arch Ophthalmol 1961;66:824–9.
56. Paton D. The conjunctival sign of sickle-cell disease. Further observations. Arch Ophthalmol 1962;68:627–32.
57. Nagpal KC, Goldberg MF, Rabb MF. Ocular manifestations of sickle hemoglobinopathies. Surv Ophthalmol 1977;21:391–411.
58. Funahashi T, Fink A, Robinson M, et al. Pathology of conjunctival vessels in sickle-cell disease. A preliminary report. Am J Ophthalmol 1964;57:713–8.
59. Chambers J, Puglisi J, Kernitsky R, et al. Iris atrophy in hemoglobin SC disease. Am J Ophthalmol 1974;77:247–9.
60. Galinos S, Rabb MF, Goldberg MF, et al. Hemoglobin SC disease and iris atrophy. Am J Ophthalmol 1973;75:421–5.
61. Bergren RL, Brown GC. Neovascular glaucoma secondary to sickle cell retinopathy. Am J Ophthalmol 1992;113:718–9.
62. Goldberg MF. The diagnosis and treatment of secondary glaucoma after hyphema in sickle cell patients. Am J Ophthalmol 1979;87:43–9.
63. Goldberg MF. Sickled erythrocytes, hyphema,and secondary glaucoma IV. The rate and percentage of sickling of erythrocytes in rabbit aqueous humor, in vitro and in vivo. Ophthalmic Surg 1979;10:62–9.
64. Goldberg MF. Sickled erythrocytes, hyphema, and secondary glaucoma I. The diagnosis and treatment of sickled erythrocytes in human hyphemas. Ophthalmic Surg 1979;10:17–31.
65. Goldberg MF, Dizon R, Raichand M. Sickled erythrocytes, hyphema, and secondary glaucoma II. Injected sickle cell erythrocytes into human, monkey, and guinea pig anterior chambers: the introduction of sickling and secondary glaucoma. Ophthalmic Surg 1979;10:32–51.
66. Deutsch TA, Weinreb RN, Goldberg MF. Indications for surgical management of hyphema in patients with sickle cell trait. Arch Ophthalmol 1984;102: 566–9.
67. Karaman K, Culic S, Erceg I, et al. Treatment of post-traumatic trabecular meshwork thrombosis and secondary glaucoma with intracameral tissue plasminogen activator in previously unrecognized sickle cell anemia. Coll Antropol 2005;29(Suppl 1):123–6.
68. Henry MD, Chapman AZ. Vitreous hemorrhage and retinopathy associated with sickle cell disease. Am J Ophthalmol 1954;38:204–9.
69. Hannon JF. Vitreous hemorrhages associated with sickle cell-hemoglobin C disease. Am J Ophthalmol 1956;42;707–12.
70. Condon PI, Serjeant GR. Ocular findings in homozygous sickle cell anemia in Jamaica. Am J Ophthalmol 1972;73:533–43.
71. Condon PI, Serjeant GR. Ocular findings in hemoglobin SC disease in Jamaica. Am J Ophthalmol 1972;74:921–31.
72. Condon PI, Serjeant GR. Ocular findings in sickle cell thalassemia in Jamaica. Am J Ophthalmol 1972;74:1105–9.
73. Nagpal KC, Goldberg MF, Asdourian G, et al. Dark-without-pressure fundus lesions. Br J Ophthalmol 1975;59;476–9.
74. Goldberg MF. Retinal vaso-occlusion in sickling hemoglobinopathies. Birth Defects Orig Artic Ser 1976;12:475–515.
75. Condon PI, Serjeant GR. Behaviour of untreated proliferative sickle retinopathy. Br J Ophthalmol 1980;64:404–11.
76. Kimmel AS, Magargal LE, Tasman WS. Proliferative sickle retinopathy and neovascularization at the disc: regression following treatment with peripheral scatter laser photocoagulation. Ophthalm Surg 1986;17:20–2.
77. Ober RR, Michels RG. Optic disk neovascularization in hemoglobin SC disease. Am J Ophthalmol 1978;85:711–4.
78. Raichand M, Goldberg MF, Nagpal KC, et al. Evolution of neovascularization in sickle cell retinopathy. A prospective fluorescein angiographic study. Trans Am Ophthalmol Soc 1992;90:481–504.
79. Goldbaum MH. Retinal depression sign indicating a small retinal infarct. Am J Ophthalmol 1978;86:45–55.
80. Sanders RJ, Brown GC, Rosenstein RB, et al. Foveal avascular zone diameter and sickle cell disease. Arch Ophthalmol 1991;109:812–5.

81. Witkin AJ, Rogers AH, Ko TH, et al. Optical coherence tomography demonstration of macular infarction in sickle cell retinopathy. Arch Ophthalmol 2006;124:747–747.
82. Hoang QV, Chau FY, Shahidi M, et al. Central macular splaying and outer retinal thinning in asymptomatic sickle cell patients by spectral-domain optical coherence tomography. Am J Ophthalmol 2011;151:990–4.
83. Murthy RK, Grover S, Chalam K. Temporal macular thinning on spectral-domain optical coherence tomography in proliferative sickle cell retinopathy. Arch Ophthalmol 2011;129:247–9.
84. Raichland M, Dizon RV, Nagpal KC, et al. Macular holes associated with proliferative sickle cell retinopathy. Arch Ophthalmol 1987;96:1592–6.
85. Moriarty BJ, Acheson RW, Serjeant GR. Epiretinal membranes in sickle cell disease. Br J Ophthalmol 1987;71:466–9.
86. Schubert HD. Schisis in sickle cell retinopathy. Arch Ophthalmol 2005;123: 1607–9.
87. Frank RN, Cronin MA. Posterior pole neovascularization in a patient with hemoglobin SC disease. Am J Ophthalmol 1979;88:680–2.
88. Clarkson JG. The ocular manifestations of sickle cell disease: a prevalence and natural history study. Trans Am Ophthalmol Soc 1992;90:481–504.
89. Clarkson JG, Altman RD. Angioid streaks. Surv Ophthalmol 1982;26:235–46.
90. Condon PI, Serjeant GR. Ocular findings in elderly cases of homozygous sickle cell disease in Jamaica. Br J Ophthalmol 1976;60:361–4.
91. Aessopos A, Farmakis D, Loukopoulos D. Elastic tissue abnormalities resembling pseudoxanthoma elasticum in beta thalassemia and the sickling syndromes. Blood 2002;99:30–5.
92. Welch RB, Goldberg MF. Sickle-cell hemoglobin and its relation to fundus abnormality. Arch Ophthalmol 1966;75:353–62.
93. Fine LC, Petrovic V, Irvine AR, et al. Spontaneous central retinal artery occlusion in hemoglobin SC disease. Am J Ophthalmol 2000;130:680–1.
94. Lutty GA, Merges C, Crone S, et al. Immunohistochemical insights into sickle cell retinopathy. Curr Eye Res 1994;13:1251–38.
95. McLeod DS, Goldberg MF, Lutty GA. Dual-perspective analysis of vascular formations in sickle cell retinopathy. Arch Ophthalmol 1993;111:1234–45.
96. Liang JC, Jampol LM. Spontaneous peripheral chorioretinal neovascularization in association with sickle cell anemia. Br J Ophthalmol 1983;67:107–10.
97. Condon PI, Jampol LM, Ford SM, et al. Choroidal neovascularization induced by photocoagulation in sickle cell disease. Br J Ophthalmol 1981;65:192–7.
98. Romayananda N, Goldberg MF, Green WR. Histopathology of sickle cell retinopathy. Trans Am Acad Opthalmol Otol 1973;77:652–76.
99. Gagliano DA, Goldberg MF. The evolution of salmon-patch hemorrhages in sickle cell retinopathy. Arch Ophthalmol 1989;107:1814–5.
100. Serjeant GR, Serjeant BE. The eyes. In: Serjeant GR, Serjeant BE, editors. Sickle cell disease. 3rd ed. Oxford: Oxford University Press; 2001. p. 366–92.
101. Emerson GG, Lutty GA. Effects of sickle cell disease on the eye: clinical features and treatment. Hematol Oncol Clin North Am 2005;19:957–63.
102. Lutty GA, McLeod DS, Pachinis A, et al. Retinal and choroidal neovascularization in a transgenic mouse model of sickle cell disease. Am J Pathol 1994; 145:490–7.
103. McLeod DS, Merges C, Fukushima A, et al. Histopathologic features of neovascularization in sickle cell retinopathy. Am J Ophthalmol 1997;124:455–72.
104. Goldberg MF. Natural history of untreated proliferative sickle retinopathy. Arch Ophthalmol 1971;85:428–37.
105. Curtis AS, Seehar GM. The control of cell division by tension or diffusion. Nature 1978;274:52–3.
106. van Meurs JC. Evolution of a retinal hemorrhage in a patient with sickle-cell hemoglobin C disease. Arch Ophthalmol 1995;113:1074–5.
107. Condon PI, Whitelocke RA, Bird AC, et al. Recurrent visual loss in homozygous sickle cell disease. Br J Ophthalmol 1985;69:700–6.
108. Penman AD, Talbot JF, Chuang EL, et al. New classification of peripheral retinal vascular changes in sickle cell disease. Br J Ophthalmol 1994;681–9.
109. Sayag D, Binaghi M, Souied EH, et al. Retinal photocoagulation for proliferative sickle cell retinopathy: A prospective clinical trial with new sea fan classification. Eur J Ophthalmol 2008;18:248–54.
110. Downes SM, Hambleton IR, Chuang EL, et al. Incidence and natural history of proliferative sickle cell retinopathy: observations from a cohort study. Ophthalmol 2005;1869–75.
111. Fox PD, Dunn DT, Morris JS, et al. Risk factors for proliferative sickle retinopathy. Br J Ophthalmol 1990;74:172–6.
112. Moriarty BJ, Acheson RW, Condon PI, et al. Patterns of visual loss in untreated sickle cell retinopathy. Eye 1988;2:330–5.
113. Condon P, Jampol LM, Farber MD, et al. A randomized clinical trial of feeder vessel photocoagulation of proliferative sickle cell retinopathy.II. Update and analysis of risk factors. Ophthalmology 1984;91:1496–8.
114. Rednam KR, Jampol LM, Goldberg MF. Scatter retinal photocoagulation for proliferative sickle cell retinopathy. Am J Ophthalmol 1982;93:594–9.
115. Shaikh S. Intravitreal bevacizumab (Avastin) for the treatment of proliferative sickle retinopathy. Indian J Ophthalmol 2008;56:259.
116. Siquiera RC, Costa RA, Scott IU, et al. Intravitreal bevacizumab (Avastin) injection associated with regression of retinal neovascularization caused by sickle cell retinopathy. Acta Ophthalmol Scand 2006;84:834–5.
117. Bove JR. Transfusion-transmitted diseases: current problems and challenges. Prog Hematol 1986;14:123–47.
118. Pulido JS, Flynn HW, Clarkson JG, et al. Pars plana vitrectomy in the management of the complications of proliferative sickle retinopathy. Arch Opthalmol 1988;106:1553–7.
119. Williamson TH, Rajput R, Laidlaw DAH, et al. Vitreoretinal management of the complications of sickle cell retinopathy by observation or pars plana vitrectomy. Eye 2009;23:1314–20.
120. Diallo JW, Kuhn D, Hayman-Gawrilow P, et al. Contribution of indocyanine green angiography in sickle cell retinopathy. J Fr Ophthalmol 2009;32:430–5.

Radiation Retinopathy

Leigh Spielberg, Patrick De Potter, Anita Leys

Chapter 58

INTRODUCTION

Radiation retinopathy (RR) is a slowly progressive, delayed-onset occlusive microangiopathy of the retinal vasculature that occurs with variable latency after exposure of the retina to ionizing radiation. First described by Stallard in 1933,[1] the term encompasses all retinal vascular changes, including ischemic and proliferative RR (PRR) and radiation maculopathy. It is a potentially devastating sequela of exposure of the eye to any source of radiation, including local plaque radiation treatment (brachytherapy), external-beam radiation treatment (ERBT), proton beam radiation, helium ion radiotherapy and gamma knife radiotherapy of the eye, ocular adnexa, orbit, and head and neck structures.[2–6] Radiotherapy offers an alternative to enucleation for patients with retinoblastoma, choroidal melanoma, and ocular metastases,[7–9] as well as life-saving treatment of orbital, sinus, and intracranial tumors. Since the Collaborative Ocular Melanoma Study showed similar survival rates after radiotherapy and enucleation, the shift towards globe-salvaging therapeutic strategies has increased the use of radiation and consequently increased its complications, with reports of the incidence of RR ranging from 3% to over 20%.[10,11] The current interest in use of radiation in the treatment of neovascular age-related macular degeneration (AMD) might further increase the risk of this complication.[12]

The risk of RR is related to characteristics of the radiation treatment itself, the presence of systemic disease, and exposure to radiation sensitizers such as chemotherapy. Fundoscopic findings can be highly variable, ranging from scattered retinal hemorrhages, microaneurysms, and cotton-wool spots to macular edema, large-vessel occlusion, extensive ischemic retinopathy and maculopathy and consequent retinal and ocular neovascularization. Within the retina, the posterior pole is particularly sensitive to this pathology,[13] with grave implications for visual prognosis. Further, RR has a long latency and may not be clinically detectable for 8 years or more.[14]

Although RR has a variable course, it is frequently fulminant, with a tendency for the vasculopathy to decrease vision progressively by affecting the macular microvasculature. Further, the structural damage is usually irreversible, particularly in cases with macular nonperfusion and ischemia.

ETIOLOGY, PATHOGENESIS, AND HISTOPATHOLOGY

RR can be described as a progressive obliterative arteritis that initiates a characteristic pattern of degenerative and proliferative vascular changes and microvascular dysfunction. Radiotherapy is the most frequent cause. Radiotherapy generates its effective tumoricidal effects both directly, via injury to the DNA of rapidly dividing cells, and indirectly, via the production of free radicals. However, these processes damage vascular and interstitial support structures of both pathological and healthy tissue. Histopathologically, ionizing radiation of the retina induces an acute transudative as well as a slowly progressive occlusive vasculopathy.[15] The initial pathologic change, and the fundamental abnormality, is retinal vascular endothelial cell injury and loss[15–18] and associated inflammation,[19] which occurs primarily in capillaries, followed by capillary closure, clearly visible with fluorescein angiography (FA),[14,20–22] retinal ischemia, nerve tissue necrosis, and fibrovascular proliferation.[13,18,21,23,24]

The loss of capillary cellularity leads to the development of microaneurysms, and hemodynamic alterations produce fenestrated telangiectatic retinal vessels. Larger retinal vessels become involved later in the course of the retinopathy, with diameter reduction of up to 75% in major retinal arteries and veins demonstrated in animal models.[19] Closure of blood vessels is the single most characteristic finding on FA. Ghost vessels are later visible ophthalmoscopically. Central retinal artery occlusion has also been described as a consequence of high-dose irradiation,[25] as has interruption of the choroidal circulation.[26,27] The choriocapillaris also suffers, and hypoperfusion is detectable several months after treatment,[27] leading to choroidopathy and chorioretinal atrophy. The widespread vascular occlusion induces the production of vascular endothelial growth factor (VEGF),[18] leading to neovascularization and an increase in vascular permeability, both of which result in vascular leakage and tissue edema.[28] Uveal effusion can also be present.

The disappearance of choriocapillaris, retinal pigment epithelium (RPE), photoreceptors and retinal nerve fibers, along with leukocyte invasion, has been demonstrated histologically.[29] Areas devoid of photoreceptor cells correspond with areas of pigment dispersion with reduced numbers of melanocytes. There is a thickening of arteriolar and capillary walls and endothelial cell loss. In contrast to diabetic retinopathy, in which pericytes are initially affected, RR exhibits an early loss of endothelial cells. However, pericytes can be affected in severely damaged capillaries.

On optical coherence tomography (OCT) images, significant thinning of the inner plexiform, inner nuclear, and outer plexiform layers is visible, suggesting that radiation-induced damage is confined to the inner layers of the retina.[30] However, secondary functional changes may occur in the outer retina.[31]

NATURAL HISTORY AND CLINICAL FEATURES

RR displays clinical and angiographic features that are virtually identical to those seen in diabetic retinopathy.[32] This is to be expected, since both radiation and diabetes primarily damage the retinal capillaries. Ophthalmoscopically, microaneurysms are the first to appear and are near-universally present,[33] closely followed by intraretinal hemorrhages, macular capillary dilation and nonperfusion, and nerve fiber layer infarcts (cotton-wool spots; Fig. 58.1).[14] Retinal edema, hard exudates, telangiectasia, and perivascular sheathing may follow in variable sequence and latency. Hard exudates have been found to be more prevalent after brachytherapy (Fig. 58.2), whereas retinal hemorrhages and microaneurysms are more commonly found after EBRT.[13] The telangiectatic-like vessels are a feature of established retinopathy and are likely to represent collateral vasculature at the edges of capillary occlusion.[14] Confluent areas of capillary closure lead to the development of large areas of retinal capillary nonperfusion.

The fluorescein angiographic hallmarks of the condition are the presence of severe retinal capillary nonperfusion, capillary dilation, and microaneurysms, frequently in combination with macular edema or ischemia.[13] Central macular chorioretinal anastomosis has also been described.[34] Neovascularization may develop later (Fig. 58.1), and does so in approximately 32% of eyes with RR.[35] This development is referred to as PRR, and its presence is ominous. Analogous to proliferative diabetic retinopathy, it suggests profound ischemia and carries a worse prognosis for long-term visual acuity. If left untreated, it can lead to neovascular glaucoma, vitreous hemorrhage, and tractional retinal detachment caused by fibrovascular

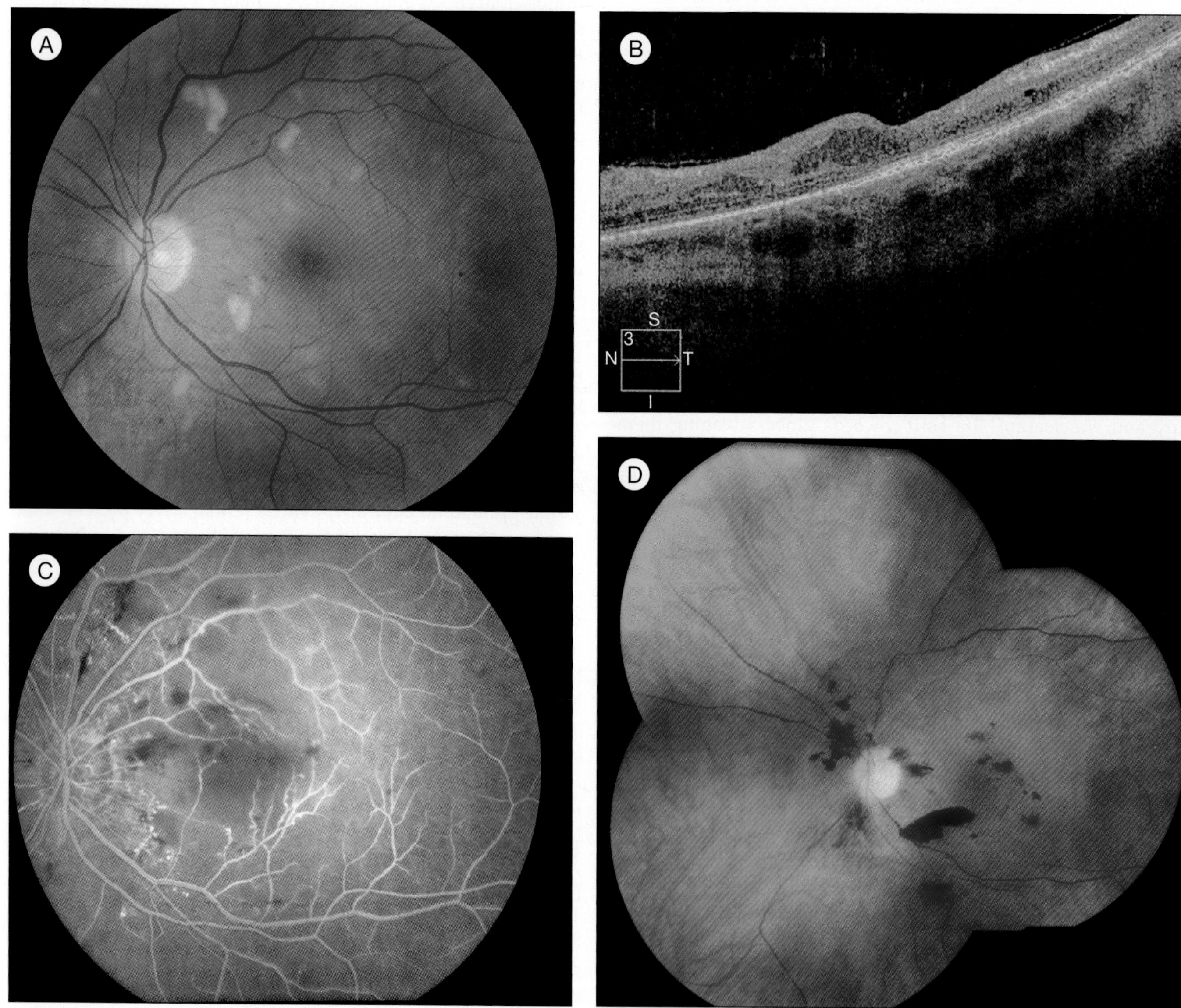

Fig. 58.1 A 32-year-old woman was treated with four cycles of rituximab and fractionated external-beam radiation therapy (20 × 2 Gy) for a non-Hodgkin lymphoma of the left maxillary sinus. Swelling of lids, ptosis, conjunctival redness, and dry-eye symptoms were the first ocular complications. Shortly thereafter, loss of visual acuity was noted due to radiation retinopathy and optic neuropathy with numerous cotton-wool spots, retinal hemorrhages, and pallor of the optic disc (A). Macular edema (B) as well as progressive capillary nonperfusion (C) were noted subsequently. A single intravitreal steroid injection was administered. Two years after radiotherapy, and 15 months after diagnosis of the radiation retinopathy, subhyaloidal and vitreous hemorrhages due to optic disc neovascularization and widespread retinal nonperfusion (D) were observed. Neither rubeosis iridis nor increased intraocular pressure was observed. However, final visual acuity was reduced to counting fingers.

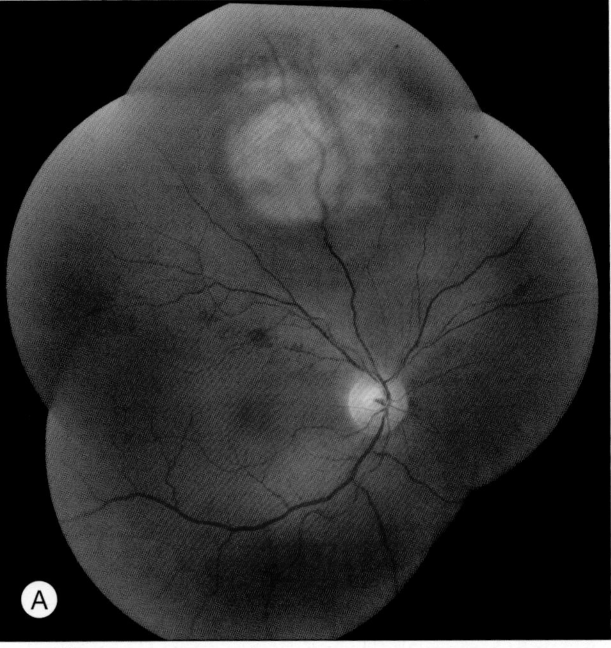

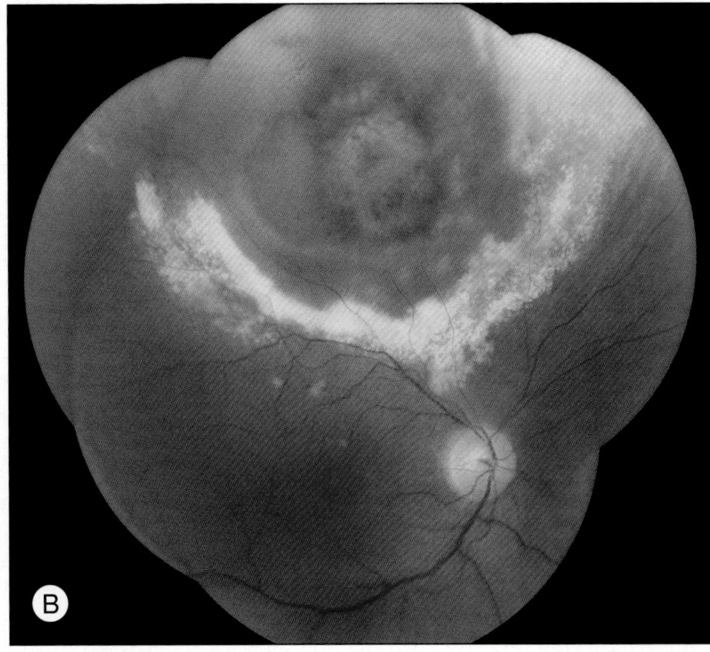

Fig. 58.2 (A) Large mushrooom-shaped choroidal melanoma before I^{125} plaque radiotherapy. (B) Radiation retinopathy is documented 14 months after treatment with supramacular cotton-wool spots, exudative retinal detachment and hard exudates threatening the macula.

Table 58.1 Findings in 87 eyes with radiation retinopathy

Complication	Incidence
Nonproliferative radiation retinopathy	68%
Proliferative radiation retinopathy	32%
Clinically significant macular edema	76%
Macular ischemia	76%
Radiation optic neuropathy	55%
Cataract	52%
Vitreous hemorrhage	24%
Glaucoma	12%
Radiation keratopathy	10%
Tractional retinal detachment	5%

(Adapted from Kinyoun JL. Long-term visual acuity results of treated and untreated radiation retinopathy (an AOS thesis). Trans Am Ophthalmol Soc 2008;106:325–35.)

proliferation similar to that seen in diabetic retinopathy. However, in contrast to diabetic retinopathy and other retinal vasculopathies, neovascularization does not typically extend through the internal limiting membrane into the vitreous.[18] Nevertheless, vitreous hemorrhage can occur and its presence is associated with a poor prognosis for both vision and globe salvage, as well as for ghost cell or neovascular glaucoma. It also impedes the clinician's ability to monitor the retinopathy and to employ laser photocoagulation to treat progression (Table 58.1).

CLASSIFICATION

There is currently no standard method of classification for RR, although several methods have been developed. These can be categorized as clinical or ophthalmoscopic, fluorescein angiographic and OCT. Finger and Kurli proposed a four-stage, prognosis-related classification that uses ophthalmoscopic and fluorescein angiographic findings to classify macular and extramacular changes.[36] In this system, stage 1 includes extramacular ischemic changes, stage 2 includes macular ischemic changes, stage 3 includes additional macular edema and retinal neovascularization, and stage 4 encompasses vitreous hemorrhage and at least 5 disc areas of retinal ischemia, whether macular or extramacular. The Early Treatment Diabetic Retinopathy Study (ETDRS) definition of clinically significant macular edema has been applied to macular edema associated with radiation damage. In these cases, it is referred to as clinically significant radiation macular edema, which follows the ETDRS definitions: retinal thickening within 500 mm of the fovea; edema-associated hard exudates within 500 mm of the fovea; and one or more zones of retinal thickening ≥1 disc area, any part of which is within 1 disc diameter of the fovea.[37] FA allows the clinician to determine the condition of the macula, allowing maculopathy to be subdivided into ischemic and nonischemic variants, which has a significant impact on the visual outcome. FA also allows for the classification of macular edema, which is useful if grid or focal laser photocoagulation is to be administered. OCT is increasingly used to guide diagnosis and treatment decisions for macular edema in various retinal disorders.[38] Horgan et al. proposed a five-point OCT-based grading scale based on standard reference OCT images: grade 1, extrafoveolar, noncystoid edema; grade 2, extrafoveolar cystoid edema; grade 3, foveolar noncystoid edema; grade 4, mild-to-moderate foveolar cystoid edema; and grade 5, severe foveolar cystoid edema.[39] This study demonstrated OCT evidence of macular edema as early as 4 months after plaque radiotherapy for uveal melanoma, with a peak incidence at 12–18 months, and that it is associated with significant vision loss. The use of OCT is important, because macular edema is visible on OCT approximately 5 months earlier than clinically detectable radiation maculopathy.[39] The classification of RR into PRR and nonproliferative (NPRR) subtypes is also of great prognostic importance. A recent retrospective study reported an incidence of PRR of 5.8% at 5 years and 7% at 10 and 15 years in 3841 eyes treated with plaque radiotherapy for uveal melanoma.[40]

RISK FACTORS

Risk factors for the development of RR can be divided into internal (inherent/patient) and external (iatrogenic) factors. The primary patient factor is concomitant vascular disease such as diabetes mellitus.[41] Since both diabetes and radiation primarily damage the retinal capillaries, this synergistic effect is to be expected, as the capillaries experience an early loss of pericytes due to diabetes and endothelial cell loss due to radiation. Destruction of these two cell types leaves little cellular structural support for capillaries and thus results in capillary closure, aneurysms, vessel leakage, and hemorrhage. Indeed, it has been suggested that concomitant diabetes mellitus is also a poor prognostic indicator for visual acuity, increasing the risk of visual loss by nearly 300%.[42] This is in part due to the fact that diabetes mellitus is associated with an increased incidence and severity of neovascular complications, including neovascular glaucoma[43] and radiation papillopathy[44] following radiotherapy.[45] Other vascular disorders predisposing to RR are arterial hypertension and coronary artery disease.[46] Tumor characteristics likely to lead to a worse prognosis include large tumors and close proximity to the macula and optic disc.[47]

Chemotherapy, whether or not concurrent/concomitant with the radiation therapy, also increases the risk,[13,48] as may pregnancy.[49] Chemotherapy increases the vulnerability of the retinal vasculature to radiation damage, possibly via an increase in oxygen-derived free radicals.[23] It also increases the risk of proliferative (or neovascular) RR, which carries a worse prognosis than the nonproliferative type.[50] The concomitant administration of chemotherapy increases the risk of visual complications,[13,23,48,51–53] potentiates the development of RR at lower radiation doses,[13] and may shorten the latent period between exposure and retinopathy.[48,52,54]

INCIDENCE AND DOSIMETRY

The most important external or iatrogenic risk factors relate to the radiation itself. These are radiation type, treatment modality (external beam versus brachytherapy or plaque), total radiation dose and the fractionation schedule of that dosage, the total elapsed time in the course of irradiation treatment, and errors in treatment technique and/or dosage calculations.[53,55]

Radiation type

If a large enough dose is applied, any type of radiation can result in retinopathy and its associated complications. RR is found in 87% of patients after plaque radiotherapy for juxtapapillary melanomas, and radiation maculopathy in 89% after proton beam irradiation. However, neither of these radiation types is as highly associated with severe sight-limiting complications (such as rubeosis and neovascular glaucoma) as gamma knife treatment, which may lead to complete loss of vision in nearly 50%.[5]

Treatment modality

An important factor to be considered is the surveillance of patients whose eyes are exposed to EBRT. In contrast to patients treated with retinal plaques for choroidal melanoma, who are periodically evaluated by retinal specialists and ocular oncologists, patients treated with EBRT are less likely to be regularly evaluated with dilated ophthalmoscopic examinations several years after treatment. Considering the progressive pathophysiology of RR, delays in diagnosis and treatment can result in long-term macular edema leading to ischemia, fibrosis, and irreversible vision loss.

Total radiation dose

The association between dose and RR is well established.[25] However, a precise threshold has been difficult to determine. The condition does not usually occur at total doses <45 Gy unless an additional risk factor such as diabetes is present.[55,56] In a study of 68 eyes that underwent EBRT for primary extracranial head and neck tumors, the dose–response curve for retinopathy was characterized by a dramatic increase in incidence between 45 and 55 Gy.[56] Nearly all patients receiving higher doses developed retinopathy. A more recent retrospective review suggests that the incidence can be significantly reduced by hyperfractionated (twice-daily doses of 1.1–1.2 Gy) EBRT.[55] However, above 70 Gy, the overall incidence of retinopathy approaches 40%.

Fractionation schedule

During EBRT, increased fraction size correlates with an increased incidence of retinal complications.[13,23,53,57,58] A dose per fraction below 1.9 Gy/fraction has been shown to decrease the incidence of retinopathy.[56] This is referred to as hyperfractionation, which theoretically allows the retina enough time to repair single-strand DNA breaks before a second nearby insult can occur.[55] This reduces late toxicity to the retina. However, for brachytherapy, which is primarily used for the treatment of choroidal melanoma, fractionation is not possible, since the radiation is delivered continuously at a predetermined dose for a certain period of time.

Volume of retina irradiated

The volume of retina irradiated has also been shown to be a significant predictor of retinopathy. Eyes receiving more than 50 Gy to greater than 60% of the retina have been shown to be more likely to develop RR.[25]

Total elapsed time

The latency between radiotherapy and the onset of clinically significant retinopathy can range from 1 month to 15 years, but it most commonly occurs between 6 months and 3 years. High-dose, single-fraction treatment regimens are associated with a more rapid onset.[59]

DIFFERENTIAL DIAGNOSIS AND DIAGNOSTIC EVALUATION

RR can occur many years after radiation therapy. Because of this potential delay, RR may not be recognized as the cause of visual loss. Further, due to the ophthalmoscopic and angiographic similarities, RR may be misdiagnosed as diabetic or hypertensive retinopathy. However, a dilated ophthalmic examination combined with a careful history, including questioning of the patient and a thorough review of the treatment records to determine whether the eyes were included in the field of radiation, will usually lead to the diagnosis. The diagnosis should be considered following cephalic radiation for any reason, including treatment for orbital inflammatory disease such as thyroid disease[60] and orbital pseudotumor,[61] sinus malignancies and periocular cutaneous lesions. A feature of RR that distinguishes it from diabetic retinopathy is the atrophy of the RPE sometimes seen after radiation treatment.

Bone marrow transplant retinopathy can mimic RR, and it can be very difficult to distinguish the two unless affected patients have a history of exposure to one (e.g., radiation) and not the other (e.g., bone marrow transplantation).[62] Other potential causes of the observed retinal abnormalities include multiple branch retinal artery occlusions, multiple retinal venous occlusive episodes or retinal telangiectasia from other causes. Severe anemia, leukemia, and human immunodeficiency virus (HIV)/acquired immunodeficiency syndrome (AIDS) must be excluded before the diagnosis of RR can be definitively made.

Although the diagnosis can usually be made clinically, further evaluation should be considered. Fluorescein and indocyanine green angiography can be useful to define the extent of retinal ischemia and vascular anomalies.[63,64] If macular pathology is suspected, OCT should be carried out to determine the degree of macular edema, since macular thickness on OCT correlates with visual acuity for up to 2 years after plaque treatment.[39]

PREVENTION AND TREATMENT

There is no widely accepted treatment protocol for RR. Treatment has until now been based on its clinical, histopathologic, and angiographic similarities with diabetic retinopathy, a disease for which large randomized controlled studies have already been successfully conducted. Indeed, several groups have applied treatment guidelines of the ETDRS to eyes with RR, with favorable results.[21,65] Further, the Branch Retinal Vein Occlusion study provided strong evidence that laser photocoagulation can decrease the probability of vision loss due to macular edema and vitreous hemorrhage in patients with regional retinal ischemia.[66] Although the proven, currently available therapeutic options are limited both in number and in success rate, and its management remains challenging, once RR has developed, all efforts should be made to minimize its impact on the patient's visual acuity. Nevertheless, once macular ischemia has developed, the likelihood of visual improvement is very low.

Retinal laser photocoagulation remains the gold standard in the treatment of most forms of ischemic retinopathies. It has shown definite promise in the treatment of RR since 1981.[67] Since then, various studies have demonstrated the utility of this modality in inducing regression of plaque-associated RR,[68,69] although no large randomized, controlled studies have yet been completed. The rationale behind laser photocoagulation is that the destruction of oxygen-consuming photoreceptor cells and RPE decreases the intraocular VEGF concentrations, thereby inhibiting active retinal neovascularization.[70] Treatment has been shown to be anatomically beneficial by decreasing macular edema, neovascularization, and vitreous hemorrhages. However, the visual acuity results of treatment have been disappointing. This may be due to differences between RR and diabetic retinopathy. First, it seems that there is more widespread capillary nonperfusion in RR than in diabetic retinopathy. Second, RR follows acute injury, whereas diabetic retinopathy is due to a long-term metabolic insult. Third, the optic nerve is affected more frequently and severely in RR than in diabetic retinopathy, likely contributing to more vision loss. Fourth, the damage to the RPE and choroid is more severe in radiation retinopathy than in diabetic retinopathy.[17,71–73] Attempts to improve visual acuity results might include development of a protocol to identify affected patients as early as possible so that treatment can be instituted before vision loss due to macular edema or proliferative retinopathy has occurred. Indeed, even prophylactic treatment may be of benefit. Finger et al. reported the use of laser photocoagulation to obliterate the ischemic zone caused by ophthalmic plaque brachytherapy.[36] They observed regression of early-stage RR in 64% of treated eyes and found that only 18.75% of the "high-risk" patients who were treated prophylactically with sector scatter laser later developed RR. Typical laser settings include a 200 μm spot size, 0.1–0.2 ms duration, and 100–300 mW.[74] Laser photocoagulation has also been used for the treatment of macular edema secondary to RR. Although macular ischemia is currently not treatable, the frequently associated macular edema may respond to photocoagulation. Hykin et al. reported a visual acuity improvement of at least one line on the Snellen chart in 42% of affected eyes at 6 months, although the difference between treated patients and controls was not significant at 12 and 24 months.[74]

Corticosteroids have both angiostatic and vascular antipermeability properties that have been harnessed in the treatment of neovascular AMD, diabetic retinopathy, and macular edema due to various conditions.[75] This treatment modality has recently been tested for RR. Intravitreal triamcinolone has been reported to be of both visual and anatomic benefit in the treatment of both radiation maculopathy[76,77] and optic neuropathy.[78] However, when compared with intravitreal injection, periocular triamcinolone is associated with lower rates of steroid-induced glaucoma,[79] cataracts, retinal detachment, and endophthalmitis.[80,81] In a prospective, randomized, controlled trial with 163 patients newly diagnosed with uveal melanoma undergoing iodine-125 plaque radiotherapy, Horgan et al. found prophylactic periocular injection of triamcinolone acetonide (40 mg in 1 mL), administered at the time of plaque radiotherapy and 4 and 8 months later, to be both safe and beneficial in reducing the risk of macular edema, moderate vision loss, and poor visual acuity.[82]

During the past several years, the focus has shifted to anti-VEGF agents for the treatment of intraocular neovascularization and vascular permeability. The discovery of VEGF-A's role in the pathogenesis of neovascular ocular disease provided a strong rationale for the use of anti-VEGF agents.[83] These agents have been proven in large trials to be effective for neovascular AMD[84] and diabetic retinopathy.[85] Finger et al. first reported the efficacy of intravitreal bevacizumab therapy for the treatment of radiation maculopathy and optic neuropathy.[86] This led to the regression of retinal edema, hemorrhages, exudates, and neovascularization after ophthalmic plaque radiation therapy. Since this early report, many reports have been published, suggesting the crucial role of intravitreal injection of both bevacizumab[87] and ranibizumab[83,88] in the treatment of radiation maculopathy[89] and optic neuropathy[86] due to plaque brachytherapy[90] and EBRT.[91] Anti-VEGF agents have also been used to treat the secondary complications of RR, namely neovascular glaucoma and exudative retinal detachment.[83,92] Systemic administration of bevacizumab might be beneficial in the treatment of macular edema after EBRT.[93] However, systemic bevacizumab has been reported to carry a risk of systemic thromboembolic events.[94] In contrast, intravitreal administration, which requires a much smaller dose, minimizes systemic risks but increases ocular risks.[95] Whether it is most effective to administer anti-VEGF agents prophylactically or only upon development of pathology has not yet been conclusively determined. However, a small study by Gupta et al. suggested that patients with shorter duration of macular edema benefited more than those with long-standing retinal disease.[89] Further, the optimal administration schedule has not yet been determined. Pharmaceutical companies have begun sponsoring studies to study this issue in depth; a recent phase I, open-label, Genentech-sponsored study of 5 patients with RR-related macular edema showed visual acuity improvement and decreased foveal thickness after monthly injections of ranibizumab for at least 4 months.[88] In sum, most of the published studies suggest that anti-VEGF agents may have a role in the treatment of RR and its secondary complications. Further studies, such as the Treatment of Radiation Retinopathy (TORR) trial, are necessary to delineate the best administration schedules. The TORR trial will determine whether treatment with intravitreal ranibizumab (0.5 mg) or intravitreal triamcinolone acetonide (4.0 mg) is associated with improved visual acuity at 1 year, as compared to natural history. Results of this trial are expected in late 2012.[96]

Of course, prevention would be ideal. Reduced risk of human error in dosage calculations, improved shielding techniques and increased surveillance of patients at risk for developing RR are desirable goals. Further, patients should be thoroughly informed of the possible consequences of radiation therapy, particularly in cases in which the treatment is being administered for nonlethal pathology such as Graves orbitopathy.

PROGNOSIS

The visual prognosis is largely dependent on the extent and location of capillary nonperfusion[97] as well as the presence of neovascularization. If the perifoveal capillary net is involved, the prognosis for central vision is grave, due to either retinal atrophy or persistent macular edema, as well as from neovascularization, which occurs at the interface of perfused and nonperfused retina as well as on the optic nerve head. PRR, present in approximately one-third of eyes with RR, is likely to carry an inferior long-term visual prognosis (mean visual acuity 20/440) than the nonproliferative type (mean visual acuity 20/100), although this retrospective study had a very different follow-up duration for PRR (109 months) and NPRR (27 months).[98] The same study reported macular edema to be more common in PRR (85.7%) than in NPRR (71.2%). Shields et al. found predictors of poor visual acuity at long-term follow-up following plaque radiotherapy included patient age ≥60 years, tumor base ≥10 mm, tumor thickness >8 mm, radiation dose to the tumor base of ≥33300 cGy, and increasing radiation dose to the optic disc.[99] Tumor location is also of great importance, with tumors located posterior to the equator at increased risk for radiation maculopathy and loss of central vision.[100]

CONCLUSION

There are two quite distinct situations that should be considered by ophthalmologists treating patients at risk for RR. In the first situation, patients will have been treated with plaque brachytherapy. They may develop capillary nonperfusion in the retinal sector containing the plaque, as well as exudative lesions that can threaten the macula. Patients must thus be followed up closely and potentially treated prophylactically with sector laser if indicated. In these cases, the patients will likely be closely followed and the developing RR will be identified and managed shortly thereafter.

The second situation involves patients who will have been treated by nonophthalmologists for extraocular tumors with techniques besides brachytherapy. These patients are at great risk for remaining undiagnosed or diagnosed late because they are less likely to have been followed as closely as patients treated for intraocular disease. A nonophthalmologist is likely to take action only when the patient complains of visual loss, which often means that the retinopathy has progressed to an advanced stage. Moreover, many patients will only develop retinopathy years after the radiation therapy, long after they have been discharged from the care of the physician who administered the radiation. Indeed, an ophthalmologist may not be consulted until vision loss has been detected by patients.

The ophthalmologist must consider this diagnosis when confronted with a patient with retinovascular disease with cotton-wool spots, microaneurysms, exudative changes, and capillary dropout that looks like more common conditions, particularly diabetic retinopathy, but with a medical history that includes radiation therapy which may have damaged the posterior segment of the eye.

REFERENCES

1. Stallard HB. Radiant energy as (a) a pathogenic and (b) a therapeutic agent in ophthalmic disorders. Br J Ophthalmol Suppl 1933;6:1–126.
2. Finger PT, Chin KJ, Duvall G, Palladium-103 for Choroidal Melanoma Study Group. Palladium-103 ophthalmic plaque radiation therapy for choroidal melanoma: 400 treated patients. Ophthalmology 2009;116:790–6.
3. Krema H, Somani S, Sahgal A, et al. Stereotactic radiotherapy for treatment of juxtapapillary choroidal melanoma: 3-year follow-up. Br J Ophthalmol 2009;93:1172–6.
4. Gragoudas ES, Seddon JM, Egan K, et al. Long-term results of proton beam irradiated uveal melanomas. Ophthalmology 1987;94:349–53.
5. Haas A, Pinter O, Papaefthymiou G, et al. Incidence of radiation retinopathy after high-dosage single-fraction gamma knife radiosurgery for choroidal melanoma. Ophthalmology 2002;109:909–13.
6. Levy RP, Fabrikant JI, Frankel KA, et al. Heavy-charged-particle radiosurgery of the pituitary gland: Clinical results of 840 patients. Stereotact Funct Neurosurg 1991;57:22–35.
7. Finger PT, Chin KJ, Duvall G. Palladium-103 ophthalmic plaque radiation therapy for choroidal melanoma: 400 treated patients. Ophthalmology 2009;116:790–6.
8. Finger PT. Radiation therapy for orbital tumors: Concepts, current use, and ophthalmic radiation side effects. Surv Ophthalmol 2009;54:545–68.
9. Finger PT, Pro MJ, Schneider S, et al. Visual recovery after radiation therapy for bilateral subfoveal acute myelogenous leukemia (AML). Am J Ophthalmol 2004;138:659–62.
10. Shields CL, Naseripour M, Cater J, et al. Plaque radiotherapy for large posterior uveal melanomas (> or = 8 mm thick) in 354 consecutive patients. Ophthalmology 2002;109:1838–49.
11. Gunduz K, Shields CL, Shields JA, et al. Radiation retinopathy following plaque radiotherapy for posterior uveal melanoma. Arch Ophthalmol 1999;117:609–14.
12. Evans JR, Sivagnanavel V, Chong V. Radiotherapy for neovascular age-related macular degeneration. Cochrane Database Syst Rev 2010;(5):CD004004.
13. Brown GC, Shields JA, Sanborn G, et al. Radiation retinopathy. Ophthalmology 1982;89:1494–501.
14. Amoaku WM, Archer DB. Cephalic radiation and retinal vasculopathy. Eye 1990;4:195–203.
15. Archer DB, Amoaku WMK, Gardinar TA. Radiation retinopathy: Clinical, histopathological, ultrastructural and experimental correlations. Eye 1991;5:239–51.

16. Irvine AR, Alvarado JA, Wara WM, et al. Radiation retinopathy: An experimental model for the ischemic-proliferative retinopathies. Trans Am Ophthalmol Soc 1981;79:103–22.
17. Egbert PR, Fajarado LF, Donaldson SS, et al. Posterior ocular abnormalities after irradiation for retinoblastoma: A histopathological study. Br J Ophthalmol 1980;64:660–65.
18. Irvine RA, Wood IS. Radiation retinopathy as an experimental model for ischemic proliferative retinopathy and rubeosis iridis. Am J Ophthalmol 1987;103:790–97.
19. Hiroshiba N, Ogura Y, Sasai K, et al. Radiation-induced leukocyte entrapment in the rat retinal microcirculation. Invest Ophthalmol Vis Sci 1999;40:1217–22.
20. Hayreh SS. Post-radiation retinopathy: A fluorescence fundus angiographic study. Br J Ophthalmol 1970;54:705–14.
21. Kinyoun JL, Chittum ME, Wells CG. Photocoagulation treatment of radiation retinopathy. Am J Ophthalmol 1988;105:470–8.
22. Archer DB, Amoaku WM, Gardiner TA. Radiation retinopathy – clinical, histopathological, ultrastructural and experimental correlations. Eye 1991;5:239–51.
23. Wara WM, Irvine AR, Neger RE, et al. Radiation retinopathy. Int J Radiat Oncol Biol Phys 1979;5:81–3.
24. Irvine AR, Alvarado JA, Wara WM, et al. Radiation retinopathy: An experimental model for the ischemic-proliferative retinopathies. Trans Am Ophthalmol Soc 1981;79:103–22.
25. Takeda A, Shigematsu N, Suzuki S, et al. Late retinal complications of radiation therapy for nasal and paranasal malignancies: relationship between irradiated-dose area and severity. Int J Radiat Oncol Biol Phys 1999;44:599–605.
26. Archer DB, Gardiner TA. Ionizing radiation and the retina. Curr Opin Ophthalmol 1994;5:59–65.
27. Midena E, Segato T, Valenti M, et al. The effect of external eye irradiation on choroidal circulation. Ophthalmology 1996;103:1651–60.
28. Ferrara N. Vascular endothelial growth factor: Basic science and clinical progress. Endocr Rev 2004;25:581–611.
29. Krebs IP, Krebs W, Merriam JC, et al. Radiation retinopathy: electron microscopy of retina and optic nerve. Histol Histopathol 1992;7:101–10.
30. Raman R, Pal SS, Krishnan T, et al. High-resolution optical coherence tomography correlates in ischemic radiation retinopathy. Cutan Ocul Toxicol 2010;29:57–61.
31. Levitz LM. The use of optical coherence tomography to determine the severity of radiation retinopathy. Ophthalmic Surg Lasers Imaging 2005;36:410–1.
32. Gass J. Stereoscopic atlas of macular diseases, diagnosis and treatment. 3rd ed. St Louis: Mosby; 1987. p. 404–5.
33. Li M, Qiu G, Luo W, et al. Clinical investigation of radiation retinopathy fundus and fluorescein angiographic features. Yan Ke Xue Bao 1999;15:183–6.
34. Berker N, Aslan O, Batman C, et al. Choroidal neovascular membrane in radiation retinopathy. Clin Experiment Ophthalmol 2006;34:625–6.
35. Kinyoun JL. Long-term visual acuity results of treated and untreated radiation retinopathy (an AOS thesis). Trans Am Ophthalmol Soc 2008;106:325–35.
36. Finger PT, Kurli M. Laser photocoagulation for radiation retinopathy after ophthalmic plaque radiation therapy. Br J Ophthalmol 2005;89:730–8.
37. Early Treatment of Diabetic Retinopathy Study Group. Photocoagulation for macular edema. Early Treatment Diabetic Retinopathy Study Report Number 1. Arch Ophthalmol 1985;103:1796–1806.
38. Catier A, Tadayoni R, Paques M, et al. Characterization of macular edema from various etiologies by optical coherence tomography. Am J Ophthalmol 2005;140:200–6.
39. Horgan N, Shields CL, Mashayekhi A, et al. Early macular morphological changes following plaque radiotherapy for uveal melanoma. Retina 2008;28:263–73.
40. Bianciotto C, Shields CL, Pirondini C, et al. Proliferative radiation retinopathy after plaque radiotherapy for uveal melanoma. Ophthalmology 2010;117:1005–12.
41. Viebahn M, Barricks ME, Osterloh MD. Synergism between diabetic and radiation retinopathy: case report and review. B J Ophthalmol 1991;75:629–32.
42. Packer S, Rotman M. Radiotherapy of choroidal melanoma with iodine 125. Int Ophthalmol Clin 1980;20:135–42.
43. Conway R, Poothullil A, Daftari I, et al. Estimates of ocular and visual retention following treatment of extra-large uveal melanomas by proton beam radiotherapy. Arch Ophthalmol 2006;124:839–43.
44. Rudoler SB, Corn BW, Shields CL, et al. External beam irradiation for choroid metastases: identification of factors predisposing to long-term sequelae. Int J Radiat Oncol Biol Phys 1997;38:251–6.
45. Gunduz K, Shields CL, Shields JA, et al. Plaque radiotherapy of uveal melanoma with predominant ciliary body involvement. Arch Ophthalmol 1999;117:170–7.
46. Wakelkamp IM, Tan H, Saeed P, et al. Orbital irradiation for Graves' ophthalmopathy: Is it safe? A long-term follow-up study. Ophthalmology 2004;111:1557e62.
47. Stack R, Elder M, Abdelaal A, et al. New Zealand experience of I125 brachytherapy for choroidal melanoma. Clin Experiment Ophthalmol 2005;33:490–4.
48. Chan RC, Shukovsky LJ. Effects of irradiation on the eye. Radiology 1976;120:673–5.
49. Kumar B, Palimar P. Accelerated radiation retinopathy in diabetes and pregnancy. Eye 2004;14:107–8.
50. Kinyoun JL, Lawrence BS, Barlow WE. Proliferative radiation retinopathy. Arch Ophthalmol 1996;114:1097–100.
51. Bagan SM, Hollenhorst RW. Radiation retinopathy after irradiation of intracranial lesions. Am J Ophthalmol 1979;88:694–69.
52. Lopez PF, Steinberg P, Dabbs CK, et al. Bone marrow transplant retinopathy. Am J Ophthalmol 1991;112:635–46.
53. Chacko DC. Considerations in the diagnosis of radiation injury. JAMA 1981;245:1255–58.
54. Bagan SM, Hollenhorst RW. Radiation retinopathy after irradiation of intracranial lesions. Am J Ophthalmol 1979;88:694–69.
55. Monroe AT, Bhandare N, Morris CG, et al. Preventing radiation retinopathy with hyperfractionation. Int J Radiat Oncol Biol Phys 2005;61:856–64.
56. Parsons JT, Bova FJ, Fitzgerald CR, et al. Radiation retinopathy after external-beam irradiation: Analysis of time-dose factors. Int J Radiat Oncol Biol Phys 1994;30:765–773.
57. Nikoskelainen E, Joensuu H. Retinopathy after irradiation for Graves' ophthalmopathy (letter). Lancet 1989;2:690–1.
58. Miller M, Goldberg S, Bullock J. Radiation retinopathy after standard radiotherapy for thyroid-related ophthalmopathy. Am J Ophthalmol 1991;112:600–1.
59. Durkin SR, Roos D, Higgs B, et al. Ophthalmic and adnexal complications of radiotherapy. Acta Ophthalmol Scand 2007;85:240–50.
60. Bradley EA, Gower EW, Bradley DJ, et al. Orbital radiation for graves ophthalmopathy: a report by the American Academy of Ophthalmology. Ophthalmology 2008;115:398–409.
61. Eng TY, Boersma MK, Fuller CD, et al. The role of radiation therapy in benign diseases. Hematol Oncol Clin North Am 2006;20:523–57.
62. Viebahn M, Barricks ME, Osterloh MD. Synergism between diabetic and radiation retinopathy: case report and review. Br J Ophthalmol 1991;75:629–32.
63. Spaide RF, Borodoker N, Shah V. Atypical choroidal neovascularization in radiation retinopathy. Am J Ophthalmol 2002;133:709–11.
64. Spaide RF, Leys A, Hermann-Delamazure B, et al. Radiation-associated choroidal neovasculopathy. Ophthalmology 1999;106:2254–60.
65. Kinyoun JL, Zamber RW, Lawrence BS, et al. Photocoagulation treatment for clinically significant radiation macular oedema. Br J Ophthalmol 1995;70:144–9.
66. Branch Vein Occlusion Study Group. Argon laser scatter photocoagulation for prevention of neovascularization and vitreous hemorrhage in branch vein occlusion. A randomized clinical trial. Arch Ophthalmol 1986;104:34–41.
67. Chaudhuri PR, Austin DJ, Rosenthal AR. Treatment of radiation retinopathy. Br J Ophthalmol 1981;65:623–5.
68. Augsburger JJ, Roth SE, Magargal LE, et al. Panretinal photocoagulation for radiation-induced ocular ischemia. Ophthalmic Surg 1987;18:589–93.
69. Finger PT. Radiation therapy for choroidal melanoma. Surv Ophthalmol 1997;42:215–32.
70. Barnstable CJ, Tombran-Tink J. Neuroprotective and anti-angiogenic actions of PEDF in the eye: molecular targets and therapeutic potential. Prog Ret Eye Res 2004;23:561–77.
71. Hidayat AA, Fine BS. Diabetic choroidopathy: light and electron microscopic observations of seven cases. Ophthalmology 1985;92:512–22.
72. Takahashi K, Kishi S, Muraoka K, et al. Radiation choroidopathy with remodeling of the choroidal venous system. Am J Ophthalmol 1998;125:367–73.
73. Flyczkowski AW, Hodes BL, Walker J. Diabetic choroidal and iris vasculature scanning electron microscopy findings. Int Ophthalmol 1989;13:269–79.
74. Hykin PG, Shields CL, Shields JA, et al. The efficacy of focal laser therapy in radiation-induced macular edema. Ophthalmology 1998;105:1425–9.
75. Ciulla TA, Walker JD, Fong DS, et al. Corticosteroids in posterior segment disease: an update on new delivery systems and new indications. Curr Opin Ophthalmol 2004;15:211–20.
76. Sutter FK, Gillies MC. Intravitreal triamcinolone for radiation-induced macular edema. Arch Ophthalmol 2003;121:1491–3.
77. Shields CL, Demirci H, Dai V, et al. Intravitreal triamcinolone acetonide for radiation maculopathy after plaque radiotherapy for choroidal melanoma. Retina 2005;25:868–74.
78. Shields CL, Demirci H, Marr BP, et al. Intravitreal triamcinolone acetonide for acute radiation papillopathy. Retina 2006;26:537–44.
79. Iwao K, Inatani M, Kawaji T, et al. Frequency and risk factors for intraocular pressure elevation after posterior sub-Tenon capsule triamcinolone acetonide injection. J Glaucoma 2007;16:251–6.
80. Gillies MC, Sutter FK, Simpson JM, et al. Intravitreal triamcinolone for refractory diabetic macular edema: Two-year results of a double-masked, placebo-controlled, randomized clinical trial. Ophthalmology 2006;113:1533–8.
81. Conti SM, Kertes PJ. The use of intravitreal corticosteroids, evidence-based and otherwise. Curr Opin Ophthalmol 2006;17:235–44.
82. Horgan N, Shields CL, Mashayekhi A, et al. Periocular triamcinolone for prevention of macular edema after plaque radiotherapy of uveal melanoma: a randomized controlled trial. Ophthalmology 2009;116:1383–90.
83. Dunavoelgyi R, Zehetmayer M, Simader C, et al. Rapid improvement of radiation-induced neovascular glaucoma and exudative retinal detachment after a single intravitreal ranibizumab injection. Clin Exp Ophthalmol 2008;35:878–80.
84. CATT Research Group. Ranibizumab and bevacizumab for neovascular age-related macular degeneration. N Engl J Med 2011;364:1897–908.

85. Mitchell P, Bandello F, Schmidt-Erfurth U, et al. The RESTORE study: ranibizumab monotherapy or combined with laser versus laser monotherapy for diabetic macular edema. Ophthalmology 2011;118:615.
86. Finger PT, Chin K. Anti-vascular endothelial growth factor bevacizumab (Avastin) for radiation retinopathy. Arch Ophthalmol 2007;125:751–6.
87. Finger PT. Radiation retinopathy is treatable with anti-vascular endothelial growth factor bevacizumab (Avastin). Int J Radiat Oncol Biol Phys 2008;70: 974–7.
88. Finger PT, Chin KJ. Intravitreous ranibizumab (lucentis) for radiation maculopathy. Arch Ophthalmol 2010;128:249–52.
89. Gupta A, Muecke JS. Treatment of radiation maculopathy with intravitreal injection of bevacizumab (Avastin). Retina 2008;28:964–8.
90. Wen JC, McCannel TA. Treatment of radiation retinopathy following plaque brachytherapy for choroidal melanoma. Curr Opin Ophthalmol 2009;20: 200–4.
91. Finger PT, Mukkamala SK. Intravitreal anti-VEGF bevacizumab (Avastin) for external beam related radiation retinopathy. Eur J Ophthalmol 2011;21: 446–51.
92. Vasquez LM, Somani S, Altomare F, et al. Intracameral bevacizumab in the treatment of neovascular glaucoma and exudative retinal detachment after brachytherapy in choroidal melanoma. Can J Ophthalmol 2009;44:106–7.
93. Solano JM, Bakri SJ, Pulido JS. Regression of radiation-induced macular edema after systemic bevacizumab. Can J Ophthalmol 2007;42:748–9.
94. Michels S, Rosenfeld PJ, Puliafito CA, et al. Systemic bevacizumab (Avastin) therapy for neovascular age-related macular degeneration twelve-week results of an uncontrolled open-label clinical study. Ophthalmology 2005; 112:1035–47.
95. Rosenfeld PJ, Schwartz SD, Blumenkranz MS, et al. Maximum tolerated dose of a humanized anti-vascular endothelial growth factor antibody fragment for treating neovascular age-related macular degeneration. Ophthalmology 2005; 112:1048–53.
96. http://clinicaltrials.gov/ct2/show/NCT00811200.
97. Noble KG, Kupersmith MJ. Retinal vascular remodelling in radiation retinopathy. Br J Ophthalmol 1984;68:475–8.
98. Kinyoun JL. Long-term visual acuity results of treated and untreated radiation retinopathy (an AOS thesis). Trans Am Ophthalmol Soc 2008;106:325–35.
99. Shields CL, Shields JA, Cater J, et al. Plaque radiotherapy for uveal melanoma: long-term visual outcome in 1106 consecutive patients. Arch Ophthalmol 2000;118:1219–28.
100. Finger PT. Tumour location affects the incidence of cataract and retinopathy after ophthalmic plaque radiation therapy. Br J Ophthalmol 2000;84: 1068–70.

For additional online content visit http://www.expertconsult.com

Ocular Ischemic Syndrome

Gary C. Brown, Sanjay Sharma

Chapter 59

In 1963, Kearns and Hollenhorst[1] reported on the ocular symptoms and signs occurring secondary to severe carotid artery obstructive disease. They called the entity "venous stasis retinopathy" and noted that it occurred in approximately 5% of patients with severe carotid artery insufficiency or thrombosis. Some confusion has since arisen with this term because it has also been used to designate mild central retinal venous obstruction.[2] A number of additional alternative names have been proposed, including ischemic ocular inflammation,[3] ischemic oculopathy,[4] and the ocular ischemic syndrome.[5,6] Histopathologic examination of eyes with the entity generally does not reveal inflammation,[7,8] and therefore the descriptive term the present authors and Dr. Larry Magargal have thought preferable is the ocular ischemic syndrome.[5,6]

DEMOGRAPHICS AND INCIDENCE

The mean age of patients with the ocular ischemic syndrome is about 65 years, with a range generally from the fifties to the eighties. No racial predilection has been identified, and males are affected more than females by a ratio of about 2:1. Either eye can be affected, and in approximately 20% of patients, ocular involvement is bilateral. The incidence of the disease has not been extensively studied, but from the work of Sturrock and Mueller[9] an annual estimate of 7.5 cases/million persons can be made. This number may be falsely low, since it is possible that a number of cases are misdiagnosed.

ETIOLOGY

In general, a 90% or greater stenosis of the ipsilateral carotid arterial system is present in eyes with the ocular ischemic syndrome.[5] It has been shown that a 90% carotid stenosis reduces the ipsilateral central retinal artery perfusion pressure by about 50%.[10,11] The obstruction can occur within the common carotid or internal carotid artery. In about 50% of cases, the affected vessel is 100% occluded, while in 10% there is bilateral 100% carotid artery obstruction.[5]

Occasionally, obstruction of the ipsilateral ophthalmic artery can also be responsible.[5,12,13] Rarely, an isolated obstruction of the central retinal artery alone can mimic the dilated retinal veins and retinal hemorrhages seen in eyes with the ocular ischemic syndrome.[14]

Atherosclerosis within the carotid artery is the cause for the great majority of cases of the ocular ischemic syndrome.[5] Dissecting aneurysm of the carotid artery has been reported as a cause,[15] as has giant cell arteritis.[16] Hypothetically, entities such as fibromuscular dysplasia,[17] Behçet disease,[18] trauma,[19] and inflammatory entities that cause carotid artery obstruction could lead to the ocular ischemic syndrome.

CLINICAL PRESENTATION

Visual loss

Greater than 90% of patients with the ocular ischemic syndrome relate a history of visual loss in the affected eye(s).[5] In two-thirds of cases, it occurs over a period of weeks, but it is abrupt in approximately 12%. In this latter group, with sudden visual loss, there is often a cherry-red spot present on funduscopic examination (Fig. 59.1).

Prolonged light recovery

Prolonged recovery following exposure to a bright light has been described in patients with severe carotid artery obstruction.[20] Concurrent attenuation of the visual evoked response has also been observed in these cases after light exposure. The phenomenon has been attributed to ischemia of the macular retina. In cases of bilateral, severe carotid artery obstruction, the visual

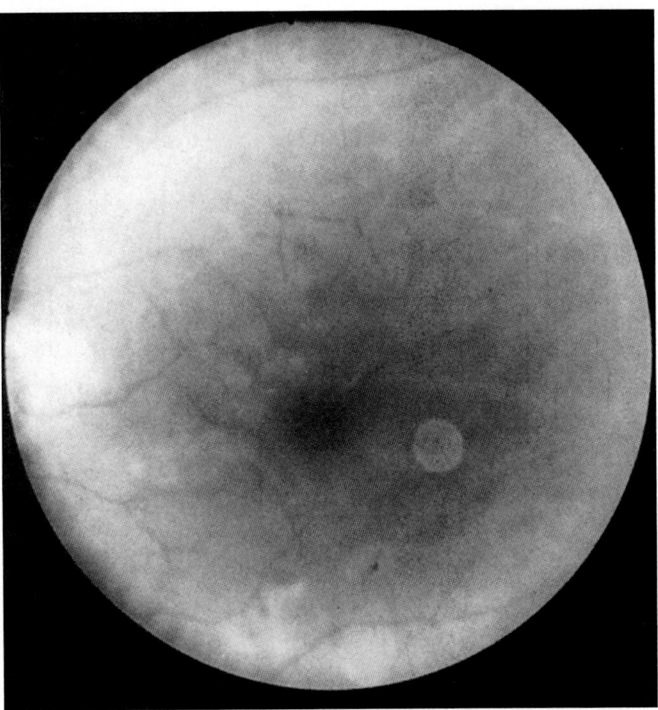

Fig. 59.1 Cherry-red spot in the left eye of a 66-year-old man with rubeosis iridis, a 100% ipsilateral common carotid artery obstruction, and a history of rapid visual loss.

loss after exposure to bright light occurs in both eyes, mimicking occipital lobe ischemia due to vertebrobasilar disease.[21]

Scintillating scotomas

Dissection of the internal carotid artery has been reported to cause scintillating scotomas that resemble a migraine aura.[22] While these could theoretically be associated with the classic ocular ischemic syndrome, they have not been observed by the authors.

Amaurosis fugax

A history of amaurosis fugax is elicited in about 10% of ocular ischemic syndrome patients.[5] Amaurosis fugax, or fleeting loss of vision for seconds to minutes, is thought to most commonly be caused by emboli to the central retinal arterial system, although vasospasm may also play a role.[23] Although the majority of people with amaurosis fugax alone do not have the ocular ischemic syndrome, it can be an indicator of concomitant, ipsilateral carotid artery obstructive disease. About one-third of patients with amaurosis fugax have an ipsilateral carotid artery obstruction of 75% or greater.[24] Rarely, it has been associated with a stenosis of the ophthalmic artery.[24]

Pain

Pain is present in the affected eye or orbital region in about 40% of cases,[5] and has been referred to as "ocular angina." Most often, it is described as a dull ache. It can occur secondary to neovascular glaucoma, but in those cases in which the intraocular pressure is normal, the cause may be ischemia to the globe and/or ipsilateral dura.

Visual acuity

The presenting visual acuities of patients with the ocular ischemic syndrome are bimodally distributed, with 43% of affected eyes having vision ranging from 20/20 to 20/50, and 37% having counting fingers or worse vision.[25] Absence of light perception is generally not seen early, but can develop in the later stages of the disease, usually secondary to neovascular glaucoma. Among all eyes with the ocular ischemic syndrome after one year of follow-up, including those with and without treatment, approximately 24% remain in the 20/20–20/50 group and 58% have counting fingers vision or worse.

External collaterals

Prominent collateral vessels are occasionally seen on the forehead (Fig. 59.2). These vessels connect the external carotid system on one side of the head to that on the other. These vascular collaterals should not be mistaken for the enlarged tender vessels seen with giant cell arteritis, since temporal artery biopsy may shut down this important source of collateral blood flow to the brain.

Anterior segment changes

Neovascularization of the iris is encountered in approximately two-thirds of eyes with the ocular ischemic syndrome at the time of presentation[5] (Fig. 59.3). Nevertheless, only slightly over half of these eyes have or develop an increase in intraocular pressure, even if the anterior chamber angle is closed by fibrovascular tissue. Impaired ciliary body perfusion, with a subsequent decrease in aqueous production, probably accounts for this phenomenon.

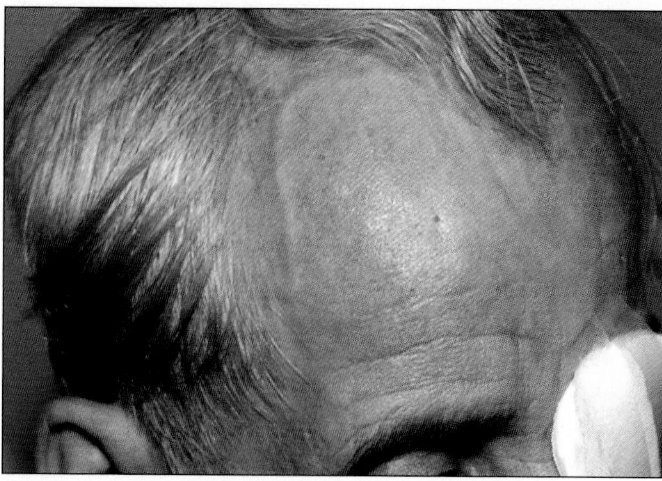

Fig. 59.2 Prominent collateral arteries from the right external carotid arterial system to the left external arterial system in a patient with a 100% common left carotid artery stenosis.

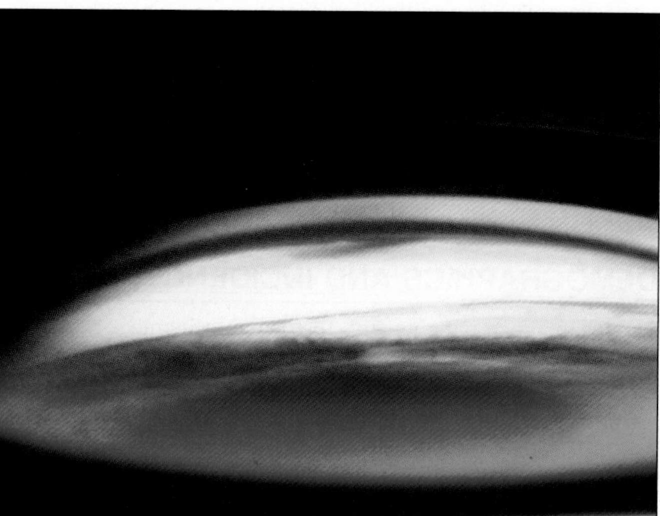

Fig. 59.3 Gonioscopy of neovascularization of the iris and angle in an eye with the ocular ischemic syndrome. A red arc of fibrovascular tissue is present, closing the anterior chamber angle.

Flare in the anterior chamber is usually present in eyes with rubeosis iridis. An anterior chamber cellular response is seen in almost one-fifth of eyes with the ocular ischemic syndrome,[5] but it rarely exceeds grade 2^+, on a 0 to 4^+ range, as per the Schlaegel classification.[26] Keratic precipitates can be present, but are typically small.

In unilateral cases, there is generally little difference between the degree of lens opacification in each eye. As the disease advances, however, cataractous lens changes can develop. In advanced cases, the lens may become mature.

Posterior segment findings

The retinal arteries are usually narrowed and the retinal veins are most often dilated, but not tortuous (Fig. 59.4). The venous dilation may be accompanied by beading, but usually not to the extent seen in eyes with marked preproliferative or proliferative diabetic retinopathy. Dilation of the veins is probably a nonspecific response to the ischemia from the inflow obstruction.

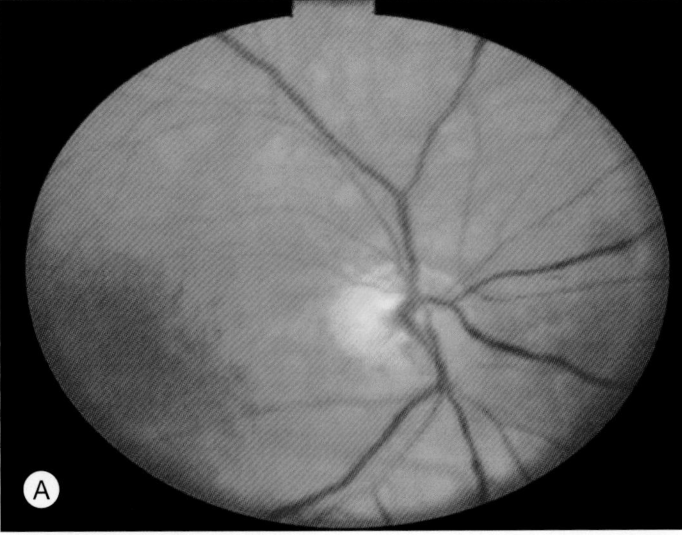

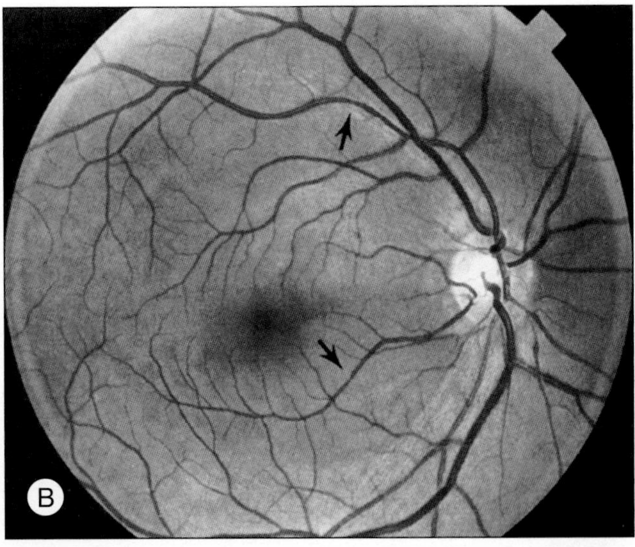

Fig. 59.4 (A) Narrowed, beaded retinal arteries and dilated, beaded, but not tortuous, retinal veins in an ocular ischemic syndrome eye. (B) Focal narrowing of the retinal arteries (arrows) in the right eye of a 55-year-old man with ocular ischemic syndrome and bilateral internal carotid artery obstructions. (Panel B reproduced with permission from Brown GC, Magargal LE. The ocular ischemic syndrome. Clinical, fluorescein angiographic and carotid angiographic features. Int Ophthalmol 1988;11:239–51.)

Nevertheless, in some eyes both the retinal arteries and veins are narrowed. In contrast, eyes with central retinal vein obstruction usually also have dilated retinal veins, but they are often tortuous. The fact that the ocular ischemic syndrome occurs secondary to impaired inflow, while central retinal vein obstruction is usually associated with compromised outflow resulting from thrombus formation at or near the lamina cribrosa, may account for this difference.[27]

Retinal hemorrhages are seen in about 80% of affected eyes. They are most commonly present in the midperiphery, but can also extend into the posterior pole (Fig. 59.5, Fig. 59.6 online). While dot and blot hemorrhages are the most common variant, superficial retinal hemorrhages in the nerve fiber layer are occasionally seen. The hemorrhages probably arise secondary to leakage from the smaller retinal vessels, which have sustained endothelial damage as a result of the ischemia. Similar to the case with diabetic retinopathy, they may also result from the rupture of microaneurysms. In general, the hemorrhages seen with the ocular ischemic syndrome are less numerous than those accompanying central retinal vein obstruction. They are almost never confluent.

Microaneurysms are frequently observed outside the posterior pole, but can be seen in the macular region also. Hyperfluorescence with fluorescein angiography (Fig. 59.7) differentiates these abnormalities from hypofluorescent retinal hemorrhages. Retinal telangiectasia has also been described.[28]

Posterior segment neovascularization can occur at the optic disc or on the retina. Neovascularization of the disc (Fig. 59.8) is encountered in about 35% of eyes, while neovascularization of the retina is seen in about 8%.[5] Vitreous hemorrhage arising from traction upon the neovascularization by the vitreous gel has been reported to occur in 4% of eyes with the ocular ischemic syndrome in a retrospective study.[5] Rarely, the neovascularization can progress to severe preretinal fibrovascular proliferation (Fig. 59.9 online). Neovascularization of the retina (Fig. 59.10 online) is encountered in 8% of eyes with ocular ischemia. It is usually present concomitant with neovascularization of the disc.

A cherry-red spot is seen in approximately 12% of eyes with the ocular ischemic syndrome (see Fig. 59.1).[5] It can occur secondary to inner layer retinal ischemia from embolic obstruction of the central retinal artery, but probably more often develops when the intraocular pressure exceeds the perfusion pressure within the central retinal artery, particularly in eyes with neovascular glaucoma.

Additional posterior segment signs[5] include cotton-wool spots (Fig. 59.11 online) in 6% of eyes, spontaneous retinal arterial pulsations in 4% (Fig. 59.12), and cholesterol emboli within the retinal arteries in 2%. In contrast to spontaneous retinal venous pulsations, which are a normal variant and located at the base of the large veins on the optic disc, the arterial pulsations are usually more pronounced, and may extend a disc diameter or more out from the optic disc into the surrounding retina. Anterior ischemic optic neuropathy (Fig. 59.13) has also been reported in ocular ischemic syndrome eyes.[5,29,30] Acquired arteriovenous communications of the retina are rarely seen.[31]

A list of the anterior and posterior segment signs found with the ocular ischemic syndrome is shown in Table 59.1.[1-5,9]

ANCILLARY STUDIES

Fluorescein angiography

The intravenous fluorescein angiographic signs[5] associated with the ocular ischemic syndrome are listed in Table 59.2.

Delayed arm-to-choroid and arm-to-retina circulation times are frequently observed in the ocular ischemic syndrome. However, these measurements may be difficult to assess, since they depend upon whether the dye was injected in the antecubital fossa or hand, and also on the rate of injection. The observation of a well-demarcated, leading edge of fluorescein dye within a retinal artery after an intravenous injection is a distinctly unusual finding. It can be seen in eyes with the ocular ischemic syndrome, secondary to hypoperfusion (Fig. 59.14).

Normally, the choroidal filling is completed within 5 seconds after the first appearance of dye. Sixty percent of eyes with the

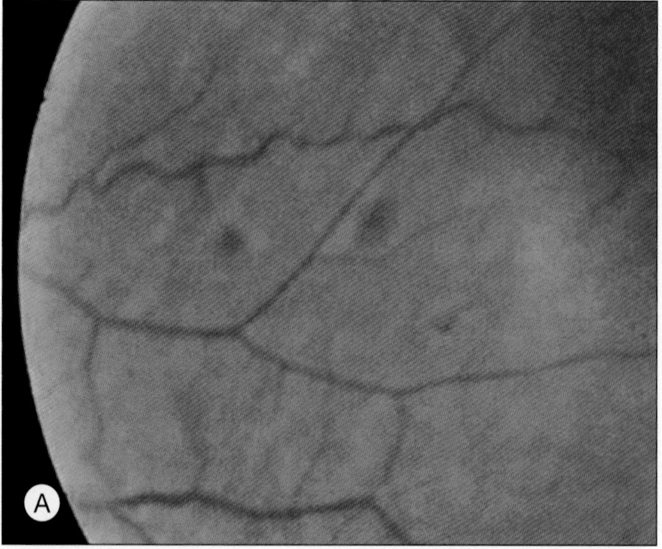

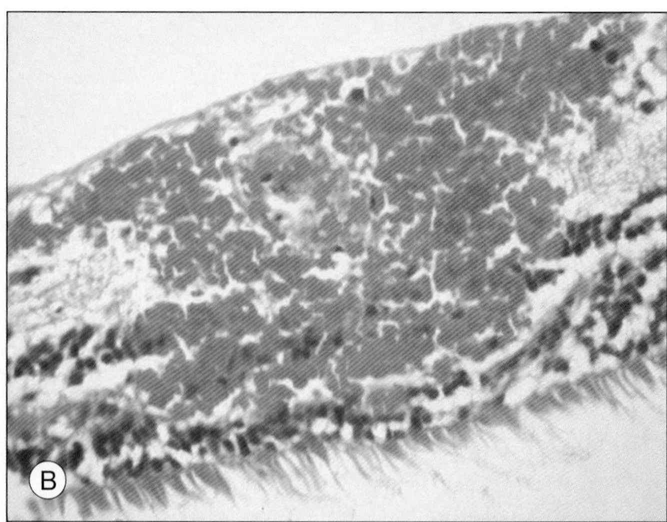

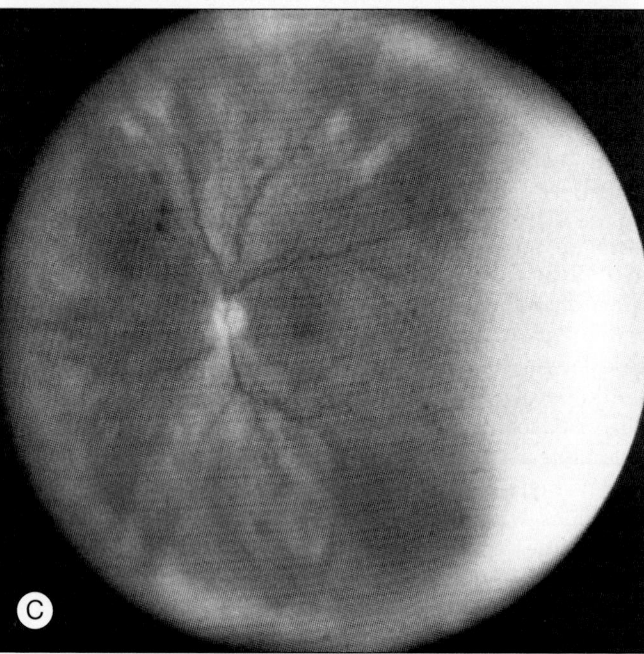

Fig. 59.5 (A) Round retinal hemorrhages in the midperiphery of an eye with the ocular ischemic syndrome. (B) Histopathologic correlate of a retinal hemorrhage in an ocular ischemic syndrome eye demonstrates blood throughout the retina (hematoxylin–eosin ×60). (Photograph courtesy of Dr W. Richard Green.) (C) Wide angle photograph demonstrating retinal hemorrhages in the midperiphery in an eye with the ocular ischemic syndrome.

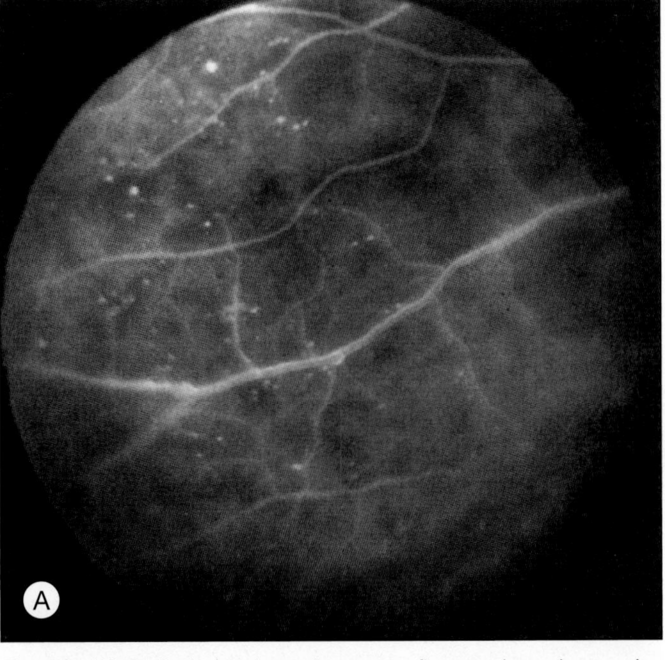

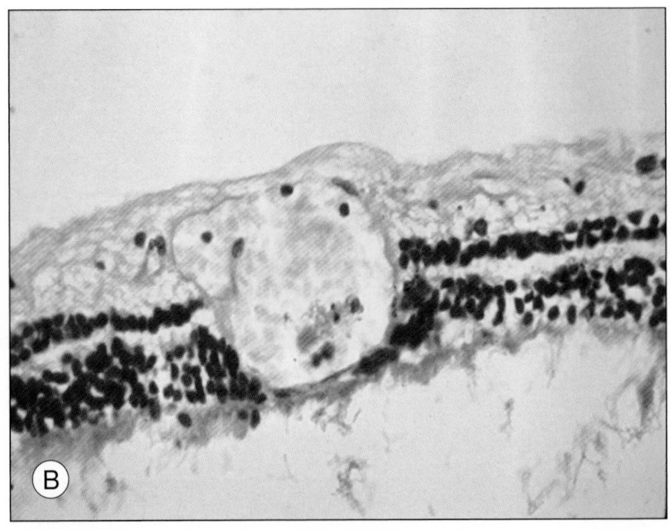

Fig. 59.7 (A) Ocular ischemic syndrome eye: fluorescein angiogram demonstrating numerous hyperfluorescent microaneurysms in the midperipheral retina. (Reproduced with permission from Brown GC, Magargal LE. The ocular ischemic syndrome. Clinical, fluorescein angiographic and carotid angiographic features. Int Ophthalmol 1988;11:239–51.) (B) Histopathologic correlation of a microaneurysm in an eye with the ocular ischemic syndrome discloses that the anomaly traverses the entire retina (periodic-acid Schiff ×60). (Courtesy of Dr W. Richard Green.)

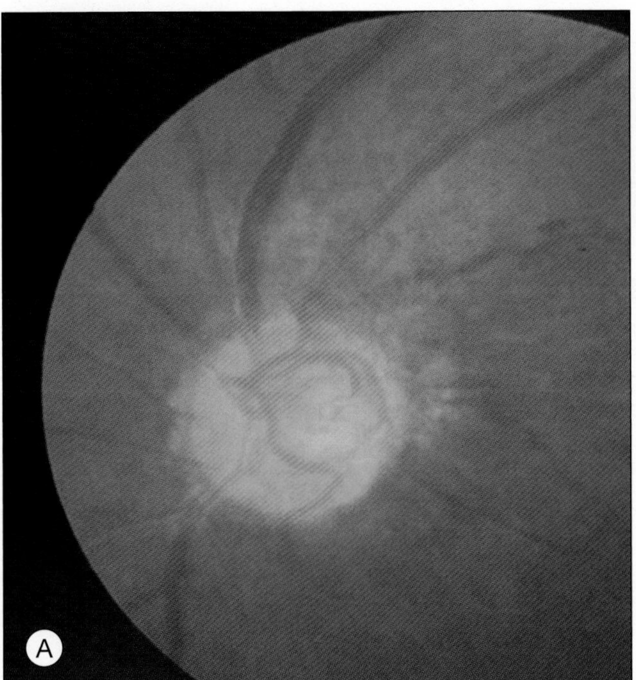

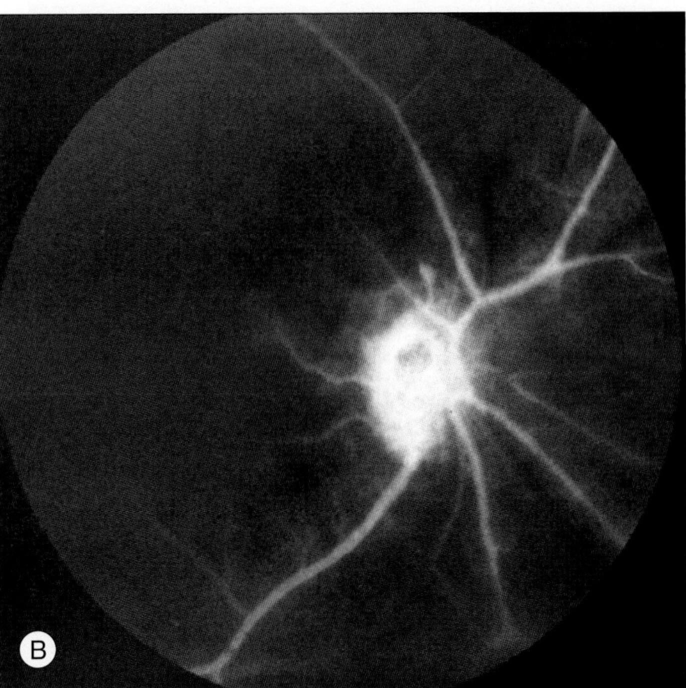

Fig. 59.8 (A) Neovascularization of the disc in an eye with the ocular ischemic syndrome. (B) Fluorescein angiogram of the eye in panel (A) reveals marked hyperfluorescence resulting from leakage of dye from new vessels. (Reproduced with permission from Brown GC, Magargal LE, Simeone FA, et al. Arterial obstruction and ocular neovascularization. Ophthalmology 1982;89:139–46. Copyright © 1982 American Academy of Ophthalmology.)

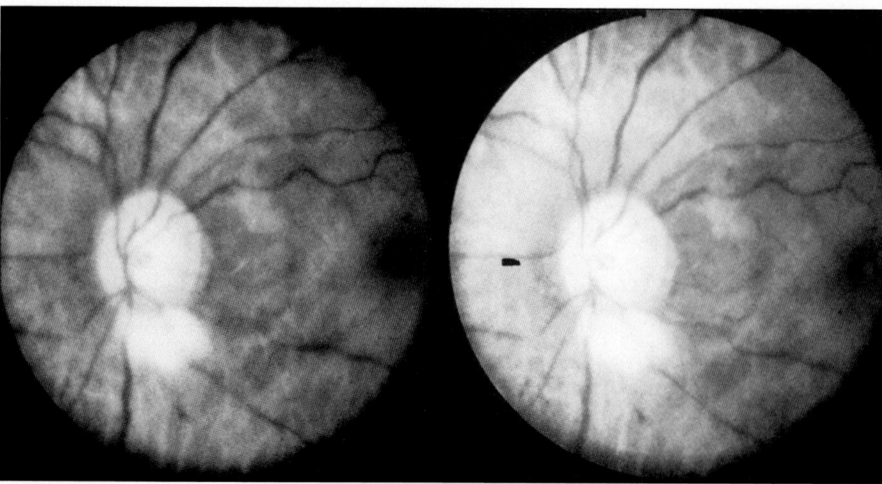

Fig. 59.12 Photographs taken several seconds apart in a fundus affected by the ocular ischemic syndrome. Closure of the retinal arteries can be seen on the right. (Reproduced with permission from Brown GC, Magargal LE. The ocular ischemic syndrome. Clinical, fluorescein angiographic and carotid angiographic features. Int Ophthalmol 1988;11:239–51.)

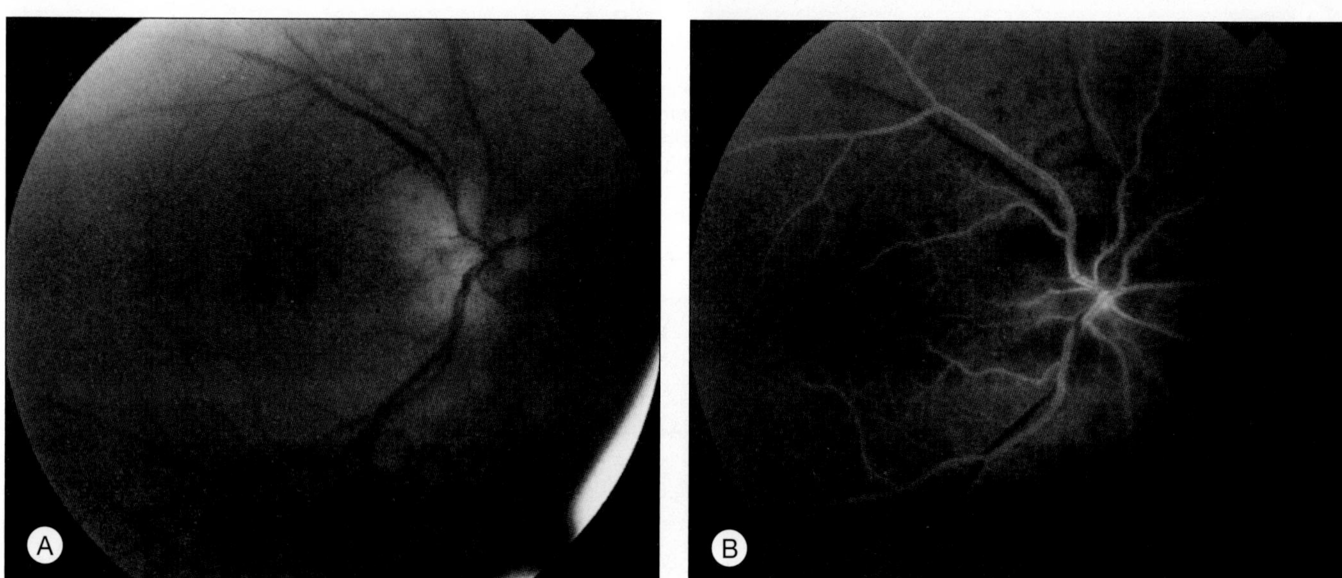

Fig. 59.13 (A) Pale optic disc resulting from ischemic optic neuropathy in a 67-year-old man with a 100% right internal carotid artery obstruction. Midperipheral retinal hemorrhages and rubeosis iridis were also present. (B) Fluorescein angiogram of the eye in panel (A) at 81 seconds after injection. The nerve head is hypofluorescent. (Reproduced with permission from Brown GC. Anterior ischemic optic neuropathy occurring in association with carotid artery obstruction. J Clin Neuroophthalmol 1986;6:39–42.)

Table 59.1 Anterior and posterior segment signs seen in eyes with the ocular ischemic syndrome

Anterior segment	
Rubeosis iridis	67%
Neovascular glaucoma	35%
Uveitis (cells and flare)	18%
Posterior segment	
Narrowed retinal arteries	Most
Dilated retinal veins	Most
Retinal hemorrhages	80%
Neovascularization	37%
Optic disc	35%
Retina	8%
Cherry red spot	12%
Cotton-wool spot(s)	6%
Spontaneous retinal arterial pulsations	4%
Vitreous hemorrhage	4%
Cholesterol emboli	2%
Ischemic optic neuropathy	2%

(Adapted from Brown GC, Magargal LE. The ocular ischemic syndrome. Clinical, fluorescein angiographic and carotid angiographic features. Int Ophthalmol 1988;11:239–51.)

Table 59.2 Fluorescein angiographic signs seen in eyes with the ocular ischemic syndrome

Delayed and/or patchy choroidal filling	60%
Prolonged retinal arteriovenous transit time	95%
Retinal vascular staining	85%
Macular edema	17%
Other signs	
Retinal capillary nonperfusion	
Optic nerve head hyperfluorescence	
Microaneurysmal hyperfluorescence	

ocular ischemic syndrome demonstrate patchy and/or delayed choroidal filling (Fig. 59.15). In some instances, the filling is delayed for a minute or longer. Although not the most sensitive sign, an abnormality in choroidal filling is the most specific fluorescein angiographic sign in ocular ischemic eyes.

Prolongation of the retinal arteriovenous transit time is seen in 95% of eyes with the ocular ischemic syndrome (highly sensitive), but can also be seen in eyes with central retinal artery

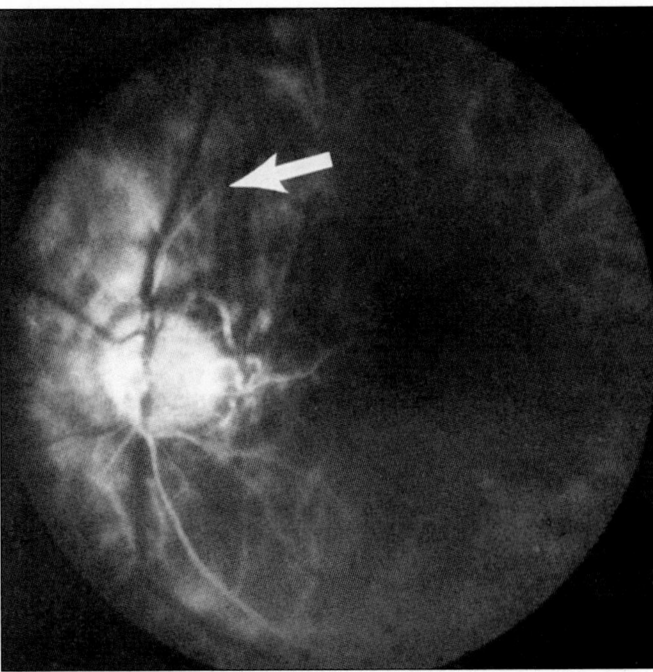

Fig. 59.14 Fluorescein angiogram of an eye with the ocular ischemic syndrome at 38 seconds after injection. A leading edge of the dye (arrow) is present within a retinal artery. (Reproduced with permission from Brown GC, Magargal LE, Simeone FA, et al. Arterial obstruction and ocular neovascularization. Ophthalmology 1982;89:139–46. Copyright © 1982 American Academy of Ophthalmology.)

obstruction and central retinal vein obstruction (low specificity). Normally, the major retinal veins in the temporal vascular arcade are completely filled within 10–11 seconds after the first appearance of dye within the corresponding retinal arteries. In extreme cases of the ocular ischemic syndrome, the retinal veins fail to fill throughout the study.

Staining of the retinal vessels in the later phases of the study is seen in about 85% of eyes (Fig. 59.16 online, Fig. 59.17). Both larger and smaller vessels can be involved, the arteries generally more so than the veins. Chronic hypoxic damage to endothelial cells may account for the staining. In contrast, staining of the retinal vessels is uncommon, with central retinal artery obstruction alone. With central retinal vein obstruction, the veins can demonstrate late staining, but the retinal arteries are generally not affected.

Macular leakage and edema evident on fluorescein angiography is seen in about one-sixth of eyes with the ocular ischemic syndrome[32] (Fig. 59.18). Hypoxia, and subsequent endothelial damage, within the smaller retinal vessels, as well as leakage from microaneurysms, may account for this phenomenon (Fig. 59.19). Dye accumulation may be mild or severe, and is usually associated with hyperfluorescence of the optic disc. The disc, however, is typically not swollen. Despite the prominent leakage with fluorescein angiography, the ophthalmoscopic cystic changes of macular edema are generally not as pronounced as those seen after ocular surgery or those associated with diabetic retinopathy.

Retinal capillary nonperfusion can be seen in some eyes (Fig. 59.20 online). The histopathologically observed absence of endothelial cells and pericytes within the retinal capillaries most likely corresponds to the areas of nonperfusion seen with fluorescein angiography.[7,8,33]

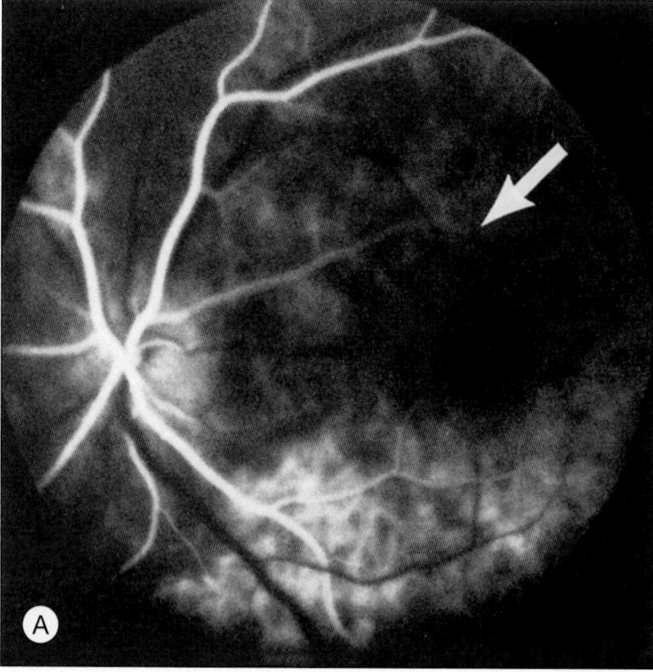

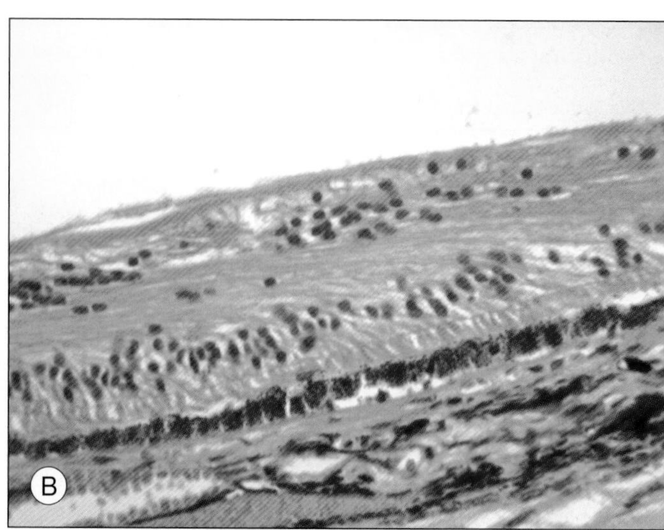

Fig. 59.15 (A) Fluorescein angiogram of an ocular ischemic syndrome eye at 44 seconds after injection shows patchy choroidal filling. A leading edge of dye (arrow) can again be seen within a retinal artery. (Reproduced with permission from Brown GC, Magargal LE. The ocular ischemic syndrome. Clinical, fluorescein angiographic and carotid angiographic features. Int Ophthalmol 1988;11:239–51.) (B) Histopathology of an ocular ischemic syndrome retina reveals a paucity of retinal ganglion cells, as well as cells in both the inner nuclear and outer nuclear layers, the latter the cell bodies for the rods and cones. These features occur secondary to panretinal ischemia from both retinal and choroidal hypoperfusion. The retinal pigment epithelial cells appear to be intact, correlating with the clinical picture that retinal pigment epithelial dropout and hyperplasia do not appear to be prominent funduscopic features associated with the ocular ischemic syndrome (hematoxylin–eosin ×60). (Courtesy of Dr W. Richard Green.)

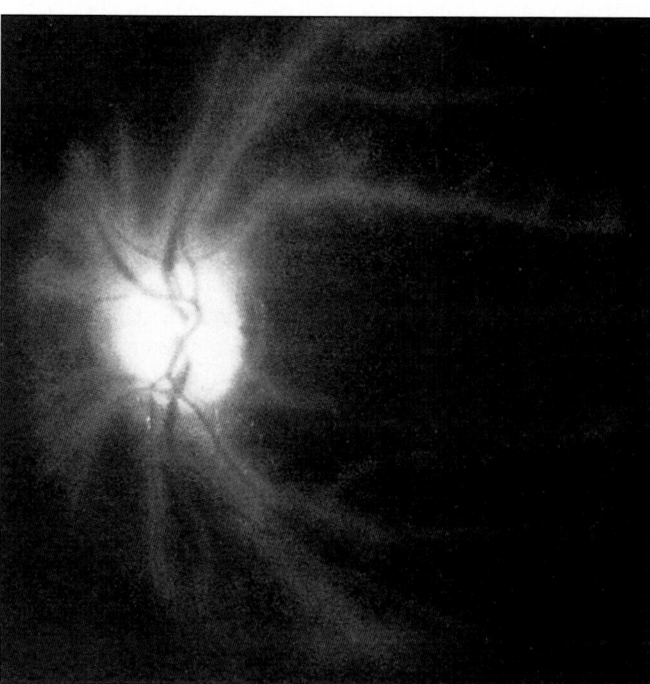

Fig. 59.17 Prominent staining of the retinal arteries in the later phases of fluorescein angiography in an eye with the ocular ischemic syndrome.

Bilateral, simultaneous, intravenous fluorescein angiography is a technique that has been reported to be helpful diagnostically in patients with a unilateral ocular ischemic syndrome.[34] However, the technique requires specialized equipment and is not generally available.

Electroretinography

The electroretinogram often discloses a diminution of the amplitude, or absence, of both the a- and b-waves in eyes with the ocular ischemic syndrome[5,6] (Fig. 59.21). The b-wave corresponds to activity of the Mueller and/or bipolar cells, and therefore to inner layer retinal function, while the a-wave correlates with activity of the photoreceptors in the outer retina.[35,36] Therefore, with central retinal artery obstruction, in which there is essentially inner layer retinal ischemia, the b-wave amplitude is characteristically decreased. With the ocular ischemic syndrome there is both retinal vascular and choroidal compromise, leading to ischemia of the inner and outer retina, respectively. Thus, both the b-wave and a-waves are affected.

Reduction in the amplitude of the oscillatory potential of the b-wave has been noted in eyes with retinal ischemia secondary to carotid artery stenosis.[37] This can be seen in patients with proven carotid artery disease, even in the presence of a normal fluorescein angiogram.

Carotid artery imaging

Carotid angiography typically discloses a 90% or greater obstruction of the ipsilateral internal or common carotid artery in persons with the ocular ischemic syndrome (Fig. 59.22). Given that noninvasive tests, such as duplex ultrasonography and oculoplethysmography, have an accuracy of approximately between 88 and 95% in detecting carotid stenosis of 75% or greater,[38–40] carotid angiography is often indicated for potential surgical cases or cases in which there is doubt about the diagnosis.

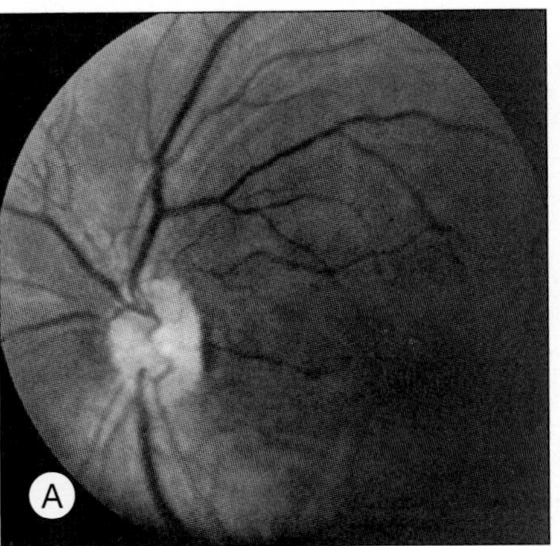

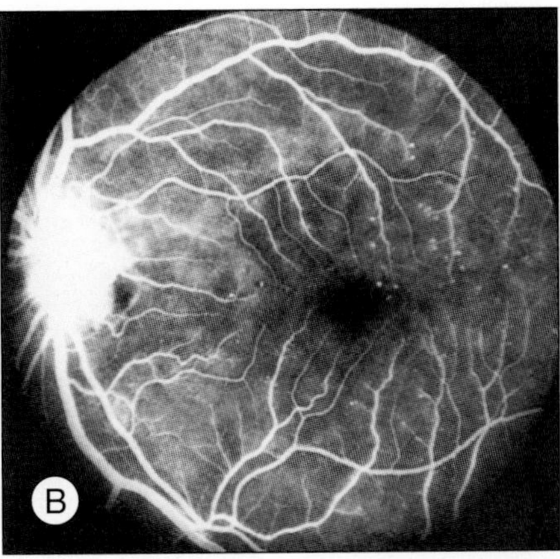

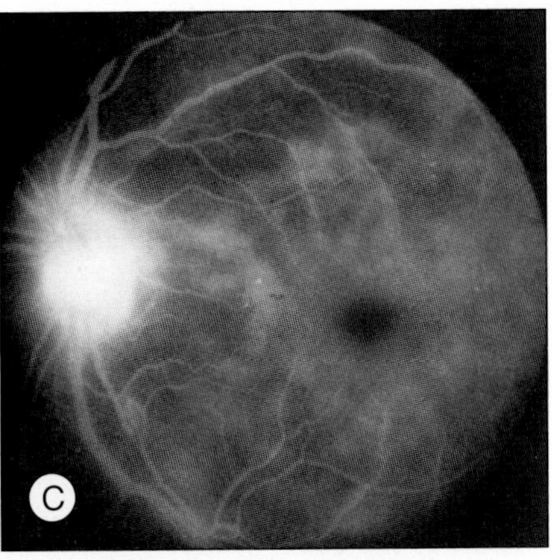

Fig. 59.18 (A) Left fundus of a 60-year-old woman with a 100% left internal carotid artery obstruction. The retinal veins are dilated, but not tortuous. (B) Fluorescein angiogram of the eye in panel (A) at more than 60 seconds after injection. A number of microaneurysms are present and the optic disc is hyperfluorescent. C, At several minutes after injection, prominent leakage of dye is evident. (Reproduced with permission from Brown GC. Macular edema in association with severe carotid artery obstruction. Am J Ophthalmol 1986;102:442; American Journal of Ophthalmology. Copyright © Ophthalmic Publishing Group.)

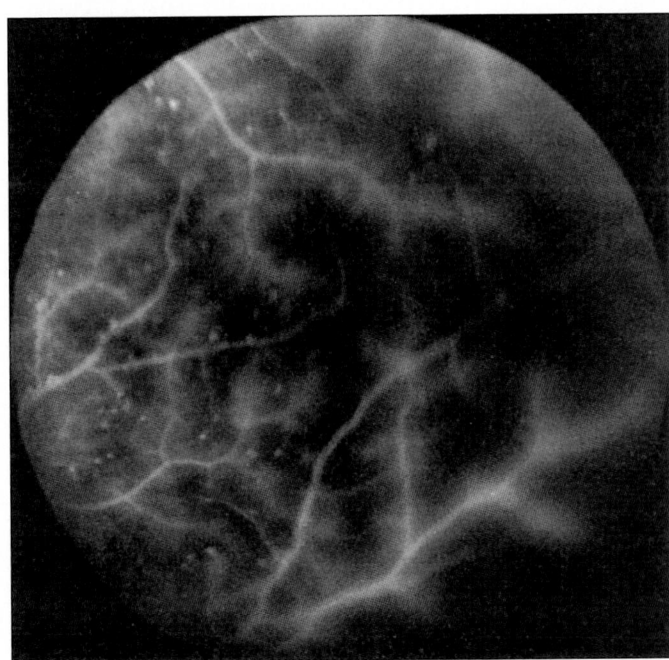

Fig. 59.19 Peripheral fluorescein angiogram of the same eye shown in Fig. 59.18. Many hyperfluorescent microaneurysms are seen, as is staining of the retinal vessels. (Reproduced with permission from Brown GC. Macular edema in association with severe carotid artery obstruction. Am J Ophthalmol 1986;102:442; American Journal of Ophthalmology. Copyright © Ophthalmic Publishing Group.)

Others

Visual evoked potentials have been used to study eyes with severe carotid artery stenosis. The recovery time of the amplitude of the major positive peak after photostress has been shown to improve in patients with severe stenosis after endarterectomy.[41]

Ophthalmodynamometry can be of benefit in detecting decreased ocular perfusion in cases of unilateral ocular ischemic syndrome.[10,42]

In the absence of an ophthalmodynamometer, Kearns[42] has advocated light digital pressure on the upper lid of the affected eye during ophthalmoscopy. Retinal arterial pulsations can usually be readily induced in eyes with the ocular ischemic syndrome. This is generally not the case in eyes with central retinal vein obstruction, an entity that can be confused with the ocular ischemic syndrome.

SYSTEMIC ASSOCIATIONS

Diseases associated in one way or another with atherosclerosis are frequently seen in conjunction with the ocular ischemic syndrome. Systemic arterial hypertension has been reported in 73% of ocular ischemic syndrome patients and concomitant diabetes mellitus has been observed in 56%.[43] In an age-matched historical control population from the Framingham Study,[44] the corresponding prevalences for systemic arterial hypertension and diabetes mellitus were 26% and 6%.

At the time of presentation, almost one-fifth of patients relate a history of having peripheral vascular disease for which previous bypass surgery was required.[43] The stroke rate for patients for people with the ocular ischemic syndrome is approximately 4% per year.[45]

A rare but serious cause of ocular ischemic syndrome is giant cell arteritis.[46] This condition has been reported to cause bilateral loss of vision, which may occur despite treatment with steroids.[47]

Mortality data[43] have shown that the 5-year death rate for patients with the ocular ischemic syndrome is 40%. The leading cause of death is cardiovascular disease, which accounts for about two-thirds of cases. Stroke is the second leading cause of death. Thus, most patients with the ocular ischemic syndrome should be considered for cardiac evaluation, in addition to a carotid workup. It is also important to note that Mizener et al. noted that in 69% of their patients, ocular ischemic syndrome was the first clinical manifestation of carotid occlusive disease, a fact that only further underscores the importance of timely systemic evaluation in these patients.[48]

DIFFERENTIAL DIAGNOSIS

The entities that are most commonly confused with the ocular ischemic syndrome include mild central retinal vein obstruction and diabetic retinopathy. Features that differentiate these

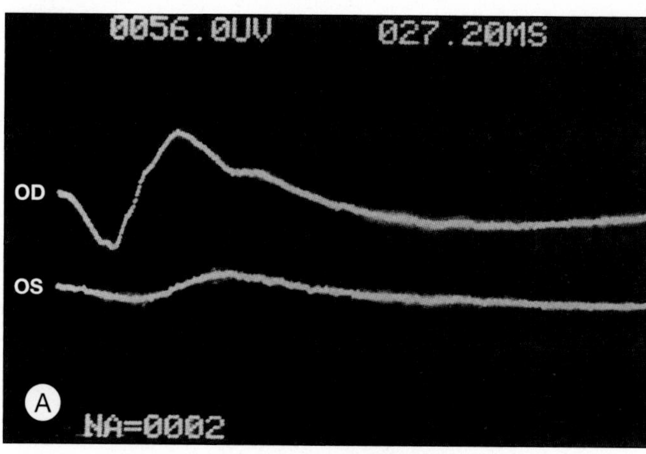

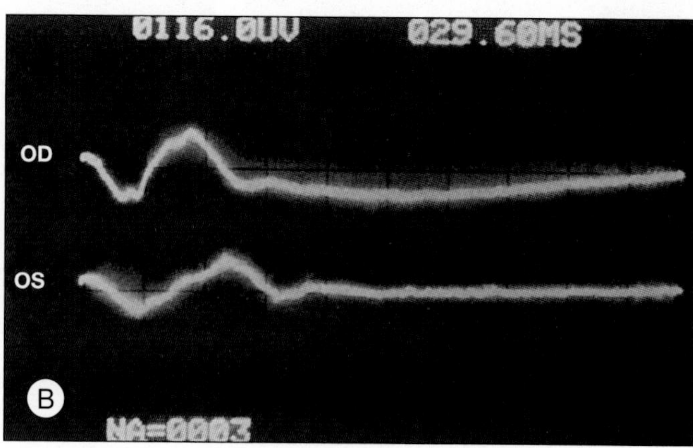

Fig. 59.21 Electroretinogram from a 62-year-old woman with ocular ischemic syndrome and a severe left carotid artery stenosis. The tracing of the right eye (OD) is seen above, and that of the left eye (OS) is seen below. (A) The a- and the b-waves are markedly diminished in the left eye before endarterectomy. (B) After left endarterectomy the amplitudes of the a- and b-waves have increased in the left eye. The vision correspondingly improved from counting fingers to 20/70.

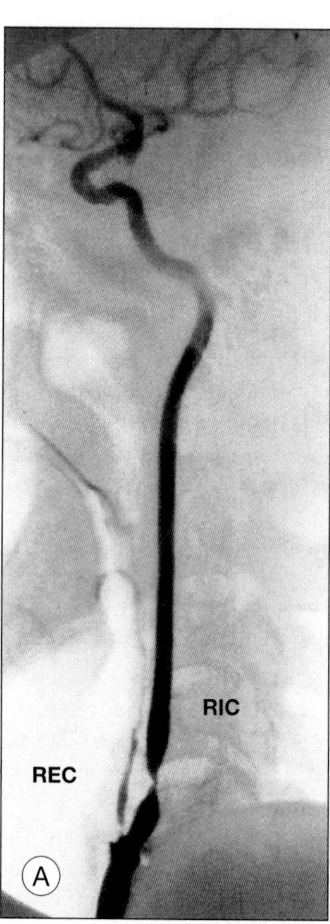

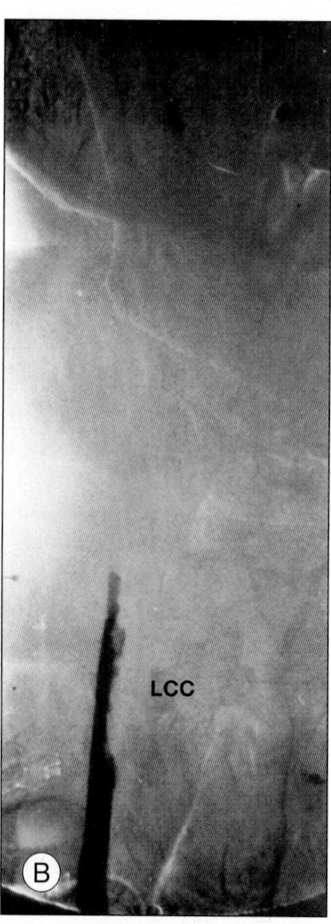

Fig. 59.22 Carotid angiography in a patient with bilateral ocular ischemic syndrome. (A) A marked stenosis is visible within the right internal carotid artery (RIC), as well as in the right external carotid artery (REC). (B) A 100% obstruction of the left common carotid artery (LCC) is present. (Reproduced with permission from Brown GC, Magargal LE. The ocular ischemic syndrome. Clinical, fluorescein angiographic and carotid angiographic features. Int Ophthalmol 1988;11:239–51.)

abnormalities are listed in Table 59.3. In contrast to the ocular ischemic syndrome, the veins in eyes with mild, or nonischemic, central retinal vein obstruction are often dilated and tortuous. Additionally, with light digital pressure on the lid it is difficult to induce retinal arterial pulsations in eyes with central retinal vein obstruction. While both entities usually have a prolonged retinal arteriovenous transit time, choroidal filling defects and prominent retinal arterial staining are usually absent on fluorescein angiography in eyes with central retinal vein obstruction.

Diabetic retinopathy can exist concomitantly with the ocular ischemic syndrome. The presence of hard exudate in the posterior pole usually suggests diabetic retinopathy, rather than the ocular ischemic syndrome.

As is the case with central retinal vein obstruction, choroidal filling defects and retinal arterial staining are generally absent on fluorescein angiography in eyes with diabetic retinopathy.

In some cases of diabetic retinopathy, the ocular ischemic syndrome can exacerbate the proliferative changes. It has not been proven that carotid stenosis is protective against the development of proliferative diabetic retinopathy.[45]

TREATMENT

With regard to vision, the natural course of the ocular ischemic syndrome is uncertain. Nonetheless, most eyes with the fully developed entity probably have a poor long-term outcome. When rubeosis iridis is present, well over 90% of eyes become legally blind within a year of discovery.[25]

Total carotid artery obstruction

When a carotid artery is 100% obstructed, endarterectomy is usually ineffective since a thrombus often propagates distally to the next major vessel. In these cases, extracranial to intracranial bypass surgery, usually from the superficial temporal artery to the middle cerebral artery, has been attempted to alleviate the obstruction. Although case reports suggest that this procedure can be of benefit initially in salvaging vision in eyes with the ocular ischemic syndrome,[49–54] as well as causing regression of neovascular glaucoma,[55] the visual prognosis at one year after the surgery is almost universally poor, despite the fact that 20% of patients have visual improvement within the first three months of surgery.[25] Additionally, the procedure has not been shown in a large randomized study to be of benefit in preventing the risk of ischemic stroke.[56]

That said, some authors have offered objective support of improvement in perfusion following endarterectomy. Costa et al. were able to demonstrate increased mean peak systolic

Table 59.3 Features that differentiate the ocular ischemic syndrome (OIS), central retinal vein obstruction (CRVO), and diabetic retinopathy

	OIS	CRVO	Diabetic retinopathy
Laterality	80% unilateral	Usually unilateral	Bilateral
Age	50s–80s	50s–80s	Variable
Fundus signs			
Venous status	Dilated (not tortuous), beaded	Dilated and tortuous	Dilated and beaded
Hemorrhages	Peripheral, dot, and blot	Nerve fiber layer, posterior pole	Posterior pole, dot, and blot
Microaneurysms	In midperiphery	Variable	Present in posterior pole
Exudate	Absent	Rare	Common
Optic disc	Normal	Swollen	Affected in papillopathy
Retinal arterial perfusion pressure	Decreased	Normal	Normal
Fluorescein angiography			
Choroidal filling	Delayed, patchy	Normal	Normal
Arteriovenous transit time	Prolonged	Prolonged	May be prolonged
Retinal vessel staining	Arterial	Venous	Usually absent

flow velocities and end diastolic velocities in the orbital vessels following surgery, with a significant reduction of the mean resistance indices in the central retinal and posterior ciliary arteries.[57]

Kawaguchi et al.[58] recently evaluated the effects of superficial temporal to middle cerebral artery (STA-MCA) bypass in a series of patients with the OIS. These authors compared a number of clinical parameters including carotid Doppler flow imaging in 32 patients who received STA-MCA as compared to nine patients with OIS who did not have STA-MCA. Prior to surgery all 32 patients had reversal of flow in their ophthalmic arteries. The mean peak systolic flow improved to 0.15 m/s at 3 months as compared to –0.26 at baseline. In addition, whereas all patients had reversal of flow in the ophthalmic artery preoperatively, 56% developed antegrade flow at the 3-month period. In the final analysis, 47% developed visual improvement following surgery and the remainder visual stability.[58]

Less than total carotid artery obstruction

Although there are no randomized studies that compare the natural history of the disease to the course after carotid endarterectomy, this surgery may also stabilize or improve vision in the eyes of patients who undergo successful endarterectomy prior to the development of rubeosis iridis.[25,59] Not withstanding, the visual results associated with this treatment are fair at best. In the series of Sivalingam et al.,[25] at the end of one year 7% of eyes with the ocular ischemic syndrome that underwent endarterectomy had visual improvement, 33% were unchanged, and 60% had worse vision. Among the 60 total ocular ischemic syndrome eyes in the group, an endarterectomy was performed for only three without rubeosis. At the end of one year follow-up the vision was better in one, stable in one, and worse in the third. Endarterectomy appears to rarely cause regression of iris neovascularization in eyes with the ocular ischemic syndrome.[60]

More recent data demonstrated that carotid revascularization surgery results in improved retinal blood in 80% of cases, although the long-term visual implications are unclear.[61] Stenting can also be undertaken in select cases to successfully restore blood flow within the carotid artery.[62,63] Rarely, bilateral external carotid obstruction can cause the ocular ischemic syndrome.[64] In this instance, external carotid endarterectomy can be considered.[64] In cases of the ocular ischemic syndrome with ipsilateral internal carotid and external carotid obstructions, it would seem that reversal of both would yield the best ocular prognosis, but this is not known with certainty at the current time.

It should be noted that eyes with the ocular ischemic syndrome will occasionally develop a severe increase in intraocular pressure after ipsilateral carotid endarterectomy.[65,66] This is most likely to occur in eyes with rubeosis iridis and anterior chamber angle compromise from fibrovascular tissue formation. Although aqueous outflow is impaired in such eyes, ciliary body perfusion and aqueous humor formation are also decreased secondary to the carotid stenosis. When the carotid obstruction is suddenly reversed, ciliary body perfusion and aqueous humor formation increase, but the outflow obstruction in the anterior chamber angle is still present. Thus, the intraocular pressure rises drastically. Ciliary body destructive procedures or glaucoma filtering surgery may be required in these cases.

Section on carotid endarterectomy in general available online.

Medical therapy

Since atherosclerosis is, by far, the most common cause of the ocular ischemic syndrome, medical therapy should be directed toward treating atherogenic disease by controlling risk factors such as systemic arterial hypertension, smoking, diabetes mellitus, and hyperlipidemia. Of considerable importance is the fact that high-dose (40 mg PO daily) rosuvastatin therapy has been shown to actually reverse coronary artery atherosclerosis, an event likely generalizable to atherosclerosis elsewhere in the body.[72] Since cardiac disease is the leading cause of death associated with the ocular ischemic syndrome, evaluation by a cardiologist should be considered.[43]

Direct ocular therapeutic modalities

Full scatter panretinal laser photocoagulation has been advocated for ocular ischemic eyes with rubeosis iridis and/or posterior segment neovascularization.[59,73,74] This generally consists of 1500–2000 500 µm burns with the argon green laser. Unlike the situation when rubeosis iridis occurs secondary to diabetic retinopathy, in which there is regression in a majority of cases with full scatter panretinal photocoagulation, approximately 36% of ocular ischemic syndrome eyes will demonstrate regression of the iris neovascularization after full scatter treatment.[25] If the anterior chamber angle is completely closed by fibrovascular tissue and there is no posterior segment neovascularization, panretinal photocoagulation is probably not indicated unless a glaucoma filtering procedure is being considered, as higher success rates of filtration surgery have been reported when PRP has been performed.[75]

While there is little in the reported literature regarding the management of macular edema secondary to this condition, Klais and Spaide reported excellent clinical resolution of fluid and dramatic improvement in vision in a patient treated with intravitreal triamcinolone acetonide.[76] Intravitreal bevacizumab has been used for the treatment of the iris neovascularization and macular edema associated with the ocular ischemic syndrome, but data are sparse.[77]

Bonus images for this chapter can be found online at http://www.expertconsult.com

Fig. 59.6 Right fundus of a 35-year-old man with a cherry-red spot, rubeosis iridis, and retinal hemorrhages in the macula. A 95% right internal carotid artery obstruction was present.

Fig. 59.9 (A) Fibrovascular proliferation overlying the optic disc and causing retinal traction in an eye with the ocular ischemic syndrome. (Reproduced with permission from Brown GC, Magargal LE. The ocular ischemic syndrome. Clinical, fluorescein angiographic and carotid angiographic features. Int Ophthalmol 1988;11:239–51.) (B) Histopathology of an eye with ischemic retinopathy demonstrates a connection of neovascularization of the optic disc on stretch (arrow) between the inferior disc and the superior vitreous gel filled with blood. Presumably, the intravitreal blood occurred as a result of rupture of the thin-walled vessels on stretch (hematoxylin–eosin ×60).

Fig. 59.10 Neovascularization of the retina (arrows) with fluorescein angiography in a nondiabetic person affected by the ocular ischemic syndrome. Retinal capillary nonperfusion (NP) can be seen. (Reproduced with permission from Brown GC, Magargal LE, Simeone FA, et al. Arterial obstruction and ocular neovascularization. Ophthalmology 1982;89:139–46. Copyright © 1982 American Academy of Ophthalmology.)

Fig. 59.11 Cotton-wool spots in the fundus of a man with the ocular ischemic syndrome. Irregularly dilated retinal veins are also evident.

Fig. 59.16 Staining of the macular vessels in the ocular ischemic syndrome. (Reproduced with permission from Brown GC, Magargal LE. The ocular ischemic syndrome. Clinical, fluorescein angiographic and carotid angiographic features. Int Ophthalmol 1988;11:239–51.)

Fig. 59.20 (A) Fluorescein angiography reveals retinal capillary nonperfusion (NP) in an ocular ischemic syndrome eye. (Reproduced with permission from Brown GC, Magargal LE. The ocular ischemic syndrome. Clinical, fluorescein angiographic and carotid angiographic features. Int Ophthalmol. 1988;11:239–51.) (B) Trypsin digest of the retinal vessels of an ocular ischemic syndrome eye reveals loss of both the endothelial cells and pericytes (hematoxylin–eosin ×200). (Courtesy of Dr W. Richard Green.)

Access the complete reference list online at http://www.expertconsult.com

1. Kearns TP, Hollenhorst RW. Venous stasis retinopathy of occlusive disease of the carotid artery. Proc Mayo Clin 1963;38:304–12.
2. Hayreh SS. So-called "central retinal vein occlusion." Venous-stasis retinopathy. Ophthalmologica 1976;172:14–37.
3. Knox DL. Ischemic ocular inflammation. Am J Ophthalmol 1965;60: 995–1002.
4. Young LHY, Appen RE. Ischemic oculopathy, a manifestation of carotid artery disease. Arch Neurol 1981;38:358–61.
5. Brown GC, Magargal LE. The ocular ischemic syndrome. Clinical, fluorescein angiographic and carotid angiographic features. Int Ophthalmol 1988;11: 239–51.
6. Brown GC, Magargal LE, Simeone FA, et al. Arterial obstruction and ocular neovascularization. Ophthalmology 1982;89:139–46.
7. Kahn M, Green WR, Knox DL, et al. Ocular features of carotid occlusive disease. Retina 1986;6:239–52.
8. Michelson PE, Knox DL, Green WR. Ischemic ocular inflammation. A clinicopathologic case report. Arch Ophthalmol 1971;86:274–80.
9. Sturrock GD, Mueller HR. Chronic ocular ischaemia. Br J Ophthalmol 1984;68:716–23.
10. Kearns TP. Ophthalmology and the carotid artery. Am J Ophthalmol 1979;88:714–22.
11. Kobayashi S, Hollenhorst RW, Sundt TM Jr. Retinal arterial pressure before and after surgery for carotid artery stenosis. Stroke 1971;2:569–75.
12. Bullock J, Falter RT, Downing JE, et al. Ischemic ophthalmia secondary to an ophthalmic artery occlusion. Am J Ophthalmol 1972;74:486–93.
13. Madsen PH. Venous-stasis insufficiency of the ophthalmic artery. Acta Ophthalmol 1965;40:940–7.
14. Magargal LE, Sanborn GE, Zimmerman A. Venous stasis retinopathy associated with embolic obstruction of the central retinal artery. J Clin Neuroophthalmol 1982;2:113–8.
15. Duker JS, Belmont JB. Ocular ischemic syndrome secondary to carotid artery dissection. Am J Ophthalmol 1988;106:750–2.
16. Hamed LM, Guy JR, Moster ML, et al. Giant cell arteritis in the ocular ischemic syndrome. Am J Ophthalmol 1992;113:702–5.
17. Effeney DJ, Krupski WC, Stoney RJ, et al. Fibromuscular dysplasia of the carotid artery. Austral NZ J Surg 1983;53:527–31.
18. Dhobb M, Ammar F, Bensaid Y, et al. Arterial manifestations in Behçet's disease: four new cases. Ann Vasc Surg 1986;1:249–52.
19. Sadun AA, Sebag J, Bienfang DC. Complete bilateral internal carotid artery occlusion in a young man. J Clin Neuroophthalmol 1983;3:63–6.
20. Donnan GA, Sharbrough FW. Carotid occlusive disease. Effect of bright light on visual evoked response. Arch Neurol 1982;39:687–9.
21. Wiebers DO, Swanson JW, Cascino TL, et al. Bilateral loss of vision in bright light. Stroke 1989;20:554–8.
22. Ramadan NM, Tietjen GE, Levine SR, et al. Scintillating scotomata associated with internal carotid artery dissection: report of three cases. Neurology 1991;41:1084–7.
23. Winterkorn JM, Teman AJ. Recurrent attacks of amaurosis fugax treated with calcium channel blocker. Ann Neurol 1991;30:423–5.
24. Aasen J, Kerty E, Russell D, et al. Amaurosis fugax: clinical, Doppler and angiographic findings. Acta Neurol Scand 1988;77:450–5.
25. Sivalingam A, Brown GC, Magargal LE. The ocular ischemic syndrome. III. Visual prognosis and the effect of treatment. Int Ophthalmol 1991;15:15–20.
26. Schlaegel T. Symptoms and signs of uveitis. In: Duane TD, editor. Clinical ophthalmology, vol. 4. Hagerstown: Harper and Row; 1983. p. 1–7.
27. Green WR, Chan CC, Hutchins GM, et al. Central retinal vein occlusion. A prospective histopathologic study of 29 eyes in 28 cases. Retina 1981;1: 27–55.
28. Campo RV, Reeser FH. Retinal telangiectasia secondary to bilateral carotid artery occlusion. Arch Ophthalmol 1983;101:1211–3.
29. Brown GC. Anterior ischemic optic neuropathy occurring in association with carotid artery obstruction. J Clin Neuro-Ophthalmol 1986;6:39–42.
30. Waybright EA, Selhorst JB, Combs J. Anterior ischemic optic neuropathy with internal carotid artery occlusion. Am J Ophthalmol 1982;93:42–7.

31. Bolling JP, Buettner H. Acquired retinal arteriovenous communications in occlusive disease of the carotid artery. Ophthalmology 1990;97:1148–52.
32. Brown GC. Macular edema in association with severe carotid artery obstruction. Am J Ophthalmol 1986;102:442–8.
33. Dugan JD, Green WR. Ophthalmic manifestations of carotid occlusive disease. Eye 1991;5:226–38.
34. Choromokos EA, Raymond LA, Sacks JG. Recognition of carotid stenosis with bilateral simultaneous retinal fluorescein angiography. Ophthalmology 1982;89:1146–8.
35. Carr RE, Siegel JM. Electrophysiologic aspects of several retinal diseases. Am J Ophthalmol 1964;58:95–107.
36. Henkes HE. Electroretinography in circulatory disturbances of the retina. II. The electroretinogram in cases of occlusion of the central retinal artery or one of its branches. Arch Ophthalmol 1954;51:42–53.
37. Coleman K, Fitzgerald D, Eustace P, et al. Electroretinography, retinal ischaemia and carotid artery disease. Eur J Vasc Surg 1990;4:569–73.
38. Bosley TM. The role of carotid noninvasive tests in stroke prevention. Semin Neurol 1986;6:194–203.
39. Castaldo JE, Nicholas GG, Gee W, et al. Duplex ultrasound and ocular pneumoplethysmography concordance in detecting severe carotid stenosis. Arch Neurol 1989;46:518–22.
40. Neale ML, Chambers JL, Kelly AT, et al. Reappraisal of duplex criteria to assess significant carotid artery stenosis with special reference to reports of the North American Symptomatic Carotid Endarterectomy Trial and the European Carotid Surgery Trial. J Vasc Surg 1994;20:642–9.
41. Banchini E, Franchi A, Magni R, et al. Carotid occlusive disease. An electrophysiological investigation. J Cardiovasc Surg 1987;28:524–7.
42. Kearns TP. Differential diagnosis of central retinal vein obstruction. Ophthalmology 1983;90:475–80.
43. Sivalingham A, Brown GC, Magargal LE, et al. The ocular ischemic syndrome II. Mortality and systemic morbidity. Int Ophthalmol 1989;13:187–91.
44. Kannel WB, Gordon T, editors. The Framingham Study. Public Health Service Publication No. NIH 77-1247, Section 6, Tables 6-9, Section 29, Tables A-22 and A-23, Section 32, p. 84–5.
45. Duker J, Brown GC, Bosley TM, et al. Asymmetric proliferative diabetic retinopathy and carotid artery disease. Ophthalmology 1990;97:869–74.
46. Casson RJ, Fleming FK, Shaikh A, et al. Bilateral ocular ischemic syndrome secondary to giant cell arteritis. Arch Ophthalmol 2001;119:306–7.
47. Hwang JM, Girkin CA, Perry JD, et al. Bilateral ocular ischemic syndrome secondary to giant cell arteritis progressing despite corticosteroid treatment. Am J Ophthalmol 1999;127:102–4.
48. Mizener JB, Podhajsky P, Hayreh SS. Ocular ischemic syndrome. Ophthalmology 1997;104:859–64.
49. Edwards MS, Chater NL, Stanley JA. Reversal of chronic ischaemia by extracranial–intracranial arterial by-pass. Neurosurgery 1980;7:480–3.
50. Higgins RA. Neovascular glaucoma associated with ocular hypoperfusion secondary to carotid artery disease. Austral J Ophthalmol 1984;12:155–62.
51. Katz B, Weinstein PR. Improvement of photostress recovery testing after extracranial–intracranial bypass surgery. Br J Ophthalmol 1986;70:277–80.
52. Kearns TP, Younge BR, Peipgras PG. Resolution of venous stasis retinopathy after carotid artery bypass surgery. Proc Mayo Clin 1980;55:342–6.
53. Kiser WD, Gonder J, Magargal LE, et al. Recovery of vision following treatment of the ocular ischemic syndrome. Ann Ophthalmol 1983;15:305–10.
54. Shibuya M, Suzuki Y, Takayasu M, et al. Effects of STA–MCA anastomosis for ischaemic oculopathy due to occlusion of the internal carotid artery. Acta Neurochir 1990;103:71–5.
55. Kearns TP, Siebert RG. The ocular aspects of carotid artery surgery. Tr Am Ophthalmol Soc 1978;76:247–65.
56. The EC/IC Bypass Study Group. Failure of extracranial–intracranial arterial bypass to reduce the risk of ischemic stroke. Results of an international randomized trial. N Eng J Med 1985;313:1191–200.
57. Costa VP, Kuzniec S, Molnar LJ, et al. The effects of carotid endarterectomy on the retrobulbar circulation of patients with severe occlusive carotid artery disease. An investigation by color Doppler imaging. Ophthalmology 1999;106:306–10.
58. Kawaguchi S, Sakaki T, Kamada K, et al. Effects of superficial temporal to middle cerebral artery bypass for ischaemic retinopathy due to internal carotid artery occlusion/stenosis. Acta Neurochir (Wien) 1994;129:166–70.
59. Johnston ME, Gonder JR, Canny CL. Successful treatment of the ocular ischemic syndrome with panretinal photocoagulation and cerebrovascular surgery. Can J Ophthalmol 1988;23:114–9.
60. Hauch TL, Busuttil RW, Yoshizumi MO. A report of iris neovascularization. An indication for carotid endarterectomy. Surgery 1984;95:358–62.
61. Cardia G, Porfido D, Guerriero S, et al. Retinal circulation after carotid artery revascularization. Angiology 2011;62:372–5.
62. Fintelman R, Rosenwasser RH, Jabbour P, et al. An old problem, a new solution. Surv Ophthalmol 2010;55:85–8.
63. Marx JL, Hreib K, Choi IS, et al. Percutaneous carotid artery angioplasty and stenting for ocular ischemic syndrome. Ophthalmology 2004 111:2284–91.
64. Alizai AM, Trobe JD, Thompson BG, et al. Ocular ischemic syndrome after occlusion of both external carotid arteries. J Neuroophthalmol 2005;25:268–7.
65. Coppeto JR, Wand M, Bear L, et al. Neovascular glaucoma and carotid artery obstructive disease. Am J Ophthalmol 1985;99:567–70.
66. Melamed S, Irvine J, Lee DA. Increased intraocular pressure following endarterectomy. Ann Ophthalmol 1987;19:304–6.
71. Rerkasem K, Rothwell PM. Carotid endarterectomy for symptomatic carotid stenosis. Cochrane Database Syst Rev 2011;Apr 13(4):CD001081.
72. Nissen SE, Nicholls SJ, Sipahi I, et al. for the ASTEROID Investigators. Effect of very high-intensity statin therapy on regression of coronary atherosclerosis: the ASTEROID trial. JAMA 2006;295:1556–65.
73. Carter JE. Panretinal photocoagulation for progressive ocular neovascularization secondary to occlusion of the common carotid artery. Ann Ophthalmol 1984;16:572–6.
74. Eggleston TF, Bohling CA, Eggleston HC, et al. Photocoagulation for ocular ischemia associated with carotid artery occlusion. Ann Ophthalmol 1980;12: 84–7.
75. Allen RC, Bellows AR, Hutchinson BT, et al. Filtration surgery in the treatment of neovascular glaucoma. Ophthalmology 1982;89:1181–7.
76. Klais CM, Spaide RF. Intravitreal triamcinolone acetonide injection in ocular ischemic syndrome. Retina 2004;24:459–61.
77. Amselem L, Montero J, Diaz-Llopis M, et al. Intravitreal bevacizumab (Avastin) injection in ocular ischemic syndrome. Am J Ophthalmol 2007;144:122–4.

Chapter 60

Coagulopathies

Sandra Liakopoulos, Florian M.A. Heussen, SriniVas R. Sadda

A variety of hereditary as well as acquired diseases belong to the group of coagulopathies – diseases that affect the blood clotting system, causing hypercoagulability and susceptibility to bleeding. Important coagulopathies include disseminated intravascular coagulation, idiopathic thrombocytopenic purpura, thrombotic thrombocytopenic purpura, and the HELLP syndrome (hemolytic anemia, elevated liver enzymes, and low platelet count). Since coagulopathies are multiorgan disease processes, ocular involvement may occur and show characteristic changes that should be recognized by ophthalmologists and retina specialists.

GENERAL CONSIDERATIONS

Disseminated intravascular coagulation

Disseminated intravascular coagulation (DIC) is often described as a secondary disease process typically associated with other disease entities.[1] The presence of DIC increases the risk of mortality beyond that associated with the primary disease.[2] A cascading activation of both procoagulants and fibrinolysis leads to simultaneous, uncontrolled hemorrhages and diffuse thrombosis of small and large vessels affecting virtually all mucocutaneous tissues and various organs, ultimately resulting in end-organ failure (see Box 60.1). As such, DIC is regarded as one of the most common causes of death. But not all presentations of DIC are lethal; it may also manifest as low-grade disease with a chronic or compensated course.

Box 60.1 Clinical manifestations of DIC

Hemorrhagic events
- Petechiae
- Purpura
- Hemorrhagic bullae
- Hematoma
- Wound bleeding

Peripheral thrombotic events
- Acral cyanosis
- Gangrene

Central/organ dysfunction
- Fever
- Hypotension
- Acidosis
- Proteinuria
- Hypoxia
- CNS dysfunction

Triggering events for DIC are manifold and range from trauma to malignancies, septicemia, obstetric complications, cardiovascular disease, inflammatory disorders, and renal disease, only to name a few. Whether DIC will pursue a fulminant or compensated course is loosely related to the disease entity with which it is associated. Chronic conditions such as cardiovascular disease, autoimmune diseases or hematologic disorders tend to be associated with a low-grade DIC, whereas more acutely presenting entities such as crush injuries are more likely to trigger a fulminant DIC. Furthermore, DIC is not restricted to a particular age range and may occur in neonates as well as elderly individuals.

The currently established theory of pathogenesis is an initial activation of the coagulation cascade following inflammation or damage to tissue and vascular endothelial cells.[3] Fibrin formation leads to microvascular or macrovascular thrombosis. Soon thereafter, fibrinolysis is upregulated and the consumption of platelets in the obstructed microcirculation causes a systemic thrombocytopenia (cell count $<100\,000/mm^3$), thereby generating an environment of simultaneous clotting and extrusion of hemorrhages. Despite a common pathophysiologic pathway, clinical manifestations of the disease may vary widely (see Box 60.1), complicating diagnosis and treatment management.

The onset of DIC is usually marked by fever, shock, acidosis and, more specifically, widespread hemorrhaging, acral cyanosis, gangrene and end-organ failure. Bleeding from more than three unrelated sites at once and a recent medical history compatible with known causes of DIC can direct the clinician towards the diagnosis. Definite diagnosis is heavily based on positive laboratory test results for platelet count, D-dimer (fibrin degradation product or FDP), antithrombin-III, protein C, prothrombin time, partial thromboplastin time, and fibrinogen.[4]

Treatment of DIC is difficult and should primarily address the underlying cause, however, removal of its cause does not necessarily alleviate the process in all cases and prognosis of a fulminant DIC is very poor. Replacement treatment such as frozen plasma transfusion or infusion of antithrombin-III, fibrinogen, and platelet-concentrates can help to limit hemorrhages. In some cases, anticoagulant treatment may be required. Further, activated protein C has been suggested to treat this condition,[5] however, the efficacy of this approach for clinically relevant outcome parameters remains unclear.[6]

Idiopathic thrombocytopenic purpura and thrombotic thrombocytopenic purpura

Thrombotic thrombocytopenic purpura (TTP) is a severe thrombotic microangiopathy caused by platelet adhesion and aggregation mediated by endothelial cell-attached ultra-large von Willebrand factor multimers (ULVWF). The underlying cause is a congenital or acquired (autoimmune) deficiency of von Willebrand factor-cleaving proteases such as ADAMTS-13.[7] TTP is more frequent in young female adults than in males or older individuals. Most presentations of the disease are idiopathic, although familial and secondary TTP have been described. Pregnancy, treatment with certain drugs (clopidogrel, cyclosporine, tacrolimus), and malignancies are associated with a higher incidence of TTP. TTP is accompanied by profound thrombocytopenia, erythrocyte fragmentation, and increased serum levels of lactatdehydrogenase (LDH).[8] Clinically it manifests with fever, renal failure, neurological symptoms, purpura, and signs of hemolytic anemia. There is often a prodromal phase that may consist of headache, dizziness, nausea, and abdominal pain, presumably caused by microinfarction of the viscera. Though there are chronic smoldering patterns of the disease, an acute and fulminant course is not uncommon and, if left untreated, can be lethal. In some cases, ocular manifestations as described below may present as the first signs of the disease; thus, prompt referral to a hematologist may be life-saving.[9] Plasmapheresis is the principal treatment for this condition and can be supplemented by immunosuppressive therapy (cyclosporine A, rituximab) in refractory cases, although relapses are generally the rule.[10] Of note, systemic treatment with bevacizumab, a monoclonal antibody to VEGF which is increasingly used via intravitreal delivery for ocular neovascular disorders, can induce a TTP-like microangiopathy.[11]

Although idiopathic thrombocytopenic purpura (ITP) also features thrombocytopenia and purpura, the underlying pathophysiology is distinctly different from TTP. In many cases, ITP is the manifestation of an autoimmune process targeting the circulating platelets, thereby causing thrombocytopenia and widespread hemorrhages. Fortunately, ITP is self-limiting in most cases and responds well to treatment with corticosteroids or other immunosuppressants. Rarely, the extremely low platelet counts seen in ITP can cause severe, live-threatening complications.

HELLP syndrome

The incidence of the HELLP syndrome (toxemia of pregnancy) is reported as being between 0.2 and 0.6% of all pregnancies.[12] Major symptoms are hemolytic anemia (H), elevated liver enzymes (EL), and low platelet count (LP). While being regarded as a microangiopathy much like TTP, it can also convert into a fulminant DIC in 20% of cases. The mortality rate is around 1.1% with adequate management, yet other serious complications such as abruptio placentae (16%), acute renal failure (7.7%), or pulmonary edema (6%) can occur more frequently.[13]

OPHTHALMIC INVOLVEMENT

Although there are many differences regarding the underlying etiology or management of the various coagulopathies discussed in this chapter, they all may present with similar ophthalmic manifestations (see Fig. 60.1). The precise frequency of ocular complications however is unknown, as many cases may remain unrecognized due to the life-threatening nature of those systemic diseases. Relatively few reports are available regarding ocular complications of DIC as most cases are diagnosed and reported after the patients have died.[14] By comparison, many more reports can be found in the literature describing ophthalmic findings in TTP and ITP.[15–17] Some groups have reported that ocular signs and symptoms occur in up to 14% of patients with TTP.[18]

The hypercoagulable state in these individuals typically leads to choriocapillaris occlusion by fibrin-platelet clots, whereas subcutanenous or subconjunctival,[19] choroidal, retinal or vitreous hemorrhages[15,17,20] are thought to be indicative of thrombocytopenia and anemia. A patchy delay in filling of the choroidal vessels on fluorescein angiography can be an early sign of ophthalmic complications. Pathophysiologically, microthrombi in the choriocapillaris cause localized ischemic injury to the retinal pigment epithelium (RPE), resulting in a dysfunction of the outer blood–retinal barrier as well as a decreased ability of the RPE to transport fluid out of the subretinal space.[21] Fluid extravasation from choroidal vessels can then pass through small disruptions of the RPE, extending into the subretinal space and manifesting as serous retinal detachments.[22] Both subretinal and intraretinal fluid accumulations have been reported.[9] Some groups observed large tears of the RPE leading to acute decrease in vision.[23] Hemorrhage in the posterior segment may vary from subclinical small intraretinal dot hemorrhages to widespread sub-RPE, subretinal or intravitreal hemorrhage resulting in dramatic decrease in vision.[15,17,20] Choroidal hemorrhage seems to be more specific and has rarely been described in conditions other than the coagulopathic disorders described in this chapter. Cotton-wool spots, typically located around the optic disc, are generally related to a secondary cause such as hypertension or other systemic disease.[24] Whereas the decrease in vision from fluid accumulation and hemorrhage may recover following resolution and resorption,[16] visual impairment due to choroidal infarction is frequently permanent.[25]

The preferential localization of fibrin-formation and occlusion in the choroidal bed at the posterior pole has not yet been fully explained. Cogan proposed the hypothesis that a sudden deceleration of the blood flow between the short posterior ciliary arteries and the choriocapillaris sinusoids greatly facilitates clot precipitation in this region.[14] Although early case reports did not demonstrate any involvement of the retinal vasculature, more recently, Lewis et al. published a case of severe DIC in meningococcemia with impaired retinal circulation.[26] The authors speculated that this may also have been due to septic emboli and not a direct effect of DIC. Schwartz et al. reported a case with bilateral central retinal artery occlusion and central retinal vein occlusion in TTP secondary to adult-onset Still's disease.[27]

There are also reports describing ocular involvement of DIC and TTP in neonates.[28] Common causes of mechanisms in this setting include placenta previa, sepsis, trauma, hepatocellular failure or infant respiratory distress syndrome (IRDS). The ocular fundi show extensive hemorrhages in the retina or the vitreous, usually with concomitant focal retinal detachments. In selected neonatal cases, anterior segment manifestations were also observed with hyphema, thrombi in the iris and the ciliary body, and subconjunctival hemorrhage.[29]

Ocular manifestations of toxemia of pregnancy are discussed in detail in Chapter 92 (Pregnancy-related disease). As the HELLP syndrome may be associated with DIC, all of the abovementioned complications may occur in this condition. Additionally, hypertensive retinal vascular changes are not uncommon. Mere presence of serous retinal detachments should not be used as an indicator of DIC, as these may also occur in pregnancy

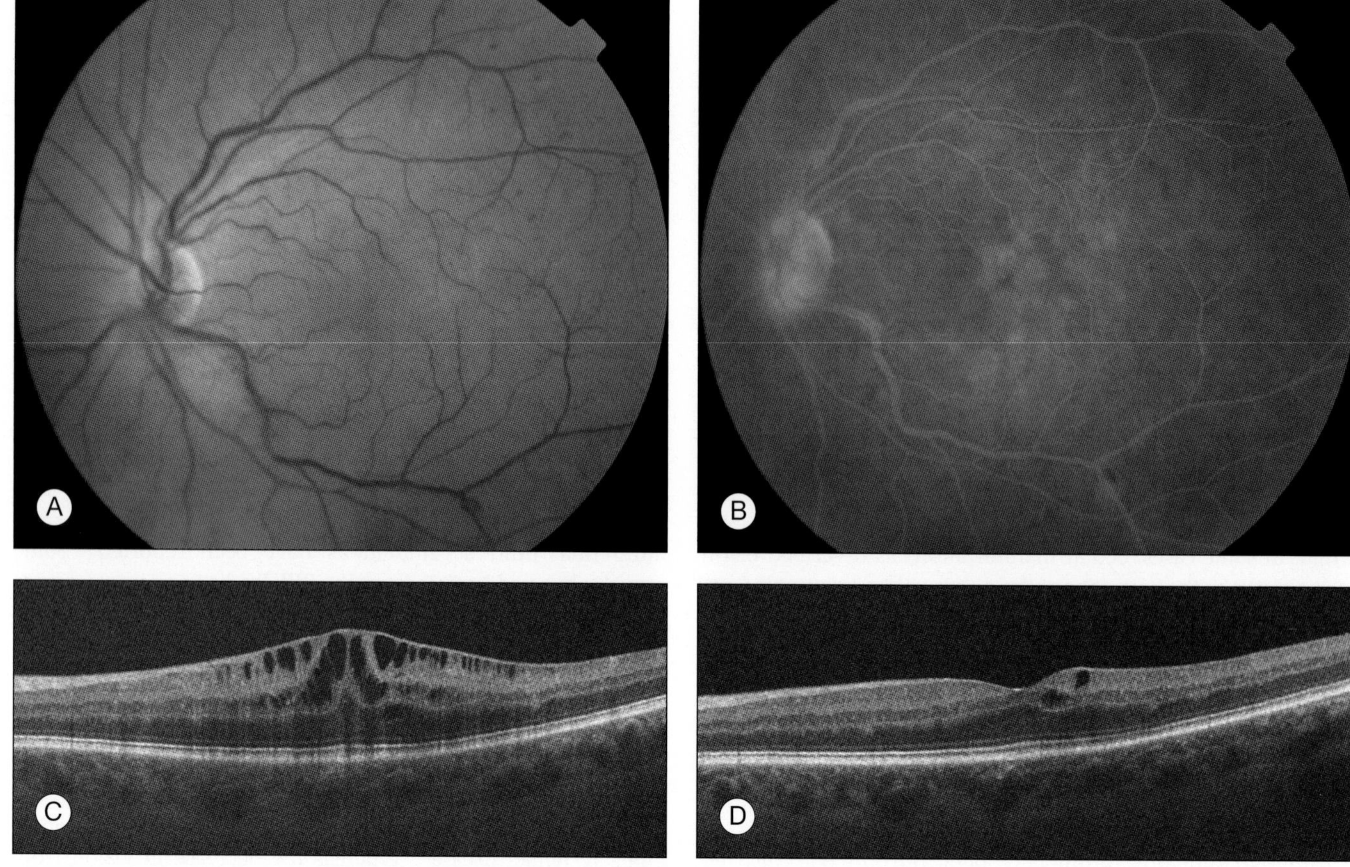

Fig. 60.1 A 75-year-old woman presented with a recent diagnosis of ITP and acute blurring of vision in her left eye with a visual acuity of 20/60. (A) Red-free photograph of the left eye illustrates a few scattered intraretinal hemorrhages in all quadrants with blurring of the inferior disc margin and loss of the foveal reflex. (B) Late-phase fluorescein angiogram demonstrates leakage from parafoveal capillaries with accumulation of dye in cystoid spaces as well as disc hyperfluoresence and focal staining of some vessels. (C) Spectral domain optical coherence tomography (SDOCT) B-scan through the foveal center shows cystoid macular edema involving multiple retinal layers. (D) SD-OCT B-scan 2 weeks following treatment with a single injection of intravitreal ranibizumab 0.5 mg. Note significant reduction in edema.

independent of the presence or absence of DIC and pregnancy-associated hypertension.[30,31]

CONCLUSION

DIC and related coagulopathies generally exhibit very similar ocular manifestations, which include widespread retinal or vitreous hemorrhage, subretinal or intraretinal fluid accumulation and choroidal infarction (see Fig. 60.1). The anterior segment is rarely involved in these disease processes. While visual loss related to these conditions is usually not the chief driver in the treatment of the underlying potentially life-threatening systemic diseases, ocular findings may be the initial presentation that enables the diagnosis of these disorders.

REFERENCES

1. Bick RL. Disseminated intravascular coagulation: current concepts of etiology, pathophysiology, diagnosis, and treatment. Hematol/Oncol Clin North Am 2003;17:149–76.
2. Gando S, Kameue T, Nanzaki S, et al. Disseminated intravascular coagulation is a frequent complication of systemic inflammatory response syndrom. Thromb Haemost 1996;75:224–8.
3. Levi M, Nieuwdorp M, vander Poll T, et al. Metabolic modulation of inflammation-induced activation of coagulation. Semin Thromb Hemost 2008;34:26–32.
4. Favaloro EJ. Laboratory testing in disseminated intravascular coagulation. Semin Thromb Hemost 2010;36:458–68.
5. Bernard GR, Vincent AL, Laterre PF, et al. Efficiacy and safety of recombinant human activated protein C for severe sepsis. N Engl J Med 2001;344:699–709.
6. Levi M, Schultz M. Coagulopathy and platelet disorders in critically ill patinets. Minerva Anestesiol 2010;76:851–9.
7. Tsai HM. Platelet activation and the formation of the platelet plug: deficiency of ADAMTS13 causes thrombotic thrombocytopenic purpura. Arterioscler Thromb Vasc Biol 2003;23:388–96.
8. Moake JL. Thrombotic microangiopathies. N Engl J Med 2002;347:589–600.
9. Hay-Smith G, Sagoo MS, Raina J. Fatal thrombotic thrombocytopenic pupura presentng with choroidal vasculopathy and serous retinal detachment. Eye 2006;20:982–4.
10. Tsai H. Current concepts in thrombotic thrombocytopenic purpura. Ann Rev Med 2006;57:419–36.
11. Eremina V, Jefferson JA, Kowalewska J, et al. VEGF inhibition and renal thrombotic microangiopathy. N Engl J Med 2008;358:1129–36.
12. Stella C, Malik K, Sibai B. HELLP syndrome: an atypical presentation. Am J Obstet Gynecol 2008;198:e6–e8.
13. Sibai BM, Ramadan MK, Usta I, et al. Maternal morbidity and mortality in 442 pregnancies with hemolysis, elevated liver enzymes, and low platelets (HELLP syndrome). Am J Obstet Gynecol 1993;169:1000–6.
14. Cogan DG. Ocular involvement in disseminated intravascular coagulopathy. Arch Ophthalmol 1975;93:1–8.
15. Majji A, Bhatia K, Mathai A. Spontaneous bilateral peripapillay, subhyalid and vitreous hemorrhage with severe anemia secondary to idiopathic thrombocytopenic purpura. Ind J Ophthalmol 2010;58:234–6.
16. Meyer CH, Callizo J, Mennel S, et al. Complete resorption of retinal hemorrhages in idiopathic thrombocytopenic purpura. Eur J Ophthalmol 2007;17:128–9.
17. Karagiannis D, Gregor Z. Valsalva retinopathy associated with idiopathic thrombocytopenic purpura and positive antiphospholipid antibodies. Eye 2006;20:1447–9.
18. Wyszynski RE, Fran KE, Grossniklaus HE. Bilateral retinal detachments in thrombotic thrombocytopenic purpura. Grafes Arch Clin Exp Ophalmol 1988;226:501–4.
19. Sodhi PK, Jose R. Subconjunctival hemorrhage: the first presenting clinical feature of idiopathic thrombocytopenic purpura. Jpn J Ophthalmol 2003;47:316–18.
20. Okuda A, Inoue M, Shinoda K, et al. Massive bilateral vitreoretinal hemorrhage in patient with chronic refractory idiopathic thrombocytopenic purpura. Graefes Arch Clin Exp Ophthalmol 2005;243:1190–3.

21. Nanayakkara P, Gans RO, Reichert-Thoen J, et al. Serous retinal detachment as an early presentation of thrombotic thrombocytopenic purpura. Eur J Intern Med 2000;11:286–8.
22. Jellie HG, Gonder JR, Canny CL, et al. Ocular involvement in thrombotic thrombocytopenic purpura: the angiographic and histopathological features. Can J Ophthalmol 1984;19:279–83.
23. Hartley KL, Benz MS. Retinal pigment epithelium tear associated with a serous detachment in a patient with thrombotic thrombocytopenic purpura and hypertension. Retina 2004;24:806–8.
24. Matsuo T, Matsuura S, Nakagawa H. Retinopathy in a patient with thrombotic thrombocytopenic purpura complicated by polymyositis. Jpn J Ophthalmol 2000;44:161–4.
25. Patel N, Riordan-Eva P, Chong V. Persistent visual loss after retinochoroidal infarction in pregnancy-induced hypertension and disseminated intravascular coagulation. J Neuroophthalmol 2005;25:128–30.
26. Lewis K, Herbert EN, Williamson TH. Severe ocular involvement in disseminated intravascular coagulation complicating meningococcaemia. Graefes Arch Clin Exp Ophthalmol 2005;243:1069–70.
27. Schwartz SG, Hickey M, Puliafito CA. Bilateral CRAO and CRVO from thrombotic thrombocytopenic purpura: OCT findings and treatment with triamcinolone acetonide and bevacizumab. Ophthal Surg Lasers Imaging 2006;37:420–2.
28. Schaffer DB. Eye findings in intrauterine infections. Clin Perinatol 1981;8: 415–43.
29. Ortiz JM, Yanoff M, Cameron JD, et al. Disseminated intravascular coagulation in infancy and in the neonate. Ocular findings. Arch Ophthalmol 1982;100: 1413–15.
30. Brismar G, Schimmelpfennig W. Bilateral exudative retinal detachment in pregnancy. Acta Ophthalmol (Copenh) 1989;67:699–702.
31. Mayo GL, Tolentino MJ. Images in clinical medicine. Central serous chorioretinopathy in pregnancy. N Engl J Med 2005;353:e6.

For additional online content visit http://www.expertconsult.com

Chapter 61

Pediatric Retinal Vascular Diseases

Thomas C. Lee, Michael F. Chiang

RETINOPATHY OF PREMATURITY

Retinopathy of prematurity (ROP) is a disease affecting the retinas of premature infants. Its key pathologic feature, local ischemia with subsequent retinal neovascularization, has common features with other proliferative disorders such as diabetic and sickle-cell retinopathy. ROP is unique in that the vascular disease is found only in infants with incompletely vascularized retinas. The spectrum of ROP disease ranges from mild cases without visual sequelae to advanced cases with bilateral irreversible blindness.

Historical perspective

Early history

ROP was first described in 1942,[1,2] and quickly became the primary cause of childhood blindness throughout the developed world.[3] Terry's original reports designated the condition retrolental fibroplasia (RLF), based on his impression that it involved a proliferation of the embryonic hyaloid system, but Owens and Owens[4] found that the hyaloid system was normal at birth and that RLF developed postnatally. As the pathogenesis and clinical manifestations became better understood, the term "retinopathy of prematurity" was adopted.

The discovery of the relationship between supplementary oxygen and ROP in the 1950s[5–9] led to rigid curtailment of oxygen supplementation in the nursery, and a dramatic decrease in ROP incidence followed. Unfortunately this had an adverse effect on infant morbidity and mortality (e.g., respiratory distress syndrome, cerebral palsy, neurologic disorders).[10–12]

Retinopathy of prematurity and contemporary nursery practices

By the early 1970s, arterial blood gas analysis had come into general use, and the oxygen requirements of premature infants with respiratory distress syndrome were better documented.[13] This enabled pediatricians to titrate the incubator oxygen concentration to more nearly meet the individual premature infant's oxygen needs.

Modern transcutaneous oxygen monitoring and continuous pulse oximetry have provided additional noninvasive tools, allowing neonatologists to monitor babies in real time more closely. These have stimulated studies, including large mutlicenter oygen restriction trials, which have found that lower target oxygen saturation levels (e.g., 85–89%) correlate with significantly improved rates of severe ROP but are also associated with increased mortality rates.[14–16] At this time, general consensus regarding target oxygen saturation levels that balance ROP risk and mortality has not been reached.

With improvements in neonatology practice, more of the smallest premature infants are now surviving. Eight percent of low-birth-weight infants survived in 1950, but with ventilators, surfactant, intravenous nutrition, and other gains in knowledge, survival has risen to 37–72%.[17–19] Clearly, infants are surviving today with more immature retinal vasculature and therefore higher ROP risk. For this reason, and because of common pathophysiology with other proliferative vascular diseases such as diabetic retinopathy, there has been mounting interest in ROP.[20–22]

The role of oxygen

Clinical findings

Results of controlled nursery studies[5,8] that suggested supplementary oxygen to be the principal cause of ROP in the epidemic of the early 1950s were confirmed, and the role of prolonged oxygen was documented in a collaborative randomized controlled trial.[9]

Since that time, attempts to delineate the critical blood oxygen levels producing ROP have not resulted in definitive conclusions. In a prospective study of 589 infants monitored by intermittent blood gas measurements, and where clinical goals were to avoid elevated arterial oxygen, the occurrence of ROP was not related to arterial oxygen levels.[23] Only the duration of oxygen exposure was a risk factor. Somewhat unexpectedly, continuous transcutaneous monitoring of blood oxygen levels was found in one study to be of no more value than intermittent monitoring in preventing visual disability.[24] It was suggested by Lucey and Dangman[25] that therapeutic oxygen, although important, has been overemphasized as a cause of ROP in contemporary neonatal practice.* They emphasized that other factors related to very low birth weight are also important, especially in view of current nursery oxygen monitoring.

Recent studies, including large mutlicenter oygen restriction trials, have found that lower target oxygen saturation levels (e.g., 85–89%) correlate with significantly improved rates of severe ROP, but are associated with increased mortality rates.[14–16] At this time, a consensus about optimal target oxygen saturation levels has not been reached.

**We agree with the conclusions in that report but do not agree with all the reasons cited by the authors. They point out that, by combining data from the early clinical studies in oxygen, approximately one-third of the "high-oxygen" group infants did not develop ROP. The failure to detect ROP in many of the high-oxygen group could be readily explained by the inability to view the peripheral fundus with the direct ophthalmoscope, the instrument used in studies in the early 1950s. As a result, patients with stages 1 and 2 ROP, particularly in zone III or peripheral zone II, could have been recorded as normal. Furthermore, because the majority of cases of stages 1 and 2 disease undergo spontaneous regression, ROP would not have been detected on follow-up examination.*

Experimental findings

In the early 1950s the laboratory kitten model, which produced lesions resembling the early stages of human ROP, was used extensively because it demonstrated selective response to oxygen by the immature retinal vessels.[6,7] In the full-term newborn kitten, the immature retinal vascularization is comparable to that of a human fetus at 6 months' gestation, thus providing the unique opportunity to study the response to oxygen of the immature retina, albeit in a full-term, healthy animal.[3] When hyperoxia studies were extended to other animal models, such as the young mouse and puppy,[6] the general concept of oxygen toxicity to immature retinal vessels was reinforced.

Investigators[26,27] have pointed out the histologic differences in the retinas of these animal models from the human but were unable to explain why progression to retinal detachment did not occur. It is noteworthy that McLeod et al. reported the production of intravitreal neovascularization with traction retinal folds in young dogs exposed to hyperoxia.[28] These findings add to the potential application of the canine model to investigate these stages of ROP (Figs 61.1 and 61.2 online).

The hyperoxic animal models demonstrated that only the incompletely vascularized retina was susceptible to oxygen's adverse effect, and that the more immature the vascularization, the greater the pathologic response to oxygen.[29] These findings supported the clinical observation that the infant with a less mature retina has greater ROP susceptibility, and that the infant with a fully vascularized retina has no risk. Accordingly, the temporal retina, the last part to vascularize, remains susceptible to ROP the longest (Fig. 61.3 online).

Mechanism of oxygen's effects on the immature retina

Primary stage of retinal vasoconstriction and vascular occlusion

The primary effect of elevated blood oxygen in any retina is vasoconstriction, which, if sustained, is followed by some degree of vascular closure. In young kittens, initial vasoconstriction occurs within several minutes after oxygen exposure. Vascular caliber is reduced by approximately 50% initially, but then rebounds to its original dimensions. Continued oxygen exposure results in gradual vasospasm during the next 4–6 hours, until the vessels are approximately 80% constricted.[30] At this stage, constriction is still reversible. However, if significantly elevated arterial oxygen partial pressure levels persist for an additional period (e.g., 10–15 hours), some immature peripheral vessels are permanently occluded.[7,23]

This occlusion progresses as the duration of hyperoxia increases, and local vascular obliteration is complete after 2–3 days of exposure. In the dog, after 4 days of exposure to hyperoxia, most capillaries are lost and only major blood vessels survive.[31]

Electron microscopic observations demonstrate selective hyperoxic injury to the endothelial cells of the most immature vessels, without obvious changes in the neuronal elements of the retina.[32]

Secondary stage of retinal neovascularization

After removal of the laboratory animal to ambient air following sustained hyperoxia, marked endothelial proliferation arises from the residual vascular complexes adjacent to retinal capillaries ablated during hyperoxia (Fig. 61.4 online). This can be demonstrated on fluorescein angiography (Fig. 61.5). Nodules of proliferating endothelial cells canalize to form new vessels that not only grow within the retina, but also erupt through the internal limiting membrane to grow on its surface, similar to the neovascularization in other proliferative retinopathies (Figs 61.6–61.9). In the dog and cat, the initial preretinal neovascular formations are like angioblastic masses with few lumens (formations sometimes called "popcorn"), which mature into neovascular formations that include vessels invested with pericytes.[33,34] Although the neovascularization may be extensive, this is generally the maximum response to oxygen in the kitten model and is followed by progressive vascular remodeling and involution

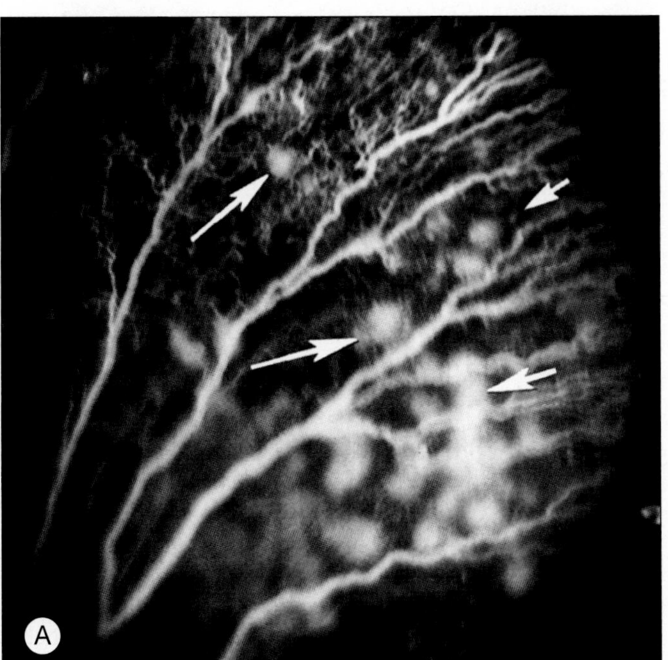

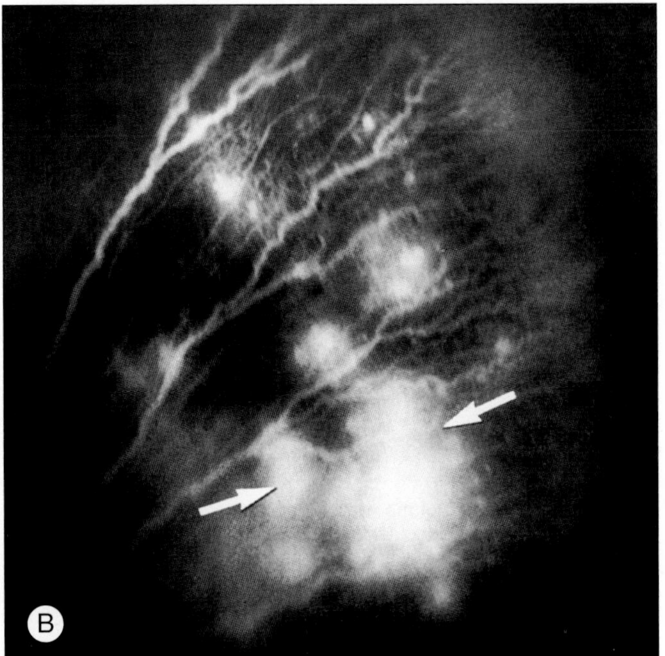

Fig. 61.5 (A) Fluorescein angiogram of a young kitten with oxygen-induced retinal neovascularization (arrows); midtransit phase of angiogram. (B) Late phase of angiogram of young kitten in A. Note dye leakage from neovascularization (arrows).

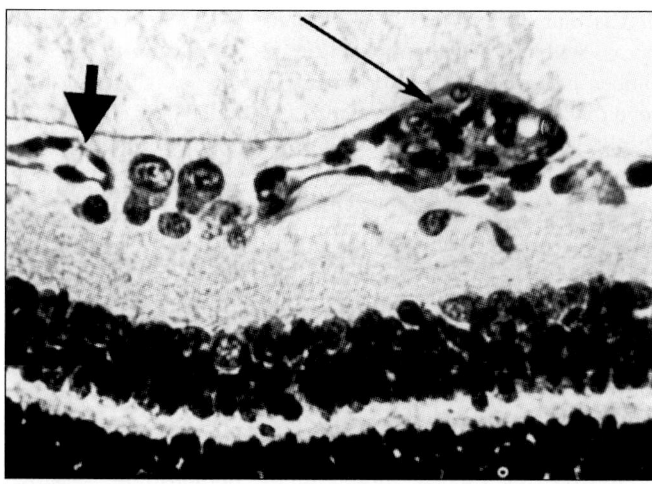

Fig. 61.6 Cross-section of the eye of a 21-day-old mouse exposed to hyperoxia. Normal capillary is seen just posterior to the area of vascular closure (short arrow); an endothelial nodule proliferating from the most anterior part of the vascularized retina is erupting through the internal limiting membrane (long arrow). (Reproduced with permission from Patz A, Eastham A, Higginbotham DH, et al. Oxygen studies in retrolental fibroplasia. II. The production of the microscopic changes of retrolental fibroplasia in experimental animals. Am J Ophthalmol 1953;36:1511–22.)

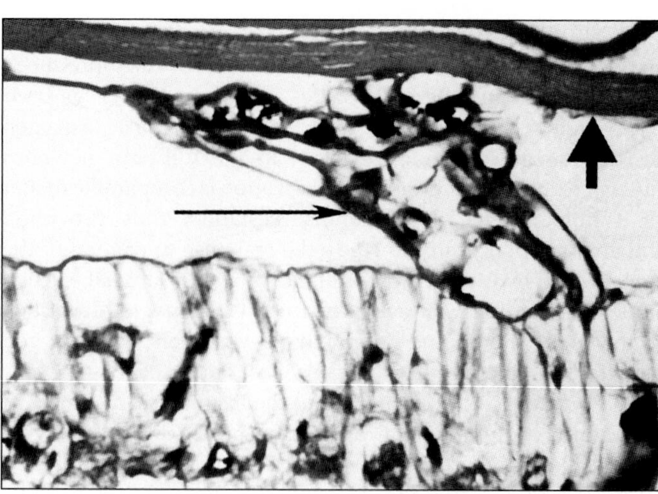

Fig. 61.8 Cross-section of the retina of a young kitten exposed to hyperoxia. Intravitreal neovascularization is seen just posterior to the zone of capillary closure (long arrow). Short arrow, lens capsule. (Reproduced with permission from Patz A. Oxygen studies in retrolental fibroplasia. IV. Clinical and experimental observations. Am J Ophthalmol 1954;38:291.)

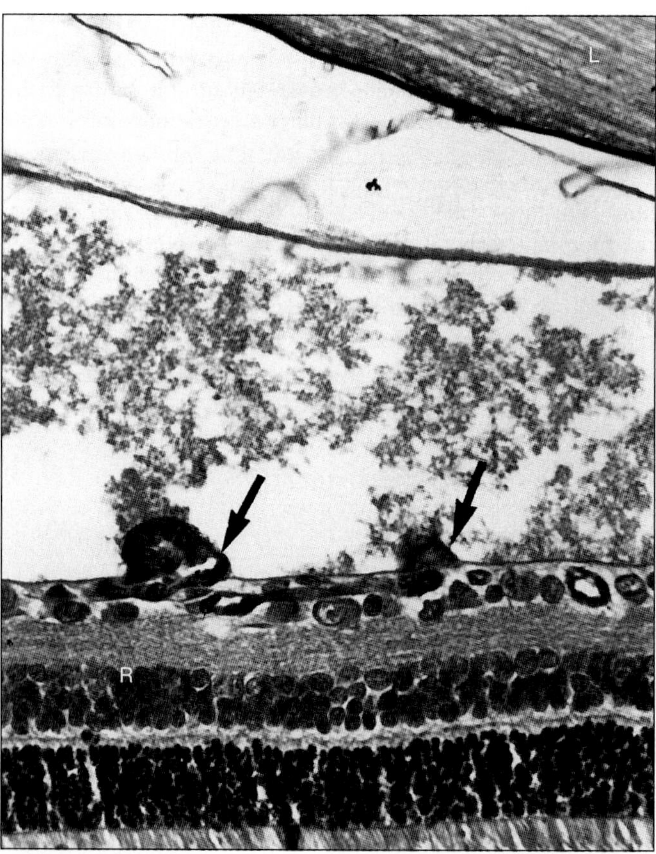

Fig. 61.7 Cross-section of the eye of a young mouse exposed to hyperoxia showing neovascularization on the surface of the retina just posterior to the zone of capillary closure (arrows). R, anterior retina; L, lens. (Reproduced with permission from Patz A. Clinical and experimental studies on retinal neovascularization. Am J Ophthalmol 1982;94:715.)

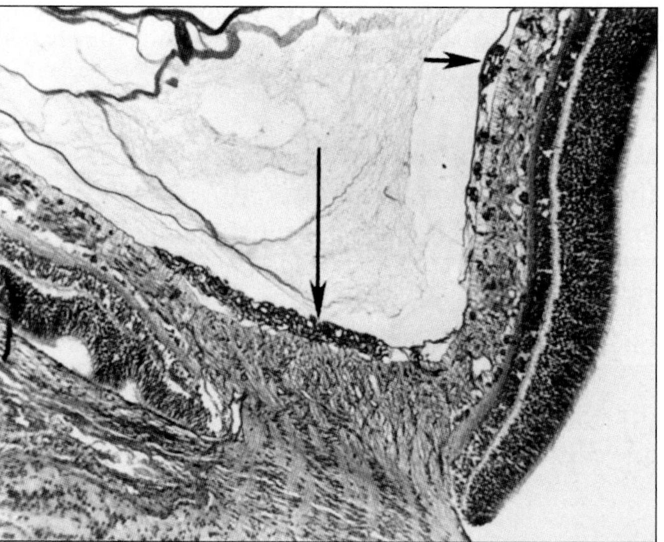

Fig. 61.9 Section of the retina of a young kitten exposed to hyperoxia. Neovascularization is seen over the surface of the disc (long arrow). Short arrow indicates small nodules of surface neovascularization. (Reproduced with permission from Patz A. Oxygen studies in retrolental fibroplasia. IV. Clinical and experimental observations. Am J Ophthalmol 1954;38:291.)

of abnormalities. The preretinal neovascularization in the dog persists and can develop into tented membranes which create tractional retinal folds in the retina (Figs 61.1 and 61.2).[28] The mouse and rat preretinal neovascular formations, however, will regress after 5 days.[30–35–37] Although regression is rapid and spontaneous in mice, the mouse model has been useful in evaluating topical[38] and systemic drugs,[39,40] experimental gene therapy strategies[41,42] and endogenous inhibitors like pigment epithelial growth factor.[43]

Oxygen exerts an important effect on the remodeling of the original primitive capillary network that develops in the retina.[44]

Capillaries regress from areas of higher oxygen concentration and grow toward areas of lower oxygen. Penn et al.[45] used experimentally alternating periods of high and low oxygen in the rat pup model to produce a more proliferative form of retinopathy. Pierce and colleagues[21] used hyperoxia and hypoxia in a mouse pup model to demonstrate the correlation of vascular endothelial growth factor (VEGF) protein production with periods of low oxygen, and its disappearance during oxygenation.

Pathogenesis

Normal retinal vasculogenesis

It is appropriate to review normal retinal vascular development as background for understanding ROP pathogenesis. Michaelson[33] originally suggested that retinal capillaries arise by budding from pre-existent arteries and veins that originate from the hyaloid vessels at the optic nerve head. Cogan[34] proposed a similar mechanism, except for the hypothesis of budding of solid endothelial cords from hyaloid vessels. Ashton[37] suggested that mesenchyme, the blood vessel precursor, grows from the optic disc through the nerve fiber layer to the periphery of the retina. Mesenchymal precursors have recently been observed far in advance of formed blood vessels in human fetal retinas.[46] On the posterior edge of the advancing mesenchyme, a "chicken-wire" meshwork of capillaries develops, and undergoes absorption and remodeling to produce mature retinal arteries and veins that are surrounded by the capillary meshwork.[37,44] Variations in capillary development may be species-specific. However, across all species studied to date, VEGF appears to be a key factor guiding vascular growth, which most closely fits the identity of Michaelson's proposed "factor X."[33] In the kitten, Chan-Ling and Stone demonstrated the role of astrocytes leading to growth of the capillary network.[47–49] Provis et al.[50] demonstrated the expression of VEGF message in the predicted location in the developing normal human retina, just anterior to the developing vessels (Fig. 61.10).

Figure 61.11 shows the normal rate of progression of the retinal vessels into the far retinal periphery in human premature infants without ROP according to their postconceptional age

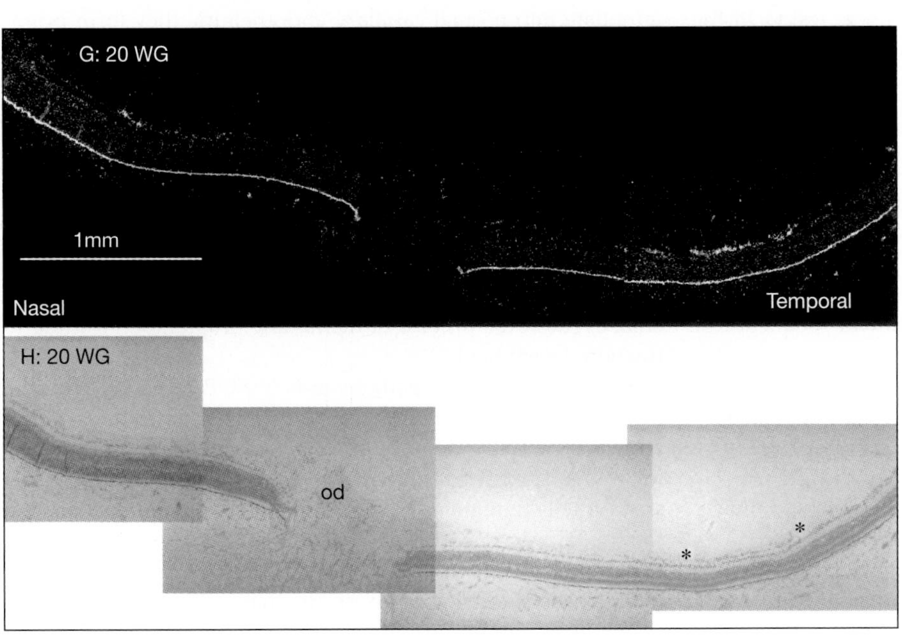

Fig. 61.10 Vascular endothelial growth factor (VEGF) mRNA expression in the human fetal retina. Bright (H) and dark-field (G) views of the retina in cross-section from a 20-week gestation human fetus. In dark-field illumination the retinal pigment epithelium is prominent. Note the greater differentiation of the retinal layers in the section to the right (temporal) of the optic disc. The vascular layer lies superficially, VEGF mRNA expression being limited to the most distal portion of that vasculature (G), indicated in the light-field image (H) by asterisks. (Reproduced with permission from Provis JM, Leech J, Diaz CM, et al. Development of the human retinal vasculature – cellular relations and VEGF expression. Exp Eye Res 1997;65:555–68.)

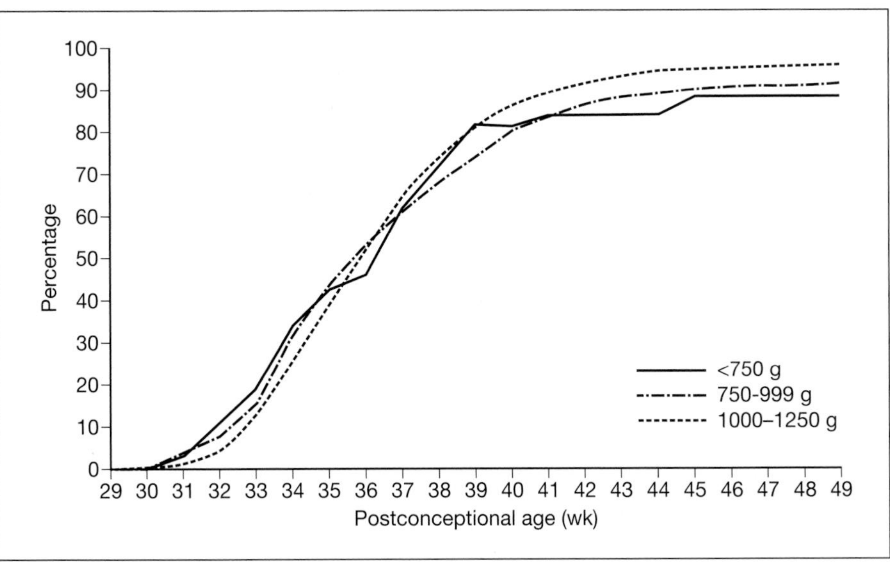

Fig. 61.11 Cumulative proportion of infants with no retinopathy of prematurity whose vessels end in zone III, by postconceptional age. (Reproduced with permission from Palmer EA, Flynn JT, Hardy RJ, et al. Incidence and early course of retinopathy of prematurity. Ophthalmology 1991;98:1628–40.)

(gestational age at birth plus chronologic age). More than 80% of prematurely born infants have been observed to develop this relatively mature retinal vasculature by the time they reach full term.

Pathogenesis of ROP

Initial changes in the developing vessels are described above, and historically this was believed to be an injury initiated by "excess" oxygen. Alon et al. demonstrated that hyperoxia caused downregulation of VEGF and death of endothelial cells, suggesting that VEGF is an endothelial survival factor.[51] In the time that follows closure of these growing vessels, the differentiating retina becomes increasingly ischemic and hypoxic and VEGF is upregulated[52,53] driving the neovascularization.[48]

Theoretically, the provision of increased oxygen should downregulate the release of such growth factor(s) and permit neovascularization to remodel and regress in an orderly fashion. Szewczyk[54] proposed this, and treated infants with significant ROP by returning them to oxygen. With no controls, it is difficult to know from his report if this success was simply due to spontaneous involution of ROP. This hypothesis was tested in the kitten model of oxygen-induced retinopathy. Systemic mild hypoxia was found to worsen the retinopathy,[55] whereas mild hyperoxia improved it.[56] With National Institutes of Health sponsorship, the multicenter Supplemental Therapeutic Oxygen for Prethreshold ROP (STOP-ROP) trial, chaired by Dale L. Phelps, found that, once the ROP was established, raising the oxygen saturation mildly did not harm the ROP, but neither was it of clear benefit.[57]

The clinical and histopathologic observations of Flynn and coworkers[58–62] led them to postulate the following sequence of events in human ROP pathogenesis:

1. Endothelial injury occurs where it has just differentiated from mesenchyme to form the primitive capillary meshwork. This is reminiscent of animal studies in which a short duration of hyperoxia resulted in capillary damage limited to the most recently differentiated vascular complexes (Fig. 61.4A). It is currently believed that environmental factors other than oxygen also are involved. For example, Brooks and associates found that nitric oxide may contribute to the vaso-obliterative stage of ROP,[63] while Alon et al. found that reduced VEGF may result in death of endothelial cells[51] because of its role as a survival factor.
2. After this injury to the vascular endothelium, the mesenchyme and mature arteries and veins survive and merge via the few remaining vascular channels to form a mesenchymal arteriovenous shunt which replaces the destroyed or damaged capillary bed.
3. The mesenchymal arteriovenous shunt is located at the demarcation between the avascular and vascularized retina. It consists of a nest of primitive mesenchymal and maturing endothelial cells that are fed by mature arteries and veins. No capillaries are found in the region of the shunt. Flynn[60] suggested that this structure represents the pathognomonic lesion of acute ROP.

Flynn described a dormant period after the injury (days to months), during which retinal findings are relatively stable. The tissues comprising the shunt may thicken, and the gray-white initial color of the structure turns from pink to salmon to red. He stated: "during this period when vasculogenic activity resumes in the retina, the fate of the eye is decided."[60] Flynn pointed out that when the cells inside the shunt divide and differentiate into normal capillary endothelium, they form primitive endothelial tubes that send forth a brush border of capillaries that grows anteriorly into the avascular retina. This represents ROP involution, which he observed to occur in more than 90% of cases at this early stage. In progressive disease, however, the primitive cells inside the shunt proliferate and erupt through the internal limiting membrane, growing on the surface of the retina and into the vitreous body. Flynn stated: "it is this lack of differentiation and destructive proliferation of cells and their invasion into spaces and tissues where they do not belong that is the chief event in the process of membrane proliferation leading to traction detachment."[60]

Foos[64–66] suggested a pathogenesis of ROP based on examination of histopathologic material. He used the terms "vanguard" and "rearguard" to describe cellular components of the developing retina. The vanguard (anterior) component contains spindle-shaped cells thought to be glia, which play a role in nourishing the immature retina during development.[67] The rearguard contains primitive endothelial cells. As the retina matures, the endothelial cells aggregate into cords that, according to Foos,[66] subsequently lumenize and become the primordial capillaries of the retina. It is from the rearguard and primitive endothelial cells that neovascularization of ROP develops (Figs 61.12 and 61.13). Foos noted that, as the developing vasculature reaches its most anterior extent and matures, the spindle cells of the vanguard

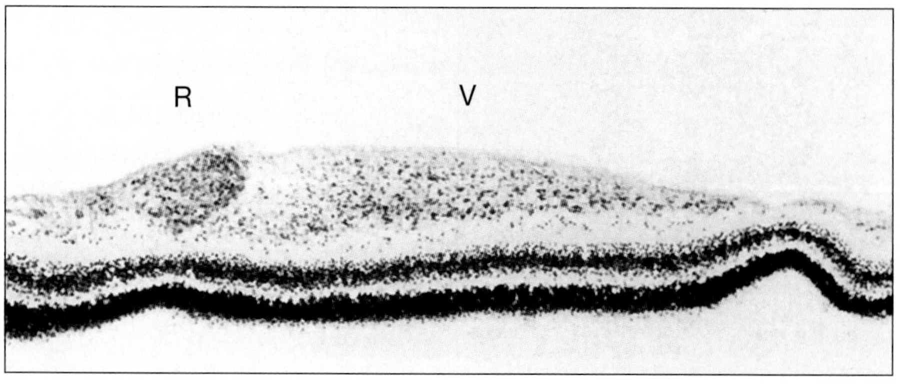

Fig. 61.12 Retinopathy of prematurity, stage 2, in a 27-week stillborn infant, showing a meridional section through the retinal ridge, with a thick layer of spindle cells that tapers anteriorly (to the right), representing the proliferative vanguard zone. Nodule of proliferating endothelial cells is seen in the rearguard zone. (Reproduced with permission from Foos RY. Retinopathy of prematurity – pathologic correlation of clinical stages. Retina 1987;7:260–76.)

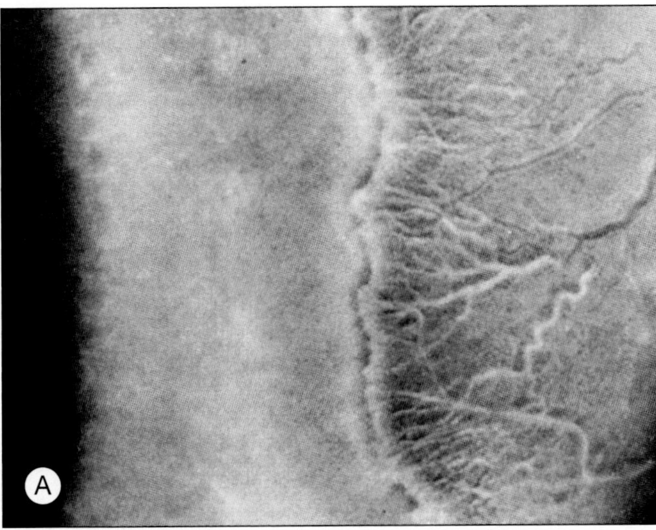

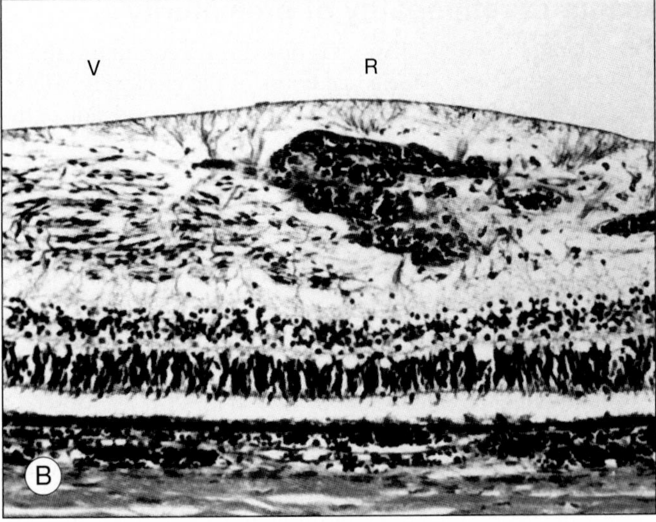

Fig. 61.13 (A) Retinopathy of prematurity, stage 2 specimen from a 29-week-old infant. Photomicrograph shows moderately elevated ridge, with tortuosity of retinal vessels posterior to ridge. (B) Photomicrograph of ridge in eye from A with posterior aspect of a thickened vanguard zone (V) and conspicuous vasodilation of rearguard zone (R), which has been characterized clinically as an arteriovenous shunt. (Reproduced with permission from Foos RY. Retinopathy of prematurity – pathologic correlation of clinical stages. Retina 1987;7:260–76.)

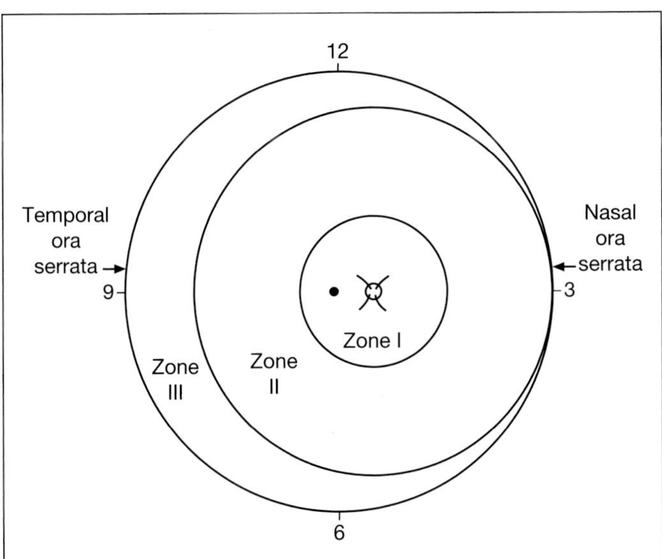

Fig. 61.14 Schematic diagram of a right eye, showing zones of the retina and clock-hours used to describe the location and extent of retinopathy of prematurity.

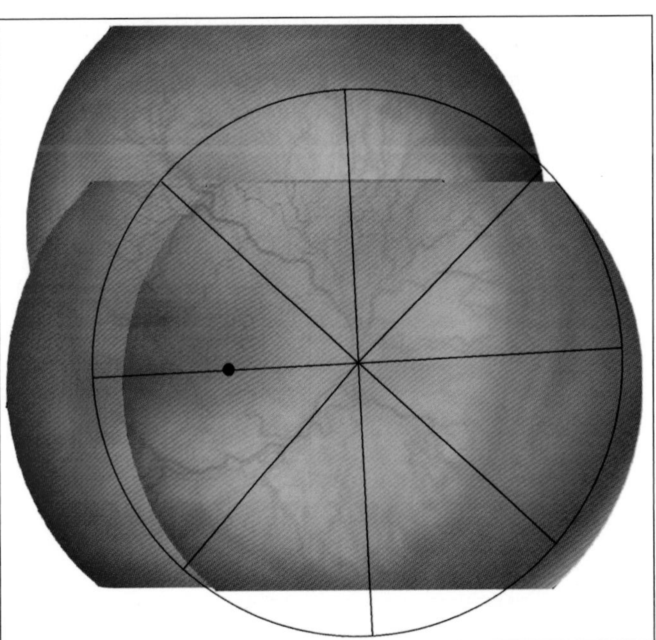

Fig. 61.15 Zone 1 grid overlaid on a montage of RetCam photos: black dot represents foveal center. Radius of circle is twice the distance from the disc to the fovea. This illustration demonstrates how retinopathy of prematurity may involve both zones I and II in the same eye.

disappear. The work of Chan-Ling et al.,[46] McLeod et al.,[68] and Provis et al.[50] showed that spindle cells are endothelial precursors and, in fetal human and neonatal dog retina,[68] the precursors organize and differentiate to form the initial retinal vasculature.[46]

International classification

The international classification of ROP divided the retina into three anteroposterior zones and describes the extent of disease by the 30° meridians (clock-hours) involved (Fig. 61.14). Retinal changes are divided into stages of severity, based on descriptive and photographic standards.[69]

Zones of involved retina

Each of the three zones of the retina is centered on the optic disc (Fig. 61.14). Zone I includes the posterior pole, and is defined as a circle, centered on the disc, whose radius is twice the distance from the disc to the macula. It subtends an arc of about 60° (Fig. 61.15). Zone II extends from the peripheral border of zone I to a concentric circle tangential to the nasal ora serrata. Temporally, this boundary corresponds approximately to the anatomic equator. Once the nasal vessels have reached the ora serrata, zone III is the remaining temporal crescent of retina anterior to zone II. Zone III, which is the farthest from the disc, is the last zone to become vascularized. It is clinically important to continue classifying ROP as zone II if there remains any active ROP or immature vessels in the nasal retina.

Extent of retinopathy of prematurity

The extent of the ROP changes is described according to the 12 30° sectors involved, labeled as hours of the clock (Fig. 61.14): the nasal side of the right eye is at 3:00, and the nasal side of the left eye is at 9:00.

Staging

Abnormal peripheral changes are divided into three stages, which may progress to retinal detachment (stages 4–5) (Figs 61.16 and 61.17).

Stage 1: demarcation line

Stage 1 is characterized by the presence of a demarcation line, the first ophthalmoscopic sign of ROP (Fig. 61.16A). This represents a structure separating the anterior, avascular retina from the posterior, vascularized retina. It appears flat and white, and lies within the plane of the retina. Abnormal branching or arcading of vessels leads up to the line. Stage 1 is relatively evanescent, generally either progressing to stage 2 or involuting to normal vascularization within several weeks. According to Garner,[70] the stage 1 demarcation line morphologically comprises two relatively distinct zones. The more anterior vanguard zone is formed by a mass of spindle-shaped cells, which are the progenitors of the differentiated vascular endothelium. As such it corresponds to the primitive mesenchyme (spindle cells) seen in normal fetal development but with a considerable increase in the number of cells. It is this hyperplasia, involving both thickening and widening, that makes the demarcation line visible.[70]

Stage 2: ridge

In stage 2, the demarcation line has grown into a ridge with height and width, which extends centripetally within the globe (Fig. 61.16B). The ridge may be white or pink and, rarely, vessels may even leave the surface of the retina to enter it. Small tufts of new vessels ("popcorn" lesions) may be seen located posterior to the ridge structure but not attached to it. The absence of fibrovascular growth from the surface of the ridge separates this stage from stage 3. According to Garner, the stage 2 retinal ridge results from the proliferation of endothelial cells "with some evidence of organization into recognizable vascular channels."[70] Flynn et al.[61] demonstrated that in this stage these channels leak fluorescein on angiographic examination.

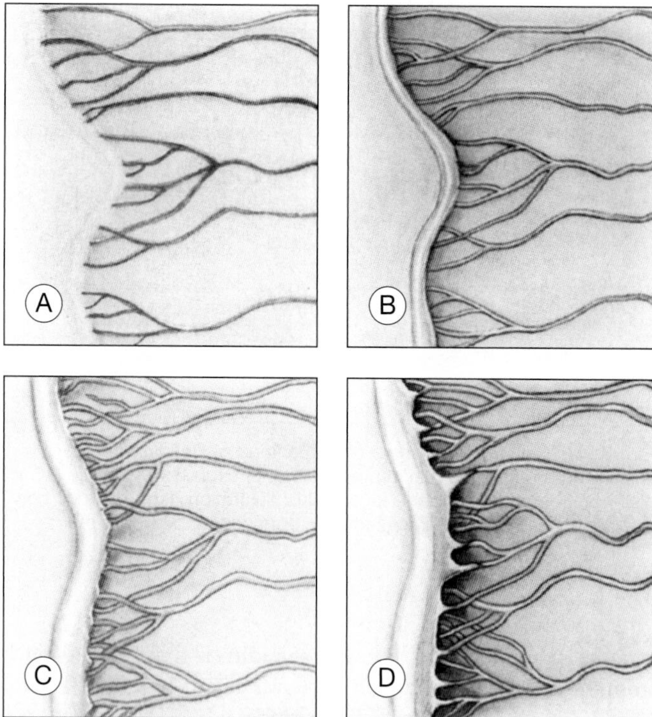

Fig. 61.16 Diagrams modified from color photographs of the international classification of retinopathy of prematurity. Vascularized, more mature retina is seen to the right and avascular retina to the left. (A) The demarcation line of stage 1. (B) The characteristic ridge of stage 2 is noted. (C) Extraretinal fibrovascular proliferative tissue of "mild" stage 3. (D) "Moderate" proliferation of extraretinal fibrovascular tissue from the ridge in more advanced stage 3. (Modified with permission from Committee for the Classification of Retinopathy of Prematurity. An international classification of retinopathy of prematurity. Arch Ophthalmol 1984;102:1130–4.)

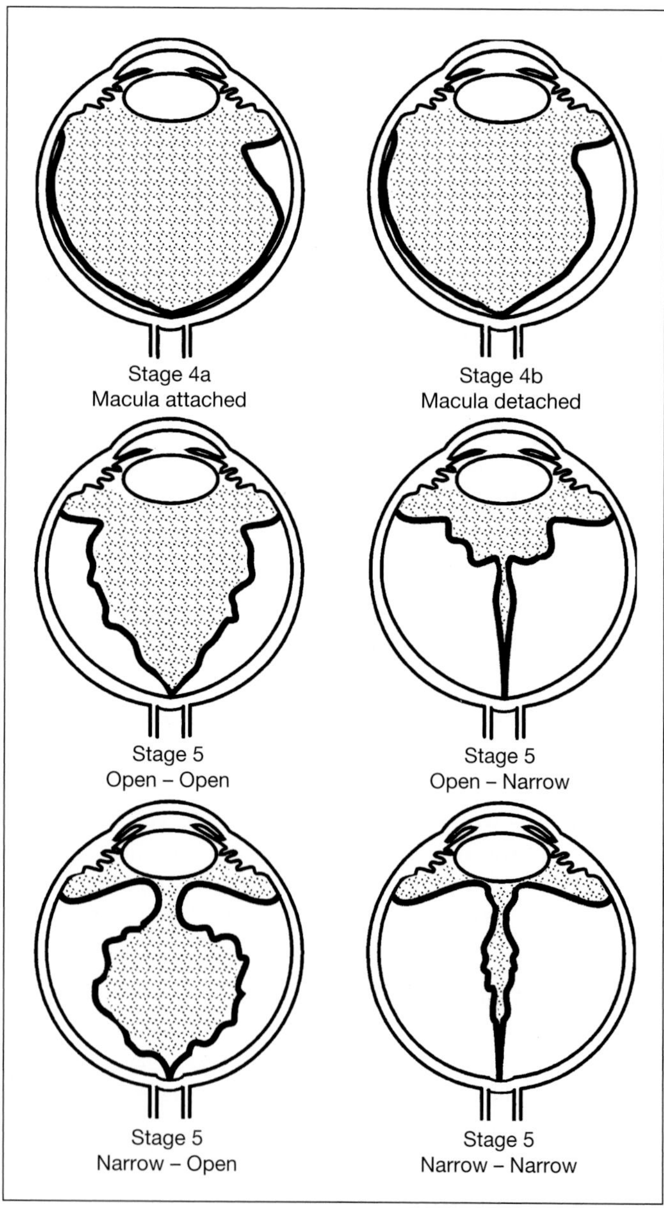

Fig. 61.17 Retinopathy of prematurity detachment configurations. Top two, stage 4a and b detachments; bottom four, stage 5. (Courtesy of Rand Spencer, MD.)

Stage 3: ridge with extraretinal fibrovascular proliferation

Stage 3 is characterized by the addition of extraretinal, fibrovascular tissue proliferating from the former ridge (Fig. 61.16C and D). This proliferating tissue is localized continuous with the posterior and interior aspect of the ridge, causing a ragged appearance of the ridge as proliferation increases into the vitreous. As in stage 2, vessels may leave the surface of the retina to enter the ridge and could be mistaken for retinoschisis or even detachment. The presence of elevated retinal vessels coursing from the retinal surface to the height of the ridge does not alone constitute a retinal detachment;[69] however, this may signify presence of vitreous traction. According to Foos,[66] the stage 3 "extraretinal vascularization" may appear placoid, polypoid, or pedunculated on histological examination. The placoid pattern is the most common and also the most important because it correlates with subsequent development of retinal detachment. Foos demonstrated that these extraretinal vessels are apparently derived from proliferating endothelial cells and not from the vasoformative mesenchymal "spindle" cells based on his factor VIII preparations. He also observed significant synchysis and condensation of the vitreous body in stage 3. Foos suggested that a condensation of the vitreous body over the ridge is related to depolymerization of hyaluronic acid and collapse of the collagenous framework into optically visible structures.[66]

"Plus" and "pre-plus" disease

Plus disease signifies a more florid form of ROP. Increasing dilation and tortuosity of the retinal vessels, iris vascular engorgement, pupillary rigidity, and vitreous haze indicate progressive vascular incompetence. When vascular changes are so marked that the posterior veins are enlarged and the arterioles tortuous, this represents plus disease, and a plus sign is added to the ROP stage number. This finding is a key sign of worse prognosis.[71] A published standard photograph selected by expert consensus, which has been used in four multicenter clinical trials and represents the minimum arteriolar tortuosity and venous dilation required for plus disease, is shown in Figure 61.18A. There has been increasing recognition of a spectrum of retinal vascular abnormalities in ROP. In 2005, the revised international classification defined an intermediate "pre-plus" categorization as abnormal arteriolar tortuosity and venous dilation of the posterior pole which is insufficient for diagnosis of plus disease.[72] Studies have shown that the diagnosis of plus disease may be subjective and qualitative, even among experts, and future definitions may be based on more quantitative measures.[73–75]

Zone I ROP

ROP located in zone I can be dangerously deceptive, in that the proliferation signifying stage 3 can appear spread out "flat" on the retina posterior to the ridge, rather than elevated.[36] In severe plus disease cases inside zone I, centripetal proliferation from the ridge may occur virtually simultaneously with detachment of the retina. Flynn and Chan-Ling examined the distinction between vasculogenesis (de novo formation of new vessels by transformation of vascular precursor cells) and angiogenesis (budding from existing vessels) with regard to the distinction of zone I and zone II ROP. They proposed that zone I ROP correlates with vasculogenesis, and is therefore less sensitive to treatment by laser or cryotherapy because the disease mechanism is not VEGF-mediated. They proposed that zone II ROP corelates with angiogenesis, is mediated by hypoxia-induced VEGF-165, and is therefore more sensitive to treatment by laser or cryotherapy.[76]

Aggressive posterior ROP

The 2005 revised international classification of ROP designated an uncommon, severe form of disease as "aggressive posterior ROP." This rapidly progressive disease variant had been previously termed "rush disease," and is characterized by its location in zone I or posterior zone II, ill-defined nature of the peripheral retinopathy, and prominent plus disease out of proportion to the peripheral findings.[72] This diagnosis can be made by a single examination without serial evaluation, and may not progress through the class stages 1–3. In fact, the peripheral disease may appear as a flat area of neovascularization at the junction of vascular and avascular retina.

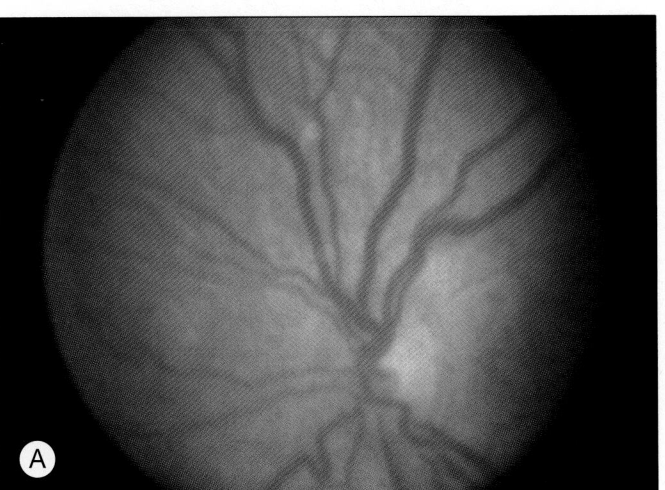

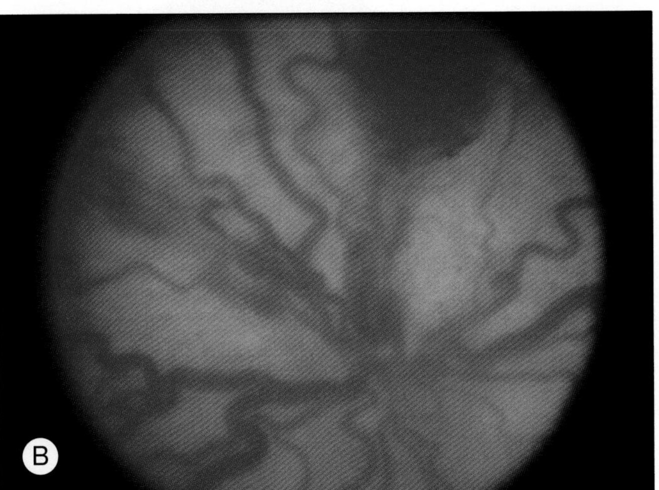

Fig. 61.18 Plus disease examples. (A) Fundus photograph of minimum dilation and tortuosity of retinal vessels considered as plus disease in National Institutes of Health studies of retinopathy of prematurity. (Reproduced with permission from Cryotherapy for Retinopathy of Prematurity Cooperative Group. Multicenter trial of cryotherapy for retinopathy of prematurity: preliminary results. Arch Ophthalmol 1988;106:471–9.) (B) Fundus appearance of an extremely severe degree of posterior pole plus disease in an eye that soon developed total retinal detachment. (Courtesy of Ophthalmic Photography, Oregon Health & Science University, Portland.)

Classification of retinal detachment

In 1987, ophthalmologists and pathologists established a second international committee, which expanded the original 1984 international classification to describe the morphology, location, and extent of retinal detachment (Fig. 61.17).[77] This classification was based on an understanding of the development of severe ROP gained from surgical experience[78] and pathology.[66] Stage 4 (subtotal) retinal detachment is usually tractional elevation added to findings in stage 3, although there may also be exudative effusion from adjacent active stage 3 neovascularization.

Stage 4A: extrafoveal retinal detachment

Typically this is a concave, traction detachment in the peripheral retina without involvement of the central macula (Fig. 61.19). Generally, these detachments are located at the sites of extraretinal fibrovascular proliferation with associated vitreous traction. Elevation may start in any zone where there was stage 3 disease that incompletely involuted following ablative treatment with laser photocoagulation or cryotherapy, and they may become circumferential. They may extend for 360° in the periphery without elevation of the macula, or they may be segmental, occupying only a portion of the periphery. The prognosis anatomically and visually is relatively good in the absence of posterior extension. Frequently these areas will reattach spontaneously, without affecting macular function.

Stage 4B: partial retinal detachment including the fovea

This can follow extension of stage 4A, or may appear as a fold from the disc through zone I to zones II and III (Fig. 61.20). Once a stage 4 detachment involves the fovea, the prognosis for recovery of good visual acuity is poor.

Stage 5: total retinal detachment

This is virtually always funnel-shaped. The classification of stage 5 detachments divides the funnel into an anterior and a posterior part (Fig. 61.17). When open both anteriorly and posteriorly, the detachment has a concave configuration and extends to the optic disc. An alternative configuration is one in which the funnel is narrow both anteriorly and posteriorly, and the detached retina is located just behind the lens. A third, less common type is one in which the funnel is open anteriorly but narrowed posteriorly. Least common is a funnel that is narrow anteriorly and open posteriorly. The configuration of the funnel-shaped detachment may be appreciated by ultrasonography.

Other factors related to retinal detachment

The classification of retinal detachment in ROP focuses attention on certain physical findings in stages 4 and 5:

1. Appearance of the retrolenticular space. This space may be occupied by heavily vascularized translucent tissue, which represents disease activity. As the disease subsides, the tissue occupying this space becomes white, with a scarcity of blood vessels. This is the appearance that gave rise to the original term "retrolental fibroplasia."
2. Peripheral trough. The presence of a peripheral red reflex in combination with apparent narrow funnel stage 5 retinal detachment indicates the presence of attached or shallowly detached avascular, stretched, and nonfunctioning peripheral retina. Occasionally, we have seen a peripheral red reflex coming from choroid beneath detached retina that has become adherent to the posterior lens capsule.
3. Anterior segment. In more severe cases of ROP, the anterior segment may become involved as follows:
   a. Shallow anterior chamber and corneal edema. A relatively shallow anterior chamber may be a normal early finding in a premature infant's eye; however, when a progressively shallow anterior chamber develops along with a retinal detachment in ROP, it has serious implications. Some cases progress to acute angle closure glaucoma or to a flat chamber and corneal decompensation. (See later section on glaucoma.)

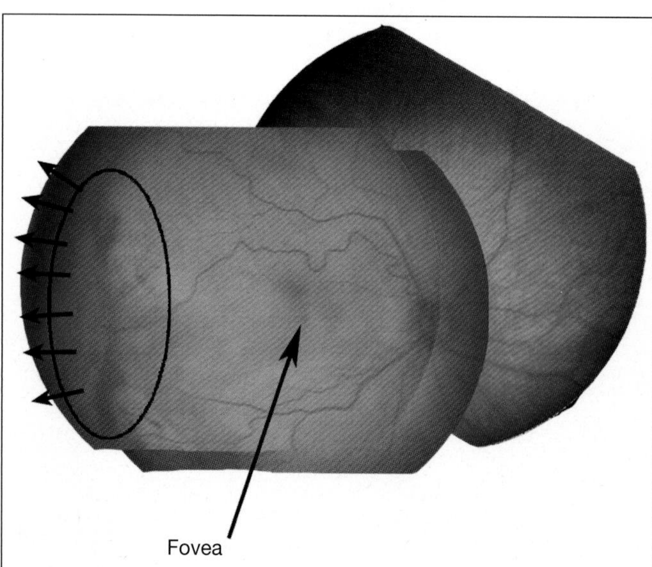

Fig. 61.19 Stage 4A retinopathy of prematurity (ROP). Fundus photo montage of right eye showing elevation of retina posterior to incompletely regressed stage 3 ROP with vitreous traction (arrows). Oval approximates area of retinal detachment.

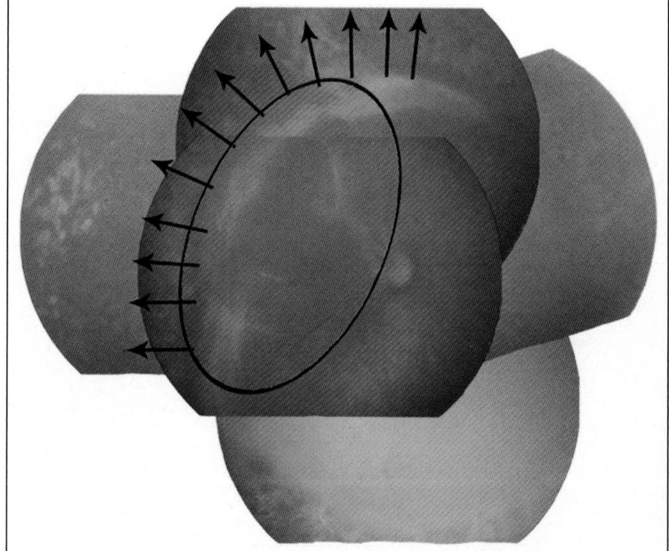

Fig. 61.20 Stage 4B retinopathy of prematurity (ROP). Fundus photo montage of right eye showing elevation of retina posterior to fibrotic ridge of incompletely regressed stage 3 ROP. Arrows away from ridge indicate vectors of vitreous traction elevating ridge and adjacent retina, including the macula. Oval approximates area of retinal detachment.

b. Iris abnormalities. Posterior synechiae, iris atrophy, and ectropion uveae are common formations in eyes with stage 4 or 5 ROP. Particularly in eyes with stage 5 disease, the iris may become rigid and the pupil difficult to dilate because of adhesions to the anterior lens capsule and persistence of the pupillary membrane with retention of its vascular network. Rarely, the pupil can seclude, leading to iris bombé and angle closure. (See later section on glaucoma.)

4. Other tissues. Subretinal blood and exudate may be identifiable by ultrasonography or optical coherence tomography, but it may be difficult to distinguish one from another. Subretinal fibrotic membranes may be present but usually are recognized only during surgery.

Involution of retinopathy of prematurity

Involution of ROP typically begins after 38 weeks' postconceptional/postmenstrual age, and may be characterized by a downgrading of staging and/or growth of retinal vessels into a more peripheral zone.[79]

Regressed rop: retinal detachment, strabismus, and amblyopia

Although active ROP usually involutes without progressing to retinal detachment, cicatricial sequelae can remain even in those cases.[80,81] The relatively stable state of the eye after retinopathy has run its course is referred to as regressed ROP. In Box 61.1 the residual changes have been classified into those affecting the retinal periphery and those affecting the posterior fundus. Retinal pigmentary changes may be mistaken for side-effects of treatment.[82]

The most serious complications of regressed ROP are late development of retinal detachment and angle closure glaucoma.

Box 61.1 Regressed retinopathy of prematurity

Peripheral changes
Vascular
Failure to vascularize peripheral retina
- Abnormal, nondichotomous branching of retinal vessels
- Vascular arcades with circumferential interconnection
- Telangiectatic vessels

Retinal
Pigmentary changes
- Vitreoretinal interface changes
- Thin retina
- Peripheral folds
- Vitreous membranes with or without attachment to retina
- Lattice-like degeneration
- Retinal breaks
- Traction or rhegmatogenous retinal detachment

Posterior changes
Vascular
Vascular tortuosity
- Straightening of blood vessels in temporal arcade
- Abnormal narrowing or widening in the angle of insertion of major temporal arcade

Retinal
Pigmentary changes
- Distortion and ectopia of macula
- Stretching and folding of retina in macular region leading to periphery
- Vitreoretinal interface changes
- Vitreous membrane
- Dragging of retina over disc

At almost any age after the neonatal period, but especially several years after birth, retinal detachment remains a risk in eyes with sequelae from ROP. Eyes with high myopia, peripheral retinal pigmentary changes or lattice-like degeneration, vitreoretinal interface changes, vitreous condensation, and stretching and folding of the retina are at special risk of developing retinal breaks and detachment. Eyes with partial retinal detachment present at about 3 months after threshold retinopathy remain at risk for progression of the detachment.[83] Overall visual outcomes for 61 eyes studied were poor: only six eyes had better than 20/200 visual acuity.[83] These patients and their parents should be alert to the symptoms of retinal detachment as soon as the child is old enough to appreciate and report them.

Patients with regressed ROP are at risk for developing strabismus and amblyopia.[84–88] In the Cryotherapy for Retinopathy of Prematurity (CRYO-ROP) study, 200 (6.6%) of 3030 infants who had weighed <1251 g at birth were strabismic at the 3-month examination. Presence of ROP was found to be a significant predictor of strabismus at 3 months. Subgroup analysis determined that the risk for strabismus increased as the zone of ROP became more posterior and the stage more severe.[89] Regular examinations and attention to refractive, visual, and extraocular muscle status are indicated for all infants who have had ROP until about age 18 months, and thereafter as clinically indicated.

In the multicenter Early Treatment for ROP (ETROP) study, the prevalence of strabismus at 6 months corrected age was 20% among infants with high-risk prethreshold ROP, and 10% among infants with low-risk prethreshold ROP. At 9 months corrected age, 30% of infants with high-risk prethreshold ROP had strabismus, and risk factors associated with development of strabismus included abnormal fixation behavior, presence of amblyopia, and outborn birth status (i.e., birth outside a study-affiliated hospital).[90] Overall, ophthalmologists should be aware of significant variability in ocular alignment early in life among infants with a history of severe ROP.

History of prematurity

In patients with a history of prematurity, particularly when there is significant myopia dating back to early childhood, careful examination is recommended to rule out any evidence of regressed ROP. This should be done regardless of the presenting age of the patient. Particular attention should be given to the temporal periphery of the retina in view of its relatively greater potential effects on macular vision.

Ocular findings of regressed retinopathy of prematurity

Myopia

In the CRYO-ROP study, 20% of infants with birth weight <1251 g were found to develop myopia in the first 2 years of life. The lower the birth weight, the higher the chance of myopia. Among infants with ROP, the incidence of myopia increased in direct relationship to the severity of ROP. For example, in patients who developed zone II, stage 3 ROP (without plus disease), 44–45% were myopic at 12 and 24 months postterm. In contrast, infants of this same birth weight group who never developed ROP had a 13% incidence of myopia.[91]

In the ETROP study, infants treated for high-risk prethreshold ROP were found to have 58% prevalence of myopia (defined as spherical equivalent ≥0.25 D) at age 6 months postterm, 68% prevalence of myopia at 9 months postterm, and little change thereafter until 3 years postnatal age. The prevalence of high myopia increased steadily between ages 6 months and 3 years. There was little difference in prevalence of myopia or high myopia between eyes with zone I versus zone II ROP, or between eyes with plus disease versus without plus disease. However, prevalence of myopia and high myopia was higher in eyes with retinal residual of ROP such as straightened temporal vessels or macular heterotopia.[92]

The exact mechanism of the myopia remains unclear. Fletcher and Brandon[93] suggested that it might be due to an elongation of the globe, alteration of the lens or the corneal curvature, or a combination of these factors. We have adopted the practice of questioning every new patient with moderate to high degrees of myopia regarding a past history of prematurity and have detected several previously unsuspected cases of regressed ROP.

Other refractive and binocular defects

Astigmatism and anisometropia are relatively common in patients with regressed ROP. In the CRYO-ROP study, 2518 infants born weighing <1251 g were refracted at 12 months postterm, and 3.3% had anisometropia. Of the 1548 who had ROP of some degree, 4.8% had anisometropia.[91] In the ETROP study, 401 infants with prethreshold ROP in one or both eyes were randomized to early treatment (laser photocoagulation at high-risk prethreshold ROP) versus conventional treatment only if threshold ROP developed. All infants were refracted at 6 and 9 months correct age, and at 2 and 3 years postnatal age. The prevalence of astigmatism was similar at each test age in the early treatment and conventional management groups. For both groups, there was an increase in prevalence of astigmatism (defined as >1.00 D) from 32% at 6 months to 42% at 3 years.[94]

Approximately 20% of ROP cases are asymmetric at the time they reach threshold for treatment, and this asymmetry may well contribute to anisometropia. Amblyopia, nystagmus, and strabismus are also common after ROP has regressed.[84,85,89,95] Taken together, these findings highlight the importance of follow-up ophthalmological examinations in infants with a history of severe ROP.

Lens and corneal changes

At the 12-month examination of the CRYO-ROP study, there was an overall incidence of cataract of 0.3% in the natural history population. The incidence of cataract among eyes with a history of zone I ROP or zone II stage 3+ ROP was approximately 2.5%.[96] At the final 6-year examination of the ETROP study, cataract or aphakia was found in 4.9% of early-treated eyes and in 7.2% of conventionally managed eyes in 271 children with symmetric ROP.[97] Kushner[95] pointed out that early development of cataract may seriously compromise vision in the presence of retinal abnormalities. Results can be satisfactory from cataract surgery in adults with a history of ROP.[98] Patients with ROP also have an increased risk of developing irregularities of corneal curvature, band keratopathy, and acute hydrops.[71]

Glaucoma in retinopathy of prematurity

Glaucoma is a serious complication of ROP in both the acute and regressed phases of the disease. The glaucoma in many of these patients is amenable to treatment.

Glaucoma in patients with advanced retinopathy

Patients with advanced retinopathy who develop a shallow anterior chamber occasionally develop acute or subacute glaucoma later. In the CRYO-ROP study, 20.3% of 195 patients with threshold ROP developed shallow anterior chambers in the control eye that did not receive cryotherapy, compared with 12% in the eye that received cryotherapy, when examined at about 12 months postterm.[99] By that time, 1.5% of those control eyes had been noted to have glaucoma.[100] This complication, which does not always look typical of iris bombé, may occur at any time: in the nursery, shortly after discharge, and throughout childhood. Where feasible, parents should be instructed to recognize the appearance of corneal haze and episcleral injection, and to seek ophthalmic consultation for these concerns. A trial of topical steroids and cycloplegic agents is recommended in suitable cases of glaucoma in the setting of ocular damage from ROP,[101] and further glaucoma management may be required.

Angle closure glaucoma in regressed retinopathy of prematurity

Eyes with regressed ROP are at increased risk of developing acute angle closure glaucoma, even in adulthood.[102,103] Kushner[101] pointed out that certain patients with mild degrees of regressed ROP have a predilection for developing ciliary block glaucoma. Because these forms of glaucoma may be treatable by surgery in selected cases, ophthalmologists and patients should be aware of these potential complications, their associated signs and symptoms, and their management.

Differential diagnosis

Although the differential diagnosis in a premature infant in a neonatal intensive care unit (NICU) is almost exclusively limited to ROP, there are several conditions that can mimic ROP out of that context in older children. Familial exudative retinopathy, incontinentia pigmenti (IP), and Norrie disease can all present with peripheral ischemic retina resulting in a tractional retinal detachment secondary to retinal neovascularization. ROP can be excluded in these cases if there is no history of prematurity. Retinoblastoma can simulate a retinal detachment, although it is exudative and has a convex as opposed to concave surface. The tumors associated with exudative detachments are typically quite large and would be seen on ultrasound. Persistent fetal vasculature (PFV) can have a similar appearance to ROP, but is usually unilateral. Coats disease is also generally unilateral and has substantial lipid exudates which are not typically seen in ROP.

Risk factors

In general, prematurity, low birth weight, a complex hospital course, and prolonged supplemental oxygen are today's established risk factors for the development of ROP.[10,72,104,105] Supplemental oxygen given for a period of weeks, without specific indication, was abundantly documented to be a major cause of ROP during the epidemic of the 1950s but is no longer the predominant factor in cases of ROP seen since the mid-1970s. Now, neonatal advances have resulted in improved survival rates of extremely low-birth-weight children. The risk of developing treatment-requiring ROP is higher in this group, with as many as 25% of children born at 750 g or less developing plus disease.[99]

The role of blood carbon dioxide levels in the development of ROP is controversial. Bauer and Widmayer,[106] following Flower's observation[107] that carbon dioxide enhanced the oxygen-induced retinal changes in beagles, conducted a retrospective analysis of infants with low birth weights. They reported that higher arterial carbon dioxide values were the most important variable in separating those infants of equal gestation who developed ROP from those without disease. Biglan et al.[108] and Brown et al.[104,109] failed to confirm this association and, indeed, found that infants with "scarring retinopathy of prematurity" had lower carbon dioxide blood levels. It is likely that this parameter, like many others, is associated with an unstable clinical course – as is ROP – but not necessarily linked with it causally.

Numerous other neonatal health factors have been reported to be associated with ROP, including cyanosis, apnea, mechanical ventilation, intraventricular hemorrhages, seizures, transfusions, septicemia, in utero hypoxia, anemia, patent ductus arteriosus, and vitamin E deficiency.[13,25,87,105–108–115] These associations require further investigation to identify causal relationships. In the CRYO-ROP natural history cohort of 4099 infants born weighing less than 1251 g, significant additional factors were identified, including white race, multiple birth, and being transported elsewhere for intensive care. Once ROP develops, greater risk is associated with ROP located in zone I, the presence of plus disease, the severity of stage, and the extent of circumferential involvement.[116,117] The risk factors studied during the CRYO-ROP study were consolidated into a mathematical model that can predict the risk of an unfavorable outcome for a particular eye that reaches prethreshold severity.[118]

Examination procedures in the nursery

General aspects and timing of the examination

The nursery surveillance carried out in the CRYO-ROP study produced definitive information concerning the early course of ROP. The "natural history" portion of this study recorded data from 4099 infants born weighing less than 1251 g. The study showed that ROP occurs on a schedule according to the infant's corrected age (postmenstrual age since mother's last menstrual period, or postconceptional age), rather than the time since birth, the so-called chronologic age (Fig. 61.21).[116] For infants in the birth weight category studied, it was found that those who develop stage 1 ROP (and no worse) do so at a median of 34.3 postmenstrual weeks. The median time for onset of stage 2 ROP that progresses no further is 35.4 weeks, and 95% of these cases have onset at 32 weeks or later. For patients with eyes

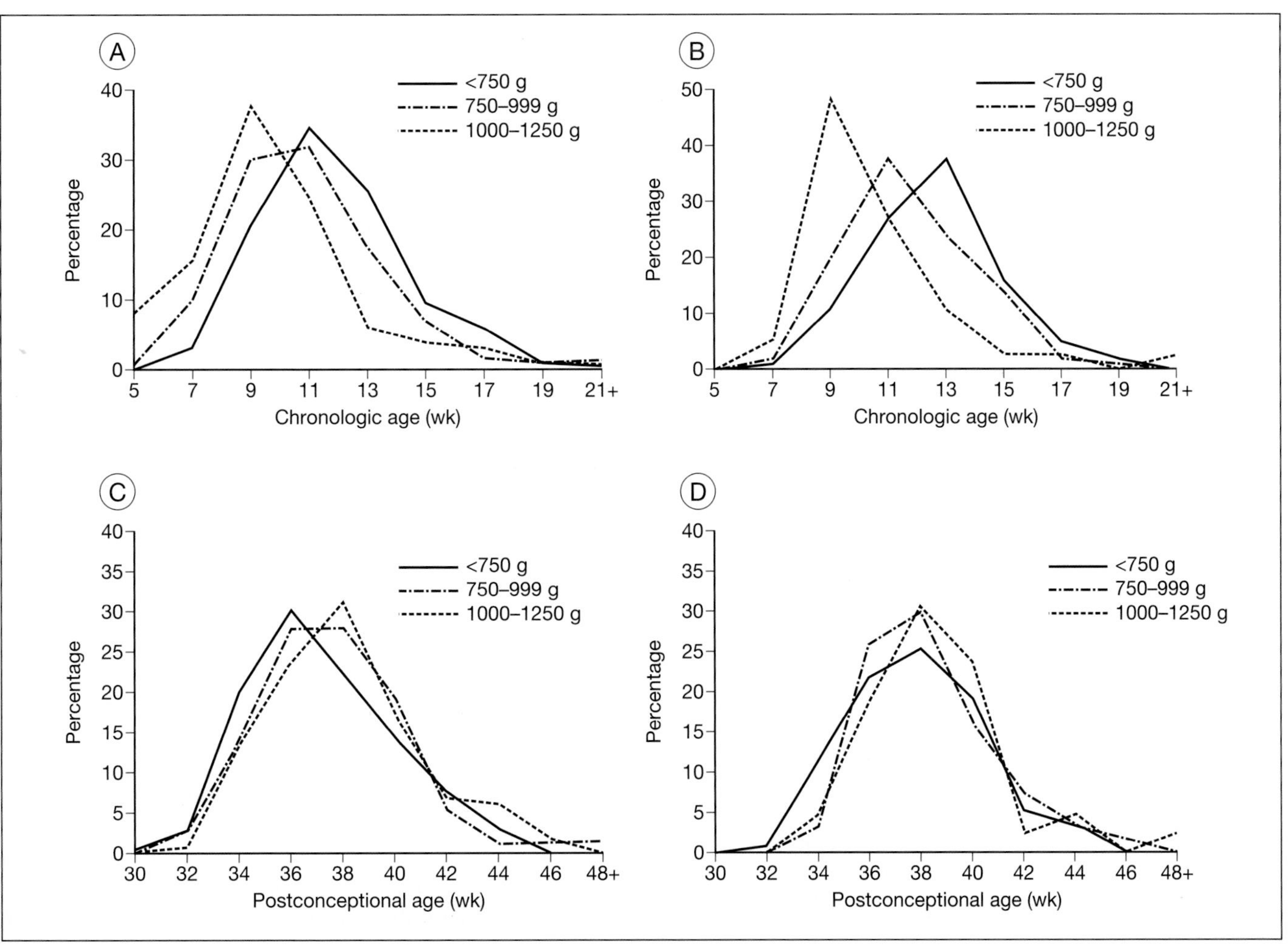

Fig. 61.21 (A) Distribution of onset of prethreshold retinopathy of prematurity (ROP) by chronologic age and by birth weight. (B) Comparable data for threshold ROP. (C) Prethreshold data by postconceptional age, for comparison with A (by chronologic age). (D) Threshold data by postconceptional age, for comparison with B (by chronologic age). (Reproduced with permission from Palmer EA, Flynn JT, Hardy RJ, et al. Incidence and early course of retinopathy of prematurity. Ophthalmology 1991;98:1628–40.)

Table 61.1 Onset of retinopathy of prematurity events in postconceptional age (weeks)

Stage	5th percentile	Median	95th percentile
1	*	34.3	39.1
2	32	35.4	40.7
Threshold	33.6	36.9	42

Not available; 17% of infants had stage 1 retinopathy of prematurity on the first examination.
(Reproduced with permission from Palmer EA, Flynn JT, Hardy RJ, et al. Incidence and early course of retinopathy of prematurity. Ophthalmology 1991;98:1628–1640.)

that reached the treatment randomization "threshold" severity of stage 3+ ROP (at least 5 contiguous or 8 interrupted clock-hours in zones I or II), the threshold was reached at a median of 36.9 weeks (90% of cases were in the range of 33.6–42.0 weeks) (Table 61.1).

Screening guidelines

Because ROP can progress to blindness during the first 3 months of life[119] and treatment is available to arrest it in many cases, a protocol has been recommended for examining the eyes of premature infants during that time span. In November 2002, Reynolds et al.[74] reported an analysis of combined data from the CRYO-ROP study ($n = 4099$) and the LIGHT-ROP study ($n = 361$) to develop screening criteria based on the evidence from those two clinical trials. The authors concluded that the initial eye examination should be performed by 31 weeks' postmenstrual age or 4 weeks from birth, whichever is later, in order to detect prethreshold retinopathy in a timely fashion. Prethreshold ROP is defined as ROP of less severity than the threshold severity in the CRYO-ROP trial, specifically as any ROP in zone I, or zone II ROP of stage 2+ or stage 3 with or without plus disease. It appeared that most risk had passed not only whenever full vascularization had been achieved, but also whenever vessels reached the nasal ora serrata without any ROP development prior to that. If the infant reaches 45 weeks' gestational age without developing prethreshold ROP or worse, the risk of visual loss from ROP is minimal.[74] The authors caution that recommendations for infants born prior to 24 weeks are by extrapolation. They also point out that the database excluded infants born weighing more than 1250 g, and some of those larger infants are at risk for ROP. Guidelines for those larger infants would need to be derived from different studies. It should also be noted that these are data from the USA, and the natural history of ROP may be different in other parts of the world. The current recommendations from the American Academies of Ophthalmology and Pediatrics are that children born at 30 weeks or less, or at less than 1500 g, should be screened for ROP. Specifically those born at a gestational age of 27 weeks or less should have their first exam at 31 weeks and children born from 28 to 32 weeks should have their first exam 4 weeks after birth. The subsequent examination schedule is determined by findings on the initial examination, as shown at the end of this chapter.[120]

Side-effects of the examination

Very-low-birth-weight infants, while they are still in a precarious general condition, must be managed with care. The stress of an indirect ophthalmoscopic examination is necessary whenever the risk of treatable disease capable of progressing to blindness exists or when information is needed to assist in the general medical evaluation.[121] Screening programs must be designed around the consideration that the procedure may be stressful for the infant.

Techniques of eye examination

Eye examinations should be performed at the request of, or with the approval of, an attending neonatologist. Pupils may be effectively dilated in most infants with Cyclomydril eye drops (cyclopentolate 0.2% and phenylephrine 1%), with the excess drops immediately blotted from the lids to minimize systemic side-effects such as hypertension and intestinal ileus.[121] The examination is performed about 25–30 minutes later using a binocular indirect ophthalmoscope and condensing lens. More heavily pigmented infants sometimes fail to respond adequately to the mydriatic drops, in which case 0.5% cyclopentolate or 1% tropicamide, or both, and 2.5% phenylephrine may be substituted and instilled twice. Most examiners generally use a lid speculum, and there are now a variety of designs suitable for premature infants (e.g., Barraquer, Sauer, Alfonso specula). The infant's hands should be physically restrained, and a nurse ordinarily assists with the exam. As a precaution against viral or chlamydial transfer, the lid speculum must be sterile for each infant and the examination lens should be wiped with an alcohol sponge between cases whenever it has touched the infant's face. The universal precaution of wearing gloves during examination is recommended.

In general, ROP severe enough to cause serious concern will be visible far enough posteriorly in the fundus to bring it into view without scleral indentation. However, to determine the final maturity of retinal vascularization requires either serial examinations past full term or, preferably, examination of the nasal retina to the ends of the growing vessels to determine whether vascularization has advanced into zone III.[77,116] For this far-nasal peripheral retinal examination, scleral indentation or eye positioning is generally needed. An aluminum-wired Calgiswab nasopharyngeal culture swab can be used as an inexpensive, sterile, and relatively gentle tool for this. The tip can be bent to any desired angle, even to resemble a fine muscle hook. Scleral depressors designed for infant examinations (e.g., Flynn depressor) are also commercially available. For scleral depression, topical anesthetic, such as proparacaine, is typically used. It is recommended that a member of the nursery staff be present during the entire examination to monitor the infant's airway, vital signs, and behavior and to deal with apnea or other adverse reactions that may occur.

Informing the patient's family

Often ROP becomes severe just as the infant is achieving medical stability, making it especially difficult on parents who have already experienced much anxiety. The ophthalmologist or neonatologist should keep families informed of the results of eye examinations. The ophthalmologist should contact the parents at the time it is first realized that the ROP is becoming severe, for example, when it develops in zone I or when zone II ROP reaches stage 3. If the parents are kept apprised of the eye condition as it develops, it may soften the emotional impact if the ROP ultimately causes vision damage, and it helps pave the way for discussion of possible surgical intervention.

Prophylaxis and therapy

The role of vitamin E

Vitamin E was considered as a potential agent to prevent ROP due to its antioxidant properties. It was evaluated by Johnson et al.[122,123] with subsequent controlled clinical trials having tested the role of large doses of vitamin E.[124–131] The results were equivocal and a report from the Institute of Medicine published in 1986 concluded: "Vitamin E as prophylaxis for retinopathy of prematurity was subject to a detailed analysis. This committee found no conclusive evidence either of benefit or harm from vitamin E administration. Risks from vitamin E appear to be minimal for premature infants provided that doses are kept moderate to achieve a blood level no higher than 3 mg/dl."[132] Currently, there is no formal recommendation on the use of vitamin E in the management of ROP.

The role of light

Historically there has been interest in a possible relationship between light and ROP. In his original descriptions of RLF, Terry[133] considered premature exposure of the eye to light as an important etiologic possibility.

Before the importance of the role of inspired oxygen levels was recognized in ROP, two studies addressed the question of the effect of light. In the late 1940s, Hepner et al.[134] patched the eyes of five premature infants from birth until they weighed 2000 g. They found that four of the five infants developed ROP and they concluded that light was not a factor in its development. In 1952, Locke and Reese[135] reported on a series of 22 premature infants (birth weight less than 2000 g) in which they had patched one eye of each baby. Both found that there was no difference in the incidence of ROP between the patched eyes and the unpatched eyes.[134,135]

To examine the relationship between light exposure and ROP more definitively, a feasibility trial of light-reducing goggles (LIGHT-ROP study), chaired by James D. Reynolds, was sponsored by the National Eye Institute in 1995 at three nurseries in the USA. Half of 409 infants with birth weights of less than 1250 g were randomly selected either to wear goggles containing 97% near-neutral density filters until 31 weeks' postconceptional age or to undergo no extraordinary light reduction. The study concluded that there is no clinically important effect of light on the occurrence or severity of ROP.[136] Neither the American Academy of Ophthalmology nor the American Academy of Pediatrics has made any recommendations about restricting ambient light from the eyes of premature infants.

Cryotherapy

From 1968, reports suggested that ablative treatment of the peripheral retina of premature infants with ROP may ameliorate the course of the disease. Those early reports suggested that photocoagulation[137,138] or cryotherapy[139,140] may accomplish this goal. Throughout the early 1980s, studies produced conflicting results and opinions regarding the efficacy and role of cryotherapy for severe ROP.[141–146] The need for a large-scale clinical trial was apparent.

The multicenter trial of cryotherapy

The CRYO-ROP study was organized in 1985 under the chairmanship of Earl A. Palmer. Supported by the National Eye Institute, the study began enrolling premature infants weighing 1250 g or less at birth in 1986. Although enrollment was scheduled to continue until mid-1988, it was stopped in January 1988 because preliminary results showed a compelling favorable effect of cryotherapy in improving the anatomic outcome for the macula of treated eyes.[99] The study has been continued for longer-term follow-up, and a final examination was carried out when the children were about 15 years old.[147]

Treatment

Infants eligible for the cryotherapy trial had stage 3 ROP, involving five or more clock-hours of retina posterior to zone III in the presence of a standardized plus disease.[69,99] Outlines of the protocol have been published,[100,116,148] as well as the manual of procedures.[149] In brief, contiguous, nonoverlapping spots of transscleral cryotherapy were directed at the entire anterior cuff of avascular retina. No infant received cryotherapy to both eyes during the study, and the eye to receive cryotherapy was randomly determined. Laser photocoagulation was not studied, since no practical laser delivery instrument had been developed at that time.

Results

The results of the CRYO-ROP study were evaluated through a masked comparison by fundus photographs of the incidence of objectively visible macular fold, retinal detachment, or retrolental mass in the eyes that received cryotherapy, with those eyes not receiving it.[150] Age-appropriate visual acuity outcomes were performed as the children grew and developed.[81,100,150] Cryotherapy was found to reduce the listed unfavorable fundus outcomes over the serial examination visits. At the 10-year outcome assessment, 247 of the original randomized cohort were examined and total retinal detachments had continued to occur in control eyes that had received cryotherapy, increasing from 38.6% at 5½ years to 41.4% at 10 years, while treated eyes remained stable at 22%. Unfavorable fundus outcomes were present in 27% of treated eyes versus 48% of control eyes, and visual acuity was 20/200 or worse in 44% of treated eyes versus 62% of control eyes.[150] By the close of the 20th century, level 3 and level 2 NICUs had become organized to provide screening ophthalmic examinations for all high-risk infants and to provide peripheral retinal ablative therapy for cases of severe ROP.

Current concepts in management of retinopathy of prematurity

Treatment techniques

Cryotherapy – special considerations

Cryotherapy was performed during the CRYO-ROP study with the use of general anesthesia in 27.5% of the patients; for the rest, cryotherapy was performed in a room within or adjacent to the NICU using local or even topical anesthesia.[99] The average number of individual freezes used in the CRYO-ROP study was 50. As with other forms of eye surgery, a number of factors are considered in determining the method of analgesia or anesthesia, including the physical arrangement of the nursery, proximity to operating or procedure rooms, experience of the anesthesiologist, current medical stability of the infant, "track record" of the infant in tolerating previous stressful procedures, experience of the cryosurgeon, and posterior extent of retinopathy.

Laser – special considerations

In an effort to reduce the time and stress accompanying cryotherapy, refinements of ablative therapeutic technique were studied – in particular, laser therapy, using the binocular laser indirect ophthalmoscope (LIO) delivery system.[151–153] During the early 1990s laser ablation gained acceptance as an alternative to cryotherapy. In general, ophthalmologists have found that the LIO delivery system is technically easier than cryotherapy and creates fewer postoperative sequelae, such as inflammation and swelling. Furthermore, it seemed apparent that the outcomes of treatment of threshold disease in zone I and posterior zone II were superior to cryotherapy, and at least equivalent to cryotherapy results for zone II disease.[152–154–161]

When LIO delivery systems became available around 1990, the only laser offered was an argon photocoagulator (488–532 nm). Subsequently, the diode laser (810 nm) photocoagulator was introduced. It has become more popular than the argon laser because of its portability and a lower incidence of postoperative cataract formation. Although circumstances may require taking patients to the operating suite for ROP laser therapy, it can also be done in the NICU, with the patient under local anesthesia and with or without the aid of conscious sedation. Subsequently, large spot laser indirect headsets became available which offered threefold increase in area covered by an individual spot.

A technique of laser treatment in the NICU is to place the infant swaddled in a blanket in an open warmer. Mydriatic drops are instilled, and treatment is performed with the aid of a neontal nurse. A neonatologist must always be available in the nursery should resuscitation be necessary. A heart rate monitor, apnea monitor, and pulse oximeter are used throughout the procedure. Topical anesthesia is instilled in the eye(s) to be treated, and a lid speculum is placed. Lidocaine 2% is injected subconjunctivally in each quadrant (0.25–0.3 cc) for local anesthesia. Approximately 10 minutes is allowed for the anesthetic to take effect. Treatment is then begun with the LIO delivery system, generally with a 28-D-condensing lens. Appropriate laser safety precautions must be taken for the protection of all personnel involved.

Photocoagulation burns are distributed in a confluent pattern to minimize skip areas. The objective of the treatment is to apply burns throughout the entire peripheral nonvascularized retina. Treatment is generally started at the anterior edge of the vascularized retina and applied out to the ora serrata utilizing a Calgiswab or similar instrument for eye positioning and scleral depression. Initial settings for the diode laser are a power of 0.2 W and a pulse duration of 0.3–0.4 seconds. This power setting is usually subthreshold for photocoagulation, and power is titrated up until a yellowish-gray reaction is observed in the retina. The power and/or pulse duration often needs to be varied from one area to another in the avascular retina.

The total number of laser applications necessary to treat a given eye will depend primarily on the size of the avascular zone in the eye. In the authors' experience, if the ROP is in mid to peripheral zone II, then 1000 laser spots may be sufficient to cover the entire nonvascularized retina. However, if the eye to be treated has vessel growth only in zone I, then it is not unusual to apply 1500–3000 laser spots for adequate coverage. Laser is usually performed during a single session in the event there is a postlaser hyphema or vitreous hemorrhage that would prevent subsequent treatment. However, circumstances such as reduced visibility or patient distress may necessitate more than one treatment session. Occasionally, inadvertently skipped areas near the ROP ridge require supplementary laser treatment, in the absence of involution.

Table 61.2 The ETROP indications for treatment

Type 1 ROP ("new threshold")	Type 2 ROP
Administer peripheral ablation treatment	Wait and watch for progression
Zone II:	Zone II:
plus disease with stage 2 or 3	stage 3 without plus disease
Zone I:	Zone I:
plus disease with stage 1, 2, or 3	stage 1 or 2 without plus disease
stage 3 without plus disease	

ETROP, Early Treatment for ROP; ROP, retinopathy of prematurity.

The Early Treatment for Retinopathy of Prematurity trial

In 1999, the National Eye Institute funded a clinical trial, under the chairmanship of William V. Good, to study optimal ROP treatment indications. In this trial, called the ETROP study, eyes were randomized to early peripheral retinal ablation or conventional management (observation until threshold criteria developed) once they achieved a high-risk level of prethreshold ROP. The ETROP study showed a significant benefit of earlier treatment intervention as measured by visual acuity outcome at a corrected age of 9 months and in the structural outcome of the retina at corrected ages of 6 and 9 months.[162] In the selected high-risk eyes that were studied, unfavorable acuity results were reduced by earlier treatment intervention to 14.5%, from 19.5% in the conventionally treated control group ($P = 0.01$). Unfavorable structural outcomes were reduced from 15.6% in the control group to 9.1% in the early treatment eyes ($P < 0.001$).

The ETROP study results, published in December 2003, produced a new clinical algorithm as a guide for treatment intervention in eyes with severe ROP.[162] Prompt treatment is indicated for eyes with type 1 ROP and continued serial observations without treatment are recommended for eyes with type 2 ROP, as shown in Table 61.2. The ETROP group cautions that plus disease should involve at least two quadrants of the fundus (usually six or more clock-hour segments) with dilation and tortuosity of the posterior retinal blood vessels meeting the published standard (Fig. 61.18A).

At the final study outcome examinations performed at age 6 years, unfavorable visual acuity outcomes in eyes with type 1 ROP were reduced by early treatment to 25.1% from 32.8% in the conventionally treated control group ($P = 0.02$). Interestingly, unfavorable visual acuity outcomes in eyes with type 2 ROP increased in the early treatment group to 23.6% from 19.4% in the conventionally treated group, although this difference was not statistically significant ($P = 0.37$).[97]

RETINAL DETACHMENT

There is a need for randomized trials of treatment approaches for retinal detachment from ROP. Current clinical thinking about the treatment of retinal detachment from ROP is discussed in Chapter 114 Retinopathy of prematurity.

The ETROP study: better outcomes, changing clinical strategy

In the ETROP trial, only 66% of the high-risk eyes selected at random to be treated conventionally went on to receive laser therapy (cryotherapy was rarely used). Secondary analysis of the large database produced a simplified revision of the indications for treatment, which was a great practical improvement over the computer-generated algorithm used to select the research subjects for the study[118] (Table 61.2).

Some of the advantages of an earlier treatment policy may be lost if newborn eye examinations do not occur, as in the ETROP study. Careful reading of the methods used in the trial[163] reveals a real impact on an intensive care unit's policy for serial ROP examinations. Therefore, consider the following schedule for infants who do not meet criteria for treatment:[120]

- 1-week or less follow-up for type 2 ROP (see Table 61.2):
  - Zone II no plus, stage 3
  - Zone I no plus, stage 1 or 2
- 1–2-week follow-up:
  - Zone II no plus, stage 2
  - Zone I immature, no ROP
  - Zone I, regressing ROP
- 2-week follow-up:
  - Zone II no plus, stage 1
  - Zone II, regressing ROP
- 2–3-week follow-up:
  - Zone III, no plus, stage 1 or 2
  - Zone II immature, no ROP
  - Zone III, regressing ROP.

Favorable signs, with respect to progression or involution of ROP, include attainment of postmenstrual age of 45 weeks without developing at least type 2 (as defined above) ROP, and either the completion of full retinal vascularization or progression of retinal vascularization into zone III without previous zone II ROP.[74]

Anti-VEGF therapy for posterior ROP

There have been numerous trials demonstrating the benefits of bevacizumab in adult patients suffering from choroidal neovascular membranes in the setting of wet age-related macular degeneration. Based on this experience, many investigators have been interested in using a similar approach for the treatment of aggressive ROP. A number of recent case series have reported that intravitreal injections of anti-VEGF antibodies (e.g., bevacizumab) are a very promising approach for the treatment of aggressive ROP, with the possibility of easier administration and improved preservation of peripheral retina compared to laser.[164–169] A prospective multicenter trial has been performed in which 150 infants with bilateral stage 3+ disease in zone I or posterior zone II were randomized to intravitreal bevacizumab (0.625 mg) versus conventional laser treatment. This showed that infants treated with bevacizumab for stage 3+ disease in zone I had significantly fewer disease recurrences and better structural outcomes at 54 weeks' postmenstrual age, although there was no difference for infants with ROP in posterior zone II.[170]

Although there is the possibility of improved treatment efficacy with bevacizumab, ROP recurrences have been reported several months postinjection.[170] Unlike laser treatment, where the regression is often durable and permanent, the potential for recurrence after bevacizumab injection emphasizes the need for prolonged follow-up examinations.

Until ROP can be prevented, it behooves physicians caring for premature infants to detect treatment-requiring cases through coordinated and timely methods. Neonatologists, ophthalmologists, discharge coordinators, and ROP coordinators must collaborate in adhering to local policies developed to benefit these infants.

OTHER PEDIATRIC RETINAL VASCULAR DISEASES

Coats disease

Coats disease arises from abnormal telangiectatic retinal vessels that result in profuse leakage, leading to retinal edema and exudative detachments. It was originally described in 1908 by George Coats, who noted that patients with this condition had unilateral telangiectatic vessels with associated lipid deposits.[171] Interestingly, none of the patients described in the original paper were children, and it was not until subsequent observations that its incidence in the pediatric population was appreciated.

Children often present initially with leukocoria. This is increasingly identified by parents who notice a glow in the setting of a flash photograph, which results from either an exudative detachment or subfoveal lipid exudate as a consequence of distant telangiectasias in the peripheral retina. The differential diagnosis includes retinoblastoma, familial exudative retinopathy, and PFV. In those cases where there are only telangiectatic vessels and subretinal lipid deposits, the diagnosis is relatively straightforward, especially if wide-angle fluorescein angiography is performed. In those cases where there is a prominent exudative detachment, discriminating between retinoblastoma and Coats disease can be challenging. One useful feature is the color of the subretinal material: an exudative detachment from retinoblastoma will often have tumor visible underneath the retina with a whitish color and a mayonnaise-like appearance. In contrast, the subretinal material in Coats disease will often appear more yellow-green with a mustard-like appearance. In addition, an eye with retinoblastoma will often have a substantial dome-shaped mass on ultrasound. The presence of telangiectatic vessels, however, is not limited to Coats disease and many exudative detachments from retinoblastoma will have similar vessels.

In 2001, Shields et al. proposed a classification system based on response to treatment. Stage 1 eyes have telangiectasias only. Stage 2 eyes have in addition exudation in either extrafoveal (2a) or subfoveal (2b) locations. Stage 3 eyes have an exudative detachment that is subtotal (3a) or total (3b). Of the stage 3a eyes, if it involves the fovea then it is stage 3a1 and if it remains outside the fovea it is stage 3a2. Stage 4 is a detachment with glaucoma, and stage 5 is end-stage disease.[172]

The primary treatment of Coats disease involves laser photocoagulation directly to telangiectatic vessels. It is helpful to have wide-angle fluorescein angiography to identify the full extent of the disease. By using a green 532-nm frequency-doubled yttrium aluminum garnet (YAG) laser indirect, it is possible to coagulate the vessels even in areas where the retina is fully detached.[173] This often requires multiple treatment sessions under anesthesia over successive months. In more recalcitrant cases, subretinal fluid drainage can help expose more retina that may be hidden anteriorly due to the extent of the detachment. In severe cases, vitrectomy with external drainage may be necessary. Prior to considering any invasive treatment, retinoblastoma must be clearly ruled out.

Little is known regarding the etiology of Coats disease. There is no clear hereditary component, and it is rarely bilateral. Although there is a mild sex predisposition toward males and it can be more common in the Asian population, there is little else that would point to an underlying cause. Interestingly, although there is often widespread ischemia due to capillary dropout, there is rarely any retinal neovascularization or vitreous hemorrhage. This is despite the high rate of neovascular glaucoma in advanced cases.

Persistent fetal vasculature

Originally labeled as persistent hyperplastic primary vitreous (PHPV), PFV is a result of incomplete regression of the vascular primary vitreous leaving a stalk of fibrovascuar tissue extending from the optic nerve to the posterior lens capsule.[174] This often leads to a white opaque membrane behind the lens, resulting in dense amblyopia. The ciliary processes are often drawn towards the center and are associated with some degree of microphthalmia. The retina around the optic nerve can be drawn up into the stalk and in some cases can involve the entire length of the stalk, making surgical amputation of the stalk a risk.

There are a number of conditions that can present with a tractional detachment, including familial exudative vitreoretinopathy (FEVR), Norrie disease, incontienta pigmenti, and retinoblastoma. PFV is almost always unilateral and can be distinguished from the hereditary conditions based on bilaterality. Also the implantation of the stalk is generally to the central posterior lens capsule, whereas in FEVR, Norrie, and incontienta pigmenti, there is not stalk but rather a fold that usually runs to the temporal ora serrata. Eyes with retinoblastoma are rarely microphthalmic and will have a mass with possible calcifications on ultrasound.

Treatment for PFV can vary from observation to surgical amputation of the stalk. In some cases, the stalk is mild and the macula can be visualized. If the retina is intact and there are macular structures, a surgical approach to clear the visual access can be helpful. In some cases, the posterior plaque is quite dense and upon removal the stalk ends up being less severe with relatively normal retinal architecture. Some have advocated surgical treatment in the setting of significantly deformed retina, even when the vision is at light perception. Amputation of the stalk is thought in these cases to prevent phthisis and allow for continued eye growth.[175]

Little is known about the pathogenesis of PFV. The primary vitreous undergoes a well-described programmed involution, and in patients with PFV, it is believed that this process is altered. Recent work suggests that astrocytes may play a role in altering how this process happens and may prevent the hayloid artery from underdoing a macrophage-mediated involution.[176]

Incontinentia pigmenti

Previously called Bloch–Sulzberger syndrome, after the two dermatologists who first recognized the condition, IP is an X-linked dominant disease with ocular, central nervous system, dermatologic, and dental abnormalities. It is associated with a mutation in the *NEMO* gene located on Xq28. The resulting protein regulates the activity of NF-κB, increasing a cell's sensitivity to apoptotic signals and resulting in increase endothelial cell death.[177]

Ocular findings include retinal ischemia with neovascularization that can lead to vitreous hemorrhage and tractional detachment. The differential diagnosis based solely on the ocular findings includes ROP, FEVR, and Norrie disease. However, unlike these diseases, the ischemia in IP does not mimic a developmental vascular pattern with distinct areas of vascularized retina posteriorly and avascular retina anteriorly. Instead, the peripheral ischemia is often accompanied by ischemia in posterior vascularized retina and in some cases the macula as well. Usually, the diagnosis of IP is made soon after birth based on the presence of the skin blisters. Approximately one in three children with IP have obvious retinal abnormalities on exam, and one in four have tractional retinal detachments.[178]

Ocular management for IP includes regular exams, including those done under anesthesia. Some have recommended monthly exams from birth to 4 months of age, and then every 3 months until the patient is 1 year old. Exams can then be performed every 6 months until 3 years of age and then every 6 months after that. Fluorescein angiography can be helpful in identifying the area and extent of ischemia. The managing physician should be careful about the presence of any ischemia, since this potentially can be progressive and may result in neovascularization and subsequent detachment. Eyes at risk for tractional detachments can be treated with laser to ischemic areas.

Familial exudative vitreoretinopathy and Norrie disease

FEVR and Norrie disease are both conditions that may result from genetic mutations affecting the Wnt pathway. They can present with similar retinal findings. These mutations result in incomplete development of the retinal vessels similar to what is seen in ROP. Patients can have peripheral avascular retina, neovascular membranes, and tractional retinal detachments. In addition to the retinal findings, Norrie disease, which is X-linked recessive, can also be associated with hearing loss and mental retardation. The differential diagnosis for both includes ROP, PFV/PHPV, and IP.

Management of any patient where FEVR or Norrie disease is being considered should include careful examination under anesthesia and, when possible, fluorescein angiography. Both conditions can have an asymmetric presentation and can mimic PFV. In these cases the presumed unaffected eye may have subtle fundoscopic abnormalities that can be overlooked in an outpatient clinic setting and even under anesthesia. Wide-angle fluorescein angiography can provide a very definitive assessment of the vasculature in both eyes and may demonstrate premature termination of the peripheral vessels and subclinical neovascularization. In eyes with ischemia and neovascularization but no detachment, laser photocoagulation to the avascular retina can induce regression and prevent a detachment. When tractional retinal detachment is present, some have advocated vitrectomy to release stress on the retina and ciliary body to reduce the likelihood of hypotony and maintain light perception vision when present.[179]

In the case of FEVR, the mutation occurs in the *FZD4* gene that encodes the frizzled-4 receptor. This receptor binds Wnt ligands

3, 5a, and 8a as well as Norrin and triggers the translocation of β-catenin to the nucleus where it can activate transcription of genes involved in cell proliferation. In Norrie disease, the mutation occurs in the *NDP* gene that produces norrin, a secreted protein that can bind frizzled-4.[180,181] Recently, another gene, *Tspan12*, was found to facilitate norrin binding to frizzled-4 and loss of *Tspan12* was found in some patients with FEVR.[182] There is currently ongoing investigation as to whether mutations in these genes may also increase the risk of developing aggressive ROP.

Bonus images for this chapter can be found online at http://www.expertconsult.com

Fig. 61.1 (A) Ophthalmoscopic examination of a 45-day-old dog exposed to 100% oxygen for the first 4 days of life disclosed a 2-mm-wide area of retinal neovascularization (arrow) extending from the disc to the temporal midperiphery. Two similar structures are present at the 2- and 5-o'clock positions. (B) Area of temporal retinal neovascularization (arrow) indicated by arrow in A shows mild folds in the retina (arrowheads) (periodic acid–Schiff and hematoxylin; ×50).

Fig. 61.2 (A) Gross appearance of the areas of neovascularization extending temporally and two smaller areas in the same 45-day-old dog shown in Figure 61.1. A denser 2 × 0.5 mm area is present inferior nasally (arrow). (B) Area from A (marked by arrow) discloses retinal neovascularization (arrow) attached to the apex of a retinal fold (periodic acid–Schiff and hematoxylin; ×125).

Fig. 61.3 Schematic diagram of retinal vessel development in humans. At 4 months' gestation, vessels grow from the disc to reach the ora serrata nasally at 8 months and the ora temporally shortly after term. The vascularization of the newborn kitten corresponds to the 6½-month-gestation human fetus. N, nasal retina; T, temporal retina; numbers refer to months' gestational age.

Fig. 61.4 (A) Schematic diagram of vascular closure of the most anterior and immature retinal vascular bed (indicated by brackets) of a young kitten exposed to hyperoxia for a relatively short period. The posterior, more mature vessels are unaffected. (B) Three weeks after removal of the subject in A to ambient air, neovascularization has developed immediately posterior to the area of capillary closure (arrow). (Panel B, reproduced with permission from Patz A. Oxygen studies in retrolental fibroplasia. IV. Clinical and experimental observations. Am J Ophthalmol 1954;38:291.)

REFERENCES

1. Terry TL. Extreme prematurity and fibroblastic overgrowth of persistent vascular sheath behind each crystalline lens. I. Preliminary report. Am J Ophthalmol 1942;25:203–4.
2. Terry TL. Fibroblastic overgrowth of persistent tunica vasculosa lentis in premature infants. II. Report of cases – clinical aspects. Arch Ophthalmol 1943;29:36–53.
3. Patz A. The role of oxygen in retrolental fibroplasias. Trans Am Ophthalmol Soc 1968;66:940–85.
4. Owens WC, Owens EU. Retrolental fibroplasia in premature infants. Am J Ophthalmol 1949;32:1–29.
5. Patz A, Hoeck LE, De La Cruz, E. Studies on the effect of high oxygen administration in retrolental fibroplasia. I. Nursery observations. Am J Ophthalmol 1952;35:1248–53.
6. Patz A, Eastham A, Higginbotham DH, et al. Oxygen studies in retrolental fibroplasia. II. The production of the microscopic changes of retrolental fibroplasia in experimental animals. Am J Ophthalmol 1953;36:1511–22.
7. Ashton N, Ward B, Serpell G. Role of oxygen in the genesis of retrolental fibroplasia: a preliminary report. Br J Ophthalmol 1953;37:513–20.
8. Lanman JT, Guy LP, Dancis J. Retrolental fibroplasia and oxygen therapy. JAMA 1954;55:223–6.
9. Kinsey VE. Retrolental fibroplasia: cooperative study of retrolental fibroplasia and the use of oxygen. Arch Ophthalmol 1956;56:481–543.
10. Bolton DPG, Cross KW. Further observations on cost of preventing retrolental fibroplasias. Lancet 1974;1:445–8.
11. Avery ME, Oppenheimer EH. Recent increase in mortality from hyaline membrane disease. J Pediatr 1960;57:553–9.
12. McDonald AD. Cerebral palsy in children of very low birth weight. Arch Dis Child 1963;38:579–88.
13. Strang LB, MacLeish MH. Ventilatory failure and right-to-left shunt in newborn infants with respiratory distress. Pediatrics 1961;28:17–27.
14. Chow LC, Wright KW, Sola A, et al. Can changes in clinical practice decrease the incidence of severe retinopathy of prematurity in very low birth weight infants? Pediatrics 2003;111:339–45.
15. SUPPORT Study Group of the Eunice Kennedy Shriver NICHD Neonatal Research Network. Target ranges of oxygen saturation in extremely preterm infants. N Engl J Med. 2010;362:1959–69.
16. Stenson B, Brocklehurst P, Tarnow-Mordi W, et al. Increased 36-week survival with high oxygen saturation target in extremely premature infants. N Engl J Med 2001;364:1680–2.
17. Finnstrom O, Olausson PO, Sedin G, et al. The Swedish national prospective study on extremely low birth weight (ELBW) infants – incidence, mortality, morbidity and survival in relation to level of care. Acta Paediatr 1998;86: 503–11.
18. National NeoKnowledge Network. Multi-institutional comparative analysis for births in 1996. Based on 1810 liveborn infants <1000 g birth weight. Wayne, Penn: MDS; 1997.
19. Strebel R, Bucher HU. [Improved chance of survival for very small premature infants in Switzerland.] Schweiz Med Wochenschr 1994;124:1653–9.
20. Smith LE. Through the eyes of a child: understanding retinopathy through ROP. The Friedenwald lecture. Invest Ophthalmol Vis Sci 2008;49:5177–82.
21. Pierce EA, Foley ED, Smith LEH. Regulation of vascular endothelial growth factor by oxygen in a model of retinopathy of prematurity. Arch Ophthalmol 1996;114:1219–28. (note: see correction of errata in Arch Ophthalmol 115:427, 1997).
22. Stone J, Maslim J. Mechanisms of retinal angiogenesis. Prog Ret Eye Res 1996;16:157–81.
23. Patz A. Current concepts of the effect of oxygen on the developing retina. Curr Eye Res 1984;3:159–63.
24. Flynn JT, Bancalari E, Bawol R, et al. Retinopathy of prematurity: a randomized, prospective trial of transcutaneous oxygen monitoring. Ophthalmology 1987;94:630–8.
25. Lucey JF, Dangman B. A reexamination of the role of oxygen in retrolental fibroplasias. Pediatrics 1984;73:82–96.
26. Gole GA. Animal models of retinopathy of prematurity. In: Silverman WA, Flynn JT, editors. Retinopathy of prematurity. Boston: Blackwell; 1985. pp. 53–96.
27. Kretzer FL, Hittner HM. Initiating events in the development of retinopathy of prematurity. In: Silverman WA, Flynn JT, editors. Retinopathy of prematurity. Boston: Blackwell; 1985. pp. 121–52.
28. McLeod DS, D'Anna SA, Lutty GA. Clinical and histopathologic features of canine oxygen-induced proliferative retinopathy. Invest Ophthalmol Vis Sci 1998;39:1918–32.
29. Ashton N, Ward B, Serpell G. Effect of oxygen on developing retinal vessels with particular reference to the problem of retrolental fibroplasias. Br J Ophthalmol 1954;38:397–432.
30. Ashton N, Cook C. Direct observation of the effect of oxygen on developing vessels: a preliminary report. Br J Ophthalmol 1954;38:433–40.
31. McLeod DS, Brownstein R, Lutty GA. Vaso-obliteration in the canine model of oxygen-induced retinopathy. Invest Ophthalmol Vis Sci 1996;37:300–11.
32. Ashton N, Pedler C. Studies on developing retinal vessels. IX. Reaction of endothelial cells to oxygen. Br J Ophthalmol 1962;16:257–76.
33. Michaelson IC. The mode of development of the vascular system of the retina with some observations on its significance for certain retinal diseases. Trans Ophthalmol Soc UK 1948;68:137–80.
34. Cogan DG. Development and senescence of the human retinal vasculature. Trans Ophthalmol Soc UK 1963;83:465–89.
35. Penn JS, Henry MM, Tolman BL. Exposure to alternating hypoxia and hyperoxia causes severe proliferative retinopathy in the newborn rat. Pediatric Res 1994;36:724–31.
36. Smith LEH, Wesolowski E, McLellan A, et al. Oxygen-induced retinopathy in the mouse. Invest Ophthalmol Vis Sci 1994;35:101–11.
37. Ashton N. Oxygen and the growth and development of retinal vessels: in vivo and in vitro studies. Am J Ophthalmol 1966;62:412–35.
38. Riecke B, Chavakis E, Bretzel R, et al. Topical application of integrin antagonists inhibits proliferative retinopathy. Horm Metab Res 2001;33:307–11.
39. Wilkinson-Berka J, Alousis N, Kelly D, et al. COX-2 inhibition and retinal angiogenesis in a mouse model of retinopathy of prematurity. Invest Ophthalmol Vis Sci 2003;44:974–9.
40. Higgins RD, Hendricks-Munoz KD, Caines VV, et al. Hyperoxia stimulates endothelin-1 secretion from endothelial cells; modulation by captopril and nifedipine. Curr Eye Res 1998;17:487–93.

41. Raisler BJ, Berns KI, Grant MB, et al. Adeno-associated virus type-2 expression of pigmented epithelium-derived factor or Kringles 1-3 of angiostatin reduce retinal neovascularization. Proc Natl Acad Sci USA 2001;99:8909–14.
42. Aurricchio A, Behling KC, Maguire A, et al. Inhibition of retinal neovascularization by intraocular viral-mediated delivery of anti-angiogenic agents. Mol Ther 2002;6:490–4.
43. Stellmach V, Crawford SE, Zhou W, et al. Prevention of ischemia-induced retinopathy by the natural ocular antiangiogenic agent pigment epithelium-derived factor. Proc Natl Acad Sci 2001;98:2593–7.
44. Phelps DL. Oxygen and developmental retinal capillary remodeling in the kitten. Invest Ophthalmol Vis Sci 1990;31:2194–200.
45. Penn JS, Tolman BAL, Henry MM. Oxygen-induced retinopathy in the rat: relationship of retinal nonperfusion to subsequent neovascularization. Invest Ophthalmol Vis Sci 1994;35:3429–35.
46. Chan-Ling T, McLeod DS, Hughes S, et al. Astrocyte–endothelial cell relationships during human retinal vascular development. Invest Ophthalmol Vis Sci 2004;45:2020–32.
47. Chan-Ling T, Tout S, Hollander H, et al. Vascular changes and their mechanisms in the feline model of retinopathy of prematurity. Invest Ophthalmol Vis Sci 1992;33:2128–47.
48. Stone J, Itin A, Chan-Ling T, et al. The roles of endothelial growth factor (VEGF) and neuroglia in retinal vascularization during normal development and in retinopathy of prematurity. J Neurochem 1995;65:121.
49. Stone J, Chan-Ling T, Pe'er J, et al. Roles of vascular endothelial growth factor and astrocyte degeneration in the genesis of retinopathy of prematurity. Invest Ophthalmol Vis Sci 1996;37:290–9.
50. Provis JM, Leech J, Diaz CM, et al. Development of the human retinal vasculature – cellular relations and VEGF expression. Exp Eye Res 1997;65: 555–68.
51. Alon T, Hemo I, Itin A, et al. Vascular endothelial growth factor acts as a survival factor for newly formed retinal vessels and has implications for retinopathy of prematurity. Nature Med 1995;1:1024–8.
52. Donahue ML, Phelps DL, Watkins RH, et al. Retinal vascular endothelial growth factor (VEGF) mRNA expression is altered in relation to neovascularization in oxygen-induced retinopathy. Curr Eye Res 1996;15:175–84.
53. Dorey CK, Aouididi S, Reynaud X, et al. Correlation of vascular permeability factor/vascular endothelial growth factor with extraretinal neovascularization in rat. Arch Ophthalmol 1996;114:1210–7.
54. Szewczyk TS. Retrolental fibroplasia and related ocular diseases: classification, etiology, and prophylaxis. Am J Ophthalmol 1953;36:1333–61.
55. Phelps DL, Rosenbaum A. Effects of marginal hypoxemia on recovery from oxygen-induced retinopathy in the kitten model. Pediatrics 1984;73:1–10.
56. Phelps DL. Reduced severity of oxygen-induced retinopathy in kittens recovered in 28% oxygen. Pediatr Res 1988;24:106–9.
57. STOP-ROP Multicenter Study Group. Supplemental therapeutic oxygen for prethreshold retinopathy of prematurity (STOP-ROP), a randomized, controlled trial. I. Primary outcomes. Pediatrics 2000;105:295–310.
58. Cantolino SJ, O'Grady GE, Herrera JA, et al. Ophthalmoscopic monitoring of oxygen therapy in premature infants: fluorescein angiography in acute retrolental fibroplasias. Am J Ophthalmol 1971;72:322–31.
59. Flynn JT. Acute proliferative retrolental fibroplasia: evolution of the lesion. Graefes Arch Clin Exp Ophthalmol 1975;195:101–11.
60. Flynn JT. Retinopathy of prematurity. Pediatr Clin North Am 1987;34: 1487–515.
61. Flynn JT, Cassady J, Essner D, et al. Fluorescein angiography in retrolental fibroplasia: experience from 1969–1977. Ophthalmology 1979;86:1700–23.
62. Flynn JT, O'Grady GE, Herrera J. Retrolental fibroplasia: I. Clinical observations. Arch Ophthalmol 1977;95:217–23.
63. Brooks SE, Gu X, Samuel S, et al. Reduced severity of oxygen-induced retinopathy in eNOS-deficient mice. Invest Ophthalmol Vis Sci 2001;42: 222–8.
64. Foos RY. Acute retrolental fibroplasias. Graefes Arch Clin Exp Ophthalmol 1975;95:87–100.
65. Foos RY. Chronic retinopathy of prematurity. Ophthalmology 1985;92: 563–74.
66. Foos RY. Retinopathy of prematurity – pathologic correlation of clinical stages. Retina 1987;7:260–76.
67. Cogan DG, Kuwabara T. Accessory cells in vessels of the perinatal human retina. Arch Ophthalmol 1986;104:747–52.
68. McLeod DS, Lutty GA, Wajer SD, et al. Visualization of a developing vasculature. Microvasc Res 1987;33:257–69.
69. Committee for the Classification of Retinopathy of Prematurity. An international classification of retinopathy of prematurity. Arch Ophthalmol 1984;102:1130–4.
70. Garner A. The pathology of retinopathy of prematurity. In: Silverman WA, Flynn JT, editors. Retinopathy of prematurity. Boston: Blackwell; 1985. pp. 19–52.
71. Hittner HM, Rhodes LM, McPherson AR. Anterior segment abnormalities in cicatricial retinopathy of prematurity. Ophthalmology 1979;86:803–16.
72. International Committee for the Classification of Retinopathy of Prematurity. The International Classification of Retinopathy of Prematurity revisited. Arch Ophthalmol 2005;123:991–9.
73. Chiang MF, Jiang L, Gelman R, et al. Interexpert agreement of plus disease diagnosis in retinopathy of prematurity. Arch Ophthalmol 2007;125:875–80.
74. Reynolds JD, Dobson V, Quinn GE, et al. Evidence-based screening criteria for retinopathy of prematurity: natural history data from the CRYO-ROP and LIGHT-ROP studies. Arch Ophthalmol 2002;120:1470–6.
75. Wallace DK, Quinn GE, Freedman SF, et al. Agreement among pediatric ophthalmologists in diagnosing plus and pre-plus disease in retinopathy of prematurity. JAAPOS 2008;12:352–6.
76. Flynn JT, Chan-Ling T. Retinopathy of prematurity: two distinct mechanisms that underlie zone 1 and zone 2 disease. Am J Ophthalmol 2006;142:46–59.
77. International Committee for Classification of the Late Stages of Retinopathy of Prematurity. An international classification of retinopathy of prematurity: II. The classification of retinal detachment. Arch Ophthalmol 1987;105:906–12.
78. Machemer R. Description and pathogenesis of late stages of retinopathy of prematurity. Ophthalmology 1985;92:1000–4.
79. Repka MX, Palmer EA. Involution of retinopathy of prematurity. Arch Ophthalmol 2000;118:645–9.
80. Cryotherapy for Retinopathy of Prematurity Cooperative Group. The natural ocular outcome of premature birth and retinopathy: status at one year. Arch Ophthalmol 1994;112:903–12.
81. Cryotherapy for Retinopathy of Prematurity Cooperative Group. Multicenter trial of cryotherapy for retinopathy of prematurity: Snellen acuity and structural outcome at 5½ years. Arch Ophthalmol 1996;114:417–24.
82. Fishburne BC, Winthrop KL, Robertson JE. Atrophic fundus lesions associated with untreated retinopathy of prematurity. Am J Ophthalmol 1997;124:247–9.
83. Gilbert WS, Quinn GE, Dobson V, et al. Partial retinal detachment at 3 months after threshhold retinopathy of prematurity. Arch Ophthalmol 1996;114: 1085–91.
84. Kushner BJ. Strabismus and amblyopia associated with regressed retinopathy of prematurity. Arch Ophthalmol 1982;100:256–61.
85. Schaffer DB, Quinn GE, Johnson L. Sequelae of arrested mild retinopathy of prematurity. Arch Ophthalmol 1984;102:373–6.
86. Cats BP, Tan KEWP. Prematures with and without regressed retinopathy of prematurity: comparison of long-term (6–10 years) ophthalmological morbidity. J Pediatr Ophthalmol Strabismus 1989;26:271–5.
87. Robinson R, O'Keefe M. Follow-up study on premature infants with and without retinopathy of prematurity. Br J Ophthalmol 1993;77:91–4.
88. Snir M, Nissenkorn I, Sherf I, et al. Visual acuity, strabismus, and amblyopia in premature babies with and without retinopathy of prematurity. Ann Ophthalmol 1988;20:256–8.
89. Bremer D, Fellows RR, Palmer EA, et al. Strabismus in premature infants in the first year of life. Arch Ophthalmol 1998;116:329–33.
90. Vanderveen DK, Coats DK, Dobson V, et al. Prevalence and course of strabismus in the first year of life for infants with prethreshold retinopathy of prematurity: findings from the Early Treatment for Retinopathy of Prematurity Study. Arch Ophthalmol 2006;124:766–73.
91. Quinn GE, Dobson V, Repka MX, et al. Development of myopia in infants with birth weights less than 1251 grams. Ophthalmology 1992;99:329–40.
92. Quinn GE, Dobson V, Davitt BV, et al. Progression of myopia and high myopia in the Early Treatment for Retinopathy of Prematurity Study: findings to 3 years of age. Ophthalmology 2008;115:1058–64.
93. Fletcher MC, Brandon S. Myopia of prematurity. Am J Ophthalmol 1955;40:474–81.
94. Davitt BV, Dobson V, Quinn GE, et al. Astigmatism in the Early Treatment for Retinopathy of Prematurity Study. Ophthalmology 2009;116:332–9.
95. Kushner BJ. The sequelae of regressed retinopathy of prematurity. In: Silverman WA, Flynn JT, editors. Retinopathy of prematurity. Boston: Blackwell; 1985. pp. 239–48.
96. Summers GC, Phelps DL, Tung B, et al. Ocular cosmesis in retinopathy of prematurity. Arch Ophthalmol 1992;110:1092–7.
97. Early Treatment for Retinopathy of Prematurity Cooperative Group. Final visual acuity results in the Early Treatment for Retinopathy Study. Arch Ophthalmol 2010;128:663–71.
98. Krolicki TJ, Tasman W. Cataract extraction in adults with retinopathy of prematurity. Arch Ophthalmol 1995;113:173–7.
99. Cryotherapy for Retinopathy of Prematurity Cooperative Group. Multicenter trial of cryotherapy for retinopathy of prematurity: preliminary results. Arch Ophthalmol 1988;106:471–9.
100. Cryotherapy for Retinopathy of Prematurity Cooperative Group. Multicenter trial of cryotherapy for retinopathy of prematurity: one-year outcome-structure and function. Arch Ophthalmol 1990;108:950–5.
101. Kushner BJ. Ciliary block glaucoma in retinopathy of prematurity. Arch Ophthalmol 1982;100:1078–9.
102. Pollard ZF. Secondary angle-closure glaucoma in cicatricial retrolental fibroplasia. Am J Ophthalmol 1980;89:651–3.
103. Smith J, Shivitz I. Angle-closure glaucoma in adults with cicatricial retinopathy of prematurity. Arch Ophthalmol 1984;102:371–2.
104. Brown DR, Biglan AW, Stretavsky MAM. Screening criteria for the detection of retinopathy of prematurity in patients in a neonatal intensive care unit. J Pediatr Ophthalmol Strabismus 1987;24:212–4.
105. Clark C, Gibbs JAH, Maniello R, et al. Blood transfusions: a possible risk factor in retrolental fibroplasias. Acta Paediatr Scand 1981; 70:535–9.
106. Bauer CR, Widmayer SM. A relationship between $PaCO_2$ and retrolental fibroplasia (RLF). Pediatr Res 1981; 15:649.
107. Flower RW. A new perspective on the pathogenesis of retrolental fibroplasia: the influence of elevated arterial CO_2. Retinopathy of Prematurity Conference 1981;Dec 4–6.
108. Biglan AW, Brown DR, Reynolds JD, et al. Risk factors associated with retrolental fibroplasias. Ophthalmology 1981;91:1504–11.
109. Brown DR, Milley JR, Ripepi U, et al. Retinopathy of prematurity – risk factors in a five-year cohort of critically ill premature neonates. Am J Dis Child 1987;141:154–60.

110. Kretzer FL, Hittner HM, Johnson AT, et al. Vitamin E and retrolental fibroplasia: ultrastructural support of clinical efficacy. Ann NY Acad Sci 1982; 393:145–66.
111. Aranda JV, Clark TE, Maniello R, et al. Blood transfusions (BT): possible potentiating risk factor in retrolental fibroplasia (RLF). Pediatr Res 1975;9:362.
112. Bossi E, Koerner F, Zulauf M. Retinopathy of prematurity (ROP): risk factors – a statistical analysis with matched pairs. Retinopathy of Prematurity Conference 1981;Dec 4–6.
113. Procianoy RS, Garcia-Prats JA, Hittner HM, et al. An association between retinopathy of prematurity and interventricular hemorrhage in very low birth weight infants. Acta Paediatr Scand 1981;70:473–7.
114. Sacks M, Schaffer DB, Anday EK, et al. Retrolental fibroplasia and blood transfusion in very low birth-weight infants. Pediatrics 1981;68:770–44.
115. Hammer ME, Mullen PW, Ferguson JG, et al. Logistic analysis of risk factors in acute retinopathy of prematurity. Am J Ophthalmol 1986;102:1–6.
116. Palmer EA, Flynn JT, Hardy RJ, et al. Incidence and early course of retinopathy of prematurity. Ophthalmology 1991;98:1628–40.
117. Schaffer DB, Palmer EA, Plotsky DF, et al. Prognostic factors in the natural course of retinopathy of prematurity. Ophthalmology 1993;100:230–6.
118. Hardy RJ, Palmer EA, Dobson V, et al. Risk analysis of prethreshold retinopathy of prematurity. Arch Ophthalmol 2003;121:1697–701.
119. Palmer EA. Optimal timing of examination for acute retrolental fibroplasia. Ophthalmology 1981;88:662–8.
120. Section on Ophthalmology American Academy of Pediatrics, American Academy of Ophthalmology, American Association for Pediatric Ophthalmology and Strabismus. Screening examination of prematurity infants for retinopathy of prematurity. Pediatrics 2006;117:572–6. Erratum in: Pediatrics 2006;118:1324.
121. Palmer EA. Risks of dilating a child's pupils. Trans Pac Coast Oto Ophthalmol Soc 1982;63:141–5.
122. Johnson L, Schaffer D, Boggs TR. The premature infant, vitamin E deficiency, and retrolental fibroplasia. Am J Clin Nutr 1974;27:1158–71.
123. Johnson LH, Schaffer DB, Goldstein DE, et al. Influence of vitamin E treatment (Rx) and adult blood transfusions on mean severity of retrolental fibroplasia (MS-RLF) in premature infants. Pediatr Res 1977;11:535.
124. Hittner HM, Godio LB, Rudolph AJ, et al. Retrolental fibroplasia: efficacy of vitamin E in a double-blind clinical study of preterm infants. N Engl J Med 1981;305:1365–71.
125. Phelps DL. Vitamin E and retinopathy of prematurity. In: Silverman WA, Flynn JT, editors. Retinopathy of prematurity. Boston: Blackwell; 1985. pp. 181–206.
126. Phelps DL, Rosenbaum AL, Isenberg SJ, et al. Tocopherol efficacy and safety for preventing retinopathy of prematurity: a randomized, controlled, double-masked trial. Pediatrics 1987;79:489–500.
127. Finer NN, Schindler RF, Peters KL, et al. Vitamin E and retrolental fibroplasia: improved visual outcome with early vitamin E. Ophthalmology 1983;90: 428–35.
128. Puklin JE, Simon RM, Ehrenkranz RA. Influence on retrolental fibroplasia of intramuscular vitamin E administration during respiratory distress syndrome. Ophthalmology 1982;89:96–103.
129. Milner RA, Watts JL, Paes B, et al. Retrolental fibroplasia in 1500 gram neonates: part of a randomized clinical trial of the effectiveness of vitamin E. Retinopathy of Prematurity Conference 1981;Dec 4–6.
130. Johnson L, Bowen F, Herman N, et al. The relationship of prolonged elevation of serum vitamin E levels to neonatal bacterial sepsis (SEP) and necrotizing enterocolitis (NEC). Pediatr Res 1983;17:319.
131. Schaffer DB, Johnson L, Quinn GE, et al. Vitamin E and retinopathy of prematurity: follow-up at one year. Ophthalmology 1985;92:1005–11.
132. Institute of Medicine. Report of a study: vitamin E and retinopathy of prematurity. Washington, DC: National Academy; 1986.
133. Terry TL. Fibroplastic overgrowth of the persistent tunica vasculosa lentis in premature infants. IV. Etiologic factors. Arch Ophthalmol 1943;29:54–65.
134. Hepner WR, Krause AC, Davis ME. Retrolental fibroplasia and light. Pediatrics 1949;3:824–8.
135. Locke JC, Reese AB. Retrolental fibroplasia: the negative role of light, mydriatics, and the ophthalmoscopic examinations in its etiology. Arch Ophthalmol 1952;48:44–7.
136. Reynolds JD, Hardy RJ, Kennedy KA, et al. Lack of efficacy of light reduction in preventing retinopathy of prematurity. N Engl J Med 1998;338:1572–6.
137. Nagata M, Kobayashi Y, Fukuda H. Photocoagulation for the treatment of the retinopathy of prematurity (first report). J Clin Ophthalmol 1968;22:419.
138. Oshima K, Ikui H, Kano M, et al. Clinical study and photocoagulation of retinopathy of prematurity. Folia Ophthalmol Jpn 1971;22:700–7.
139. Payne JW, Patz A. Treatment of acute proliferative retrolental fibroplasia. Trans Am Acad Ophthalmol Otolaryngol 1972;76:1234–46.
140. Yamashita Y. Studies on retinopathy of prematurity. III. Cryocautery for retinopathy of prematurity. Rinsho Ganka 1972;26:385–93.
141. Palmer EA, Biglan AW, Hardy RJ. Retinal ablative therapy for active proliferative retinopathy of prematurity: history, current status, and prospects. In: Silverman WA, Flynn JT, editors. Retinopathy of prematurity. Boston: Blackwell; 1985. pp. 207–28.
142. Kingham JD. Acute retrolental fibroplasia. II. Treatment by cryosurgery. Arch Ophthalmol 1978;96:2049–53.
143. Kalina RE. Treatment of retrolental fibroplasia. Surv Ophthalmol 1980;24: 229–36.
144. Hindle NW. Cryotherapy for retinopathy of prematurity to prevent retrolental fibroplasias. Can J Ophthalmol 1982;17:207–12.
145. Mousel DK. Cryotherapy for retinopathy of prematurity: a personal retrospective. Ophthalmology 1985;92:375–8.
146. Tasman W, Brown GC, Schaffer DB, et al. Cryotherapy for active retinopathy of prematurity. Ophthalmology 1986;93:580–5.
147. Palmer EA, Hardy RJ, Dobson V, et al. 15-year outcomes following threshold retinopathy of prematurity: final results from the multicenter trial of cryotherapy for retinopathy of prematurity. Arch Ophthalmol 2005;123: 311–8.
148. Palmer EA, Phelps DL. Multicenter trial of cryotherapy for retinopathy of prematurity. Pediatrics 1986;77:428–9.
149. Cryotherapy for Retinopathy of Prematurity Cooperative Group. Manual of Procedures. Archived at the National Technical Information Service, Springfield, Va: US Department of Commerce, NTIS accession no. PB88–16350; 1988.
150. Cryotherapy for Retinopathy of Prematurity Cooperative Group. Multicenter trial of cryotherapy for retinopathy of prematurity: ophthalmological outcomes at 10 years. Arch Ophthalmol 2001;119:1110–8.
151. Landers MB, Semple HC, Ruben JB, et al. Argon laser photocoagulation for advanced retinopathy of prematurity. Am J Ophthalmol 1990;110:429–31.
152. Landers III MB, Toth CA, Semple CS, et al. Treatment of retinopathy of prematurity with argon laser photocoagulation. Arch Ophthalmol 1992;110: 44–7.
153. McNamara JA, Tasman WS, Brown GC, et al. Laser photocoagulation for retinopathy of prematurity. Ophthalmology 1991;98:576–80.
154. O'Keefe M, Burke J, Algawi K, et al. Diode laser photocoagulation to the vascular retina for progressively advancing retinopathy of prematurity. Br J Ophthalmol 1995;79:1012–4.
155. Hammer ME, Pusateri TJ, Hess JB, et al. Threshold retinopathy of prematurity. Transition from cryopexy to laser treatment. Retina 1995;15:486–9.
156. Capone Jr A, Diaz-Rohena R, Sternberg Jr P, et al. Diode-laser photocoagulation for zone 1 threshold retinopathy of prematurity. Am J Ophthalmol 1993; 116:444–50.
157. Hunter DG, Repka MX. Diode laser photocoagulation for threshold retinopathy of prematurity. A randomized study. Ophthalmology 1993;100: 238–44.
158. McNamara JA, Tasman W, Vander JF, et al. Diode laser photocoagulation for retinopathy of prematurity. Preliminary results. Arch Ophthalmol 1992;110: 1714–6.
159. Fleming TN, Runge PE, Charles ST. Diode laser photocoagulation for prethreshold, posterior retinopathy of prematurity. Am J Ophthalmol 1992;114: 589–92.
160. DeJoyce MH, Ferrone PJ, Trese MT. Diode laser ablation for threshold retinopathy of prematurity. Arch Ophthalmol 2000;118:365–7.
161. White JE, Repka MX. Randomized comparison of diode laser photocoagulation versus cryotherapy for threshold retinopathy of prematurity. Three-year outcome. J Pediatr Ophthalmol Strabismus 1997;34:83–7.
162. Early Treatment for Retinopathy of Prematurity Cooperative Group. Revised indications for treatment of retinopathy of prematurity: results of the early treatment for retinopathy of prematurity randomized trial. Arch Ophthalmol 2003;121:1684–96.
163. Early Treatment for Retinopathy of Prematurity Cooperative Group. Multicenter trial of early treatment for retinopathy of prematurity: study design. Controlled Clin Trials 2004;25:311–25.
164. Quiroz-Mercado H, Martinez-Castellanos MA, Hernandez-Rojas ML, et al. Antiangiogenic therapy with intravitreal bevacizumab for retinopathy of prematurity. Retina 2008;28(3 Suppl):S19–25. Erratum in: Retina 2009; 29:127.
165. Travassos A, Teixeira S, Ferreira P, et al. Intravitreal bevacizumab in aggressive posterior retinopathy of prematurity. Ophthalmic Surg Lasers Imaging 2007;38:233–7.
166. Lalwani GA, Berroca AM, Murray TG, et al. Off-label use of intravitreal bevacizumab (Avastin) for salvage treatment in progressive threshold retinopathy of prematurity. Retina 2008;28(Suppl):S13–18.
167. Kusaka S, Shima C, Wada K, et al. Efficacy of intravitreal injection of bevacizumab for severe retinopathy of prematurity: a pilot study. Br J Ophthalmol 2008;92:1450–5.
168. Law JC, Recchia FM, Morrison DG, et al. Intravitreal bevacizumab as adjunctive treatment for retinopathy of prematurity. JAAPOS 2010;14:6–10.
169. Wu WC, Yeh PT, Chen SN, et al. Effects and complications of bevacizumab use in patients with retinopathy of prematurity: a multicenter study in Taiwan. Ophthalmology 2011;118:176–83.
170. Mintz-Hittner HA, Kennedy KA, Chuang AZ, et al. Efficacy of intravitreal bevacizumab for stage 3+ retinopathy of prematurity. N Engl J Med 2011;364: 603–15.
171. Coats G. Forms of retinal disease with massive exudation. R Lond Ophthalmic Hosp Rep 1908;17:440–525.
172. Shields JA, Shields CL, Honavar SG, et al. Clinical variations and complications of Coats disease in 150 cases: the 2000 Sanford Gifford memorial lecture. Am J Ophthalmol 2001;131:561–71.
173. Shapiro MJ, Chow CC, Karth PA, et al. Effects of green diode laser in the treatment of pediatric Coats disease. Am J Ophthalmol 2011;151:725–31.e2.
174. Goldberg MF. Persistent fetal vasculature (PFV): an integrated interpretation of signs and symptoms associated with persistent hyperplastic primary vitreous (PHPV). LIV Edward Jackson memorial lecture. Am J Ophthalmol 1997;124:587–626.
175. Shaikh S, Trese MT. Lens-sparing vitrectomy in predominantly posterior persistent fetal vasculature syndrome in eyes with nonaxial lens opacification. Retina 2003;23:330–4.

176. Zhang C, Asnaghi L, Gongora C, et al. A developmental defect in astrocytes inhibits programmed regression of the hyaloid vasculature in the mammalian eye. Eur J Cell Biol 2011;90:440–8.
177. Jin DY, Jeang KT. Isolation of full-length cDNA and chromosomal localization of human NF-κB modulator NEMO to Xq28. J Biomed Sci 1999;6:115–20.
178. O'Doherty M, Mc Creery K, Green AJ, et al. Incontinentia pigmenti – ophthalmological observation of a series of cases and review of the literature. Br J Ophthalmol 2011;95:11–6.
179. Walsh MK, Drenser KA, Capone Jr A, et al. Early vitrectomy effective for Norrie disease. Arch Ophthalmol. 2010;128:456–60.
180. Chen ZY, Battinelli EM, Fielder A, et al. A mutation in the Norrie disease gene (NDP) associated with X-linked familial exudative vitreoretinopathy. Nat Genet 1993;5:180–3.
181. Xu Q, Wang Y, Dabdoub A, et al. Vascular development in the retina and inner ear: control by norrin and frizzled-4, a high-affinity ligand-receptor pair. Cell 2004;116:883–95.
182. Junge HJ, Yang S, Burton JB, et al. TSPAN12 regulates retinal vascular development by promoting Norrin- but not Wnt-induced FZD4/beta-catenin signaling. Cell 2009;139:299–311.

Chapter 62

Telescreening for Retinopathy of Prematurity

Michael F. Chiang

LIMITATIONS OF TRADITIONAL CARE

Traditional screening for retinopathy of prematurity (ROP) involves indirect ophthalmoscopy at the bedside in the neonatal intensive care unit (NICU). Although this has been effective at identifying infants with severe treatment-requiring disease,[1–3] there are important limitations. Ophthalmoscopic examinations are logistically difficult, require significant travel time and coordination, and are physiologically stressful for infants.[4] Findings are documented using hand-drawn sketches, which are subjective and qualitative (Fig. 62.1). In addition, there may be variability in diagnosis of critical features such as zone I and plus disease, even among experts,[5,6] and there is enormous medicolegal liability. Surveys have found that the number of retinal specialists and pediatric ophthalmologists willing to manage ROP is decreasing for these reasons.[7] Meanwhile, more infants are at risk for disease because of increasing premature birth rates and improved neonatal survival throughout the world.

TELEMEDICINE AS AN EMERGING APPROACH

Telemedicine is an emerging approach with potential to improve the quality, delivery, and cost of care compared to traditional strategies. This may be particularly important in developing nations and other areas with limited accessibility to care. In this approach, clinical data and images are captured from the infant's eyes by trained personnel in the NICU. Data are transmitted for review by a remote ophthalmologist, who sends management recommendations to the consulting physician. Examples of wide-angle images taken with a commercially available camera (RetCam; Clarity Medical Systems, Pleasanton, CA) are shown in Fig. 62.2. It has been shown that trained neonatal nurses can capture high-quality retinal images,[8,9] and that imaging may cause less physiological stress to infants than ophthalmoscopy with scleral depression.[10]

In a telemedicine approach, the availability of archived retinal images would provide other advantages. Infant photographs could be directly compared to references such as the published standard photograph for plus disease,[1] and may be transmitted securely to experts for second opinions. Images provide objective documentation of clinical findings, improve recognition of disease progression, enhance communication, and create infrastructure for education and research.[11]

EVALUATION STUDIES

Accuracy

Diagnostic accuracy of telemedicine for ROP has been evaluated since the late 1990s. Virtually all studies have used wide-angle digital images captured by a neonatal nurse, ophthalmologist, or ophthalmic photographer. Although these studies have varied in design and outcome measure, most have compared the

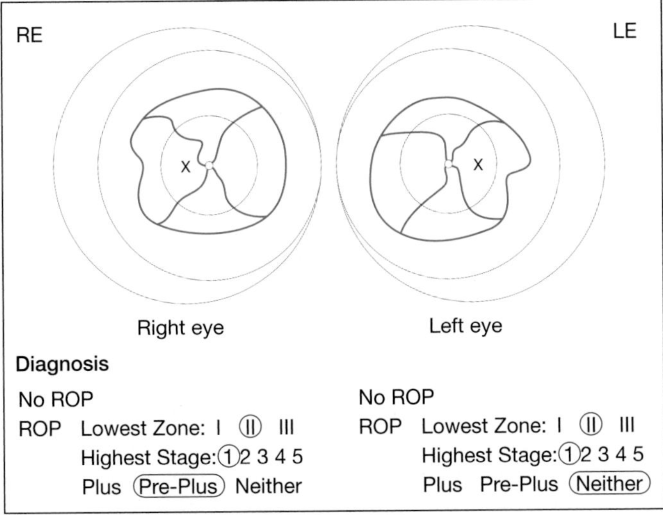

Fig. 62.1 Documentation of traditional indirect ophthalmoscopy using annotated examination template. Limitations include subjective and qualitative documentation, and difficulty identifying change during serial examinations.

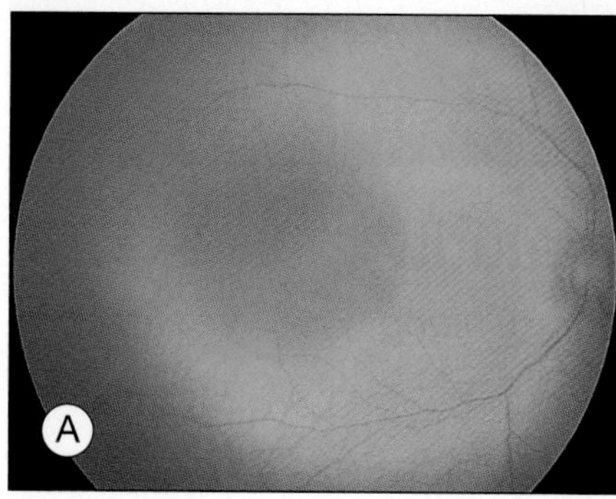

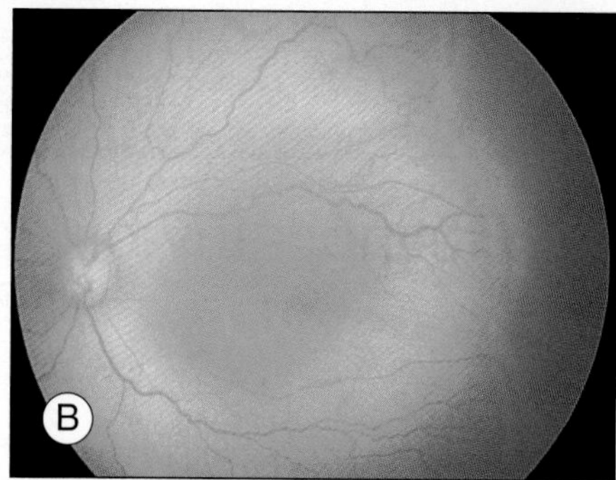

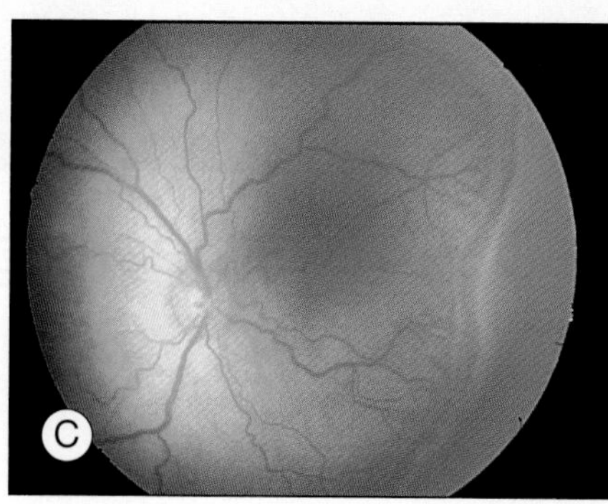

Fig. 62.2 Examples of ROP images captured by a trained neonatal nurse during routine screening using a wide-angle camera (RetCam; Clarity Medical Systems, Pleasanton, CA). Images demonstrate retinas with (A) no ROP, (B) type 2 ROP based on the presence of stage 3 disease in zone II, and (C) type 1 treatment-requiring ROP based on the presence of plus disease as well as posterior stage 3 disease.

diagnostic performance of telemedicine to a reference standard of dilated ophthalmoscopy. Schwartz et al. (19 eyes from 10 infants) examined the accuacy of telemedicine in a selected group of infants at 30–32 weeks postmenstrual age (PMA), all of whom had moderate or severe ROP. The sensitivity and specificity of telemedicine for detecting prethreshold or worse ROP were 89% and 100%, respectively.[12]

Since that time, research has involved larger and broader cohorts of consecutively enrolled infants. For diagnosis of any ROP regardless of severity, studies have demonstrated sensitivity of 46%–97% and specificity 49%–100% compared to a reference standard of indirect ophthalmoscopy[8,13,14] (Table 62.1). Generally, lower accuracy has been found while examining infants at lower PMA, and when detecting presence of mild ROP (e.g. peripheral stage 1). This is presumably because younger infants have milder disease with more subtle diagnostic features, and because it may be technically more difficult to image smaller eyes with increased media opacities.[15]

Other studies have examined accuracy of telemedicine for detecting clinically significant ROP (Table 62.2). Ells et al. (371 exams from 36 infants) found sensitivity 100% and specificity 96% for diagnosis of "referral-warranted ROP"* during serial examinations throughout an infant's hospital course.[18] Wu et al. (serial exams from 43 infants) performed telemedicine screening for prethreshold or worse ROP, and found sensitivity 100% and specificity 98%.[19] Chiang et al. (163 exams from 64 infants) reported sensitivity 72%–83% and specificity 90%–99% for detection of type 2 or worse ROP, and sensitivity 85%–90% and specificity 95%–97% for detection of treatment-requiring ROP.[13] The multicenter prospective Photo-ROP Study (300 exams from 51 infants) found sensitivity 92% and specificity 37% for detection of "clinically significant ROP"† during weekly examinations throughout an infant's hospital course.[20]

In a prospective study, Chiang et al. (248 exams from 67 infants) examined the effect of PMA and disease severity on telemedicine accuracy. At 31–33 weeks PMA, the sensitivity and specificity by three expert graders was 71%–86% and 93%–97% respectively for detection of type 2 or worse ROP, and the specificity for detection of treatment-requiring ROP was 94%–100%. At 35–37 weeks PMA, sensitivity and specificity by three graders were 91%–97% and 98%–100% respectively for detection of any ROP, 100%–100% and 85%–94% respectively for detection of type 2 or worse ROP, and 100%–100% and 81%–94% respectively for detection of treatment-requiring ROP.[8] The finding of higher accuracy in older infants was in agreement with previous studies.[15]

Dhaliwal et al. (245 exams from 81 infants) conducted a masked, double-observer prospective longitudinal cohort study. Two pediatric ophthalmologists were randomized to perform examinations using either telemedicine or ophthalmoscopy. Sensitivity of telemedicine for detecting stage 3 or worse ROP was

Table 62.1 Diagnostic accuracy of telescreening for detection of any ROP using images captured by wide-angle camera.* Reference standard was standard indirect ophthalmoscopy

Study	Outcome measures	Sensitivity/specificity
Roth et al., 2001[14]	Any ROP	0.82/0.94
Yen et al., 2002[15]	Any ROP at 32–34 wks PMA	0.46/1.00
	Any ROP at 38–40 wks PMA	0.76/1.00
Chiang et al., 2006[13]	Any ROP	0.82–0.86/0.49–0.96
Shah et al., 2006[16]	Any ROP	0.86/0.92
Chiang et al., 2007[8]	Any ROP at 31–33 wks PMA	0.73–0.94/0.89–0.97
	Any ROP at 35–37 wks PMA	0.91–0.97/0.98–1.00
Dhaliwal et al., 2009[17]	Any ROP at 34 wks PMA or 4–6 wks CA	0.60/0.91

**RetCam; Clarity Medical Systems, Pleasanton, CA.*
PMA, postmenstrual age; CA, chronological age.

*"Referral-warranted ROP" was defined as any ROP in zone I, plus disease, or stage 3 ROP.

†Clinically significant ROP was defined as: (a) zone 1, any ROP, without vascular dilation or tortuosity; (b) zone II, stage 2, with up to one quadrant of vascular dilation and tortuosity; (c) zone II, stage 3, with up to one quadrant of vascular dilation and tortuosity; (d) any vascular dilation and tortuosity noted in eyes for which ridge characteristics were not interpretable (not imaged or poor image quality); or (e) any ROP noted in eyes for which disc features (plus disease) were not interpretable (not imaged or poor image quality).

Table 62.2 Diagnostic accuracy of telescreening for detection of clinically significant ROP using images captured by wide-angle camera.* Reference standard was standard indirect ophthalmoscopy

Study	Outcome measures	Sensitivity/specificity
Ells et al., 2003[18]	Any ROP zone I, presence of plus disease, or presence of any stage 3 ROP at any time during hospital course	1.00/0.96
Chiang et al., 2006[13]	Type 2 or worse ROP	0.72–0.83/0.90–0.99
	Treatment-requiring ROP	0.85–0.90/0.95–0.97
Wu et al., 2006[19]	Prethreshold or worse ROP	1.00/0.98
Chiang et al., 2007[8]	Type 2 or worse ROP at 31–33 wks PMA	0.71–0.86/0.93–0.97
	Type 2 or worse ROP at 35–37 wks PMA	1.00/0.85–0.94
	Treatment requiring ROP at 31–33 wks PMA	NA/0.94–1.00
	Treatment requiring ROP at 35–37 wks PMA	1.00/0.81–0.94
Photo-ROP Cooperative Group, 2008[20]	"Clinically significant ROP"	0.92/0.37
Dhaliwal et al., 2009[17]	Stage 3 ROP at 34 wks PMA or 4–6 wks CA	0.57/0.98
	Presence of plus disease	0.80/0.98
Lorenz et al., 2009[21]	Suspected treatment-requiring ROP: threshold ROP in zone II, prethreshold in zone I, or disease possibly requiring treatment but not reliably classified from images	1.00/NA
Silva et al., 2011[9]	Referral-warranted ROP: type 2 or worse	1.00/0.99
Dai et al., 2011[22]	Treatment-requiring ROP	1.00/0.98

**RetCam; Clarity Medical Systems, Pleasanton, CA. For definition of "clinically significant ROP", see text.*
PMA, postmenstrual age; CA, chronological age; NA, not applicable.

57%, and specificity was 98% compared to ophthalmoscopy. Sensitivity for detecting plus disease was 80%, and specificity was 98%. Absolute agreement between ophthalmoscopy and telemedicine was 96% for detection of stage 3, and 97% for detection of plus disease.[17] Dai et al. (422 exams from 108 infants) conducted a study in which all infants received telemedicine imaging and ophthalmoscopy by a pediatric ophthalmologist. Images were reviewed independently by a masked grader. Using ophthalmoscopy as the reference standard, sensitivity of telemedicine for detecting treatment-requiring ROP (i.e., type 1 or worse) was 100% and specificity was 98%. The positive predictive value of telemedicine for detecting treatment-requiring ROP was 86%, and the negative predictive value was 100%.[22]

Scott et al. compared the accuracy of telemedicine vs ophthalmoscopy using a study design in which these two methods were performed by the *same* experts in 67 consecutive infants. There was substantial to near-perfect agreement between these methods, with absolute intra-grader agreement of 86% (178/206 eyes) and kappa values of 0.66–0.85 between ophthalmoscopy and telemedicine. Among the 14% (28/206 eyes) intra-expert discrepancies, some cases provided photographic evidence that ophthalmoscopy failed to recognize mild ROP that was detected by telemedicine. There were also discrepancies involving presence of zone I and plus disease, in which telemedicine may have provided theoretical advantages by allowing examiners to review their diagnoses, make more exact measurements of anatomical landmarks, and directly compare images to standard photographs.[23]

Image quality

Several studies have examined the quality of images captured by nurses, ophthalmic photographers, or ophthalmologists. Ells et al. found that wide-angle images were captured successfully in 96% of examinations, and that 94% of image sets could be graded remotely. In the remaining 6%, readable photographs were obtained within 1–4 weeks.[18] Wu et al. found that 79% of initial retinal images and 78% of repeated images were acceptable.[19] The Photo-ROP cooperative group found that 92% of image sets were acceptable.[20] Chiang et al. reported that telemedicine graders reported an "unknown" diagnosis because of inadequate image quality or insufficient retinal coverage in 0%–41% of exams at 31–33 weeks PMA, and in 0%–7% of exams at 35–37 weeks PMA.[8] Lorenz et al. reported that, among 6460 telemedicine imaging sessions conducted at five NICUs over a six-year period, nearly 98% were of adequate quality.[21] Heavy fundus pigmentation, corneal and vitreous haze, smaller palpebral fissures, and limited dilation may be associated with decreased image quality.[8,13,16,19]

Cost-effectiveness, speed, and satisfaction

Economic and practical factors must be considered for long-term viability of telemedicine systems. Two studies have compared the cost-effectiveness of telemedicine versus ophthalmoscopy for ROP management using decision tree models created from published results involving disease incidence, diagnostic accuracy, and treatment outcomes. One study, performed in the United States, found that telemedicine is more cost-effective than traditional ophthalmoscopy ($3193 per quality-adjusted life year [QALY] compared to $5617/QALY).[24] The second study, performed in the United Kingdom, modeled five possible strategies for ROP surveillance using telemedicine and ophthalmoscopy, and found that telemedicine using image capture and grading by visiting nurses (£175 per infant examined) and telemedicine using image capture by visiting nurses and image grading by remote ophthalmologists (£201/infant examined) were more cost-effective than traditional ophthalmoscopy at the NICU bedside (£321/infant examined).[25]

Other studies have examined logistical factors such as examination time and acceptability to patients. Richter et al. found that telemedicine examinations required significantly less physician time than ophthalmoscopy (1.02–1.75 minutes per telemedicine exam versus 4.17–6.63 minutes per ophthalmoscopic exam).[26] Lee et al. developed and validated a survey instrument to assess attitudes toward digital imaging and telemedicine by parents, and found high acceptance of these technologies. Families did, however, report that face-to-face contact with physicians was important.[27]

EVALUATION OF OPERATIONAL ROP TELEMEDICINE PROGRAMS

Real-world telemedicine programs have been implemented in several centers, typically relying on trained neonatal technicians or nurses to capture images and transfer data for interpretation by remote ophthalmologists. Infants identified with clinically significant disease are either examined locally by an ophthalmologist, or transferred for further evaluation.

A telemedicine program involving five German NICUs has been operational since 2001. In this program, all premature infants at risk for ROP are screened with wide-angle imaging and also examined by local ophthalmologists. All suspected treatment-requiring ROP stages were detected with 100% sensitivity, and the overall positive predictive value for treatment-requiring ROP was 88.2% after 6460 examinations in 1222 infants.[21]

A similar program involving four NICUs, in which nurses are trained to capture serial images, has been used for routine telemedicine management at Stanford University since 2005.[9] Infants felt to have referral-warranted (i.e. type 2 or worse) or treatment-requiring (i.e. type 1 or worse) ROP based on telemedicine were referred for complete ophthalmoscopic evaluation. Within one week of NICU discharge, all infants in this program received a mandatory ophthalmoscopic examination by the same retinal specialist. The sensitivity of telemedicine for identifying referral-warranted and treatment-requiring ROP was reported to be 100%, the positive predictive value of telemedicine for identifying treatment-requiring ROP was 90%, and the negative predictive value was 100%. No known cases of treatment-requiring ROP were missed, and there were no adverse outcomes such as retinal detachment.[9]

BARRIERS AND CHALLENGES

Despite technological advances to support telemedicine for ROP management, its widespread adoption has been limited by factors such as medical licensure and lack of consistent insurance coverage and reimbursement policies.[28] The level of diagnostic accuracy required for implementation of real-world ROP telemedicine systems is unclear, given concerns about medicolegal liability. Furthermore, it is difficult to rigorously assess accuracy because there may be variability in the reference standard of indirect ophthalmoscopy. Capturing images with sufficient diagnostic quality may not always be practical, particularly in the peripheral retinas of younger infants, warranting re-evaluation either by repeat imaging or ophthalmoscopy. Finally, implementation of telemedicine for ROP requires approval of physicians and financial investments for new equipment and information technologies.

FUTURE DIRECTIONS

Telemedicine has potential benefits for ROP management, education, and research. Studies have demonstrated that it has very high accuracy for detection of clinically significant ROP, particularly in older infants. An ongoing study is examining the validity, reliability, feasibility, safety, and cost-effectiveness of an ROP telemedicine system to detect referral-warranted ROP with a multicenter design,[29] and a centralized image-reading center.

Attention should be given to training protocols, and to the assignment of roles and responsibilities for neonatology and ophthalmology personnel. Rules must be defined for cases in which image quality is inadequate, and when digital imaging is impractical because of systemic illness, infection contact precautions, or other reasons. Development of image capture protocols will help standardize the process of ROP telemedicine diagnosis, analogous to what has been done in diseases such as diabetic retinopathy (Chapter 50, Telescreening for diabetic retinopathy). Reading center software, which helps optimize workflow and mitigate risk, should be easily accessible for ophthalmologists and hospitals.[30] The success from several operational programs suggests that this is practical, but the maintenance of large sustainable ROP telemedicine programs will require generalizable solutions to these challenges.

Disclosure

M.F.C. is an unpaid member of the Scientific Advisory Board for Clarity Medical Systems (Pleasanton, CA).

REFERENCES

1. Multicenter trial of cryotherapy for retinopathy of prematurity. Preliminary results. Cryotherapy for Retinopathy of Prematurity Cooperative Group. Pediatrics 1988;81:697–706.
2. Early Treatment for Retinopathy of Prematurity Cooperative Group. Revised indications for the treatment of retinopathy of prematurity: results of the early treatment for retinopathy of prematurity randomized trial. Arch Ophthalmol 2003;121:1684–94.
3. Section on Ophthalmology American Academy of Pediatrics, American Academy of Pediatrics. Screening examination of premature infants for retinopathy of prematurity. Pediatrics 2006;117:572–6. Erratum in Pediatrics 2006;118:1324.
4. Laws DE, Morton C, Weindling M, et al. Systemic effects of screening for retinopathy of prematurity. Br J Ophthalmol 1996;80:425–8.
5. Chiang MF, Jiang L, Gelman R, et al. Interexpert agreement of plus disease diagnosis in retinopathy of prematurity diagnosis. Arch Ophthalmol 2007;125:875–80.
6. Chiang MF, Thyparampil PJ, Rabinowitz D. Interexpert agreement in identification of macular location in infants at risk for retinopathy of prematurity. Arch Ophthalmol 2010;128:1153–9.
7. Ocular Surgery News U.S. Edition [Internet] 2006 [cited 2010 Nov 1]. Survey: Physicians being driven away from ROP treatment. http://www.osnsupersite.com/view/asp?rID=18018.
8. Chiang MF, Wang L, Busuioc M, et al. Telemedical retinopathy of prematurity diagnosis: accuracy, reliability, and image quality. Arch Ophthalmol 2007;125:1531–8.
9. Silva RA, Murakami Y, Lad EM, et al. Stanford University network for diagnosis of retinopathy of prematurity (SUNDROP): 36-month experience with telemedicine screening. Ophthalmic Surg Lasers Imaging 2011;42:12–9.
10. Mukherjee AN, Watts P, Al-Madfai H, et al. Impact of retinopathy of prematurity screening examination on cardiorespiratory indices: a comparison of indirect ophthalmoscopy and RetCam imaging. Ophthalmology 2006;113:1547–52.
11. Chiang MF, Gelman R, Martinez-Perez ME, et al. Image analysis for retinopathy of prematurity diagnosis. J AAPOS 2009;13:438–45.
12. Schwartz SD, Harrison SA, Ferrone PJ, et al. Telemedical evaluation and management of retinopathy of prematurity using a fiberoptic digital fundus camera. Ophthalmology 2000;107:25–8.
13. Chiang MF, Keenan JD, Starren J, et al. Accuracy and reliability of remote retinopathy of prematurity diagnosis. Arch Ophthalmol 2006;124:322–7.
14. Roth DB, Morales D, Feuer WJ, et al. Screening for retinopathy of prematurity employing the RetCam 120: sensitivity and specificity. Arch Ophthalmol 2001;119:268–72.
15. Yen KG, Hess D, Burke B, et al. Telephotoscreening to detect retinopathy of prematurity: preliminary study of the optimum time to employ digital fundus camera imaging to detect ROP. J AAPOS 2002;6:64–70.

16. Shah PK, Narendran V, Saravanan VR, et al. Screening for retinopathy of prematurity: a comparison between binocular indirect ophthalmoscopy and RetCam 120. Indian J Ophthalmol 2006;54:35–8.
17. Dhaliwal C, Wright E, Graham C, et al. Wide-field digital retinal imaging versus binocular indirect ophthalmoscopy for retinopathy of prematurity screening: a two-observer prospective, randomised comparison. Br J Ophthalmol 2009;93:355–9.
18. Ells AL, Holmes JM, Astle WF, et al. Telemedicine approach to screening for severe retinopathy of prematurity: a pilot study. Ophthalmology 2003;110: 2113–7.
19. Wu C, Petersen RA, VanderVeen DK. RetCam imaging for retinopathy of prematurity screening. J AAPOS 2006; 10:107–11.
20. Photographic Screening for Retinopathy of Prematurity (PHOTO-ROP) Cooperative Group. The photographic screening for retinopathy of prematurity study (PHOTO-ROP): primary outcomes. Retina 2008;28:S47–54.
21. Lorenz B, Spasovska K, Elflein H, et al. Wide-field digital imaging based telemedicine for screening for acute retinopathy of prematurity (ROP). Six-year results of a multicentre field study. Graefes Arch Clin Exp Ophthalmol 2009;247:1251–62.
22. Dai S, Chow K, Vincent A. Efficacy of wide-field digital retinal imaging for retinopathy of prematurity screening. Clin Experiment Ophthalmol 2011;39: 23–9.
23. Scott KA, Kim DY, Wang L, et al. Telemedical diagnosis of retinopathy of prematurity: intraphysician and agreement between ophthalmoscopic examination and image-based interpretation. Ophthalmology 2008;115:1222–8
24. Jackson KM, Scott KE, Graff-Zivin J, et al. Cost-utility analysis of telemedicine and ophthalmoscopy for retinopathy of prematurity management. Arch Ophthalmol 2008; 126:493–9.
25. Castillo-Riquelme MC, Lord J, Moseley MJ, et al. Cost-effectiveness of digital photographic screening for retinopathy of prematurity in the United Kingdom. Int J Technol Assess Health Care 2004; 20:201–13.
26. Richter GM, Sun G, Lee TC, et al. Speed of telemedicine vs ophthalmoscopy for retinopathy of prematurity diagnosis. Am J Ophthalmol 2009;148:136–42.
27. Lee JY, Du YE, Coki O, et al. Parental perceptions toward digital imaging and telemedicine for retinopathy of prematurity management. Graefes Arch Clin Exp Ophthalmol 2010; 248:141–7.
28. Grigsby J, Sanders JH. Telemedicine: where it is and where it's going. Ann Intern Med 1998;129:123–7.
29. ClinicalTrials.gov [Internet]. US National Institutes of Health 2011 [cited 2011 June 28]. Telemedicine approaches to evaluating acute-phase ROP. Available from: http://clinicaltrials.gov/ct2/show/NCT01264276.
30. Focus-ROP Remote Disease Management [Internet]. 2011 [reviewed 2011 Jan 12; cited 2011 May 6]. Cast a wide safety net for retinopathy of prematurity (ROP) Available from: http://www.focusrop.com/.

Chapter 63

Epidemiology and Risk Factors for Age-Related Macular Degeneration

Johanna M. Seddon, Lucia Sobrin

Age-related macular degeneration (AMD) is the leading cause of irreversible blindness.[1] The disease adversely affects quality of life and activities of daily living, causing many affected individuals to lose their independence in their retirement years. AMD is estimated to affect more than 8 million individuals in the USA;[2] the advanced form of the disease affects more than 1.75 million individuals.[1] Despite the introduction of new therapies for prevention and treatment of AMD, the prevalence of AMD is expected to increase by 97% by the year 2050.[3]

The only proven treatment available for the dry or nonexudative forms of this disease, comprising 85% of cases, is an antioxidant/mineral supplement which can slow the progression of the disease by 25% over 5 years.[4] For the wet form of the disease, anti-vascular endothelial growth factor (VEGF) treatments have been very effective in preventing severe vision loss. Still, preventive measures are needed to reduce the burden of this disease. Smoking is the most consistently identified modifiable risk factor.[5–6] Obesity, sunlight exposure, and nutritional factors including antioxidants and dietary fat intake may also affect AMD incidence and progression.[4,7–14] There has also been great progress in identifying the genetic variants that impact risk of AMD.[15–29] The knowledge of genetic risk variants for the disease coupled with knowledge of nongenetic risk factors have improved the ability to predict which patients will develop advanced forms of the disease.[23,30–32] Although much progress has been made over the past two decades, finding the causes and mechanisms of this condition remains a challenge.

CLASSIFICATION

Macular degenerative changes have typically been classified into two clinical forms, dry or wet, both of which can lead to visual loss. The wet form is also called advanced wet, exudative or neovascular. In the early or intermediate dry forms visual loss is infrequent, and when it occurs it is usually gradual. Ophthalmoscopy reveals yellow subretinal deposits called drusen, or retinal pigment epithelial (RPE) irregularities, including hyperpigmentation or hypopigmentary changes. Larger drusen may become confluent and evolve into drusenoid RPE detachments. These drusenoid RPE detachments often progress to geographic atrophy and less frequently to neovascular AMD. Geographic atrophy involving the center of the macula, which is the advanced dry form, leads to visual loss. Each of these signs can be further subdivided according to the number or size of the lesions. In the wet form, vision loss can appear to occur suddenly, when a choroidal neovascular membrane leaks fluid or blood into the subpigment epithelial or subretinal space. Serous RPE detachments with or without coexisting choroidal neovascularization (CNV) are also classified as the wet form. Exudative serous RPE detachments often, but not always, advance to the neovascular stage. This phenotypic heterogeneity, or wide range of clinical findings, has led to the use of various definitions of AMD and also to some difficulties with comparisons among studies.

It is important for investigators to standardize definitions of a disease and its subtypes to enhance comparability and to promote collaborative efforts. Toward this goal, an international classification and grading system for AMD was recommended, although it is not universally applied.[33] In this system age-related maculopathy (ARM) or early AMD is defined as the presence of drusen and RPE irregularities, and the terms late ARM and advanced AMD are limited to the occurrence of geographic atrophy and neovascular disease, the forms most often associated with greater visual loss. Clinical manifestations of AMD can be subcategorized according to the specific type of AMD, which for example can yield a four- or five-step grading system.[34–35] The Clinical Age-Related Maculopathy grading System (CARMS)[34] is useful for clinical management and genetic epidemiologic research and has been used in several studies.[11,13,23,25–27,29,36–39] Alternative and more detailed systems have been used in some of the population-based studies described below.[40–41] New subcategories of AMD will evolve as genetic and epidemiologic studies provide further insight into the pathogenesis of this disease. An updated classification under the auspices of the Beckman Initiative for Macular Research is underway.

PREVALENCE

Prevalence is the total number of cases in the population, divided by the number of individuals in the population. Population-based studies that have provided information on the prevalence of AMD within the USA include the National Health and Nutrition Examination Survey (NHANES),[42–43] the Framingham Eye Study (FES),[44] the Chesapeake Bay Watermen Study,[40] the Beaver Dam Eye Study (BDES),[45] the Baltimore Eye Survey,[46] and the Salisbury Eye Evaluation Project.[47] Population-based studies outside the USA include the Rotterdam Study in the Netherlands,[48] the Blue Mountains Eye Study (BMES) in Australia,[49] the Barbados Eye Study,[50] and a study in Italy.[51] Prevalence rates are quite variable for all types of AMD combined, because of differences in definitions of AMD, but are more consistent for "advanced AMD."

The BDES was a census of the population of Beaver Dam, Wisconsin.[45] This study found that the early forms are much more common than the late stages of AMD, and both types increase in frequency with increasing age. The prevalence of late AMD was 1.6% overall; exudative maculopathy was present in at least one eye in 1.2% of the population; and geographic atrophy was present in 0.6%. The prevalence of late AMD rose to 7.1% in persons who were 75 or older.

Total prevalence of AMD in the USA was also estimated in 2004 using pooled findings from seven large population-based studies both inside and outside the USA, and applying those prevalence rates to the USA population.[1] This meta-analysis by the Eye Diseases Prevalence Group calculated the overall prevalence of neovascular AMD and/or geographic atrophy to be 1.47% of the USA population aged 40 years or older. The most recent NHANES, conducted from 2005 to 2008, sampled approximately 5500 persons.[43] The total prevalence of any AMD in this civilian noninstitutionalized USA population aged 40 years or older was 6.5% (7.2 million people), and 809 000 persons were estimated to have the late stage of AMD.[43]

Studies conducted outside the USA have found similar or lower rates of AMD compared to those conducted inside the USA. In the Rotterdam Study, fundus photographs of 6251 participants aged 55–98 years were reviewed for drusen, pigmentary changes, and atrophic or neovascular AMD.[48] The prevalence of AMD was observed to be slightly lower in that study compared with the BDES in Wisconsin. In the BMES in Australia, the authors also found lower prevalence of all lesions related to AMD in each age stratum.[49] After adjusting for age, differences were significant for both soft drusen and retinal pigmentary abnormalities; they were lower but not significantly different for geographic atrophy and exudative disease. In a population-based study of 354 participants in rural southern Italy, the prevalence rates of AMD were also lower than those found in the USA.[51] Methodological differences between studies may exist, but the lower prevalence rates found in these countries may also reflect genetic or environmental differences compared with the US population.

INCIDENCE

Incidence is a measure of the risk of developing some new condition within a specified period of time. A few studies have been done to evaluate the incidence of AMD. The FES used the age-specific prevalence data to estimate 5-year incidence rates of AMD, according to the definition of AMD in that study. These estimates were 2.5%, 6.7%, and 10.8% for individuals who were 65, 70, and 75 years of age, respectively.[52] The BDES determined the 5-year cumulative incidence of developing early and late AMD in a population of 3583 adults (age range 43–86 years).[53] Incidence of early AMD increased from 3.9% in individuals aged 43–54 years to 22.8% in persons 75 years of age and older. The overall 5-year incidence of late AMD was 0.9%. Persons 75 years of age or older had a 5.4% incidence rate of late AMD. The Visual Impairment Project of Melbourne, Australia, described the 5-year incidence of early AMD lesions in a population of 3271 participants aged 40 years and older.[54] The overall 5-year incidence of AMD was 0.49%, and overall incidence of early AMD was 17.3% in this population. As with the BDES, incidence of AMD increased with age – up to 6.3% for people aged 80 years and older at baseline. The Barbados Eye Study described a 4-year incidence of early macular changes as 5.2% in a black population, with an extremely low incidence of exudative AMD.[55] The differences in prevalence and incidence rates by race/ethnicity are discussed below. One report suggests that the incidence of advanced AMD in the USA may be on the decline, possibly due in part to changes in lifestyle habits of the American public over the past 40 years.[56]

QUALITY OF LIFE

The psychologic costs associated with AMD underscore the growing importance of this disease on the expanding older adult population. For this reason it is important to incorporate a functional component into studies of AMD. Instruments such as the National Eye Institute Visual Function Questionnaire and the Macular Disease Dependent Quality of Life Questionnaire have been used in AMD studies.[57–58] Patients with visual loss resulting from AMD often report AMD as their worst medical problem and have a diminished quality of life.[59–60] More recently in one study of well-being, patients with AMD had lower scores than patients with chronic obstructive pulmonary disease and acquired immunodeficiency syndrome (AIDS); the lower quality of life in patients with AMD was related to greater emotional distress, worse self-reported general health, and greater difficulty carrying out daily activities. Not only is AMD associated with a higher rate of depression in the community-dwelling adult population when compared to the unaffected adult population,[61–62] but depression also exacerbates the effects of AMD.[63]

SOCIODEMOGRAPHIC RISK FACTORS

Age

All studies demonstrate that the prevalence, incidence, and progression of all forms of AMD rise steeply with increasing age. There was a 17-fold increased risk of AMD comparing the oldest to the youngest age group in the Framingham Study.[44] In the Watermen Study, the prevalence of moderate to advanced AMD doubled with each decade after age 60.[40] In the BDES, approximately 30% of individuals 75 years of age or older had early AMD; of the remainder, 23% developed early AMD within 5 years.[45,53] By age 75 years and older in that study, 7.1% had late AMD, compared with 0.1% in the age group 43–54 years and 0.6% among persons aged 55–64 years. Pooled data in a prevalence paper showed similar rates, with dramatic increases in rates for both men and women older than 80 years.[1]

Gender

Several studies[1,44–45,48] have shown no overall difference in the frequency of AMD between men and women, after controlling for age. However, in NHANES III, men, regardless of race and age, had a lower prevalence of AMD than women.[42] Incidence rates within the Beaver Dam population also suggest a gender difference. After adjusting for age, women aged 75 years or older had approximately twice the incidence of early AMD compared with men.[53] A study using reported incidence of exudative AMD in the USA among Medicare beneficiaries supported the Beaver Dam results.[64] In the BMES, there were consistent, though not significant, gender differences in prevalence for most lesions of AMD, with women having higher rates for soft, indistinct drusen, but not for retinal pigmentary abnormalities.[49] A case–control study in the Age-Related Eye Disease Study (AREDS) also found women had a higher risk for intermediate drusen.[65] Residual confounding by age in the broad age category "75 and older" may partially explain the differences between studies since there are more women than men in that age group. Additional research is needed, however, to assess these associations.

Race/ethnicity

Ophthalmologists observe visual loss caused by CNV less frequently among US ethnic minority groups compared with Caucasians. In the Baltimore Eye Survey, AMD accounted for 30% of bilateral blindness among whites and for 0% among African Americans.[66] Data from a population-based study of blacks in Barbados, West Indies,[50,55] revealed that incidence of AMD and signs of AMD changes occurred commonly but at a lower frequency than in predominantly white populations in other studies. Hispanics also have a lower prevalence of advanced AMD than non-Hispanics. Late-stage AMD was significantly less frequent among Hispanics vs. non-Hispanic whites in Beaver Dam (OR = 0.07; 95% CI = 0.01–0.49).[67] The Los Angeles Latino Eye Study indicates Latinos have a relatively high rate of early AMD but not late AMD.[68] Among persons aged 40–79 years, the age-specific prevalence of late AMD in Asians was comparable with that reported from white populations, but early AMD signs were less common among Asians.[69]

Overall, the literature to date suggests that early AMD is common among blacks and Hispanics, although less common than among non-Hispanic whites, whereas advanced AMD is much less common in these groups compared with non-Hispanic whites. Furthermore, differences in prevalence rates between non-Hispanic whites in different regions of the USA suggest that ethnicity is an important determinant of AMD.

Socioeconomic status

Less education and lower income have been shown to be related to increased morbidity and mortality from a number of diseases,[70] and there are mixed findings for AMD. The Eye Disease Case Control Study (EDCCS), a National Eye Institute-sponsored multicenter study, was designed to study risk factors for several types of maculopathy, including neovascular AMD.[71] Persons with higher levels of education had a slightly reduced risk of neovascular AMD, but the association did not remain statistically significant after multivariate modeling.[71] Education was also inversely related to AMD in case–control and prospective studies based on the AREDS population even in multivariate analyses.[30,65] In the BDES, no association was found between education, income, employment status, or marital status and maculopathy.[72] Furthermore, no associations were noted in another case–control study[73] or in the FES,[44] although different definitions of macular degeneration were used in those reports, compared with the more recent studies. It is possible that education is a surrogate marker for behaviors and lifestyles related to AMD.

OCULAR RISK FACTORS

Refractive error

Several case–control studies have shown an association between AMD and hyperopia.[65,71,73–75] The potential problem with some of these studies is the clinical setting in which they were conducted. Because ophthalmology practices tend to contain a disproportionate number of myopic patients, controls selected from such practices would tend to have a higher prevalence of myopia than that of the general population. Population-based data from the BMES, less likely to have such potential bias, has also suggested a weak association between hyperopia and early AMD, but not late AMD.[76] The population-based Rotterdam Study also showed an association between hyperopia and both incident and prevalent AMD.[77] This association, therefore, might implicate structural and mechanical differences that render some eyes predisposed to maculopathy.[78]

Iris color

Higher levels of ocular melanin may be protective against light-induced oxidative damage to the retina, since melanin can act as a free radical scavenger and may have an antiangiogenesis function. To date, the literature is inconclusive about the relationship between iris color and AMD. Darker irides have been found to be protective in some studies[73,79–83] but not in others.[71,84–88] Differences between studies may be partly related to the use of different definitions of disease, different number and types of other factors evaluated simultaneously, and residual confounding by ethnicity in some studies.

Lens opacities, cataracts, and cataract surgery

Data regarding the relationship between cataracts and AMD are inconsistent. FES investigators found no relationship,[89] whereas data from the NHANES did support a relationship between AMD and lens opacities.[90] In the BDES, in which photographs of the lens and macula were graded, nuclear sclerosis was associated with increased odds of early AMD (OR 1.96; 95% CI 1.3–3.0) but not of late AMD. Neither cortical nor posterior subcapsular cataracts were related to AMD.[91] A case–control study of 1844 cases and 1844 controls indicated that lens opacities or cataract surgery were associated with an increased risk of AMD.[74]

Although AMD-affected individuals reported better visual function and quality of life after cataract surgery,[92] a history of cataract surgery has been found to be associated with an increased risk for advanced AMD in some earlier studies.[93] Investigators have postulated that this association might arise because the cataractous lens can block damaging ultraviolet light. Inflammatory changes after cataract surgery may also cause progression of early to late AMD. In the BDES, previous cataract surgery at baseline was associated with a statistically significant increased risk for progression of AMD (OR 2.7) and for development of late AMD (OR 2.8; 95% CI 1.03–7.6).[85] In more recent prospective studies, however, including the large AREDS study cohort, there was no evidence to support a higher rate of progression of AMD in patients who underwent cataract surgery.[94–95]

Cup-to-disc ratio

The EDCCS demonstrated that eyes with larger cup-to-disc ratios had a reduced risk of exudative AMD. This effect persisted even after multivariate modeling,[71] adjusting for known and potential confounding factors. Whether this finding, which is consistent with the association between AMD and hyperopic refractive error mentioned earlier, is meaningful in terms of the mechanisms associated with the development of AMD awaits further study.

BEHAVIORAL AND LIFESTYLE FACTORS

Smoking

The preponderance of epidemiologic evidence indicates a strong positive association between both wet and dry AMD and smoking. Two large prospective cohort studies have evaluated the relationship between smoking and wet AMD and dry AMD associated with visual loss.[5,96] Seddon et al. reported that women in the Nurses' Health Study who currently smoked 25 or more cigarettes per day had a relative risk (RR) of 2.4 (95% CI 1.4–4), and women who were past smokers had an RR of 2.0 (95% CI 1.2–3.4) for developing AMD compared with women who never smoked.[5] There was a dose–response relationship between AMD and pack-years of smoking, and risk remained elevated for many years after smoking cessation. Results were consistent for various definitions of AMD, including wet AMD and dry AMD, with different levels of visual loss, and for different definitions of smoking. It was estimated that 29% of the AMD cases in that study could be attributable to smoking.[5] These results were supported by a study among men participating in the Physicians' Health Study.[96] Several other studies have also shown an increased risk for AMD among smokers.[65,97–99] Smoking is an important, independent, modifiable risk factor for AMD.

Mechanisms by which smoking may increase the risk of developing AMD include its adverse effect on blood lipids by decreasing levels of high-density lipoprotein (HDL) and increasing platelet aggregability and fibrinogen, increasing oxidative stress and lipid peroxidation, and reducing plasma levels of antioxidants.[5] In animal models, nicotine has been shown to increase the size and severity of experimental CNV, suggesting that non-neuronal nicotinic receptors may also play a part in the effect of smoking on advanced AMD.[100] Statistical interactions between smoking and either the Complement Factor H (*CFH*) Y402H or *ARMS2/HTRA1* genotypes have not been confirmed (see "Genetics factors" below).[101–102]

Antioxidants, vitamins, and minerals

The role of antioxidant vitamins in the pathogenesis of AMD has received a great deal of attention. Antioxidants, which include vitamin C (ascorbic acid), vitamin E (alpha-tocopherol), and the carotenoids (including alpha-carotene, beta-carotene, cryptoxanthin, lutein, and zeaxanthin), may be relevant to AMD because of their physiologic functions and the location of some of these nutrients in the retina. Lutein and zeaxanthin, in particular, are associated with macular pigment.[103–105] Trace minerals such as zinc, selenium, copper, and manganese may also be involved in antioxidant functions of the retina. Antioxidants could prevent oxidative damage to the retina, which could in turn prevent development of AMD.[10,106] Damage to retinal photoreceptor cells could be caused by photo-oxidation or by free radical-induced lipid peroxidation.[107–108] This could lead to impaired function of the RPE and eventually to degeneration involving the macula. The deposit of oxidized compounds in healthy tissue may result in cell death because they are indigestible by cellular enzymes.[108–109] Antioxidants may scavenge, decompose, or reduce the formation of harmful compounds.

The AREDS confirmed that antioxidant and zinc supplementation can decrease the risk of AMD progression and vision loss.[4] This study included a double-blind clinical trial in 11 centers around the USA, randomly assigning 3640 participants to take daily oral supplements of antioxidants, zinc, antioxidants and zinc, or placebo. Both zinc alone and antioxidants and zinc together significantly reduced the odds of developing advanced AMD in participants with intermediate signs of AMD (see Chapter 65, Age-related macular degeneration: Non-neovascular early AMD, intermediate AMD, and geographic atrophy) in at least one eye. The zinc supplement included zinc (80 mg) as zinc oxide, and copper (2 mg) as cupric oxide; the antioxidant supplement included vitamin C (500 mg), vitamin E (400 IU), and beta-carotene (15 mg). If the AREDS formulation were used to treat the 8 million individuals in the USA who are at increased risk for developing advanced AMD, the AREDS group authors estimate that more than 300,000 would avoid advanced AMD and the associated vision loss during the next 5 years.[2] AREDS-type supplements are a cost-effective way of reducing visual loss due to the progression of AMD.[110] The effect of dietary antioxidants on the incidence of early AMD has not been established and there are questions about the effect of beta-carotene supplements on AMD since there is none in the retina, and high doses of zinc could have side-effects.

Diets high in antioxidant-rich fruits and vegetables may be related to a lower risk of exudative AMD. The first study launched to evaluate diet and AMD, the Dietary Intake Study, ancillary to the EDCCS, showed an inverse association between exudative AMD and dietary intake of carotenoids from foods.[10] In that study reported in 1994, a diet rich in green leafy vegetables containing the carotenoids lutein and zeaxanthin was associated with a reduction in the risk of exudative AMD. Intake of 6 mg of lutein per day was associated with a significant 43% reduction in risk of AMD.[10] A prospective double-masked study involving lutein and antioxidant supplementation in a group of 90 individuals showed that visual function was improved with 10 mg of lutein or a lutein/antioxidant formula.[111] In a British study of 380 men and women, lower plasma levels of zeaxanthin were also found to be associated with an increased risk of AMD.[112] A cross-sectional study using previously collected NHANES I data found a weak protective effect with increased consumption of fruits and vegetables rich in vitamin A.[113] A prospective follow-up study has shown that fruit intake is inversely associated with exudative AMD. Participants who consumed three or more servings of fresh fruit per day have an RR of 0.64 (95% CI 0.44–0.93) compared to those who consumed less than 1.5 servings per day.[7] The early evidence regarding lutein was recently supported by analyses of diet data from AREDS.[114] AREDS2, an ongoing trial of lutein, zeaxanthin, and omega 3 fatty acids and assessment of omission of beta-carotene and use of much lower doses of zinc for the prevention of AMD progression, may provide additional data regarding optimal vitamin supplement regimens for AMD patients.

Alcohol intake

Studies that have examined the relationship between AMD and alcohol consumption have yielded mixed results. In the EDCCS, no significant relationship between alcohol intake and exudative AMD was noted in univariate analyses,[71] but an inverse association could not be ruled out in multivariate analyses. Another case–control study found a suggestion of a nonlinear trend with higher risk of AMD in persons who had five drinks or more per day and a lower risk in persons who had one or two drinks per day compared with nondrinkers.[115] In a case–control study using NHANES I data, moderate wine consumption was associated with a decreased risk of developing AMD, although the analysis did not control for the potential confounding effects of smoking.[116] In a large prospective study, no support was found for a protective association between moderate alcohol consumption and risk of AMD, although there was a suggestion of a modest increased risk of AMD in heavier drinkers.[117] The BDES found heavy drinkers were more likely to develop late AMD,[98] whereas the BMES found an increased risk of early AMD only in current spirits drinkers.[118] The evidence to date suggests that alcohol intake does not have a large effect on the development of AMD.

Obesity and physical activity

There is an association between AMD and overall obesity[13,119–122] and abdominal adiposity.[13] In a prospective cohort study of 261 individuals with some sign of nonadvanced AMD in at least one eye,[13] individuals with a body mass index (BMI) between 25 and 29 had an RR of 2.32 (95% CI 1.32–4.07) for progression to advanced AMD when compared to those with a BMI of less than 25. Those with a BMI of at least 30 had an RR of 2.35 (95% CI 1.27–4.34) compared to the lowest category (BMI <25), after controlling for other factors. Similarly, the highest tertile of waist circumference had a twofold increased risk compared to the lowest tertile, and the highest tertile of waist-to-hip ratio had an RR of 1.84 compared to the lowest tertile. Thus, both overall and abdominal obesity were related to AMD progression. Vigorous physical activity three times a week reduced the risk of AMD progression by 25% compared to no physical activity.[13] Obesity and physical activity are modifiable factors that may alter an individual's risk of AMD incidence and progression. In one study, the susceptibility to advanced AMD associated with *CFH* Y402H was modified by body mass index (BMI), and both higher BMI and current and past smoking increased risk of advanced AMD within the same genotype category (see "Genetics factors" below).[101]

Sunlight exposure

The literature to date regarding the association between sunlight exposure and AMD is conflicting. Overall, the data do not support a strong association between ultraviolet radiation exposure and risk of AMD, although a small effect cannot be ruled out. In the BDES,[123] increased time spent outdoors in the summer was associated with a twofold increased risk of advanced AMD. The 5-year[124] and 10-year[125] incidence of early AMD in the BDES confirmed this association, although the 10-year incidence study showed few significant associations between environmental light and incidence and progression of early AMD. The EDCCS[71] and the Pathologies Oculaires Liées à l'Age (POLA) study in France[126] showed no significant association between advanced AMD and sunlight exposure. Sensitivity to sunburn may also be a risk factor. An Australian case–control study noted an association between sun-sensitive skin and risk of neovascular AMD.[127] Conflicting results in these studies exemplify the difficulties encountered when studying this complex exposure. These include challenges in measuring acute and chronic lifetime exposure and the effect of potential confounding variables, such as sun sensitivity and sun avoidance behaviors. Furthermore, studies have evaluated different populations with different stages of AMD and people with varying intensity of exposures.

Medications

The use of certain medications may be associated with AMD, although studies have yielded mixed results. Some studies have shown borderline statistically significant associations between increased risk of early AMD with use of antihypertensive medication, especially beta-blockers.[128] Other studies have shown a decreased rate of CNV among AMD patients taking aspirin[129] or cholesterol-lowering drugs such as statins.[129–130] The prospective Rotterdam Study, however, did not find a relationship between cholesterol-lowering drugs and risk of AMD.[131] The use of statins, in particular, may be associated with decreased CNV because of their anti-inflammatory and antioxidant properties.[132] Increased levels of C-reactive protein in patients with AMD have implicated a role for inflammation in the pathophysiology of the disease,[133] and it may be the anti-inflammatory effects of statins that affect risk, rather than the medication's cholesterol-lowering effect. The potential link between anticholesterol medications is more intriguing given the recent finding that the lipase C (*LIPC*) gene, a gene that influences high density lipoprotein (HDL) level, and other genes involved in cholesterol pathways, including cholesterylester transfer protein (*CETP*), are associated with AMD.[27–28] The effects of hormone replacement therapy and AMD are discussed below, in the section on hormonal and reproductive factors.

CARDIOVASCULAR-RELATED FACTORS

Cardiovascular diseases

It is important to study possible cardiovascular risk factors not only to understand the epidemiology of AMD, but also because anti-VEGF therapies have associated cardiovascular risks. Some studies have suggested an association between AMD and clinical manifestations of cardiovascular disease (CVD).[134–137] The presence of atherosclerotic lesions, determined by ultrasound, was examined in relation to risk of macular degeneration in a large population-based study conducted in the Netherlands.[137] Results obtained from this cross-sectional study showed a 4.5-fold increased risk of late AMD (defined as geographic atrophy or neovascular macular degeneration) associated with plaques in the carotid bifurcation and a twofold increased risk associated with plaques in the common carotid artery. Lower-extremity arterial disease (as measured by the ratio of the systolic blood pressure (SBP) level of the ankle to the SBP of the arm) was also associated with a 2.5-times increased risk of AMD.

In addition, a case–control study found a relationship between AMD and a history of one or more CVDs.[73] The NHANES I study reported a positive association between AMD and cerebrovascular disease, but positive associations with other vascular diseases did not reach statistical significance.[113] A Finnish study reported a significant correlation between occurrence of AMD and the severity of retinal arteriosclerosis.[138] However, other studies found that individuals who reported a history of cerebrovascular disease did not have a significantly greater risk of AMD.[71,97,139] On the other hand, many CVD risk factors are associated with AMD.

Blood pressure and hypertension

The role of blood pressure in the etiology of AMD remains unclear. There was a small and consistent statistically significant relationship between AMD and systemic hypertension in two cross-sectional population-based studies.[113,140] A case–control study found that individuals with AMD were significantly more likely to be taking antihypertensive medication.[141] Also, a significant relationship was found between AMD and diastolic blood pressure measured several years before the eye examination in the FES[142] and in a small Israeli study.[143] The BDES reported that SBP was associated with incidence of RPE depigmentation,[144] 10-year incidence of advanced AMD lesions, and progression of AMD.[134] That study has also shown that arteriovenous nicking, a retinal vascular characteristic associated with hypertension, is associated with an increased incidence of AMD.[145] The Rotterdam Study showed a relationship between elevated SBP and incidence of AMD.[136] In the Macular Photocoagulation Study, there was an increased incidence of exudative AMD associated with hypertension in the second eye of individuals with exudative AMD in one eye at baseline (RR 1.7; 95% CI 1.2–2.4).[146] In another case–control study, dry AMD was not associated with hypertension, but exudative AMD was significantly associated with both hypertension and antihypertensive medication use.[128] In a study evaluating lipid biomarkers and the hepatic lipase gene, there was a higher risk of advanced AMD for hypertension defined as over 160 mmHg systolic or 100 mmHg diastolic (OR 2.5, 95% CI 1.1–6.0) compared with normal levels.[147] Other cross-sectional[97,137,148] and case–control studies,[71] as well as one prospective study[139] (in which duration of hypertension was not taken into account) did not show an increased risk of AMD associated with current hypertension or systolic or diastolic blood pressure. Evidence suggests a possible mild to moderate association between elevated blood pressure and AMD. Assessment of this relationship could be enhanced by evaluating the duration of hypertension and its subsequent effects on onset and progression of maculopathy in large study populations with a sufficient number of subjects with advanced stages of AMD.

Cholesterol levels and dietary fat intake

There is some evidence linking cholesterol level to AMD, but not all results are consistent. The EDCCS reported a statistically significant fourfold increased risk of exudative AMD associated with the highest serum cholesterol level (>4.88 mmol/l) and a twofold increased risk in the middle-cholesterol-level group, compared with the lowest-cholesterol-level group, controlling for other factors.[71] A positive association was found between risk of AMD and increasing HDL levels in both the population-based POLA study[120] and the Rotterdam Study.[149] A case–control study showed that higher HDL cholesterol levels tended to reduce the risk of AMD.[147] The BDES found that early AMD was related to low total serum cholesterol levels in women and men older than 75. Furthermore, men with early AMD had higher HDL and lower total cholesterol-to-HDL ratios.[97,144] Slightly, but not significantly, increased risk of wet AMD was seen with increasing triglyceride level in the EDCCS.[71] This finding was not seen in the Rotterdam Study[137] or the BDES[97] (both of which had small numbers of exudative AMD cases and therefore limited power).

The genes involved in the HDL cholesterol pathway that have been associated with AMD have had discordant effects between the HDL-increasing alleles and the protective or risk effects for AMD. An HDL-raising allele of the *LIPC* gene was associated with a reduced risk of AMD whereas an HDL-increasing allele of *CETP* increased risk for AMD.[27-28] Furthermore, in one study, mean HDL level was lower in advanced AMD cases compared with controls, and this association was independent of *LIPC* genotype.[147] In turn, *LIPC* genotype was associated with advanced AMD independent of HDL level and other factors including dietary lutein, smoking, BMI, and genotypes at other established AMD genes.[147] The mechanisms through which genetic variants in the HDL cholesterol pathway exert their effect on AMD risk require further investigation.

An association between dietary fat intake and AMD was first reported in 1994.[14] Dietary fat intake was associated with an elevated risk of exudative AMD in the Dietary Ancillary Study of EDCCS.[12] This association was primarily caused by vegetable fat rather than animal fat. An inverse, protective association was found for higher consumption of docosahexaenoic acid and eicosapentaenoic acid omega-3 fatty acids in the multivariate model.[12] Also reported were positive associations between risk of AMD and total fat, vegetable, monounsaturated, and polyunsaturated fats and linoleic acid.[12] All of these relationships were strengthened in a prospective longitudinal study of progression to advanced forms of AMD.[11] A high intake of fish and omega-3 fatty acids reduced the risk when linoleic acid intake was low.[11,12] Prospective data from participants in the Women's Health Study confirmed that regular consumption of omega-3 fatty acids and fish was beneficial and they were associated with significantly decreased risk of incident early AMD.[150] Nuts have also been shown to decrease the risk of AMD progression.[11] In the BDES, individuals with greater saturated fat and cholesterol intake also had increased risk for early AMD.[151] However, no relationship was found between AMD and dietary fat intake in NHANES III.[152] Recent analyses of dietary data from AREDS support the previous observations of a beneficial effect of higher intake of omega-3 fatty acids.[153]

In summary, serum cholesterol levels may be related to exudative AMD, and the relationship with dietary fat is more consistent. The mechanisms through which variants in HDL-related genes affect AMD risk is not simply through their influence on serum HDL level. Dissection of the mechanisms through which HDL mediates AMD risk may illuminate additional treatment strategies. The consistent association between AMD and dietary fat and the possible association with cholesterol intake may indicate a relationship with atherosclerosis.[135,154]

Diabetes and hyperglycemia

Many studies have investigated the relationship between diabetes and/or hyperglycemia and AMD, and most have found no significant relationships. Only a few studies suggested a possible positive association.[42,155] One difficulty with these studies is the uncertainty of diagnosing AMD in the presence of diabetic retinopathy. Also, many studies of AMD exclude persons with diabetic retinopathy. This could result in attenuated relationships between AMD and diabetes in published studies.

HORMONAL AND REPRODUCTIVE FACTORS

There is evidence to support a small protective effect of hormone therapy on AMD,[71,156-157] but associations with pregnancies[71,158] or menopause[158,159] are more mixed. The EDCCS showed a marked decrease in the risk of neovascular AMD among postmenopausal women who used estrogen therapy,[71] as did a cross-sectional study.[156] No relationship was found in the BDES between years of estrogen therapy and exudative AMD (OR 0.9 (per 1 year of therapy); 95% CI 0.8–1.1) or any of the less severe forms of AMD among women.[158] However, this study had limited power to detect a potential effect of estrogen therapy on advanced AMD. The POLA study did not show an association between AMD and hormone therapy, hysterectomy, or oophorectomy.[160] Some studies,[161-162] including the BMES,[159] reported no relationship between AMD and hormone replacement therapy or early menopause. However, the BMES did describe a small but significant decrease in risk of early AMD with increasing number of years between menarche and menopause. The evidence is sparse, but a protective effect of estrogen on

AMD is possible and potentially important, and further research is warranted.

INFLAMMATORY FACTORS

Studies have suggested that inflammation plays a role in the pathogenesis of drusen and AMD.[133,135,163–165] Examination of tissue samples has shown that "cellular debris" from RPE cells becomes trapped in the RPE basal lamina and Bruch's membrane, potentially causing a chronic inflammatory response which may prompt drusen formation.[163] Drusen contain proteins that are associated with chronic and acute inflammatory responses[164] and other age-related diseases, including amyloid P component and complement proteins.[165] Inflammation is also associated with angiogenesis and may play a role in the neovascularization seen in the advanced forms of AMD.

A study of 930 individuals has shown that serum levels of the systemic inflammatory marker, C-reactive protein, are significantly elevated in individuals with advanced AMD.[133] This study showed that, after adjusting for variables such as age, gender, BMI, and smoking, the odds ratio for AMD comparing the highest and lowest quartiles of C-reactive protein was 1.65 (95% CI 1.07–2.55, P for trend = 0.02). In stratified analyses, the highest levels of C-reactive protein were associated with a twofold increased risk among both smokers and nonsmokers. High-sensitivity CRP and single nucleotide polymorphisms (SNPs) in the *CFH* gene are independently associated with risk of AMD in the Age Related Eye Disease Ancillary Study. Higher C-reactive protein level tends to confer a higher risk of AMD within most genotype groups.[166] These elevated levels suggest that reducing inflammation may slow the progression of AMD. Some studies raise the possibility that medications with anti-inflammatory properties, such as statins[129–130, 132] and triamcinolone,[167] may be beneficial.

The existence of multiple, complement-related AMD risk alleles has lent further support to the inflammatory pathogenesis theory for AMD and shed light on the role of uncontrolled alternative complement pathway activation in this disease (see "Genetic factors" below). CFH inhibits the alternative complement pathway by blocking formation of and accelerating the decay of alternative pathway C3 convertases; it also serves as a cofactor for the Factor-1-mediated cleavage and inactivation of C3b.[168] The Y402H SNP is within the CFH binding site for heparin and C-reactive protein. Binding to these sites increases the affinity of CFH for C3b, which in turn increases the ability of CFH to inhibit complement's effects.

As a result of the complement-related genetic discoveries, various complement-modulating agents are currently in clinical trials for the treatment of AMD.[169] Phase 1 clinical trials examining intravitreal compstatin/POT-4, a C3 inhibitor, in the treatment of wet AMD have been completed, and trials for dry AMD are underway. Systemic administration of the anti-C5 antibody, eculizumab, is being investigated for geographic atrophy. Intravitreal use of ARC1905, a C5 inhibitor, is being examined for the treatment of both dry and wet AMD in phase 1 clinical trials. An intravitreal antibody against Complement Factor D has also completed phase 1 clinical trials for geographic atrophy.

GENETIC FACTORS

AMD is a common, polygenic disease in which multiple genetic variants, each adding a small to moderate amount of increased risk, contribute to disease in addition to environmental factors.[170] The risk of developing the disease is threefold higher in people who have a family member with AMD than in those without a first-degree relative with AMD.[171–72] Since 2005, several genetic variants have been consistently associated with AMD. The common coding variant Y402H in the *CFH* gene was the first; the odds ratio associated with being homozygous for the risk variant for all categories of AMD is estimated to be between 2.45 and 3.33.[15–18,23,39,173] The odds ratios are higher, between 3.5 and 7.4, for advanced dry and wet forms of AMD. Several other genes in the alternative complement cascade have also been consistently shown to impact AMD risk. These include another variant in *CFH*,[23] Factor B (*BF*)/Complement Component 2 (*C2*),[22–3] Complement Component 3 (*C3*),[24–5] and Complement Factor I (*CFI*).[26]

Several genes not involved in the complement cascade have also been implicated. Variation in the *ARMS2/HTRA1* locus on chromosome 10 has been convincingly associated with AMD with an effect size similar to or greater than that of *CFH*.[19–21,174] The function of this gene is not completely understood but there is evidence that it confers greater risk for wet AMD as compared with geographic atrophy.[175] *LIPC* and tissue inhibitor of metalloproteinase 3 (*TIMP3*) were associated with AMD in large genome-wide association studies.[27–28] *LIPC* is involved in HDL cholesterol metabolism and *TIMP3* is implicated in a Mendelian, early-onset form of macular degeneration, Sorsby's fundus dystrophy.[176] Most recently, new variants near the collagen type X alpha 1 precursor/fyn related kinase (*COL10A1/FRK*) genes and in *VEGFA* were discovered to be associated with advanced AMD,[29] supporting the previous association noted with the gene *COL8A1*[27] and emphasizing the importance of extracellular matrix biology and angiogenesis in AMD.[29] The genetic variants discovered to date explain about half of the classical sibling risk of AMD, and commercial genetic testing for some AMD risk variants is currently available. Knowledge of genetic variation at risk loci increases the ability to predict AMD progression above and beyond knowledge of demographics, ocular factors, smoking history, and BMI.[31-32] However, there is no consensus yet on how genetic testing should be integrated into clinical practice. Further validation of genetic testing for predicting AMD development and progression will occur as additional genetic risk variants are discovered. Eventually, genotyping may become a useful tool for identifying individuals who are at higher risk for disease and thus may benefit from more intense monitoring and/or preventive treatment strategies and may help with designing clinical trials.[32]

A few pharmacogenetic studies have been published to date. These focus mainly on the association of the *CFH* and/or *ARMS2/HTRA1* polymorphisms to patients' responses to either anti-VEGF therapy, photodynamic therapy (PDT), or antioxidant supplements. One retrospective cohort study found that patients witht the *CFH* Y204H CC genotype had worse visual outcomes with intravitreal bevacizumab than did those with the *CFH* TC and TT genotypes; they found no pharmacogenetic relationship with *ARMS2/HTRA1*.[177] This relationship between *CFH* genotype and poorer visual acuity outcomes with intravitreal bevacizumab was corroborated by a prospective study.[178] Another retrospective study looking only at *CFH* locus found that patients who were homozygous for the Y402H risk allele have a 37% significantly higher risk of requiring additional intravitreal ranibizumab injections.[179] In a retrospective analysis of the interaction between *CFH* and *ARMS2/HTRA1* variants and treatment response to antioxidants and zinc, an interaction between *CFH* Y402H genotype and supplementation with antioxidants plus zinc and zinc alone was observed.[31,180] There were no significant treatment interactions with *ARMS2/HTRA1*. The association between *CFH* and *ARMS2/HTRA1* variants and response to PDT are mixed with some studies showing association to *CFH* only,[181] other studies showing no association to *CFH*,[182–183] and one study in an Asian population showing an association to both.[184] Results from several well-powered, ongoing pharmacogenetic studies are needed to clarify whether genetic make-up influences response to treatment in AMD.

CONCLUSION

AMD is a multifactorial disease that affects a large segment of the population and research to date has yielded some preventive measures and a few effective treatments for the advanced wet form of the disease. Several modifiable risk factors have been identified, including smoking, dietary intake of omega-3 fatty acids and vegetables and fruit with antioxidants including lutein and zeaxanthin, as well as, exercise, and maintaining a healthy weight. Population-based studies have shown mixed effects of sunlight exposure, medication use, and alcohol intake. The understanding of the genetic architecture of AMD has increased significantly over the past decade and underscores the roles of inflammation, HDL cholesterol metabolism, angiogenesis and degradation of extracellular matrix in the etiology of this disease. Discovery of a rare, penetrant, pathogenic mutation in the CFH gene,[185] which causes earlier onset age-related macular degeneration, points the way for future genetic studies of this disease.

REFERENCES

1. Friedman DS, O'Colmain BJ, Munoz B, et al. Prevalence of age-related macular degeneration in the United States. Arch Ophthalmol 2004;122:564–72.
2. Bressler NM, Bressler SB, Congdon NG, et al. Potential public health impact of Age-Related Eye Disease Study results: AREDS report no. 11. Arch Ophthalmol 2003;121:1621–4.
3. Rein DB, Wittenborn JS, Zhang X, et al. Forecasting age-related macular degeneration through the year 2050: the potential impact of new treatments. Arch Ophthalmol 2009;127:533–40.
4. AREDS Research Study Group. A randomized, placebo-controlled, clinical trial of high-dose supplementation with vitamins C and E, beta carotene, and zinc for age-related macular degeneration and vision loss: AREDS report no. 8. Arch Ophthalmol 2001;119:1417–36.
5. Seddon JM, Willett WC, Speizer FE, et al. A prospective study of cigarette smoking and age-related macular degeneration in women. JAMA 1996;276:1141–6.
6. Tomany SC, Wang JJ, Van Leeuwen R, et al. Risk factors for incident age-related macular degeneration: pooled findings from 3 continents. Ophthalmology 2004;111:1280–7.
7. Cho E, Seddon JM, Rosner B, et al. Prospective study of intake of fruits, vegetables, vitamins, and carotenoids and risk of age-related maculopathy. Arch Ophthalmol 2004;122:883–92.
8. Antioxidant status and neovascular age-related macular degeneration. Eye Disease Case-Control Study Group. Arch Ophthalmol 1993;111:104–9.
9. Mares-Perlman JA, Brady WE, Klein R, et al. Serum antioxidants and age-related macular degeneration in a population-based case-control study. Arch Ophthalmol 1995;113:1518–23.
10. Seddon JM, Ajani UA, Sperduto RD, et al. Dietary carotenoids, vitamins A, C, and E, and advanced age-related macular degeneration. Eye Disease Case-Control Study Group. JAMA 1994;272:1413–20.
11. Seddon JM, Cote J, Rosner B. Progression of age-related macular degeneration: association with dietary fat, transunsaturated fat, nuts, and fish intake. Arch Ophthalmol 2003;121:1728–37.
12. Seddon JM, Rosner B, Sperduto RD, et al. Dietary fat and risk for advanced age-related macular degeneration. Arch Ophthalmol 2001;119:1191–9.
13. Seddon JM, Cote J, Davis N, et al. Progression of age-related macular degeneration: association with body mass index, waist circumference, and waist-hip ratio. Arch Ophthalmol 2003;121:785–92.
14. Seddon J, et al. Dietary fat intake and age-related macular degeneration. Invest Ophthalmol Vis Sci 1994;35: ARVO abstract 2003.
15. Klein RJ, Zeiss C, Chew EY, et al. Complement factor H polymorphism in age-related macular degeneration. Science 2005;308:385–9.
16. Edwards AO, Ritter 3rd R, Abel KJ, et al. Complement factor H polymorphism and age-related macular degeneration. Science 2005;308:421–4.
17. Haines JL, Hauser MA, Schmidt S, et al. Complement factor H variant increases the risk of age-related macular degeneration. Science 2005;308:419–21.
18. Hageman GS, Anderson DH, Johnson LV, et al. A common haplotype in the complement regulatory gene factor H (HF1/CFH) predisposes individuals to age-related macular degeneration. Proc Natl Acad Sci U S A 2005;102:7227–32.
19. Rivera A, Fisher SA, Fritsche LG, et al. Hypothetical LOC387715 is a second major susceptibility gene for age-related macular degeneration, contributing independently of complement factor H to disease risk. Hum Mol Genet 2005;14:3227–36.
20. Dewan A, Liu M, Hartman S, et al. HTRA1 promoter polymorphism in wet age-related macular degeneration. Science 2006;314:989–92.
21. Yang Z, Camp NJ, Sun H, et al. A variant of the HTRA1 gene increases susceptibility to age-related macular degeneration. Science 2006;314:992–3.
22. Gold B, Merriam JE, Zernant J, et al. Variation in factor B (BF) and complement component 2 (C2) genes is associated with age-related macular degeneration. Nat Genet 2006;38:458–62.
23. Maller J, George S, Purcell S, et al. Common variation in three genes, including a noncoding variant in CFH, strongly influences risk of age-related macular degeneration. Nat Genet 2006;38:1055–9.
24. Yates JR, Sepp T, Matharu BK, et al. Complement C3 variant and the risk of age-related macular degeneration. N Engl J Med 2007;357:553–61.
25. Maller JB, Fagerness JA, Reynolds RC, et al. Variation in complement factor 3 is associated with risk of age-related macular degeneration. Nat Genet 2007;39:1200–1.
26. Fagerness JA, Maller JB, Neale BM, et al. Variation near complement factor I is associated with risk of advanced AMD. Eur J Hum Genet 2009;17:100–4.
27. Neale BM, Fagerness J, Reynolds R, et al. Genome-wide association study of advanced age-related macular degeneration identifies a role of the hepatic lipase gene (LIPC). Proc Natl Acad Sci U S A 2010;107:7395–400.
28. Chen W, Stambolian D, Edwards AO, et al. Genetic variants near TIMP3 and high-density lipoprotein-associated loci influence susceptibility to age-related macular degeneration. Proc Natl Acad Sci U S A 2010;107:7401–6.
29. Yu Y, Bhangale T, Fagerness J, et al. Common variants near *FRK/COL10A1* and *VEGFA* are associated with advanced age-related macular degeneration. Hum Mol Genet 2011;20(18):3699–709.
30. Seddon JM, Francis PJ, George S, et al. Association of CFH Y402H and LOC387715 A69S with progression of age-related macular degeneration. JAMA 2007;297:1793–800.
31. Seddon JM, Reynolds R, Maller J, et al. Prediction model for prevalence and incidence of advanced age-related macular degeneration based on genetic, demographic, and environmental variables. Invest Ophthalmol Vis Sci 2009;50:2044–53.
32. Seddon JM, Reynolds R, Yu Y, et al. Risk models for progression to advanced age-related macular degeneration using demographic, environmental, genetic and ocular factors. Ophthalmology 2011;118(11):2203–11.
33. Bird AC, Bressler NM, Bressler SB, et al. An international classification and grading system for age-related maculopathy and age-related macular degeneration. The International ARM Epidemiological Study Group. Surv Ophthalmol 1995;39:367–74.
34. Seddon JM, Sharma S, Adelman RA. Evaluation of the clinical age-related maculopathy staging system. Ophthalmology 2006;113:260–6.
35. The Age-Related Eye Disease Study (AREDS): design implications. AREDS report no. 1. Control Clin Trials 1999;20:573–600.
36. Seddon JM, Santangelo SL, Book K, et al. A genomewide scan for age-related macular degeneration provides evidence for linkage to several chromosomal regions. Am J Hum Genet 2003;73:780–90.
37. Sobrin L, Reynolds R, Yu Y, et al. ARMS2/HTRA1 Locus can confer differential susceptibility to the advanced subtypes of age-related macular degeneration. Am J Ophthalmol 2010;151:345–52.
38. Sobrin L, Maller JB, Neale BM, et al. Genetic profile for five common variants associated with age-related macular degeneration in densely affected families: a novel analytic approach. Eur J Hum Genet 2010;18:496–501.
39. Raychaudhuri S, Ripke S, Li M, et al. Associations of CFHR1-CFHR3 deletion and a CFH SNP to age-related macular degeneration are not independent. Nat Genet 2010;42:553–5.
40. Bressler NM, Bressler SB, West SK, et al. The grading and prevalence of macular degeneration in Chesapeake Bay watermen. Arch Ophthalmol 1989;107:847–52.
41. Klein R, Davis MD, Magli YL, et al. The Wisconsin age-related maculopathy grading system. Ophthalmology 1991;98:1128–34.
42. Klein R, Rowland ML, Harris MI. Racial/ethnic differences in age-related maculopathy. Third National Health and Nutrition Examination Survey. Ophthalmology 1995;102:371–81.
43. Klein R, Chou CF, Klein BE, et al. Prevalence of age-related macular degeneration in the US population. Arch Ophthalmol 2011;129:75–80.
44. Leibowitz HM, Krueger DE, Maunder LR, et al. The Framingham Eye Study monograph: An ophthalmological and epidemiological study of cataract, glaucoma, diabetic retinopathy, macular degeneration, and visual acuity in a general population of 2631 adults, 1973–1975. Surv Ophthalmol 1980;24:335–610.
45. Klein R, Klein BE, Linton KL. Prevalence of age-related maculopathy. The Beaver Dam Eye Study. Ophthalmology 1992;99:933–43.

46. Friedman DS, Katz J, Bressler NM, et al. Racial differences in the prevalence of age-related macular degeneration: the Baltimore Eye Survey. Ophthalmology 1999;106:1049–55.
47. West SK, Munoz B, Rubin GS, et al. Function and visual impairment in a population-based study of older adults. The SEE project. Salisbury Eye Evaluation. Invest Ophthalmol Vis Sci 1997;38:72–82.
48. Vingerling JR, Dielemans I, Hofman A, et al. The prevalence of age-related maculopathy in the Rotterdam Study. Ophthalmology 1995;102:205–10.
49. Mitchell P, Smith W, Attebo K, et al. Prevalence of age-related maculopathy in Australia. The Blue Mountains Eye Study. Ophthalmology 1995;102:1450–60.
50. Schachat AP, Hyman L, Leske MC, et al. Features of age-related macular degeneration in a black population. The Barbados Eye Study Group. Arch Ophthalmol 1995;113:728–35.
51. Pagliarini S, Moramarco A, Wormald RP, et al. Age-related macular disease in rural southern Italy. Arch Ophthalmol 1997;115:616–22.
52. Podgor MJ, Leske MC, Ederer F. Incidence estimates for lens changes, macular changes, open-angle glaucoma and diabetic retinopathy. Am J Epidemiol 1983;118:206–12.
53. Klein R, Klein BE, Jensen SC, et al. The five-year incidence and progression of age-related maculopathy: the Beaver Dam Eye Study. Ophthalmology 1997;104:7–21.
54. Mukesh BN, Dimitrov PN, Leikin S, et al. Five-year incidence of age-related maculopathy: the Visual Impairment Project. Ophthalmology 2004;111: 1176–82.
55. Leske MC, Wu SY, Hyman L, et al. Four-year incidence of macular changes in the Barbados Eye Studies. Ophthalmology 2004;111:706–11.
56. Klein R, Knudtson MD, Lee KE, et al. Age-period-cohort effect on the incidence of age-related macular degeneration: the Beaver Dam Eye Study. Ophthalmology 2008;115:1460–7.
57. Clemons TE, Chew EY, Bressler SB, et al. National Eye Institute Visual Function Questionnaire in the Age-Related Eye Disease Study (AREDS): AREDS report no. 10. Arch Ophthalmol 2003;121:211–7.
58. Mitchell J, Wolffsohn J, Woodcock A, et al. The MacDQoL individualized measure of the impact of macular degeneration on quality of life: reliability and responsiveness. Am J Ophthalmol 2008;146:447–54.
59. Alexander MF, Maguire MG, Lietman TM, et al. Assessment of visual function in patients with age-related macular degeneration and low visual acuity. Arch Ophthalmol 1988;106:1543–7.
60. Mangione CM, Gutierrez PR, Lowe G, et al. Influence of age-related maculopathy on visual functioning and health-related quality of life. Am J Ophthalmol 1999;128:45–53.
61. Brody BL, Gamst AC, Williams RA, et al. Depression, visual acuity, comorbidity, and disability associated with age-related macular degeneration. Ophthalmology 2001;108:1893–900; discussion 900–1.
62. Casten RJ, Rovner BW, Tasman W. Age-related macular degeneration and depression: a review of recent research. Curr Opin Ophthalmol 2004;15: 181–3.
63. Rovner BW, Casten RJ, Tasman WS. Effect of depression on vision function in age-related macular degeneration. Arch Ophthalmol 2002;120:1041–4.
64. Javitt JC, Zhou Z, Maguire MG, et al. Incidence of exudative age-related macular degeneration among elderly Americans. Ophthalmology 2003;110: 1534–9.
65. Risk factors associated with age-related macular degeneration. A case-control study in the age-related eye disease study: Age-Related Eye Disease Study Report no. 3. Ophthalmology 2000;107:2224–32.
66. Sommer A, Tielsch JM, Katz J, et al. Racial differences in the cause-specific prevalence of blindness in east Baltimore. N Engl J Med 1991;325:1412–7.
67. Cruickshanks KJ, Hamman RF, Klein R, et al. The prevalence of age-related maculopathy by geographic region and ethnicity. The Colorado–Wisconsin Study of Age-Related Maculopathy. Arch Ophthalmol 1997;115:242–50.
68. Varma R, Fraser-Bell S, Tan S, et al. Prevalence of age-related macular degeneration in Latinos: the Los Angeles Latino eye study. Ophthalmology 2004;111:1288–97.
69. Kawasaki R, Yasuda M, Song SJ, et al. The prevalence of age-related macular degeneration in Asians: a systematic review and meta-analysis. Ophthalmology 2010;117:921–7.
70. Adler NE, Boyce WT, Chesney MA, et al. Socioeconomic inequalities in health. No easy solution. JAMA 1993;269:3140–5.
71. Risk factors for neovascular age-related macular degeneration. The Eye Disease Case–Control Study Group. Arch Ophthalmol 1992;110:1701–8.
72. Klein R, Klein BE, Jensen SC, et al. The relation of socioeconomic factors to age-related cataract, maculopathy, and impaired vision. The Beaver Dam Eye Study. Ophthalmology 1994;101:1969–79.
73. Hyman LG, Lilienfeld AM, Ferris FL 3rd, et al. Senile macular degeneration: a case–control study. Am J Epidemiol 1983;118:213–27.
74. Chaine G, Hullo A, Sahel J, et al. Case–control study of the risk factors for age related macular degeneration. France-DMLA Study Group. Br J Ophthalmol 1998;82:996–1002.
75. Maltzman BA, Mulvihill MN, Greenbaum A. Senile macular degeneration and risk factors: a case–control study. Ann Ophthalmol 1979;11:1197–201.
76. Wang JJ, Mitchell P, Smith W. Refractive error and age-related maculopathy: the Blue Mountains Eye Study. Invest Ophthalmol Vis Sci 1998;39:2167–71.
77. Ikram MK, van Leeuwen R, Vingerling JR, et al. Relationship between refraction and prevalent as well as incident age-related maculopathy: the Rotterdam Study. Invest Ophthalmol Vis Sci 2003;44:3778–82.
78. Friedman E, Ivry M, Ebert E, et al. Increased scleral rigidity and age-related macular degeneration. Ophthalmology 1989;96:104–8.
79. Frank RN, Puklin JE, Stock C, et al. Race, iris color, and age-related macular degeneration. Trans Am Ophthalmol Soc 2000;98:109–15; discussion 15–7.
80. Holz FG, Piguet B, Minassian DC, et al. Decreasing stromal iris pigmentation as a risk factor for age-related macular degeneration. Am J Ophthalmol 1994;117:19–23.
81. Mitchell P, Smith W, Wang JJ. Iris color, skin sun sensitivity, and age-related maculopathy. The Blue Mountains Eye Study. Ophthalmology 1998;105: 1359–63.
82. Sandberg MA, Gaudio AR, Miller S, et al. Iris pigmentation and extent of disease in patients with neovascular age-related macular degeneration. Invest Ophthalmol Vis Sci 1994;35:2734–40.
83. Weiter JJ, Delori FC, Wing GL, et al. Relationship of senile macular degeneration to ocular pigmentation. Am J Ophthalmol 1985;99:185–7.
84. Gibson JM, Shaw DE, Rosenthal AR. Senile cataract and senile macular degeneration: an investigation into possible risk factors. Trans Ophthalmol Soc U K 1986;105 (Pt 4):463–8.
85. Klein R, Klein BE, Jensen SC, et al. The relationship of ocular factors to the incidence and progression of age-related maculopathy. Arch Ophthalmol 1998;116:506–13.
86. Tomany SC, Klein R, Klein BE. The relationship between iris color, hair color, and skin sun sensitivity and the 10-year incidence of age-related maculopathy: the Beaver Dam Eye Study. Ophthalmology 2003;110:1526–33.
87. Wang JJ, Jakobsen K, Smith W, et al. Five-year incidence of age-related maculopathy in relation to iris, skin or hair colour, and skin sun sensitivity: the Blue Mountains Eye Study. Clin Experiment Ophthalmol 2003;31:317–21.
88. West SK, Rosenthal FS, Bressler NM, et al. Exposure to sunlight and other risk factors for age-related macular degeneration. Arch Ophthalmol 1989;107: 875–9.
89. Sperduto RD, Hiller R, Seigel D. Lens opacities and senile maculopathy. Arch Ophthalmol 1981;99:1004–8.
90. Liu IY, White L, LaCroix AZ. The association of age-related macular degeneration and lens opacities in the aged. Am J Public Health 1989;79:765–9.
91. Klein R, Klein BE, Wang Q, et al. Is age-related maculopathy associated with cataracts? Arch Ophthalmol 1994;112:191–6.
92. Lundstrom M, Brege KG, Floren I, et al. Cataract surgery and quality of life in patients with age related macular degeneration. Br J Ophthalmol 2002;86:1330–5.
93. Freeman EE, Munoz B, West SK, et al. Is there an association between cataract surgery and age-related macular degeneration? Data from three population-based studies. Am J Ophthalmol 2003;135:849–56.
94. Chew EY, Sperduto RD, Milton RC, et al. Risk of advanced age-related macular degeneration after cataract surgery in the Age-Related Eye Disease Study: AREDS report no. 25. Ophthalmology 2009;116:297–303.
95. Dong LM, Stark WJ, Jefferys JL, et al. Progression of age-related macular degeneration after cataract surgery. Arch Ophthalmol 2009;127:1412–9.
96. Christen WG, Glynn RJ, Manson JE, et al. A prospective study of cigarette smoking and risk of age-related macular degeneration in men. JAMA 1996;276:1147–51.
97. Klein R, Klein BE, Franke T. The relationship of cardiovascular disease and its risk factors to age-related maculopathy. The Beaver Dam Eye Study. Ophthalmology 1993;100:406–14.
98. Klein R, Klein BE, Tomany SC, et al. Ten-year incidence of age-related maculopathy and smoking and drinking: the Beaver Dam Eye Study. Am J Epidemiol 2002;156:589–98.
99. Delcourt C, Diaz JL, Ponton-Sanchez A, et al. Smoking and age-related macular degeneration. The POLA Study. Pathologies Oculaires Liées à l'Age. Arch Ophthalmol 1998;116:1031–5.
100. Suner IJ, Espinosa-Heidmann DG, Marin-Castano ME, et al. Nicotine increases size and severity of experimental choroidal neovascularization. Invest Ophthalmol Vis Sci 2004;45:311–7.
101. Seddon JM, George S, Rosner B, et al. CFH gene variant, Y402H, and smoking, body mass index, environmental associations with advanced age-related macular degeneration. Hum Hered 2006;61:157–65.
102. Francis PJ, George S, Schultz DW, et al. The LOC387715 gene, smoking, body mass index, environmental associations with advanced age-related macular degeneration. Hum Hered 2007;63:212–8.
103. Bone RA, Landrum JT, Guerra LH, et al. Lutein and zeaxanthin dietary supplements raise macular pigment density and serum concentrations of these carotenoids in humans. J Nutr 2003;133:992–8.
104. Krinsky NI, Landrum JT, Bone RA. Biologic mechanisms of the protective role of lutein and zeaxanthin in the eye. Annu Rev Nutr 2003;23:171–201.
105. Bernstein PS, Delori FC, Richer S, et al. The value of measurement of macular carotenoid pigment optical densities and distributions in age-related macular degeneration and other retinal disorders. Vision Res 2010;50:716–28.
106. Evereklioglu C, Er H, Doganay S, et al. Nitric oxide and lipid peroxidation are increased and associated with decreased antioxidant enzyme activities in patients with age-related macular degeneration. Doc Ophthalmol 2003;106: 129–36.
107. Anderson RE, Kretzer FL, Rapp LM. Free radicals and ocular disease. Adv Exp Med Biol 1994;366:73–86.
108. Anderson RE, Rapp LM, Wiegand RD. Lipid peroxidation and retinal degeneration. Curr Eye Res 1984;3:223–7.
109. Young RW. Pathophysiology of age-related macular degeneration. Surv Ophthalmol 1987;31:291–306.
110. Hopley C, Salkeld G, Wang JJ, et al. Cost utility of screening and treatment for early age related macular degeneration with zinc and antioxidants. Br J Ophthalmol 2004;88:450–4.

111. Richer S, Stiles W, Statkute L, et al. Double-masked, placebo-controlled, randomized trial of lutein and antioxidant supplementation in the intervention of atrophic age-related macular degeneration: the Veterans LAST study (Lutein Antioxidant Supplementation Trial). Optometry 2004;75: 216–30.
112. Gale CR, Hall NF, Phillips DI, et al. Lutein and zeaxanthin status and risk of age-related macular degeneration. Invest Ophthalmol Vis Sci 2003;44: 2461–5.
113. Goldberg J, Flowerdew G, Smith E, et al. Factors associated with age-related macular degeneration. An analysis of data from the first National Health and Nutrition Examination Survey. Am J Epidemiol 1988;128:700–10.
114. SanGiovanni JP, Chew EY, Clemons TE, et al. The relationship of dietary carotenoid and vitamin A, E, and C intake with age-related macular degeneration in a case-control study: AREDS report no. 22. Arch Ophthalmol 2007;125:1225–32.
115. Vinding T, Appleyard M, Nyboe J, et al. Risk factor analysis for atrophic and exudative age-related macular degeneration. An epidemiological study of 1000 aged individuals. Acta Ophthalmol (Copenh) 1992;70:66–72.
116. Obisesan TO, Hirsch R, Kosoko O, et al. Moderate wine consumption is associated with decreased odds of developing age-related macular degeneration in NHANES-1. J Am Geriatr Soc 1998;46:1–7.
117. Cho E, Hankinson SE, Willett WC, et al. Prospective study of alcohol consumption and the risk of age-related macular degeneration. Arch Ophthalmol 2000;118:681–8.
118. Smith W, Mitchell P. Alcohol intake and age-related maculopathy. Am J Ophthalmol 1996;122:743–5.
119. Klein BE, Klein R, Lee KE, et al. Measures of obesity and age-related eye diseases. Ophthalmic Epidemiol 2001;8:251–62.
120. Delcourt C, Michel F, Colvez A, et al. Associations of cardiovascular disease and its risk factors with age-related macular degeneration: the POLA study. Ophthalmic Epidemiol 2001;8:237–49.
121. Schaumberg DA, Christen WG, Hankinson SE, et al. Body mass index and the incidence of visually significant age-related maculopathy in men. Arch Ophthalmol 2001;119:1259–65.
122. Smith W, Mitchell P, Leeder SR, et al. Plasma fibrinogen levels, other cardiovascular risk factors, and age-related maculopathy: the Blue Mountains Eye Study. Arch Ophthalmol 1998;116:583–7.
123. Cruickshanks KJ, Klein R, Klein BE. Sunlight and age-related macular degeneration. The Beaver Dam Eye Study. Arch Ophthalmol 1993;111: 514–8.
124. Cruickshanks KJ, Klein R, Klein BE, et al. Sunlight and the 5-year incidence of early age-related maculopathy: the beaver dam eye study. Arch Ophthalmol 2001;119:246–50.
125. Tomany SC, Cruickshanks KJ, Klein R, et al. Sunlight and the 10-year incidence of age-related maculopathy: the Beaver Dam Eye Study. Arch Ophthalmol 2004;122:750–7.
126. Delcourt C, Carriere I, Ponton-Sanchez A, et al. Light exposure and the risk of age-related macular degeneration: the Pathologies Oculaires Liées à l'Age (POLA) study. Arch Ophthalmol 2001;119:1463–8.
127. Darzins P, Mitchell P, Heller RF. Sun exposure and age-related macular degeneration. An Australian case–control study. Ophthalmology 1997;104: 770–6.
128. Hyman L, Schachat AP, He Q, et al. Hypertension, cardiovascular disease, and age-related macular degeneration. Age-Related Macular Degeneration Risk Factors Study Group. Arch Ophthalmol 2000;118:351–8.
129. Wilson HL, Schwartz DM, Bhatt HR, et al. Statin and aspirin therapy are associated with decreased rates of choroidal neovascularization among patients with age-related macular degeneration. Am J Ophthalmol 2004;137: 615–24.
130. Hall NF, Gale CR, Syddall H, et al. Risk of macular degeneration in users of statins: cross-sectional study. BMJ 2001;323:375–6.
131. van Leeuwen R, Vingerling JR, Hofman A, et al. Cholesterol lowering drugs and risk of age related maculopathy: prospective cohort study with cumulative exposure measurement. BMJ 2003;326:255–6.
132. Hall NF, Martyn CN. Could statins prevent age-related macular degeneration? Expert Opin Pharmacother 2002;3:803–7.
133. Seddon JM, Gensler G, Milton RC, et al. Association between C-reactive protein and age-related macular degeneration. JAMA 2004;291:704–10.
134. Klein R, Klein BE, Tomany SC, et al. The association of cardiovascular disease with the long-term incidence of age-related maculopathy: the Beaver Dam Eye Study. Ophthalmology 2003;110:1273–80.
135. Snow KK, Seddon JM. Do age-related macular degeneration and cardiovascular disease share common antecedents? Ophthalmic Epidemiol 1999;6: 125–43.
136. van Leeuwen R, Ikram MK, Vingerling JR, et al. Blood pressure, atherosclerosis, and the incidence of age-related maculopathy: the Rotterdam Study. Invest Ophthalmol Vis Sci 2003;44:3771–7.
137. Vingerling JR, Dielemans I, Bots ML, et al. Age-related macular degeneration is associated with atherosclerosis. The Rotterdam Study. Am J Epidemiol 1995;142:404–9.
138. Hirvela H, Luukinen H, Laara E, et al. Risk factors of age-related maculopathy in a population 70 years of age or older. Ophthalmology 1996;103:871–7.
139. Vinding T. Age-related macular degeneration. An epidemiological study of 1000 elderly individuals. With reference to prevalence, funduscopic findings, visual impairment and risk factors. Acta Ophthalmol Scand Suppl 1995:1–32.
140. Sperduto RD, Hiller R. Systemic hypertension and age-related maculopathy in the Framingham Study. Arch Ophthalmol 1986;104:216–9.
141. Delaney Jr WV, Oates RP. Senile macular degeneration: a preliminary study. Ann Ophthalmol 1982;14:21–4.
142. Kahn HA, Leibowitz HM, Ganley JP, et al. The Framingham Eye Study. II. Association of ophthalmic pathology with single variables previously measured in the Framingham Heart Study. Am J Epidemiol 1977;106: 33–41.
143. Vidaurri JS, Pe'er J, Halfon ST, et al. Association between drusen and some of the risk factors for coronary artery disease. Ophthalmologica 1984;188: 243–7.
144. Klein R, Klein BE, Jensen SC. The relation of cardiovascular disease and its risk factors to the 5-year incidence of age-related maculopathy: the Beaver Dam Eye Study. Ophthalmology 1997;104:1804–12.
145. Klein R, Klein BE, Tomany SC, et al. The relation of retinal microvascular characteristics to age-related eye disease: the Beaver Dam eye study. Am J Ophthalmol 2004;137:435–44.
146. Risk factors for choroidal neovascularization in the second eye of patients with juxtafoveal or subfoveal choroidal neovascularization secondary to age-related macular degeneration. Macular Photocoagulation Study Group. Arch Ophthalmol 1997;115:741–7.
147. Reynolds R, Rosner B, Seddon JM. Serum lipid biomarkers and hepatic lipase gene associations with age-related macular degeneration. Ophthalmology 2010;117:1989–95.
148. Klein R, Klein BE, Marino EK, et al. Early age-related maculopathy in the cardiovascular health study. Ophthalmology 2003;110:25–33.
149. van Leeuwen R, Klaver CC, Vingerling JR, et al. Cholesterol and age-related macular degeneration: is there a link? Am J Ophthalmol 2004;137:750–2.
150. Christen WG, Schaumberg DA, Glynn RJ, et al. Dietary Ω-3 fatty acid and fish intake and incident age-related macular degeneration in women. Arch Ophthalmol 2011;129:921–9.
151. Mares-Perlman JA, Brady WE, Klein R, et al. Dietary fat and age-related maculopathy. Arch Ophthalmol 1995;113:743–8.
152. Heuberger RA, Mares-Perlman JA, Klein R, et al. Relationship of dietary fat to age-related maculopathy in the Third National Health and Nutrition Examination Survey. Arch Ophthalmol 2001;119:1833–8.
153. SanGiovanni JP, Chew EY, Agron E, et al. The relationship of dietary omega-3 long-chain polyunsaturated fatty acid intake with incident age-related macular degeneration: AREDS report no. 23. Arch Ophthalmol 2008;126:1274–9.
154. Friedman E. Dietary fat and age-related maculopathy. Arch Ophthalmol 1996;114:235–6.
155. Klein R, Klein BE, Moss SE. Diabetes, hyperglycemia, and age-related maculopathy. The Beaver Dam Eye Study. Ophthalmology 1992;99:1527–34.
156. Snow KK, Cote J, Yang W, et al. Association between reproductive and hormonal factors and age-related maculopathy in postmenopausal women. Am J Ophthalmol 2002;134:842–8.
157. Snow KK, Seddon JM. Age-related eye diseases: impact of hormone replacement therapy, and reproductive and other risk factors. Int J Fertil Womens Med 2000;45:301–13.
158. Klein BE, Klein R, Jensen SC, et al. Are sex hormones associated with age-related maculopathy in women? The Beaver Dam Eye Study. Trans Am Ophthalmol Soc 1994;92:289–95; discussion 95–7.
159. Smith W, Mitchell P, Wang JJ. Gender, oestrogen, hormone replacement and age-related macular degeneration: results from the Blue Mountains Eye Study. Aust N Z J Ophthalmol 1997;25(Suppl 1):S13–5.
160. Defay R, Pinchinat S, Lumbroso S, et al. Sex steroids and age-related macular degeneration in older French women: the POLA study. Ann Epidemiol 2004;14:202–8.
161. Abramov Y, Borik S, Yahalom C, et al. The effect of hormone therapy on the risk for age-related maculopathy in postmenopausal women. Menopause 2004;11:62–8.
162. Klein R, Deng Y, Klein BE, et al. Cardiovascular disease, its risk factors and treatment, and age-related macular degeneration: Women's Health Initiative Sight Exam ancillary study. Am J Ophthalmol 2007;143:473–83.
163. Anderson DH, Mullins RF, Hageman GS, et al. A role for local inflammation in the formation of drusen in the aging eye. Am J Ophthalmol 2002;134: 411–31.
164. Johnson LV, Leitner WP, Staples MK, et al. Complement activation and inflammatory processes in Drusen formation and age related macular degeneration. Exp Eye Res 2001;73:887–96.
165. Mullins RF, Russell SR, Anderson DH, et al. Drusen associated with aging and age-related macular degeneration contain proteins common to extracellular deposits associated with atherosclerosis, elastosis, amyloidosis, and dense deposit disease. FASEB J 2000;14:835–46.
166. Seddon JM, Gensler G, Rosner B. C-reactive protein and CFH, ARMS2/HTRA1 gene variants are independently associated with risk of macular degeneration. Ophthalmology 2010;117:1560–6.
167. Becerra EM, Morescalchi F, Gandolfo F, et al. Clinical evidence of intravitreal triamcinolone acetonide in the management of age-related macular degeneration. Curr Drug Targets 2011;12:149–72.
168. Soames CJ, Sim RB. Interactions between human complement components factor H, factor I and C3b. Biochem J 1997;326(Pt 2):553–61.
169. Gehrs KM, Jackson JR, Brown EN, et al. Complement, age-related macular degeneration and a vision of the future. Arch Ophthalmol 2010;128:349–58.
170. Seddon JM, Sobrin, L. Epidemiology of age-related macular degeneration. In: Albert D, Miller J, Azar D, et al., editors. Albert & Jakobiec's Principles and practice of ophthalmology. Philadelphia: W.B. Saunders; 2007. p. 413–22.
171. Seddon JM, Ajani UA, Mitchell BD. Familial aggregation of age-related maculopathy. Am J Ophthalmol 1997;123:199–206.

172. Klaver CC, Wolfs RC, Assink JJ, et al. Genetic risk of age-related maculopathy. Population-based familial aggregation study. Arch Ophthalmol 1998;116: 1646–51.
173. Hughes AE, Orr N, Esfandiary H, et al. A common CFH haplotype, with deletion of CFHR1 and CFHR3, is associated with lower risk of age-related macular degeneration. Nat Genet 2006;38:1173–7.
174. Jakobsdottir J, Conley YP, Weeks DE, et al. Susceptibility genes for age-related maculopathy on chromosome 10q26. Am J Hum Genet 2005;77: 389–407.
175. Sobrin L, Reynolds R, Yu Y, et al. ARMS2/HTRA1 locus can confer differential susceptibility to the advanced subtypes of age-related macular degeneration. Am J Ophthalmol 2011;151(2):345–52.
176. Weber BH, Vogt G, Pruett RC, et al. Mutations in the tissue inhibitor of metalloproteinases-3 (TIMP3) in patients with Sorsby's fundus dystrophy. Nat Genet 1994;8:352–6.
177. Brantley Jr MA, Fang AM, King JM, et al. Association of complement factor H and LOC387715 genotypes with response of exudative age-related macular degeneration to intravitreal bevacizumab. Ophthalmology 2007;114:2168–73.
178. Nischler C, Oberkofler H, Ortner C, et al. Complement factor H Y402H gene polymorphism and response to intravitreal bevacizumab in exudative age-related macular degeneration. Acta Ophthalmol 2011;89:e344–9.
179. Lee AY, Raya AK, Kymes SM, et al. Pharmacogenetics of complement factor H (Y402H) and treatment of exudative age-related macular degeneration with ranibizumab. Br J Ophthalmol 2009;93:610–3.
180. Klein ML, Francis PJ, Rosner B, et al. CFH and LOC387715/ARMS2 genotypes and treatment with antioxidants and zinc for age-related macular degeneration. Ophthalmology 2008;115:1019–25.
181. Brantley Jr MA, Edelstein SL, King JM, et al. Association of complement factor H and LOC387715 genotypes with response of exudative age-related macular degeneration to photodynamic therapy. Eye (Lond) 2009;23:626–31.
182. Chowers I, Cohen Y, Goldenberg-Cohen N, et al. Association of complement factor H Y402H polymorphism with phenotype of neovascular age related macular degeneration in Israel. Mol Vis 2008;14:1829–34.
183. Feng X, Xiao J, Longville B, et al. Complement factor H Y402H and C-reactive protein polymorphism and photodynamic therapy response in age-related macular degeneration. Ophthalmology 2009;116:1908–12 e1.
184. Tsuchihashi T, Mori K, Horie-Inoue K, et al. Complement factor H and high-temperature requirement A-1 genotypes and treatment response of age-related macular degeneration. Ophthalmology 2011;118:93–100.
185. Raychaudhuri S, Iartchouk O, Chin K, et al. A rare penetrant mutation in CFH confers high risk of age-related macular degeneration. Nat Genet 2011;43: 1232–36.

Pathogenetic Mechanisms in Age-Related Macular Degeneration

Chapter 64

Alan C. Bird

INTRODUCTION

Age-related macular degeneration (AMD) can be divided into early and late stages. In early disease visual acuity is good and in the fundus focal deposits are seen in Bruch's membrane, called drusen. The distribution and size of drusen varies from one patient to another, although their attributes are highly concordant between eyes of an individual. There may also be pigmentary changes at the level of the retinal pigment epithelium (RPE).

The three forms of late AMD cause loss of central vision. In most communities the most common is choroidal neovascularization (CNV), in which blood vessels grow inwards into or through Bruch's membrane. Detachment of the retinal pigment epithelium (PED), in which there is accumulation of fluid between the RPE and Bruch's membrane, is relatively uncommon. In geographic atrophy (GA) there is well-defined loss of RPE and photoreceptor cells.

It is generally considered that GA is the default pathway of the disease process and that CNV occurs as a reactive event during the evolution of change. The treatment of CNV is well established and is described elsewhere in this book. There is no well-recognized treatment whereby the disease mechanisms during transition from early AMD to GA can be modified.

The structures involved in the disease process are the photoreceptor cells in the outer retina, the retinal pigment epithelium (RPE), Bruch's membrane and the capillary bed in the inner choroid (choriocapillaris). In AMD changes occur in all these tissues throughout the eye, although they are most marked at the macula that subserves central vision in which there is a high density of cones. The changes in each of these tissues represent a potential target for treatment based on the current understanding of the relevant pathogenic mechanisms. In this chapter the logic of the various therapeutic approaches will be discussed.

STRUCTURAL CHANGES

Choroid

In the young, the choroidal capillary bed is formed of a sinusoidal complex in which the capillary bed is fenestrated and lacks tight junctions. It is believed that the nature of the choriocapillaris is determined largely by the constitutive expression of vascular endothelial growth factor (VEGF) outwards toward the choroid by the RPE.[1–5] In one morphometric study it was found that the density of the choriocapillaris is decreased with age in eyes without AMD[6] and choroidal casts have shown that the capillary bed may become tubular.[7] With advanced AMD, loss or narrowing of the choriocapillaris occurs.[8–11]

A clue as to possible clinical detection of change in the choriocapillaris came from studies of Sorsby fundus dystrophy, a monogenic disorder characterized by major thickening of Bruch's membrane and a prolonged choroidal filling phase on fluorescein angiography.[12] It was thought that the diffusely thickened Bruch's membrane represented a barrier to diffusion of VEGF towards the choroid resulting in changes in the capillary bed to a tubular state such that acquisition of fluorescence of the inner choroid is irregular and delayed.[13,14] This angiographic sign has also been identified in patients with AMD.[15] It is not known whether this sign indicates only change in circulation, or if slow egress of dye through the fenestrae and diffusion through tissues also contributes to this angiographic abnormality. The potential significance of this clinical sign has been established by demonstrating discrete areas of scotopic threshold elevation of up to 3.4 log units and slow dark adaptation which corresponded closely to regions of choroidal perfusion abnormality.[16,17] Loss of photopic function was less marked. Subsequent studies have also shown that the recovery from bleaching is prolonged[18] and the functional loss has an impact on daily tasks.[19]

Therapeutic implications

It is most likely that modification of the choroid in AMD is a response to alteration of neighboring tissues rather representing an intrinsic change, although the consequent reduction of metabolic supply to the outer retina may play a contributory role in the generating of disease. However, the possibility that choroidal changes occur independently of changes in other tissues cannot be excluded. This is not seen as a good target for therapy currently.

Bruch's membrane

A direct relationship between aging and thickness of Bruch's membrane has been established both by electron and light microscopy,[20,21] but in one study the correlation coefficients (R^2) were only 0.57 and 0.32, respectively, with great variation in the elderly.[22] Thus about half of the change in thickness must be explained by factors other than age, such as genetic or environmental influences.

Several studies on the nature of the deposits have been undertaken. Consequent upon discussion of the pathogenesis of PEDs it was hypothesized that reduction of the hydraulic conductivity of Bruch's membrane would hamper movement of water towards the choroid thus causing it to accumulate in the sub-RPE space.[23] This demands that Bruch's membrane contain a high lipid content that would increase the resistance of fluid flow. A series of investigations followed to test this hypothesis and support was derived from both histopathological, biochemical, biophysical, and clinical observations. A study of frozen tissue undertaken using histochemical staining on human eyes with an age range between 1 and 95 years showed accumulation of lipids with age that varied greatly both in the quantity and form of lipids in the elderly.[24] Some eyes stained for neutral lipids alone, some stained predominantly for phospholipids, and others stained equally for both neutral lipids and phospholipids. To confirm these conclusions, material extracted by universal lipid solvents from tissue of eye-bank fresh eyes was analyzed by thin layer and gas chromatography.[25,26] After separation, the chemical species were identified by mass spectroscopy which included fatty acids, cholesterol, triglycerides, and phospholipids. This study confirmed the conclusion that the quantity of total lipid in Bruch's membrane increases with age. Little or no lipid was extracted from specimens from donors younger than 50 years of age. In specimens from donors older than 50 years, the increase was exponential. Eyes from donors over the age of 60 years showed wide variation of total lipid extracted from donors of similar age, and that the ratios of phospholipids to neutral fats was different from one specimen to another. The ratio of neutral lipids to phospholipids did not correlate with the total quantity of lipid. The finding that the major lipid species were phospholipids and fatty acids rather than cholesterol and cholesterol esters, and that only 50% of the phospholipids was phosphatidylcholine led to the conclusion that the lipids were of a cellular (presumably RPE), rather than plasma origin.[26] Curcio, using different extraction methods, reported that cholesterol and cholesterol esters were the major lipids rather than phospholipids. As in the previous study, however, it was concluded that the lipids were of RPE origin on the basis of the nature of the cholesterol.[27] Unlike atheroma, there was little free cholesterol.

Finally, measurements of hydraulic conductivity of Bruch's membrane showed that it becomes reduced with age,[28,29] and after the age of 50 years there is a close direct linear relationship between resistance of fluid flow and lipid content.

Clinical observations were sought to support the concept that the biochemical content as well as thickness of Bruch's membrane influenced subsequent clinical behavior. It was hypothesized that drusen that are hyperfluorescent on fluorescein angiography must be hydrophilic allowing free diffusion of water-soluble sodium fluorescein into the abnormal deposit and that there would be binding of dye to polar molecules. In contrast, if the drusen were hypofluorescent it would imply that they are hydrophobic due to the presence of neutral lipids. This conclusion was supported by histological observations in which it was shown that *in vitro* binding of sodium fluorescein correlated well with the biochemical contents of drusen as shown by histochemistry.[30] Drusen rich in neutral lipids did not bind fluorescein whereas those with little lipid content bound fluorescein strongly.

It would be predicted that the highest resistance to water flow in Bruch's membrane would be found in eyes destined to suffer tears of the detached RPE in which there is sufficient tangential stress in the detached tissues to cause them to rupture. The determination that a tear in one eye implied high risk of a similar event occurring in the fellow eye[31] provided the opportunity to test the concept. A comparison was made of the drusen in the fellow eye of a tear with those of the fellow eye of one with visual loss due to subretinal neovascularization. It was shown that the drusen were larger, more confluent, and less fluorescent on angiography in the former group than in the latter.[32] Thus, there is good reason to believe that thickening and lipid accumulation in Bruch's membrane would hamper movement of metabolites and water between the RPE and choroid.

There is considerable lipid trafficking through Bruch's membrane and lipids are believed to accumulate as they fail to pass freely through a thickened Bruch's membrane. This demands that Bruch's membrane becomes thicker as a prerequisite for this lipid accumulation. Analysis has been undertaken of proteins in aging Bruch's membrane since this is likely to initiate the thickening. Recent studies have shown that several of the proteins associated with the immune system such as C3, C5b-C9 and CFH are present in high quantity in Bruch's membrane in AMD.[33] These observations serve to underline the potential significance of a disordered immune system to AMD. However, unlike inflammation elsewhere there is no infiltration by inflammatory cells. Beta-amyloid has also been identified.[34] In the inner part of Bruch's membrane there are high levels of vitronectin.[35,36] The origin of the proteins is in doubt given that there is RPE expression of some of the constituents although a major contribution may come from plasma. The state of the proteins is unknown but circumstantial evidence suggests that they are oligomerized[37] and that this may be generated by high levels of zinc or other metallic ions. In Bruch's membrane the levels of zinc are very high.[38] The levels of bioavailable zinc are many times that necessary to cause oligomerization of CFH in vitro[37] and the high risk variant of CFH would predictably oligomerize more readily than the low-risk variant. Thus the proteins may not have the biological properties of the monomers.

Further insight into the possible mechanisms of accumulation of material in Bruch's membrane was derived from observation in the $CFH^{-/-}$ mouse.[39] It is acknowledged that a gene knockout is not necessarily homologous with a polymorphism, that the immune system in mouse is dissimilar from human and mouse does not have a macula. However, if reduction of CFH activity is important, as has been concluded from genetic studies, the observations may help in understanding AMD. In this mouse there is thickening of the renal glomerulus basement membrane, but surprisingly, Bruch's membrane was thinner than in age-matched mice. This implies that dysregulation of the immune system alone may not explain thickening Bruch's membrane and that the presence of the CFH protein is important to the process.

Therapeutic implications

If thickening of Bruch's membrane and impedance of metabolic exchange and fluid movement is important to the pathogenesis of AMD, several therapeutic approaches might be considered. Reduction of the availability of the constituent proteins may slow the disease process, such as might be achieved with the chronic use of anti-inflammatory agents. Once thickening is established, mobilizing lipids or breaking down the oligomers may be achieved with the use of antibodies or possibly zinc buffers, as has been suggested in Alzheimer disease.[40] There might be potential risks in rapid generation of monomers.[41] Alternatively, the lipids might be mobilized. All these approaches would increase hydraulic conductivity and improve metabolic exchange between the RPE and choriocapillaris. In addition, it may induce an increase in choroidal circulation and in the density of fenestrae.

The retinal pigment epithelium

Accumulation of residual bodies that fluoresce can be used as an index of age change in the RPE. A quadratic relationship exists between age, and both autofluorescence and residual body quantity as measured by autofluorescence imaging as seen by light microscopy and electron microscopy, respectively.[22] The slowing of accumulation in the elderly was not surprising since the population of photoreceptors decreases in late life.[42] The relationship between age and autofluorescence, however, is not close, with an adjusted R^2 of only 0.45, and for residual bodies the R^2 was 0.50,[22] reflecting the wide variation in the eyes from elderly donors. Thus 50% of the variation in either autofluorescence or residual bodies is not explained by aging, the suspicion being that genetic or environmental factors would play a role in determining the variance. Most surprising was the relationship between autofluorescence and residual body volume. The relationship was direct, which would have been expected since it is from the residual bodies that the autofluorescence is derived. However, the R^2 was only 0.26. In retrospect, the variation between specimens should not have been surprising since only a small proportion of the material in residual bodies fluoresces, and this proportion may be influenced by circumstances such as vitamin A content in diet.[43] If rodents are given a diet low in vitamin A the residual bodies do not fluoresce. In littermates given a diet high in vitamin A the residual content of the RPE is similar but they fluoresce brightly. From this observation it might be concluded that those with high autofluorescence levels had a diet high in vitamin A.

The clinical relevance of these finding is underlined by the ability now to image RPE autofluorescence in vivo through the efforts of Fitzke and von Rückmann.[44] This is achieved using a confocal scanning laser ophthalmoscope with an excitation wavelength of 488 nm generated by an argon laser. Emission is recorded above 500 nm by inserting a barrier filter. The evidence that the signal originates from lipofuscin in the RPE is derived from the work of Delori and coworkers.[45] It has been shown that in early AMD the distribution of autofluorescence varies from one patient to another. In about half of cases of early AMD autofluorescence is homogeneous, whereas in the remainder diffusely irregular or focally increased autofluorescence is seen.[46] Drusen do not appear to explain the differences, since apart from serogranular drusen at the fovea, drusen in AMD do not autofluoresce significantly. It has been shown that in bilateral early AMD the pattern is symmetrical, implying that the autofluorescence characteristics reflect the form of disease in an individual that may be determined by the genetic or environmental influences. In patients with unilateral visual loss from AMD, focal increased autofluorescence in the good eye is associated with GA in the other eye, and predicts the development of GA in the good eye. This impression was reinforced by the observation that a high level of autofluorescence is found around the perimeter of GA, and that this area becomes atrophic within one year,[47] whereas cases without marginal hyperautofluorescence tend not to have progression of their GA.

The underlying molecular mechanisms by which changes in the RPE result in the development of GA have been subject to debate. It has been argued that the cytoplasmic volume occupied by the residual bodies may interfere with cell metabolism.[48] It has been shown that lipofuscin is a free radical generator and that may cause cell damage.[49] In addition, there is evidence for toxic effects of individual lipofuscin compounds. A2-E, a Schiff-base product of retinaldehyde and ethanolamine, has surfactant-like properties on biomembranes that have been shown in one study to increase intralysosomal pH by inhibition of the ATP-dependent lysosomal proton pump that in turn would inhibit activity of lysosomal hydrolases.[50] Furthermore, A2-E has been shown to cause leakage of lysosomes in vitro.[51] Release of lysosomal content may cause further RPE cell dysfunction and cell death. Another study failed to confirm a rise in lysosomal pH, possibly because lower quantities of lipofuscin were used, but it did show that lipid degradation was reduced.[52] Thus, both studies imply that lipofuscin reduces the activity of phagolysosomal enzymes.

The possible consequences of reduced RPE lysosomal degradation have been investigated in vivo. Interference with degradation of lysosomes was achieved in 11-week-old Sprague–Dawley rats by injection of 5 µl of a lysosomal protease inhibitor, E-64 (2.22 µM) intravitreally.[53] A single injection of E-64 caused a transient accumulation of phagolysosome-like inclusion bodies in the RPE. Furthermore, 2 or 3 injections on alternate days caused progressive accumulation of these inclusions associated with changes in intracellular organelles such as loss of smooth endoplasmic reticulum and RPE cell conformation. This was accompanied by shortening and loss of photoreceptor outer segments without prior dysmorphic changes, photoreceptor loss, reduction of fenestrae in the choroidal capillaries, and invasion of Bruch's membrane by fibroblasts and pericytes. Intravitreal injection of vehicle for comparison induced no structural changes.

It was considered likely that the changes in the RPE reflected reduced metabolism of lipids and reduction of basolateral VEGF expression caused the loss of fenestrae. The shortening and loss of the outer segments was thought to be due to impaired morphogenesis of disc membranes rather than a direct effect of E-64 on photoreceptor cells, because there was no vesiculation of disk membranes. The shortening of the OS could be explained by the lack of available lipids due to the inability of the RPE to break down the contents of the phagosome. The findings imply greater dependence upon the availability of products of phagosomal degradation for OS renewal than was previously considered, and that acquisition of plasma-derived material is insufficient to sustain this process fully. The ability of the RPE to recycle lipids has been well illustrated.[54,55] The observed changes in rats are similar in many respects to age changes in RPE, photoreceptor, and choroid in humans, although there are major differences between such an acute experiment, and the consequences of lifelong metabolic activity, and species differences between rat and human.

Thus, both experimental evidence and clinical observations illustrate potential pathogenetic mechanisms of geographic atrophy and explain the association of geographic atrophy with focal increased autofluorescence if the latter is witness to the inability to recycle phagosomal contents.

Another potential intriguing consequence of the presence of lipofuscin is the demonstration that photodegradation products of the fluorophore induce the complement cascade that may be relevant to Bruch's membrane thickening.[56]

Measurement of visual function over areas of increased autofluorescence showed loss of scotopic function that was much greater than photopic, and that the loss was as great as 3.5 log units.[57] The question as to whether the loss is due to cell loss or cell dysfunction was not addressed.

Therapeutic implications

If increased lipofuscin is important to genesis of GA, it would argue against dietary supplementation with vitamin A. Efforts are now underway to reduce the accumulation of lipofuscin therapeutically by restricting the availability of vitamin A to the retina. Initial results have shown the potential benefits of this approach in the ABCA4 knockout mouse.[58] Agents that increase lysosomal activity or lower phagolysosomal pH might also be effective. On theoretical grounds light restriction might also be helpful.

Outer retina

Relative to other structures there is less information on physical changes in the neuroretina in AMD. From early histological studies it was concluded that photoreceptor cell loss occurs progressively in early AMD although it was thought that this may occur as a consequence of RPE dysfunction.[59,60] Clinical studies have served to support this conclusion that photoreceptor loss occurs early. Two representative papers describe ocular coherence tomography in patients with geographic atrophy.[61,62] Areas of the fundus beyond the edge of atrophy in which the retina appeared normal by ophthalmoscopy apart from drusen were imaged to determine the thickness of the photoreceptor layer. In some subjects there was an abrupt change from the lack of photoreceptor cells in the area of atrophy, to a normal thickness outer nuclear layer. In the majority, however, there was evidence of major photoreceptor loss for a considerable distance beyond the edge. As a consequence of these observations it appears to be likely that the functional losses in early AMD are due in part or completely to cell loss rather than cell dysfunction. The magnitude of functional loss implies major photoreceptor loss in early AMD.

Observations in the CFH knockout mouse may also be relevant to cell loss in AMD.[39] It had been shown that visual function was reduced when compared with age-matched mice despite the lack of expected Bruch's membrane thickening. In these mice the photoreceptor outer segments were dysmorphic and there was increased C3 expression in the outer retina. The relevance of C3 to outer segment morphology or of the genetic risk factors to presence of C3 are unknown. As a result of these observations it was concluded that the consequences of the high-risk CFH polymorphism may not be restricted to its influence upon Bruch's membrane. Of possible relevance is that RPE expression of CFH in vitro appears to be apical into the outer retina rather than through the basolateral domain into the choroid.[63] These observations raise the possibility that there is a role played by the immune system in photoreceptor physiology, and that disturbance of these may cause demise of photoreceptor cells that is unrelated to changes in Bruch's membrane or the RPE.

Therapeutic implications

Preservation of the photoreceptor cells might be best achieved by improving RPE function by reduction of accumulation of lipofuscin that may be achieved through manipulation of A2E formation in the photoreceptor outer segment. Restriction of vitamin A availability presumably would achieve this end. Neuroprotective agents might be of benefit as has been hypothesized in the treatment of glaucoma.[64] Similarly, such an approach might slow or prevent photoreceptor cell loss and this has been attempted with the use of a slow release device that uses cells embedded in a matrix that express CNTF.[65] There is early indication that this may be successful in the management of retinitis pigmentosa.[66]

This chapter is by no means exhaustive and additional factors have been considered that are not tissue-specific, such as free radical damage and mitochondrial dysfunction.[67,68] There is a large body of circumstantial evidence to support each although neither is proven. If mitochondrial dysfunction were important it would affect photoreceptors more than other cells since they require large quantities of oxygen to maintain the dark current.

CONCLUSION

In age-related macular degeneration changes occur in the choroid, Bruch's membrane, the RPE, and outer retina. Both genetic and environmental influences have been identified as conferring risk of disease and presumably initiate disease through their cumulative effect. However, there is doubt as to tissues primarily affected by these factors. It is most likely that the balance of changes in the various tissues would vary from one case to another given that many factors confer risk and that they vary from one case to another. Thus in some individuals Bruch's membrane thickening may be the most threatening change whereas it may be the RPE alterations in others. It is also possible that photoreceptor loss may not be due to dysfunction of either the RPE or Bruch's membrane in some cases but is a consequence of an abnormality limited to the outer retina. If correct, therapy directed to one aspect of the disorder should be reserved to those in whom the specific tissue is the primary threat to photoreceptor survival. To achieve this goal it would be necessary to have knowledge of changes to the various tissues involved. Hints or even proof might come from genetic research.

The photoreceptor population could be assessed using imaging such as optical coherence tomography, or visualization of the photoreceptor cells with adaptive optics. The same objective could be achieved using psychophysics means such as visual field recording, microperimetry or fine matrix mapping. Assessment of the concentration of bleachable rhodopsin using reflectometry might be the most effective method of determining the population of viable photoreceptor cells.[69,70] Whatever testing device is used it would be important to test the scotopic as well as the photopic system. The health of the RPE might be assessed by measuring absolute levels of autofluorescence. There is some doubt as to whether or not the thickness of Bruch's membrane could be measured in vivo, but it is likely that the state of the choroid is determined by access of VEGF expressed outward by the RPE. Thus choroidal thickness and choriocapillaris flow would be influenced by the biophysical properties of Bruch's membrane. Both these have been measured recently although variation in normal subjects has yet to be fully established. Characterization of disease in this way would be important in selecting patients for a specific therapeutic approach and in monitoring the response to treatment. It is true that the tissues are metabolically interdependent and modulation of age change in one tissue may have secondary benefits on its neighbors.

REFERENCES

1. Korte GE, Repucci V, Henkind P. RPE destruction causes choriocapilary atrophy. Invest Ophthalmol Vis Sci 1984;25:1135–45.
2. Blaauwgeers HG, Holtkamp GM, Rutten H, et al. Polarized vascular endothelial growth factor secretion by human retinal pigment epithelium and localization of vascular endothelial growth factor receptors on the inner choriocapillaris. Evidence for a trophic paracrine relation. Am J Pathol 1999;155:421–8.
3. Kannan R, Zhang N, Sreekumar PG, et al. Stimulation of apical and basolateral VEGF-A and VEGF-C secretion by oxidative stress in polarized retinal pigment epithelial cells. Mol Vis 2006;12:1649–59.
4. Saint-Geniez M, Kurihara T, Sekiyama E, et al. An essential role for RPE-derived soluble VEGF in the maintenance of the choriocapillaris. Proc Natl Acad Sci U S A 2009;106:18751–6.

5. McLeod DS, Grebe R, Bhutto I, et al. Relationship between RPE and choriocapillaris in age-related macular degeneration. Invest Ophthalmol Vis Sci 2009;50:4982–91.
6. Ramrattan RS, van der Schaft TL, Mooy CM, et al. Morphometric analysis of Bruch's membrane, the choriocapillaris, and the choroid in aging. Invest Ophthalmol Vis Sci 1994;35:2857–64.
7. Olver J. Quoted by AC Bird in: Therapeutic targets in age-related macular disease. J Clin Invest 2010;120:3033–41.
8. Hogan MJ. Macular diseases, pathogenesis: electron microscopy of Bruch's membrane. Trans Am Acad Ophthalmol 1965;69:683–90.
9. Green WR, Key SN. Senile macular degeneration: a histopathological study. Trans Am Ophthalmol Soc 1977;75:180–250.
10. Sarks SH. Changes in the region of the choriocapillaris in aging and degeneration. 23rd Concilium Ophthalmol, Kyoto; 1978 p. 228–38.
11. Tso MOM. Pathogenetic factors of aging macular degeneration. Ophthalmology 1985;92:628–35.
12. Polkinghorne PJ, Capon MR, Berninger TA, et al. Sorsby's fundus dystrophy: a clinical study. Ophthalmology 1989;96:1763–8.
13. Meves H. Die pathologisch-anatomischen gefassveranderungen des Auges bei der beningen und malingen Nephrosklerose. Graefes Arch Ophthalmol 1948;168:287.
14. Friedman E, Smith TR, Kuwabara T, et al. Choroidal vascular patterns in hypertension. Arch Ophthalmol 1964;71:842.
15. Pauleikhoff D, Chen JC, Chisholm IH, et al. Choroidal perfusion abnormalities in age related macular disease. Am J Ophthalmol 1990;109:211–7.
16. Chen JC, Fitzke FW, Pauleikhoff D, et al. Functional loss in age-related Bruch's membrane change with choroidal perfusion defect. Invest Ophthalmol Vis Sci 1992;33:334–40.
17. Steinmetz RL, Haimovici R, Jubb C, et al. Symptomatic abnormalities of dark adaptation in patients with age-related Bruch's membrane change. Br J Ophthalmol 1993;77:549–54.
18. Owsley C, Jackson GR, White M, et al. Delays in rod-mediated dark adaptation in early age-related maculopathy. Ophthalmology 2001;108:1196–202.
19. Scilley K, Jackson GR, Cideciyan AV, et al. Early age-related maculopathy and self-reported visual difficulty in daily life. Ophthalmology 2002;109:1235–42.
20. Green WR, Key SN. Senile macular degeneration: a histopathological study. Trans Am Ophthalmol Soc 1977;75:180–250.
21. Ramrattan RS, van der Schaft TL, Mooy CM, et al. Morphometric analysis of Bruch's membrane, the choriocapillaris, and the choroid in aging. Invest Ophthalmol Vis Sci 1994;35:2857–64.
22. Okubo A, Rosa RH, Bunce KV, et al. The relationships between age changes in retinal pigment epithelium and Bruch's membrane. Invest Ophthalmol Vis Sci 1999;40:443–9.
23. Bird AC, Marshall J. Retinal pigment epithelial detachments in the elderly. Trans Ophthalmol Soc UK 1986;105:674–82.
24. Pauleikhoff D, Harper CA, Marshall J, et al. Aging changes in Bruch's membrane: a histochemical and morphological study. Ophthalmology 1990;97:171–8.
25. Holz FG, Sheraidah G, Pauleikhoff D, et al. Analysis of lipid deposits extracted from macular and peripheral Bruch's membrane. Arch Ophthalmol 1994;112:402–6.
26. Sheraidah G, Steinmetz R, Maguire J, et al. Correlation between lipids extracted from Bruch's membrane and age. Ophthalmology 1993;100:47–51.
27. Li CM, Chung BH, Presley JB, et al. Lipoprotein-like particles and cholesteryl esters in human Bruch's membrane: initial characterization. Invest Ophthalmol Vis Sci 2005;46:2576–86.
28. Moore DJ, Hussain AA, Marshall J. Age related variation in the hydraulic conductivity of Bruch's membrane. Invest Ophthalmol Vis Sci 1995;36:1290–7.
29. Starita C, Hussain AA, Patmore A, et al. Localization of the site of major resistance to fluid transport in Bruch's membrane. Invest Ophthalmol Vis Sci 1997;38:762–7.
30. Pauleikhoff D, Zuels S, Sheraidah G, et al. Correlation between biochemical composition and fluorescein binding of deposits in Bruch's membrane. Ophthalmology 1992;99:1548–53.
31. Chuang EL, Bird AC. Bilaterality of tears of the retinal pigment epithelium. Br J Ophthalmol 1988;72:918–20.
32. Chuang EL, Bird AC. The pathogenesis of tears of the retinal pigment epithelium. Am J Ophthalmol 1988;105:185–90.
33. Hageman GS, Luthert PJ, Victor Chong NH, et al. An integrated hypothesis that considers drusen as biomarkers of immune-mediated processes at the RPE-Bruch's membrane interface in aging and age-related macular degeneration. Prog Retin Eye Res 2001;20:705–32.
34. Yoshida T, Ohno-Matsui K, Ichinose S, et al. The potential role of amyloid beta in the pathogenesis of age-related macular degeneration. J Clin Invest 2005;115:2793–800.
35. Hageman GS, Mullins RF, Russell SR, et al. Vitronectin is a constituent of ocular drusen and the vitronectin gene is expressed in human retinal pigmented epithelial cells. FASEB J 1999;13:477–84.
36. Wasmuth S, Lueck K, Baehler H, et al. Increased vitronectin production by complement-stimulated human retinal pigment epithelial cells. Invest Ophthalmol Vis Sci 2009;50:5304–9.
37. Nan R, Gor J, Lengyel I, et al. Uncontrolled zinc- and copper-induced oligomerisation of the human complement regulator factor H and its possible implications for function and disease. J Mol Biol 2008;384:1341–52.
38. Lengyel I, Flinn JM, Peto T, et al. High concentration of zinc in sub-retinal pigment epithelial deposits. Exp Eye Res 2007;84:772–80.
39. Coffey PJ, Gias C, McDermott CJ, et al. Complement factor H deficiency in aged mice causes retinal abnormalities and visual dysfunction. Proc Natl Acad Sci U S A 2007;104:16651–6.
40. Lovell MA. A potential role for alterations of zinc and zinc transport proteins in the progression of Alzheimer's disease. J Alzheimers Dis 2009;16:471–83.
41. Li W, Chen S, Ma M, et al. Complement 5b-9 complex-induced alterations in human RPE cell physiology. Med Sci Monit 2010;16:17–23.
42. Curcio CA, Medeiros NE, Millican CL. Photoreceptor loss in age-related macular degeneration. Invest Ophthalmol Vis Sci 1996;37:1236–49.
43. Katz ML, Norberg M. Influence of dietary vitamin A on autofluorescence of leupeptin-induced inclusions in the retinal pigment epithelium. Exp Eye Res 1992;54:239–46.
44. von Rückmann A, Fitzke FW, Bird AC. Distribution of fundus autofluorescence with a scanning laser ophthalmoscope. Br J Ophthalmol 1995;79:407–12.
45. Delori FC, Dorey CK, Staurenghi G, et al. In vivo fluorescence of the ocular fundus exhibits retinal pigment epithelial lipofuscin characteristics. Invest Ophthalmol Vis Sci 1995;36:718–29.
46. Lois N, Coco R, Hopkins J, et al. Fundus autofluorescence in patients with age-related macular degeneration and high risk characteristics. Am J Ophthalmol 2002;133:341–9.
47. Holz FG, Bellman C, Staudt S, et al. Fundus autofluorescence and development of geographic atrophy in age-related macular degeneration. Invest Ophthalmol Vis Sci 2001;42:1051–6.
48. Feeney-Burns L, Eldred GE. The fate of the phagosome: conversion to "age-pigment" and impact in human retinal pigment epithelium. Trans Ophthalmol Soc UK 1984;103:416–21.
49. Rozanowska M, Korytowski W, Rozanowski B, et al. Photoreactivity of aged human RPE melanosomes: a comparison with lipofuscin. Invest Ophthalmol Vis Sci 2002;43:2088–96.
50. Holz FG, Schutt F, Kopitz J, et al. Inhibition of lysosomal degradative functions in RPE cells by a retinoid component of lipofuscin. Invest Ophthalmol Vis Sci 1999;40:737–43.
51. Schutt F, Bergmann M, Holz FG, et al. Isolation of intact lysosomes from human RPE cells and effects of A2-E on the integrity of the lysosomal and other cellular membranes. Graefes Arch Clin Exp Ophthalmol 2002;240:983–8.
52. Lakkaraju A, Finnemann SC, Rodriguez-Boulan E. The lipofuscin fluorophore A2E perturbs cholesterol metabolism in retinal pigment epithelial cells. Proc Natl Acad Sci U S A 2007;104:11026–31.
53. Okubo A, Sameshima M, Unoki K, et al. Ultrastructural changes associated with accumulation of inclusion bodies in rat retinal pigment epithelium. Invest Ophthalmol Vis Sci 2000;41:4305–12.
54. Wiegand RD, Koutz CA, Stinson AM, et al. Conservation of docosahexaenoic acid in rod outer segments of rat retina during n-3 and n-6 fatty acid deficiency. J Neurochem 1991;57:1690–9.
55. Stinson AM, Wiegand RD, Anderson RE. Recycling of docosahexaenoic acid in rat retinas during n-3 fatty acid deficiency. J Lipid Res 1991;32: 2009–17.
56. Zhou J, Kim SR, Westlund BS, et al. Complement activation by bisretinoid constituents of RPE lipofuscin. Invest Ophthalmol Vis Sci 2009;50:1392–9.
57. Scholl HPN, Bellmann C, Dandekar SS, et al. Photopic and scotopic fine matrix mapping of retinal areas of increased fundus autofluorescence in patients with age related macular degeneration. Invest Ophthalmol Vis Sci 2004;45:574–83.
58. Radu RA, Mata NL, Nusinowitz S, et al. Treatment with isotretinoin inhibits lipofuscin accumulation in a mouse model of recessive Stargardt's macular degeneration. Proc Natl Acad Sci U S A 2003;100:4742–7.
59. Hogan MJ. Role of the retinal pigment epithelium in macular disease. Trans Am Acad Ophthalmol Otolaryngol 1972;76:64–80.
60. Sarks SH. Ageing and degeneration in the macular region: a clinico-pathological study. Br J Ophthalmol 1976;60:324–41.
61 Wolf-Schnurrbusch UEK, Enzmann V, Brinkmann CK, et al. Morphological changes in patients with geographic atrophy assessed with a novel spectral OCT-SLO combination. Invest Ophthalmol Vis Sci 2008;49:3095–9.
62. Fleckenstein M, Issa PC, Helb HM, et al. High-resolution spectral domain-OCT imaging in geographic atrophy associated with age-related macular degeneration. Invest Ophthalmol Vis Sci 2008;49:4137–44.
63. Kim YH, He S, Kase S, et al. Regulated secretion of complement factor H by RPE and its role in RPE migration. Graefes Arch Clin Exp Ophthalmol 2009;247:651–9.
64. Fu QL, Li X, Yip HK, et al. Combined effect of brain-derived neurotrophic factor and LINGO-1 fusion protein on long-term survival of retinal ganglion cells in chronic glaucoma. Neuroscience 2009;162:375–82.
65. Zhang K, Hopkins JJ, Heier JS, et al. Ciliary neurotrophic factor delivered by encapsulated cell intraocular implants for treatment of geographic atrophy in age-related macular degeneration. Proc Natl Acad Sci U S A 2011;108:6241–5.
66. Talcott KE, Ratnam K, Sundquist SM, et al. Longitudinal study of cone photoreceptors during retinal degeneration and in response to ciliary neurotrophic factor treatment. Invest Ophthalmol Vis Sci 2011;52:2219–26.
67. Beatty S, Koh H, Phil M, et al. The role of oxidative stress in the pathogenesis of age-related macular degeneration. Surv Ophthalmol 2000;45:115–34.
68. Brennan LA, Kantorow M. Mitochondrial function and redox control in the aging eye: role of MsrA and other repair systems in cataract and macular degenerations. Exp Eye Res 2009;88:195–203.
69. Kemp CM, Jacobson SG, Faulkner DJ. Two types of visual dysfunction in autosomal dominant retinitis pigmentosa. Invest Ophthalmol Vis Sci 1988;29:1235–41.
70. Chuang EL, Sharp DM, Fitzke FW, et al. Retinal dysfunction in central serous retinopathy. Eye 1987;1:20–5.

Chapter 65

Age-Related Macular Degeneration: Non-neovascular Early AMD, Intermediate AMD, and Geographic Atrophy

Susan B. Bressler, Neil M. Bressler

INTRODUCTION

Age-related macular degeneration (AMD) has been the leading cause of legal blindness in patients aged 65 or over,[1] and it has been the most common overall cause of blindness in the western world. Using data from the 2000 census, it has been estimated that in the USA more than 8 million people have specific AMD features that put them at risk for progression to advanced AMD and vision loss.[2,3] Over a 5-year period about 1.3 million of these individuals are predicted to develop the advanced forms of AMD, namely neovascular AMD or foveal geographic atrophy (GA).[2] In addition, hundreds of thousands of people aged 75 and over are anticipated to join the pool of people at increased risk of developing advanced AMD over subsequent 5-year periods.[4] The prevalence of AMD continues to rise as a result of the increasing percentage of elderly persons and the improved management of other eye diseases.[3] Prevalence of AMD has also increased steadily in the UK, accounting for approximately 50% of registered blindness in England and Wales that cannot be explained by the increasing age of the population alone.[5] In addition, macular degeneration is the commonest reason that patients with lesser handicaps attend low-vision clinics.

Within the past 5 years new and improved treatments for the neovascular form of advanced AMD have been adopted throughout the developed world. Therefore, in the years ahead the overall burden of vision loss associated with AMD is anticipated to decline substantially.[6] The same progress has not been made for treatment of advanced non-neovascular AMD (GA); as such, the importance of atrophic AMD as a leading cause of vision impairment is expected to increase.

The advanced forms of AMD are those that are frequently associated with visual acuity loss and they are divided into non-neovascular atrophic (dry) type and neovascular (wet) type. In atrophic AMD, gradual disappearance of the retinal pigment epithelium (RPE) results in one or more patches of atrophy that slowly enlarge and coalesce. Affected areas have no visual function, since loss of the RPE is associated with fallout of photoreceptors. Gass[7] applied the term "geographic atrophy of the retinal pigment epithelium" to this presentation, which is the natural end-result of AMD in the absence of clinical evidence of choroidal neovascularization (CNV). This chapter is devoted to the clinical and pathologic features that may lead to this development, as well as their management.

Senile macular degeneration was first reported as a clinical entity in 1885 by Otto Haab,[8] who described a variety of pigmentary and atrophic changes in the macular region, causing progressive impairment of central vision in patients over the age of 50. Subsequent observers referred to the different fundus manifestations of the disease as separate entities, resulting in a variety of descriptive eponyms. A review of dominantly inherited drusen[9] found, however, that only Doyne's honeycomb familial choroiditis and malattia levantinese were disorders that could be distinguished from each other by clinical criteria, and these entities are considered to be a separate category. A major step toward a better understanding of the disease was taken when Gass[10] clarified that drusen, senile macular degeneration, and senile disciform macular degeneration represented a single disease.

In the 1990s it had been proposed that the features should be termed either early or late age-related maculopathy (ARM),[11,12] to suggest that early ARM was not necessarily a pathologic state, with the term age-related macular degeneration (AMD) being reserved for late ARM and encompassing geographic atrophy and neovascular AMD. Since many epidemiologic studies are based on the International Epidemiological Age-related Maculopathy Study Group[11] description, it is described here. However, more recent descriptions of AMD from the Age-Related Eye Disease Study Group[13] have provided longitudinal information to understand features associated with an increased risk of developing advanced forms of AMD and are used in the description of the clinical management of AMD that follows.

In the International Epidemiological Age-related Maculopathy Study Group[11] definitions used in many epidemiologic studies, early ARM was defined as a degenerative disorder in individuals ≥50 years of age, characterized by the presence of any of the following lesions:

- Soft drusen (intermediate >63 μm, ≤125 μm; large >125 μm) drusen. When occurring alone, soft, indistinct drusen are considered more likely to indicate AMD than soft, distinct drusen,[4,14,15] and drusen over 125 μm have greater importance than smaller drusen.[16,17]
- Areas of hyperpigmentation associated with drusen but excluding pigment surrounding hard drusen.
- Areas of depigmentation or hypopigmentation associated with drusen. These areas, which commonly occur as drusen fade, are most often more sharply demarcated than drusen, but do not permit exposure of the underlying choroidal vessels.
- Visual acuity is not used to define ARM or AMD because advanced changes may be present without anatomically affecting the fovea.

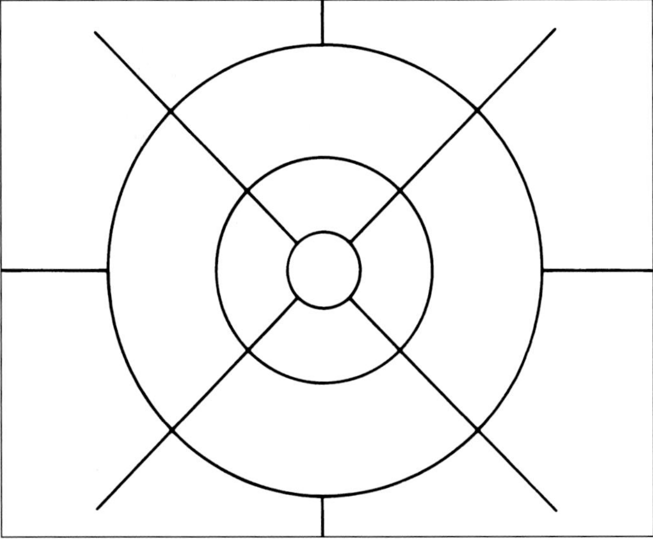

Fig. 65.1 Standard grid for classification of age-related macular degeneration. For a 30-degree fundus camera the diameters of the central, middle, and outer circles are 1000 μm, 3000 μm, and 6000 μm, respectively. These circles represent the central, inner, and outer subfields. The diagonal lines help to center the grid on the macula. (Reproduced with permission from Klein R, Davis MD, Magli YL, et al. The Wisconsin age-related maculopathy grading system. Ophthalmology 1991;98:1128–34.)

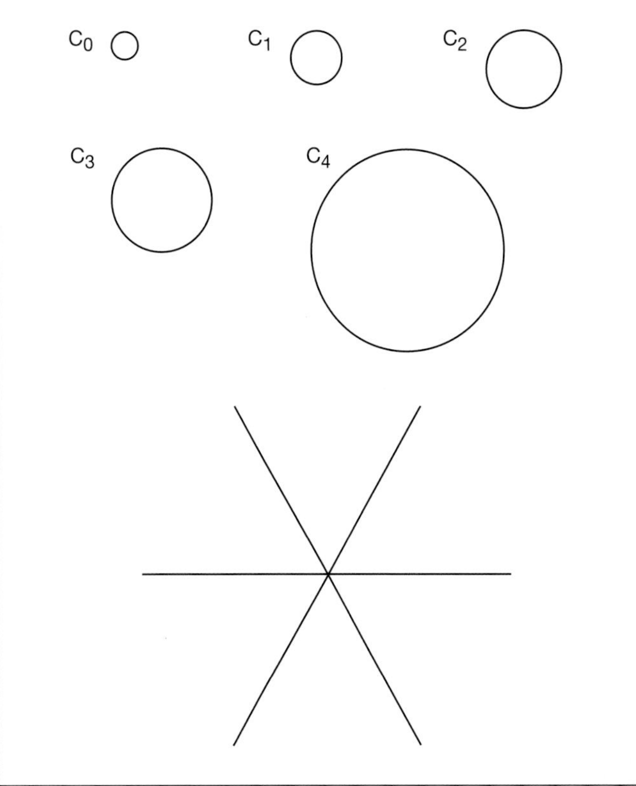

Fig. 65.2 Standard circles C0, C1, C2, C3, and C4 that are used to grade the size of specified lesions. They are reduced on a transparent sheet to range from 1/24 to 1/3 disc diameter, thereby representing 63 μm, 125 μm, 175 μm, 250 μm, and 500 μm. Circle C0 is used to differentiate small from medium drusen, circle C1 is used to differentiate medium from large drusen, and circle C2 indicates the minimum area on which to base a definition of geographic atrophy. The diagonal lines facilitate locating the central point and estimating size of lesions. (Reproduced with permission from Bird AC, Bressler NB, Bressler SB, et al. An international classification and grading system for age-related maculopathy and age-related macular degeneration. Surv Ophthalmol 1995;39:367–74.)

This definition of early ARM excluded small, hard drusen alone, pigment changes alone, and even pigment changes surrounding small, hard drusen for two reasons: (1) hard drusen become an almost constant finding in the fifth decade; and (2) a number of diverse processes can cause pigment abnormalities that may not be possible to distinguish from early ARM, so the inclusion of soft drusen makes the definition more specific to ARM and AMD.[14] However, eyes with numerous small, hard drusen or eyes with pigment abnormalities in the absence of obvious drusen can also progress to soft drusen.

Grading systems have been devised to permit comparison of severity over time in the size, number, and extent of drusen.[11,18–20] Drusen extent is measured by mentally sweeping all drusen present in the area of interest into a condensed zone and estimating the area of that zone. Grids and standard circles prepared on transparent sheets are overlaid to one film image of a pair of stereoscopic color fundus transparencies to assist in the grading process. Alternatively, a digital version of the same grids and circles is superimposed on a digital fundus image. Because of the 3× magnification of the 30-degree fundus camera, 4.7 mm on the grid corresponds to approximately 1500 μm, the diameter of the optic disc in the average fundus. Figure 65.1 illustrates the standard grid used when applying the Wisconsin Age-Related Maculopathy Grading System.[20] This same grid is used in most fundus grading systems of AMD from color photographs. The diameters of the circles within the standard grid are respectively 1000 μm, 3000 μm, and 6000 μm. The central and middle circles combined define the inner macula, which is two disc diameters across. The outer circle defines the macula itself. Figure 65.2 illustrates smaller standard circles, which are used to grade the size and area of specified lesions.[11]

These grading systems are applied to color images and are intended primarily for epidemiologic studies and clinical trials. However, fluorescein angiography often provides additional insight into the natural history of the disease, as do pathologic studies,[21–25] which have demonstrated aging and degeneration to be a continuum based on diffuse morphologic changes at the level of the RPE under the macula, as distinct from focal abnormalities such as drusen. These diffuse changes comprise two types of sub-RPE or basal deposits separated by the RPE basement membrane. On the internal aspect lies a layer of abnormal basement membrane material, referred to as the basal laminar deposit (BLD); on the external aspect of the basement membrane is a layer of membranous debris, referred to as the basal linear deposit.[22] This latter deposit may build up into a type of soft drusen specific for AMD. However, although significant diffuse changes correlate with a decline in visual acuity,[23] they are difficult to see in the fundus, making a histologic definition of AMD based on basal laminar and basal linear deposits unworkable in a clinical setting.

AGING

One of the difficulties in establishing the pathologic changes in AMD is separating the effects of age from those of disease. Aging is a fundamental biologic phenomenon that occurs even in the absence of disease, each cell having a genetically programmed lifespan. Tissues that do not undergo mitotic division to replace this cell fallout, such as the central nervous system and the retina, have a high incidence of aging manifestations, particularly after 75 years of age. This age-related deterioration indicates a reduced anatomic reserve capacity in older subjects.

The aging eye – clinical findings

The normal aged fundus usually demonstrates loss of the foveal and foveolar reflexes. This may be due to fallout of cells from the inner retinal layers, shallowing of the walls of the foveal pit, and enlargement of the capillary-free zone.[26] A few small, hard drusen are almost always present.[12,14,16,18]

Irregularity of retinal pigmentation gives rise to a fine granularity, and the fundus commonly demonstrates a tigroid background. This senile tigroid fundus (see Fig. 65.3A) is increasingly apparent with advancing age but remains compatible with normal vision. It is unrelated to skin pigmentation and differs from the tigroid fundus in youth in that the choroidal vessels become visible under the macula. There is commonly also a peripapillary halo of atrophy in which the exposed vessels may be sheathed and the intervascular spaces appear pale. Studies using blue-field stimulation[27] and scanning laser Doppler flowmetry[28] have shown a decrease in blood flow in the retinal macular capillaries of older individuals, and a lower number of perifoveal arterioles and venules have also been reported.[29] These findings are consistent with enlargement of the capillary-free zone[26] and loss of ganglion cells.[30]

Many aspects of visual function, not just visual acuity, show a decline with age, including dark adaptation, stereopsis, contrast sensitivity, sensitivity to glare, and visual field tests.[31,32] Color perception and foveal cone pigment densities show a decline.[33] The limits of normal aging are therefore difficult to define in terms of visual performance.

The aging eye – morphologic changes

The evolution of the aging process is easier to appreciate by studying morphologic changes. The RPE, Bruch's membrane, and choriocapillaris must function efficiently to serve as the nutritional complex for the photoreceptors. In a normal eye (Fig. 65.4A), the complement of photoreceptors is normal, the RPE forms a regular layer, Bruch's membrane is not unduly thickened, and the choroid consists of the usual three layers of vessels. Each of these tissues has at one time been regarded as primarily at fault in macular degeneration. Therefore it is first necessary to consider the changes developing in these structures during life (Fig. 65.4B).

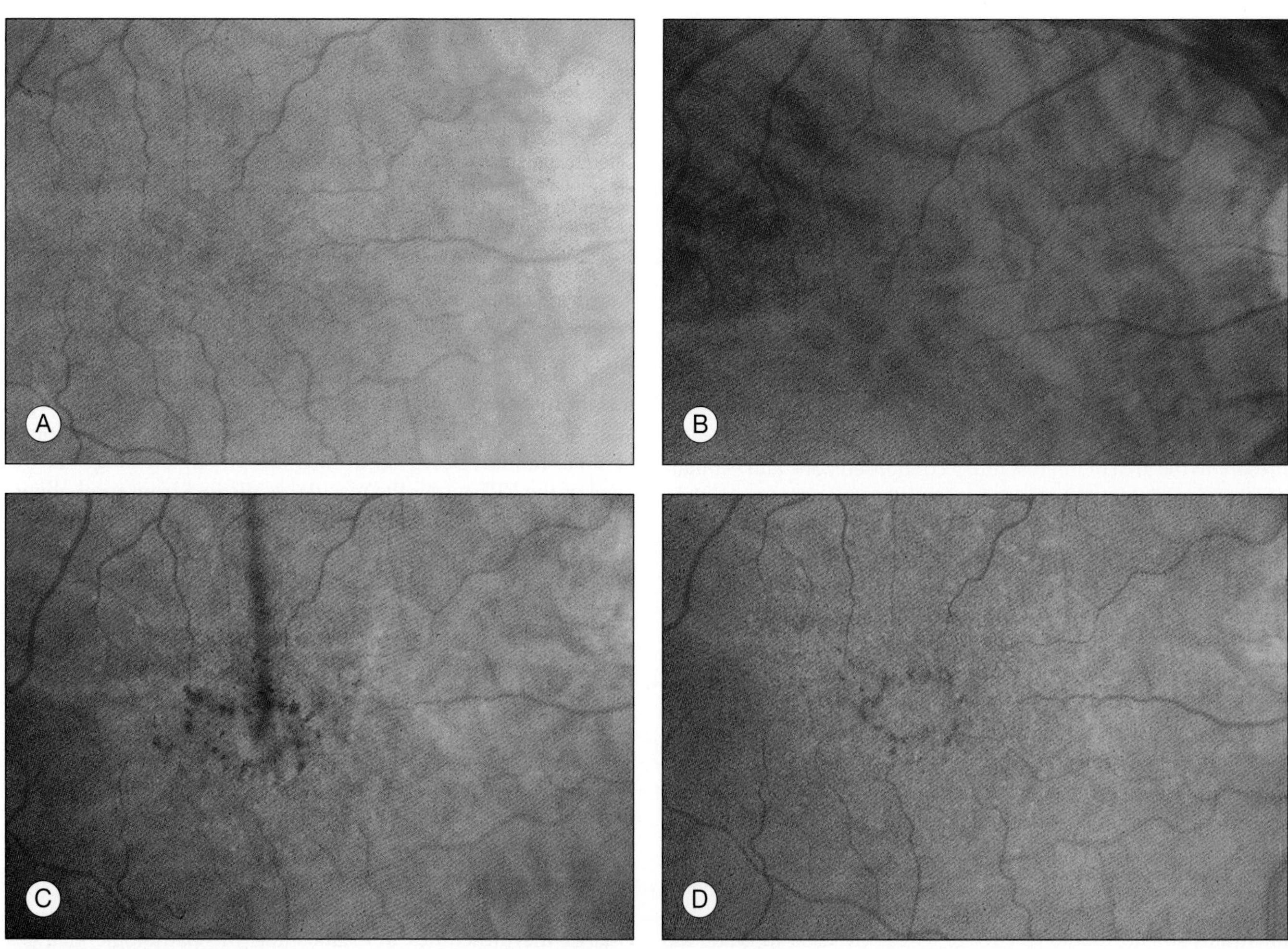

Fig. 65.3 Evolution of age-related macular degeneration, apparently unrelated to drusen, developing into geographic atrophy over 16 years. (A) At age 68, the patient has a normal left fundus with senile tigroid pattern (vision 20/15). (B) At age 73, small drusen-like dots are present, ≤63 μm in size (vision 20/20). (C) At age 77, a ring of pigment clumps is developing around the center of the fovea. (D) At age 79, the pigment clumping around fixation has increased; vision is still 20/20. The choroidal vascular pattern is more prominent. (Reproduced with permission from Sarks JP, Sarks SH, Killingsworth M. Evolution of geographic atrophy of the retinal pigment epithelium. Eye 1988;2:552–77.)

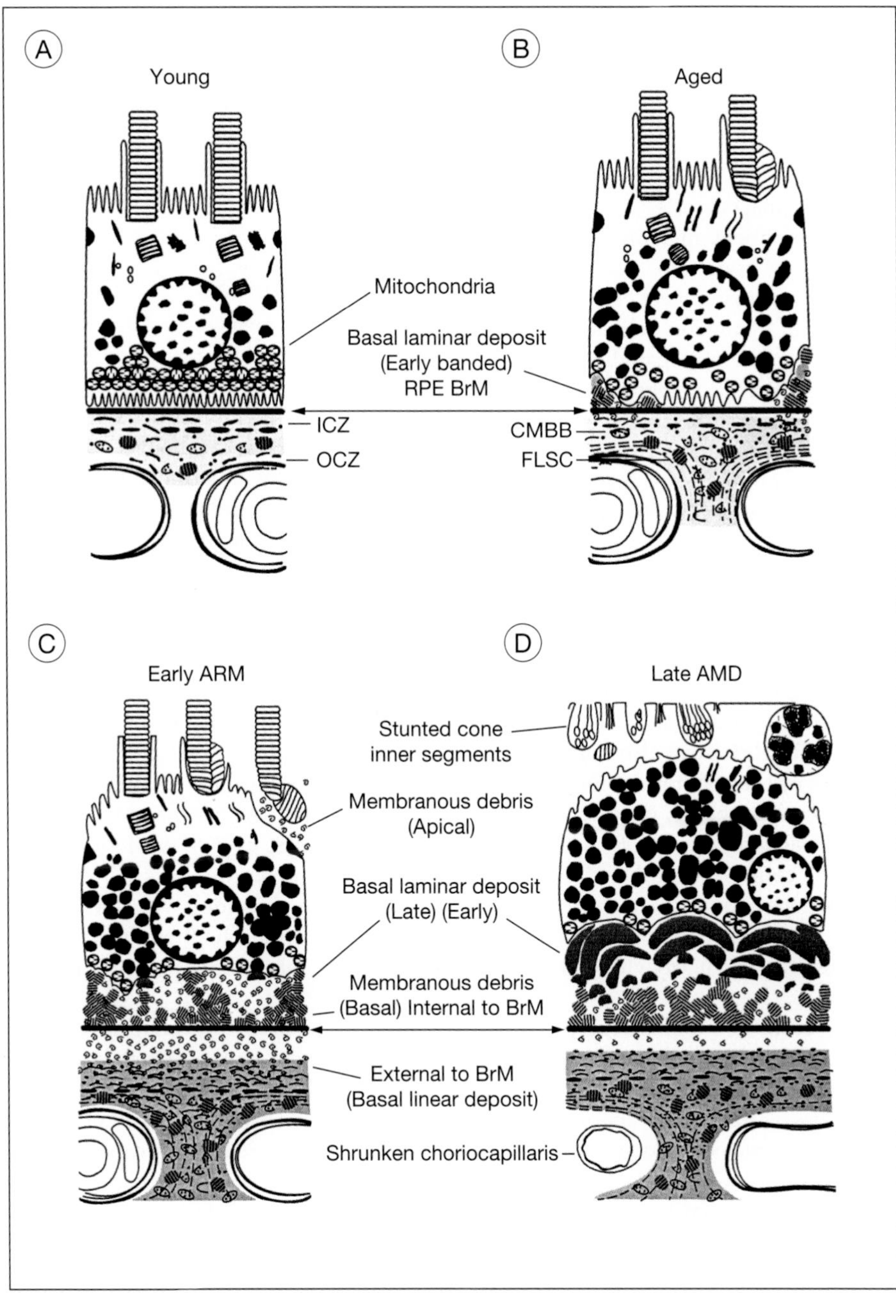

Fig. 65.4 Diagram depicting the ultrastructural features of aging and the evolution of age-related macular degeneration (AMD) in the retinal pigment epithelium (RPE) and Bruch's membrane (BrM). Bruch's membrane is defined as an inner and outer collagenous zone (ICZ and OCZ) separated by an elastic layer but excluding the basement membranes of the RPE and choriocapillaris, instead of as a five-layered structure. The principal distinguishing feature of each stage is the quantity and type of basal laminar deposit (BLD) present at the base of the RPE. (A) Young. The BLD is absent. Mitochondria lie at the base of the cell. The pigment granules comprise elliptical melanin granules in the apical part of the cell and the incompletely degraded products of phagolysosomal digestion, or lipofuscin, toward the base. (B) Aged. Patches of the early, or striated, type of BLD appear on the inner aspect of the RPE basement membrane, where the basal infoldings of the cells are reduced. Also, fewer apical microvilli are present, and elongated rod outer segments attest to impaired phagocytosis. Progressive accumulation of lipofuscin causes the RPE cells to enlarge. Coated membrane-bound bodies (CMBB) accumulate in Bruch's membrane and, together with an increase in fibrous long-spacing collagen (FLSC), cause thickening of the OCZ. (C) Early age-related macular degeneration (AMD). The early type of BLD now forms a continuous layer. Membranous debris in the form of coiled lipid membranes is found: (1) at the apex of the RPE, where there is more distortion of outer segments; (2) at the base of the RPE interspersed among the strands of BLD, where it may form basal mounds; (3) as a layer between the RPE basement membrane and the ICZ (basal linear deposit), where it may build up into soft drusen; and (4) within the collagenous zones. CMBB and FLSC accumulating in Bruch's membrane can be seen in the intercapillary pillars extending to the level of the outer surface of the choroidal capillaries. (D) Late age-related macular degeneration. A thick layer of late BLD is present, predominantly of the amorphous type. Being a later development, the amorphous layer lies on the internal aspect of the early type and appears to be formed in waves as the base of the RPE retracts. The retinal pigment cells are engorged with lipofuscin and become rounder, with loss of both apical microvilli and basal infoldings. Cell fallout occurs, and necrotic portions of cells containing membrane-bound granules are liberated into the subretinal space. The photoreceptor outer segments disappear, leaving stunted cone inner segments. The membranous debris disappears, resulting in "empty spaces" between the strands of early BLD internal to the basement membrane and the regression of any soft drusen present external to the basement membrane. The choroidal capillaries undergo disuse atrophy.

Photoreceptors

The cone density at the foveal center does not appear to alter significantly during the first eight decades.[30,34,35] A significant loss beyond the ninth decade has been reported, but it is not invariable.[36]

In the rods the outer segments become convoluted, possibly as an expression of impaired phagocytosis.[37] This may lead to the accumulation of outer-segment material at the apical surface of the RPE.[36] Fallout of rods can also be demonstrated, with the fastest rate occurring between the second and fourth decades. Cells in the ganglion cell layer show a similar rate of decrease, so the rod and ganglion cell layer densities maintain a constant ratio.[30] Rod photoreceptors and cells in the ganglion cell layer therefore appear to be more vulnerable than cones to loss during aging. In fact, this may be the initial subclinical stage of AMD because the spatial population of parafoveal rods decreases by 30% during adulthood, and AMD often commences in a similar parafoveal distribution.[34,38]

Retinal pigment epithelium

Each pigment epithelial cell must continue to engulf spent photoreceptor discs on a diurnal basis for life, the rods being digested by day and the cones by night,[39] and any undigested residual bodies remain as lipofuscin.[40] The RPE must also remove material from other retinal pigment cells or photoreceptors that may be eliminated, a burden that increases sharply once degeneration of these tissues commences. Finally, because the RPE is a nondividing tissue, autophagy alone could lead to the accumulation of lipofuscin in the same way that it builds up in the neurons of the central nervous system, which have no photoreceptors to phagocytose. The RPE is therefore particularly vulnerable to cell encumbrance.

Damage to molecules may occur in the photoreceptor outer segments as a result of free radical chain reactions initiated by radiation or oxygen metabolism. After phagocytosis, the lysosomal enzymes may fail to "recognize" these abnormal molecules, with a consequent failure of molecular degradation[41] and accumulation of lipofuscin. Free radicals also damage the cells' own molecules, and there is evidence that enzymatic inactivation occurs, particularly cathepsin D, which is the main lysosomal protease responsible for rod outer-segment digestion.[42] There is also an increase of complex granules of melanolysosomes and melanolipofuscin, which are thought to be melanin granules undergoing repair or degradation.

The accumulation of lipofuscin in the RPE, which can be demonstrated as early as the second decade of life,[43] reduces the cytoplasmic space. As the cell volume available to the organelles diminishes, the capacity to deal with photoreceptors is reduced. The issue of whether lipofuscin accumulation has significant deleterious effects on the RPE, and consequently on overall retinal function, continues to be of great interest.[44,45] Since lipofuscin is the predominant fluorophore responsible for fundus autofluorescence, the in vivo imaging and mapping of retinal autofluorescence using the confocal scanning laser ophthalmoscope[46] or fundus spectrophotometer[47] may prove helpful in estimating the risk for progression to AMD.

A certain loss of RPE cells occurs with age, particularly in the periphery. For the fovea this decrease in cell density has been estimated to be about 0.3% per year.[48] The ratio of photoreceptors to RPE cells remains the same,[30,36] the average cone-to-RPE ratio at the center of fovea being approximately 24:1. Photoreceptors and RPE cells therefore show a parallel loss during aging. However, the most notable changes in the RPE develop at the base of the cells, where there is loss of basal infoldings and deposition of patches of abnormal basement membrane material (Fig. 65.4B). (This BLD is described under "Onset and progress of age-related macular degeneration", below.)

Bruch's membrane

Although anatomists regard Bruch's membrane as a five-layered structure, pathologic processes are more readily understood if one uses the definition proposed by Gass[49] that excludes the basement membranes of the RPE and choriocapillaris. Bruch's membrane can then be thought of as a sheet-like condensation of the innermost portion of the choroidal stroma that consists of an inner and outer collagenous zone separated by the elastic layer. In this way the location of drusen, RPE detachments, and sub-RPE neovascular membranes can be described more accurately than by using the all-embracing term "within Bruch's membrane." Also, thickening of Bruch's membrane then refers to the collagenous layers alone, which focuses on a possible etiologic role for Bruch's membrane in AMD, rather than on the actual manifestations of the disease mentioned above.

A linear relationship exists between the thickness of Bruch's membrane and age, the membrane increasing in thickness from 2 μm in the first decade of life to 4.7 μm by the 10th decade.[50] The debris that accumulates within the collagenous and elastic layers, which coincides with the buildup of lipofuscin in the RPE and is similarly first detected early in life on electron microscopy, takes three main forms:

1. A general increase in collagen. The 64 nm banded fibers found in increasing numbers in the collagenous layers with age are believed to be fibrillar type I collagen.[51] Clumps of fibrous long-spacing collagen with band periodicity of about 120 nm are found primarily in the outer collagenous layer or embedded in the basement membrane of the choriocapillaris.[52,53] Fibrous long-spacing collagen is thought to be a combination of collagen and proteoglycans or glycoprotein and may be formed by depolymerization of native collagen fibrils.[52] Other components that have been identified include collagen types III, IV, and V, fibronectin, chondroitin sulfate, dermatan sulfate, and proteoglycans.[51,54] A significant linear decline in solubility of Bruch's membrane collagen occurs with age and may be due to increase in crosslinking.[51]
2. Rounded, coated membrane-bound bodies (Fig. 65.4B, Fig. 65.5). Since these are found as early as the second decade,[55] it has been suggested that this material may result from the shedding of unwanted basal cytoplasm through the basement membrane of the RPE.[56] The actual separation of the bodies from the cells appears to have been demonstrated,[57] but it is such a rare finding that their derivation remains uncertain. These membrane-bound bodies then rupture, spilling their content of coated vesicles and granular material into Bruch's membrane and, together with fragments of the coated membrane wall, the resulting debris accounts for most of the thickening of Bruch's membrane with age.[58] However, most of the debris is found

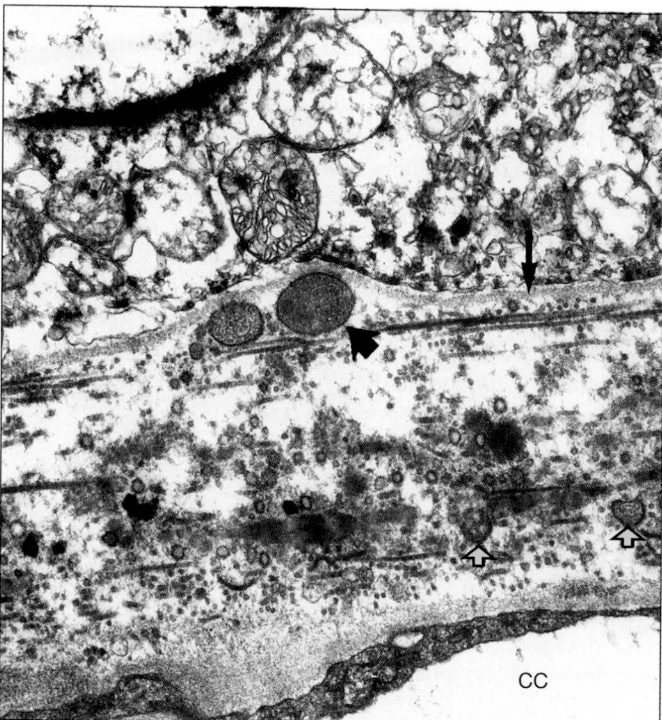

Fig. 65.5 Electron micrograph shows accumulation of debris in Bruch's membrane. The patient was 62 years of age and had 20/20 vision; however, this process can be detected as early as the second decade. Coated membrane-bound bodies (short arrow) are apparently trapped between the basement membrane of the RPE and the inner collagenous zone (entrapment sites). Others lie in the outer collagenous layer (yellow arrows). Some have ruptured, releasing vesicular and granular material and fragments of the coated membrane. Bruch's membrane is normally defined as a five-layered structure, but it may be more appropriate not to regard the basement membrane of the RPE (long arrow) or of the choriocapillaris (CC) as part of the membrane (×11 800). (Courtesy of M.C. Killingsworth.)

in the outer collagenous zone and even on the outer side of the choroidal capillaries, suggesting that it may also be derived from the choroid.[53]

3. Mineralized deposits, which primarily affect the elastic lamina. The degeneration of elastin may be initiated by actinic damage.[24] The corresponding histologic findings in Bruch's membrane, which become evident in the fifth decade, comprise thickening, hyalinization, and patchy basophilia.[23,25] This diffuse deposition in the collagenous zones also extends down the intercapillary pillars and can be correlated with an increase in the lipid content of Bruch's membrane after the fourth decade.[59–61] The lipids consist largely of phospholipids, triglycerides, fatty acids, and free cholesterol. There is little cholesterol ester, which would have been expected to predominate if the lipids had been derived from the bloodstream, suggesting that the source of the material is the RPE.[59] However, the specific inclusions seen with electron microscopy cannot be correlated with any particular type of lipid.[62]

Peroxidized lipids have been identified in Bruch's membrane, the total amount increasing exponentially with age. The peroxidized lipids identified were derived from long-chain polyunsaturated fatty acids, particularly docosahexanoic acid and linolenic acid, which are polyunsaturated fatty acids found in photoreceptor outer segments. Lipid peroxides have been shown to induce neovascularization by inducing expression of a cascade of angiogenic cytokines.[63]

Changes in hydraulic conductivity

Hydraulic conductivity is the measurement of the bulk flow of fluid through a test membrane in response to applied pressure. Bruch's membrane would be expected to show increasing resistance to flow with age because it exhibits a linear increase in thickness[50] and a significant accumulation of lipid after the fourth decade.[61,62,64] However, studies undertaken on Bruch's membrane have shown that the decrease in hydraulic conductivity is exponential, being greatest in the first four decades of life.[65,66] It is unclear why this occurs before age 40. It has therefore been suggested that remodeling of collagen occurs as a result of increased cross-linkage, and this may cause an increase in rigidity of the membrane and reduced pore size, with entrapment of passing protein molecules.[67] After age 40 the increasing lipid content would be expected to have an increasing effect on hydraulic conductivity, while in the 60s a further reduction would result from the diffuse deposits that appear beneath the RPE.

The excimer laser has been used to remove progressively ultrathin shavings of Bruch's membrane to determine in which layer the major barrier to the flow of water lies. This demonstrated that the greatest resistance throughout life resides within the inner collagenous zone.[66] Serial ultrathin sections cut parallel to the plane of Bruch's membrane to estimate the porosity at sequential levels confirmed that the inner collagenous zone presented the lowest porosity. Calculations based on the pore radii and length further confirmed that the inner collagenous zone also had the lowest flow rate. However, ultrastructural studies would appear to indicate that it is mainly the outer collagenous zone that increases in thickness with age, with the inner collagenous zone remaining constant.[58] Clearly, further studies are required, as only a limited number of younger eyes have been examined.

The debris that accumulates in Bruch's membrane is probably the result, rather than the cause, of degeneration of the RPE. Nevertheless, the associated reduction in permeability may in turn further compromise the RPE.

Choroid

A decrease in choroidal blood flow with age can be demonstrated by laser Doppler flowmetry and is mainly due to a decrease in choroidal blood volume rather than in velocity of flow.[68] This is consistent with histologic changes in aged eyes. Comparing normal maculas in the first and 10th decades, the density of the choroidal capillaries (combined length of capillary lumina per unit length) decreased in a linear fashion by 45%, and the anteroposterior diameter by 34%.[50]

The middle layer of medium-sized vessels decreases with age, resulting in a progressive decrease in thickness of the choroid from 200 μm at birth to 80 μm by the age of 90 years.[50] The resulting thinning of the choroid throws the remaining larger vessels into greater prominence, accounting for the senile tigroid fundus. This clinical appearance has generally been attributed to unmasking of the choroidal vessels by attenuation and loss of pigment from the retinal pigment cells. However, senile choroidal atrophy appears to contribute more significantly to the increased visibility of the vessels.

ONSET AND PROGRESS OF AGE-RELATED MACULAR DEGENERATION

Clinical features in the absence of drusen

The lipofuscin-laden RPE cells that disappear with age are phagocytosed by their neighbors. The fundi usually retain a normal appearance during this process, but in older eyes the number of cells shed may be sufficient to become visible in the fundus as a diffuse mottling of small pigment clumps or as a microreticular pattern of small lines, more obvious on fluorescein angiography. The progress of AMD is thus closely related to the degree of pigmentary disturbance evident in the fundus, and this may occur in the absence of typical drusen.

The patient illustrated in Figs 65.3 and 65.6 shows this evolution to geographic atrophy over a 17-year time span. The first change detected was the presence of scattered, small drusen-like dots, 25–50 µm in size (Fig. 65.3B). A ring of small pigment clumps then developed around the fovea (Fig. 65.3C, D), but vision remained 20/20, demonstrating the difficulty of determining when, on the basis of visual acuity alone, pigment changes become pathologic. This is due to the fact that the foveal center is often spared for many years. Hyperpigmentation is accompanied by hypopigmentation, with geographic atrophy (Fig. 65.6) then spreading into the area of attenuated RPE (incipient atrophy).

Morphologic changes

The morphologic alterations (see Fig. 65.4C) considered thus far in the photoreceptors, RPE, Bruch's membrane, and choroid are progressive throughout life. However, by the seventh decade other changes have appeared at the base of the RPE that have no counterpart in earlier life. These comprise the deposition of basement membrane-like material and shedding of membranous debris. Although these changes first develop in a patchy distribution while the fundus and vision are still normal, their diffuse occurrence is the principal feature of AMD.[23,69,70]

Basal laminar deposit – early form

The BLD lies beneath the RPE, between the plasma membrane and the basement membrane, in contrast to typical drusen, which lie external to the basement membrane. It can be demonstrated consistently by the seventh decade,[23] but has been found even in the fifth decade.[25] It first appears in a patchy distribution over thickened or basophilic segments of Bruch's membrane, over intercapillary pillars, or over small drusen, suggesting a

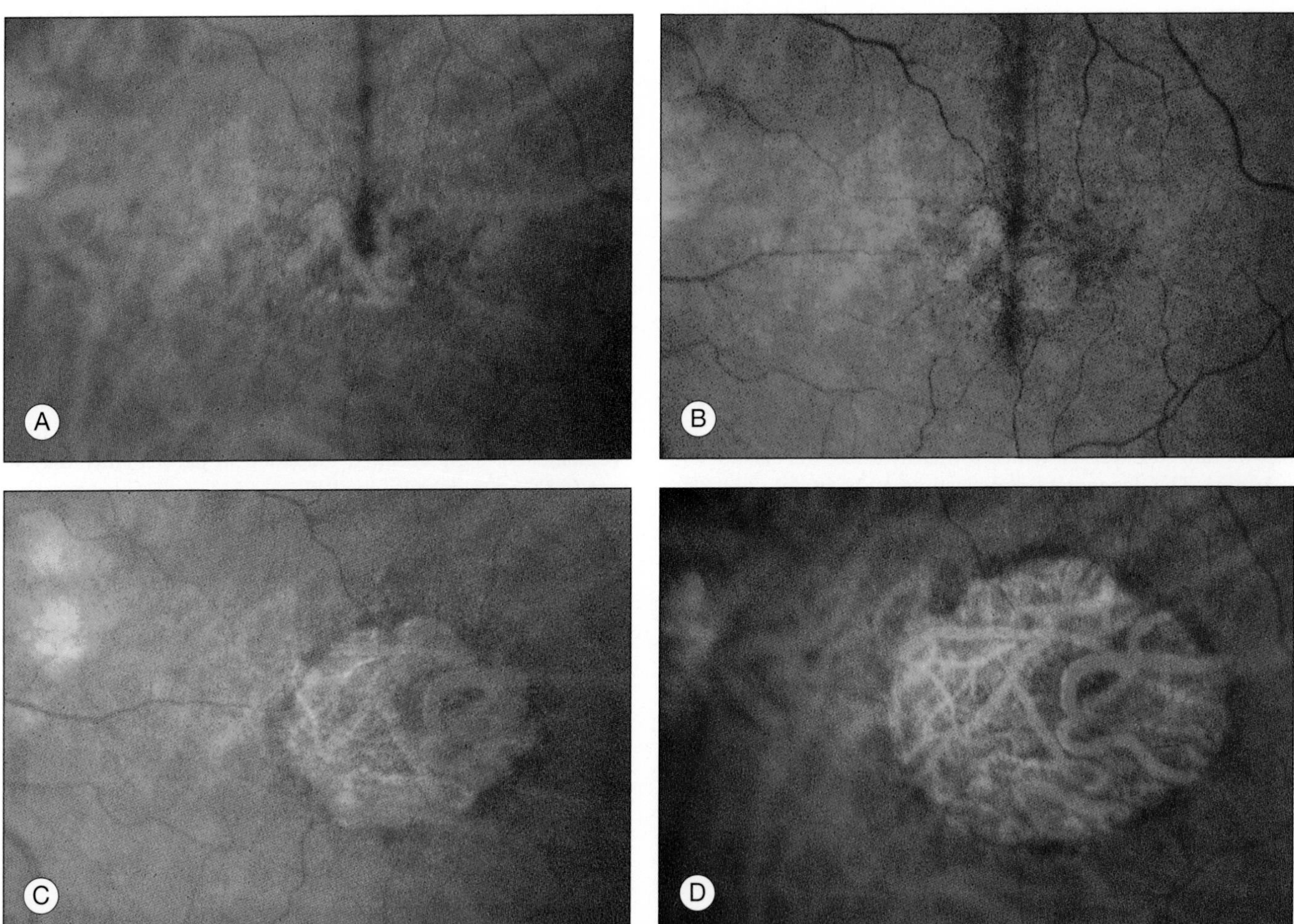

Fig. 65.6 Same patient as in Fig. 65.3. (A and B, red-free) At age 81, patient fixing between two small areas of atrophy that have developed. Pigment clumping and drusen-like dots are spreading outward. This surrounding incipient atrophy corresponds to the area of geographic atrophy that developed subsequently (D); vision is still 20/30. (C) At age 82, atrophy involves fixation, and dots have faded. Vision has dropped to 20/200. (D) At age 84, area of atrophy has almost doubled; vision is 20/400. Choroidal atrophy causes exposed vessels to appear white. Patient died at age 85. Pathology of this eye is shown in Fig. 65.8. (Reproduced with permission from Sarks JP, Sarks SH, Killingsworth M. Evolution of geographic atrophy of the retinal pigment epithelium. Eye 1988;2:552–77.)

potential response to altered filtration at these sites. It can be quantified histologically[25] as class 1 (small, solitary patches), class 2 (a thin continuous layer), and class 3 (a thick layer, at least half the height of the RPE).

Histologically the deposit exists in two different forms, early and late, according to the stage of degeneration. The early BLD is a pale-staining eosinophilic material that stains blue with picro-Mallory and shows faint anteroposterior striations (Fig. 65.7). On electron microscopy the BLD consists of three phenotypes: fibrillar, amorphous, and polymerized. The fibrillar phenotype appears to be the earliest manifestation and may only be detected by electron microscopy as irregular nodules lying on the original basement membrane. The polymerized form resembles the fibrous long-spacing collagen seen in Bruch's membrane and is also found in the cornea, trabecular meshwork, and other tissues in the body.[53] It projects internally from the original RPE basement membrane[71] (Fig. 65.8) and accounts for the striations, or bush-like appearance, seen histologically.

The similarity of the BLD to basement membrane and its proximity to rough endoplasmic reticulum at the base of the cells suggest it is a secretory product of the RPE.[71,72] It reacts with antibodies against type IV collagen, heparan sulfate proteoglycans, and laminin,[54,55,72,73] but the BLD is biochemically distinct from the RPE basement membrane, and a faulty, degradative process rather than enhanced synthesis may account for its accumulation in aged maculas.[54,55]

Membranous debris

Coiled membrane fragments continuous with the plasma membrane of the RPE appear together with the BLD, but they are not found unless BLD is also present[24] (Fig. 65.8). This material has the bilayered structure of phospholipids and is not to be confused with the coated membrane-bound bodies described earlier in Bruch's membrane. Whereas by light microscopy the BLD was regarded as the hallmark of macular degeneration, by electron microscopy it is this membranous debris that correlates more closely with the degree of degeneration. These membranes are found in three locations, as described in the following paragraphs.

Internal to the retinal pigment epithelium basement membrane

The coils appear to be extruded from the base of the cells, which have lost their infoldings, although they may alternatively result from a free-energy process in which lipid molecules are deposited by the RPE into Bruch's membrane and coalesce. The membranes form layers and then basal mounds internal to the RPE basement membrane (Fig. 65.4C, Fig. 65.9), which may account for the drusen-like dots noted clinically (Fig. 65.3B). The membranes are not demonstrated in conventional histologic sections, since the mounds manifest only as small, unstained spaces within the BLD (Fig. 65.10). As the mounds enlarge and fuse, the RPE shows more derangement and cell dropout.

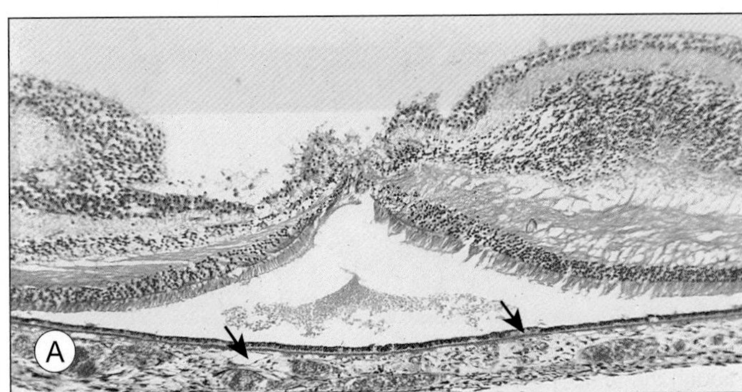

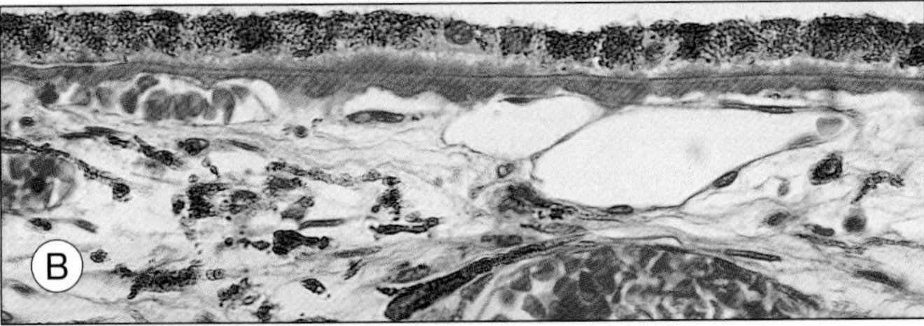

Fig. 65.7 (A) Section through the macula of a 79-year-old man. Fundus appeared normal, and vision was 20/30. Early form of basal laminar deposit is seen as continuous, blue-staining layer beneath the retinal pigment epithelium. Unstained spaces (right arrow) would correspond to membranous debris on electron microscopy. Arrow at left indicates area magnified in panel B (×75). (B) Basal laminar deposit is most developed over a thicker segment of Bruch's membrane. Hyalinization of Bruch's membrane extends down intercapillary pillars (picro-Mallory stain; ×500). (Reproduced with permission from Sarks SH. Aging and degeneration in the macular region: a clinico-pathological study. Br J Ophthalmol 1976;60:324–41.)

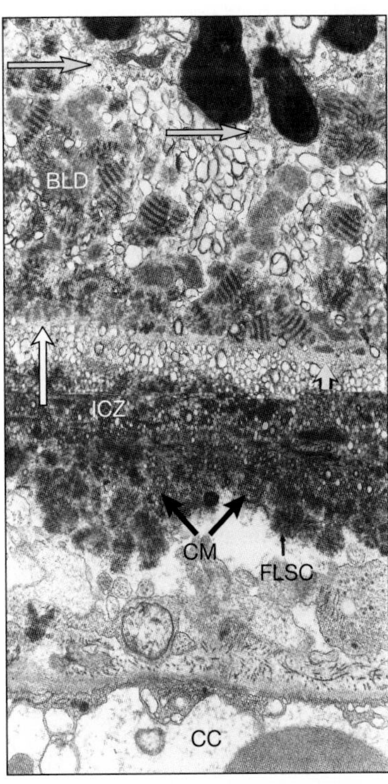

Fig. 65.8 Electron micrograph illustrating changes developing between retinal pigment epithelium and choriocapillaris (CC) in age-related maculopathy corresponding to Fig. 65.4C. Horizontal yellow arrows indicate the basal plasma membrane of the RPE. Early-type basal laminar deposit (BLD) projects inward from the RPE basement membrane (white arrows) and comprises mainly banded material resembling fibrous long-spacing collagen. Coiled membranes with a bilayered structure of lipids lie among the clumps of BLD and appear to pass through the basement membrane to lie between it and the inner collagenous zone (ICZ), as well as filtering into the membrane itself. Identifiable structures within Bruch's membrane include fragments of coated membrane (CM) and fibrous long-spacing collagen (FLSC) (×11 780). (Reproduced with permission from Killingsworth MC, Sarks JP, Sarks SH. Macrophages related to Bruch's membrane in age-related macular degeneration. Eye 1990;4:613–21.)

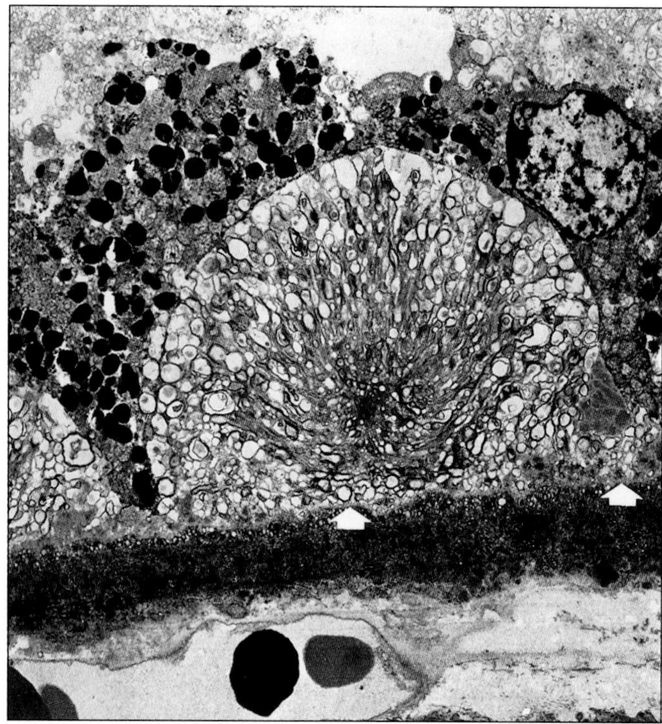

Fig. 65.9 Basal mound lying internal to RPE basement membrane. Electron micrograph shows build-up of coiled membranous debris separating the grossly abnormal RPE from its basement membrane. These collections are referred to as "basal mounds" and may account for the drusen-like dots noted clinically. Only a very thin layer of membranous debris lies external to the basement membrane (arrows), so there are no soft drusen (×1680). (Courtesy of M.C. Killingsworth.)

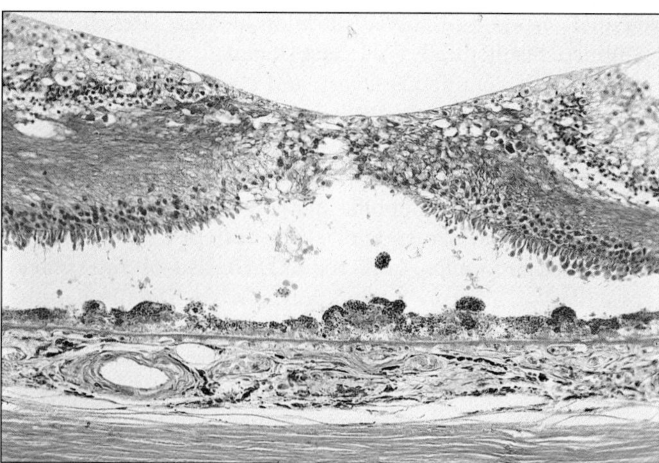

Fig. 65.10 Section through the macula of an 83-year-old man in whom pigment changes were evident clinically. Stretches of attenuated, hypopigmented RPE alternate with clumps from which hyperpigmented cells are shed into the subretinal space. Basal laminar deposit is thicker and comprises both early and late forms. Small, unstained patches beneath the RPE would correspond to mounds of membranous debris on electron microscopy (×525). (Reproduced with permission from Sarks SH. Aging and degeneration in the macular region: a clinico-pathological study. Br J Ophthalmol 1976;60:324–41.)

*External to the RPE basement membrane (basal linear deposit[22])**

Membranes appear to pass through the basement membrane to form a layer between the basement membrane and the inner collagenous layer of Bruch's membrane (Fig. 65.8). In this location the debris may build up into the soft drusen specific for AMD[73] (see Fig. 65.26). The debris also appears to disturb the normal attachment of the RPE to Bruch's membrane, creating a cleavage plane, and it is in this plane that RPE detachments due to blood and serous fluid lie and into which early choroidal new vessels grow.[74] The membranes even appear to percolate into the collagenous zones of Bruch's membrane.

At the apex of the retinal pigment epithelium

Morphologically similar membranous debris is also found over the apex of the RPE, lying in the subretinal space and presumably representing outer-segment material that has not been phagocytosed (Fig. 65.11).

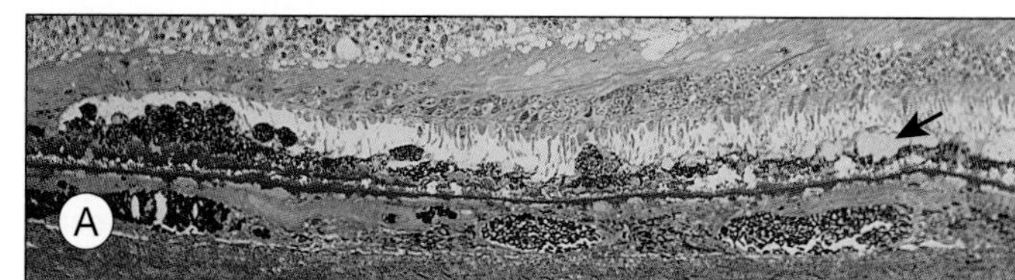

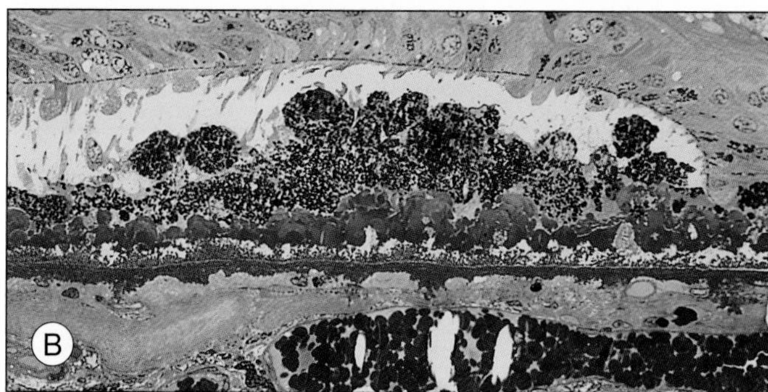

Fig. 65.11 Same eye as in Figs 65.5 and 65.6. Section passes through the temporal margin of the area of geographic atrophy. (A) Photoreceptors become fewer and outer segments wider and stunted as they approach the edge. Vacuolated appearance under the RPE is due to disappearance of membranous debris. Collections of membranous debris can be seen on the internal (apical) surface of RPE (arrow), possibly due to failure of phagocytosis (×150). (B) Hyperpigmented edge noted clinically corresponds to a double layer of RPE, the inner layer representing necrotic hyperpigmented cells in the process of being eliminated. Late amorphous form of BLD lies internal to striated form and has a multilaminar appearance, suggesting formation in successive waves according to the level of RPE (see Fig. 65.4D). Photoreceptors disappear, and external limiting membrane terminates on BLD (methylene blue and basic fuscin; ×500). (Reproduced with permission from Sarks JP, Sarks SH, Killingsworth M. Evolution of geographic atrophy of the retinal pigment epithelium. Eye 1988;2:552–77.)

Membranous debris is therefore seen in three different locations: (1) in the subretinal space, (2) between the RPE and its basement membrane, and (3) external to the basement

**A uniform terminology for the diffuse deposits is gaining acceptance. The original observations by light microscopy distinguished only one deposit. This was referred to as the basal linear deposit and it proved a useful histologic marker for the stage of the disease.[23] Subsequent electron microscopic studies showed that this deposit lies internal to the RPE basement membrane, so the name was changed to basal laminar deposit, but another layer could also be demonstrated lying external to the basement membrane. Green and Enger[22] suggested retaining the term basal laminar deposit for the material internal to the basement membrane, but resurrecting basal linear deposit for the diffuse layer of vesicular and granular material on the external aspect. Unfortunately the acronym BLD could then be applied to either deposit, so recently the term basement membrane deposit (BMD) has been proposed for the basal laminar deposit. Until the terminology and the abbreviations become standardized, this chapter will continue to apply the abbreviation BLD for the basal laminar deposit and use the terms membranous debris, or the unabbreviated basal linear deposit, when referring to the material external to the basement membrane. These definitions replace older terms such as diffuse thickening of the inner aspect of Bruch's membrane and diffuse drusen.[21,74,75]* membrane, but it is always dependent on the presence of intact outer segments.

Basal laminar deposit – late form (diffuse thickening of the internal aspect of Bruch's membrane)

With progressive degeneration of the RPE, another form of basal laminar material appears. On light microscopy it forms a thick, hyalinized layer that stains red with picro-Mallory, similar to hyalinized Bruch's membrane, and that is more periodic acid–Schiff-positive than the earlier, banded form. Being a later development, it forms a distinct layer on the internal surface of the earlier form (Fig. 65.4D) and may approximate the thickness of the normal RPE, occasionally displaying nodular elevations on its internal surface[75] (Fig. 65.12).

On electron microscopy, the later form of the BLD has a flocculent appearance and consists mainly of amorphous material. It may be uplifted with the attenuated RPE over the membranous mounds and appears to be formed in waves according to the level of the base of the cell at the time (Fig. 65.11). It indicates the altered metabolism of a severely stressed RPE and occurs typically over regressing drusen (see Fig. 65.30).

Clinically the BLD has not yet been identified in the fundus with any certainty, but the presence of the late form can be inferred by the presence of significant pigment changes and, since there is an associated reduction of the choriocapillary bed, by noting delayed choroidal perfusion during fluorescein angiography.

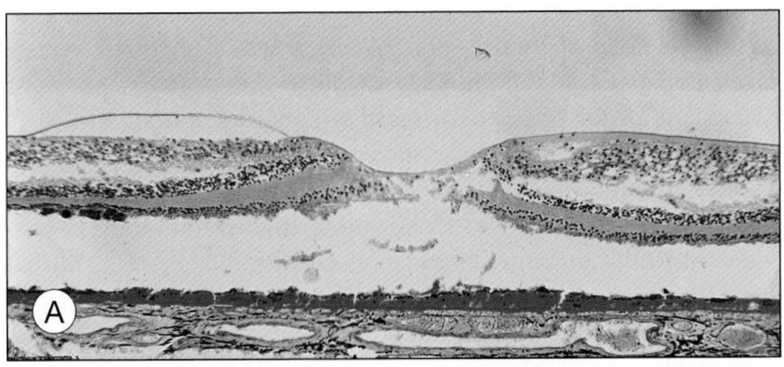

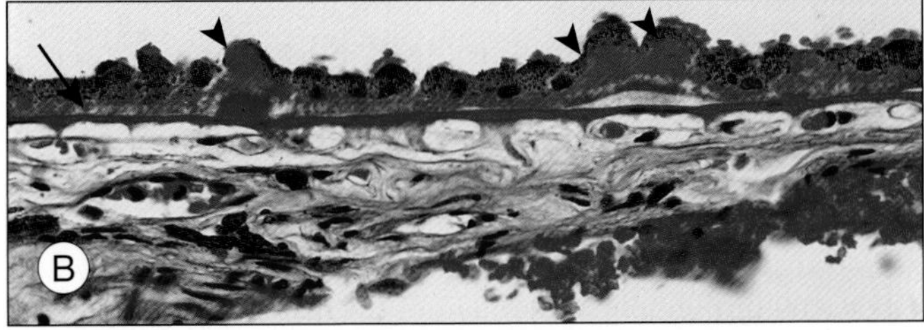

Fig. 65.12 (A) Incipient atrophy, showing an unusually thick layer of late BLD, which has also been referred to as diffuse thickening of the inner aspect of Bruch's membrane. This material is hyalinized and periodic acid–Schiff-positive; on electron microscopy it would have a corresponding amorphous appearance. The retinal pigment epithelium forms a very attenuated layer over the surface and seems about to disappear (periodic acid–Schiff; ×45). (B) Parafoveal area from the same eye shows the different deposits. The two forms of the BLD are seen: the blue-staining, early form (long arrow) and, on its inner surface, nodular collections of the late hyalinized form (arrowheads), also referred to as "basal laminar drusen." External to the BLD lie two typical drusen; beneath the short arrow at left is a small hard druse; beneath the two short arrows at right is a soft druse (picro-Mallory stain; ×500). (Reproduced with permission from Sarks SH. Aging and degeneration in the macular region: a clinico-pathological study. Br J Ophthalmol 1976;60:324–41.)

Retinal pigment epithelium and photoreceptors

Lipofuscin and complex melanolipofuscin granules continue to accumulate in the retinal pigment cells, which enlarge and lose their regular shape. The external or basal surface of the cell shows loss of the basal infoldings (with a consequent reduction in surface area) and becomes increasingly separated from its basement membrane by thickening of the BLD and more membranous debris. Occasional cells undergo lipoidal degeneration.[76] Finally the hyperpigmented cells resulting from this phagocytic overload round off, so only a few stubby apical microvilli remain, and they lose their ability to phagocytose. Lipofuscin is packed into large degenerate retinal pigment cells or membrane-bound bodies and shed (Fig. 65.4D).

The corresponding pigment abnormalities in the fundus may be classified[11] as increased pigmentation (or hyperpigmentation) and depigmentation (or hypopigmentation). Focal hyperpigmentation correlates histologically with localized areas of RPE cell hypertrophy, which may be accompanied by clumps of hyperpigmented cells in the sub-RPE space, in the subretinal space (see Fig. 65.10), and even migrating to the outer nuclear layer. With the advent of spectral domain (SD) ocular coherence tomography (OCT)[77] and ultrahigh resolution (UHR) OCT,[78,79] deposits have been demonstrated, in vivo, with moderate to intense hyperreflectivity in these various planes and correspond to hyperpigmentation on clinical examination or on fundus photographs. It is common for eyes with drusen to have these intraretinal deposits directly above the drusen, and although the outer nuclear layer is more common, some migration has even occurred into more anterior retinal layers.[79] Focal hypopigmentation correlates with attenuated, depigmented RPE cells surrounding the hyperpigmented cells.[75] A careful review of SD OCT images in areas of hypopigmentation show attenuated signal from the RPE layer.

The sequence of events leading to pigment disturbance and, ultimately, atrophy seems to be the same irrespective of the cause. When a retinal pigment cell dies, the products are phagocytosed by its neighbors. These cells in turn become filled with lipofuscin and round off, losing their ability to phagocytose. As the cells are discarded, the nearby cells migrate and increase in surface area in an attempt to maintain the integrity of the blood–retinal barrier. This results in thinned, hypopigmented cells adjacent to focal hyperpigmentation. Finally, these cells can no longer stretch to fill the gap and atrophy results. Hyperpigmentation therefore precedes hypopigmentation, and this in turn is the prelude to the development of patches of atrophy.[80]

Another instance where pigment figures precede atrophy occurs over long-standing drusenoid pigment epithelial detachments (PEDs). However, atrophy is likely to occur only after the cell population is already depleted, and, in younger patients with focal hyperpigmentation related to drusen or in patients with pattern dystrophies of the RPE, patches of attenuated RPE may be present for many years without progressing to atrophy.

Progressive derangement of the RPE is accompanied by dropout of photoreceptors, with a reduction in the number of nuclei in the outer nuclear layer. The inner segments tend to become shorter and more bulbous. The outer segments may terminate in collections of membranes over the apical surface of the RPE (Fig. 65.11).

Bruch's membrane and choroid

Hyalinization and densification of Bruch's membrane extend down the intercapillary pillars and may even surround the choriocapillaris. The choroidal capillaries, already separated by widening of the intercapillary pillars, become further narrowed by retraction away from Bruch's membrane, and this is accompanied by a loss of fenestrations. Patent capillaries now begin to occupy less space than the intercapillary distances under the macula, in keeping with the reduced requirements of the attenuated RPE.

Macrophages, giant cells, fibroblasts, and occasional lymphocytes are found in relation to the outer surface of Bruch's membrane in the space formerly occupied by the choroidal capillaries.[81] Segments of the membrane begin to thin, and cell processes are occasionally observed splitting off and even enveloping small fragments of the membrane.[71] The choroidal capillaries in the vicinity may show signs of activation, and new vessels still confined entirely to the choroid have been identified.[82] This chronic, low-grade inflammatory reaction, which possibly develops in response to the membranous debris liberated by degenerating RPE, is often found in the choroid near breaks in Bruch's membrane,[83] and it appears to be a link in the chain of events leading to CNV. As such mechanisms that decrease inflammation are actively being investigated as a means of altering both the atrophic and neovascular pathways of advanced AMD.

DRUSEN

Clinical grading

Drusen type

Drusen are broadly divided into hard and soft, with soft drusen being further subdivided into soft indistinct or soft distinct. Soft drusen are generally larger than hard drusen and have a soft or amorphous appearance. They appear to have a thickness when viewed stereoscopically and tend to become confluent, so they show greater variation in size and shape than hard drusen.

Drusen size

Clinically, drusen size can be compared to the width of a major vein at the disc edge (approximately 125 μm). Small drusen are those less than 0.5 vein width (<63 μm), and since size and morphology are generally correlated, these are considered to be hard.[12,18] Drusen ≥125 μm (Fig. 65.2, circle C1) are large, and these are typically considered to be soft based on the appearance of their perimeter. Drusen between ≥63 μm and <125 μm may be termed medium or intermediate in size and are more frequently classified as soft drusen as well.

Extent of fundus involvement

This may be assessed by noting drusen number, the area of fundus involved,[20,84] and the density of drusen (discrete, touching, or confluent). The area occupied by drusen yields important prognostic significance as it is a cornerstone in the Age-Related Eye Disease Study (AREDS) severity scale. Drusen area is identified by mentally condensing all drusen located in the zone of interest into a single area and estimating the size of that area by comparison to standard grid areas measured in disc area (DA) equivalents.[84] Automated detection of total drusen area on digital fundus images remains under development and may eventually replace, partially or in full, grading by trained readers.

Drusen distribution

Detailed natural history studies have focused on the drusen characteristics for drusen that are located within 1 or 2 disc diameters of the foveal center (see Fig. 65.1).[12,84–88] Different patterns of drusen distribution have been reported,[15] and it is the superior and temporal quadrants that have been associated with greatest area of drusen involvement and highest prevalence of soft, indistinct drusen or reticular drusen.

Drusen symmetry

Comparisons of the distribution, number, and type of drusen between the two eyes of an individual tend to show a remarkable symmetry, which often leads to similar outcomes in both eyes.[15,17,25,89] The drusen type which are most commonly present in both eyes of an individual are reticular drusen and soft, indistinct drusen.[17]

Drusen color

Drusen color varies from white, to pale yellow to bright yellow. As drusen regress they lose their coloration and may be associated with glistening areas of calcification and areas of RPE atrophy or depigmentation.

Clinical grading of AMD severity

Despite their apparently significant role in the evolution of AMD, diffuse deposits detected on histopathology are difficult to study clinically. However, prognostic significance is ascribed to the clinical presence of drusen, the white-to-yellow clinically apparent deposits described above that lie deep to the retina, representing accumulation of the materials described in the preceding sections of this chapter. While it was previously recognized that patients with at least medium-size, soft, or confluent drusen are predisposed to develop advanced stages of AMD,[19,87] more recent natural history data from the AREDS has suggested a somewhat more detailed description of non-neovascular AMD to characterize prognosis. In addition, this terminology is also relevant to the management of non-neovascular AMD.[13] In this classification features are evaluated within 3000 μm of the center of the macula (Fig. 65.1) and eyes can be classified into one of four groups:

Group 1: An eye is graded as *no AMD* if there are no drusen or only a few (~5–15) small drusen in the absence of any other stage of AMD.

Group 2: An eye is considered to have *early* stage AMD if there are extensive (>15) small drusen, or a few (approximately <20) medium-size indistinct drusen (soft borders) or pigment abnormalities (increased pigmentation or depigmentation but not geographic atrophy) and no other stage of AMD.

Group 3: The *intermediate* stage of AMD refers to the presence of at least one large druse, but can also be applied to the eye with numerous medium-size drusen (approximately 20 or more when the drusen boundaries are amorphous and approximately 65 or more when the drusen boundaries are distinct, sharp or hard) or to the presence of geographic atrophy that does not extend under the center of the macula (noncentral GA).

Group 4: The *advanced* stage of AMD is reserved for the presence of geographic atrophy extending under the center of the macula or presence of neovascular AMD.

In addition to providing this simplified classification of AMD (no AMD, early AMD, intermediate AMD, and advanced AMD), the AREDS investigators also devised a simplified clinical scale defining risk categories for development of advanced AMD.[88] A scoring system tabulates a person score by assigning 1 risk factor to each eye of an individual for the presence of at least 1 large druse and 1 risk factor for the presence of any pigment abnormality. Drusen are to be scored only within 2 disc diameters of the foveal center, and pigment abnormalities consist of either increased pigment thought to be attributed to AMD, RPE depigmentation, or areas of noncentral geographic atrophy. Risk factors are summed across both eyes, resulting in a 5-step scale (0–4) on which the 5-year risk of developing advanced AMD in at least one eye can be approximated. Risk of progression escalates as follows: total score 0, 0.5% risk; 1 factor, 3%; 2 factors, 12%; 3 factors, 25%, and 4 factors, 50%. Modifications of the scale award persons without any large drusen 1 risk factor if medium-size drusen are present in both eyes and individuals with advanced AMD in their first eye receive a score of 2 for that eye when tabulating the person score to estimate the risk for their fellow eye.

Grading in scientific studies

While the grading of drusen described above is relevant to management and relatively easy to apply in clinical practice, a means of more specific grading of drusen for scientific studies is desirable, ideally without requiring fluorescein angiography. The system proposed by the International Epidemiology Study Group,[11] which is based on stereoscopic color fundus photographs, grades for the predominant drusen type, the most severe drusen type, drusen numbers, largest drusen size, area involved by drusen, drusen confluence, and drusen disappearance (see Fig 65.1, 65.2).

A more recent detailed fundus photographic severity scale to be used in research settings has been presented by the AREDS investigators.[84] Baseline photographs and annual photographs beginning at year 2 of follow-up from AREDS participants were graded for drusen characteristics (size, type, area), pigmentary abnormalities (increased pigment, depigmentation, geographic atrophy) and presence of abnormalities consistent with neovascular AMD. Relationships between various baseline characteristics and development of advanced AMD at the 5-year exam were explored to develop a 9-step severity scale that sorts the 5-year risk of advanced AMD from less than 1% in step 1 to about 50% in step 9. About half the eyes that had at least a 3-step progression between baseline and the 5 year exam showed stepwise progression through intervening severity levels at intervening visits. The second Age-Related Eye Disease Study (AREDS2), which is presently underway, aims to validate this scale in a separate cohort of patients at high risk for AMD progression. If validated, progression along this scale may be considered as a surrogate outcome for progression to advanced AMD in future studies.

Imaging of drusen

Fluorescence of drusen

Drusen have a variety of constituents that range from being hydrophobic to those that are hydrophilic. Fluorescein is a hydrophilic dye, which diffuses into hydrophilic areas. As such, some drusen routinely bind the dye and hyperfluoresce in late stage angiography. About 50% of drusen present within an eye will stain with fluorescein.[90] Although drusen that stain with fluorescein appear across the spectrum of drusen sizes, drusen that stain are, on average, larger than drusen that do not stain. When considering fluorescein-stained drusen, drusen area appears similar to that which is appreciated on color photographs.

During indocyanine green angiography, hard drusen become hyperfluorescent 2–3 minutes after dye administration, and this persists through the middle and late phases. Soft drusen are either hypofluorescent (darker than the background fluorescence) throughout the angiogram with a thin hyperfluorescent rim or remain isofluorescent (indistinguishable from background fluorescence).[91,92]

Autofluorescence

On autofluorescence imaging, large drusen may or may not be apparent depending upon the alterations in the RPE overlying the druse.[64] There may be a pattern of decreased autofluorescence in the center of the druse often surrounded by a ring of subtle increased autofluorescence.[93] However, areas of emerging RPE atrophy in eyes with drusen may be more apparent on autofluorescence as compared to clinical examination, as regions in which autofluorescence is completely absent.[64]

Ocular coherence tomography (OCT)

Cross-sectional imaging of drusen in eyes with non-neovascular AMD is possible in vivo with OCT, particularly in the era of high speed and high resolution SD-OCT instrumentation. A wide variety of drusen patterns have been identified which may reflect the diversity in chemical and histologic features of drusen. The most common pattern consists of a convex, homogeneous, medium internal reflective deposit without overlying hyperreflective foci.[94] Half of the soft indistinct drusen found on color photographs manifested this pattern; however, the other half had significant variability in their OCT patterns. Calcified drusen differed in that the deposit was predominantly hyporeflective, nonhomogeneous with or without a core and more apt to have overlying foci of hyperreflectivity. The hyperreflective foci are suspected to represent retinal pigment migration. At this time it is unknown how drusen subtypes identified on OCT relate to ultrastructural drusen characteristics or to clinical prognosis. Further study is underway in an ancillary study within the second age-related eye disease study that may elucidate the prognostic rule of OCT of drusen.

Automated evaluation of drusen location, total macular area, and total volume involved is under development with segmentation software for use on various OCT instruments and maybe a useful tool to monitor disease progression in the future.[95,96] Studies have also demonstrated focal thinning of the photoreceptor layer immediately overlying drusen, loss of photoreceptor outer segments, and normal inner retinal thickness.[77] These qualitative and quantitative changes may ultimately predict vision dysfunction.

Pathologic considerations

Typical age-related drusen are deposits of extracellular material, which typically lie between the basement membrane of the RPE cells and the inner collagenous zone of Bruch's membrane (Fig. 65.13). In contrast, diffuse thickening of the inner aspect of Bruch's membrane and cuticular drusen,[22,53] also called basal laminar drusen,[97] describe material internal to the basement membrane and appear to be similar to the late, amorphous form of BLD (Fig. 65.12). Basal laminar drusen are attributed to internal nodularity of the RPE basement membrane and can produce a starry-sky appearance on fluorescein angiography, which can be impossible to distinguish clinically from myriads of small, hard drusen (Fig. 65.14). However, the condition can usually be recognized when a myriad of small drusen have a somewhat translucent appearance with retroillumination in an individual in their 40s or 50s, sometimes with a vitelliform detachment of yellowish material. (The latter will progressively accumulate fluorescein but should not be confused with progressive fluorescein leakage from CNV.) Another type of small, yellow lesion resembling drusen, but which is nonfluorescent, has been found to be due to lipoidal degeneration of individual retinal pigment cells.[76] The discussion which follows is confined to typical drusen external to the basement membrane.

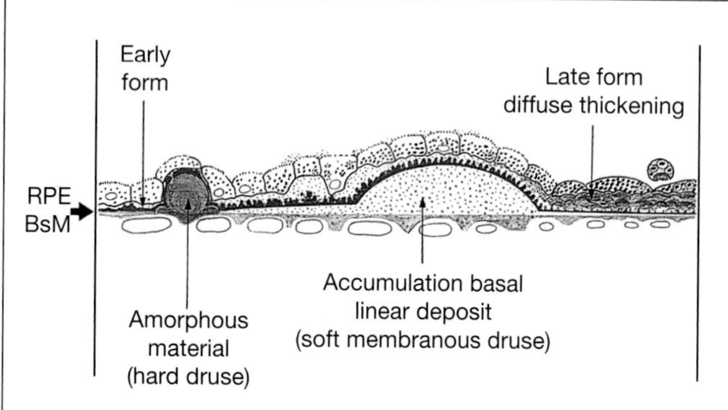

Fig. 65.13 Diagram showing the relationship to the retinal pigment epithelium (RPE) basement membrane (BsM) of the deposits accumulating under the RPE during the evolution of age-related macular degeneration. The basal laminar deposit lies internal to the BsM, and typical drusen lie external. The BLD exists in an early striated form (shown in blue) and late amorphous form (shown in brown). Membrane coils are found both internal to BsM, as mounds at the base of the RPE, and external to the BsM, as the BLD, where it may form soft, membranous drusen. Hard drusen consist predominantly of amorphous material.

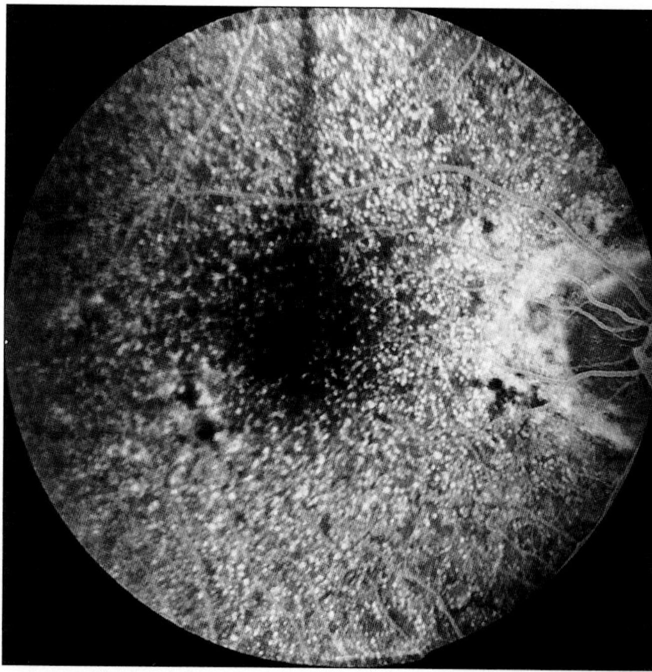

Fig. 65.14 Scattered, small, hard drusen in generalized distribution. Fluorescein angiogram of the right eye of a 59-year-old man. The whole posterior pole is studded with drusen, mostly of the discrete, small, hard variety, in the region of 25–75 μm. A few larger drusen, up to 150 μm across, have resulted from the fusion of several smaller drusen, and small reticular pigment figures are developing in relation to these larger drusen. Vision was still 20/20. The drusen were not obvious on ophthalmoscopy because most were only 30 μm tall. The patient died 6 months later. The pathology is shown in Fig. 65.16. (Reproduced with permission from Sarks JP, Sarks SH, Killingsworth MC. Evolution of soft drusen in age-related macular degeneration. Eye 1994;8:269–83.)

The clinical classification of drusen mentioned above is based on ophthalmoscopic appearance, but fluorescein angiography and histopathologic examination add further information and suggest two main paths of development. Small, hard drusen with a hyalinized structure are the predominant type in younger persons, and some larger soft drusen show evidence of their derivation from clusters of these small drusen.[73] A clinicopathologic correlation study of 353 normal and aged eyes without AMD showed that, in the absence of the diffuse deposits, all the drusen were of the hyalinized variety.[98] Other drusen, however, develop de novo in the seventh decade, when the diffuse layer of membranous debris (basal linear deposit) appears, and these latter are specific for AMD. To these may be added a third presumed mechanism, the addition of proteinaceous fluid in those drusen ≥250 μm that resemble serous PEDs. Other authors have identified five distinct morphologic classes of drusen at the ultrastructural level. No attempt was made to correlate these classes of drusen to clinical phenotypes described in the literature. However, class 1 corresponds to hard drusen and class 2 to soft drusen with the same composition as the basal linear deposit.[99] Therefore, until the complete life cycle of drusen can be recognized clinically, a classification of drusen must remain part clinical and part morphologic.

Clinicopathologic classification

1. Small, hard (hyalinized) drusen.
2. Soft (pseudosoft), cluster-derived drusen.
3. True soft drusen, which have three morphologic subtypes:
   a. Granular
   b. Fluid, including drusenoid PEDs
   c. Membranous (accumulation of basal linear deposit).
4. Reticular drusen (pseudodrusen ditto).
5. Regressing (fading) drusen.

Small, hard (hyalinized, nodular[75]) drusen

Clinical features

Small, hard drusen are not visible in the fundus until they measure 30–50 μm, the width of two to three retinal pigment cells. They are difficult to see in lightly pigmented fundi but use of red-free light may facilitate identification. They may be visible with fluorescein angiography, even when as small as 25 μm, fluorescing brightly in the mid-venous phase and fading soon after the background choroidal fluorescence (Fig. 65.14).

Small, hard drusen may first be noted within 1 disc diameter of the fovea[15] but when numerous they are most common on the temporal side of the fovea. They tend to occur in clusters, and histopathologic specimens show that where hard drusen can be demonstrated clinically, there are often numerous intervening drusen too small to be seen (see Fig. 65.15). Another common pattern consists of a wide band outside the vascular arcades and passing on the nasal side of the disc, with sparing of the inner macula. Toward the equator they assume a linear arrangement

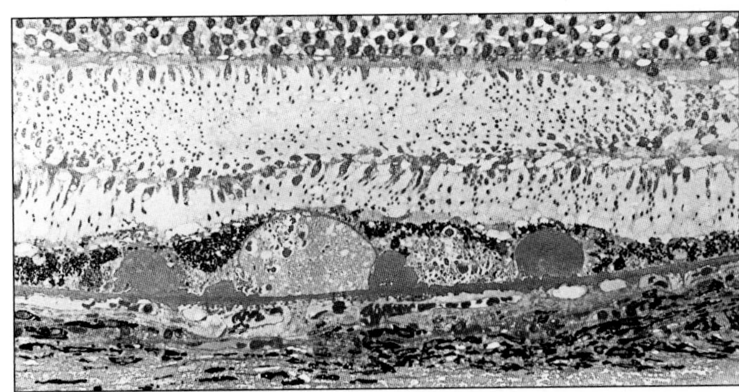

Fig. 65.15 Electron micrograph shows a parafoveal cluster of small, hard drusen measuring 250 μm in diameter, the drusen touching and fusing. Larger drusen inside the cluster are breaking down into globules of hyaline material, leaving small, hyalinized drusen around the perimeter. The smallest drusen would not be seen clinically, but they can be assumed to be present around the larger, visible drusen. Retinal pigment epithelium over the larger drusen is thinned. Fundus had shown only a few drusen clusters. Vision was 20/20 2 years before death at age 81; lens opacities and dementia precluded further documentation. The cluster would appear as a single deposit, and fluorescein angiography (not performed) would be expected to demonstrate brightly staining, small drusen around a more homogeneous center (methylene blue and basic fuchsin; ×290).

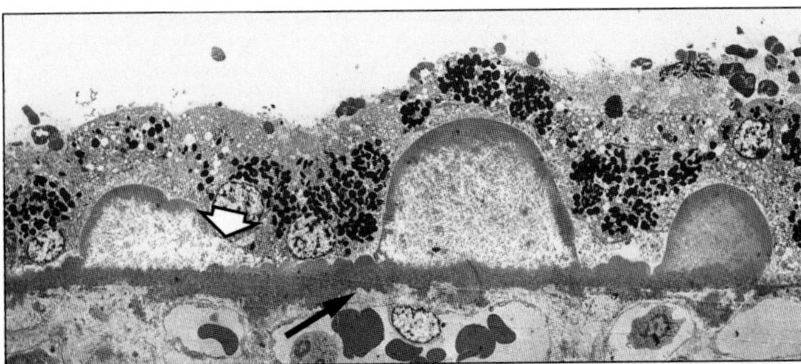

Fig. 65.16 Electron micrograph of small, hard drusen present in the eye shown in Fig. 65.14. Druse at far right demonstrates greater electron density around the margin than in the center. Larger druse in middle shows dispersion of contents except for a peripheral shell of amorphous material, with the outline of the druse remaining sharp. Druse at left is similar but has lost rim of amorphous material on one side (arrowhead), and this edge is spreading out on Bruch's membrane. Note that the inner surface of Bruch's membrane is raised into a row of small, rounded, electron-dense elevations, or microdrusen (arrow), which also lie beneath the larger drusen. Similar extensions occur on the choroidal side of the membrane (near arrow). Despite the presence of numerous drusen, there was no basal laminar deposit or membranous debris in this eye (the patient was only 62 years of age) (×7315). (Reproduced with permission from Sarks JP, Sarks SH, Killingsworth MC. Evolution of soft drusen in age-related macular degeneration. Eye 1994;8:269–83.)

in relation to a polygonal pattern of hyperpigmented lines, giving rise to the picture of reticular (honeycomb) degeneration of the pigment epithelium.

Formation

Small, hard drusen histologically are globular deposits of hyalinized material with staining properties similar to hyalinized Bruch's membrane and have an amorphous appearance on electron microscopy. They have been identified in the macula in 83% of postmortem eyes.[100]

Certain preceding changes in Bruch's membrane may determine their formation.[98] In eyes with only a few drusen, small hyalinized plaques of densification in Bruch's membrane are observed, sometimes with extensions into the outer collagenous zone and even on to its choroidal surface. Another early change, seen only by electron microscopy, appears as coated membrane-bound bodies, both ruptured and intact (see Fig. 65.5), similar to those found within the outer collagenous zone. However, here they appear "trapped" between the elevated RPE basement membrane and the inner collagenous zone. It has been proposed that they develop by the shedding of unwanted basal cytoplasm through the basement membrane of the RPE[56] by a process likened to apoptosis (from the Greek: "a falling off, as the petals of a flower"), but the process of evagination and pinching-off of cytoplasm from the base of the RPE is so difficult to find that it has not been established to be a mechanism by which drusen form, and the term entrapment sites[98] seems preferable to shedding sites. These entrapment sites are found at all ages and have also been detected in primate eyes, probably indicating a normal aging phenomenon.

In eyes with many small, hard drusen the preceding thickenings in Bruch's membrane are more extensive, appearing as a row of microdrusen, or rounded elevations 2 μm in diameter, and composed of very dense amorphous material[73] (Fig. 65.16). Hyalinized drusen form over these changes and as they grow they become hemispherical or almost globular. When small, hard drusen grow larger than about 63 μm, the amorphous contents become less compact and paler-staining, a process that begins in the lower part of the druse. Single hard drusen rarely exceed 125 μm, and further enlargement is the result of the fusion of several drusen. As the RPE over the drusen degenerates, the contents become increasingly dispersed (Fig. 65.16) or, especially in older patients, coarsely granular (Fig. 65.5). When the drusen finally fade, the basement membrane of the overlying RPE becomes infolded and collapses on to Bruch's membrane, usually leaving a small patch of clinical hypopigmentation.

Significance

Population-based studies[12,14,16,18,101] all reported that one or more drusen were found commonly – in 95.5% of the population aged over 43 years[12] to 98.8% of those over 49 years[14] – with small, hard drusen less than 63 μm being the most frequent type in all age groups. Pathologic studies[22] support the conclusion that the presence of a few small, hard drusen is not a risk factor for AMD. However, several studies[4,101] have found that if a threshold number of small, hard drusen is exceeded, the eye is more likely to develop larger drusen. Longitudinal clinical studies of at least 5 years' duration suggest advanced AMD rarely develops in eyes with only small, hard drusen at baseline, regardless of the total area involved.[4,13]

Soft (pseudosoft) cluster-derived drusen

Initially the small, hard drusen in a cluster may remain discrete, or even may be touching, but individual drusen can still be distinguished on ophthalmoscopy. As the drusen become so closely packed together, the cluster appears as a single larger deposit that clinically appears soft, but the small drusen can usually still be made out in red-free light or on fluorescein angiography (Fig. 65.17). These fused drusen are up to 250 μm, depending on the number of drusen in the cluster. If sufficiently elevated, they may tent up the retina and cause a reddish halo

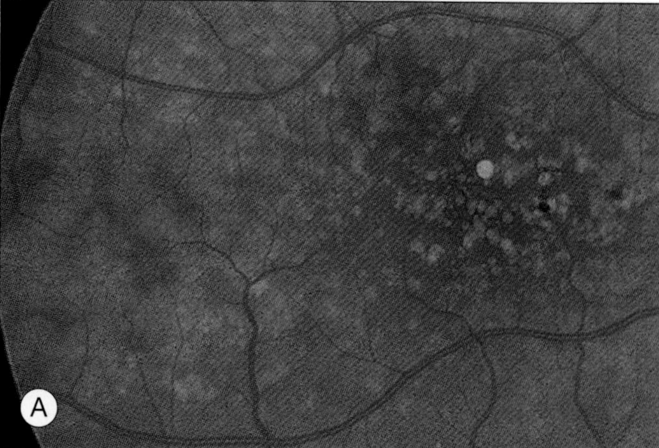

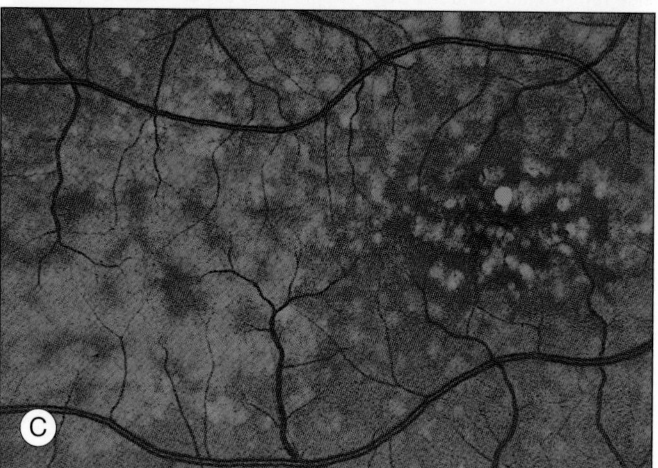

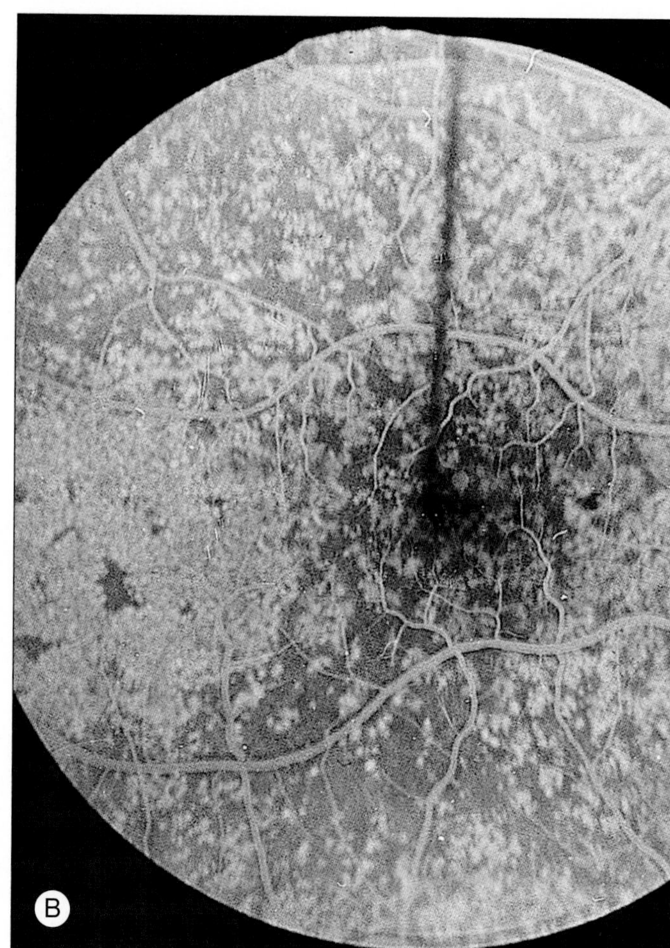

Fig. 65.17 Soft, cluster-derived drusen (pseudosoft drusen). Right fundus of a 50-year-old man with 20/20 vision (A). Groups of mainly small, hard drusen associated with hyperpigmentation are seen at the fovea. Large, soft, confluent drusen appear to be located temporal to the fovea, but in red-free light (C), and particularly on fluorescein angiography (B), the soft drusen can be seen to consist of closely packed clusters of small, hard drusen.

around the base, which is a favorable sign because it reflects the hard, abruptly elevated margins and the integrity of the surrounding retina (Fig. 65.18). On fluorescein angiography they remain brightly fluorescent, although staining is not uniform. These clusters of fused, small, hard drusen occur in middle age, and the prognosis is generally good, with the drusen slowly regressing over many years and leaving a focal patch of atrophy (Fig. 65.18). It is of interest that this cycle may be completed in younger persons before the BLD and membranous debris characteristic of AMD have developed. Hard drusen therefore appear to occur independently of the intermediate or advanced stage of AMD.

True soft drusen

These soft drusen are not visibly derived from small, hard drusen. At least three separate processes may contribute to their formation, but since all may be present in the same druse, they often cannot be distinguished from one another clinically. Moreover, the contents of soft drusen are easily lost during histopathologic processing, so not all the constituents will have been identified. In the following discussion, true soft drusen are subdivided according to their apparent pathogenesis.

Granular soft drusen (synonyms: serogranular drusen, semisolid drusen,[102] localized detachment of the basal linear deposit[22])

Clinically, most of these drusen are about 250 μm and have a yellow, solid appearance, their confluence resulting in crescentic or sinuous shapes (Fig. 65.19). Histologically, they have a coarsely granular structure, consisting of membrane-bound globules of amorphous material, small membrane fragments, and other cellular debris. The presence of microdrusen and the proximity of some of these drusen to hyalinized drusen (Fig. 65.15) suggest that the granular contents represent, in part, cluster-derived drusen in which the original hard drusen have broken down (Fig. 65.20). A thin layer of this granular material would appear to resemble the soft drusen described by Green and Enger[22] (see Fig. 65.8), as localized detachment of the RPE and basal linear deposit, in an eye with diffuse basal linear deposit.

Not all these drusen can be seen to be derived from the breakdown of hard drusen, but when this does occur the drusen in the center of the cluster seem to be affected first (Fig. 65.15), and small, hard drusen may remain identifiable around the perimeter of the cluster. The detection of this heterogeneous composition, either on fluorescein angiography or in histologic sections,

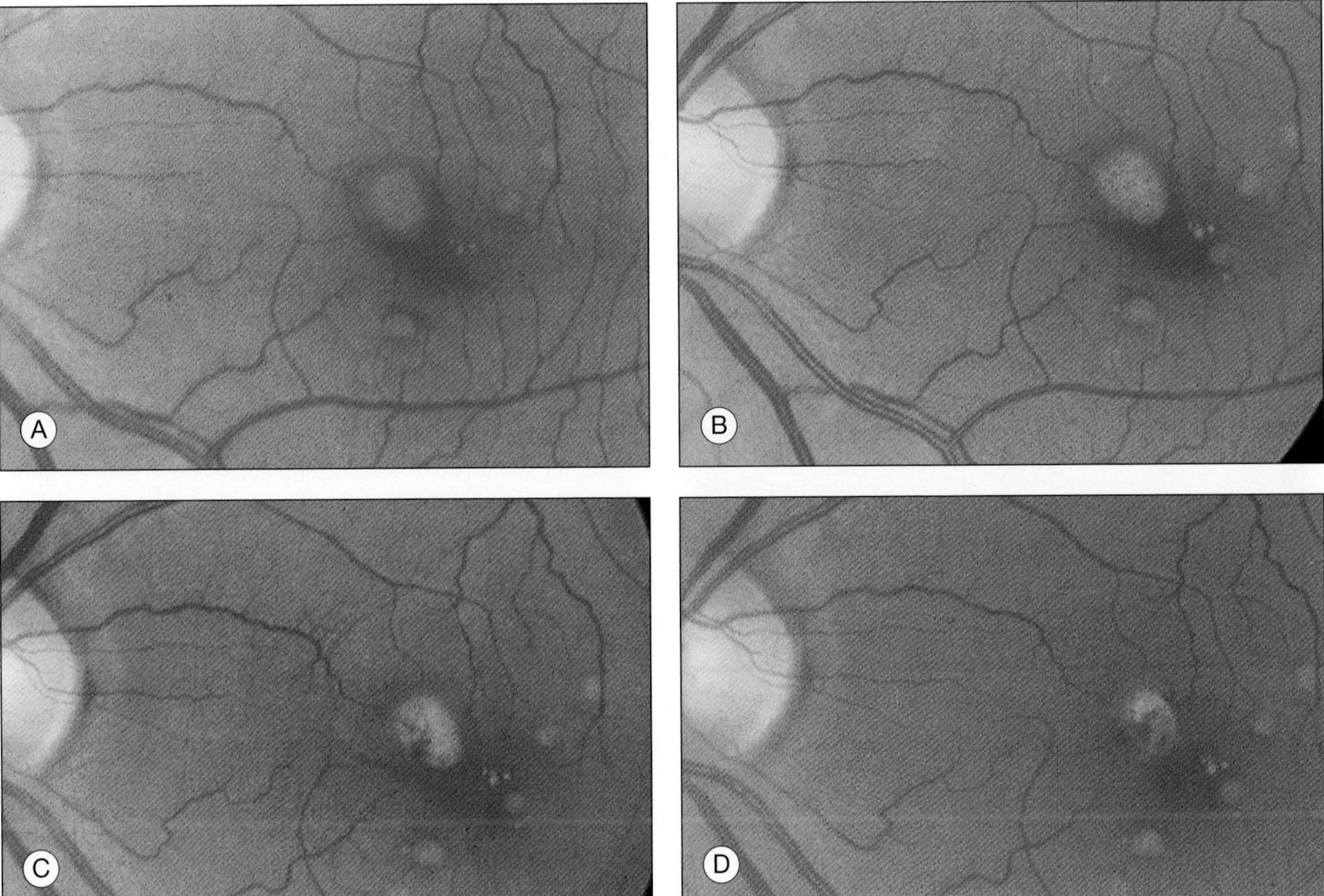

Fig. 65.18 Patient illustrating large pseudosoft druse with halo around base, apparently derived from a fused cluster of small, hard drusen. Photographs trace the regression of the druse over 9 years. The druse was located just above fixation, and vision remained unaffected. (A) At age 48, druse is surrounded by a red halo. (B) At age 52, the druse appears whiter, and pigment stippling is present over the surface. (C) At age 54, the halo fades as the druse becomes shallower. (D) At age 57, hyperpigmentation is preceding the formation of a patch of atrophy. The atrophy remains localized in younger persons in whom the retinal pigment epithelium between the drusen is normal. (Reproduced with permission from Sarks SH. Drusen patterns predisposing to geographic atrophy of the retinal pigment epithelium. Aust J Ophthalmol 1982;10:91–7.)

led to the designation semisolid.[102] Calcified particles may also be found and, as these deposits are commonly observed around an area of atrophy, they appear to be in the early stages of regression.

Soft, fluid (serous) drusen and drusenoid pigment epithelial detachments

Soft, confluent drusen larger than 500 μm, and even some over 250 μm, may have an accumulation of serous fluid if the lipoidal debris in Bruch's membrane has created a hydrophobic barrier[103] and interferes with the retinal pigment epithelial pump. This may be important in causing hard drusen to become soft and in fostering the enlargement and confluence of drusen.[49] As a result some larger drusen appear to have a fluid consistency, even appearing blister-like and being translucent on retroillumination.

Further confluence leads to larger soft drusen that resemble serous PEDs (Fig. 65.21), often retaining a scalloped outline representing the original drusen. This subset of serous PEDs was characterized as the "drusen form"[104] when they were noted to have different ophthalmoscopic and angiographic features, as well as better short-term vision prognosis. The term drusen or drusenoid[75] RPE detachments may arbitrarily be applied to drusen over 500 μm but often are used to describe those with an even larger diameter. Generally they remain less than one disc diameter in size. This evolution occurs at times on a background of small, hard drusen; Fig. 65.21 shows how the small drusen become incorporated into the larger fluid deposits. In the outer macula the brightly fluorescent small drusen remain discrete. In the inner macula they form clusters in which the individual drusen become progressively more difficult to distinguish. These now fill more slowly on the fluorescein angiogram but often show a few brightly fluorescent highlights around the edge of the deposits. Those drusen clusters closest to the fovea can become completely homogeneous during fluorescein angiography. Hyperpigmentation gradually develops over the surface, often in the form of a radiating pigment figure. With fluorescein angiography the drusenoid PEDs are shallowly elevated and manifest faint late fluorescence similar to the filling of the surrounding fluid drusen. The overlying hyperpigmentation creates hypofluorescent figures on the anterior surface of the PED.

Drusenoid PEDs are compatible with good visual acuity at presentation (20/40 or better), although they may be responsible for metamorphopsia. However, as overlying hyperpigmentation and hypopigmentation develop, the contents appear whiter and more inspissated, and visual acuity may begin to decline.

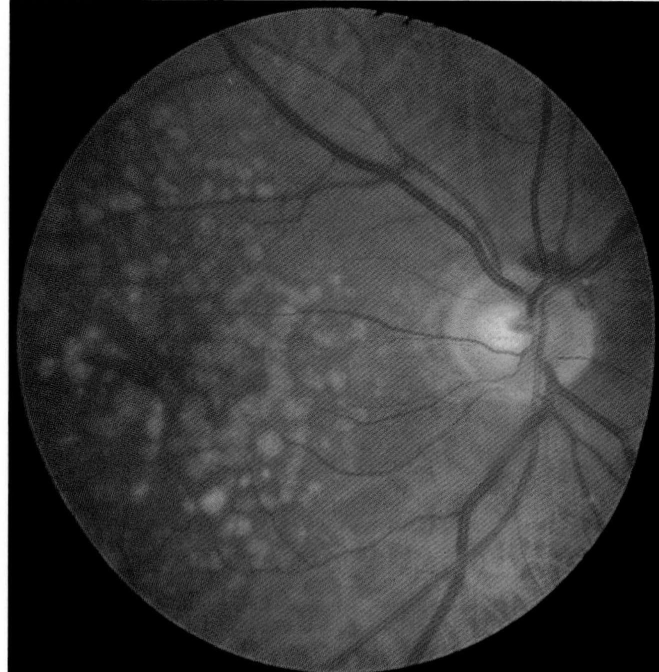

Fig. 65.19 Soft drusen of granular structure. Numerous soft, yellow drusen of solid appearance in the right eye of a 72-year-old man. Confluence of soft drusen results in a sinuous pattern. Patient died 3 years later, and corresponding histopathology (see Fig. 65.20) demonstrated a granular structure derived from broken down small, hard drusen. (Reproduced with permission from Sarks SH. Drusen and their relationship to senile macular degeneration. Aust J Ophthalmol 1980;8:117–30.)

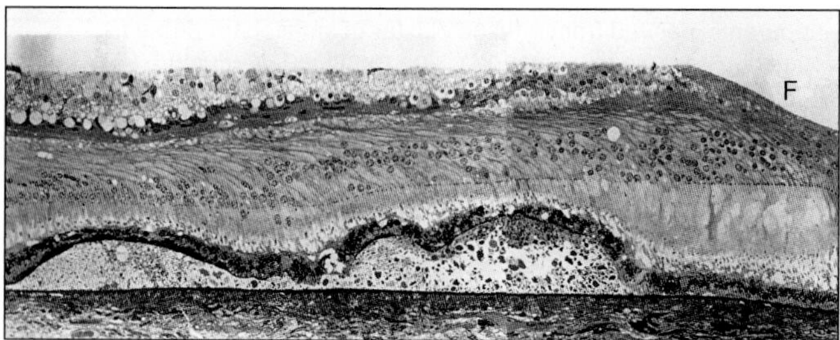

Fig. 65.20 Semithin section through edge of fovea (F) of eye shown in Fig. 65.19 demonstrates confluence of three soft drusen. Drusen have a granular structure, comprising variably sized globules of amorphous material, some membrane-bound. This material appeared to be derived from the breakdown of small hard drusen, several of which were still present around the edge of these drusen. Note that, as the contents break down, drusen tend to lose sharp margins and nodular surface elevations present in fused clusters (see Figs 65.12 and 65.13). The fellow eye demonstrated similar drusen, but many were regressing (methylene blue and basic fuchsin; ×115). (Reproduced with permission from Sarks JP, Sarks SH, Killingsworth MC. Evolution of soft drusen in age-related macular degeneration. Eye 1994;8: 269–83.)

Once heavy clumping has appeared, the drusenoid PED generally begins to collapse within a couple of years, and atrophy may rapidly evolve with greater consequences on visual acuity (Fig. 65.22).[80,104–106]

Within the AREDS, 288 eyes with drusenoid PEDS (in the absence of advanced AMD) were followed for a median of 8 years, among which 42% developed advanced AMD within 5 years.[107] About half of these events were central geographic atrophy and the other half neovascular AMD. Rates of progression to advanced AMD and rates of vision loss were higher in this group of participants than those with large drusen and pigmentary alterations. Those that did not develop advanced AMD still tended to show evidence of progression with development of calcification, pigmentary changes (typically hypopigmentation), and non-central GA. Five years after presentation of the drusenoid PED, visual acuity declined in those with incident-advanced AMD by a mean of 26 letters (~ 5 lines) and even by 8 letters among those without progression to advanced AMD.

Disappearance of drusen following prophylactic laser photocoagulation

Although longitudinal studies have shown that drusen may spontaneously develop and resolve, another indication of the fluid nature of drusenoid PEDs is the rapidity with which they resolve after photocoagulation. Drusenoid PEDs occur most commonly within the fovea and sometimes these flatten following gentle photocoagulation to their margin. Laser burns have been shown to cause a focal reduction in age-related lipid deposits in Bruch's membrane, which may alter the egress of fluid. Alternatively, a cellular mechanism may also be invoked, since laser induces inflammation with occasional cellular intrusions into the membrane.[108]

Based on these findings, as well as case series providing evidence of drusen resorption following photocoagulation, a number of trials evaluated photocoagulation in eyes with drusen to decrease progression to advanced AMD and vision loss. The most definitive assessment, the Complications of Age-Related Macular Degeneration Prevention Trial (CAPT), did not find that low-intensity laser treatment prevented vision loss among individuals with bilateral evidence of large drusen and vision of at least 20/40. A total of 1052 participants had 1 eye randomly assigned to grid photocoagulation as close as 1000 µm and as far as 2500 µm from the foveal center while the other eye was assigned to observation. About 20% of eyes in the treated and the observed group lost at least 3 lines of acuity by the 5-year follow-up examination.[108] The cumulative 5-year incidence of choroidal neovascularization was about 13% in each group; whereas each group had similar rates of geographic atrophy at roughly 7.5%.

Soft (membranous) drusen (localized accumulation of the basal linear deposit[22])

Soft membranous drusen often appear paler and shallower than the yellow granular drusen (Fig. 65.23). They are usually smaller than 250 µm, most commonly 63–175 µm. These drusen are common in intermediate or advanced AMD. Since they represent focal accentuations of a continuous layer of debris, their margins are usually indistinct and they readily become confluent. Histologically these drusen are pale-staining and faintly periodic acid–Schiff-positive, with a finely granular or ground-glass appearance; they may even appear optically empty. However, on electron microscopy they contain tightly packed membrane coils (Figs 65.24, 65.25). A small amount of amorphous material may be present within the coils, so their contents have also been described as vesicular and granular electron-dense, lipid-rich material.[22,75] This membranous debris is morphologically similar to that which forms basal mounds internal to the RPE basement membrane, and continuity between the mounds and drusen through the basement membrane can at times be observed (Fig. 65.25). Similar material has also been found in autosomal dominant drusen.[52]

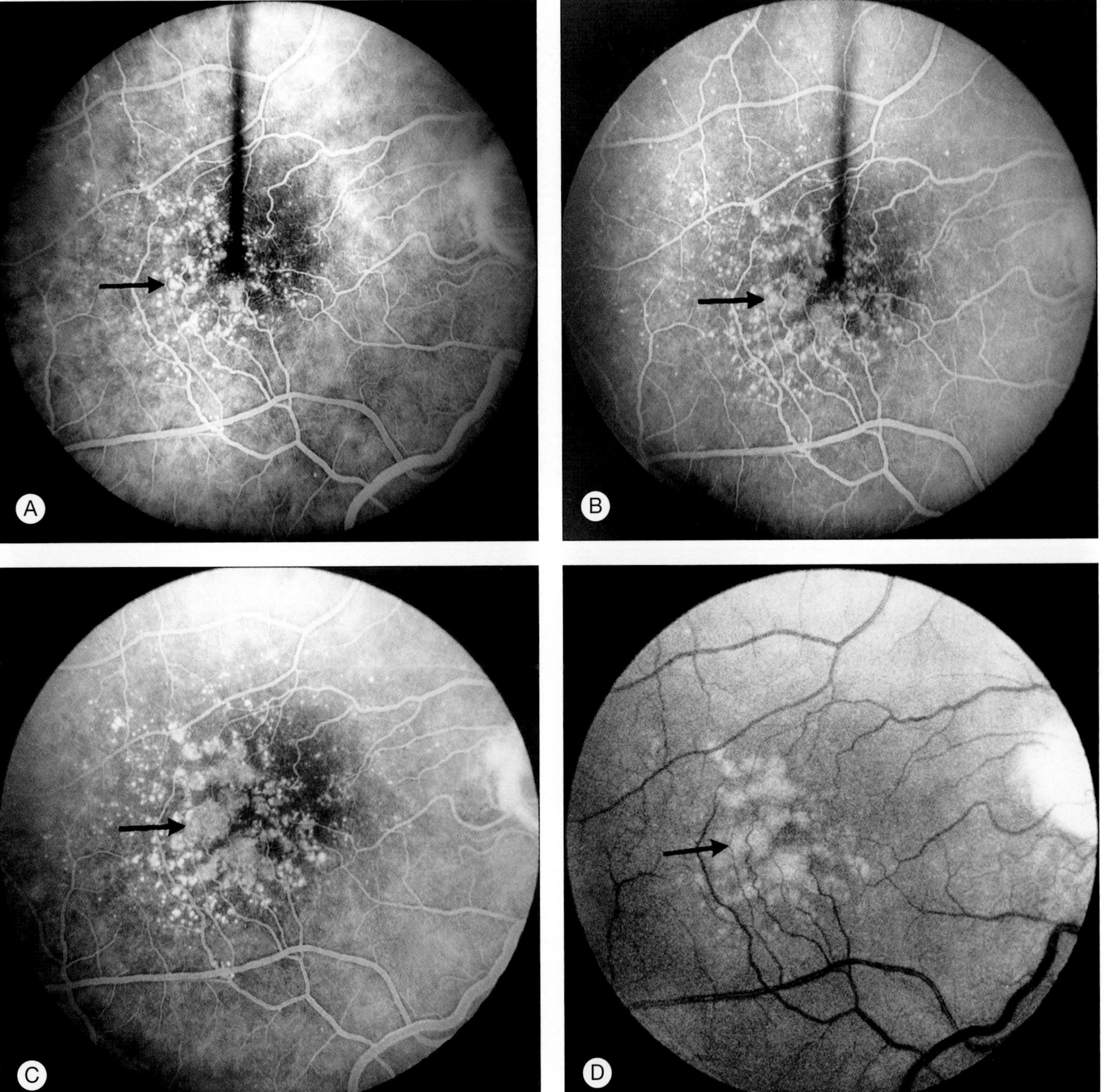

Fig. 65.21 Patient showing evolution of clusters of small, hard drusen into larger, soft, confluent drusen (arrows), presumably due to the addition of serous fluid. Fluorescein angiograms of the right eye of a man at age 55 (A), 58 (B), and 61 (C). The drusen farthest from the fovea remain discrete. In the inner macula they form clusters in which the individual drusen are more difficult to distinguish owing to confluence and breakdown. The more central clusters have become completely homogeneous on fluorescein angiography. (D) Red-free photograph at age 61 shows corresponding clinical picture. Homogenized clusters have a soft, yellow appearance. Visual acuity remained 20/20, although the patient had been aware of some deterioration, the other eye being amblyopic.

Membranous drusen have a high risk of CNV and are often found in advance of choroidal neovascular membranes in pathologic specimens, unlike granular drusen, which more often occur around areas of atrophy. They are significant because they are not simply a focal pathology but are part of a diffuse layer of debris external to the basement membrane that opens a cleavage plane for the spread of new vessels. The BLD over these drusen is usually the early type because membranous material declines as late BLD appears. Although these soft drusen develop de novo, small, hard drusen are commonly also present and then become incorporated into the membranous drusen; their amorphous contents break down (Fig. 65.26).

This debris coincides with a macrophage response in the choroid, and segments of thinning of Bruch's membrane may be found, with signs of activation in the adjacent choroidal capillaries.[82] This occurs preferentially beneath hard drusen, possibly

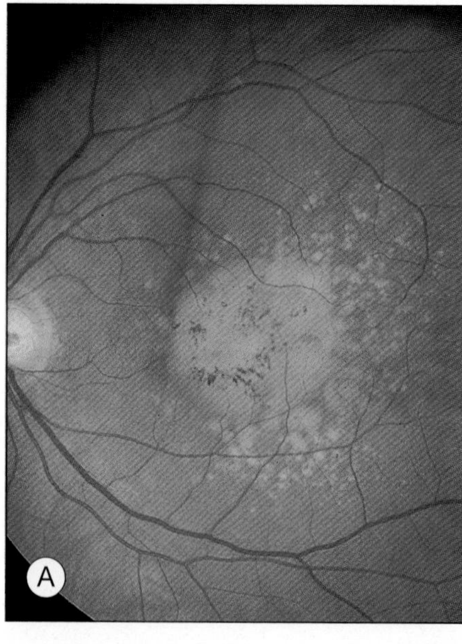

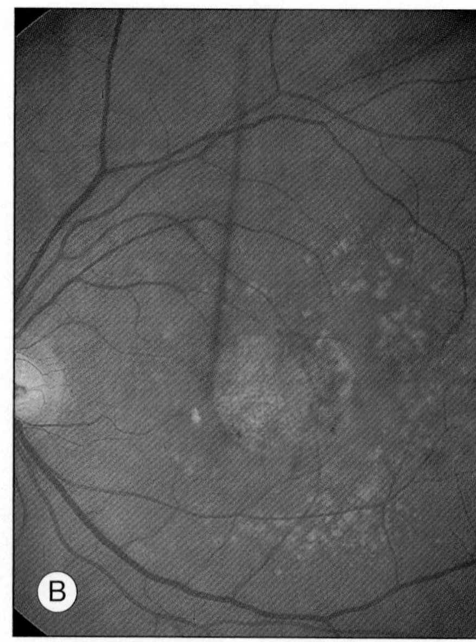

Fig. 65.22 Development of geographic atrophy after collapse of a pigment epithelial detachment. (A) Left eye of a 65-year-old woman with a PED that had been observed to develop from the confluence of soft, fluid drusen. It subsequently developed into an avascular, true PED that demonstrated bright hyperfluorescence. Hyperpigmentation developed over the surface (vision 20/50). (B) Three years later the PED had collapsed, leaving an area of geographic atrophy abutting on fixation (vision 20/100).

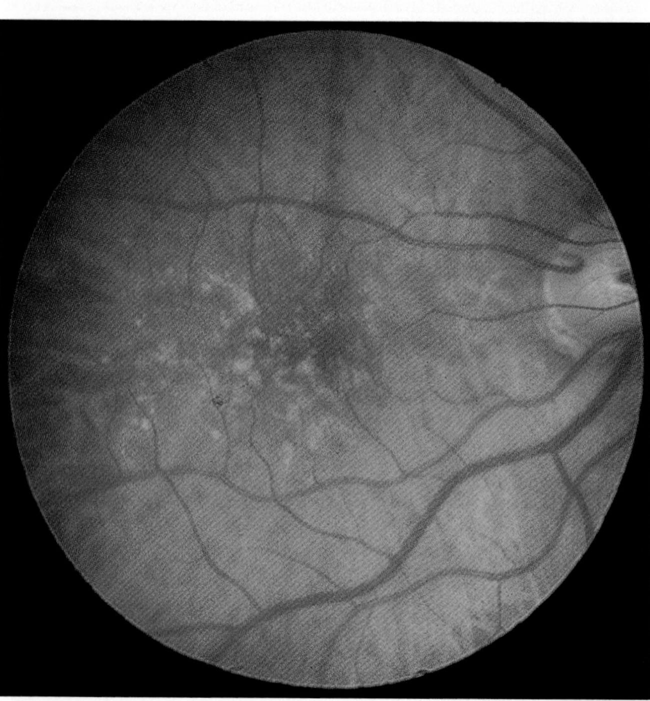

Fig. 65.23 Soft, indistinct drusen composed of membranous debris. The right eye of a 71-year-old man shows small, hard drusen and medium-sized soft drusen of smudgy appearance. This eye developed a hemorrhagic disciform lesion shortly before the patient died at age 75. The left eye had similar drusen and also proved to contain an early active neovascular membrane. The morphology of the drusen in the left eye is illustrated in Figs. 65.24–65.26. (Reproduced with permission from Sarks JP, Sarks SH, Killingsworth MC. Evolution of soft drusen in age-related macular degeneration. Eye 1994;8:269–83.)

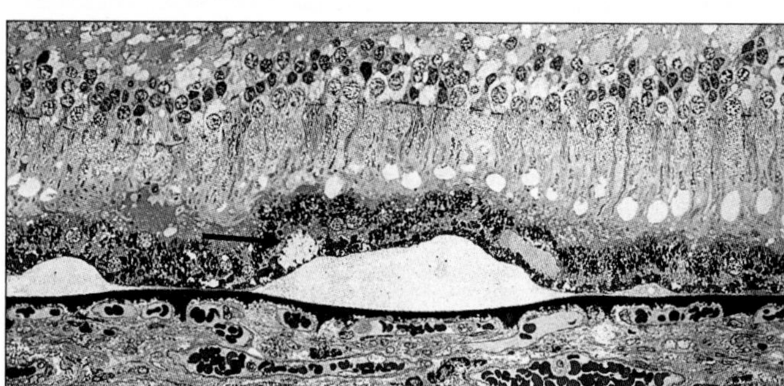

Fig. 65.24 Semithin section showing medium-sized soft drusen from the left eye of the patient illustrated in Fig. 65.23. Since these deposits are focal accentuations of a continuous layer of debris, their margins are ill defined and they readily become confluent. It is into this plane that choroidal new vessels grow; a neovascular membrane was present nearby. Drusen appear empty or very finely granular at this magnification. The arrow points to a small basal mound of similar appearance, lying above the druse. Higher magnification is shown in Fig. 65.25 (methylene blue and basic fuchsin; ×240). (Reproduced with permission from Sarks JP, Sarks SH, Killingsworth MC. Evolution of soft drusen in age-related macular degeneration. Eye 1994;8:269–83.)

because the RPE remains anchored to these for a time, while becoming increasingly separated from Bruch's membrane elsewhere by the membranous debris. An ischemic stimulus induced in the outer retina by this separation may cause the RPE to release diffusible angiogenic factors that would reach the choroid in greatest concentration where the RPE remains attached to Bruch's membrane (Fig. 65.26).

Reticular pseudodrusen,[109] reticular drusen,[14,20] subretinal drusenoid deposits[110,111]

These drusen are characterized by a yellowish interlacing network about 250 μm in diameter[20] that resembles soft confluent drusen. These first appear in the superior outer macula (Fig. 65.27) and the network may slowly extend into other quadrants and also peripherally. The transition with normal retina often appears to be marked by a scalloped line breaking up into islands. The pattern does not fluoresce on fluorescein angiography, being best observed in red-free light (blue channel color light) or the near infrared light of the scanning laser ophthalmoscope. Despite the clinical resemblance to soft confluent drusen, SD-OCT correlation shows deposits of material above (rather than below) the RPE in the subretinal space.[110] The material can be configured as relatively flat aggregates to conical mounds that

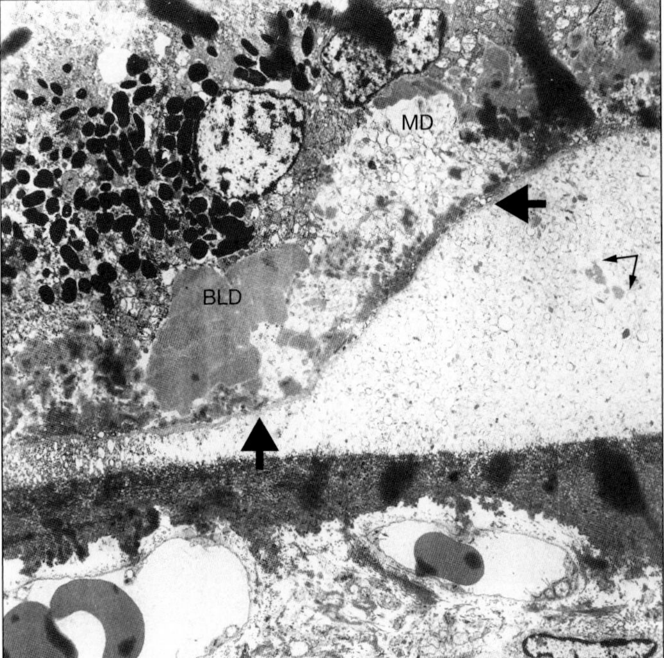

Fig. 65.25 Electron micrograph corresponding to the area indicated in Fig. 65.24 shows formation of a soft druse made up of coiled lipid membranes lying external to the basement membrane of the retinal pigment epithelium (arrows). The membranes appear first at the base of the RPE, where they may form basal mounds (MD). At the site of the right-hand arrow, some membranes can be seen within the basement membrane of the RPE and appear to be entering the soft druse from the basal mound. Some of the coils appear empty, and others contain amorphous material (double arrow). These drusen are specific for age-related macular degeneration, since they are only found after membranous debris develops. BLD, Basal laminar deposit (×2210). (Reproduced with permission from Sarks JP, Sarks SH, Killingsworth MC. Evolution of soft drusen in age-related macular degeneration. Eye 1994;8:269–83.)

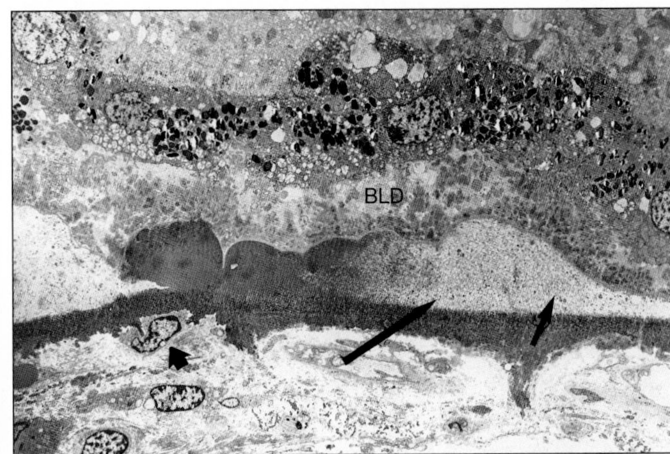

Fig. 65.26 Electron micrograph of the same eye in Figs 65.23–65.25 shows a cluster of subclinical, small, hard drusen apparently becoming eroded by membranous debris and breaking down into small membrane-bound particles (central arrow). At right (shorter arrow), druse consists of more characteristic membranous debris. This scenario suggests that small, hard drusen become incorporated into soft drusen once membranous debris develops. Early-type basal laminar deposit (BLD) lies over drusen. Note that the BLD and retinal pigment epithelium remain anchored at the site of hard drusen but are separated from Bruch's membrane on either side by soft drusen. This may permit a retinal stimulus to evoke the maximum cellular response in the choroid directly beneath these drusen. Small arrow at left points to macrophage-type cell adjacent to outer surface of Bruch's membrane, where retina remains attached (×1260). (Courtesy of M.C. Killingsworth.)

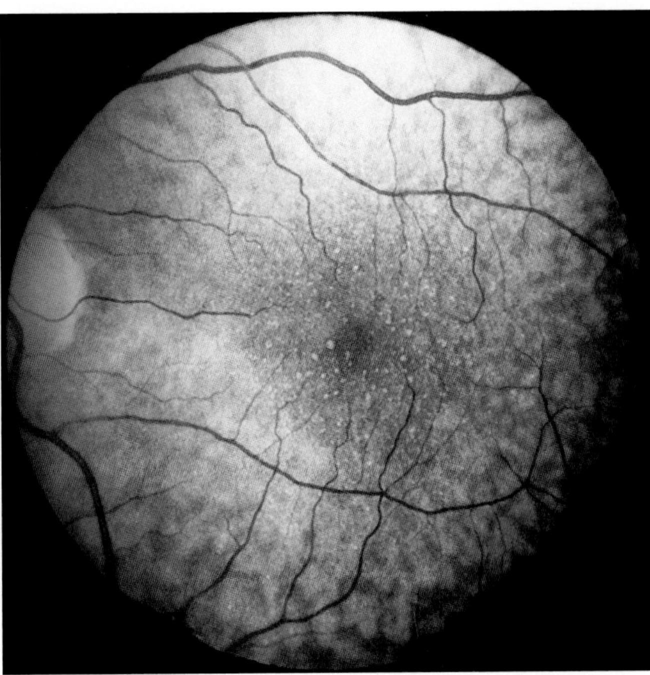

Fig. 65.27 Reticular pseudodrusen, a yellowish, lobular pattern in the outer macular region, in a 65-year-old woman with a disciform scar in the other eye. Pseudodrusen are not visible on fluorescein angiography and are best observed with red-free light. Delayed choroidal perfusion was present, and the appearance presumably results from choroidal ischemia. Vision was 20/30, and small, soft, distinct drusen are scattered over the fovea. This picture suggests a very high risk of choroidal neovascularization.

extend to the region between the inner and outer photoreceptor segments, and appears to be far more extensive when visualized with OCT as compared to color photographs.[111] Histologically, the composition of these subretinal deposits has been similar to that of soft drusen with membranous debris, cholesterol, cholesterol esters, and complement.[112] Although eyes with soft drusen may also contain reticular drusen, each "drusen" type may exert an independent risk for late AMD progression, with the magnitude of risk being far greater for soft drusen than reticular drusen.[111,113]

Regressing (fading) drusen (localized detachment of the basal laminar deposit within an area of retinal pigment epithelium and photoreceptor atrophy[22])

All drusen types may in time disappear,[4,16,101] but this does not necessarily signify a return to a more normal state, since areas of drusen may be replaced by more severe manifestations of AMD. A proportion of eyes show changes in the appearance of the macula that might be considered "improved" but whether this is associated with a decreased risk of the advanced stage of AMD remains to be seen. It is doubtful that the RPE remains unaffected, and fluorescein angiography may show increased transmission of fluorescence where drusen have faded.

Drusen begin to regress when the overlying RPE fails, often assuming a whiter and harder appearance (see Fig. 65.18). It has been suggested that the drusen have reverted to a previous type,[4] but hardening of the drusen in this situation is caused by inspissation of the contents and is associated with more

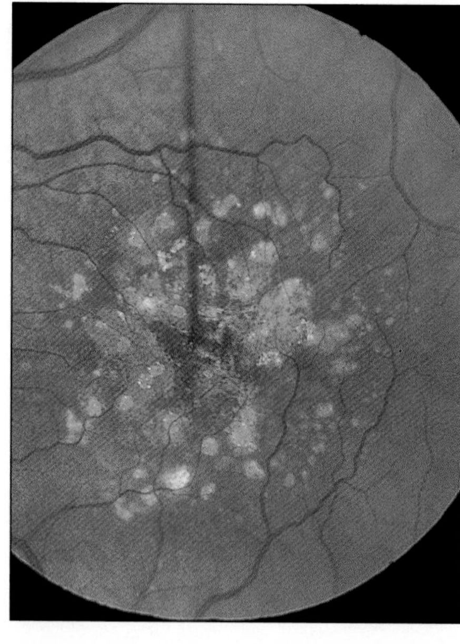
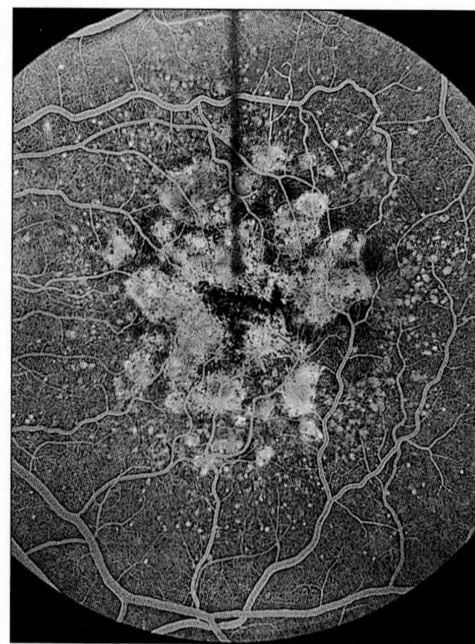

Fig. 65.28 Regressing drusen, showing multifocal pattern of atrophy, in a patient 69 years of age. The separate patches of atrophy have spread into the surrounding retina, and many have coalesced to produce the geographic pattern. The drusen within these areas have disappeared, and only calcified particles remain. Vision was 20/40, and although still capable of fixing on the small central island of retina, the patient was unable to read along a line.

advanced degeneration of the RPE, with hyperpigmentation and hypopigmentation often developing over the surface of the druse. Later the margins become irregular and foci of calcification may appear, especially after the age of 60 years. Ultimately the drusen fade, leaving multifocal patches of RPE atrophy that reflect their original distribution and often spare fixation (Fig. 65.28). Glistening calcium deposits may remain in these atrophic areas for many years.

Histopathologically, both RPE and photoreceptors overlying regressing drusen disappear, leaving a thick layer of late-type amorphous BLD over the apex (Fig. 65.29). Regressing drusen therefore not only have a reduced input of membranous debris due to loss of overlying RPE, but also show evidence of its removal by macrophages. Material not removed becomes invaded by glial cells or collagen fibers or undergoes dystrophic calcification. Regression of soft drusen therefore closes the cleavage plane created by membranous debris and, if CNV occurs, it remains localized (Fig. 65.2).

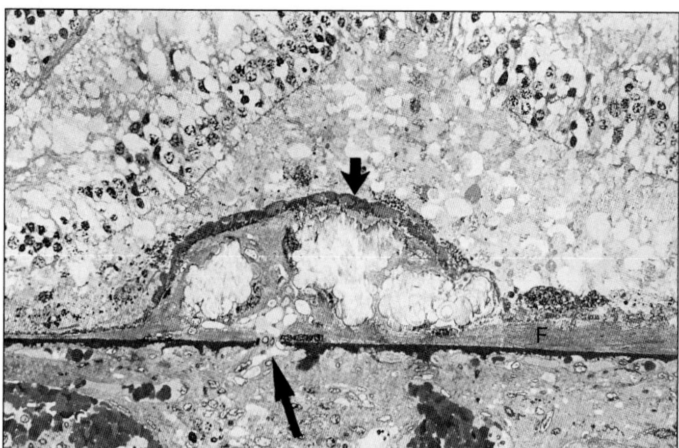

Fig. 65.29 Example of regressing druse in an area of geographic atrophy. The druse is covered by late, amorphous basal laminar deposit (short arrow) and has dystrophic calcification. A clinically unsuspected small vessel passes through a gap in Bruch's membrane beneath the druse (long arrow), but the surrounding atrophy has inhibited its further spread. A layer of fibrous tissue (F) lies on Bruch's membrane, with fibroblasts replacing macrophages as new vessels become less active (methylene blue and basic fuchsin; ×240). (Reproduced with permission from Sarks JP, Sarks SH, Killingsworth M. Evolution of geographic atrophy of the retinal pigment epithelium. Eye 1988;2:552–77.)

Outcome of drusen

The cumulative incidence of advanced AMD in individuals with bilateral drusen has been reported in several prospective studies. Among 126 patients attending an ophthalmology clinic in England the 3-year cumulative incidence of neovascular AMD was 14%; whereas the incidence of GA was 5%.[106] Two significant risk factors for progression to these new lesions were the presence of confluent drusen or focal hyperpigmentation within 1600 µm of the center of the fovea. In the Beaver Dam study 197 persons had signs of "early ARM" in both eyes at baseline, among which 7% progressed to neovascular AMD and 5% to GA within 5 years.[4]

In patients who have developed CNV in the first eye, in the fellow eye at risk the presence of five or more drusen, or one or more large drusen, were two factors associated independently with an increased risk of developing CNV in the second eye within 5 years.[86] Another prospective study followed[103] patients with unilateral neovascular AMD and drusen only in the fellow eye for up to 9 years. Yearly incidence rates for the development of CNV or geographic atrophy in the fellow were between 5% and 14%. The risk of CNV peaked at 4 years and decreased thereafter. Longer follow-up was associated with a slightly increased incidence of geographic atrophy. The risk of CNV in patients with AMD was heralded by an increase in the number, size, and confluence of drusen (in decreasing order of significance). This risk eventually declines and is followed by later increased risk of geographic atrophy.[114]

Most recently, the AREDS Group[2,13] reported that the risk of progressing to the advanced stage of AMD within 5 years was extremely low for individuals with early AMD (about 1%), approximately 6% for individuals with intermediate AMD in only 1 eye, approximately 25% for individuals with intermediate AMD in both eyes, and approximately 43% for the second eye of individuals who already have advanced AMD in their first eye (Fig. 65.30A). Patients with early or intermediate AMD, or those who already have lost vision in their first eye from advanced AMD often want an assessment of their risk of progression at the time of their clinical examination. As discussed earlier, the AREDS group developed a simple grading scale that lends itself to quantifying patient risk, even in a busy clinical practice. Each eye of a person is scored individually, assigning one point for each risk factor present (large drusen, pigmentary abnormalities). A cumulative person score ranging from 0 to 4 is calculated. If an eye has either form of advanced AMD then that eye receives a score of 2 and the person score would range from 2 to 4. Individuals who do not have large drusen in either eye but manifest bilateral medium drusen receive 1 point and earn additional points if pigmentary abnormalities are present. Each total score has been associated with an escalating estimated 5-year risk that ranges from 0.5% to 50% that at least 1 eye will progress to advanced AMD.[88]

Histochemistry

Drusen contain neutral fats and phospholipids,[115] as well as glycoconjugates containing specific carbohydrate residues. The latter were found in all classes of drusen, suggesting that both hard and soft drusen may have a similar origin.[116] Many hard and soft drusen contain specific cores with a carbohydrate-rich composition confined to distinct domains. These cores are positioned centrally within the drusen and are typically juxtapositioned to Bruch's membrane. Some researchers have suggested that they may represent an early nucleation site around which other drusen-associated molecules including lipid are subsequently deposited.[83,117]

Other distinct components common to all phenotypes of hard and soft drusen include apolipoprotein E, immunoglobulins, factor X, amyloid P component, complement C5 and C5b-9 terminal complexes, fibrinogen, and thrombospondin.[116] Vitronectin is a major constituent of both hard and soft drusen, and vitronectin mRNA is expressed locally in the RPE, suggesting that vitronectin may participate in the pathogenesis of AMD.[118] A number of these drusen-associated constituents are participants in humoral and cellular immunity, including a number of acute-phase reactants, plasma proteins that rapidly elevate in response to inflammatory stimuli.

The membranous debris appears to bleb from the surface of the RPE and pass through the RPE basement membrane to form

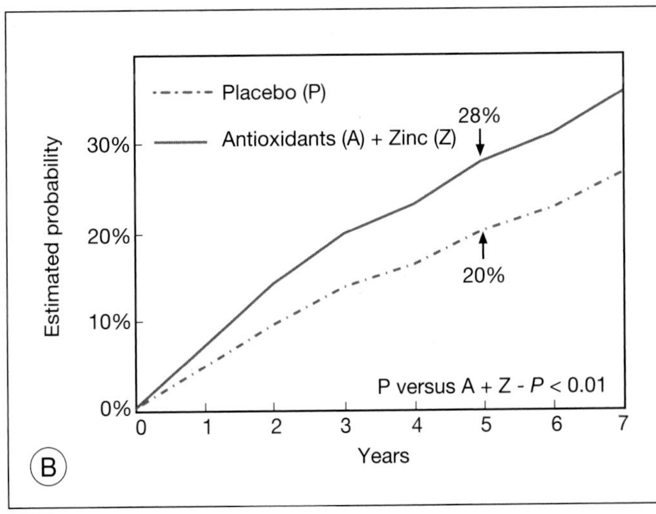

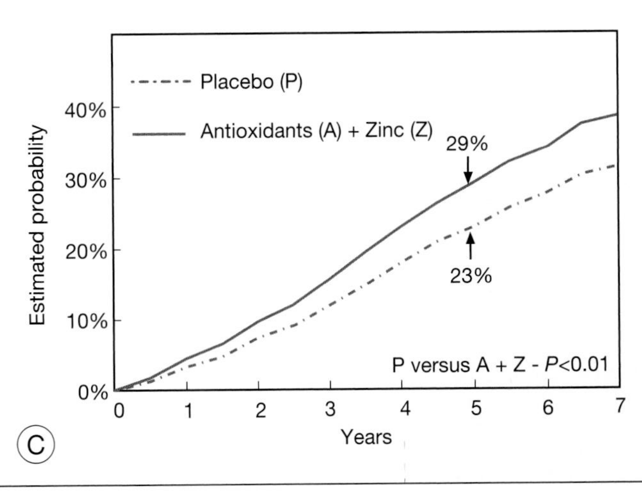

Fig. 65.30 Results of the Age-Related Eye Disease Study (AREDS) trial. Risk of progressing to advanced age-related macular degeneration (AMD) within 5 years for patients with early AMD and intermediate AMD and unilateral advanced AMD (B). The effect of treatment with antioxidants and zinc for eyes with intermediate AMD or unilateral advanced AMD is also shown in (B). (C) Effect of antioxidants and zinc on vision loss in patients with intermediate or monocular advanced AMD within 5 years.

soft drusen specific for intermediate or advanced AMD. Ultrastructurally, this material resembles the extracellular lipid found in developing atheromatous plaque.[69,70] The debris probably arises indirectly at least from peroxidized lipid[63] derived from the photoreceptor outer segments, since membranous debris disappears with loss of photoreceptors.

The outer segments of the photoreceptors are rich in polyunsaturated fatty acids and subject to light and oxygen damage, promoting free radical production. This, combined with environmental factors (e.g., smoking) and inherited risk factors, may promote RPE damage and membrane production.

INCIPIENT ATROPHY (NONGEOGRAPHIC ATROPHY[18])

Incipient atrophy is a stage that may immediately precede geographic atrophy. Although not as sharply demarcated as actual geographic atrophy, areas of RPE thinning or depigmentation (incipient atrophy) can nevertheless be recognized. The affected retina appears pinker than the normal fundus background, and any drusen present appear whiter and harder before fading. Fluorescein angiography demonstrates diffuse hyperfluorescence, not as bright as an area of geographic atrophy (see Fig. 65.31), and it is commonly associated with a reticular pattern of hyperpigmentation (Fig. 65.32) inducing hypofluorescence on angiography. The areas of associated hyperpigmentation may be more easily delineated on autofluorescence as areas lacking fundus autofluorescence (FAF) due to absorption of the exciting light by melanin granules. Alternatively, the associated hyperpigmentation may appear as an increase in FAF if melanolipofuscin has accumulated in the pigmented sites.[119] The areas of hypopigmentation generally are associated with decreased FAF, suggesting the absence of RPE cells or degenerated RPE cells with reduced lipofuscin content.

Pathology

It has been shown that the character of the material liberated by the RPE reflects the stage of degeneration. The debris made up of coiled membranes (basal linear deposit) appears when the cells are also elaborating the early form of BLD. As degeneration develops, there is initially a marked increase in the quantity of both these diffuse deposits. However, with more advanced fallout of photoreceptors, the amount of membranous debris produced declines, and both the basal mounds internal to the basement membrane and the soft drusen fade, and the BLD is now the late amorphous type. Multinucleated giant cells and mononuclear inflammatory cells are observed lying on Bruch's membrane at the margin of areas of geographic atrophy and may play a role in clearing the debris from necrotic cells at this site.[119] Therefore, as the late type of BLD increases, the quantity of membranous debris is reduced, which is particularly noticeable at the edge of an area of atrophy (see Fig. 65.11).

CHOROIDAL PERFUSION IN AGE-RELATED MACULAR DEGENERATION

The retina has the highest oxygen uptake in the body, most of which is provided by the choroid, but as AMD advances, the cross-sectional area of the choriocapillary bed progressively decreases. Histologic measurements made in eyes with (1) continuous BLD, (2) geographic atrophy, and (3) disciform scarring showed that the choriocapillary density, defined as the combined length of patent capillary lumina parallel to Bruch's membrane, was respectively 63%, 54%, and 43% of normal. The corresponding figures for the choriocapillary diameter measured perpendicular to Bruch's membrane were 81%, 73%, and 75% of normal.[50] Laboratory studies have suggested that decreased foveolar choroidal blood flow is associated with AMD, in particular increased drusen extent, and that abnormal choroidal circulatory measurements may predict risk of progression of the disease.[120] Not surprisingly, therefore, one hypothesis of the pathogenesis of AMD relates to ischemia. The macula is the watershed zone where branches of the short posterior ciliary arteries meet, and an area where multiple watershed zones meet is an area of poor vascularity and therefore most vulnerable to ischemic disorders. Moreover, the distribution of diffuse deposits beneath the RPE is often closely related to regions of choroidal capillary dropout.[121]

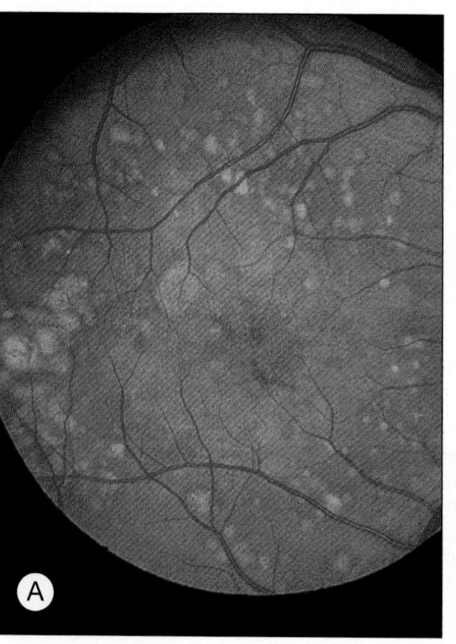

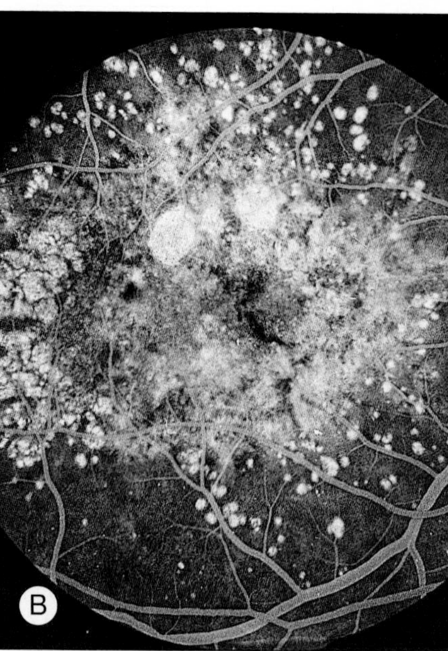

Fig. 65.31 Example of geographic atrophy developing in a 47-year-old man due to excessive numbers of drusen (A). Fluorescein angiogram (B) revealed numerous, mostly small, hard drusen, although many aggregated into clusters. Drusen are fading centrally in an area of incipient atrophy of the retinal pigment epithelium, which appears as a pinker area of the fundus, showing diffuse hyperfluorescence. Geographic atrophy commences as rounded, more circumscribed, brighter window defects within the incipient atrophy. Vision was still 20/15.

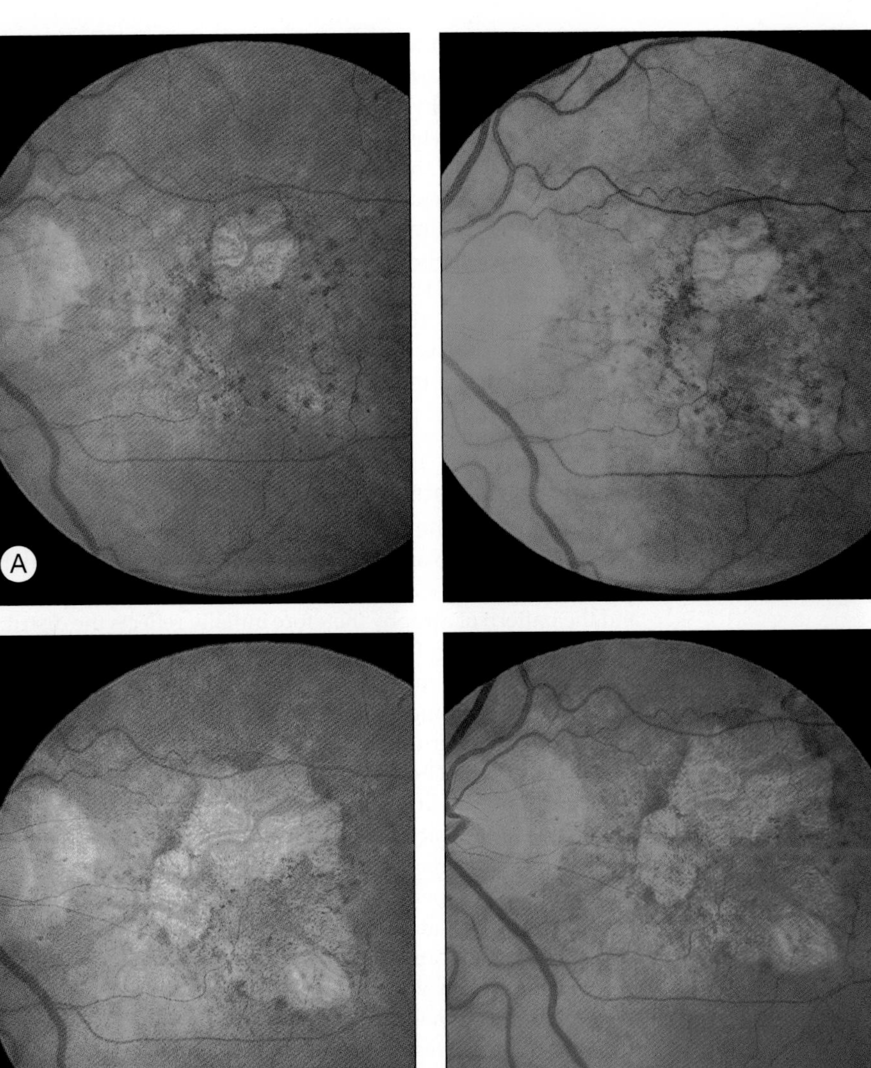

Fig. 65.32 An eye illustrating the spread of geographic atrophy unrelated to drusen. (A) At age 68, atrophy was developing in relation to a ring of incipient atrophy, showing reticular pigmentation, located around the perimeter of the fovea. (B) One year later atrophy was progressing around the ring, but vision was still 20/30.

Relationship to age-related macular degeneration

Choroidal perfusion abnormalities have been found in patients with the intermediate and advanced forms of AMD and interpreted as a clinical sign for diffuse aging changes in Bruch's membrane,[122] especially in eyes with soft drusen.[123] A prolonged choroidal filling time, as evidenced by patchy and slow filling of the choroid in the early phase of fluorescein angiography, was found in 40% of eyes with AMD, and this was corroborated by indocyanine green angiography, by means of which a distinct area of reduced fluorescence of the choriocapillaris was noted in the middle phase in 44% of eyes.[124] A prolonged choroidal filling phase may therefore be a marker for loss of the choriocapillaris and the presence of diffuse deposits.

It was first reasoned,[125] and then confirmed,[126] that the RPE modulates the choroidal vasculature by secreting a diffusible growth factor. Since intermediate AMD is associated with a continuous layer of debris internal to Bruch's membrane that may present a barrier to metabolic exchange between the RPE and the choriocapillaris, and since the RPE cells are degenerate, less growth factor would be expected to reach the choriocapillaris. This may be the reason why the choriocapillaris is initially slow to fill, then loses its endothelial fenestrations and ultimately atrophies. Hence the narrowing of the choriocapillaris, rather than causing the disease, may represent a disuse atrophy secondary to degeneration of the RPE. The alternative view, that impaired choroidal perfusion is responsible for dysfunction of the RPE, is supported by the use of color Doppler imaging, which demonstrated increased pulsatility and decreased velocity in the short posterior ciliary arteries. This suggested greater scleral rigidity in AMD, which increases the resistance of the choroid to the flow of blood.[127]

Functional effects

In patients with AMD and delayed choroidal perfusion on fluorescein angiography, discrete areas of scotopic threshold elevation can be recorded that correspond to regions of choroidal perfusion abnormality.[128] It is interesting that these patients reported easy fatigability when doing close work,[128] the need for increased light intensity to read, fading of vision and slow recovery of vision after exposure to bright light,[128,129] and a central scotoma noticeable in the dark.[129] Delayed choroidal perfusion has also been linked to a prolonged foveal cone electroretinogram implicit time.[130] Since the diffuse deposits, especially the late amorphous BLD, are associated with some loss of RPE and photoreceptors, these deposits may account for the functional disturbances, as well as the perfusion abnormality.[129]

Prognostic value

Eyes with prolonged choroidal filling have been found to be at greater risk of visual loss, compared with eyes with normal choroidal filling. Whereas the proportion of eyes that develop CNV is the same in the two groups, the difference is caused by a higher incidence of geographic atrophy in the eyes with prolonged choroidal filling.[131] In eyes with drusen, a reduced retinal sensitivity may similarly predict the development of advanced AMD, especially drusenoid PEDs,[132] which may be followed by geographic atrophy.

A prolonged choroidal filling phase was also found to be associated with more evidence of atrophy of the RPE in the fellow eye[124] and, together with reduced foveal sensitivity, may therefore be a predictor that geographic atrophy will develop. Areas of incipient atrophy around a region of geographic atrophy, a region where the late form of the BLD is maximally developed with an associated fallout of RPE and photoreceptors, would also be expected to have reduced retinal sensitivity under dark-adapted conditions, so in addition it may be possible to predict the rate and spread of geographic atrophy.[133]

GEOGRAPHIC ATROPHY

Geographic atrophy is the end-result of the non-neovascular form of AMD and is currently defined[11] as any sharply delineated round or oval area of hypopigmentation or depigmentation or apparent absence of the RPE, in which choroidal vessels are more visible than in surrounding areas and which must be at least 175 μm in diameter (see Fig. 65.2, circle C2). Other wider dimensions have been proposed, although most studies specify dimensions between 175 μm and 350 μm as an area to reliably be considered geographic atrophy. It should be noted that for epidemiologic purposes an eye that shows any evidence of CNV in the setting of atrophy is classified as neovascular AMD, even if atrophy predominates. This stems from the difficulty inherent in determining the pathologic sequence that led to the development of the atrophic areas.

Evolution

Drusen-unrelated atrophy

This is an extension of AMD as considered thus far. Stippling of the RPE and small drusen often coexist, but atrophy does not begin in relation to individual drusen. Instead, the atrophy often begins around the perimeter of the fovea in a band of microreticular hyperpigmentation[80,134] (Fig. 65.32), although this is not always the case (see Figs 65.3 and 65.6).

Spread continues into retina affected by incipient atrophy and is more rapid when the ring of pigment clumps is pronounced. It tends to expand in a horseshoe-like fashion around the central fovea or develops simultaneously in several areas around the foveal perimeter.[80,134–137] The nasal or temporal side of the ring is usually the last part to close, completing the bull's-eye that may spare fixation for several years.

The reason atrophy tends to skirt fixation may be determined by the manner in which lipofuscin accumulates at the posterior pole. This parallels the distribution of rods in the human retina and reflects the greater vulnerability to fallout of rods than cones.[34] In the central rod-free area the lipofuscin content in the pigment epithelium is lower;[138] a sharp increase occurs on the foveal slope.[35] This sparing of the central fovea may also be attributable to the distribution of macular pigment. In humans this consists of two major carotenoids, lutein and zeaxanthin, which are thought to function as antioxidants and as blue-light filters, to potentially protect the macula from phototoxic damage.[138,139]

Drusen-related atrophy

Most cases of geographic atrophy occur in eyes with prominent drusen and develop as the drusen regress.[7,74] Degeneration of the RPE is usually more advanced immediately anterior to drusen, and the pattern of atrophy therefore initially reflects the distribution of the drusen. In younger patients such foci of atrophy remain discrete for many years (see Fig. 65.18), but when AMD affects the intervening RPE, the patches enlarge and coalesce in an irregular manner (Fig. 65.28).

Within the AREDS, 95 eyes monitored prospectively developed areas of GA at least 4 years into the trial. In each eye, drusen were found at the site of later development of GA; in fact, drusen >125 μm preceded GA in 96% of these eyes, confluent drusen in 94%, hyperpigmentation in 96%, drusen >250 μm in 83%, hypopigmentation in 82%, and refractile deposits presumed to be calcification in 23%.[140] The time from lesion appearance to onset of GA varied by lesion type, ranging from 6 years for confluent drusen to 2.5 years for hypopigmentation or refractile deposits. Progression from drusen to hyperpigmentation to regression of drusen to hypopigmentation was the most common sequence of these manifestations.

This pattern of evolution similarly tends to be more advanced around the perimeter of the fovea and spreads into the center. At the time of presentation single or multifocal lobules of atrophy may be present, and foveal involvement can be a presenting feature. In some cases the only evidence that atrophy evolved in a multifocal distribution in relation to drusen may be some scattered calcified deposits and a few small outlying islands of atrophy. In those younger patients with widespread drusen, there is an initial diffuse pigmentary disturbance (nongeographic atrophy), within which focal patches of geographic atrophy then develop (see Fig. 65.31).

Following pigment epithelial detachments

Geographic atrophy may follow collapse of an RPE detachment (see Fig. 65.22), especially those drusenoid RPE detachments formed by the confluence of large soft confluent drusen.[104,107] Vision may be only mildly compromised for as long as the RPE detachment is intact. Ultimately the RPE that lies on the anterior border of the drusenoid detachment may fail, leading to loss of vision and/or a scotoma, flattening of the detachment, and a rapidly developing area of atrophy. If an RPE detachment is complicated by a rip, the resulting retraction of the pigment epithelium leaves a sharply demarcated area of denuded RPE in which there is increased visualization of the choroidal vessels. Such an area may mimic an area of geographic atrophy. However, if the RPE is recent, two features are present to help differentiate the area as a rip: marked subretinal and intraretinal fluid overlying the area, and intense early fluorescence on a fluorescein angiogram.

Pathology

The changes causing an area of atrophy to expand are best studied at the junctional zone (see Fig. 65.11), where in vivo studies have demonstrated increased lipofuscin-induced autofluorescence.[64] Here the lipofuscin content of the RPE is maximal, presumably the result of both autophagy and outer-segment phagocytosis, and engulfment of discarded RPE and their photoreceptor cells. The few surviving photoreceptors comprise grossly abnormal cones with widened inner segments and absent outer segments, with no evidence of phagocytosis. The photoreceptors and the RPE then disappear together.

The heaping up of necrotic RPE cells as they are shed into the subretinal space accounts for the hyperpigmented edge commonly noted clinically around an area of atrophy. These pigment-laden cells have been referred to as macrophages, but certain features point to their pigment epithelial origin. Some have a few distorted apical villi or remain associated with basal laminar material; they may contain abundant smooth endoplasmic reticulum, and they occasionally demonstrate cell junctions with the underlying pigment epithelial cells. However, although the RPE seems capable of phagocytosing the debris released as a result of the normal cell deletion that occurs with age, an excessive amount of debris may attract macrophages and giant cells.

Within the area of atrophy itself there is absence of photoreceptors, RPE, and choriocapillaris; the loss of RPE precedes the loss of the choroidal capillaries. An occasional surviving whorl of persisting photoreceptors may be observed converging on a group of degenerating pigment cells, but only if there are some surviving choroidal capillaries. The outer nuclear layer disappears, causing the outer plexiform layer to rest directly on the BLD. The outer plexiform layer is thinned and vacuolated, but the inner nuclear layer is less affected.

Once there is loss of RPE and photoreceptors, the membranous material (basal linear deposit) disappears, but the BLD, particularly the late amorphous form, can be traced throughout the area of atrophy for a long time. Obliteration of the choriocapillaris is followed by erosion of the intercapillary pillars of Bruch's membrane, and in long-standing cases the membrane becomes thinner. Fibroblasts and macrophage processes are found in contact with the outer surface of the membrane, commonly splitting off fragments or even passing through small breaks.

Choroidal atrophy

In long-standing geographic atrophy, there are fewer large choroidal vessels, and the exposed choroidal arteries may display white sheathing of their walls or even appear bloodless. This picture was formerly called senile choroidal sclerosis, but on histologic examination the white fibrotic appearance does not result from sclerosis; the majority of arteries show only fibrous replacement of the media without thickening of the walls and with retention of wide lumina.

The appearance is instead an expression of choroidal atrophy;[22] loss of the choriocapillaris and the middle layer of vessels throws the remaining larger vessels into greater prominence. The white sheathing is due to the disproportionate thickening of the vessel walls by becoming flattened in the thinned choroid, but in many cases it also reflects a reduced blood column.

Since choroidal atrophy is a normal aging change, the white sheathing of the exposed choroidal arteries develops much more rapidly in patients over 80 years of age. In many patients with senile tigroid fundi and good vision, even the unexposed choroidal vessels assume this whiter appearance (see Fig. 65.3).

Imaging geographic atrophy

Fluorescein angiography

Areas of geographic atrophy are recognized as lobules of hyperfluorescence that appear during the transit phase of fluorescein angiography, often with visualization of the choroidal vessels passing through the region. There may be a surrounding rim of blocked fluorescence. In late phase images the areas may decrease in intensity, but some staining may persist. These sharply demarcated areas are never as intensely fluorescent as an RPE rip.

Fundus autofluorescence

The actual GA lesion appears as a sharply defined and homogeneous area of hypoautofluorescence on fundus autofluorescence (FAF) imaging due to the loss of RPE and therefore lipofuscin accumulation. The high contrast difference between areas absent of FAF and those that retain FAF has led to FAF images being used to monitor presence, configuration, and size of GA lesions within longitudinal clinical studies. What is more variable within an eye, or between eyes, is the FAF pattern in the "junctional" area of the atrophic and nonatrophic tissue. In the junctional area various patterns of high-intensity FAF have been noted such as banded, focal, patchy, and diffuse. In the diffuse patterns the increase in FAF may be present at the margin of the GA and elsewhere in the posterior pole. Existing atrophy enlarges, or new atrophy occurs exactly where there previously has been increased FAF; therefore presence and pattern of increased FAF in these eyes may have prognostic significance for GA progression.[119] A high degree of symmetry has been noted for the pattern of increased FAF in patients with bilateral GA, in contrast to the marked interindividual variations in these patterns. This suggests a genetic determinant that may be affecting this behavior. Evidence is emerging that the specific pattern of increased FAF in the junctional zone is associated with the growth rate of GA, such that some clinical trials are presently requiring these "high-risk" patterns of banded or diffuse FAF be present at entry.[119]

Optical coherence tomography

Using SD-OCT line scans, areas of GA show absence of several structures including the external limiting membrane (ELM), inner/outer-segment (IS-OS) junctions, and the RPE and Bruch's membrane complex (Fig. 65.33).[141] As a result of these alterations there is choroidal signal enhancement or choroidal hyperreflectivity. This group of OCT alterations corresponds to the same area with severe reduction of FAF signal on FAF images. Junctional regions between GA and the surrounding macular show abrupt breaks in the IS/OS junction and RPE/Bruch's membrane complex and curved endings of the ELM as it merges with the atrophic region. Areas of increased FAF in eyes with GA have been shown to correspond to outer plexiform layer clumps,

Enlargement of GA has also been monitored with serial SD-OCT imaging with the following observations: progressive loss of the outer hyperreflective SD-OCT bands (those which are described above in a cross-sectional examination), thinning

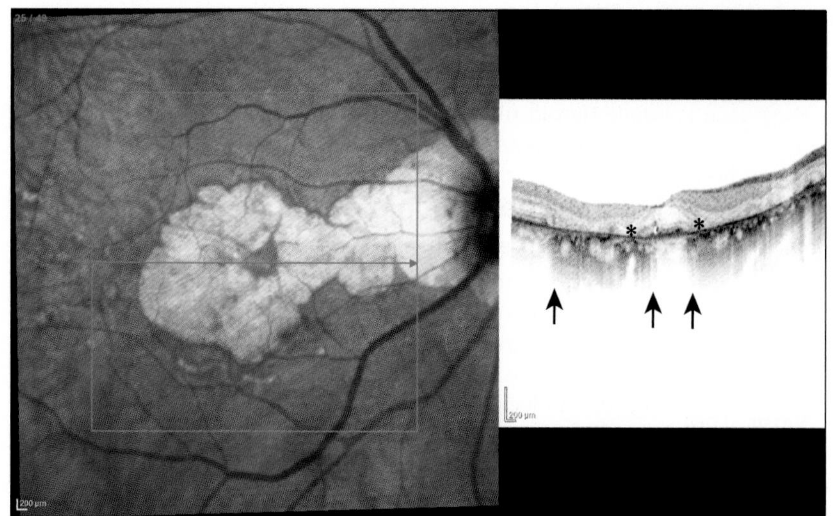

Fig. 65.33 Heidelberg Spectralis OCT image in an eye with a large ring of geographic atrophy sparing the fovea. This shows two areas of geographic atrophy on either side of a preserved island of tissue in the fovea. Arrows denote enhanced signal from the choroid which corresponds to the area of GA. (Arrows mark where the temporal area of GA begins and ends and where the nasal area of GA begins. The nasal area of GA continues to the nasal end of the image.) Immediately anterior to the zone of enhanced choroidal signal there is attenuation or loss of the following layers: Bruch's membrane, RPE, IS–OS junctions, and the ELM. Note the curved endings of the ELM at the lateral margins of the preserved foveal island as it merges with the atrophic region (asterisks).

of the outer nuclear layer, and approach of the outer plexiform layer toward Bruch's membrane. Sequential measurements of retinal thickness at the borders of GA manifest a median loss of 14 µm per year, whereas lateral spread can also be quantitated on these scans, with a median growth of 107 µm per year.[141]

SD-OCT instruments also construct a fundus image, and areas of GA are readily identified on these images as confluent, sharply defined areas of pigment alteration. Comparison of GA size as reflected on these images and those of FAF shows relatively little variation.

Clinical significance of geographic atrophy

The 15-year cumulative incidence of GA among individuals age 43–86 with early signs of AMD at the baseline examination in the Beaver Dam Eye Study is 14%. However, concentrating on the oldest sector of our population, those 85 and older, the cumulative incidence of GA is four times greater than that of neovascular AMD.[142] As individuals live longer, the number of people affected by the advanced form of non-neovascular AMD will continue to climb.

Two case studies[10,143] found that geographic atrophy accounts for only 12–21% of eyes with severe visual loss due to AMD. However, visual acuity does not always reflect the level of vision impairment associated with GA, since a large area of atrophy may spare fixation but still cause the patient difficulty with reading a line of print. The reading rate is slowed not only by the paracentral scotomas, but also because eyes with geographic atrophy demonstrate abnormal foveal dark-adapted sensitivity, reduced visual acuity in dim illumination, and reduced contrast sensitivity.[135] Magnifying aids rarely help these reading difficulties because the image will be enlarged on to nonfunctioning retina.

In one study central fixation was not completely lost until atrophy occupied more than 80% of the fovea, and this occurred about 5 years earlier in drusen-related atrophy as compared with drusen-unrelated atrophy.[80] Even when fixation is affected, vision may vary depending on the patient's ability to find a surviving island of retina within the atrophic area, or the least affected portion of retina outside the area.[144] There seems to be a preference to fix with the scotoma to the right,[137] favoring the ability to see the beginning of a line rather than the end. Visual retraining may enable a patient to use the closest viable area of retina.

Prognosis

Once geographic atrophy has developed, its growth can be monitored by color fundus photographs or FAF images. Annual linear growth rate can be estimated at about 2 mm^2 per year based on 181 eyes followed for a median period of 6 years within AREDS.[145] Factors reported to influence the rate and direction of further spread are the number, distribution, and regression of drusen, the baseline size of the atrophic lesion, the extent of incipient atrophy, and the growth of GA in the contralateral eye. For eyes presenting with noncentral GA, the median time between presentation and foveal involvement is 2.5 years.[145]

Prognostication therefore requires each case to be assessed individually, but in one study the average interval from onset of geographic atrophy to legal blindness was about 9 years.[136] In another study an interval of just over 5 years elapsed from the time atrophy first encroached into the fovea until vision fell to 20/200; fixation was lost earlier in the drusen-related group.[80] In a third study the average rate of expansion in one direction was 139 µm per year and 8% of affected eyes had significant visual loss (from 20/50 or better to 20/100 or worse) per year.[134] In another series in which visual acuity was 20/50 or better at baseline, 50% of eyes lost three or more lines of acuity, and 25% lost six or more lines of acuity at 2-year follow-up.[135] Within the AREDS cohort over 400 eyes progressed to foveal GA. Mean acuity prior to foveal involvement was 20/50, with a drop of 4 letters when the fovea became involved, culminating in a mean decrease of 22 letters 5 years following foveal involvement.[145] Areas of atrophy continue to enlarge over time, even if large at baseline and even after the fovea becomes involved. The combination of reduced visual acuity with enlargement of atrophy, occurring bilaterally in most patients, can lead to significant impairment of visual function.[144]

Geographic atrophy and choroidal neovascularization

Geographic atrophy tends to be a bilateral disease. In one series of over 200 patients with geographic atrophy, the fellow eye was affected in over 50% of cases, and there was a tendency to symmetry between the two eyes, the area of atrophy being only about 20% smaller in the fellow eye.[80]

Histologic studies have shown that eyes with geographic atrophy may also contain small areas of CNV and that CNV is more frequently bilateral than clinical impressions suggest.[22,23] In about 25% of persons with unilateral GA, the fellow eye has evidence of neovascular disease or a disciform process, and these are the patients who are most at risk of developing CNV in the second eye despite the presence of geographic atrophy in this eye. Clinical evidence of CNV may be subtle in these eyes with small areas of elevated RPE accompanied by subretinal blood and fluid. Fluorescein angiography is difficult to interpret in these eyes due to the extensive pigmentary abnormalities causing hyper- and hypofluorescent regions. The CNV may have a classic or occult pattern. In a study of 152 patients with geographic atrophy and no CNV in at least one eye in which patients were followed annually, among patients with CNV in the fellow eye, 18% developed CNV in the study eye that initially manifested GA by 2 years and 34% by 4 years. In contrast, for patients with bilateral geographic atrophy at baseline, the risk for developing CNV was relatively low: 2% by 2 years and 11% by 4 years.[144] As geographic atrophy enlarges in the first eye, the risk of subsequently developing clinically obvious CNV decreases in both eyes.[80,135,146]

INTERMEDIATE STAGE OF AGE-RELATED MACULAR DEGENERATION AND CATARACT

In this aged population, the question of cataract extraction commonly arises, requiring an estimation of the postoperative visual acuity and of how long it may be expected to last. A preoperative fluorescein angiogram and OCT can potentially identify areas of visually significant atrophy or raise suspicion regarding simultaneous presence of neovascular AMD, either one of which may affect postoperative vision function and management. Even when atrophy is suspected on examination, angiography, or OCT indistinct landmarks and poor image quality can make it difficult to tell where the center of the fovea lies[80] and whether various layers of the neurosensory retina are intact.

Despite the presence of AMD, most individuals can derive vision benefits following cataract surgery when lens opacity is presumed to contribute to visual impairment. During the AREDS, 1939 eyes underwent cataract surgery. Although eyes without AMD had the largest magnitude of visual acuity improvement (about 8 letters), those with mild AMD had a mean improvement of 6 letters, moderate AMD eyes gained 4 letters, and even those with advanced AMD gained 2 letters when assessed at their first annual study visit that followed cataract surgery.[147] These improvements (which were significantly different than preoperative levels in each group) were maintained for at least one year following the surgery. The magnitude of vision improvement following cataract surgery in eyes with neovascular AMD may be even greater than that reported by AREDS, particularly in the present era of anti-VEGF management of neovascular AMD. An analysis of individuals who underwent cataract surgery while participating in the two pivotal phase III trials of ranibizumab for assorted neovascular lesion compositions, showed that the average visual acuity improvement in eyes assigned to the ranibizumab treatment arms was approximately a 10-letter increase from an average level of about 20/125 immediately preceding surgery to 20/80 3 months after surgery.[148]

The other common concern is whether the insult of cataract surgery accelerates progression of pre-existing AMD. A combined analysis of two population-based surveys (the Beaver Dam and Blue Mountains Eye studies) suggested that cataract surgery increased the risk of incident neovascular AMD by a factor of 5 within 5 years of surgery.[149] Although this may have reflected easier visualization of the fundus after surgery and identification of pre-existing neovascular AMD, damage due to photic injury or inflammation at the time of surgery is hypothesized to "trigger" AMD progression. More recent information from AREDS used a variety of analytical methods to explore development of neovascular AMD or central GA following cataract surgery and no clear deleterious effect of any concerning magnitude was identified.[150]

The best evidence at this time suggests that patients with AMD can derive vision benefits from cataract surgery and that cataract surgery does not appear to increase the risk that AMD will progress. Ophthalmologists should be cognizant of the possibility that advanced AMD (especially geographic atrophy in a blonde fundus or CNV with minimal subretinal fluid, hemorrhage, lipid, or scarring) might not be readily apparent through a cataract, despite preoperative imaging. Pre-existing advanced AMD might be a cause of vision loss which is mistakenly attributed to the cataract before surgery and it may remain a cause of continued vision loss after cataract surgery. Furthermore, the patient may presume that loss of vision following cataract surgery, which is really due to progression of AMD that was pre-existing and unrelated to cataract surgery, was due to progression of AMD caused by the cataract surgery because of the temporal relationship of loss of vision soon after cataract surgery. Careful examination for the advanced stage of AMD before cataract surgery in any individual at risk for AMD, therefore, is important. Potential clues that advanced AMD may exist posterior to the cataract include the presence of advanced AMD in the contralateral eye, pigmentary abnormalities in the macula (which may be associated with less visible atrophy or CNV), or glistening from calcification (which is usually associated with geographic atrophy).

AGE-RELATED MACULAR DEGENERATION AND AGE

Reference has already been made to the physiologic visual decline with age. If AMD is present in addition, subjective tests, such as the time for visual recovery after exposure to a glare source,[32] become increasingly abnormal. The incidence and progression of AMD are closely related to age. Over a 5-year period,[4] compared to persons 43–54 years, persons 75 years of age and over were more than 10 times as likely to develop earlier stages of AMD and more than 40 times as likely to develop drusen 250 μm in diameter. The 5-year incidence of soft indistinct drusen, increased retinal pigment, and depigmentation was strongly associated with age, the most marked increase being found in people aged 75 and over.[4,101] This accelerated deterioration in older persons coincides with the accumulation of the diffuse deposits and makes prognostication in younger persons difficult.

MANAGEMENT OF NON-NEOVASCULAR AMD

The management of non-neovascular AMD begins with the recognition that most people with intermediate AMD, while at risk of progressing to advanced AMD, have no symptoms. Since it is estimated that approximately 8 million of the 60 million people aged 55 or older residing in the United States have the intermediate stage of AMD,[3,13] usually without symptoms, annual ophthalmologic examination of all people in this age group should include an evaluation of the retina to determine the presence and stage of AMD. If subretinal or intraretinal fluid, hemorrhage, lipid, or elevation of the RPE is noted then neovascular AMD maybe present and fluorescein angiography and OCT is indicated to determine the management, as outlined in Chapter 66 Neovascular (exudative or "wet") age-related macular degeneration.

If neovascular AMD is not suspected, then the stage of AMD in each eye should be determined. If there is no AMD or only early AMD as the most advanced feature of AMD in both eyes, then no intervention is indicated at that time. Specifically, AREDS could find no evidence that using a dietary supplement of antioxidants and minerals, reduced the risk of progression to advanced AMD or even to intermediate AMD among individuals with early AMD. These individuals may be appropriately counseled that they are at very low risk of visually significant disease within the next 5 years. However, those with early AMD may be invited to undergo annual reassessments to check for progression to intermediate AMD as about one-third of AREDS participants with early AMD progressed to intermediate AMD during the first 5 years of follow-up.[13]

If intermediate AMD is noted in at least one eye, then the individual should consider using a dietary supplement such as that used in AREDS, provided the individual's physicians know of no contraindication to using this formulation of antioxidants (daily dose of 500 mg vitamin C, 400 international units of vitamin E, and 15 mg beta carotene) and zinc (daily dose of 80 mg zinc oxide with 2 mg cupric oxide added to reduce the risk of a copper-deficiency anemia). Individuals with at least unilateral intermediate AMD or unilateral advanced AMD who were assigned to this formulation within AREDS had a decreased risk of progression to advanced AMD (Fig. 65.30B) and a decreased risk of vision loss (Fig. 65.30C) through at least 10 years. Although there is minimal risk associated with the use of these supplements (Tables 65.1 and 65.2), a thorough discussion of the modest treatment benefit and the minimal risks should be held. Cigarette smokers should be advised that higher doses of beta-carotene in other randomized trials resulted in a definite, although small, increased risk of developing lung cancer with concomitant adverse effects on mortality.[151,152] The discussion should also include the present fact that other formulations, such as those containing lutein or omega-3 long-chain polyunsaturated fatty acids, have not been proven effective in randomized clinical trials and the risks associated with other formulations are presently unknown. Individuals should be reminded that micronutrients, such as beta-carotene, were not suspected to be harmful and concern only arose about its use after careful investigations were performed. The AREDS2 study, is expected to report results in 2013 that should clarify the role of oral supplementation with lutein, zeaxanthin, and omega-3 fatty acids among individuals with bilateral intermediate AMD or those with unilateral advanced AMD with large drusen in the healthier contralateral eye.

Table 65.1 Safety – antioxidants

Condition	No antioxidants (%)	Antioxidants (%)
Hospitalization for mild/moderate symptoms	10.1	7.4
Hospitalization for infections	0.8	1.6
Circulatory	0.8	0.3
Skin, subcutaneous tissue	1.0	2.2
Change in skin color	6.0	8.3
Chest pain	23.1	20.2

Table 65.2 Safety – zinc oxide

Condition	No zinc (%)	Zinc (%)
Hospitalization for mild/moderate symptoms	7.8	9.7
Hospitalization for genitourinary	4.9	7.5
Hospitalization for genitourinary problems in men	4.4	8.6
Circulatory	0.3	0.9
Anemia	10.2	13.2
Difficulty swallowing pills	15.3	17.8

If a person has unilateral advanced AMD (either central GA or neovascular AMD/disciform scar), the fellow eye is at high risk of progression to advanced AMD, especially if large drusen and pigment abnormalities are present in this eye. Irrespective of the specific non-neovascular AMD manifestations in this healthier eye, a dietary supplement such as that used in AREDS should be considered, as explained above, to decrease anatomic progression and functional impairment. If advanced AMD is noted in one eye, and the fellow eye also has advanced AMD, the physician may consider an AREDS type supplement if visual acuity is relatively good (20/100 or better) in at least one eye in the presence of CNV. This consideration is based on AREDS data which showed a decreased risk of at least 3 additional lines of visual acuity in the eye with neovascular AMD among the advanced AMD participants with unilateral CNV at baseline. However, this observation only applied to eyes with CNV and acuity of at least 20/100 at baseline (Table 65.3).

Modeling of data from AREDS and epidemiologic surveys of the US population reporting prevalence rates of AMD have

Table 65.3 Effect of treatment on risk of moderate vision loss from baseline in eyes with neovascular age-related macular degeneration at baseline

	Odds ratio	99% CI	*P* value
Baseline visual acuity 20/100 or better (*n* = 260)*			
Antioxidant vs no antioxidant	0.54	0.30–0.95	0.005
Zinc vs no zinc	0.99	0.56–1.74	0.96
Antioxidant vs placebo	0.35	0.15–0.81	0.001
Zinc vs placebo	0.65	0.28–1.50	0.18
Antioxidant + zinc vs placebo	0.53	0.23–1.24	0.05
Baseline visual acuity 20/200 or better (*n* = 352)†			
Antioxidant vs no antioxidant	0.66	0.40–1.07	0.03
Zinc vs no zinc	1.10	0.67–1.79	0.62
Antioxidant vs placebo	0.56	0.27–1.13	0.03
Zinc vs placebo	0.93	0.46–1.89	0.79
Antioxidant + zinc vs placebo	0.72	0.36–1.46	0.24

CI, confidence interval.
**167 participants had moderate vision loss.*
†206 participants had moderate vision loss.

suggested that approximately 300 000 individuals would avoid development of advanced AMD in at least one eye over 5 years if all 8 million people at risk of AMD progression were identified, educated in regards to supplement use, and were compliant in their use of an AREDS type supplement. Nevertheless, an additional 1 million people will still develop advanced AMD, of whom approximately two-thirds will develop the neovascular stage. With the availability of new and substantially more effective treatments for neovascular AMD, early diagnosis of neovascular AMD has become increasingly important to stabilize vision at levels as close to normal as possible. Therefore, individuals with intermediate AMD or unilateral advanced AMD are invited to return to their ophthalmologist for the following reasons: (1) to evaluate their AMD status and receive further updates on AMD management; (2) to identify any asymptomatic neovascular AMD for which prompt treatment affects final vision outcome; (3) to review the regular need and methods for periodic monitoring to increase the chance that the individual will identify progression to the neovascular stage when the neovascular lesion is small, before significant visual acuity has been lost, when treatment has been shown to be more likely to be most effective; and (4) to be reminded to promptly contact their ophthalmologist if symptoms of progression are suspected.

There are a small number of clinical trials underway testing other therapies for non-neovascular AMD. Additional information is included in Chapter 67 (Pharmacotherapy of age-related macular degeneration).

Although an Amsler grid has not been shown to be very sensitive at detecting neovascular AMD,[153-156] many physicians recommend its use to individuals at risk of AMD progression. More recently, a perimetry device, the Preferential Hyperacuity Perimeter (PreView PHP, Carl Zeiss Meditec, Dublin, CA) was shown to have twice the sensitivity of an Amsler grid test in individuals with neovascular AMD.[156] Additional studies have demonstrated that the device could differentiate eyes with recent-onset neovascular AMD from those with intermediate AMD with both a high sensitivity (82%) and high specificity (88%). These findings make it likely that individuals identified as having progressed to neovascular AMD by PHP testing will indeed have progressed.[157] Based on this information, a similar device (ForeseePHP 2.05 Notal Vision, Ltd, Tel Aviv, Israel), was evaluated within a nested case–control study as part of the Carotenoids and co-antioxidants in patients with Age-Related Maculopathy (CARMA) clinical trial. Eyes that progressed to CNV before the device was incorporated into the clinic exam had larger magnitude losses in visual acuity and larger lesion size at time of CNV detection than eyes that progressed to CNV during use of the PHP during the office exam.[158] The same technology has now been developed into a home monitoring device (ForeseeHome, Notal Vision, Ltd, Tel Aviv, Israel) and a large-scale randomized clinical trial is underway comparing use of this ForseeHome comprehensive solution to our standard care practices for patient symptom monitoring. The primary objective of this endeavor is to learn whether patients can successfully use this device and experience early detection of disease progression as indicated by less vision loss at time of CNV diagnosis and smaller lesion size at presentation relative to standard care methods of patient monitoring. Even with the potential for devices such as this to improve our ability to detect disease progression early on, it is unlikely that all cases that progress will be detected by this method; therefore, periodic examinations for asymptomatic progression and reassessment of a patient's functional needs is still indicated.

Finally, if advanced AMD is noted in one or both eyes, or if there is vision impairment from lesser degrees of atrophic disease such as foveal nongeographic atrophy, then rehabilitation with a low-vision service should be considered. These experienced eye care and social service professionals can determine what services or devices might help the individual cope with the visual loss from AMD. It is hopeful that future research will elucidate further the causes, treatments, and prevention of drusen, atrophy, and CNV, as well as additional ways to rehabilitate the individual who has lost vision from AMD.

REFERENCES

1. Ferris FL III. Senile macular degeneration: review of epidemiologic features. Am J Epidemiol 1983;118:132–51.
2. The Age-Related Eye Disease Study Research Group. Potential public health impact of AREDS results: AREDS report no. 11. Arch Ophthalmol 2003;121:1621–4.
3. The Eye Diseases Prevalence Research Group. Prevalence of age-related macular degeneration in the United States. Arch Ophthalmol 2004;122:567–72.
4. Klein R, Klein BEK, Jensen SC, et al. The five-year incidence and progression of age-related maculopathy. Ophthalmology 1997;104:7–21.
5. Evans J, Wormold R. Is the incidence of registrable age-related macular degeneration increasing? Br J Ophthalmol 1996;80:9–14.
6. Campbell JP, Bressler SB, Bressler NB. Impact of availability of anti-VEGF therapy on vision impairment and blindness due to neovascular AMD. Arch Ophthalmol 2012;130:794–5.
7. Gass JDM. Drusen and disciform macular detachment and degeneration. Arch Ophthalmol 1973;90:206–17.
8. Haab O. Erkrankungen der Macula Lutea. Centralblat Augenheilkd 1885;9:384–91. (Cited by Duke-Elder S. System of ophthalmology, vol. 9. London: Kimpton; 1966.)
9. Piguet B, Haimovici R, Bird AC. Dominantly inherited drusen represent more than one disorder: a historical review. Eye 1995;9:34–41.
10. Gass JDM. Pathogenesis of disciform detachment of the neuroepithelium (parts I and III). Am J Ophthalmol 1967;63:573–711.
11. Bird AC, Bressler NB, Bressler SB, et al. An international classification and grading system for age-related maculopathy and age-related macular degeneration. Surv Ophthalmol 1995;39:367–74.
12. Klein R, Klein BEK, Linton KLP. Prevalence of age-related maculopathy: the Beaver Dam Eye Study. Ophthalmology 1992;99:933–43.
13. The Age-Related Eye Disease Study Research Group. A randomized, placebo-controlled, clinical trial of high-dose supplementation with vitamins C and E, beta carotene, and zinc for age-related macular degeneration and vision loss: AREDS report no. 8. Arch Ophthalmol 2001;119:1417–36.
14. Mitchell P, Smith W, Attebo K, et al. Prevalence of age-related maculopathy in Australia. Ophthalmology 1995;102:1450–60.
15. Wang Q, Chappell RJ, Klein R et al. Patterns of age-related maculopathy in the macular area, the Beaver Dam Eye Study. Invest Ophthalmol Vis Sci 1996;37:2234–42.
16. Vingerling JR, Dielemans I, Hofman A, et al. The prevalence of age-related maculopathy in the Rotterdam study. Ophthalmology 1995;102:205–10.
17. Wang JJ, Mitchell P, Smith W, et al. Bilateral involvement by age-related maculopathy lesions in a population, the Blue Mountains Eye Study. Br J Ophthalmol 1998;82:743–7.
18. Bressler NM, Bressler SB, West SK, et al. The grading and prevalence of macular degeneration in Chesapeake Bay watermen. Arch Ophthalmol 1989;107:847–52.
19. Gregor Z, Bird AC, Chisholm IH. Senile disciform macular degeneration in the second eye. Br J Ophthalmol 1977;61:141–7.
20. Klein R, Davis MD, Magli YL, et al. The Wisconsin age-related maculopathy grading system. Ophthalmology 1991;98:1128–34.
21. Green WR, McDonnell PJ, Yeo JH. Pathologic features of senile macular degeneration. Ophthalmology 1985;92:615–27.
22. Green WR, Enger C. Age-related macular degeneration histopathologic studies: the 1992 Lorenz E. Zimmerman lecture. Ophthalmology 1993;100:1519–35.
23. Sarks SH. Aging and degeneration in the macular region: a clinico-pathological study. Br J Ophthalmol 1976;60:324–41.
24. Spraul CW, Grossniklaus HE. Characteristics of drusen and Bruch's membrane in postmortem eyes with age-related macular degeneration. Arch Ophthalmol 1997;115:267–73.
25. van der Schaft TL, Mooy CM, de Bruijn WC, et al. Histologic features of the early stages of age-related macular degeneration. A statistical analysis. Ophthalmology 1992;99:278–86.
26. Laatikainen L, Karinkari J. Capillary-free area of the fovea with advancing age. Invest Ophthalmol Vis Sci 1977;161:1154–7.
27. Grunwald JE, Piltz J, Patel N, et al. Effect of aging on retinal macular micro-circulation: a blue-field simulation study. Invest Ophthalmol Vis Sci 1994;34:3609–13.
28. Groh MJM, Michelson G, Langhans MJ, et al. Influence of age on retinal and optic nerve head blood circulation. Ophthalmology 1996;103:529–34.
29. Ibrahim YWM, Bots ML, Mulder PGH, et al. Number of perifoveal vessels in aging, hypertension, and atherosclerosis: the Rotterdam Study. Invest Ophthalmol Vis Sci 1998;39:1049–53.
30. Gao H, Hollyfield JG. Aging of the human retina: differential loss of neurons and retinal pigment epithelial cells. Invest Ophthalmol Vis Sci 1992;33:1–17.
31. Rubin GS, West SK, Munoz B, et al. A comprehensive assessment of visual impairment in a population of older Americans, the SEE study. Invest Ophthalmol Vis Sci 1977;38:557–68.
32. Sandberg MA, Gaudio AR. Slow photostress recovery and disease severity in age-related macular degeneration. Retina 1995;15:407–12.
33. Liem AT, Keunen JE, van Norren D. Clinical applications of fundus reflection densitometry. Surv Ophthalmol 1996;41:37–50.
34. Curcio CA, Millican CL, Allen KA, et al. Aging of the human photoreceptor mosaic: evidence for selective vulnerability of rods in central retina. Invest Ophthalmol Vis Sci 1993;34:3278–96.
35. Dorey CK, Wu G, Ebenstein D, et al. Cell loss in the aging retina: relationship to lipofuscin accumulation and macular degeneration. Invest Ophthalmol Vis Sci 1989;30:1691–9.
36. Feeney-Burns L, Burns RP, Gao C. Age-related macular changes in humans over 90 years old. Am J Ophthalmol 1990;109:265–78.
37. Marshall J, Grindle J, Ansell PL, et al. Convolution in human rods: an ageing process. Br J Ophthalmol 1979;63:181–7.
38. Curcio CA, Medeiros NE, Millican CL. Photoreceptor loss in age-related macular degeneration. Invest Ophthalmol Vis Sci 1996;37:1236–49.
39. Young RW. The Bowman Lecture, 1982. Biological renewal: applications to the eye. Trans Ophthalmol Soc UK 1982;102:42–75.
40. Feeney-Burns L, Berman ER, Rothman H. Lipofuscin of human retinal pigment epithelium. Am J Ophthalmol 1980;90:783–91.
41. Young RW. Pathophysiology of age-related macular degeneration. Surv Ophthalmol 1987;31:291–306.
42. Rakoczy PE, Baines M, Kennedy C, et al. Correlation between autofluorescent debris accumulation and the presence of partially processed forms of cathepsin D in cultured retinal pigment epithelial cells challenged with rod outer segments. Exp Eye Res 1996;63:159–67.
43. Feeney-Burns L, Hilderbrand ES, Eldridge S. Aging human RPE: morphometric analysis of macular, equatorial, and peripheral cells. Invest Ophthalmol Vis Sci 1984;25:195–200.
44. Beatty S, Boulton M, Henson D, et al. Macular pigment and age-related macular degeneration. Br J Ophthalmol 1999;83:867–77.
45. Kennedy CJ, Rakoczy PE, Constable IJ. Lipofuscin of the retinal pigment epithelium: a review. Eye 1995;9:763–71.
46. von Ruckmann A, Fitzke FW, Bird AC. In vivo fundus autofluorescence in macular dystrophies. Arch Ophthalmol 1997;115:609–15.
47. Delori FC, Dorey CK, Staurenghi G, et al. In vivo fluorescence of the ocular fundus exhibits retinal pigment epithelium lipofuscin characteristics. Invest Ophthalmol Vis Sci 1995;36:718–29.
48. Panda-Jonas S, Jonas JB, Jakobczyk-Zmija M. Retinal pigment epithelial cell count, distribution, and correlations in normal human eyes. Am J Ophthalmol 1996;121:181–9.
49. Gass JDM. Stereoscopic atlas of macular diseases: diagnosis and treatment. 4th ed. St Louis: Mosby; 1997.
50. Ramrattan RS, van der Schaft TL, Mooy CM, et al. Morphometric analysis of Bruch's membrane, the choriocapillaris, and the choroid in aging. Invest Ophthalmol Vis Sci 1994;35:2857–64.
51. Karwatowski WSS, Jeffries TE, Duance VC, et al. Preparation of Bruch's membrane and analysis of the age-related changes in the structural collagens. Br J Ophthalmol 1995;79:944–52.
52. Holz FG, Owens SL, Marks J, et al. Ultrastructural findings in autosomal dominant drusen. Arch Ophthalmol 1997;115:788–92.
53. van der Schaft TL, de Bruijn WC, Mooy CM, et al. Is basal laminar deposit unique for age-related macular degeneration? Arch Ophthalmol 1991;109:420–5.
54. Marshall GE, Konstas AGP, Reid GG, et al. Type IV collagen and laminin in Bruch's membrane and basal linear deposit in the human macula. Br J Ophthalmol 1992;76:607–14.
55. Feeney-Burns L, Ellersieck MR. Age-related changes in the ultrastructure of Bruch's membrane. Am J Ophthalmol 1985;100:686–697.
56. Burns RP, Feeney-Burns L. Clinico-morphologic correlations of drusen of Bruch's membrane. Trans Am Ophthalmol Soc 1980;78:206–25.
57. Ishibashi T, Sorgente N, Patterson R, et al. Aging changes in Bruch's membrane of monkeys: an electron microscopic study. Ophthalmologica 1986;192:179–90.
58. Killingsworth MC. Age-related components of Bruch's membrane in the human eye. Graefes Arch Clin Exp Ophthalmol 1987;225:406–12.
59. Holz FG, Sheraidah G, Pauleikhoff D, et al. Analysis of lipid deposits extracted from human macular and peripheral Bruch's membrane. Arch Ophthalmol 1994;112:402–6.
60. Klein R, Klein BEK, Jensen SC, et al. The relationship of ocular factors to the incidence and progression of age-related maculopathy. Arch Ophthalmol 1998;116:506–13.
61. Sheraidah G, Steinmetz R, Maguire J, et al. Correlation between lipids extracted from Bruch's membrane and age. Ophthalmology 1993;100:47–52.
62. Pauleikhoff D, Harper CA, Marshall J, et al. Aging changes in Bruch's membrane: a histochemical and morphologic study. Ophthalmology 1990;97:171–8.
63. Spaide RF, Ho-Spaide WC, Browne R, et al. Characterization of peroxidized lipids in Bruch's membrane. Retina 1999;19:141–7.

64. Holz FG, Bellmann C, Margaritidis M, et al. Patterns of increased in vivo fundus autofluorescence in the junctional zone of geographic atrophy associated with age-related macular degeneration. Graefes Arch Clin Exp Ophthalmol 1999;237:145–52.
65. Moore DJ, Hussain AA, Marshall J. Age-related variation in the hydraulic conductivity of Bruch's membrane. Invest Ophthalmol Vis Sci 1995;36: 1290–7.
66. Starita C, Hussain AA, Patmore A, et al. Localization of the site of major resistance to fluid transport in Bruch's membrane. Invest Ophthalmol Vis Sci 1997;38:762–7.
67. Marshall J, Hussain AA, Starita C, et al, editors. The retinal pigment epithelium: function and disease. New York: Oxford University Press; 1998.
68. Grunwald JE, Hariprasad SM, Dupont J. Effect of aging on foveolar choroidal circulation. Arch Ophthalmol 1998;116:150–4.
69. Curcio CA, Millican CL. Basal linear deposit and large drusen are specific for early age-related maculopathy. Arch Ophthalmol 1999;117:329–39.
70. Zarbin MA. Age-related macular degeneration: review of pathogenesis. Eur J Ophthalmol 1998;8:199–206.
71. Löffler KU, Lee WR. Basal linear deposit in the human macula. Graefes Arch Clin Exp Ophthalmol 1986;224:493–501.
72. van der Schaft TL, Mooy CM, de Bruijn WC, et al. Immunohistochemical light and electron microscopy of basal laminar deposit. Graefes Arch Clin Exp Ophthalmol 1994;232:40–6.
73. Sarks JP, Sarks SH, Killingsworth MC. Evolution of soft drusen in age-related macular degeneration. Eye 1994;8:269–83.
74. Green WR, Key SN III. Senile macular degeneration: a histopathologic study. Trans Am Ophthalmol Soc 1977;75:180–254.
75. Bressler NM, Silva JC, Bressler SB, et al. Clinicopathologic correlation of drusen and retinal pigment epithelial abnormalities in age-related macular degeneration. Retina 1994;14:130–42.
76. El Baba F, Green WR, Fleischmann J, et al. Clinicopathologic correlation of lipidization and detachment of the retinal pigment epithelium. Am J Ophthalmol 1986;101:576–83.
77. Shuman SG, Koreishi AF, Farsui S, et al. Photoreceptor layer thinning over drusen in eyes with age-related macular degeneration imaged in vivo with sepctral-domain optical coherence tomography. Ophthalmology 2009;116: 488–96.
78. Pieroni CG, Witkin AJ, Ko TH, et al. Ultrahigh resolution optical coherence tomography in non-exudative age related macular degeneration. Br J Ophthalmolo 2006;90:191–7.
79. Ho J, Witkin AJ, Liu J, et al. Documentation of intraretinal retinal pigment epithelium migration via high-speed ultrahigh-resolution optical coherence tomography. Ophthalmology 2011;118:687–93.
80. Sarks JP, Sarks SH, Killingsworth M. Evolution of geographic atrophy of the retinal pigment epithelium. Eye 1988;2:552–77.
81. Penfold PL, Killingsworth MC, Sarks SH. Senile macular degeneration: the involvement of immunocompetent cells. Graefes Arch Clin Exp Ophthalmol 1985;223:69–76.
82. Sarks JP, Sarks SH, Killingsworth MC. Morphology of early choroidal neovascularisation in age-related macular degeneration. Eye 1997;11: 515–22.
83. Killingsworth MC, Sarks JP, Sarks SH. Macrophages related to Bruch's membrane in age-related macular degeneration. Eye 1990;4:613–21.
84. The Age-Related Eye Disease Study Research Group. The Age-Related Eye Disease Study severity scale for age-related macular degeneration: AREDS report no. 17. Arch Ophthalmol. 2005;123:1484–98.
85. Eye Disease Case-Control Study Group. Risk factors for neovascular age-related macular degeneration. Arch Ophthalmol 1992;110:1701–8.
86. Macular Photocoagulation Study Group. Risk factors for choroidal neovascularization in the second eye of patients with juxtafoveal or subfoveal choroidal neovascularization secondary to age-related macular degeneration. Arch Ophthalmol 1997;115:741–7.
87. Bressler NM, Bressler SB, Seddon JM, et al. Drusen characteristics in patients with exudative versus nonexudative age-related macular degeneration. Retina 1988;8:108–14.
88. The Age-Related Eye Disease Study Research Group. A simplified severity scale for age-related macular degeneration: AREDS no. 18. Arch Ophthalmol 2005;123:1570–4.
89. Barondes M, Pauleikhoff D, Chisholm IC, et al. Bilaterality of drusen. Br J Ophthalmol 1990;74:180–2.
90. Friedman D, Parker JS, Kimble JA, et al. Quantification of fluorescein-stained drusen associated with age-related macular degeneration. Retina 2011;31(10): 1–6.
91. Chang AA, Guyer DR, Orlock DR, et al. Age-dependent variations in the drusen fluorescence on indocyanine green angiography. Clin Experiment Ophthalmol 2003;31(4):300–4.
92. Arnold JJ, Quaranta M, Soubrane G, et al. Indocyanine green angiography of drusen. Am J Ophthalmol 1997;124:344–56.
93. Delori FC, Fleckner MR, Goger DG, et al. Autofluorescence distribution associated with drusen in age-related macular degeneration. Invest Ophthalmol Vis Sci 2000;41(2):496–504.
94. Khanifar AA, Koreishi AF, Izatt JA, et al. Drusen ultrastructure imaging with spectral domain optical coherence tomography in age-related macular degeneration. Ophthalmology 2008;115:1883–90.
95. Schlanitz FG, Baumann B, Spaliek T, et al. Performance of automated drusen detection by polarization-sensitive optical coherence tomography. Invest Ophthalmol Vis Sci 2011;51:4571–9.
96. Jain N, Farsiu S, Khanifar AA, et al. Quantitative comparison of drusen segmented on SD-OCT versus drusen delineated on color fundus photographs. Invest Ophthalmol Vis Sci 2010;51:4875–83.
97. Gass JDM, Jallow S, Davis B. Adult vitelliform macular detachment occurring in patients with basal laminar drusen. Am J Ophthalmol 1985;99: 445–59.
98. Sarks SH, Arnold JJ, Killinsworth MC, et al. Early drusen formation in the normal and aging eye and their relationship to age-related maculopathy: a clinicopathological study. Br J Ophthalmol 1999;83:358–68.
99. Hageman GS, Mullins RF. Molecular composition of drusen as related to substructural phenotype. Mol Vis 1999;5:28–37.
100. Coffey AJH, Brownstein S. The prevalence of macular drusen in postmortem eyes. Am J Ophthalmol 1986;102:164–71.
101. Bressler NM, Munoz B, Maguire MG, et al. Five-year incidence and disappearance of drusen and retinal pigment epithelial abnormalities, Chesapeake Bay watermen study. Arch Ophthalmol 1995;113:301–8.
102. Sarks SH. Drusen and their relationship to senile macular degeneration. Aust J Ophthalmol 1980;8:117–30.
103. Bird AC. Pathogenesis of retinal pigment epithelial detachment in the elderly: the relevance of Bruch's membrane change: Doyne lecture. Eye 1991;5: 1–12.
104. Casswell AG, Kohen D, Bird AC. Retinal pigment epithelial detachments in the elderly: classification and outcome. Br J Ophthalmol 1985;69: 397–403.
105. Hartnett ME, Weiter JJ, Garsd A, et al. Classification of retinal pigment epithelial detachments associated with drusen. Graefes Arch Clin Exp Ophthalmol 1992;230:11–9.
106. Holz FG, Wolfensberger TJ, Piguet B, et al. Bilateral macular drusen in age-related macular degeneration: prognosis and risk factors. Ophthalmology 1994;101:1522–8.
107. Cukras C, Agron E, Klein ML, et al; for the Age-Related Eye Disease Study Research Group. Natural history of drusenoid pigment epithelial detachment in age-related macular degeneration: Age-Related Eye Disease Study Report No. 28. Ophthalmology 2010;117:489–499.
108. Complications of Age-Related Macular Degeneration Prevention Trial Research Group. Laser treatment in patients with bilateral large drusen. The Complications of Age-Related Macular Degeneration Prevention Trial. Ophthalmology 2006;113:1974–86.
109. Arnold JJ, Sarks SH, Killingsworth MC, et al. Reticular pseudodrusen: a risk factor in age-related maculopathy. Retina 1995;15:183–91.
110. Zweifel SA, Spaide RF, Curio CA, et al. Reticular pseudodrusen are subretinal deposits. Ophthalmology 2010;117:303–12.
111. Zweifel SA, Imamura Y, Spaide TC, et al. Prevalence and significance of subretinal drusenoid deposits (reticular psuedodrusen) in age-related macular degeneration. Ophthalmology 2010;117:1775–81.
112. Rudolf M, Malek G, Messinge JD, et al. Sub-retinal drusenoid deposits in human retina: organization and composition. Exp Eye Res 2008;87: 402–8.
113. Pumariega NM, Smith RT, Sohrab MA, et al. A prospective study of reticular macular disease. Ophthalmology 2011;118(8):1619–26.
114. Sarraf D, Gin T, Yu F, et al. Long-term drusen study. Retina 1999;19:513–19.
115. Pauleikhoff D, Zuels S, Sheraidah GS, et al. Correlation between biochemical composition and fluorescein binding of deposits in Bruch's membrane. Ophthalmology 1992;99:1548–53.
116. Mullins RF, Johnson LV, Anderson DH, et al. Characterization of drusen-associated glycoconjugates. Ophthalmology 1998;104:288–98.
117. Mullins RF, Hageman GS. Human ocular drusen possess novel core domains with a distinct carbohydrate composition. J Histochem Cytochem 1999;47: 1533–9.
118. Hageman GS, Mullins RF, Russell SR, et al. Vitronectin is a constituent of ocular drusen and the vitronectin gene is expressed in human retinal pigmented epithelial cells. FASEB J 1999;13:477–84.
119. Schmitz-Valckenberg A, Fleckenstein M, Scholl H, et al. Fundus autofluorescence and progression of age-related macular degeneration. Surv Ophthalmol 2009;54:96–117.
120. Berenberg TL, Metelitsina TI, Madow B, et al. The association between drusen extent and foveolar choroidal bloodflow in age-related macular degeneration. Retina 2011;31(10):1–7.
121. McLeod DS, Lutty GA. High-resolution histologic analysis of the human choroidal vasculature. Invest Ophthalmol Vis Sci 1994;35:3799–811.
122. Pauleikhoff D, Chen JC, Chisholm IH, et al. Choroidal perfusion abnormality with age-related Bruch's membrane change. Ophthalmology 1990;109: 211–17.
123. Staurenghi G, Bottoni F, Lonati C, et al. Drusen and choroidal filling defects: a cross-sectional survey. Ophthalmologica 1992;205:178–86.
124. Pauleikhoff D, Spital M, Radermacher M, et al. Regression of the choriocapillaris in age-related macular degeneration. Invest Ophthalmol Vis Sci 1997; 38(Suppl.):967.
125. Henkind P, Gartner S. The relationship between retinal pigment epithelium and the choriocapillaris. Trans Ophthalmol Soc UK 1983;103:444–47.
126. Glaser BM. Extracellular modulating factors and the control of intraocular neovascularization. Arch Ophthalmol 1988;106:603–7.
127. Friedman E, Krupsky S, Lane AM, et al. Ocular blood flow velocity in age-related macular degeneration. Ophthalmology 1995;102:640–6.
128. Chen JC, Fitzke FW, Pauleikhoff D, et al. Functional loss in age-related Bruch's membrane change with choroidal perfusion defect. Invest Ophthalmol Vis Sci 1992;33:334–40.

129. Steinmetz RL, Haimovici R, Jubb C, et al. Symptomatic abnormalities of dark adaptation in patients with age-related Bruch's membrane change. Br J Ophthalmol 1993;77:549–54.
130. Remulla JFC, Gaudio AR, Miller S, et al. Foveal electroretinograms and choroidal perfusion characteristics in fellow eyes of patients with unilateral neovascular age-related macular degeneration. Br J Ophthalmol 1995;79: 558–61.
131. Piguet B, Palmvang TB, Chisholm IH, et al. Evolution of age-related macular degeneration with choroidal perfusion abnormality. Am J Ophthalmol 1992; 113:657–63.
132. Sunness JS, Massof RW, Johnson MA, et al. Diminished foveal sensitivity may predict the development of advanced age-related macular degeneration. Ophthalmology 1989;96:375–81.
133. Sunness JS, Johnson MA, Massof RW, et al. Retinal sensitivity over drusen and nondrusen areas: a study using fundus perimetry. Arch Ophthalmol 1988;106:1081–4.
134. Schatz H, McDonald HR. Atrophic macular degeneration: rate of spread of geographic atrophy and visual loss. Ophthalmology 1989;96:1541–51.
135. Sunness JS, Rubin GS, Applegate CA, et al. Visual function abnormalities and prognosis in eyes with age-related geographic atrophy of the macula and good visual acuity. Ophthalmology 1997;104:1677–91.
136. Maguire P, Vine AK. Geographic atrophy of the retinal pigment epithelium. Am J Ophthalmol 1986;102:621–5.
137. Sunness JS, Applegate CA, Haselwood D, et al. Fixation patterns and reading rates in eyes with central scotomas from advanced atrophic age-related macular degeneration and Stargardt's disease. Ophthalmology 1996;103: 1458–66.
138. Weiter JJ, Delori F, Dorey CK. Central sparing in annular macular degeneration. Am J Ophthalmol 1988;106:286–92.
139. Snodderly DM. Evidence for protection against age-related macular degeneration by carotenoids and antioxidant vitamins. Am J Clin Nutr 1995;62 (Suppl):1448–61.
140. Klein MK, Ferris FL, Armstrong J, et al. AREDS Research Group. Retinal precursors and the development of geographic atrophy in age-related macular degeneration. Ophthalmology 2008;115;1026–31.
141. Fleckenstein M, Schmitz-Valckenberg S, Adrion C, et al. Tracking progression with spectral-domain optical coherence tomography in geographic atrophy caused by age-related macular degeneration. Invest Ophthalmol Vis Sci 2010;51:3846–52.
142. Klein R, Klein BE, Knudston MD, et al. Fifteen-year cumulative incidence of age-related macular degeneration: the Beaver Dam Eye Study. Ophthalmology 2007;114:253–62.
143. Hyman LG, Lilienfeld AM, Ferris FL III, et al. Senile macular degeneration: a case-control study. Am J Epidemiol 1983;118:213–27.
144. Sunness JS, Gonzalez-Baron J, Applegate CA, et al. Enlargement of atrophy and visual acuity loss in the geographic atrophy form of age-related macular degeneration. Ophthalmology 1999;106:1768–79.
145. AREDS Research Group. Change in area of geographic atrophy in the Age-Related Eye Disease Study: AREDS report no. 26. Arch Ophthalmol 2009; 127(9):1168–74.
146. Sunness JS, Gonzalez-Baron J, Bressler NM, et al. The development of choroidal neovascularization in eyes with geographic atrophy form of age-related macular degeneration. Ophthalmology 1999;106:910–19.
147. Forooghian F, Agron E, Clemons TE, et al for the AREDS Research Group. Visual acuity outcomes after cataract surgery in patients with age-related macular degeneration: Age-Related Eye Disease Study report no. 27. Ophthalmology 2009;116:2093–100.
148. Rosenfeld PJ, Shapiro H, Ehrlich JA, et al, on behalf of the MARINA and ANCHOR Study Groups. Cataract surgery in ranibizumab-treated patients with neovascular age-related macular degeneration from the phase 3 ANCHOR and MARINA Trials. Am J Ophthalmol 2011;152:793–8.
149. Wang JJ, Klein R, Smith W, et al. Cataract surgery and the 5-year incidenceof late-stage age-related maculopathy. Pooled findings form the Beaver Dam and Blue Mountains Eye Studies. Ophthalmology 2003;110:1960–7.
150. Chew EY, Sperduto RD, Milton RC, et al. Risk of advanced age-related macular degeneration after cataract surgery in the Age-Related Eye Disease Study: AREDS report no. 25. Ophthalmology 2009;116:297–303.
151. The Alpha-Tocopherol, Beta Carotene Cancer Prevention StudyGroup. The effect of vitamin E and beta carotene on the incidence of lung cancer and other cancers in male smokers. N Engl J Med 1994;330:1029–35.
152. Omenn GS, Goodman GE, Thornquist MD, et al. Risk factors for lung cancer and for intervention effects in CARET, the Beta-Carotene and Retinol Efficacy Trial. J Natl Cancer Inst 1996;88(21):1550–9.
153. Fine AM, Elman MJ, Ebert JE, et al. Earliest symptoms caused by neovascular membranes in the macula. Arch Ophthalmol 1986;104:513–14.
154. Achard OA, Safran AB, Duret FC, et al. Role of the completion phenomenon in the evaluation of Amsler grid results. Am J Ophthalmol 1995;120:322–9.
155. Schuchard RA. Validity and interpretation of Amsler grid report. Arch Ophthalmol 1993;111:776–80.
156. Goldstein M, Loewenstein A, Barak A, et al. Results of a multicenter clinical trial to evaluate the preferential hyperacuity perimeter for detection of age-related macular degeneration. Retina 2005;25:296–303.
157. Preferential Hyperacuity Perimetry (PHP) Research Group. Preferential Hyperacuity Perimeter (PreView PHPTM) for detecting choroidal neovascularization study. Ophthalmology 2005;112:1758–65.
158. Lai Y, Grattan J, Shi Y, et al. Functional and morphologic benefits in early detection of neovascular age-related macular degeneration using the preferential hyperacuity perimeter. Retina 2011;31(8):1620–6.

Neovascular (Exudative or "Wet") Age-Related Macular Degeneration

Chapter 66

Neil M. Bressler, Susan B. Bressler

EPIDEMIOLOGY

Age-related macular degeneration (AMD) is the major cause of severe visual loss in older adults[1] if left untreated.[2] Most AMD patients have macular drusen or retinal pigment epithelial abnormalities or both.[3] Approximately 10% of AMD patients manifest the neovascular form of the disease.[4] Neovascular AMD includes choroidal neovascularization (CNV) and associated manifestations such as retinal pigment epithelial detachment (PED), retinal pigment epithelial tears, fibrovascular disciform scarring, and vitreous hemorrhage.[3] In the absence of antivascular endothelial growth factor (anti-VEGF) therapy, the vast majority of people with severe vision loss (20/200 or worse in either eye) from AMD have the neovascular form.[4]

RISK FACTORS

The prevalence of AMD-associated vision loss in at least one eye increases with age. For example, AMD was the leading cause of blindness in white (prevalence 2.7 per 1000; 95% CI 1.2–5.4) but not black subjects randomly selected to participate in the Baltimore Eye Survey. In this study, AMD resulting in blindness affected 3% of all white subjects 80 years of age or older.[5]

AMD may be a multifactorial syndrome with different causative factors damaging the macula and resulting in common clinical manifestations that are recognized clinically as AMD. Risk factors implicated in clinical and laboratory studies include drusen, visible (but not ultraviolet) injury, micronutrient deficiency as measured in blood serum levels or by dietary history, cigarette smoking, family history (genetic predisposition[6]), and cardiovascular risk factors (including systemic hypertension).[7,8] More detailed information regarding the epidemiology of AMD is reviewed in Chapter 63 (Epidemiology and risk factors for age-related macular degeneration).

CLINICAL (INCLUDING BIOMICROSCOPIC) PRESENTATION

Overview

Blurred vision and distortion, especially distorted near vision, are the symptoms most patients with CNV notice first.[3,9] Patients also may complain of decreased vision, micropsia, metamorphopsia, or a scotoma; however, many times they volunteer no symptoms or report only vague visual complaints.[8] Symptoms generally arise from subretinal fluid, intraretinal fluid, blood, or destruction of photoreceptors and the retinal pigment epithelium (RPE) by fibrous or fibrovascular tissue.[10-13] In some cases, areas of distortion or scotoma can be mapped out on an Amsler grid. Visual acuity, although frequently decreased, may not always be affected. Functional vision generally declines in accordance with Snellen visual acuity. Thus patients with poor Snellen acuity generally report decreased ability to perform functional tasks (e.g., face recognition, telling time) with the affected eye.[14]

In some patients with AMD, CNV may appear as a gray–green elevation of tissue deep to the retina with overlying detachment of the neurosensory retina (Fig. 66.1). The gray–green color may arise from hyperplastic RPE in response to the CNV,[15] as has typically been seen in patients, usually younger individuals, with ocular histoplasmosis syndrome (OHS), pathologic myopia, and other conditions complicated by CNV. This gray–green appearance is not always present in older individuals with AMD. Often, the presence of blood or lipid or a sensory retinal detachment in an elderly patient with vision loss indicates the presence of CNV. The CNV capillary network may become more apparent when the overlying RPE has atrophied. Occasionally, a shallow neurosensory detachment may be the only presenting sign of underlying CNV. Elevated RPE, also termed a pigment epithelial detachment (PED), even without overlying subretinal

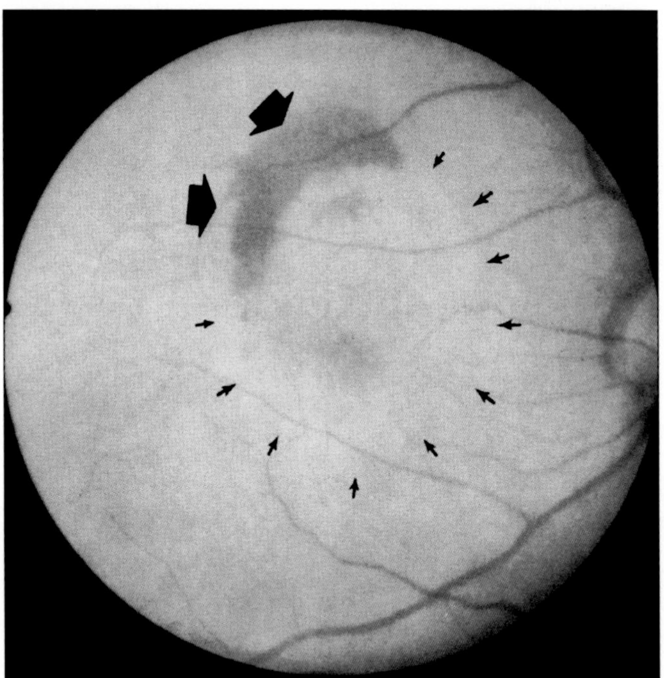

Fig. 66.1 Fundus photograph of choroidal neovascularization. Note area of hemorrhage (large arrows), as well as neurosensory retinal detachment (small arrows). (Reproduced with permission from Elman MJ. Age-related macular degeneration. Int Ophthalmol Clin 1986;26: 117–44.)

fluid, may also suggest the presence of CNV to be identified subsequently by a fluorescein angiogram. RPE folds beneath a shallow RPE elevation usually indicate the presence of CNV.[16] These subtle clinical findings can easily be missed without careful stereoscopic slit-lamp biomicroscopic examination, facilitated with a contact lens.

Retinal pigment epithelial detachments

Retinal PEDs appear clinically as sharply demarcated, dome-shaped elevations of the RPE (Fig. 66.2). They usually transilluminate if they are filled with serous fluid only. Often, there is accompanying RPE atrophy and "pigment figure" formation. Pigment figures, a reticulated pattern of increased pigmentation extending radially over the PED, indicate chronicity of disease and probably have no prognostic significance. Although an overlying sensory retinal detachment may be a clue to the presence of CNV beneath a PED,[17] sometimes a shallow neurosensory detachment may occur as a result of breakdown of the physiologic RPE pump or from disruption of the tight junctions between adjacent RPE cells in the absence of CNV. Unlike a PED, the borders of a neurosensory detachment are not sharply demarcated. The presence of a PED may or may not be a feature of CNV. The fluorescein angiographic pattern (see subsequent discussion) can differentiate a drusenoid PED,[18] which does not have CNV, from a fibrovascular PED, which is a form of occult CNV,[19] as well as from a serous PED, which may or may not overlie an area with CNV.[19] Several clinical signs suggest the presence of CNV underlying an area of PED identified biomicroscopically, including overlying sensory retinal detachment and lipid, blood, and chorioretinal folds radiating from the PED.[3] Blood within or surrounding a PED implies the presence of CNV (Fig. 66.3). When confined to the sub-RPE space, the blood may appear as a discretely elevated, green or dark-red mound. The hemorrhage can dissect through the RPE into the subsensory retinal space or into the retina. Rarely, blood may pass through the retina into the vitreous cavity, causing extensive vitreous hemorrhage. The Submacular Surgery Trials (SST) Research Group suggested that this event was more likely in predominantly hemorrhagic lesions that were large (>12 disc areas) or associated with very poor visual acuity (worse than 20/1280 Snellen equivalent).[20]

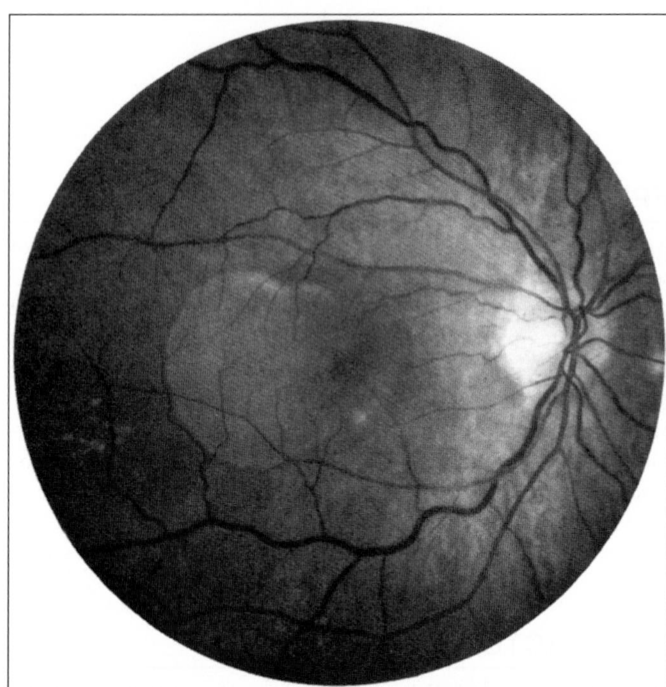

Fig. 66.2 Fundus photograph in which a round, sharply demarcated mound indicates the detached retinal pigment epithelium. (Reproduced with permission from Bressler NM, Bressler SB, Fine SL. Age-related macular degeneration. Surv Ophthalmol 1988;32:375–413.)

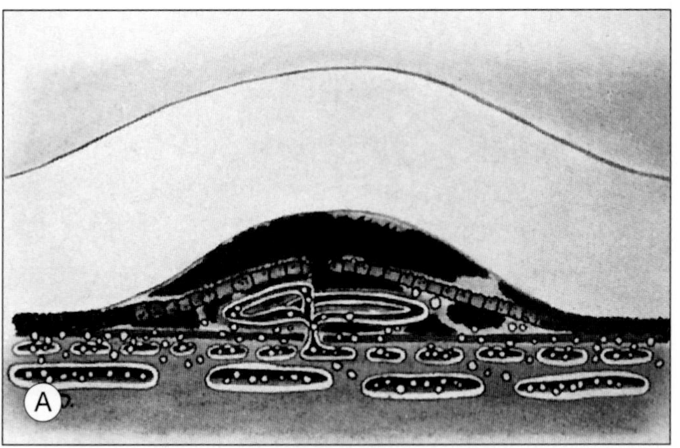

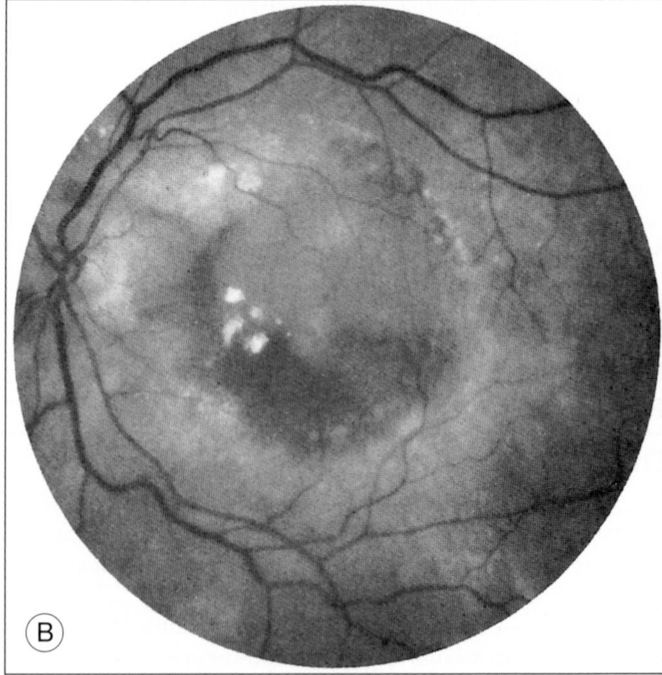

Fig. 66.3 Hemorrhagic retinal pigment epithelial detachment. (A) Sketch of hemorrhagic detachment in which the blood has also dissected underneath the sensory retina. (B) Fundus photograph of hemorrhagic pigment epithelial detachment. (Reproduced with permission from Bressler NM, Bressler SB, Fine SL. Age-related macular degeneration. Surv Ophthalmol 1988;32:375–413.)

Breakthrough vitreous hemorrhage

In most cases of neovascular AMD, the peripheral visual field remains unaffected. If bleeding breaks through the retina into the vitreous cavity, however, patients may complain of severe and sudden visual loss involving the peripheral visual field, as well as the central field. This may be accompanied by pain believed to result from stretching of the nerve fibers within the choroid.[21]

Massive subretinal hemorrhage

Massive subretinal hemorrhage is an unusual complication of neovascular AMD. If – extremely rarely – total hemorrhagic retinal detachment occurs, secondary angle closure glaucoma may develop. These patients may report sudden visual loss followed by pain.[22] Anticoagulation therapy may contribute to massive subretinal hemorrhage. In one report,[23] 19% of AMD patients with massive subretinal hemorrhage were taking sodium warfarin or aspirin. Although sodium warfarin therapy may have contributed to the massive subretinal hemorrhage, the antiplatelet therapy was likely a chance association because several Macular Photocoagulation Study (MPS) reports did not observe any increased risk of hemorrhage associated with the use of aspirin.[24–26] Furthermore, comparing baseline characteristics in study participants with predominantly choroidal neovascular lesions in the SST Group N Trial[27] with participants with predominantly hemorrhagic lesions,[20] no difference in use of aspirin was detected. Recent epidemiology studies found an association of aspirin use with neovascular AMD, but this finding does not necessarily confirm or refute an association of aspirin with the development of predominantly hemorrhagic lesions or massive subretinal hemorrhages.[28]

We believe the strongest evidence suggests that patients with AMD who need to follow a regimen of aspirin therapy should continue to do so without unnecessary fear they will increase their risk of vitreous hemorrhage.

Retinal pigment epithelial tears

RPE dehiscence or tears have been described as a complication associated with CNV, often in an eye with a serous or fibrovascular PED, and secondary to or unassociated with laser photocoagulation.[29–33] One report[34] suggested that CNV underlying a detached RPE can contribute to RPE tear formation. Tears occur at the junction of attached and detached RPE, perhaps when the PED can no longer resist the stretching forces from the fluid in the sub-RPE space emanating from the underlying occult CNV (Fig. 66.4) or from the contractile forces of the underlying fibrovascular tissue that may be intimately associated or entwined with the overlying RPE. When the RPE tears, the free edge of the RPE retracts and rolls toward the mound of fibrovascular tissue. Acutely, a serous detachment of the sensory retina may be caused by the leaking of fluid from the exposed choriocapillaris.[18] This is rarely seen after a few days following the tear.

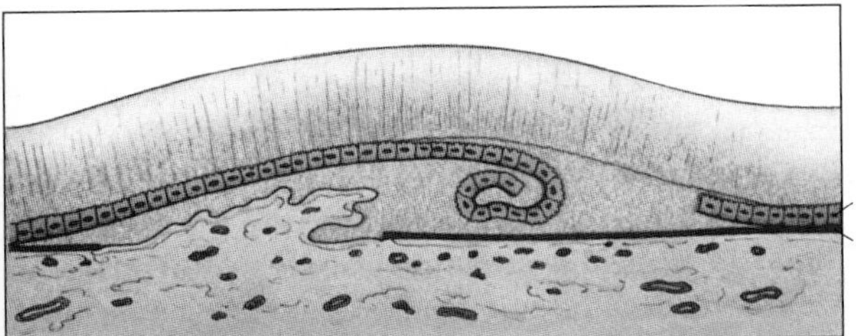

Fig. 66.4 Sketch of tear or rip of the retinal pigment epithelium (RPE), showing contracted RPE tear. Cc + C, choriocapillaris and choroid. (Reproduced with permission from Bressler NM, Bressler SB, Fine SL. Age-related macular degeneration. Surv Ophthalmol 1988;32:375–413.)

Disciform scars

Histologically, CNV usually is accompanied by fibrous tissue, even when no fibrous tissue is readily apparent on initial presentation to an ophthalmologist.[10,35,36] This fibrous tissue may be accompanied by CNV (fibrovascular tissue) or not (fibroglial tissue).[10] The fibrous tissue complex may be beneath the RPE (usually proliferating within the inner aspect of an abnormally thickened Bruch's membrane), and has been termed type I, or between the RPE and the photoreceptors, termed type II.[34] While some people speculate that these types differentiate classic CNV from occult CNV,[37,38] there is little evidence to support that these histologic types are *always* differentiated by histopathologic correlation.[39] Often, over time, the plane of the RPE is destroyed by the fibrovascular or fibroglial tissue, so the location of the CNV with respect to the RPE can no longer be identified readily. When the fibrous tissue becomes apparent clinically, the CNV and fibrous tissue complex may be termed a disciform scar.

Clinically, disciform lesions may vary in color, although typically they appear white to yellow. Hyperpigmented areas may be present depending on the degree of RPE hyperplasia within the scar tissue. Disciform fibrovascular scars may continue to grow, with neovascularization recurring along the edge, invading previously unaffected areas (Fig. 66.5). Varying degrees of subretinal hemorrhage and lipid may overlie or surround the scar. Occasionally, fibrovascular scars may precipitate massive transudation of fluid, mimicking a retinal detachment. The scars may be accompanied by massive lipid, as might be seen in retinal telangiectasis from Coats disease, and hence are sometimes called a "senile Coats response" in AMD. Disciform scars occasionally masquerade as choroidal tumors when much pigment is seen.[34] Not infrequently, anastomoses are observed between the retina and the fibrovascular tissue.[13] As a rule, most fibrovascular scars involve the fovea and cause severe visual loss. However, surviving islands of intact photoreceptor cells noted histologically may explain the better visual performance than would be predicted from the morphologic appearance alone in some scars. Reading vision, rarely better than 20/200, becomes severely compromised in most cases with extensive scars.

FLUORESCEIN ANGIOGRAPHIC FEATURES

Overview

Whenever one suspects CNV for which treatment might be indicated, one should consider obtaining stereoscopic fluorescein angiography promptly (Fig. 66.6), even in an era of optical coherence tomography (OCT). The treating ophthalmologist is about to embark on a recommendation for treatment involving drugs which carry risks, potentially large expenses, and requiring many years of follow-up. Although the clinical picture may be "obviously" CNV, other lesions masquerading for CNV can exist (see below) having a fluorescein angiogram at the time of diagnosis reduces the possibility that an error in diagnosis will be made. In addition, fluorescein angiography frequently allows

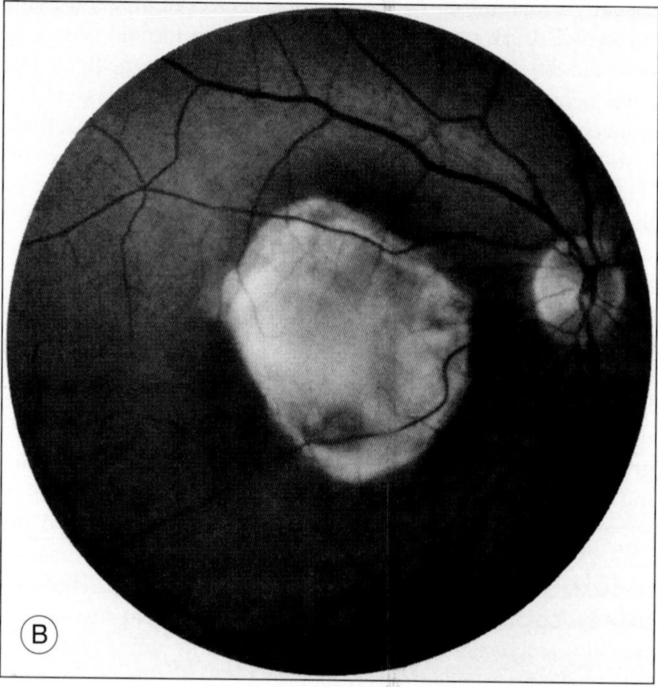

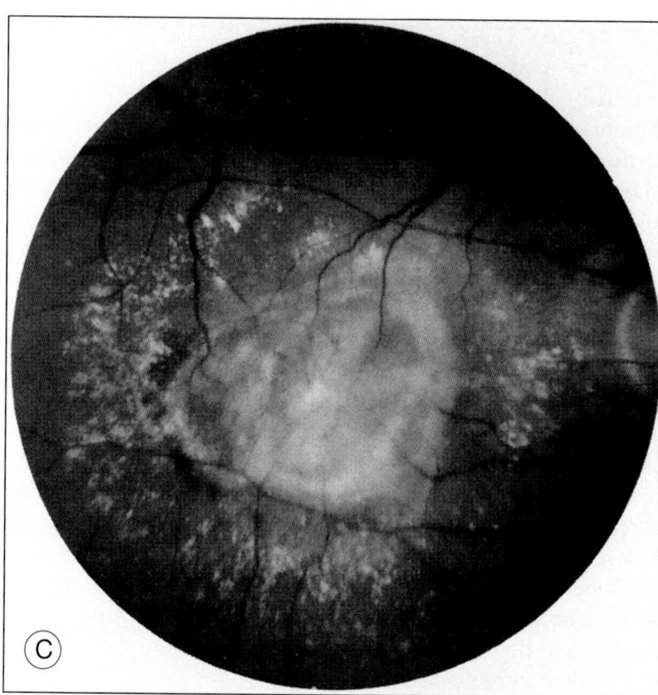

Fig. 66.5 Disciform scar. (A) Sketch demonstrating that most of the sensory retina, pigment epithelium, and inner choroid has been replaced by a fibrovascular scar. (B) Fundus photograph of a disciform scar after choroidal neovascularization. (C) Fundus photograph of a disciform scar in which continued subretinal fluid and lipid from persistent choroidal neovascularization at the periphery of the fibrous tissue can be seen. (Reproduced with permission from Bressler NM, Bressler SB, Fine SL. Age-related macular degeneration. Surv Ophthalmol 1988;32:375–413.)

one to determine the pattern (classic or occult), boundaries (well defined or poorly defined), composition (e.g., predominantly CNV, predominantly classic CNV, predominantly CNV with a minimally classic composition, predominantly CNV with an occult with no classic composition, predominantly hemorrhagic), and location of the neovascular lesions with respect to the geometric center of the foveal avascular zone (FAZ). Although many physicians no longer refer to CNV composition, entry criteria for many and even most of the treatment trials cited later in this chapter relied in part on lesion composition. If one chooses to treat only patients who would have been eligible for, e.g., the MARINA trial, baseline angiography is necessary. High-quality stereoscopic fluorescein angiograms, together with meticulous slit-lamp biomicroscopic examination (ideally with a contact lens examination using topical anesthesia and hard contact lens wetting solution to avoid degradation of any subsequent image acquisition that might occur if an ophthalmic demulcent is used), facilitate detecting obvious and subtle features of CNV on angiography.[14,19,40] It should be noted that the descriptive terms below refer to patterns of fluorescence on fluorescein angiography that have been shown to be reliable and reproducible in multicenter clinical trials,[19,41,42] and in practice, and are not related to terms based on other imaging such as OCT, indocyanine green angiography, histopathology, or immunohistochemistry.

Classic choroidal neovascularization

The fluorescein angiographic appearance of classic CNV consists of a discrete, well-demarcated focal area of hyperfluorescence that can be discerned in the early phases of the angiogram, sometimes before dye has completely filled the retinal vessels during choroidal filling.[19,41,42] Although fluorescein can occasionally be observed within the actual capillary network of CNV in the early phase of the angiogram (Fig. 66.7A), the ability to visualize the appearance of actual new vessels is not needed to diagnose classic CNV and is not a specific feature of classic versus occult CNV.[19,41–43] Since both classic and occult patterns of CNV contain new vessels histologically, early-phase angiography

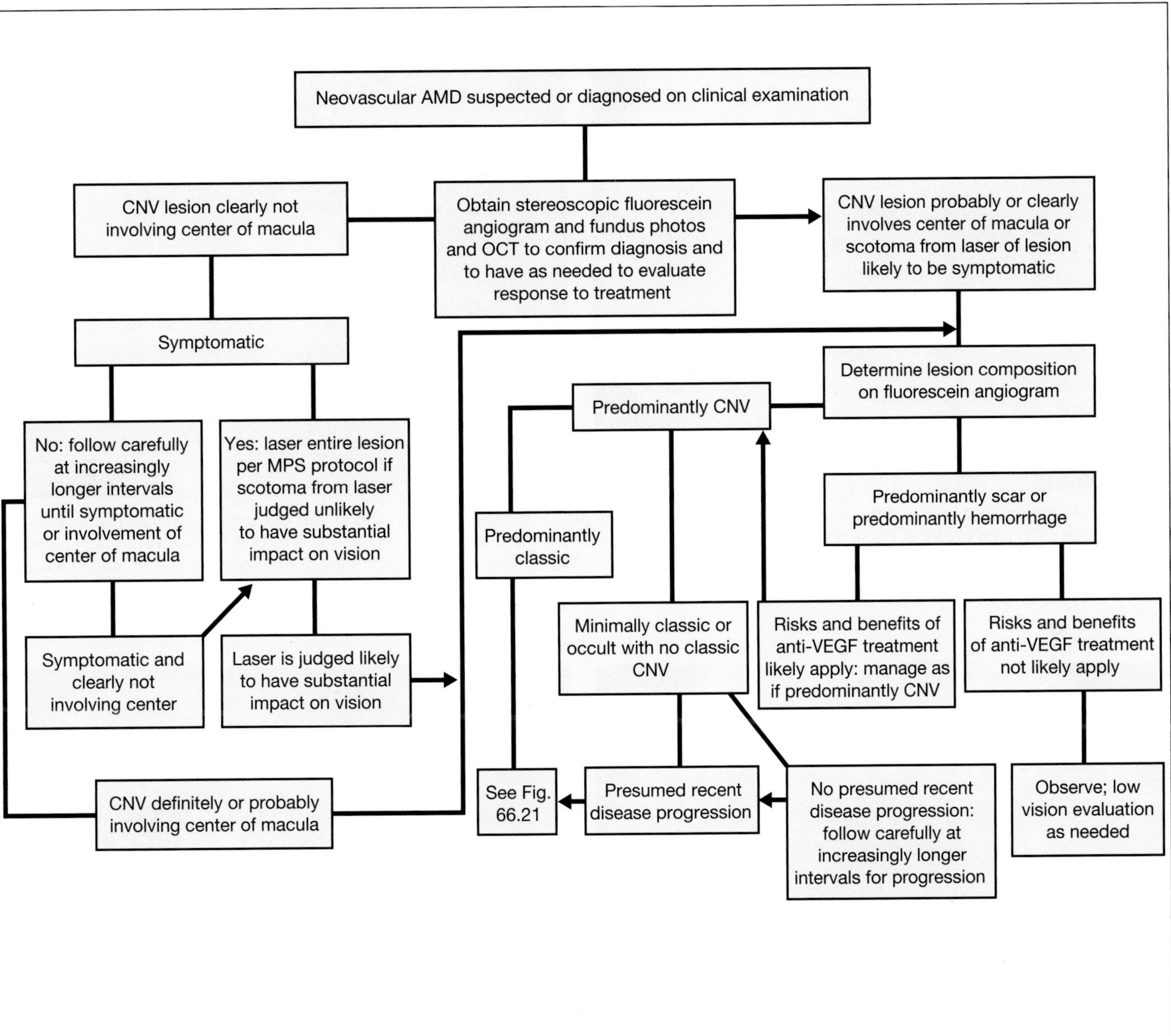

Fig. 66.6 Algorithm for management of neovascular age-related macular degeneration suspected or diagnosed on clinical examination. AMD, age-related macular degeneration; CNV, choroidal neovascularization; OCT, optical coherence tomography; MPS, Macular Photocoagulation Study; VEGF, vascular endothelial growth factor. (© Neil M. Bressler, MD, Johns Hopkins University, 2011.)

may be able to demonstrate these vessels in either pattern. As the angiogram is evaluated within the area of classic CNV, hyperfluorescence increases in intensity and extends beyond the boundaries of the hyperfluorescent area identified in earlier phases of the angiogram through mid- and late-phase frames. Fluorescein may also pool in subsensory retinal fluid overlying the classic CNV (Fig. 66.7B), best seen when visualizing early- and late-phase frames of classic CNV on stereoscopic images. This presentation of classic CNV is in contrast to the appearance of an area of RPE atrophy on fluorescein angiography. RPE atrophy, like classic CNV, is hyperfluorescent during the early phase of the angiogram (Fig. 66.8A). The increased fluorescence through the atrophic patch results from increased transmission of fluorescein through an overlying RPE with a reduced amount of pigment that normally obscures the choroidal blush (sometimes termed a window, or transmission, defect). Unlike the increase in extent and intensity of hyperfluorescence due to leakage from the fluorescence of classic CNV, RPE atrophy does not show leakage of fluorescein at its boundaries through the mid- and late-phase frames. The fluorescence fades after several minutes (Fig. 66.8B), without leakage of fluorescein beyond the boundaries of hyperfluorescence defined in the early stages. Two other lesions in AMD that may show an area of discrete hyperfluorescence in the early phase of the angiogram include a serous PED and a rip or tear of the RPE (angiographic features that differentiate these abnormalities from classic CNV are discussed later). Neither one of these latter abnormalities should show fluorescein leakage in later phases of the angiogram at the boundary of the hyperfluorescence noted in earlier phases.

Occult choroidal neovascularization

Occult CNV refers to two hyperfluorescent patterns on fluorescein angiography.[19,41,42] The first pattern, termed a fibrovascular pigment epithelial detachment (FVPED), is best appreciated with stereoscopic views, usually at approximately 1–2 min after dye injection. It appears as an irregular elevation of the RPE,

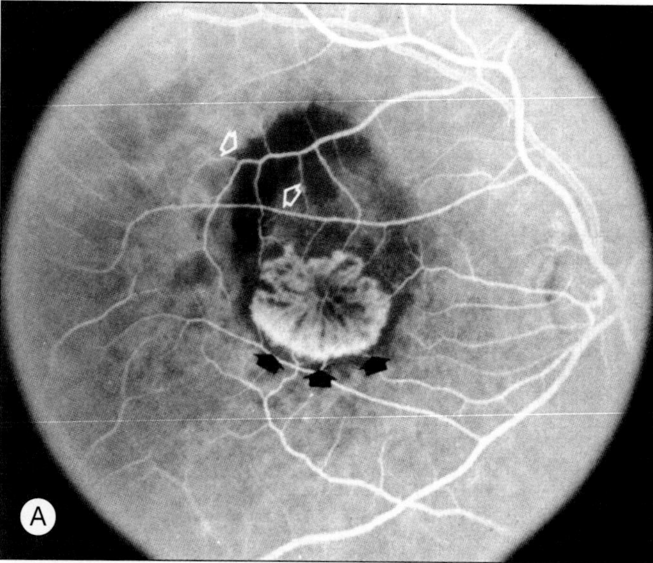

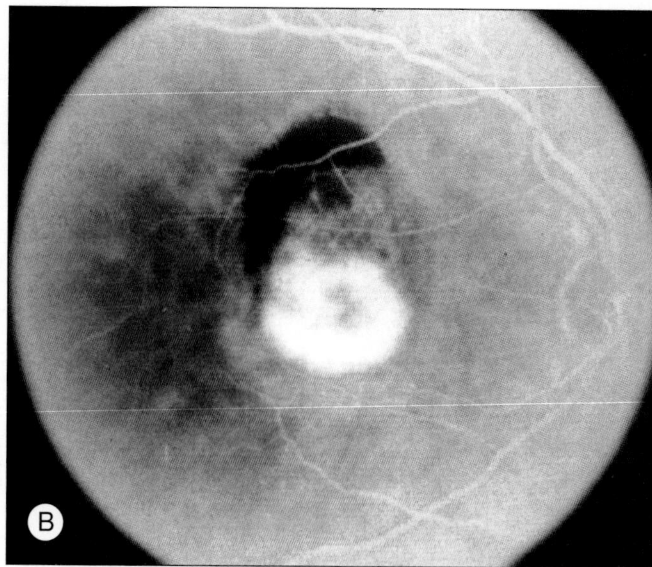

Fig. 66.7 (A) Early transit phase of fluorescein angiogram showing fine net of vessels corresponding to part of choroidal neovascular lesion (black arrows). (B) Late phase of the fluorescein angiogram, demonstrating an increase in the degree and size of fluorescence. In both panels (A) and (B) there is blocked fluorescence resulting from overlying hemorrhage (white arrows). (Reproduced with permission from Elman MJ. Age-related macular degeneration. Int Ophthalmol Clin 1986;26:117–44.)

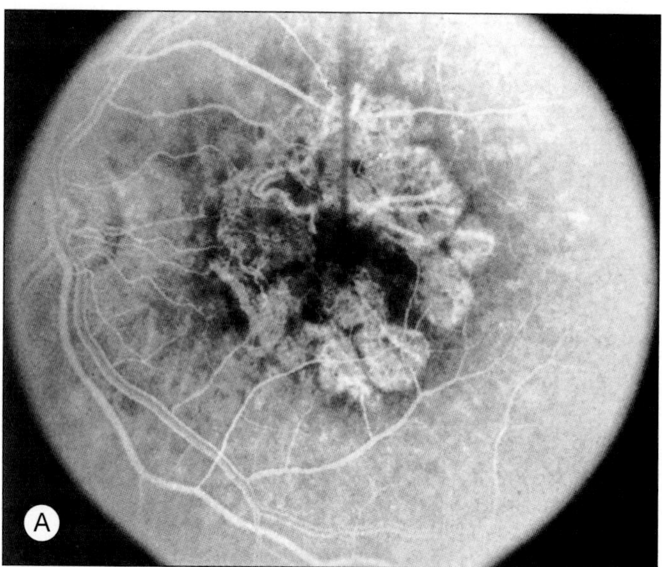

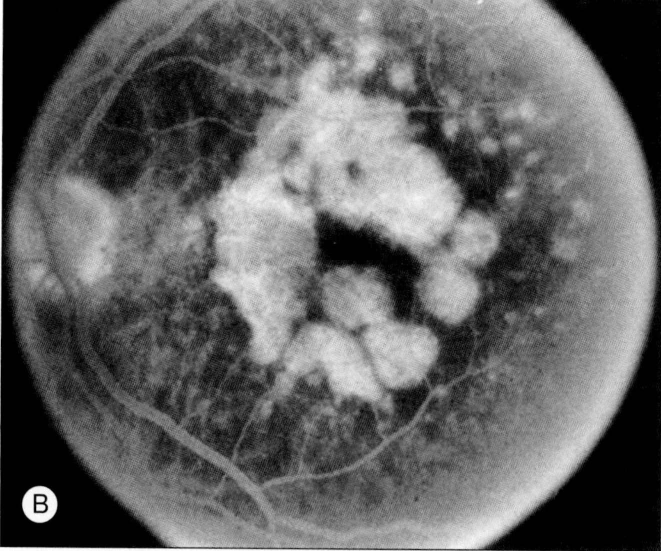

Fig. 66.8 (A) Transit phase of fluorescein angiogram, showing hyperfluorescence corresponding to atrophic zones of the retinal pigment epithelium (transmission, or window, defect) and easily visualized choroidal vessels (too large to be vessels of choroidal neovascularization). (B) Hypofluorescence does not increase in size and fades with the later phases of the angiogram. This is in contrast to the pattern seen in choroidal neovascularization (Fig. 66.5). (Reproduced with permission from Elman MJ. Age-related macular degeneration. Int Ophthalmol Clin 1986;26:117–44.)

often stippled with hyperfluorescent dots (Fig. 66.9). The boundaries may or may not show leakage in the late-phase frames as fluorescein collects within the fibrous tissue or pools in the subretinal space overlying the FVPED. The exact boundaries of a FVPED can usually be determined most accurately only when fluorescence sharply outlines the elevated RPE. The amount of elevation depends on the quality of the stereoscopic photographs and the thickness of the fibrovascular tissue. Stereoscopic pairs of fluorescein angiogram frames can sometimes facilitate identification of the boundaries of the elevated RPE, although not always, as the elevation can slope gradually down to the normal level of the RPE. The second pattern, late leakage of an undetermined source (Fig. 66.10), refers to late choroidal-based leakage in which there is no clearly identifiable classic CNV or FVPED in the early or mid-phase of the angiogram to account for an area of leakage in the late phase. Often this pattern of occult CNV can appear as speckled hyperfluorescence with pooling of dye in the subretinal space overlying the speckles. Usually the boundaries of this type of CNV cannot be determined precisely, and a lesion with this component should not be considered for photocoagulation treatment if it contributes to poorly demarcated boundaries of the lesion.

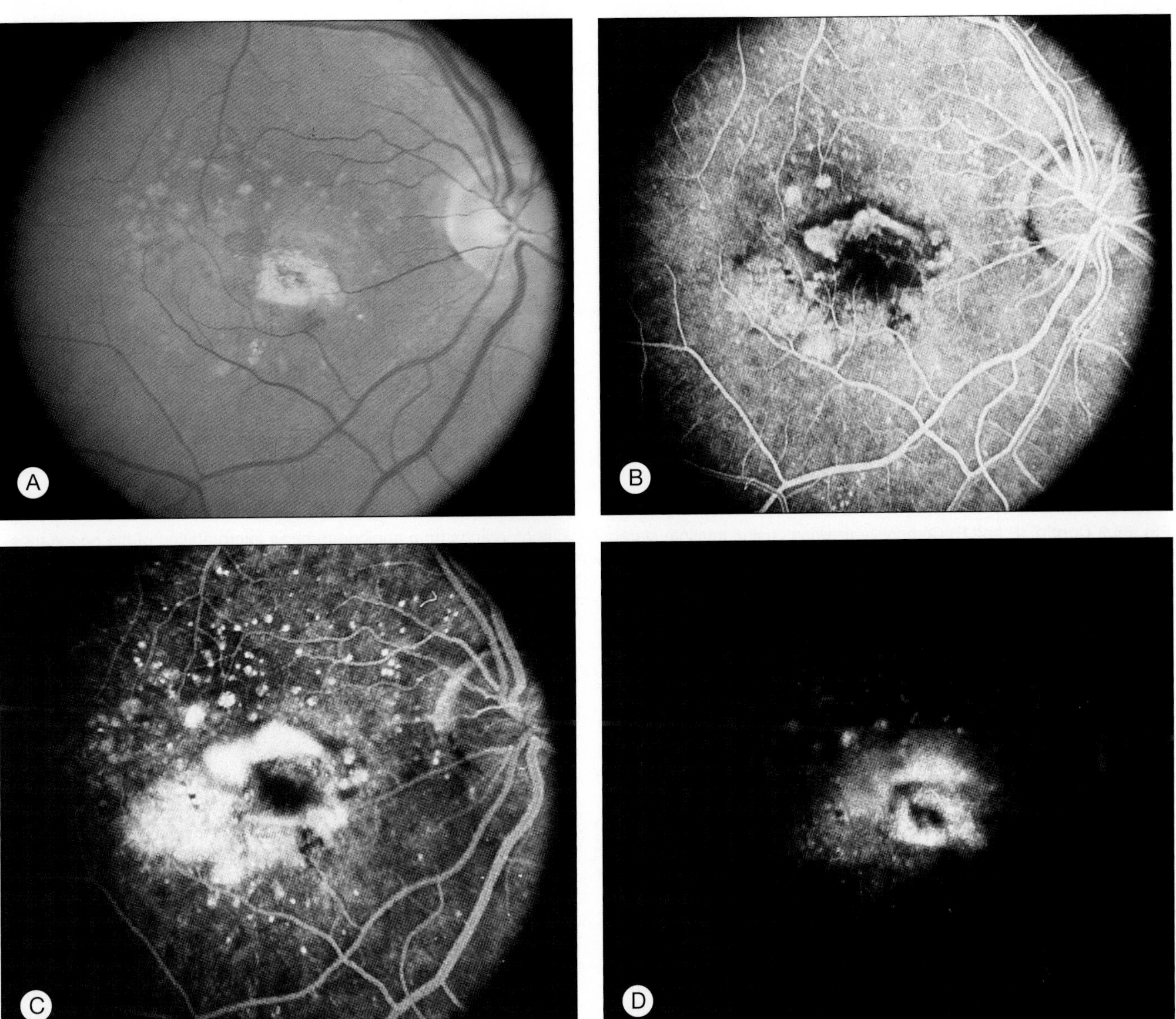

Fig. 66.9 Classic and occult choroidal neovascularization (CNV) with well-demarcated borders. (A) Color photograph shows scar from prior photocoagulation surrounded by several clues to suggest recurrent CNV, including subretinal hemorrhage, subretinal lipid, irregular elevation of retinal pigment epithelium (RPE) below the area of prior laser treatment, and overlying subretinal fluid. (B) Early phase of fluorescein angiogram shows area of classic CNV, scar from prior laser treatment, and irregular elevation of RPE with stippled hyperfluorescence representing fibrovascular pigment epithelial detachment (PED) inferior and temporal to the scar. (C) Stereoscopic photograph of the same eye 1 min after fluorescein injection. Note fluorescein leakage already apparent from classic CNV and increased intensity of stippled hyperfluorescence corresponding to fibrovascular PED. The boundaries of the fibrovascular PED remain well demarcated. (D) Angiogram taken 10 min after fluorescein injection shows persistence of fluorescein staining and leakage within a sensory retinal detachment overlying the lesion. It is difficult to determine the precise demarcation of fluorescence outlining the elevated RPE from these photographs alone. Although a fairly well-demarcated border can be seen in (C), the intensity of fluorescence at the boundary of elevated RPE is quite irregular in these late-phase photographs, with some areas fading relative to fluorescence of remaining areas of elevated RPE (D).

Continued

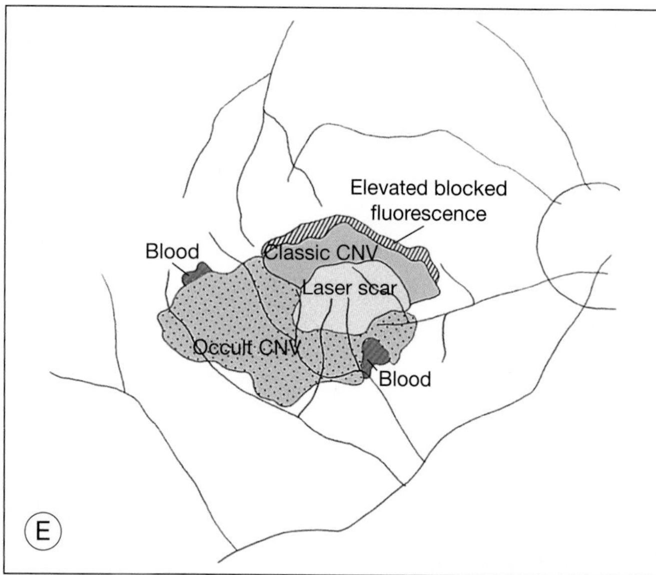

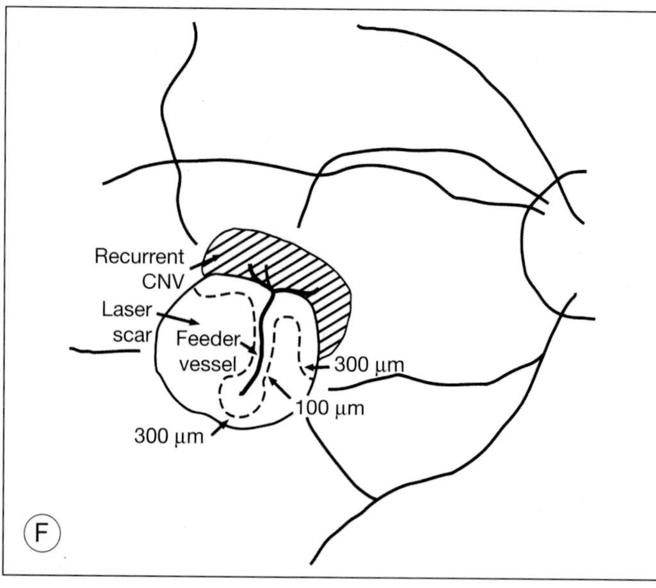

Fig. 66.9 Cont'd (E and F) Composite drawings using multiple stereoscopic photographs from angiogram show interpretation of the boundaries of the lesion. At each clock-hour, the boundary of the lesion is clearly demarcated; the lesion included classic CNV, which occupies the foveal center. (Reproduced with permission from Macular Photocoagulation Study Group. Subfoveal neovascular lesions in age-related macular degeneration: guidelines for evaluation and treatment in the Macular Photocoagulation Study. Arch Ophthalmol 1991;109:1242–57.)

Other terms relevant to interpreting fluorescein angiography of choroidal neovascularization

The terms lesion component versus lesion are important to differentiate in the discussion of fluorescein interpretation and treatment of CNV.[19,41,42] Lesion component is classic or occult CNV or any of four angiographic features that could obscure the boundaries of classic or occult CNV. These four features include: (1) blood that is visible on color fundus photographs and thick enough to obscure the normal choroidal fluorescence; (2) hypofluorescence due to hyperplastic pigment or fibrous tissue, or blood not visible on color fundus photographs; (3) a serous detachment of the RPE (Fig. 66.11); and (4) scar from CNV which either stains or blocks fluorescence (depending on the extent of RPE within the scar). The first two of these four features block the angiographic view of the choroid, making it impossible to determine whether CNV is located in the area of this component. The bright, reasonably uniform, early hyperfluorescence associated with a serous detachment of the RPE (described later) may obscure hyperfluorescence from classic or occult CNV and therefore interfere with the ability to judge whether CNV extends under the area of the serous detachment. The term lesion, in contrast, refers to the entire complex of lesion components.

The terms well-defined (synonymous with well-demarcated) and poorly defined (synonymous with poorly demarcated or ill-defined) refer to a description of the boundaries of the entire lesion (not of individual lesion components). In a well-defined lesion, the entire boundary for 360 degrees is well demarcated (for example, Figs 66.9, 66.12, 66.13). If the entire boundary is not well demarcated for 360 degrees, then the lesion is poorly defined (for example, Fig. 61.9). Thus the terms well-defined and classic should not be used interchangeably, nor should poorly defined and occult. Well-defined and poorly defined describe lesion boundaries (for a lesion that may be composed of classic CNV, or occult CNV, or both). Classic and occult CNV refer to patterns of fluorescence. In addition, the term poorly defined should not be used to describe situations in which blood blocks the ability to see fluorescence from CNV,[19,41,42] even though earlier publications had alluded to descriptions incorporating this possibility.[44]

The term predominantly CNV indicates that at least 50% of the lesion is composed of either classic CNV or occult CNV, or both, while the term predominantly hemorrhagic indicates that at least 50% of the lesion is composed of hemorrhage.[41,42] These terms are critical in the management of AMD (Fig. 66.14), since treatments for CNV with anti-VEGF therapy, or less frequently, with laser photocoagulation, photodynamic therapy (PDT), or surgery, have been tested only in lesions that are predominantly CNV or predominantly hemorrhagic. After determining whether a lesion's composition is predominantly CNV, it should be determined whether the lesion is predominantly classic, rather than minimally classic or occult with no classic. If predominantly classic, then treatment could be considered with or without evidence of presumed recent disease progression (defined as evidence of blood associated with CNV, or definite visual acuity loss within 3 months, or definite growth of the lesion within 3 months). If minimally classic or occult with no classic, treatment has been shown to be beneficial compared with no treatment only with evidence of presumed recent disease progression, although a therapeutic trial of anti-VEGF therapy might be considered if visual acuity loss already had occurred and one believed that visual acuity improvement might occur with anti-VEGF therapy because of the presence of intraretinal or subretinal fluid judged to be contributing to visual acuity loss and judged likely to resolve with visual acuity improvement following initiation of anti-VEGF therapy.

Retinal pigment epithelium detachments in age-related macular degeneration

Various changes in an eye with AMD may result in elevation or detachment of the RPE, as seen on stereoscopic biomicroscopic or angiographic evaluation. The term RPE detachment or retinal

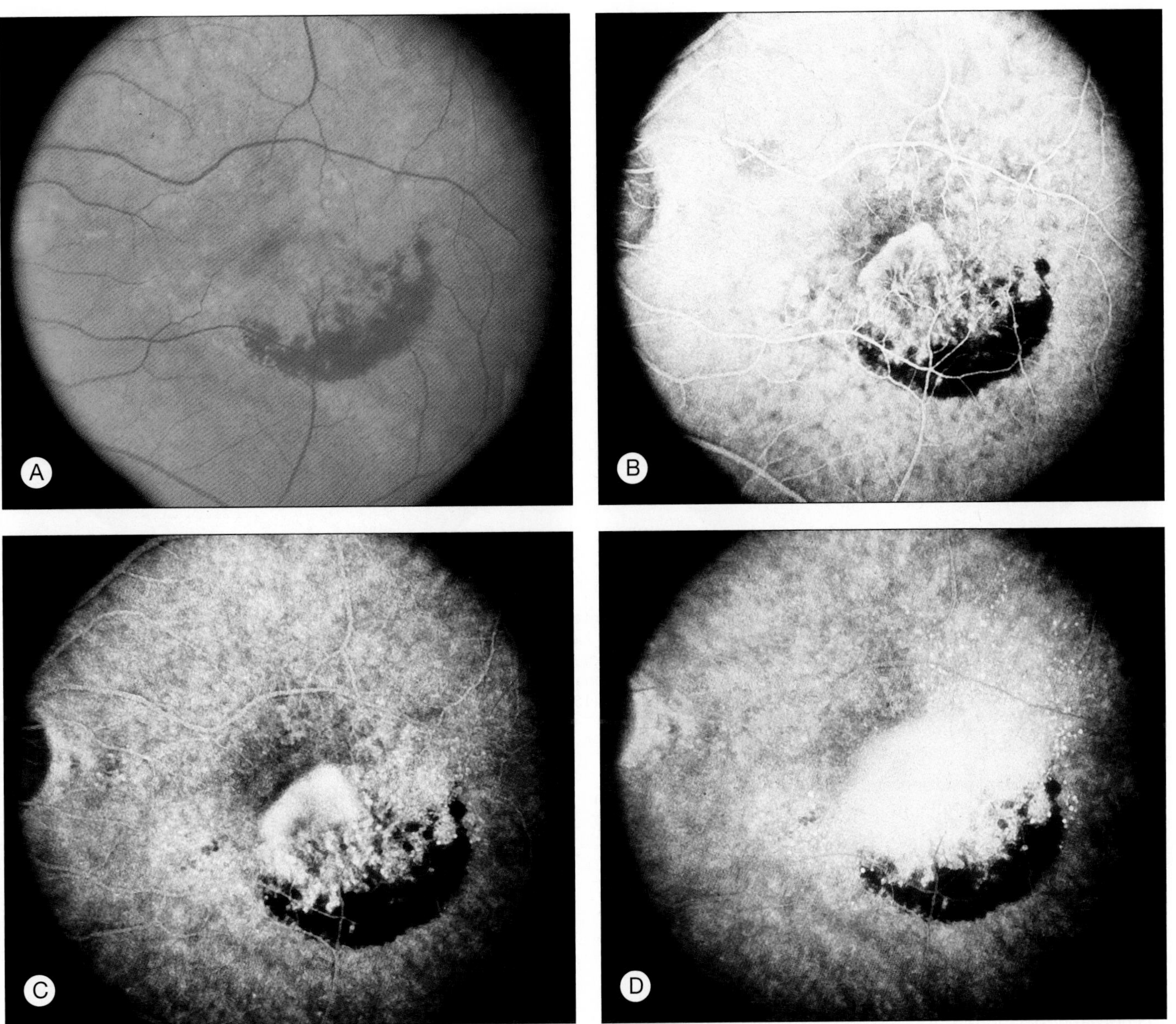

Fig. 66.10 Occult choroidal neovascularization (CNV) with poorly demarcated boundaries accompanied by classic CNV. (A) Subretinal fluid and hemorrhage in eye with drusen. (B) Early phase of fluorescein angiogram shows both feeder vessels to classic CNV and fibrovascular pigment epithelial detachment (PED). Blocked fluorescence due to thick blood obscures inferior boundary of occult CNV. (C) Mid-phase stereoscopic photographs of angiogram show leakage from classic CNV. (D) Late phase of angiogram shows other areas of late leakage of undetermined source with no discernible, discrete, well-demarcated area of hyperfluorescence from classic CNV or fibrovascular PED detectable in early or mid-phase frames of angiogram that might be considered a source of late leakage. (Reproduced with permission from Macular Photocoagulation Study Group. Subfoveal neovascular lesions in age-related macular degeneration: guidelines for evaluation and treatment in the Macular Photocoagulation Study. Arch Ophthalmol 1991;109:1242–57.)

pigment epithelial detachment (retinal PED) secondary to AMD in the ophthalmic literature remains confusing because various RPE detachments may have quite different compositions, fluorescein angiographic appearances, prognoses, and management. Fortunately, these various RPE detachments can usually be differentiated on the basis of fluorescein angiographic patterns of fluorescence. The patterns include the following: (1) fibrovascular PEDs,[19] which are a subset of occult CNV (see Figs 66.9 and 66.10); (2) serous detachments of the RPE[45] (see Fig. 66.11); (3) hemorrhagic detachments of the RPE, in which blood from a choroidal neovascular lesion is noted beneath or exterior to the RPE (see Fig. 66.3); and (4) drusenoid RPE detachments,[9] in which large areas of confluent, soft drusen are noted. It is potentially difficult to differentiate between fibrovascular PEDs and serous PEDs. Using descriptions from the MPS Group, fibrovascular PEDs (as a subset of occult CNV) have been distinguished from a typical serous detachment of the RPE, in that the former do not have uniform, bright hyperfluorescence in the early phase. Instead, they show a stippled fluorescence along the surface of the RPE by the middle phase of the angiogram and may show pooling of dye in the overlying subsensory retinal space in the late phase (see Fig. 66.9). Serous PEDs show uniform, bright hyperfluorescence in the early phase, with a smooth contour to the RPE by the middle phase, and little, if any, leakage at the borders of the PED by the late phase (see Fig. 66.11). The fluorescent pattern of a serous PED obscures the ability to

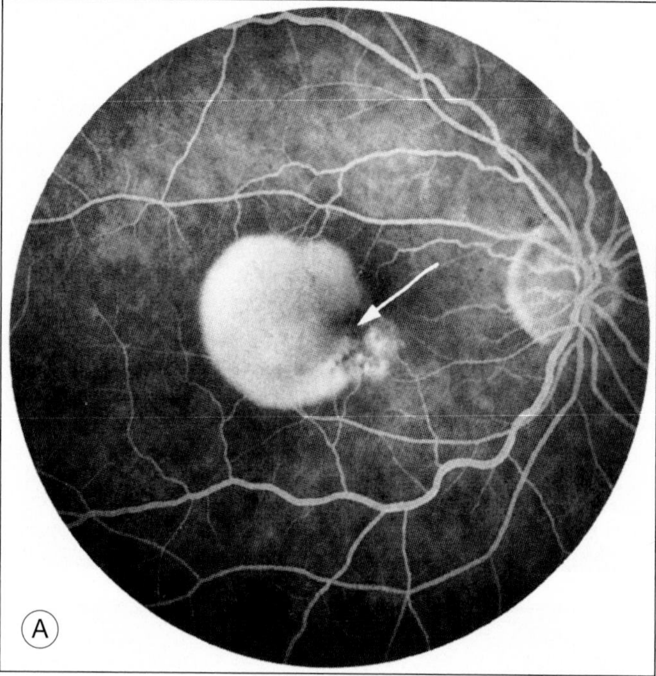

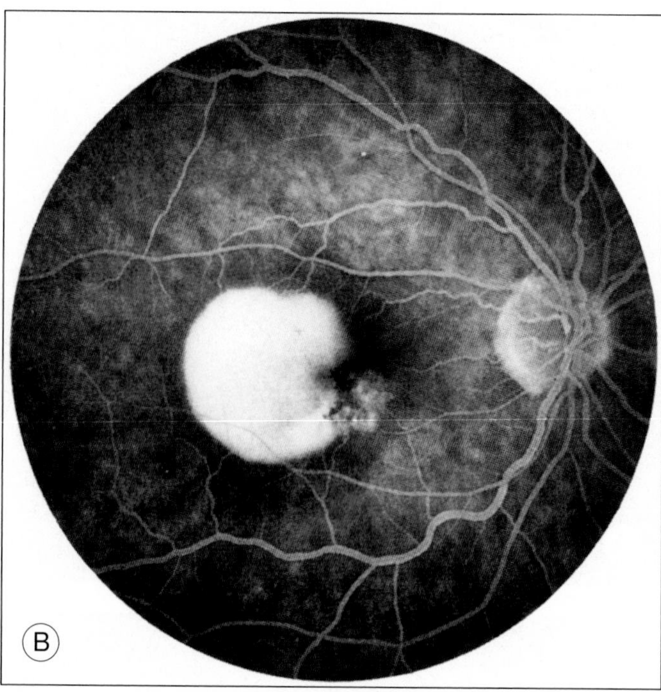

Fig. 66.11 Fluorescein angiogram of serous retinal pigment epithelial detachment. (A) Early transit phase of a fluorescein angiogram demonstrates uniform fluorescence under the dome of the detachment. Note the deformation of the otherwise round detachment by a notch of the hyperfluorescence (arrow). (B) Later phase of the fluorescein angiogram demonstrates persistent hyperfluorescence that does not extend beyond the margins of the hyperfluorescence seen in the early transit phase. (Reproduced with permission from Bressler NM, Bressler SB, Fine SL. Age-related macular degeneration. Surv Ophthalmol 1988;32:375–413.)

determine whether classic or occult CNV exists within or beneath the area of the serous PED. In contrast, a fibrovascular PED is an area of occult CNV.

A hemorrhagic detachment of the RPE will block choroidal fluorescence because of the mound-like collection of blood beneath the RPE (see Fig. 66.3). Occasionally a hemorrhagic detachment of the RPE may be mistaken for a choroidal melanoma, but usually hemorrhagic detachments of the RPE do not demonstrate low internal reflectivity, as is seen characteristically in choroidal melanomas.

One other feature of AMD that appears as an elevated or detached RPE is a drusenoid RPE detachment,[18] which represents extensive areas of large, confluent drusen. Drusenoid RPE detachments can be distinguished from serous detachments of the RPE in that drusenoid RPE detachments fluoresce faintly during the transit and do not progress to bright hyperfluorescence in the late phase of the angiogram. In contrast, serous detachments of the RPE fluoresce brightly in the early-transit phase and remain brightly hyperfluorescent in the late phase. In addition, serous detachments will usually have a smoother, sharper boundary compared with drusenoid RPE detachments. Drusenoid RPE detachments can be distinguished from fibrovascular PEDs in occult CNV by noting that fibrovascular PEDs show areas of stippled hyperfluorescence with persistence of staining or leakage within a sensory retinal detachment overlying the area in the late phase of the angiogram. RPE detachments due to large, soft, confluent drusen are usually smaller, shallower, and more irregular in outline than are fibrovascular PEDs. In addition, the drusenoid RPE detachments often have reticulated pigment clumping overlying the large, soft, confluent drusen, a scalloped border, and have less fluorescence in late-phase frames as compared with earlier-phase frames.

Other angiographic features

Speckled hyperfluorescence

Speckled fluorescence (Fig. 66.15A) in the absence of fluorescein leakage consists of several punctuate spots of hyperfluorescence, usually within 500 μm of each other that are apparent between 2 and 5 minutes after fluorescein injection and cannot be detected in early phase frames in contrast to drusen.[46] The fluorescence of these spots persisted or increased in intensity by the late phase of the angiogram (Fig. 66.15B), in contrast to drusen or atrophy of the retinal pigment epithelium which do not remain brightly hyperfluorescent by the late phase of the angiogram. Typically, clusters of speckles would appear at the edge of the CNV lesion, rather than the typical distribution of drusen throughout the macular area. This angiographic feature was previously reported to be associated with recurrent CNV.[46] If speckled hyperfluorescence is noted in the presence of fluorescein leakage in the late phase frames in the absence of elevation of the RPE, then the pattern would be considered to meet the definition of late leakage of an undetermined source, a type of occult CNV.

Fading choroidal neovascularization

CNV may occasionally be recognized in the early- or middle-transit phase of the angiogram with fading in the late phase, so little fluorescein staining or leakage can be discerned in the late phase within an area that was presumed to harbor CNV on the basis of its early-phase features[19] (Fig. 66.16). A vascular pattern of the fibrovascular tissue can occasionally be discerned in early-phase frames.[43] Most ophthalmologists are reluctant to treat areas of CNV that fade. These areas are usually not associated with overlying subretinal fluid (in conjunction with the lack of fluorescein leakage on angiography), so one can only presume

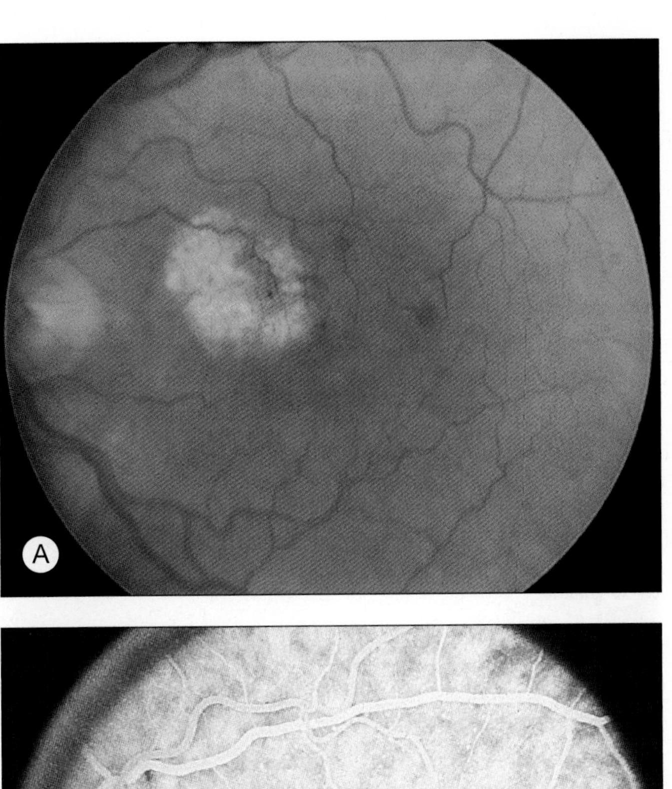

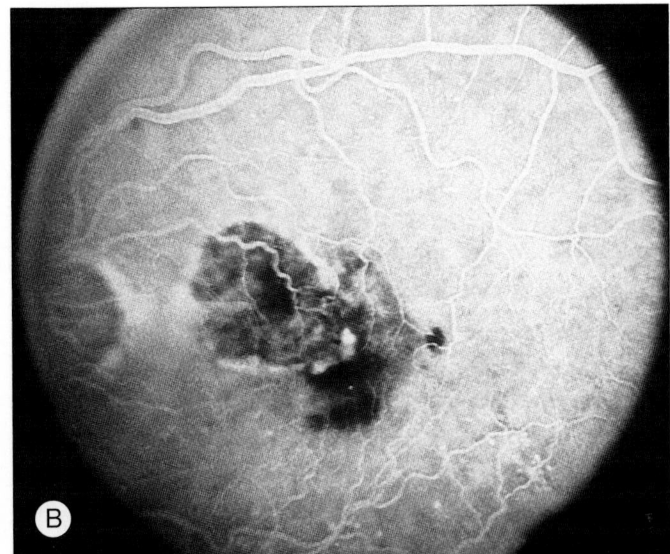

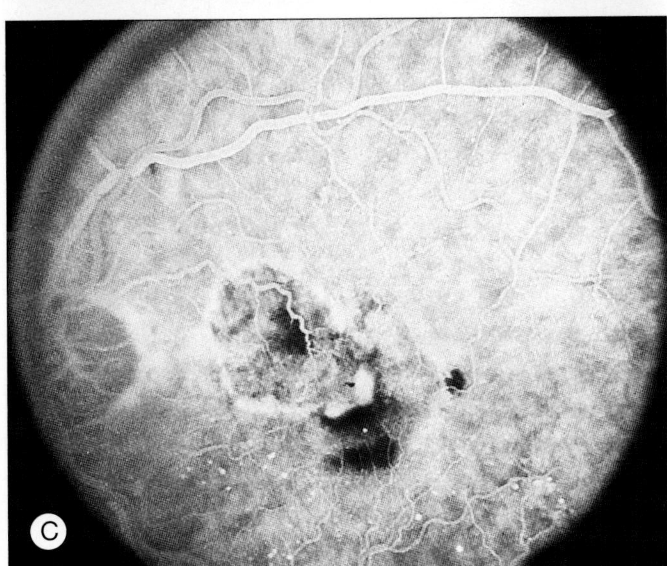

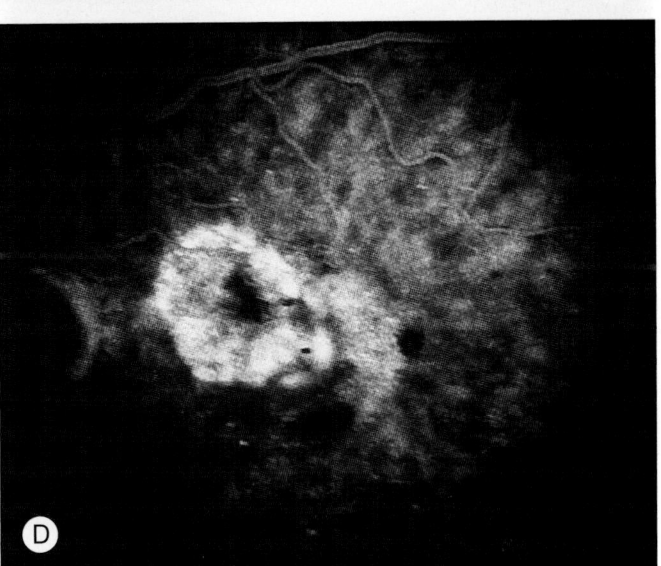

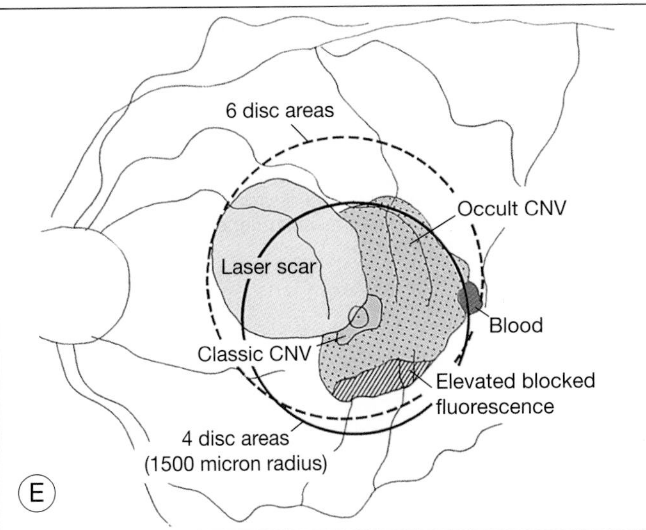

Fig. 66.12 Classic and occult choroidal neovascularization (CNV) and elevated blocked fluorescence (EBF) with well-demarcated borders. (A) Recurrent subfoveal CNV. Note small area of hemorrhage temporal to recurrence. (B) Early phase of fluorescein angiogram shows sharp demarcation of hyperfluorescence of classic CNV. (C) Mid-phase photograph of angiogram with fluorescein leakage from classic CNV and sharply demarcated hyperfluorescence of elevated retinal pigment epithelium due to fibrovascular pigment epithelial detachment and indicative of occult CNV. Elevated blocked fluorescence still obscures choroidal fluorescence and possibly the inferior boundary of CNV. (D) Late phase of angiogram demonstrates fluorescein leakage from both classic and occult neovascularization. Note hardly discernible EBF. (E) Composite drawing using multiple stereoscopic photographs of angiogram shows interpretation of boundaries of lesion. Since each lesion component (classic CNV, occult CNV, blood, and EBF) has well-demarcated boundaries, boundaries of entire lesion are considered well demarcated. (Reproduced with permission from Macular Photocoagulation Study Group. Subfoveal neovascular lesions in age-related macular degeneration: guidelines for evaluation and treatment in the Macular Photocoagulation Study. Arch Ophthalmol 1991;109:1242–57.)

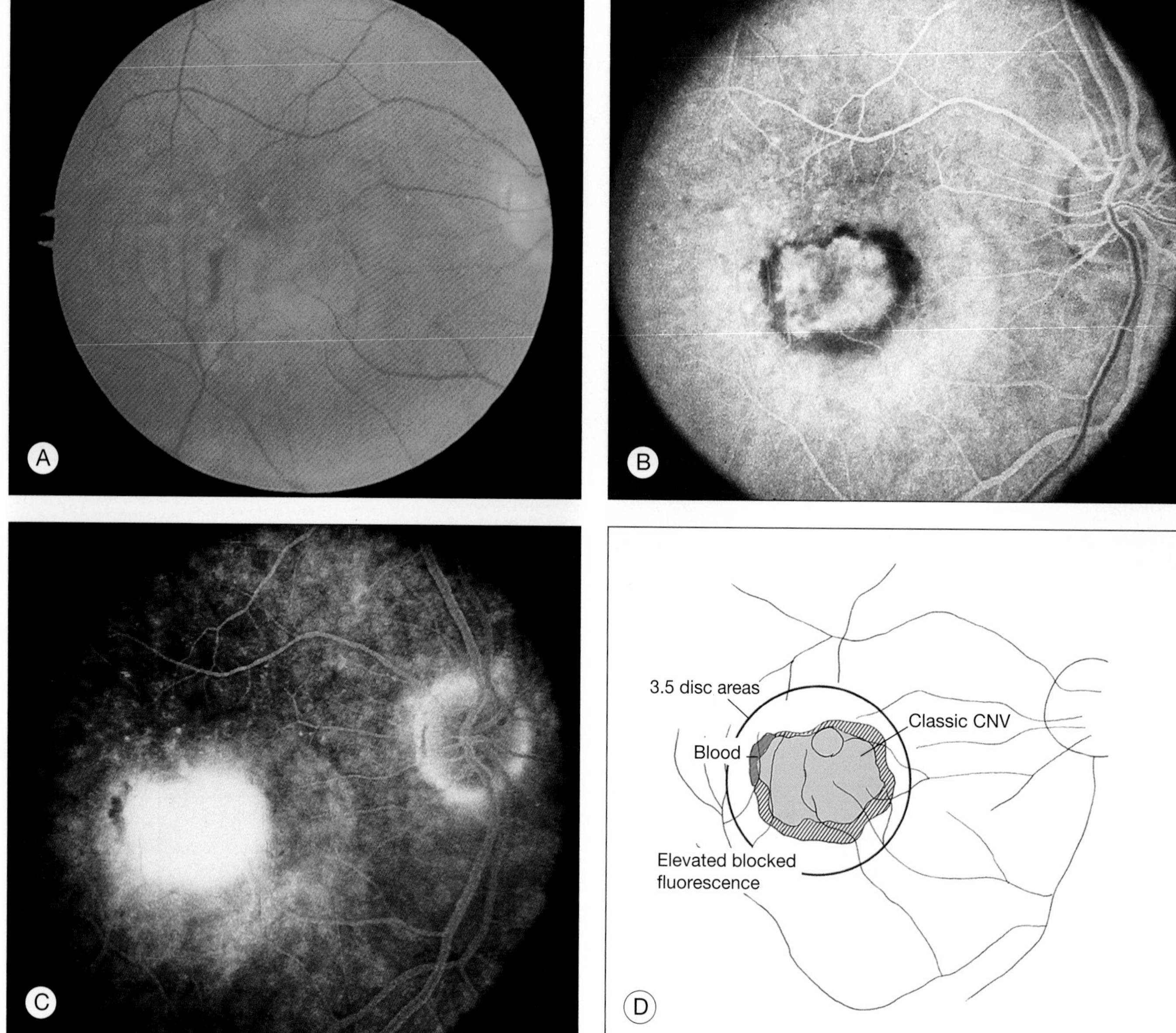

Fig. 66.13 (A) Subfoveal choroidal neovascularization (CNV) and contiguous blood. (B) Early phase of fluorescein angiogram shows classic CNV with blocked fluorescence corresponding to contiguous blood that obscures boundaries of CNV along temporal border. Remaining blocked fluorescein surrounding CNV (elevated when viewed stereoscopically) was probably due to the fibrous component of CNV. (C) Late phase of fluorescein angiogram demonstrates that borders of CNV, blood, and elevated blocked fluorescence (green, red, and blue, respectively, in (D) were derived from viewing the entire stereoscopic fluorescein angiogram taken according to study protocol. (D) Drawing demonstrates that combined areas of blood and elevated blocked fluorescence that obscured borders of CNV did not exceed area of visible CNV. (Reproduced with permission from Macular Photocoagulation Study Group. Subfoveal neovascular lesions in age-related macular degeneration: guidelines for evaluation and treatment in the Macular Photocoagulation Study. Arch Ophthalmol 1991;109:1242–57.)

that this region may proceed to disciform scarring. Perhaps these areas represent CNV histologically, but without evidence of subretinal fluid or late leakage, one cannot be certain that this pattern definitively represents CNV, and laser treatment of this area may damage the retina unnecessarily.

Feeder vessels

These vessels may be identified as choroidal vessels apparent during the transit phase of the angiogram and connected unequivocally to leaking choroidal capillaries[19] (see Fig. 66.9). Although feeder vessels have been described as extending from a laser-treated area to recurrent CNV across the perimeter of the laser-treated areas, feeder vessels may also be seen in untreated eyes (see Fig. 66.10). In the latter situation, peripheral, untreated areas of CNV may be connected by feeder vessels to more central areas of CNV that are evolving toward natural scar formation.

Retinal lesion anastomosis ("retinal angiomatous proliferans" or "chorioretinal anastomosis")

Retinal vessels can anastomose with CNV from AMD.[47] The vessels can be seen dividing at right angles from the surface of the retina to the neovascular lesion (as may be seen with idiopathic parafoveal telangiectasis).

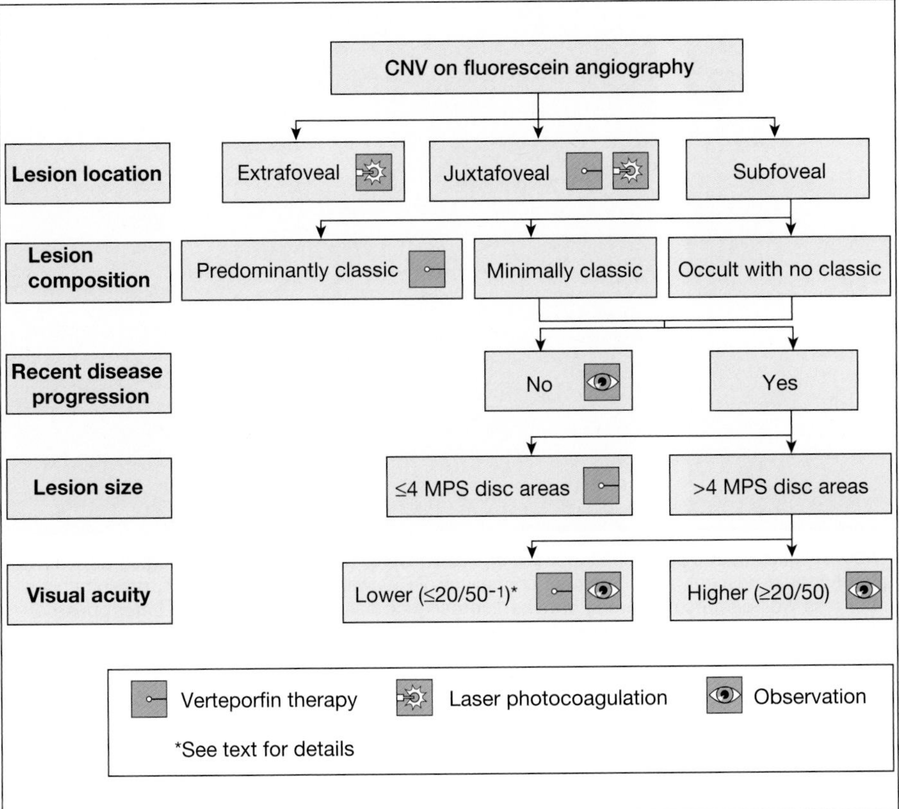

Fig. 66.14 Algorithm for verteporfin therapy or laser photocoagulation or observation for symptomatic patients with age-related macular degeneration, pathologic myopia, or other causes of choroidal neovascularization (CNV) in which the natural course is likely worse without treatment. MPS, Macular Photocoagulation Study, and now largely replaced by anti-VEGF therapy as outlined in Fig. 66.21.

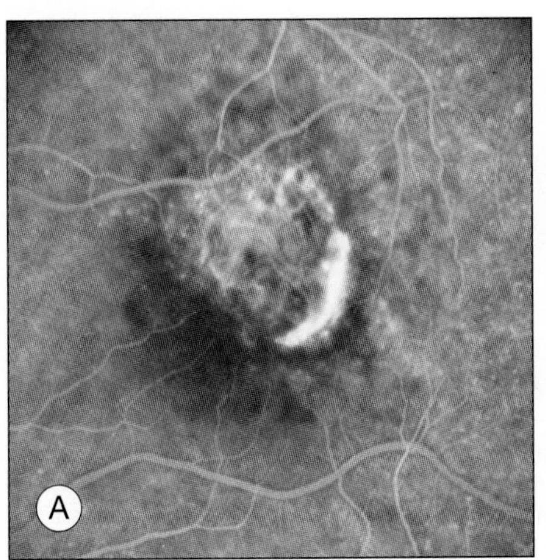

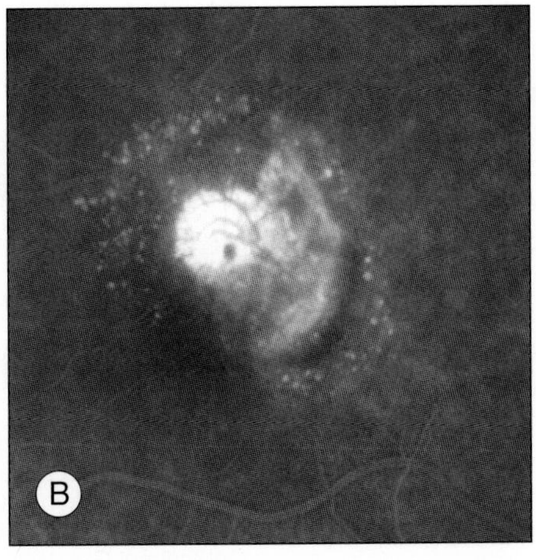

Fig. 66.15 (A and B) Example of speckled fluorescence noted in an eye with choroidal neovascularization. Multiple punctuate spots of hyperfluorescence within 500 μm of each other are apparent in a late phase frame (B) but cannot be detected in early phase frame (A). Note the typical appearance of clusters of speckles at the edge of the CNV lesion. (© Neil M. Bressler, MD, Johns Hopkins University, 2011.)

Loculated fluid

This fluid consists of a well-demarcated area of hyperfluorescence that appears to represent pooling of fluorescein in a compartmentalized space anterior to the choroidal neovascular leakage, usually seen in the late phase of the angiogram.[48] Although the loculated fluid may conform to a pattern of typical cystoid macular edema, it can also pool within an area deep to the sensory retina in a shape that does not bear any resemblance to cystoid macular edema.

Retinal pigment epithelial tears

RPE tears have a characteristic fluorescein angiographic appearance.[49] The denuded RPE displays marked early hyperfluorescence. Later, staining of the choroid and sclera may be observed, but fluorescein generally does not leak from the denuded area. The folded pigment epithelial mound blocks fluorescence; However, this area may leak later during the angiogram, presumably from underlying CNV. Tears may occur following development of a serous PED in the absence of CNV. In addition, tears may occur following development of CNV, sometimes accompanied by large areas of hemorrhage. Tears in any of these situations may occur without any antecedent treatment or may occur soon after laser photocoagulation or PDT.

Disciform scars

Fibrovascular scars frequently hyperfluoresce from both fluorescein leakage and staining. One may also notice chorioretinal anastomoses or, more precisely, retinal anastomoses into fibrovascular tissue (also called retinal angiomatous proliferans[47] or chorioretinal anastomoses or retinal lesion anastomoses). Some

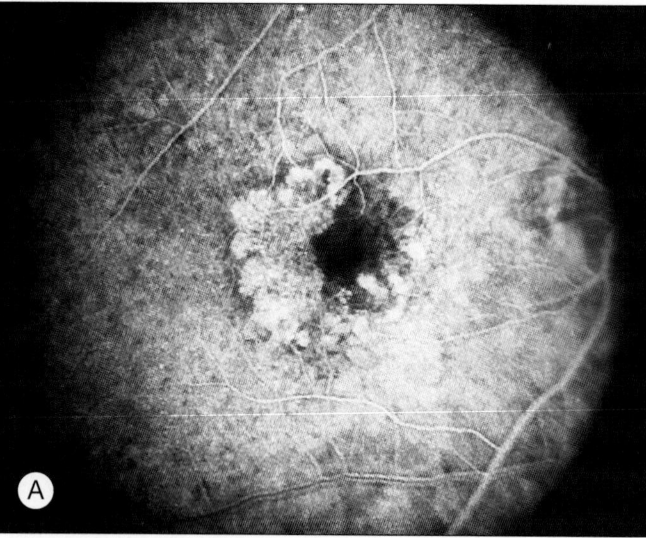

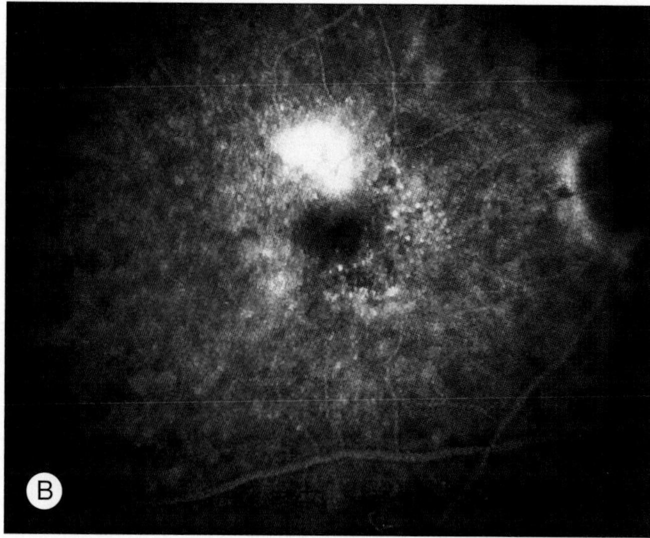

Fig. 66.16 Fading fluorescence of occult choroidal neovascularization (CNV) contiguous with classic CNV. (A) Early phase of angiogram shows classic CNV with contiguous areas of slightly elevated hyperfluorescent retinal pigment epithelium (RPE) with a vascular pattern, presumably a fibrovascular pigment epithelial detachment, and other less well-demarcated areas of hyperfluorescence nasal to the fovea. (B) Later phase of angiogram shows fluorescein leakage from classic CNV. However, areas of elevated hyperfluorescent RPE on early phase of angiogram (left) begin to fade, and vascular pattern is no longer apparent. Faded area is not considered a lesion component because hyperfluorescence does not meet minimal leakage/staining standard for occult CNV. (Reproduced with permission from Macular Photocoagulation Study Group. Subfoveal neovascular lesions in age-related macular degeneration: guidelines for evaluation and treatment in the Macular Photocoagulation Study. Arch Ophthalmol 1991;109:1242–57.)

descriptions of these vessels have suggested that they can develop prior to the development of CNV (as is seen in the subretinal neovascularization that can develop in an individual with idiopathic parafoveal telangiectasis). Theoretically, these descriptions seem plausible if sufficient VEGF production, which typically would be involved in the development of CNV, first led to the development of proliferation of retinal capillaries. However, there is no evidence that these vessels develop in the absence of CNV from AMD on histopathology. Furthermore, most cases show evidence of CNV in the presence of these anastomoses of retinal vessels with the neovascular lesion, and those cases that do not show obvious CNV often have difficult angiograms to interpret to state with certainty that CNV is not present. The area of anastomosis, when noted before development of extensive visible scar tissue, often shows a bright area of fluorescence in the early phase, occasionally accompanied by a small area of intraretinal hemorrhage. While some reports have suggested that the natural history of lesions with these anastomoses is worse than the natural history without these anastomoses, there is no strong evidence to support this impression at this time.

PATHOGENESIS

Choroidal neovascularization

Histopathology

CNV appears as a neovascular sprout growing under or through the RPE through breaks in Bruch's membrane[13] (Figs 66.17, 66.18). Usually this occurs in association with evidence of fibroblasts, myofibroblasts, lymphocytes, and macrophages.[50] Various growth factors are suspected to be involved in the development of this CNV, such as vascular endothelial growth factor (VEGF).[51] However, while drugs designed to interfere with VEGF have been shown to reduce the risk of vision loss,[52–57] vision loss still occurred in many treated cases, and it is not yet clear how much

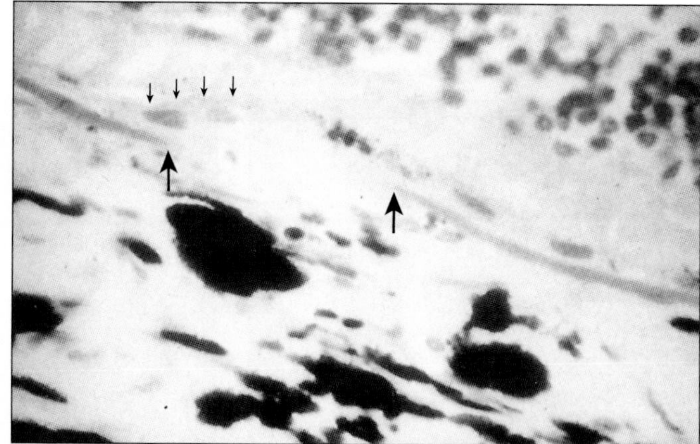

Fig. 66.17 Photomicrograph of choroidal neovascularization (outlined by small arrows) beneath the retinal pigment epithelium growing through a break in Bruch's membrane (large arrows). (Reproduced with permission from Elman MJ. Age-related macular degeneration. Int Ophthalmol Clin 1986;26:117–44.)

these drugs produce an antiangiogenic effect or an antipermeability effect. Following penetration of the inner aspect of Bruch's membrane, the new vessels proliferate laterally between the RPE and Bruch's membrane.[13] As these neovascular twigs mature, they develop a more organized vascular system stemming from a trunk of feeder vessels off the choroid, as well as proliferation of fibrous tissue. The endothelial cells in the arborizing neovascular tufts lack the barrier function of more mature endothelial cells. Hence these new vessels can leak fluid (and fluorescein) in the neurosensory, subsensory, and RPE layers of the retina. Proteins and lipids may accompany this process and precipitate in any layer of the retina. In addition, the fragile vessels are prone to hemorrhage. Occasionally, blood may extend through all the layers of the retina, breaking through into the vitreous cavity.

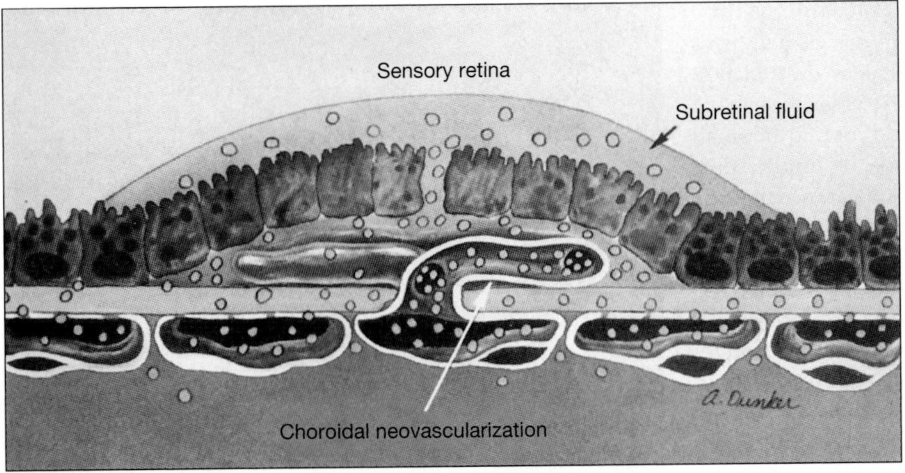

Fig. 66.18 Sketch of choroidal neovascularization showing ingrowth of vessels from the choriocapillaris, through a break in Bruch's membrane, into the subretinal pigment epithelial space. (Reproduced with permission from Bressler NM, Bressler SB, Fine SL. Age-related macular degeneration. Surv Ophthalmol 1988;32:375–413.)

Ultimately, a fibrovascular scar results, usually causing disruption and death of the overlying sensory retinal tissue accompanied by severe visual loss.

Associated factors

The stimulus for vascular ingrowth of choroidal vessels remains unknown, but several theories have been advanced. Soft drusen have been associated histopathologically with CNV. The soft drusen represent focal accumulation of membranous debris (ultrastructurally termed basal linear deposits) accumulated as a diffuse, shallow layer between the RPE basement membrane and the inner aspect of Bruch's membrane.[11–13,58–63] This material should not be confused with basal laminar deposit, which is material that collects between the RPE plasma membrane and the basement membrane of the RPE and accumulates with age but may not lead to vision loss from CNV or geographic atrophy and therefore may not be part of AMD.[58,59] The term should also not be confused with basal laminar drusen, also called cuticular drusen. (Basal laminar, or cuticular, drusen usually present in midlife with a myriad of small, translucent drusen that appear like a starry sky on a fluorescein angiogram and may be associated with vitelliform macular detachments: see below.[3,64]) Some investigators believe that soft drusen represent extracellular matrix material produced by the RPE.[58,65] Deposition of this material may suggest a widespread RPE abnormality.[20] The diffusely thickened area is weakly attached, allowing the development of localized detachments seen clinically as soft drusen. These localized detachments can coalesce into larger drusenoid or serous RPE detachments.[12] Alternatively, drusen may act as an indirect angiogenic factor by attracting macrophages from the choroid.[50]

Breaks in Bruch's membrane permit ingrowth of new vessels from the choriocapillaris. However, these breaks can also be seen without ingrowth of choroidal new vessels. Some investigators have suggested that endothelial cells of growing CNV may actually produce the break in Bruch's membrane rather than grow through pre-existing breaks in Bruch's membrane.[66] An inflammatory component seen in association with AMD may play a role in the development of CNV.[67] Eyes with AMD show an increased prevalence of lymphocytes, fibroblasts, and macrophages within Bruch's membrane as compared with control eyes without AMD. However, these findings are not specific to eyes with neovascular AMD.[67,68] The presence of macrophages and lymphocytes near breaks in Bruch's membrane suggests that leukocytes may be involved in the induction of CNV growth and the release of collagenases from endothelial cells. It is postulated that leukocytes may initially stimulate neovascular proliferation, promote the release of factors leading to breakdown of Bruch's membrane, and even affect (with pericytes) the dilation of new vessels.[69] Whether these inflammatory cells act as mediators of the degenerative changes seen in Bruch's membrane or directly stimulate new vessel growth remains unknown. Finally, as mentioned above, other angiogenic factors, such as VEGF or a platelet-derived growth factor (PDGF),[51,53,70] may contribute to the ingrowth of new vessels from the choroid through Bruch's membrane into the sub-RPE space. Growth factors leading to neovascular formation may arise from an imbalance between stimulating and inhibiting chemical modulators. The RPE has been implicated as the source of these factors, but RPE cells may also act indirectly through the attraction of macrophages.[71]

DIFFERENTIAL DIAGNOSIS

Choroidal neovascularization

CNV may arise in association with a number of conditions other than AMD, such as OHS, pathologic myopia, angioid streaks (especially when associated with pseudoxanthoma elasticum), choroidal ruptures, and idiopathic causes. Whether AMD is present when CNV arises in patients older than 50 years without drusen is controversial.

CNV may masquerade as central serous chorioretinopathy. Although the classic case of central serous chorioretinopathy shows a "smokestack" configuration on fluorescein angiography, the more common presentation is a dot of hyperfluorescence that merely increases in size and intensity of fluorescence, much like a small area of CNV. One must strongly consider CNV in patients aged 50 and older who have typical central serous chorioretinopathy. In these cases the increased age contrasts to the third to fifth decades, when central serous chorioretinopathy is most commonly seen. Presentation of central serous chorioretinopathy in an elderly patient with drusen can be difficult to distinguish and should alert one to the possibility of CNV, necessitating careful follow-up. If CNV is indeed present, growth of the area of hyperfluorescence might be detected while treatment may still be beneficial.

Basal laminar, or cuticular, drusen may be complicated by foveal detachments of vitelliform material in one or both eyes that may mimic neovascular AMD. Contact lens examination with transillumination of the fundus in these cases reveals an appearance similar to that of pigskin, with a myriad of small drusen. Angiographically, literally hundreds of bright spots appear very early during the angiogram, an appearance that has been described as a "starry sky." These patients are usually asymptomatic until they accumulate vitelliform lesions in the fovea. The ensuing foveal detachment by this material, which can be unilateral or bilateral, simulates the foveal detachment that occurs with subfoveal CNV. The hyperfluorescence usually progressively fills the area of vitelliform material, rather than showing one area of bright fluorescence early that leaks late in classic CNV. Unlike subfoveal CNV, which most often progresses to a disciform scar with visual acuity of 20/200 or worse, eyes with a foveal detachment secondary to cuticular drusen resolve without scarring. The retina then may or may not have an area of RPE atrophy about one to two disc areas in size. Foveal acuity with atrophy is more often in the range of 20/80 to 20/125, in contrast to the more severe visual loss that accompanies true subfoveal CNV. Patients with cuticular drusen can still develop typical drusen associated with AMD or CNV.

Pattern dystrophies of the RPE may also have vitelliform detachments in which the angiographic pattern can mimic CNV. When one identifies any condition with a vitelliform detachment, it is critical to determine if the late-phase bright fluorescence is progressive fluorescein staining of the vitelliform material or leakage of fluorescein from CNV. The former would not benefit from laser photocoagulation, whereas the latter might. As discussed earlier, usually the fluorescence from a vitelliform detachment shows one or more areas of hyperfluorescence in the early phase of the angiogram with progressive hyperfluorescence of the entire area of yellow vitelliform material by the late phase. In contrast, a diffuse area of hyperfluorescence in the late phase that corresponds to classic CNV (rather than the stippled fluorescence of occult CNV) should show an area of bright hyperfluorescence in the early phase that is only slightly smaller than the area of hyperfluorescent leakage in the late phase.

Vitreous hemorrhage

If a new patient has vitreous hemorrhage in one eye and signs of AMD in the other eye, other causes of vitreous hemorrhage must first be ruled out. Common causes of vitreous hemorrhage include retinal tear formation and retinal vascular diseases such as diabetic retinopathy or branch vein occlusion. Ultrasonography usually differentiates breakthrough vitreous hemorrhage secondary to neovascular AMD or retinal vascular causes from that caused by a tumor (Fig. 66.19).

NATURAL HISTORY

Most prospective natural history data of CNV comes from control (untreated) groups of individuals participating in randomized clinical trials. As such, the natural-history information is specific to the eligibility criteria of those trials and is not necessarily reflective of the natural history of the universe of choroidal neovascular lesions in the population, and precludes precise comparisons of natural histories from one study to another. With this caveat in mind, the natural history from these trials is reviewed to provide some evidence regarding the outcome of these lesions without treatment.

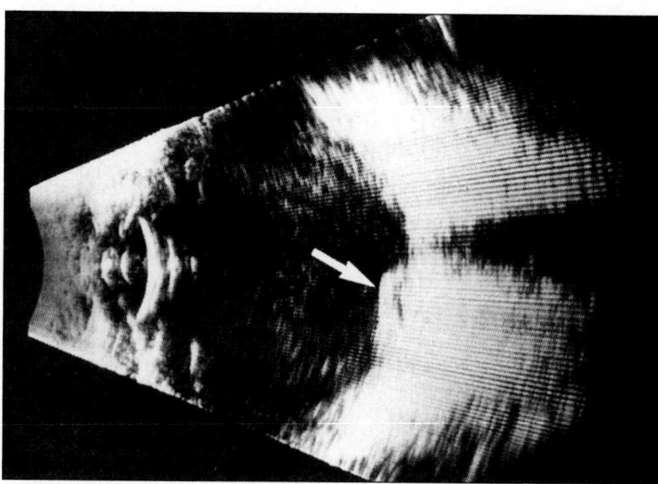

Fig. 66.19 Ultrasound image of a vitreous hemorrhage associated with neovascular age-related macular degeneration in which a relatively flat and broad-based posterior pole lesion (arrow) with a fairly homogeneous pattern and with no choroidal excavation is seen. (Reproduced with permission from Bressler NM, Bressler SB, Fine SL. Age-related macular degeneration. Surv Ophthalmol 1988;32:375–413.)

Well-defined extrafoveal and juxtafoveal choroidal neovascularization

Patients assigned to observation in the MPS trials provide natural-history information on cases that met criteria for these studies. When lesions have well-defined boundaries, the CNV lesion can be classified according to the location of the most posterior boundary of the lesion with respect to the center of the FAZ on the fluorescein angiogram. CNV lesions located more than 200 μm from the FAZ center are termed extrafoveal; those between 1 and 199 μm from the center are juxtafoveal; CNV lesions extending under the center of the FAZ are termed subfoveal. In contrast to other pathologic conditions predisposing to CNV (e.g., OHS and pathologic myopia) in eyes with AMD, CNV presents more frequently under the FAZ center. In addition, subfoveal CNV from AMD tends to be larger on initial presentation than when seen in other conditions.[72] In a retrospective review of fluorescein angiograms of AMD ordered at a community hospital over a 9.5-year period, only 8% (19/244) of the CNV lesions were extrafoveal.[73] Other retrospective reports not derived solely from a retinal referral practice have suggested that most patients with CNV from AMD present to an ophthalmologist with subfoveal CNV with poorly demarcated boundaries.[72,74] However, there is no information from population-based studies to describe precisely how many choroidal neovascular lesions are subfoveal versus not subfoveal, and for those that are not subfoveal, how many are well demarcated on laser photocoagulation. Furthermore, there are no studies to determine how many cases that are subfoveal are predominantly classic, and if not predominantly classic, how many have presumed recent disease progression after developing.

In the MPS, 62% of untreated eyes with well-defined, extrafoveal CNV (posterior boundary of lesion located at least 200 μm from the FAZ center) lost 6 or more lines of visual acuity by 3 years of follow-up.[75] By 5 years, this percentage was similar at 64%.[76] Furthermore, in nearly 75% of the untreated eyes, the

CNV extended under the FAZ center.[77] For juxtafoveal lesions, 49% of untreated eyes had lost 6 or more lines of visual acuity by 3 years of follow-up.[26]

Subfoveal choroidal neovascularization

For subfoveal lesions, the MPS reported that 48% of untreated eyes with well-defined subfoveal CNV that was predominantly CNV and included a component of classic CNV in which the entire lesion was no greater than 3.5 MPS disc areas lost 6 or more lines of vision from baseline by 48 months.[24,78] Similar outcomes were noted for untreated eyes with recurrent subfoveal CNV with similar features as for new subfoveal lesions except the total size of the lesion plus any area of prior treatment was to be no greater than 6 MPS disc areas.[25,78] A broader group of subfoveal lesions in the Treatment of Age-related macular degeneration with Photodynamic therapy (TAP) investigation described the natural history in subfoveal lesions that were predominantly CNV with evidence of classic CNV and a lesion size no greater than 9 disc areas in which 62% lost 3 or more lines at 2 years after entry, including 30% losing 6 or more lines of visual acuity.[79] With increasing size of predominantly classic lesions on presentation, the average visual acuity is more likely to be worse by 2 years.[80] Similar natural history outcomes were noted for untreated eyes with occult with no classic CNV with presumed recent disease progression,[54] in which almost half of the eyes lost 3 or more lines at 2 years after entry, including 23% losing 6 or more lines of visual acuity.

A variety of studies have shown that cases of predominantly CNV with a composition that is occult with no classic CNV, or minimally classic CNV have a more heterogeneous outcome.[44,80–85] Most of this information is from series in clinical trials with presumed recent disease progression. Some cases may remain stable for years without visual loss, whereas other cases may develop severe visual loss at a rate similar to the deterioration noted for cases of classic CNV only. Furthermore, increasing size of minimally classic or occult with no classic lesions is not associated with a worse natural history outcome.[80]

Up to 50% of the cases with no classic CNV may develop classic CNV within a year of presentation.[44,81,82,86] Cases that develop some classic CNV may be more likely to have severe visual acuity loss.[81,82,86] Results from several clinical trials suggest that the natural history of lesions with classic CNV but no occult CNV is worse than the natural history of lesions with classic and occult CNV or occult with no classic CNV.[82,84,87] It is likely that the natural history of lesions with classic and occult CNV may lie somewhere between the natural course of lesions with classic CNV only and occult CNV only.[82]

Natural course of large subfoveal subretinal hemorrhage in age-related macular degeneration

Some eyes with subfoveal subretinal hemorrhage associated with AMD have poor outcomes.[88–90] However, the visual acuity of other eyes does not deteriorate or may improve spontaneously.[88,90] Such findings underscore the importance of evaluating the role of therapeutic interventions for these cases, such as surgery[91,92] to remove subretinal hemorrhage and associated CNV, in randomized clinical trials.[93] The SST Group B Trial of relatively large, predominantly hemorrhagic subfoveal lesions demonstrated that 41% of untreated eyes remained stable or improved, although 36% had severe visual acuity loss after enrollment into the trial. Furthermore, this trial suggested that 18% of large subfoveal subretinal hemorrhages will progress to a vitreous hemorrhage as blood dissects from the subretinal space through the retina and into the vitreous.[27]

Retinal pigment epithelial tears

Patients with RPE tears involving the foveal center may initially maintain good vision but usually develop severe visual loss. However, cases with RPE tears through the fovea and preservation of good visual acuity have been reported.[94] Unfortunately, there is a substantial risk of AMD-related visual loss in the fellow eye. Schoeppner and associates[95] reported a cumulative risk of visual loss in the fellow eye of patients who had an RPE tear in the eye as 37% at 1 year, 59% at 2 years, and 80% at 3 years of follow-up. Visual loss usually arose from development of a PED, RPE tear, or CNV.

LASER PHOTOCOAGULATION TREATMENT

Laser treatment of well-defined choroidal neovascular lesions

While laser photocoagulation has been shown to be beneficial for well-defined lesions not involving the foveal center or very small lesions involving the foveal center with a component of classic CNV, failure to cover the entire lesion increases the likelihood of recurrent CNV[96–98] and, for extrafoveal and juxtafoveal lesions, of additional visual acuity loss,[96,98,99] and treatment will destroy retinal tissue (and corresponding function).[98] Therefore, such treatment generally is reserved for cases that are extrafoveal and in which it is judged that a scotoma from the laser is preferred over proceeding with anti-VEGF therapy.

Preparation for laser photocoagulation treatment

Before photocoagulation treatment, patients with a potentially treatable CNV lesion should be informed that laser treatment will create a permanent blank area, or blind spot, corresponding to the area of retina to be treated. The postoperative vision will correlate with the extent of central retina destroyed with laser photocoagulation treatment. Whereas patients with binocular macular vision and a treated lesion away from the center of the FAZ frequently remain unaware of this treatment scotoma unless they cover the untreated fellow eye, patients with a central scotoma in the fellow eye usually are aware immediately of the laser-induced scotoma in the treated eye. Because laser treatment may cause hemorrhage or increase sensory retinal detachment during the immediate postoperative period, all patients should be warned that they may experience increased distortion and decreased vision after treatment and that this may persist for several weeks. In addition, the ophthalmologist must emphasize that laser treatment is not a cure for AMD; rather, laser photocoagulation treatment is designed to obliterate the neovascular complex and thereby reduce the risk of additional severe visual loss in the future. Furthermore, the treating ophthalmologist must recall that, even under the best conditions in the MPS, many of the treated eyes had recurrent CNV in which anti-VEGF therapy likely would be indicated.

Following the treatment protocol established by the MPS (discussed below), a recent fluorescein angiogram (if possible, less than 72–96 hours old) should be used to guide the ophthalmologist during treatment. Because the CNV may grow, a fluorescein angiogram older than a few days may no longer depict the extent of CNV accurately. A suitable frame from the angiogram is displayed near the laser console top. The angiogram thus displayed permits rapid and accurate orientation of critical retinal vascular and CNV landmarks. With a cooperative patient, an ophthalmologist with adequate experience in the treatment of CNV should be able to treat using topical anesthesia.

Macular Photocoagulation Study photocoagulation techniques

Using a 200 μm spot size and duration of at least 0.2 s, a test burn is placed along the lesion's perimeter to determine the necessary power setting. Then, the lesion is outlined with laser burns. Ideally, one should start at the inferior edge of a lesion and work superiorly, as if case intraoperative bleeding occurs and tracks inferiorly, obscuring retinal landmarks, this area will have been treated. To obliterate the CNV, the burns should be sufficiently intense to produce retinal whitening. Finally, the center of the CNV is obliterated (Fig. 66.20).

To ensure adequate treatment, the MPS protocol required that the entire CNV lesion be covered by a uniformly intense area of whitening extending 100 μm beyond the angiographically visible lesion. Excessive treatment can contribute to visual loss. However, failure to cover the CNV in its entirety could lead to increased persistence within 6 weeks of treatment.[96–98]

Rarely, choroidal hemorrhage occurs as a treatment complication. Generally, choroidal hemorrhage stops spontaneously. If not, it can usually be controlled by applying pressure to the globe with the contact lens while treating the area of hemorrhage with repetitive laser spots, employing a larger spot size and

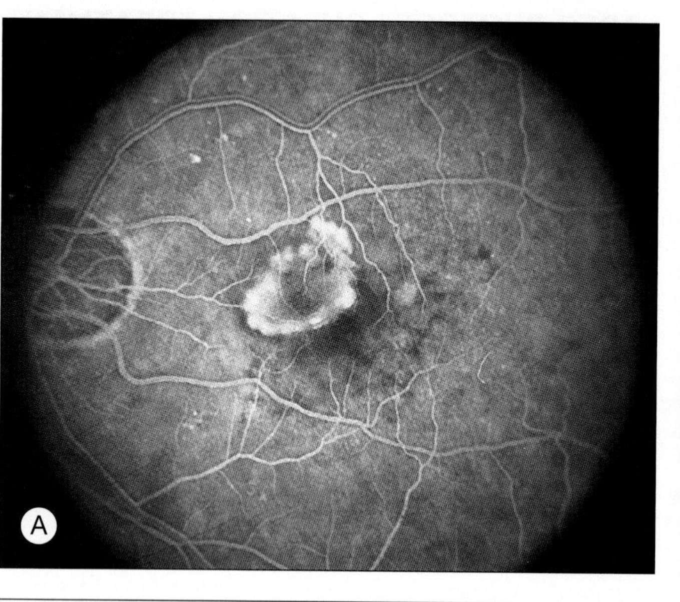

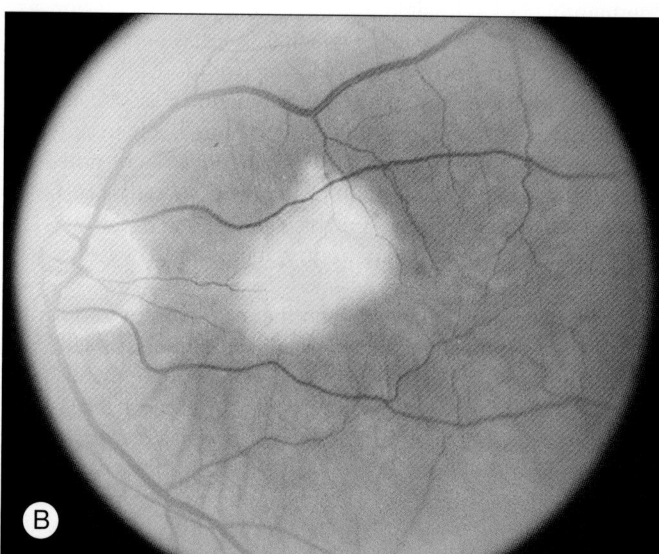

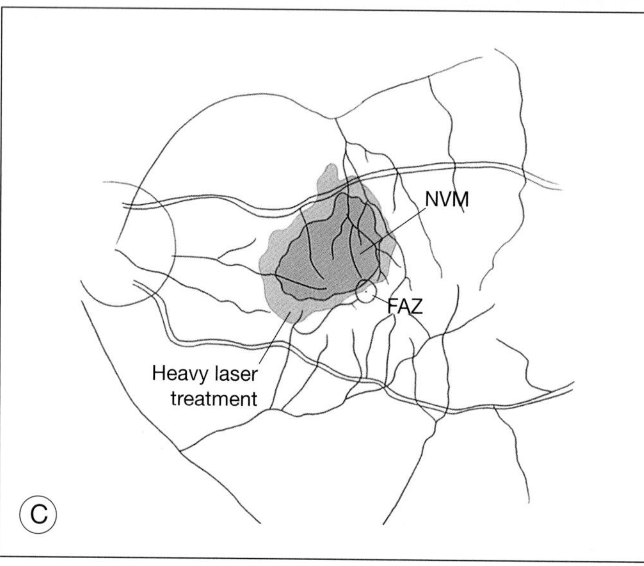

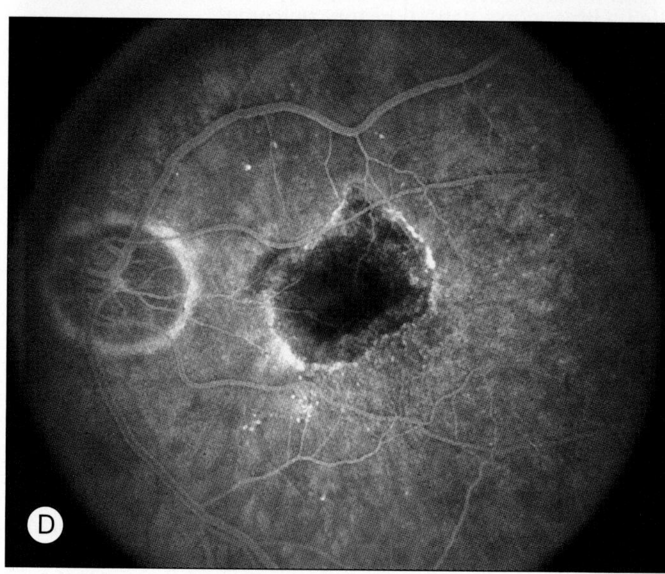

Fig. 66.20 Juxtafoveal choroidal neovascularization lesion. (A) Fluorescein angiogram shows choroidal neovascularization (CNV) in which the posterior edge of the CNV is more than 200 μm from the foveal center and is associated with blocked fluorescence on the posterior edge of the lesion within 200 μm of the foveal center. (B) Red-free photograph of same eye demonstrating that, except for a small amount of blood superonasal to the neovascular lesion, the blocked fluorescence is not due to subretinal blood visible on photograph. (C) Drawing of CNV or neovascular membrane (NVM) in which blocked fluorescence is represented by hatched area surrounding the neovascular lesion. (Reproduced with permission from Macular Photocoagulation Study Group. Subfoveal neovascular lesions in age-related macular degeneration: guidelines for evaluation and treatment in the Macular Photocoagulation Study. Arch Ophthalmol 1991;109:1242–57.)

longer duration than might have been used for CNV treatment. Long burns (0.5–1.0 s) and large spot sizes (200 µm or larger) decrease the chances of additional choroidal hemorrhage.

No visible wavelength appears to have a significant advantage over other wavelengths. Small differences in convenience of achieving the end-point of a uniform white burn might be seen with red or yellow wavelengths when penetrating through the increased yellow color of the lens nucleus in the older age group afflicted with CNV secondary to AMD, but any significant difference of clinical importance has not been shown. When treating CNV that lies under a major retinal vessel, the laser burns should straddle the retinal vessel to reduce the possibility of causing hemorrhage or damaging the vessel by thermal vasculitis. No evidence has suggested that this technique compromised the effectiveness of treatment.

When treating CNV that is contiguous with the optic nerve, it should be kept in mind that laser treatment directly over the optic nerve can cause thermal necrosis of disc tissue and nerve fiber bundle defects. Therefore one should consider refraining from treatment within 100–200 µm of the optic nerve. Similarly, when treating a peripapillary area of CNV, one may want to consider treatment only when at least 1½ clock-hours of papillomacular bundle on the temporal side of the disc is uninvolved with CNV so that at least 1½ clock-hours of papillomacular bundle can be spared of treatment, as was done in several of the MPS trials. Treatment to nasal or peripapillary lesions that met criteria for MPS trials will likely not lead to severe visual loss from damage to the nerve fiber layer that serves the central macula if the treatment guidelines outlined previously are followed.[100] In these situations, the MPS group reported that severe visual acuity loss was noted after treatment only when recurrent CNV extended through the center of the fovea.[100] This finding suggests that, in the absence of subfoveal recurrence, severe visual loss only from nerve fiber layer damage after this treatment approach must be a rare complication.

On rare occasions, an area of extrafoveal CNV is contiguous to a serous detachment of the RPE in which the serous detachment extends under the center of the FAZ. There have been case reports in which only the extrafoveal CNV in these lesions is treated, resulting in prompt flattening of the RPE detachment with improvement of vision in selected cases.[101] Nevertheless, with follow-up, many of these eyes have acquired recurrent CNV with extensive scarring and visual loss. In these situations, one should consider the possibility that the extrafoveal CNV is associated with a subfoveal fibrovascular PED – a pattern of occult CNV in which treatment of the extrafoveal CNV alone has not been shown to be of any benefit. In such cases, anti-VEGF therapy typically would be indicated.

Evaluations following laser photocoagulation

A follow-up evaluation that includes best-corrected vision, biomicroscopy of the fundus, and fluorescein angiography is obtained 2–3 weeks after treatment. Follow-up earlier than 2 weeks is often difficult to evaluate because swelling and leakage from the treatment itself may obscure persistent or recurrent CNV. At follow-up, an angiogram should be scrutinized for the presence of leakage at the periphery of the laser-treated area to identify the presence of persistent or recurrent CNV, while an OCT can be scrutinized for intraretinal or subretinal fluid. Simultaneous projection of the fluorescein angiogram during biomicroscopy may help differentiate areas of atrophy, which stain, from areas of recurrent leakage with subretinal fluid. If no residual or recurrent CNV is noted at this time, a similar evaluation is repeated 2 to 4 weeks later because the risk of recurrent CNV is so high within the first 6 weeks to 12 months after treatment. By 6 weeks after treatment, a patient should be encouraged to monitor the central vision of the treated eye daily for clarity of distance and near vision, as well as for any distortion, blurry vision, or increase in scotoma. These latter symptoms might indicate leakage from persistent or recurrent CNV and are an indication for prompt examination. The ophthalmologist's office staff should also be aware that these patients may need prompt re-evaluation if such symptoms develop and not necessarily schedule such patients for the "next available opening" 2 or 3 weeks later. Furthermore, although the risk of recurrent CNV after treatment in eyes with AMD is high, results showing the benefits of treating selected cases of recurrent subfoveal CNV make follow-up warranted for identifying these recurrences before they become too large.

Clinical examination probably cannot replace fluorescein angiography in detecting all recurrent CNV after laser treatment or PDT (as described below) or anti-VEGF therapy (as described below). In one prospective evaluation in which recurrent CNV was not suspected on biomicroscopy within approximately 1 year after laser photocoagulation to CNV, definite or questionable recurrent CNV was identified on the fluorescein angiogram 12% of the time.[40] Most of these recurrent cases that were not identified on biomicroscopy alone were treated promptly after review of the fluorescein angiogram. This study also showed that questionable recurrences that showed focal staining along the edge of the laser lesion and speckled hyperfluorescence were the patterns that were most likely to progress to definite recurrence.[14]

Since many recurrences occur within 3–6 months after treatment, an evaluation, including fluorescein angiography, is again repeated at 3–4 and 6–8 months after treatment. Subsequent evaluations, probably with angiography, at 9–12 months after treatment appear to be indicated for CNV secondary to AMD that has been treated because many recurrences develop between 6 and 12 months after treatment. After 2 years, recurrences are unusual; follow-up every 6–12 months without angiography (unless signs or symptoms suggest a recurrence) is probably sufficient.

Complications of laser photocoagulation

Immediate complications from treatment of CNV are uncommon. Rates of choroidal hemorrhage, which can occur when attempting to achieve a white burn, may be minimized by avoiding a spot size less than 200 µm and an exposure time shorter than 0.2 s. Macular pucker, observed with some frequency after argon blue–green laser treatment, is rarely clinically significant and is far less common when employing argon green or krypton red wavelengths.[73] Rates of inadvertent treatment of the foveola in extrafoveal or juxtafoveal lesions, the most serious treatment complication, are rare now that anti-VEGF therapy or PDT is used for these lesions.

Delayed perfusion of choroidal vessels, thought to result from vascular spasm, has been reported following the use of the krypton red laser.[102] In most cases, normal choroidal perfusion returns rapidly without any permanent visual sequelae. The krypton red laser has also been implicated in RPE tears arising from treatment of CNV.[33] However, RPE tears may be observed spontaneously and after treatment of CNV using any wavelength, particularly in patients with associated RPE detachments, either serous or fibrovascular.

Visual acuity might decline several years after treatment with late remodeling and enlargement of the area of RPE disturbance. Such occurrences may be less frequent now that anti-VEGF therapy, or less commonly, PDT, is used to treat most CNV, while laser is reserved for lesions that are relatively far away from the center of the macula. These areas of enlargement of RPE abnormalities following thermal laser have been reported by Morgan and Schatz[103] to increase in size by 50–100 μm over serial follow-up. In their series, 4 (3%) of 174 eyes lost vision when the area of disturbance extended into the fovea. The peripheral zone of atrophy in a laser-treated area may correspond with the runoff or spread of the laser burn during the treatment. "Runoff" refers to the border of less-intense whitening surrounding the area of heavy treatment; it probably represents less severe damage to the RPE, retina, and choroid.

PHOTODYNAMIC THERAPY

Until 1999, no treatment other than laser photocoagulation had been shown to reduce the risk of vision loss in patients with CNV from AMD in large-scale, randomized clinical trials. The TAP Study Group,[79,104] reported that PDT with verteporfin (Visudyne) can reduce the risk of moderate and severe visual acuity loss for at least 2 years in patients who present with subfoveal lesions in AMD with a predominantly classic lesion composition (in which the area of classic CNV is at least 50% of the area of the lesion). The results were even better in the absence of occult CNV.[87] The therapy also reduced the risk of contrast sensitivity loss at a level likely to be beneficial for a patient's visual function.[105] For occult with no classic lesions, the Verteporfin In Photodynamic therapy (VIP) Trial in AMD showed that PDT could reduce the risk of moderate and severe visual acuity loss by 2 years after randomization compared with a sham treatment.[85] While the primary outcome for the VIP trial, avoiding at least 15 letters (or 3 lines) of visual acuity loss at 1 year after randomization, was not statistically significantly different between the PDT and control group, the totality of the vision results (including avoiding 3 lines of loss at 2 years, avoiding 6 lines of loss at 1 and 2 years, mean visual acuity loss at 1 and 2 years, percentage 20/200 or worse) support considering this therapy for selected occult with no classic lesions. Specifically, occult with no classic lesions for which therapy was shown to reduce the risk of vision loss included lesions with recent disease progression (having blood associated with CNV, or definite loss of visual acuity within the past 3 months, or growth of the lesion on fluorescein angiography). Furthermore, therapy appeared to be beneficial for relatively small occult with no classic lesions or larger lesions with relatively poorer levels of visual acuity. While minimally classic lesions evaluated within a subgroup of classic-containing lesions in the TAP investigation showed no benefit of therapy, subsequent retrospective analyses of relatively small minimally classic lesions[85] and a small randomized clinical trial of relatively smaller minimally classic lesions,[106] showed a treatment benefit.

PDT involves the use of an intravenously injected photosensitizing drug combined with a low-intensity laser light to cause damage of choroidal neovascular tissue through a photochemical reaction by the light-activated drug that appears to result in direct cellular injury, including damage to vascular endothelial cells and vessel thrombosis.[107,108] An important advantage of this therapy is the potentially selective destruction of the CNV tissue. Retinal and choroidal tissue surrounding the CNV may be minimally disturbed, thus maintaining function of surrounding and overlying sensory retina, RPE, and choroid. Three multicenter, randomized clinical trials using benzoporphyrin-derivative monoacid verteporfin as the photosensitizing agent are currently underway to evaluate the effectiveness of this therapy, with additional trials evaluating other drugs, which have yet to show benefit in randomized clinical trials. When complexed with low-density lipoprotein (LDL) and injected intravenously, verteporfin may be taken up selectively by rapidly proliferating endothelial cells that have an increased number of LDL receptors active in their plasma membranes. Infrared laser light of low power (to avoid thermal damage) is used to irradiate the neovascular complex after verteporfin injection. Although the treatment can result in cessation of fluorescein dye leakage from CNV without significant visual loss at 1 and 4 weeks after treatment, fluorescein leakage from CNV is often apparent by 12 weeks after treatment,[107] with fewer and fewer treated cases showing fluorescein leakage with each subsequent follow-up after treatment is given.

Results of photodynamic therapy treatment

Preparation for photodynamic therapy

Before PDT, patients with a potentially treatable CNV lesion should be informed that PDT will not likely improve vision (in contrast to anti-VEGF therapy, described below, in which approximately one-third of patients experience substantial visual acuity gain). Nevertheless, although PDT does not reduce the chance of improving vision compared with no treatment, it does reduce the risk of substantial visual acuity loss. Patients should understand that most individuals lose some vision after PDT, usually within the first 12 months, although this may not be true for patients with a polypoidal choroidal vasculopathy pattern of CNV in AMD, as suggested in small studies within an Asian population.[109] Patients also should understand that there is a small risk of acute severe visual acuity decrease (loss of at least 4 lines of visual acuity compared with pretreatment levels within 7 days of treatment). Such events can occur from sudden hemorrhages (sometimes associated with tears or rips of the RPE), or choroidal perfusion abnormalities (sometimes associated with extensive subretinal fluid accumulation).[87]

Following the treatment protocol established by the TAP Investigation and VIP Trial, a recent fluorescein angiogram (if possible, less than 2 weeks old) should be used to guide the ophthalmologist during treatment. Because the CNV may grow or bleed, the treating ophthalmologist should confirm with careful biomicroscopic examination on the day of treatment that the lesion has not changed on that day if different from the day of the fluorescein angiogram. A suitable frame from the fluorescein angiogram can be displayed near the laser console. Once the area of the entire lesion is determined, one can determine the greatest linear dimension (GLD) of the lesion. The spot size to be used to activate the verteporfin should be approximately 1 mm greater than the GLD of the lesion on the retina. The ophthalmologist then enters the magnification of the lens to be used for applying laser light to activate verteporfin on the laser console before entering the spot size to be applied to the retina. Then the ophthalmologist should enter the spot size to be applied to the retina (that is, the GLD of the lesion on the retina, plus 1 mm). The ophthalmologist should confirm that the laser is set to a standard fluence rate shown to be beneficial (50 J/cm^2), which should indicate 83 s at 600 mW/cm^2. While some ophthalmologists have considered that a reduced fluence (25 J/cm^2) might reduce the chance of acute severe visual acuity loss, there is no strong evidence to support this hypothesis; thus, using the standard fluence which has been shown to be beneficial in large-scale randomized clinical trials has the strongest evidence to support its safety and efficacy in the clinical setting.

The patient receiving PDT also should be warned of potential side-effects, including photosensitivity reactions, which are usually transient and mild, occurring in 2% of treated eyes. Verteporfin-treated patients should avoid significant light exposure for up to 2 days, when almost all photosensitivity reactions were reported in clinical trials (although the product insert for the drug recommends avoiding significant light exposure for up to 5 days). The physician or nurse overseeing the infusion of verteporfin over 10 min should watch for extravasations that might not cause pain during the extravasation but can cause significant pain or edema at the injection site or, rarely, skin damage if exposed to sunlight. The patient also should understand that any extravasations should be covered from sunlight until the drug is believed to have been completely resorbed. Transient visual disturbance (20% of the time) and infusion-related back pain (2% of the time), not noted to be of any lasting significance, may also be seen. Post-treatment follow-up will require identification of fluorescein leakage following previous PDT to judge when and where retreatment should be applied or whether anti-VEGF therapy should be considered if any visual acuity loss, worsening of intraretinal or subretinal fluid on OCT, or growth of the lesion on fluorescein angiography is noted.

Follow-up after photodynamic therapy

Any decreased vision within 5 weeks after treatment may need prompt evaluation. If a change in the biomicroscopic examination is noted compared with the pretreatment appearance, OCT and fluorescein angiography may be indicated to try to understand why decreased vision has occurred, for example, due to growth of the lesion, additional fluid accumulation, bleeding, choroidal perfusion abnormalities, tears of the RPE, or other causes. Additional treatment for growth of the lesion earlier than 5–6 weeks has not been studied extensively, so that if deterioration occurs, switching to anti-VEGF therapy likely is warranted. Even if no change in vision is noted by 12 weeks after treatment, re-examination should occur at that time. If no fluorescein leakage from CNV is noted at that time, then no additional treatment is needed, although re-examination in another 6–12 weeks is warranted to see if leakage develops subsequently. If fluorescein leakage is noted and visual acuity has not improved, then switching to anti-VEGF therapy likely is warranted. If improvement in visual acuity has occurred but fluorescein leakage persists, then either switching to anti-VEGF therapy or continuing PDT treatment might be considered. If retreatment with PDT is considered, it should be applied using the GLD on the area of leakage and any contiguous blood plus 1 mm when determining the spot size. This follow-up approach should be repeated indefinitely until the situation has stabilized (because there is minimal leakage associated with a relatively flat scar and no change in visual acuity, biomicroscopic appearance, or fluorescein angiographic appearance for at least 6 months). Usually, if therapy is not switched to anti-VEGF treatments, patients will need two to three PDT treatments in the first year, and possibly one to two treatments in the second year.

PHARMACOLOGIC THERAPY WITH ANTI-VEGF PRODUCTS AND OVERALL MANAGEMENT APPROACH TO CNV IN AMD[110]

Based on the results from several clinical trials evaluating anti-VEGF therapies for CNV in AMD,[54–57] a current approach to management of subfoveal CNV in AMD in which the CNV is the predominant component (that is, the area of any classic CNV plus any occult CNV is at least 50% of the area of the lesion) is summarized in Fig. 66.21. For lesions that are predominantly scar or predominantly a serous PED, it is unknown if any treatment is beneficial. For lesions that are predominantly hemorrhagic (area of blood at least 50% of the area of the lesion), anti-VEGF therapy might be considered to reduce the risk of additional severe visual acuity loss although it is not known if such therapy might increase the chance of visual acuity improvement compared with no treatment.[111]

Recombinant interferon-alpha-2a administered systemically is a weak inhibitor of angiogenesis that is commercially available. When tested in a randomized clinical trial, however, the treatment was found to be of no benefit, and possibly harmful, compared to placebo treatment.[112] This outcome, which confirmed the variable course of untreated subfoveal CNV in AMD, especially within the first year after presentation, underscores the need for randomized clinical trials in any evaluation of pharmacologic or other therapies for CNV in AMD.

Pegaptanib sodium, a modified oligonucleotide that binds to an isoform of vascular endothelial growth factor (VEGF), has been studied in two recent phase II/III multicenter trials involving 1186 patients randomized 1:1:1:1 to sham, or 0.3 mg, 1 mg, or 3 mg of pegaptanib intraocular injections. Injections were given every 6 weeks. The trials enrolled patients with subfoveal CNV due to AMD with lesions smaller than 12 disc areas, of which at least 50% of the lesion had to be CNV (i.e., the lesion was predominantly CNV). In addition, there could not be atrophy or fibrosis in the center of the macula. Individuals with minimally classic or occult with no classic lesion compositions required evidence of recent disease progression.[113] For the primary endpoint of the proportion of patients losing less than 3 lines of visual acuity by week 54, a combined analysis found an absolute difference of 15% in favor of treatment (70% vs 55%; P <0.001) for the 294 patients receiving pegaptanib 0.3 mg. No dose response was seen in the pegaptanib studies; pegaptanib at 1.0 mg or 3.0 mg was less effective than at 0.3 mg for all outcomes. Although the incidence of endophthalmitis was low when expressed on a per-injection basis, the need to administer treatment at 6-week intervals increases this risk. During the 12 months of the studies, 1.3% of pegaptanib recipients had endophthalmitis; of these, few (8%) lost 6 or more lines of visual acuity. This anti-VEGF therapy largely has been replaced based on the more favorable results utilizing ranibizumab,[54,55] bevacizumab,[56] and aflibercept.[57]

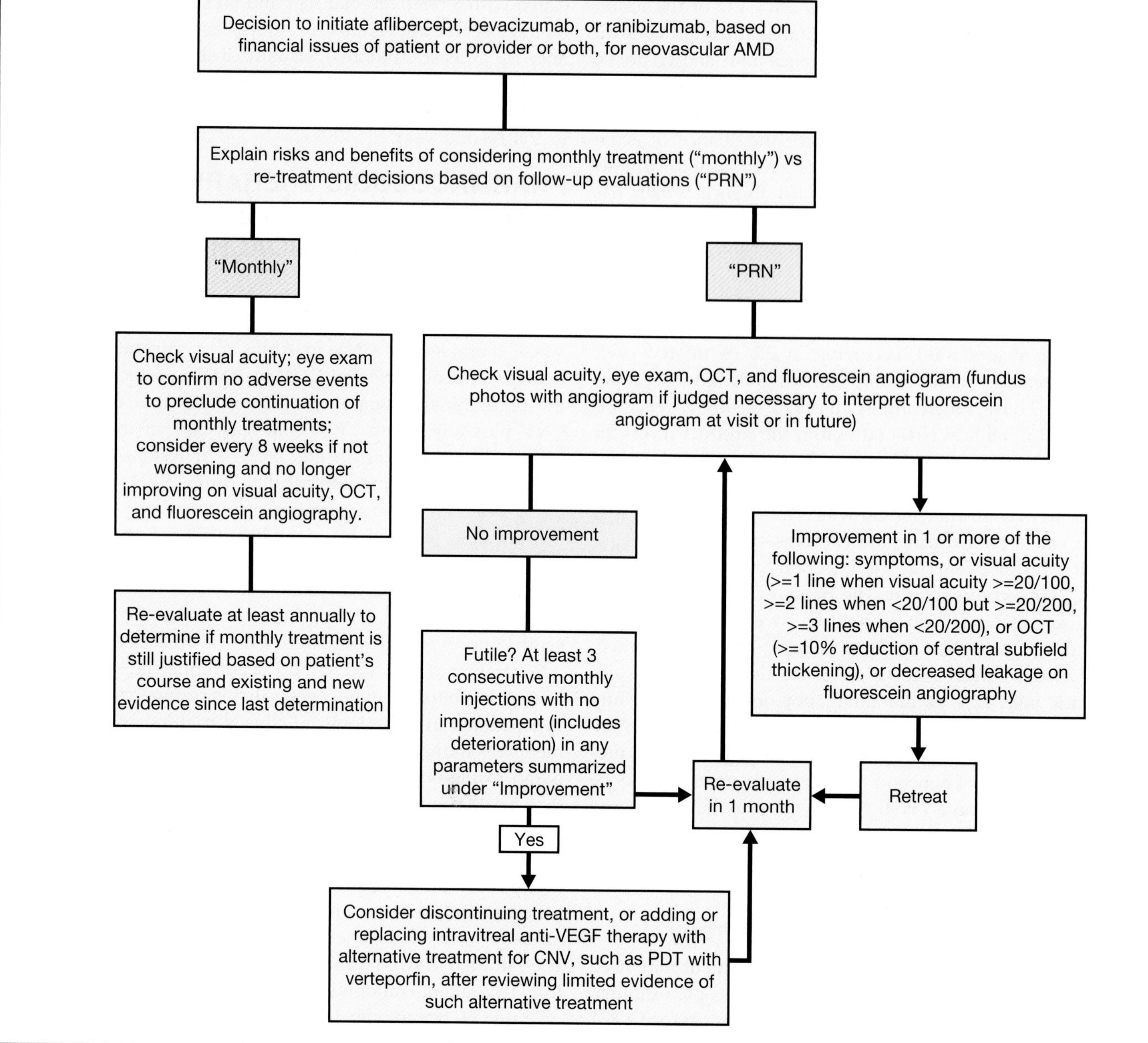

Fig. 66.21 Follow-up after initiating anti-VEGF therapy for neovascular age-related macular degeneration. AMD, age-related macular degeneration; OCT, optical coherence tomography; VEGF, vascular endothelial growth factor; CNV, choroidal neovascularization; PDT, photodynamic therapy. (© Neil M. Bressler, MD, Johns Hopkins University, 2011.)

Efficacy of ranibizumab vs PDT with verteporfin for predominantly classic subfoveal CNV lesions

Trial participants in the ANCHOR study had CNV lesions that were to be predominantly classic CNV (at least 50% of the total area of the lesion was classic CNV).[55] Unlike eligibility requirements for the MARINA study (see following section), participants were not required to have presumed recent disease progression (usually defined as presence of blood, documented recent loss of visual acuity, or documented recent growth of the choroidal neovascular lesion). Participants received ranibizumab monthly for 24 months.

Mean visual acuity letter score at baseline was 47.1 (approximate Snellen equivalent of 20/125^{+2}) in the 0.5 mg ranibizumab group. For the primary outcome (visual acuity decline of fewer than 15 letters from baseline at 12 months), 96.4% of the 0.5 mg group (n = 140) and 64.3% of the verteporfin group (n = 143) avoided this loss (P <0.001).[55] These outcomes were maintained at 24 months for most subjects, with 89.9% of the 0.5 mg group and 65.7% of the verteporfin group avoiding a loss of 3 lines or greater. Investigators also reported that visual acuity improved by 15 letters or more in 40.3% of the 0.5 mg group, as compared with 5.6% of the verteporfin group (P <0.001) at 12 months[55] and 41.0% of the 0.5 mg group gained 3 or more lines of visual acuity versus only 6.3% of the verteporfin group at 24 months. Differences in the mean visual acuity from baseline visual acuity were noted as early as 1 month, when 8.4 letters of improvement occurred in the 0.5 mg ranibizumab group compared with 0.5 letters in the PDT group (P <0.001).[55]

At 12 months, mean visual acuity improved by 11.3 letters in the 0.5 mg ranibizumab group but decreased by a mean of 9.5 letters in the verteporfin group (*P* <0.001).[55] At 24 months, mean visual acuity improved by 10.7 letters in the 0.5 mg ranibizumab group but decreased by 9.8 letters in the verteporfin group.

Although PDT produced outcomes that likely were better than the natural course of the disease, the 24-month data reinforced the conclusions of the 12-month data previously published and indicated that the increased chance of avoiding 15 or more letter loss and of gaining 15 or more letters with monthly intravitreal ranibizumab persisted through at least 2 years compared with standard applications of PDT.

Efficacy of ranibizumab vs sham treatment for minimally classic or occult with no classic subfoveal choroidal neovascular lesions and presumed recent disease progression

In a phase 3, double-blind, sham-controlled, randomized clinical trial, eligibility criteria included subfoveal CNV with lesion composition on FA that was minimally classic or occult with no classic component accompanied by presumed recent disease progression.[54] Mean visual acuity letter score at baseline was 53.7 ($20/80^{-1}$) in the 0.5 mg ranibizumab group.[54] Using the primary outcome of visual acuity decline of fewer than 15 letters from baseline as a measure of efficacy, 94.6% of those in the 0.5 mg ranibizumab group and 62.2% of those in the sham-injection group met the primary goal (*P* <0.001) after 12 months of treatment.[54] At 24 months, 90.0% of those in the 0.5 mg ranibizumab group and 52.9% of those in the sham-injection group met the primary goal (*P* <0.001).[54]

At 12 months, visual acuity improved by 15 or more letters in 33.8% of the 0.5 mg ranibizumab group, as compared with 5% of the sham-injection group (*P* <0.001).[54] Participants in the 0.5 mg ranibizumab group achieved mean increases in visual acuity of 7.2 letters, whereas the sham-injection group lost an average of 10.4 letters (*P* <0.001).[54] At 24 months, participants in the 0.5 mg ranibizumab group gained a mean of 6.6 letters of visual acuity, compared with a mean loss of 14.9 letters in the sham-injection group (*P* <0.001).[54]

In addition to experiencing improvements in objectively measurable visual outcomes, at 12 and 24 months, patients treated with ranibizumab were more likely to improve with respect to self-reported vision-related quality of life (QOL)[114–116] regardless of whether the better- or worse-seeing eye was treated. This information is complementary to the visual acuity outcomes described above because although most physicians and patients make decisions based on functional parameters such as a patient's ability to read, watch television, and avoid dependence on others because of vision, the primary outcome measure in most recent trials evaluating treatments for neovascular AMD has been visual acuity in the treated eye.[54,55] Although changes in visual acuity on an eye chart are important in understanding treatment effects, measures of visual acuity do not always completely capture the degree of visual function. Clinicians may assume that visual function or patient's perception of visual function improves along with visual acuity; however, this is not always the case.[117] Among MARINA participants, scores on the National Eye Institute Visual Function Questionnaire-25 (NEI VFQ-25) relating to activities that require both near vision (such as sewing) and distance vision (such as watching television) were more likely to improve by 10 or more points, a clinically relevant amount, in the ranibizumab group than in the sham-injection group (*P* <0.001).[118] In addition, ranibizumab-treated patients were less likely to perceive themselves as being dependent on others because of their vision.[118] Similar results were confirmed in the ANCHOR trial.

Safety of ranibizumab

Safety issues with ranibizumab intravitreal injections include local ocular adverse events (AEs) from the drug or the injection, as well as potential systemic AEs of the drug. Ocular AEs may be categorized as common but not serious and rare but potentially serious. AEs that are common but not serious include subconjunctival hemorrhage, vitreous floaters from medication or vitreous hemorrhage, and discomfort from antiseptic used to prepare the cornea before the injection. Endophthalmitis is a rare but potentially serious ocular AE that may develop after any intravitreal injection, regardless of what is being injected. Just how much preparation is necessary to minimize the development of postinjection infections is controversial. Based on data from the Diabetic Retinopathy Clinical Research Network, there is little evidence to support the need for pretreatment or post-treatment topical antibiotics.[119] Some clinicians use sterile gloves and drapes. All clinicians seem to agree that the use of a lid speculum and povidone-iodine treatment of lids, lashes, and the area to receive the injection are generally recommended to minimize postinjection colonization with normal flora. Other rare but serious ocular AEs include inflammation (as opposed to infection), vitreous hemorrhage, retinal tear or detachment, and increased intraocular pressure, which in the trials was listed as a serious AE (SAE) but might not always be considered an SAE by a treating ophthalmologist.

Systemic AEs can be a concern; VEGF inhibitors that cross into the general circulation can compromise functions that rely on VEGF outside of the eye, such as wound healing and the formation of new blood vessels around the heart or brain in cases of ischemia. Patients with AMD already are at higher risk of cardiovascular disease than the general population by virtue of their age, and patients with such risk did not have to be excluded from participating in ANCHOR or MARINA. Consequently, participants in clinical trials of VEGF inhibitors were carefully monitored for possible increases in blood pressure, occurrence of myocardial infarction/stroke, and nonocular hemorrhages.

There was no evidence that ranibizumab 0.5 mg was associated with increases in either diastolic or systolic blood pressure. In fact, treatment-related hypertension emerged in a larger proportion of PDT patients (12 of 143, or 8.4%) than among ranibizumab 0.5 mg patients (9 of 140, or 6.4%).[55] Among participants in the MARINA trial, approximately 16% in both the ranibizumab 0.5 mg and sham-injection groups developed hypertension.[54]

Nonocular hemorrhages include events such as cerebral or gastrointestinal bleeding. In the ANCHOR trial, nonocular hemorrhage was more frequent in the 0.5 mg ranibizumab group (6.4%) than in the PDT group (2.1%). In the MARINA trial, the cumulative frequency of nonocular hemorrhage by month 24 was 5.5% (13 of 236) in the sham-injection group, compared with 8.8% (21 of 239) in the 0.5 mg ranibizumab group.

Since ranibizumab is a recombinant monoclonal antibody (mAb) that contains both mouse- and human-derived segments, the human segments are engineered into the monoclonal antibody to minimize the chance that the patient's immune system will react against the mAb. Nevertheless, some patients treated with ranibizumab may develop antibodies to it. Thus, ranibizumab trials included routine testing of participants for antiranibizumab antibodies using an electrochemiluminescent assay.

In the ANCHOR trial, 8% of ranibizumab 0.5 mg subjects and 1.5% of subjects with PDT had low levels of antibodies to ranibizumab at baseline. At trial conclusion, 3.9% of ranibizumab 0.5 mg subjects had developed antibodies to ranibizumab, compared with 0% in the PDT group. In the MARINA trial, none of the subjects in the 0.5 mg ranibizumab group and 0.5% of those in the sham-injection group had antibodies to ranibizumab at baseline. After 24 months, 6.3% of subjects treated with ranibizumab 0.5 mg and 1.1% of those in the sham-injection group developed antibodies to ranibizumab.

The clinical implications of baseline and postexposure immunoreactivity to ranibizumab are unclear. Although the numbers were small, subjects in the ANCHOR trial who were immunoreactive were more likely to develop inflammation than those who were not.

With respect to cardiovascular or cerebrovascular events, during the ANCHOR trial, 1 subject in the PDT group (0.7%) and 3 subjects in the ranibizumab 0.5 mg group (2.1%) developed nonfatal myocardial infarctions, although the events occurred at times that were unrelated to treatment. The frequency of stroke (1 in each group) and cerebral infarction (0 in each group) in the ANCHOR trial were too low to draw meaningful conclusions.

At 24 months, the overall frequency of cardiovascular systemic events in the MARINA trial was similar in the 0.5 mg ranibizumab and sham-injection groups. There were only small differences in the frequency of thromboembolic events between the sham-injection group (3.8%) and the ranibizumab 0.5 mg group (4.6%). The frequency of death (2.5%) was the same in the ranibizumab 0.5 mg and sham-injection groups. Two individuals in each group died of stroke.

Although event rates for these cerebrovascular or cardiovascular events appear to be low with ranibizumab, ophthalmologists should ensure that patients understand the theoretic potential for these risks. Additional studies over time may help to refine understanding of the magnitude, if any, of this risk.

Impact of noninferiority results on frequency of treatment and the role of aflibercept or bevacizumab in place of ranibizumab

The Comparison of Age-related Macular Degeneration Treatments Trial (CATT) protocol was designed to answer two important questions relevant to treatment of CNV in AMD: (1) does bevacizumab (Avastin) injected every 4 weeks provide visual acuity results which are equivalent (strictly speaking, which are noninferior) to ranibizumab (Lucentis) injected every 4 weeks with an acceptable safety profile; and (2) does either bevacizumab or ranibizumab when provided as needed result in visual acuity outcomes equivalent to those following ranibizumab provided every 4 weeks. Here, "as needed" means that an initial injection is given with subsequent examinations of the eye every 4 weeks; reinjection is given at the time of any examination at which any disease activity is noted. Activity includes subretinal or intraretinal fluid or thickening on OCT, new or persistent hemorrhage from CNV, persistent fluorescein leakage from CNV or growth of CNV on fluorescein angiography, or visual acuity loss since the most recent injection.

The major outcomes during the first year which are relevant to these important questions included the following: (1) visual acuity outcomes when using bevacizumab every 4 weeks were equivalent (not inferior) to those when using ranibizumab every 4 weeks; (2) visual acuity outcomes when using ranibizumab as needed, based on examinations every 4 weeks, were equivalent to those when ranibizumab was given every 4 weeks; (3) visual acuity outcomes when bevacizumab as needed was compared with ranibizumab every 4 weeks were inconclusive, i.e., possibly equivalent but also possibly inferior; (4) CATT participants assigned to ranibizumab as needed received an average of approximately seven treatments in the first year and those assigned to bevacizumab as needed received an average of approximately eight treatments; (5) although no difference between ranibizumab and bevacizumab participants was identified with respect to proportions of participants who had myocardial infarction, cerebrovascular accidents, or endophthalmitis, the combined bevacizumab groups had a higher rate of systemic serious AEs than the combined ranibizumab groups (24% for bevacizumab, 19% for ranibizumab) – of note, the point estimates for these systemic serious adverse events was higher in the bevacizumab as-needed group than the bevacizumab every-4-weeks group; and (6) the average cost of drug per patient for the first year was $23400 in the ranibizumab every-4-weeks group, $13800 in the ranibizumab as-needed group, and $595 in the bevacizumab every-4-weeks group. Two-year data confirmed that every-4-week bevacizumab was equivalent to ranibizumab, the increased risk of serious systemic adverse events with bevacizumab was sustained and still requires further study, and the average visual acuity in both the bevacizumab-as-needed and ranibizumab-as-needed groups continued to decline from year 1 to year 2.[120]

The 1-year results from another trial comparing bevacizumab and ranibizumab, and continuous and discontinuous treatment[121] confirmed that the bevacizumab group appeared to have a slightly smaller mean gain in visual acuity at 1 year compared with the ranibizumab group (when combining both continuous and discontinuous treatment groups), and the discontinuous group (which required three consecutive monthly injections whenever treatment was resumed) appeared to have only a slightly smaller gain in mean visual acuity when compared with the continuous group (combining the ranibizumab and bevacizumab groups). Two-year data are anticipated in 2013.

Yet another set of trials confirmed that aflibercept (Eyelea) given every 4 weeks for three doses followed by every 8 weeks through 48 weeks gave equivalent outcomes to ranibizuamb-every-4 weeks.[57] In the second year of these trials, when either aflibercept or ranibizumab was given at least every 12 weeks as well as when retreatment was judged to be indicated based on clinical parameters, including OCT, evaluated every 4 weeks, showed a small decline in the average visual acuity for each of the groups.

Potential implications of anti-VEGF noninferiority trials results on clinical practice

Based on the information summarized above and published from other randomized controlled trials, the following implications should be considered.

If treatment with bevacizumab is to be initiated in an eye with CNV due to AMD, the patient should be informed that when using bevacizumab, treatment every 4 weeks for at least the next year, without dependence on OCT or other imaging, has been shown by CATT to be equivalent to the current "gold standard" of ranibizumab every 4 weeks. If treatment with bevacizumab every 4 weeks is to be given, the patient also should be informed that the 2-year CATT results show an increase in serious systemic AEs with intravitreal bevacizumab for which the causes are not yet understood fully. The ophthalmologist should keep in mind that comparison of visual acuity outcomes when bevacizumab or ranibizumab from treatment initiation, or aflibercept starting 1 year after treatment initiation, was given as needed, with examinations every 4 weeks, visual acuity outcomes appeared, on average, to be slightly worse. While a slightly worse outcome may not be clinically relevant one year after treatment initiation, it becomes relevant if the decline in the average visual acuity continues, as it appears to do at least from 1 to 2 years after treatment initiation. Very importantly, the ophthalmologist and patient must keep in mind that from the societal perspective, use of bevacizumab leads to very large cost savings in the management of this condition.

Ranibizumab as needed with examinations every 4 weeks, including OCT, to detect features that suggest the need for retreatment, provides equivalent visual acuity outcomes to the current gold standard of ranibizumab every 4 weeks at 1 year but not necessarily by 2 years, or thereafter. Aflibercept every 4 weeks for three doses followed by every 8 weeks to 1 year also provides equivalent results to ranibizumab-every-4 weeks; when the group given this regimen received an as-needed regimen starting at 1 year, the average visual acuity declined by 2 years, although not by a clinically relevant amount. However, if this decline were to continue during treatment 3 or 5 years after initiating therapy, the decline could be clinically relevant.

The results should be interpreted with the finding that as-needed ranibizumab or aflibercept costs about $13 000 more at least for the first year than every-4-week bevacizumab, and every-4-week ranibizumab costs about $10 000 more than ranibizumab as needed. Whether the greater costs of ranibizumab or aflibercept are worth the possibility that a small percentage of patients *might* have substantially better vision or that a larger number of patients might have slightly better vision or a slightly higher risk of systemic AEs, or clusters of endophthalmitis when not compounded properly, are beyond the scope of this chapter. However, these trials provide important data for both private (commercial) and government-sponsored insurances to make decisions on utilization of funds from the perspective of the public health and societal costs for patients who cannot pay for the costs of these very beneficial treatments which, when indicated and available, could reduce at least 75%[2,122] of the prevalence of blindness from what was the leading cause of blindness just a decade ago.

Follow-up after deciding to initiate anti-VEGF therapy for neovascular AMD

Figure 66.21 provides one approach[123] to consider if monthly anti-VEGF therapy with bevacizumab or ranibizumab, or 3 monthly doses of aflibercept followed by every-2-months aflibercept, is not employed. The approach considers repeating therapy as long as improvement is noted on subjective symptoms, visual acuity, biomicroscopic examination, OCT, or fluorescein angiography. The approach errs on the side of treatment since failure to treat when VEGF is present could result in irreversible visual acuity loss from fibrosis involving the retina or RPE.

EARLY IDENTIFICATION OF CHOROIDAL NEOVASCULARIZATION

It has become critically important to identify, while potentially still at a treatable stage, those eyes at high risk for visual loss. Unfortunately, the likelihood of finding a case that will benefit from treatment appears to be time-dependent. Fluorescein angiographic studies have suggested growth of CNV lesions at an average rate of 10–18 μm per day.[124,125] Grey and colleagues[126] reported that patients with acute visual loss from AMD are more likely to have extrafoveal CNV if they are examined within the first month after the onset of symptoms.

Clearly, identifying lesions before they extend under the foveal center, when visual acuity loss may be minimal, is worthwhile. Furthermore, identifying lesions while visual acuity is relatively good might result in better levels of final visual acuity since most cases treated with anti-VEGF therapy avoid substantial visual acuity loss but fewer than 50% have substantial visual acuity gain. Studies are underway to determine if devices designed for home detection of CNV are worthwhile in identifying CNV before other symptoms herald its onset.

PREVENTION OF CHOROIDAL NEOVASCULARIZATION

The Age-Related Eye Disease Study (AREDS) suggested that dietary supplements of vitamins C, E, beta-carotene, and zinc can reduce the chance of CNV developing in eyes with large drusen, especially when retinal pigment epithelial abnormalities were present and when these features were in both eyes. The Complications of Age-related Macular Degeneration Prevention Trial (CAPT) was not able to demonstrate that light laser photocoagulation, which has been associated with a decreased visualization of drusen,[127] can prevent the development of complications of AMD associated with visual loss, including CNV and geographic atrophy.

RISK OF FELLOW-EYE INVOLVEMENT

When one eye has developed CNV, it is important to monitor the other eye for CNV, especially since substantial loss of vision in the first eye is highly likely.[128] Development of CNV in the second eye can be devastating, since patients may have functioned quite well with good vision in their remaining eye but would be abruptly confronted for the first time with severe lifestyle impairment with development of CNV in both eyes. Often, they may not have planned for this eventuality despite proper counseling at the time of the first eye involvement. It is therefore paramount to discover and treat CNV as soon as possible to maximize the possibility of detecting treatable lesions. Because patients may be aware of symptoms only when the fovea has become involved, it would be useful to stratify risk based on fundus appearance and perhaps employ more aggressive monitoring strategies in those deemed at high risk.

The investigators of the MPS Group have studied the eyes of 670 patients enrolled in the trials of laser therapy for extrafoveal, juxtafoveal, and subfoveal CNV to identify fundus characteristics that might be predictive of CNV development in the uninvolved fellow eyes.[129–131] Follow-up ranged from 3 to 5 years and revealed an overall incidence of 35%, which is consistent with previously reported figures. Application of life table estimation methods to this data yielded cumulative incidence rates of 10%, 28%, and 42% at 1, 3, and 5 years respectively. Three characteristics of the central macula and one systemic factor were associated independently with increased risk of developing CNV: the presence of five or more drusen, one or more large drusen, focal hyperpigmentation, and systemic hypertension. A substantial difference in prognosis was seen depending on the number of risk factors present. Estimated 5-year incidence rates ranged from 7% for the subgroup with no risk factors to 87% for the subgroup with all four risk factors. Similarly, in AREDS, subjects enrolled with advanced AMD (either neovascular AMD or central atrophy of the RPE) in one eye only at study entry had a 43% chance of developing advanced AMD in the fellow eye by 5 years.[132] The type of CNV present in the affected eye, classic versus occult, appeared to have no effect on the rate of CNV development in the fellow eye. It must be stressed that these figures do not apply to patients with non-neovascular abnormalities only in both eyes. They are, however, very important in counseling the AMD patient who has just experienced the initial development of CNV in one eye with respect to prognosis and frequency of follow-up to try to protect the vision in the other eye.

ADDITIONAL THERAPIES

Submacular surgery

Studies have shown that visual acuity outcomes with submacular surgery are no different compared with observation for subfoveal CNV in patients with AMD in which a majority of the lesion is CNV and there is evidence of classic CNV.[27] However, for lesions that are predominantly hemorrhagic (at least 50% of the lesion is blood), submacular surgery can reduce the risk of additional severe visual acuity loss compared with observation, although many patients undergoing surgery lost at least two lines of visual acuity.[20] Specifically, 21% of patients undergoing removal of hemorrhage lost 6 or more lines of visual acuity compared with 36% assigned to observation. Almost half of the patients who were phakic at the time of undergoing submacular surgery had cataract surgery by 2 years. Furthermore, there was a relatively high risk of rhegmatogenous retinal detachment, especially when the lesion was greater than 16 disc areas or the visual acuity was very poor after enrollment. For this reason, submacular surgery for predominantly hemorrhagic lesions could be considered for lesions that were no greater than 16 disc areas if identified before visual acuity was very poor. More details on the findings of the trials investigating surgery for CNV in patients with AMD are included in the surgery volume of this book.

Although there is no strong evidence to support benefits of submacular surgery,[27,93,104,133] except for reducing the risk of additional severe visual acuity loss in selected cases of predominantly hemorrhagic lesions, alternative surgical approaches under investigation for managing CNV and its neovascular complications include macular translocation and mechanical displacement of relatively large submacular hemorrhages using intraocular gas injection. Macular translocation can be accomplished by vitrectomy combined with retinotomy or by vitrectomy combined with external sclerochoroidal foreshortening.[134] After translocation has been accomplished and the CNV lesion is no longer subfoveal, laser photocoagulation is applied with sparing of the foveal center from photocoagulation. The American Academy of Ophthalmology published an Ophthalmic Procedure Preliminary Assessment of this technique,[135] highlighting the need for large-scale case series and randomized trials before widespread acceptance of this approach should be considered.

When AMD-related CNV is associated with a large submacular hemorrhage, intraocular injection of gas and face-down positioning may allow for mechanical displacement of the blood and at least temporary recovery of visual acuity.[136] The improvement may not have long-term benefit if the underlying neovascular lesion and its accompanying destruction of the retina, not the blood, determines the ultimate visual outcome. More experience is needed to evaluate the safety and benefit of these surgical approaches.

Indocyanine green angiography

Indocyanine green is a dye that is more highly protein-bound than sodium fluorescein and that fluoresces in the near-infrared wavelength. These properties were suggested to be useful in the evaluation and management of CNV (see Chapter 2, Indocyanine green angiography). Three basic patterns of fluorescence have been reported in indocyanine green angiography of CNV judged to be occult on fluorescein angiography: a small, focal "hot spot" (a bright area of fluorescence more than one disc area that usually shows by the mid-phase of the angiogram), a plaque (a well-demarcated area of fluorescence more than one disc area in size that emerges relatively late in the angiogram), and ill-defined fluorescence.[137,138] Because the hot spot is small and may be extrafoveal in location, attention is drawn to it as a possible treatment site. Pilot studies utilizing photocoagulation of this site have reported improvement or stabilization of visual acuity, as well as resolution of "exudative features."[137–140] However, similar outcomes have been observed in eyes with occult CNV that have not received any treatment.[82,139] For example, a reanalysis of data used in the MPS juxtafoveal trial suggested that eyes with occult only CNV may have a more favorable natural course than eyes with classic CNV only. It is possible that the outcome of treating hot spots is no better than that of the natural course of these lesions. As described previously, eyes with both classic and occult CNV did not benefit from photocoagulation of the classic component alone. Treatment of the entire neovascular complex appears to be necessary. Treatment of a "hot spot" alone, identified on indocyanine green and associated with a larger area judged to be occult CNV on fluorescein angiography, may be similar to the unsuccessful strategy of treating just the classic CNV in an eye with both classic and occult CNV on fluorescein angiography. Until carefully designed, randomized clinical trials are conducted that show that indocyanine green-guided laser therapy of AMD-related CNV results in a better visual outcome than no treatment, one cannot know for sure if this particular intervention is beneficial.[141] The role of ICG angiography in the setting of polypoidal choroidal vasculopathy patterns of CNV also is discussed further in Chapter 71 (Polypoidal choroidal vasculopathy).

Radiation therapy

The use of radiation therapy for CNV in AMD is based on the possibility that radiation can damage rapidly proliferating neovascular tissue. Studies have been inconsistent in documenting a benefit to this approach, either using external beam, plaques, or use of a probe with local irradiation.[142–144]

Other pharmacologic therapies and combination therapies

A variety of other pharmacologic therapies, delivery devices for pharmacologic therapies, and combinations of therapies are under investigation,[145,146] but given the public health importance and biologic variability of visual acuity outcomes with CNV in AMD, changes in the management of CNV in AMD should be influenced strongly by large-scale, appropriately designed randomized clinical trials with adequate follow-up that show benefit before new therapies are incorporated into standard practice.

PATIENT EDUCATION AND REHABILITATION

Patient education is an extremely important part of the management of patients with AMD. All patients over the age of 50 who have drusen should be made aware of the importance of regular central visual acuity testing in each eye to facilitate early detection of CNV. Although the Amsler grid is often recommended, it is not particularly sensitive or specific; frequently, changes in near or distance vision herald underlying neovascularization not detected by the patient on an Amsler grid.[9] Therefore patients experiencing any change in vision in eyes at risk for neovascularization should be encouraged to contact their ophthalmologist promptly. Although patients should be counseled about the risk of severe central visual loss, they should also be reassured that AMD almost never leads to total blindness. Patients at risk should be informed that, in its more severe neovascular form, central visual tasks can be severely and permanently impaired. In light of the therapeutic implications of prompt anti-VEGF therapy when indicated, the importance of quickly reporting new visual symptoms must be stressed to all patients. At the same time, they should be reassured that no harm will come by continuing to read or perform routine visual tasks. On the contrary, patients should be encouraged to continue reading and to pursue vigorously any visual activity that they enjoy.

Treatment does not end in the physician's office when the diagnosis is established or when anti-VEGF therapy is applied. Visual rehabilitation forms an integral part of patient care in AMD. Patients with central visual impairment should be evaluated and educated in the use of visual aids such as magnifiers. Magnification and improved contrast sensitivity through bright illumination are particularly helpful. To arrive at the best magnifying aid, one starts with a complete low visual evaluation. In addition, the patient should be counseled on available low-vision materials such as large-print newspapers, magazines, and books. Large-print materials or electronically magnified text permit many people who are unable to read normal print to continue reading for a considerable period of time. Many newspapers and periodicals are currently published in large-print editions or electronically as available through the internet. The local library can assist with the selection of magazines and books available in large print. The Library of Congress in Washington, DC, maintains a list of books and magazines available on loan without cost on virtually every subject. The combination of bright illumination, powerful magnification, high contrast, and large type allows all but the most severely impaired patients to continue reading, albeit on a more limited scale. Reading skills frequently need to be re-learned in a painstakingly slow process. Nevertheless the ability to continue reading, even on a limited basis, may provide tremendous psychologic support to these patients. Some patients with AMD may find the use of a closed-circuit television viewer helpful for reading. This machine uses a projection device to magnify one or several words on to a television screen. Unfortunately, this instrument is large and fairly expensive; thus it is generally purchased by people with sufficient economic means who use it primarily in one location such as at work or at home. For those patients who are unable to take advantage of large-print materials or who cannot use magnification devices, talking books or tapes are available. These may be borrowed through local libraries or from the Library of Congress. Audiotapes of popular books are also sold at many bookstores.

Patients with severe visual loss require early referral to an appropriate agency for low vision so that they can take advantage of community support services. Information can be obtained from the Directory of Agencies serving the visually handicapped in the USA through the American Foundation for the Blind. The American Foundation for the Blind also provides information regarding other aids such as talking books and clocks and watches that audibly tell time.

Because AMD can place severe restrictions on many activities such as driving and rapid reading of small print, visual rehabilitation efforts are directed toward preserving the patient's independence as much as possible. Toward this end, social service consultations are invaluable. In addition, in-house evaluations by agencies designed to assist the visually impaired are useful in helping with activities of daily living. Simple recommendations, such as using brightly colored utensils on a white or black background in the kitchen, as well as suggestions on improving existing lighting, can be of tremendous benefit. Similar ideas aimed at increasing contrast may improve the quality of life for these patients. Patients often become frustrated because of their inability to perform certain fine visual tasks, such as reading and sewing. Unable to recognize faces from across the room, patients with visual loss from AMD may feel isolated and withdraw from social contact. In the absence of any external tell-tale signs of blindness, friends and relatives may attribute the lack of recognition to a sudden "snobbishness" rather than to visual impairment. Patient and family alike should be educated about these problems. In particular, patients should be encouraged to become more outgoing, which in turn fosters recognition of others through speech rather than vision. Discussion of the patient's problems by the physician often helps to relieve patients of much of their burdens.

Ophthalmologists must recognize that older patients can have difficulty coping with the new onset of severe visual loss. Patients may resist efforts to use magnifying devices for a variety of reasons, including denial and secondary gain. Often tremulousness interferes with the patient's ability to use certain aids. All these conditions may increase the tendency to depression or anxiety that many patients with visual loss have, including patients with AMD. In addition to caring for the eye, the ophthalmologist should serve as the patient's advocate, marshaling his or her resources for the patient's benefit. This includes compassionate support, educating the patient and family, and making appropriate referrals to maintain the patient's quality of life. With complete care of the patient, many individuals at risk for, or suffering severe visual loss from, neovascular AMD can continue to enjoy fulfilling lives.

Disclosure

The Johns Hopkins University School of Medicine receives research grants from Bayer, Genentech, Lumenis, Novartis, Regeneron, Optovue, QLT, Carl Zeiss Meditec for N.M.B.'s effort in research activities with those industries.

REFERENCES

1. Eye Diseases Prevalence Research Group. Prevalence of age-related macular degeneration in the United States. Arch Ophthalmol 2004;122:564–72.
2. Bressler NM, Doan QV, Varma R, et al. Estimated cases of legal blindness and visual impairment avoided using ranibizumab for choroidal neovascularization. Arch Ophthalmol 2011;129:709–17.
3. Bressler NM, Bressler SB, Fine SL. Age-related macular degeneration. Surv Ophthalmol 1988;32:375–413.
4. Ferris FL III, Fine SL, Hyman LA. Age-related macular degeneration and blindness due to neovascular maculopathy. Arch Ophthalmol 1984;102:1640–2.
5. Sommer A, Tielsch JM, Katz J, et al. Racial differences in the cause-specific prevalence of blindness in east Baltimore. N Engl J Med 1991;325:1412–7.
6. Schultz DW, Klein M, Humpert AJ, et al. Analysis of the ARMD1 locus: evidence that a mutation in HEMICENTIN-1 is associated with age-related macular degeneration in a large family. Hum Mol Genet 2003;12:3315–23.
7. Hyman L, Schachat AP, He Q, et al. Hypertension, cardiovascular disease, and age-related macular degeneration. Age-Related Macular Degeneration Risk Factors Study Group. Arch Ophthalmol 2000;118:351–8.
8. Loewenstein A, Bressler NM, Bressler SB. Epidemiology of RPE disease. In: Marmor MF, Wolfensberger TJ, editors. Retinal pigment epithelium: current aspects of function and disease. New York: Oxford University Press; 1999.
9. Fine AM, Elman MJ, Ebert JE, et al. Earliest symptoms caused by neovascular membranes in the macula. Arch Ophthalmol 1986;104:513–14.
10. Bressler SB, Silva JC, Bressler NM, et al. Clinicopathologic correlation of occult choroidal neovascularization in age-related macular degeneration. Arch Ophthalmol 1992;110:827–32.
11. Green WR, Key SN. Senile macular degeneration: a histopathologic study. Trans Am Ophthalmol Soc 1977;75:180–254.
12. Green WR, McDonnell PH, Yeo JH. Pathologic features of senile macular degeneration. Ophthalmology 1985;92:615–27.
13. Green WR, Enger C. Age-related macular degeneration histopathologic studies. The 1992 Lorenz E. Zimmerman lecture. Ophthalmology 1993;100:1519–35.
14. Dyer DS, Brant AM, Schachat AP, et al. Questionable recurrent choroidal neovascularization: angiographic features and outcome. Am J Ophthalmol 1995;120:497–505.
15. Doyle WJ, Davidorf FH, Makley TA, et al. Histopathology of an active lesion of ocular histoplasmosis. Ophthalm Forum 1984;2:105–11.
16. Schatz H, McDonald HR, Johnson RN. Retinal pigment epithelial folds associated with retinal pigment epithelial detachment in macular degeneration. Ophthalmology 1990;97:658–65.
17. Elman MJ, Fine SL, Murphy RP, et al. The natural history of serous retinal pigment epithelium detachments in patients with age-related macular degeneration. Ophthalmology 1986;93:224–30.
18. Bird AC, Marshal J. Retinal pigment epithelial detachment in the elderly. Trans Ophthalmol Soc UK 1986;105:674–82.
19. Macular Photocoagulation Study Group. Subfoveal neovascular lesions in age-related macular degeneration: guidelines for evaluation and treatment in the Macular Photocoagulation Study. Arch Ophthalmol 1991;109:1242–57.
20. Bressler NM, Bressler SB, Childs AL, et al. Submacular Surgery Trials (SST) Research Group. Surgery for hemorrhagic choroidal lesions of age-related macular degeneration: ophthalmic findings. SST report no. 13. Ophthalmology 2004;111:1993–2006.
21. Taylor HR, West S, Munoz B, et al. The long-term effects of visible light on the eye. Arch Ophthalmol 1992;110:99–104.
22. Wood WJ, Smith TR. Senile disciform macular degeneration complicated by massive hemorrhagic retinal detachment and angle closure glaucoma. Retina 1983;3:296–303.
23. el Baba F, Jarrett WH II, Harbin IS, et al. Massive hemorrhage complicating age-related macular degeneration. Ophthalmology 1986;93:1281–592.
24. Macular Photocoagulation Study Group. Laser photocoagulation of subfoveal neovascular lesions in age-related macular degeneration: results of a randomized clinical trial. Arch Ophthalmol 1991;109:1220–31.
25. Macular Photocoagulation Study Group. Laser photocoagulation of subfoveal neovascular lesions in age-related macular degeneration: results of a randomized clinical trial. Arch Ophthalmol 1991;109:1232–41.
26. Macular Photocoagulation Study Group. Laser photocoagulation of juxtafoveal choroidal neovascularization: 5-year results from randomized clinical trials. Arch Ophthalmol 1994;111:500–9.
27. Hawkins BS, Bressler NM, Miskala PH, et al. Submacular Surgery Trials (SST) Research Group. Surgery for subfoveal choroidal neovascularization of age-related macular degeneration: ophthalmic findings. SST report no. 11. Ophthalmology 2004;111:1967–80.
28. De Jong PTVM, Chakravarthy U, Rahu M, et al. Associations between aspirin use and aging macula disorder. The European Eye Study. Ophthalmology 2012; in press.
29. Cantrill HL, Ramsay RC, Knoblock WH. Rips in the pigment epithelium. Arch Ophthalmol 1983;101:1074–9.
30. Decker WL, Sanborn GF, Ridley M, et al. Retinal pigment epithelial tears. Ophthalmology 1983;90:507–12.
31. Green SN, Yarian D. Acute tears of the retinal pigment epithelium. Retina 1983;3:16–20.
32. Hoskin A, Bird AC, Sehow K. Tears of detached retinal pigment epithelium. Br J Ophthalmol 1981;65:417–22.
33. Yeo JH, Marcus S, Murphy RP. Retinal pigment epithelial tears: patterns and prognosis. Ophthalmology 1988;95:813.
34. Gass JDM. Stereoscopic atlas of macular disease and treatment, 4th ed. St Louis: Mosby; 1997.
35. Grossniklaus HE, Green WR, for the Submacular Surgery Trials Research Group. Histopathologic and ultrastructural findings of surgically-excised choroidal neovascularization. Arch Ophthalmol 1998;116:745–9.
36. Grossniklaus HE, Miskala PH, Green WR, et al. Submacular Surgery Trials (SST) Research Group. Histopathological and ultrastructural features of surgically-excised subfoveal choroidal neovascularization and associated tissue. SST report no. 7. Arch Ophthalmol 2005;123:914–21.
37. Grossniklaus HE, Green WR. Choroidal neovascularization. Am J Ophthalmol 2004;137:496–503.
38. Lafaut BA, Bartz-Schmidt KU, Vanden Broecke C, et al. Clinicopathologic correlation in exudative age related macular degeneration: histological differentiation between classic and occult choroidal neovascularization. Br J Ophthalmol 2000;84:239–43.
39. Submacular Surgery Trials Research Group. Comparison of two-dimensional reconstructions of surgically-excised subfoveal choroidal neovascularization with fluorescein angiographic features: SST report no. 15. Ophthalmology 2006;113:279.
40. Sykes SO, Bressler NM, Maguire MG, et al. Detecting recurrent choroidal neovascularization: comparison of clinical examination with and without fluorescein angiography. Arch Ophthalmol 1994;111:1561–6.
41. Treatment of Age-Related Macular Degeneration with Photodynamic Therapy (TAP) and Verteporfin in Photodynamic Therapy Study Groups. Photodynamic therapy of subfoveal choroidal neovascularization with verteporfin: fluorescein angiographic guidelines for evaluation and treatment – TAP and VIP report no. 2. Arch Ophthalmol 2003;121:1253–68.
42. Solomon SD, Bressler SB, Hawkins BS, et al. Submacular Surgery Trials (SST) Research Group. Guidelines for interpreting retinal photographs in the Submacular Surgery Trials (SST). SST report no. 8. Retina 2005;25:253–68.
43. Koenig F, Soubrane G, Coscas G. Angiographic aspects of senile macular degeneration: spontaneous course. J Fr Ophtalmol 1984;7:93–8.
44. Frost L, Bressler NM, Bressler SB, et al. Natural course of poorly defined choroidal neovascularization associated with age-related macular degeneration. Invest Ophthalmol 1988;29(Suppl):120.
45. Hyman L, Lilienfeld AM, Ferris FL III, et al. Senile macular degeneration: a case-control study. Am J Epidemiol 1983;118:213–27.
46. Dyer DS, Brant AM, Schachat AP, et al. Angiographic features and outcome of questionable recurrent choroidal neovascularization. Am J Ophthalmol 1995;120:497–505.
47. Yannuzzi LA, Negrao S, Iida T, et al. Retinal angiomatous proliferation in age-related macular degeneration. Retina 2001;21:416–34.
48. Bressler NM, Bressler SB, Alexander J, et al. Loculated fluid: a previously undescribed angiographic finding in macular degeneration. Arch Ophthalmol 1991;109:211–15.
49. Chuang EL, Bird AC. The pathogenesis of tears of the retinal pigment epithelium. Am J Ophthalmol 1988;105:285–90.
50. Killingsworth MC, Sarks JP, Sarks SH. Macrophages related to Bruch's membrane in age-related macular degeneration. Eye 1990;4:613–21.
51. Ambati J, Ambati BK, Yoo SH, et al. Age-related macular degeneration: etiology, pathogenesis, and therapeutic strategies. Surv Ophthalmol 2003;48:257–93.
52. Gragoudas ES, Adamis AP, Cunningham Jr ET, et al. for the VEGF Inhibition Study in Ocular Neovascularization Clinical Trial Group. Pegaptanib for neovascular age-related macular degeneration. N Engl J Med 2004;351:2805–16.
53. Genentech [Internet]. Preliminary phase III data show Lucentis maintained or improved vision in nearly 95 percent of patients with wet age-related macular degeneration. http://www.gene.com/gene/news/press-releases/; Press release May 23, 2005 [cited June 2005].
54. Rosenfeld PJ, Brown DM, Heier JS, et al. Ranibizumab for neovascular age-related macular degeneration. N Engl J Med 2006;355:1419–31.
55. Brown DM, Kaiser PK, Michels M, et al. Ranibizumab versus verteporfin for neovascular age-related macular degeneration. N Engl J Med 2006;355:1432–44.

56. The CATT Research Group. Ranibizumab and bevacizumab for neovascular age-related macular degeneration. N Engl J Med 2011;364:1897–908.
57. Aflibercept Product Insert. 11/2011. http://www.regeneron.com/Eylea/eylea-fpi.pdf [accessed 2012 July 4].
58. Bressler NM, Silva JC, Bressler SB, et al. Clinicopathologic correlation of drusen and retinal pigment epithelial abnormalities in age-related macular degeneration. Retina 1994;14:130–42.
59. Curcio CA, Millican CL. Basal linear deposit and large drusen are specific for early age-related macular degeneration. Arch Ophthalmol 1999;117:329–39.
60. Sarks SH. Aging and degeneration in the macular region: a clinicopathological study. Br J Ophthalmol 1976;60:324–41.
61. Sarks SH. Drusen and their relationship to senile macular degeneration. Aust J Ophthalmol 1980;8:117–30.
62. Sarks SH, Penfold PL, Killingsworth MC, et al. Patterns in macular degeneration. In: Ryan SJ, Dawson AK, Little HL, editors. Retinal diseases. Orlando, FL: Grune & Stratton; 1985.
63. Sarks SH, Van Driel D, Maxwell L, et al. Softening of drusen and subretinal neovascularization. Trans Ophthalmol Soc UK 1980;100:414–22.
64. Kenyon KR, Maumenee AE, Ryan SJ, et al. Diffuse drusen and associated complications. Am J Ophthalmol 1985;100:119–28.
65. Eagle RC. Mechanisms of maculopathy. Ophthalmology 1984;91:613–25.
66. Heriot WJ, Henkind P, Bellhorn RW, et al. Choroidal neovascularization can digest Bruch's membrane: a prior break is not essential. Ophthalmology 1984;91:1603–8.
67. Loffer KU, Lee WR. Basal linear deposit in the human macula. Graefes Arch Clin Exp Ophthalmol 1986;224:493–501.
68. Penfold PL, Killingsworth MC, Sarks SH. Senile macular degeneration: the involvement of immunocompetent cells. Graefes Arch Clin Exp Ophthalmol 1985;223:69–76.
69. Penfold PL, Provis JM, Billson FA. Age-related macular degeneration: ultrastructural studies of the relationship of leukocytes to angiogenesis. Graefes Arch Clin Exp Ophthalmol 1987;225:70–6.
70. Campochiaro PA, Hackett SF, Vinores SA, et al. Platelet-derived growth factor is an autocrine growth stimulator in retinal pigmented epithelial cells. J Cell Sci 1994;107:2459–69.
71. Glaser BM. Extracellular modulating factors and the control of intraocular neovascularization. Arch Ophthalmol 1988;106:603–7.
72. Bressler NM, Bressler SB, Gragoudas ES. Clinical characteristics of choroidal neovascular membranes. Arch Ophthalmol 1987;105:209–13.
73. Berkow JW. Subretinal neovascularization in senile macular degeneration. Am J Ophthalmol 1984;97:143–7.
74. Moisseiev J, Alhalel A, Masuri R, et al. The impact of the Macular Photocoagulation Study results on the treatment of exudative age-related macular degeneration. Arch Ophthalmol 1995;113:185–9.
75. Macular Photocoagulation Study Group. Argon laser photocoagulation for neovascular maculopathy: 3-year results from randomized clinical trials. Arch Ophthalmol 1986;104:694–701.
76. Macular Photocoagulation Study Group. Argon laser photocoagulation for neovascular maculopathy after 5 years: results from randomized clinical trials. Arch Ophthalmol 1991;109:1109–14.
77. Macular Photocoagulation Study Group. Argon laser photocoagulation for senile macular degeneration: results of a randomized clinical trial. Arch Ophthalmol 1982;100:912–18.
78. Macular Photocoagulation Study Group. Laser photocoagulation of subfoveal neovascular lesions of age-related macular degeneration: updated findings from two clinical trials. Arch Ophthalmol 1993;111:1200–9.
79. Treatment of Age-Related Macular Degeneration with Photodynamic Therapy (TAP) Study Group. Photodynamic therapy of subfoveal choroidal neovascularization in age-related macular degeneration with verteporfin: Two year results of 2 randomized clinical trials – TAP report no. 2. Arch Ophthalmol 2001;119:198–207.
80. Treatment of Age-Related Macular Degeneration with Photodynamic Therapy (TAP) Study Group. Effect of lesion size, visual acuity, and lesion composition on visual acuity change from baseline with and without verteporfin therapy in choroidal neovascularization secondary to age-related macular degeneration: TAP and VIP report no. 1. Am J Ophthalmol 2003;136:407–18.
81. Bressler NM, Maguire MG, Murphy PL, et al. Macular scatter ("grid") laser treatment of poorly demarcated subfoveal choroidal neovascularization in age-related macular degeneration: results of a randomized pilot trial. Arch Ophthalmol 1996;114:1456–64.
82. Macular Photocoagulation Study Group. Occult choroidal neovascularization: influence on visual outcome in patients with age-related macular degeneration. Arch Ophthalmol 1996;114:400–12.
83. Soubrane G, Coscas G, Francais C, et al. Occult subretinal new vessels in age-related macular degeneration: natural history and early laser treatment. Ophthalmology 1990;97:649–57.
84. Tani PM, Buettner H, Robertson DM. Massive vitreous hemorrhage and senile macular choroidal degeneration. Am J Ophthalmol 1980;90:525–33.
85. Verteporfin in Photodynamic Therapy (VIP) Study Group. Photodynamic therapy of subfoveal choroidal neovascularization in age-related macular degeneration with verteporfin: Two year results of a randomized clinical trial including lesions with occult but no classic neovascularization – VIP report no. 2. Am J Ophthalmol 2001;131:541–60.
86. Treatment of Age-Related Macular Degeneration with Photodynamic Therapy (TAP) Study Group. Natural history of minimally classic subfoveal choroidal neovascular lesions in the Treatment of Age-related macular degeneration with Photodynamic therapy (TAP) Investigation: Outcomes potentially relevant to management – TAP report no. 6. Arch Ophthalmol 2004;122:325–9.
87. Treatment of Age-Related Macular Degeneration with Photodynamic Therapy (TAP) Study Group. Verteporfin therapy of subfoveal choroidal neovascularization in patients with age-related macular degeneration: additional information regarding baseline lesion composition's impact on vision outcomes – TAP Report No. 3. Arch Ophthalmol 2002;120:1443–54.
88. Avery RL, Fekrat S, Hawkins BS, et al. Natural history of subfoveal subretinal hemorrhage in age-related macular degeneration. Retina 1996;16:183–9.
89. Bennett SR, Folk JC, Blodi CF, et al. Factors prognostic of visual outcome in patients with subretinal hemorrhage. Am J Ophthalmol 1990;109:33–7.
90. Berrocal MH, Lewis ML, Flynn HW Jr. Variations in the clinical course of submacular hemorrhage. Am J Ophthalmol 1996;122:486–93.
91. Hanscom TA, Diddie KP. Early surgical drainage of macular subretinal hemorrhage. Arch Ophthalmol 1987;105:1722–3.
92. Lewis H, Jaffe GJ, Blumenkranz MS. Management of submacular hemorrhage with vitreoretinal surgery and subretinal injection of tissue plasminogen activator. Invest Ophthalmol Vis Sci 1992;33:898.
93. Bressler NM. Submacular surgery: are randomized trials necessary? Arch Ophthalmol 1995;113:1557–60.
94. Bressler NM, Finkelstein D, Sunness JS, et al. Retinal pigment epithelial tears through the fovea with preservation of good visual acuity. Arch Ophthalmol 1990;108:1694–7.
95. Schoeppner G, Chuang EL, Bird AC. The risk of fellow eye visual loss with unilateral retinal pigment epithelial tears. Am J Ophthalmol 1989;108:683–5.
96. Macular Photocoagulation Study Group. Persistent and recurrent neovascularization after krypton laser photocoagulation for neovascular lesions of age-related macular degeneration. Arch Ophthalmol 1990;108:825–33.
97. Macular Photocoagulation Study Group. Persistent and recurrent choroidal neovascularization after laser photocoagulation for subfoveal choroidal neovascularization of age-related macular degeneration. Arch Ophthalmol 1994;112:489–99.
98. Macular Photocoagulation Study Group. The influence of treatment coverage on the visual acuity of eyes treated with krypton laser for juxtafoveal choroidal neovascularization. Arch Ophthalmol 1995;113:190–4.
99. Macular Photocoagulation Study Group. Recurrent choroidal neovascularization after argon laser photocoagulation for neovascular maculopathy. Arch Ophthalmol 1986;104:503–12.
100. Macular Photocoagulation Study Group. Laser photocoagulation for neovascular lesions nasal to the fovea associated with ocular histoplasmosis or idiopathic causes. Arch Ophthalmol 1995;113:56–61.
101. Maguire JI, Benson WE, Brown GC. Treatment of foveal pigment epithelial detachments with contiguous extrafoveal choroidal neovascular membranes. Am J Ophthalmol 1990;109:523–9.
102. Cohen SMZ, Fine SL, Murphy RP, et al. Transient delay in choroidal filling after krypton red laser photocoagulation for choroidal neovascular membranes. Retina 1983;3:284–90.
103. Morgan CM, Schatz H. Atrophic creep of the retinal pigment epithelium after focal macular photocoagulation. Ophthalmology 1989;96:96–103.
104. Treatment of Age-Related Macular Degeneration with Photodynamic Therapy (TAP) Study Group. Verteporfin (Visudyne) therapy of subfoveal choroidal neovascularization in age-related macular degeneration: 1-year results of two randomized clinical trials, TAP report no 1. Arch Ophthalmol 1999;117:1329–45.
105. Rubin GS, Bressler NM, Treatment of Age-related Macular Degeneration with Photodynamic Therapy (TAP) Study Group. Effects of verteporfin therapy on contrast sensitivity; results from the Treatment of Age-related Macular Degeneration with Photodynamic therapy (TAP) Investigation: TAP report no. 4. Retina 2002;22:536–44.
106. Visudyne® In Minimally Classic Choroidal Neovascularization Study Group. Verteporfin therapy of subfoveal minimally classic choroidal neovascularization in age-related macular degeneration: 2-year results of a randomized clinical trial. Arch Ophthalmol 2005;123:448–57.
107. Miller JW, Schmidt-Erfurth U, Sickenberg M, et al. Photodynamic therapy for choroidal neovascularization due to age-related macular degeneration with verteporfin: results of a single treatment in a phase I and II study. Arch Ophthalmol 1999;117:1161–73.
108. Schmidt-Erfurth U, Miller JW, Sickenberg M, et al. Photodynamic therapy of choroidal neovascularization due to age-related macular degeneration with verteporfin: results of retreatments in a phase I and II study. Arch Ophthalmol 1999;117:1177–87.
109. Phase IV EVEREST PCV trial. Clinical trials identifier NCT00674323.
110. Bressler NM. Update on treatment of neovascular age-related macular degeneration: focus on antiangiogenesis in clinical practice. Ophthalmology 2009;116(Suppl), S15–23.
111. Chang MA, Do DV, Bressler SB, et al. Prospective one-year study of ranibizumab for predominantly hemorrhagic choroidal neovascular lesions in age-related macular degeneration. Retina 2010;30:1171–6.
112. Pharmacological Therapy for Macular Degeneration Study Group. Interferon alfa-2a is ineffective for patients with choroidal neovascularization secondary to age-related macular degeneration: results of a prospective, randomized, placebo-controlled clinical trial. Arch Ophthalmol 1997;115:865–72.
113. Gragoudas ES, Adamis AP, Cunningham ET Jr, et al. VEGF, Inhibition Study in Ocular Neovascularization Clinical Trial Group. Pegaptanib for neovascular age-related macular degeneration. N Engl J Med 2004;351:2805–16.

114. Chang TS, Bressler NM, Fine JT, et al. Improved vision-related function after ranibizumab treatment of neovascular age-related macular degeneration. Arch Ophthalmol 2007;125:1460–9.
115. Bressler NM, Chang TS, Fine JT, et al. for the Anti-VEGF Antibody for the Treatment of Predominantly Classic Choroidal Neovascularization in Age-Related Macular Degeneration (ANCHOR) Research Group. Improved vision-related function after ranibizumab vs photodynamic therapy. Arch Ophthalmol 2009;127:13–21.
116. Bressler NM, Chang TS, Suñer IJ, et al. for the MARINA and ANCHOR Research Groups. Vision-related function after ranibizumab treatment by better- or worse-seeing eye: clinical trial results from MARINA and ANCHOR. Ophthalmology 2010;117:747–56.
117. Miskala PH, Bressler NM, Meinert CL. Relative contributions of reduced vision and general health to NEI-VFQ scores in patients with neovascular age-related macular degeneration. Arch Ophthalmol 2004;122:758–66.
118. Chang TS, Bressler NM, Fine JT, et al. Improved vision-related function after ranibizumab treatment of neovascular age-related macular degeneration. Arch Ophthalmol 2007;125:1460–9.
119. BhavsarARGoogeJMStockdaleCRet alRisk of endophthalmitis after intravitreal drug injection when topical antibiotics are not required: The DRCR.net Diabetic Retinopathy Clinical Research Network Laser-Ranibizumab-Triamcinolone Clinical Trialsfor the Diabetic Retinopathy Clinical Research NetworkArch Ophthalmol127200915813
120. Comparison of Age-Related Macular Degeneration Treatments Trials (CATT) Research Group. Ranibizumab and bevacizumab for treatment of neovascular age-related macular degeneration: two-year results. Ophthalmology 2012;119:1388–98.
121. The IVAN Study Investigators Writing Committee: Chakravarthy U, Harding SP, Rogers CA, et al. Ranibizumab versus bevacizumab to treat neovascular age-related macular degeneration: one-year findings from the IVAN Randomized Trial. Ophthalmology 2012; in press.
122. Campbell JP, Bressler SB, Bressler NM. Impact of availability of anti-VEGF therapy on vision impairment and blindness due to neovascular AMD. Arch Ophthalmol 2012; in press.
123. Bressler NM. Retina Times 2010. (published online by the American Society of Retina Specialists)
124. Klein ML, Jorizzo PA, Watzke RC. Growth features of choroidal neovascular membranes in age-related macular degeneration. Ophthalmology 1989;96:1416–9.
125. Vander JF, Morgan CM, Schatz H. Growth rate of subretinal neovascularization in age-related macular degeneration. Ophthalmology 1989;96:1422–6.
126. Grey RHB, Bird AC, Chisholm IH. Senile disciform macular degeneration: features indicating suitability for photocoagulation. Br J Ophthalmol 1986;104:702–5.
127. Choroidal Neovascularization Prevention Trial Research Group. Laser treatment in eyes with large drusen. Ophthalmology 1998;105:11–23.
128. Thomas MS, Grand MG, Williams DF, et al. Surgical management of subfoveal choroidal neovascularization. Ophthalmology 1992;99:952–66.
129. Bressler SB, Maguire MG, Bressler NM et al. Relationship of drusen and abnormalities of the retinal pigment epithelium to the prognosis of neovascular macular degeneration. The Macular Photocoagulation Study Group. Arch Ophthalmol 1990;108:1442–7.
130. Macular Photocoagulation Study Group. Five-year follow-up of fellow eyes of patients with age-related macular degeneration and unilateral extrafoveal choroidal neovascularization. Arch Ophthalmol 1993;111:1189–99.
131. Macular Photocoagulation Study Group. Risk factors for choroidal neovascularization in the second eye of patients with juxtafoveal or subfoveal choroidal neovascularization secondary to age-related macular degeneration. Arch Ophthalmol 1997;115:741–7.
132. The Age-Related Eye Disease Study Research Group. A randomized, placebo-controlled, clinical trial of high-dose supplementation with vitamins C and E, beta carotene, and zinc for age-related macular degeneration and vision loss: AREDS report no. 8. Arch Ophthalmol 2001;119:1417–36.
133. Berger AS, Kaplan HJ. Clinical experience with the surgical removal of subfoveal neovascular membranes. Ophthalmology 1992;99:969–76.
134. deJuan E Jr, Loewenstein A, Bressler NM, et al. Translocation of the retina for management of subfoveal choroidal neovascularization. II. A preliminary report in humans. Am J Ophthalmol 1998;125:635–46.
135. American Academy of Ophthalmology. Macular translocation. Ophthalmic procedure preliminary assessment. Ophthalmology 2000;107:1015–8.
136. Hassan AS, Johnson MW, Regillo CD, et al. Management of submacular hemorrhage with intravitreal tPA injection and pneumatic displacement. Invest Ophthalmol Vis Sci 1998;39(Suppl):227.
137. Regillo CD, Benson WE, Maguire JI, et al. Indocyanine green angiography and occult neovascularization. Ophthalmology 1994;101:280–8.
138. Yannuzzi LA, Slakter JS, Sorenson JA, et al. Digital indocyanine green videoangiography and choroidal neovascularization. Retina 1992;12:191–223.
139. Guyer DR, Yannuzzi LA, Ladas I, et al. Indocyanine green-guided laser photocoagulation of focal spots at the edge of plaques of choroidal neovascularization. Arch Ophthalmol 1996;114:693–7.
140. Regillo CD, Blade KA, Custis PH, et al. Evaluating persistent and recurrent choroidal neovascularization: the role of indocyanine green angiography. Ophthalmology 1998;105:1821–6.
141. Bressler NM, Bressler SB. Indocyanine green angiography: can it help preserve the vision of our patients? Arch Ophthalmol 1996;114:747–9.
142. Bergink GJ, Hoyng CB, van der Maazen RW, et al. A randomized controlled clinical trial on the efficacy of radiation therapy in the control of subfoveal choroidal neovascularization in age-related macular degeneration: radiation versus observation. Graefes Arch Clin Exp Ophthalmol 1998;236:321–5.
143. Holz FG, Unnebrink K, Engenhart-Cabillic R, et al. Results of a prospective, randomized, controlled, double-blind multicenter trial on external beam radiation therapy for subfoveal choroidal neovascularization secondary to ARMD (RAD-study). Invest Ophthalmol Vis Sci 1999;40(Suppl):2115.
144. Spaide RF, Guyer DR, McCormick B, et al. External beam radiation therapy for choroidal neovascularization. Ophthalmology 1998;105:24–30.
145. Kaiser PK, Boyer DS, Cruess AF, et al. on behalf of the DENALI Study Group. Verteporfin plus ranibizumab for choroidal neovascularization in age-related macular degeneration. Twelve-month results of the DENALI study. Ophthalmology 2012;119:1001–10.
146. Larsen M, Schmidt-Erfurth U, Lanzetta P, et al. Verteporfin plus ranibizumab for choroidal neovascularization in age-related macular degeneration. Twelve-month MONT BLANC study results. Ophthalmology 2012; in press.

Chapter 67

Pharmacotherapy of Age-Related Macular Degeneration

Mark S. Blumenkranz, Loh-Shan Leung, Daniel F. Martin, Philip J. Rosenfeld, Marco A. Zarbin

INTRODUCTION

Age-related macular degeneration (AMD) is a spectrum of related diseases that have in common the progressive decline of vision as a consequence of dysfunction of the central retina and its underlying supporting elements, principally the retinal pigment epithelium (RPE) and choroid in older adults.[1] Although the disease is seen in all racial and ethnic groups, it is more commonly encountered in females and light-skinned individuals and typically presents after the seventh decade.[2–5] The disease has been traditionally classified into early and late stages.[1]

The early stages consist of alterations in the coloration of the macular pigment epithelium, both hypo- and hyperpigmentation, and the presence of drusen of greater than 125 μm in diameter. The early phases have been variously referred to as atrophic, nonexudative, preangiogenic, or dry AMD (Fig. 67.1). In contrast, exudative or neovascular AMD is typically a later-onset phenomenon, occurring in eyes with high-risk characteristics, including the presence of extensive soft drusen, Bruch's membrane thickening, and focal hyperpigmentation. This phase of the disease is characteristically accompanied by rapid loss of vision over a period of 6–12 months and the development of a central disciform fibrotic scar. Without intervention, the visual acuity generally decreases to the range 20/200 or worse over the 12 months following the onset of this phase.[3,5] In light of major improvements in therapy for this condition in the past 5–10 years, previously employed forms of treatment including thermal laser photocoagulation and surgery are now viewed to have limited benefit for this condition, particularly when it presents with involvement of the center of the fovea.[6–10] In recent years, AMD therapy has become increasingly targeted toward specific molecular pathways. The discovery of multiple genes and markers for AMD and neovascularization has identified a significant number of new targets for pharmacotherapy.

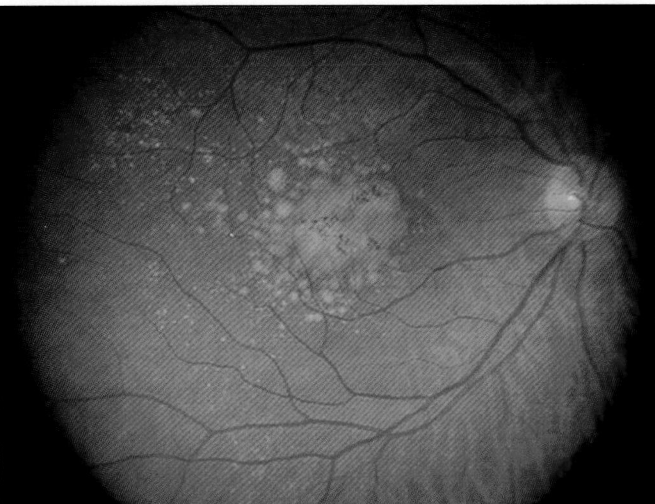

Fig. 67.1 Color fundus photograph of the right eye of a patient with early age-related macular degeneration. Note the extensive drusen throughout the posterior pole, some of which appear calcific and others large and soft. The patient has not yet progressed to the stage of either geographic atrophy or choroidal neovascularization.

Relevant to the purpose of this chapter, it is important to understand that the mechanisms of vision loss in AMD differ according to the stage, and that different stages may be amenable to different points of attack.[2,5] Importantly, at least two separate and distinct mechanisms for vision loss occur in exudative AMD: (1) proliferation of new vessels accompanied by secondary fibrosis and disorganization of the pigment epithelium and outer retina, which is a somewhat gradual process; (2) secondary alterations in the permeability of retinal and choroidal vessels accompanied by retinal pigment epithelial dysfunction leading to the accumulation of serous or serosanguineous fluid beneath the RPE, neurosensory retina, or within the retina itself, and are associated with more acute visual dysfunction. Preventing the vision loss associated with advanced forms of nonexudative disease has proven more challenging. In recent years an increased understanding of the mechanisms underlying drusen formation, pigment epithelial senescence, and loss of photoreceptors and choriocapillaris has made it more feasible to address therapeutically the visual dysfunction arising from the atrophic form of the disease (Fig. 67.2).

ETIOLOGIC FACTORS

A variety of factors are thought to play a role in the development of AMD, including genetic susceptibility and a host of potentially modifiable environmental factors, including comorbidities, diet, medications, and light exposure.[11]

Genetic susceptibility

Over the past decade, high resolution genome scans for susceptibility loci in populations enriched for either choroidal neovascularization (CNV), geographic atrophy (GA), or both suggest susceptibility loci on numerous chromosomes. A number of candidate genes and their functions are listed in Table 67.1.[2,12–15] An exhaustive discussion of the genetics and postulated mechanisms of ARMD is beyond the scope of this chapter; however, several genes deserve mention.

A significant breakthrough in the study of AMD genetics came in 2005, when it was discovered that single nucleotide

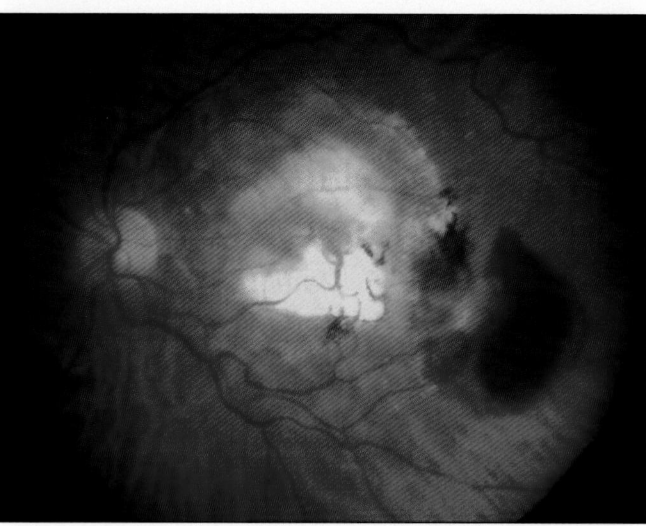

Fig. 67.2 Color photograph of the left eye of another patient with the severe form of late exudative age-related macular degeneration. Note the extensive scarring beneath the sensory retina, hemorrhage, and lipid exudation.

polymorphisms (SNPs) in the regulation of the complement activation locus (RCA) of chromosome 1q31.3 increased the risk of AMD. The RCA locus contains the gene encoding complement factor H (CFH). The tyr402his protein polymorphism increased the risk of AMD between 2.7- and 7.4-fold and appeared to account for between 43% and 50% of the attributable risk of AMD. Additionally, it has been found that CFH genotypes may influence an individual's response to certain treatment modalities and medications, including bevacizumab, photodynamic therapy with verteporfin, as well as AREDS (Age-Related Eye Disease Study) nutritional supplementation.[16–20] CFH is responsible for downregulating activation of the complement system, including c5b-9, known as the membrane attack complex (MAC). MAC is thought to be important in the immune-mediated damage to Bruch's membrane and an important pathogenic component of drusen.[21,22]

It is clear that both immune dysregulation and inflammation play key roles in the development and progression of AMD. Two recent studies found protective associations against the development of advanced AMD in those with genetic polymorphisms

Table 67.1 Candidate genes for AMD

Location	Gene	Function	Strength of association
1p22.1	*ABCA4*	ATP binding/ATPase	Possible
1q25–1q32	*HMCN1*	Extracellular matrix	Possible
1q31.3	*CFH*	Complement component	Established
3p21.3	*CX3CR1*	Chemokine receptor regulator of immune response	Probable
4q35.1	*TLR3*	Toll-like receptor: activator of inflammatory cytokine response to viral dsRNA	Possible
6p12	*VEGFA*	Regulator of angiogenesis and vascular permeability	Possible
6p21.3	*C2*	Complement component (classical pathway)	Probable
6p21.3	*CFB*	Complement component (alternate pathway)	Probable
6q24–q14	*ELOVL4*	Photoreceptor-specific elongation enzyme of long-chain fatty acids	Possible
9p24	*VLDLR*	VLDL transporter	Possible
9q32–q33	*TLR4*	Activates inflammatory immunity in response to bacterial lipopolysaccharide	Possible
10q26.13	*HTRA1*	Serine protease	Locus established, individual gene contributions unknown
10q26.13	*PLEKHA1*	Phospholipid-binding protein	
10q26.13	*ARMS2*	Unknown	
12p11–p13	*LRP6*	Wnt signaling protein	Possible
14q32.12	*FBLN5*	ECM protein, promotes endothelial cell adhesion	Possible
19p13.3	*C3*	Complement component	Probable
19q13.2	*APOE*	Lipoprotein binding, internalization, metabolism	Established
22q12.3	*TIMP3*	Metalloproteinase inhibitor (extracellular matrix protein)	Possible

of the complement components C2 (OR 0.35–0.46) and complement factor B (CFB) (OR 0.35–0.44), while C3 (OR 2.66–3.9) was strongly associated with the development of GA.[13,23] Figure 67.3 illustrates other complement components implicated in the pathogenesis of AMD. Additionally, elevated levels of the acute phase reactant CRP have been found to correlate with neovascular AMD. It is still unclear how genotypic variations in complement lead to an increased inflammatory state and the AMD phenotype. However, clinicopathologic specimens demonstrate the presence of inflammatory cells in Bruch's membrane, and of bioactive fragments of C3 (C3a) and C5 (C5a) in drusen of AMD eyes and elevated VEGF expression in RPE cells.[24,25] The inflammatory cascade is further characterized by retinal microglial activation and choroidal macrophage infiltration.[26,27]

The gene products for tissue inhibitor for metalloproteinase 3 (TIMP-3, chromosome 22) and EFEMP1 (chromosome 2, encoding an elastin-related protein, fibulin 3), which act to inhibit the stimulatory effects of VEGF on vascular cells, have been independently associated with advanced AMD in genome scans mentioned previously.[28,29] Multiple distinct alleles in exon 5 of the gene encoding TIMP-3 have been causally linked to an autosomal dominant form of exudative macular degeneration with strong phenotypic similarities to exudative AMD,[30–32] although it is not thought to account for the majority of patients with exudative AMD.[33] TIMP-3 is also found in increasing quantities and is associated with thickening of Bruch's membrane during aging, including within drusen and the RPE.[34–36] An Arg to Trp mutation in EFEMP1 is thought to cause the abnormal accumulation of extensive drusen in malattia leventinese, an inherited macular degenerative disease with phenotypic characteristics closely correlated with advanced nonexudative AMD.[34,37] The increased frequency of genome alterations coding for these two proteins (TIMP-3 and fibulin), which are important in the regulation of the extracellular matrix, particularly Bruch's membrane, provides support for the hypothesis proposed by Blumenkranz that generalized increased susceptibility of elastic fibers to photic degeneration is an important risk factor for choroidal neovascularization.[3]

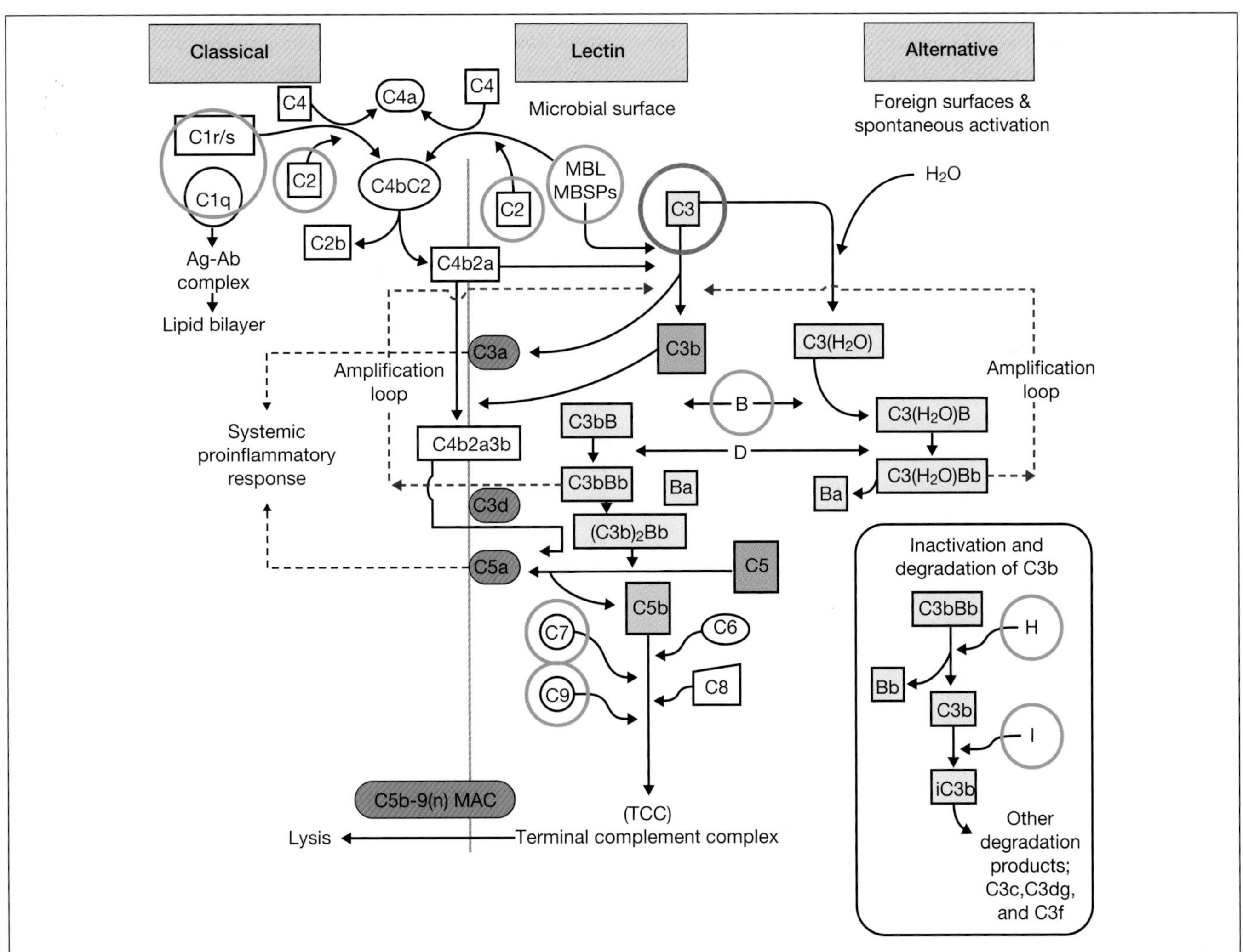

Fig. 67.3 AMD-associated mutations in the complement cascade. Four major activation pathways for the complement system are known, and three of these are illustrated. (The fibrinolytic-activated intrinsic pathway is not shown.) Activation of the complement system plays an important role in immunity. Inappropriate complement activation can damage tissue. Multiple complement components have been linked to AMD (green circles), including drusen, GA, and CNVs. Complement C3 (red circle) is the key point of convergence of all activation pathways. (Reproduced with permission from Zarbin M, Rosenfeld, PJ. Review of emerging treatments for age-related macular degeneration. In: Stratton RD, Hauswirth WW, Gardner TW, editors. Oxidative stress in applied basic research and clinical practice: Studies in retinal and choroidal disorders. New York: Humana Press; 2012.)

Early onset macular retinal degenerations such as Stargardt disease, characterized by the accumulation of lipofuscin within the RPE, have shed light on both the pathophysiology of RPE apoptosis and potential therapeutic avenues.[38,39] While initial reports also suggested that the ABCR gene linked to Stargardt disease might also be a dominant susceptibility locus for AMD, subsequent investigators have been unable to confirm this apparent increased frequency.[40,41] Nonetheless, increased amounts of lipofuscin are present in both Stargardt disease and in the earlier stages of the nonexudative AMD, and both diseases are characterized by GA in their later stages, suggesting that an understanding of the common pathways expressed by these two different diseases may provide some pharmacologic insights. Biochemical studies on the lipofuscin found in both Stargardt disease and AMD confirm that the principal component is N-retinylidene-N-retinylethanolamine (A2E), which accumulates in cells of the RPE and results in RPE apoptosis, photoreceptor death, and vision loss.[22,42,43] This process is thought to be initiated by light activation of rhodopsin in the course of normal visual transduction as the first reactant in A2E biosynthesis. Isotretinoin (Accutane, discussed later), which slows the synthesis of 11-*cis* retinaldehyde and regeneration of rhodopsin, is able to slow the accumulation of lipofuscin in ABCR knockout mice and also aged wild-type mice.[42] This suggests that compounds with mechanisms of action similar to isotretinoin, which is structurally related to vitamin A, may represent another therapeutic avenue for the slowing or prevention of AMD.[22,39,41-43]

There is additional discussion of AMD genetic susceptibility in Chapter 64 (Pathogenetic mechanisms in age-related macular degeneration.)

ENVIRONMENTAL FACTORS

Diet

The principal environmental factors thought to be associated with age-related macular degeneration include diet, history of smoking, light exposure, and use of supplemental medications. Recent AREDS reports have established a relationship between dietary intake of omega-3 long-chain polyunsaturated fatty acids and reduced risk of neovascular AMD (OR 0.61), as well as progression from drusen to GA.[44-46] A large case control study suggested that higher dietary intake of carotenoids, particularly lutein and zeaxanthin, was associated with a lower risk of AMD, with the highest quintile having a 43% reduction compared with those in the lowest quintile. In that study no reduction could be found with the use of oral vitamin A, vitamin E or vitamin C.[47] Subsequent studies suggest that the use of foods, particularly fruits rich in antioxidants and carotenoids, when consumed at the level of three servings or more per day, result in a pooled multivariate reduced relative risk of 0.64 compared with persons who consumed less than 1.5 servings per day.[2] However, there have been a number of studies that have demonstrated little to no benefit with dietary regimens.[28,48-50,51]

Smoking*

Most studies have consistently implicated smoking as a statistically significant risk factor for the development of late-stage AMD.[2,54] In a meta-analysis of three pooled studies from the United States, The Netherlands, and Australia, smoking was one of only two significant associations identified with incident AMD along with total serum cholesterol. Current smoking is associated with a 4.55-fold increased risk of neovascular AMD (vs. "never" smokers) and a 2.54-fold increased risk of atrophic AMD (vs. "never" smokers).[55] Based on a pooled analysis of data, the risks of both neovascular and atrophic AMD seem to decrease once one stops smoking.[55]

*Selected text adapted with kind permission of Springer Science+Business Media.[52,53]

Light exposure

Although there is a considerable body of compelling experimental data to suggest that increased retinal irradiance is positively correlated with an increased likelihood of advanced AMD, the epidemiological evidence supporting this hypothesis is modest.[3,56,57] In the Beaver Dam eye study, participants exposed to summer sun for more than five hours a day during selected periods of time were at increased risk for increased retinal pigment (relative risk 3.17) and early AMD (relative risk 2.14) after 10 years of follow-up compared with those exposed to less than 2 hours per day.[57]

The underlying rationale for the hypothesis that increased light stress predisposes to AMD rests on the role of oxidative stress inherent with photo bleaching of the photoreceptors and, to a lesser extent, pigment epithelium. In particular, reactive oxygen intermediates (ROI) including hydrogen peroxide, singlet oxygen, and other short-lived species, which arise as the byproducts of cellular metabolism, are known to have a toxic effect on cellular membranes.[48] It is felt that the cumulative effects of chronic low levels of these species result in profound damage to the retina and pigment epithelium through lipid peroxidation, mitochondrial DNA damage and induction of apoptosis.[2,48] Experimental studies have confirmed the deleterious effect of chronic light and in particular blue and ultraviolet light on the RPE in part through the creation of A2E oxiranes, a major component of lipofuscin. The presence of natural antioxidants derived from dietary sources including lutein, zeaxanthin, lycopene, and ascorbate are thought to mitigate the effects of photooxidation by quenching free radicals and other intermediate species.[48] It has been hypothesized that this represents one, but not the only mechanism of action, of the antioxidants in the AREDS study.[58]

Use of medications

Meta-analyses of pooled prospective studies suggest that certain medications may be associated with an increased or decreased risk of age-related macular degeneration. Antihypertensive medications, particularly beta-blockers, are associated with modest increased risk, whereas hormone replacement therapy in women, and tricyclic antidepressants, confer some relative protection.[59] These observations may be able to be further exploited in the development of new classes of drugs in addition to avoiding potentially harmful drug interactions.

The reader is referred to Chapter 63 (Epidemiology and risk factors for age-related macular degeneration).

SYSTEMIC RISK FACTORS

As previously noted, there appears to be a strong association between levels of ocular inflammation or systemic inflammatory disease and age-related macular degeneration. It has long been known that there is a relationship between VEGF and inflammation.[2,60] Inflammatory foci and white cells are commonly seen in

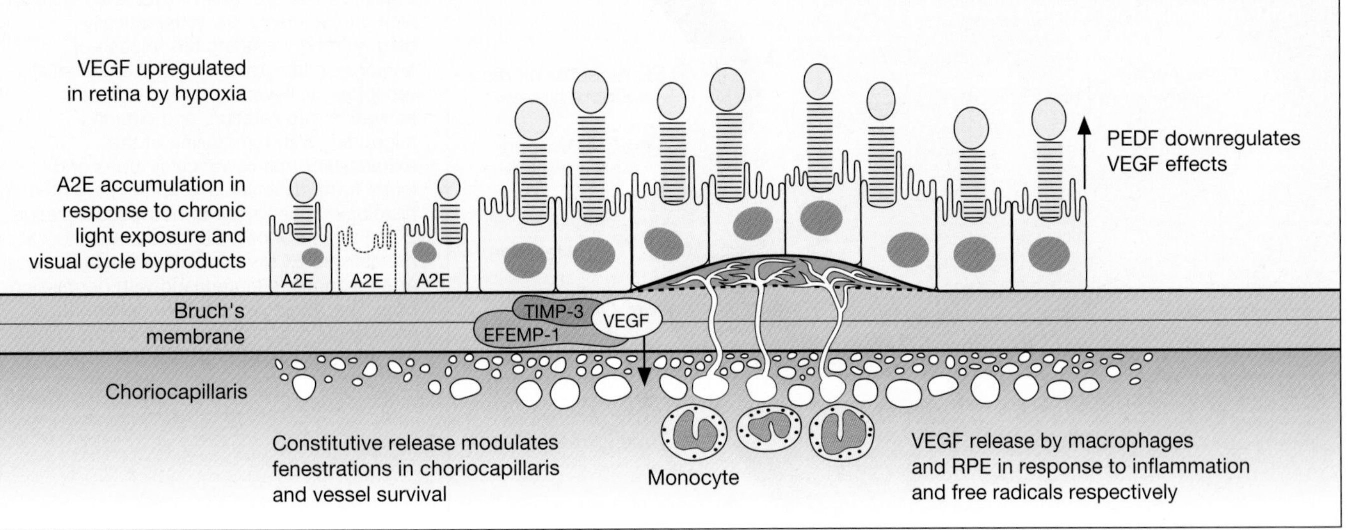

Fig. 67.4 Schematic diagram of pathogenic mechanisms associated with atrophic and exudative age-related macular degeneration. Normal constitutive release of VEGF, which is responsible for maintenance of fenestrations and other desirable permeability effects on the normal choriocapillaris through basal lateral secretion in an outward direction, appears to be effectively counterbalanced by the apical secretion of cytokines inhibitory for angiogenesis, including PEDF. This results in the relative avascularity of the outer retina as seen in the diagram on the right. In response to chronic light exposure and oxidation of phospholipids associated with the visual cycle, A2E and other oxidative byproducts accumulate in the retinal pigment epithelium, accounting for the characteristic autofluorescence seen on fundus photography. They also result in senescence of the pigment epithelium and apoptotic death associated with secondary atrophic effects on the overlying photoreceptors and underlying choriocapillaris, seen on the left in the diagram. The accumulation of increased lipoproteins as well as other glycoproteins including TIMP-3 and EFEMP-1 contribute to the thickening of Bruch's membrane, characteristically seen in patients with more advanced forms of the disease (seen centrally). Low-grade inflammation, chemoattraction of monocytes, and proangiogenic signals both from the pigment epithelium and inflammatory cells lead to vascular ingrowth from the choroid through defects in calcific and fragmented Bruch's membrane.

the choroid in autopsy specimens of patients with CNV.[61–65] To the extent that inflammation does have a causative effect on the development of AMD, therapy aimed at reducing inflammation through complement inhibition or regulation, immunomodulation or stabilization of intracellular organelles such as lysosomes and resultant proteolysis, may be successful pharmacologic strategies. In animal models, intravitreal triamcinolone acetonide has been shown to inhibit preretinal and choroidal neovascularization induced by laser injury.[66] There is increasing evidence of the linkage between VEGF, inflammation, and intracellular adhesion molecule 1 (ICAM-1) (Fig. 67.4). Triamcinolone modulates permeability and intracellular adhesion and ICAM-1 expression in cell culture, and it has further been shown that upregulation of ICAM-1 and invasion by CD18 positive leucocytes follows laser injury and precedes neovascularization.[67,68] Comparable laser injury in ICAM-1 knockout mice demonstrated considerable reduction in neovascularization, confirming the likely participation of this class of molecules in VEGF-mediated angiogenesis. Other therapies that target CD18-positive leucocytes or ICAM-1 are likely to be beneficial in reducing the angiogenic stimulus associated with inflammation and aging.

THE PATHOPHYSIOLOGY OF EXUDATIVE AMD: THE CRUCIAL ROLE OF CYTOKINES

Definition and steps in angiogenesis

Angiogenesis refers to the creation of new blood vessels from existing blood vessels, and therefore is contrasted from the process of vasculogenesis seen characteristically in utero in which vessels are created de novo. The angiogenesis cascade has been characterized as occurring in multiple sequenced steps (adapted from The Angiogenesis Foundation, www.angio.org/understanding/process.php [current as of February 15, 2012]):

1. Release of angiogenic growth factors by diseased tissue.
2. Binding of the angiogenic growth factors to adjacent existing vascular endothelial cells (EC).
3. Activation of EC to produce molecules, including enzymes.
4. Dissolution of the surrounding basement membrane by activated enzymes.
5. Proliferation and migration of EC.
6. Adhesion molecules (integrins) help to serve as framework for advancing EC.
7. Further dissolution of tissue and remodeling with matrix metalloproteinases.
8. Formation of vascular tubes by EC.
9. Formation of blood vessel loops from EC tubes.
10. Stabilization of new blood vessels by smooth muscle cells and pericytes. Antiangiogenic therapies currently under investigation are thought to inhibit angiogenesis at various steps in this process (Fig. 67.5).

VEGF and other positive and negative modulators of angiogenesis

Regardless of the inciting stimulus involved in the development of pathologic neovascularization, it is now well established that VEGF plays a principal role, including not only the neovascular forms of age-related macular degeneration, but also diabetic retinopathy, iris neovascularization, and retinopathy of prematurity. Additionally, other cytokines may play an important role as well, including fibroblast growth factor (FGF), pigment epithelial-derived factor (PEDF), the integrins, angiopoietins, and matrix metalloproteinase inhibitors.[2,30,69–72]

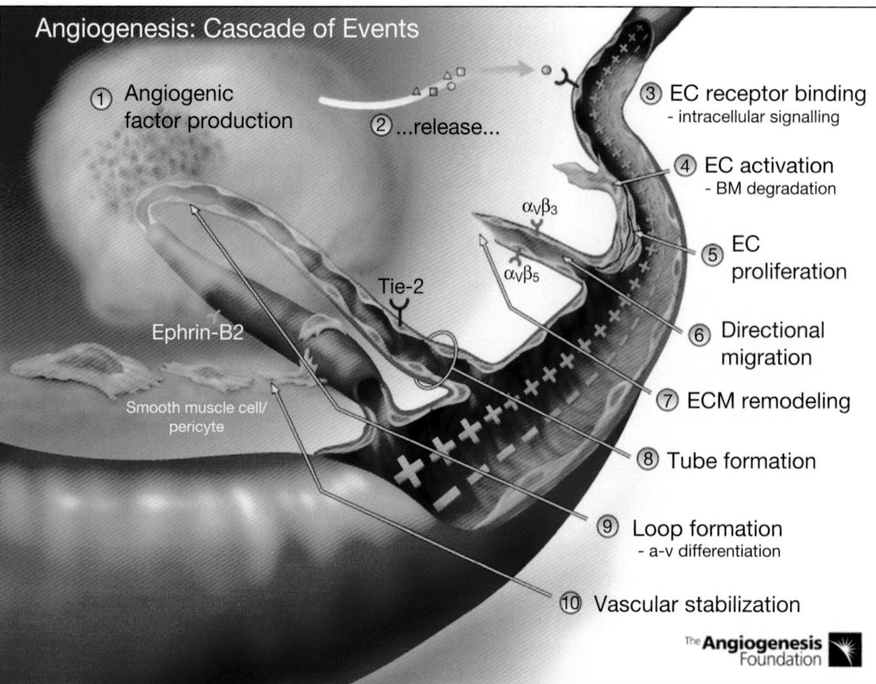

Fig. 67.5 The cascade of events associated with angiogenesis are schematically diagrammed, including the release of angiogenic factors, binding by endothelial receptors, followed by endothelial cell activation, proliferation, and directed migration. With remodeling of the extracellular matrix, vascular tubes and loops form, associated eventually with the histologic appearance of neovascularization. EC, endothelial cell; BM, basement membrane; ECM, extracellular matrix; a-v, arteriovenous. (Reproduced with permission from The Angiogenesis Foundation. http://www.angio.org/understanding/process.php [current as of 2012 Feb 15].)

VEGF undoubtedly represents the putative factor X first postulated by Michaelson associated with pathologic neovascularization.[2] First described as a vasopermeability factor associated with tumors, the molecule has since been cloned and well characterized.[73,74] VEGF has two important characteristics relevant to its role in the pathogenesis of the neovascular forms of age-related macular degeneration: (1) induction of angiogenesis through endothelial proliferation, migration, and new capillary formation, and (2) enhancement of vascular permeability.

Vascular permeability

VEGF produces important increases in hydraulic conductivity of isolated microvessels that are mediated by increased calcium influx and likely changes in levels of nitric oxide caused by induction of nitric oxide synthetase (NOS). While VEGF is both necessary and sufficient when administered exogenously to induce both these effects in vitro and in vivo, it is also well known that a number of other growth factors participate in this process. Some represent steps in a cascade initiated by VEGF while others act upstream.[75,76] The chemical structure of VEGF is that of a heparin-binding homodimeric glycoprotein of 45 kDa.[73] VEGF has significant homology to platelet-derived growth factor (PDGF). The human VEGF gene is organized into eight exons separated by seven introns and is localized in chromosome 6p21.3. Although there is only a single gene for VEGF-A, alternate post-translational exon splicing results in the generation of between four and six different isoforms having 121, 145, 165, 183, 189, and 206, amino acids respectively after signal sequence cleavage[72,73] (Fig. 67.6). $VEGF_{165}$ exists in both soluble and bound forms[73] (Figs 67.6, 67.7), and is thought to be predominantly responsible for pathologic neovascularization.

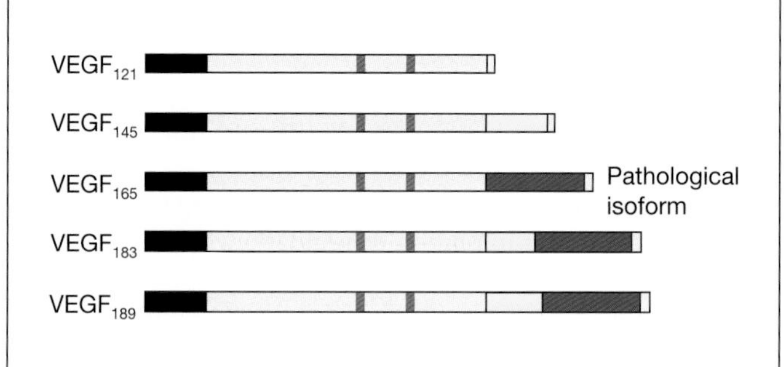

Fig. 67.6 Multiple isoforms of VEGF exist in nature and appear to participate to a differential degree in the normal events of vasculogenesis, as well as the pathologic events of angiogenesis occurring in response to local stimuli. Although there is only a single gene for VEGF, alternate splicing as well as post-transcriptional modification by plasminogen in the extracellular matrix accounts for a variety of isoforms that determine the relative balance between normal vascular homeostasis and pathologic neovascularization. The shorter amino acid length isoforms $VEGF_{121}$ and $VEGF_{145}$ are principally found in soluble form, whereas the longer spliced lengths 183, 189, and 206 are principally tissue fixed and bound by heparin. $VEGF_{165}$ is thought to stimulate pathologic neovascularization and exists both in soluble and tissue-fixed configurations.

Although VEGF inhibitors share in common an attempt to mitigate the proliferative and permeability effects of VEGF on normal and neovascular tissue, there are likely to be differences in both efficacy and safety related to the choice of agents for several reasons. From a theoretical standpoint, since $VEGF_{165}$ is the principal isoform involved in pathologic neovascularization, it has been argued that leaving the other three principal isoforms intact (121, which is principally diffusible in soluble form, and 189 and 206 which are principally matrix-bound through high affinity heparin binding sites), avoids the possibility of interference with normal homeostatic mechanisms associated with constitutive VEGF expression. Indeed, previous animal studies suggested that blockade of $VEGF_{164}$ in the mouse (equivalent to $VEGF_{165}$ in humans) is as effective as nonselective antibody-mediated VEGF blockade in preventing pathologic neovascularization in a hypoxia-induced angiogenesis model, while not interfering with normal physiologic development of

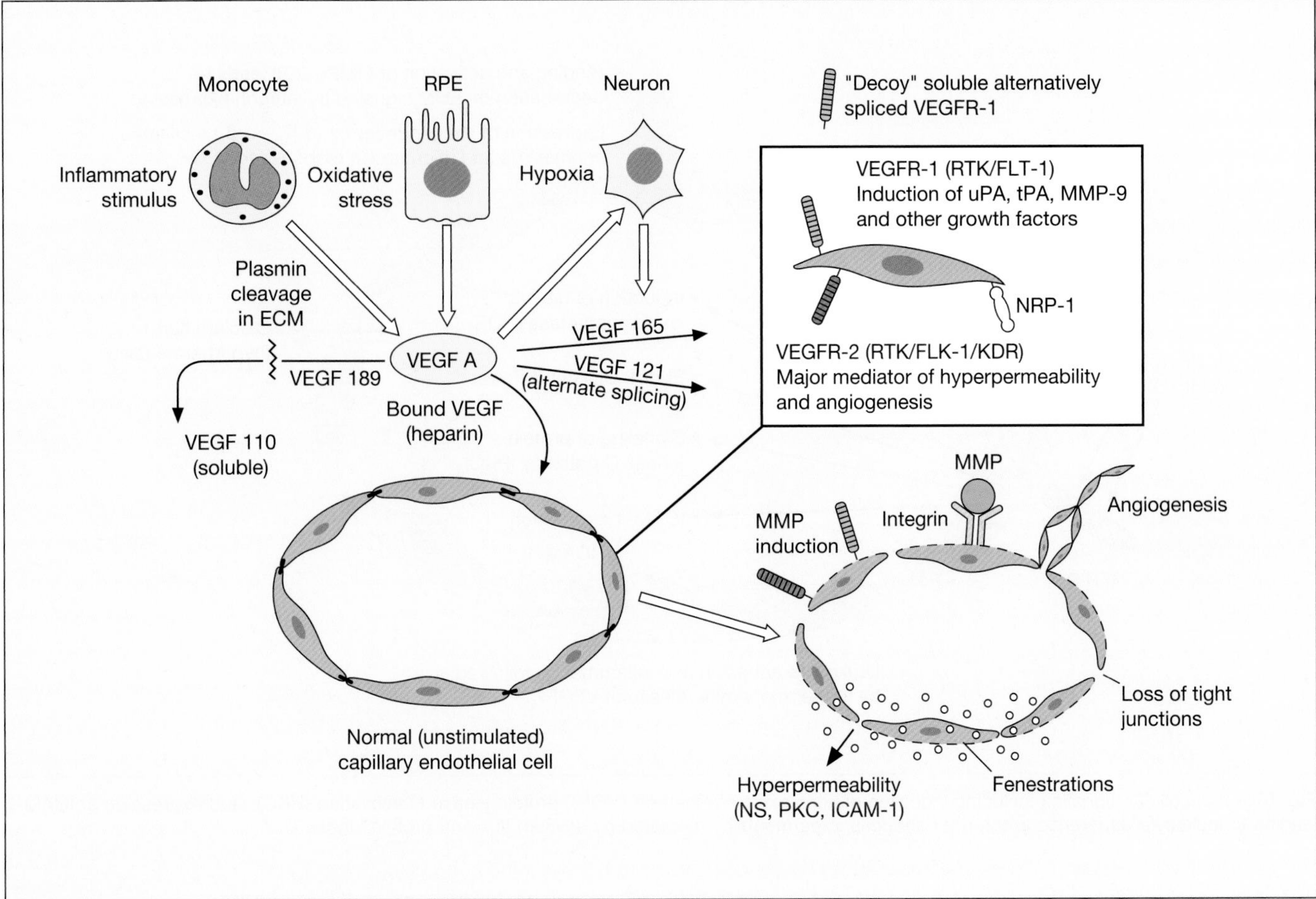

Fig. 67.7 Pathways of VEGF expression and effects on vascular cells are demonstrated schematically. A variety of cells contribute to VEGF release, including monocytes, retinal pigment epithelial cells and neurons responding to inflammation, oxidative stress, and hypoxia respectively. These and other cell types produce predominantly VEGF-A which is expressed in various isoforms through transcriptional and post-translational steps. $VEGF_{165}$ and $VEGF_{121}$ are the predominant forms, with $VEGF_{189}$ being cleaved in the extracellular matrix to $VEGF_{110}$, a soluble form by activated plasmin. Each of these molecules, but principally $VEGF_{165}$, bind to endothelial cells through specific receptors VEGFR-1 and VEGFR-2. A sequence of events is set in motion through subsequent intracellular messaging systems as well as extracellular events that result in the loss of tight junctions between individual endothelial cells, the formation of fenestrations within endothelial cells and calcium-mediated permeability channels resulting in loss of the normal inner and outer blood–retinal barriers. Additionally matrix metalloproteinase activation occurs through its interaction with integrin receptors alpha v beta 3 and alpha v beta 5, which are found on the surface of endothelial cells exclusively following induction of the cell through activation with the VEGFR-1.

retinal vasculature.[60,77] However, it has become apparent with widespread use of bevacizumab and ranibizumab (monoclonal antibodies against multiple VEGF isoforms) that nonselective blockade has few untoward effects on normal retinal vascular physiology.

VEGF receptors

VEGF exerts its effects on cells through two highly related receptor tyrosine kinases (RTKs) VEGFR-1 and VEGFR-2.[73] VEGFR-1 also termed FLT-1 (FMS-like tyrosine kinase) was described first, but its role remains open to debate. Like VEGF, VEGFR-1 is upregulated by a hypoxia-inducing factor (HIF)-dependent mechanism. The receptor undergoes weak tyrosine autophosphorylation in response to VEGF. It is thought not to be primarily a mitogenic stimulus but rather a "decoy" receptor, which downregulates the activity of VEGF by sequestering and rendering the factor less available to VEGFR-2 (Fig 67.7, 67.8). This factor may be most important during embryogenesis rather than during pathologic neovascularization as well as in hematopoietic bone marrow-derived cells and neural signaling.[73,78]

VEGFR-2 (KDR in humans or FLK-1 in mice)

VEGFR-2 binds VEGF with lower affinity relative to VEGFR-1, but is felt to be the major mediator of the mitogenic, angiogenic, and permeability enhancing effects of VEGF. The binding site for VEGF on VEGFR-2 has been mapped to the second and third IgG-like domains and it undergoes dimerization and strong ligand-dependent tyrosine phosphorylation resulting in a mitogenic chemotactic and pro-survival signal. It appears to have at least two separate tyrosine phosphorylation sites. VEGFR-2 is thought to be critical as a survival factor with apoptosis occurring in its absence.

A large body of evidence exists to support the critical and probably rate-limiting role of VEGF in neovascular forms of age-related macular degeneration. High messenger RNA levels and increased VEGF receptor levels are observed in areas of CNV in primates as well as in the extracted neovascular membranes of patients removed at surgery and following autopsy.[2,63] Additionally there are strong indications that elevated levels of VEGF are the proximal cause for the hyperpermeability seen not only in

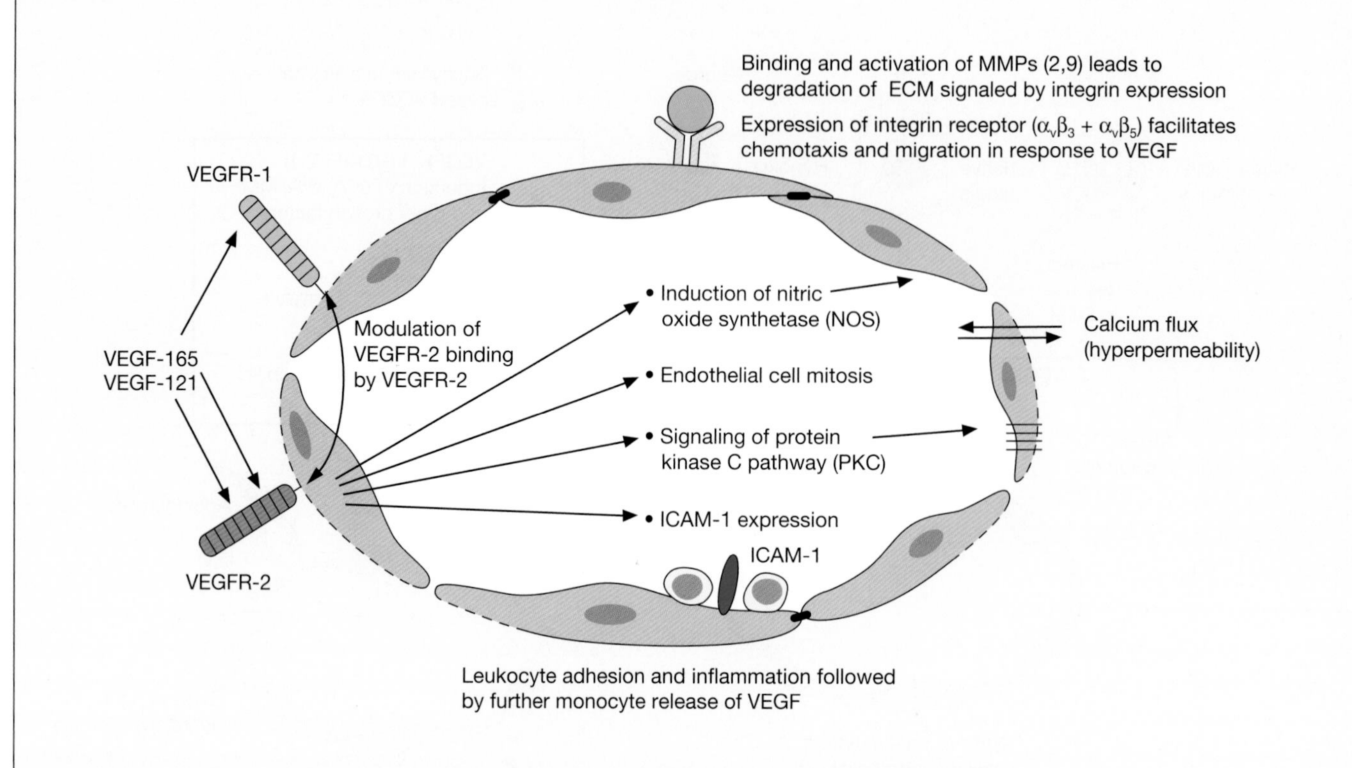

Fig. 67.8 Intracellular signaling including induction of nitric oxide synthetase (NOS), protein kinase C activation (PKC), and expression of ICAM-1 leading to leukocyte adherence and further changes in permeability mediated by calcium flux and protein kinase C.

diabetic macular edema, but in patients with subsensory and intraretinal fluid associated with CNV as well. The permeability changes resulting from VEGFR-2 are thought to be mediated to a large extent by endothelial nitric oxide synthetase-based generation of increased nitric oxide levels, and associated changes in calcium flux (Fig. 67.8). These alterations can be reversed either by direct blockade of VEGF, the receptor, or NOS using a knockout model.[2,74,75] Inactivation of soluble VEGF by monoclonal antibodies directed against it, or inhibition of ICAM also appear to be effective as well. In addition to either the indirect inhibition of VEGF effects through modulation of ICAM, or indirect effects on nitric oxide phosphorylase, nitric oxide synthetase, or protein kinase C, another modulator of permeability, there are several other methods by which VEGF effects can be blocked in the eye and elsewhere. These include the use of a class of molecules termed aptamers, which are chemically synthesized single strand nucleic acids, either RNA or DNA, that bind to target molecules with high selectivity and affinity leaving non-targeted protein functions intact.[79,80] Other methods of direct inhibition of VEGF include inhibition of its tyrosine kinase receptors (VEGFR-1 and -2), either by systemic administration or gene transfer. Several laboratories have described the use of small-interfering RNA (siRNAs) in effectively downregulating gene regulation[81] (see subsequent sections).

Other cytokines and regulators of angiogenesis

A number of cytokines have been identified that either upregulate VEGF or VEGF-associated effects, or act in an inhibitory capacity. In some instances, the same compounds may perform both functions depending upon the other extracellular signals present in the milieu as well as post-transcriptional or post-translational events, including cleavage by proteases, or binding by soluble receptors such as the family of tyrosine kinases.[2] Accordingly, any of this class of normally occurring compounds can be considered either in their native form, through splice or cleavage products, or chemical substitution to be potential therapeutic compounds in the treatment of pathologic neovascularization. Examples of stimulatory cytokines in addition to vascular endothelial growth factor include basic and acidic fibroblast growth factor, the angiopoietins, transforming growth factor (TGF), IL-8, and platelet-derived growth factor (PDGF). Naturally occurring inhibitory factors include interferon alpha, thrombospondin 1, angiostatin, endostatin, hemopexin-like domain of matrix metalloproteinase 2 (PEX), and pigment epithelial-derived factor (PEDF).[2,82–90] Additionally, it is likely there are many other naturally occurring compounds as well, as yet not recognized or well characterized biochemically. The relative balance between naturally occurring stimulatory and inhibitory factors is thought to contribute to the tight control of ocular vascular homeostasis, and may explain the differential ability of normal vascular as well as neovascular tissue to respond exquisitely both spatially and temporally to various stimuli.

NATURALLY OCCURRING UPREGULATORS OF ANGIOGENESIS

Fibroblast growth factor and integrins

Basic fibroblast growth factor (bFGF/FGF2) has been found to be elevated in excised choroidal neovascular membranes from patients undergoing surgery for AMD, and is capable of inducing pathologic neovascularization when implanted within the eye or adjacent to the retina.[69,70] Laser models of choroidal neovascularization are accompanied by upregulation of bFGF-associated mRNA, which precedes the development of histologically identifiable new vessels. While bFGF is sufficient when inserted exogenously in creating choroidal neovascularization, it is not necessary; *BFGF* gene knockout animals are also capable of developing laser-induced CNV bFGF upregulation of angiogenesis is thought to be in part mediated by adhesion-mediated signals including expression of the cell membrane-associated integrins such as the alpha v beta 3 integrin.[2,69,70] Although the alpha v beta 3 and another integrin, alpha v beta 5, appear to differentially represent the stimulatory effects of bFGF and VEGF respectively in laboratory studies, there is conflicting evidence as to whether these pathways are distinct. As a result, considered therapeutic approaches to integrin inhibition may be directed at downstream events such as intracellular signaling in addition to targeted inhibition of the individual receptors through monoclonal antibodies or related mechanisms.

Platelet-derived growth factor

Platelet-derived growth factor (PDGF) is a homo- or heterodimeric glycoprotein that stimulates pericyte and vascular smooth muscle cell recruitment in angiogenesis, which are essential in the maintenance and survival of new vessels. The PDGF receptors (PDGFR-A and PDGFR-B) are tyrosine kinases, and are expressed differentially on different cell types, with PDGFR-B being more extensively expressed in endothelial cells, vascular smooth muscle cells, and fibroblasts, among others.[91,92] In the absence of PDGFR-B signaling, vascular pericytes detach, and the integrity of vessel is lost. Immature vessels are highly sensitive to the withdrawal of VEGF prior to pericyte recruitment and coverage; conversely, when pericyte coverage is complete, new vessels are resistant to VEGF withdrawal. This is the so-called plasticity window, during which time vessels can regress rapidly with changes in exposure to growth factors.[93,94] PDGF blockade in animal models of corneal neovascularization has resulted in prevention and regression of new vessels.[95,96] PDGF blockade alone or combined with VEGF inhibition (taking advantage of the plasticity window) may thus serve as a potent inhibitor of neovascular AMD.

Angiopoietins

Angiopoietins, which are also highly specific for endothelial cells, perform a variety of other regulatory activities related to supporting cells and the extracellular matrix. A laboratory study suggests that two different isoforms, Angiopoietin 1 and Angiopoietin 2, appear to have differential and counteracting effects on the vasculature. Angiopoietin 2, which is upregulated by both hypoxia and VEGF, binds to an endothelial cell receptor TIE2 and enhances VEGF-mediated retinal neovascularization, but does not by itself stimulate endothelial cells or proliferation in vitro.[2,97] Angiopoietin 1 appears to play a maturation role and is associated with nonleaky behavior and may have potential therapeutic benefit through its inhibition of inflammatory pathways.[2]

Matrix metalloproteinases and tissue inhibitors of metalloproteinases

Expression of matrix metalloproteinases (MMPs) and their associated RNA, particularly MMP-2 and MMP-9, have been associated with pathologic neovascularization. Both matrix metalloproteinases, which are bound to the integrin receptors alpha v beta 3 and alpha v beta 5 on endothelial cells, are activated by VEGF and other regulatory cytokines and act to digest the extracellular matrix and thereby facilitate the spreading and chemotaxis of actively proliferating endothelial cells as they aggregate to form new capillaries.[2] Matrix metalloproteinases (MMPs) appear to be modulated and principally downregulated by naturally occurring tissue inhibitors of metalloproteinases (TIMPs) of which TIMP-1, TIMP-2, and TIMP-4 are thought to be soluble, and TIMP-3 principally extracellular matrix-bound. TIMP-3 is thought to play an important and possibly critical role in the natural modulation of matrix metalloproteinase regulation in Bruch's membrane, and is found in increased amounts in drusen and thickened basement membranes associated with age-related macular degeneration.[36,98] Mutations in exon-5 of the TIMP-3 molecule are associated with Sorsby's fundus dystrophy,[31,32,35] and an experimental model that either delivers increased amounts of TIMP-3 or induces overexpression of TIMP-3 by gene therapy demonstrates potent antiangiogenic effects for this molecule.[99,100]

NATURALLY OCCURRING DOWNREGULATORS OF ANGIOGENESIS

A variety of naturally occurring cytokines are known to have a downregulatory effect on angiogenesis and VEGF-mediated effect on cells.

Pigment epithelial-derived factor

Pigment epithelial-derived factor (PEDF), which is secreted by the pigment epithelium in vivo as well as in cell culture, has been shown to be biochemically identical to the product of the wild type of retinoblastoma tumor suppressor gene (RB) and is thought to induce differentiation of retinoblastoma cells, inhibit microglial growth, and other important regulatory functions in addition to its effects on angiogenesis.[56] Its relevance to AMD is likely related to its role in counterbalancing VEGF. In a study of donor human eyes with and without AMD, relative VEGF and PEDF levels were measured using immunoreactivity assays. Interestingly, VEGF levels were not significantly different between the two groups of eyes, even in the presence of advanced exudative change. In contrast, PEDF levels were much lower in the RPE and choroid of eyes with AMD, suggesting that it is lower levels of PEDF in the ocular milieu that may contribute to the formation of choroidal neovascularization.[101] Results from in vitro studies have suggested that the role of PEDF is regulation or inhibition of VEGF receptor signaling, rather than direct VEGF antagonism.[102]

Other cytokines

Another interesting class of regulatory cytokines that appear to have an inhibitory effect on angiogenesis relate to the class of aminoacyl-tRNA synthetases, which are associated with the first step of protein synthesis. Tryptophanyl-tRNA synthetase (TrpRS, a homolog of TyrRS) has no effect in its native form on angiogenesis or angiogenesis signaling. In contrast, an alternatively spliced fragment reported to be stimulated by interferon-alpha and lacking a portion of the amino terminal fragment, has potent antiangiogenic effects in both in vitro and in vivo.[103]

Thrombospondin 1 (TSP-1) has been described as both an up- and downregulator of VEGF. Under specified conditions TSP-1, which is produced by platelets and monocytes, enhances simulated VEGF release and is dependent upon binding to alpha v beta 5 and alpha v beta 1 integrins. In separate studies, TSP-1 has also been noted to inhibit endothelial cell proliferation, migration, and angiogenesis. VEGF and TSP-1 appear to participate in a feedback loop and its potential role as a therapeutic agent remains uncertain.[2] Angiostatin, is a 38 kDa internal fragment of plasminogen that encompasses the first four cringles of the molecule. It shows inhibitory effects on vascular endothelial proliferation in vitro and in vivo, particularly within tumors.[90,104] Endostatin, a cleavage product of collagen XVIII, is structurally related to and shares homology with angiostatin, and inhibits tumor-associated angiogenesis.[89] Each of these classes is further discussed in the following section as they relate to preclinical or clinical studies.

AGENTS CURRENTLY IN USE OR UNDER INVESTIGATION: NON-NEOVASCULAR AMD

Antioxidants, vitamins, and cofactors

The rationale for the use of antioxidants, multivitamins and other cofactors is based upon several lines of evidence, including the essential role of vitamin A in the visual transduction cycle, the known and predicted effects of oxidative stress resulting in reactive oxygen intermediates, and the requirement of certain critical metal ions including zinc in the functioning of critical proteases and other naturally occurring defense mechanisms against oxidative injury. Prior to the release of the data from the AREDS study, there remained some controversy as to whether antioxidant multivitamin therapy was efficacious, with some studies suggesting a protective effect, and others not.[49,50,105]

Age-Related Eye Disease Study (AREDS) and related supplements

The AREDS was a large, well-designed multicenter randomized clinical trial, which evaluated the effect of high-dose vitamin C and E, beta-carotene, and zinc supplements on AMD progression and visual acuity. A total 4757 persons were enrolled and stratified into one of four categories of increasing severity of disease. Due to the low rate of progression of category 1, consisting of drusen area of less than five small drusen of 63 μm or less, statistical analysis was only performed on the remaining 3640 patients with categories 2, 3, 4. Only the latter two (categories 3 and 4) were ultimately found to be at more than a trivial risk for progression. Patients in category 2 with at least one intermediate size druse, but not extensive drusen, had only a 1.3% probability of progression to advanced AMD by year 5 and no meaningful inference could be drawn regarding their risk with or without intervention. Patients in category 3 had either extensive intermediate drusen, large drusen, or non-central geographic atrophy, and patients in category 4 had visual acuity of less than 20/32 due to AMD in one eye related either to geographic atrophy involving the center of the macula or choroidal neovascularization in the fellow eye, but not the study eye, which had visual acuity 20/32 or better. The average follow-up of the 3640 enrolled study participants aged 55–80 was 6.3 years, and by comparison with placebo, patients treated with antioxidants plus zinc demonstrated a statistically significant odds reduction for the development of advanced AMD (OR 0.72, 99% CI 0.52–0.98). The odds ratio for zinc alone and antioxidants alone were 0.75 and 0.8, respectively, and the odds reduction estimates increased when only patients with category 3 or category 4 drusen were included, reducing to 0.66, 0.71, and 0.76 for antioxidants plus zinc, zinc alone, and antioxidants alone respectively. These data are further reflected in Fig. 67.9.

Based upon these findings, and extrapolation of the US population at risk, it has been estimated that of the 8 million persons in the United States at least age 55 or greater with AMD, if those at highest risk including categories 3 and 4 were to receive therapy with the formulation employed in the AREDS trial, as many as 300 000 of the 1.3 million at highest risk for advancement might avoid progression to the severe forms of the disease.[106] Additionally, based upon recent epidemiologic data, exclusion of beta-carotene is recommended for persons with a current history of smoking, or a long smoking history based upon a theoretical increased risk of lung cancer.

The macular carotenoids thought to be the principal contributors to the yellow coloration of the macula include lutein and zeaxanthin. One study suggested that a high dietary intake of these carotenoids protected against AMD, resulting in a 43% reduction in risk for AMD when the upper quartile of use was compared with the lowest quartile.[47] Recent AREDS reports have supported these findings, showing in cohort studies that those with a high level of dietary intake of lutein and zeaxanthin were less likely to have advanced AMD, as well as large or extensive intermediate drusen.[107] High dietary intake of ω-3 long-chain polyunsaturated fatty acids were also found by the AREDS

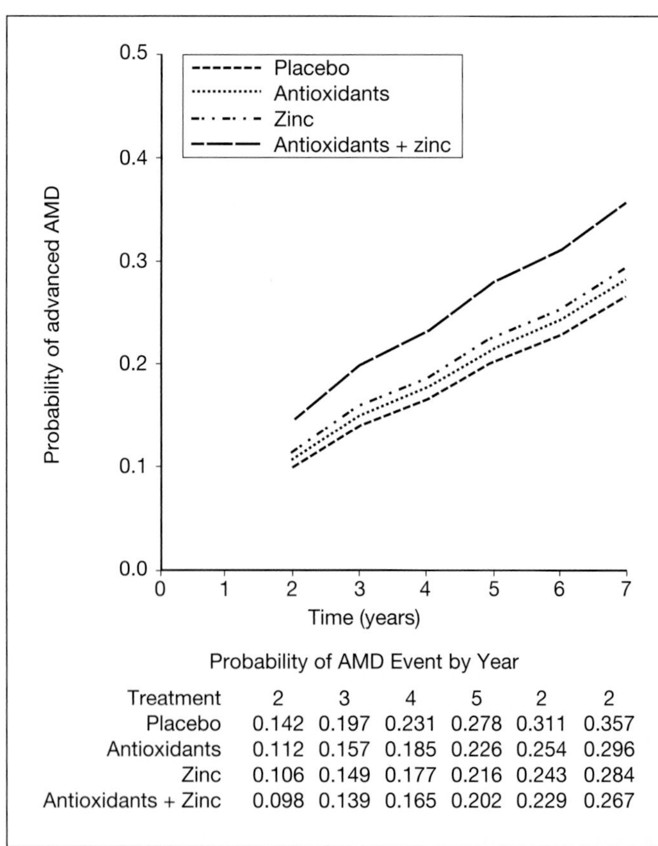

Probability of AMD Event by Year

Treatment	2	3	4	5	2	2
Placebo	0.142	0.197	0.231	0.278	0.311	0.357
Antioxidants	0.112	0.157	0.185	0.226	0.254	0.296
Zinc	0.106	0.149	0.177	0.216	0.243	0.284
Antioxidants + Zinc	0.098	0.139	0.165	0.202	0.229	0.267

Fig. 67.9 Repeated-measures estimates of the probability of loss in the visual acuity score of at least 15 letters in at least one study eye of participants within categories 3 and 4. (Reproduced with permission AREDS report no. 8: from A randomized, placebo-controlled, clinical trial of high-dose supplementation with vitamins C and E, beta carotene, and zinc for age-related macular degeneration and vision loss. Arch Ophthalmol 2001;119:1417–36.)

investigators to be inversely related to progression to both GA as well as neovascular AMD.[44–46] The critical dependence of the naturally occurring antioxidant enzymes (superoxide dismutase, catalase, and glutathione peroxidase) as well as the matrix metalloproteinases, on copper, zinc and manganese, provides a potential mechanism by which AREDS supplementation of both copper and zinc could be beneficial. The naturally occurring antioxidants such as vitamin E and vitamin C might have a beneficial effect on the progression of AMD as well.[48] At present no definitive recommendations can be made regarding dietary supplementation with lutein and zeaxanthin, as well as ω-3 long-chain polyunsaturated fatty acids. However, the AREDS2 randomized multicenter phase III clinical trial (NCT00345176) is currently underway, and is designed to address: (1) the role of lutein (10 mg)/zeaxanthin (2 mg) and ω-3 long-chain polyunsaturated fatty acids (350 mg docosahexaenoic acid (DHA)/650 mg eicosapentaenoic acid (EPA)) in the prevention of development of GA or CNV; and (2) the effect of possible deletion of β-carotene and lowering the daily zinc oxide dose from 80 mg to 25 mg. The AREDS study is discussed also in Chapter 65 (Age-related macular degeneration: Non-neovascular early AMD, intermediate AMD, and geographic atrophy).

Visual cycle inhibitors*

Visual cycle modulators are intended to reduce the accumulation of toxic fluorophores such as A2E in RPE cells. Fenretinide (ReVision Therapeutics, Inc.) treatment causes a dose-dependent, reversible reduction in circulating retinal binding protein (RBP) and retinol by displacing retinol from RBP, as well as interfering with RBP binding to transthyretin (TTR), thus facilitating their elimination via glomerular filtration. In ABCA4$^{-/-}$ mice, fenretinide reduces RPE lipofuscin and A2E accumulation, although it causes modest delays in dark adaptation.[108] Notably, however, despite low blood retinol levels, RPB$^{-/-}$ mice acquire normal vision by 5 months of age when given a vitamin A-sufficient diet.[109,110] Thus, it is not clear that blockade of vitamin A transport to RPE by inhibition of vitamin A binding to RBP will block vitamin A uptake by the RPE during long-term administration unless dietary vitamin A is restricted also. Patients in a phase IIb clinical trial of fenretinide received placebo, 100 mg, or a 300 mg daily dose for 24 months (NCT00429936). At the conclusion of the two-year study, an exploratory and ad hoc analysis of the data revealed that 15 (18.3%) of 82 patients in the placebo arm progressed to CNV, compared with 15 (9.2%) of 164 patients receiving fenretinide at either dose (P = 0.039). In the 300 mg fenretinide dose cohort, analysis of GA lesion growth by color fundus photography showed a trend for slowing of lesion growth, particularly among patients who had RBP and retinol levels reduced by more than 50%. Although fenretinide can affect dark adaptation[111–118] and ERG readings,[119–122] and is associated with symptoms of dry eye, [116,117] it was generally well tolerated in this study.

Accutane (13-*cis*-retinoic acid) inhibits the conversion of all-trans-retinyl esters (in retinosomes) to 11-*cis*-retinol and the conversion of 11-*cis*-retinol to 11-*cis*-retinal by retinol dehydrogenase and also reduces lipofuscin accumulation in ABCA4$^{-/-}$ mice.[42,123] This oral agent is associated with a high incidence of nyctalopia.[124] Another drug known as ACU-4429 (Acucela) is an orally administered compound that inhibits conversion of all-trans-retinyl ester to 11-*cis*-retinol via blockade of RPE65. ACU-4429 also reduces lipofuscin and A2E accumulation in the RPE of ABCA4$^{-/-}$ mice. A phase I clinical trial (NCT00942240) in 46 healthy volunteers was completed successfully.[125] The most common adverse events were vision-related, occurring in 50% of patients receiving the medication, which included dyschromatopsia (32%), unspecified visual disturbance (29%), night blindness (18%), blurred vision (11%), and photophobia (8%). All adverse events were mild or moderate in intensity and were transient in nature, resolving within a few days after onset. There was dose-dependent suppression of the ERG b-wave as expected. A dose escalation phase II study is underway in patients with GA (NCT01002950).

*Selected text adapted with kind permission of Springer Science+Business Media.[52,53]

Complement modulators*

In general, complement modulating agents work by replacing a defective complement component; by inhibiting the activation of convertases; by promoting the decay of convertases; or by blocking effector molecules (Fig. 67.10).[126] The following examples illustrate some of the promise as well as the challenges associated with manipulation of the complement pathway.

Inhibition of C5 blocks terminal complement activity, but proximal complement functions remain intact, e.g., C3a anaphylatoxin production, C3b opsonization, and immune complex and apoptotic body clearance. ARC1905 (Ophthotech Corp.) is an anti-C5 aptamer delivered by intravitreal injection. It binds C5 with high affinity (KD = ~700 pM) and prevents cleavage to C5a and C5b. ARC1905 is in a phase I trial (NCT00950638) for patients with GA. Eculizumab (SOLIRIS, Alexion Pharmaceuticals) is a humanized monoclonal antibody that binds to and prevents cleavage of C5 and is administered intravenously. Eculizumab is FDA-approved for the treatment of paroxysmal nocturnal hemoglobinuria and is in phase II trials (NCT00935883) for treatment of nonexudative AMD, including patients with high-risk drusen or GA. C5a receptor blockade – e.g., JPE1375 (Jerini); PMX025 (Arana Therapeutics); Neutrazimab (G2 Therapies) – might have both advantages and disadvantages over direct C5a inhibition. C5a receptor blockade might inhibit some important inflammatory pathways,[24] although without disabling membrane attack complex formation.

Factor D is the rate-limiting enzyme in the activation of the complement alternative pathway. It plays an important role in the positive feedback loop that results in the amplification of proinflammatory effectors.[127] FCFD45145 (Genentech/Roche) is a monoclonal antibody fragment (Fab) directed against Factor D. A 108-patient placebo-controlled phase I clinical trial (NCT00973011) of intravitreal therapy for GA is complete, and the medication was well tolerated up to a 10 mg dose. Patients were treated monthly or every other month during an 18-month period. A phase II study (NCT01229215) is underway.

Replacement of complement factor H should inhibit inflammation in AMD patients with risk-enhancing mutations in CFH. This approach, which probably would require genetic screening prior to treatment, involves restoration of complement homeostasis so there is no increased risk of infection with therapy. Replacement of defective CFH is being developed by Alexion. TT30 is a recombinant fusion protein comprising complement

*Selected text adapted with kind permission of Springer Science+Business Media.[52,53]

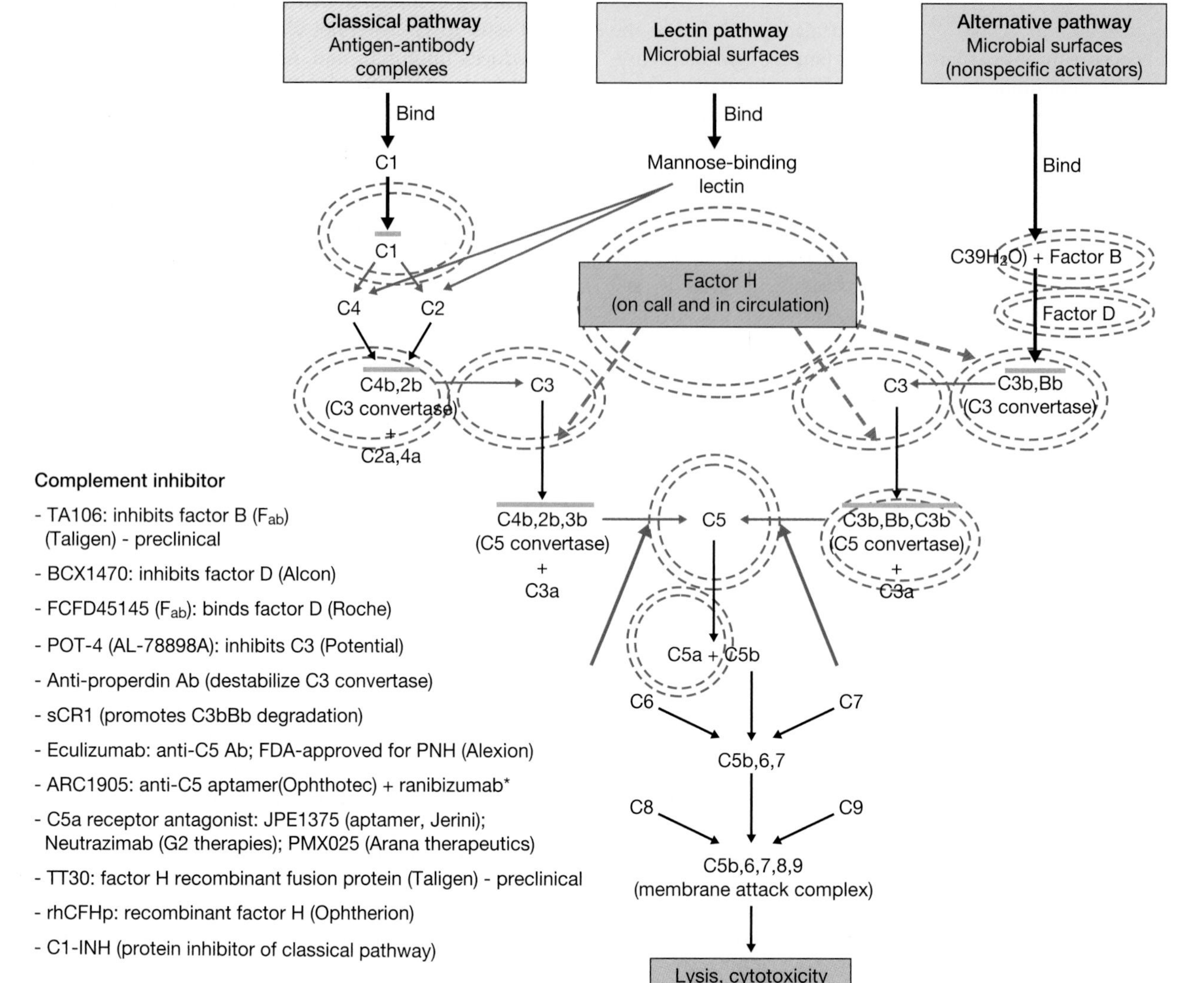

Fig. 67.10 Numerous compounds that modulate the complement pathway are in development for or in clinical trials for AMD treatment. Red circles indicate the parts of the complement pathway that are being modified. The complement pathway illustrated is adapted from Donoso et al.[126] (Reproduced from Zarbin MA, Rosenfeld PJ. Pathway-based therapies for age-related macular degeneration: an integrated survey of emerging treatment alternatives. Retina 2010;30:1350–67 with permission of Springer Science+Business Media.)

receptor type 2 and the regulatory domain of factor H. The receptor domain of TT30 binds iC3b/C3d-coated cells, delivering the regulatory domain of CFH to areas where complement regulation is necessary.[127] Preclinical testing is underway. Alexion is also exploring factor B inhibition using a humanized antibody fragment (TA106).

The differential expression of complement components in different ocular tissues presents difficulty in determining the optimal route of administration of these agents. For example, factor D is deposited diffusely in the human retina as well as in the choroid,[128] while factors B, H, C3, C5, and C5b-9 are found primarily in the choroid, Bruch's membrane, and/or subjacent to the RPE.[128,129] Thus, intravitreal injection may not be the ideal route of delivery for all the complement inhibitors under study.

Another approach to complement modulation is the silencing of genes by preventing mRNA expression, as deletion of genes closely related to CFH (i.e., CFHR1 and CFHR3) appears to be strongly protective against AMD.[130] However, short-interfering RNA (siRNA) therapies in the eye may be toxic, and it seems that the deletion of CFHR1 and CFHR3 protect against development of AMD at least in part because the deletion tags a protective haplotype and does not occur in association with the Y402H single nucleotide polymorphism.[131] See below for further discussion of siRNAs and other complement inhibitors for exudative AMD.

AGENTS CURRENTLY IN USE OR UNDER INVESTIGATION: NEOVASCULAR AMD

VEGF inhibitors

A variety of methods are now available to directly inhibit the $VEGF_{165}$ molecule as well as its various other isoforms. These include the use of monoclonal antibodies directed at one or more isoforms, oligonucleotides with chain-specific sequences corresponding to the VEGF protein, and molecules directed at one or more of the VEGF receptors, including native decoys, tyrosine kinase inhibitors, fusion proteins, and TIE2 receptors. Finally, because VEGF is thought to initiate a cascade of intracellular signals initially, and subsequently extracellular events, it is possible to inhibit VEGF effects either through prevention of secretion of the molecule, direct inhibition of the molecule in the extracellular space, blockade of the receptors, or through interruption in the downstream intracellular signaling pathways leading to both intra- and extracellular events.[132] In addition to the sections that follow, the interested reader is referred to Chapter 66 (Neovascular (exudative or "wet") age-related macular degeneration).

Direct VEGF inhibitors

Monoclonal antibody: bevacizumab (Avastin)

Bevacizumab is a humanized monoclonal antibody (IgG1) against human VEGF-A that selectively inhibits all isoforms and bioactive proteolytic breakdown products of VEGF-A (Fig. 67.11).[133] Bevacizumab is an immunoglobulin G molecule that is comprised of amino acid sequences which are about 93% human and 7% murine. Preclinical studies in animal models of various tumor cell lines as well as different forms of ocular neovascularization indicated that the fully sized antibody had excellent efficacy against the primary permeability and proliferative effects of VEGF isoforms. Following extensive clinical testing, it was found to be effective in slowing tumor growth through its effects on angiogenesis.[73] Bevacizumab was FDA-approved in 2004 as a treatment for metastatic colorectal cancer when given intravenously at a dose of 5 mg/kg and infused every 2 weeks in combination with 5-fluorouracil. Bevacizumab was shown to increase survival, response rate, and duration of response compared with conventional therapy consisting of irinotecan, fluorouracil, and leukovorin for metastatic colorectal cancer.[134] Additional phase III clinical trials with bevacizumab have since resulted in FDA-approval for the treatment of lung, kidney, and brain cancers.

In 2004, a study investigating the use of systemic bevacizumab in patients with exudative AMD (Systemic Avastin for Neovascular AMD – SANA) was initiated at the Bascom Palmer Eye Institute. This study was the first demonstration that bevacizumab was effective for this disease. In this open-label, uncontrolled study, 18 patients underwent two to three intravenous infusions of bevacizumab (5 mg/kg) to evaluate the potential safety and efficacy of systemic bevacizumab over 6 months.[135,136] Although clinical trials using intravitreal pegaptanib and ranibizumab for CNV were underway, the prior use of bevacizumab for ocular disease in humans using any route had previously been untested. While no serious adverse events were observed, and only a mild transient increase in blood pressure was identified, the SANA study was too small to establish the safety of

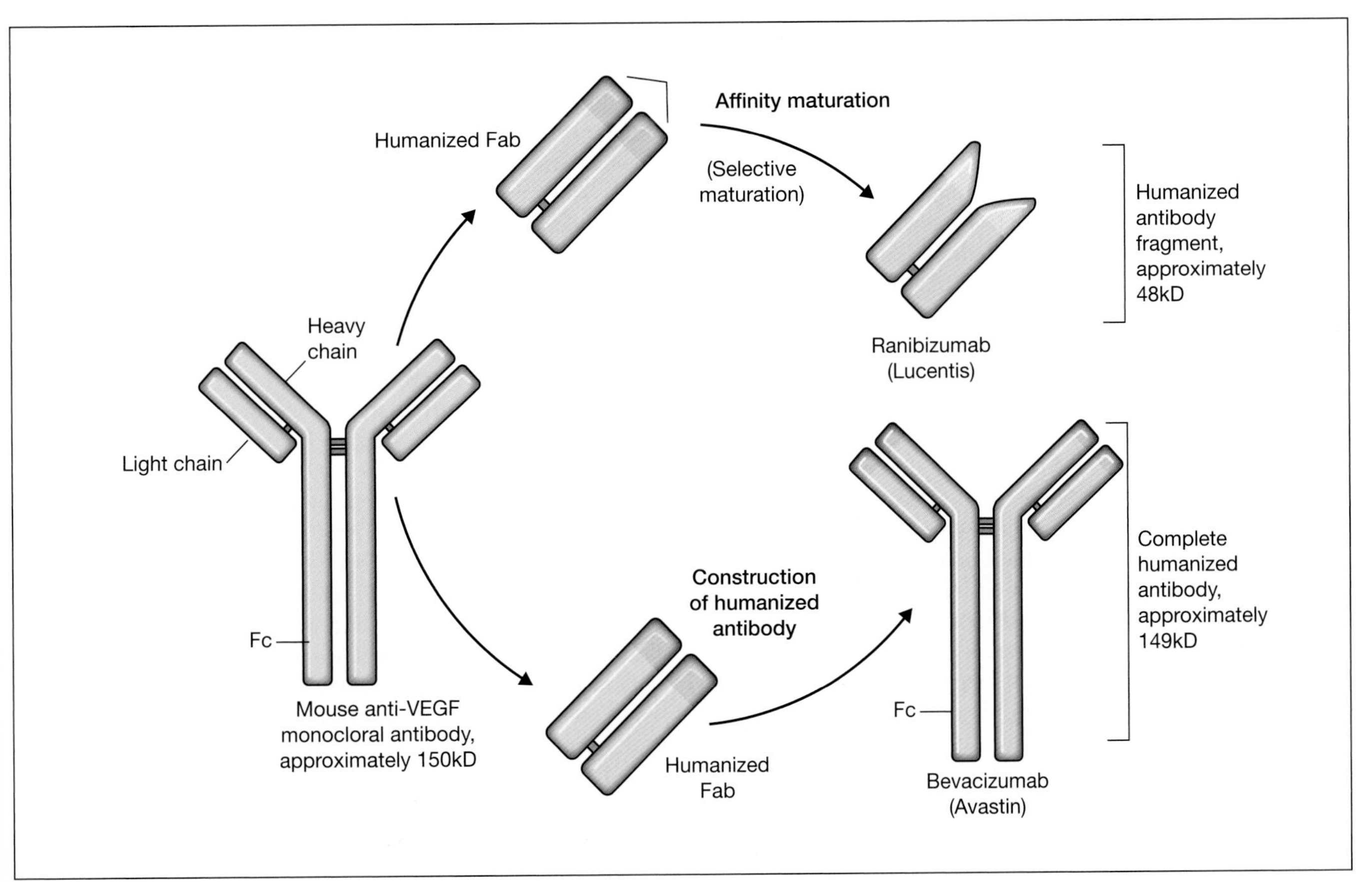

Fig. 67.11 Relationship between ranibizumab and bevacizumab. Ranibizumab is a recombinant humanized monoclonal IgG1 kappa-isotype antibody fragment (with a molecular weight of about 48 kD). It is produced in an *Escherichia coli* expression system (and thus is not glycosylated) and is designed for intraocular use. Bevacizumab is a recombinant humanized monoclonal IgG1 antibody (with a molecular weight of about 149 kD). It is produced in a Chinese-hamster-ovary mammalian-cell expression system (and thus is glycosylated) and is designed for intravenous infusion. Both the antibody fragment and the full-length antibody bind to and inhibit all the biologically active forms of vascular endothelial growth factor (VEGF) A and are derived from the same mouse monoclonal antibody. However, ranibizumab has been genetically engineered through a process of selective mutation to increase its affinity for binding and inhibiting the growth factor. The Fab domain of ranibizumab differs from the Fab domain of bevacizumab by six amino acids, five on the heavy chain (four of which are in the binding site) and one on the light chain. Not all the intermediate Fabs between the mouse monoclonal antibody and ranibizumab are shown. (Reproduced with permission from the Massachusetts Medical Society from Steinbrook R. The price of sight – ranibizumab, bevacizumab, and the treatment of macular degeneration. N Engl J Med 2006;355:1409–12.)

bevacizumab. However, significant improvements in visual acuity and OCT central retinal thickness measurements were observed comparable to the changes observed in the early phase Lucentis trials.

While systemic bevacizumab (5 mg/kg) was shown to reduce leakage from CNV, decrease OCT central retinal thickness measurements, and significantly improve vision in exudative AMD, the intravenous use of bevacizumab for exudative AMD was never widely adopted, because the intravitreal approach used up to 500-fold less drug, is much less expensive, and is perceived to be safer due to the smaller dose of drug. In the first-reported case of intravitreal bevacizumab,[137] a patient with recurrent CNV secondary to AMD, who had previously been treated with verteporfin photodynamic therapy (PDT) in combination with triamcinolone acetonide followed by treatment with pegaptanib injections, was shown to improve with a decrease in OCT central retinal thickness, subretinal fluid, as well as improvement of subjective visual distortion within 1 week of a single injection of 1.0 mg bevacizumab.

The bevacizumab used for this injection was the commercially available form available as 100 mg and 400 mg preservative-free, single-use vials in volumes of 4 ml or 16 ml (25 mg/ml). The 100 mg product is formulated in 240 mg α(alpha),α(alpha)-trehalose dihydrate, 23.2 mg sodium phosphate (monobasic, monohydrate), 4.8 mg sodium phosphate (dibasic, anhydrous), 1.6 mg polysorbate 20, and was diluted in water prior to intravenous infusion. For off-label intravitreal use, bevacizumab was not diluted, but rather dispensed into individual syringes for intravitreal injection and the volume (dose) of injection ranged from 0.05 ml (1.25 mg) to 0.1 ml (2.5 mg).

Initially, there was concern that a molecule as large as the 149 kDa bevacizumab may not penetrate the retina and effectively treat CNV compared with ranibizumab, which is one-third the size. However, it became apparent that bevacizumab could penetrate the retina based upon the empiric observations of decreased subretinal fluid on OCT examination and improved visual acuities in treated patients. Subsequently, Han et al. were the first to show that a full-length immunoglobulin the size of bevacizumab was capable of penetrating the rabbit retina after an intravitreal injection.[138] Sharar et al. used qualitative immunofluorescence to confirm that intravitreal bevacizumab was able to completely penetrate the retina by 24 hours and was essentially absent at 4 weeks after an injection.[139] Moreover, Dib et al. demonstrated bevacizumab molecules in the subretinal space of all six eyes studied two hours after an intravitreal bevacizumab injection of 0.05 ml (1.25 mg), confirming the initial observations that the molecule could rapidly diffuse through the retina.[140]

The ocular pharmacokinetics of various other monoclonal antibodies injected into the vitreous cavity of monkeys and rabbits demonstrated a half-life of about 5.6 days.[141,142] Studies of bevacizumab in rabbits and monkeys suggest a half-life in the range of 4–6 days.[143–145] A human study reported that a single dose of intravitreal bevacizumab had a half-life of 3 days and was likely to provide complete intravitreal VEGF blockade for a minimum of 4 weeks.[146] One human study suggested a half-life of 6.7 days and yet another study has reported a half-life of as long as 9.8 days.[147,148] It is likely that human ocular pharmacokinetics of bevacizumab varies from patient to patient, depending on factors such as the extent of vitreous liquefaction and the phakic status of the eye.

Since the first case of intravitreal bevacizumab for the treatment of exudative AMD was reported, numerous retrospective studies and a few small prospective studies using a dose range between 1.0 and 2.5 mg have been published, all demonstrating clinically significant improvement in mean visual acuity, reduction in fluorescein angiographic leakage, and resolution of OCT-visualized edema in up to 90% of bevacizumab-treated patients. These reports also supported the apparent clinical safety of bevacizumab. As of the time of writing (February 2012), despite the subsequent approval of ranibizumab in 2006, the off-label use of intravitreal bevacizumab has become the most common treatment for exudative AMD in the United State.[149,150] In addition, it has also become frequently used for wide range of other forms of macular new vessels including pathologic high myopia, multifocal choroiditis, and ocular histoplasmosis; it has also been used successfully for treatment of clinically significant macular edema from diabetic retinopathy, retinal venous occlusions, and retinopathy of prematurity.[151–159] It is being explored for treatment of other macular conditions not associated with new vessels or known elevated VEGF levels, including central serous choroidopathy and uveitides, although its efficacy in those conditions is not yet firmly established. Prior to the release of the Comparison of Age-Related Macular Degeneration Treatments Trial (CATT, discussed below), most of the early pilot studies were small (less than 100 patients) and uncontrolled, with different retreatment criteria and outcome measures; most physicians have frequently extrapolated the results from the phase III ranibizumab trials for these indications to bevacizumab.[160] However, two randomized, controlled studies deserve mention.

The ABC trial compared intravitreal bevacizumab (three loading doses every 6 weeks, followed by additional injections at 6-week intervals as needed) to standard therapy, defined at the time of recruitment as verteporfin PDT for predominantly classic CNV, or pegaptanib injection or sham injection for minimally classic or occult CNV. A total of 131 patients were recruited and randomized 1:1 to receive either bevacizumab or standard therapy. A significantly higher proportion of the bevacizumab group improved by 15 letters compared with the standard therapy group (32% vs 3%, $P < 0.001$), irrespective of lesion type. Additionally, more patients lost fewer than 15 letters in the bevacizumab group (91% vs 67%, $P < 0.001$), and a larger proportion of bevacizumab patients achieved 6/12 or better vision by week 54 of the study. By study end, mean change in vision was +7.0 letters in the bevacizumab group, versus −9.4 letters in the standard care group. Serious ocular and nonocular adverse events were rare in all groups, with no serious intraocular infections in any of the intervention groups. Two myocardial infarctions, one fatal, occurred in the bevacizumab group.[161] This study represented the first level 1 evidence of the efficacy of bevacizumab for the treatment of AMD.

A small randomized study conducted at the Veterans Affairs Boston Healthcare System Hospital compared bevacizumab and ranibizumab directly. A total of 28 patients were randomized in a 2:1 ratio to receive bevacizumab or ranibizumab, of which 22 patients completed one year of follow-up. Injections were given monthly for 3 months, followed by additional injections given on the basis of OCT findings primarily, or vision or clinical exam. Visual and anatomic results were similar between the two groups: patients receiving bevacizumab improved an average of 7.6 letters, compared with 6.3 letters in the ranibizumab group ($P = 0.74$). The change in central macular thickness as determined by OCT was −50 µm in the bevacizumab group, versus −91 µm in the ranibizumab group ($P = 0.29$). The number of ranibizumab injections administered was significantly lower than the number of bevacizumab injections (4 vs 8, $P = 0.001$). The authors hypothesized two possible reasons: (1) tachyphylaxis to bevacizumab; or (2) a more robust early anatomic response to ranibizumab, leading to a higher number of bevacizumab injections given on an as-needed basis determined primarily by OCT findings.[162] This study, although small in size, was the first head-to-head trial of bevacizumab and ranibizumab, and demonstrated the similar efficacy of bevacizumab to ranibizumab.

Antigen binding fragment: ranibizumab (Lucentis)

Ranibizumab is a humanized anti-VEGF-A recombinant Fab fragment that has been affinity matured to increase its binding affinity for VEGF-A (see Fig. 67.11). Ranibizumab binds within the VEGFR-binding domain of all biologically active isoforms of VEGF-A. Two randomized, double-masked, pivotal phase III clinical trials have demonstrated that monthly intravitreal injections of ranibizumab are an effective and safe treatment for subfoveal CNV in AMD patients.[163,164]

The MARINA study assessed the response of minimally classic or occult CNV to ranibizumab.[163] Patients (n = 716) were assigned randomly to receive sham injection (n = 238), 0.3 mg (n = 238), or 0.5 mg (n = 240) ranibizumab. After 4 months of follow-up, approximately 90% of ranibizumab-treated patients had lost less than 15 letters on the Bailey – Lovie (ETDRS) chart as compared to 53% of the sham-injected patients. This treatment response was independent of lesion size, initial visual acuity, or whether the lesion was classified as minimally classic or occult with no classic CNV on fluorescein angiography. Vision improved by at least 15 letters in approximately 33% of patients receiving 0.5 mg ranibizumab at 24 months of follow-up versus 4% in the sham-injected patients (Fig. 67.12).[165] Approximately 1% of patients receiving intravitreal ranibizumab developed endophthalmitis. The risk of cataract was approximately 0.2%. There were no cases of retinal detachment among patients receiving intravitreal therapy. Despite the theoretical risk of systemic vascular complications, there was no imbalance among treated and control groups regarding hypertension, and the risk of myocardial infarction among sham-injected, 0.3 mg, and 0.5 mg cohorts was 1.7%, 2.5%, and 1.3%, respectively. The risk of stroke among the three groups was 0.8%, 1.3%, and 2.5%, respectively. The risk of nonocular hemorrhage was 5.5%, 9.2%, and 8.8% in each of the three cohorts, respectively. None of these differences was statistically significant, although the authors recognized that the study was not powered to detect small differences.

The ANCHOR study assessed the response of patients with predominantly classic CNV as determined by fluorescein angiography.[164] Patients ($n = 423$) were randomly assigned to receive verteporfin-PDT plus sham injection (n = 143) or sham PDT plus injection of either 0.3 mg (n = 140) or 0.5 mg (n = 140) ranibizumab. At 12 months follow-up, approximately 95% of ranibizumab-treated patients lost less than 15 letters of vision versus 64% in the verteporfin active-treatment control group. Forty percent of patients treated with 0.5 mg ranibizumab gained at least 15 letters vision versus 6% in the verteporfin treatment cohort. At month 24, the visual benefit from ranibizumab remained statistically ($P < 0.0001$ vs PDT) and clinically significant: 89.9–90.0% of ranibizumab-treated patients had lost <15 letters from baseline (vs 65.7% of PDT patients); 34–41.0% had gained ≥15 letters (vs 6.3% of PDT group); and, on average, visual acuity was improved from baseline by 8.1–10.7 letters (versus a mean decline of 9.8 letters in the PDT groups).[166] Changes in lesion anatomic characteristics on fluorescein angiography also favored ranibizumab (all comparisons $P < 0.0001$ vs PDT). Overall, there was no imbalance among groups in rates of serious ocular and nonocular adverse events. In the pooled ranibizumab groups, 3 (1.1%) of 277 patients developed presumed endophthalmitis in the study eye (rate per injection = 3/5921, or 0.05%). Retinal detachment was observed in one patient in both the verteporfin (0.7%) and 0.3 mg ranibizumab (0.7%) cohorts. There were no cases of lens injury. The risk of hypertension was the same in all cohorts. The risk of myocardial infarction among verteporfin, 0.3 mg ranibizumab, and 0.5 mg ranibizumab cohorts was 0.7%, 0.7%, and 2.1%, respectively. The risk of stroke or cerebral infarction was 0.7% in each of the three cohorts. The risk of nonocular hemorrhage was 2.1%, 5.1%, and 6.4% in each of the three cohorts. Immunoreactivity to ranibizumab before treatment was 1.5%, 3.2%, and 0.8% among the verteporfin, 0.3 mg ranibizumab, and 0.5 mg ranibizumab cohorts, respectively. Immunoreactivity was present in 1.6%, 1.6%, and 3.9% of patients in each of these cohorts, respectively, after 12 months of treatment. (The concern regarding immunoreactivity is that patients who develop an immune response might exhibit increased intraocular inflammation following intravitreal injection and consequently might not respond to the medication as well as patients who do not exhibit such a response. In practice, most retina surgeons have not observed this phenomenon and the drug has been minimally immunogenic in the doses tested.[167])

In both the MARINA and ANCHOR trials, visual acuity improvement seemed to reach a plateau by the 4-month time point (Fig. 67.12). Because monthly injections were considered inconvenient and daunting for some patients and their family members, and entailed risk as well as considerable expense, studies were undertaken to evaluate alternative treatment regimens. The PIER and EXCITE studies provided useful information in this regard.[168,169] In PIER, a phase IIIb multicenter, randomized, double-masked trial, patients with subfoveal CNV were randomly assigned to sham injection (n = 63), 0.3 mg ranibizumab (n = 60), or 0.5 mg ranibizumab (n = 61). Patients received sham or ranibizumab injections every 4 weeks for three doses followed by additional treatment every 3 months. By month 12, mean changes from baseline visual acuity were −16.3, −1.6, and −0.2 letters for the sham, 0.3 mg, and 0.5 mg groups, respectively ($P \leq 0.0001$, each ranibizumab dose vs sham). Ranibizumab arrested CNV growth and reduced leakage from CNV. The treatment effect declined, however, in the ranibizumab groups during quarterly dosing. At month 3, for example, the mean changes from baseline vision had been gains of +2.9 and +4.3 letters for the 0.3 mg and 0.5 mg doses, respectively. During study year 2, eligible sham-group patients crossed over to 0.5 mg ranibizumab quarterly. Later in year 2, all eligible randomized patients rolled over to 0.5 mg ranibizumab monthly dosing. The ranibizumab-treated patients showed an improvement in mean visual acuity during the first three months of the study, but this improvement was not sustained. Nonetheless, the 0.5 mg ranibizumab cohort had a mean visual acuity change that was 16 letters better than that of the sham cohort by month 12 ($P < 0.0001$). By month 24, visual acuity had decreased an

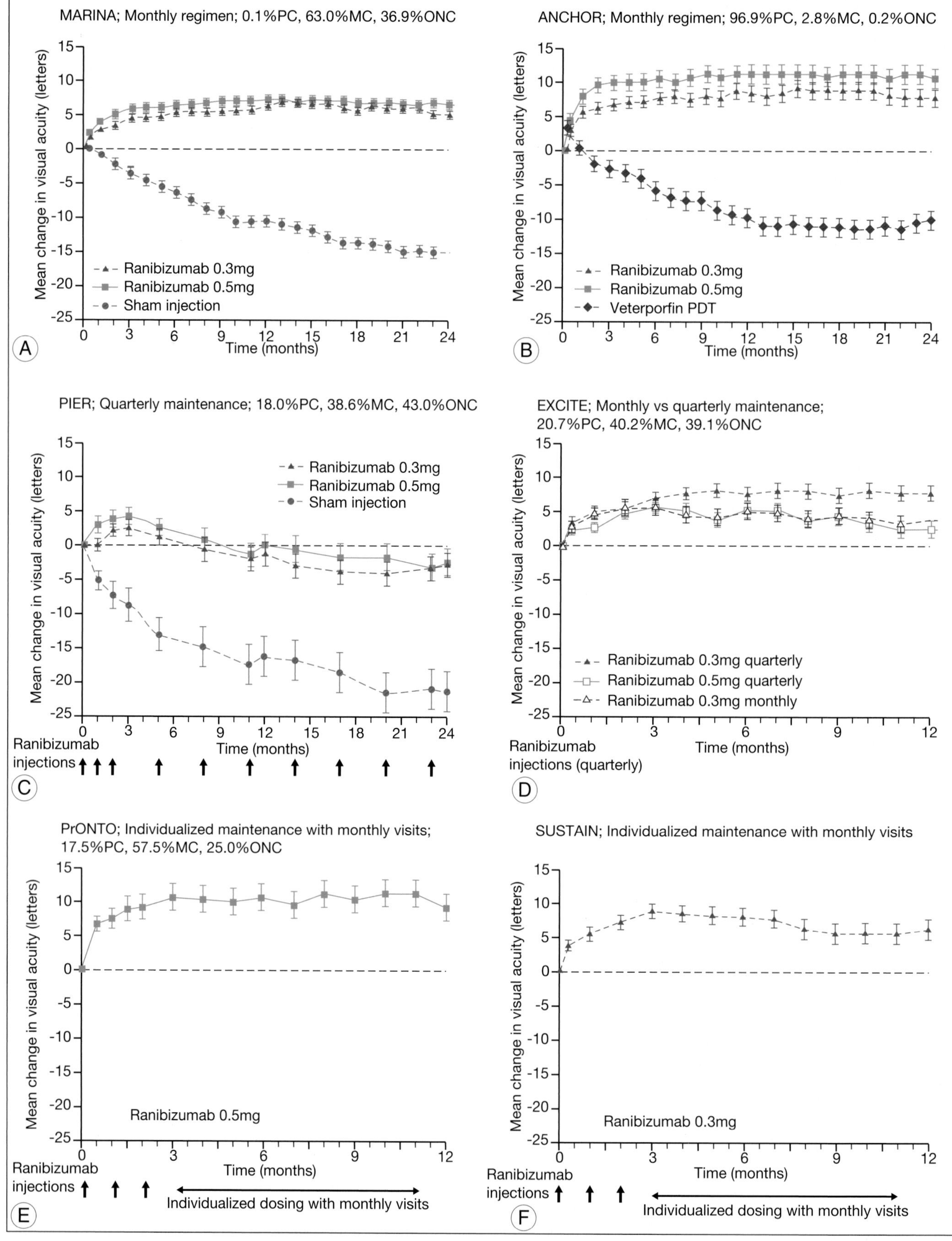

Fig. 67.12 Mean change from baseline in best-corrected visual acuity by month for (A) MARINA, (B) ANCHOR, (C) PIER, (D) EXCITE, (E) PrONTO, (F) SUSTAIN. (Panel A Copyright © 2006 Massachusetts Medical Society. All rights reserved. Panel B reproduced with permission from Brown DM, Michels M, Kaiser PK, et al. Ranibizumab versus verteporfin photodynamic therapy for neovascular age-related macular degeneration: 2-year results of ANCHOR Study. Ophthalmology 2009;116:57–65, Copyright 2009, with permission from Elsevier. Panel C reproduced with permission from Regillo, et al. Ranibizumab (Lucentis) in treatment of neovascular age-related macular degeneration (AMD): 2-year results of PIER study, poster PO459 presented at the AAO 2007. Panel E reproduced with permission from Fung AE, Lalwani GA, Rosenfeld PJ, et al. An optical coherence tomography-guided, variable dosing regimen with intravitreal ranibizumab (Lucentis) for neovascular age-related macular degeneration. Am J Ophthalmol 2007;143:566–83, Copyright 2007, with permission from Elsevier. Compilation reproduced with permission from Mitchell P, Korobelnik JF, Lanzetta P, et al. Ranibizumab (Lucentis) in neovascular age-related macular degeneration: evidence from clinical trials. Br J Ophthalmol 2010;94:2–13.)

average of 21.4, 2.2, and 2.3 letters from baseline in the sham, 0.3 mg, and 0.5 mg groups ($P < 0.0001$ for each ranibizumab group vs sham). The visual acuity of sham patients who crossed over to ranibizumab decreased over time, with an average loss of 3.5 letters 10 months after crossover. The visual acuity of patients in the 0.3 mg and 0.5 mg cohorts who rolled over to monthly ranibizumab injections increased for an average gain of 2.2 and 4.1 letters, respectively, 4 months after transition. These data indicate that injecting patients with ranibizumab every 3 months (after an induction phase of three monthly injections) does not produce the same chance for visual benefit as monthly injection, at least during the first 12 months of therapy. Ranibizumab appeared to provide additional visual benefit to treated patients who rolled over to monthly dosing, but not to patients who began receiving ranibizumab after >14 months of sham injections.

The EXCITE study, was a 12-month, multicenter, randomized, double-masked, active-controlled, phase IIIb study designed to demonstrate the noninferiority of a quarterly treatment versus monthly intravitreal ranibizumab treatment regimen in patients with AMD-associated CNV.[170] Patients with primary or recurrent subfoveal CNV secondary to AMD (353 patients), including those with predominantly classic, minimally classic, or occult (no classic component) lesions, were enrolled. Patients were randomized (1:1:1) to 0.3 mg quarterly, 0.5 mg quarterly, or 0.3 mg monthly doses of ranibizumab. Treatment comprised three consecutive monthly injections followed by a 9-month maintenance phase (either monthly or quarterly injection). In the per-protocol population (293 patients), visual acuity increased from baseline to month 12 by 4.9, 3.8, and 8.3 letters in the 0.3 mg quarterly (104 patients), 0.5 mg quarterly (88 patients), and 0.3 mg monthly (101 patients) dosing groups, respectively. Similar results were observed in the intent-to-treat (ITT) population (353 patients). The mean decrease in CRT from baseline to month 12 in the ITT population was −96.0 μm in the 0.3 mg quarterly, −105.6 μm in the 0.5 mg quarterly, and −105.3 μm in the 0.3 mg monthly group. At month 12, the visual acuity gain in the monthly treatment cohort was higher than that of the quarterly regimens. The noninferiority of a quarterly regimen was not achieved with reference to 5.0 letters.

The SUSTAIN study is a 12-month, phase III, multicenter, open-label, single-arm study involving 513 ranibizumab-naive patients with AMD-associated CNV.[171] In this study, patients received three initial monthly injections of ranibizumab (0.3 mg) and thereafter pro re nata (PRN) retreatment for 9 months based on prespecified retreatment criteria. Patients switched to 0.5 mg ranibizumab after approval in Europe. The average number of retreatments from months 3 to 11 was 2.7. Mean best-corrected visual acuity increased steadily from baseline to month 3 to reach +5.8 letters, decreased slightly from month 3 to 6, and remained stable from month 6 to 12, reaching +3.6 at month 12. The mean change in CRT was −101.1 μm from baseline to month 3 and −91.5 μm from baseline to month 12.

In summary, data from the ANCHOR, MARINA, PIER, EXCITE, and SUSTAIN studies indicated that after a loading dose period of three monthly injections, subsequently monthly ranibizumab injections give superior visual acuity outcomes compared to quarterly or PRN injections (Fig. 67.13).

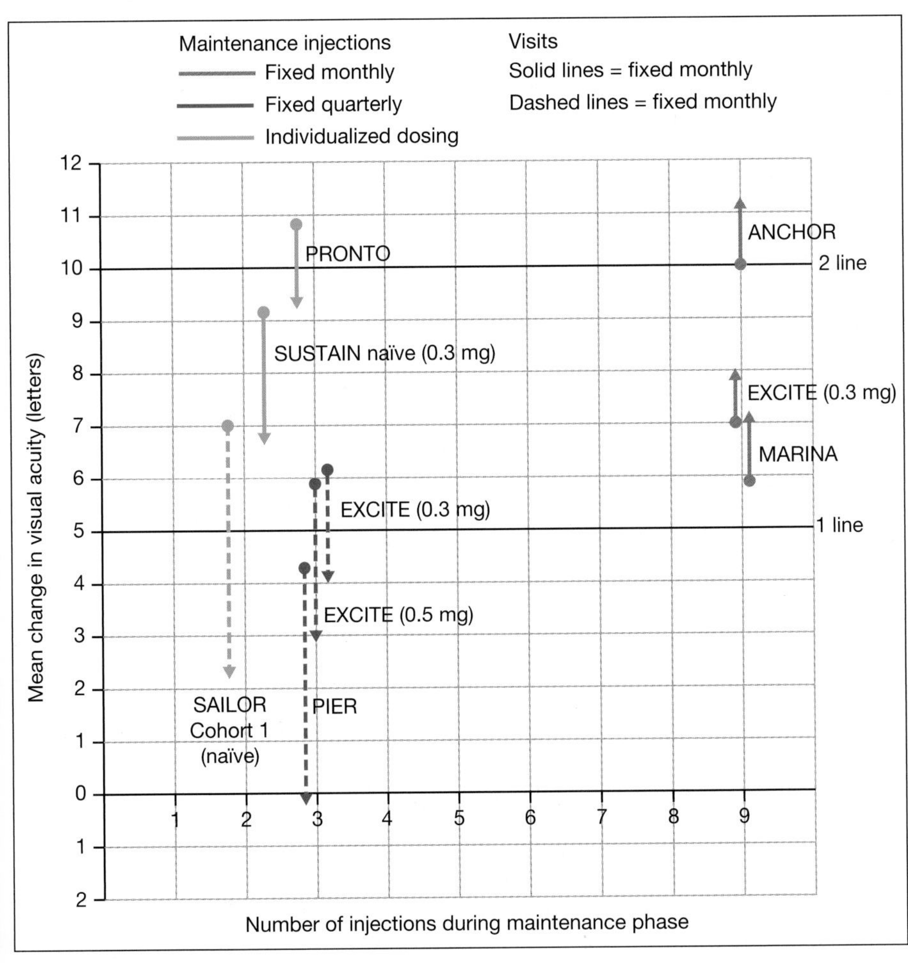

Fig. 67.13 Mean change in visual acuity from baseline at the end of the loading phase (•) and at 12 months (arrowhead) against the number of injections during 9 months of the maintenance phase (ranibizumab 0.5 mg data unless indicated). (Reproduced with permission from Mitchell P, Korobelnik JF, Lanzetta P, et al. Ranibizumab (Lucentis) in neovascular age-related macular degeneration: evidence from clinical trials. Br J Ophthalmol 2010;94:2–13.)

In the PrONTO (Prospective OCT Imaging of Patients with Neovascular AMD Treated with Intraocular Lucentis) study, patients (n = 40) received 0.5 mg ranibizumab at entry, month 1, and month 2.[172] Optical coherence tomography (OCT) measurements were obtained at baseline and at least monthly after injection (more frequently during the first two months after entry). Fluorescein angiograms were obtained at baseline and every 3 months thereafter. Retreatment with ranibizumab was done only if one or more of the following conditions was observed: (1) OCT central thickness (CRT) increased 100 μm; (2) ≥5 letter visual loss associated with subretinal fluid (as judged with OCT); (3) new onset classic CNV; (4) new macular hemorrhage; (5) persistent subretinal or intraretinal fluid was present 1 month after the previous injection. One day after the first injection, there was a decrease in the mean OCT thickness of 47 μm. By month 12, the mean visual acuity improved by 9.3 letters (P <0.001), and the mean central thickness decreased by 178 μm compared with baseline (P <0.001). Mean visual acuity improvement was 9.3 letters, and the mean central thickness had decreased by 178 μm. The average number of injections over the first year was 5.6. Visual acuity improved ≥15 letters in 35% of patients, and once macular fluid resorbed completely, the mean interval before another injection was 4.5 months. During the second year, the retreatment criteria were amended to include retreatment if any qualitative increase in the amount of fluid was detected using OCT.[173] Forty patients were enrolled and 37 completed the 2-year study. At month 24, the mean visual acuity improved by 11.1 letters (P < .001) and the OCT-CRT decreased by 212 μm (P < 0.001). Visual acuity improved by 15 letters or more in 43% of patients. These visual acuity and OCT outcomes were achieved with an average of 9.9 injections over 24 months. The PrONTO Study data suggested that OCT-guided variable-dosing regimens with intravitreal ranibizumab were capable of achieving visual acuity outcomes comparable to those from the phase III clinical studies, but with fewer intravitreal injections.

Although the risk of arterial thromboembolic events was not increased to a statistically significant degree among ranibizumab-treated patients in these phase III studies (overall risk ~2.1% in ranibizumab-treated patients during year 1 vs ~1.1% among controls), some concerns were expressed about relative safety compared with alternative therapies, efficacy aside, as the studies were not powered for statistical significance between the two different ranibizumab doses. Year 2 data from the MARINA study indicate the overall rate of antiplatelet trialists' collaboration (APTC)-defined arterial thromboembolic events, which includes nonfatal myocardial infarction, nonfatal stroke, and death from a vascular or unknown cause,[174] was 4.6%, 4.6%, and 3.8% among the 0.5 mg ranibizumab, 0.3 mg ranibizumab, and control cohorts, respectively. Year 2 data from the ANCHOR study indicate the overall rate of APTC arterial thromboembolic events was 5%, 4.4%, and 4.2% in the 0.5 mg, 0.3 mg, and verteporfin-PDT cohorts, respectively. The PIER[168,169] and EXCITE[170] studies had similar results in this regard.

The SAILOR study was a phase IIIb study whose objectives are to evaluate the safety of 0.3 mg and 0.5 mg Lucentis in patients with AMD-associated subfoveal CNV. In cohort 1 of this study, the dose was randomly assigned and administered once a month for 3 months and thereafter as needed based on retreatment criteria. In SAILOR, there was a numerically higher rate of cerebrovascular stroke with 0.5 mg ranibizumab compared with 0.3 mg ranibizumab (1.2 vs 0.7%), which was not statistically significant in patients with a history of stroke.[175] In the SUSTAIN study, a total of 249 patients (48.5%) reported ocular adverse events, 5 patients (1.2%) with ocular serious adverse events involving the study eye (retinal hemorrhage, cataract, retinal pigment epithelial tear, reduced visual acuity, vitreous hemorrhage), 19 patients (3.7%) with arteriothromboembolic events were observed, with 8 deaths (1.5%).[171] The most frequent adverse events in the study eye were reduced visual acuity (18.5%), retinal hemorrhage (7.2%), increased intraocular pressure (7.0%), and conjunctival hemorrhage (5.5%). Overall, the ocular and systemic risks associated with ranibizumab use appear to be low and within a reasonable range when taking into account the associated likelihood of visual improvement in properly selected patients (Table 67.2).[165]

Comparison of Age-related Macular Degeneration Treatments Trial (CATT)

Despite a relative lack of level 1 evidence prior to 2011, bevacizumab had become the most widely used agent for AMD in the world due to a number of factors, including its low cost compared to ranibizumab, similarity in therapeutic mechanism, and its availability to physicians prior to the FDA approval of ranibizumab. A large amount of data from retrospective reviews, interventional case series, and anecdotal reports have provided physicians with evidence to support the continued off-label use of bevacizumab. However, in the absence of a large, randomized clinical controlled trial comparing bevacizumab to ranibizumab, the current gold standard, several questions have arisen:

1. Does one treatment offer superior visual outcomes to another?
2. What is the optimal treatment regimen and interval?
3. Is the safety profile of bevacizumab comparable to that of ranibizumab, which has been subjected to rigorous phase I - phase IV evaluation?

The CATT was designed to address these questions.[150]

The CATT is a multicenter, randomized clinical trial, that enrolled 1208 patients with previously untreated subfoveal CNV due to AMD, as determined by leakage on fluorescein angiogram and fluid on time domain OCT. The primary outcome measure in the study was visual acuity change. The study designers also elected to examine the proportion of patients with a 15-letter difference in vision, number of injections, fluid and thickness on OCT, lesion size on fluorescein angiography, incidence of ocular and systemic adverse events, and annual treatment cost as secondary treatment endpoints. Patients were randomized to one of four groups: (1) ranibizumab 0.5 mg monthly (every 28 days); (2) bevacizumab 1.25 mg monthly; (3) ranibizumab as needed (when signs of active neovascularization were present); (4) bevacizumab as needed (with similar indications for retreatment as group 3). The study was designed to determine noninferiority of one treatment group with respect to each of the remaining three groups, using a statistically robust 99.2% confidence interval and a noninferiority limit of 5 letters on the ETDRS chart.

Visual acuity data were available for 1105 patients at one year. The six pairwise comparisons showed the following:

Table 67.2 Summary of key ocular and non-ocular adverse events in ranibizumab clinical trials

	MARINA (24-month data)			ANCHOR (12-month data)			PIER (12-month data)			EXCITE (12-month data)			SUSTAIN (12-month data)
	Ranibizumab 0.3 mg (n = 238)	Ranibizumab 0.5 mg (n = 240)	Sham control (n = 238)	Ranibizumab 0.3 mg (n = 137)	Ranibizumab 0.5 mg (n = 140)	Verteporfin control (n = 143)	Ranibizumab 0.3 mg (n = 59)	Ranibizumab 0.5 mg (n = 61)	Sham control (n = 63)	Ranibizumab 0.3 mg control (n = 101)	Ranibizumab 0.3 mg (n = 104)	Ranibizumab 0.5 mg (n = 88)	Ranibizumab 0.3 mg (n = 69; interim data)
Key serious ocular adverse events													
Presumed endophthalmitis	2 (0.8)	3 (1.3)	0	0	2 (1.4)	0	0	0	0	0	0	0	0
Culture positive	0	0	0	0	1 (0.7)	0	0	0	0	0	0	0	0
Culture negative	1 (0.4)	3 (1.3)	0	0	0	0	0	0	0	0	0	0	0
Culture not done	1 (0.4)	0	0	0	1 (0.7)	0	0	0	0	0	0	0	0
Uveitis	3 (1.3)	3 (1.3)	0	0	1 (0.7)	0	0	0	0	0	0	0	0
Retinal detachments	0	0	1 (0.4)	1 (0.7)	0	1 (0.7)	0	0	0	0	1 (0.8)	0	0
Retinal tear	1 (0.4)	1 (0.4)	0	0	0	0	0	0	0	0	0	2 (1.7)	0
Retinal hemorrhage	NA	NA	NA	NA	NA	NA	1 (1.7)	0	2 (3.2)	0	0	1 (0.8)	1 (1.4)
Detachment of RPE	NA	NA	NA	NA	NA	NA	NA	NA	NA	0	0	0	1 (1.4)
Vitreous hemorrhage	1 (0.4)	1 (0.4)	2 (0.8)	1 (0.7)	0	0	0	0	0	0	0	0	0
Key nonocular adverse events													
Hypertension	41 (17.2)	39 (16.3)	18 (16.1)	3 (2.2)	9 (6.4)	12 (8.4)	4 (6.8)	6 (9.8)	5 (8.1)	8 (7.0)	10 (8.3)	6 (5.1)	3 (4.3)

Continued

Table 67.2 Summary of key ocular and non-ocular adverse events in ranibizumab clinical trials—Cont'd

	MARINA (24-month data)			ANCHOR (12-month data)			PIER (12-month data)			EXCITE (12-month data)			SUSTAIN (12-month data)
	Ranibizumab 0.3 mg (*n* = 238)	Ranibizumab 0.5 mg (*n* = 240)	Sham control (*n* = 238)	Ranibizumab 0.3 mg (*n* = 137)	Ranibizumab 0.5 mg (*n* = 140)	Verteporfin control (*n* = 143)	Ranibizumab 0.3 mg (*n* = 59)	Ranibizumab 0.5 mg (*n* = 61)	Sham control (*n* = 63)	Ranibizumab 0.3 mg control (*n* = 101)	Ranibizumab 0.3 mg (*n* = 104)	Ranibizumab 0.5 mg (*n* = 88)	Ranibizumab 0.3 mg (*n* = 69; interim data)
Key arterial thromboembolic events (nonfatal)													
Myocardial infarction	6 (2.5)[*]	3 (1.3)[†]	4 (1.7)	1 (0.7)	3 (2.1)	1 (0.7)	0	0	0	1 (0.9)	1 (0.8)	0	0
Stroke	3 (1.3)[‡]	6 (2.5)[†§]	2 (0.8)[¶,**]	0	1 (0.7)	1 (0.7)	0	0	0	1 (0.9)	0	0	0
Cerebral infarction	NA	NA	NA	1 (0.7)	0	0	NA	NA	NA	0	0	1 (0.8)	0
Death													
Vascular cause	3 (1.3)[‡,††]	3 (1.3)[‡‡]	4 (1.7)[§§]	1 (0.7)[¶¶]	2 (1.4)[***]	1 (0.7)[¶¶]	0	0	0	1 (0.9)[†††]	0	1(0.8)[‡‡‡]	0
Nonvascular cause	2 (0.8)	3 (1.3)	2 (0.8)	2 (1.5)	0	1 (0.7)	0	0	0	1 (0.9)	0	1 (0.8)	0
Nonocular hemorrhage	22 (9.2)	21 (8.8)	13 (5.5)	7 (5.1)	9 (6.4)	3 (2.1)	2 (3.4)	4 (6.6)	3 (4.8)	NA	NA	NA	NA

NA, not available; RPE, retinal pigment epithelium.
[*]*One patient had two episodes.*
[†]*One patient had a myocardial infarction and a hemorrhagic stroke, both non-fatal.*
[‡]*One patient had a non-fatal ischemic stroke and died of an unknown cause.*
[§]*One patient had a cerebral ischemic incident that was categorized as an ischemic stroke.*
[¶]*One patient in the sham group received a single ranibizumab 0.5 mg dose in error approximately 8 months before the onset of stroke.*
[**]*One patient had a second episode of stroke, which resulted in death.*
[††]*Two patients died from myocardial infarction and one from an unknown cause.*
[‡‡]*One patient died from a small-bowel infarct and two from stroke.*
[§§]*Two patients died from stroke, one from congestive heart failure and one from an unknown cause.*
[¶¶]*One patient died from cardiac arrest.*
[***]*One patient died from cardiac failure and one from worsening of chronic heart failure.*
[†††]*One patient died from cerebral hemorrhage.*
[‡‡‡]*One patient died from cardiorespiratory arrest.*
(Reproduced with permission from Mitchell P, Korobelnik JF, Lanzetta P, et al. Ranibizumab (Lucentis) in neovascular age-related macular degeneration: evidence from clinical trials. Br J Ophthalmol 2010;94:2–13.)

1. Bevacizumab monthly injections (8.0 letters gained) and ranibizumab monthly injections (+8.5 letters) yielded equivalent visual outcomes.
2. Bevacizumab given as needed (+5.9 letters) was also equivalent to ranibizumab given as needed (+6.8 letters).
3. Ranibizumab given as needed was equivalent to ranibizumab given monthly.
4. Ranibizumab given as needed was also equivalent to bevacizumab given monthly.
5. Bevacizumab given as needed was neither inferior nor not-inferior (inconclusive) to bevacizumab given monthly.
6. Bevacizumab given as needed was neither inferior nor not-inferior (inconclusive) to ranibizumab given monthly.

Detailed visual and anatomic outcome data are shown in Fig. 67.14 and Table 67.3.

Secondary visual outcomes were similarly equivalent, with 91.5% (bevacizumab as needed) to 95.4% (ranibizumab as needed) of patients not having a decrease in vision of 15 letters or more from baseline, and 24.9% (ranibizumab as needed) to 34.2% (ranibizumab monthly) experiencing a gain of at least 15 letters. Anatomic outcomes showed that all groups had substantial decreases in retinal thickness as measured by OCT at 1 year, although the monthly ranibizumab group experienced a greater decrease in thickness (196 ± 176 μm) than those patients receiving bevacizumab as needed (152 ± 178 μm, $P = 0.03$). The mean number of injections given in the as-needed groups was 7.7 ± 3.5 (bevacizumab) and 6.9 ± 3.0 (ranibizumab) out of 13 possible, translating to an average yearly cost of $385 vs $13 800, respectively. The average cost to patients given monthly injections was $595 for bevacizumab and $23 400 for ranibizumab (Table 67.3).

Table 67.3 CATT one-year outcomes: primary outcome (visual acuity) and additional outcomes

Outcome	Ranibizumab		Bevacizumab		
	Monthly *n* = 284	As needed *n* = 285	Monthly *n* = 265	As needed *n* = 271	*P* value
ETDRS letter score (Snellen equivalent), no. (%)					
83–97 (20/12–20/20)	42 (14.8)	38 (13.3)	45 (17.0)	40 (14.8)	
68–82 (20/25–20/40)	149 (52.5)	141 (49.5)	134 (50.6)	127 (46.9)	
53–67 (20/50–20/80)	52 (18.3)	66 (23.2)	47 (17.7)	57 (21.0)	
38–52 (20/100–20/160)	23 (8.1)	23 (8.1)	21 (7.9)	24 (8.9)	
≤37 (≤20/200)	18 (6.3)	17 (6.0)	18 (6.8)	23 (8.5)	
Mean letter score (±SD)	68.8 ± 17.7	68.4 ± 16.4	68.4 ± 18.2	66.5 ± 19.0	0.45
Change from baseline vision, no. (%)					
≥15 letter increase	97 (34.2)	71 (24.9)	83 (31.3)	76 (28.0)	
5–14 letter increase	90 (31.7)	103 (36.1)	98 (37.0)	90 (33.2)	
≤4 letter change	62 (21.8)	75 (26.3)	50 (18.9)	59 (21.8)	
5–14 letter decrease	19 (6.7)	23 (8.1)	18 (6.8)	23 (8.5)	
≥15 letter decrease	16 (5.6)	13 (4.6)	16 (6.0)	23 (23.8)	
Mean change (letters±SD)	8.5 ± 14.1	6.8 ± 13.1	8.0 ± 15.8	5.9 ± 15.7	0.16
OCT foveal thickness (μm)*					
Mean total thickness†	266 ± 125	294 ± 139	300 ± 149	308 ± 127	0.002
Mean change from baseline‡	−196 ± 176	−168 ± 186	−164 ± 181	−152 ± 178	0.03
Mean number of injections	**11.7 ± 1.5**	**6.9 ± 3.0**	**11.9 ± 1.2**	**7.7 ± 3.5**	**<0.001**
Average annual cost/patient	**$23 400**	**$13 800**	**$595**	**$385**	

SD, standard deviation; OCT, optical coherence tomography
**The total foveal thickness includes the retina, subretinal fluid, choroidal neovascularization, and retinal pigment epithelial elevation.*
†Data were missing for 4 patients in the ranibizumab-monthly group, 4 patients in the ranibizumab-as-needed group, 4 patients in the bevacizumab-monthly group, and 5 patients in the bevacizumab-as-needed group.
‡Data were missing for 4 patients in the ranibizumab-monthly group, 7 patients in the ranibizumab-as-needed group, 5 patients in the bevacizumab-monthly group, and 6 patients in the bevacizumab-as-needed group.
(Reproduced with permission from Martin DF, Maguire MG, Ying GS, et al. Ranibizumab and bevacizumab for neovascular age-related macular degeneration. N Engl J Med 2011;364:1897–908.)

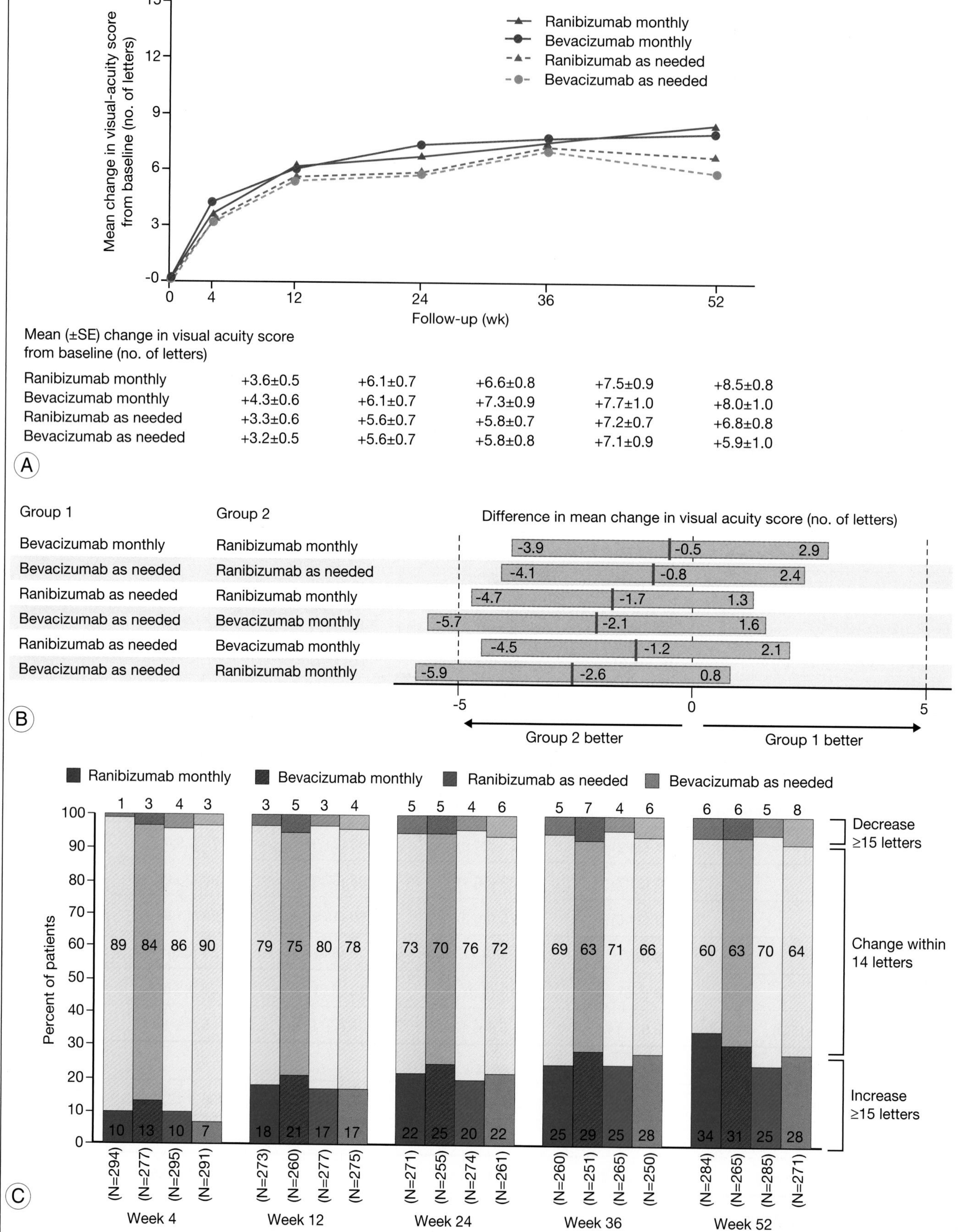

Fig. 67.14 (A) Mean change in the visual acuity score during the first year of follow-up. (B) Differences between pairs of study groups in the mean change from baseline to 1 year in the visual acuity score. The red vertical lines indicate means, and the gray bars 99.2% confidence intervals. Negative values reflect a greater mean increase in group 2. Confidence intervals within –5 and +5 letters (dashed vertical lines) indicate that the two groups are equivalent. Confidence intervals extending beyond the noninferiority limit of –5 letters indicate that the comparison of the two groups is inconclusive with respect to noninferiority. (C) Proportions of patients in each group with a decrease of 15 letters or more, a change within 14 letters, or an increase of 15 letters or more from baseline values during the first study year. (Reproduced with permission from Martin DF, Maguire MG, Ying GS, et al. Ranibizumab and bevacizumab for neovascular age-related macular degeneration. N Engl J Med 2011;364:1897–908.)

Deaths occurred in 2.0% of the entire study group over the one-year period, with no significant difference among any of the groups. The occurrence of arteriothrombotic events was 2–3% for each group, also without significant differences. Venous thrombotic events occurred in 4 out of 286 patients receiving bevacizumab monthly (P = 0.08 difference between all groups) but occurred infrequently in all groups. When serious systemic adverse events were pooled among drug-specific groups, they occurred in 24.1% of patients receiving bevacizumab, vs 19.0% of those receiving ranibizumab (P=0.04). Endophthalmitis occurred in 0.05% of the total number of injections, without a significant difference between medication groups. All other serious ocular adverse events occurred with rare frequency (Table 67.4).

The impact of the one-year CATT study results was significant, establishing the equivalent visual outcomes of ranibizumab and bevacizumab when given monthly. Although bevacizumab as needed, when compared to ranibizumab or bevacizumab monthly, yielded inconclusive results, all other groups showed similar efficacy. Rosenfeld proposed in explanation that the treatment effect for bevacizumab may be less durable in some patients; thus, giving more frequent injections might improve visual outcomes in that subgroup.[176] Importantly, the first-year study results also appeared to establish that as-needed ranibizumab (as well as monthly bevacizumab) was as effective as monthly ranibizumab, which not only has significant implications for treatment cost, but also for the cumulative risk of injection-associated adverse events as well as patient anxiety surrounding treatment administration. Interestingly, although the effect of the medication on retinal thickness was more prominent for ranibizumab, this did not translate to better vision as compared to bevacizumab. Finally, the study authors recognized that the CATT was insufficiently powered to determine a difference in infrequently occurring systemic and ocular adverse events, and although bevacizumab was associated with a higher overall rate of systemic adverse events, these events involved organ systems not typically associated with systemic anti-VEGF therapy. In particular, the rate of arteriothrombotic and venous thrombotic events was no different between the two medications, and was low in all groups. Additionally, the risk of adverse events was not noted to correlate with increased exposure to medication, with a higher rate of occurrence in patients receiving injections on an as-needed basis.

Interested readers might also refer to the one-year interim report from the IVAN study. The efficacy and safety of ranibizumab and bevacizumab intravitreal injections to treat neovascular age-related macular degeneration were compared, and participants were randomize to four groups: ranibizumab or bevacizumab, given either every month (continuous) or as needed (discontinuous), with monthly review. The authors concluded: "The comparison of visual acuity at 1 year between bevacizumab and ranibizumab was inconclusive. Visual acuities with continuous and discontinuous treatment were equivalent. Other outcomes are consistent with the drugs and treatment regimens having similar efficacy and safety."[176a]

Table 67.4 CATT first-year serious adverse events*

Event type	Ranibizumab Monthly n = 301	Ranibizumab As needed n = 298	Bevacizumab Monthly n = 286	Bevacizumab As needed n = 300	P value By group	P value By drug
Systemic events						
Death (all causes)	4 (1.3)	5 (1.7)	4 (1.4)	11 (3.7)	0.18	0.22
Arteriothrombotic event	7 (2.3)	6 (2.0)	6 (2.1)	8 (2.7)	0.97	0.85
Nonfatal myocardial infarction‡	2 (0.7)	3 (1.0)	2 (0.7)	1 (0.3)	0.78	0.73
Nonfatal stroke	3 (1.0)	1 (0.3)	2 (0.7)	2 (0.7)	0.88	1.00
Death from vascular causes	2 (0.7)	2 (0.7)	2 (0.7)	5 (1.7)	0.57	0.38
Venous thrombotic event	0	2 (0.7)	4 (1.4)	1 (0.3)	0.08	0.28
Transient ischemic attack	1 (0.3)	2 (0.7)	0	3 (1.0)	0.48	1.00
Hypertension	0	0	2 (0.7)	0	0.06	0.24
One or more systemic event	53 (17.6)	61 (20.5)	64 (22.4)	77 (25.7)	0.11	0.04
Ocular events						
Endophthalmitis	2 (0.7)	0	4 (1.4)	0	0.03	0.45
Pseudoendophthalmitis	1 (0.3)	0	0	0	1.00	1.00

*Multiple events in the same category counted only once.
‡Includes deaths following myocardial infarction, stroke, or cardiac arrest.
(Reproduced with permission from Martin DF, Maguire MG, Ying GS, et al. Ranibizumab and bevacizumab for neovascular age-related macular degeneration. N Engl J Med 2011;364:1897–908.)

The second year results of CATT, published in mid-2012, described the visual impact of switching from monthly to as-needed treatment after the first year, as well as any differences in disease activity or progression, as demonstrated by fluid on OCT, leakage on fluorescein angiography, and lesion size. In addition, the use of high-resolution spectral-domain OCT in year two allowed for comparison between standard and high-resolution imaging in the detection of disease activity.[177]

At week 52 of the study, the study groups were modified such that monthly treatment groups were reassigned at random to either maintain monthly dosing or switch to as-needed dosing of the same medication. The existing as-needed groups maintained the same dosing regimen. Comparisons in the second year were not made between each drug regimen group, as the reassignment resulted in a larger number of groups, and consequently reduced group size and statistical power. Rather, the analysis compared bevacizumab with ranibizumab, and monthly with as-needed dosing groups overall.

In patients maintaining the same dosing regimen (either monthly or as needed) through the two-year study period, vision change remained similar, with monthly ranibizumab showing the greatest visual improvement (+8.8 letters), followed by monthly bevacizumab (+7.8), as-needed ranibizumab (+6.7), and as-needed bevacizumab (+5.0). There was no significant difference when comparing all ranibizumab groups with all bevacizumab groups (which showed a 1.4-letter smaller gain relative to ranibizumab), but as-needed therapy showed less vision improvement by 2.4 letters relative to monthly therapy (P = 0.046). Secondary visual outcomes were also similar, including the final mean acuity (Snellen equivalent about 20/40 in all groups), the proportion gaining or losing 15 letters, and the proportion with 20/20 or better or 20/200 or worse final vision. Of note, those receiving bevacizumab as needed required more injections over the course of the study (14.1 total injections) than those receiving ranibizumab as needed (12.6), a significant difference consistent with the higher proportion of visits with detectable fluid.

Anatomic outcomes showed improved retinal thickness in patients treated monthly as compared to those treated as needed (29 µm difference, P = 0.005). Additionally, the proportion of patients without fluid as detected by OCT was lower in both the ranibizumab group as well as the monthly group (up to 45.5% in the monthly ranibizumab group); similarly, the proportion of patients with no fluorescein leakage was higher in patients treated monthly, and lesion area remained stable in these patients while growing in the as-needed group. However, the study also found that the proportion of monthly patients developing geographic atrophy was significantly higher in patients receiving monthly treatment as compared to the as-needed group, with the highest rate in those receiving ranibizumab monthly. (Vision and anatomic outcomes are detailed in Fig. 67.15 and Table 67.5).

In contrast to patients maintaining monthly therapy through two years, those switching to as-needed therapy at week 52 lost from 1.8 (ranibizumab) to 3.6 (bevacizumab) letters after year one (P = 0.03 when comparing monthly to as-needed therapy), resulting in very similar visual outcomes to patients maintained on as-needed therapy since study enrollment for both medications. Final visual acuity was similar for all groups, without significant differences between bevacizumab and ranibizumab, or between monthly and as-needed therapy. Anatomically, retinal thickness increased significantly, with a range of +19 µm (ranibizumab) to +31 µm (bevacizumab) in patients who were reassigned to as-needed therapy. The proportion of patients without fluid on OCT was significantly higher in patients who switched regimens, as well as in patients receiving bevacizumab. As in patients receiving the same regimen through year two, the proportion demonstrating dye leakage was higher in switched patients. Although the lesion area was not significantly different in either group, the rate of development of geographic atrophy was higher in ranibizumab patients as well as those receiving monthly dosing (Table 67.6).

In contrast to the first year of the study, when all study patients underwent testing with time domain OCT only, in year two 22.6% of scans were performed with high-resolution spectral domain OCT. Treatment decisions in the second year were consistent with reading center interpretation of OCT fluid in 68.5% of the ranibizumab group and 69.6% of the bevacizumab group; 95% of these cases resulted in undertreatment (the reading center interpreted fluid, yet the patient did not receive injection). The use of spectral domain OCT did not appear to increase the consistency between treating physicians and the reading center, with 70.1% agreement in the spectral domain group versus 68.7% in the time domain group.

As reported in the first year of results, the rate of systemic adverse events was significantly higher in the bevacizumab group than in the ranibizumab group, at 39.9% as compared to 31.7% overall, and 24.4% vs. 18.0% in the second year alone. Again, this difference persisted after excluding vascular events previously associated with systemic anti-VEGF drugs (P = 0.02), while the difference in events previously associated with anti-VEGF therapy approached statistical significance (P = 0.07). In addition, as noted in the first year, over the course of two years, patients treated as needed had a higher rate of systemic serious adverse events than those treated monthly (risk ratio of 1.30, P = 0.009), although this difference in the second year alone was not significant. There was no difference between drugs in the proportion of patients who died (6.1% vs 5.3%) or in the number of arteriothrombotic (5.0% vs 4.7%) or venous thrombotic events (1.7% vs 0.5%). Endophthalmitis occurred in 7 patients receiving bevacizumab and 4 patients receiving ranibizumab (P = 0.38), with 10 of these 11 cases occurring in patients receiving monthly therapy (Table 67.7).

The second year of the CATT was not designed to determine the relative efficacy of each dosing regimen for each medication. However, one may conclude the following:

1. In contrast to the first-year results, longer-term follow-up suggests that as-needed therapy is somewhat less effective than monthly therapy overall in terms of visual gain.
2. Visual acuity and visual gain are associated with, but do not closely mirror retinal thickness or the presence of fluid.
3. One year of monthly therapy does not appear to confer lesion stability when subsequently changing to as-needed therapy.
4. When given as needed, bevacizumab is required more frequently, on average 1.5 more injections over the two-year period.
5. Geographic atrophy occurs with greater frequency in patients receiving monthly therapy.
6. Spectral domain OCT does not appear to increase the accuracy of identifying retinal fluid by the treating physician.

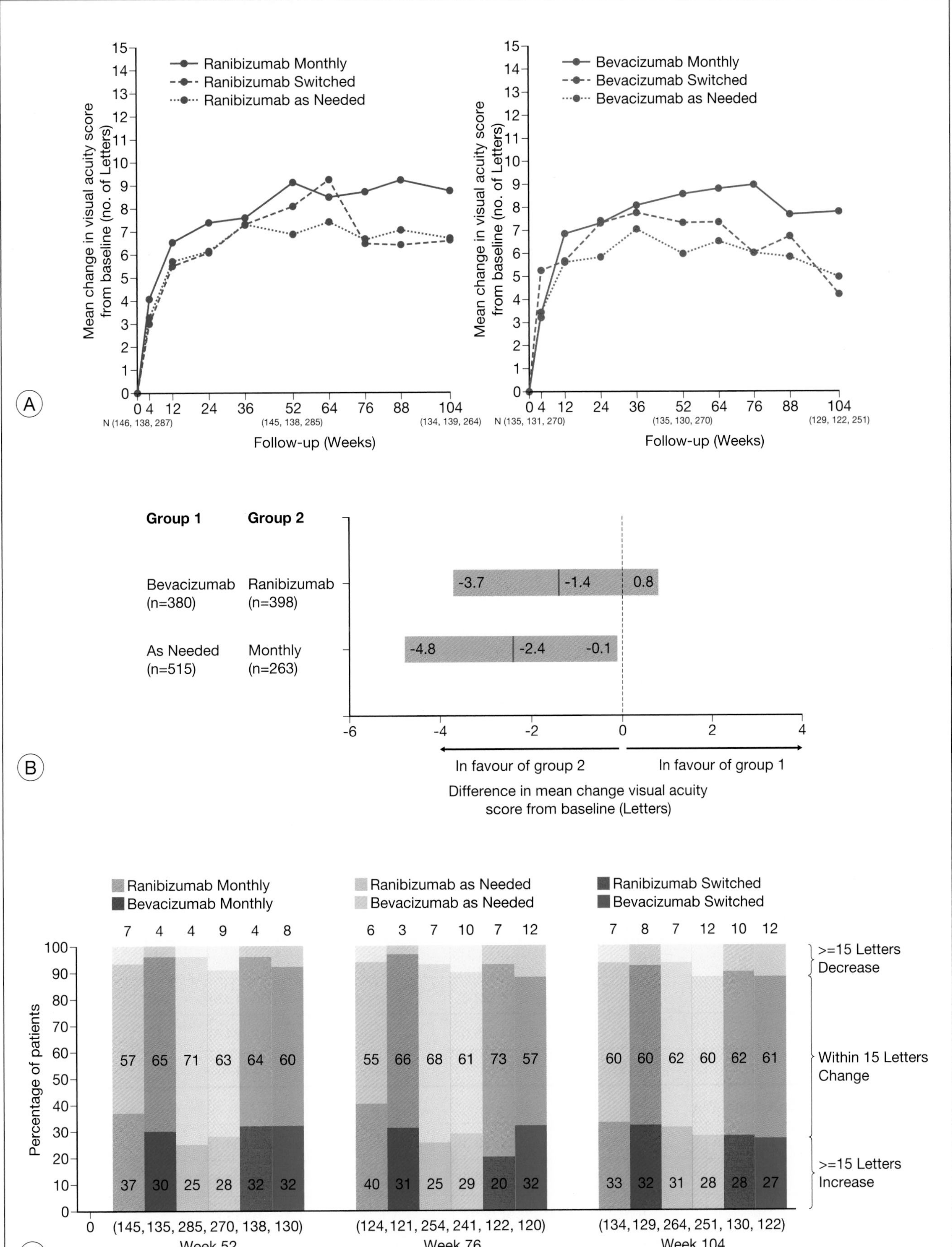

Fig. 67.15 (A) The mean change in visual acuity from enrollment over time by dosing regimen within drug group ranibizumab (left) and bevacizumab (right). (B) Differences in mean change in visual acuity at 2 years and 95% confidence intervals in patients treated with the same dosing regimen for 2 years. (C) The 3-line change in visual acuity from enrollment by treatment group and follow-up time. (Reproduced with permission from Martin DF, Maguire MG, Fine SL, et al. Ranibizumab and bevacizumab for treatment of neovascular age-related macular degeneration: two-year results. *Ophthalmology* 2012. Corrected proof published online 2012 May 2. http//:www.ophsource.org/periodicals/ophtha/article/S0161-6420(12)00321-1/ [cited 2012 June 8].)

Table 67.5 CATT 2-year outcomes: patients treated with the same dosing regimen for 2 years

Outcome	Ranibizumab Monthly $n = 134$	As needed $n = 264$	Bevacizumab Monthly $n = 129$	As needed $n = 251$	*P* value	
					By drug	By regimen
Visual acuity score: letters (Snellen equivalent), no. (%)						
83–97 (20/12–20)	24 (17.9)	44 (16.7)	17 (13.2)	35 (13.9)		
68–82, (20/25–40)	67 (50.0)	123 (46.6)	61 (47.3)	121 (48.2)		
53–67 (20/50–80)	23 (17.2)	59 (22.3)	31 (24.0)	46 (18.3)		
38–52 (20/100–160)	11 (8.2)	23 (8.7)	14 (10.9)	28 (11.2)		
≤37 (≤20/200)	9 (6.7)	15 (5.7)	6 (4.7)	21 (8.4)		
Mean letters (SD)	68.5 (18.9)	68.5 (15.3)	68.2 (16.1)	66.0 (19.9)	0.17	0.41
Change in visual acuity score from baseline (letters), no. (%)						
≥15 increase	44 (32.8)	81 (30.7)	41 (31.8)	71 (28.3)		
5–14 increase	49 (36.6)	78 (29.5)	36 (27.9)	79 (31.5)		
≤4 change	22 (16.4)	62 (23.5)	31 (24.0)	49 (19.5)		
5–14 decrease	10 (7.5)	24 (9.1)	11 (8.5)	23 (9.2)		
≥15 decrease	9 (6.7)	19 (7.2)	10 (7.8)	29 (11.6)		
Mean (SD)	8.8 (15.9)	6.7 (14.6)	7.8 (15.5)	5.0 (17.9)	0.21	0.046
No. treatments, 2 yr. mean (SD)	22.4 (3.9)	12.6 (6.6)	23.4 (2.8)	14.1 (7.0)	0.01*	—
Mean cost of drug/patient	$44 800	$25 200	$1170	$705		
Total thickness at fovea (μm)						
Mean (SD)†	267 (143)	293 (129)	274 (137)	306 (134)	0.26	0.005
Mean change (SD) from baseline‡	−190 (172)	−166 (190)	−180 (196)	−153 (189)	0.38	0.08
Retinal thickness and subfoveal fluid thickness (μm)						
Mean (SD)†	162 (81)	167 (75)	166 (79)	169 (83)	0.63	0.53
Mean change (SD) from baseline‡	−91 (152)	−78 (131)	−84 (133)	−84 (145)	0.86	0.54
Fluid on OCT, no. (%)						
None	61 (45.5)	59 (22.3)	39 (30.2)	35 (13.9)	0.0003	<0.0001
Present	69 (51.5)	198 (75.0)	87 (67.4)	212 (84.5)		
Unknown/missing	4 (3.0)	7 (2.7)	3 (2.3)	4 (1.6)		
Dye leakage on angiogram, no. (%)						
None	102 (76.1)	183 (69.3)	97 (75.2)	161 (64.1)	0.24	0.002
Present	24 (17.9)	75 (28.4)	27 (20.9)	81 (32.3)		
Unknown/missing	8 (6.0)	6 (2.3)	5 (3.9)	9 (3.6)		
Area of lesion, mm²						
Mean (SD)§	6.7 (7.8)	8.5 (7.4)	7.8 (8.5)	8.6 (8.3)	0.44	0.04
Mean change (SD) from baseline‖	−0.4 (6.8)	1.9 (6.5)	1.6 (5.9)	3.0 (7.0)	0.006	0.0003

Table 67.5 CATT 2-year outcomes: patients treated with the same dosing regimen for 2 years—Cont'd

Outcome	Ranibizumab Monthly $n = 134$	As needed $n = 264$	Bevacizumab Monthly $n = 129$	As needed $n = 251$	*P* value	
					By drug	By regimen
Geographic atrophy, no. (%)[¶]						
None	90 (70.3)	205 (84.0)	99 (80.5)	200 (85.8)	0.13	0.007
Nonfoveal	27 (21.1)	28 (11.5)	17 (13.8)	20 (8.6)		
Foveal	6 (4.7)	9 (3.7)	5 (4.1)	10 (4.3)		
Unknown/missing	5 (3.9)	2 (0.8)	2 (1.6)	3 (1.3)		

SD, standard deviation; OCT, optical coherence tomography. The dashes indicate that calculation of a P value is not appropriate. The treatment groups are defined by dosing regimen; therefore, the role of random variation in producing a difference by regimen is not relevant because by definition they are different.
[*]Comparison restricted to as needed groups.
[†]Number of unknown in each group unknown or missing: 3, 3, 3, 1.
[‡]Number in each group unknown or missing: 3, 3, 6, 2.
[§]Includes choroidal neovascularization, hemorrhage, blocked fluorescence, serous pigment epithelium detachment, scar, geographic atrophy, nongeographic atrophy or tear of the retinal pigment epithelium, adjacent to the location of choroidal neovascularization at baseline. Number in each group unknown or missing: 12, 8, 16, 18.
[‖]Number in each group unknown or missing: 16, 12, 22, 27.
[¶]Areas of hypopigmentation or hyperfluorescence of ≥250 μm diameter having ≥2 of the following characteristics: circular shape, sharp borders, visible choroidal vessels. Areas meeting this definition surrounding a scar were not considered geographic atrophy. Excluded those with geographic atrophy at enrollment: 6 (4.4%), 6 (4.7%), 20 (7.8%), 18 (7.2%).
(Reproduced with permission from Martin DF, Maguire MG, Fine SL, et al. Ranibizumab and bevacizumab for treatment of neovascular age-related macular degeneration: two-year results. Ophthalmology 2012. Corrected proof published online 2012 May 2. http//:www.ophsource.org/periodicals/ophtha/article/S0161-6420(12)00321-1/ [cited 2012 June 8].)

Table 67.6 CATT 2-year outcomes: patients whose dosing regimen was reassigned at 1 year

Outcome	Ranibizumab		Bevacizumab		*P* value	
	Monthly $n = 134$	Switched $n = 130$	Monthly $n = 129$	Switched $n = 122$	Drug	Regimen
Visual acuity score, letters (Snellen equivalent), no. (%)						
83–97 (20/12–20)	24 (17.9)	22 (16.9)	17 (13.2)	23 (18.9)		
68–82 (20/25–40)	67 (50.0)	61 (46.9)	61 (47.3)	54 (44.3)		
53–67 (20/50–80)	23 (17.2)	23 (17.7)	31 (24.0)	19 (15.6)		
38–52 (20/100–160)	11 (8.2)	13 (10.0)	14 (10.9)	11 (9.0)		
≤37, ≤20/200	9 (6.7)	11 (8.5)	6 (4.7)	15 (12.3)		
Mean letters (SD)	68.5(18.9)	67.7 (18.5)	68.2 (16.1)	65.0 (21.8)	0.39	0.23
Change in visual acuity score, from 1 yr, letters, no. (%)*						
≥15 increase	4 (3.0)	6 (4.6)	8 (6.2)	2 (1.7)		
5–14 increase	34 (25.6)	19 (14.6)	21 (16.3)	17 (14.0)		
≤4 change	58 (43.6)	66 (50.8)	63 (48.8)	61 (50.4)		
5–14 decrease	28 (21.1)	27 (20.8)	27 (20.9)	26 (21.5)		
≥15 decrease	9 (6.8)	12 (9.2)	10 (7.8)	15 (12.4)		
Mean (SD)	−0.3 (11.1)	−1.8 (11.2)	−0.6 (10.3)	−3.6 (12.1)	0.29	0.03
No. of treatments, yr 2, mean (SD)	10.5 (3.1)	5.0 (3.8)	11.3 (2.3)	5.8 (4.4)	0.11[†]	—
Cost of drug/patient	$21 000	$10 000	$565	$290		

Continued

Table 67.6 CATT 2-year outcomes: patients whose dosing regimen was reassigned at 1 year—Cont'd

	Ranibizumab		Bevacizumab		*P* value	
Outcome	Monthly $n = 134$	Switched $n = 130$	Monthly $n = 129$	Switched $n = 122$	Drug	Regimen
Total thickness at fovea, μm						
Mean (SD)‡	267 (143)	295 (135)	274 (137)	334 (190)	0.09	0.001
Mean change (SD) from1 yr§	1 (78)	31 (78)	–9 (94)	19 (114)	0.18	0.0004
Retinal thickness and subfoveal fluid thickness, μm						
Mean (SD)‡	162 (81)	162 (63)	166 (79)	189 (116)	0.04	0.14
Mean change (SD) from 1 yr§	12 (51)	10 (46)	–5 (61)	16 (92)	0.35	0.12
Fluid on OCT						
None	61 (45.5)	25 (19.2)	39 (30.2)	22 (18.0)	0.03	<0.0001
Present	69 (51.5)	100 (76.9)	87 (67.4)	97 (79.5)		
Unknown/missing	4 (3.0)	5 (3.8)	3 (2.3)	3 (2.5)		
Dye leakage on angiogram						
None	102 (76.1)	88 (67.7)	97 (75.2)	80 (65.6)	0.59	0.01
Present	24 (17.9)	37 (28.5)	27 (20.9)	36 (29.5)		
Unknown/missing	8 (6.0)	5 (3.8)	5 (3.9)	6 (4.9)		
Area of lesion, mm²						
Mean (SD)‖	6.7 (7.8)	9.0 (8.1)	7.8 (8.5)	8.2 (7.8)	0.80	0.06
Mean change (SD) from 1 yr¶	0.7 (4.5)	1.7 (5.3)	1.1 (4.0)	1.8 (5.7)	0.63	0.08
Geographic atrophy, no. (%)#						
None	90 (70.3)	97 (80.8)	99 (80.5)	97 (86.7)	0.05	0.02
Nonfoveal	27 (21.1)	16 (13.3)	17 (13.8)	6 (5.4)		
Foveal	6 (4.7)	4 (3.3)	5 (4.1)	6 (5.4)		
Unknown/missing	5 (3.9)	3 (2.5)	2 (1.6)	3 (2.7)		

SD, standard deviation; OCT, optical coherence tomography. The dashes indicate that calculation of a P value is not appropriate. The treatment groups are defined by dosing regimen; therefore, the role of random variation in producing a difference by regimen is not relevant because by definition they are different.
**Number in each group unknown or missing: 1, 0, 0, 1.*
†Comparison restricted to as-needed groups.
‡Number in each group unknown or missing: 3, 3, 3, 1.
§Number in each group unknown or missing: 5, 3, 4, 5.
‖See Table 67.5 for definition. Number in each group unknown or missing: 12, 8, 8, 6.
¶Number in each group unknown or missing: 22, 17, 15, 14.
#See Table 67.5 for definition. Excluded those with geographic atrophy at baseline: 6, 10, 6, 10.
(Reproduced with permission from Martin DF, Maguire MG, Fine SL, et al. Ranibizumab and bevacizumab for treatment of neovascular age-related macular degeneration: two-year results. Ophthalmology 2012. Corrected proof published online 2012 May 2. http//:www.ophsource.org/periodicals/ophtha/article/S0161-6420(12)00321-1/ [cited 2012 June 8].)

7. Endophthalmitis occurs at similar rates in ranibizumab- and bevacizumab-treated patients, although (as one may expect) it is appears to be associated with an increased rate of injections, occurring most often in patients treated monthly.
8. The increased rate of systemic serious adverse events in bevacizumab persisted in the second year. The authors remained unsure of the reason for the increased risk ratio of systemic adverse events. As in the first year, the rate of vascular events previously associated with anti-VEGF therapy was similar in both groups.

The two-year CATT results certainly support the continued off-label use of bevacizumab for exudative AMD. In addition, it appears that monthly dosing results in better and more sustained visual outcomes than as-needed dosing. However, any treatment regimen should still be made with careful

Table 67.7 CATT adverse events within 2 years of enrollment

Event type	Ranibizumab (*n* = 599), no. (%)	Bevacizumab (*n* = 586), no. (%)	*P* value*
Systemic serious			
Death, all causes	32 (5.3)	36 (6.1)	0.62
Arteriothrombotic events	28† (4.7)	29 (5.0)	0.89
Nonfatal stroke	8 (1.3)	8 (1.4)	1.00
Nonfatal myocardial infarction	9 (1.5)	7 (1.2)	0.80
Vascular death	12 (2.0)	14 (2.4)	0.70
Venous thrombotic events	3 (0.5)	10 (1.7)	0.054
Hypertension	3 (0.5)	4 (0.7)	0.72
One or more serious event	190 (31.7)	234 (39.9)	0.004
Previously associated with anti-VEGF treatment‡			
Yes	45 (7.5)	62 (10.6)	0.07
No	170 (28.4)	202 (34.5)	0.02
MedDRA system organ class§			
Cardiac disorders	47 (7.8)	62 (10.6)	0.11
Infections	41 (6.8)	54 (9.2)	0.14
Nervous system disorders	34 (5.7)	36 (6.1)	0.81
Injury and procedural complications	23 (3.8)	35 (6.0)	0.11
Neoplasms benign and malignant	27 (4.5)	22 (3.8)	0.56
Gastrointestinal disorders	11 (1.8)	28 (4.8)	0.005
Any other system organ class	81 (13.5)	104 (17.8)	0.046
Ocular event, study eye			
Endophthalmitis	4 (0.7)	7 (1.2)	0.38
Pseudo-endophthalmitis	1 (0.2)	1 (0.2)	1.00

VEGF, vascular endothelial growth factor; MedDRA, Medical Dictionary for Regulatory Activities.
**Fisher exact test.*
†One patient had both a nonfatal stroke and a nonfatal myocardial infarction.
‡Arteriothrombotic events, systemic hemorrhage, congestive heart failure, venous thrombotic events, hypertension, and vascular death.
§Data are listed only for system organ classes with 35 or more events.
(Reproduced with permission from Martin DF, Maguire MG, Fine SL, et al. Ranibizumab and bevacizumab for treatment of neovascular age-related macular degeneration: two-year results. Ophthalmology 2012. Corrected proof published online 2012 May 2. http//:www.ophsource.org/periodicals/ophtha/article/S0161-6420(12)00321-1/ [cited 2012 June 8].)

consideration, given the cost of monthly therapy (roughly 60–80% higher than that of as-needed therapy for each medication), as well as the increased risk of geographic atrophy, which over a treatment course of many years may result in significant visual loss.

Soluble receptor: aflibercept (VEGF-TRAP EYE)

Aflibercept (VEGF-TRAP EYE, *EYLEA*™) is a product of Regeneron Pharmaceuticals. It is soluble fusion protein which combines ligand-binding elements taken from the extracellular components of VEGF receptors 1 and 2 fused to the Fc portion of IgG1,[178] It has at least a 200-fold higher affinity for VEGF than ranibizumab,[179] and aflibercept is thought to penetrate all layers of the retina.[180] Unlike bevacizumab and ranibizumab that inhibit just VEGF-A, aflibercept also binds VEGF-B and PlGF.[179,181] Aflibercept has undergone phase I and II clinical trials in wet AMD, and recently concluded phase III clinical testing. The phase I study, known as CLEAR-IT 1 (*CL*inical *E*valuation of *A*nti-angiogenesis in the *R*etina *I*ntravitreal *T*rial), showed safety and a functional and anatomical improvement with a dose of 0.5 and 2 mg.[182] The phase II trial, known as Clear-IT 2, evaluated the biologic effects and safety of aflibercept during a 12-week fixed-dosing period in patients with exudative AMD followed by PRN dosing out to 1 year.[183,184] Patients were randomized

1:1:1:1:1 to aflibercept during the fixed-dosing phase (day 1 to week 12): 0.5 or 2 mg every 4 weeks on day 1 and at weeks 4, 8, and 12; or 0.5, 2, or 4 mg every 12 weeks on day 1 and at week 12. At week 12, treatment with aflibercept resulted in a significant mean decrease in central retinal thickness from baseline in all groups combined ($P < 0.0001$). The reduction with the 2 mg every 4 weeks and 0.5 mg every 4 weeks regimens was significantly greater than each of the quarterly dosing regimens. Visual acuity increased significantly by a mean of 5.7 letters at 12 weeks in the combined group ($P < 0.0001$), with the greatest mean gain of >8 letters in the monthly dosing groups.

In the PRN dosing phase of the study out to week 52, the decrease in central retinal thickness observed at week 12 versus baseline remained significant at weeks 12–52 (–130 μm from baseline at week 52) and CNV size regressed from baseline. After achieving a significant improvement in visual acuity during the 12 weeks, PRN dosing for 40 weeks maintained improvements in visual acuity out to 52 weeks (5.3-letter gain; $P < 0.0001$). The most robust improvements and consistent maintenance of visual acuity generally occurred in patients initially dosed with 2 mg every 4 weeks for 12 weeks. These patients demonstrated a gain of 9 letters at 52 weeks. Overall, a mean of 2 injections was administered after the 12-week fixed-dosing phase, and the mean time to first reinjection was 129 days. Nineteen percent of patients received no injections and 45% received 1 or 2 injections. During the year-long study, PRN dosing with VEGF-TRAP EYE at weeks 16–52 maintained the significant anatomic and vision improvements established during the 12-week fixed-dosing phase with a low frequency of reinjection, and the drug was generally safe and well tolerated.

Based on the phase II results, aflibercept appeared to be a new anti-VEGF treatment requiring fewer intravitreal injections compared with ranibizumab and bevacizumab. This possibility is being tested in the recently completed phase III VIEW 1 and VIEW 2 studies (*V*EGF Trap-Eye: *I*nvestigation of *E*fficacy and Safety in *W*et AMD) in which aflibercept is being compared with the standard monthly dosing regimen of 0.5 mg ranibizumab (NCT00509795). In these two parallel phase III studies, patients with exudative AMD are randomized 1:1:1:1 to aflibercept 0.5 mg monthly, aflibercept 2 mg monthly, aflibercept 2 mg every 2 months (following three monthly loading doses), or ranibizumab administered 0.5 mg every month during the first year of the studies. As-needed (PRN) dosing with both agents, with a dose administered at least every 3 months (but not more often than monthly), is being evaluated during the second year of each study. The primary endpoint was statistical noninferiority in the proportion of patients who maintained (or improved) vision over 52 weeks compared to ranibizumab.

After 1 year, there was no difference in the outcomes when the three aflibercept groups were compared with the ranibizumab group.[185,186] This was true with respect to visual acuity, OCT central retinal thickness, and safety outcomes. The most important outcome for patients and clinicians was the observation that aflibercept 2 mg dosed every 2 months was equivalent to ranibizumab dosed monthly suggesting that aflibercept could be dosed less frequently. The phase III main results manuscript is expected to be published in 2012.

KH902

KH902 (Chengdu Kanghong Biotechnology) is also a fusion protein that combines ligand-binding elements taken from the extracellular domains of VEGF receptors 1(Flt-1) and 2 (KDR) to the Fc portion of IgG1.[187] However, compared with aflibercept (VEGF TRAP-EYE), KH902 also includes the extracellular domain 4 of VEGF receptor 2(KDRd4) which may stabilize the three-dimensional structure and increase the efficiency of dimerization.[188] KH902 has a much higher affinity for VEGF due to this additional extracellular domain and may have a longer half-life in the vitreous.[187,189] In vivo experiments have shown that intravitreal KH902 was able to inhibit leakage and growth of CNV in rhesus monkeys without signs of toxicity at doses of 300 and 500 μg.[187] In a phase I, dose escalation study, intravitreal injections of KH902 up to a dose of 3.0 mg were well tolerated in 28 patients. On day 42 after a single injection, the mean change in visual acuity from baseline was +19.6 letters with no subjects losing 1 letter or more and 57% of patients gaining 15 letters or more from baseline. The mean change in center-point retinal thickness from baseline was –77.2 μm and the mean decrease in CNV area was 12.6%. No safety concerns were detected after a single, intravitreal injection. A phase III trial is currently underway in China.

Adeno-associated viral vector (AAV) gene transduction

As previously discussed, the angiogenic effects of VEGF are mediated through the endothelial receptor tyrosine kinases, VEGFR-1 (also called Flt-1) and VEGFR-2 (Flk-1/KDR),[73] with Flt-1 having a tenfold-higher affinity for VEGF.[190] A naturally existing soluble form of Flt-1 (sFlt-1) has no transmembrane domains, and thus has no signal transduction properties, instead forming a heterodimer with Flt-1 and Flk-1 extracellular domains.[191] This molecule has provided a unique target for gene therapy using an adeno-associated viral (AAV) vector.

AAV vectors are particular suited for gene therapy in part because of their low immunogenicity and pathogenicity, and ability to induce long-term gene expression in the eye. They have been used with success for gene transduction of PEDF for animal models of CNV,[192] and have been tested in human trials for RPE65-associated Leber congenital amaurosis.[193–195]Moreover, for a soluble gene product such as sFlt-1, gene therapy may be especially effective, as transduction need not be cell-specific.[188]

AAV-mediated sFlt-1 (and related fusion protein) gene therapy has been successful in a number of animal models, including rodent and primate.[190,196–199] Lai et al. tested gene transfer using an injected AAV vector with full-length sFlt-1 on both mice and monkeys.[190] In the mouse, they found a marked decrease in hyperfluorescence on fluorescein angiography in sFlt-1 transduced eyes when compared to noninjected and control AAV-Green Fluorescent Protein (GFP)-injected eyes. Morphologically, they found that more extensive CNV-induced photoreceptor loss occurred in the noninjected and control eyes when compared to sFlt-1 eyes. Electroretinographic studies showed no significant loss of function as a result of sFlt-1 transduction. Primate studies showed similarly encouraging results, including prevention of CNV induced by laser, without evidence of toxicity on histology. Importantly, there was long-term expression of transduced gene products, with detection of sFlt-1 mRNA at up to 17 months after injection. A similar recent primate study tested an AAV vector tied to a gene for a novel fusion protein of a single domain of sFlt-1 and a human IgG1 heavy chain Fc fragment (termed sFLT01), finding both long-term expression over 5 months, as well as inhibition of CNV in a dose-dependent fashion.[198] A phase I clinical rial is currently recruiting for AAV2-sFLT01 gene therapy for neovascular AMD (NCT01024998).

Oligonucleotide aptamer (pegaptanib – Macugen)

The first VEGF inhibitor approved for use in macular degeneration was pegaptanib. Although it has largely been replaced by the monoclonal anti-VEGF antibodies bevacizumab and ranibizumab, it represented the first targeted molecular therapy for macular degeneration, and therefore is of particular historical interest. Pegaptanib is an aptamer, or a short single-stranded nucleic acid sequence of specified strand shape and length, which has a high degree of specificity and affinity for a target polypeptide.[200] In the case of pegaptanib, a large library of RNA sequences ranging from 10^{14} to 10^{15} sequences are incubated with the target molecule, VEGF isoform 165. The molecule is capable of selectively binding only $VEGF_{165}$, and not the other isoforms or other receptors and providing sustained inhibition for in excess of 20 days in vitro corresponding to a desired intraocular concentration in excess of the minimal inhibitory concentration necessary to inhibit $VEGF_{165}$ for a period of approximately 6 weeks.[201]

Phase II/III double-masked, multicenter clinical trials were conducted in humans in the United States and in Europe concurrently.[202] A total of 1186 patients were randomized to one of three treatment doses or sham. Results showed lower risk of moderate and severe vision loss with pegaptanib vs control, with a favorable safety profile. As stated previously, pegaptanib is currently used infrequently for the treatment of exudative AMD, except in the context of combination therapy, or in some cases, maintenance therapy following induction with ranibizumab or bevacizumab.[203]

Small interfering RNA (siRNA)

RNA interference is the process of sequence-specific post-transcriptional gene silencing in animals and plants, which is initiated by double-stranded RNA (dsRNA) that is homologous in sequence to the silent gene. Confronted with double-stranded RNA eukaryotic cells respond by destroying their own messenger RNA (mRNA) that shares these sequences with the double-strand.[204] The process appears to be mediated by 21 and 22 nucleotide siRNAs that are generated by ribonuclease 3 cleavage from longer dsRNAs. siRNA differs from an aptamer in being double- rather than single-stranded RNA; mechanistically, the presence of siRNA results in the inhibition of protein synthesis. In this context, neovascularization is theoretically prevented because VEGF mRNA is destroyed prior to translation, in contrast to the inhibition through the binding of free $VEGF_{165}$ by an aptamer such as pegaptanib. In testing this hypothesis, siRNA specific for human vascular endothelial growth factor (VEGF) and an enhanced green fluorescent protein (EGFP) were designed and tested as active molecule and negative control in both in vitro cell lines chemically induced to simulate hypoxia as well as in a laser-induced model of CNV in mice. siRNA was delivered by coinjection with recombinant viruses carrying small hVEGF cDNA to induce expression of the appropriate siRNA in the subretinal space. Production of siRNA was confirmed by the expression of EGFP in the subretinal space with positive controls, and as evidence of VEGF transgene expression, which resulted in significant inhibition of CNV compared with negative controls after laser photocoagulation.[204] Conventionally injected siRNA at dosages of 70, 150 or 350μg in a 0.05 ml volume with a vehicle serving as a negative

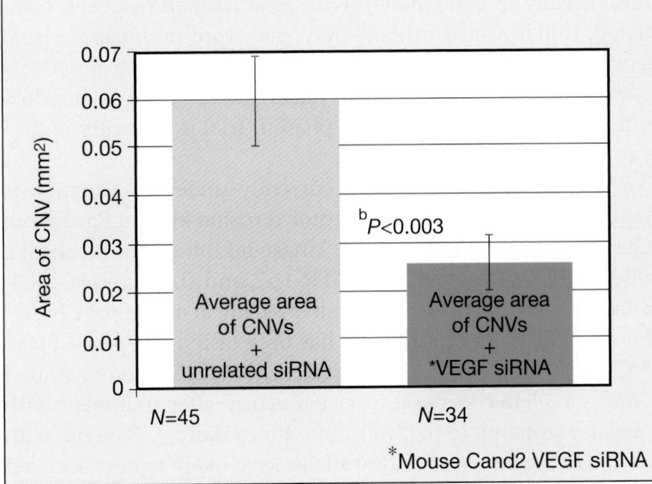

Fig. 67.16 Effects of siRNA treatment in murine model of choroidal neovascularization. (Reproduced with permission from Reich SJ, Fosnot J, Kuroki A, et al. Small interfering RNA (siRNA) targeting VEGF effectively inhibits ocular neovascularization in a mouse model. Mol Vis 2003;9:210–6.)

control was successful in reducing CNV in a primate model following standardized laser injury between 15 and 36 days after treatment in conjunction with reduced permeability, angiographically and reduced lesion sizes measured by planimetric methods in a masked fashion[81] (Fig. 67.16).

A recent phase I study of Sirna-027, a siRNA molecule targeting a conserved region of VEGFR-1, has been conducted. Twenty-six patients were divided into cohorts of 3–6, each receiving sequentially escalating doses of 200–1600 μg in order to determine the maximally tolerated dose. The study authors reported no dose-limiting toxicity, and few medication-specific adverse events. Additionally, visual acuity improved by a mean of +5.5 letters, and stabilized or improved in the vast majority of study participants. Foveal thickness as measured by OCT showed improvement of up to 20.3% in one cohort. The study illustrated the therapeutic principle, as well as showing a favorable safety profile of siRNAs for the treatment of neovascular AMD.[205] Two other molecules have also undergone clinical trials. RTP801i-14 (PF-04523655, Quark/Pfizer), a small inhibitory RNA (siRNA) that targets VEGF production via the REDD1/mTOR/HIF1-alpha pathway, is currently in a phase II study (NCT00713518) as adjunctive therapy to ranibizumab for treatment of AMD-associated CNV.

Interestingly, recent evidence suggests that the effect of siRNAs on CNV may in fact be a class effect of the molecule, and not contingent upon sequence specificity of the dsRNA.[206–208] The effect is instead postulated to occur through a toll-like receptor, TLR3, expressed on the endothelial cell surface, and mediated by the interferon-gamma and IL-12 cytokines.[208] How this may influence further study of siRNA pharmacotherapy is unclear.

Intracellular signaling blockers

PDGF/PDGFR inhibitors*

Currently, an anti-PDGF-B pegylated aptamer, E10030, is under study. A phase I trial in which the aptamer was administered

*Selected text adapted with kind permission of Springer Science+Business Media.[52,53]

intravitreally in combination with ranibizumab has been completed. Initial results in this safety trial were promising: visual acuity improved by 21–27 letters at 8 weeks, with 59% of patients showing moderate visual improvement at 12 weeks, versus 36% of the ranibizumab cohort.[209] A phase II trial is currently underway (NCT01089517).

Another therapeutic avenue currently under examination is the inhibition of the PDGF receptor tyrosine kinase. Pazopanib (GlaxoSmithKline) is a tyrosine kinase inhibitor that blocks the action of PDGFR, as well as VEGFR-1, -2, and -3, kit, and FGFR-1. It has been shown to be effective in preclinical models of CNV.[210] It is administered topically and has been tested in a phase I trial (NCT01154062). A phase II study (NCT00612456) demonstrated a mean 4.3-letter increase in visual acuity after treatment with topical pazopanib (5 mg/ml) three times daily.[211] Patients with the *CFH* TT genotype (i.e., the alleles least likely to be associated with AMD) exhibited the best response, both from the standpoint of visual acuity as well as reduction in retinal thickness. PTK787 (Vatalanib, Novartis) is an oral protein kinase inhibitor that targets all known VEGFRs, including VEGFR-1, -2, and -3, PDGFR, and kit and has been tested previously as a treatment for CNV in phase I/II clinical studies (NCT00138632).

Additionally, a tetravalent, bispecific antibody against VEGF-A and PDGFR-B is in development and has shown activity both in vitro as well as in a mouse model of tumorigenesis.[212] This may have therapeutic potential for the treatment of AMD as well.

TrpRS

Another class of compounds that appear to play an important role in intracellular signaling following VEGF stimulation are the human aminoacyl-t-RNA synthetases. These molecules, which catalyze the first step of protein synthesis by aminoacylation of transfer RNA appear to have novel cytokine functions in addition to their role in protein synthesis. The catalytic core domain of tryptophanyl-tRNA synthetase (TrpRS) is a close homolog of the catalytic domain of tyrosine RS (TyrRS).[103] In normal human cells the TrpRS exists as two forms. The major form is a full-length protein, which is stimulated by interferon gamma and has no cytokine activity. The other is truncated TrpRS (miniTrpRS) in which most of the extra amino terminal domain is deleted through alternate splicing of the mRNA. In addition to its production by alternative splicing, shorter fragment lengths of TrpRS can also be created by PMN Elastase cleavage of full human length TrpRS into two forms of mini TrpRS, both of which show cytokine-related activity. When cells are induced with $VEGF_{165}$ and then treated with TrpRS, migration is inhibited by the miniTrp fraction, but not the full-length fraction. Following digestion with leukocyte elastase, the smaller of the two mini-TrpRS (T2-TrpRS) in which the entire amino terminal domain has been deleted, appears to be the most potent antiangiogenesis agent with dose-dependent angiostatic activity. The role of TrpRS is complex and incompletely understood. The mechanism of action of this molecule (which is bound to endothelial cells within the retina) appears to be not as an intrinsic inhibitor, but as a downregulator of VEGF-induced pathways, suggesting it represents a portion of the downstream signal cascade following VEGF stimulation, along with NOS, and expression of surface integrins.[213] Additionally, in a mouse model of oxygen-induced retinopathy, T2-TrpRS induced nonpathologic revascularization of areas of retina with oxygen-induced vascular obliteration even when expressed at levels insufficient to cause regression of neovascular tufts.[214] The study authors hypothesized that T2-TrpRS may act primarily to enhance revascularization of the retina, hence reducing the hypoxic stimulus leading to pathologic neovascularization, although they recognized that this was an unlikely explanation given the apparent potent angiostatic activity of the molecule. This dual nature of T2-TrpRS may be useful especially in eyes prone to hypoxia or vascular insufficiency, including in patients with advanced age. Study of the TrpRS class of molecules is still in preclinical stages.

Protein kinase C inhibitors

Protein kinase C (PKC) isoforms, particularly the beta isoform, are thought to play an important regulatory role in intracellular signaling following VEGF stimulation of endothelial and other cells through phosphorylation mechanisms.[215] Most of the work detailing the interaction between VEGF effects on vascular permeability and PKC-β has been performed in experimental diabetic retinopathy and in preliminary human trials, and ongoing clinical studies of the PKC-β inhibitor ruboxistaurin in diabetes have shown promising results. Experience using PKC in experimental CNV is limited; however, one protein kinase C inhibitor, PKC412, has been tested in a porcine model of CNV. PKC412, which blocks several isoforms of PKC, was administered to pigs via a periocular injection within microspheres containing either 25% or 50% drug. Ten to 20 days following laser rupture and injection, experimentally produced CNV at Bruch's membrane laser rupture sites were smaller in eyes receiving drug than those receiving control microspheres without drugs. Additionally, 20 days following periocular injection, high levels of the inhibitor were measured in the choroid, vitreous, and retina for eyes with 50% loading and to a lesser extent with 25% loading.[216]

Complement inhibitors*

Complement inhibitors are thought to be a promising class of agents for the treatment of both atrophic and exudative AMD. POT-4 (AL-78898A, Alcon/Potentia Pharmaceuticals), a cyclic peptide derivative of Compstatin 13 amino acids in length, is a C3 inhibitor administered by intravitreal injection. Gel-like deposits form in the vitreous when POT-4 is injected at high concentrations (>0.45 mg dose), which may last as long as 6 months, thus providing a sustained-release delivery system. A phase I study of POT-4 in AMD eyes with CNV was completed successfully without any safety concerns at doses up to 1.05 mg (NCT00473928), although the systemic effects of intravitreal administration are unknown. A phase II study is currently underway (NCT01157065). C3 inhibition should block complement activation arising from many of the currently described complement pathway mutations, as the classical, lectin, fibrinolytic, and alternative pathways all generate the bioactive fragments C3a and C5a and the membrane attack complex (C5b,6,7,8,9) via C3 cleavage (see Fig. 67.3). This targets a relatively large population of AMD patients; however, the broad degree of complement inhibition may theoretically increase risk of intravitreal injection-associated endophthalmitis. In a murine model, it seems that C3 deficiency does not increase the risk of *Staphylococcus aureus* endophthalmitis.[217] In contrast, in a guinea-pig model, complement depletion with cobra venom factor does

*Selected text adapted with kind permission of Springer Science+Business Media.[52,53]

seem to increase the risk of *S. aureus*, *S. epidermidis*, and *Pseudomonas aeruginosa* endophthalmitis.[209,218,219] Other treatments related to complement factors are being examined in the context of nonexudative AMD and have been discussed previously.

NATURALLY OCCURRING INHIBITORY POLYPEPTIDES AND INDUCIBLE CLEAVAGE PRODUCTS

While the protein miniTrpRS might also be considered in this category, a broader category is reserved for those agents that are thought to be naturally secreted into the extracellular space rather than acting as intracellular signals and include normal inducible homeostatic regulators. An example is PEDF, which is thought to modulate neuronal differentiation in the outer retina following apical secretion by the pigment epithelium in addition to its downregulation of VEGF effects on endothelial cells. In addition to these compounds, there are pathologically expressed circulating molecules that are formed as a result of cleavage by specific proteases from larger pre-existing polypeptides that have intrinsic antiangiogenic potency, including angiostatin and endostatin.[220]

Pigment epithelial-derived factor

Pigment epithelial-derived factor (PEDF) was first purified in the conditioned media of human retinal pigment epithelial cells that induced neuronal differentiation as well as inhibiting microglial growth. The protein shares sequence and structural homology with the serum proteinase inhibitor family (Serpen). It acts in counterpoint to VEGF, inhibiting signaling pathways of the VEGF receptors.[101,102] One of its most striking abilities is the capacity to inhibit endothelial cell migration in a dose-dependent manner with a greater degree of potency than either angiostatin, thrombospondin-1 or endostatin. It has been possible to use adenovirus vector-mediated gene transfer of cDNA constructs to iris pigment epithelium (IPE) resulting in autologous IPE cells gaining the capacity to support the choriocapillaris and outer retina in vivo.[221] Iris pigment epithelial cells overexpressing PEDF have been found to be capable of rescuing photoreceptors in RCS rats, reducing laser-induced CNV, and partially reversing the effects of ischemic retinopathy in various animal models.[87] An open-label phase I study of AdPEDF.11 in patients with CNV was designed to test both the safety and feasibility of adenoviral gene transfer for retinal diseases.[222] In the 28 patients administered the gene vector, there were no serious adverse events, and only transient intraocular pressure rise and intraocular inflammation without evidence of adenoviral infection. Additionally, although the study was not designed to determine efficacy, there appeared to be a trend toward visual stability in patients receiving a 10^8 particle units (PU) or higher dose of the vector, as well as stability in lesion size in patients receiving $\geq 10^8$ PU, compared with increase in size in those receiving 10^6–$10^{7.5}$ PU. The study authors concluded that gene transformation using an adenoviral vector was both safe and viable for future study.

Pathologically expressed circulating molecules

Angiostatin and endostatin

Angiostatin is an internal proteolytic fragment of a known protein, plasminogen, expressed in association with tumor growth in the serum such that it inhibits primary metastatic tumor growth by blocking tumor angiogenesis. Angiostatin does not appear to have a specific gene locus resulting in transcription, but rather represents a cryptic fragment produced in response to pathologic rather than physiologic conditions, such as primary tumor growth. The molecule has a molecular weight of 38 kDa and inhibits endothelial cell proliferation in vitro and angiogenesis in vivo.[104] It appears that tumor cells do not themselves express angiostatin or other fragments of plasminogen. Rather gelatinase A, also known as matrix metalloproteinase-2, which is produced by rapidly growing tumor cells such as experimental Lewis lung carcinoma, performs the proteolysis of plasminogen.[90] When administered systemically, angiostatin can cause regression of a wide variety of malignant tumors through its inhibitory effects on angiogenesis. Adenoassociated viral (AAV) vectors causing overexpression of angiostatin in a murine model of CNV were effective in causing regression. Expression of the angiostatin gene in chorioretinal tissue for up to 150 days was possible as was reduction in the average size of CNV lesions in treated eyes as compared with control eyes. There were no significant adverse events reported in the animal model using target gene therapy.[86,223]

Another compound from this class, endostatin, is thought to represent a proteolytic fragment of 20 kD created by digestion of the C terminal fragment of collagen XVIII.[89] Endostatin inhibits both endothelial cell proliferation in vitro and angiogenesis and tumor growth in vivo and is capable of being delivered by a variety of methods including sustained delivery or adenoviral vector.[88] Zinc binding of endostatin is thought to be essential for its antiangiogenic activity and metal chelating agents can induce internal degradation of endostatin with associated loss of activity.[224] Full-length human type 18 collagen cDNAs that encode 1516 or 336 residue alpha chains exhibit homology with endostatin. Incorporated with adenoviral vectors and administered intravenously, endostatin levels have been demonstrated to rise, with concomitant reduction in CNV size in experimental models. The zinc requirement for endostatin may be one component of the apparent beneficial effect of zinc in the AREDS trial.[88] Recently, there has been enthusiasm for lentiviral vectors for the delivery of angiostatin or endostatin genes, and a vector has been developed for the delivery of both simultaneously.[224,225] Animal models of CNV have demonstrated significant reduction in area and hyperpermeability, without any significant adverse events. This has led to a dose-escalating phase I clinical trial testing the safety of subretinal administration of Retinostat, a vector that delivers both the endostatin and angiostatin genes (NCT01301443). This study is underway at the time of writing.

EXTRACELLULAR MATRIX MODULATORS

A variety of targets exist outside the cell in the extracellular matrix (ECM) for therapeutic intervention. Some, such as the alpha v beta 3 and alpha v beta 5 integrins, are expressed on the cell surface in response to VEGF stimulation and participate in the adhesion of regulatory molecules as well as the interaction with metalloproteinases responsible for degradation of the ECM, facilitating migration and sprouting of new vessels.[226] Others, such as the naturally occurring tissue inhibitors of metalloproteinase (TIMP) or other synthetic metalloproteinase inhibitors may precede the VEGF activation step and represent both early and late targets for intervention.

Integrin antagonists

Examination of tissues from eyes with pathologic neovascularization indicate that at least two cytokine-dependent pathways of angiogenesis exist and both may be important in pathologic neovascularization. In in vivo models of angiogenesis induced by basic fibroblast growth factor (bFGF) or tumor necrosis factor-alpha (TNF-α), the cell surface-expressed integrin alpha v beta 3 predominates, whereas in models initiated by VEGF transforming growth factor-alpha (TGF-α), or phorbol ester the pathway is characterized by dependence on and expression of the related cytokine alpha v beta 5.[69,70] These findings are further confirmed by evidence that inhibition of protein kinase C (using the specific inhibitor calphostin C) blocked angiogenesis induced by VEGF and TGF-α, but had only a small effect on bFGF or TNF-α-mediated angiogenesis. This suggests the specificity of the two pathways: (1) that dependent on alpha v beta 3 and relatively independent of PKC; and (2) the second potentiated by alpha v beta 5, and dependent upon both VEGF stimulation and PKC activation.[69,70]

Therapeutically, several alternative methods for the inhibition of alpha v beta 3 and alpha v beta 5 expression exist. In immunohistochemical examination of tissues removed from eyes with pathologic neovascularization, it appears that for the purposes of inhibiting choroidal rather than retinal neovascularization, selective inhibition of the alpha v beta 3 pathway may be preferred. When neovascular membranes removed from patients with CNV secondary to age-related macular degeneration were examined, only the expression of alpha v beta 3 was observed whereas both alpha v beta 3 and alpha v beta 5 were present on vascular cells and tissues from patients with proliferative diabetic retinopathy.

A cyclic peptide antagonist (cyclo RGDv) of alpha v beta 3 and alpha v beta 5 was capable of dramatically reducing retinal vessel blood growth compared with a control peptide in a neonatal mouse model of retinopathy of prematurity. Other molecules in preclinical studies, including XJ735 (a selective alpha v beta 3 antagonist), and XK002, a combined antagonist of alpha v beta 3 and alpha v beta 5, also inhibit retinal neovascularization in a murine model.[227] Cyclic RGDfV peptide was found to represent an antagonist of vitronectin receptor type integrins by other groups.[2]

Another approach rather than specific receptor binding with polypeptide molecules is the use of selective monoclonal antibodies directed against cell surface integrins. Specific mouse monoclonal antibodies to integrins alpha v beta 3 (LM609) and alpha v beta 5 (P1F6) have been prepared, and in addition to demonstrating the presence of expressed integrins on vascular cell surfaces, have also been used therapeutically to inhibit neovascularization. Antibodies directed against alpha v beta 3 appeared to selectively block bFGF-induced angiogenesis whereas antibodies directed against antibeta 1 and alpha v beta 5 had dramatically less effect and appeared to spare pre-existing preformed vessels.[69,70] Other approaches have included the conjugation of mitomycin C dextran to a monoclonal anti-integrin alpha v beta 3 antibody, which was more effective than the use of a mouse monoclonal alone in a rat model of laser-induced CNV.[228] Yet another strategy involves the targeting of an proapoptotic peptide domain to a homing target that localizes to the alpha v beta 3/beta 5 integrins expressed preferentially in neovascular endothelial cells, thus inducing apoptosis in the newly forming vessels. This strategy takes advantage of the expression pattern of the alpha v beta 3/beta 5 integrins without specifically targeting their function or downstream effects, and has proven effective in a mouse model of retinopathy of prematurity.[229]

The integrin alpha 5 beta 1 has also been identified as a significant player in choroidal neovascularization.[230-232] It has been found to be significantly expressed in laser-induced CNV in animal models, and an inhibitor of alpha 5 beta 1 have been show to reverse corneal neovascularization as well as hypoxia-induced retinal neovascularization.[233,234] Currently, antagonists to alpha 5 beta 1 have shown mixed results in the inhibition or reversal of CNV in animal models. There is currently a phase I trial underway evaluating Volociximab, an anti-alpha 5 beta 1 monoclonal antibody already being tested for cancer therapy, for exudative AMD (NCT00782093).[235]

MMP inhibitors

The naturally occurring class of tissue inhibitors of metalloproteinase (TIMP), particularly TIMP-3, are thought to be critically important in the homeostasis of the extracellular matrix and thereby to factors contributing to the development of CNV. As discussed earlier, large quantities of TIMP-3 have been found with increasing age in Bruch's membrane where it is thought to be a normal structural component and particularly in areas where there is pathologic thickening of Bruch's membrane.[30,36,98] The carboxy terminus of TIMP-3, unlike the soluble TIMP-1, TIMP-2, and TIMP-4, is exclusively membrane-bound, while the amino terminus appears to inhibit MMPs 2 and 9, which are known to be expressed in choroidal new vessels membranes removed from patients with subfoveal CNV.[99] TIMP-3 naturally inhibits VEGF and is capable of reducing angiogenesis in vitro and in vivo including CAM assays and also when overexpressed by selective gene therapy in rat eyes undergoing laser photocoagulation for the induction of CNV.[99,100] Pharmacologic therapies directed at replacement or modification of TIMP-3 and potentially other related compounds may have utility as a pharmacologic strategy not only for regulation of the extracellular matrix in response to VEGF stimulation late, but also potentially earlier in regulating the homeostatic mechanisms that lead to Bruch's membrane thickening and the other inducible factors for CNV preceding VEGF activation (Fig. 67.17).[236]

Matrix metalloproteinase inhibitors (MMPI) have been tested for their ability to inhibit pathologic ocular neovascularization. AG3340, a synthetic MMP2,9 inhibitor was shown to significantly inhibit neovascularization in a mouse model of retinopathy of prematurity leading to a human phase II/III trial.[237] However, the study was unable to confirm any inhibitory effect of the small molecular weight binding inhibitor of MMP-2 MMP-9 in any dose tested either with regards to lesion size, or final visual acuity and efforts were halted. Other MMP inhibitors continue to be tested in preclinical studies.

OTHER MOLECULES

A variety of molecules with varying mechanisms of action are undergoing preliminary evaluation. Combretastatin A-4a naturally occurring agent from tree bark that binds tubulin and causes necrosis and shrinkage of tumors by inhibition of the blood supply is capable of suppressing experimental CNV in response to photocoagulation.[25,238] Preliminary trials of a phosphate prodrug of combretastatin A4 (fosbretabulin, OXiGENE)

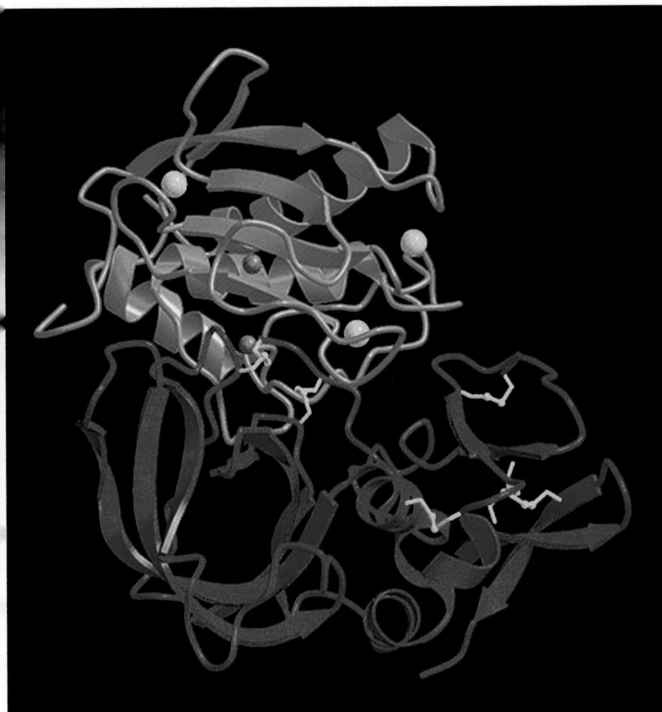

Fig. 67.17 Computerized rendering of TIMP-1 interacting as its active NH site with MMP-3 catalytic domain. (Reproduced with permission from Gomis-Ruth FX, Maskos K, Betz M, et al. Mechanism of inhibition of the human matrix metalloproteinase stromelysin-1 by TIMP-1. Nature 1997;389:77–81.)

are underway in humans to test its efficacy in early stage neovascularization AMD.

Squalamine

Squalamine is an antiangiogenic amino sterol derived from shark liver which inhibits iris neovascularization when administered by intravenous injection, although it is ineffective when administered by intravitreal injection.[239,240] Squalamine also induces regression of experimental retinopathy of prematurity in a mouse model[241] and has been tested in a phase I study of CNV in patients with no safety concerns expressed leading to several phase II trials. Initial visual results were promising, with improvement or stability in those patients receiving higher doses of the drug. Interestingly, the fellow non-study eyes with advanced macular degeneration also showed significant improvement after drug administration. A phase III study was initiated; however, it was terminated.

THE ROLE OF STEROIDS AND OTHER IMMUNOMODULATORS

Steroids

Steroids have long known to be associated with neovascularization reduction by mechanisms that were not clearly understood. Folkman and colleagues were the first to suggest that the antiangiogenic effects of steroids could be separated into two categories: (1) those related to anti-inflammatory effects paralleling convention glucocorticoid and mineralocorticoid activity; and (2) a separate structural configuration of the pregnan nucleus conferring distinct antiangiogenic capability.[83,84] Although preclinical studies suggested benefit in terms of VEGF-stimulated vascular permeability and angiogenesis, and while steroids have long been used with success for diabetic macular edema, clinical studies employing conventional steroids alone for AMD have shown relatively unimpressive effects on the natural history of the disease. In the era of anti-VEGF therapy, steroid therapy is largely an adjunct; however, steroid monotherapy is still being examined in continuing clinical trials. At this time, a sustained release fluocinolone implant (Iluvien, Alimera Pharmaceuticals) is in phase II clinical trials for both choroidal neovascularization (NCT00605423) as well as geographic atrophy in AMD (NCT00695318). Additionally, there has been enthusiasm for potential beneficial effects associated with the use of intravitreal triamcinolone combined with conventional photodynamic therapy (PDT) using verteporfin for subfoveal CNV[242–252] (discussed below in a separate section on combination therapy).

Rapamycin

Rapamycin (sirolimus) is a macrocyclic, naturally occurring lactone that was initially isolated from the species *Streptomyces hygroscopicus* and given its name from Rapa Nui (Easter Island) during the course of a search for novel antifungal agents. Rapamycin is structurally related to the immunosuppressive agent FK506 (tacrolimus), which has been used extensively for the prevention of organ transplant rejection. Rapamycin requires direct interaction with at least two intracellular proteins to exert its action of arresting cell phase progression. FK binding protein (FKBP12) forms a rapamycin FK complex, which in turn binds to and inhibits the activity of the mammalian target of rapamycin (mTOR) through which it exerts its intracellular affects. Other FKBPs have been identified and interact with heat shock proteins. When bound to mTOR, phosphorylation does not occur, and the cells' mitotic ability is blocked in addition to other effects involving protein kinase C delta, and IL-2 dependent functions that control the progression of T cells into the S phase.[253]

Rapamycin inhibits primary metastatic tumor growth by inhibition with angiogenesis through direct inhibition of vascular endothelial growth factors as well as endothelial cell responses to VEGF.[254] Additionally, rapamycin, through its intrinsic immunomodulatory effects, may reduce macrophage chemotaxis and activation with concomitant reduction in release of VEGF and other angiogenic cytokines.

In experimental models, rapamycin has been shown to inhibit the development of ocular neovascularization in rats in response to subretinal matrigel placement orally at a dose of 2.5 mg per kilograms per day, or as an intraocular injection. Inhibition was also seen in a murine model of retinopathy of prematurity and laser-induced neovascularization when administered by an intraperitoneal route in doses of 2–4 mg per kilogram per day.[255]

A recent phase I/II pilot study has been conducted, comparing the effectiveness of adjunctive systemic administration of one of three immunosuppressive agents (including rapamycin) when combined with anti-VEGF treatment (either ranibizumab or bevacizumab), against anti-VEGF therapy alone.[256] The prospective randomized, unmasked trial assigned patients 1:1:1:1 to receive either intravenous daclizumab, intravenous infliximab, oral rapamycin tablets, or observation for a study duration of 6 months. All patients were administered intravitreous bevacizumab (1.25 mg/0.05 mL or 2.5 mg/1.0 mL) or ranibizumab (0.5 mg) at intervals determined by the treating physician based on the presence of intraretinal or subretinal fluid on OCT imaging. The primary study outcome was the number of injections required in each group over the study period, which was also compared to the number of injections required prior to joining the study. There was a decrease in the number of injections in patients receiving daclizumab as well as rapamycin, although the study was small, and differences were not significant. However, the results do suggest that there may be a role for immunomodulators in the treatment of AMD. There is currently a phase I/II study underway examining subconjunctival administration of sirolimus for the treatment of geographic atrophy (NCT00766649).

PHOTODYNAMIC THERAPY

Pharmacology of photodynamic sensitizers

Photodynamic therapy actually represents the combination of a pharmacologic therapy and a laser-based therapy in a two-step process capable of successfully treating subfoveal CNV. Photosensitizers have biophysical properties well suited to the thrombotic closure of abnormal neovascularization while preserving normal physiologic vessels. Most agents possess strong absorption properties in the far-red spectral region (660–780 nm), where light has the greatest penetration through blood and tissue. Photosensitizers also selectively bind to abnormal neovascularization through its expression of increased numbers of lipoprotein receptors contrasted with normal mature vessels, thus achieving the desirable feature of selectivity. Most photosensitizing molecules, including verteporfin, which has been approved for human use, as well as a number of agents under clinical evaluation, are structurally related to porphyrins (Fig. 67.18). Porphyrins are fused tetrapyrrolic macromolecules found in nature as pigments such as protoporphyrin IX, the nonprotein portion of hemoglobin.

Other molecules undergoing evaluation although not yet approved for use in humans include Tin-ethyl-etiopurpurin (Purlytin), monotexafin lutetium (optrin, Lu-tex), Npe6, and ATX-S10. Their chemical formulas are listed in Fig. 67.18. Purlytin was subjected to a large multicenter phase II/III clinical trial, which demonstrated a trend towards efficacy in selected subgroups, although it failed to meet the preapproved regulatory efficacy endpoint.

Lu-tex underwent a phase I dose escalation trial, in humans, which demonstrated its ability to achieve photodynamic closure, although associated with a greater degree of surrounding choroidal damage than verteporfin and also associated with peripheral paresthesias and occasional periocular pain in selected patients and the trial was discontinued. A phase I dose-ranging study of NPE6 was terminated. ATX-S10 has been the subject of continuing preclinical studies and at the time of this writing no human trials are under way.[257]

Verteporfin (Visudyne)

The benzoporphyrin derivative monoacid verteporfin (Visudyne) consists of two isomers that differ in the location of the carboxylic acid and methyl ester on the lower pyrrole rings of the chlorine macrocycle. Because verteporfin is hydrophobic, it requires formulation within liposomes, which in addition to improving penetration into cells and delivery by an intravenous route, also may actually further enhance its selectivity. Verteporfin is activated with a monochromatic laser light in the range of approximately 689–691 nm. The molecule is well tolerated following intravenous administration and cutaneous light sensitivity is kept to a minimum compared with other molecules, which either have longer periods of photosensitization, or less favorable therapeutic indices.

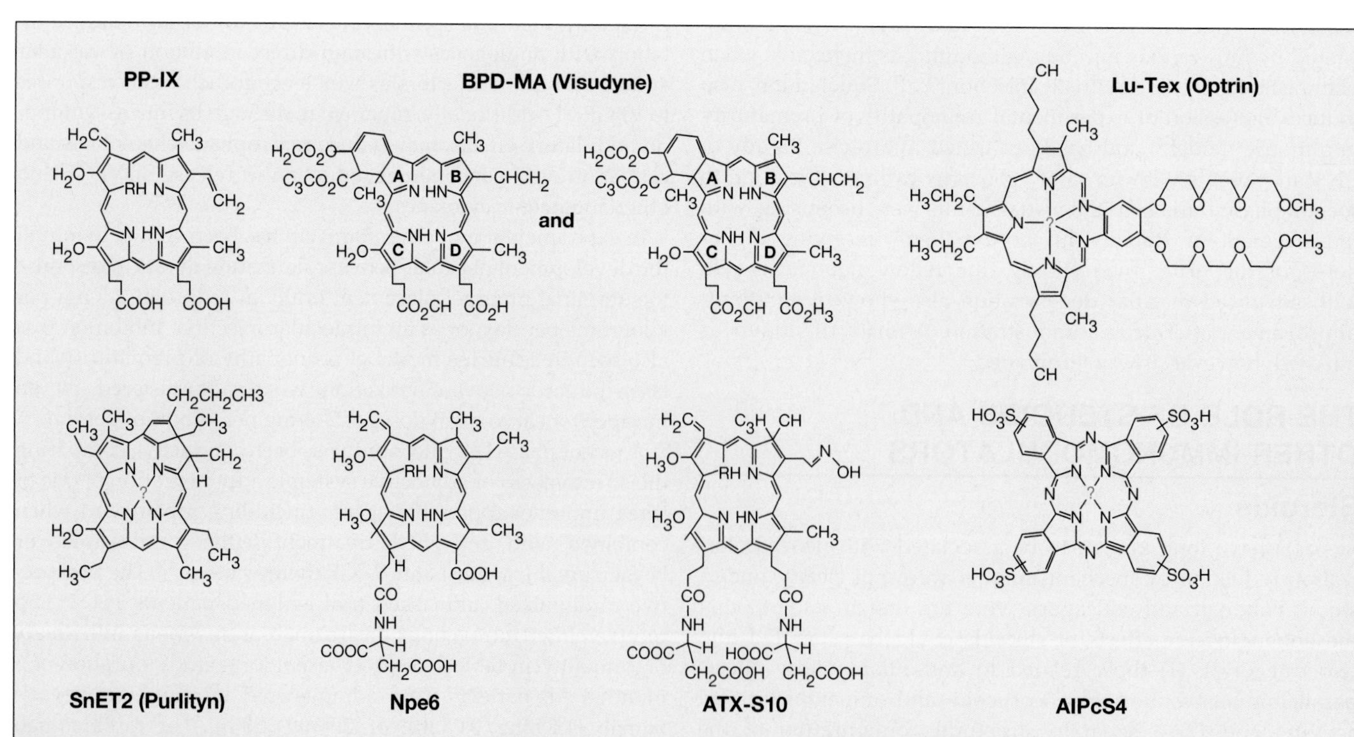

Fig. 67.18 Structural formulae of photodynamic therapy agents either approved (verteporfin) or under investigation for use in humans. (Reproduced with permission from Woodburn KW, Engelman CJ, Blumenkranz MS. Photodynamic therapy for choroidal neovascularization: a review. Retina 2002;22:391–405.)

Verteporfin photodynamic therapy (PDT) was the first photosensitizer approved for the treatment of exudative AMD. The technique involves infusion of 6 mg/m^2 verteporfin over a 10 minute period followed by laser irradiation using a 689 nm diode laser (light dose: 50 J/cm^2; power density: 600 mW/cm^2; duration: 83 seconds) 15 minutes after the start of the infusion. Verteporfin demonstrated safety and efficacy in selectively localizing to choroidal neovascular membranes in preclinical trials in nonhuman primates. The mechanism of action is postulated to occur by activation of verteporfin to a triplet state following laser irradiation, resulting in the creation of singlet and reactive oxygen species that induces endothelial cellular damage and, ultimately, occlusion of the neovascular membranes through activation of the clotting cascade.[258–262] Unfortunately, the generation of free radicals necessary for the photothrombotic effect, may also serve as a proangiogenic stimulus, possibly accounting for the apparent benefit associated with concomitant administration of steroids.

Verteporfin PDT was demonstrated to be safe and effective for treatment of CNV due to AMD in phase I and II testing.[263,264] The Treatment of Age-related macular degeneration with Photodynamic Therapy (TAP) Study demonstrated that patients with CNV due to AMD demonstrated a beneficial effect following verteporfin PDT. The greatest benefit was seen among the subset of patients with predominantly classic subfoveal CNV due to AMD, with 67% of verteporfin-treated eyes versus 39% of placebo-treated eyes prevented from progressing to moderate visual loss – loss of 15 or more letters on the Early Treatment Diabetic Retinopathy Study (ETDRS) scale or approximately 3 lines of vision – $P < 0.001$. Lesions that were less than 50% classic did not demonstrate a treatment benefit. These results were valid through 2- and 3-year follow-up.[265,266] Further discussion of the role of verteporfin in AMD is covered in Chapter 66 (Neovascular (exudative or "wet") age-related macular degeneration). Presently, verteporfin PDT is approved for the treatment of AMD lesions that are predominantly classic subfoveal CNV, or for occult or minimally classic subfoveal CNV less than 4 disc diameters in size.[202,265,267]

COMBINATION THERAPIES*

The principles of combination therapy have been well established in the treatment of infectious diseases such as HIV,[268] or in cancer therapy. The combination of VEGF blockade (e.g., with bevacizumab) with chemotherapy or radiation therapy, for example, results in a greater antitumor effect than with either treatment alone.[269,270] Combining AMD treatments with differing mechanisms of action may have synergistic effects that might result in: (1) better visual outcome; (2) reduced frequency of treatment; (3) greater patient convenience (e.g., subconjunctival versus intravitreal injection); (4) lower risk of adverse events such as endophthalmitis; and/or (5) less likelihood of "escape" (a phenomenon in which cells (e.g., infectious agents or tumor cells) develop alternative pathways that allow them to overcome the inhibition of a pathway essential for their survival or growth). A number of variations have been examined, including retrospective and prospective trials of verteporfin photodynamic therapy with anti-VEGF therapy and/or intraocular or periocular triamcinolone or dexamethasone.[242–245,247–251,271–277] The efficacy and safety of verteporfin PDT has been demonstrated in multicenter, double-masked, randomized placebo-controlled studies.[202,278] However, PDT may affect the choriocapillary bed surrounding the CNV,[279] resulting in upregulation of VEGF that might further potentiate CNV growth.[280] Thus, adding an anti-VEGF agent to PDT has theoretical merit. Combining anti-VEGF therapy and photodynamic therapy (with or without steroid) is thought to reduce the number of treatments needed to stabilize the CNV, although this benefit has not been observed in all studies.[281]

Large, multicenter, randomized studies (DENALI (NCT00433017), MONT BLANC (NCT00433017), RADICAL (NCT00492284) have been completed, and 12-month results published in 2012 indicate that the combination of anti-VEGF therapy and PDT has shown no great advantage over anti-VEGF therapy alone. The phase IIIb DENALI study involved the combination of verteporfin PDT (Visudyne, Novartis Pharma AG, QLT, Inc.) with ranibizumab (Lucentis, Genentech/Roche). Three ranibizumab loading doses were followed by additional injections on a monthly as-needed basis in patients ($n = 321$) with subfoveal CNV of all lesion types secondary to AMD. Verteporfin PDT was administered on day 1 and at 3-month intervals as needed. At month 12, patients in the standard fluence combination group gained on average 5.3 letters from baseline, and patients in the reduced fluence combination group gained on average 4.4 letters. Patients in the ranibizumab monthly monotherapy group gained on average 8.1 letters at month 12. DENALI ($n = 255$) did not demonstrate noninferiority in terms of visual acuity gain for verteporfin PDT ranibizumab combination therapy compared with ranibizumab monthly monotherapy. On average, patients in the combination groups required 2.2 (standard fluence) or 2.8 (reduced fluence) additional ranibizumab injections after the mandatory three loading doses as compared to an average of 7.6 additional injections in the ranibizumab monthly monotherapy cohort.[282]

Similarly, in the MONT BLANC study, patients were randomized 1:1 to as-needed (PRN) combination (standard-fluence verteporfin 6 mg/m2 PDT and ranibizumab 0.5 mg) or PRN ranibizumab monotherapy (sham infusion PDT with ranibizumab 0.5 mg) following a loading dose of three injections. At month 12, visual improvement was +2.5 letters in the combination therapy group and +4.4 letters in the ranibizumab monotherapy group ($P = 0.0048$). The noninferiority limit of 7 letters was met; however, other endpoints, including the proportion of patients with a treatment-free interval of >/=3 months (96 vs 92%, $P = 0.036$) and the number of ranibizumab retreatments (1.9 vs 2.2, $P = 0.1373$) were similar, suggesting that adding verteporfin PDT does not reduce the number of ranibizumab injections required.[283]

The RADICAL study, a phase II trial, included 162 patients randomized to one of four treatment arms: double therapy of PDT with reduced-fluence verteporfin PDT (25 J/cm^2: 300 mW/cm^2 for 83 seconds) followed by ranibizumab ($n = 43$), reduced-fluence verteporfin PDT (25 J/cm^2: 300 mW/cm^2 for 83 seconds) followed by ranibizumab-dexamethasone triple therapy ($n = 39$), very low-fluence verteporfin PDT (15 J/cm^2: 180 mW/cm^2 for 83 seconds) followed by ranibizumab dexamethasone triple therapy ($n = 39$), or ranibizumab monotherapy ($n = 41$). At 24 months follow-up, mean visual acuity change from baseline was not statistically different among the treatment groups. Through 24 months, patients in the triple therapy half-fluence group had a

*Selected text adapted with kind permission of Springer Science+Business Media.[52,53]

mean of 4.2 retreatment visits compared with 8.9 for patients who received ranibizumab monotherapy ($P < 0.001$). At month 24, mean visual acuity in the triple therapy half-fluence group improved 1.8 letters fewer (95% CI 11.1 letters fewer to 7.6 letters better) compared with the ranibizumab monotherapy group ($P = 0.71$).[284]

Anti-VEGF therapy is also being combined with macular radiation therapy. Two different radiation approaches are currently in clinical trials: the internal approach, which requires a pars plana vitrectomy and the introduction of a radioactive (beta-radiation) probe (Epi-Rad90™ Ophthalmic System, NeoVista, Inc., NCT00454389),[285,286] and the office-based external approach (X-ray radiation),[287] which is delivered through the inferior sclera (IRay, Oraya Therapeutics Inc., NCT01016873). Detailed discussion of radiation therapy for AMD is beyond the scope of this chapter, but the rationale for combining anti-VEGF therapy and irradiation is that the anti-inflammatory, antineovascular, and antifibrotic effects of radiation therapy might logically be combined with the dehydrating effects of anti-VEGF therapy. Combination intraocular epiretinal irradiation and ranibizumab appears to result in a reduced need for intravitreal injection (with comparable visual outcome) compared with intravitreal ranibizumab therapy alone.[285,286] Phase III (NCT00454389, CABERNET) and phase IV (NCT01006538, MERLOT) studies are underway.

CONCLUSION

A variety of molecules, specifically targeted to different pathologic pathways in AMD, have been identified for their therapeutic potential. Additionally, our understanding of the genetic basis for AMD continues to increase rapidly, which has led to a systematic and rational basis for pharmacotherapy. A number of associated genes and alleles have been identified that confer risk or are protective against the disease, and as the related pathways are elaborated, we are able not only to target these pathways with great specificity, but also to identify those individuals who are most likely to benefit from a particular therapy. Research is actively being pursued in preclinical models both in academic laboratories and in the pharmaceutical industry, including a large number of early stage clinical trials in recent years. It is anticipated that agents that can modulate and inhibit various stages of the disease, and especially including those multiple stages relating to RPE function, the visual transduction cycle, metalloproteinase homeostasis, and VEGF inhibition, will find prominent roles either alone or in combination, such as photodynamic therapy and combined with other drug therapies. It is increasingly likely that not only treatments targeted at specific molecular pathways, but also gene transformation and replacement, are likely to become increasingly important tools in addition to standard VEGF inhibitors and other classes of small molecules and specific monoclonals in the management of this disease.

REFERENCES

1. Bird AC, Bressler NM, Bressler SB, et al. An international classification and grading system for age-related maculopathy and age-related macular degeneration. The International ARM Epidemiological Study Group. Surv Ophthalmol 1995;39:367–74.
2. Ambati J, Ambati BK, Yoo SH, et al. Age-related macular degeneration: etiology, pathogenesis, and therapeutic strategies. Surv Ophthalmol 2003;48: 257–93.
3. Blumenkranz MS, Russell SR, Robey MG, et al. Risk factors in age-related maculopathy complicated by choroidal neovascularization. Ophthalmology 1986;93:552–8.
4. Ferris 3rd FL. Senile macular degeneration: review of epidemiologic features. Am J Epidemiol 1983; 118:132–51.
5. Ferris 3rd FL, Fine SL, Hyman L. Age-related macular degeneration and blindness due to neovascular maculopathy. Arch Ophthalmol 1984;102:1640–2.
6. Bressler NM, Hawkins BS, Sternberg Jr P, et al. Are the submacular surgery trials still relevant in an era of photodynamic therapy? Ophthalmology 2001;108:435–6.
7. Argon laser photocoagulation for senile macular degeneration. Results of a randomized clinical trial. Arch Ophthalmol 1982;100:912–8.
8. Argon laser photocoagulation for neovascular maculopathy. Three-year results from randomized clinical trials. Macular Photocoagulation Study Group. Arch Ophthalmol 1986;104:694–701.
9. Laser photocoagulation of subfoveal neovascular lesions of age-related macular degeneration. Updated findings from two clinical trials. Macular Photocoagulation Study Group. Arch Ophthalmol 1993;111:1200–9.
10. Slakter JS, Yannuzzi LA, Sorenson JA, et al. A pilot study of indocyanine green videoangiography-guided laser photocoagulation of occult choroidal neovascularization in age-related macular degeneration. Arch Ophthalmol 1994; 112:465–72.
11. Leibowitz HM, Krueger DE, Maunder LR, et al. The Framingham Eye Study monograph: An ophthalmological and epidemiological study of cataract, glaucoma, diabetic retinopathy, macular degeneration, and visual acuity in a general population of 2631 adults, 1973–1975. Surv Ophthalmol 1980;24: 335–610.
12. Patel N, Adewoyin T, Chong NV. Age-related macular degeneration: a perspective on genetic studies. Eye (Lond) 2008;22:768–76.
13. Francis PJ, Hamon SC, Ott J, et al. Polymorphisms in C2, CFB and C3 are associated with progression to advanced age related macular degeneration associated with visual loss. J Med Genet 2009;46:300–7.
14. Seddon JM, Gensler G, Rosner B. C-reactive protein and CFH, ARMS2/HTRA1 gene variants are independently associated with risk of macular degeneration. Ophthalmology 2010;117:1560–6.
15. Conley YP, Jakobsdottir J, Mah T, et al. CFH, ELOVL4, PLEKHA1 and LOC387715 genes and susceptibility to age-related maculopathy: AREDS and CHS cohorts and meta-analyses. Hum Mol Genet 2006;15:3206–18.
16. Brantley Jr MA, Fang AM, King JM, et al. Association of complement factor H and LOC387715 genotypes with response of exudative age-related macular degeneration to intravitreal bevacizumab. Ophthalmology 2007;114:2168–73.
17. Brantley Jr MA, Edelstein SL, King JM, et al. Association of complement factor H and LOC387715 genotypes with response of exudative age-related macular degeneration to photodynamic therapy. Eye (Lond) 2009;23:626–31.
18. Tsuchihashi T, Mori K, Horie-Inoue K, et al. Complement factor H and high-temperature requirement A-1 genotypes and treatment response of age-related macular degeneration. Ophthalmology 2011;118:93–100.
19. Feng X, Xiao J, Longville B, et al. Complement factor H Y402H and C-reactive protein polymorphism and photodynamic therapy response in age-related macular degeneration. Ophthalmology 2009;116:1908–12 e1.
20. Klein ML, Francis PJ, Rosner B, et al. CFH and LOC387715/ARMS2 genotypes and treatment with antioxidants and zinc for age-related macular degeneration. Ophthalmology 2008;115:1019–25.
21. Klein RJ, Zeiss C, Chew EY, et al. Complement factor H polymorphism in age-related macular degeneration. Science 2005;308:385–9.
22. Edwards AO, Ritter 3rd R, Abel KJ, et al. Complement factor *H. polymorphism* and age-related macular degeneration. Science 2005;308:421–4.
23. Chen Y, Zeng J, Zhao C, et al. Assessing susceptibility to age-related macular degeneration with genetic markers and environmental factors. Arch Ophthalmol 2011;129:344–51.
24. Nozaki M, Raisler BJ, Sakurai E, et al. Drusen complement components C3a and C5a promote choroidal neovascularization. Proc Natl Acad Sci U S A 2006;103:2328–33.
25. Hageman GS, Luthert PJ, Victor Chong NH, et al. An integrated hypothesis that considers drusen as biomarkers of immune-mediated processes at the RPE-Bruch's membrane interface in aging and age-related macular degeneration. Prog Retin Eye Res 2001;20:705–32.
26. Patel M, Chan CC. Immunopathological aspects of age-related macular degeneration. Semin Immunopathol 2008;30:97–110.
27. Penfold PL, Madigan MC, Gillies MC, et al. Immunological and aetiological aspects of macular degeneration. Prog Retin Eye Res 2001;20:385–414.
28. Albig AR, Schiemann WP. Fibulin-5 antagonizes vascular endothelial growth factor (VEGF) signaling and angiogenic sprouting by endothelial cells. DNA Cell Biol 2004;23:367–79.
29. Klenotic PA, Munier FL, Marmorstein LY, et al. Tissue inhibitor of metalloproteinases-3 (TIMP-3) is a binding partner of epithelial growth factor-containing fibulin-like extracellular matrix protein 1 (EFEMP1). Implications for macular degenerations. J Biol Chem 2004;279:30469–73.
30. Fariss RN, Apte SS, Olsen BR, et al. Tissue inhibitor of metalloproteinases-3 is a component of Bruch's membrane of the eye. Am J Pathol 1997; 150:323–8.
31. Felbor U, Stohr H, Amann T, et al. A second independent Tyr168Cys mutation in the tissue inhibitor of metalloproteinases-3 (TIMP3) in Sorsby's fundus dystrophy. J Med Genet 1996;33:233–6.
32. Lin RJ, Blumenkranz MS, Binkley J, et al. A novel His158Arg mutation in TIMP3 causes a late-onset form of Sorsby fundus dystrophy. Am J Ophthalmol 2006;142:839–48.
33. De La Paz MA, Pericak-Vance MA, Lennon F, et al. Exclusion of TIMP3 as a candidate locus in age-related macular degeneration. Invest Ophthalmol Vis Sci 1997;38:1060–5.

34. Marmorstein LY, Munier FL, Arsenijevic Y, et al. Aberrant accumulation of EFEMP1 underlies drusen formation in Malattia Leventinese and age-related macular degeneration. Proc Natl Acad Sci U S A 2002;99: 13067–72.
35. Chong NH, Alexander RA, Gin T, et al. TIMP-3, collagen, and elastin immunohistochemistry and histopathology of Sorsby's fundus dystrophy. Invest Ophthalmol Vis Sci 2000;41:898–902.
36. Kamei M, Hollyfield JG. TIMP-3 in Bruch's membrane: changes during aging and in age-related macular degeneration. Invest Ophthalmol Vis Sci 1999; 40:2367–75.
37. Stone EM, Lotery AJ, Munier FL, et al. A single EFEMP1 mutation associated with both Malattia Leventinese and Doyne honeycomb retinal dystrophy. Nat Genet 1999;22:199–202.
38. Mata NL, Weng J, Travis GH. Biosynthesis of a major lipofuscin fluorophore in mice and humans with ABCR-mediated retinal and macular degeneration. Proc Natl Acad Sci U S A 2000;97:7154–9.
39. Zhang K, Garibaldi DC, Kniazeva M, et al. A novel mutation in the ABCR gene in four patients with autosomal recessive Stargardt disease. Am J Ophthalmol 1999;128:720–4.
40. Allikmets R. Further evidence for an association of ABCR alleles with age-related macular degeneration. The International ABCR Screening Consortium. Am J Hum Genet 2000;67:487–91.
41. Bernstein PS, Leppert M, Singh N, et al. Genotype-phenotype analysis of ABCR variants in macular degeneration probands and siblings. Invest Ophthalmol Vis Sci 2002;43:466–73.
42. Radu RA, Mata NL, Nusinowitz S, et al. Treatment with isotretinoin inhibits lipofuscin accumulation in a mouse model of recessive Stargardt's macular degeneration. Proc Natl Acad Sci U S A 2003;100:4742–7.
43. Radu RA, Mata NL, Bagla A, et al. Light exposure stimulates formation of A2E oxiranes in a mouse model of Stargardt's macular degeneration. Proc Natl Acad Sci U S A 2004;101:5928–33.
44. SanGiovanni JP, Chew EY, Clemons TE, et al. The relationship of dietary lipid intake and age-related macular degeneration in a case-control study: AREDS report no. 20. Arch Ophthalmol 2007;125:671–9.
45. SanGiovanni JP, Chew EY, Agron E, et al. The relationship of dietary omega-3 long-chain polyunsaturated fatty acid intake with incident age-related macular degeneration: AREDS report no. 23. Arch Ophthalmol 2008;126: 1274–9.
46. Sangiovanni JP, Agron E, Meleth AD, et al. ω-3 Long-chain polyunsaturated fatty acid intake and 12-y incidence of neovascular age-related macular degeneration and central geographic atrophy: AREDS report 30, a prospective cohort study from the Age-Related Eye Disease Study. Am J Clin Nutr 2009;90:1601–7.
47. Seddon JM, Ajani UA, Sperduto RD, et al. Dietary carotenoids, vitamins A, C, and E, and advanced age-related macular degeneration. Eye Disease Case-Control Study Group. JAMA 1994;272:1413–20.
48. Beatty S, Koh H, Phil M, et al. The role of oxidative stress in the pathogenesis of age-related macular degeneration. Surv Ophthalmol 2000;45:115–34.
49. Cho E, Stampfer MJ, Seddon JM, et al. Prospective study of zinc intake and the risk of age-related macular degeneration. Ann Epidemiol 2001;11: 328–36.
50. Cho E, Seddon JM, Rosner B, et al. Prospective study of intake of fruits, vegetables, vitamins, and carotenoids and risk of age-related maculopathy. Arch Ophthalmol 2004;122:883–92.
51. Heuberger RA, Mares-Perlman JA, Klein R, et al. Relationship of dietary fat to age-related maculopathy in the Third National Health and Nutrition Examination Survey. Arch Ophthalmol 2001;119:1833–8.
52. Zarbin MA, Rosenfeld PJ. Pathway-based therapies for age-related macular degeneration: an integrated survey of emerging treatment alternatives. Retina 2010;30:1350–67.
53. Zarbin M, Rosenfeld, PJ. Review of emerging treatments for age-related macular degeneration. In: Stratton RD Hauswirth WW, Gardner TW, editors. Oxidative stress in applied basic research and clinical practice: Studies in retinal and choroidal disorders. New York: Humana Press; 2012.
54. Tomany SC, Wang JJ, Van Leeuwen R, et al. Risk factors for incident age-related macular degeneration: pooled findings from 3 continents. Ophthalmology 2004;111:1280–7.
55. Thornton J, Edwards R, Mitchell P, et al. Smoking and age-related macular degeneration: a review of association. Eye (Lond) 2005;19:935–44.
56. Darzins P, Mitchell P, Heller RF. Sun exposure and age-related macular degeneration. An Australian case–control study. Ophthalmology 1997;104: 770–6.
57. Tomany SC, Cruickshanks KJ, Klein R, et al. Sunlight and the 10-year incidence of age-related maculopathy: the Beaver Dam Eye Study. Arch Ophthalmol 2004;122:750–7.
58. A randomized, placebo-controlled, clinical trial of high-dose supplementation with vitamins C and E, beta carotene, and zinc for age-related macular degeneration and vision loss: AREDS report no. 8. Arch Ophthalmol 2001;119: 1417–36.
59. van Leeuwen R, Tomany SC, Wang JJ, et al. Is medication use associated with the incidence of early age-related maculopathy? Pooled findings from 3 continents. Ophthalmology 2004;111:1169–75.
60. Ishida S, Usui T, Yamashiro K, et al. VEGF164-mediated inflammation is required for pathological, but not physiological, ischemia-induced retinal neovascularization. J Exp Med 2003;198:483–9.
61. Arroyo JG, Michaud N, Jakobiec FA. Choroidal neovascular membranes treated with photodynamic therapy. Arch Ophthalmol 2003;121:898–903.
62. Ghazi NG, Jabbour NM, De La Cruz ZC, et al. Clinicopathologic studies of age-related macular degeneration with classic subfoveal choroidal neovascularization treated with photodynamic therapy. Retina 2001;21:478–86.
63. Grossniklaus HE, Ling JX, Wallace TM, et al. Macrophage and retinal pigment epithelium expression of angiogenic cytokines in choroidal neovascularization. Mol Vis 2002;8:119–26.
64. Schnurrbusch UE, Welt K, Horn LC, et al. Histological findings of surgically excised choroidal neovascular membranes after photodynamic therapy. Br J Ophthalmol 2001;85:1086–91.
65. Moshfeghi DM, Kaiser PK, Grossniklaus HE, et al. Clinicopathologic study after submacular removal of choroidal neovascular membranes treated with verteporfin ocular photodynamic therapy. Am J Ophthalmol 2003;135: 343–50.
66. Ciulla TA, Criswell MH, Danis RP, et al. Intravitreal triamcinolone acetonide inhibits choroidal neovascularization in a laser-treated rat model. Arch Ophthalmol 2001;119:399–404.
67. Penfold PL, Wen L, Madigan MC, et al. Triamcinolone acetonide modulates permeability and intercellular adhesion molecule-1 (ICAM-1) expression of the ECV304 cell line: implications for macular degeneration. Clin Exp Immunol 2000;121:458–65.
68. Sakurai E, Taguchi H, Anand A, et al. Targeted disruption of the CD18 or ICAM-1 gene inhibits choroidal neovascularization. Invest Ophthalmol Vis Sci 2003;44:2743–9.
69. Friedlander M, Theesfeld CL, Sugita M, et al. Involvement of integrins alpha v beta 3 and alpha v beta 5 in ocular neovascular diseases. Proc Natl Acad Sci U S A 1996;93:9764–9.
70. Friedlander M, Brooks PC, Shaffer RW, et al. Definition of two angiogenic pathways by distinct alpha v integrins. Science 1995;270:1500–2.
71. Miller JW. Vascular endothelial growth factor and ocular neovascularization. Am J Pathol 1997;151:13–23.
72. Robinson CJ, Stringer SE. The splice variants of vascular endothelial growth factor (VEGF) and their receptors. J Cell Sci 2001;114:853–65.
73. Ferrara N. Vascular endothelial growth factor: basic science and clinical progress. Endocr Rev 2004;25:581–611.
74. Senger DR, Galli SJ, Dvorak AM, et al. Tumor cells secrete a vascular permeability factor that promotes accumulation of ascites fluid. Science 1983; 219:983–5.
75. Fukumura D, Gohongi T, Kadambi A, et al. Predominant role of endothelial nitric oxide synthase in vascular endothelial growth factor-induced angiogenesis and vascular permeability. Proc Natl Acad Sci U S A 2001;98:2604–9.
76. Sennlaub F, Courtois Y, Goureau O. Inducible nitric oxide synthase mediates retinal apoptosis in ischemic proliferative retinopathy. J Neurosci 2002;22: 3987–93.
77. Usui T, Ishida S, Yamashiro K, et al. VEGF164(165) as the pathological isoform: differential leukocyte and endothelial responses through VEGFR1 and VEGFR2. Invest Ophthalmol Vis Sci 2004;45:368–74.
78. Mayerhofer M, Valent P, Sperr WR, et al. BCR/ABL induces expression of vascular endothelial growth factor and its transcriptional activator, hypoxia inducible factor-1alpha, through a pathway involving phosphoinositide 3-kinase and the mammalian target of rapamycin. Blood 2002;100:3767–75.
79. Elbashir SM, Harborth J, Lendeckel W, et al. Duplexes of 21-nucleotide RNAs mediate RNA interference in cultured mammalian cells. Nature 2001;411: 494–8.
80. El-Hashemite N, Walker V, Zhang H, et al. Loss of Tsc1 or Tsc2 induces vascular endothelial growth factor production through mammalian target of rapamycin. Cancer Res 2003;63:5173–7.
81. Tolentino MJ, Brucker AJ, Fosnot J, et al. Intravitreal injection of vascular endothelial growth factor small interfering RNA inhibits growth and leakage in a nonhuman primate, laser-induced model of choroidal neovascularization. Retina 2004;24:660.
82. Dawson DW, Volpert OV, Gillis P, et al. Pigment epithelium-derived factor: a potent inhibitor of angiogenesis. Science 1999;285:245–8.
83. Folkman J, Ingber DE. Angiostatic steroids. Method of discovery and mechanism of action. Ann Surg 1987;206:374–83.
84. Folkman J, Weisz PB, Joullie MM, et al. Control of angiogenesis with synthetic heparin substitutes. Science 1989;243:1490–3.
85. Fung WE. Interferon alpha 2a for treatment of age-related macular degeneration. Am J Ophthalmol 1991;112:349–50.
86. Lai CC, Wu WC, Chen SL, et al. Suppression of choroidal neovascularization by adeno-associated virus vector expressing angiostatin. Invest Ophthalmol Vis Sci 2001;42:2401–7.
87. Mori K, Duh E, Gehlbach P, et al. Pigment epithelium-derived factor inhibits retinal and choroidal neovascularization. J Cell Physiol 2001;188:253–63.
88. Mori K, Ando A, Gehlbach P, et al. Inhibition of choroidal neovascularization by intravenous injection of adenoviral vectors expressing secretable endostatin. Am J Pathol 2001;159:313–20.
89. O'Reilly MS, Boehm T, Shing Y, et al. Endostatin: an endogenous inhibitor of angiogenesis and tumor growth. Cell 1997;88:277–85.
90. O'Reilly MS, Wiederschain D, Stetler-Stevenson WG, et al. Regulation of angiostatin production by matrix metalloproteinase-2 in a model of concomitant resistance. J Biol Chem 1999;274:29568–71.
91. Hellstrom M, Kalen M, Lindahl P, et al. Role of PDGF-B and PDGFR-beta in recruitment of vascular smooth muscle cells and pericytes during embryonic blood vessel formation in the mouse. Development 1999;126:3047–55.
92. Tolentino MJ. Current molecular understanding and future treatment strategies for pathologic ocular neovascularization. Curr Mol Med 2009;9: 973–81.

93. Benjamin LE, Golijanin D, Itin A, et al. Selective ablation of immature blood vessels in established human tumors follows vascular endothelial growth factor withdrawal. J Clin Invest 1999;103:159–65.
94. Benjamin LE, Hemo I, Keshet E. A plasticity window for blood vessel remodelling is defined by pericyte coverage of the preformed endothelial network and is regulated by PDGF-B and VEGF. Development 1998;125:1591–8.
95. Dell S, Peters S, Muther P, et al. The role of PDGF receptor inhibitors and PI3-kinase signaling in the pathogenesis of corneal neovascularization. Invest Ophthalmol Vis Sci 2006;47:1928–37.
96. Perez-Santonja JJ, Campos-Mollo E, Lledo-Riquelme M, et al. Inhibition of corneal neovascularization by topical bevacizumab (Anti-VEGF) and Sunitinib (anti-VEGF and anti-PDGF) in an animal model. Am J Ophthalmol 2010;150:519–28 e1.
97. Oshima Y, Deering T, Oshima S, et al. Angiopoietin-2 enhances retinal vessel sensitivity to vascular endothelial growth factor. J Cell Physiol 2004;199: 412–7.
98. Crabb JW, Miyagi M, Gu X, et al. Drusen proteome analysis: an approach to the etiology of age-related macular degeneration. Proc Natl Acad Sci U S A 2002;99:14682–7.
99. Anand-Apte B, Pepper MS, Voest E, et al. Inhibition of angiogenesis by tissue inhibitor of metalloproteinase-3. Invest Ophthalmol Vis Sci 1997;38:817–23.
100. Takahashi T, Nakamura T, Hayashi A, et al. Inhibition of experimental choroidal neovascularization by overexpression of tissue inhibitor of metalloproteinases-3 in retinal pigment epithelium cells. Am J Ophthalmol 2000;130:774–81.
101. Bhutto IA, McLeod DS, Hasegawa T, et al. Pigment epithelium-derived factor (PEDF) and vascular endothelial growth factor (VEGF) in aged human choroid and eyes with age-related macular degeneration. Exp Eye Res 2006;82:99–110.
102. Amaral J, Becerra SP. Effects of human recombinant PEDF protein and PEDF-derived peptide 34-mer on choroidal neovascularization. Invest Ophthalmol Vis Sci 2010;51:1318–26.
103. Otani A, Slike BM, Dorrell MI, et al. A fragment of human TrpRS as a potent antagonist of ocular angiogenesis. Proc Natl Acad Sci U S A 2002;99:178–83.
104. Cao Y, Xue L. Angiostatin. Semin Thromb Hemost 2004;30:83–93.
105. Newsome DA, Swartz M, Leone NC, et al. Oral zinc in macular degeneration. Arch Ophthalmol 1988;106:192–8.
106. Bressler NM, Bressler SB, Congdon NG, et al. Potential public health impact of Age-Related Eye Disease Study results: AREDS report no. 11. Arch Ophthalmol 2003;121:1621–4.
107. SanGiovanni JP, Chew EY, Clemons TE, et al. The relationship of dietary carotenoid and vitamin A, E, and C intake with age-related macular degeneration in a case-control study: AREDS report no. 22. Arch Ophthalmol 2007;125:1225–32.
108. Radu RA, Han Y, Bui TV, et al. Reductions in serum vitamin A arrest accumulation of toxic retinal fluorophores: a potential therapy for treatment of lipofuscin-based retinal diseases. Invest Ophthalmol Vis Sci 2005;46: 4393–401.
109. Quadro L, Blaner WS, Salchow DJ, et al. Impaired retinal function and vitamin A availability in mice lacking retinol-binding protein. EMBO J 1999;18: 4633–44.
110. Vogel S, Piantedosi R, O'Byrne SM, et al. Retinol-binding protein-deficient mice: biochemical basis for impaired vision. Biochemistry 2002;41:15360–8.
111. Decensi A, Torrisi R, Bruno S, et al. Randomized trial of fenretinide in superficial bladder cancer using DNA flow cytometry as an intermediate end point. Cancer Epidemiol Biomarkers Prev 2000;9:1071–8.
112. Follen M, Atkinson EN, Schottenfeld D, et al. A randomized clinical trial of 4-hydroxyphenylretinamide for high-grade squamous intraepithelial lesions of the cervix. Clin Cancer Res 2001;7:3356–65.
113. Camerini T, Mariani L, De Palo G, et al. Safety of the synthetic retinoid fenretinide: long-term results from a controlled clinical trial for the prevention of contralateral breast cancer. J Clin Oncol 2001;19:1664–70.
114. Garaventa A, Luksch R, Lo Piccolo MS, et al. Phase I trial and pharmacokinetics of fenretinide in children with neuroblastoma. Clin Cancer Res 2003;9:2032–9.
115. Puduvalli VK, Yung WK, Hess KR, et al. Phase II study of fenretinide (NSC 374551) in adults with recurrent malignant gliomas: A North American Brain Tumor Consortium study. J Clin Oncol 2004;22:4282–9.
116. Mariani L, Formelli F, De Palo G, et al. Chemoprevention of breast cancer with fenretinide (4-HPR): study of long-term visual and ophthalmologic tolerability. Tumori 1996;82:444–9.
117. Conley B, O'Shaughnessy J, Prindiville S, et al. Pilot trial of the safety, tolerability, and retinoid levels of N-(4-hydroxyphenyl) retinamide in combination with tamoxifen in patients at high risk for developing invasive breast cancer. J Clin Oncol 2000;18:275–83.
118. Caruso RC, Zujewski J, Iwata F, et al. Effects of fenretinide (4-HPR) on dark adaptation. Arch Ophthalmol 1998;116:759–63.
119. Kaiser-Kupfer MI, Peck GL, Caruso RC, et al. Abnormal retinal function associated with fenretinide, a synthetic retinoid. Arch Ophthalmol 1986; 104:69–70.
120. Decensi A, Torrisi R, Polizzi A, et al. Effect of the synthetic retinoid fenretinide on dark adaptation and the ocular surface. J Natl Cancer Inst 1994;86: 105–10.
121. Decensi A, Fontana V, Fioretto M, et al. Long-term effects of fenretinide on retinal function. Eur J Cancer 1997;33:80–4.
122. Marmor MF, Jain A, Moshfeghi D. Total rod ERG suppression with high dose compassionate Fenretinide usage. Doc Ophthalmol 2008;117:257–61.
123. Radu RA, Mata NL, Nusinowitz S, et al. Isotretinoin treatment inhibits lipofuscin accumulation in a mouse model of recessive Stargardt's macular degeneration. Novartis Found Symp 2004;255:51–63;discussion 7, 177–8.
124. Sieving PA, Chaudhry P, Kondo M, et al. Inhibition of the visual cycle in vivo by 13-cis retinoic acid protects from light damage and provides a mechanism for night blindness in isotretinoin therapy. Proc Natl Acad Sci U S A 2001;98:1835–40.
125. Kubota R, Boman NL, David R, et al. Safety and effect on rod function of Acu-4429, a novel small-molecule visual cycle modulator. Retina 2012;32: 183–8.
126. Donoso LA, Kim D, Frost A, et al. The role of inflammation in the pathogenesis of age-related macular degeneration. Surv Ophthalmol 2006;51:137–52.
127. Emlen W, Li W, Kirschfink M. Therapeutic complement inhibition: new developments. Semin Thromb Hemost 2010;36:660–8.
128. Anderson DH, Radeke MJ, Gallo NB, et al. The pivotal role of the complement system in aging and age-related macular degeneration: hypothesis re-visited. Prog Retin Eye Res 2010;29:95–112.
129. Anderson DH, Mullins RF, Hageman GS, et al. A role for local inflammation in the formation of drusen in the aging eye. Am J Ophthalmol 2002;134: 411–31.
130. Hughes AE, Orr N, Esfandiary H, et al. A common CFH haplotype, with deletion of CFHR1 and CFHR3, is associated with lower risk of age-related macular degeneration. Nat Genet 2006;38:1173–7.
131. Schmid-Kubista KE, Tosakulwong N, Wu Y, et al. Contribution of copy number variation in the regulation of complement activation locus to development of age-related macular degeneration. Invest Ophthalmol Vis Sci 2009; 50:5070–9.
132. Campochiaro PA. Ocular neovascularisation and excessive vascular permeability. Expert Opin Biol Ther 2004;4:1395–402.
133. Steinbrook R. The price of sight–ranibizumab, bevacizumab, and the treatment of macular degeneration. N Engl J Med 2006; 355:1409–12.
134. Hurwitz H, Fehrenbacher L, Novotny W, et al. Bevacizumab plus irinotecan, fluorouracil, and leucovorin for metastatic colorectal cancer. N Engl J Med 2004;350:2335–42.
135. Michels S, Rosenfeld PJ, Puliafito CA, et al. Systemic bevacizumab (Avastin) therapy for neovascular age-related macular degeneration twelve-week results of an uncontrolled open-label clinical study. Ophthalmology 2005;112:1035–47.
136. Moshfeghi AA, Rosenfeld PJ, Puliafito CA, et al. Systemic bevacizumab (Avastin) therapy for neovascular age-related macular degeneration: twenty-four-week results of an uncontrolled open-label clinical study. Ophthalmology 2006;113:2002e1–12.
137. Rosenfeld PJ, Moshfeghi AA, Puliafito CA. Optical coherence tomography findings after an intravitreal injection of bevacizumab (avastin) for neovascular age-related macular degeneration. Ophthalmic Surg Lasers Imaging 2005;36:331–5.
138. Han DP. Intravitreal human immune globulin in a rabbit model of *Staphylococcus aureus* toxin-mediated endophthalmitis: a potential adjunct in the treatment of endophthalmitis. Trans Am Ophthalmol Soc 2004;102: 305–20.
139. Shahar J, Avery RL, Heilweil G, et al. Electrophysiologic and retinal penetration studies following intravitreal injection of bevacizumab (Avastin). Retina 2006;26:262–9.
140. Dib E, Maia M, Longo-Maugeri IM, et al. Subretinal bevacizumab detection after intravitreous injection in rabbits. Invest Ophthalmol Vis Sci 2008;49: 1097–100.
141. Mordenti J, Thomsen K, Licko V, et al. Intraocular pharmacokinetics and safety of a humanized monoclonal antibody in rabbits after intravitreal administration of a solution or a PLGA microsphere formulation. Toxicol Sci 1999;52:101–6.
142. Mordenti J, Cuthbertson RA, Ferrara N, et al. Comparisons of the intraocular tissue distribution, pharmacokinetics, and safety of 125I-labeled full-length and Fab antibodies in rhesus monkeys following intravitreal administration. Toxicol Pathol 1999;27:536–44.
143. Bakri SJ, Kitzmann AS. Retinal pigment epithelial tear after intravitreal ranibizumab. Am J Ophthalmol 2007;143:505–7.
144. Miyake T, Sawada O, Kakinoki M, et al. Pharmacokinetics of bevacizumab and its effect on vascular endothelial growth factor after intravitreal injection of bevacizumab in macaque eyes. Invest Ophthalmol Vis Sci 2010;51:1606–8.
145. Nomoto H, Shiraga F, Kuno N, et al. Pharmacokinetics of bevacizumab after topical, subconjunctival, and intravitreal administration in rabbits. Invest Ophthalmol Vis Sci 2009;50:4807–13.
146. Beer PM, Wong SJ, Hammad AM, et al. Vitreous levels of unbound bevacizumab and unbound vascular endothelial growth factor in two patients. Retina 2006;26:871–6.
147. Krohne TU, Eter N, Holz FG, et al. Intraocular pharmacokinetics of bevacizumab after a single intravitreal injection in humans. Am J Ophthalmol 2008;146:508–12.
148. Zhu Q, Ziemssen F, Henke-Fahle S, et al. Vitreous levels of bevacizumab and vascular endothelial growth factor-A in patients with choroidal neovascularization. Ophthalmology 2008;115:1750–5, 5 e1.
149. Brechner RJ, Rosenfeld PJ, Babish JD, et al. Pharmacotherapy for neovascular age-related macular degeneration: an analysis of the 100% 2008 medicare fee-for-service part B claims file. Am J Ophthalmol 2011;151:887–95 e1.
150. Martin DF, Maguire MG, Ying GS, et al. Ranibizumab and bevacizumab for neovascular age-related macular degeneration. N Engl J Med 2011;364: 1897–908.

151. Arevalo JF, Maia M, Garcia-Amaris RA, et al. Intravitreal bevacizumab for refractory pseudophakic cystoid macular edema: the Pan-American Collaborative Retina Study Group results. Ophthalmology 2009;116:1481–7, 7 e1.
152. Caccavale A, Romanazzi F, Imparato M, et al. Central serous chorioretinopathy: a pathogenetic model. Clin Ophthalmol 2011;5:239–43.
153. Cervantes-Castaneda RA, Giuliari GP, Gallagher MJ, et al. Intravitreal bevacizumab in refractory uveitic macular edema: one-year follow-up. Eur J Ophthalmol 2009;19:622–9.
154. Ehrlich R, Ciulla TA, Maturi R, et al. Intravitreal bevacizumab for choroidal neovascularization secondary to presumed ocular histoplasmosis syndrome. Retina 2009;29:1418–23.
155. El Matri L, Kort F, Bouraoui R, et al. Intravitreal bevacizumab for the treatment of choroidal neovascularization secondary to angioid streaks: one year of follow-up. Acta Ophthalmol 2010 89:641–6.
156. Gregori NZ, Rattan GH, Rosenfeld PJ, et al. Safety and efficacy of intravitreal bevacizumab (avastin) for the management of branch and hemiretinal vein occlusion. Retina 2009;29:913–25.
157. Mintz-Hittner HA, Kennedy KA, Chuang AZ. Efficacy of intravitreal bevacizumab for stage 3+ retinopathy of prematurity. N Engl J Med 2011;364: 603–15.
158. Nakanishi H, Tsujikawa A, Yodoi Y, et al. Prognostic factors for visual outcomes 2-years after intravitreal bevacizumab for myopic choroidal neovascularization. Eye (Lond) 2011;25:375–81.
159. Wu L, Arevalo JF, Berrocal MH, et al. Comparison of two doses of intravitreal bevacizumab as primary treatment for macular edema secondary to branch retinal vein occlusions: results of the Pan American Collaborative Retina Study Group at 24 months. Retina 2009;29:1396–403.
160. Chiang A, Regillo CD. Preferred therapies for neovascular age-related macular degeneration. Curr Opin Ophthalmol 2011;22:199–204.
161. Tufail A, Patel PJ, Egan C, et al. Bevacizumab for neovascular age related macular degeneration (ABC Trial): multicentre randomised double masked study. BMJ 2010;340:c2459.
162. Subramanian ML, Ness S, Abedi G, et al. Bevacizumab vs ranibizumab for age-related macular degeneration: early results of a prospective double-masked, randomized clinical trial. Am J Ophthalmol 2009;148:875–82.
163. Rosenfeld PJ, Brown DM, Heier JS, et al. Ranibizumab for neovascular age-related macular degeneration. N Engl J Med 2006;355:1419–31.
164. Brown DM, Kaiser PK, Michels M, et al. Ranibizumab versus verteporfin for neovascular age-related macular degeneration. N Engl J Med 2006;355: 1432–44.
165. Mitchell P, Korobelnik JF, Lanzetta P, et al. Ranibizumab (Lucentis) in neovascular age-related macular degeneration: evidence from clinical trials. Br J Ophthalmol 2010; 94:2–13.
166. Brown DM, Michels M, Kaiser PK, et al. Ranibizumab versus verteporfin photodynamic therapy for neovascular age-related macular degeneration: Two-year results of the ANCHOR study. Ophthalmology 2009;116:57–65.
167. Rosenfeld PJ, Schwartz SD, Blumenkranz MS, et al. Maximum tolerated dose of a humanized anti-vascular endothelial growth factor antibody fragment for treating neovascular age-related macular degeneration. Ophthalmology 2005;112:1048–53.
168. Regillo CD, Brown DM, Abraham P, et al. Randomized, double-masked, sham-controlled trial of ranibizumab for neovascular age-related macular degeneration: PIER Study year 1. Am J Ophthalmol 2008;145:239–48.
169. Abraham P, Yue H, Wilson L. Randomized, double-masked, sham-controlled trial of ranibizumab for neovascular age-related macular degeneration: PIER study year 2. Am J Ophthalmol 2010;150:315–24.
170. Schmidt-Erfurth U, Eldem B, Guymer R, et al. Efficacy and safety of monthly versus quarterly ranibizumab treatment in neovascular age-related macular degeneration: the EXCITE study. Ophthalmology 2011;118:831–9.
171. Holz FG, Amoaku W, Donate J, et al. Safety and efficacy of a flexible dosing regimen of ranibizumab in neovascular age-related macular degeneration: the SUSTAIN study. Ophthalmology 2011;118:663–71.
172. Fung AE, Lalwani GA, Rosenfeld PJ, et al. An optical coherence tomography-guided, variable dosing regimen with intravitreal ranibizumab (Lucentis) for neovascular age-related macular degeneration. Am J Ophthalmol 2007;143: 566–83.
173. Lalwani GA, Rosenfeld PJ, Fung AE, et al. A variable-dosing regimen with intravitreal ranibizumab for neovascular age-related macular degeneration: year 2 of the PrONTO Study. Am J Ophthalmol 2009;148:43–58.
174. Collaborative overview of randomised trials of antiplatelet therapy – I: Prevention of death, myocardial infarction, and stroke by prolonged antiplatelet therapy in various categories of patients. Antiplatelet Trialists' Collaboration. BMJ 1994;308:81–106.
175. Schmidt-Erfurth U. Clinical safety of ranibizumab in age-related macular degeneration. Expert Opin Drug Saf 2010;9:149–65.
176. Rosenfeld PJ. Bevacizumab versus ranibizumab for AMD. N Engl J Med 2011;364:1966–7.
176a. IVAN Study Investigators. Ranibizumab versus bevacizumab to treat neovascular age-related macular degeneration: one-year findings from the IVAN randomized trial. Ophthalmology 2012. Corrected proof published online 2012 May 11. http//:www.ophsource.org/periodicals/ophtha/article/S0161-6420(12)00358-2/ [cited 2012 June 8].
177. Martin DF, Maguire MG, Fine SL, et al. Ranibizumab and bevacizumab for treatment of neovascular age-related macular degeneration: two-year results. Ophthalmology 2012. Corrected proof published online 2012 May 2. http//: www.ophsource.org/periodicals/ophtha/article/S0161-6420(12)00321-1/ [cited 2012 June 8].
178. Holash J, Davis S, Papadopoulos N, et al. VEGF-Trap: a VEGF blocker with potent antitumor effects. Proc Natl Acad Sci U S A 2002;99:11393–8.
179. Chappelow AV, Kaiser PK. Neovascular age-related macular degeneration: potential therapies. Drugs 2008;68:1029–36.
180. Cao J, Song H, Renard RA, et al. Systemic or intravitreal administration of VEGF Trap suppresses vascular leak and leukostasis in the retinas of diabetic rats. Invest Ophthalmol Vis Sci 2006;47.
181. Rudge JS, Thurston G, Davis S, et al. VEGF trap as a novel antiangiogenic treatment currently in clinical trials for cancer and eye diseases, and VelociGene- based discovery of the next generation of angiogenesis targets. Cold Spring Harb Symp Quant Biol 2005;70:411–8.
182. Nguyen QD, Shah SM, Browning DJ, et al. A phase I study of intravitreal vascular endothelial growth factor trap-eye in patients with neovascular age-related macular degeneration. Ophthalmology 2009;116:2141–8.
183. Brown DM, Heier JS, Ciulla T, et al. Primary endpoint results of a phase II study of vascular endothelial growth factor trap-eye in wet age-related macular degeneration. Ophthalmology 2011;118:1089–97.
184. Heier JS, Boyer D, Nguyen QD, et al. The 1-year results of CLEAR-IT 2, a phase 2 study of vascular endothelial growth factor trap-eye dosed as-needed after 12-week fixed dosing. Ophthalmology 2011;118:1098–106.
185. http://investor.regeneron.com/releasedetail.cfm?ReleaseID=532099. v. 2012 [cited 2012 Feb 15].
186. http://files.shareholder.com/downloads/REGN/1026966568x0x440864/8BEB55ED-1AA6-43DB-8783-EA5C0C4C78DE/REGN_Angiogenesis_Final_021311.pdf. v. 2012 [cited 2012 Feb 15].
187. Zhang M, Zhang J, Yan M, et al. Recombinant anti-vascular endothelial growth factor fusion protein efficiently suppresses choridal neovasularization in monkeys. Mol Vis 2008;14:37–49.
188. Suto K, Yamazaki Y, Morita T, et al. Crystal structures of novel vascular endothelial growth factors (VEGF) from snake venoms: insight into selective VEGF binding to kinase insert domain-containing receptor but not to fms-like tyrosine kinase-1. J Biol Chem 2005;280:2126–31.
189. Zhang M, Yu D, Yang C, et al. The pharmacology study of a new recombinant human VEGF receptor-fc fusion protein on experimental choroidal neovascularization. Pharm Res 2009;26:204–10.
190. Lai CM, Shen WY, Brankov M, et al. Long-term evaluation of AAV-mediated sFlt-1 gene therapy for ocular neovascularization in mice and monkeys. Mol Ther 2005;12:659–68.
191. Kendall RL, Wang G, Thomas KA. Identification of a natural soluble form of the vascular endothelial growth factor receptor, FLT-1, and its heterodimerization with KDR. Biochem Biophys Res Commun 1996;226:324–8.
192. Mori K, Gehlbach P, Yamamoto S, et al. AAV-mediated gene transfer of pigment epithelium-derived factor inhibits choroidal neovascularization. Invest Ophthalmol Vis Sci 2002;43:1994–2000.
193. Maguire AM, Simonelli F, Pierce EA, et al. Safety and efficacy of gene transfer for Leber's congenital amaurosis. N Engl J Med 2008;358:2240–8.
194. Bainbridge JW, Smith AJ, Barker SS, et al. Effect of gene therapy on visual function in Leber's congenital amaurosis. N Engl J Med 2008;358:2231–9.
195. Cideciyan AV, Hauswirth WW, Aleman TS, et al. Human RPE65 gene therapy for Leber congenital amaurosis: persistence of early visual improvements and safety at 1 year. Hum Gene Ther 2009;20:999–1004.
196. Bainbridge JW, Mistry A, De Alwis M, et al. Inhibition of retinal neovascularisation by gene transfer of soluble VEGF receptor sFlt-1. Gene Ther 2002;9:320–6.
197. Gehlbach P, Demetriades AM, Yamamoto S, et al. Periocular gene transfer of sFlt-1 suppresses ocular neovascularization and vascular endothelial growth factor-induced breakdown of the blood-retinal barrier. Hum Gene Ther 2003;14:129–41.
198. Lukason M, DuFresne E, Rubin H, et al. Inhibition of choroidal neovascularization in a nonhuman primate model by intravitreal administration of an AAV2 vector expressing a novel anti-VEGF molecule. Mol Ther 2011;19: 260–5.
199. Igarashi T, Miyake K, Masuda I, et al. Adeno-associated vector (type 8)-mediated expression of soluble Flt-1 efficiently inhibits neovascularization in a murine choroidal neovascularization model. Hum Gene Ther 2010;21:631–7.
200. Jellinek D, Green LS, Bell C, et al. Inhibition of receptor binding by high-affinity RNA ligands to vascular endothelial growth factor. Biochemistry 1994;33:10450–6.
201. Gragoudas ES, Adamis AP, Cunningham ET et al. Pegaptanib for neovascular age-related macular degeneration. N Engl J Med 2004;351:2805–16.
202. Verteporfin therapy of subfoveal choroidal neovascularization in age-related macular degeneration: two-year results of a randomized clinical trial including lesions with occult with no classic choroidal neovascularization – verteporfin in photodynamic therapy report 2. Am J Ophthalmol 2001;131: 541–60.
203. Friberg TR, Tolentino M, Weber P, et al. Pegaptanib sodium as maintenance therapy in neovascular age-related macular degeneration: the LEVEL study. Br J Ophthalmol 2010;94:1611–7.
204. Reich SJ, Fosnot J, Kuroki A, et al. Small interfering RNA (siRNA) targeting VEGF effectively inhibits ocular neovascularization in a mouse model. Mol Vis 2003;9:210–6.
205. Kaiser PK, Symons RC, Shah SM, et al. RNAi-based treatment for neovascular age-related macular degeneration by Sirna-027. Am J Ophthalmol 2010;150: 33–9.
206. Ashikari M, Tokoro M, Itaya M, et al. Suppression of laser-induced choroidal neovascularization by nontargeted siRNA. Invest Ophthalmol Vis Sci 2010;51:3820–4.

207. Gu L, Chen H, Tuo J, et al. Inhibition of experimental choroidal neovascularization in mice by anti-VEGFA/VEGFR2 or non-specific siRNA. Exp Eye Res 2010;91:433–9.
208. Kleinman ME, Yamada K, Takeda A, et al. Sequence- and target-independent angiogenesis suppression by siRNA via TLR3. Nature 2008;452:591–7.
209. Ni Z, Hui P. Emerging pharmacologic therapies for wet age-related macular degeneration. Ophthalmologica 2009;223:401–10.
210. Takahashi K, Saishin Y, King AG, et al. Suppression and regression of choroidal neovascularization by the multitargeted kinase inhibitor pazopanib. Arch Ophthalmol 2009;127:494–9.
211. Charters L. Pazopanib explored for neovascular age-related macular degeneration. Ophthalmology Times 2010;Mar 1: 34.
212. Mabry R, Gilbertson DG, Frank A, et al. A dual-targeting PDGFRbeta/VEGF-A molecule assembled from stable antibody fragments demonstrates anti-angiogenic activity in vitro and in vivo. MAbs 2010;2:20–34.
213. Wakasugi K, Slike BM, Hood J, et al. A human aminoacyl-tRNA synthetase as a regulator of angiogenesis. Proc Natl Acad Sci U S A 2002;99:173–7.
214. Banin E, Dorrell MI, Aguilar E, et al. T2-TrpRS inhibits preretinal neovascularization and enhances physiological vascular regrowth in OIR as assessed by a new method of quantification. Invest Ophthalmol Vis Sci 2006;47:2125–34.
215. Aiello LP. The potential role of PKC beta in diabetic retinopathy and macular edema. Surv Ophthalmol 2002;47(Suppl 2):S263–9.
216. Saishin Y, Silva RL, Callahan K, et al. Periocular injection of microspheres containing PKC412 inhibits choroidal neovascularization in a porcine model. Invest Ophthalmol Vis Sci 2003;44:4989–93.
217. Engelbert M, Gilmore MS. Fas ligand but not complement is critical for control of experimental *Staphylococcus aureus* endophthalmitis. Invest Ophthalmol Vis Sci 2005;46:2479–86.
218. Giese MJ, Mondino BJ, Glasgow BJ, et al. Complement system and host defense against staphylococcal endophthalmitis. Invest Ophthalmol Vis Sci 1994;35:1026–32.
219. Aizuss DH, Mondino BJ, Sumner HL, et al. The complement system and host defense against Pseudomonas endophthalmitis. Invest Ophthalmol Vis Sci 1985;26:1262–6.
220. Brooks SE, Gu X, Samuel S, et al. Reduced severity of oxygen-induced retinopathy in eNOS-deficient mice. Invest Ophthalmol Vis Sci 2001;42:222–8.
221. Semkova I, Kreppel F, Welsandt G, et al. Autologous transplantation of genetically modified iris pigment epithelial cells: a promising concept for the treatment of age-related macular degeneration and other disorders of the eye. Proc Natl Acad Sci U S A 2002;99:13090–5.
222. Campochiaro PA, Nguyen QD, Shah SM, et al. Adenoviral vector-delivered pigment epithelium-derived factor for neovascular age-related macular degeneration: results of a phase I clinical trial. Hum Gene Ther 2006;17:167–76.
223. Lai YK, Shen WY, Brankov M, et al. Potential long-term inhibition of ocular neovascularisation by recombinant adeno-associated virus-mediated secretion gene therapy. Gene Ther 2002;9:804–13.
224. Kachi S, Binley K, Yokoi K, et al. Equine infectious anemia viral vector-mediated codelivery of endostatin and angiostatin driven by retinal pigmented epithelium-specific VMD2 promoter inhibits choroidal neovascularization. Hum Gene Ther 2009;20:31–9.
225. Balaggan KS, Binley K, Esapa M, et al. EIAV vector-mediated delivery of endostatin or angiostatin inhibits angiogenesis and vascular hyperpermeability in experimental CNV. Gene Ther 2006;13:1153–65.
226. Brooks PC, Clark RA, Cheresh DA. Requirement of vascular integrin alpha v beta 3 for angiogenesis. Science 1994;264:569–71.
227. Luna J, Tobe T, Mousa SA, et al. Antagonists of integrin alpha v beta 3 inhibit retinal neovascularization in a murine model. Lab Invest 1996;75:563–73.
228. Kamizuru H, Kimura H, Yasukawa T, et al. Monoclonal antibody-mediated drug targeting to choroidal neovascularization in the rat. Invest Ophthalmol Vis Sci 2001;42:2664–72.
229. Lahdenranta J, Sidman RL, Pasqualini R, et al. Treatment of hypoxia-induced retinopathy with targeted proapoptotic peptidomimetic in a mouse model of disease. FASEB J 2007;21:3272–8.
230. Umeda N, Kachi S, Akiyama H, et al. Suppression and regression of choroidal neovascularization by systemic administration of an alpha5beta1 integrin antagonist. Mol Pharmacol 2006;69:1820–8.
231. Zahn G, Vossmeyer D, Stragies R, et al. Preclinical evaluation of the novel small-molecule integrin alpha5beta1 inhibitor JSM6427 in monkey and rabbit models of choroidal neovascularization. Arch Ophthalmol 2009;127:1329–35.
232. Wang W, Wang F, Lu F, et al. The anti-angiogenic effects of integrin $\alpha5\beta1$ inhibitor (ATN-161) in vitro and in vivo. Invest Ophthalmol Vis Sci 2011;52:7213–20.
233. Maier AK, Kociok N, Zahn G, et al. Modulation of hypoxia-induced neovascularization by JSM6427, an integrin alpha5beta1 inhibiting molecule. Curr Eye Res 2007;32:801–12.
234. Muether PS, Dell S, Kociok N, et al. The role of integrin alpha5beta1 in the regulation of corneal neovascularization. Exp Eye Res 2007;85:356–65.
235. Kuwada SK. Drug evaluation: Volociximab, an angiogenesis-inhibiting chimeric monoclonal antibody. Curr Opin Mol Ther 2007;9:92–8.
236. Gomis-Ruth FX, Maskos K, Betz M, et al. Mechanism of inhibition of the human matrix metalloproteinase stromelysin-1 by TIMP-1. Nature 1997;389:77–81.
237. Garcia C, Bartsch DU, Rivero ME, et al. Efficacy of Prinomastat (AG3340), a matrix metalloprotease inhibitor, in treatment of retinal neovascularization. Curr Eye Res 2002;24:33–8.
238. Nambu H, Nambu R, Melia M, et al. Combretastatin A-4 phosphate suppresses development and induces regression of choroidal neovascularization. Invest Ophthalmol Vis Sci 2003;44:3650–5.
239. Genaidy M, Kazi AA, Peyman GA, et al. Effect of squalamine on iris neovascularization in monkeys. Retina 2002;22:772–8.
240. Jones SR, Kinney WA, Zhang X, et al. The synthesis and characterization of analogs of the antimicrobial compound squalamine: 6 beta-hydroxy-3-aminosterols synthesized from hyodeoxycholic acid. Steroids 1996;61:565–71.
241. Higgins RD, Yan Y, Geng Y, et al. Regression of retinopathy by squalamine in a mouse model. Pediatr Res 2004;56:144–9.
242. Spaide RF, Sorenson J, Maranan L. Combined photodynamic therapy with verteporfin and intravitreal triamcinolone acetonide for choroidal neovascularization. Ophthalmology 2003;110:1517–25.
243. Spaide RF, Sorenson J, Maranan L. Photodynamic therapy with verteporfin combined with intravitreal injection of triamcinolone acetonide for choroidal neovascularization. Ophthalmology 2005;112:301–4.
244. Chan A, Blumenkranz MS, Wu KH, et al. Photodynamic therapy with and without adjunctive intravitreal triamcinolone acetonide: a retrospective comparative study. Ophthalmic Surg Lasers Imaging 2009;40:561–9.
245. Chaudhary V, Mao A, Hooper PL, et al. Triamcinolone acetonide as adjunctive treatment to verteporfin in neovascular age-related macular degeneration: a prospective randomized trial. Ophthalmology 2007;114:2183–9.
246. Luttrull JK, Spink CJ. Prolongation of choroidal hypofluorescence following combined verteporfin photodynamic therapy and intravitreal triamcinolone acetonide injection. Retina 2007;27:688–92.
247. Maberley D. Photodynamic therapy and intravitreal triamcinolone for neovascular age-related macular degeneration: a randomized clinical trial. Ophthalmology 2009;116:2149–57.
248. Hatta Y, Ishikawa K, Nishihara H, et al. Effect of photodynamic therapy alone or combined with posterior subtenon triamcinolone acetonide or intravitreal bevacizumab on choroidal hypofluorescence by indocyanine green angiography. Retina 2010;30:495–502.
249 Kovacs KD, Quirk MT, Kinoshita T, et al. A retrospective analysis of triple combination therapy with intravitreal bevacizumab, posterior sub-tenon's triamcinolone acetonide, and low-fluence verteporfin photodynamic therapy in patients with neovascular age-related macular degeneration. Retina 2011;31:446–52.
250. Liggett PE, Colina J, Chaudhry NA, et al. Triple therapy of intravitreal triamcinolone, photodynamic therapy, and pegaptanib sodium for choroidal neovascularization. Am J Ophthalmol 2006;142:1072–4.
251. Arias L, Garcia-Arumi J, Ramon JM, et al. Photodynamic therapy with intravitreal triamcinolone in predominantly classic choroidal neovascularization: one-year results of a randomized study. Ophthalmology 2006;113:2243–50.
252. Arias L, Garcia-Arumi J, Ramon JM, et al. Optical coherence tomography analysis of a randomized study combining photodynamic therapy with intravitreal triamcinolone. Graefes Arch Clin Exp Ophthalmol 2008;246:245–54.
253. Napoli KL, Taylor PJ. From beach to bedside: history of the development of sirolimus. Ther Drug Monit 2001;23:559–86.
254. Guba M, von Breitenbuch P, Steinbauer M, et al. Rapamycin inhibits primary and metastatic tumor growth by antiangiogenesis: involvement of vascular endothelial growth factor. Nat Med 2002;8:128–35.
255. Dejneka NS, Kuroki AM, Fosnot J, et al. Systemic rapamycin inhibits retinal and choroidal neovascularization in mice. Mol Vis 2004;10:964–72.
256. Nussenblatt RB, Byrnes G, Sen HN, et al. A randomized pilot study of systemic immunosuppression in the treatment of age-related macular degeneration with choroidal neovascularization. Retina 2010;30:1579–87.
257. Woodburn KW, Engelman CJ, Blumenkranz MS. Photodynamic therapy for choroidal neovascularization: a review. Retina 2002;22:391–405;quiz 527–8.
258. Flower RW, von Kerczek C, Zhu L, et al. Theoretical investigation of the role of choriocapillaris blood flow in treatment of subfoveal choroidal neovascularization associated with age-related macular degeneration. Am J Ophthalmol 2001;132:85–93.
259. Husain D, Kramer M, Kenny AG, et al. Effects of photodynamic therapy using verteporfin on experimental choroidal neovascularization and normal retina and choroid up to 7 weeks after treatment. Invest Ophthalmol Vis Sci 1999;40:2322–31.
260. Husain D, Miller JW, Michaud N, et al. Intravenous infusion of liposomal benzoporphyrin derivative for photodynamic therapy of experimental choroidal neovascularization. Arch Ophthalmol 1996;114:978–85.
261. Kramer M, Miller JW, Michaud N, et al. Liposomal benzoporphyrin derivative verteporfin photodynamic therapy. Selective treatment of choroidal neovascularization in monkeys. Ophthalmology 1996;103:427–38.
262. Miller JW, Walsh AW, Kramer M, et al. Photodynamic therapy of experimental choroidal neovascularization using lipoprotein-delivered benzoporphyrin. Arch Ophthalmol 1995;113:810–8.
263. Miller JW, Schmidt-Erfurth U, Sickenberg M, et al. Photodynamic therapy with verteporfin for choroidal neovascularization caused by age-related macular degeneration: results of a single treatment in a phase 1 and 2 study. Arch Ophthalmol 1999;117:1161–73.
264. Schmidt-Erfurth U, Miller JW, Sickenberg M, et al. Photodynamic therapy with verteporfin for choroidal neovascularization caused by age-related macular degeneration: results of retreatments in a phase 1 and 2 study. Arch Ophthalmol 1999;117:1177–87.

265. Photodynamic therapy of subfoveal choroidal neovascularization in pathologic myopia with verteporfin. 1-year results of a randomized clinical trial – VIP report no. 1. Ophthalmology 2001;108:841–52.
266. Blumenkranz MS, Bressler NM, Bressler SB, et al. Verteporfin therapy for subfoveal choroidal neovascularization in age-related macular degeneration: three-year results of an open-label extension of 2 randomized clinical trials – TAP Report no. 5. Arch Ophthalmol 2002;120:1307–14.
267. Blinder KJ, Bradley S, Bressler NM, et al. Effect of lesion size, visual acuity, and lesion composition on visual acuity change with and without verteporfin therapy for choroidal neovascularization secondary to age-related macular degeneration: TAP and VIP report no. 1. Am J Ophthalmol 2003;136:407–18.
268. Mathis S, Khanlari B, Pulido F, et al. Effectiveness of protease inhibitor monotherapy versus combination antiretroviral maintenance therapy: a meta-analysis. PLoS One 2011;6:e22003.
269. Klement G, Baruchel S, Rak J, et al. Continuous low-dose therapy with vinblastine and VEGF receptor-2 antibody induces sustained tumor regression without overt toxicity. J Clin Invest 2000;105:R15–24.
270. Lee CG, Heijn M, di Tomaso E, et al. Anti-vascular endothelial growth factor treatment augments tumor radiation response under normoxic or hypoxic conditions. Cancer Res 2000;60:5565–70.
271. Piermarocchi S, Sartore M, Lo Giudice G, et al. Combination of photodynamic therapy and intraocular triamcinolone for exudative age-related macular degeneration and long-term chorioretinal macular atrophy. Arch Ophthalmol 2008;126:1367–74.
272. Roth DB, Kulkarni KM, Walsman S, et al. Intravitreal triamcinolone acetonide preceding photodynamic therapy for exudative age-related macular degeneration. Ophthalmic Surg Lasers Imaging 2009;40:467–71.
273. Sacu S, Michels S, Prager F, et al. Randomised clinical trial of intravitreal Avastin vs photodynamic therapy and intravitreal triamcinolone: long-term results. Eye (Lond) 2009;23:2223–7.
274. Augustin AJ, Puls S, Offermann I. Triple therapy for choroidal neovascularization due to age-related macular degeneration: verteporfin PDT, bevacizumab, and dexamethasone. Retina 2007;27:133–40.
275. Bakri SJ, Couch SM, McCannel CA, et al. Same-day triple therapy with photodynamic therapy, intravitreal dexamethasone, and bevacizumab in wet age-related macular degeneration. Retina 2009;29:573–8.
276. Kaiser PK, Boyer DS, Garcia R, et al. Verteporfin photodynamic therapy combined with intravitreal bevacizumab for neovascular age-related macular degeneration. Ophthalmology 2009;116:747–55.
277. Forte R, Bonavolonta P, Benayoun Y, et al. Intravitreal ranibizumab and bevacizumab in combination with full-fluence verteporfin therapy and dexamethasone for exudative age-related macular degeneration. Ophthalmic Res 2011; 45:129–34.
278. Azab M, Boyer DS, Bressler NM, et al. Verteporfin therapy of subfoveal minimally classic choroidal neovascularization in age-related macular degeneration: 2-year results of a randomized clinical trial. Arch Ophthalmol 2005;123:448–57.
279. Schmidt-Erfurth U, Michels S, Barbazetto I, et al. Photodynamic effects on choroidal neovascularization and physiological choroid. Invest Ophthalmol Vis Sci 2002;43:830–41.
280. Schmidt-Erfurth U, Schlotzer-Schrehard U, Cursiefen C, et al. Influence of photodynamic therapy on expression of vascular endothelial growth factor (VEGF), VEGF receptor 3, and pigment epithelium-derived factor. Invest Ophthalmol Vis Sci 2003;44:4473–80.
281. Lim JY, Lee SY, Kim JG, et al. Intravitreal bevacizumab alone versus in combination with photodynamic therapy for the treatment of neovascular maculopathy in patients aged 50 years or older: 1-year results of a prospective clinical study. Acta Ophthalmol 2012;90:61–7.
282. Kaiser PK, Boyer DS, Cruess AF, et al. Verteporfin plus ranibizumab for choroidal neovascularization in age-related macular degeneration: Twelve-month results of the DENALI Study. Ophthalmology 2012;119:1001–10.
283. Larsen M, Schmidt-Erfurth U, Lanzetta P, et al. Verteporfin plus ranibizumab for choroidal neovascularization in age-related macular degeneration: Twelve-month MONT BLANC Study Results. Ophthalmology 2012;119: 992–1000.
284. RADICAL demonstrated fewer retreatment visits for AMD combination therapy. Retina Today: Bryn Mawr Communications LLC, 2010.
285. Avila MP, Farah ME, Santos A, et al. Twelve-month short-term safety and visual-acuity results from a multicentre prospective study of epiretinal strontium-90 brachytherapy with bevacizumab for the treatment of subfoveal choroidal neovascularisation secondary to age-related macular degeneration. Br J Ophthalmol 2009;93:305–9.
286. Avila MP, Farah ME, Santos A, et al. Twelve-month safety and visual acuity results from a feasibility study of intraocular, epiretinal radiation therapy for the treatment of subfoveal CNV secondary to AMD. Retina 2009;29: 157–69.
287. Moshfeghi DM, Kaiser PK, Gertner M. Stereotactic low-voltage x-ray irradiation for age-related macular degeneration. Br J Ophthalmol 2011;95:185–8.

Chapter 68

Myopic Macular Degeneration

Kyoko Ohno-Matsui, Yasushi Ikuno, Miho Yasuda, Toshinori Murata, Taiji Sakamoto, Tatsuro Ishibashi

Pathologic myopia is a major cause of legal blindness and low vision worldwide,[1-5] and its prevalence is increasing in modern society, presumably due to an increase of near activities. In patients with pathologic myopia, various kinds of myopic macular degeneration develop in the posterior fundus, and these are the cause of visual impairment.[6,7] There are new ideas concerning the pathogenesis of pathologic myopia and novel treatments for myopic macular degeneration. Although myopic macular degeneration had been an incurable degenerative disorder, the recent application of photodynamic therapy (PDT) with verteporfin and anti-vascular endothelial growth factor (VEGF) therapy has enabled treatment of myopic choroidal neovascularization (CNV). With these advances, myopic macular degeneration is now a curable disorder in some patients to some extent. Importantly, a novel pathology called "myopic macular retinoschisis" has been described using optical coherence tomography (OCT).[8] The OCT examinations showed that retinoschisis was present in some eyes with pathologic myopia before the development of myopic macular holes. With the description of myopic macular retinoschisis, vitrectomy has been actively performed to reduce the chance of progression to more serious conditions like macular holes or macular retinal detachment.

EPIDEMIOLOGY

Myopia is more common among Asian populations, especially in East Asian countries, than among white, black, or Hispanic people. The prevalence of myopia (spherical equivalent (SE) < −0.5 or −1.0 D) is reported to range from 17% to 43% among Asian populations.[9-17] Among white populations in Europe, the USA, and Australia, it is reported to be between 13% and 27%.[18-21] In Hispanic and black populations, it is reported to be 17% and 21%, respectively.[19, 22] The prevalence of high myopia (SE < −5.0 or −6.0 D) is also greater in Asian populations, ranging from 1.7% to 9.1%, than that in white, Hispanic, and black populations (2.0%, 2.4%, and 1.0%, respectively) (Table 68.1).[9-22]

Pathologic myopia is one of the major causes of visual impairment and blindness worldwide. For example, myopic macular degeneration is the leading cause of blindness in Japan, the second most common cause in Denmark[4] and in China,[23] and the third cause of blindness in Latinos 40 years and older in USA.[3,] Myopic macular degeneration was the leading cause of impaired vision for persons aged between 55 and 75 years in the Netherlands.[3,23,24] In Italy and Taiwan, it is the second most common cause of low vision.[25,26] The impact of myopic retinopathy on visual impairment is of great concern because it is often bilateral and irreversible, and it frequently affects individuals during their most productive years.[7,27]

To date, three population-based studies have estimated the prevalence of myopic retinopathy. The Blue Mountains Eye Study in Australia, which focused on a white population, reported that the prevalence of myopic retinopathy was 1.2%.[27] In the Beijing Eye Study in China and the Hisayama Study in Japan, the prevalence was 3.1% and 1.7%, respectively.[28a] Study participants' characteristics, methodology, and study design (for example, the definition of myopic retinopathy) were different between those studies, therefore the precise racial difference in myopic retinopathy prevalence is unknown. But it may be higher in East Asian populations than in white populations and the prevalence of high myopia is probably higher as well (Table 68.2).

The prevalence of myopic retinopathy is increased with advancing age in those population-based studies. Histological studies have shown a decreased density of photoreceptors, ganglion cells, retinal pigment epithelium (RPE), and optic nerve fibers with age.[29,30] Several studies using OCT have examined subjects with healthy eyes with neither high myopia nor hyperopia and reported a negative relationship between retinal thickness and age.[31,32] In addition to the axial elongation of the eyeball in highly myopic eyes, increasing age may contribute to the pathogenesis of myopic retinopathy by causing retinal thinning.

Although it is reported that men have longer axial length than women,[33,34] many hospital-based studies showed higher prevalence of myopic retinopathy in women than in men.[35-37] For example, Hayashi et al. showed that, of 429 consecutive patients with pathologic myopia, 147 were men and 282 were women, which is about twice as many cases in women as in men.[7] Comparable findings were also observed in population-based studies. In the Blue Mountains Eye Study, the prevalence of myopic retinopathy in men was 0.06% and that in women was 0.4%. In the Hisayama Study, the prevalence of myopic retinopathy in men and in women was 1.2% and 2.2%, respectively. The Beijing Eye Study did not report the prevalence of myopic retinopathy by sex, but the numbers of female/male subjects with and without myopic retinopathy were 75/57 and 570/489, respectively. It suggests that not only greater axial length but other risk factors such as genetic factors and lifestyle risk factors may contribute to the pathogenesis of myopic retinopathy.

PATHOGENESIS

Hereditary or genetic factors play important roles in the development of pathologic myopia. There is a large international linkage study on familial high myopia, in which linkage analyses were performed on 1201 samples from Asian, African American,

Table 68.1 Comparison of prevalence of myopia in population-based studies

Study	Country	Age (years)	Myopia <–0.5D (%)	Myopia <–1.0D (%)	High myopia <–5.0D (%)	High myopia <–6.0D (%)
Beaver Dam Eye Study	United States (white subjects)	≥43	27.4			
Baltimore Eye Survey	United States (white subjects)	≥40	24.8			2.0
Baltimore Eye Survey	United States (black subjects)	≥40	21.0			1.0
Los Angeles Latino Eye Study	United States (Latino subjects)	≥40		16.8		2.4
Blue Mountains Eye Study	Australia (white subjects)	≥49	14.4			
Visual Impairment Project	Australia (white subjects)	≥40	16.9	12.8		
Andhra Pradesh Eye Disease Study	India (Indian subjects)	≥40	28.2			
Sumatra, Indonesia	Indonesia (Indonesian subjects)	≥40	34.1	22.4		1.7
Tanjong Pagar	Singapore (Chinese subjects)	≥40	38.7	31.9	9.1	
Singapore Malay Eye Survey	Singapore (Malay subjects)	≥40	26.2	20.2	3.9	
National Survey	Bangladesh (Bangladeshi subjects)	≥30	25.5	19.7	3.0	
Meiktila Eye Study	Myanmar (Burmese subjects)	≥40		42.7		6.5
Mongolia	Mongolia (Mongolian subjects)	≥40	17.2		2.7	
Beijing Eye Study	China (Chinese subjects)	≥40	21.8	16.9	3.3	
Tajimi Study	Japan (Japanese subjects)	≥40	41.8	32.4	8.2	5.5
Hisayama Study	Japan (Japanese subjects)	≥40	37.7		5.7	3.6

and Caucasian families, finding that the MYP1, MYP3, MYP6, MYP11, MYP12, and MYP14 loci were replicated.[38] Recent genomewide studies identified susceptibility loci at 15q14 and 15q25 for myopia.[39,40] However, the genetic influence on the development of myopic macular degeneration is not clear. The genetic risk factors of age-related macular degeneration related to rs11200638 of HTRA1, and rs1061170 (Y402H) of complement factor H did not appear to contribute significantly to the development of CNV in a highly myopic elderly Japanese population.[41] It was reported that the responsiveness of myopic CNV to PDT had a correlation with common coagulation balance gene polymorphisms.[42]

Various factors, such as aging, and biomechanical factors in addition to hereditary factors, have been considered to contribute to the development of myopic macular degeneration in highly myopic eyes.[43–45] Excessive axial elongation and posterior staphyloma (defined below) formation are critical features of pathologic myopia and these are considered important for the development and progression of myopic macular degeneration.[44] Large-scale studies show that a peripapillary crescent, chorioretinal atrophy, and posterior staphyloma are significantly related to increased axial length.[28,44] Above all, the incidence, size, and type of peripapillary crescent have the strongest correlation with the axial length;[6,44] more than 95% of eyes with an axial length of 26.5 mm or more have a peripapillary crescent, while 0% of eyes with an axial length of 21.4 mm or less have a peripapillary crescent.[44] Chorioretinal atrophy has also been related directly to increased axial length.

In addition to the influence of biomechanical factors, aging is an important factor for the development of posterior staphyloma and subsequent myopic macular degeneration. A posterior staphyloma is rarely found in highly myopic patients younger than 40 years of age.[46] The posterior staphyloma develops as patients age, and this accelerates the further mechanical extension of the posterior fundus and causes the development of myopic macular degeneration. The incidence of myopic chorioretinal atrophy increases with age, and these changes are rarely seen in persons less than 20 years old.[6,44] Childhood high myopes do not develop myopic macular degeneration or posterior staphyloma.[47]

The development of myopic CNV and lacquer cracks is not directly correlated with axial length. The incidence of myopic

Table 68.2 Comparison of prevalence of myopic retinopathy in population-based studies

Study	Participants	Prevalence of myopic retinopathy	Definition of myopic retinopathy	
Blue Mountains Eye Study (Australia)	n = 3653 Age ≥49 years	1.2%	Staphyloma	0.7%
			Chorioretinal atrophy	0.2%
			Fuchs spot	0.1%
			Lacquer cracks	0.2%
Beijing Eye Study (China)	n = 4319 Age ≥40 years	3.1%	Staphyloma	1.6%
			Chorioretinal atrophy	3.1%
			Fuchs spot	0.1%
			Lacquer cracks	0.2%
Hisayama Study (Japan)	n = 1890 Age ≥40 years	4.6%	Diffuse chorioretinal atrophy	1.7%
			Patchy chorioretinal atrophy	0.4%
			Lacquer cracks	0.2%
			Macular atrophy	0.4%

CNV peaks in the fourth decade. There may be biological mechanisms of neovascular membrane formation other than axial elongation or aging.[6] Steidl and Pruett[48] reported that eyes with a shallow staphyloma had the high frequency of CNV. They suggested that it is possible that eyes with a shallow staphyloma may be healthier and more metabolically active with well-perfused chorioretinal tissue and good capacity to respond to injury by neovascular ingrowth. It appears that the influence of aging and mechanical factors is rather complicated and different lesions may have different pathogenetic influences.

HISTOPATHOLOGY

The sclera

Scleral thinning and localized ectasia of the posterior sclera are characteristic changes of the eyes with pathologic myopia. Microscopically, the normal sclera consists of interwoven bands or bundles of collagen fibers.[43] These are usually well integrated and in longitudinal section present a relatively homogeneous appearance throughout their extent. The architectural changes in the longitudinal fibers in pathologic myopia consist of thinning of the collagen bundles, a reduction in refringence of the bundle edges, and the loss of longitudinal fiber striations. The cross-sectional fibers demonstrate dissociation such that the individual fibers separate from one another. There is also a reduction in the size of the individual dissociated fibers. The more advanced examples of architectural disorganization are found in and about the regions of the posterior pole and peripapillary sclera. It has also been reported that the elastic fibers within the sclera showed a definite decrease in the number of fibers.

Electron microscopic analyses showed that a predominance of collagen fibrils of small diameter, usually averaging below 60–70 nm, was found.[43] Fibrils of a very fine diameter were also observed. Also, the cross-sectioned fibrils showed a marked increase in the prevalence of fissured or "star-shaped" forms. Most of the ultramicroscopic alterations seen in the myopic sclera indicate a derangement of the growth and organization of the fibrils. These may be products of defective fibrillogenesis. These aspects of development are thought to be under the control of the acidic glycosaminoglycan composition of the interfibrillar substance. It is also conceivable that this picture corresponds to abnormal fibril growth in the presence of an accentuated breakdown or catabolism of the sclera.

Choroid and retinal pigment epithelium

The degenerative changes found in pathologic myopia initially appear to involve the choriocapillaris – Bruch's membrane – RPE complex. The changes subsequently affecting the choroid were essentially degenerative and atrophic. Thinning of the choroid and loss of the choriocapillaris were reported. Choroidal vascular occlusions are a prominent feature of the disease, and this process appears to affect the smaller-diameter vessels initially. The choroidal vessels appear to be fewer and to have thinner walls than seen normally. There is a generalized loss of the normal connective tissue framework of the choroid with some degree of compaction of the vessels. Although the large-sized choroidal vessels tend to be most resistant, these, too, may undergo occlusion in the late stages of the disease. Recent studies using enhanced-depth imaging of OCT or high-penetrance OCT also showed significant thinning of the choroid in highly myopic eyes.[49]

The RPE cells are seen to be flatter and larger than usual, a possible consequence of passive expansion. Hyperpigmentation, hypopigmentation, and multilayered clumping of the RPE cells may also be seen. Bruch's membrane may show a variety of changes, including thinning, splitting, and rupture. These ruptures of Bruch's membrane can be seen clinically as "lacquer cracks."

ANIMAL MODELS

Rhesus monkeys, chickens, fish, tree shrews, marmosets, and guinea pigs have long been used as animal models of experimental myopia by inducing form deprivation myopia by lid suture or by wearing plastic goggles (Figs 68.1 and 68.2).[50–52] Chicks have long been the main animal model for experimental myopia because myopia accompanying a dramatic increase of the axial length can be induced easily by wearing plastic goggles in about 2 weeks.[53] Therefore, many studies were performed using chick models of experimental myopia; these studies identified responsible factors which cause excessive eye growth. However the sclera of chickens differs from that of humans. The chicken has the classic vertebrate sclera, consisting of a layer of cartilage surrounded by layers of fibrous connective tissue, whereas in most mammals, including primates and rodents, the cartilage has been lost.

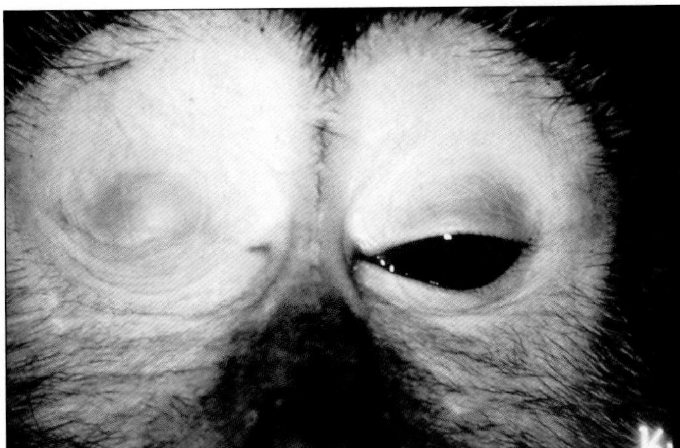

Fig. 68.1 Monkey model of experimental myopia. Form deprivation myopia is induced by lid fusion in neonate monkeys. (Courtesy of Prof. Takashi Tokoro.)

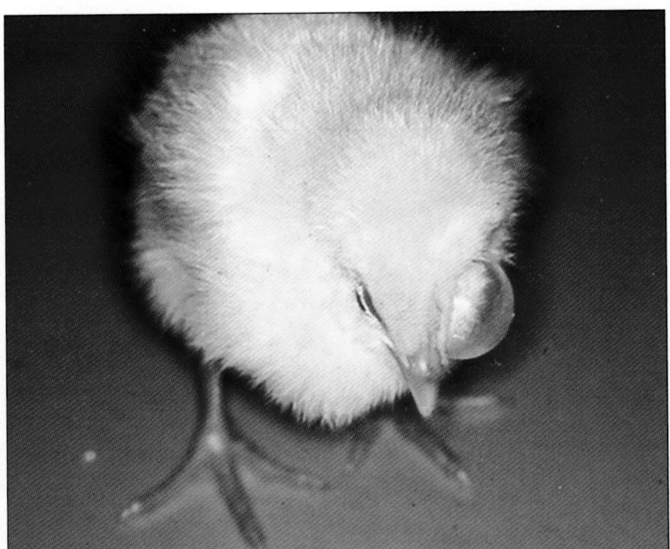

Fig. 68.2 Chick models of experimental myopia. One eye is covered by plastic goggle to induce blurred image on the retina. (Courtesy of Prof. Takashi Tokoro.)

Based on the benefit of having similar scleral components, mice have commonly been used as examples of experimental myopia (Fig. 68.3),[54,55] although there is some drawback that the induced myopia is not as severe as in chickens because mice are not "visual animals." Mouse model advantages also include the availability of numerous knockout mutants, more advanced gene microarrays for screening the transcriptome, and a completely sequenced genome.

The transcriptome of neurosensory retina without RPE was analyzed with Affymetrix GeneChip mouse genome 430 2.0 arrays after unilateral retinal image degradation by use of frosted goggles in mice,[56] and some genes were identified as being altered, including a downregulation of the early growth response 1 (*Egr*-1) gene. The refractions of homozygous *Egr*-1 knockout mice were some 4–5 D less hyperopic relative to the wild type.[58] Zebrafish have also been considered as a model of experimental myopia. Downregulation of zebrafish lumican gene expression manifested ocular enlargement resembling axial myopia due to disruption of the collagen fibril arrangement in the sclera and resulted in scleral thinning.[58] The lumican gene, which encodes one of the major keratan sulfate proteoglycans in the vertebrate cornea and sclera, has been linked to axial myopia in humans. Veth and colleagues[59] have used zebrafish to identify a genetically complex, recessive mutant that shows risk factors for glaucoma, including adult-onset severe myopia, elevated intraocular pressure, and progressive retinal ganglion cell pathology. Positional cloning and analysis of a noncomplementing allele indicated that nonsense mutations in low-density lipoprotein receptor-related protein 2 (lrp2) underlie the mutant phenotype.

FEATURES OF THE MYOPIC FUNDUS

We understand "pathologic myopia" to mean myopia which develops retinal pathology due to axial elongation. Posterior staphyloma is one pathology in pathologic myopia and not all eyes with pathologic myopia have staphyloma (especially in younger patients). Posterior staphyloma tends to develop at around the age of 40 and is discussed below.

Myopic conus

Myopic conus is one of the earliest features which develop in the posterior fundus of highly myopic eyes. Due to a mechanical

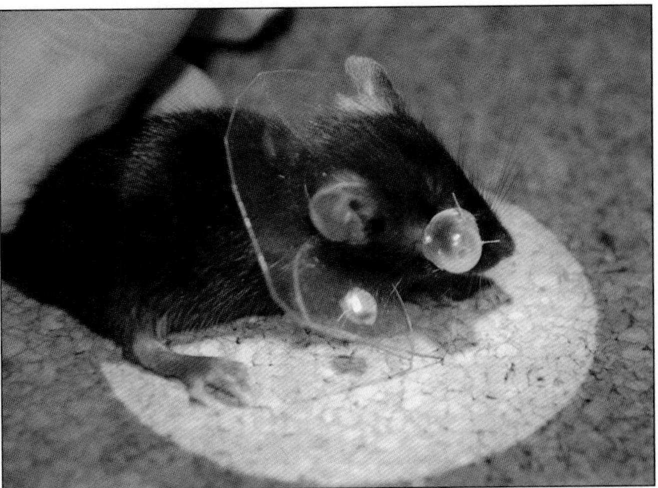

Fig. 68.3 Mouse models of experimental myopia. One eye is covered by plastic goggle to induce blurred image on the retina.

expansion in the peripapillary sclera, the optic disc in eyes with pathologic myopia is surrounded by a concentric area of depigmentation, the so-called myopic conus. The myopic crescent usually appears as a white, sharply defined area where the inner surface of the sclera is seen distinctly (Fig. 68.4). According to its range, the myopic conus is divided into the temporal conus, the nasal conus, the inferior conus, and the annular conus (Fig. 68.4). Sometimes the myopic conus becomes remarkably large. The myopic conus and tesselated fundus are the earliest lesions which develop in eyes with pathologic myopia, and these lesions can be observed even in children and young individuals.[47] When we perform indocyanine green angiography, we see the Zinn – Haller arterial ring in the middle of the myopic conus in eyes with a large annular conus (Fig. 68.5).[60,61] The inner zone of myopic conus might develop as a result of mechanical stretching, and the outer zone might be the result of a secondary circulatory disturbance and mechanical stretching.

Posterior staphyloma

A posterior staphyloma is an outward protrusion of all layers of the posterior eye globe and is considered a hallmark lesion of pathological myopia. There are 10 different types of staphyloma according to Curtin (Fig. 68.6).[62] Types I through V are basic staphylomas, and types VI through X are compound staphylomas. A posterior staphyloma is not common in children with pathologic myopia, and the incidence of staphyloma is

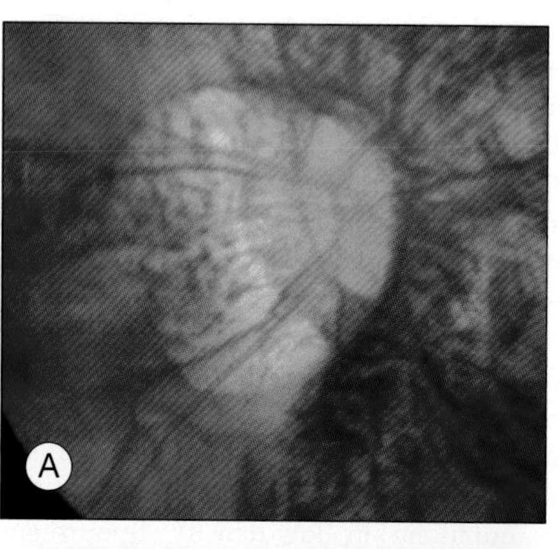

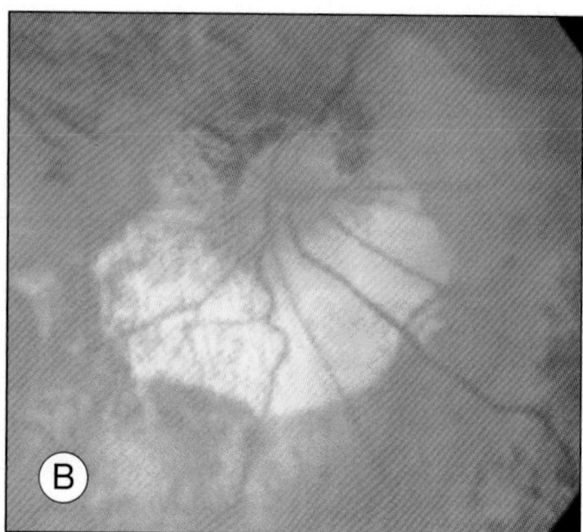

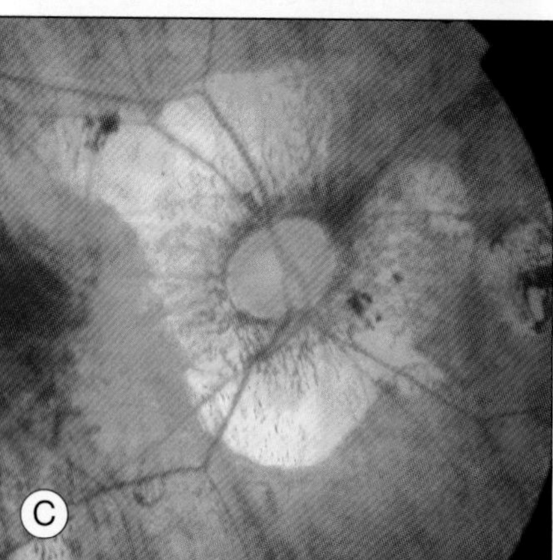

Fig. 68.4 Various types of myopic conus. (A) Temporal conus; (B) inferior conus; (C) annular or ring conus.

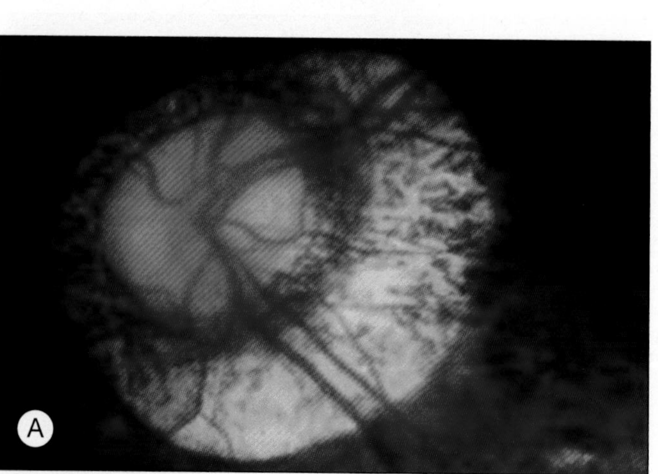

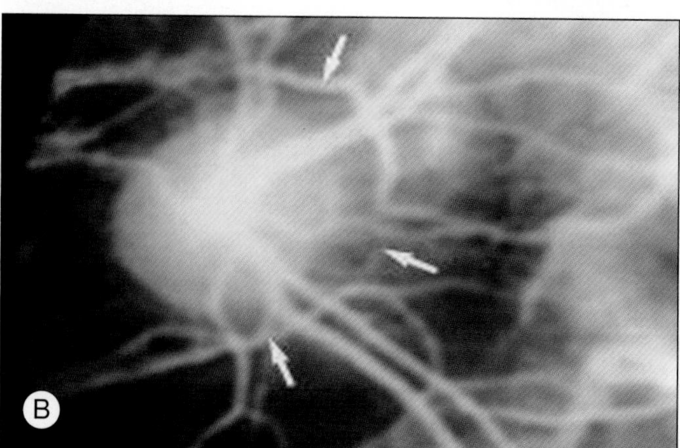

Fig. 68.5 Zinn – Haller arterial ring observed within myopic conus. (A) Disc photograph shows ring conus. The conus seems to be divided into a pigmented inner zone and white outer zone. (B) Indocyanine green angiography shows the circular course of intrascleral branches of short posterior ciliary arteries (arrows).

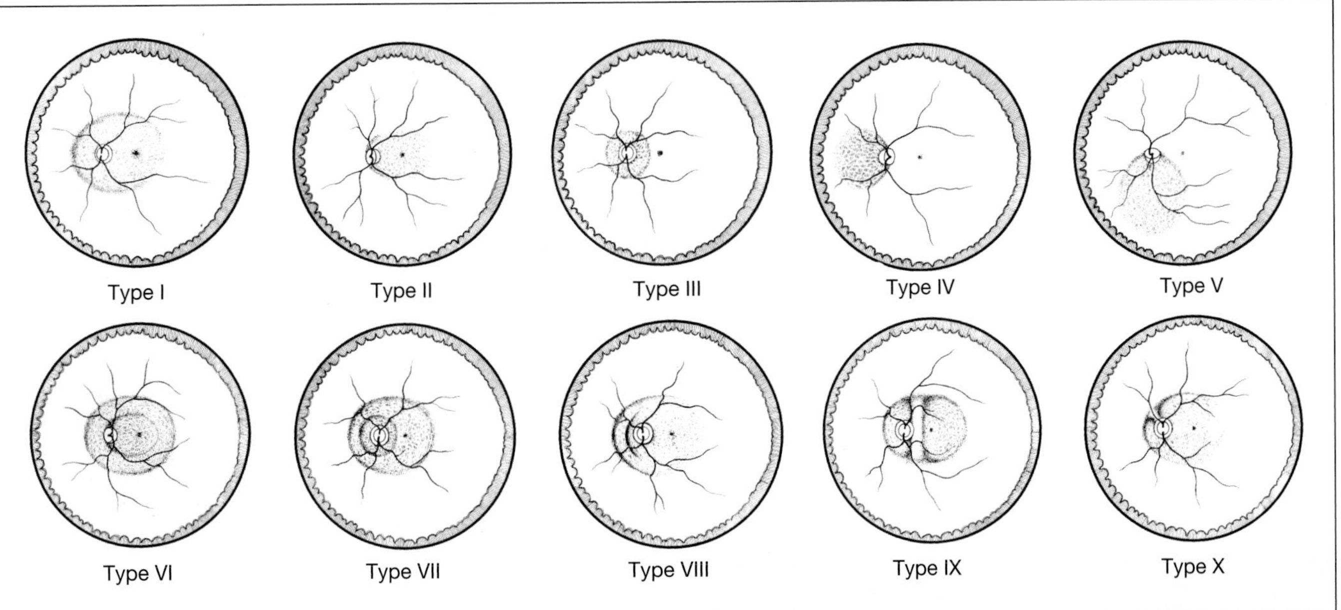

Fig. 68.6 Classification of posterior staphyloma according to Curtin.

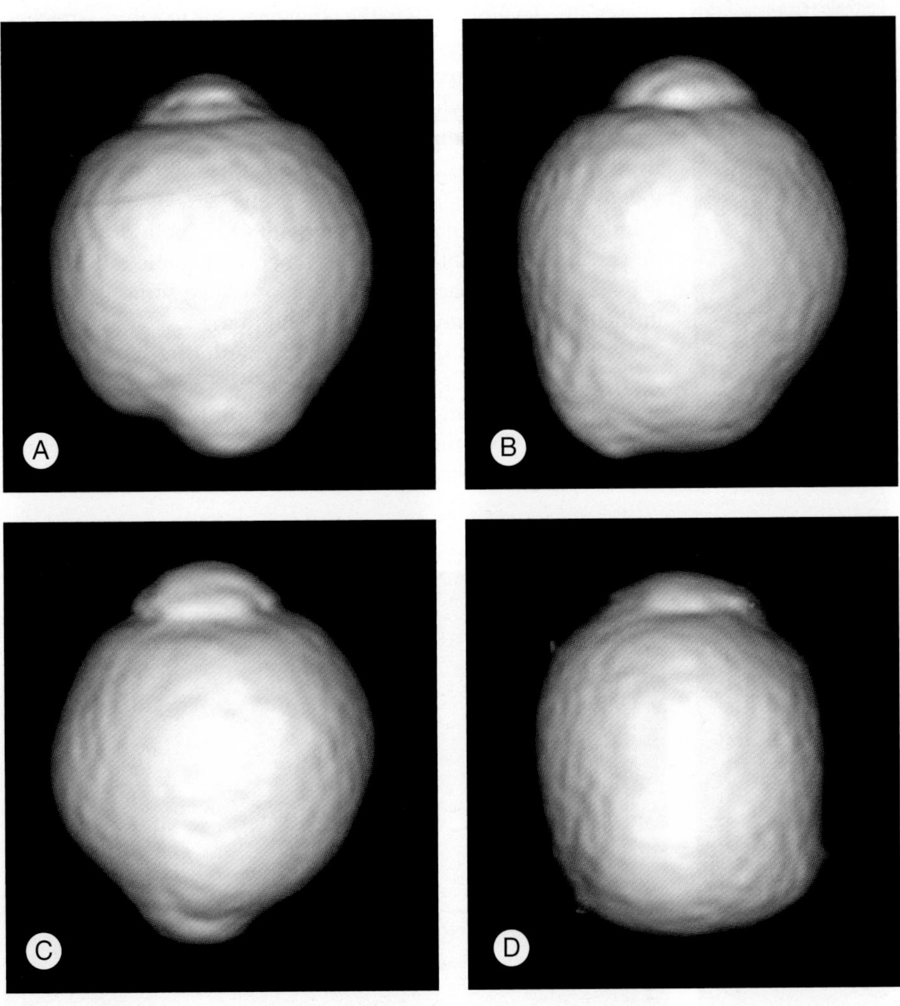

Fig. 68.7 Classification of eye shape of highly myopic eyes based on three-dimensional magnetic resonance imaging analyses by Moriyama and Ohno-Matsui. These are the images of the right eye viewed from inferiorly. (A) Nasally distorted type; (B) temporally distorted type; (C) cylinder type; (D) barrel type.

significantly higher in older patients (96.7% in those ≥50 years of age) than in younger patients (80.7% in those <50 years).[46] Earlier studies on human cadaver eyes suggested the possibility that eyes with pathologic myopia were not simply elongated but were deformed and did not have a spherical shape.

With the development of three-dimensional magnetic resonance imaging analysis of human globes in highly myopic patients, it is possible to demonstrate distinctly different shapes of eyes with pathologic myopia (Fig. 68.7).[63] This clearly supports the idea that pathologic myopia is a disease accompanied by deformity of the globe. The eye is an exact optical device and the fact that its shape is different from normal spherical shape could cause serious visual problems. The correlation between specific eye shape in eyes with pathologic myopia and its effect on visual impairment are now being investigated.

Myopic chorioretinal atrophy

Two types of myopic chorioretinal atrophy develop in the posterior fundus. According to Tokoro, there is diffuse chorioretinal atrophy and patchy chorioretinal atrophy.[6] Diffuse chorioretinal atrophy is observed as yellowish-white and ill-defined chorioretinal atrophy (Fig. 68.8), and patchy chorioretinal atrophy is observed as grayish-white and well-defined chorioretinal atrophy (Fig. 68.9). Different from diffuse chorioretinal atrophy, the patchy chorioretinal atrophy is caused by complete loss of choriocapillaris and there is a corresponding absolute scotoma.

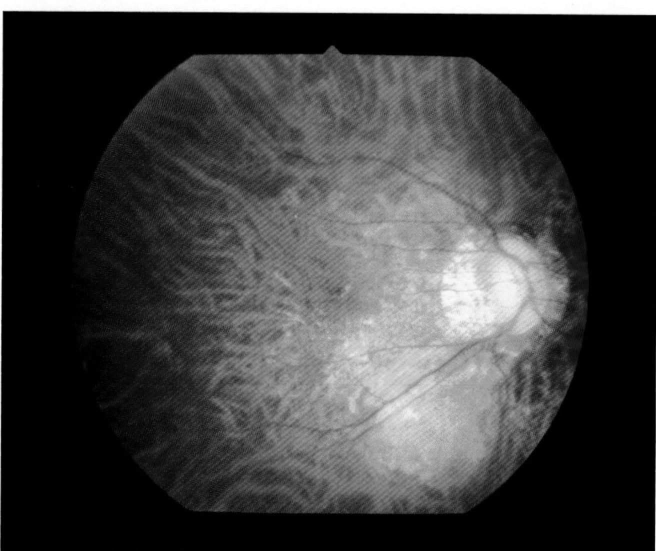

Fig. 68.8 Diffuse chorioretinal atrophy. The posterior fundus appears yellowish.

Lacquer cracks

Lacquer cracks are linear ruptures of Bruch's membrane in the macular area of highly myopic eyes and are observed as yellowish linear lesions in the macula (Fig. 68.10). Lacquer cracks are more easily detected by fluorescein angiography, fundus autofluorescence imaging, and indocyanine green angiography.[64,65] With time, lacquer cracks increase in number and also increase their width.[66] When new lacquer cracks develop, the choriocapillaris is also damaged and subretinal bleeding may occur.[67] Subretinal bleeding without CNV is a visible sign of new lacquer crack formation, and after absorption of bleeding, lacquer cracks appear as yellowish linear lesions. Lacquer cracks are known as precursor lesions of myopic CNV.[65,68] Often, CNV tends to develop along the foveal edge of chorioretinal atrophy which was formed by increased width of lacquer cracks.

Myopic chorodial neovascularization

Macular CNV is a one of the most frequent complications that reduce the central vision in patients with pathologic myopia (Fig. 68.11). Myopic CNV develops in 10% of highly myopic patients,[68] and 30% of the patients who have a CNV in one eye eventually develop CNV in the other eye. Due to a thin, stretched fundus, the bleeding does not usually overlie the CNV and thus, CNV is easily observed ophthalmoscopically. Myopic CNV is almost always so-called classic CNV and CNV shows distinct hyperfluorescence throughout the entire angiographic phase. Especially for small CNV, fluorescein angiography is a powerful tool to detect CNV.

Indocyanine green angiography and OCT, both of which are powerful tools to detect CNV in other angiogenic eye diseases (e.g., age-related macular degeneration) have some limitations in the detection of myopic CNV. Due to the low activity of the CNV, myopic CNV does not show hyperfluorescence by indocyanine green angiography in most cases. OCT shows CNV as an elevated lesion in the subretinal space; however most eyes with myopic CNV do not show exudative changes like retinal edema or retinal detachment. Thus, OCT does not differentiate

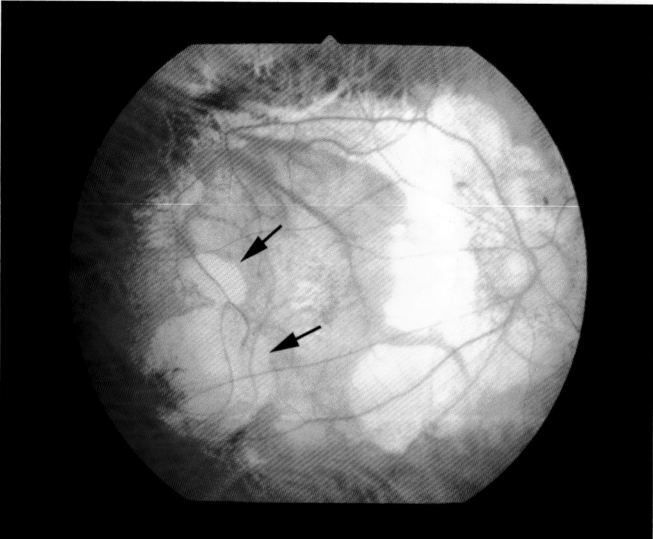

Fig. 68.9 Patchy chorioretinal atrophy. Well-delineated white lesion is observed (arrows).

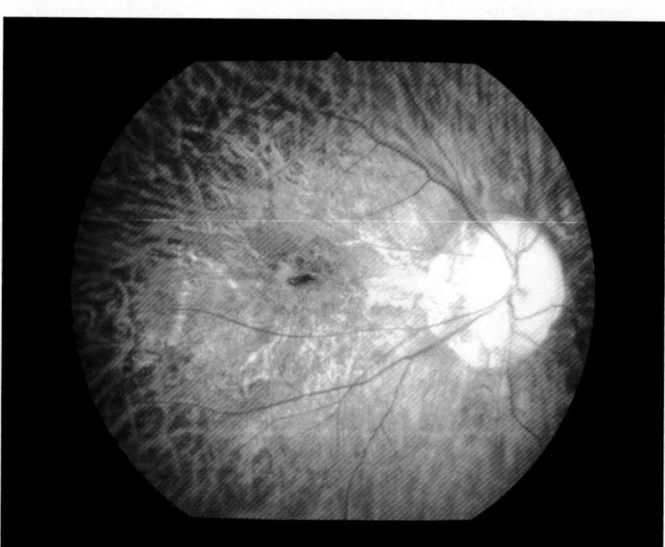

Fig. 68.10 Lacquer cracks. Multiple yellowish linear lesions are observed in the macula.

subretinal bleeding with or without CNV in eyes with pathologic myopia.

Myopic macular retinoschisis or myopic foveoschisis

Myopic macular retinoschisis (also known as myopic foveoschisis[69] or myopic traction maculopathy[70]) was first identified using OCT by Takano and Kishi in 1999.[8] Myopic macular retinoschisis is found in 9% of highly myopic eyes with posterior staphyloma,[71] and 50% of patients progress to more serious complications like full-thickness macular hole or macular retinal detachment within 2 years.[72] Myopic macular retinoschisis is considered to be caused by various factors. The rigidity of the internal limiting membrane (ILM) can induce significant traction on the retina.[4] OCT examinations of serial sections along the entire posterior vascular arcade showed that the paravascular abnormalities, such as paravascular lamellar holes,[73] vascular microfolds,[73-75] and paravascular retinal cysts,[73] are frequently found in eyes with myopic macular retinoschisis. Although the mechanism of the development of this condition is not fully clear, the glial cells like astrocytes which exist abundantly around the retinal vessels can migrate and proliferate through the paravascular lamellar holes. These cells can produce collagen and facilitate the proliferative and contractile response of ILM. Studies have shown that vitrectomy is useful to treat myopic macular retinoschisis in some patients (Fig. 68.12).[69,76] The need for ILM peeling remains controversial; however, it is appropriate to consider when apparent ILM traction is recognized on preoperative OCT images.

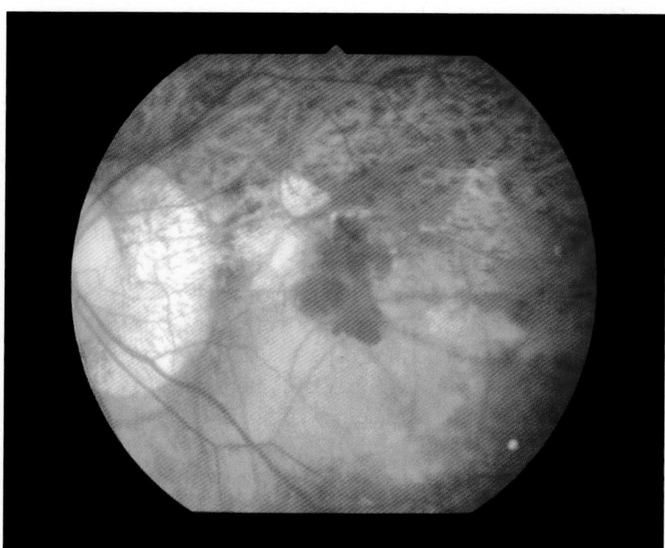

Fig. 68.11 Myopic choroidal neovascularization.

Natural course and treatment of myopic CNV

Myopic CNV is not intensely active, and thus has a tendency to regress spontaneously, and progresses from an active phase (Fig. 68.13A) to a scar phase (Fig. 68.13B). In the scar phase, the CNV is covered by proliferated RPE cells and is observed as a dark pigmented spot (Fuchs spot). After CNV regression, well-defined chorioretinal atrophy gradually develops and enlarges around the Fuchs spot and this causes a progressive visual decrease in the long term. This phase is called atrophic CNV (Fig. 68.13C).

The prognosis of myopic CNV is poor. A natural history study with 10-year follow-up showed that, at the onset of CNV, 70% had a visual acuity better than 20/200, and 22% had a visual acuity better than 20/40. Three years after the onset of CNV, 56% retained a visual acuity of better than 20/200. At 5 and 10 years after onset, however, visual acuity dropped to 20/200 or less in 89% and 96%, respectively (Fig. 68.14).[37,77] The mechanism by which chorioretinal atrophy develops and enlarges around the regressed CNV in eyes with pathologic myopia is not clear. Because chorioretinal atrophy around the CNV affects the final visual outcome of eyes with myopic CNV, we need to determine the effect of treatment against myopic CNV on chorioretinal atrophy development.

Anti-VEGF therapy and PDT with verteporfin (Visudyne) have recently been used to treat myopic CNV. The Verteporfin in the Photodynamic Therapy Study Group study, a randomized, prospective, clinical trial performed to confirm the safety and efficacy of the treatment of myopic CNV with PDT, reported a significantly better visual outcome at 12 months;[78] however, the visual increase was not significant at 24 months,[79] indicating that the long-term efficacy of PDT is not confirmed. PDT acts by producing selective choriocapillaris endothelial damage, which stabilizes the myopic CNV. Recently, a long-term study

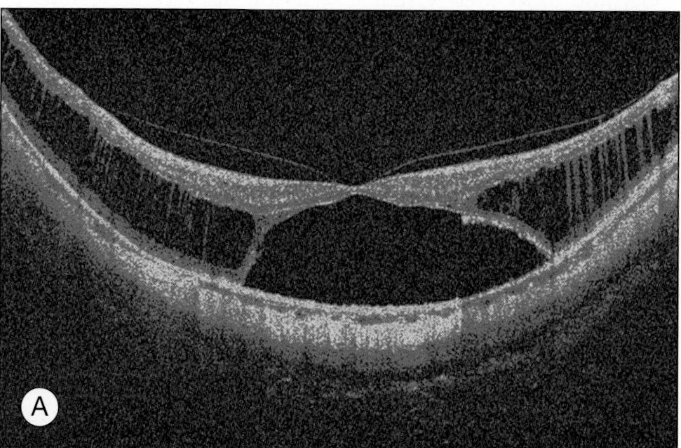

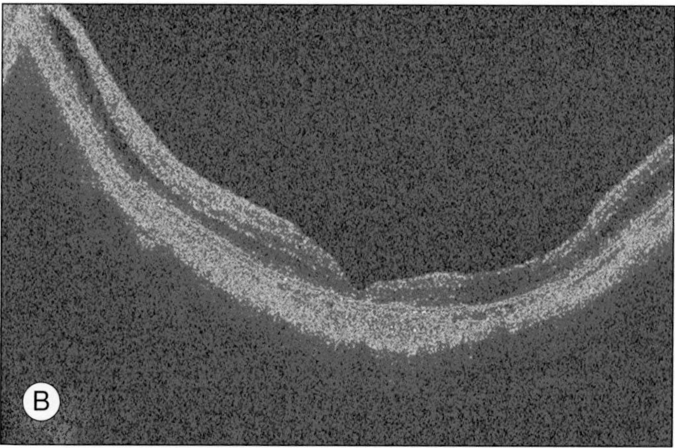

Fig. 68.12 Myopic macular retinoschisis. (A) Horizontal optical coherence tomography scan across the central fovea shows macular retinoschisis accompanying macular retinal detachment. (B) Six months after vitrectomy, the macular retinoschisis as well as retinal detachment is resolved.

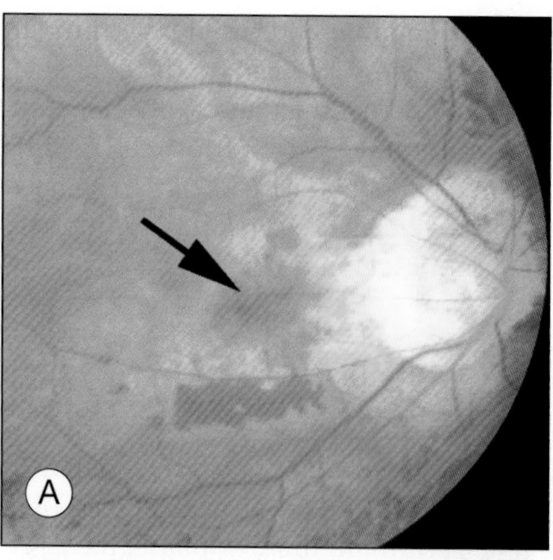

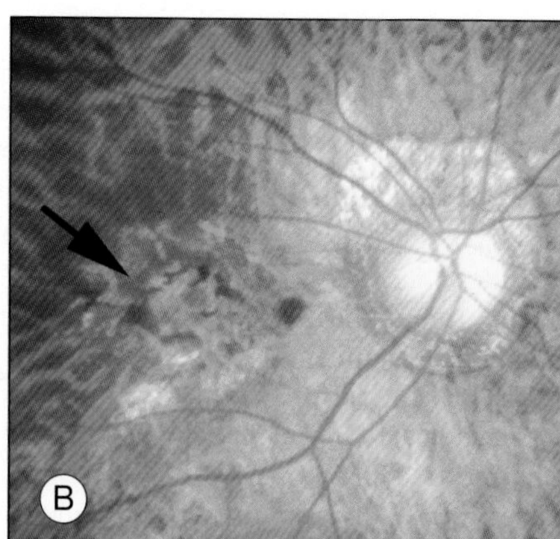

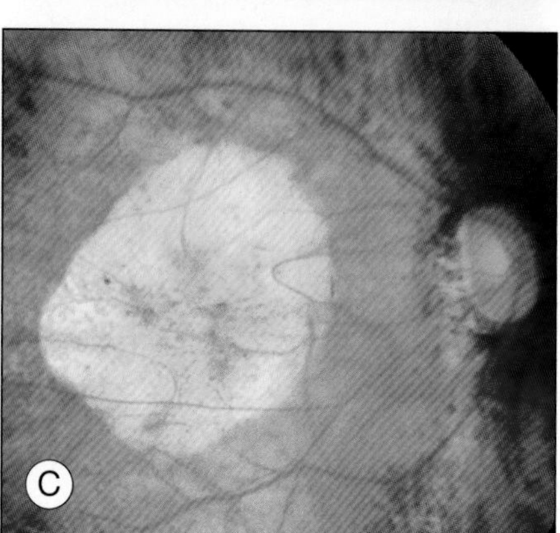

Fig. 68.13 Natural course of myopic choroidal neovascularization (CNV). (A) Active phase. The CNV (arrow) is surrounded by the hemorrhage. (B) Scar phase. The pigmented Fuchs spot is observed. (C) Atrophic phase. The scarred CNV is surrounded by well-delineated chorioretinal atrophy.

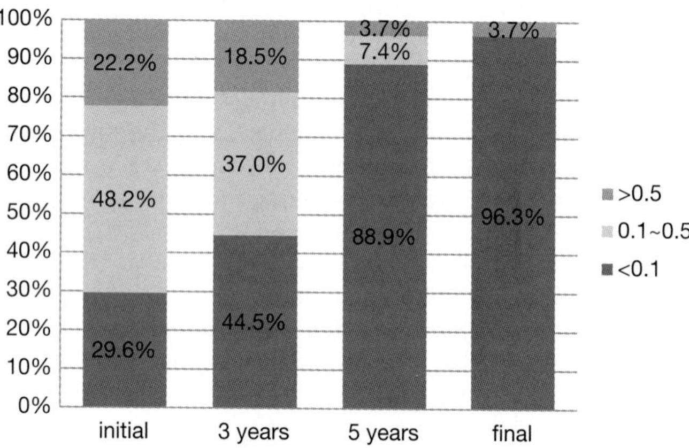

Fig. 68.14 The natural course of distribution of the best-corrected visual acuity (BCVA) in patients with myopic choroidal neovascularization (CNV). The BCVA progressively declines in the long term after onset of CNV. (Reproduced with permission from Yoshida T, Ohno-Matsui K, Yasuzumi K, et al. Myopic choroidal neovascularization: a 10-year follow-up. Ophthalmology 2003;110:1297–305.)

evaluating the effectiveness of PDT on myopic CNV showed that better visual outcome was associated with better initial best-corrected visual acuity (BCVA) and larger lesions in younger patients treated by PDT.[80] Also, 71% of the highly myopic eyes with juxtafoveal CNV had BCVA of 0.5 or better at 4 years after PDT.[35]

Currently, bevacizumab (Avastin) and ranibizumab (Lucentis) are the most commonly used intravitreal anti-VEGF agents. It has been reported that 40% of patients have a significant (three lines or more) visual improvement at 1-year follow-up.[36,81] The duration of symptoms, baseline visual acuity, and location of the CNV are factors that are predictive of the final visual acuity.[81,82] CNV sometimes recurs, typically within 6 months of the initial injection.[83] The number of treatments during the first year may depend on the loading dose regimen; however, the number of required treatments has been reported to range from 2.4 to 4.9 times annually.[81–83] Several prospective and retrospective investigations have shown that anti-VEGF therapies offer more beneficial effects for visual outcomes compared with PDT.[84–86] The influence of anti-VEGF therapies on the development of chorioretinal atrophy around myopic CNV needs to be evaluated to prove the long-term effectiveness of this treatment, since the outcome of 2-year results is not consistent.[85,87–90]

CONCLUSION

Pathologic myopia is a major cause of visual impairment worldwide, and associated visual loss is due to various lesions of myopic macular degeneration which develop secondary to posterior staphyloma formation and progressive thinning of the RPE – choroid with age in addition to an increase in axial length. Among various lesions of myopic macular degeneration, myopic CNV can be treated by the application of anti-VEGF therapy or PDT. Also, the advance of OCT technology has enabled the evaluation of pathogenic mechanism of myopic macular retinoschisis and vitrectomy has been proven useful to treat this condition. Further studies evaluating the long-term outcome of anti-VEGF therapy for myopic CNV and vitrectomy to manage myopic macular retinoschisis are expected.

REFERENCES

1. Krumpaszky HG, Ludtke R, Mickler A, et al. Blindness incidence in Germany. A population-based study from Wurttemberg-Hohenzollern. Ophthalmologica 1999;213:176–82.
2. Munier A, Gunning T, Kenny D, et al. Causes of blindness in the adult population of the Republic of Ireland. Br J Ophthalmol 1998;82:630–3.

3. Cotter SA, Varma R, Ying-Lai M, et al., Causes of low vision and blindness in adult Latinos: the Los Angeles Latino Eye Study. Ophthalmology 2006;113: 1574–82.
4. Buch H, Vinding T, La Cour M, et al. Prevalence and causes of visual impairment and blindness among 9980 Scandinavian adults: the Copenhagen City Eye Study. Ophthalmology 2004;111:53–61.
5. Iwase A, Araie M, Tomidokoro A, et al. Prevalence and causes of low vision and blindness in a Japanese adult population: the Tajimi study. Ophthalmology 2006;113:1354–62.
6. Tokoro T. Types of fundus changes in the posterior pole. In: Tokoro T, editor. Atlas of posterior fundus changes in pathologic myopia. Tokyo: Springer-Verlag; 1998. p. 5–22.
7. Hayashi K, Ohno-Matsui K, Shimada N, et al. Long-term pattern of progression of myopic maculopathy: a natural history study. Ophthalmology 2010;117:1595–611, 1611 e1–4.
8. Takano M, Kishi S. Foveal retinoschisis and retinal detachment in severely myopic eyes with posterior staphyloma. Am J Ophthalmol 1999;128:472–6.
9. Dandona R, Dandona L, Naduvilath TJ, et al. Refractive errors in an urban population in Southern India: the Andhra Pradesh Eye Disease Study. Invest Ophthalmol Vis Sci 1999;40:2810–8.
10. Saw SM, Chan YH, Wong WL, et al. Prevalence and risk factors for refractive errors in the Singapore Malay Eye Survey. Ophthalmology 2008;115:1713–9.
11. Wong TY, Foster PJ, Hee J, et al. Prevalence and risk factors for refractive errors in adult Chinese in Singapore. Invest Ophthalmol Vis Sci 2000;41: 2486–94.
12. Saw SM, Gazzard G, Koh D, et al. Prevalence rates of refractive errors in Sumatra, Indonesia. Invest Ophthalmol Vis Sci 2002;43:3174–80.
13. Bourne RR, Dineen BP, Ali SM, et al. Prevalence of refractive error in Bangladeshi adults: results of the National Blindness and Low Vision Survey of Bangladesh. Ophthalmology 2004;111:1150–60.
14. Gupta A, Casson RJ, Newland HS, et al. Prevalence of refractive error in rural Myanmar: the Meiktila Eye Study. Ophthalmology 2008;115:26–32.
15. Wickremasinghe S, Foster PJ, Uranchimeg D, et al. Ocular biometry and refraction in Mongolian adults. Invest Ophthalmol Vis Sci 2004;45:776–83.
16. Xu L, Li J, Cui T, et al. Refractive error in urban and rural adult Chinese in Beijing. Ophthalmology 2005;112:1676–83.
17. Sawada A, Tomidokoro A, Araie M, et al. Refractive errors in an elderly Japanese population: the Tajimi study. Ophthalmology 2008;115:363–70 e3.
18. Wang Q, Klein BE, Klein R, et al. Refractive status in the Beaver Dam Eye Study. Invest Ophthalmol Vis Sci 1994;35:4344–7.
19. Katz J, Tielsch JM, Sommer A. Prevalence and risk factors for refractive errors in an adult inner city population. Invest Ophthalmol Vis Sci 1997;38:334–40.
20. Attebo K, Ivers RQ, Mitchell P. Refractive errors in an older population: the Blue Mountains Eye Study. Ophthalmology 1999;106:1066–72.
21. Wensor M, McCarty CA, Taylor HR. Prevalence and risk factors of myopia in Victoria, Australia. Arch Ophthalmol 1999;117:658–63.
22. Tarczy-Hornoch K, Ying-Lai M, Varma R. Myopic refractive error in adult Latinos: the Los Angeles Latino Eye Study. Invest Ophthalmol Vis Sci 2006;47: 1845–52.
23. Xu L, Wang Y, Li Y, et al. Causes of blindness and visual impairment in urban and rural areas in Beijing: the Beijing Eye Study. Ophthalmology 2006;113:1134 e1–11.
24. Klaver CC, Wolfs RC, Vingerling JR, et al. Age-specific prevalence and causes of blindness and visual impairment in an older population: the Rotterdam Study. Arch Ophthalmol 1998;116:653–8.
25. Cedrone C, Culasso F, Cesareo M, et al. Incidence of blindness and low vision in a sample population: the Priverno Eye Study, Italy. Ophthalmology 2003;110:584–8.
26. Hsu WM, Cheng CY, Liu JH, et al. Prevalence and causes of visual impairment in an elderly Chinese population in Taiwan: the Shihpai Eye Study. Ophthalmology 2004;111:62–9.
27. Vongphanit J, Mitchell P, Wang JJ. Prevalence and progression of myopic retinopathy in an older population. Ophthalmology 2002;109:704–11.
28. Liu HH, Xu L, Wang YX, et al. Prevalence and progression of myopic retinopathy in Chinese adults: the Beijing Eye Study. Ophthalmology 2010;117: 1763–8.
28a. Asakuma T, Yasuda M, Ninomiya T, et al. Prevalence and risk factors for myopic retinopathy in a Japanese population: The Hisayama Study. Ophthalmology 2012, May 10 [Epub ahead of print]. PMID: 22578442.
29. Panda-Jonas S, Jonas JB, Jakobczyk-Zmija M. Retinal photoreceptor density decreases with age. Ophthalmology 1995;102:1853–9.
30. Gao H, Hollyfield JG. Aging of the human retina. Differential loss of neurons and retinal pigment epithelial cells. Invest Ophthalmol Vis Sci 1992;33:1–17.
31. Eriksson U, Alm A. Macular thickness decreases with age in normal eyes: a study on the macular thickness map protocol in the Stratus OCT. Br J Ophthalmol 2009;93:1448–52.
32. Alamouti B, Funk J. Retinal thickness decreases with age: an OCT study. Br J Ophthalmol 2003;87:899–901.
33. Lim LS, Saw SM, Jeganathan VS, et al. Distribution and determinants of ocular biometric parameters in an Asian population: the Singapore Malay eye study. Invest Ophthalmol Vis Sci 2010;51:103–9.
34. Fotedar R, Wang JJ, Burlutsky G, et al. Distribution of axial length and ocular biometry measured using partial coherence laser interferometry (IOL Master) in an older white population. Ophthalmology 2010;117:417–23.
35. Hayashi K, Ohno-Matsui K, Shimada N, et al. Long-term results of photodynamic therapy for choroidal neovascularization in Japanese patients with pathologic myopia. Am J Ophthalmol 2010.
36. Gharbiya M, Giustolisi R, Allievi F, et al. Choroidal neovascularization in pathologic myopia: intravitreal ranibizumab versus bevacizumab – a randomized controlled trial. Am J Ophthalmol 2010;149:458–64 e1.
37. Yoshida T, Ohno-Matsui K, Yasuzumi K, et al. Myopic choroidal neovascularization: a 10-year follow-up. Ophthalmology 2003;110:1297–305.
38. Li YJ, Guggenheim JA, Bulusu A, et al. An international collaborative family-based whole-genome linkage scan for high-grade myopia. Invest Ophthalmol Vis Sci 2009;50:3116–27.
39. Solouki AM, Verhoeven VJ, van Duijn CM, et al. A genome-wide association study identifies a susceptibility locus for refractive errors and myopia at 15q14. Nat Genet 2010;42:897–901.
40. Hysi PG, Young TL, Mackey DA, et al. A genome-wide association study for myopia and refractive error identifies a susceptibility locus at 15q25. Nat Genet 2010;42:902–5.
41. Nakanishi H, Gotoh N, Yamada R, et al. ARMS2/HTRA1 and CFH polymorphisms are not associated with choroidal neovascularization in highly myopic eyes of the elderly Japanese population. Eye (Lond) 2010;24:1078–84.
42. Parmeggiani F, Gemmati D, Costagliola C, et al. Impact of coagulation-balance gene predictors on efficacy of photodynamic therapy for choroidal neovascularization in pathologic myopia. Ophthalmology 2010;117:517–23.
43. Curtin BJ. Basic science and clinical management. In: Curtin BJ, editor. The myopias. New York: Harper and Row; 1985. p. 177.
44. Curtin BJ, Karlin DB. Axial length measurements and fundus changes of the myopic eye. I. The posterior fundus. Trans Am Ophthalmol Soc 1970;68: 312–34.
45. Tokoro T. Lacquer crack lesions and simple bleeding. In: Tokoro T, editor. Atlas of posterior fundus changes in pathologic myopia. Tokyo: Springer; 1998. pp. 101–23.
46. Hsiang HW, Ohno-Matsui K, Shimada N, et al. Clinical characteristics of posterior staphyloma in eyes with pathologic myopia. Am J Ophthalmol 2008; 146:102–10.
47. Kobayashi K, Ohno-Matsui K, Kojima A, et al. Fundus characteristics of high myopia in children. Jpn J Ophthalmol 2005;49:306–11.
48. Steidl SM, Pruett RC. Macular complications associated with posterior staphyloma. Am J Ophthalmol 1997;123:181–7.
49. Fujiwara T, Imamura Y, Margolis R, et al. Enhanced depth imaging optical coherence tomography of the choroid in highly myopic eyes. Am J Ophthalmol 2009;148:445–50.
50. Wiesel TN, Raviola E. Myopia and eye enlargement after neonatal lid fusion in monkeys. Nature 1977;266:66–8.
51. Raviola E, Wiesel TN. An animal model of myopia. N Engl J Med 1985;312: 1609–15.
52. Wallman J, Turkel J, Trachtman J. Extreme myopia produced by modest change in early visual experience. Science 1978;201:1249–51.
53. Troilo D. Experimental studies of emmetropization in the chick. Ciba Found Symp, 1990;155:89–102; discussion 102–14.
54. Tkatchenko TV, Shen Y, Tkatchenko AV. Mouse experimental myopia has features of primate myopia. Invest Ophthalmol Vis Sci 2010;51:1297–303.
55. Barathi VA, Boopathi VG, Yap EP, et al. Two models of experimental myopia in the mouse. Vision Res 2008;48:904–16.
56. Brand C, Schaeffel F, Feldkaemper MP. A microarray analysis of retinal transcripts that are controlled by image contrast in mice. Mol Vis 2007;13: 920–32.
57. Schippert R, Burkhardt E, Feldkaemper M, et al. Relative axial myopia in Egr-1 (ZENK) knockout mice. Invest Ophthalmol Vis Sci 2007;48:11–7.
58. Yeh LK, Liu CY, Kao WW, et al. Knockdown of zebrafish lumican gene (zlum) causes scleral thinning and increased size of scleral coats. J Biol Chem 2010; 285:28141–55.
59. Veth KN, Willer JR, Collery RF, et al. Mutations in zebrafish lrp2 Result in adult-onset ocular pathogenesis that models myopia and other risk factors for glaucoma. PLoS Genet 2011;7:e1001310.
60. Yasuzumi K, Ohno-Matsui K, Yoshida T, et al. Peripapillary crescent enlargement in highly myopic eyes evaluated by fluorescein and indocyanine green angiography. Br J Ophthalmol 2003;87:1088–90.
61. Ohno-Matsui K, Morishima N, Ito M, et al. Indocyanine green angiography of retrobulbar vascular structures in severe myopia. Am J Ophthalmol 1997;123: 494–505.
62. Curtin BJ The posterior staphyloma of pathologic myopia. Trans Am Ophthalmol Soc 1977;75:67–86.
63. Moriyama M, Ohno-Matsui K, Hayashi K, et al. Topographical analyses of shape of eyes with pathologic myopia by high-resolution three dimensional magnetic resonance imaging. Ophthalmology 2011;118:1626–47.
64. Ohno-Matsui K, Morishima N, Ito M, et al. Indocyanine green angiographic findings of lacquer cracks in pathologic myopia. Jpn J Ophthalmol 1998;42: 293–9.
65. Ikuno Y, Sayanagi K, Soga K, et al. Lacquer crack formation and choroidal neovascularization in pathologic myopia. Retina 2008;28:1124–31.
66. Ohno-Matsui K, Tokoro T. The progression of lacquer cracks in pathologic myopia. Retina 1996;16:29–37.
67. Ohno-Matsui K, Ito M, Tokoro T. Subretinal bleeding without choroidal neovascularization in pathologic myopia. A sign of new lacquer crack formation. Retina 1996;16:196–202.
68. Ohno-Matsui K, Yoshida T, Futagami S, et al. Patchy atrophy and lacquer cracks predispose to the development of choroidal neovascularisation in pathological myopia. Br J Ophthalmol 2003;87:570–3.
69. Ikuno Y, Sayanagi K, Ohji M, et al. Vitrectomy and internal limiting membrane peeling for myopic foveoschisis. Am J Ophthalmol 2004;137:719–24.

70. Panozzo G, Mercanti A Optical coherence tomography findings in myopic traction maculopathy. Arch Ophthalmol 2004;122:1455–60.
71. Baba T, Ohno-Matsui K, Futagami S, et al. Prevalence and characteristics of foveal retinal detachment without macular hole in high myopia. Am J Ophthalmol 2003;135:338–42.
72. Shimada N, Ohno-Matsui K, Baba T, et al. Natural course of macular retinoschisis in highly myopic eyes without macular hole or retinal detachment. Am J Ophthalmol 2006;142:497–500.
73. Shimada N, Ohno-Matsui K, Nishimuta A, et al. Detection of paravascular lamellar holes and other paravascular abnormalities by optical coherence tomography in eyes with high myopia. Ophthalmology 2008;115:708–17.
74. Shimada N, Ohno-Matsui K, Nishimuta A, et al. Peripapillary changes detected by optical coherence tomography in eyes with high myopia. Ophthalmology 2007;114:2070–6.
75. Ikuno Y, Gomi F, Tano Y Potent retinal arteriolar traction as a possible cause of myopic foveoschisis. Am J Ophthalmol 2005;139:462–7.
76. Kobayashi H, Kishi S. Vitreous surgery for highly myopic eyes with foveal detachment and retinoschisis. Ophthalmology 2003;110:1702–7.
77. Yoshida T, Ohno-Matsui K, Ohtake Y, et al. Long-term visual prognosis of choroidal neovascularization in high myopia: a comparison between age groups. Ophthalmology 2002;109:712–9.
78. Photodynamic therapy of subfoveal choroidal neovascularization in pathologic myopia with verteporfin. 1-year results of a randomized clinical trial – VIP report no. 1. Ophthalmology 2001;108:841–52.
79. Blinder KJ, Blumenkranz MS, Bressler NM, et al. Verteporfin therapy of subfoveal choroidal neovascularization in pathologic myopia: 2-year results of a randomized clinical trial – VIP report no. 3. Ophthalmology 2003;110:667–73.
80. Ruiz-Moreno JM, Amat P, Montero JA, et al. Photodynamic therapy to treat choroidal neovascularisation in highly myopic patients: 4 years' outcome. Br J Ophthalmol 2008;92:792–4.
81. Ikuno Y, Sayanagi K, Soga K, et al. Intravitreal bevacizumab for choroidal neovascularization attributable to pathological myopia: one-year results. Am J Ophthalmol 2009;147: 94–100 e1.
82. Calvo-Gonzalez C, Reche-Frutos J, Donate J, et al. Intravitreal ranibizumab for myopic choroidal neovascularization: factors predictive of visual outcome and need for retreatment. Am J Ophthalmol 2011;151:529–34.
83. Chan WM, Lai TY, Liu DT, et al. Intravitreal bevacizumab (Avastin) for myopic choroidal neovascularisation: 1-year results of a prospective pilot study. Br J Ophthalmol 2009;93:150–4.
84. Hayashi K, Ohno-Matsui K, Teramukai S, et al. Comparison of visual outcome and regression pattern of myopic choroidal neovascularization after intravitreal bevacizumab or after photodynamic therapy. Am J Ophthalmol 2009;148:396–408.
85. Ikuno Y, Nagai Y, Matsuda S, et al. Two-year visual results for older Asian women treated with photodynamic therapy or bevacizumab for myopic choroidal neovascularization. Am J Ophthalmol 2010;149:140–6.
86. Parodi MB, Iacono P, Papayannis A, et al. Laser photocoagulation, photodynamic therapy, and intravitreal bevacizumab for the treatment of juxtafoveal choroidal neovascularization secondary to pathologic myopia. Arch Ophthalmol 2010.
87. Baba T, Kubota-Taniai M, Kitahashi M, et al. Two-year comparison of photodynamic therapy and intravitreal bevacizumab for treatment of myopic choroidal neovascularisation. Br J Ophthalmol 2010;94:864–70.
88. Ruiz-Moreno JM, Montero JA. Intravitreal bevacizumab to treat myopic choroidal neovascularization: 2-year outcome. Graefes Arch Clin Exp Ophthalmol 2010;248:937–41.
89. Hayashi K, Shimada N, Moriyama M, et al. Two year outcomes of intravitreal bevacizumab for choroidal neovascularization in Japanese patients with pathological myopia. Retina (in press).
90. Voykov B, Gelisken F, Inhoffen W, et al. Bevacizumab for choroidal neovascularization secondary to pathologic myopia: Is there a decline of the treatment efficacy after 2 years? Graefes Arch Clin Exp Ophthalmol 2010;248:543–50.

Angioid Streaks

Linda A. Lam

Chapter 69

INTRODUCTION

The appearance of angioid streaks was initially described by Doyne in 1889 as irregular and radiating lines extending from the optic nerve to the peripheral retina found in an eye with retinal hemorrhages after blunt trauma.[1] The term "angioid streaks" originated as the ophthalmoscopic appearance of the lines was similar to that of blood vessels.[2] Histopathologic studies found that angioid streaks represent irregular dehiscences in the collagenous and elastic portion of Bruch's membrane.[3,4] Associations have been found between angioid streaks and systemic conditions such as pseudoxanthoma elasticum (Grönbald-Strandberg syndrome),[5,6,7] osteitis deformans (Paget's disease),[5,8–10] blood dyscrasias such as sickle-cell anemia,[5,11–13] fibrodysplasia hyperelastica (Ehlers–Danlos syndrome),[5,14] and acromegaly.[5,15] However, angioid streaks may also occur in patients without associated systemic disease.[16] Patients with angioid streaks usually are asymptomatic unless complications such as macular choroidal neovascularization develop.[5,16] In cases of macular involvement the prognosis is often poor, with most eyes progressing to legal blindness without treatment.[5,6,16] Multiple therapeutic strategies have been used to treat choroidal neovascularization secondary to angioid streaks, including argon laser photocoagulation,[17–19] transpupillary thermotherapy,[20] photodynamic therapy,[21,22] macular translocation surgery,[23–25] intravitreal anti-vascular endothelial growth factor treatments with pegabtanib,[26] bevacizumab,[27–33] or ranibizumab,[33–38] and combination therapy.[39]

HISTOPATHOLOGY

Angioid streaks represent discrete irregular breaks in Bruch's membrane, and are often associated with atrophic changes of the overlying retinal pigment epithelium (RPE) and calcific degeneration.[4] Klein proposed a dual mechanism for the development of Bruch's membrane, including (1) a primary abnormality in the fibers of Bruch's membrane and (2) increased deposits of metal salts or an increasing tendency for their pathologic deposition.[3] The deposition of calcium may cause Bruch's membrane to be more brittle and to develop choroidal rupture.[4] Recent immunohistochemical studies show significant calcium deposition and infiltration of vascularized tissue above the RPE from Bruch's membrane in the area of choroidal neovascularization in an eye with angioid streaks.[40]

Tissue metalloproteinase, specifically MMP-9, was found in high concentrations in the excised Bruch's membrane in an area of choroidal neovascularization in an eye with angioid streaks. MMP-9 is known to induce basement membrane destruction and angiogenesis.[40]

In the early stages, angioid streaks are partial breaks of the thickened and calcified Bruch's membrane with thinning of the RPE, events that do not cause anatomic changes in the overlying retinal layers.[41] Subsequently a full-thickness defect of the Bruch's membrane may occur followed by atrophy of the choriocapillaris, RPE, and photoreceptors. Fibrovascular proliferation from the choroid may occur through the Bruch's membrane break resulting in choroidal neovascularization and subsequent development of a disciform scar.[4,10,41] This process usually results in slowly progressive macular changes and vision loss. Sudden vision loss can result, however, from a serous or hemorrhagic detachment around the areas of choroidal neovascularization.[4,10] Sudden loss of central vision may occur following mild trauma leading to choroidal rupture and submacular hemorrhage resulting from the brittleness of Bruch's membrane.[4,10]

SYSTEMIC ASSOCIATIONS

Angioid streaks have been most commonly associated with systemic conditions such as pseudoxanthoma elasticum (Grönbald–Strandberg syndrome),[5–7] osteitis deformans (Paget's disease),[5,8–10] fibrodysplasia hyperelastica (Ehlers–Danlos syndrome),[5,14] acromegaly,[5,15] Marfan syndrome,[6] and blood dyscrasias such as sickle-cell anemia,[11,12] thalassemia,[6] and spherocytosis.[6] Angioid streaks have also been described in patients with the following conditions: alpha-beta-lipoproteinemia, acquired hemolytic anemia, hemochromatosis, hypertension, diabetes, hypercalcinosis, hyperphosphatemia, diffuse lipomatosis, Sturge–Weber syndrome, tuberous sclerosis, neurofibromatosis, microsomia, epilepsy, senile elastosis, cutaneous calcinosis, and trauma[5,6,16] (Box 69.1).

In a large study examining associated systemic diagnosis in 50 patients with angioid streaks, half of the patients were found to have a related systemic condition.[5] Seventeen of the 25 patients were diagnosed also with pseudoxanthoma elasticum (PXE), 5 patients with Paget's disease, and 3 patients had sickle-cell disease.[5] The remaining half of the patients with angioid streaks did not demonstrate associated systemic disease.[5]

The most common systemic association of angioid streaks is PXE, an inherited disorder associated with degeneration of the elastic fibers in the dermatologic, gastrointestinal, cardiovascular, and ocular tissues. PXE accounts for 59–87% of cases with angioid streaks.[7] In PXE, the primary finding is elastic fiber degeneration in connective tissue, followed by a secondary calcium deposition.[4,10] In addition to angioid streaks, eyes also demonstrate a so-called "peau d'orange" pigmentary change, reticular pigmentary dystrophy affecting the macula, atrophic lesions of the RPE, crystalline bodies, and optic disc drusen (in

Box 69.1 Systemic conditions associated with angioid streaks

Pseudoxanthoma elasticum (Grönbald–Strandberg syndrome)
Osteitis deformans (Paget's disease)
Fibrodysplasia hyperelastica (Ehlers–Danlos syndrome)
Acromegaly
Marfan syndrome
Sickle cell anemia
Thalassemia
Spherocytosis
Acquired hemolytic anemia
Hemochromatosis
Alpha-beta-lipoproteinemia
Hypertension
Diabetes
Hypercalcinosis
Hyperphosphatemia
Diffuse lipomatosis
Sturge–Weber syndrome
Neurofibromatosis
Tuberous sclerosis
Microsomia
Epilepsy
Cutaneous calcinosis
Trauma

21% of patients with PXE and angioid streaks).[42] By 20 years after first diagnosis, angioid streaks develop in almost all patients with PXE.[16]

In patients with Paget's disease, extensive Bruch's membrane calcification and angioid streaks followed by choroidal neovascularization and disciform scarring may develp.[9,10] About 10% of patients with advanced Paget's disease develop angioid streaks.[9,10]

Similar significant calcium depositions at Bruch's membrane have been identified using histochemical and electron microscopic studies in patients with sickle-cell hemoglobinopathies.[13] The presence of iron–calcium complexes at the level of Bruch's membrane was previously suggested as an etiology for angioid streaks in patients with hemoglobinopathy; however, histopathologic studies demonstrate no increased iron deposition at the Bruch's membrane.[42] Compared to PXE, a smaller proportion of patients develop choroidal neovascularization and subsequent visual loss.[6]

OCULAR MANIFESTATIONS AND CLINICAL COURSE

Angioid streaks usually originate from the optic nerve and may either radiate out or surround it concentrically and appear as irregular lines of varying width.[6] The subretinal lines can range in diameter from 50 to 500 μm.[16] The color of angioid streaks varies based on the fundus pigmentation and tends to be reddish in light-colored individuals and brown-colored in darker-pigmented individuals[16] (see Fig. 69.1A–D).

Angioid streaks have not been reported in newborns, and few cases have been described in individuals under 10 years of age.[6] Angioid streaks remain over time and do not regress, and the streaks may increase in length and width over time.[43] New streaks may form adjacent to old lesions. Over time, the adjacent RPE and choriocapillaris may develop atrophy.[43]

Most patients with angioid streaks are asymptomatic unless the macula is involved, with the development of traumatic rupture of the Bruch's membrane or choroidal neovascularization (Figs 69.1B, 69.2A,B). If the macula is involved, patients may report metamorphopsia or blurred vision.

Patients may demonstrate breaks of Bruch's membrane after mild head or eye injuries, due to the brittleness of the calcified Bruch's membrane. Rupture of Bruch's membrane after trauma may be followed by subretinal hemorrhages. Up to 15% of patients with angioid streaks develop significant visual loss after mild head injury.

The most common and significant complication of angioid streaks is the development of choroidal neovascularization (CNV). Choroidal neovascularization is often bilateral and occurs in 72–86% of eyes with angioid streaks.[16] CNV is usually bilateral but asymmetric, with an interval of approximately 18 months between the development of CNV in initial and fellow eye.[7]

Patients with PXE have a higher risk of CNV development compared to patients with other systemic diseases. By age 50, the majority of patients with PXE demonstrate reduced vision less than 20/200.

OCULAR IMAGING AND DIAGNOSIS

Fluorescein angiography (FA)

Usually the diagnosis of angioid streaks is made on fundoscopic examination, but fluorescein angiography may be helpful to detect the streaks and associated choroidal neovascularization when the findings are subtle. Irregular hyperfluorescence of the angioid streaks occurs during early phase angiography followed by varying degrees of staining during the later phases.[4] In some individuals with deeply pigmented choroidal tissue, the angioid streaks may be difficult to detect angiographically; whereas in lightly pigmented individuals, fluorescein angiography may aid in the identification of the angioid streaks before ophthalmoscopic detection[4] (Fig. 69.2C).

Fundus autofluorescence (FAF)

Autofluorescence imaging uses light emission from lipofuscin in RPE cells and is considered to reflect RPE metabolic activity. Angioid streaks can show increased or decreased fundus autofluorescence. Autofluorescence often demonstrates RPE atrophy more extensive than that seen on fundus ophthalmoscopy or fluorescein angiography; therefore, FAF may be a useful non-invasive tool to monitor the progression of the RPE changes related to angioid streaks and choroidal neovascularization[6] (see Figs 69.1C,D). FAF in eyes with angioid streaks has also been similar to the FAF images from eyes with pattern dystrophy. FAF demonstrated large areas of confluent hypoautofluorescence, demonstrating widespread loss of RPE cells in eyes with PXE.[44]

Indocyanine green angiography (ICGA)

A study incorporating the use of multiple modalities (FA, ICGA, FAF, and confocal near-infrared reflectance) in patients with angioid streaks and PXE has suggested a centrifugal spread of progressive calcification of Bruch's membrane that begins at the posterior pole and progresses toward the retinal periphery.[45] A central area of decreased fluorescence centered on the posterior pole on late-phase ICGA, while eccentric areas demonstrated a normal fluorescence on late-phase ICGA.[45]

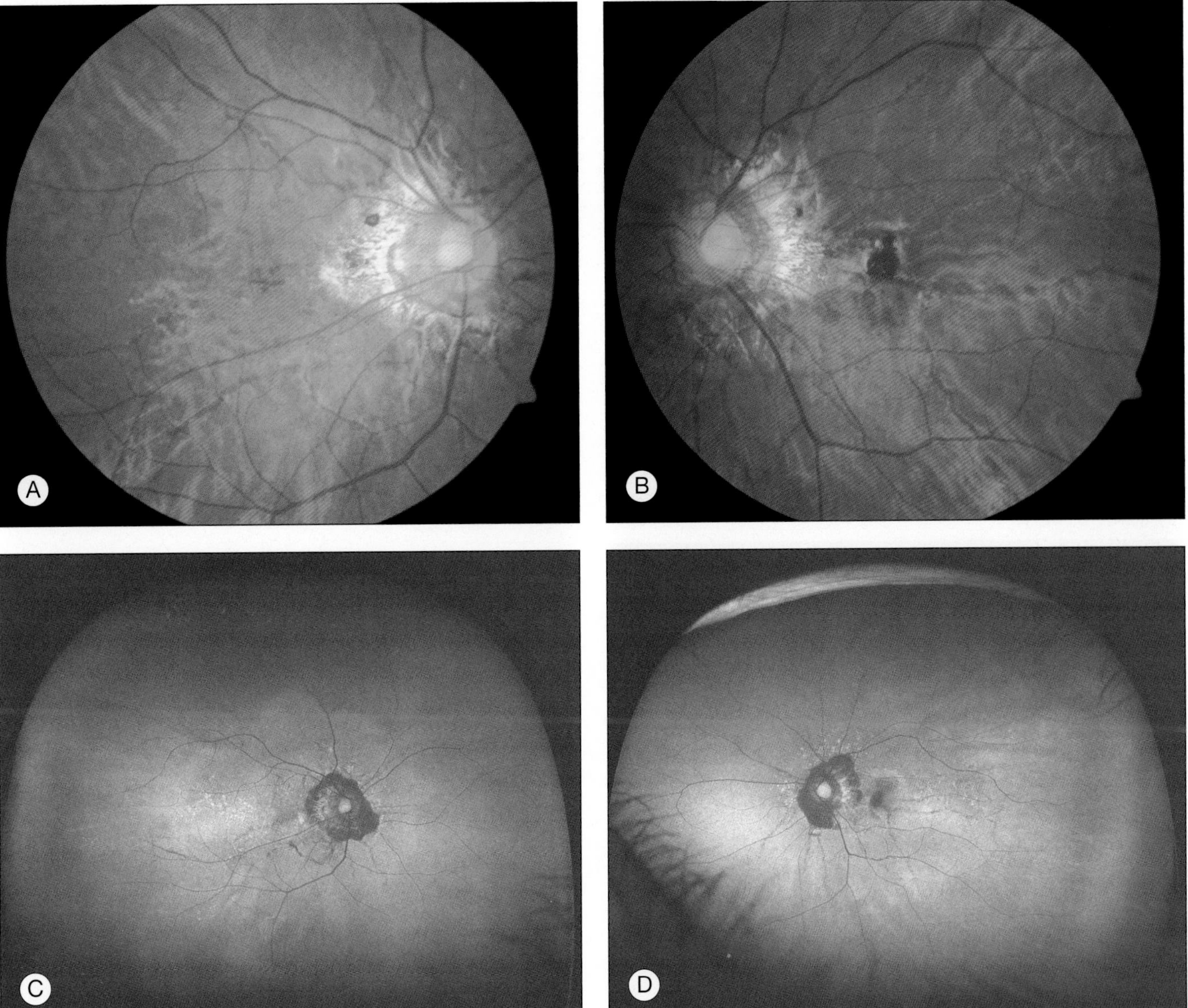

Fig. 69.1 A 63-year-old Asian woman with pseudoxanthoma elasticum and angioid streaks. Wide-field imaging of the right (A) and left (B) eyes shows angioid streaks (darker lines) radiating out from the optic disc. A hyperpigmented scar just nasal to the fovea developed after laser photocoagulation (A). The laser treatment was given prior to the use of intravitreal anti-VEGF therapy. Fundus autofluorescence imaging demonstrates the angioid streaks in the right (C) and left (D) eye. Spectral domain optical coherence tomography in this patient is shown in Fig. 69.3.

Spectral domain optical coherence tomography (SD-OCT)

In eyes with advanced fundus pathology, such as large areas of atrophy and fibrosis, the underlying Bruch's membrane breaks cannot be detected on fundus photography, fluorescein angiography, or fundus autofluorescence imaging.[46] SD-OCT can detect abnormalities in Bruch's membrane as well as subretinal fibrosis and deposits that can be difficult to discern in areas of atrophy on FAF, FA, or ICGA[46] (Fig. 69.3).

THERAPY

There is no known prophylaxis except perhaps eye protection to reduce trauma. Treatment strategies are only directed to the eyes with choroidal neovascularization (CNV). Untreated CNV results in poor visual outcomes in the majority of published reports. One study found a final visual acuity of 20/640 in a group of 26 untreated eyes with either active CNV or disciform scar secondary to angioid streaks.[19]

Laser photocoagulation

Results from laser photocoagulation in the treatment of macular CNV demonstrate a high recurrence rate of up to 77% and poor overall visual outcomes.[17-19] Thermal laser was one of the first therapies used for the treatment of macular CNV (see Fig. 69.1B). In one case series, the eyes treated with laser for macular CNV developed further CNV growth and vision loss.[8] However, other studies suggested that laser treatment for extrafoveal CNV related to angioid streaks resulted in better visual outcomes than untreated eyes.[17] Prophylactic treatment of angioid streaks prior to development of CNV is not recommended.[42] Although the outcome following treatment is poor, there has been the sense that visual loss at least is somewhat delayed. Most retina specialists advise focal laser therapy if there is discrete extrafoveal CNV.

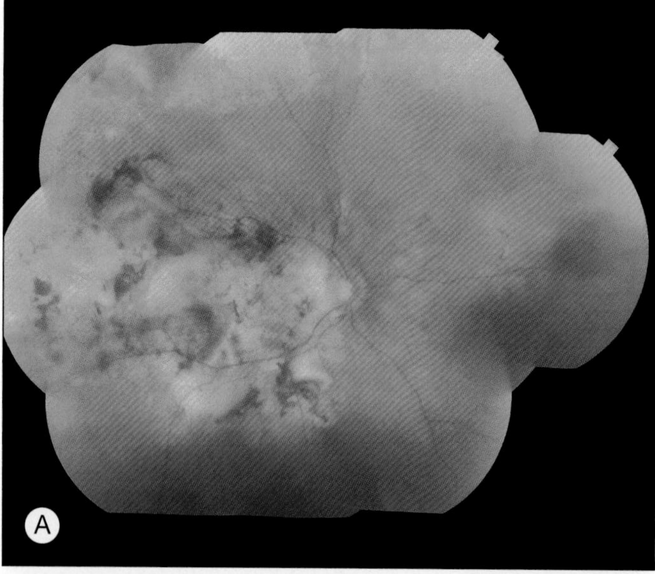

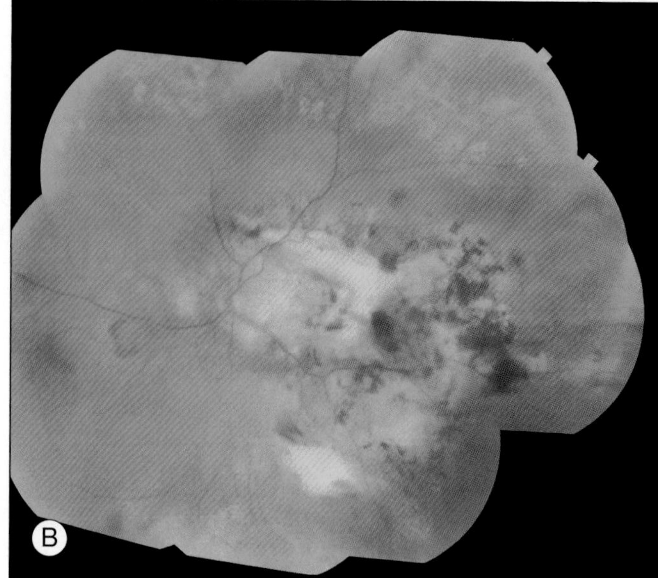

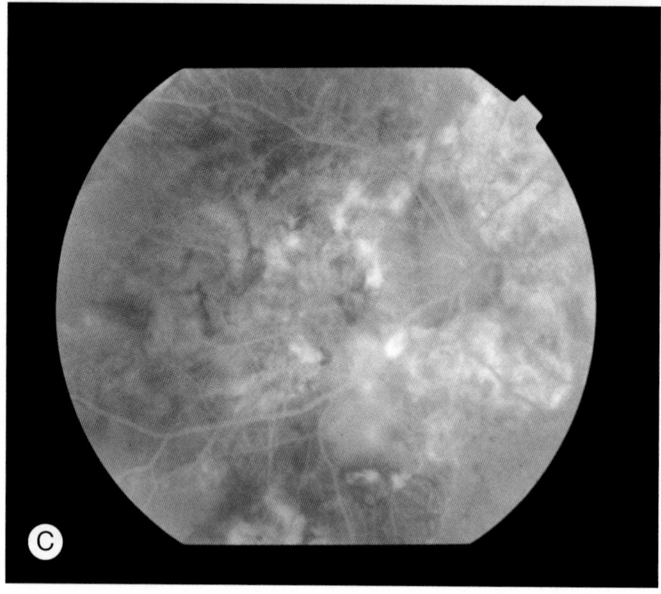

Fig. 69.2 An 86-year-old Caucasian woman with angioid streaks. Extensive disciform scar is found in the macula in both eyes (A,B), with new choroidal neovascularization and subretinal hemorrhage in the peripheral nasal retina in the left eye (B). Fluorescein angiography demonstrates extensive pigmentary changes and disciform scarring in the right eye (C). She underwent multiple intravitreal bevacizumab injections in the right eye and her visual acuity had improved from 20/100^{-2} to 20/60. In the left eye the visual acuity was 20/400.

Transpupillary thermotherapy

Using a diode laser beam with 810 nm wavelength, transpupillary thermotherapy (TTT) may have better penetration to the choriocapillaris and may be less damaging to the RPE. TTT employs a diode with a lower threshold to avoid producing a thermal burn. However, a retrospective study investigating the use of TTT in treatment of subfoveal choroidal neovascularization found no significant long-term benefit in reducing the growth of the CNV or in visual improvement.[20]

Photodynamic therapy

Data from both retrospective and prospective case series of eyes treated with photodynamic therapy (PDT) demonstrate variability in visual outcomes after treatment.[47] Several early reports investigating PDT use in eyes with angioid streaks suggest a reduction of CNV progression compared to natural history alone.[21,47] A retrospective, placebo-controlled case series found a greater reduction in mean visual acuity over the mean follow-up period of 18 months in untreated (from 20/160 to 20/640) versus PDT-treated eyes (from 20/126 to 20/500).[21] However, another study found mean visual acuity decreased after PDT treatment from 20/400 to 20/600.[48] Extension of an initial study with two additional years of follow-up identified progressive decrease in visual acuity following PDT treatment.[49]

Macular translocation

Prior to the use of anti-vascular endothelial growth factor (VEGF) treatments for CNV, macular translocation was an option for CNV treatment. Translocation is a surgical technique used to move the macular neuroretina to lie on top of an area of RPE without previous choroidal neovascularization. Several techniques have been described, including a limited translocation, as well as a 360° translocation where the entire retina is rotated. Varying short-term visual acuity improvement has been reported in a few studies employing macular translocation for CNV related angioid streaks, but the number of eyes treated (less than 10) was limited.[24,25]

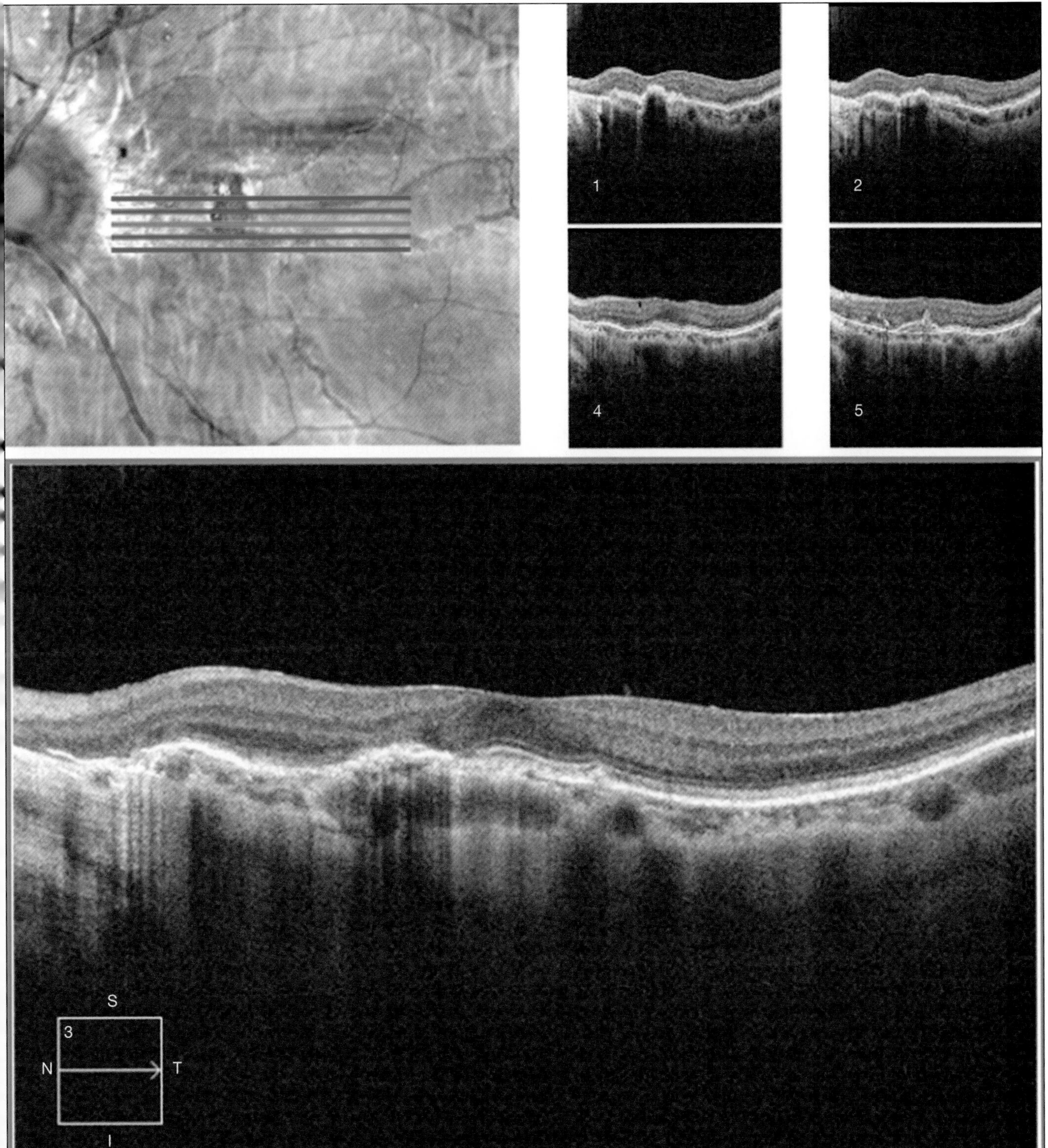

Fig. 69.3 Same patient as Fig. 69.1. Spectral domain optical coherence tomography demonstrates chorioretinal atrophy corresponding to the laser scar nasal to the fovea in the left eye, which has a best corrected visual acuity of 20/25. Visual acuity in the right eye was 20/25.

Anti-VEGF treatment

Laser photocoagulation, TTT, and PDT have not been as successful in reducing the degree of visual loss compared with the visual outcomes following anti-VEGF therapy. Treatments with anti-VEGF therapies such as with both bevacizumab[27–33] and ranibizumab[33–38] have demonstrated a marked reduction in the rate of visual acuity loss in the treated eyes compared with that in untreated eyes but again, follow-up is short and randomized trials lacking.

Bevacizumab

The majority of eyes with CNV secondary to angioid streaks treated with intravitreal bevacizumab demonstrated an improvement or stabilization in mean visual acuity on long-term follow-up ranging from 12 to 28 months.[27–33] Several retrospective case series reported stabilization or improvement of visual acuity after bevacizumab treatment for CNV related to angioid streaks in 87–100% of eyes with a follow-up ranging from 12 to 28 months.[27–31] Mean visual acuity improved by 3 or more lines in 44–62% of eyes by 12 months after bevacizumab treatment.[28,30]

In a study involving patients with angioid streaks secondary to PXE, the mean visual acuity improved from 20/80 to 20/40 with an average of 6.5 injections over a mean follow-up of 28 months.[27] In the same study, eyes with early disease demonstrated better visual outcomes, with a mean visual acuity of 20/25 compared to a final mean visual acuity of 20/63 in eyes with advanced disease.[27]

Eyes with CNV were initially treated with intravitreal bevacizumab and were followed every 4–6 weeks.[27–31] Retreatment with another bevacizumab injection was given if CNV activity was detected, such as decreased visual acuity, new or persistent leakage on FA, retinal hemorrhage, or sub- or intraretinal fluid was found on OCT.[27,30]

Multiple studies with at least 12-month follow-up reported a mean of approximately four bevacizumab injections (1.25–1.5 mg) were given over 12–18 months to treat the CNV secondary to angioid streaks.[28,29,31] Recurrent CNV is common, occurring in 33% of eyes by 19 months in one case series.[31] Not only can CNV recur at the same location, but new CNV can also develop in a different location requiring retreatment.[31]

Angiographic resolution of the CNV was found in 67% of the eyes by 19 months.[31] At final follow-up between 12 and 19 months, several studies have shown a reduction of central retinal thickness by 67–103 μm after bevacizumab treatment.[28,30]

Despite a majority of eyes demonstrating stable or improved visual acuity at the final follow-up in studies using bevacizumab to treat CNV secondary to angioid streaks, 8–13% of eyes demonstrate further decreased visual acuity.[27,30,31] In the eyes with visual loss after undergoing bevacizumab treatment, the visual decline is postulated to be related to atrophic macular changes and not from active choroidal neovascularization.[27,30]

Ranibizumab

Similar to the visual outcomes in bevacizumab trials, the majority of eyes treated with intravitreal ranibizumab demonstrated improved or stable visual outcomes at final follow-up, ranging from 3 months to 24 months.[34–38] In several prospective and retrospective case series reports, final visual acuity outcomes were stable or improved in 66–93% of eyes treated with ranibizumab (0.3–0.5 mg).[34,35,37,38] While the majority of eyes treated with intravitreal ranibizumab maintained or improved vision, 7–33% of eyes treated with ranibizumab lost vision by the end of the study.[34–38]

In two prospective studies, all eyes were given either three or four monthly loading doses of ranibizumab.[37,38] Then an "as needed" treatment protocol was used: another ranibizumab injection was given if CNV activity was detected, such as decreased visual acuity, new or persistent leakage on FA, retinal hemorrhage, or sub- or intraretinal fluid was found on OCT. An average of 5–7 ranibizumab injections was given in two prospective trials with a follow-up of 14–16 months, respectively.[37,38] One prospective trial found that 78% of eyes needed retreatment after the first three loading doses of ranibizumab.[38] Angiographic resolution of the CNV after ranibizumab treatment was reported in 66% of eyes.[35] On OCT testing, a mean decrease of 107 μm was shown in one prospective study at one year.[37]

Combination therapy

One prospective trial investigated the outcomes using combination reduced fluence PDT (25 J/cm^2) and intravitreal ranibizumab (0.5 mg) for treatment-naïve eyes with CNV related to angioid streaks.[39] At 12 months of follow-up, 9 of the 10 eyes demonstrated stable or improved vision, with 6 eyes showing visual acuity gains of two or greater lines. One eye had more than 3 lines of decreased vision at the end of the study.[39] Given the small sample size of this study, further investigations involving combination therapies are needed before determining its added benefit over monotherapy with anti-VEGF treatment alone.

CONCLUSION

Calcification and degeneration in Bruch's membrane account for the fundus and histopathologic appearance of angioid streaks. Angioid streaks are associated with multiple systemic conditions, including PXE, Paget's disease, Ehlers–Danlos syndrome, and various blood dyscrasias such as sickle cell anemia. Angioid streaks may not significantly affect vision if they remain extramacular or if choroidal neovascularization does not develop. However, choroidal neovascularization has been reported to occur in the majority of eyes with angioid streaks and is often bilateral. Treatments with laser photocoagulation, photodynamic therapy, and macular translocation have not resulted in sustained visual improvement. However, significant improvement in visual outcomes has been found after using anti-VEGF therapy with bevacizumab and ranibizumab. Whether the early favorable results are sustained with longer follow-up requires study. Combination therapy may also serve a role in future treatment for choroidal neovascularization secondary to angioid streaks.

REFERENCES

1. Doyne RW. Choroidal and retinal changes. The results of blows on the eyes. Trans Ophthalmol Soc UK 1889;9:128.
2. Knapp H. On the formation of dark angioid streaks as unusual metamorphosis of retinal hemorrhage. Arch Ophthalmol 1892;26:289–92.
3. Klein BA. Angioid streaks: a clinical and histopathologic study. Am J Ophthalmol 1947;30:955–68.
4. Gass JDM. Pathogenesis of disciform detachment of the neuroepithelium. VI. Disciform detachment secondary to heredodegenerative, neoplastic and traumatic lesions of the choroid. Am J Ophthalmol 1967;63:289–711.
5. Clarkson JG, Altman RD. Angioid streaks. Surv Ophthalmol 1982;26:235–46.
6. Finger RP, Issa PC, Ladewig MS, et al. Pseudoxanthoma elasticum. Surv Ophthamol 2009;54:272–85.
7. Connor Jr PJ, Juergens JL, Perry HO, et al. Pseudoxanthoma elasticum and angioid streaks: A review of 106 cases. Am J Med 1961;30:537–43.
8. Clarkson JG. Paget's disease and angioid streaks: One complication less? Br J Ophthalmol 1991;75:511.
9. Dabbs TR, Skjodt K. Prevalence of angioid streaks and other ocular complications of Paget's disease of bone. Br J Ophthalmol 1990;74:579–82.
10. Gass JDM, Clarkson JG. Angioid streaks and disciform macular detachment in Paget's disease (osteitis deformans). Am J Ophthalmol 1973;75:576–86.
11. Condon PI, Serjeant GR. Ocular findings in elderly cases of homozygous sickle-cell disease in Jamaica. Br J Ophthalmol 1976;60:361–4.
12. Geeraets WJ, Guerry III D. Angioid streaks and sickle-cell disease. Am J Ophthalmol 1960;49:450–70.
13. Jampol LM, Acheson R, Eagle Jr RC, et al. Calcification of Bruch's membrane in angioid streaks with homozygous sickle cell disease. Arch Ophthalmol 1987; 105:93–8.
14. Green WR, Friedman-Kien A, Banfield WG. Angioid streaks in Ehlers–Danlos syndrome. Arch Ophthalmol 1966;76:197–204.
15. Paton D. Angioid streaks and acromegaly. Am J Ophthalmol 1963;56:841–2.
16. Georgalas I, Papconstantinou D, Koutsandrea C, et al. Angioid streaks, clinical course, complications, and current therapeutic management. Ther Clinical Risk Mgmt 2009;5:81–9.

17. Gelisken O, Hendrikske F, Deutman AF. A long-term follow-up study of laser coagulation of neovascular membranes in angioid streaks. Am J Ophthalmol 1988;105:299–303.
18. Lim JI, Bressler NM, Marsh MJ, et al. Laser treatment of choroidal neovascularization in patients with angioid streaks. Am J Ophthalmol 1993;116: 414–23.
19. Pece A, Avanza P, Galli L, et al. Laser photocoagulation of choroidal neovascularization in angioid streaks. Retina 1997;17:12–6.
20. Ozdek S, Bozan E, Gurelik G, et al. Transpupillary thermotherapy for the treatment of choroidal neovascularization secondary to angioid streaks. Can J Ophthalmol 2007;42:95–100.
21. Karacorlu M, Karacorlu S. Ozdemir H, et al. Photodynamic therapy with verteporfin for choroidal neovascularization in patients with angioid streaks. Am J Ophthalmol 2002;134:360–6.
22. Menchini U, Virgili G, Introini U, et al. Outcomes of choroidal neovascularization in angioid streaks after photodynamic therapy. Retina 2004;24:763–71.
23. Mennel S, Schmidt JC, Meyer CH. Therapeutic strategies in choroidal neovascularization secondary to angioid streaks. Am J Ophthalmol 2003;136:580–2.
24. Roth DB, Estafanous M, Lewis H. Macular translocation for subfoveal choroidal neovascularization in angioid streaks. Am J Ophthalmol 2001;131:390–2.
25. Thomas MA, Dickinson JD, Melberg NS, et al. Visual results after surgical removal of subfoveal choroidal neovascular membranes. Ophthalmology 1994;101:1384–96.
26. Cekic O, Gocmez E, Kocabora MS. Management of CNV in angioid streaks by intravitreal use of specific anti-VEGF aptamer (pegaptanib sodium): Long-term results. Curr Eye Res 2011;36:492–5.
27. Finger RP, Issa PC, Schmitz-Valckenberg S, et al. Long-term effectiveness of intravitreal bevacizumab for choroidal neovascularization secondary to angioid streaks in pseudoxanthoma elasticum. Retina 2011;10:1–11.
28. El Matri L, Kort F, Bouraoui R, et al. Intravitreal bevacizumab for the treatment of choroidal neovascularization secondary to angioid streaks: one year of follow-up. Acta Ophthalmol 2011;89(7):641–6.
29. Teixeira A, Mattos T, Velletri R, et al. Clinical course of choroidal neovascularization secondary to angioid streaks treated with intravitreal bevacizumab. Ophthal Surg Lasers Imaging 2010;41:546–9.
30. Wiegand TW, Rogers AH, McCabe F, et al. Intravitreal bevacizumab treatment of choroidal neovascularization in patients with angioid streaks. Br J Ophthalmol 2009;93:47–51.
31. Sawa M, Gomi F, Tsujikawa M, et al. Long-term results of intravitreal bevacizumab injection for choroidal neovascularization secondary to angioid streaks. Am J Ophthalmol 2009;148:594–0.
32. Chang LK, Spaide RF, Brue C, et al. Bevacizumab treatment for subfoveal choroidal neovascularization from causes other than age-related macular degeneration. Arch Ophthalmol 2008;126:941–5.
33. Myung J, Bhatnagar P, Spaide RF, et al. Long-term outcomes of intravitreal antivascular endothelial growth factor therapy for the management of choroidal neovascularization in pseudoxanthoma elasticum. Retina 2010;30:748–55.
34. Carneiro AM, Silva RM, Veludo MJ, et al. Ranibizumab treatment for choriodal neovascularization from causes other than age-related macular degeneration and pathological myopia. Ophthalmologica 2011;225:81–8.
35. Mimoun G, Tilleul J, Leys A, et al. Intravitreal ranibizumab for choroidal neovascularization in angioid streaks. Am J Ophthalmol 2010;150:692–700.
36. Heier JS, Brown D, Ciulla T, et al. Ranibizumab for choroidal neovascularization secondary to causes other than age-related macular degeneration: a phase I clinical trial. Ophthalmology 2011;118:111–8.
37. Ladas ID, Kotsolis AI, Ladas DS, et al. Intravitreal ranibizumab for macular choroidal neovascularization secondary to angioid streaks: one-year results of a prospective study. Retina 2010;30:1185–9.
38. Vadala M, Pece A, Cipolla S, et al. Angioid streak-related choroidal neovascularization treated by intravitreal ranibizumab. Retina 2010;30:903–90.
39. Artunay O, Yuzbasioglu E, Rasier R, et al. Combination treatment with intravitreal injection of ranibizumab and reduced fluence photodynamic therapy for choroidal neovascularization secondary to angioid streaks: preliminary clinical results of 12-month follow-up. Retina 2011;10:1–8.
40. Kazato Y, Shimada H, Nakashizuka H. et al. Immunohistochemical findings of a Bruch's membrane defect and active choroidal neovascularization in angioid streaks. Jpn J Ophthalmol 2011;54:172–4.
41. Dreyer R, Green WR. The pathology of angioid streaks: a study of twenty-one cases. Trans Pa Acad Ophthalmol Otolaryngol 1978;31:158–67.
42. Gass HD. Stereoscopic atlas of macular diseases: Diagnosis and treatment. 4th ed. St Louis: Mosby; 1997. p. 118–25.
43. Shilling JS, Black RK. Prognosis and therapy of angioid streaks. Trans Ophthalmol Soc UK 1975;95:301–6.
44. Sawa M, Ober MD, Freund KB, et al. Fundus autofluorescence in patients with pseudoxanthoma elasticum. Ophthalmology 2006;113:814–20.
45. Issa PC, Finger RP, Gotting C, et al. Centrifugal fundus abnormalities in pseudoxanthoma elasticum. Ophthalmology 2010;117:1406–14.
46. Issa PC, Finger RP, Holz FG, et al. Multimodal imaging including spectral domain OCT and confocal near infrared reflectance for characterization of outer retinal pathology in pseudoxanthoma elasticum. IOVS 2009;50:5913–8.
47. Chan WM, Lim TH, Pece A, et al. Verteporfin PDT for non standard indications: a review of current literature. Graefes Arch Clin Exp Ophthalmol 2010;248:613–26.
48. Shaikh S, Ruby AJ, Williams GA. Photodynamic therapy using verteporfin for choroidal neovascularization in angioid streaks. Am J Ophthalmol 2003;136: 1–6.
49. Browning AC, Amoaku WM, Chung AK, et al. Photodynamic therapy for angioid steaks. Ophthalmology 2007;114:1592.

Chapter 70

Ocular Histoplasmosis

Justis P. Ehlers, Barbara S. Hawkins, Andrew P. Schachat

HISTORICAL PERSPECTIVE

In 1942 Reid provided the first description of histoplasmosis-associated ophthalmic abnormalities from a patient with acute disseminated histoplasmosis.[1] Following Reid's description, additional reports surfaced of atrophic chorioretinal lesions associated with positive histoplasmin skin testing.[2-4] In 1959 Woods and Wahlen[4] published a series of 62 patients with granulomatous uveitis. Nineteen of these patients "showed a peculiar and consistent pattern of ocular lesions" that included both discrete atrophic, sparsely pigmented or unpigmented, peripheral lesions (frequently referred to as "histo spots") and later cystic lesions in the macula. Skin testing for histoplasmin was positive in all of these 19 patients. Woods and Wahlen concluded that previous benign systemic histoplasmosis was responsible for the ocular findings in these 19 patients.[4] A few years later Schlaegel and Kenney[5] demonstrated that atrophic lesions around the optic nerve were also part of the clinical spectrum of ocular histoplasmosis syndrome (OHS), often called ocular histoplasmosis or presumed ocular histoplasmosis syndrome (POHS).

CLINICAL FEATURES OF OCULAR HISTOPLASMOSIS

The symptoms associated with ocular histoplasmosis are wide-ranging and are dependent on the pathology present. Atrophic lesions are typically asymptomatic. The presence of choroidal neovascularization (CNV) often results in variable vision loss and metamorphosia.

A clinical diagnosis of ocular histoplasmosis is based on the presence of at least two of the following fundus lesions in one or both eyes in the absence of ocular inflammation:[6,7]

- Discrete, focal, atrophic (i.e., punched-out) choroidal scars in the macula or the periphery, smaller in size than the optic disc (histo spots) (Fig. 70.1).
- Peripapillary chorioretinal scarring (i.e., peripapillary atrophy) (Fig. 70.2).
- CNV or associated sequelae (hemorrhagic retinal detachment, fibrovascular disciform scar) (Figs 70.3–70.5).

Most often both eyes have typical lesions, although the appearance may not be symmetric at initial presentation. The early granulomatous stage of ocular histoplasmosis, as described by Woods and Whalen, is rarely seen clinically.[4,6] The initial focal scars are probably too small to be seen with the ophthalmoscope. Gass[6] has postulated that lymphocytic infiltration of the surrounding tissue produces enlargement of the lesion over a period of years and thus allows it to become clinically detectable.

Differential diagnosis

The differential diagnosis of ocular histoplasmosis includes a wide spectrum of disorders:

- **Multifocal choroiditis with panuveitis.** Characterized by multiple chorioretinal scars with similar findings to ocular histoplasmosis. Significant anterior and/or posterior

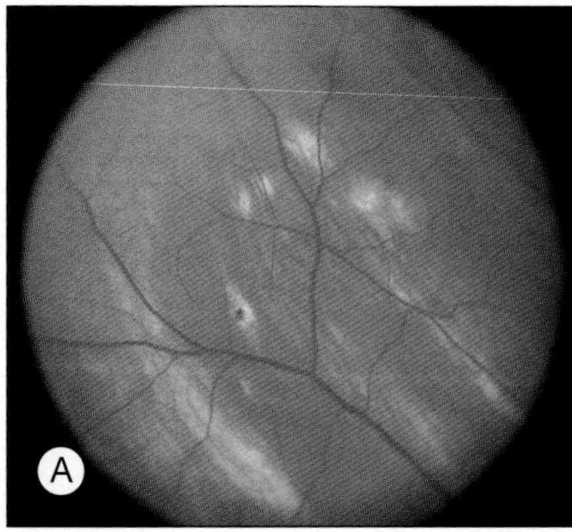

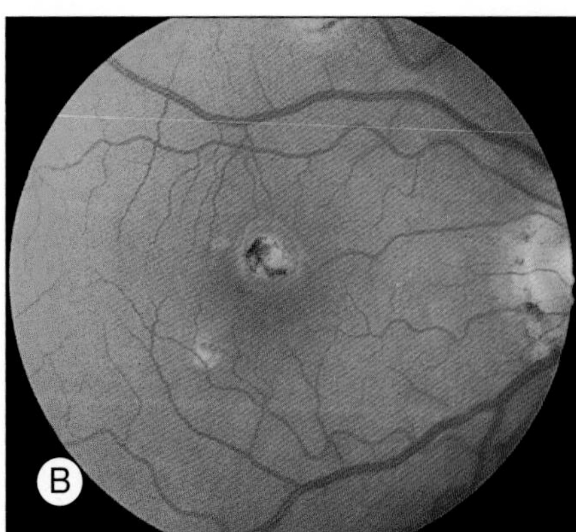

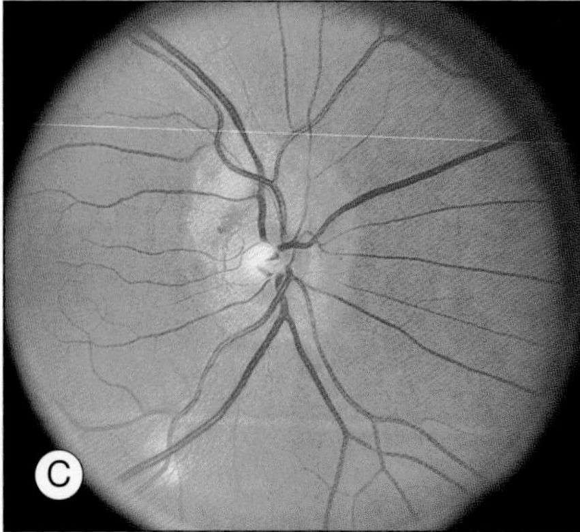

Fig. 70.1 Chorioretinal scars (i.e., "histo spots") characteristic of ocular histoplasmosis. (A) Peripheral histo spots. (B) Macular histo spots. Larger lesion with pigment proliferation may represent spontaneously regressed choroidal neovascularization (CNV). (C) Histo spots and peripapillary scarring. The peripapillary lesion superotemporal and within the peripapillary scarring probably represents spontaneously regressed CNV.

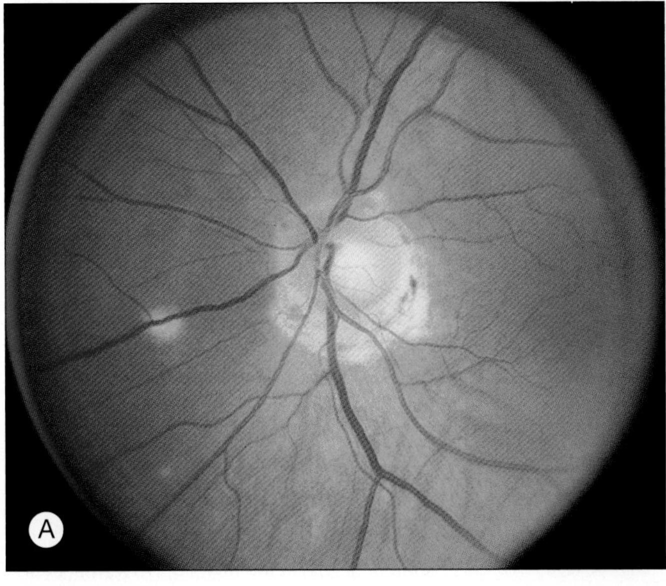

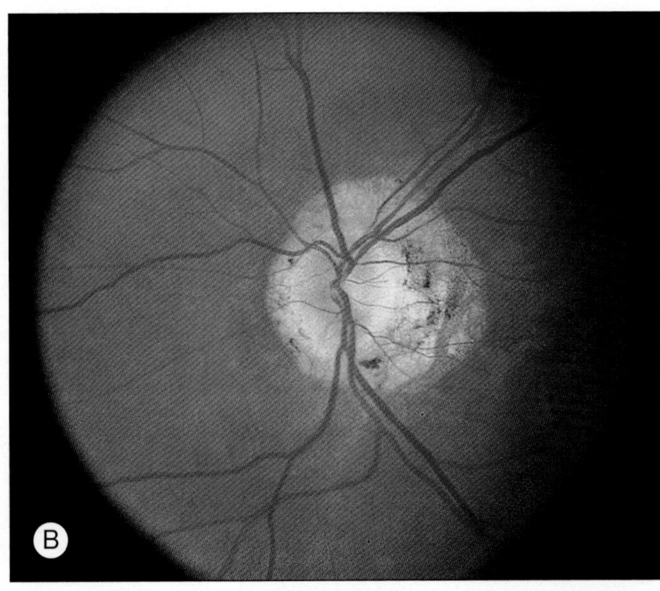

Fig. 70.2 Two examples of peripapillary scarring.

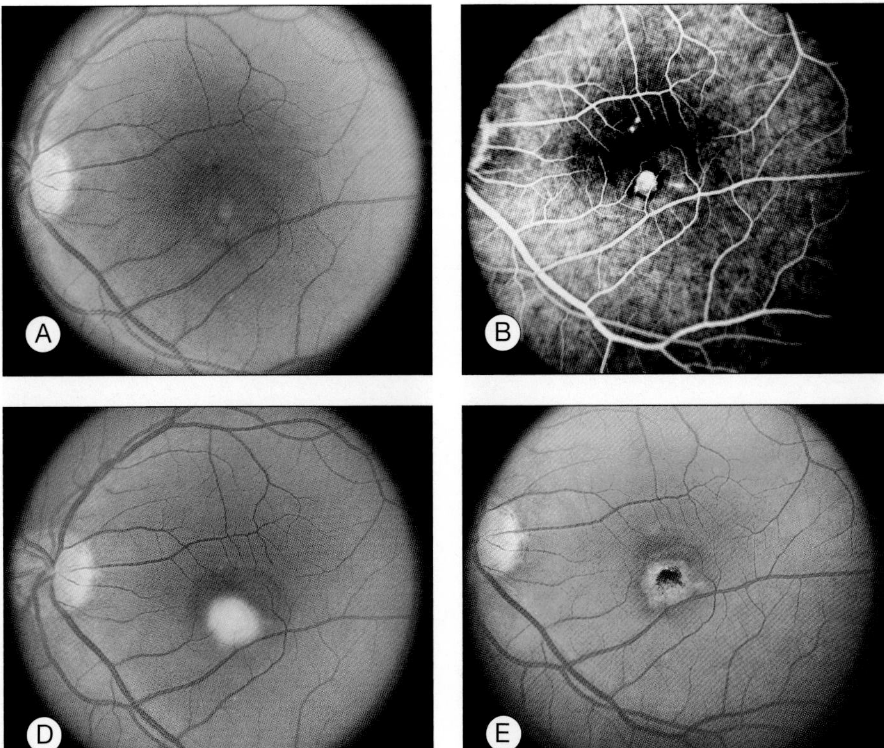

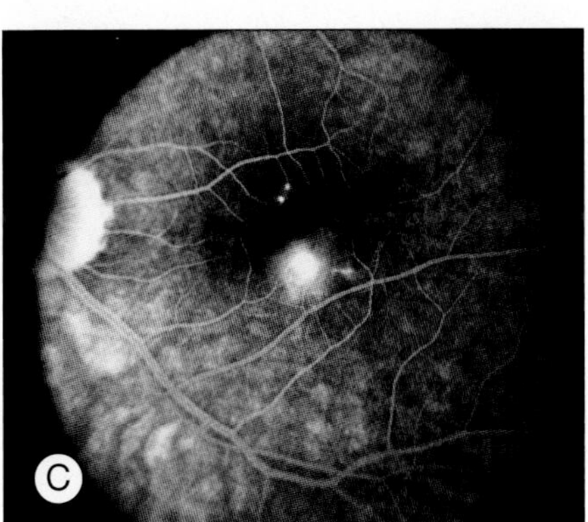

Fig. 70.3 (A) Choroidal neovascularization (CNV) secondary to ocular histoplasmosis with subretinal fluid in the macula. (B) Early frame of fluorescein angiogram shows extrafoveal CNV. (C) Late frame of fluorescein angiogram shows increased leakage of fluorescein dye. (D) Color photograph taken 1 day after laser photocoagulation shows whitening of retina from treatment. (E) Treatment scar 2 years after laser photocoagulation; no evidence of recurrent CNV.

inflammation present in the active phase, and there may have associated CNV. One study examined distinguishing features of multifocal choroiditis compared to ocular histoplasmosis.[8] Findings that were more characteristic of multifocal choroiditis included progressive growth of lesions, bridging scars, progressive proliferation of pigment, myopic disc changes, clustering of lesions (e.g., macula, equator), disc swelling, subretinal fibrosis, and narrowed/sheathed vessels.[8] These features may be particularly important in distinguishing quiescent multifocal choroiditis from ocular histoplasmosis (see Chapter 76, White spot syndromes and related diseases).

- **Myopic degeneration.** Peripapillary atrophy and CNV may be seen in patients with myopic degeneration. Small white focal areas of chorioretinal atrophy along with linear atrophic areas (e.g., lacquer cracks) may also be present in the posterior pole (see Chapter 68, Myopic macular degeneration).
- **Multiple evanescent white-dot syndrome (MEWDS).** White lesions of the retinal pigment epithelium (RPE)/outer retina may be present with associated granularity of the fovea. Often the vision is transiently decreased with an associated enlarged blind spot. Mild inflammation may be present. Scarring and permanent chorioretinal lesions are not usually

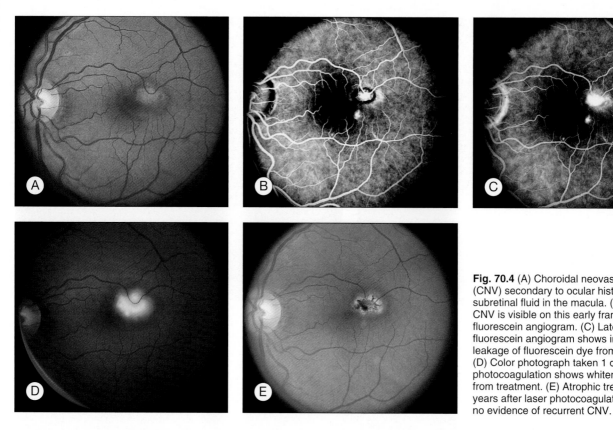

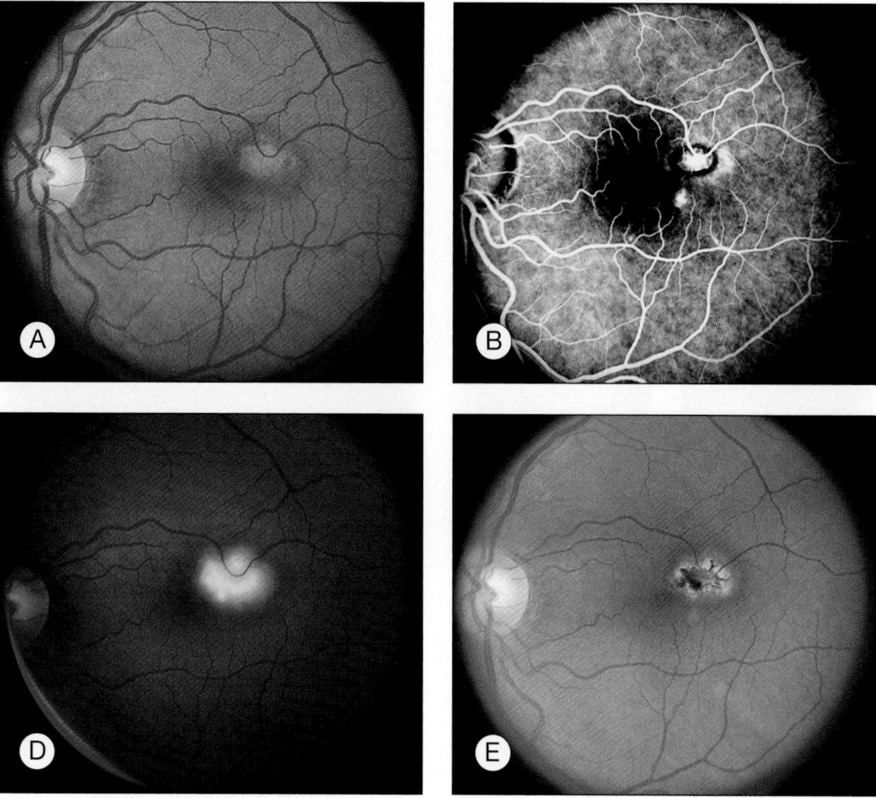

Fig. 70.4 (A) Choroidal neovascularization (CNV) secondary to ocular histoplasmosis with subretinal fluid in the macula. (B) Extrafoveal CNV is visible on this early frame of a fluorescein angiogram. (C) Late frame of fluorescein angiogram shows increased leakage of fluorescein dye from the CNV. (D) Color photograph taken 1 day after laser photocoagulation shows whitening of retina from treatment. (E) Atrophic treatment scar 2.5 years after laser photocoagulation; no evidence of recurrent CNV.

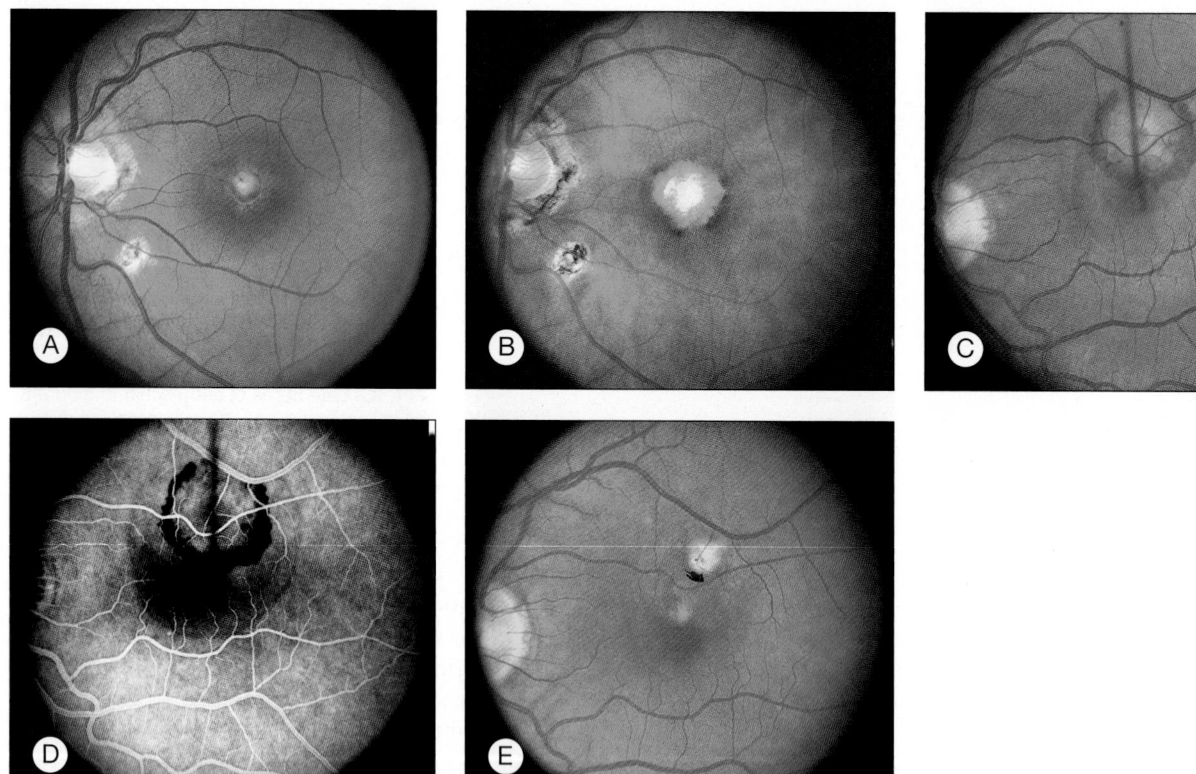

Fig. 70.5 The Macular Photocoagulation Study Group demonstrated that laser treatment of eligible choroidal neovascular lesions was better than no treatment with respect to delaying or preventing loss of visual acuity. However, some CNV regresses spontaneously. These two patients did not have laser treatment of their choroidal neovascularization (CNV), which involuted spontaneously. (A) Juxtafoveal CNV in first patient. (B) Disciform scar 4 years later. (C) This patient had extrafoveal CNV with a rim of hemorrhage visible on the photograph. (D) CNV, hemorrhage, and fluid are all visible on this early frame of a fluorescein angiogram. (E) A small scar with pigment proliferation is visible 4 years later. Visual acuity returned to 20/20 3 months after enrollment and remained at 20/20 throughout the 5-year follow-up period.

observed (see Chapter 76, White spot syndromes and related diseases).

- **Idiopathic CNV.** A diagnosis of exclusion. Particularly in younger individuals, idiopathic CNV is seen in the absence of other signs of ocular histoplasmosis, age-related macular degeneration (AMD), angioid streaks, and other CNV-related conditions.
- **Choroidal rupture with CNV.** A history of trauma is usually present. A partially circumferential concentric chorioretinal macular scar is typically present and is associated with the CNV. Peripapillary atrophy and associated peripheral chorioretinal atrophy is not present (see Chapter 91, Traumatic chorioretinopathies).
- **Punctate inner choroidopathy.** Minimal to mild inflammation may be present. Atrophic scars may be associated with CNV. Spots are usually smaller than those seen with ocular histoplasmosis. Predominantly seen in women. Peripapillary atrophy is usually not present. Acute symptoms (e.g., photopsias) are usually associated with the initial diagnosis of the white lesions and may correlate with location of lesions (see Chapter 76, White spot syndromes and related diseases).
- **Neovascular AMD.** Typically in older patients (i.e., >50 years). Drusen present. Areas of focal atrophy may be present in the macula but the atrophy is not usually seen in the periphery. Peripapillary atrophy is often not present (see Chapter 66, Neovascular (exudative or "wet") age-related macular degeneration).
- **Sarcoidosis.** Scattered active inflammatory choroidal lesions may be present. Usually accompanied by anterior/posterior inflammation. CNV and peripapillary atrophy not typically present. Elevated angiotensin-converting enzyme may be seen. Often associated with hilar adenopathy on chest X-ray or CT scan of the chest (see Chapter 78, Sarcoidosis).

RELATIONSHIP OF OCULAR DISEASE TO SYSTEMIC INFECTION

Systemic infection with *Histoplasma capsulatum* via the respiratory tract is thought to be the initial event prior to the development of ocular histoplasmosis. Although a definitive causal relationship between *H. capsulatum* and the ocular disorder has not been demonstrated to satisfy Koch's postulates completely,[9,10] continuing experimental work with primates,[11,12] may eventually satisfy this requirement.

Several observations support a causal relationship between *H. capsulatum* and the ocular histoplasmosis syndrome:

- Almost all patients diagnosed as having ocular histoplasmosis in the USA have lived some or all of their lives in an endemic area.[13,14]
- Positive histoplasmin skin testing occurs more frequently in patients with ocular histoplasmosis compared with controls.[14–16]
- Activation of lesions of ocular histoplasmosis has been reported following histoplasmin skin testing.[2–4,16–18]
- DNA from *H. capsulatum* has been isolated from an enucleated eye previously diagnosed with ocular histoplasmosis.[19]

Other observations can be used to question the causal relationship between *H. capsulatum* and the ocular syndrome. In the UK and Europe, a clinical syndrome nearly identical to ocular histoplasmosis may occur.[20–24] These patients have never lived in or visited an endemic area, however, and only a small proportion of Europeans are positive reactors to histoplasmin skin testing.[20–25] Additionally, *H. capsulatum* has not been identified in the UK.[25] Certainly, the possibility exists that an alternate organism may result in a similar ocular syndrome in these areas.[22] Systemic antifungal treatment with amphotericin B has not been shown to be effective for the treatment of the ocular disorder.[26]

Clinical features of systemic infection

Goodwin[27] classified systemic infection based on the immune status of the host and exposure type. The usual histoplasmosis infection is a relatively mild illness with flu-like respiratory symptoms. Most patients do not seek medical care. Studies in Tennessee have demonstrated that almost 90% of children of 13 years of age had positive reactions to histoplasmin skin tests.[28] A great deal of variation has been observed in the distribution of positive reactors by neighborhood of residence.[29,30] Rarely, more severe, even fatal cases of disseminated infection may occur, but these are usually associated with immune system deficiencies, such as acquired immunodeficency syndrome (AIDS). Occasionally, epidemics of systemic disease outbreak may occur which are often associated with high levels of environmental exposure (e.g., excavations, construction projects in old buildings, work in chicken or other fowl habitats, or exposure in bat-inhabited caves).[31–46]

EPIDEMIOLOGY OF OCULAR HISTOPLASMOSIS

Geographic distribution of *H. capsulatum* in the USA

The Ohio and Mississippi river valleys make up the largest part of the "histo belt," where 60% or more of lifelong residents have positive histoplasmin skin testing.[47] Comstock described the major endemic histoplasmosis area as a triangle with its apices in Eastern Nebraska, Central Ohio, and Southwestern Mississippi.[29]

Prevalence and incidence

The prevalence of asymptomatic ocular histoplasmosis in endemic areas (e.g., Ohio, Maryland) within the USA ranges from 1.6 to 5.3%.[14,15,48] The disciform lesion prevalence rates in the same areas were 0.0 to 0.1% of the endemic populations.[14,15,48] In those eyes that had atrophic spots, the prevalence of disciform lesions was 4.5%.[48]

The incidence rate of neovascular disciform lesions and atrophic lesions is largely unknown. The development of initial neovascular disciform lesions has been reported at around 2 per 100 000 population per year.[49] Studies examining the incidence rate of neovascular lesions in fellow eyes have shown a rate of 0.0 to 12% per year.[50–54]

Age

The median age of patients with vision-threatening disciform lesions has typically been reported to be in the fourth and fifth decade, with an age range of 10 to 81 years old.[13,17,49,55–58] The median age of persons who have atrophic scars has been reported to be in the fourth, fifth, and sixth decades of life by various investigators.[15,59] These reports are of the age at detection, however, and not necessarily the age of development of the atrophic lesion. It is likely that these lesions develop earlier in life and are only coincidentally discovered during ophthalmic examinations for causes of visual symptoms that may or may not be related to ocular histoplasmosis.

Gender and race

There is no gender predilection for ocular histoplasmosis. The vast majority of disciform lesions occur in Caucasians with only around a dozen cases reported among African Americans.[60] Interestingly, histo spots and positive skin tests have been reported in some studies to have similar prevalence among Caucasians and African Americans.[15,61] Other studies have found a much higher prevalence in Caucasians (i.e., nearly 100% of all cases) as compared to Hispanics or African Americans.[14,16,48,55]

Histocompatibility antigens and genetic predisposition

In disciform lesions, both human leukocyte antigen (HLA)-B7 and HLA-DRw2 have been reported to be two to four times more common among cases than controls.[62–64] For histo spots, HLA-DRw2 was twice as common among cases as among controls, but less difference was seen between the groups in regards to HLA-B7.[64,65] These findings suggest an underlying genetic susceptibility or predisposition for development of ocular histoplasmosis. It is unclear whether this genetic predisposition specifically reflects the susceptibility to ocular histoplasmosis or to infection by *H. capsulatum*. Although these associations exist, routine testing for HLA typing in connection with ocular histoplasmosis is not typically performed owing to the lack of significant positive and negative predictive values.

PATHOGENESIS

Numerous theories regarding the pathogenesis of ocular histoplasmosis have been proposed. The most widely accepted theory involves focal infection of the choroid at the time of systemic infection. The focal inflammatory/infectious process results in an atrophic scar that disrupts Bruch's membrane. Alternatively, the infection may involve the retinal pigment epithelium and choriocapillaris and may progress rapidly to subretinal hemorrhage, exudation, and a fibrovascular disciform scar (Fig. 70.6).

CNV formation may be promoted by multiple factors at the site of the atrophic scar. Disruption of Bruch's membrane provides access to the subretinal space for neovascularization.[66] The fragile vessels are prone to hemorrhage and exudation, often ultimately resulting in disorganization of the RPE and neurosensory retina and, ultimately, a fibrovascular scar.

The initiator for CNV development is unknown. The results from HLA typing suggest a possible genetic predisposition for progression from atrophic scars to disciform lesions in ocular histoplasmosis.[62–65] Other hypotheses have attributed these phenomena to a larger initial inoculum of the fungus,[11,67] reinfection,[4,68] hypersensitivity,[4,14] and the presence of other factors that compromise the vascular system[14,69,70] or the immune system.[71] CNV development has also been associated with proangiogenic factors such as vascular endothelial growth factor.[72]

Studying ocular histoplasmosis with animal models has been difficult. Histoplasmosis is known to occur in many species of animals.[73–77] However, efforts to develop an animal model for ocular histoplasmosis have been hampered by two major factors: (1) nonprimates do not have a macula with its special anatomic, physiologic, and neurologic characteristics; and (2) decades are believed to elapse between initial infection with *H. capsulatum* and the development of characteristic macular lesions. The most promising animal models are primates, in which systemic infection and ocular lesions have been produced.[11,12]

NATURAL HISTORY OF OCULAR HISTOPLASMOSIS AND PUBLIC HEALTH IMPLICATIONS

Histo spots outside the macular area are typically asymptomatic, although visual symptoms occasionally have been reported that correlate with the location of the atrophic scars.[78] Active CNV may result in sudden decrease in vision secondary to hemorrhage or exudation. The vision loss in this disease often occurs in middle-aged individuals who are in the most active and productive stage of their life.[13,17,49,55–58] Spontaneous recovery of central vision has been reported in the Macular Photocoagulation Study (MPS)[51,56] and by other investigators.[79–81]

Two studies have addressed the public health importance of ocular histoplasmosis as a cause of visual impairment. One study in Tennessee found that ocular histoplasmosis was responsible for 2.8% of visual impairment among applicants for aid for the blind.[49] In Maryland a study comparing the 15-year incidence of visual impairment in those persons with histo spots to those persons without histo spots found that there was no difference in the rates of visual impairment.[50] The Submacular Surgery Trials Research Group found that individuals with unilateral and bilateral CNV cases had significant deficits in visual function, similar to patients with neovascular age-related macular degeneration (AMD).[82] Not surprisingly, the study showed that patients with bilateral CNV had significantly worse functional impairment of all groups, but those with unilateral involvement also had significant functional deficits.[82]

TREATMENT

Numerous approaches for ocular histoplasmosis management have been suggested, including avoidance of stress, avoidance of aspirin, avoidance of the Valsalva maneuver, hyposensitization to histoplasmin, use of immunosuppressive agents, and photocoagulation.[9] Histoplasmin desensitization,[83] amphotericin B,[17,26] and other prophylactic interventions[84,85] have been tried by many investigators and discarded. No treatment is known to prevent inactive lesions from giving rise to exudative or hemorrhagic neovascular complexes that typically end in disciform macular scars. Systemic corticosteroids also have been suggested, particularly in cases of "active" histo spots and subfoveal CNV.[6] in the era of anti-vascular endothelial growth factor (VEGF) and photodynamic therapy (PDT), however, the use of systemic corticosteroids even in subfoveal cases is now mainly of historic interest. Whether there is a role to manage active histo spots is unclear since many or perhaps most spontaneously involute.

Laser photocoagulation

Initiated in 1979, the Macular Photocoagulation Study (MPS) Group demonstrated the effectiveness of laser treatment in comparison to no treatment two randomized clinical trials for patients with well-defined extrafoveal or juxtafoveal CNV.[56,57,86,87] The first trial enrolled 262 patients with well-demarcated extrafoveal CNV.[57,86] The posterior border of these lesions could not

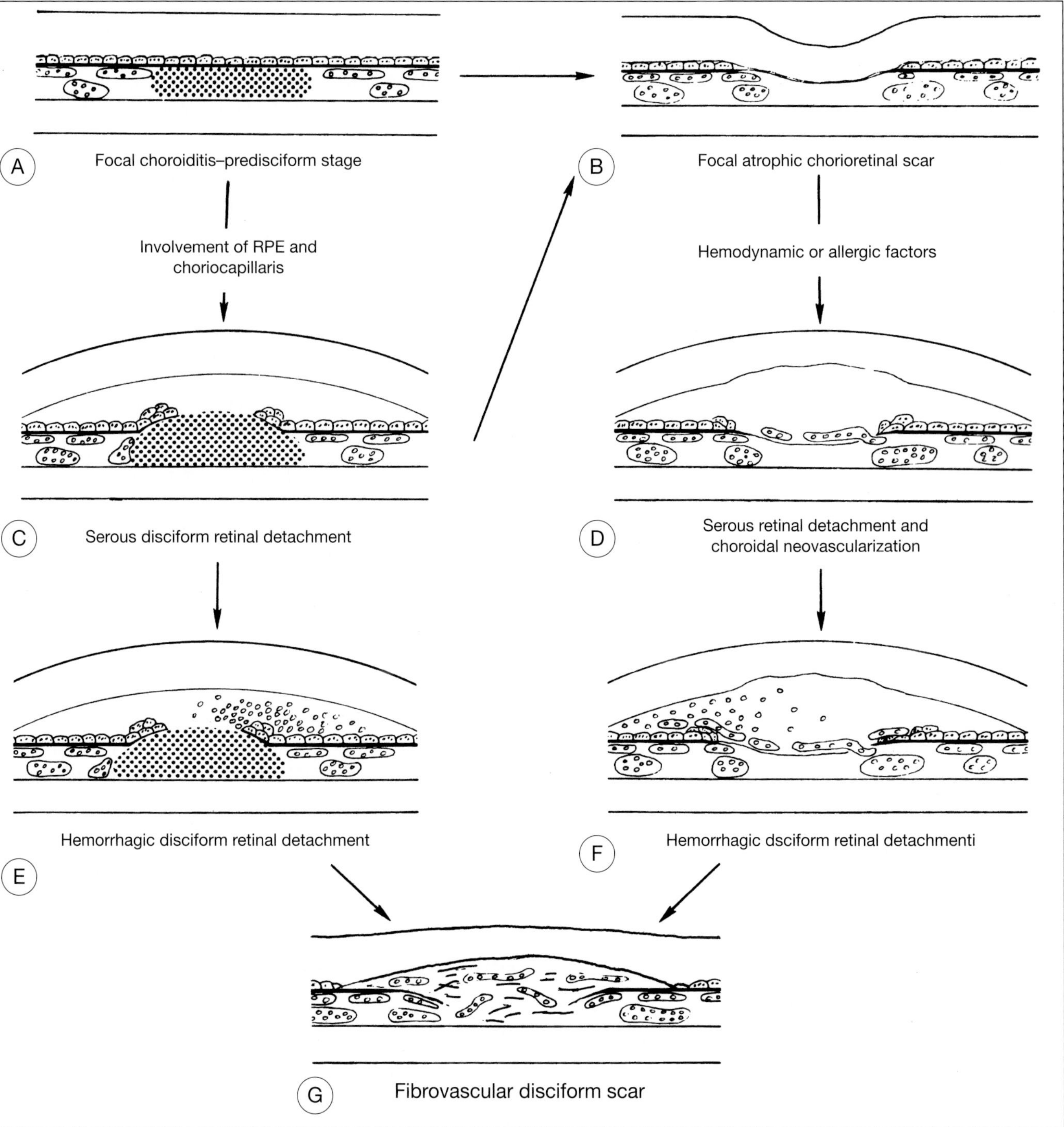

Fig. 70.6 Hypothesized mechanism of the pathogenesis of disciform lesions of ocular histoplasmosis. Focal choroiditis (A) damages the choriocapillaris, retinal pigment epithelium (RPE), and Bruch's membrane and produces an exudative detachment of the retina (B) or hemorrhage into the subretinal space (C). Any of these three stages may resolve, leaving either a focal area of atrophy of the retinal pigment epithelium, Bruch's membrane, and choroid (D) or, in the case of subretinal hemorrhage, a disciform scar (G). Either in the absence of further inflammation or under the influence of recurrent episodes of inflammation, the choroidal blood vessels surrounding an atrophic chorioretinal scar (D) may decompensate and cause serous exudation, choroidal neovascularization, and transient serous detachment of the retina (E). This process in turn may result in a hemorrhagic detachment of the retina (F) that resolves as a disciform scar (G). (Reproduced with permission from Gass JDM. Stereoscopic atlas of macular diseases, vol. 1: Diagnosis and treatment. St Louis: Mosby; 1987. p 6.)

be closer than 200 μm from the center of the foveal avascular zone; initial best-corrected visual acuity of the affected eye was 20/100 or better. Eligible eyes were randomly assigned to argon laser treatment or to no treatment. The eyes were re-examined twice each year, at which time best-corrected VA was measured and color photographs were taken. Fluorescein angiograms were taken at time of study entry, 6 and 12 months after enrollment, and annually thereafter.

In 1983, the MPS Data and Safety Monitoring Committee halted enrollment after concluding that argon laser photocoagulation was beneficial in preventing or delaying large loss of visual acuity compared to observation without treatment. From

18 months through 5 years, a 6 or more line loss of VA was experienced in 10% of treated eyes compared to 40% of untreated controls. Median VA at baseline was 20/25 and after five years dropped to 20/40 in the treated group compared to 20/80 in controls.[86] In the laser-treated group, 26% of eyes had persistence of CNV or recurrence of CNV at the scar edge, and 7% developed a new CNV not contiguous with the laser scar.[86]

In 1981 a second trial was initiated by the MPS Group for patients with juxtafoveal CNV.[87] In this trial, best-corrected VA at entry was permitted to be as poor as 20/400 in the study eye. A total of 289 eyes were randomized between krypton laser treatment and no treatment. Five years after the trial began, the MPS Data and Safety Monitoring Committee again halted enrollment after concluding that eyes treated with krypton laser were less likely to lose visual acuity than untreated eyes. A 6- or more line loss was seen in 11% of the treated eyes compared to about 30% of the controls.[87] Approximately one-third of treated patients had persistent or recurrent CNV contiguous with the zone of laser treatment; and new, noncontiguous areas of CNV developed in 2% of treated eyes.[87] A subgroup analysis by the MPS group of CNV located between the fovea and optic nerve showed that there was no contraindication to treatment of these lesions in the papillomacular bundle with laser.[88] A subset of the MPS Group piloted laser photocoagulation for subfoveal CNV secondary to ocular histoplasmosis but observed no short-term benefit compared to observation.[89]

In view of the very good results with extrafoveal CNV and even juxtafoveal CNV from the MPS studies, laser photocoagulation therapy should be seriously considered for these lesions. Additionally, when compared to anti-VEGF therapy, laser photocoagulation is not as expensive and avoids many of the ocular and possible systemic risks of intravitreal injections with anti-VEGF agents. If subfoveal recurrence or primary subfoveal disease develops, photodynamic therapy or anti-VEGF treatment should be considered (see below).

Photodynamic therapy

The treatment of subfoveal CNV secondary to ocular histoplasmosis with photodynamic therapy (PDT) was first suggested in 2002.[90] Since that small study, numerous studies have been published examining the use of PDT for ocular histoplasmosis. In fact, PDT is now approved by the United States Food and Drug Administration (FDA) for the treatment of subfoveal CNV secondary to ocular histoplasmosis.

Most of the studies performed for PDT with ocular histoplasmosis have been retrospective case series. In a 2003 retrospective review of 38 eyes with juxtafoveal CNV treated with PDT, treated eyes were more than twice as likely to have visual improvement or stabilization compared to the natural history group in the corresponding MPS clinical trial. Visual acuity improved or stabilized in 69% of eyes, with 44% of eyes improving at least 2 lines. Nearly 40% of eyes had undergone submacular surgery prior to PDT.[91] In 2004 a retrospective review of 11 eyes, of which 5 had juxtafoveal CNV and 6 had subfoveal CNV, documented similar findings. Eighty percent of eyes showed vision stabilization or improvement in the juxtafoveal group. Sixty percent of eyes with juxtafoveal lesions achieved a final visual acuity of 20/40 or better. Eyes with subfoveal lesions had similar results with 83% of eyes having stabilization or improvement in vision. Fifty percent of eyes with subfoveal CNV also had a final visual acuity of 20/40 or better.[92] In 2005 a retrospective review of 23 eyes with juxtafoveal CNV associated with ocular histoplasmosis found that approximately 82% of eyes had visual stabilization (less than 2 line loss) or improvement. Thirty percent of eyes gained more than 2 lines of vision. Approximately, 60% of patients required only a single PDT session. Following PDT, submacular surgery was performed in 16% of patients due to CNV progression.[93]

In 2006 a retrospective review of young patients undergoing PDT for CNV secondary to etiologies other than AMD included 6 patients with ocular histoplasmosis with subfoveal CNV. The mean pretreatment acuity in these eyes was 20/50 and the mean final visual acuity was 20/50. Three of these eyes (50%) required at least one retreatment session with PDT. One of 6 patients improved by more than 1 line of VA. Four eyes (67%) maintained their visual acuity (i.e., less than 2 lines lost or gained), and one eye gained more than 2 lines of VA and one eye lost 2 lines.[94]

An uncontrolled prospective trial evaluating PDT for subfoveal CNV secondary to POHS included 26 eyes. Examination of 22 eyes 2 years following initial treatment revealed that 45% of eyes had gained 1.5 lines or more. Eighteen percent of eyes lost 1.5 lines or more, including 9% of eyes that lost 3 or more lines of VA. The mean number of treatments was 2.9 during the first year and 1 during the second year. After 2 years, only 15% of eyes had persistent angiographic leakage.[95]

Anti-VEGF therapy

Over the last several years, the use of anti-VEGF agents has transformed the landscape in the treatment of CNV-related disease, particularly neovascular AMD. Case reports and case series suggest that anti-VEGF agents may also be effective in the treatment of CNV secondary to ocular histoplasmosis (Fig. 70.7). In 2007 the first case report was published documenting a

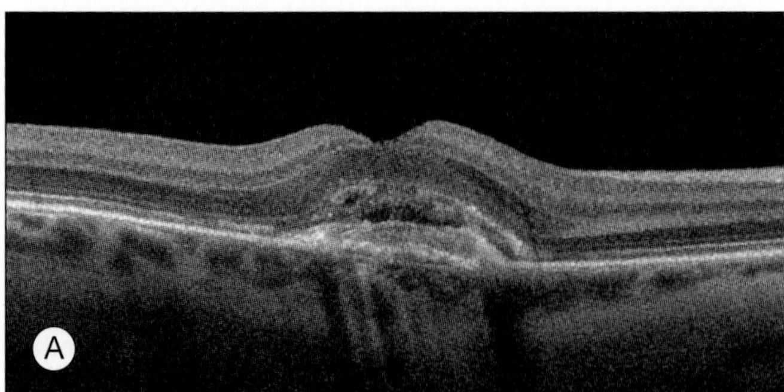

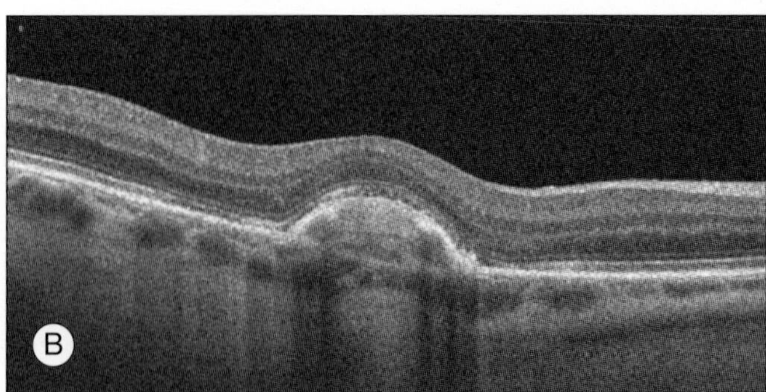

Fig. 70.7 Optical coherence tomography images of subfoveal choroidal neovascularization (CNV). CNV is visible in the subfoveal area with overlying subretinal fluid (A). Following intravitreal bevacizumab therapy, the subretinal fluid is significantly improved although the CNV remains (B).

23-year-old female with sudden vision loss to 20/200 with subfoveal CNV. After a single intravitreal injection of bevacizumab, the visual acuity improved to 20/30 by 6 months follow-up.[96] Of course, the control arms of the MPS studies discussed above show that spontaneous involution can occur, but following this case report, retrospective consecutive case series were published examining the use of the intravitreal bevacizumab for the treatment of CNV in ocular histoplasmosis. One study examined intravitreal bevacizumab in 24 treatment-naïve eyes. The mean age was 43 years and the average number of injections was 6.8 per year. After 3 months, visual acuity improved from a mean baseline visual acuity of 20/114 to 20/55 (i.e., approximately 3-lines). Fifty-eight percent of eyes had 20/40 or better vision at final follow-up compared to 21% at baseline. Nine patients had 12 month follow-up and improved from a mean baseline visual acuity of 20/150 to 20/45 (i.e., approximately 6 lines). No significant complications were reported.[97]

A second study examined the use of bevacizumab in 28 eyes with CNV secondary to histoplasmosis. All patients included had active CNV with subfoveal fluid and either juxtafoveal or subfoveal CNV. Previous or concurrent PDT was allowed in this study. Seven patients were treatment naïve, 16 were PDT failures, and 5 patients were treated with combination PDT/bevacizumab therapy. The mean age was 46 years and mean follow-up was 5 months. Overall, the mean initial visual acuity was 20/88 and the mean final visual acuity was 20/54. Stability of visual acuity (<1.5 line loss) was seen in 93% of patients. Additionally, 43% of eyes experienced a 3 or more line gain. Both of the studies examining bevacizumab were retrospective with significant methodologic shortcomings and the results should be interpreted with caution.[98]

A phase I randomized 12-month clinical trial evaluated ranibizumab for the treatment of CNV secondary to conditions other than AMD has been conducted. This study randomized eyes to monthly ranibizumab or 3-monthly injections followed by an as needed (prn) dosing schedule at monthly visits. Nine eyes (of 30) with ocular histoplasmosis were included in this trial, 4 in the monthly arm and 5 in the prn arm. Prior treatment with other therapeutic modalities was allowed. Subgroup analysis was not performed for each diagnosis included. As a group, mean lines of change from baseline was +7.4 in the monthly injection arm and +5.0 in the prn group. A 3-line or more gain in visual acuity was seen in 66.7% of the monthly arm patients and in 57% in the prn arm. There were no statistically significant differences between the groups at any time point. No serious ocular or systemic adverse events were observed but larger sample sizes are needed to detect infrequent severe adverse events.[99]

Further research is needed to define better the role of anti-VEGF therapy in the management of CNV secondary to ocular histoplasmosis. Early research suggests that it may have an important role in the management of this condition.

Combination therapy

Similar to AMD, combination therapy is also being considered for the treatment of CNV secondary to ocular histoplasmosis. Combination therapy may reduce the need for ongoing intravitreal injections. PDT or laser photocoagulation may provide a more enduring effect, compared to anti-VEGF therapy alone. Adding anti-VEGF therapy may reduce the required spot size needed for either laser modality. In 2010, a small retrospective case series examining combination anti-VEGF agents with PDT included three eyes with CNV secondary to ocular histoplasmosis. Treatment consisted of PDT and intravitreal bevacizumab initiated concurrently with retreatment with PDT every 10–12 weeks and with bevacizumab every 4–6 weeks. Retreatment was based on persistent edema or subretinal fluid. Three of 3 (100%) eyes improved 2 lines or more at final follow-up.[100] As outlined in the previous section, a retrospective case series utilizing bevacizumab for CNV secondary to ocular histoplasmosis included 5 eyes that were treated with concurrent PDT therapy. Subgroup analysis of these five patients revealed that all five eyes experienced stabilization or improvement in visual acuity with a mean gain of 2.4 lines.[98]

Intravitreal triamcinolone

Given the possible underlying inflammatory pathogenic mechanisms of ocular histoplasmosis, the use of intravitreal steroids may be of use in the treatment of CNV secondary to ocular histoplasmosis. A retrospective case series examined the use of intravitreal triamcinolone in 10 eyes with CNV secondary to ocular histoplasmosis (5 subfoveal and 5 juxtafoveal) was conducted with a median follow-up of 17 months. Visual acuity improved or stabilized in 80% of eyes, including 30% that gained 1 line or more. Twenty percent of eyes lost 1–3 lines of visual acuity, and no eyes lost more than 3 lines of vision. Cataract progression and increased intraocular pressure were concerning ocular side effects.[101]

Submacular surgery and macular translocation

Prior to PDT and anti-VEGF therapy, submacular surgery for CNV secondary to ocular histoplasmosis was an important treatment alternative for many patients with significant vision loss.[102–104] As with many treatment modalities for CNV, recurrence of CNV is a major issue. In fact, the recurrence rate after submacular surgery is higher than recurrence following laser photocoagulation.[105] In 1997 the National Eye Institute and the National Institutes of Health initiated the Submacular Surgery Trials group H trial in order to compare functional outcomes and quality of life between patients assigned to surgery versus those assigned to observation (Fig. 70.8). The trial included 225 patients non-AMD with subfoveal CNV and visual acuity of 20/50 to 20/800. Of the 225 patients, 192 patients had ocular histoplasmosis. At 2 years, vision had improved or remained stable in 20% more patients treated with surgery than with observation.[106] This outcome difference was not statistically significant. Subgroup analyses revealed that nearly all of the benefit seen with surgery was in those eyes with 20/100 or worse baseline visual acuity. In this subset of 92 eyes, 76% of surgery eyes remained stable or improved compared to 50% of eyes that were observed. Additionally, quality-of-life scores improved more with surgery.[107]

Macular translocation has also been utilized for the treatment of patients with bilateral vision loss associated with ocular histoplasmosis.[108] One report described three cases of ocular histoplasmosis treated with 360-degree macular translocation. Two of the 3 eyes showed improvement in visual acuity. Two of the 3 cases developed recurrent CNV, and 2 of the 3 cases developed chronic cystoid macular edema.[108] Limited macular translocation for ocular histoplasmosis has also been reported, but the specific visual acuity results were not separated from the larger study which included predominantly AMD cases so that conclusions

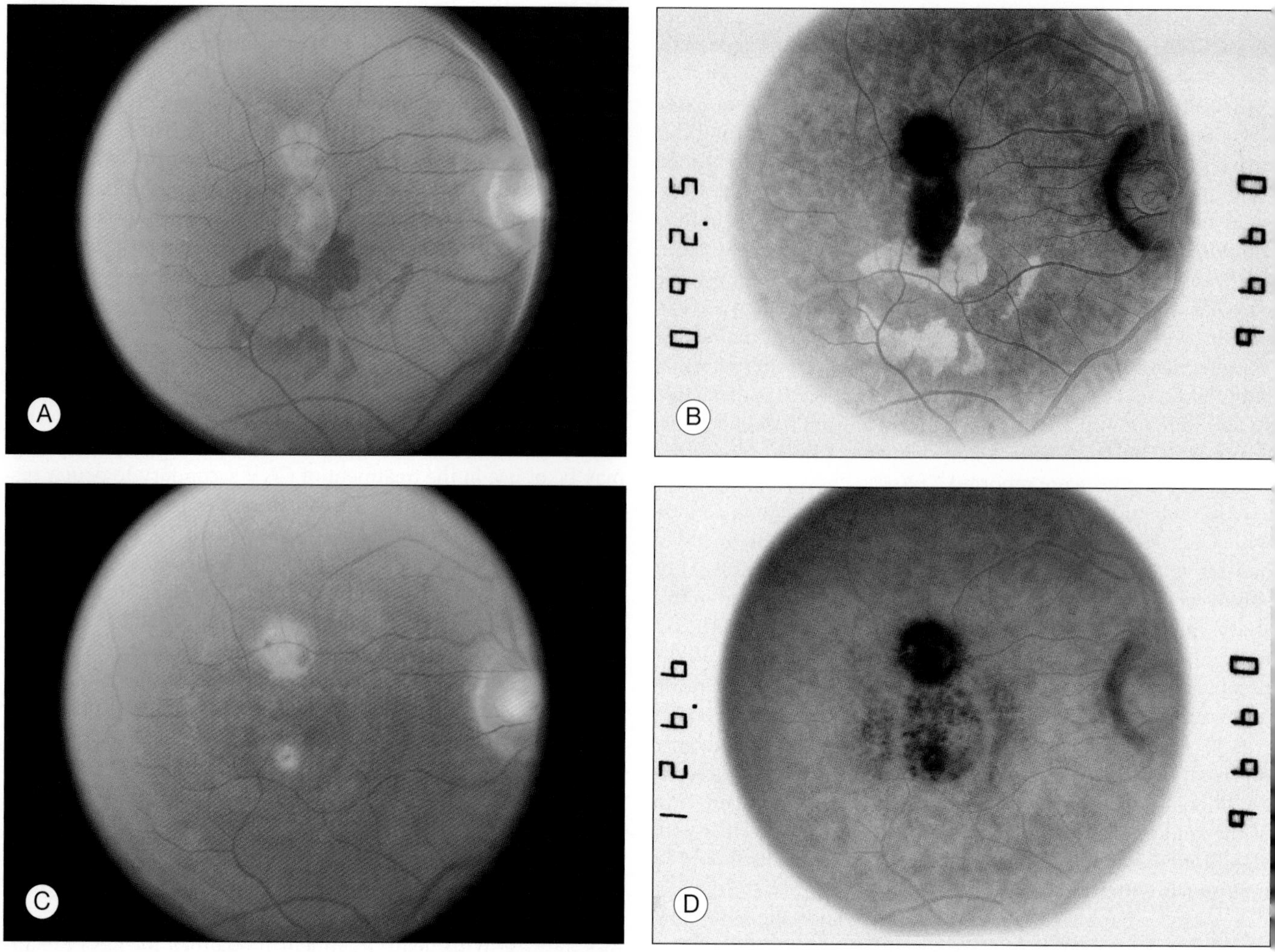

Fig. 70.8 Eye with subfoveal choroidal neovascularization (CNV) treated with submacular surgery in the Submacular Surgery Trials (group H trial). Color photograph (A) and early frame of fluorescein angiogram (B) shows subfoveal CNV in an eye with characteristic lesions of ocular histoplasmosis. Color photograph (C) and early frame of fluorescein angiogram (D) taken 6 months after submacular surgery show a well-demarcated postoperative disturbed area of the retinal pigment epithelium.

cannot be drawn regarding the effectiveness of limited translocation for ocular histoplasmosis.[109] Although surgical intervention remains a viable option in select situations, anti-VEGF therapy and PDT are now the mainstays of treatment for subfoveal and juxtafoveal CNV secondary to ocular histoplasmosis and laser photocoagulation is the typical treatment advised for extrafoveal CNV.

REFERENCES

1. Reid JD, Scherer JH, Herbut PA, et al. Systemic histoplasmosis diagnosed before death and produced experimentally in guinea pigs. J Lab Clin Med 1942;27:419–34.
2. Krause AC, Hopkins WG. Ocular manifestation of histoplasmosis. Am J Ophthalmol 1951;39:564–6.
3. Schlaegel TF. Granulomatous uveitis: an etiologic survey of 100 cases. Trans Am Acad Ophthalmol Otolaryngol 1958;62:813–25.
4. Woods AC, Wahlen HE. The probable role of benign histoplasmosis in the etiology of granulomatous uveitis. Trans Am Ophthalmol Soc 1959;57:318–43.
5. Schlaegel TF, Kenney D. Changes around the optic nerve head in presumed ocular histoplasmosis. Am J Ophthalmol 1966;62:454–8.
6. Gass JDM. Stereoscopic atlas of macular diseases. Vol. 1, Diagnosis and treatment. St Louis, MO: Mosby; 1987.
7. Patz A, Fine SL. Presumed ocular histoplasmosis. In: Yanuzzi LA, Gitter KA, Schatz H, editors. The macula: a comprehensive text and atlas. Baltimore: Williams & Wilkins; 1979.
8. Parnell JR, Jampol LM, Yannuzzi LA, et al. Differentiation between presumed ocular histoplasmosis syndrome and multifocal choroiditis with panuveitis based on morphology of photographed fundus lesions and fluorescein angiography. Arch Ophthalmol 2001;119:208–12.
9. Schlaegel TF. Ocular histoplasmosis. New York: Grune & Stratton; 1977.
10. Wong VG, Kwon-Chung KJ, Hill WB. Koch's postulates and experimental ocular histoplasmosis. Int Ophthalmol Clin 1975;15:139–45.
11. Smith RE. Natural history and reactivation studies of experimental ocular histoplasmosis in a primate model. Trans Am Ophthalmol Soc 1982;80:695–757.
12. Jester JV, Smith RE. Subretinal neovascularization after experimental ocular histoplasmosis in a subhuman primate. Am J Ophthalmol 1985;100:252–8.
13. Van Metre TE, Maumenee AE. Specific ocular uveal lesions in patients with evidence of histoplasmosis. Arch Ophthalmol 1964;71:314–24.
14. Ganley JP. Epidemiologic characteristics of presumed ocular histoplasmosis. Acta Ophthalmol 1973;(Suppl. 119):1–63.
15. Asbury T. The status of presumed ocular histoplasmosis: including a report of a survey. Trans Am Ophthalmol Soc 1966;4:371–400.
16. Schlaegel TF, Weber JC, Helveston E, et al. Presumed histoplasmic choroiditis. Am J Ophthalmol 1967;63:919–25.
17. Makley TA, Long JW, Suie T, et al. Presumed histoplasmic chorioretinitis with special emphasis on the present modes of therapy. Trans Am Acad Ophthalmol Otolaryngol 1965;69:443–57.
18. McCulloch C. Histoplasmosis. Trans Can Ophthalmol Soc 1963;26:107–25.
19. Spencer WH, Chan C-C, Shen DF, et al. Detection of *Histoplasma capsulatum* DNA in lesions of chronic ocular histoplasmosis syndrome. Arch Ophthalmol 2003;121:1551–5.
20. Braunstein RA, Rosen DA, Bird AC. Ocular histoplasmosis syndrome in the United Kingdom. Br J Ophthalmol 1974;58:893–8.
21. Craandijk A. Focal macular choroidopathy. Doc Ophthalmol 1979;48:1–99.
22. Bottoni FG, Deutman AF, Aandekerk AL. Presumed ocular histoplasmosis syndrome and linear streak lesions. Br J Ophthalmol 1989;73:528–35.
23. Suttorp-Schulten MSA, Bollemeijer JG, Bos PJM, et al. Presumed ocular histoplasmosis in the Netherlands – an area without histoplasmosis. Br J Ophthalmol 1997;81:7–11.

24. Ongkosuwito JV, Kortbeek LM, Van der Lelij A, et al. Aetiological study of the presumed ocular histoplasmosis syndrome in the Netherlands. Br J Ophthalmol 1999;83:535–9.
25. Edwards PQ, Billings EL. Worldwide pattern of skin sensitivity to histoplasmin. Am J Trop Med Hyg 1971;20:288–319.
26. Giles CL, Falls HF. Further evaluation of amphotericin-B therapy in presumptive histoplasmosis chorioretinitis. Am J Ophthalmol 1961;51:588–98.
27. Goodwin RA, Shapiro JL, Thurman GH, et al. Disseminated histoplasmosis: clinical and pathologic correlations. Medicine 1980;95:1–33.
28. Zeidberg LD, Dillon A, Gass RS. Some factors in the epidemiology of histoplasmin sensitivity in Williamson county, Tennessee. Am J Public Health 1951;41:80–9.
29. Comstock GW, Vicens CN, Goodman NL, et al. Differences in the distribution of sensitivity to histoplasmin and isolations of *Histoplasma capsulatum*. Am J Epidemiol 1968;88:195–209.
30. Zeidberg LD. The microdistribution of histoplasmin sensitivity in an endemic area. Public Health Monogr 1956;39:190–7.
31. Burke DS, Churchill FE, Gaydos JC, et al. Epidemic histoplasmosis in patients with undifferentiated fever. Mil Med 1982;147:466–7.
32. Ryder KW, Jay SJ, Kiblawi SO, et al. Serum angiotensin converting enzyme activity in patients with histoplasmosis. JAMA 1983;249:1888–9.
33. Weber TR, Grosfeld JL, Kleiman MB, et al. Surgical implications of endemic histoplasmosis in children. J Pediatr Surg 1983;18:486–91.
34. Weinberg GA, Kleiman MB, Grosfeld JL, et al. Unusual manifestations of histoplasmosis in childhood. Pediatrics 1983;72:99–105.
35. Wheat U, Stein L, Corya BC, et al. Pericarditis as a manifestation of histoplasmosis during two large urban outbreaks. Medicine 1983;62:110–9.
36. Brodsky AL, Gregg MB, Loewenstein MS, et al. Outbreak of histoplasmosis associated with the 1970 Earth Day activities. Am J Med 1973;54:333–42.
37. Schwarz J, Salfelder K, Viloria JE. *Histoplasma capsulatum* in vessels of the choroid. Ann Ophthalmol 1977;9:633–6.
38. Schlech WF, Wheat U, Ho JL, et al. Recurrent urban histoplasmosis, Indianapolis, Indiana, 1980–1981. Am J Epidemiol 1983;118:301–12.
39. Waldman RJ, England AC, Tauxe R, et al. A winter outbreak of acute histoplasmosis in northern Michigan. Am J Epidemiol 1983;117:68–75.
40. Wilcox KR, Waisbren BA, Martin J. The Walworth, Wisconsin, epidemic of histoplasmosis. Ann Intern Med 1958;49:388–418.
41. Younglove RM, Terry RM, Rose NJ, et al. An outbreak of histoplasmosis in Illinois associated with starlings. Illinois Med J 1968;134:259–63.
42. Larrabee WF, Ajello L, Kaufman L. An epidemic of histoplasmosis on the isthmus of Panama. Am J Trop Med Hyg 1978;27:281–5.
43. Loosli CG, Grayston JT, Alexander ER, et al. Epidemiological studies of pulmonary histoplasmosis in a farm family. Am J Hyg 1952;55:392–401.
44. Bartlett PC, Vonbehren LA, Tewari RP, et al. Bats in the belfry: an outbreak of histoplasmosis. Am J Public Health 1982;72:1369–72.
45. Morse DL, Gordon MA, Matte T, et al. An outbreak of histoplasmosis in a prison. Am J Epidemiol 1985;122:253–61.
46. Sorley DL, Levin ML, Warren JW, et al. Bat-associated histoplasmosis in Maryland bridge workers. Am J Med 1979;67:623–6.
47. Edwards LB, Acquaviva FA, Livesay VT, et al. An atlas of sensitivity to tuberculin, PPD-B, and histoplasmin in the United States. Am Rev Respir Dis 1969;99:1–132.
48. Smith RE, Ganley JP. An epidemiologic study of presumed ocular histoplasmosis. Trans Am Acad Ophthalmol Otolaryngol 1971;75:994–1005.
49. Feman SS, Podgorski SF, Penn MK. Blindness from presumed ocular histoplasmosis in Tennessee. Ophthalmology 1982;89:1295–8.
50. Hawkins BS, Ganley JP. Risk of visual impairment attributable to ocular histoplasmosis. Arch Ophthalmol 1994;112:655–66.
51. Macular Photocoagulation Study Group. Five-year follow-up of fellow eyes of individuals with ocular histoplasmosis and unilateral extrafoveal or juxtafoveal choroidal neovascularization. Arch Ophthalmol 1996;114:677–88.
52. Lewis ML, Schiffman JC. Long-term follow-up of the second eye in ocular histoplasmosis. Ophthalmol Clin 1983;23:125–35.
53. Watzke RC, Claussen RW. The long-term course of multifocal choroiditis (presumed ocular histoplasmosis). Am J Ophthalmol 1981;91:750–60.
54. Sawelson H, Goldberg RE, Annesley WH, et al. Presumed ocular histoplasmosis syndrome: the fellow eye. Arch Ophthalmol 1976;94:221–4.
55. Gass JDM, Wilkinson CP. Follow-up study of presumed ocular histoplasmosis. Trans Am Acad Ophthalmol Otolaryngol 1972;76:672–94.
56. Macular Photocoagulation Study Group. Krypton laser photocoagulation for neovascular lesions of ocular histoplasmosis: results of a randomized clinical trial. Arch Ophthalmol 1987;105:1499–507.
57. Macular Photocoagulation Study Group. Argon laser photocoagulation for ocular histoplasmosis: results of a randomized clinical trial. Arch Ophthalmol 1983;101:1347–57.
58. Schlaegel TF, Weber JC. Follow-up study of presumed ocular histoplasmic choroiditis. Am J Ophthalmol 1971;71:1192–5.
59. Smith RE, Ganley JP, Knox DL. Presumed ocular histoplasmosis. II. Patterns of peripheral and peripapillary scarring in persons with nonmacular disease. Arch Ophthalmol 1972;87:251–7.
60. Baskin MA, Jampol LM, Huamonte FU, et al. Macular lesions in blacks with the presumed ocular histoplasmosis syndrome. Am J Ophthalmol 1980;89:77–83.
61. Edwards PQ, Palmer CE. Sensitivity to histoplasmin among negro and white residents of different communities in the USA. Bull WHO 1964;30:575–85.
62. Godfrey WA, Sabates R, Cross DE. Association of presumed ocular histoplasmosis with HLA-B7. Am J Ophthalmol 1978;85:854–8.
63. Braley RE, Meredith TA, Aaberg TM, et al. The prevalence of HLA-B7 in presumed ocular histoplasmosis. Am J Ophthalmol 1978;85:859–61.
64. Meredith TA, Smith RE, Duquesnoy RJ. Association of HLA-DRw2 antigen with presumed ocular histoplasmosis. Am J Ophthalmol 1980;89:70–6.
65. Meredith TA, Smith RE, Braley RE, et al. The prevalence of HLA-B7 in presumed ocular histoplasmosis in patients with peripheral atrophic scars. Am J Ophthalmol 1978;86:325–8.
66. Weingeist TA, Watzke RC. Ocular involvement by *Histoplasma capsulatum*. Int Ophthalmol Clin 1983;23:33–47.
67. Smith RE, Macy JI, Parrett C, et al. Variations in acute multifocal histoplasmic choroiditis in the primate. Invest Ophthalmol Vis Sci 1978;17:1005–18.
68. Davidorf FH. The role of T-lymphocytes in the reactivation of presumed ocular histoplasmosis scars. Int Ophthalmol Clin 1975;15:111–24.
69. Gamble CN, Aronson SB, Brescia FB. Experimental uveitis. 1. The production of recurrent immunologic (Auer) uveitis and its relationship to increased uveal vascular permeability. Arch Ophthalmol 1970;84:321–30.
70. Aronson SB, Fish MB, Pollycove M, et al. Altered vascular permeability in ocular inflammatory disease. Arch Ophthalmol 1971;85:455–66.
71. Kaplan HJ, Waldrep JC. Immunological basis of presumed ocular histoplasmosis. Int Ophthalmol Clin 1983;23:19–31.
72. Kwak N, Okamoto N, Wood JM, et al. VEGF is major stimulator in model of choroidal neovascularization. Invest Ophthalmol Vis Sci 2000;41:3158–64.
73. De Monbreun WA. The dog as a natural host for *Histoplasma capsulatum*: report of a case of histoplasmosis in this animal. Am J Trop Med 1939;19:565–87.
74. Emmons CW, Morlan HB, Hill EL. Histoplasmosis in rats and skunks in Georgia. Public Health Rep 1949;64:1423–30.
75. Akun RS. Histoplasmosis in a cat. J Am Vet Med Assoc 1950;117:43–4.
76. Menges RW. Histoplasmin sensitivity in animals. Public Health Monogr 1956;39:210–5.
77. Menges RW, Furcolow ML, Hinton A. The role of animals in the epidemiology of histoplasmosis. Public Health Monogr 1956;39:277–81.
78. Rivers MB, Pulido JS, Folk JC. Ill-defined choroidal neovascularization within ocular histoplasmosis scars. Retina 1992;12:90–5.
79. Orlando RG, Davidorf FH. Spontaneous recovery phenomenon in the presumed ocular histoplasmosis syndrome. Int Ophthalmol Clin 1983;23:137–49.
80. Jost BF, Olk RJ, Burgess DR. Factors related to spontaneous visual recovery in the ocular histoplasmosis syndrome. Retina 1987;7:1–8.
81. Campochiaro PA, Morgan KM, Conway BP, et al. Spontaneous involution of subfoveal neovascularization. Am J Ophthalmol 1990;109:668–75.
82. Submacular Surgery Trials Research Group. Health- and vision-related quality of life among patients with ocular histoplasmosis or idiopathic choroidal neovascularization at time of enrollment in a randomized trial of submacular surgery. SST report no. 5. Arch Ophthalmol 2005;123:78–88.
83. Kaiser RJ, Torsch T, O'Connor PR. Prognostic criteria in macular histoplasmic choroiditis. Int Ophthalmol Clin 1975;15:41–9.
84. Makley TA, Long JW, Suie T. Therapy of chorioretinitis presumed to be caused by histoplasmosis. Int Ophthalmol Clin 1975;15:181–95.
85. Schlaegel TF. Corticosteroids in the treatment of ocular histoplasmosis. Int Ophthalmol Clin 1983;23:111–23.
86. Macular Photocoagulation Study Group. Argon laser photocoagulation for neovascular maculopathy: five-year results from randomized clinical trials. Arch Ophthalmol 1991;109:1109–14.
87. Macular Photocoagulation Study Group. Laser photocoagulation for juxtafoveal choroidal neovascularization: five-year results from randomized clinical trials. Arch Ophthalmol 1994;112:500–9.
88. Macular Photocoagulation Study Group. Laser photocoagulation for neovascular lesions nasal to the fovea: results from clinical trials for lesions secondary to ocular histoplasmosis and idiopathic causes. Arch Ophthalmol 1995;113:56–61.
89. Fine SL, Wood WJ, Isernhagen RD, et al. Laser treatment of subfoveal neovascular membranes of ocular histoplasmosis. Arch Ophthalmol 1993;111:19–20.
90. Saperstein DA, Rosenfeld PJ, Bressler NM, et al. Photodynamic therapy of subfoveal choroidal neovascularization with verteporfin in the ocular histoplasmosis syndrome. One-year results of an uncontrolled, prospective case series. Ophthalmology 2002;109:1499–505.
91. Busquets MA, Shah GK, Wickens J, et al. Ocular photodynamic therapy with verteporfin for choroidal neovascularization secondary to ocular histoplasmosis syndrome. Retina 2003;23:299–306.
92. Liu JC, Boldt HC, Folk JC, et al. Photodynamic therapy of subfoveal and juxtafoveal choroidal neovascularization in ocular histoplasmosis syndrome: a retrospective case series. Retina 2004;24:863–70.
93. Shah GK, Blinder KJ, Hariprasad SM, et al. Photodynamic therapy for juxtafoveal choroidal neovascularization due to ocular histoplasmosis syndrome. Retina 2005;25:26–32.
94. Lam A, Lee HC, Ho AC, et al. Photodynamic therapy in young patients. Ophthalmic Surg Lasers Imaging 2006;37:182–9.
95. Rosenfeld PJ, Saperstein DA, Bressler NM, et al. Verteporfin in Ocular Histoplasmosis Study Group. Photodynamic therapy with verteporfin in ocular histoplasmosis:uncontrolled, open-label 2-year study. Ophthalmology 2004;111:1725–33.
96. Adán A, Navarro M, Casaroli-Marano RP, et al. Intravitreal bevacizumab as initial treatment for choroidal neovascularization associated with presumed ocular histoplasmosis syndrome. Graefes Arch Clin Exp Ophthalmol 2007;245:1873–5.

97. Ehrlich R, Ciulla TA, Maturi R, et al. Intravitreal bevacizumab for choroidal neovascularization secondary to presumed ocular histoplasmosis syndrome. Retina 2009;29:1418–23.
98. Schadlu R, Blinder KJ, Shah GK, et al. Intravitreal bevacizumab for choroidal neovascularization in ocular histoplasmosis. Am J Ophthalmol 2008;145: 875–8.
99. Heier JS, Brown D, Ciulla T, et al. Ranibizumab for choroidal neovascularization secondary to causes other than age-related macular degeneration: a phase I clinical trial. Ophthalmology 2011;118:111–8.
100. Han DP, McAllister JT, Weinberg DV, et al. Combined intravitreal anti-VEGF and verteporfin photodynamic therapy for juxtafoveal and extrafoveal choroidal neovascularization as an alternative to laser photocoagulation. Eye (Lond) 2010;713–6.
101. Rechtman E, Allen VD, Danis RP, et al. Intravitreal triamcinolone for choroidal neovascularization in ocular histoplasmosis syndrome.Am J Ophthalmol 2003;136:739–41.
102. Thomas MA, Kaplan HJ. Surgical removal of subfoveal neovascularization in the presumed ocular histoplasmosis syndrome. Am J Ophthalmol 1991;111: 1–7.
103. Thomas MA, Grand MG, Williams DF, et al. Surgical management of subfoveal choroidal neovascularization. Ophthalmology 1992;99:952–68.
104. Thomas MA, Dickinson JD, Melberg NS, et al. Visual results after surgical removal of subfoveal choroidal neovascular membranes. Ophthalmology 1994;101:1384–96.
105. Melberg NS, Thomas MA, Dickinson JD, et al. Managing recurrent neovascularization after subfoveal surgery in presumed ocular histoplasmosis syndrome. Ophthalmology 1996;108:1064–8.
106. Submacular Surgery Trials Research Group. Surgical removal vs observation for subfoveal choroidal neovascularization, either associated with the ocular histoplasmosis syndrome or idiopathic. I. Ophthalmic findings from a randomized clinical trial: Submacular Surgery Trials (SST) group H trial: SST report no. 9. Arch Ophthalmol 2004;122:1597–611.
107. Submacular Surgery Trials Research Group. Surgical removal vs observation for subfoveal choroidal neovascularization, either associated with the ocular histoplasmosis syndrome or idiopathic. II. Quality-of-life findings from a randomized clinical trial: SST group H trial: SST report no. 10. Arch Ophthalmol 2004;122:1616–28.
108. Ehlers JP, Maldonado R, Sarin N, et al. Treatment of non-age-related macular degeneration submacular diseases with macular translocation surgery. Retina 2011;31:1337-46.
109. Ng EW, Fujii GY, Au Eong KG, et al. Macular translocation in patients with recurrent subfoveal choroidal neovascularization after laser photocoagulation for nonsubfoveal choroidal neovascularization. Ophthalmology 2004;111: 1889–93.

Polypoidal Choroidal Vasculopathy

Chapter 71

Xiaoxin Li

INTRODUCTION

Polypoidal choroidal vasculopathy (PCV) is an exudative maculopathy with features similar to neovascular age-related macular degeneration (AMD) with hemorrhage, pigment epithelial detachment (PED), and neurosensory detachment. The pathogenesis of PCV is mostly unknown. It remains controversial as to whether PCV represents a subtype of neovascular age-related macular degeneration.

PCV is more common in non-white populations (including blacks, Hispanics, and Asians).[1] The incidence of PCV in Chinese and Japanese patients in exudative AMD has been reported to be much higher than in Caucasians.[2–7] The true prevalence and consequences may be underestimated if indocyanine green angiography (ICGA) is not performed. The widespread availability of ICGA has improved the diagnosis of PCV.

Polypoidal choroidal vasculopathy was first described as polypoidal, subretinal, vascular lesions associated with serous and hemorrhagic detachments of the retinal pigment epithelium (RPE) in a series of patients (10/11 were women) by Yannuzzi et al. at the Annual Meeting of the American Academy of Ophthalmology in 1982.[8] The entitity was initially called idiopathic polypoidal choroidal vasculopathy (IPCV). Kleiner et al. in 1984[9] described a peculiar hemorrhagic disorder of the macula, characterized by recurrent subretinal and subretinal pigment epithelium bleeding in middle-aged black women, which they termed posterior uveal bleeding syndrome (PUBS).[10] Later, a study from the same group of authors showed an expanded clinical spectrum for PCV, affecting various ages, both genders, and several racial populations.[11] For the remainder of the chapter, I will use the PCV nomenclature; the IPCV and PUBS terms are mentioned for historical benefit.

The past decade has witnessed dramatic improvements in the understanding of exudative maculopathy and recognition of the importance of PCV, especially in the Asia–Pacific regions. A PCV Roundtable meeting panel of experts suggest that PCV is defined angiographically as the presence of single or multiple focal nodular areas of hyperfluorescence arising from the choroidal circulation within the first 6 minutes after injection of indocyanine green, with or without an associated choroidal interconnecting vascular network. The presence of orange–red subretinal nodules with corresponding indocyanine green hyperfluorescence is pathognomonic of PCV.[12] The implication of the definition is obvious but bears repetition. The definition of PCV relies on ICGA. Retina specialists who do not generally utilize ICGA tend not to diagnose PCV. Later in the chapter, there is a clinical definition of PCV as well.

PATHOGENESIS

PCV is regarded as a primary abnormality of the choroidal circulation, characterized by an inner choroidal vascular network of vessels ending in an aneurysmal bulge or outward projection, often visible as a reddish-orange, spheroid, polyp-like structure. PCV primarily involves the inner choroidal vasculature that is well differentiated from the middle and larger choroid vessels by histology.[13]

Histopathological features have been reported by Kuroiwa from surgically excised specimens from five patients with PCV, who had been diagnosed by ICGA. The results indicated that arteriosclerosis appears to be an important pathological feature in the choroidal vessels of PCV subjects.[14] In another histopathologic report, by Nakashizuka et al., who examined specimens surgically extracted from five eyes of five PCV patients, the pathologic findings revealed little granulation tissue formation in any of the specimens; on the other hand, all the specimens exhibited a massive exudative change and leaking, all the vessels exhibited hyalinization, and choriocapillaris had disappeared, even in the cases in which RPE had been preserved.[15] This group also demonstrated by immunohistochemistry that PCV is not the same as choroidal neovascularization (CNV). CD-34 is a marker of vascular endothelial expression and CD-34 staining revealed discontinuity in the vascular endothelium, smooth muscle actin (SMA) was negative in hyalinized vessels, and there was disruption and injury of smooth muscle cells causing dilation of vessels. VEGF antibody was negative in vascular endothelial cells. These histopathologic findings indicated that hyalinization of choroidal vessels, like arteriosclerosis, was characteristic of PCV.[15]

The genetic studies with CNV and PCV have been controversial in published papers.[16,17] Recently, we investigated the relationship between CNV of AMD and PCV by performing a series of meta-analyses. We found that many genes have common associations with PCV and CNV. For example, the pooled odds ratio (OR) between SNP rs10490924 (TT:GG, within the *ARMS2* gene, previously identified as LOC387715)[18] and CNV is 4.23 (95% CI 3.535.06), while the pooled OR between this SNP and PCV is 5.13 (95%CI 3.40–7.75) (data unpublished). SNP rs9332739 within complement factor 3 (C3) gene also have a common association with CNV (GG:CC, pooled OR 2.12, 95%CI 1.81–2.47) and PCV (pooled OR 3.52, 95%CI 1.43–8.69). Moreover, a similar trend was found in complement factor H (CFH, rs1061170, CC:TT) and SERPING1 (C1 inhibitor, rs2511989 GG:AA). The elastin gene identified by Kondo et al. in 2008 was shown to disrupt the elastic area of the Bruch's membrane. He found that a common elastin gene (ELN) variant was significantly associated with susceptibility to PCV.[19]

Furthermore, a series of meta-analyses was performed to investigate the pooled OR between the risk factors for CNV and PCV. We found that CNV and PCV have many common risk factors, such as smoking and diabetes. For example, the pooled OR between smoking and CNV is 1.78 (95%CI 1.52–2.09),[20] while the pooled OR between smoking and PCV is 1.51 (95% CI 1.06–2.16, data unpublished). The pooled OR between diabetes and CNV is 1.66 (95% CI 1.05–2.63),[20] while the pooled OR between diabetes and PCV is 1.94 (95% CI 1.29–2.92, data unpublished). However, the pooled OR between hypertension and CNV is 1.02 (95% CI 0.77–1.35),[20] while the pooled OR between hypertension and PCV is 1.60 (95% CI 1.17–2.18, data unpublished). Therefore, hypertension is only associated with PCV. This is consistent with pathology findings: the PCV lesion has thickened and hyalinized vessel walls, which is similar to that seen in hypertension.[21]

CLINICAL FEATURES

Demographics

The prevalence of PCV in presumed neovascular AMD was reported as 7.8% in US,[1] 4.0% in Belgian,[22] 9.8% in Italian,[23] 8.2% in Greeek.[24] 23.0–54.7% in Japanese,[25] 22.3% in Chinese,[26] and 24.6%[27] in Korean populations. The prevalence varies with age.[28] In summary, PCV is more prevalent in blacks, Japanese and other Asians than in whites, while the incidence of AMD is very high in whites, and low in blacks. The incidence of both diseases is high in Asians.

Although early reports suggested that PCV was a condition predominantly of middle-aged women,[11] and that typically PCV presents one to two decades earlier than classical AMD, it is most commonly diagnosed in patients between the ages of 50 and 65.[29] However, the age of the subjects was reported with a mean of 66.1 ± 9.6 years in a Chinese population.[28] Caucasian patients usually present with PCV at an older age.[30] It has subsequently been established that PCV occurs in both genders (and more commonly in Asian men than women).[27] Although women are involved more often than men in some reports, more men still have manifestations of the disorder among Chinese patients.[26,28,30,31] PCV is usually a bilateral disease. The majority of the patients with evidence of PCV in one eye eventually develop similar lesions in the fellow eye.

The natural course of PCV is variable: it may be relatively stable or there may be repeated bleeding and leakage with vision loss and chorioretinal atrophy, with or without fibrotic scarring. Reddish-orange nodules alone, or nodules and small subretinal hemorrhage and absence of hard exudates, may still allow a benign clinical course and stable vision.[32,33]

The association of PCV with other conditions is not certain. PCV with severe thrombocytopenia and massive hemorrhage has been reported,[34] and PCV has also been associated with sickle cell disease and irradiation.[35] Some experts believe it is advisable to screen PCV patients for hypertension and platelet count, but hypertension is common in older patients and is already monitored during medical visits, and the platelet data are not firmly established. The role of hereditary and environmental factors in its etiology is inconclusive and needs further study.

Clinical findings

Clinically, PCV is characterized by protruding orange-red elevated lesions, often with nodular elevations of the RPE, that can be seen during routine fundus examination using ophthalmoscopy and contact lens slit-lamp biomicroscopy. The nodular elevations of the RPE are easily visible by optical coherence tomography (OCT). PCV is also characterized by polypoidal lesions only observed when using ICGA. The lesions appear as polyp-like or grape-like clusters (Fig. 71.1).[11,15] The nodular lesions are associated with serous exudation and hemorrhage that may lead to detachment of the RPE and sometimes the neurosensory retina.[32] Associated features are recurrent subretinal hemorrhage and vitreous hemorrhage (Fig. 71.2).

Polypoidal lesions are located mainly in the macular area, although this may be ascertainment bias since ICGA tends to look at that area. In one report, 69.5% polypoidal lesions were located in the macular area, 15% PCV lesions were located under the temporal retinal vascular arcade, and 4.5% PCV lesions were located peripapillary (within one disc diameter of the disc edge). PCV lesions were also located in the midperipheral area.[28]

PCV lesions may be active or inactive (Fig. 71.3). PCV is considered as active if there is clinical, OCT or fluorescein angiography (FA) evidence of any one of the following: vision loss of 5 or more letters (ETDRS chart); subretinal fluid with or without

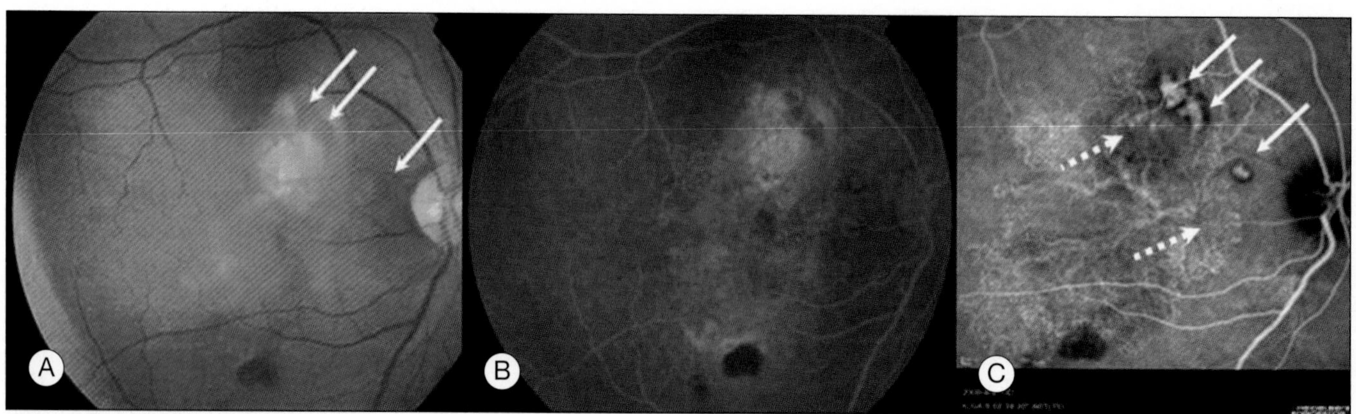

Fig. 71.1 (A) Color photograph of a 53-year-old male with blurred vision in the right eye for 2 years; visual acuity was 20/200. There are protruded orange–red elevated lesions (arrows) in the superior area of the macula. (B) Fluorescein angiogram of the same fundus showing occult choroidal neovascularization. (C) ICGA at 6 minutes 3 seconds reveals a branching vascular network in the central macula and polypoidal lesions with hypofluorescent halo (arrows) connecting to a branching vascular network (dashed arrows) and corresponding to the orange–red subretinal nodules.

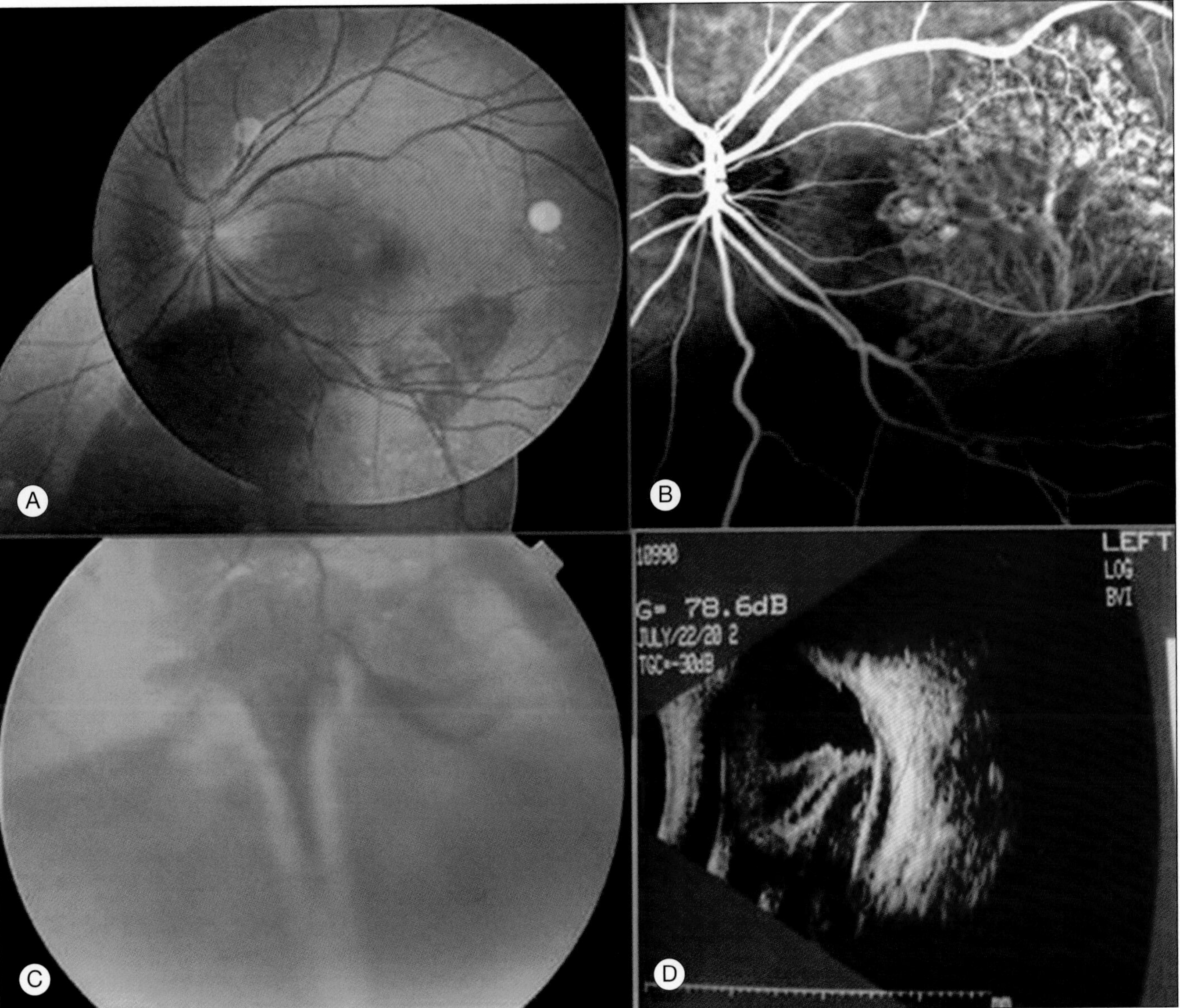

Fig. 71.2 (A) Color photograph of a 65-year-old man with blurred vision for 18 months. There is a large area of a protruding orange–red elevated lesion on the temporal side of the fovea. (B) ICGA from the same fundus. (C) One month later the vision dropped to hand motions and the color photograph showed hemorrhagic retinal detachment inferior to the fovea. (D) One week later subretinal hemorrhages and bleeding into the vitreous cavity was demonstated on B-scan ultrasonography.

intraretinal fluid; pigment epithelial detachment; subretinal hemorrhage; or fluorescein leakage (Box 71.1). There are currently no universally recognized criteria for defining disease activity in PCV; treatment should be initiated for active and symptomatic PCV and can be considered for active, asymptomatic PCV.[12]

Choroidal vascular hyperpermeability, reportedly a characteristic finding in central serous chorioretinopathy (CSC), might play a role in the pathogenesis of PCV. PCV with angioid streaks secondary to pseudoxanthoma elasticum has also been reported in one patient.[36,37]

Some patients with PCV may develop CNV. PCV can induce ischemic changes, inflammation, sick RPE and breaks in Bruch's membrane. These changes can contribute to the development of CNV, and fibrosis and scarring may ensue.[38]

Angiographic features

PCV is better visualized by ICGA than by FA, because indocyanine green absorbs and emits near-infrared light, which readily penetrates the RPE, enhancing viewing of choroidal lesions. Also the binding affinity of indocyanine green to plasma proteins means that it does not leak from the choriocapillaris in the same way as fluorescein, so choroidal lesions are less obscured.[39] PCV primarily involves the inner choroidal vasculature.[22,40] In recent years ICGA has been accepted as the gold standard for the diagnosis of PCV, and as one of the specific criteria to distinguish PCV, retinal angiomatous proliferation, and typical AMD as types of neovascular AMD.[3] The ICGA characteristics of PCV (summarized in Box 71.2) include: a branching network of inner choroidal vessels,[3,21,40–43] and nodular polypoidal aneurysms or

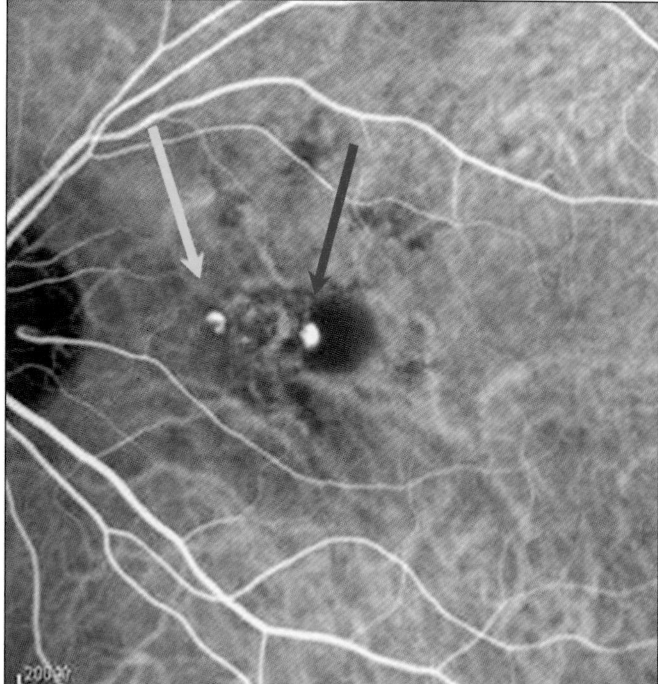

Fig. 71.3 ICGA of a 73-year-old man with polypoidal choroidal vasculopathy and a 7-month history of decreased visual acuity in his left eye. There are two polyps in the macular region. The yellow arrowhead identifies an inactive polyp, while the red arrowhead points to an active polyp with surrounding hypofluorescence.

Box 71.1 Characteristics of active PCV

- Neurosensory detachment
- Pigment epithelium detachment
- Subretinal lipid exudation
- FA evidence of activity is leaking hyperfluorescence, mostly in an "occult" pattern
- Subretinal hemorrhage
- Polyp surrounded by fluid (hypofluorescent halo in ICGA)

PCV, Polypoidal choroidal vasculopathy; FA, fluorescence angiography; ICGA, indocyanine green angiography.

Box 71.2 ICGA characteristics of PCV

- Polypoidal lesions shown on ICGA as typical nodular hyperfluorescence, and one of the following angiographic criteria:
  - a branching network of inner choroidal vessels
  - nodular polypoidal aneurysms or dilations at the edge of these abnormal vessel networks
  - presence of hypofluorescent halo (in first 6 minutes)
- Pulsation in polyps can be observed only using video ICGA

ICGA, indocyanine green angiography; PCV, polypoidal choroidal vasculopathy.

dilations at the edge of these abnormal vessel networks, which correspond to orange subretinal nodules;[3,11,20,31,32,40–42] and the presence of single or multiple focal nodular areas of hyperfluorescence (hypofluorescent halo, see Figure 71.1C) arising from the choroidal circulation within the first 6 minutes. Pulsation in polyps and/or associated vasculature has been less extensively reported and can be observed only using video ICGA.[44,45]

ICGA should be considered to assist the diagnosis of PCV when routine ophthalmoscopic examination indicates a serosanguineous maculopathy with one of the following features: clinically visible orange–red subretinal nodules, spontaneous massive subretinal hemorrhage (if not so severe as to preclude all ICGA views), and in some cases with notched or hemorrhagic pigment epithelium detachment (PED), or a lack of response to anti-VEGF therapy. The total lesion area for PCV is the area of all polyps and the branching vascular network (BVN) as viewed by ICGA. This is important for laser and photodynamic treatment modalities.

Classification

PCV was classified by the Japanese Study Group on PCV.[42] This panel of experts proposed three categories to subclassify PCV:[12]

- **Quiescent:** polyps in the absence of subretinal or intraretinal fluid or hemorrhage.
- **Exudative:** exudation without hemorrhage, which may include sensory retinal thickening, neurosensory detachment, PED, and subretinal lipid exudation.
- **Hemorrhagic:** any hemorrhage with or without other exudative characteristics.

DIFFERENTIAL DIAGNOSIS

Neovascular age-related macular degeneration

Some authors categorize PCV as a subtype of neovascular AMD.[3] PCV has been considered to be part of or similar to AMD CNV due to similar features (Fig. 71.4A), elevated levels of vascular endothelial growth factor (VEGF), similar histology, and expression of growth factors and receptor antibodies. We view PCV as a distinct condition. It has been documented that the increased levels of VEGF in PCV are lower compared with AMD CNV or myopic CNV. The increase in VEGF levels in PCV is mild to moderate. The clinical features of the PCV are different from those of neovascular age-related macular degeneration. PCV is associated with polyp-like structures projecting from the plane of the inner choroid towards the outer retina or RPE, the RPE is mostly intact, while in neovascular AMD the neovascular tufts arising from the choroid may either invade and perforate Bruch's membrane or grow throw defects in Bruch's membrane and proliferate in either sub-RPE space (type I CNV) or in the subsensory retinal space (type II CNV).[46] The ingrowth of new vessels extending from the choroid into the sub-RPE space is the most important histopathologic change of occult CNV (Fig. 71.4B).

OCT findings (Fig. 71.4C and F) can assist in understanding the differences in the retinal structures that are affected by these two clinical entities and also may help in the differential diagnosis of PCV and neovascular AMD.[13]

Central serous chorioretinopathy

Central serous chorioretinopathy (CSC) is characterized by accumulation of transparent fluid and round, serous detachment of the macular retina. It has been thought to be due to a focal leakage from one or more defects at the level of the RPE, which allow serous fluid from the choriocapillaris to diffuse into the subretinal space. It has been hypothesized that a protracted disturbance in the microcirculation of the choriocapillaris leads to leakage of fluid into the sub-RPE space. A combination of choroidal hyperpermeability and impaired RPE function leads to

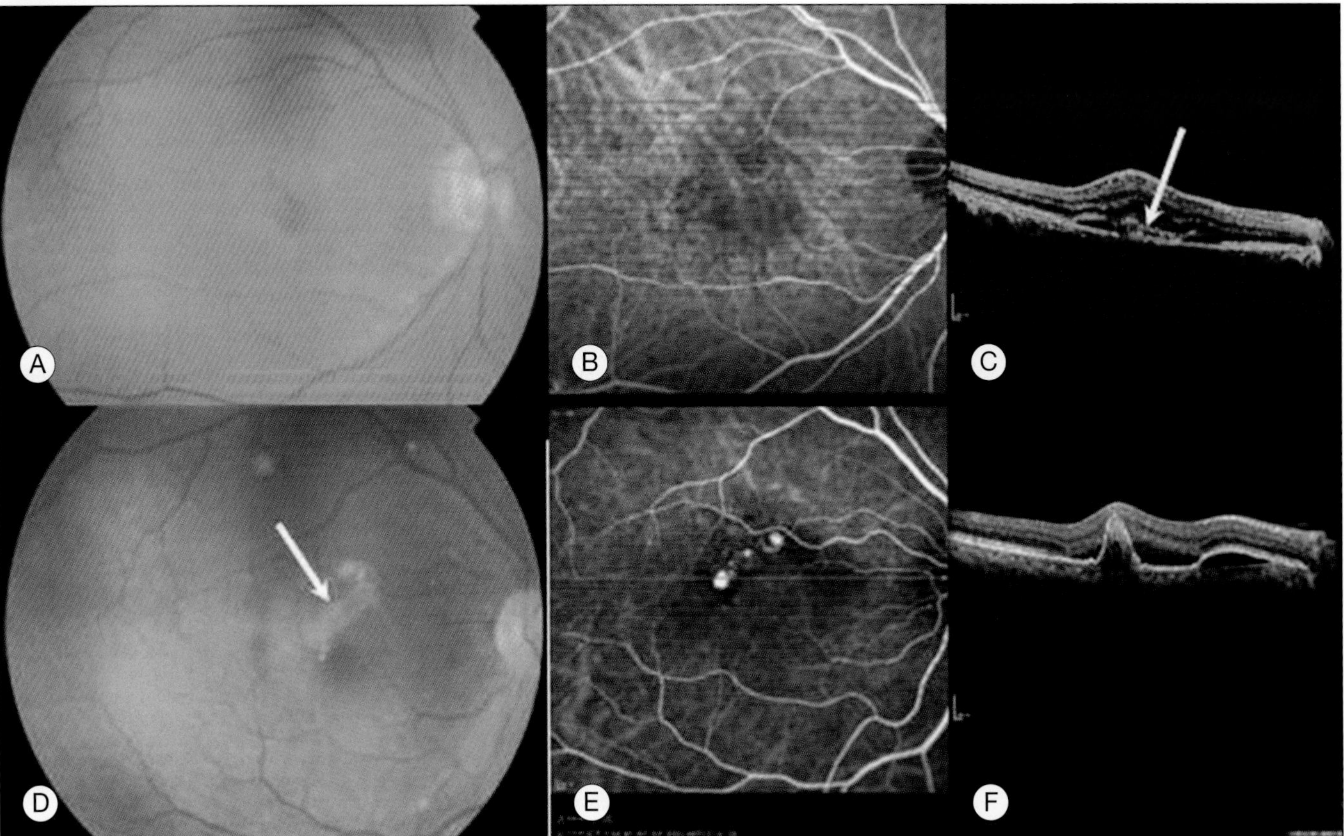

Fig. 71.4 (A) Color photograph of 72-year-old man with visual acuity 20/20. (B) ICGA demonstrates choroidal neovascularization (CNV) superior to fovea. (C) Optical coherence tomography (OCT) of the same fundus; the arrow points to the CNV component above the retinal pigment epithelium (RPE) band and the RPE band is broken. (D) Color photograph of 66-year-old woman with visual acuity 20/100, with orange–red subretinal nodules in the macular area (arrow). (E) ICGA of the same fundus showed polyps corresponding to the orange–red lesions. (F) OCT of the same fundus showed a detached RPE in a "bent back" form corresponding to the polypoidal lesion with subretinal fluid and a large area RPE detachment.

pooling of fluid in the sub-RPE space with eventual leakage through the RPE into the subretinal space. ICGA has expanded our knowledge of CSC. A consistent finding is the hyperpermeability of the choroid during ICGA in CSC. The multifocal choroid hyperfluorescence patches in the ICG demonstrate multifocal choroid vascular hyperpermeable areas.[41]

PCV masquerading as CSC has been reported. In CSC with persistent and/or recurrent exudation, a myriad of retinal pigment epithelial changes may evolve that make it difficult to differentiate it from PCV. In such patients, ICGA may be useful in differentiating these two entities. An accurate clinical diagnosis is important since CSC and PCV differ in terms of their risk factors, natural course, visual prognosis and treatment.[47]

TREATMENT

Thermal laser photocoagulation

Laser photocoagulation has been suggested to be beneficial, albeit it with short-term follow-up. The greatest benefit may be for extrafoveal PCV.[48] In some studies that analyzed reported vision outcomes, ICGA-guided laser photocoagulation was successful in stabilizing or improving vision in 55–100% of eyes; however, vision loss occurred in 13–45% of eyes.[31,48–50] Photocoagulation of the whole lesion, compared with polyps only, appears to be more efficacious.[49]

Photodynamic therapy

Verteporfin photodynamic therapy (PDT) causes regression or resolution of polyps by its angio-occlusive mechanism of action. It has been shown to achieve complete occlusion of polyps and resolution of exudative changes after less than three treatments, restricts loss of letters on the ETDRS chart to less than 15, or improved vision in 80–100% of patients after 1 year.[51,52] For treatment-naïve patients the entire PCV lesion as indicated by ICGA (polyps plus the BVN) should be treated.

Common complications reported with verteporfin-PDT therapy are subretinal hemorrhage, recurrence of PCV with leakage from the BVN, and fibrous scarring. Subretinal hemorrhage is common and can lead to vitreous hemorrhage and consequently a poor outcome.[51,52] Larger lesion size and a leaking vascular net[51] are risk factors for bleeding after PDT.

Anti-VEGF therapy

Recent studies have demonstrated that anti-VEGF agents are useful in the treatment of CNV in neovascular AMD. Since increased VEGF levels have been observed in PCV patients,[45,] anti-VEGF therapy might be theoretically beneficial for treating PCV. It was shown that intravitreal anti-VEGF helped in resolving the macular edema, polypoidal complexes decreased in 4/12 (33%) eyes by intravitreal ranibizumab,[53] and 1/11 (9.09%) eyes by intravitreal bevacizumab.[54]

Combination therapy

EVEREST is a multicenter, double-masked, ICGA-guided randomized controlled trial studying patients with symptomatic PCV. Eyes were treated with verteporfin PDT monotherapy, 0.5 mg ranibizumab monotherapy or a combination of these treatments. Both combination therapy and verteporfin PDT monotherapy were superior to ranibizumab monotherapy in achieving complete polyp regression at month 6. Improvements in best-corrected visual acuity (BCVA) and central retinal thickness (CRT) also favored combination therapy.[12]

The authors of a recent relatively large comparative case series reported that with combination verteporfin PDT plus bevacizumab there were better early BCVA outcomes than with verteporfin PDT alone (P = 0.0016 for the difference between treatments in mean BCVA change from baseline at 3 months and P = 0.048 at 12 months).[52] Combination therapy also decreased the rate of PDT-related hemorrhages compared with verteporfin PDT monotherapy (3/61 [4.9%] vs 15/85 [17.6%], respectively), but did not impact the resolution and recurrence of lesions.[55]

These trials support the selection of ICGA-guided verteporfin PDT with or without combination with ranibizumab as standard preferred treatment options.

REFERENCES

1. Yannuzzi LA, Wong DW, Sforzolini BS, et al. Polypoidal choroidal vasculopathy and neovascularized age-related macular degeneration. Arch Ophthalmol 1999;117:1503–10.
2. Wen F, Chen C, Wu D, et al. Polypoidal choroidal vasculopathy in elderly Chinese patients. Graefes Arch Clin Exp Ophthalmol 2004;242:625–9.
3. Maruko I, Iida T, Saito M, et al. Clinical characteristics of exudative age-related macular degeneration in Japanese patients. Am J Ophthal 2007;144:15–22.
4. Hwang DK, Yang CS, Lee FL, et al. Idiopathic polypoidal choroidal vasculopathy. J Chin Med Assoc 2007;70:84–8.
5. Liu Y, Wen F, Huang S, et al. Subtype lesions of neovascular age-related macular degeneration in Chinese patients. Graefes Arch Clin Exp Ophthalmol 2007;245:1441–5.
6. Yi C, Ou J, Yian H, et al. A case report of 360 idiopathic polypoidal choroidal vasculopathy. Yan ke xue bao/Eye Science 2001;17:126–9.
7. Japanese Study Group of Polypoidal Choroidal Vasculopathy. [Criteria for diagnosis of polypoidal choroidal vasculopathy.] Nippon Ganka Gakkai Zasshi 2005;109:417–27.
8. Yannuzzi LA. Idiopathic polypoidal choroidal vasculopathy. Presented at the February 1982 Macula Society Meeting, Miami, Florida.
9. Kleiner RC, Bruckner AJ, Johnson RL: Posterior uveal bleeding syndrome. Ophthalmology 1984;91:110
10. Kleiner RC, Bruckner AJ, Johnson RL. The posterior uveal bleeding syndrome. Retina 1990;10:9–17.
11. Yannuzzi LA, Sorenson J, Spaide RF, et al. Idiopathic polypoidal choroidal vasculopathy (IPCV). Retina 1990;10:1–8.
12. PCV Roundtable Participants. Polypoidal choroidal vasculopathy: evidence-based guidelines for clinical diagnosis and treatment. Submitted to *Retina*.
13. Ozawa S, Ishikawa K, Ito Y. Differences in macular morphology between polypoidal choroidal vasculopathy and exudative age-related macular degeneration detected by optical coherence tomography. Retina 2009;29:793–802.
14. Kuroiwa S, Tateiwa H, Hisatomi T, et al. Pathological features of surgically excised polypoidal choroidal vasculopathy membranes. Clin Exp Ophthalmol 2004;32:297–302.
15. Nakashizuka H, Mitsumata M, Okisaka S, et al. Clinicopathologic findings in polypoidal choroidal vasculopathy. Invest Ophthalmol Vis Sci 2008;49: 4729–37.
16. Klein RJ, Zeiss C, Chew EY, et al. Complement factor H polymorphism in age-related macular degeneration.Science 2005;308:385–9.
17. Dewan A, Liu M, Hartman S, et al. HTRA1 promoter polymorphism in wet age-related macular degeneration. Science 2006;314:989–92.
18. Kondo N, Honda S, Ishibashi K, et al. LOC387715/HTRA1 variants in polypoidal choroidal vasculopathy and age-related macular degeneration in a Japanese population. Am J Ophthalmol 2007;144:608–12.
19. Kondo N, Honda S, Ishibashi K, et al. Elastin gene polymorphisms in neovascular age-related macular degeneration and polypoidal choroidal vasculopathy. Invest Ophthalmol Vis Sci 2008;49:1101–5
20. Chakravarthy U, Wong TY, Fletcher A, et al. Clinical risk factors for age-related macular degeneration: a systematic review and meta-analysis. BMC Ophthalmol 2010;10:31.
21. Nakashizuka H, Yuzawa M. Hyalinization of choroidal vessels in polypoidal choroidal vasculopathy. Surv Ophthalmol 2011;56:278–9; author reply 279.
22. Lafaut BA, Leys AM, Snyers B, et al. Polypoidal choroidal vasculopathy in Caucasians. Graefes Arch Clin Exp Ophthalmol 2000;238:752–9.
23. Scassellati-Sforzolini B, Mariotti C, Bryan R, et al. Polypoidal choroidal vasculopathy in Italy. Retina 2001;21:121–5.
24. Ladas ID, Rouvas AA, Moschos MM, et al. Polypoidal choroidal vasculopathy and exudative age-related macular degeneration in Greek population. Eye (Lond) 2004;18:455–9.
25. Sho K, Takahashi K, Yamada H, et al. Polypoidal choroidal vasculopathy: incidence, demographic features, and clinical characteristics. Arch Ophthalmol 2003;121:1392–6.
26. Wen F, Chen C, Wu D, et al. Polypoidal choroidal vasculopathy in elderly Chinese patients. Graefes Arch Clin Exp Ophthalmol 2004;242:625–9.
27. Byeon SH, Lee SC, Oh HS, et al. Incidence and clinical patterns of polypoidal choroidal vasculopathy in Korean patients. Jpn J Ophthalmol 2008;52:57–62.
28 Hou J, Tao Y, Li XX, et al. Clinical characteristics of polypoidal choroidal vasculopathy in Chinese patients. Graefes Arch Clin Exp Ophthalmol 2011;249: 975–9.
29. Ciardella AP, Donsoff IM, Yannuzzi LA. Polypoidal choroidal vasculopathy. Ophthalmol Clin North Am 2002;15:537–54.
30. Gomi F, Sawa M, Wakabayashi T, et al. Efficacy of intravitreal bevacizumab combined with photodynamic therapy for polypoidal choroidal vasculopathy. Am J Ophthalmol 2010;150:48–54.
31. Kwok AK, Lai TY, Chan CW, et al. Polypoidal choroidal vasculopathy in Chinese patients. Br J Ophthalmol 2002;86:892–7.
32 Uyama M, Wada M, Nagai Y, et al. Polypoidal choroidal vasculopathy: natural history. Am J Ophthalmol 2002;133:639–48.
33. Okubo A, Arimura N, Abematsu N, et al. Predictable signs of benign course of polypoidal choroidal vasculopathy: based upon the long-term observation of non-treated eyes. Acta Ophthalmol 2010;88:107–14.
34. Lip PL, Hope-Ross MW, Gibson JM. Idiopathic polypoidal choroidal vasculopathy: a disease with diverse clinical spectrum and systemic associations. Eye (Lond) 2000;14(Pt 5):695–700.
35. Smith RE, Wise K, Kingsley RM. Idiopathic polypoidal choroidal vasculopathy and sickle cell retinopathy. Am J Ophthalmol 2000;129:544–6.
36. Sasahara M, Tsujikawa A, Musashi K, et al. Polypoidal choroidal vasculopathy with choroidal vascular hyperpermeability. Am J Ophthalmol 2006;142: 601–7.
37. Baillif-Gostoli S, Quaranta-El Maftouhi M, Mauget-Fa?sse M. Polypoidal choroidal vasculopathy in a patient with angioid streaks secondary to pseudoxanthoma elasticum. Graefes Arch Clin Exp Ophthalmol 2010;248:1845–8.
38. Chen Yanli, Wen Feng, Sun Zuhua, Wu Dezheng. Polypoidal choroidal vasculopathy coexisting with exudative age-related macular degeneration. Int Ophthalmol 2008;28:119–23.
39. Desmettre T, Devoisselle JM, Mordon S. Fluorescence properties and metabolic features of indocyanine green (ICG) as related to angiography. Surv Ophthalmol 2000;45:15–27.
40. Yuzawa M, Mori R, Kawamura A. The origins of polypoidal choroidal vasculopathy. Br J Ophthalmol 2005;89:602–7.
41. Spaide RF, Hall L, Haas A, et al. Indocyanine green videoangiography of older patients with central serous chorioretinopathy. Retina 1996;16:203–13.
42. Japanese Study Group of Polypoidal Choroidal Vasculopathy. [Criteria for diagnosis of polypoidal choroidal vasculopathy.] Nippon Ganka Gakkai Zasshi 2005;109:417–27.
43. Costa RA, Navajas EV, Farah ME, et al. Polypoidal choroidal vasculopathy: angiographic characterization of the network vascular elements and a new treatment paradigm. Prog Retin Eye Res 2005;24:560–86.
44. Okubo A, Hirakawa M, Ito M, et al. Clinical features of early and late stage polypoidal choroidal vasculopathy characterized by lesion size and disease duration. Graefes Arch Clin Exp Ophthalmol 2008;246:491–9.
45. Byeon SH, Lew YJ, Lee SC, et al. Clinical features and follow-up results of pulsating polypoidal choroidal vasculopathy treated with photodynamic therapy. Acta Ophthalmol 2010;88:660–8.
46. Gass JDM:Biomicroscopic and histopatholic considerations regarding the feasibility of surgical excision of subfoveal neovascular membrane. Am J Ophthalmol 1994;118:285–98.
47. Yannuzzi LA, Freund KB, Goldbaum M, et al. Polypoidal choroidal vasculopathy masquerading as central serous chorioretinopathy. Ophthalmology 2000;107:767–77.
48. Lee MW, Yeo I, Wong D, Ang CL. Argon laser photocoagulation for the treatment of polypoidal choroidal vasculopathy. Eye (Lond) 2009;23:145–8.
49. Yuzawa M, Mori R, Haruyama M. A study of laser photocoagulation for polypoidal choroidal vasculopathy. Jpn J Ophthalmol 2003;47:379–84.
50. Nishijima K, Takahashi M, Akita J, et al. Laser photocoagulation of indocyanine green angiographically identified feeder vessels to idiopathic polypoidal choroidal vasculopathy. Am J Ophthalmol 2004;137:770–3.
51. Hirami Y, Tsujikawa A, Otani A, et al. Hemorrhagic complications after photodynamic therapy for polypoidal choroidal vasculopathy. Retina 2007;27(3): 335–41.
52. Chan WM, Lam DS, Lai TY, et al. Photodynamic therapy with verteporfin for symptomatic polypoidal choroidal vasculopathy: one-year results of a prospective case series. Ophthalmology 2004;111:1576–84.
53. Kokame GT, Yeung L, Lai JC. Continuous anti-VEGF treatment with ranibizumab for polypoidal choroidal vasculopathy: 6-month results. Br J Ophthalmol 2010;94:297–301.
54. Gomi F, Ohji M, Sayanagi K, et al. One-year outcomes of photodynamic therapy in age-related macular degeneration and polypoidal choroidal vasculopathy in Japanese patients. Ophthalmology 2008;115:141–6.
55. Gomi F, Sawa M, Wakabayashi T, et al. Efficacy of intravitreal bevacizumab combined with photodynamic therapy for polypoidal choroidal vasculopathy. Am J Ophthalmol 2010;150:48–54.

Central Serous Chorioretinopathy

David T. Liu, Andrew C. Fok, Waiman Chan, Timothy Y. Lai, Dennis S. Lam

INTRODUCTION

Central serous chorioretinopathy (CSC) was first described by Albrecht von Graefe as central recurrent retinitis in 1866.[1] It is a chorioretinal disorder, incompletely understood, with systemic associations, a multifactorial etiology, as well as a complex pathogenesis. It typically affects young to middle-aged men and is characterized by serous detachment of the neurosensory retina, which is usually located at the posterior pole. It is usually idiopathic but might also be secondary to high levels of endogenous or exogenous corticosteroids. Advances in imaging, particularly in indocyanine green angiography (ICGA) and optical coherence tomography (OCT), have led to a greater understanding of the pathophysiology of CSC. Most cases of CSC are self-limiting, with spontaneous resolution and good visual prognosis. However, some patients may suffer from persistent or recurrent serous macular detachment with subsequent progressive visual loss. A greater understanding of CSC has led many to believe that CSC is not a completely benign condition. Treatments for CSC, in particular the photodynamic therapy (PDT) using lower doses and reduced fluence, and the antivascular endothelial growth factor (anti-VEGF) therapy, are evolving. Although treatment results appear to be promising, more randomized large-scale controlled studies are needed before their treatment roles can be fully delineated.

PATHOGENESIS, PREDISPOSITION, AND RISK FACTORS

The pathophysiology of CSC has yet to be fully elucidated. It has, however, been thought to involve multiple etiologies and mechanisms that ultimately lead to widespread choroidal circulation abnormalities.[2] Hyperdynamic choroidal circulation and choroidal vascular hyperpermeability are the main features that are shared among patients with CSC.[3] The resultant increase in hydrostatic pressure in the choroid causes breakdown of the retinal pigment epithelial (RPE) barrier with subsequent leakage of fluid from the choroid through defects in RPE cell tight junctions into the subretinal space.[4,5] Studies of ICGA of patients with CSC also revealed areas of hypofluorescence, indicating choriocapillary nonperfusion, which might also be one of the mechanisms that lead to choroidal venous dilation and congestion.

Horniker first suggested that psychiatric disturbances were linked to CSC in 1927.[6] He described a mechanism in which mental disturbances would lead to retinal angiospasm and subsequent macular exudation. In the subsequent 60 years, however, there was a lack of study in the literature to confirm this link between psychiatric problems and CSC. It was not until 1987 that Yannuzzi's cross-sectional study demonstrated the association of CSC with Type A behavioral pattern.[7] The mechanism was thought to be related to elevation of catecholamine levels, which might trigger vasoconstriction of choroidal vessels by stimulating the sympathetic nervous system and adrenergic receptors.

Exogenous as well as elevated endogenous corticosteroids are well-known predisposing factors for CSC.[8] Patients taking systemic steroid for diseases such as autoimmune conditions and after organ transplantation are at risk.[4,9,10] CSC has been reported to occur in up to 6% of patients receiving corticosteroids after renal transplant.[11] Other routes of exogenous corticosteroids such as intra-articular, intranasal, and topical have also been reported to put patients at risk of CSC.[12–14] Diseases associated with an increased endogenous cortisol production such as Cushing's disease and pregnancy also increase the risk of CSC.[15–19] In some cases, CSC can even be the presenting symptom of Cushing syndrome.[20] There are a number of proposed mechanisms as to how corticosteroids are related to CSC. Corticosteroids could induce choroidal vasoconstriction by reducing nitric oxide production. Direct increase in the permeability of the blood vessels might also occur, together with RPE cell tight junction damage.[21–23] Corticosteroids could reverse the polarity of RPE cells, which causes them to pump ions into the subretinal space. Fluid will then enter the subretinal space by osmosis.[24,25]

Abnormal coagulation and platelet aggregation have also been proposed to be involved in the pathogenesis of CSC.[26] Aqueous sample cytokine analysis showed that eyes with CSC have lower platelet-derived growth factor (PDGF) levels in the aqueous, suggesting that PDGF might play a role in the pathogenesis of CSC.[27] The role of VEGF in CSC has been studied and intravitreal anti-VEGF injections have been tried. However, aqueous and plasma samples from patients with CSC showed no elevation in VEGF level when compared with normal controls.[27,28]

Helicobacter pylori infection has been reported to be associated with CSC and its treatment to hasten the rate of subretinal fluid resolution.[29–31] Hypertension, smoking, antibiotic use, antihistamine use, alcohol consumption and allergic respiratory diseases have also been implicated in increasing the risk of CSC.[16,32] Obstructive sleep apnea has been postulated to be associated with CSC and its treatment has been reported to lead to the resolution of CSC.[33] A case-controlled study showed that patients with CSC have a less chance of glaucoma when compared with controls.[34] This might be related to increased choroidal blood supply to the optic nerve but the exact mechanism remains unclear. While there have been isolated case reports of patients developing CSC after rhinoplasty[35] and laser in situ keratomileusis,[36] their relationship is unclear.

CLINICAL FEATURES

Typical CSC with the classic presentations is easy to diagnose. Atypical CSC, however, has a wide range of presentations and can mimic many other ocular diseases. In order to ensure an accurate and prompt diagnosis of the condition, the demographics, clinical features, and clinical patterns should be taken into account with vigilance. When in doubt, the use of imaging techniques and other new modalities of investigation would be helpful.

Demographics

CSC predominately affects males, with a male to female ratio of approximately 6:1.[37] The age of onset is usually between 30 and 50 years but patients with chronic CSC might continue to suffer from the disease even though they are advanced in age. However, if a patient over 50 years of age presents a clinical appearance of CSC, one should be suspicious of differential diagnoses such as age-related macular degeneration (AMD) and polypoidal choroidal vasculopathy (PCV).[38] CSC appears to have a low incidence in blacks when compared to whites and Asians, but it might behave more aggressively in blacks.[39–41] At presentation, involvement is usually unilateral. However bilateral involvement is common in chronic cases and cases related to excessive endogenous or exogenous corticosteroids.

Symptoms

Common symptoms of CSC include relative central scotoma, metamorphopsia, micropsia, dyschromatopsia, and blurring of vision. The detached neurosensory retina is anteriorly displaced and causes the eye to become more hyperopic. Therefore vision is often improved with the use of a hyperopic correction lens.

Signs

Fundus examination typically shows a well-demarcated oval-shaped area of neurosensory retinal detachment in the posterior pole (Fig. 72.1). Serous pigment epithelium detachment (PED) can also occur together or independently. The diagnosis is usually obvious from examination with indirect ophthalmoscopy. However, in cases with minimal subretinal fluid or small PED, slit-lamp biomicroscopy with fundus contact lens might be useful. In these cases, the loss of the normal foveal reflex might provide a good hint. Yellow dots are frequently observed on the posterior surface of the detached retina and are postulated to be associated with phagocytosis of shed photoreceptor outer segments (Fig. 72.2).[42] Yellowish discoloration of the fovea is often seen and is caused by increased visibility of retinal xanthophyll.[4,17,39,43] The subretinal fluid is usually transparent and colorless, but occasionally it can also appear cloudy.[39,44] Fibrin can form in the subretinal and sub-RPE spaces and cause the subretinal fluid to become opaque. The fibrin usually dissolves spontaneously but rarely it could cause fibrosis and lead to permanent drop in vision. In chronic recurrent cases, RPE change and atrophy might develop. Patients with CSC can also present bullous neurosensory detachments,[10,45–48] which are usually located inferiorly as the subretinal fluid drains down from the macula by gravity. In chronic cases, an atrophic RPE tract connecting the macula to the inferior detachment might be seen. Other complications of chronic CSC include secondary choroidal neovascularization (CNV) formation, cystoid macular edema, subretinal lipid deposition, and choriocapillaris atrophy.[49]

INVESTIGATIONS

Fluorescein angiography

Fluorescein angiography (FA) in acute CSC typically shows one of two different types of leakage patterns: ink blot or smoke stack. In the former, the leakage starts as a pin point in the early phase and then concentrically diffuses out in the late phase and appears like an ink blot (Fig. 72.3). In the smoke stack appearance, the leakage again starts as a pin point in the early phase, but it gradually tracks upward and then expands to form a mushroom cloud or umbrella-like appearance (Fig. 72.4). Smoke stack appearance is less common and only appears in about 10–15% of patients with acute CSC.[50] It is caused by an increased protein concentration in the subretinal fluid. In cases in which

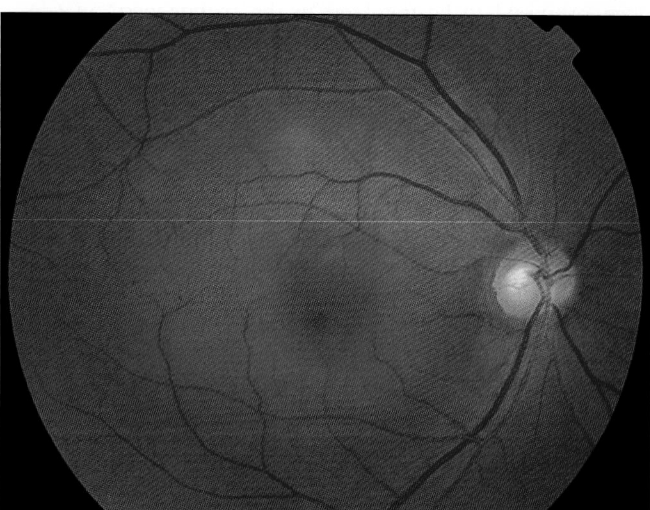

Fig. 72.1 Color fundus photograph of a patient with central serous chorioretinopathy showing neurosensory retinal detachment at the posterior pole.

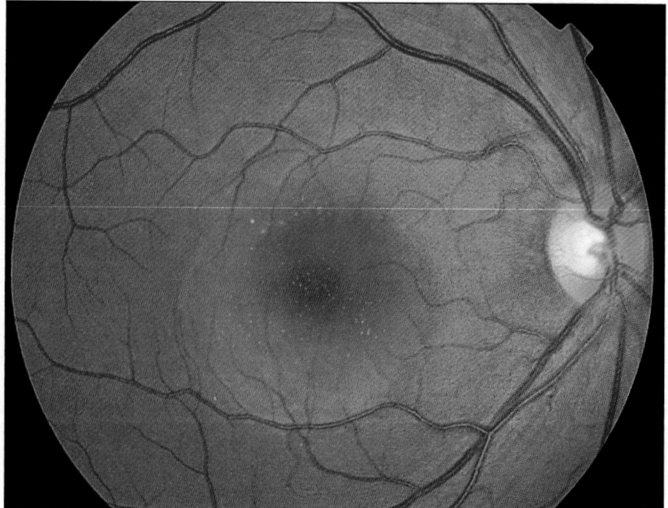

Fig. 72.2 Color fundus photograph of a patient with central serous chorioretinopathy showing neurosensory detachment of the macula. Note the presence of yellow dots on the posterior surface of the detached retina.

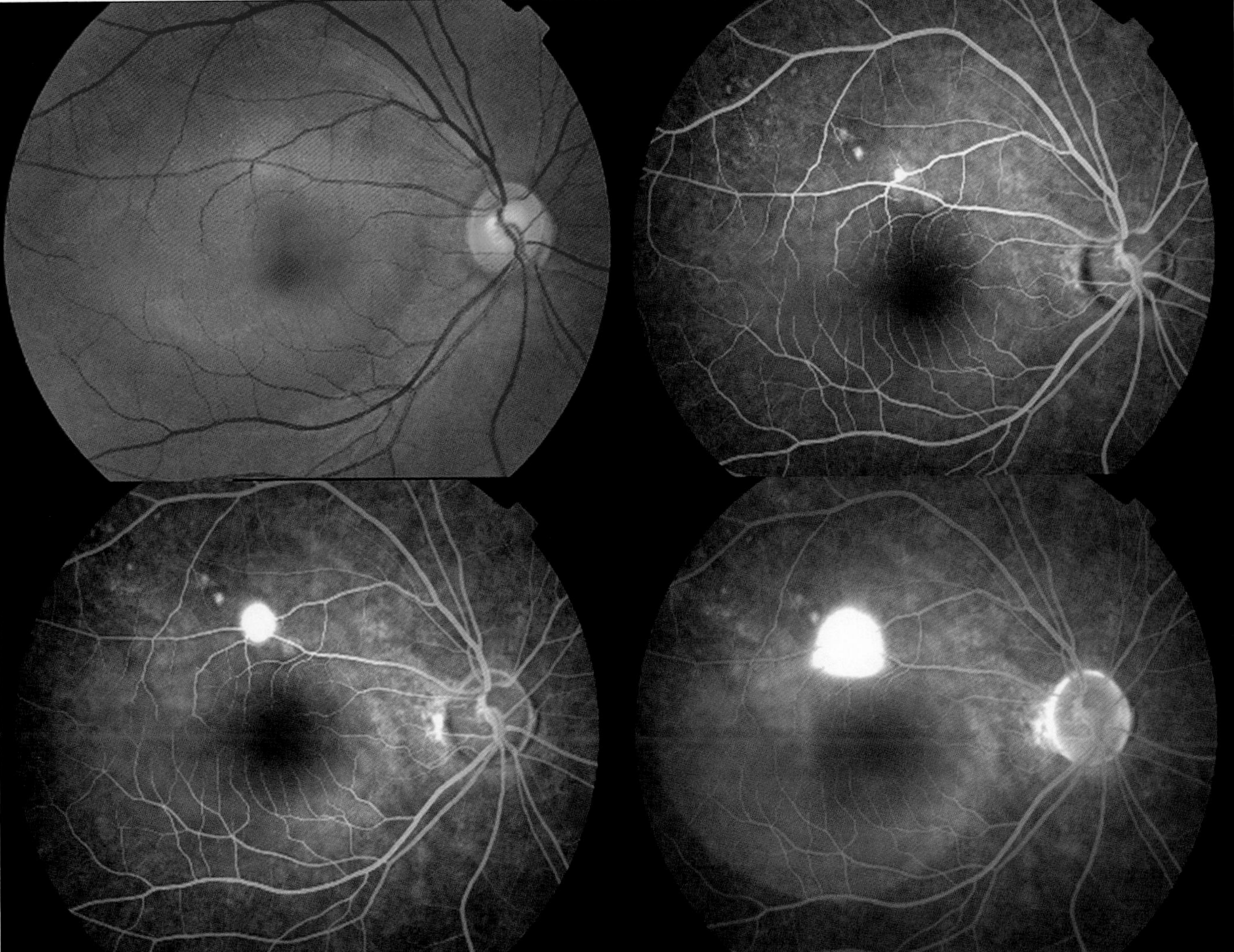

Fig. 72.3 Fluorescein angiogram shows leakage with an ink blot appearance. The hyperfluorescence starts as a pinpoint and then enlarges concentrically similar to the appearance of dropping ink onto a piece of paper.

there is PED, the FA appearance would be the pooling of dye in the sub-RPE space (Fig. 72.5). Chronic CSC might show an RPE window defect due to RPE atrophy. Multifocal CSC would show multiple sites of leakage. FA is also useful in differentiating CSC from other diagnoses such as choroidal neovascularization (CNV) and Vogt–Koyanagi–Harada disease.

Indocyanine green angiography

ICGA is one of the most important investigations in CSC because it demonstrates the choroidal vascular abnormalities and can act as a guide to treatments such as photodynamic therapy. In CSC, delay in choroidal filling is usually present. Typical features include abnormally dilated choroidal vasculature in the early phase and choroidal hyperpermeability in the late phase (Fig. 72.6).[51–54] The area of choroidal vascular abnormality is usually much more widespread than the leakage point on FA and is commonly present in the fellow eye as well. Punctate hyperfluorescent spots are often seen in the mid-phase.[55] In the later phases of ICGA, the dye usually leaks into the deeper layers of the choroid to produce hyperfluorescent patches.[39] Hypofluorescent areas can also be seen on ICGA. They represent areas of choriocapillary nonperfusion and this might be one of the mechanisms that lead to choroidal venous dilation and congestion.

Optical coherence tomography

The availability of OCT has vastly enhanced the anatomical assessment and understanding of CSC by providing cross-sectional imaging of the macula. OCT demonstrates beautifully the presence of subretinal fluid or PED and helps in differentiation between the two.[56,57] Subretinal yellow dots observed clinically, which typically show high reflectivity, can also be seen.[42] Outer nuclear layer OCT is especially useful in detecting shallow subretinal fluid and small PED, which might be difficult to identify clinically (Fig. 72.7). OCT might be able to demonstrate lesions in the fellow asymptomatic eye, such as RPE bumps and small PED.[58] Serial scans can be used to assess disease progression and treatment response (Fig. 72.8). Quantitative measurements and thickness maps can be generated and are useful for documentation as well as research purposes (Fig. 72.9). The software can also render three-dimensional images to allow better structural visualization and understanding (Fig. 72.10). Choroidal vascular hyperpermeability on ICGA is associated with an

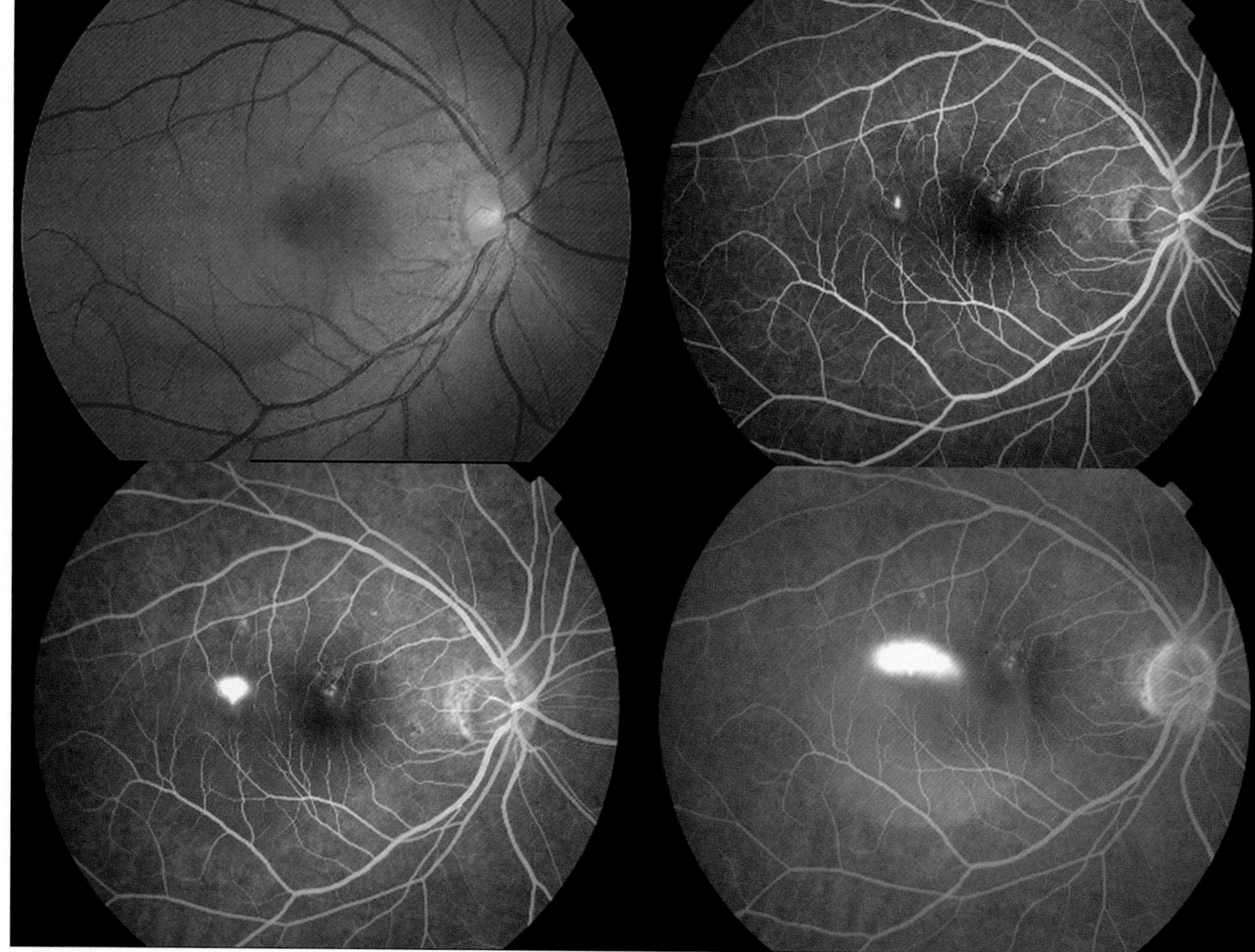

Fig. 72.4 Fluorescein angiogram shows leakage with a smoke stack appearance. The hyperfluorescence starts as a pinpoint and then migrates upward and subsequently diffuses laterally, leading to a mushroom cloud or umbrella-like appearance.

increase in subfoveal choroidal thickness on OCT.[59,60] With the introduction of enhanced depth imaging, many researchers consider that increased choroidal thickening is a hallmark of CSC. OCT can also offer valuable prognostic information. Cystoid degeneration and disruption of the outer photoreceptor layer and the inner/outer-segment junction have been reported to be associated with poor visual outcomes.[61] OCT can also assist in differentiating CSC from other diagnosis such as CNV and PCV by detecting lesions in the subretinal space (Fig. 72.11). Another reported distinguishing feature between PCV and CSC is that eyes with PCV might show thinning of the photoreceptor outer segments on OCT.[62]

Fundus autofluorescence

Fundus autofluorescence (FAF) is an adjunctive tool for the assessment of CSC. During the acute phase of the disease, FAF typically shows hypofluorescence at the leakage point and over the area of neurosensory detachment due to blockage by subretinal fluid.[63] The subretinal yellow dots observed clinically might demonstrate hyperfluorescence.[42] In chronic-recurrent CSC, hyperfluorescence is common in areas of residual neurosensory detachment. Therefore, FAF might give additional information on whether the disease is acute or chronic.[64] Moreover, the pattern of FAF has been shown to correlate with visual acuity.[65] After the resolution of subretinal fluid, areas of hyperfluorescence might become visible due to release of fluorophore materials into the subretinal space. Photopigment density has been studied with autofluorescence densitometry. It was found to be decreased in eyes with CSC and showed a delayed recovery after the resolution of subretinal fluid.[66]

Multifocal electroretinography

Multifocal electroretinography (mfERG) is useful in evaluating macular function in CSC. First- and second-order kernel mfERG response amplitudes have been shown to be reduced in patients with CSC.[67,68] Reductions in response amplitudes appear to be localized in the center for the first-order kernel mfERG but predominately affect the more peripheral retina for the second-order kernel mfERG. These suggest that while outer retinal dysfunction is localized in the center, inner retinal dysfunction might be more widespread. Unlike OCT, mfERG response amplitudes were found to correlate with visual acuity.[67,69]

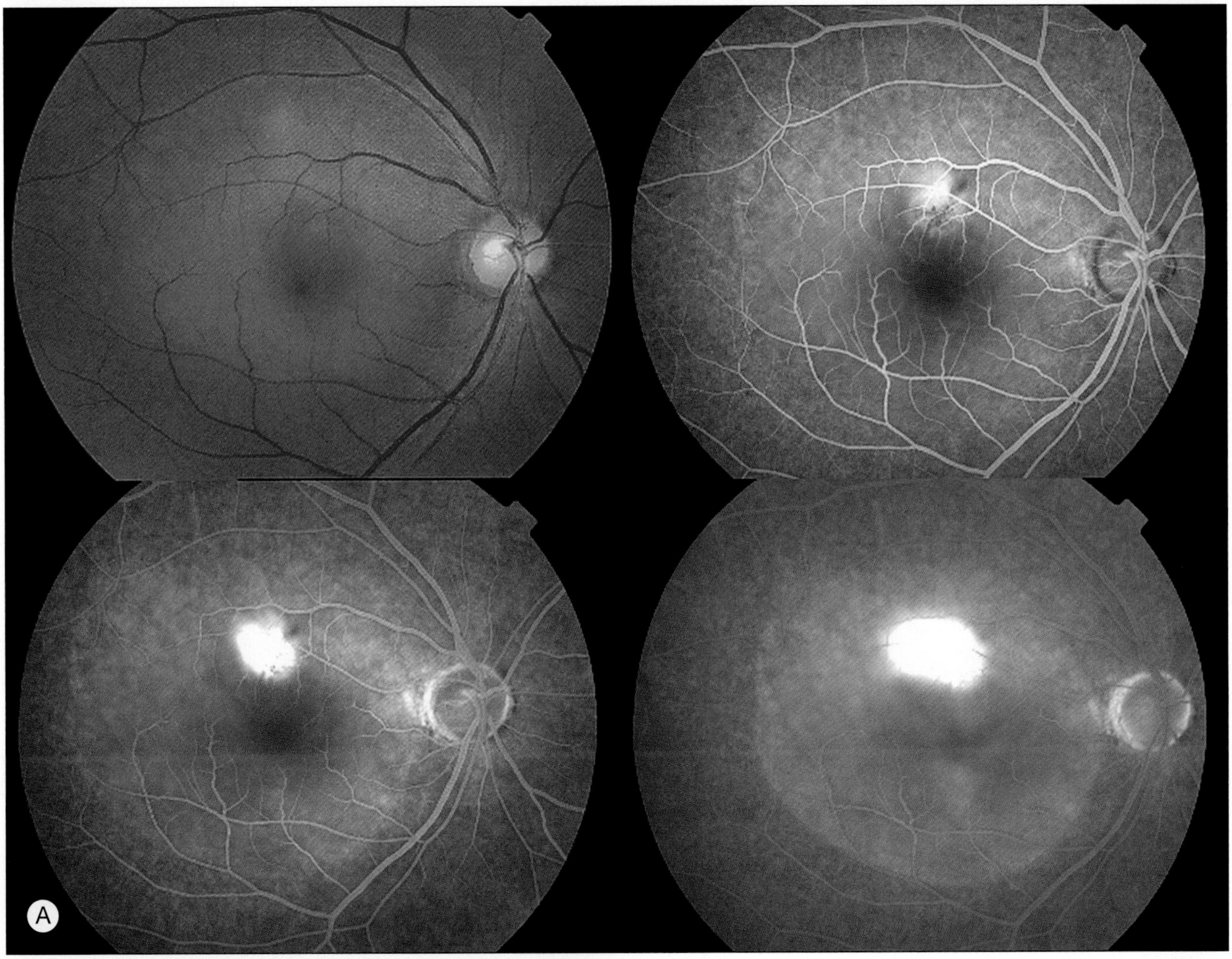

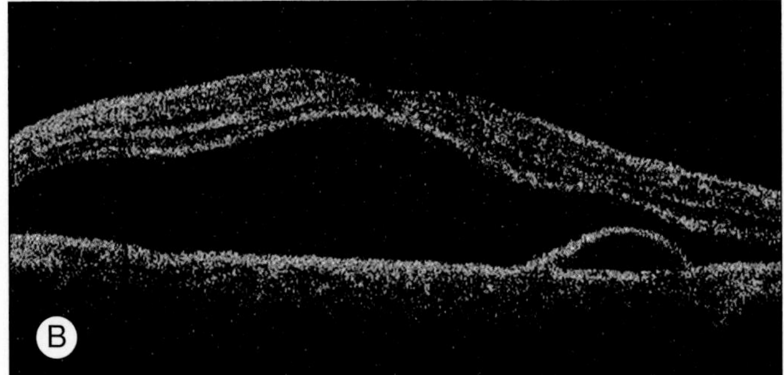

Fig. 72.5 This 42-year-old male presented with a right eye relative scotoma for 3 weeks. (A) Clinical examination showed subretinal fluid together with a pigment epithelium detachment (PED) in the macula. Fluorescein angiogram shows initial pooling of dye in the PED followed by leakage. (B) Optical coherence tomography shows the presence of subretinal fluid and PED.

Therefore mfERG and OCT can complement each other in the functional and anatomical assessments of CSC respectively.

Microperimetry

Microperimetry is useful in the assessment of macular sensitivity in patients with CSC. Macular sensitivity is reduced in both the central and paracentral areas in the active phase of the disease when there is subretinal fluid.[50] It has been shown to improve after the resolution of subretinal fluid with or without treatment.[70–72] However, more often than not there are residual focal areas with reduced sensitivity that correspond to RPE irregularities or defects of the inner/outer-segment junction on OCT.[73,74] Moreover, macular sensitivity was demonstrated to correlate with central macular thickness on OCT, which suggested the existence of structural and functional correlation.[75]

NATURAL HISTORY

The disease is usually self-limiting and 90% of the cases will show spontaneous recovery within a few months without

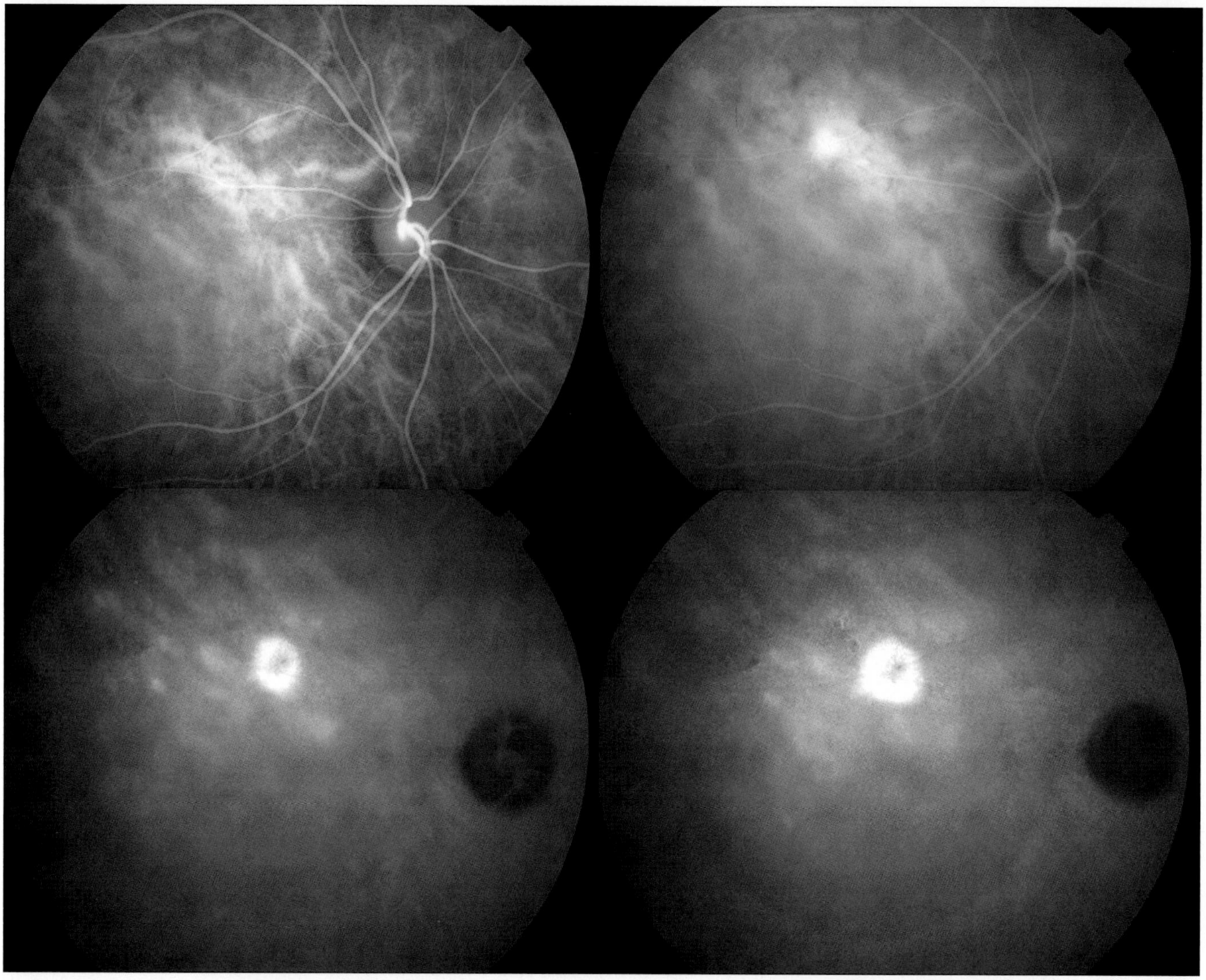

Fig. 72.6 Indocyanine green angiography demonstrates dilated choroidal vasculature in the early phase and hyperpermeability in the later phases. In the later phases, hyperfluorescent patches occur because the dye leaks into the deeper layers of the choroid.

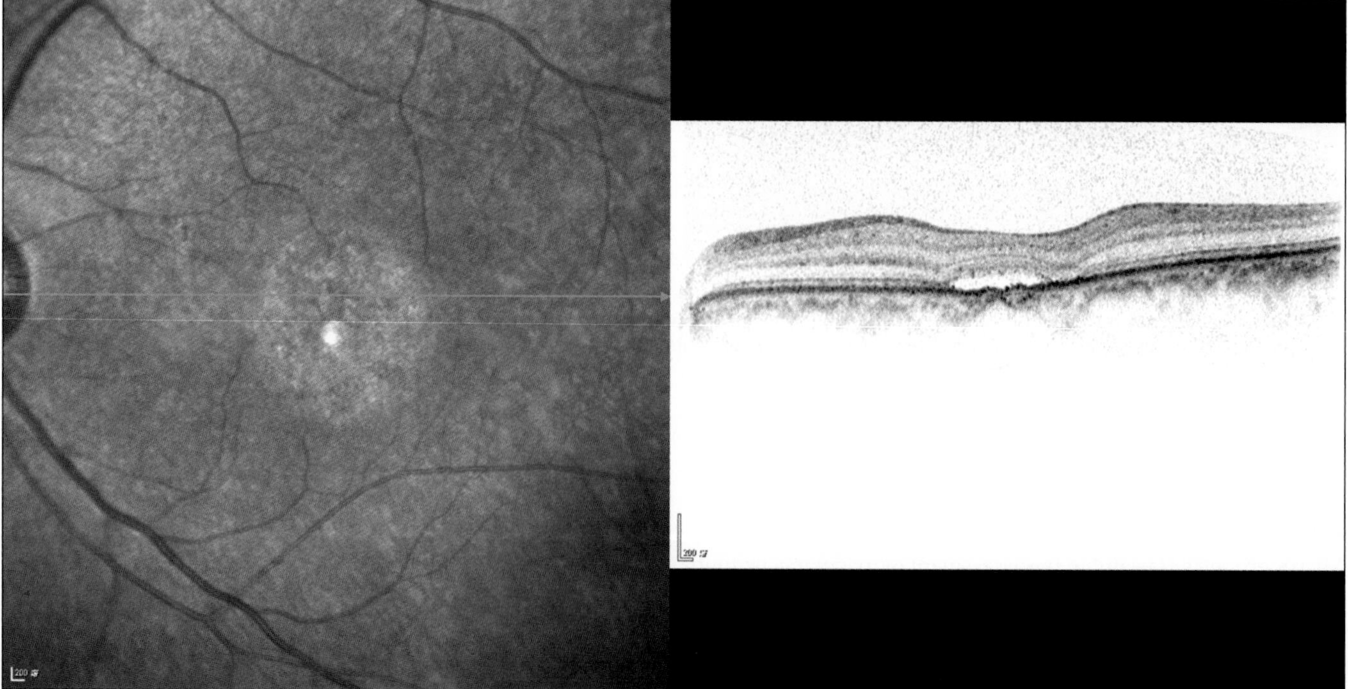

Fig. 72.7 This 37-year-old male presented with blurring of vision in the left eye for 2 weeks. Clinical examination revealed retinal pigment epithelium changes on fundal examination but no obvious subretinal fluid was seen. However, optical coherence tomography was able to clearly demonstrate the presence of subretinal fluid and confirm the diagnosis of central serous chorioretinopathy.

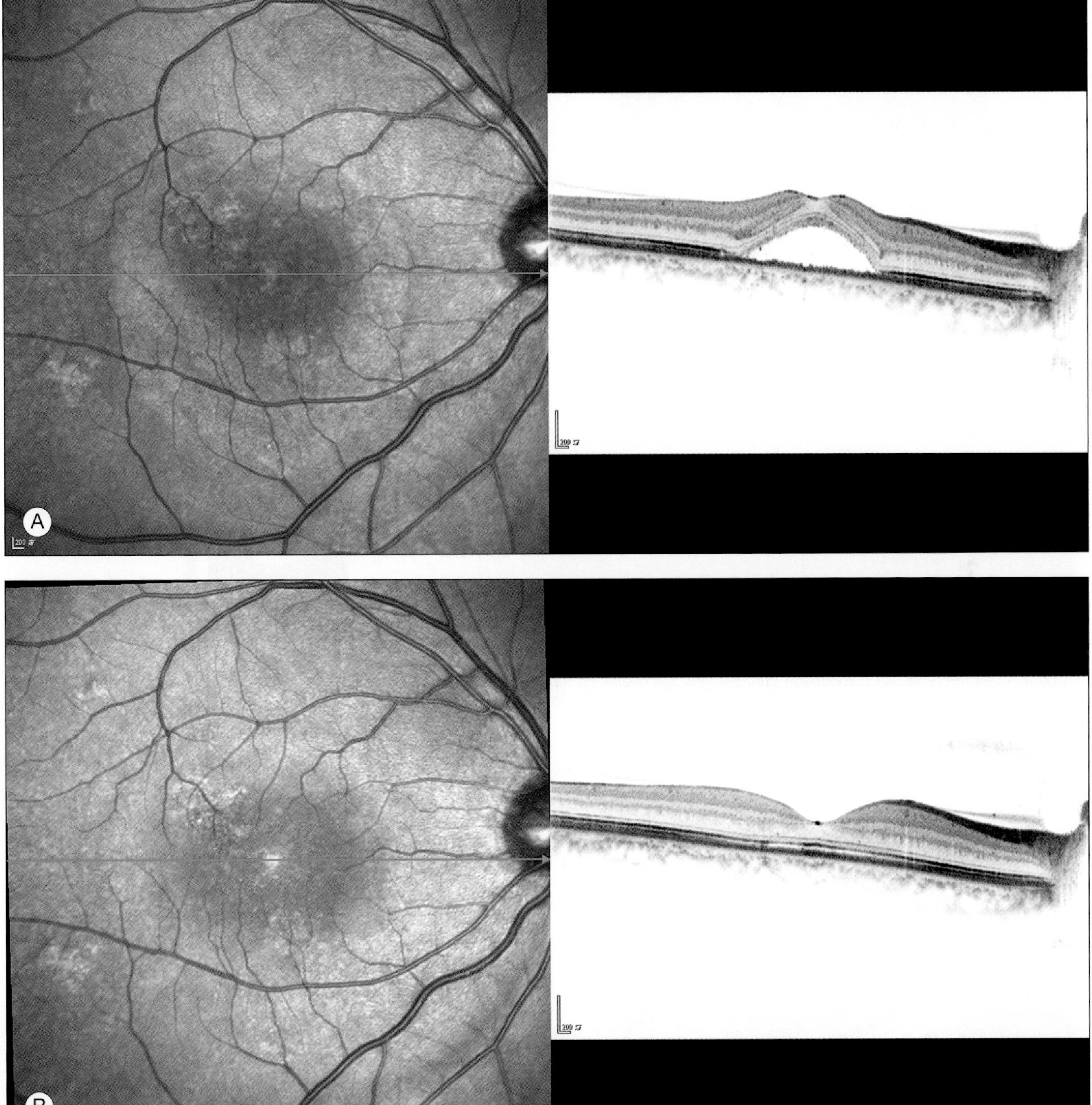

Fig. 72.8 This 33-year-old male presented with a right eye relative scotoma for 1 week. (A) Optical coherence tomography (OCT) shows neurosensory detachment of the macula. (B) His symptoms resolved three months later and OCT shows resolution of subretinal fluid and restoration of normal architecture of the macula. Different layers of the retina are seen clearly. The preservation of the photoreceptor inner/outer-segment junction is demonstrated.

significant visual loss.[37,76,77] However, some patients may develop chronic or recurrent diseases that lead to areas of RPE atrophy or hypertrophy with visual loss. Poor visual acuity on presentation and a prolonged duration of serous macular detachment appear to be associated with poor visual outcomes.[78] Up to 50% of patients might develop recurrence.[79–82] Recurrence can develop at any time and CSC recurs in about 50% of the patients within the first year. A history of psychiatric illness is associated with a higher rate of recurrence.[82] A small proportion of patients develop severe irreversible visual loss due to, for example, RPE atrophy, CNV development (in up to 6% of patients), and transformation into polypoidal choroidal vasculopathy (PCV) with exudation and hemorrhage. Adaptive optics scanning laser ophthalmoscopy was able to demonstrate reduced cone densities in eyes with resolved CSC.[83] Even patients whose visual acuity has recovered to baseline might be left with residual symptoms such as metamorphopsia, scotoma, and reduced contrast sensitivity. Therefore, CSC should not be considered a benign disease.

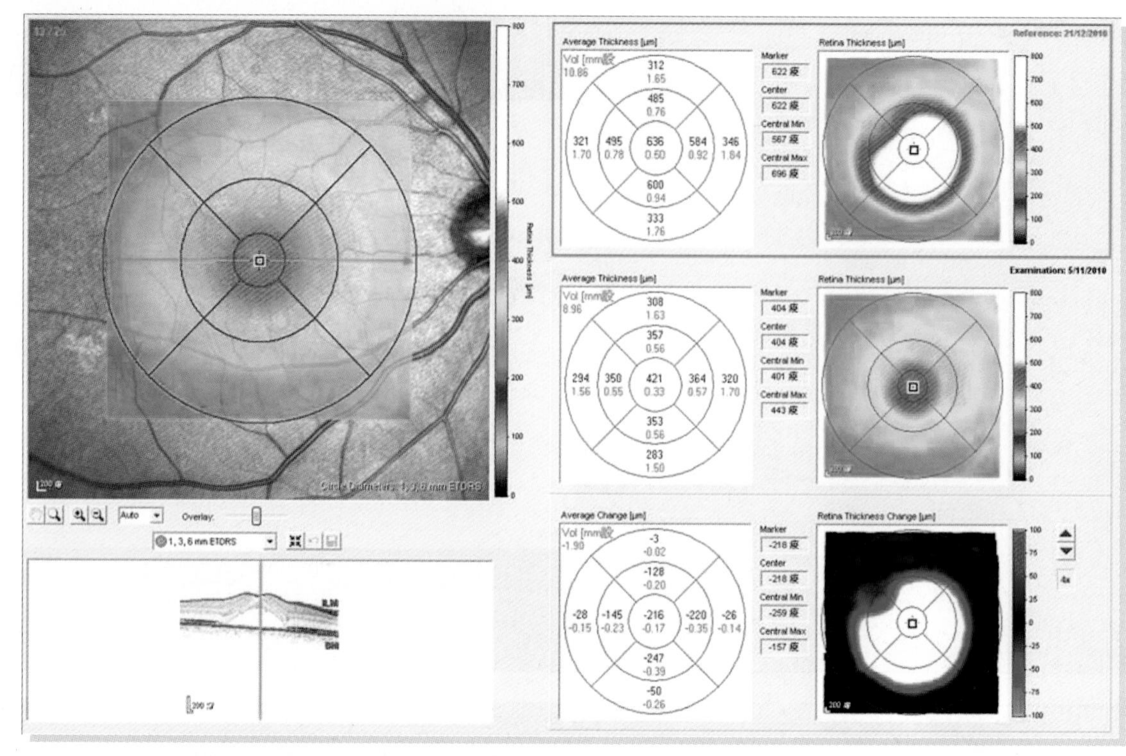

Fig. 72.9 Optical coherence tomography thickness map allows topographic and quantitative assessment of macular thickness. Previous scans can be used as reference for comparison and changes are displaced topographically and numerically. The reference scan is indicated by the red rectangle. The software and its tracking system are capable of performing serial scans at a location exactly the same as the reference scan.

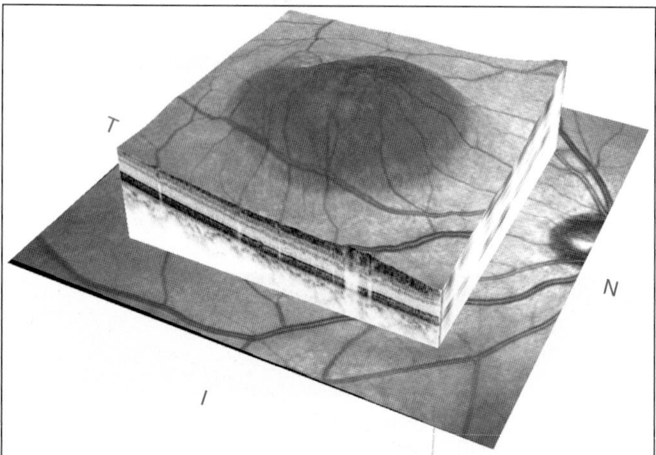

Fig. 72.10 Three-dimensional rendering of optical coherence tomography scans allows enhanced perception of the neurosensory detachment.

DIFFERENTIAL DIAGNOSIS

The diagnosis of CSC is usually clear and straightforward from clinical examination and is confirmed by FA, ICGA, and OCT. However, several diseases can mimic CSC and it is important to keep in mind the following differential diagnoses (Table 72.1).

Optic disc pit

Serous macular detachment develops in up to 45% of patients with optic disc pit. Therefore, the optic disc should always be examined closely for such a condition in cases of suspected CSC. The pit is usually located in the temporal aspect of the disc. Macular detachment usually begins with schisis of the inner retina, followed by serous detachment of the outer retina. The diagnosis is usually obvious clinically and FA would show an absence of leakage.

Age-related macular degeneration

One should be careful in making a diagnosis of CSC in patients aged 50 years or above because AMD is an important differential diagnosis. Moreover, secondary CNV can develop in patients with chronic CSC or after treatment such as laser photocoagulation. Although each of the diseases has its own characteristic FA and ICGA features, it might be difficult to differentiate between the two, especially in chronic CSC when the leakage is more diffused and ill-defined. OCT might be useful in these cases when looking for the presence of CNV.

Polypoidal choroidal vasculopathy

PCV is characterized by the development of abnormal polypoidal dilations arising from the inner choroidal circulation, which causes recurrent episodes of exudative maculopathy with serous or hemorrhagic PED. When patients present PCV with simply serous PED or serous macular detachment, it might be mistaken

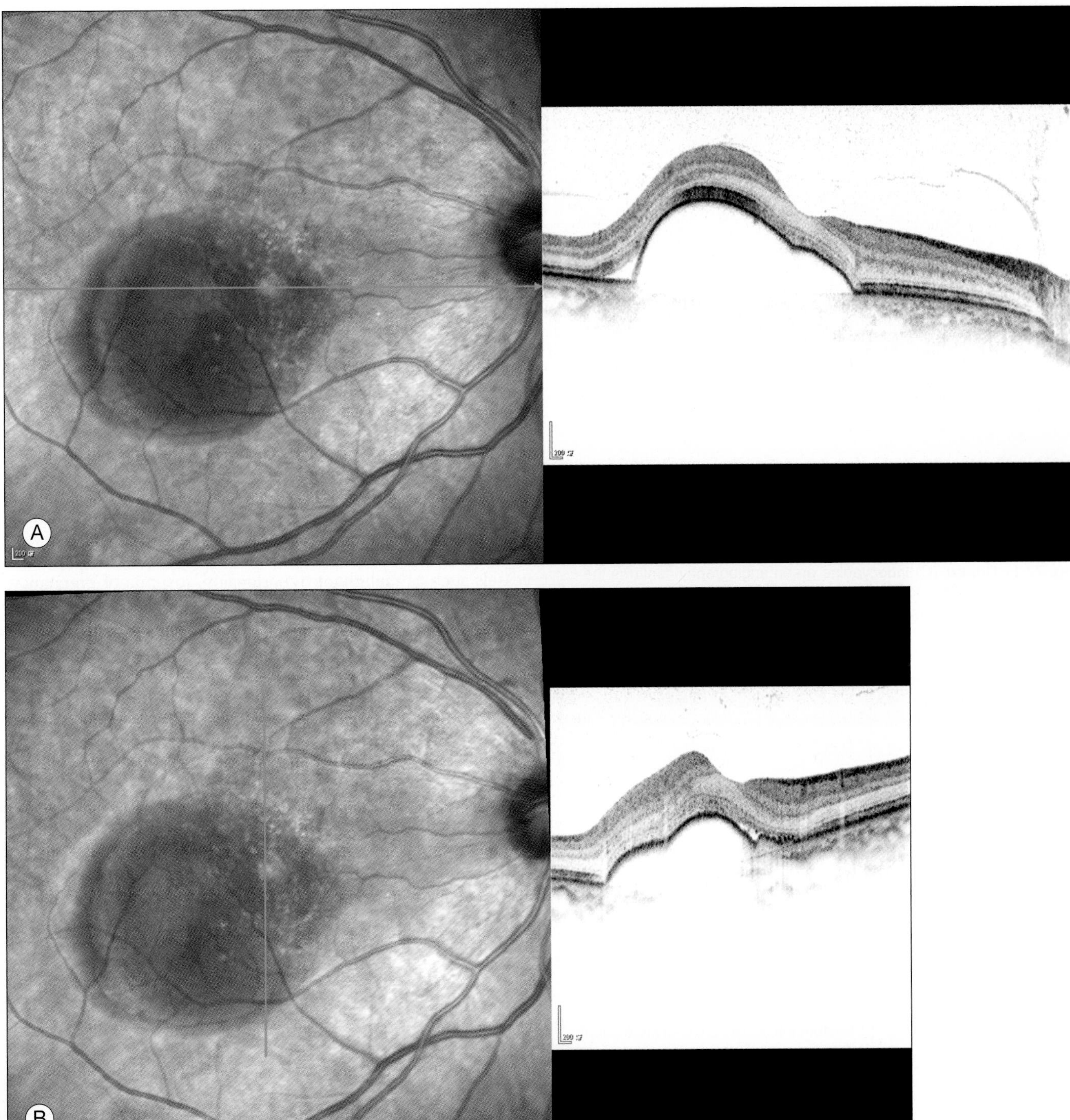

Fig. 72.11 This 50-year-old male was initially thought to have central serous chorioretinopathy causing serous pigment epithelium detachment (PED). (A) Optical coherence tomography (OCT) shows the presence of PED and adjacent subretinal fluid. (B) An OCT scan at another location reveals the presence of polyps at the edge of the PED.

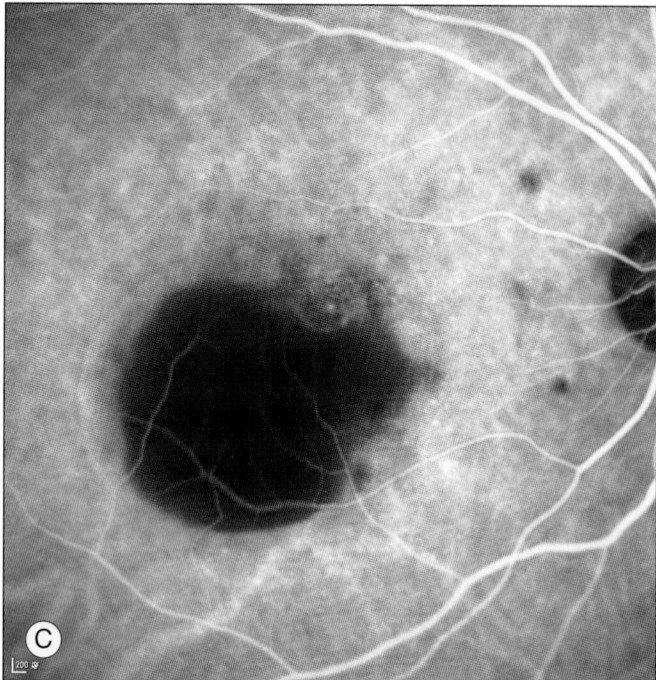

Fig. 72.11 Cont'd (C) Indocyanine green angiography confirms the presence of polyps and the patient was diagnosed with polypoidal choroidal vasculopathy.

Table 72.1 Important differential diagnoses of central serous chorioretinopathy and their differentiating features

Differential diagnosis	Differentiating features
Optic disc pit	Presence of optic disc pit, absence of leakage on FA
AMD	Older age group, CNV on FA
PCV	ICGA shows polyps and branching vascular network
Inflammatory and infectious diseases	Systemic features and bilateral involvement in VKH; ultrasonic T-sign in posterior scleritis
Autoimmune and vascular disorders	Systemic features are usually evident
Intraocular tumors	Ultrasound is useful in the detection and differentiation between different types of tumors

FA, fluorescein angiography; AMD, age-related macular degeneration; CNV, choroidal neovascularization; PCV, polypoidal choroidal vasculopathy; ICGA, indocyanine green angiography; VKH, Vogt–Koyanagi–Harada disease..

as CSC. Differential diagnosis can be made by ICGA, which demonstrates branching vascular networks and polyps.[84] OCT can also help to differentiate between the two entities. OCT is able to demonstrate polyps in PCV whereas in CSC, the subretinal space should be clean.

Inflammatory and infectious diseases

Inflammatory and infectious diseases causing serous macular detachment can be considered as a differential diagnosis of CSC. Vogt–Koyanagi–Harada (VKH) disease is a multisystem disorder with granulomatous panuveitis that often presents with serous retinal detachment. Its systemic manifestations, including neurological and dermatological signs as well as bilaterality, readily distinguish it from CSC. Patients with VKH usually show multifocal leakage on FA. In contrast to CSC, VKH is treated with systemic steroids. Posterior scleritis can also present with serous retinal detachment. Unlike CSC, patients frequently experience pain. Ultrasound scans demonstrating the characteristic T-sign can confirm the diagnosis. Other rarer inflammatory conditions causing serous macular detachment include sympathetic ophthalmia, uveal effusion syndrome, and benign reactive lymphoid hyperplasia of the choroid. Presumed ocular histoplasmosis syndrome is an infectious disease that could cause serous macular detachment. It has characteristic punched-out lesions known as histospots.

Autoimmune and vascular disorders

Autoimmune diseases such as systemic lupus erythematosus and polyarteritis nodosa that affect choroidal vessels can cause serous macular detachment. Systemic steroid is frequently used in the treatment of autoimmune diseases and this alone would also cause CSC. Non-autoimmune conditions affecting blood vessels such as malignant hypertension, toxemia of pregnancy, and disseminated intravascular coagulopathy can also present with a secondary neurosensory detachment. The mechanism is believed to be acute multifocal occlusion of choroidal blood vessels.

Intraocular tumors

Various types of choroidal tumors can mimic CSC by causing exudative macular detachment. Examples include choroidal hemangioma, choroidal melanoma, and choroidal metastasis. It is important to differentiate a malignant and potentially lethal condition from CSC. For tumors with a significant size, the diagnosis is usually obvious from clinical examination. However, small tumors, especially choroidal hemangiomas, might not be detected easily in the presence of subretinal fluid. Ultrasound scans are very useful in detecting and differentiating the nature of the tumor. OCT is not a routine investigation for tumor detection, but sometimes choroidal elevations might be detected underneath the subretinal fluid while scanning patients with suspected CSC.

TREATMENT

Observation in most cases

Since CSC has a favorable natural history, observation has been considered as an appropriate first-line approach. As high levels of endogenous or exogenous corticosteroids have been implicated as an etiology for CSC, it is important to check whether CSC patients have such problems by asking if they have had exposure to nasal sprays, intra-articular injections or other covert sources of corticosteroids. In case of high levels of endogenous and exogenous corticosteroids, correction to normal levels, when possible, can lead to resolution of detachment in 90% of the cases.[85] Lifestyle modification and other forms of psychosocial therapies may help in some CSC patients who are prone to psychological stress.[37,86] However, with a greater understanding of pathophysiology and the natural course of CSC, there are increasing doubts about the proclaimed "benign" nature of

CSC.[37,86] Foveal attenuation, cystoid macular degeneration, and damage of the foveal photoreceptor layer have been proposed to be the pathological changes contributing to irreversible visual loss in CSC.[37,86]

There has been ongoing debate regarding when active treatment should be offered to patients with CSC. It is important to note that photoreceptor atrophy in the fovea occurs as early as 4 months after onset of symptoms.[77] Therefore, it has been recommended that if symptoms persist for more than 3 months, further active treatments should be considered.[37,86] On the other hand, there are data showing that although some treatments may speed up visual recovery, no treatment has been shown to improve the final visual acuity of patients with acute CSC.[87,88] Therefore, we have to refrain from tipping the balance in favor of either observation or treatment. Treatments with known risks or side-effects should be used cautiously in acute CSC. Observation with vigilance is usually the mainstay of treatment for the good visual prognosis group: patients with good presenting visual acuity and duration of symptom presentation of less than 3 months. In the wake of increasing reports of permanent visual quality derangements including metamorphopsia, paracentral or central scotoma observed in patients having been managed conservatively by observation and reassurance,[37,86] the indication for active and timely treatment, however, may be much stronger in some susceptible individuals who suffer from chronic CSC, i.e., symptoms presenting for at least six months or indication of serous macular elevation associated with RPE atrophic areas and subtle leaks or ill-defined staining on FA.[39,89] The debate as to the best timing for treating CSC continues and further research is needed.

Treatment for selected cases

In the past few years, an array of new treatment modalities for CSC had emerged. Based on the best scientific evidence available in the literature, the efficacy and safety of these evolving treatment modalities should, however, be interpreted with caution as most of these studies have limitations like selection bias, lack of randomization, a small sample size, and short follow-up duration.[37,86]

Safety-enhanced photodynamic therapy in selected cases

Safety-enhanced photodynamic therapy (PDT) may be offered to patients with poor presenting visual acuity and with duration of symptom presentation longer than 3 months.

PDT with verteporfin

Following the success of TAP and VIP studies in the management of age-related macular degeneration, expanded indication of PDT has allowed attempted use of PDT to tackle some CSC cases.[90,91] Subsequent studies have confirmed efficacy and favorable visual outcomes of PDT to treat CSC in a majority of cases, especially if it is used under guidance of indocyanine green angiography (ICGA).[92-97] The proposed mechanisms of PDT are choriocapillaris narrowing, choroidal hypoperfusion, reduction of choroidal exudation and choroidal vascular remodeling.[96,98,99] However, the use of PDT is not without complications, especially with conventional verteporfin dosage, as well as fluence and large laser spot size, as RPE atrophy, choriocapillaris ischemia, and secondary CNV have been reported.[94,96] The use of mfERG has further revealed that PDT might cause transient impairment in retinal function after treatment.[100,101]

Conventional PDT with normal dosage and fluence

Conventional or standard PDT for treatment of neovascular age-related macular degeneration was performed using the dose of 6 mg/m^2 infusion of verteporfin (Visudyne, Novartis AG, Bülach, Switzerland). Infusion of verteporfin was performed over 15 minutes, followed by delivery of laser at 692 nm 15 minutes after commencement of the infusion. A total light energy of 50 J/cm^2, light dose rate of 600 mW/cm^2, and photosensitization time of 83 seconds was delivered to the targeted area. Pilot studies showed normalization in calibers of the dilated and congested choroidal vasculature, and a decrease in the extravascular leakage in cases treated by PDT.[96] The effect of the vascular modulation persisted and was sustained for years. With alterations in blood flow and decreased leakages in the choroidal vessels, the corresponding fluorescence leakages also stopped in the fluorescein angiography coupled with subjective and objective visual improvements in most of the patients who had received treatment for CSC. The possible development of CNV, post-treatment visual loss, and potential choroidal ischemia may have limited the widespread application of standard dosage PDT treatment for CSC patients.

Safety-enhanced PDT with reduced verteporfin dosage

In order to enhance the efficacy of PDT in treating CSC while minimizing its side-effects, various ways such as reducing the dosage of verteporfin and shortening the interval between infusion and laser application have been tried. As demonstrated by a previous study, the maximal concentration of verteporfin within the choroidal circulation is achieved 10 minutes after the infusion, when the concentration at the retinal outer segment is still relatively low.[102] Shortening the interval between the infusion and laser application might, therefore, minimize any collateral damage to adjacent retinal structures. Reducing the dosage of verteporfin infusion by half may lower the risk of retinal-choroidal complications without compromising the vascular remodeling ability of PDT as photochemical response in the choroid is dose–response-dependent.[103] Safety-enhanced PDT was performed using half the normal dose of verteporfin at 3 mg/m^2. Infusion of verteporfin was performed over 8 minutes, followed by a delivery of laser at 692 nm 10 minutes afterwards. A total light energy of 50 J/cm^2 was delivered within 83 seconds.[104,105] The treatment efficacy of this half-dose PDT was not affected while the well-proven safety issues such as impairment of retinal function associated with full-dose PDT were alleviated by the use of the half-dose regimen, as reflected by prospective studies worldwide.[72,104,105] In a study of 48 eyes from 48 patients with chronic central serous chorioretinopathy, 40 (83.3%) eyes had complete resolution of serous detachment 3 months afterwards, and 43 (89.6%) eyes, 12 months afterwards. The mean improvement in visual acuity was 1.6 lines and 45 (95.8%) eyes had stable or improved vision. Eyes without PED had significantly greater visual improvement, compared with eyes with PED. Interestingly, patients with CSC for 6 months or less, or younger than 45 years of age, were more likely to gain vision by 2 or more lines after treatment.[105] In a randomized controlled trial involving 63 patients with acute symptomatic CSC for the duration of less than 3 months, 39 patients were randomized into the verteporfin group and 19 patients were enrolled into the placebo group. Thirty-seven (94.9%) eyes in the verteporfin group, compared with 11 (57.9%) eyes in the placebo group, showed absence of macular subretinal fluid 12 months afterwards. All the 39 (100%) eyes treated with verteporfin had stable or improved vision, compared with 15 (78.9%) eyes in the placebo group. No ocular or systemic adverse event was encountered in all the treated patients.[87] The success of safety-enhanced PDT to manage CSC has given birth to more than 10 prospective, retrospective, and/or interventional case series, with or without randomization, so far.[37,86] In spite of the encouraging results and reports on the safety of half-dose PDT in the management of CSC, it is prudent to individualize management plans owing to the absence of a randomized controlled trial of a large sample size to document treatment adversity, and sporadic observations of transient impairment of multifocal ERG response with the use of half-dose PDT.[105,106]

Safety-enhanced PDT with reduced laser fluence

Drug dosage and the timing of laser application are not the only parameters that can be modified to enhance the safety of PDT. Similarly, other parameters like laser fluence and infusion time can also be changed. For instance, improved efficacy and safety profiles of low fluence PDT have been documented in the management of chronic CSC.[107–110] It should, however, be noted that a lack of quality randomized controlled trials to discern either short-term or long-term safety, coupled with reports of severe complications like RPE rip/tear, is sufficient to remind clinicians of the importance of caution and individualization when managing CSC by reduced laser fluence PDT.[111]

Historical thermal (argon) laser photocoagulation and micropulsed diode laser

The use of thermal laser photocoagulation in the management of CSC probably stems from the observation that a successful laser photocoagulation of a fluorescein-detectable pigment epithelial leak may accelerate resolution of the associated neurosensory detachment.[37,76,77,112,113] This initially promising treatment method has gone out of favor in recent years because of significant adverse effects such as permanent scotoma, enlargement of RPE scar, secondary laser-induced CNV formation, and, rarely but sinisterly, inadvertent foveal photocoagulation, especially if the leaking point is subfoveal, or parafoveal, or when more than one pigment epithelial leakage is identified.[114–117] Therefore, in the event of multiple leaking points or subfoveal leaking, safety-enhanced PDT may be considered as a viable alternative. Thermal laser photocoagulation may still have a role in the management of CSC with a discrete, solitary extrafoveal leaking point. However, it should be emphasized that thermal laser photocoagulation may not affect the final functional outcomes and the rate of recurrence.[80] This may be due to the fact that zonal hyperperfusion and hyperpermeability of the choriocapillaris, the presumptive primary alternation in CSC, are not amenable to laser photocoagulation therapy. Piccolino et al. studied 145 patients with CSC by ICGA and areas of choroidal leakage attributable to hyperpermeability of choriocapillaris were identified in 98.6% of the patients in association with active or resolved CSC.[118] Some areas of choroidal hyperpermeability and leakage did not show any significant change after a mean follow-up period of 10 months. These changes in the choroidal level persisted even after resolution of fluorescein leakage and subretinal fluid.[103] As a result, recurrence of the fluorescein leakage point may still occur over areas of choroidal hyperpermeability despite thermal laser treatment.

There has been a revival of interest in recent years in using laser, or micropulse diode laser, instead of the conventional argon laser photocoagulation, to treat CSC.[119–123] The diode laser with micropulsed emission enables subthreshold therapy without a visible burn endpoint. This may theoretically curtail the risk of structural and functional retinal damage while retaining the therapeutic efficacy of conventional laser treatment. A small case series has demonstrated the beneficial effect of using indocyanine green (ICG) dye-enhanced subthreshold diode-laser micropulse (SDM) photocoagulation.[123] Nevertheless, there are concerns over the efficacy and safety of micropulse diode laser in the face of more than one leaking point, which is more commonly encountered in chronic CSC. Randomized controlled trials involving comparison between micropulse diode laser and placebo or control groups are warranted in order to fully substantiate the observed treatment efficacy and safety of micropulse diode laser in the management of CSC.

Transpupillary thermotherapy

Several small case series have shown promising results of transpupillary thermotherapy (TTT) in treating chronic CSC cases and suggested that it may be a viable treatment alternative.[124–127] Future studies involving comparison of TTT with either standard treatment like PDT or placebo are warranted.

Intravitreal anti-VEGF therapy with or without adjuvant PDT

In the era of intravitreal pharmacology and therapeutics for macular diseases, it is not surprising that we should use intravitreal anti-VEGF to treat CSC. Several studies have demonstrated anatomic and functional improvement following either intravitreal bevacizumab or intravitreal ranibizumab injections.[110,128–133] These findings suggest that VEGF may be involved in fluid leakage in patients who have suffered from chronic CSC, despite the failure to detect changes in VEGF and interleukine-8 concentrations in aqueous humor and plasma from CSC patients after intravitreal anti-VEGF injections.[28] It has been suggested that combined PDT and intravitreal anti-VEGF has a beneficial role to play for CSC patients in a small case series but long-term efficacy and safety remain issues that warrant further studies.[134]

Anticorticosteroid treatment

Anticorticosteroid treatment was first suggested by Jampol et al.[135] This was based on the association of endogenous hypercortisolism with the development of CSC. The use of antiglucocorticoid agents including RU486 (mifepristone) and ketoconazole has not yet yielded significant results. The interest in using an anticorticosteroid to treat CSC has been revived since Packo and coworkers reported an interesting observation at the 2010 American Society of Retina Specialists Annual Meeting. They found that rifampin, a semisynthetic antituberculosis antibiotic with DNA-dependent RNA polymerase inhibitory effect, had caused resolution of macular edema and subretinal fluid in a CSC patient suspected initially to have tuberculosis. It is believed that the collateral anticorticosteroid or endogenous steroid production inhibition of rifampin may contribute to its inadvertent therapeutic efficacy in CSC. Since then, Packo et al. have used rifampin in several other patients with CSC and good results with resolution of the fluid were seen within 1–4 weeks.[136] Further research in using corticosteroid antagonists in treatment of CSC is warranted.

Management of special variants of CSC

Bullous CSC and its putative management

Bullous CSC is an uncommon form of CSC associated with a large amount of subretinal fluid and notably poor visual prognosis because of its frequent recurrence even after initial complete regression.[137] Traditional management options including observation or thermal laser photocoagulation, however, have dubious treatment benefits as the outcome of thermal laser photocoagulation is similar to the natural course of the disease in terms of disease duration and final visual acuity.[137] Ng et al. have reported the beneficial treatment effect of half-dose verteporfin PDT in the management of a case of bullous CSC with complete resolution of subretinal fluid and bullous retina detachment three months afterwards.[138]

Other potential but still exploratory systemic therapies

Systemic acetazolamide

The use of systemic acetazolamide to treat CSC came from sporadic cases and series reports claiming resolution of neurosensory retinal detachmentt after several weeks of systemic acetazolamide therapy.[139] Although acetazolamide might shorten the duration of symptoms it does not alter the final visual outcomes and the recurrence rate.[140] Prior to a good clinical trial involving systemic acetazolamide for CSC, its role remains elusive.

Antiadrenergic blockage and beta-blockers

Tatham et al. have reported two successful trials of using oral propanolol 40 mg twice a day in two CSC patients.[141] It is, however, unknown whether the resolution of neurosensory retinal detachment was due to the proposed therapeutic effect of a beta-blocker or a spontaneous recovery.

Aspirin, finasteride, anti-*Helicobacter pylori* treatment

The usefulness of low-dose aspirin (100 mg per day orally for 1 month, followed by 100 mg on alternate days for 5 months) to manage CSC was identified in a prospective study comprising 109 study subjects and 89 historic control subjects.[142] More rapid visual rehabilitation with fewer recurrences in the treated group was observed. The effectiveness of treatment with aspirin may be accounted for by its antiplatelet aggregation and profibinolytic effect against the postulated multifocal vascular occlusive disease of choriocapillaris in CSC (under the influence of plasminogen activator inhibitor-1, PAI-1).[142] A small pilot case series consisting of five chronic CSC patients who were put on finasteride, an inhibitor of dihydrotestosterone synthesis, has reported anatomical improvement and drug safety despite a lack of concomitant visual improvement.[143] Another prospective study involving 25 *H. pylori*-positive CSC patients treated with the standard *H. pylori* eradication regiment (metronidazole and amoxicillin 500 mg three times a day for 2 weeks and omeprazole once a day for 6 weeks) has demonstrated an expedition of subretinal fluid reabsorption, compared with the 25 controls.[144] No effect on final visual outcomes or recurrence rate was noted.[144] Similar to other new treatment modalities, the aforementioned new systemic treatments for CSC may require well-designed randomized controlled trials to document their long-term efficacy and safety.

CONCLUSION

Based on the current evidence in the literature, it seems that CSC is a multifactorial disease. It appears to result from a complex interaction of both known and unknown environmental and genetic factors. This ultimately leads to a bilateral disease with systemic associations. Because its generally favorable natural history provides no clear proof of the necessity and long-term efficacy of any of the treatment choices that have been mentioned earlier in this chapter, it can be concluded that treatments for CSC are still evolving. "Safety-enhanced" PDT using lower doses and reduced fluence, intravitreal anti-VEGF therapy, micropulsed diode laser treatment, and the use of corticosteroid antagonists do merit further investigation. Combination therapies involving two or more of the above modalities of treatments may have a role to play and thus warrant further research.

REFERENCES

1. Von Graefe A. Ueber central recidivierende retinitis. Graefes Arch Clin Exp Ophthalmol 1866;12:211–5.
2. Spaide RF, Goldbaum M, Wong DWK, et al. Serous detachment of the retina. Retina 2003;23:820–46.
3. Guyer DR, Yannuzzi LA, Slakter JS, et al. Digital indocyanine green videoangiography of central serous chorioretinopathy. Arch Ophthalmol 1994;112: 1057–62.
4. Gass JD. Stereoscopic atlas of macular diseases. St Louis: CV Mosby; 1987. p. 56–7.
5. Pryds A, Sander B, Larsen M. Characterization of subretinal fluid leakage in central serous chorioretinopathy. Invest Ophthalmol Vis Sci 2010;51:5853–7.
6. Horniker. Su di unaforma di retinite centrale di origine vasoneurotica. Ann Ottalmol 1927;55:578–600, 830–40, 665–63.
7. Yannuzzi LA. Type-A behavior and central serous chorioretinopathy. Retina 1987;7:111–31.
8. Zakir SM, Shukla M, Simi ZU, et al. Serum cortisol and testosterone levels in idiopathic central serous chorioretinopathy. Indian J Ophthalmol 2009;57: 419–22.
9. Friberg TR, Eller AW. Serous retinal detachment resembling central serous chorioretinopathy following organ transplantation. Graefes Arch Clin Exp Ophthalmol 1990;228:305–9.
10. Gass JD, Little H. Bilateral bullous exudative retinal detachment complicating idiopathic central serous chorioretinopathy during systemic corticosteroid therapy. Ophthalmology 1995;102:737–47.
11. Lee CS, Kang EC, Lee KS, et al. Central serous chorioretinopathy after renal transplantation. Retina 2011;31:1896–903.
12. Hurvitz AP, Hodapp KL, Jadgchew J, et al. Central serous chorioretinopathy resulting in altered vision and color perception after glenohumeral corticosteroid injection. Orthopedics 2009;32:600.
13. Haimovici R, Gragoudas ES, Duker JS, et al. Central serous chorioretinopathy associated with inhaled or intranasal corticosteroids. Ophthalmology 1997; 104:1653–60.
14. Fernandez C, Mendoza AJ, Arevalo JF. Central serous chorioretinopathy associated with topical dermal corticosteroids. Retina 2004;24:471–4.
15. Garg SP, Dada T, Talwar D, et al. Endogenous cortisol profile in patients with central serous chorioretinopathy. Br J Ophthalmol 1997;81:962–4.
16. Haimovici R, Koh S, Gagnon DR, et al. Risk factors for central serous chorioretinopathy: a case–control study. Ophthalmology 2004;111:244–9.
17. Gass JD. Central serous chorioretinopathy and white subretinal exudation during pregnancy. Arch Ophthalmol 1991;109:677–81.
18. Fastenberg DM, Ober RR. Central serous choroidopathy in pregnancy. Arch Ophthalmol 1983;101:1055–8.
19. Quillen DA, Gass DM, Brod RD, et al. Central serous chorioretinopathy in women. Ophthalmology 1996;103:72–9.
20. Iannetti L, Spinucci G, Pesci FR, et al. Central serous chorioretinopathy as a presenting symptom of endogenous Cushing syndrome: a case report. Eur J Ophthalmol 2011;21:661–4.
21. Chrousos GP, Gold PW. The concepts of stress and stress system disorders. Overview of physical and behavioral homeostasis. JAMA 1992;267:1244–52.
22. Smith TJ. Dexamethasone regulation of glycosaminoglycan synthesis in cultured human skin fibroblasts. Similar effects of glucocorticoid and thyroid hormones. J Clin Invest 1984;74:2157–63.
23. Pratt WB, Aronow L. The effect of glucocorticoids on protein and nucleic acid synthesis in mouse fibroblasts growing in vitro. J Biol Chem 1966;241: 5244–50.
24. Bastl CP. Regulation of cation transport by low doses of glucocorticoids in in vivo adrenalectomized rat colon. J Clin Invest 1987;80:348–56.
25. Sandle GI, McGlone F. Acute effects of dexamethasone on cation transport in colonic epithelium. Gut 1987;28:701–6.
26. Caccavale A, Romanazzi F, Imparato M, et al. Central serous chorioretinopathy: a pathogenetic model. Clin Ophthalmol 2011;5:239–43.
27. Shin MC, Lim JW. Concentration of cytokines in the aqueous humor of patients with central serous chorioretinopathy. Retina 2011;31:1937–43.

28. Lim JW, Kim MU, Shin MC. Aqueous humor and plasma levels of vascular endothelial growth factor and interleukin-8 in patients with central serous chorioretinopathy. Retina 2010;30:1465–71.
29. Rahbani-Nobar MB, Javadzadeh A, Ghojazadeh L, et al. The effect of *Helicobacter pylori* treatment on remission of idiopathic central serous chorioretinopathy. Mol Vis 2011;17:99–103.
30. Cotticelli L, Borrelli M, D'Alessio AC, et al. Central serous chorioretinopathy and *Helicobacter pylori*. Eur J Ophthalmol 2006;16:274–8.
31. Misiuk-Hojlo M, Michalowska M, Turno-Krecicka A. *Helicobacter pylori* –a risk factor for the developement of the central serous chorioretinopathy. Klin Oczna 2009;111:30–2.
32. Tittl MK, Spaide RF, Wong D, et al. Systemic findings associated with central serous chorioretinopathy. Am J Ophthalmol 1999;128:63–8.
33. Jain AK, Kaines A, Schwartz S. Bilateral central serous chorioretinopathy resolving rapidly with treatment for obstructive sleep apnea. Graefes Arch Clin Exp Ophthalmol 2010;248:1037–9.
34. Imamura Y, Fujiwara T, Spaide RF. Frequency of glaucoma in central serous chorioretinopathy: a case-control study. Retina 2010;30:267–70.
35. Moschos MM, Droutsas K, Margetis I. Central serous chorioretinopathy after rhinoplasty. Case Report Ophthalmol 2010;1:90–3.
36. Peponis VG, Chalkiadakis SE, Nikas SD, et al. Bilateral central serous retinopathy following laser in situ keratomileusis for myopia. J Cataract Refract Surg 2011;37:778–80.
37. Ross A, Ross AH, Mohamed Q. Review and update of central serous chorioretinopathy. Curr Opin Ophthalmol 2011;22(3):166–73.
38. Leibowitz HM, Krueger DE, Maunder LR, et al. The Framingham Eye Study monograph: An ophthalmological and epidemiological study of cataract, glaucoma, diabetic retinopathy, macular degeneration, and visual acuity in a general population of 2631 adults, 1973–1975. Surv Ophthalmol 1980;24 (Suppl):335–610.
39. Spaide RF, Campeas L, Haas A, et al. Central serous chorioretinopathy in younger and older adults. Ophthalmology 1996;103:2070–9; discussion 9–80.
40. Fukunaga K. [Central chorioretinopathy with disharmony of the autonomous nerve system.] Nippon Ganka Gakkai Zasshi 1969;73:1468–77.
41. Desai UR, Alhalel AA, Campen TJ, et al. Central serous chorioretinopathy in African Americans. J Natl Med Assoc 2003;95:553–9.
42. Maruko I, Iida T, Ojima A, et al. Subretinal dot-like precipitates and yellow material in central serous chorioretinopathy. Retina 2011;31:759–65.
43. Ie D, Yannuzzi LA, Spaide RF, et al. Subretinal exudative deposits in central serous chorioretinopathy. Br J Ophthalmol 1993;77:349–53.
44. Gass JD. Stereoscopic atlas of macular diseases: diagnosis and treatment. 4th ed. St Louis: Mosby; 1997. p. 52–70.
45. Yannuzzi LA, Shakin JL, Fisher YL, et al. Peripheral retinal detachments and retinal pigment epithelial atrophic tracts secondary to central serous pigment epitheliopathy. Ophthalmology 1984;91:1554–72.
46. Cohen D, Gaudric A, Coscas G, et al. [Diffuse retinal epitheliopathy and central serous chorioretinopathy.] J Fr Ophtalmol 1983;6:339–49.
47. Gass JD. Bullous retinal detachment. An unusual manifestation of idiopathic central serous choroidopathy. Am J Ophthalmol 1973;75:810–21.
48. Nadel AJ, Turan MI, Coles RS. Central serous retinopathy. A generalized disease of the pigment epithelium. Mod Probl Ophthalmol 1979;20:76–88.
49. Schatz H, Osterloh MD, McDonald HR, et al. Development of retinal vascular leakage and cystoid macular oedema secondary to central serous chorioretinopathy. Br J Ophthalmol 1993;77:744–6.
50. Bujarborua D, Nagpal PN, Deka M. Smokestack leak in central serous chorioretinopathy. Graefes Arch Clin Exp Ophthalmol 2010;248:339–51.
51. Prunte C, Flammer J. Choroidal capillary and venous congestion in central serous chorioretinopathy. Am J Ophthalmol 1996;121:26–34.
52. Spaide RF, Hall L, Haas A, et al. Indocyanine green videoangiography of older patients with central serous chorioretinopathy. Retina. 1996;16:203–13.
53. Iida T, Kishi S, Hagimura N, et al. Persistent and bilateral choroidal vascular abnormalities in central serous chorioretinopathy. Retina 1999;19:508–12.
54. Iida T, Spaide RF, Haas A, et al. Leopard-spot pattern of yellowish subretinal deposits in central serous chorioretinopathy. Arch Ophthalmol 2002;120: 37–42.
55. Tsujikawa A, Ojima Y, Yamashiro K, et al. Punctate hyperfluorescent spots associated with central serous chorioretinopathy as seen on indocyanine green angiography. Retina 2010;30:801–9.
56. Huang D, Swanson EA, Lin CP, et al. Optical coherence tomography. Science 1991;254:1178–81.
57. Hee MR, Puliafito CA, Wong C, et al. Optical coherence tomography of central serous chorioretinopathy. Am J Ophthalmol 1995;120:65–74.
58. Gupta P, Gupta V, Dogra MR, et al. Morphological changes in the retinal pigment epithelium on spectral-domain OCT in the unaffected eyes with idiopathic central serous chorioretinopathy. Int Ophthalmol 2010;30:175–81.
59. Maruko I, Iida T, Sugano Y, et al. Subfoveal choroidal thickness in fellow eyes of patients with central serous chorioretinopathy. Retina 2011;31(8):1603–8.
60. Imamura Y, Fujiwara T, Margolis R, et al. Enhanced depth imaging optical coherence tomography of the choroid in central serous chorioretinopathy. Retina 2009;29:1469–73.
61. Kim YY, Flaxel CJ. Factors influencing the visual acuity of chronic central serous chorioretinopathy. Korean J Ophthalmol 2011;25:90–7.
62. Ooto S, Tsujikawa A, Mori S, et al. Thickness of photoreceptor layers in polypoidal choroidal vasculopathy and central serous chorioretinopathy. Graefes Arch Clin Exp Ophthalmol 2010;248:1077–86.
63. Dinc UA, Tatlipinar S, Yenerel M, et al. Fundus autofluorescence in acute and chronic central serous chorioretinopathy. Clin Exp Optom 2011;94:452–7.
64. Framme C, Walter A, Gabler B, et al. Fundus autofluorescence in acute and chronic-recurrent central serous chorioretinopathy. Acta Ophthalmol Scand 2005;83:161–7.
65. Imamura Y, Fujiwara T, Spaide RF. Fundus autofluorescence and visual acuity in central serous chorioretinopathy. Ophthalmology 2011;118:700–5.
66. Ojima A, Iida T, Sekiryu T, et al. Photopigments in central serous chorioretinopathy. Am J Ophthalmol 2011;151:940–52,e1.
67. Lai TY, Lai RY, Ngai JW, et al. First- and second-order kernel multifocal electroretinography abnormalities in acute central serous chorioretinopathy. Doc Ophthalmol 2008;116:29–40.
68. Shimada Y, Imai D, Ota Y, et al. Retinal adaptability loss in serous retinal detachment with central serous chorioretinopathy. Invest Ophthalmol Vis Sci 2010;51:3210–5.
69. Yip YWY, Ngai JWS, Fok ACT, et al. Correlation between functional and anatomical assessments by multifocal electroretinography and optical coherence tomography in central serous chorioretinopathy. Doc Ophthalmol 2010;120:193–200.
70. Reibaldi M, Boscia F, Avitabile T, et al. Functional retinal changes measured by microperimetry in standard-fluence vs low-fluence photodynamic therapy in chronic central serous chorioretinopathy. Am J Ophthalmol 2011;151: 953–60.
71. Senturk F, Karacorlu M, Ozdemir H, et al. Microperimetric changes after photodynamic therapy for central serous chorioretinopathy. Am J Ophthalmol 2011;151:303–9.
72. Fujita K, Yuzawa M, Mori R. Retinal sensitivity after photodynamic therapy with half-dose verteporfin for chronic central serous: short-term results. Retina 2011;31:772–8.
73. Ojima Y, Tsujikawa A, Hangai M, et al. Retinal sensitivity measured with the micro perimeter 1 after resolution of central serous chorioretinopathy. Am J Ophthalmol 2008;146:77–84.
74. Kim S-W, Oh J, Huh K. Correlations among various functional and morphological tests in resolved central serous chorioretinopathy. Br J Ophthalmol Epub ahead of print May 26, 2011. PMID 21617156.
75. Dinc UA, Yenerel M, Tatlipinar S, et al. Correlation of retinal sensitivity and retinal thickness in central serous chorioretinopathy. Ophthalmologica 2010;224:2–9.
76. Aggio FB, Roisman L, Melo GB, et al. Clinical factors related to visual outcome in central serous chorioretinopathy. Retina 2010;30:1128–34.
77. Gass JD. Pathogenesis of disciform detachment of the neuroepithelium. Am J Ophthalmol 1967;63(Suppl):1–139.
78. Ficker L, Vafidis G, While A, et al. Long-term follow-up of a prospective trial of argon laser photocoagulation in the treatment of central serous retinopathy. Br J Ophthalmol 1988;72:829–34.
79. Yap EY, Robertson DM. The long-term outcome of central serous chorioretinopathy. Arch Ophthalmol 1996;114:689–92.
80. Fok AC, Chan PP, Lam DS, et al. Risk factors for recurrence of serous macular detachment in untreated patients with central serous chorioretinopathy. Ophthalmic Res 2011;46:160–3.
81. Ooto S, Hangai M, Sakamoto A, et al. High-resolution imaging of resolved central serous chorioretinopathy using adaptive optics scanning laser ophthalmoscopy. Ophthalmology 2010;117:1800–9, 1809.e1–2.
82. Spaide RF, Yannuzzi LA, Slakter JS, et al. Indocyanine green videoangiography of idiopathic polypoidal choroidal vasculopathy. Retina 1995;15:100–10.
83. Sharma T, Shah N, Rao M, et al. Visual outcome after discontinuation of corticosteroids in atypical severe central serous chorioretinopathy. Ophthalmology 2004;111:1708–14.
84. Gemenetzi M, De Salvo G, Lotery AJ. Central serous chorioretinopathy: update on pathogenesis and treatments. Eye 2010;24:1743–56.
85. Yannuzzi LA. Central serous chorioretinopathy: a personal perspective. Am J Ophthalmol 2010;149:361–3.
86. Wang MS, Sander B, Larsen M. Retinal atrophy in idiopathic central serous chorioretinopathy. Am J Ophthalmol 2002;133:787–93.
87. Chan WM, Lai TY, Lai RY, et al. Half-dose verteporfin photodynamic therapy for acute central serous chorioretinopathy: one-year results of a randomized controlled trial. Ophthalmology 2008;115:1756–65.
88. Lim JW, Ryu SJ, Shin MC. The effect of intravitreal bevacizumab in patients with acute central serous chorioretinopathy. Korean J Ophthalmol 2010;24: 155–8.
89. Yannuzzi LA, Slakter JS, Kaufman SR, et al. Laser treatment of diffuse retinal pigment epitheliopathy. Eur J Ophthalmol 1992;2:103–14.
90. Chan WM, Lai TY, Tano Y, et al. Photodynamic therapy in macular diseases of Asian populations: when East meets West. Jpn J Ophthalmol 2006;50: 161–9.
91. Chan WM, Lim TH, Pece A, et al. Verteporfin PDT for non-standard indications – a review of current literature. Graefes Arch Clin Exp Ophthalmol 2010;248:613–26.
92. Battaglia Parodi M, Da Pozzo S, Ravalico G. Photodynamic therapy in chronic central serous chorioretinopathy. Retina 2003;23:235–7.
93. Canakis C, Livir-Rallatos C, Panayiotis Z, et al. Ocular photodynamic therapy for serous macular detachment in the diffuse retinal pigment epitheliopathy variant of idiopathic central serous chorioretinopathy. Am J Ophthalmol 2003;136:750–2.
94. Cardillo Piccolino F, Eandi CM, Ventre L, et al. Photodynamic therapy for chronic central serous chorioretinopathy. Retina 2003;23:752–63.
95. Yannuzzi LA, Slakter JS, Gross NE, et al. Indocyanine green angiography-guided photodynamic therapy for treatment of chronic central serous chorioretinopathy: a pilot study. Retina 2003;23:288–98.

96. Chan WM, Lam DS, Lai TY, et al. Choroidal vascular remodelling in central serous chorioretinopathy after indocyanine green guided photodynamic therapy with verteporfin: a novel treatment at the primary disease level. Br J Ophthalmol 2003;87:1453–8.
97. Taban M, Boyer DS, Thomas EL, et al. Chronic central serous chorioretinopathy: photodynamic therapy. Am J Ophthalmol 2004;137:1073–80.
98. Schlotzer-Schrehardt U, Viestenz A, Naumann GO, et al. Dose-related structural effects of photodynamic therapy on choroidal and retinal structures of human eyes. Graefes Arch Clin Exp Ophthalmol 2002;240:748–57.
99. Schmidt-Erfurth U, Laqua H, Schlotzer-Schrehard U, et al. Histopathological changes following photodynamic therapy in human eyes. Arch Ophthalmol 2002;120:835–44.
100. Lai TY, Chan WM, Lam DS. Transient reduction in retinal function revealed by multifocal electroretinogram following photodynamic therapy. Am J Ophthalmol 2004;137:826–33.
101. Tzekov R, Lin T, Zhang KM, et al. Ocular changes after photodynamic therapy. Invest Ophthalmol Vis Sci 2006;47:377–85.
102. Haimovici R, Kramer M, Miller JW, et al. Localization of lipoprotein-delivered benzoporphyrin derivative in the rabbit eye. Curr Eye Res 1997;16:83–90.
103. Maruko I, Iida T, Sugano Y, et al. Subfoveal choroidal thickness after treatment of central serous chorioretinopathy. Ophthalmology 2010;117:1792–9.
104. Lai TY, Chan WM, Li H, et al. Safety enhanced photodynamic therapy with half dose verteporfin for chronic central serous chorioretinopathy: a short term pilot study. Br J Ophthalmol 2006;90:869–74.
105. Chan WM, Lai TY, Lai RY, et al. Safety enhanced photodynamic therapy for chronic central serous chorioretinopathy: one-year results of a prospective study. Retina 2008;28:85–93.
106. Wu ZH, Lai RY, Yip YW, et al. Improvement in multifocal electroretinography after half-dose verteporfin photodynamic therapy for central serous chorioretinopathy: a randomized placebo-controlled trial. Retina Epub ahead of print March 3, 2011; PMID 21386761.
107 Reibaldi M, Cardascia N, Longo A, et al. Standard-fluence versus low-fluence photodynamic therapy in chronic central serous chorioretinopathy: a nonrandomized clinical trial. Am J Ophthalmol 2010;149:307–15.
108. Reibaldi M, Boscia F, Avitabile T, et al. Functional retinal changes measured by microperimetry in standard-fluence vs low-fluence photodynamic therapy in chronic central serous chorioretinopathy. Am J Ophthalmol 2011;151: 953–60.
109. Shin JY, Woo SJ, Yu HG, et al. Comparison of efficacy and safety between half-fluence and full-fluence photodynamic therapy for chronic central serous chorioretinopathy. Retina 2011;31:119–26.
110. Bae SH, Heo JW, Kim C, et al. Randomized pilot study of low-fluence photodynamic therapy versus intravitreal ranibizumab for chronic central serous chorioretinopathy. Am J Ophthalmol 2011;152:784–92.
111. Kim SW, Oh J, Oh IK, et al. Retinal pigment epithelial tear after half fluence PDT for serous pigment epithelial detachment in central serous chorioretinopathy. Ophthalmic Surg Lasers Imaging 2009;40:300–3.
112. Ascaso FJ, Rojo M, Minguez E, et al. Diagnostic and therapeutic challenges. Retina 2011;31:616–22.
113. Burumcek E, Mudun A, Karacorlu S, et al. Laser photocoagulation for persistent central serous chorioretinopathy: results of long term follow-up. Ophthalmology 1997;104:616–22.
114. Robertson DM, Ilstrup D. Direct, indirect, and sham laser photocoagulation in the management of central serous chorioretinopathy. Am J Ophthalmol. 1983;95:457–66.
115. Gartner J. Long-term follow-up of an ophthalmologist's central serous retinopathy,photocoagulated by sungazing. Doc Ophthalmol 1987;66:19–33.
116. Lim JI. Iatrogenic choroidal neovascularization. Surv Ophthalmol 1999;44: 95–111.
117. Lim JW, Kang SW, Kim YT, et al. Comparative study of patients with central serous chorioretinopathy undergoing focal laser photocoagulation or photodynamic therapy. Br J Ophthalmol 2011;95:514–7.
118. Piccolino FC, Borgia L, Zinicola E, et al. Indocyanine green angiographic findings in central serous chorioretinopathy. Eye 1995;9:324–32.
119. Sivaprasad S, Elagonz M, McHugh D, et al. Micropulsed diode laser therapy: evolution and clinical applications. Surv Ophthalmol 2010;55:516–30.
120. Gupta B, Elagouz M, McHugh D, et al. Micropulse diode laser photocoagulation for central serous chorioretinopathy. Clin Exp Ophthalmol 2009;37: 801–5.
121. Chen SN, Hwang JF, Tseng LF, et al. Subthreshold diode micropulse photocoagulation for the treatment of chronic central serous chorioretinopathy with juxtafoveal leakage. Ophthalmology 2008;115:2229–34.
122. Lanzetta P, Furlan F, Morgante L, et al. Nonvisible subthreshold micropulse diode laser (810 nm) treatment of central serous chorioretinopathy. A pilot study. Eur J Ophthalmol 2008;18:934–40.
123. Ricci F, Missiroli F, Regine F, et al. Indocycnine green enhanced subthreshold diode-laser micropulse photocoagulation treatment of chronic central serous chorioretinopathy. Graefes Arch Clin Exp Ophthalmol 2009;247:597–607.
124. Hussain N, Khanna R, Hussain A, et al. Transpupillary thermotherapy for chronic central serous chorioretinopathy. Graefes Arch Clin Exp Ophthalmol 2006;244:1045–51.
125. Shukla D, Kolluru C, Vignesh TP, et al. Transpupillary thermotherapy for subfoveal leaks in central serous chorioretinopathy. Eye 2008;22:100–6.
126. Sharma T, Parikh SD. Transpupillary thermotherapy for juxtafoveal leak in central serous chorioretinopathy. Ophthalmic Surg Lasers Imaging 2010;9: 1–3.
127. Giudice GL, de Belvis V, Tavolato M, et al. Large-spot subthreshold transpupillary thermotherapy for chronic serous macular detachment. Clin Ophthalmol 2011;5:355–60.
128. Schaal KB, Hoeh AE, Scheuerle A, et al. Intravitreal bevacizumab for treatment of chronic central serous chorioretinopathy. Eur J Ophthalmol 2009;19: 613–7.
129 Lim SJ, Roh MI, Kwon OW. Intravitreal bevacizumab injection for central serous chorioretinopathy. Retina 2010;30:100–6.
130. Artunay O, Yuzbasioglu E, Rasier R, et al. Intravitreal bevacizumab in treatment of idiopathic persistent central serous chorioretinopathy: a prospective, controlled clinical study. Curr Eye Res 2010;35:91–8.
131. Inoue M, Kadonosono K, Watanabe Y, et al. Results of one-year follow-up examinations after intravitreal bevacizumab administration for chronic central serous chorioretinopathy. Ophthalmologica 2011;225:37–40.
132. Lim JW, Kim MU. The efficacy of intravitreal bevacizumab for idiopathic central serous chorioretinopathy. Graefes Arch Clin Exp Ophthalmol 2011;249:969–74.
133. Symeonidis C, Kaprinis K, Manthos K, et al. Central serous chorioretinopathy with subretinal deposition of fibrin-like material and its prompt response to ranibizumab injections. Case Report Ophthalmol 2011;2:59–64.
134. Arevalo JF, Espinoza JV. Single-session combined photodynamic therapy with verteporfin and intravitreal anti-vascular endothelial growth factor therapy for chronic central serous chorioretinopathy: a pilot study at 12-month follow-up. Graefes Arch Clin Exp Ophthalmol 2011;249:1159–66.
135. Jampol LM, Weinreb R, Yannuzzi L. Involvement of corticosteroids and catecholamines in the pathogenesis of central serous chorioretinopathy: a rationale for new treatment strategies. Ophthalmology 2002;109:1765–6.
136. Khorram D [Internet]. The Retina Blog: Rifampin for central serous chorioretinopathy [August 2010; cited 2011, July 29]. Available from: http://theretinablog.com/2010/08/30/rifampin-for-central-serous-chorioretinopathy.
137. Otsuka S, Ohba N, Nakao K. A long-term follow up study of severe variant of central serous chorioretinopathy. Retina 2002;22:25–32.
138. Ng WW, Wu ZH, Lai TY. Half-dose verteporfin photodynamic therapy for bullous variant of central serous chorioretinopathy: a case report. J Med Case Reports 2011;5:208.
139. Gonzalez C. [Serous retinal detachment. Value of acetazolamide.] J Fr Ophtalmol 1992;15:529–36.
140. Pikkel J, Beiran I, Ophir A, et al. Acetazolamide for central serous retinopathy. Ophthalmology 2002;109:1723–5.
141. Tatham A, Macfarlane A. The use of propranolol to treat central serous chorioretinopathy: an evaluation by serial OCT. J Ocul Pharmacol Ther 2006;22: 145–9.
142. Caccavale A, Romanazzi F, Imparato M, et al. Low-dose aspirin as treatment for central serous chorioretinopathy. Clin Ophthalmol 2010;4:899–903.
143. Forooghian F, Meleth AD, Cukras C, et al. Finasteride for chronic central serous chorioretinopathy. Retina 2011;31:766–71.
144. Rahbani-Nobar MB, Javadzadeh A, Ghojazadeh L, et al. The effect of *Helicobacter pylori* treatment on remission of idiopathic central serous chorioretinopathy. Mol Vis 2011;17:99–103.

Chapter 73

Uveal Effusion Syndrome and Hypotony Maculopathy

Cagri G. Besirli, Mark W. Johnson

The clinical observation of abnormal serous fluid accumulation in the outer layer of the ciliary body and choroid is called uveal effusion. This exudative detachment of the choroid and the ciliary body is also known as ciliochoroidal effusion, ciliochoroidal detachment, choroidal effusion, or choroidal detachment. These names are used interchangeably in this chapter. Uveal effusion does not refer to a specific entity, but this name is used as the common term to describe a pathoanatomic condition caused by several ocular and systemic disorders. Uveal effusion is frequently associated with nonrhegmatogenous retinal detachment, secondary to the chronic accumulation of protein-rich fluid in the choroid and the breakdown of the retinal pigment epithelial fluid barrier. The term "idiopathic uveal effusion syndrome" or "uveal effusion syndrome" in short refers to the presence of ciliochoroidal effusion in an eye with no other known associated ocular or systemic disorder. Uveal effusion syndrome typically occurs spontaneously in an otherwise healthy middle-aged man.

Hypotony maculopathy refers to the structural changes in the macular region and related visual dysfunction that may develop in an eye with low intraocular pressure. In addition to the changes in the macular region, hypotony may be associated with other posterior-segment abnormalities, including optic nerve swelling, vascular tortuosity, and chorioretinal folds. The vision loss may be profound in the setting of persistent ocular hypotony, but visual improvement is typical after intraocular pressure is restored.

UVEAL EFFUSION SYNDROME

Introduction

Spontaneous exudative detachment of the choroid and ciliary body was first reported by Schepens and Brockhurst in 1963[1]; these authors used the term "uveal effusion" in their description of this disorder. Almost two decades later, Gass and Jallow in 1982 coined the term "idiopathic uveal effusion syndrome" to describe idiopathic serous detachment of the choroid, ciliary body, and retina.[2] Uveal effusion syndrome is a rare ocular disorder that typically manifests itself in an otherwise healthy middle-aged male. In their original report, Schepens and Brockhurst described 17 patients, only one of whom was female. The diagnosis of uveal effusion syndrome is based on characteristic clinical findings and exclusion of other known causes of uveal effusion. Bilateral involvement is common and unilateral cases tend to occur in older males. In addition to the accumulation of serous fluid in the ciliary body and choroid, nonrhegmatogenous retinal detachment with marked shifting of the subretinal fluid are commonly observed in patients with uveal effusion syndrome. Retinal detachment often begins inferiorly, as in other causes of exudative retinal detachment. Other ocular findings include dilation of the episcleral blood vessels, blood in Schlemm's canal, normal intraocular pressure, mild vitreous cells, leopard-spot retinal pigment epithelial alterations, elevation of the subretinal fluid protein levels, and elevation of the cerebrospinal fluid protein. Without treatment, a protracted clinical course with remissions and exacerbations over many months to years may cause significant visual decline and morbidity. Unlike other causes of ciliochoridal effusion, patients with idiopathic uveal effusion syndrome respond poorly to nonsurgical treatment, including corticosteroids or antimetabolites. Similarly, surgical treatment of nonrhegmatogenous retinal detachment in uveal effusion syndrome using conventional techniques, including scleral buckling or pars plana vitrectomy, fails to reattach the neurosensory retina secondary to persistent serous exudation. In most cases, successful reattachment of the nonrhegmatogenous retinal detachment requires a scleral-thinning procedure, including quadrantic partial-thickness sclerectomies and sclerostomies.

Pathophysiology of ciliochoroidal effusions

General mechanisms

Since idiopathic uveal effusion syndrome represents only a small percentage of ciliochoroidal effusions, it is important to discuss the general mechanisms of serous accumulation in the ciliary body and choroid. Most cases of ciliochoroidal effusion can be classified into one of the following pathophysiologic categories: (1) hydrodynamic; (2) inflammatory; (3) neoplastic; or (4) associated with abnormal sclera.[3] Under physiologic conditions, a normal eye has equilibrium between the transmural hydrostatic pressure gradient, defined as the difference between the intravascular blood pressure and intraocular pressure, and the colloid osmotic pressure gradient of the choriocapillaris (Fig. 73.1). Albumin is the most abundant protein in the choroidal capillaries and is the primary driver of the colloid osmotic pressure. This pressure gradient draws fluid into blood vessels and maintains relative dehydration of the suprachoroidal space due to a low extravascular colloid concentration.[4] Fenestrated capillaries of the choroid allow albumin to escape into the extravascular space. To maintain the colloid osmotic gradient, albumin leaves the choroid across the sclera and this transscleral protein flow is facilitated by intraocular pressure.[5–7]

The fluid equilibrium across the layers of the choroid may be disturbed by several factors affecting one or more components of this intricate system.[3] Ocular hypotony decreases the driving

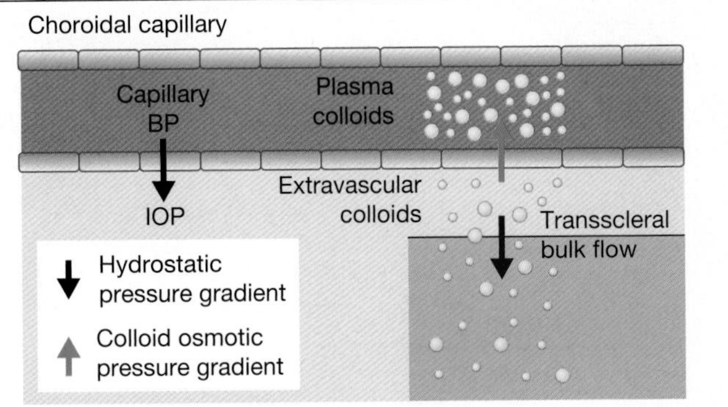

Fig. 73.1 In normal choroidal capillaries, the transmural hydrostatic pressure gradient is in equilibrium with the colloid osmotic pressure gradient. Colloids escaping the fenestrated capillaries move across the sclera by bulk flow, driven by intraocular pressure (IOP). BP, blood pressure. (Courtesy of Biomedical Communications, University of Michigan.)

force for transscleral protein flow and increases the transmural hydrostatic pressure gradient. These changes then facilitate the accumulation of protein and fluid in the suprachoroidal space. Elevated uveal venous pressure increases the transmural hydrostatic pressure gradient and leads to increased fluid movement into the extravascular space. Vascular competence may be compromised by inflammation, which then increases capillary protein permeability and accumulation of protein in the extravascular space. This reduces the colloid osmotic pressure gradient and the absorption of extravascular fluid into the capillaries. Abnormal scleral composition or thickness may increase resistance to transscleral protein outflow and accumulation of protein-rich fluid in the suprachoroidal space. These alterations are more likely to affect the choroidal fluid dynamics when two or more are present simultaneously. Indeed, the creation of ciliochoroidal effusion in animal models requires experimental alteration of two or more pathophysiologic factors.[8,9]

Idiopathic and nanophthalmic uveal effusion

In patients with uveal effusion syndrome or the closely related condition of nanophthalmos, abnormal sclera, referred to here as scleropathy, is the most likely primary ocular anomaly affecting choroidal fluid dynamics. In nanophthalmos, scleropathy is congenital in origin and associated with other ocular abnormalities. Acquired scleropathy may be secondary to a systemic disorder, such as the accumulation of amyloid in systemic amyloidosis or mucopolysaccharide in Hunter syndrome.[10,11] In uveal effusion syndrome, scleropathy appears to be secondary to the abnormal accumulation of glycosaminoglycan-like deposits and thickening of the sclera in the absence of any known systemic disorder.[12–14] Ward et al. reported that electron microscopy of excised sclera showed increased glycosaminoglycan-like deposits between the scleral fibers.[14] In a following report, Forrester and colleagues performed histochemical studies on scleras excised from patients with uveal effusion syndrome and showed deposition of the glycosaminoglycan proteodermatan sulfate and a smaller amount of proteochondroitin sulfate, indicating a primary defect in scleral proteodermatan metabolism and representing a form of ocular mucopolysaccharidosis.[12] Histologic similarities between scleras isolated from eyes with uveal effusion syndrome and nanophthalmos were demonstrated by Uyama et al., who found disorganized scleral fibers and proteoglycan deposits in 6 nanophthalmic eyes and 11 non-nanophthalmic eyes with uveal effusion syndrome.[13] As discussed above, abnormal scleral composition increases resistance to transscleral protein outflow, which in turn leads to the accumulation of protein in the extravascular space of the choroid and higher colloid osmotic pressure. This results in reduced movement of fluid from the suprachoroidal space into the choroidal capillaries and leads to serous ciliochoroidal effusion. In vitro experimental evidence is consistent with this model, as chondroitinase ABC digestion, which removes glycosaminoglycans, improves scleral transport in human cadaver eyes.[15]

Ciliochoroidal effusion and nonrhegmatogenous retinal detachment can be successfully treated in patients with uveal effusion syndrome by quadrantic partial-thickness sclerectomies.[16,17] The disappearance of serous fluid after partial-thickness sclerectomies is consistent with the hypothesis that abnormally thickened sclera prevents outflow of protein and suggests that the removal of excess extravascular protein may be improved by reducing scleral thickness and resistance. Under normal conditions, eyes with congenital or acquired scleropathies may have enough redundancy in choroidal protein transport mechanisms to achieve physiologic fluid equilibrium and dehydration of the suprachoroid. However, when choroidal fluid dynamics are further stressed by additional pathologic factors, such as compression of the vortex veins, these compensatory mechanisms may no longer be sufficient to overcome the effect of increased colloids in the suprachoroidal space, which may then lead to increased extravascular fluid retention and ciliochoroidal detachment.

Vortex vein compression was first suggested by Schaffer in 1975 as a possible mechanism of uveal effusion in nanophthalmic eyes following glaucoma filtration surgery.[18] Relative obstruction of venous outflow secondary to compressed vortex veins may cause congestion of the choriocapillaris and alter the transmural hydrostatic pressure gradient, favoring increased retention of fluid in the suprachoroidal space. Brockhurst reported successful reattachment of the retina and resolution of ciliochoroidal effusion in nanophthalmic eyes after surgical decompression of the vortex veins.[19] Additional evidence for the role of increased intravascular pressure secondary to reduced ocular venous drainage in uveal effusion was provided by Casswell and colleagues, who reported resolution of retinal detachment after vortex vein decompression in patients with uveal effusion syndrome.[20] As proposed by Gass, compression of the vortex veins by an abnormally thickened sclera may contribute to increased fluid retention and serous exudation in the choroid and ciliary body in uveal effusion syndrome.[16]

Clinical features

Ciliochoroidal detachments in uveal effusion syndrome are brown-orange, solid-appearing elevations with smooth, convex surfaces (Fig. 73.2). Transillumination of the globe confirms the serous nature of the exudation. Choroidal detachments do not undulate appreciably with ocular movements, and this helps to distinguish them from rhegmatogenous retinal detachments. In early or mild cases, the diagnosis is suggested when the ora serrata is visible without the use of scleral depression secondary to shallow elevation of the pars plana and peripheral choroid (Fig. 73.3). As the effusion progresses, annular or lobular choroidal detachment may be seen. The characteristic four-lobed configuration results from the attachment of the

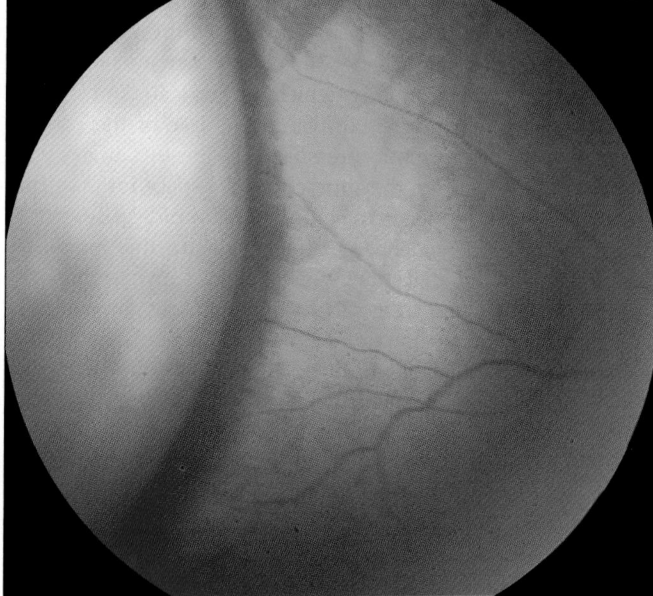
Fig. 73.2 Ciliochoroidal effusion demonstrating the characteristic solid-appearing choroidal elevation with a smooth, convex surface.

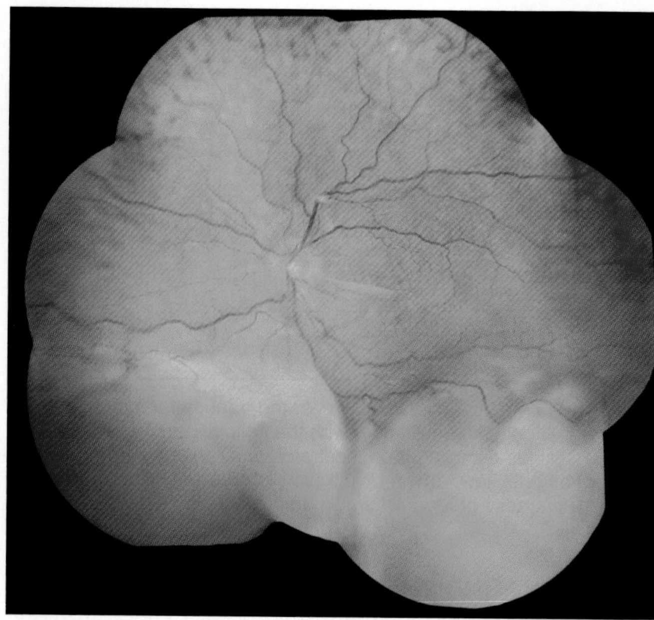
Fig. 73.4 Nonrhegmatogenous retinal detachment in a patient with uveal effusion. Location of the subretinal fluid is dependent on gravity. Leopard-spot retinal pigmentation is apparent superiorly.

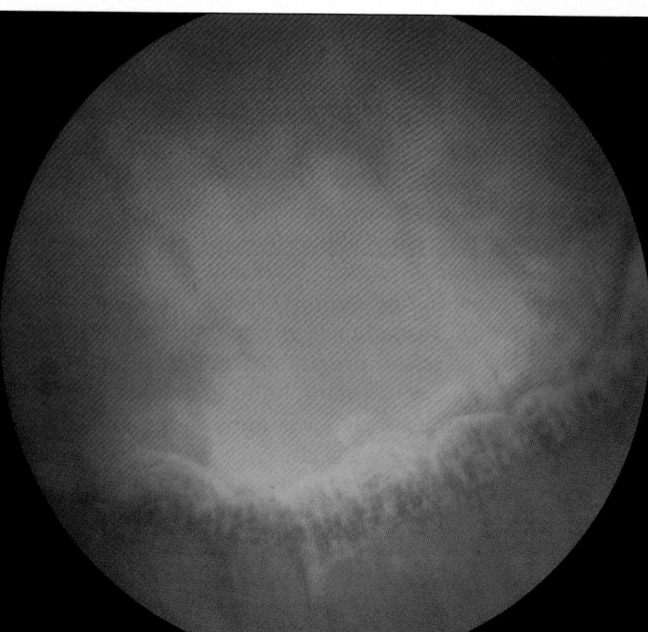
Fig. 73.3 Visible ora serrata without the use of scleral depression secondary to shallow elevation of the pars plana and peripheral choroid in an eye with ciliochoroidal effusion.

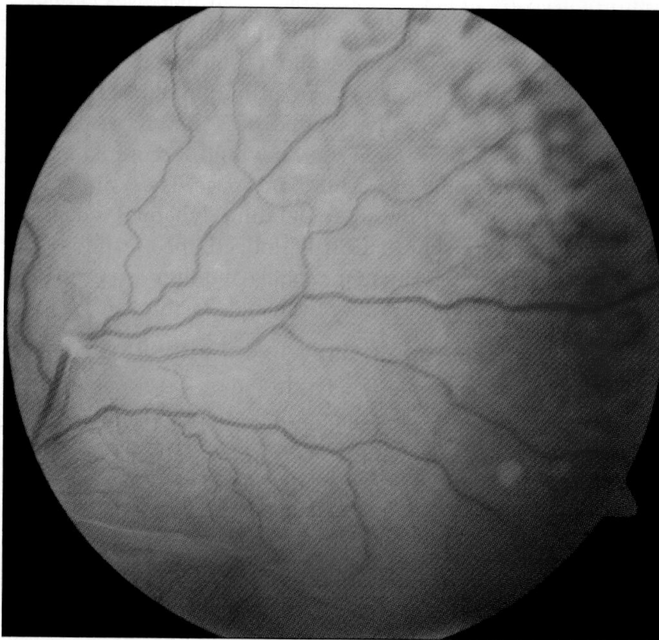
Fig. 73.5 Leopard-spot retinal pigmentation in uveal effusion syndrome.

choroid to the sclera at the vortex vein ampullae. The fluid accumulation is always greater anteriorly, as the anterior connecting fibers attaching choroid to the sclera are long and tangentially oriented, unlike the posterior fibers that are short and run more directly from uvea to sclera.[21]

Long-standing uveal effusion causes decompensation of the retinal pigment epithelial fluid barrier, resulting in increased protein and fluid accumulation in the subretinal space and development of nonrhegmatogenous retinal detachment (Fig. 73.4). There is greater absorption of fluid from the subretinal space compared with protein outflow, which results in rising protein concentration and marked shifting of subretinal fluid with changes in head position. Progressive subretinal fluid accumulation may lead to total retinal detachment. Chronic serous effusion and subretinal fluid accumulation may result in diffuse depigmentation and multifocal hyperplasia of the retinal pigment epithelium, forming the characteristic clinical finding of leopard spots in the fundus (Figs 73.4 and 73.5).

Anterior-segment examination in a patient with uveal effusion syndrome may reveal dilation of the episcleral blood vessels. Blood may be present in the Schlemm's canal on gonioscopy. The anterior chamber is free of any signs of inflammation and the presence of anterior-chamber cell should increase suspicion of another ocular disorder with secondary uveal effusion. Mild vitreous cells may be present. Intraocular pressure is normal in patients with uveal effusion syndrome and hypotony would indicate the presence of an alternative etiology. Elevation of subretinal fluid protein levels has been documented.[2,22,23] Although not commonly tested today, earlier studies of patients with uveal effusion syndrome demonstrated increased cerebrospinal fluid pressure and protein levels in some cases.[1,2]

Diagnostic studies

In addition to the clinical examination, ancillary studies are important for the diagnosis of uveal effusion syndrome and, more importantly, for the exclusion of other more common etiologies of ciliochoroidal effusion.

Ophthalmic ultrasound

B-scan ultrasound examination typically shows a smooth, thick, dome-shaped membrane with little aftermovement.[24] Ciliochoroidal effusion may be distinguished from retinal detachment by extension of the detachment anterior to the ora serrata. Highly bullous ciliochoroidal detachments may extend posteriorly and insert near the edge of the optic nerve. A-scan evaluation demonstrates a thick, 100% spike at tissue sensitivity, which at low sensitivity can often be seen to be double-peaked.[24] In early presentations of uveal effusion syndrome, the only evidence for ciliochoroidal effusion may be subtle degrees of supraciliary effusion on high-frequency ultrasound biomicroscopy. Diffuse, high-reflective thickening of the posterior choroid may be seen (Fig. 73.6). Low-reflective choroidal thickening should raise the suspicion for an infiltrative process secondary to an inflammatory or neoplastic condition.[24]

Angiography and optical coherence tomography

The diagnostic value of fluorescein and indocyanine green angiography and optical coherence tomography is limited in uveal effusion syndrome and serves mostly to exclude other etiologies. Angiography may demonstrate a leopard-skin appearance of hyperfluorescence and hypofluorescence (Fig. 73.7). The presence of focal fluorescein leaks and focal pigment epithelial detachments should increase the suspicion for idiopathic central serous chorioretinopathy as the underlying diagnosis. Multiple pinpoint leaks may indicate the presence of an inflammatory or neoplastic choroidal infiltration. Indocyanine green angiography shows diffuse granular choroidal hyperfluorescence in the early phase, indicating marked hyperpermeability of the choroidal vessels.[13] This choroidal hyperfluorescence persists into the late-phase angiogram and becomes more diffuse, demonstrating increased accumulation of fluid in the choroid. Spectral-domain optical coherence tomography may show focal thickening of the retinal pigment epithelium layer corresponding to the areas of leopard spots.[25]

Differential diagnosis

Uveal effusion syndrome is a diagnosis of exclusion. The differential diagnosis may be categorized by primary pathogenic factors causing ciliochoroidal effusion (Table 73.1). As discussed above, serous effusions in the ciliary body and choroid generally require the simultaneous presence of multiple pathogenic factors.

Congenital and acquired scleropathies

As discussed above, congenital or acquired scleropathy with abnormal thickening of the sclera significantly alters

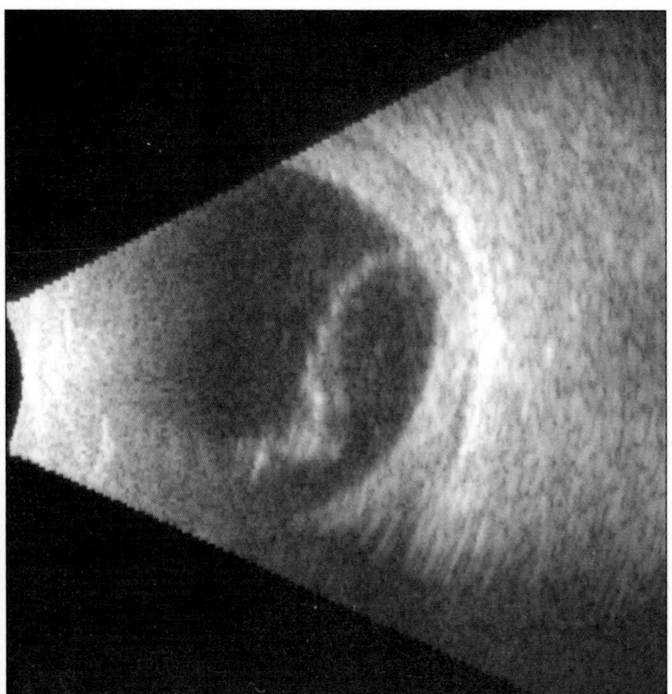

Fig. 73.6 B-scan ultrasound of an eye with uveal effusion syndrome shows choroidal thickening and inferior nonrhegmatogenous retinal detachment.

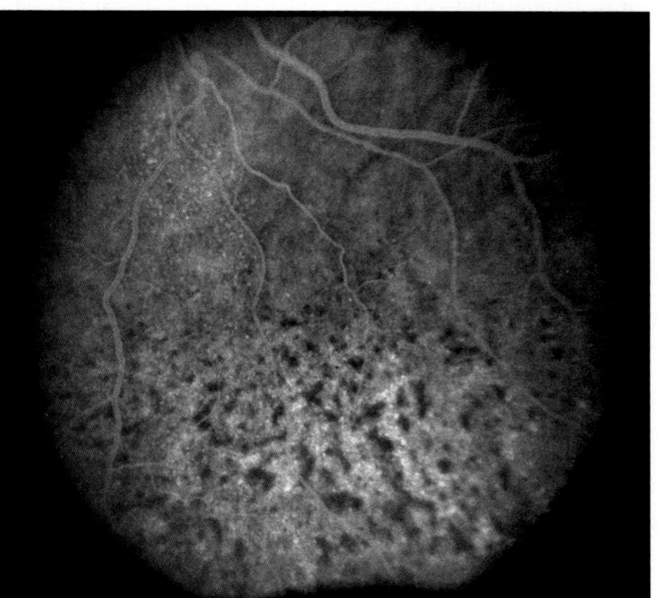

Fig. 73.7 Fluorescein angiogram of a patient with uveal effusion syndrome demonstrating leopard-skin appearance of hyperfluorescence and hypofluorescence.

Table 73.1 Differential diagnosis of ciliochoroidal effusions

Scleropathies
Congenital Uveal effusion syndrome Nanophthalmos
Acquired Amyloidosis Mucopolysaccharidosis
Hydrodynamic factors
Ocular hypotony Wound leak Overfiltration Cyclodialysis Penetrating ocular trauma Rhegmatogenous retinal detachment Ciliary body dysfunction
Elevated uveal venous pressure Arteriovenous fistula Sturge–Weber syndrome Idiopathic prominent episcleral vessels Vortex vein compression Valsalva maneuver
Malignant hypertension
Inflammatory factors After trauma or surgery After photocoagulation or cryotherapy Drug reaction Uveitis Scleritis Orbital cellulitis Idiopathic orbital inflammation
Neoplastic conditions Metastatic carcinoma Malignant melanoma Lymphoproliferative and melanocytic choroidal infiltration

the choroidal fluid dynamics and may cause uveal effusion, especially in the presence of other pathogenic factors such as vortex vein compression with reduced venous outflow and elevated uveal venous pressure. Uveal effusion syndrome and nanophthalmos can be considered in the same spectrum of diseases with a congenital primary scleral abnormality. Secondary scleral abnormalities are seen in association with systemic disorders, including amyloidosis or mucopolysaccharidosis.[10,11]

Uveal effusion in patients with nanophthalmos is remarkably similar to that seen in the idiopathic uveal effusion syndrome. Nanophthalmos is a pure form of microphthalmia characterized by small eyes and extremely thick sclera with no other identifiable ocular or systemic abnormalities. The axial length is generally less than 20 mm and high hyperopia (> +7.00 D) is typical. Other findings include small corneal diameter, shallow anterior chamber, high lens-to-eye volume ratio, and strong predisposition to develop angle closure glaucoma.[26] Uveal effusion and nonrhegmatogenous retinal detachment may occur spontaneously and are frequently induced by intraocular surgery in nanophthalmic eyes.[26,27] The detection of nanophthalmos is important prior to any planned intraocular procedure since prophylactic use of sclerectomies may prevent significant postoperative complications secondary to uveal effusion.

Hydrodynamic effusions

Hydrodynamic factors associated with ciliochoroidal effusion include ocular hypotony, elevated uveal venous pressure, and malignant hypertension. Long-standing low intraocular pressure induces uveal effusion and may in turn be worsened by ciliary body detachment. The most common reason for hypotony is glaucoma filtering or drainage device surgery, especially in the early postoperative period. Resuturing the scleral flap, scleral patch grafting, autologous blood injection, and other methods have been described in the literature to reverse postoperative hypotony.[28–30] Hypotony and uveal effusion complicating anterior-segment surgery are usually secondary to a wound leak or inadvertent filtering bleb. Other ocular disorders that may lead to hypotony and secondary ciliochoroidal effusion include cyclodialysis, penetrating ocular trauma, rhegmatogenous retinal detachment, and ciliary body dysfunction.

Elevated uveal venous pressure and increased transudation from choroidal vessels may be seen in the setting of carotid-cavernous sinus fistula or dural arteriovenous fistulas. When an intracranial fistula is suspected in a patient with uveal effusion, nonrhegmatogenous retinal detachment, and other associated findings, neuroimaging should be obtained. Patients with idiopathic prominent episcleral vessels or Sturge–Weber syndrome have elevated episcleral venous pressure and likely secondary increase in choriocapillaris pressure, which predisposes them to a higher risk of significant ciliochoroidal effusion during intraocular surgery when the intraocular pressure drops to zero.[31] Compression of the vortex veins and reduction of ocular venous outflow may lead to uveal effusion after scleral buckling surgery.

Malignant hypertension secondary to severe renal disease or pregnancy may lead to ciliochoroidal effusion and nonrhegmatogenous retinal detachment, which usually resolve with blood pressure control.

Inflammatory factors

In addition to causing hypotony, penetrating trauma may induce marked intraocular inflammation, which leads to increased vascular permeability. Chronic low-grade inflammation with increased permeability of the choriocapillaris may also be seen after intraocular surgery. Transient vascular leakage and serous ciliochoroidal fluid accumulation may be seen after thermal injury from panretinal photocoagulation or transscleral cryotherapy. Inflammation of the uveal tract secondary to autoimmune or infectious etiologies may be complicated by ciliochoroidal effusion and nonrhegmatogenous retinal detachment. A uveitic syndrome is usually suspected in these patients based on other ocular findings. A painful or red eye in a patient with uveal effusion may be secondary to scleritis, idiopathic orbital inflammation, or orbital cellulitis. A buckle infection should always be in the differential diagnosis of uveal effusion in a patient with scleral inflammation after scleral buckling surgery.

Neoplastic effusions

Choroidal metastatic tumors or malignant melanoma may infrequently present with ciliochoroidal effusion and nonrhegmatogenous retinal detachment. The diagnosis may only be apparent after an ophthalmic ultrasound in cases with extensive choroidal and subretinal fluid accumulation. In addition to solid tumors of the eye, neoplastic infiltrations and secondary uveal thickening may cause nonrhegmatogenous retinal detachment and occasional serous uveal effusion in lymphoproliferative disorders or melanocytic proliferation.

Treatment of idiopathic uveal effusion syndrome

Most patients with idiopathic uveal effusion syndrome become symptomatic of their disease when the subretinal fluid from the inferior nonrhegmatogenous retinal detachment progresses superiorly and causes macular detachment. Macular damage can also occur from repeated episodes wherein subretinal fluid shifts into the macula while the patient is lying down. Some patients may initially be misdiagnosed and treated medically for other causes of exudative retinal detachment, which fails to restore vision. Surgical treatment is required to prevent further macular damage by facilitating the resolution of subretinal fluid. In patients with known idiopathic uveal effusion syndrome and an otherwise asymptomatic eye (e.g., fellow eye of a patient with a unilateral presentation), prophylactic treatment with a scleral-thinning procedure should be considered prior to any intraocular surgery in order to prevent postoperative ciliochoroidal effusion and nonrhegmatogenous retinal detachment.

Scleral thinning procedures

Gass first described sclerectomy with sclerostomy for the treatment of uveal effusion syndrome in 1983.[16] The idea of using this procedure in patients with uveal effusion syndrome arose after an unsuccessful attempt at vortex vein decompression in another patient. Gass operated on both eyes of a patient with thick sclera and uveal effusion and amputated or ruptured the vortex veins during attempted decompression. Despite the occurrence of suprachoroidal hemorrhage in both eyes, ciliochoroidal and nonrhegmatogenous detachment resolved in both eyes postoperatively. This observation led him to hypothesize that the excision of large scleral flaps at the sites of vortex veins was responsible for the successful outcome. To test this hypothesis, he performed quadrantic partial-thickness sclerectomies and sclerostomies without vortex vein decompression or drainage of subretinal fluid in both eyes of a patient with long-standing uveal effusion and bullous nonrhegmatogenous retinal detachment. Complete resolution of ciliochoroidal and subretinal fluid occurred 10–12 weeks after surgery.[16] In 1990, Johnson and Gass expanded on this initial result in a retrospective study of 23 eyes of 20 patients with uveal effusion syndrome who underwent a scleral-thinning procedure without vortex vein decompression.[17] The investigators observed complete resolution of subretinal and supraciliochoroidal fluid in 96% of eyes after one or two procedures. The mean time for resolution of uveal effusion and nonrhegmatogenous retinal detachment was 2.4 months. Other investigators reported similar results using scleral-thinning procedures for treatment of uveal effusion and nonrhegmatogenous retinal detachment associated with Hunter syndrome, nanophthalmos, and uveal effusion syndrome.[11,13,20,32,33]

The surgical procedure for scleral thinning involves the creation of 5 × 7 mm, one-half to two-thirds thickness sclerectomies in each quadrant, centered 1–2 mm anterior to the equator and placed outside the meridian of each vortex vein to avoid its intrascleral course (Fig. 73.8).[16,17] The long axis of the sclerectomy is oriented circumferentially. An approximately 2-mm linear sclerostomy may be created in the center of each sclerectomy bed and enlarged with a 1–2-mm scleral punch. Similar scleral-thinning techniques have been reported by others treating nanophthalmic or idiopathic uveal effusion.[13,34]

Pars plana vitrectomy

The extent of visual improvement after scleral-thinning procedures may be limited by photoreceptor and retinal pigment epithelial damage secondary to chronic retinal detachment. In the series reported by Johnson and Gass, visual acuity improved by two or more Snellen lines in 56% of eyes, remained stable in 35% of eyes, and worsened in 9% of eyes.[17] Overall visual acuity was 20/400 or better in 96% of eyes and 20/40 or better in 35% of eyes. Among the 12 of 23 eyes whose final visual acuity was worse than 20/40, the primary vision-limiting factor was atrophic photoreceptor and retinal pigment epithelial damage due to chronic retinal detachment. The mean time for retinal reattachment following scleral-thinning surgery in this series was 2.4 months. To facilitate rapid retinal reattachment and prevent ongoing damage to photoreceptors and the retinal pigment epithelium, Schneiderman and Johnson performed pars plana vitrectomy and internal drainage of subretinal fluid at the time of quadrantic partial-thickness sclerectomies in a 73-year-old man with uveal effusion syndrome and total retinal detachment.[35] This patient's vision improved from hand motions to 20/70 1 year postoperatively. This combined approach of sclerectomies and pars plana vitrectomy for macula-off nonrhegmatogenous retinal detachment in uveal effusion syndrome allows immediate approximation of the photoreceptors and the retinal pigment epithelium and prevents further photoreceptor cell death. An alternative approach is external drainage of the subretinal fluid,[22] which presents significant risk of subretinal hemorrhage, profound ocular hypotony, and difficulty accessing the posteriorly shifting subretinal fluid.

Vortex vein decompression

In 1980, Brockhurst reported successful use of scleral-thinning procedure with vortex vein decompression in the treatment of nanophthalmic ciliochoroidal effusion.[19] He described the isolation of the intrascleral portion of the vortex vein and decompressing all four veins. Since scleral-thinning procedures alone are successful in the treatment of uveal effusion syndrome, vortex vein decompression for the treatment of ciliochoroidal effusion in uveal effusion syndrome or nanophthalmos is no longer performed by most vitreoretinal surgeons.

Conclusion

Idiopathic uveal effusion syndrome is a rare condition which typically presents in otherwise healthy middle-aged males with spontaneous detachment of the ciliary body and the peripheral choroid. This condition is frequently associated with nonrhegmatogenous retinal detachment with marked shifting of subretinal fluid due to its exceptionally high protein content. Other ocular findings include dilation of the episcleral blood vessels, blood in Schlemm's canal, normal intraocular pressure, mild vitreous cells, and leopard-spot pigment epithelial alterations. Current evidence indicates that congenital scleropathy manifesting with abnormal accumulation of glycosaminoglycan-like deposits and thickening of the sclera is the primary pathologic anomaly in patients with uveal effusion syndrome. The diagnosis of uveal effusion syndrome is based on characteristic clinical findings and exclusion of the other known causes of

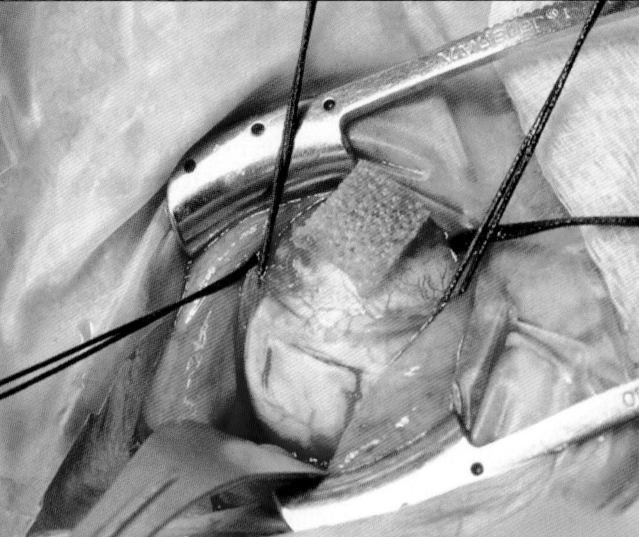

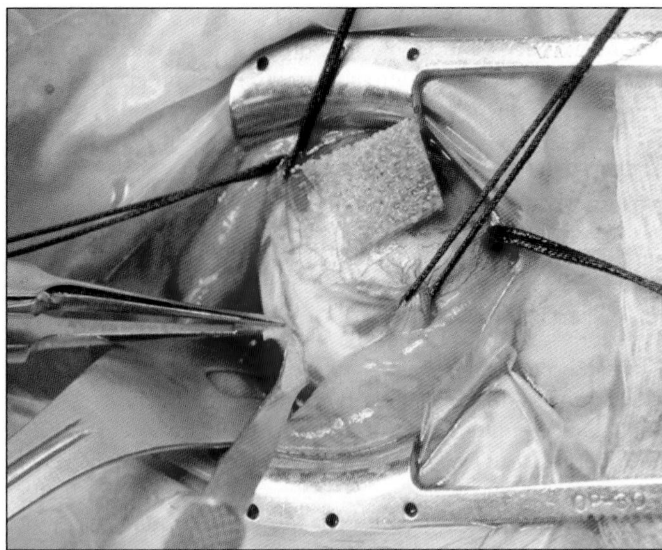

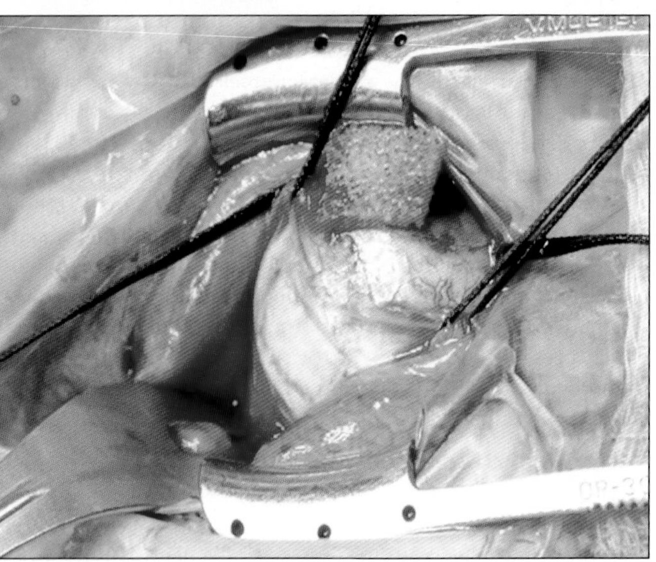

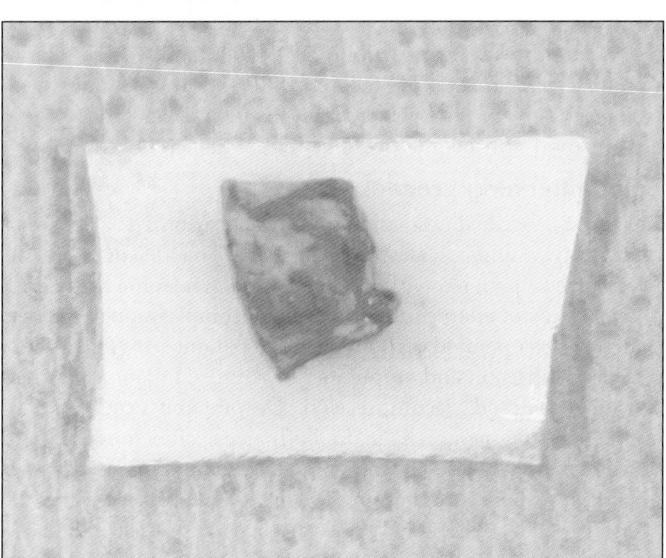

Fig. 73.8 Scleral-thinning procedure for uveal effusion syndrome. Borders of the sclerectomy are outlined with partial-thickness scleral incisions (top left). One-half to two-thirds thickness lamellar scleral dissection is performed (top right), creating a scleral window (bottom left) and an excised section of abnormally thick sclera (bottom right).

ciliochoroidal effusion and nonrhegmatogenous retinal detachment. The natural course is usually prolonged with remissions and exacerbations, and without treatment, patients may experience permanent loss of vision. Treatment is primarily surgical and requires quadrantic partial-thickness sclerectomies and sclerostomies.

HYPOTONY MACULOPATHY

Introduction

Loss of central vision may develop in patients with reduced intraocular pressure following trauma or ocular surgery. One of the causes of reduced vision in the setting of hypotony is significant folding of the choroid, neurosensory retina, and retinal pigment epithelium in the posterior pole, termed hypotony maculopathy by Gass in 1972.[36–38] The initial description of fundus changes associated with hypotony dates back to the 1950s, when Dellaporta described patients with reduced vision following glaucoma procedures or perforating eye injuries.[36] He noted that hypotony was associated with several fundus abnormalities, including optic nerve swelling, vascular tortuosity, and chorioretinal folds.[36] The incidence of hypotony maculopathy significantly increased after the introduction of antimetabolites in glaucoma-filtering surgery.[39–41] Younger age, myopia, and male gender are significant risk factors for the development of hypotony maculopathy after glaucoma procedures.[40–42]

Clinical features

Posterior-segment examination in patients with hypotony maculopathy shows irregular folding of the neurosensory retina, retinal pigment epithelium, and choroid (Fig. 73.9). These folds are initially broad and indistinct and tend to radiate outward in a branching fashion from the optic disc temporally and appear concentric or irregular nasally. Around the center of the fovea, retinal folds may be arranged in a stellate pattern. The elevated crests of the folds appear yellow with dark narrow troughs in between. Reduction of the ocular anteroposterior diameter causes relative hyperopia. Marked optic disc edema may be

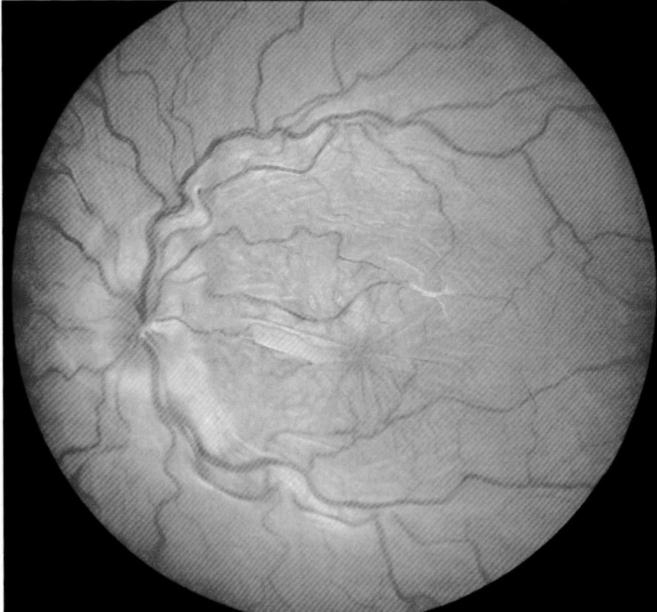

Fig. 73.9 Chorioretinal folds and optic disc edema in a patient with hypotony maculopathy.

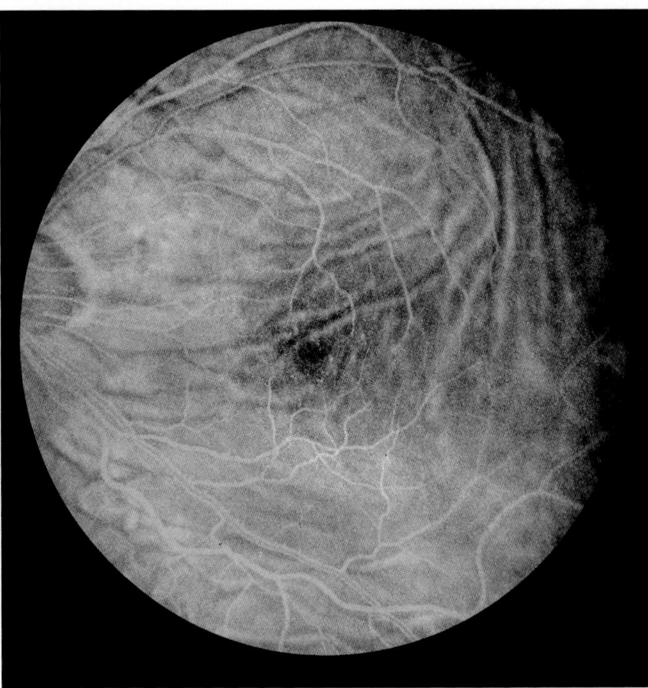

Fig. 73.10 Fluorescein angiogram in hypotony maculopathy demonstrates hyperfluorescent streaks corresponding to the crest of the chorioretinal folds.

present. Retinal vasculature is typically tortuous and may be engorged in some eyes. Anterior-segment examination may show a shallow anterior chamber if there is ciliochoroidal effusion. As the intraocular pressure returns to the normal range, the choroidal folds flatten and may disappear. If the hypotony was chronic, permanent retinal pigment epithelial changes may cause pigmented lines in the fundus.

Diagnosis

Fluorescein angiography

Fluorescein angiography is useful in demonstrating chorioretinal folds, especially in mild cases with a normal-appearing fundus examination. In the initial stages of hypotony, fluorescein angiography demonstrates an irregular increase in background choroidal fluorescence corresponding to the crest of the choroidal folds (Fig. 73.10). This produces hyperfluorescent streaks that may be seen in the early arterial phase. The hyperfluorescence of these streaks are multifactorial: (1) thinning of the retinal pigment epithelium on the crest of the folds; (2) pooling of the choroidal fluorescein under the crest; and (3) shorter course of the incident blue and reflected yellow-green light during angiography. The troughs of the folds are occupied by compressed retinal pigment epithelial cells, which reduce the transmission of the background choroidal fluorescence and cause hypofluorescence on angiography. Leakage of fluorescein may be seen in the capillaries of the optic nerve and there is typically no leakage in the retinal capillaries.[43] In long-standing hypotony, angiography may show permanent alterations in the retinal pigment epithelium. The chorioretinal folds may be differentiated from the folds of the neurosensory retina, which do not alter the background fluorescence.

Ocular ultrasound

B-scan ultrasonography typically shows flattening and thickening of the sclera and choroid in the posterior pole[44] (Fig. 73.11). Anterior-segment evaluation with ultrasound biomicroscopy may be useful for the identification of the underlying etiology of hypotony. The presence of a cyclodialysis cleft or anterior ciliary detachment may only be apparent on ultrasound biomicroscopy.[45,46]

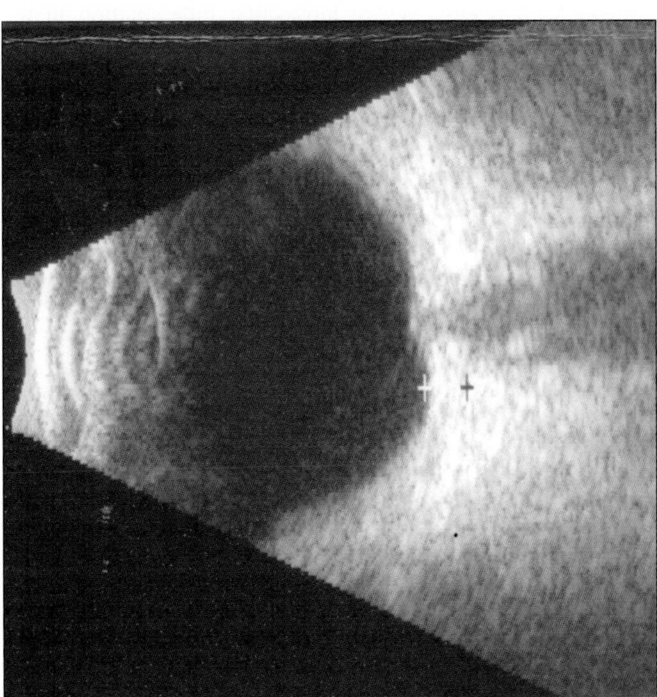

Fig. 73.11 B-scan ultrasonography in a patient with low intraocular pressure showing characteristic flattening and thickening of the sclera and choroid in the posterior pole.

Optical coherence tomography

In patients with low intraocular pressure and reduced visual acuity, optical coherence tomography imaging of the posterior pole can help to demonstrate subtle chorioretinal folds of the macula that may otherwise be difficult to detect on biomicroscopy[47–49] (Fig. 73.12). High-resolution optical coherence tomography may detect chorioretinal folding in early hypotony, which may not show any changes in the background choroidal fluorescence during fluorescein angiography.[48] However, the clinical significance of subtle chorioretinal folds detected only by optical coherence tomography in a patient with unchanged vision is unclear. Optical coherence tomography in a patient with symptomatic hypotony maculopathy and stereotypical biomicroscopic findings typically shows prominent chorioretinal folds (Fig. 73.12).

Pathogenesis

Hypotony

The reduction of intraocular pressure may be secondary to decreased aqueous production or increased aqueous outflow. In most cases, both a reduction in aqueous production and an increase in aqueous outflow are present in a hypotonous eye. Table 73.2 lists various etiologies of decreased intraocular pressure, some of which will be briefly discussed below.

Decreased aqueous production

Reduced aqueous production is an uncommon etiology of hypotony. The factors that lead to decreased aqueous production may be inflammatory, vascular, or structural. Ciliary body inflammation may compromise the production of aqueous in patients with uveitis. Severe intraocular inflammation in the immediate postoperative period following intraocular surgery may decrease aqueous secretion. Trauma may be associated with significant iridocyclitis and hypotony, which may be worsened by increased aqueous outflow due to a cyclodialysis cleft or globe rupture. Decreased ocular perfusion in patients with vasculitis or arterial occlusion may cause ciliary body ischemia. Other causes of decreased aqueous production include ciliary body detachment secondary to ciliochoroidal effusion, trauma, or proliferative vitreoretinopathy.

Increased aqueous outflow

When the aqueous production is no longer sufficient to match the increased outflow, hypotony develops. Most cases of ocular hypotony are secondary to increased aqueous outflow. Under physiologic conditions, the aqueous leaves the eye primarily through the trabecular meshwork and Schlemm's canal in a pressure-dependent manner, with much smaller amounts exiting through uveoscleral outflow. Several factors may increase aqueous outflow, including wound leak after anterior-segment surgery and excessive aqueous filtration after glaucoma filtering or drainage device surgery. After the introduction of antimetabolites in glaucoma-filtering procedures, the incidence of hypotony increased.[39] Antimetabolites inhibit subconjunctival healing and scarring, which would otherwise limit the overfiltration rate. With the introduction of sutureless small-gauge vitrectomy technology, vitreoretinal surgeons encounter ocular hypotony with increasing frequency in their postoperative patients.[50] Ocular trauma may be associated with scleral rupture and wound leak. Postoperative or traumatic cyclodialysis creates a free communication between the anterior chamber and the suprachoroidal space, increasing the uveoscleral outflow.

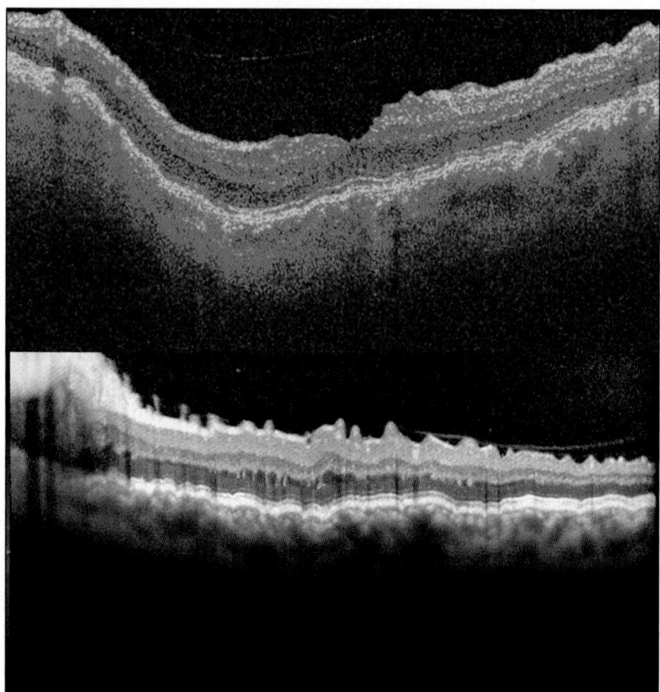

Fig. 73.12 High-resolution optical coherence tomography may demonstrate subtle (top panel) or prominent (bottom panel) chorioretinal folding in hypotony maculopathy.

Table 73.2 Causes of hypotony
Postoperative • Wound leak • Overfiltration
Ocular trauma Cyclodialysis Perforating injury
Inflammatory Iridocyclitis
Retinal detachment
Ciliochoroidal detachment
Ciliary body hypoperfusion Carotid occlusion Giant cell arteritis
Photocoagulation or cryoablation of the ciliary body
Excessive reduction of intraocular pressure by pharmacologic agents
Systemic Hyperosmotic agents Dehydration Uremia Diabetic ketoacidosis Myotonic dystrophy

Mechanism of maculopathy

Chorioretinal folds form in the hypotonous eye due to scleral shrinkage and reduction of the inner surface area of the sclera. This loss of surface area then leads to folding of the inner portion of choroid and the outer retina.[51–54] Maculopathy develops when the neurosensory retina is thrown into a series of stellate folds around the center of the fovea. This central stellate retinal wrinkling is caused by the thickened posterior scleral wall and the choroid displacing the normally thick retina surrounding the thin foveola.[43] The folding of the neurosensory retina is the primary cause of vision loss in hypotony maculopathy. The risk of hypotony maculopathy is highest in young myopic patients, and this may indicate that the sclera is more vulnerable to swelling and contraction in young patients.

Mechanism of optic disc edema

Reduced intraocular pressure may lead to broad areas of choroidal swelling and retinal folding around the optic nerve and this may cause disc edema.[43] Another proposed mechanism is the anterior bowing of the lamina cribrosa and constriction of axonal bundles in the lamina scleralis, causing reduced orthograde and retrograde axoplasmic transport and swelling of the optic nerve.[55] Disc edema may be less impressive in eyes with preexisting optic nerve disease and loss of axons.

Differential diagnosis

The finding of chorioretinal folds may be seen in any condition that reduces the inner surface area of the sclera secondary to thickening or shrinkage (Table 73.3).

Idiopathic chorioretinal folds

Horizontal macular chorioretinal folds as well as folds radiating from the optic nerve may be seen in young hyperopic patients on routine evaluation.[52,56] These idiopathic chorioretinal folds are usually confined to the area around the macula and optic nerve, but may at times involve most of the posterior pole. Patients usually do not report any visual dysfunction. The appearance of the folds is usually symmetric in both eyes, but may occasionally be seen unilaterally. As the name indicates, the etiology of these chorioretinal folds is unknown and may be secondary to the shrinkage of the fibrous tunic of the eye after an inflammatory process during early years of life.[43]

Retrobulbar mass lesions

Any space-occupying mass in the orbit may cause scleral edema, choroidal congestion, and chorioretinal folds.[57,58] A mass in the extraconal space may induce astigmatism, whereas intraconal location of a tumor may lead to acquired hyperopia.[57] Both benign and malignant tumors have been reported to present with chorioretinal folds.

Table 73.3 Differential diagnosis of hypotony maculopathy
Idiopathic chorioretinal folds
Retrobulbar mass lesions
Scleral inflammation
Scleral buckle
Choroidal tumors
Choroidal neovascularization
Focal chorioretinal scars
Optic nerve head disorders
Retinal folds

Scleral inflammation

Scleral inflammation with edema, thickening, and choroidal congestion may lead to the development of chorioretinal folds. Thyroid eye disease, idiopathic orbital inflammation, and other autoimmune or infectious uveitic diseases presenting with scleritis may have associated chorioretinal folds.[43,59,60]

Scleral buckle

Thickening of the sclera in the posterior slope of a scleral buckle may cause occasional chorioretinal folds in patients who underwent rhegmatogenous retinal detachment repair.

Choroidal tumors

Malignant melanoma or metastatic lesions of the choroid may cause vascular congestion, choroidal edema, and scleral thickening, leading to chorioretinal folds surrounding the tumor.[43]

Choroidal neovascularization

Spontaneous or laser-induced contraction of subretinal pigment epithelial choroidal neovascular membrane may induce the formation of chorioretinal folds that radiate away from the membrane.[61]

Focal chorioretinal scars

Focal scars of the choroid and the retina may sometimes cause contraction and induce chorioretinal folds radiating towards the center of the scar.[62]

Optic nerve head disorders

Idiopathic intracranial hypertension and papilledema may be associated with chorioretinal folds. These folds are usually horizontal in the macula and converge on the nasal side of the swollen optic nerve.[63,64] Chorioretinal folds have also been seen in patients with unexplained optic atrophy.[65] In some patients with increased intracranial pressure, chorioretinal folds may present in the absence of any detectable papilledema and a lumbar puncture with an opening pressure may need to be performed to rule out idiopathic intracranial hypertension.[66]

Retinal folds

Retinal folds may be mistaken for chorioretinal folds in some eyes. Usually, folds of the neurosensory retina are narrow and seen radiating away from a focal inner retinal contraction caused by macular pucker or outer retinal contraction secondary to a chorioretinal scar (Fig. 73.13).[43] Fluorescein angiography is helpful in differentiating retinal folds from chorioretinal folds, since folds of the neurosensory retina do not change the fluorescence pattern and are not seen on angiography.

Treatment

The effective treatment of hypotony maculopathy requires correcting the underlying ocular abnormality and restoring normal intraocular pressure. Since postoperative hypotony accounts for a significant portion of hypotony maculopathy patients, treatment is typically managed by an anterior-segment surgeon. Injection of viscoelastic or fluid into the anterior chamber to increase intraocular pressure produces short-lived effects. Wound leaks after anterior-segment surgery need to be addressed immediately with a bandage contact lens or suturing the wound to prevent further aqueous loss. Ocular inflammation requires treatment with a topical or oral corticosteroid. Posttraumatic cyclodialysis cleft may require laser or surgical closure to normalize intraocular pressure. Overfiltration after glaucoma

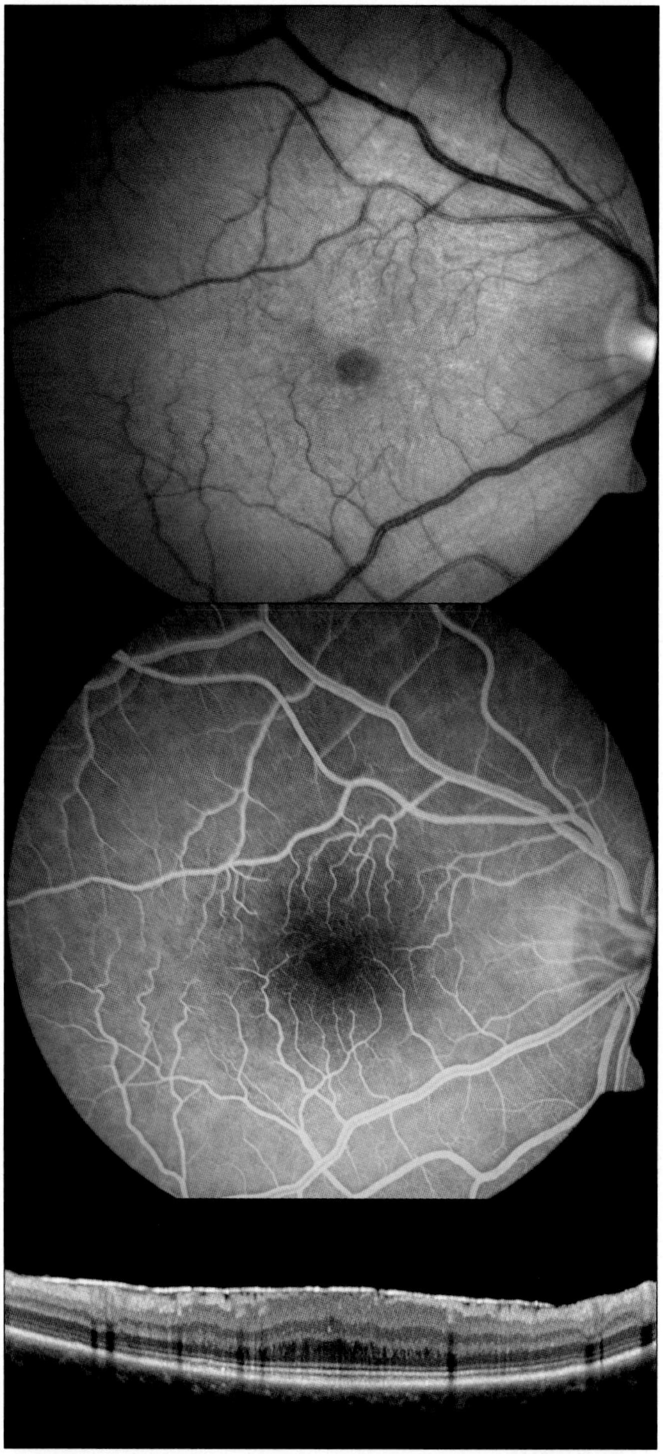

Fig. 73.13 Red-free photo of the posterior pole (top panel) and high-resolution optical coherence tomography (bottom panel) demonstrate fine, subtle retinal folds associated with an epiretinal membrane. Fluorescein angiogram shows no fluorescence changes associated with these folds (middle panel).

surgery may require resuturing the scleral flap, donor scleral patch graft placement, or autologous blood injection.[28–30,67]

Chorioretinal folds may resolve following the restoration of normal intraocular pressure. In cases of chronic hypotony, the retinal pigment epithelium will show permanent changes, including hyperpigmentation at the troughs of the folds, causing irregularly dark, pigmented lines in the posterior pole detected by fluorescein angiography.[43] The choroid and the sclera return to normal thickness and the tortuosity and engorgement of the retinal vessels disappear.

Early detection of hypotony maculopathy is important for implementing the necessary measures to restore normal intraocular pressure and recovery of vision. The prognosis for visual recovery depends on the duration of the hypotony and the chronicity of the chorioretinal folds. Prolonged folding of the choroid and the neurosensory retina may cause irreversible structural changes in the macula and poor visual recovery after normalization of the intraocular pressure. However, significant visual improvement may still occur in some patients after treatment of chronic hypotony.[68] Duker and Schuman reported that pars plana vitrectomy and mechanical flattening of the posterior pole with intraoperative instillation of perfluorocarbon liquid significantly improved visual acuity in a patient who had minimal visual recovery after increasing the intraocular pressure with previous bleb revision.[69] The efficacy of this approach has not been confirmed in larger patient cohorts.

Conclusion

Hypotony maculopathy is characterized by folding of the choroid, neurosensory retina, and retinal pigment epithelium in the posterior pole in an eye with low intraocular pressure. The folding of the neurosensory retina is believed to be the primary cause of vision loss. In addition to chorioretinal folds, acquired hyperopia, optic disc edema, and tortuous retinal vasculature may be associated with hypotony maculopathy. Fluorescein angiography demonstrates an irregular increase in background choroidal fluorescence corresponding to the crest of the chorioretinal folds. B-scan ultrasonography shows flattening and thickening of the sclera and choroid in the posterior pole. High-resolution optical coherence tomography allows early detection of chorioretinal folding that may be difficult to diagnose on clinical examination. Early detection and treatment are important for preventing permanent structural changes in the retina and maximizing visual recovery.

REFERENCES

1. Schepens CL, Brockhurst RJ. Uveal effusion. 1. Clinical picture. Arch Ophthalmol 1963;70:189–201.
2. Gass JD, Jallow S. Idiopathic serous detachment of the choroid, ciliary body, and retina (uveal effusion syndrome). Ophthalmology 1982;89:1018–32.
3. Johnson MW. Uveal Effusion. In: Guyer DR, Yannuzzi LA, Chang S, et al, editors. Retina–vitreous–macula. Philadelphia: W.B. Saunders; 1999. p. 658–68.
4. Toris CB, Pederson JE, Tsuboi S, et al. Extravascular albumin concentration of the uvea. Invest Ophthalmol Vis Sci 1990;31:43–53.
5. Brubaker RF, Pederson JE. Ciliochoroidal detachment. Surv Ophthalmol 1983;27:281–9.
6. Inomata H, Bill A. Exit sites of uveoscleral flow of aqueous humor in cynomolgus monkey eyes. Exp Eye Res 1977;25:113–8.
7. Alm A Bill A. Ocular circulation. In: Moses RA, Hart WM Jr, editors. Adler's physiology of the eye. St Louis: Mosby; 1987. p. 199.
8. Aaberg TM, Maggiano JM. Choroidal edema associated with retinal detachment repair: experimental and clinical correlation. Mod Probl Ophthalmol 1979;20:6–15.
9. Hawkins WR, Schepens CL. Choroidal detachment and retinal surgery. Am J Ophthalmol 1966;62:813–9.
10. Liew SC, McCluskey PJ, Parker G, et al. Bilateral uveal effusion associated with scleral thickening due to amyloidosis. Arch Ophthalmol 2000;118: 1293–5.
11. Vine AK. Uveal effusion in Hunter's syndrome. Evidence that abnormal sclera is responsible for the uveal effusion syndrome. Retina 1986;6:57–60.
12. Forrester JV, Lee WR, Kerr PR, et al. The uveal effusion syndrome and transscleral flow. Eye (Lond) 1990;4:354–65.
13. Uyama M, Takahashi K, Kozaki J, et al. Uveal effusion syndrome: clinical features, surgical treatment, histologic examination of the sclera, and pathophysiology. Ophthalmology 2000;107:441–9.
14. Ward RC, Gragoudas ES, Pon DM, et al. Abnormal scleral findings in uveal effusion syndrome. Am J Ophthalmol 1988;106:139–46.

15. Boubriak OA, Urban JP, Bron AJ. Differential effects of aging on transport properties of anterior and posterior human sclera. Exp Eye Res 2003;76:701–13.
16. Gass JD. Uveal effusion syndrome. A new hypothesis concerning pathogenesis and technique of surgical treatment. Retina 1983;3:159–63.
17. Johnson MW, Gass JD. Surgical management of the idiopathic uveal effusion syndrome. Ophthalmology 1990;97:778–85.
18. Calhoun FP, Jr. The management of glaucoma in nanophthalmos. Trans Am Ophthalmol Soc 1975;73:97–122.
19. Brockhurst RJ. Vortex vein decompression for nanophthalmic uveal effusion. Arch Ophthalmol 1980;98:1987–90.
20. Casswell AG, Gregor ZJ, Bird AC. The surgical management of uveal effusion syndrome. Eye (Lond) 1987;1:115–9.
21. Moses RA. Detachment of ciliary body – anatomical and physical considerations. Invest Ophthalmol 1965;4:935–41.
22. Brockhurst RJ, Lam KW. Uveal effusion. II. Report of a case with analysis of subretinal fluid. Arch Ophthalmol 1973;90:399–401.
23. Gass JD. Uveal effusion syndrome: a new hypothesis concerning pathogenesis and technique of surgical treatment. Trans Am Ophthalmol Soc 1983;81:246–60.
24. Green RL, Byrne SF. Diagnostic ophthalmic ultrasound. In: Ryan SJ, editor. Retina. St. Louis: Mosby; 1989.
25. Okuda T, Higashide T, Wakabayashi Y, et al. Fundus autofluorescence and spectral-domain optical coherence tomography findings of leopard spots in nanophthalmic uveal effusion syndrome. Graefes Arch Clin Exp Ophthalmol 2010;248:1199–202.
26. Singh OS, Simmons RJ, Brockhurst RJ, et al. Nanophthalmos: a perspective on identification and therapy. Ophthalmology 1982;89:1006–12.
27. Brockhurst RJ. Nanophthalmos with uveal effusion. A new clinical entity. Arch Ophthalmol 1975;93:1989–99.
28. Cohen SM, Flynn HW Jr, Palmberg PF, et al. Treatment of hypotony maculopathy after trabeculectomy. Ophthalmic Surg Lasers 1995;26:435–41.
29. Haynes WL, Alward WL. Rapid visual recovery and long-term intraocular pressure control after donor scleral patch grafting for trabeculectomy-induced hypotony maculopathy. J Glaucoma 1995;4:200–1.
30. Haynes WL, Alward WL. Combination of autologous blood injection and bleb compression sutures to treat hypotony maculopathy. J Glaucoma 1999;8: 384–7.
31. Bellows AR, Chylack LT, Jr., Epstein DL, et al. Choroidal effusion during glaucoma surgery in patients with prominent episcleral vessels. Arch Ophthalmol 1979;97:493–7.
32. Allen KM, Meyers SM, Zegarra H. Nanophthalmic uveal effusion. Retina 1988;8:145–7.
33. Good WV, Stern WH. Recurrent nanophthalmic uveal effusion syndrome following laser trabeculoplasty. Am J Ophthalmol 1988;106:234–5.
34. Faulborn J, Kolli H. Sclerotomy in uveal effusion syndrome. Retina 1999;19: 504–7.
35. Schneiderman TE, Johnson MW. A new approach to the surgical management of idiopathic uveal effusion syndrome. Am J Ophthalmol 1997;123:262–3.
36. Dellaporta A. Fundus changes in postoperative hypotony. Am J Ophthalmol 1955;40:781–5.
37. Gass JDM. Hypotony maculopathy. In: Bellows JC, editor. Contemporary ophthalmology, honoring Sir Stewart Duke-Elder. Baltimore: Williams & Wilkins; 1972. p. 343–66.
38. Hovanesian JA, Higginbotham EJ, Lichter PR, et al. Long-term visual outcome of ocular hypotension after thermosclerostomy. Am J Ophthalmol 1993;115: 603–7.
39. Costa VP, Wilson RP, Moster MR, et al. Hypotony maculopathy following the use of topical mitomycin C in glaucoma filtration surgery. Ophthalmic Surg 1993;24:389–94.
40. Jampel HD, Pasquale LR, Dibernardo C. Hypotony maculopathy following trabeculectomy with mitomycin C. Arch Ophthalmol 1992;110:1049–50.
41. Stamper RL, McMenemy MG, Lieberman MF. Hypotonous maculopathy after trabeculectomy with subconjunctival 5-fluorouracil. Am J Ophthalmol 1992; 114:544–53.
42. Fannin LA, Schiffman JC, Budenz DL. Risk factors for hypotony maculopathy. Ophthalmology 2003;110:1185–91.
43. Gass JDM. Hypotony maculopathy. Stereoscopic atlas of macular diseases: diagnosis and treatment. St. Louis: Mosby; 1997. p. 294–5.
44. Cappaert WE, Purnell EW, Frank KE. Use of B-sector scan ultrasound in the diagnosis of benign choroidal folds. Am J Ophthalmol 1977;84:375–9.
45. Chan TK, Talbot JF, Rennie IG, et al. The application of ultrasonic biomicroscopy in the management of traumatic hypotony. Eye (Lond) 2000;14(Pt 5): 805–7.
46. Roters S, Engels BF, Szurman P, et al. Typical ultrasound biomicroscopic findings seen in ocular hypotony. Ophthalmologica 2002;216:90–5.
47. Budenz DL, Schwartz K, Gedde SJ. Occult hypotony maculopathy diagnosed with optical coherence tomography. Arch Ophthalmol 2005;123:113–4.
48. Lima VC, Prata TS, Castro DP, et al. Macular changes detected by Fourier-domain optical coherence tomography in patients with hypotony without clinical maculopathy. Acta Ophthalmol (Copenh) 2011;89:e274–277.
49. Martinez de la Casa JM, Garcia Feijoo J, Castillo Gomez A, et al. [Hypotony maculopathy diagnosed by optical coherence tomography.] Arch Soc Esp Oftalmol 2003;78:567–9.
50. Thompson JT. Advantages and limitations of small gauge vitrectomy. Surv Ophthalmol 2011;56:162–72.
51. Cangemi FE, Trempe CL, Walsh JB. Choroidal folds. Am J Ophthalmol 1978;86:380–7.
52. Leahey AB, Brucker AJ, Wyszynski RE, et al. Chorioretinal folds. A comparison of unilateral and bilateral cases. Arch Ophthalmol 1993;111:357–9.
53. Newell FW. Choroidal folds. The seventh Harry Searls Gradle memorial lecture. Am J Ophthalmol 1973;75:930–42.
54. Newell FW. Fundus changes in persistent and recurrent choroidal folds. Br J Ophthalmol 1984;68:32–5.
55. Minckler DS, Bunt AH. Axoplasmic transport in ocular hypotony and papilledema in the monkey. Arch Ophthalmol 1977;95:1430–6.
56. Kalina RE, Mills RP. Acquired hyperopia with choroidal folds. Ophthalmology 1980;87:44–50.
57. Friberg TR, Grove AS Jr. Choroidal folds and refractive errors associated with orbital tumors. An analysis. Arch Ophthalmol 1983;101:598–603.
58. Shields JA, Shields CL, Rashid RC. Clinicopathologic correlation of choroidal folds: secondary to massive cranioorbital hemangiopericytoma. Ophthal Plast Reconstr Surg 1992;8:62–8.
59. Krist D, Wenkel H. Posterior scleritis associated with *Borrelia burgdorferi* (Lyme disease) infection. Ophthalmology 2002;109:143–5.
60. Haruyama M, Yuzawa M, Kawamura A, et al. Indocyanine green angiographic findings of chorioretinal folds. Jpn J Ophthalmol 2001;45:293–300.
61. Diskin J, Maguire AM, Margherio RR. Choroidal folds induced with diode endolaser. Arch Ophthalmol 1992;110:754.
62. Johnson RN, Schatz H, McDonald HR. Photic maculopathy: early angiographic and ophthalmoscopic findings and late development of choroidal folds. Case report. Arch Ophthalmol 1987;105:1633–4.
63. Bird AC, Sanders MD. Choroidal folds in association with papilloedema. Br J Ophthalmol 1973;57:89–97.
64. Lavinsky J, Lavinsky D, Lavinsky F, et al. Acquired choroidal folds: a sign of idiopathic intracranial hypertension. Graefes Arch Clin Exp Ophthalmol 2007;245:883–8.
65. Sarraf D, Schwartz SD. Bilateral choroidal folds and optic neuropathy: a variant of the crowded disk syndrome? Ophthalmology 2003;110:1047–52.
66. Griebel SR, Kosmorsky GS. Choroidal folds associated with increased intracranial pressure. Am J Ophthalmol 2000;129:513–6.
67. Schwartz GF, Robin AL, Wilson RP, et al. Resuturing the scleral flap leads to resolution of hypotony maculopathy. J Glaucoma 1996;5:246–51.
68. Delgado MF, Daniels S, Pascal S, et al. Hypotony maculopathy: improvement of visual acuity after 7 years. Am J Ophthalmol 2001;132:931–3.
69. Duker JS, Schuman JS. Successful surgical treatment of hypotony maculopathy following trabeculectomy with topical mitomycin C. Ophthalmic Surg 1994; 25:463–5.

Chapter 74

Sympathetic Ophthalmia

Daniel Vítor Vasconcelos-Santos, Narsing A. Rao

INTRODUCTION

Sympathetic ophthalmia, also known as sympathetic ophthalmitis and sympathetic uveitis, is a rare bilateral diffuse granulomatous uveitis that occurs a few days to several decades after penetrating accidental or surgical trauma to an eye. Both the traumatized eye, commonly referred to as the "exciting" eye, and the fellow eye, referred to as the "sympathizing" eye, are affected. Injury to and/or incarceration of uveal tissue has been a feature of nearly all cases of sympathetic ophthalmia. The clinical signs and symptoms are usually detected in the sympathizing eye within the first 3 months after trauma to the fellow eye.[1,2]

The notion that injury to one eye may have repercussion in the contralateral eye probably dates back to ancient times, with Hippocrates (460–370 BC), but has also been reported by Agathias, in a compilation from Constantius Cephalis (1000 AD).[1,3] However it was William Mackenzie, in 1830, who provided the first comprehensive clinical description and pioneered the use of the term "sympathetic ophthalmia" to describe this entity.[1,3] Ernst Fuchs, in 1905, thoroughly detailed the characteristic histopathologic features.[4] The pathogenesis of sympathetic ophthalmia has, however, remained an enigma despite years of study, although the two most commonly held views were that it represented an autoimmune response or was infectious. There is now some experimental evidence implicating the development of an autoimmune delayed hypersensitivity reaction to melanocytes or tyrosinase peptide antigen as a possible pathogenetic mechanism.

EPIDEMIOLOGY

Sympathetic ophthalmia is a relatively rare disease, although exact figures are difficult to determine because the onset or the diagnosis, or both, are often delayed for months to years after the initial injury. In addition, definite histopathologic confirmation of the diagnosis is made in only about one-third of suspected cases, but may be established histopathologically in others not suspected clinically.[2] In 1972, Liddy and Stuart[5] reported an incidence of sympathetic ophthalmia of 0.19% following penetrating injuries and 0.007% following intraocular surgery. Among the general population, sympathetic ophthalmia has been estimated to affect 0.03 per 100 000 persons per year[6] and possibly corresponds to 1–2% of all uveitis cases.[7] Surgical procedures that may lead to sympathetic ophthalmia include cataract extraction, iridectomy, paracentesis, cyclodialysis, synechialysis, retinal detachment repair, keratectomy, vitrectomy, evisceration, laser cyclophotocoagulation, and others.[2,3]

Although advances in modern surgical techniques may be contributing to a lower incidence of sympathetic ophthalmia, this is probably being partially offset by more aggressive surgical management of severely traumatized eyes, which in the past would have been promptly enucleated. In fact, the epidemiology of sympathetic ophthalmia has been changing, and more cases are now being associated with intraocular surgery,[6–8] in contrast to accidental penetrating trauma.[3] Pars plana vitrectomy is one of the leading surgical procedures associated with sympathetic ophthalmia,[9] with an estimated risk of around 0.01%;[10] cases have been recently reported even after the advent of small-gauge sutureless vitrectomy surgery.[11,12] For these reasons, sympathetic ophthalmia should not be considered a disappearing disease and thus should not be neglected.

Some studies have shown a male preponderance, but this is believed to be a reflection of the higher incidence of accidental trauma in males. Indeed, when only cases of surgical trauma are considered, the ratio is similar. In Winter's series of 257 cases of sympathetic ophthalmia, there was no difference in age incidence.[13] Other authors have reported relative peaks in childhood and early adult years, thought to reflect a higher incidence of accidental trauma in these ages, and an additional peak in the sixth and seventh decades, thought to represent an increased incidence of surgical procedures among persons in this age group.[14]

PATHOGENESIS

The exact cause of sympathetic ophthalmia is unknown. Clinical studies have shown that the predominant predisposing factors are accidental penetrating trauma, accounting for approximately 60–70% of cases, and penetrating surgical trauma, accounting for nearly 30%. Recent studies have pointed to an inversion of this proportion, with many cases now being associated with surgical rather than accidental trauma.[6,7,9] A small percentage of cases are the result of contusion injuries with occult scleral rupture and perforating corneal ulcers. The common denominator in the overwhelming majority of cases is the presence of a penetrating injury in which wound healing is complicated by incarceration of the iris, ciliary body, or choroid.[2]

Historically, the pathogenesis of sympathetic ophthalmia has been suspected to be infectious. However no organisms have ever been isolated from cases of sympathetic ophthalmia, and infective agents have not induced the disease in laboratory animals. Cases associated with severe infectious keratitis in the absence of a corneal perforation are probably associated with exposure of the uveal antigens to the immune system, through a disrupted hemato-ocular barrier.[15,16] Sympathetic ophthalmia

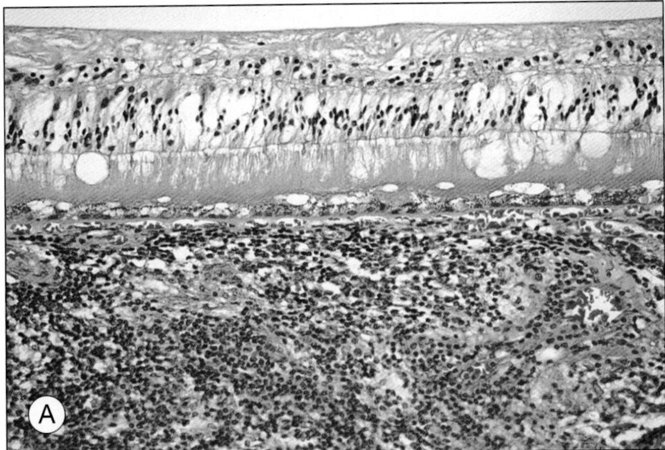

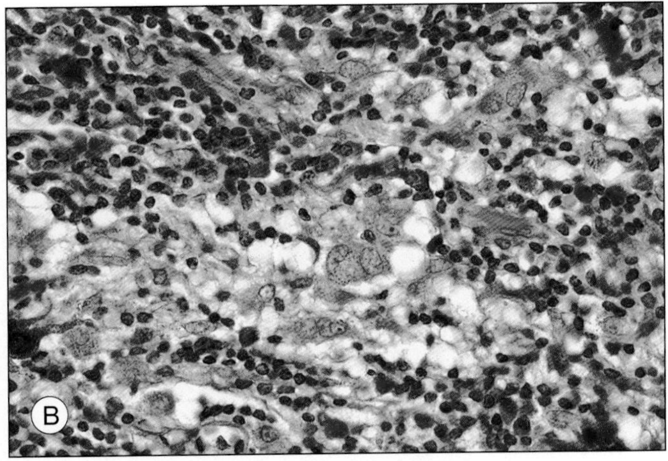

Fig. 74.1 Histopathological aspects of sympathetic ophthalmia. (A) Note granulomatous inflammation of the choroid with focal serous detachment of the retina (hematoxylin and eosin, ×130). (B) Multinucleated giant cells and epithelioid histiocytes have pigment in their cytoplasm (hematoxylin and eosin, ×565).

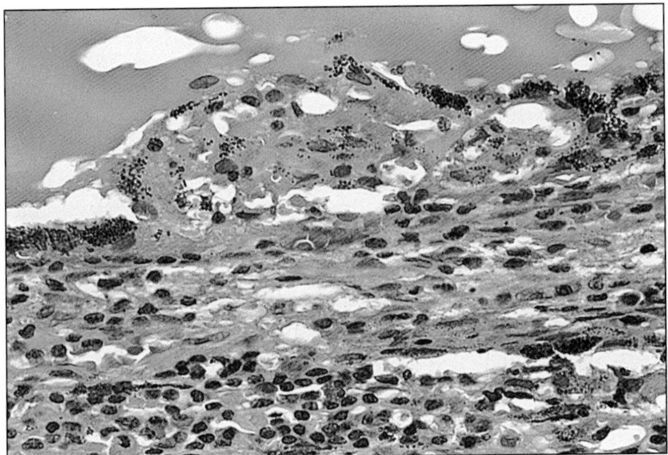

Fig. 74.2 Histopathologically, the Dalen–Fuchs nodule is characterized by focal collections of epithelioid cells at the level of Bruch's membrane (hematoxylin and eosin, ×250).

may also develop in the setting of posttraumatic or postoperative infectious endophthalmitis and it is possible that such infection may potentiate the development of sympathetic ophthalmia in these cases[17] and not prevent it, in contrast to what had previously been suggested.[1,18,19] Most cases of sympathetic ophthalmia however develop in the absence of intraocular infection.[14]

Several investigators have proposed an immunologic basis for sympathetic ophthalmia, in which a T-cell-mediated autoimmune response against an antigenic protein from the uvea, particularly a uveal tyrosinase peptide, may be involved.[20–24] Marak[25,26] and Wong and colleagues[20] demonstrated enhanced transformation of peripheral lymphocytes from patients with histologically confirmed sympathetic ophthalmia when exposed to homologous uveal-retinal extracts in tissue culture, suggesting that these patients have lymphocytes that are sensitized to some component(s) of uveal-retinal antigen. When antigens extracted from the retina are injected into guinea pigs, intraocular inflammation similar to sympathetic ophthalmia develops in these animals.[26] Some studies indeed suggest that sympathetic ophthalmia may result from altered T-cell response to one of the soluble proteins associated with the retinal photoreceptor membranes, particularly the retinal S antigen, or to other retinal or choroidal melanocyte antigens.[21–23,26,27] However, recent studies reveal that T-cell immune response to tyrosinase peptide may play a role in the development of sympathetic ophthalmia, as in Vogt–Koyanagi–Harada disease.[22,28–30]

There may be a genetic predisposition to the development of sympathetic ophthalmia. Human leukocyte antigen (HLA) association has been reported in sympathetic ophthalmia, including HLA-A11, HLA-B40, HLA-DR4/DRw53, and HLA-DR4/DQw3 haplotypes.[31,32] Studies from Asia and Europe found a significant correlation between HLA-DRB1*4 and HLA-DQB1*04 and the development of sympathetic ophthalmia.[33–35] A similar association was also seen in patients with Vogt–Koyanagi–Harada disease. Finally, genetic background may also correlate to disease severity, either through some of those predisposing HLA haplotypes such as HLA-DRB1[33] or through cytokine polymorphisms such as in interleukin-10, modifying the immune response and the risk of disease recurrence.[36]

IMMUNOPATHOLOGY

In sympathetic ophthalmia the immunopathologic alterations are similar in both the exciting and sympathizing eyes and typically consist of a diffuse granulomatous inflammation of the uveal tract, made up of lymphocytes, plasma cells, and nests of epithelioid histiocytes; pigment is often present within these epithelioid cells and also within giant cells (Fig. 74.1). In the majority of cases, the inflammatory process does not involve the choriocapillaris or the retina. Absence of necrosis is another characteristic feature. The choroid is diffusely involved and thickened by an infiltration of predominantly lymphocytes, collections of epithelioid cells, and a few giant cells; neutrophils are rarely seen. Plasma cells may be present, particularly in patients treated with corticosteroids. Eosinophils can also be found and are frequently concentrated in the inner choroid, particularly in heavily pigmented individuals. Nodular clusters of epithelioid cells containing pigment are often seen lying between the retinal pigment epithelium (RPE) and Bruch's membrane; these appear clinically as the drusen-like, yellow-white dots known as Dalen–Fuchs nodules (Fig. 74.2).[1,2,4,13,14,37,38] Infiltration of the pars plana of the ciliary body occurs early in the course of disease, and the inflammatory cells from this site may spill over into the vitreous

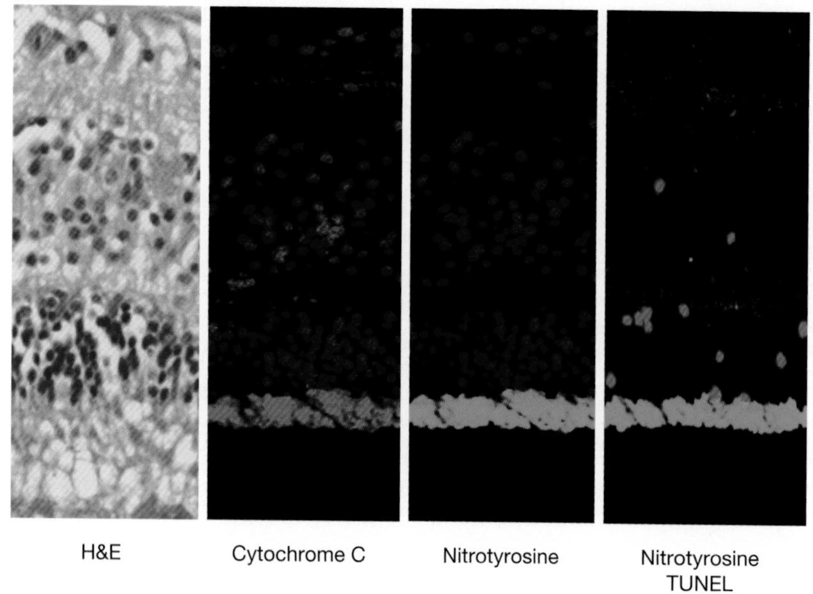

Fig. 74.3 Mitochondrial oxidative stress and apoptosis in the human retina with sympathetic ophthalmia. Cytochrome C and nitrotyrosine are immunolocalized in the inner segments (IS) of the photoreceptors. Apoptotic neurons marked by terminal deoxynucleotidyl transferase-mediated dUTP nick end labeling (TUNEL) assay are detected primarily in the outer nuclear layer (ONL), and also in the inner nuclear layer (INL), but not in the ganglion cell layer (GCL). The corresponding hematoxylin and eosin (H&E)-stained section is seen on the left.[45]

cavity. Similar inflammatory cell infiltration in the iris may result in the clinical appearance of a thickened iris.

The retina is usually free of inflammatory infiltrates. However, few enucleated eyes of sympathetic ophthalmia show collections of mononuclear cells around the blood vessels, and occasional involvement in the areas overlying the Dalen–Fuchs nodules, and in the pars plana region. Other pathologic changes include scleral involvement with inflammatory infiltrates around the emissary veins and extension of the granulomatous process into the optic nerve and surrounding meningeal sheaths, the sites where melanocytes are also present.[1,4,14,39] Some of the eyes with characteristic histologic features of sympathetic ophthalmia but also with breaks in the lens capsule may additionally reveal features of phacoanaphylaxis, with zonal granulomatous inflammation around the lens material.[39] Even though typical features of sympathetic ophthalmia include nonnecrotizing granulomatous uveitis, there are cases exhibiting atypical features such as nongranulomatous choroiditis or chorioretinal adhesions with the inflammatory process involving the choriocapillaris, as seen in chronic Vogt–Koyanagi–Harada disease.[13,39]

Immunohistochemical studies have revealed infiltration of predominantly T lymphocytes in the uveal tract.[37,40] B lymphocytes may also be present, especially in longstanding disease.[41,42] Among the T lymphocytes, both helper (CD4+) and suppressor/cytotoxic (CD8+) cells have been observed,[37,40] driving a Th1 response with secretion of proinflammatory cytokines such as interferon-γ and interleukin-2.[43] These cells are probably recruited to the eye by the selective expression of intercellular adhesion proteins in the uveal tract (particularly some integrins),[44] as well as some other molecules in macrophages and RPE cells, including chemokines, such as monocyte chemotactic protein-1 (CCL2/MCP-1) and stromal cell-derived factor-1 (CXCL12/SDF-1), and metalloproteinases, such as gelatinase-B.[42] Relative preservation of the choriocapillaries in the acute phase of the disease process may be associated with secretion of anti-inflammatory cytokines by the RPE.[27] A recent study has interestingly shown CD4+ T lymphocytes and melanin-laden macrophages expressing HLA-DR underneath the conjunctiva in the exciting eye, suggesting that antigen processing and presentation may initially take place at that site, further leading to activation of lymphocytes and to the granulomatous response.[45]

Even though the retina seems to be relatively spared in the pathologic process of sympathetic ophthalmia, tumor necrosis factor (TNF)-α-mediated mitochondrial oxidative stress has recently been localized in the outer retina of enucleated human globes with the disease (Fig. 74.3). This was associated with apoptosis of photoreceptors and probably such photoreceptor damage could be a mechanism leading to vision loss in sympathetic ophthalmia.[46]

CLINICAL FINDINGS

The clinical onset of sympathetic ophthalmia is typically heralded by the development of an apparently mild intraocular inflammation in the sympathizing eye and worsening of inflammation in the exciting eye. The interval between the time of injury and the onset of inflammation in the sympathizing eye has been reported to be as short as 5 days and as long as 66 years after trauma.[1,3,47] In general, however, sympathetic ophthalmia rarely develops sooner than 2 weeks after trauma, with 80% of cases occurring within 3 months and 90% within 1 year of the penetrating injury.[2,7,9] The peak incidence occurs between 4 and 8 weeks after accidental trauma, while cases following surgical trauma may have a more delayed onset.[48]

Symptoms in the sympathizing eye include mild pain, photophobia, and increased lacrimation, blurring of vision, visual fatigue, or even paresis of accommodation. The exciting eye may have a decrease in vision and an increase in photophobia. Moreover, both eyes may show ciliary injection and a partially dilated and poorly responsive pupil.[1,2,8,9]

The clinical signs are variable and can be either insidious or fairly rapid in onset. Anterior-segment changes are those of an anterior uveitis, with ciliary injection, keratic precipitates, flare, and inflammatory cells in the anterior chamber. Thickening of the iris and even iris nodules may also be seen and posterior synechiae are common. Posterior-segment findings in sympathetic ophthalmia include inflammatory cell infiltration of the vitreous, hyperemia and edema of the optic disc, diffuse edema

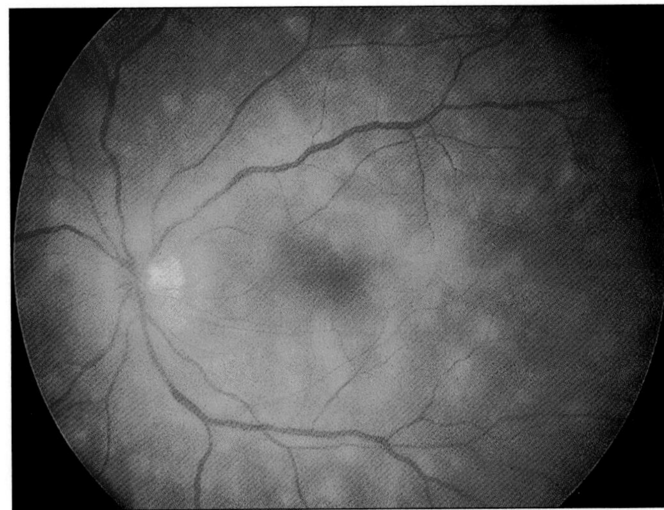

Fig. 74.4 Multiple choroidal granulomas in sympathetic ophthalmia.

and exudative detachment of the retina, as well as small yellow-white deposits beneath the RPE, so-called Dalen–Fuchs nodules.[1,2,8,9,13,14] Bullous serous detachments may also be seen in the peripheral retina. Occasionally, multiple deep ill-defined yellowish lesions may be present, corresponding to choroidal granulomas (Fig. 74.4). Inflammatory scleral involvement is rarely seen clinically, but is a common finding on microscopic examination of enucleated eyes. With time, patients may develop depigmentation of the choroid leading to the so-called sunset glow fundus, as well as RPE changes, as seen in individuals with chronic Vogt–Koyanagi–Harada disease.[49,50] Although less commonly than in Vogt–Koyanagi–Harada disease, extraocular involvement - including meningismus, dysacusis, vitiligo, poliosis, and alopecia - may also be present in patients with sympathetic ophthalmia.[2,49,51]

DIAGNOSIS

The diagnosis of sympathetic ophthalmia is essentially clinical.[1,2,9] No serologic or immunologic tests are available to aid in the diagnosis. Even though there are no systematized diagnostic criteria, the presence of penetrating ocular trauma (either accidental or surgical) is a fundamental feature. Bilateral intraocular inflammation should also be present, and may be accompanied by exudative retinal detachments and/or optic disc edema early in the disease process, or by choroidal depigmentation (sunset glow fundus) and RPE changes in chronic cases, similarly to Vogt–Koyanagi–Harada disease.[52] However, variations in this clinical presentation can challenge or delay the diagnosis. Some imaging studies, such as fluorescein angiography, indocyanine green angiography, B-scan ultrasound, as well as optical coherence tomography (OCT), may be helpful to disclose or delineate better some supportive features of sympathetic ophthalmia.

Fluorescein angiography may typically show multiple progressively fluorescent dots at the level of the RPE (pinpoint leakage; Fig. 74.5), as well as disc leakage, as also seen in Vogt–Koyanagi–Harada disease. Coalescence of the dye from these foci occurs in the areas of exudative detachment.[2,53,54] Less frequently there may also be early focal blockage of the background choroidal fluorescence, a finding also noted in acute posterior multifocal placoid pigment epitheliopathy.[55] On indocyanine green angiography, numerous hypofluorescent patches may be visible during the intermediate phase, presumably corresponding to the choroidal granulomas. Some of these may become isofluorescent at the later phases.[56–58]

Ultrasound examination may reveal choroidal thickening and also areas of exudative retinal detachment, being particularly useful in the exciting eyes with opaque media.[9,17] Usually the choroidal thickening is more prominent around the optic disc and less in the anterior choroid. OCT can nicely delineate the foci of exudative retinal detachment, their resolution following appropriate therapy (Fig. 74.6), as well as other progressive changes in the neurosensory retina and in the RPE.[55,59,60]

Especially in those severely traumatized eyes that later require enucleation, histopathologic examination may help to make or confirm the diagnosis.[2,14,17,39]

DIFFERENTIAL DIAGNOSIS

Sympathetic ophthalmia must be differentiated from several infectious and also other noninfectious uveitides, including syphilis, tuberculosis, sarcoidosis, multifocal choroiditis, and panuveitis. Other bacterial and fungal infections can also produce a granulomatous anterior and/or posterior uveitis, being usually differentiated by history and associated clinical findings. Infectious endophthalmitis must always be considered following any penetrating trauma to the eye. In particular, less virulent microorganisms such as *Propionibacterium acnes* and some fungi may lead to a picture of chronic endophthalmitis, which should be distinguished from sympathetic ophthalmia. Reactivation of a preexisting uveitis after injury or the development of a posttraumatic iritis or iridocyclitis can also occur.[2,9]

Phacoanaphylatic endophthalmitis can also closely simulate the clinical picture of sympathetic ophthalmia and these two entities may even coexist in the same eye. Although unilaterality can be a clue, phacoanaphylaxis may also be bilateral but such bilaterality is rare. The incidence of phacoanaphylaxis in cases of sympathetic ophthalmia has been estimated to range between 4 and 25%. Unlike sympathetic ophthalmia, in bilateral phacoanaphylaxis the eye first involved is usually quiet by the time inflammation begins in the fellow eye. Moreover ultrasound examination usually reveals predominant thickening of the anterior uveal tract in phacoanaphylactic endophthalmitis, in contrast to sympathetic ophthalmia, in which such thickening is more pronounced in the posterior uveal tract. A careful slit-lamp examination should always be carried out to search for ruptured lens capsule and fragments of lens cortex in the anterior chamber. In phacoanaphylactic endophthalmitis, lens extraction can be curative, thereby avoiding unnecessary enucleation.[17,61]

Vogt–Koyanagi–Harada syndrome is a bilateral granulomatous panuveitis, often associated with a prodrome of meningeal and auditory symptoms. The disease may have clinical and histopathologic features identical to sympathetic ophthalmia in both the acute and in the chronic phase. However, findings such as vitiligo and alopecia are more common in Vogt–Koyanagi–Harada syndrome than in sympathetic ophthalmia. A history of penetrating trauma is helpful in this differential diagnosis.[2,49,50]

COURSE AND COMPLICATIONS

Untreated sympathetic ophthalmia runs a long, variable, and complicated course, marked initially by episodes of active intraocular inflammation followed by quiescent periods that can last

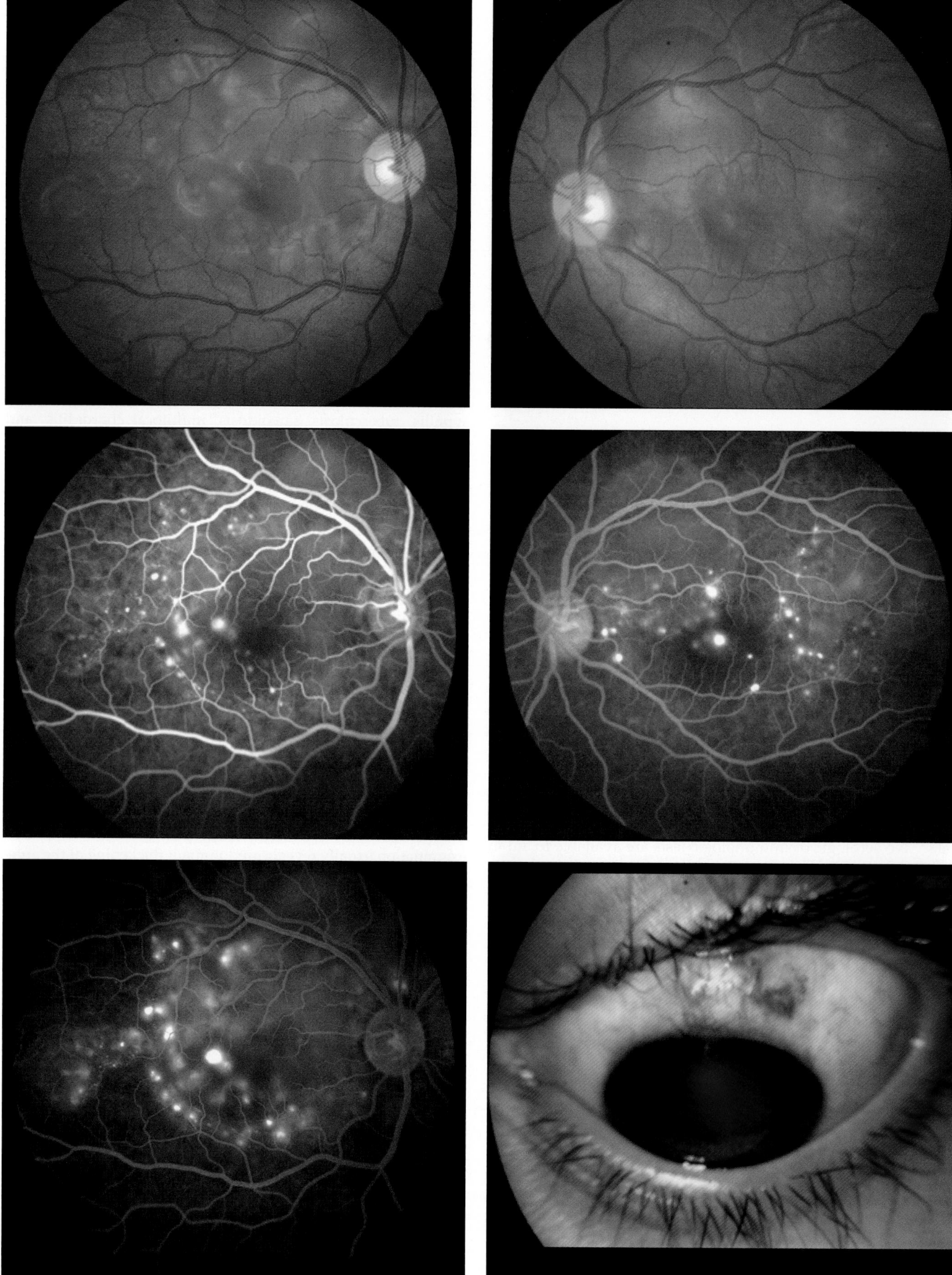

Fig. 74.5 Fundus and angiographic features of sympathetic ophthalmia following a penetrating scleral injury in the left eye. Foci of exudative retinal detachment are seen in the posterior pole of both eyes. Fluorescein angiography reveals multiple pinpoint leaks at the level of the retinal pigment epithelium.

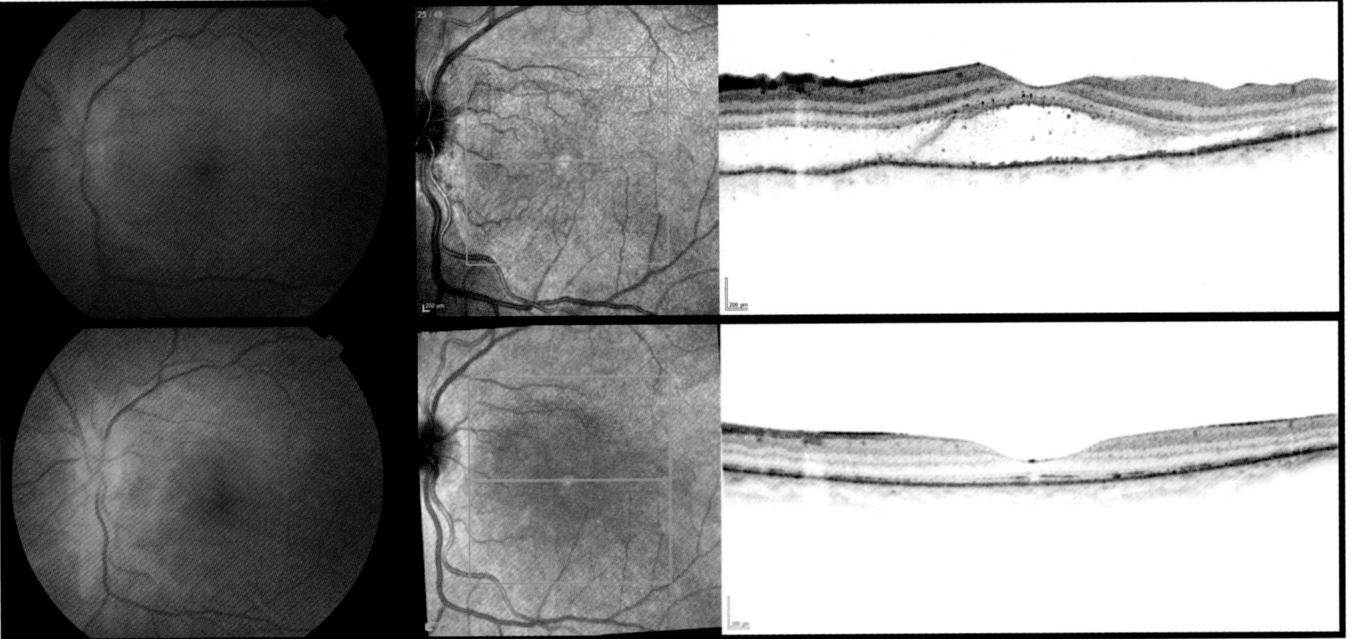

Fig. 74.6 Fundus and tomographic features of sympathetic ophthalmia before (top) and 2 months after (bottom) appropriate treatment with high-dose oral corticosteroid. Complete resolution of the exudative retinal detachment is seen. (Courtesy of Centro Brasileiro de Ciências Visuais, Belo Horizonte, Brazil.)

months to several years. With time, the disease may become chronically active, eventually producing irreversible ocular damage and even phthisis bulbi. Long-term complications of sympathetic ophthalmia include cataract, secondary ocular hypertension or hypotony, glaucoma, persistent cystoid macular edema or retinal detachment, chorioretinal scarring (including epiretinal membrane formation), choroidal neovascularization, subretinal fibrosis, and optic atrophy.[2,14,62] In spite of treatment, the overall risk of developing any of these ocular complications reaches 40% per patient per year, with around half of the patients losing vision to <20/40 and roughly one-fourth eventually becoming legally blind.[48]

THERAPY

Although corticosteroids have not been shown to be effective in the prevention of sympathetic ophthalmia, they do constitute the mainstay of its therapy.[2,6,8] Large doses of corticosteroids should be given early in the course of the disease and continued for at least 6 months. For the first week, 1.5–2.0 mg/kg of body weight of oral prednisone (or equivalent) is given daily and then gradually tapered over several months, following clinical response of the uveitis. Alternatively, pulse therapy with intravenous methylprednisolone (up to 1 g daily for 3 days), as well as supplementation with sub-Tenon's injection of triamcinolone acetonide (20–40 mg), may be considered. Topical corticosteroids and mydriatic/cycloplegic agents are used adjunctively as needed. Special care should be taken to monitor side-effects of the systemic corticosteroids, including periodic measurement of blood pressure, body weight, lipids, blood glucose, as well as gastroduodenal protection and prophylaxis of osteoporosis (with calcium and vitamin D supplementation).[63]

In a number of patients, medical problems or systemic or ophthalmologic complications may prevent the long-term use of high doses of steroids. In these patients, supplemental treatment with immunosuppressive agents (azathioprine, 2–4 mg/kg/day; cyclosporine, 2.5–5 mg/kg/day; mycophenolate mofetil, 1–1.5 g bid; methotrexate, 15–25 mg/week) has been shown to suppress inflammation effectively, allow reduction of corticosteroid therapy to nontoxic levels (<10 mg/day), and, in some cases, induce disease remission. These drugs are usually started as monotherapy, but can be combined or switched in case of lack of adequate response.[6,8] Careful monitoring of their side-effects every 4–6 weeks, with the supervision of an internist, is recommended. Bone marrow suppression, renal and/or hepatic toxicity can occur with prolonged use of these agents.[63] The alkylating agents cyclophosphamide (2–3 mg/kg/day) and chlorambucil (0.1–0.2 mg/kg/day) are reserved for more severe and refractory cases.[63,64] These agents require careful monitoring for side-effects, including hemorrhagic urinary bladder inflammation and development of malignancies.

Biologicals, particularly anti-TNF agents such as infliximab and adalimumab, may also be used in cases of sympathetic ophthalmia that are unresponsive to conventional immunomodulatory agents and, in this setting, favorable results have been anecdotally reported in the recent literature.[65,66] However the long-term safety of these agents is still uncertain.[67]

Intraocular corticosteroids, either administered as intravitreal injections (triamcinolone acetonide 4 mg) or as slow-release devices, such as fluocinolone or dexamethasone intravitreal implants, may also be used, especially in individuals who cannot tolerate the systemic medications.[68–70] Special concern should be given to the high risk of cataract and secondary glaucoma associated with these intravitreal devices.

PREVENTION

The prevention of sympathetic ophthalmia entails careful microsurgical wound toilet and prompt closure of all penetrating injuries. Every attempt should be made to save any eye with a reasonable prognosis for useful vision, but in those eyes with barely discernible or no visual function, and with demonstrable disorganization of the ocular contents, enucleation within 2 weeks after injury is possibly the only way to definitely prevent the development of sympathetic ophthalmia.[3] At one time it was believed that the use of steroids following penetrating injury would in some instances prevent the development of sympathetic ophthalmia; this has not been proved to be the case.

Enucleation of the exciting eye once sympathetic ophthalmia has commenced has been a topic of considerable controversy. Some studies suggest that early enucleation of the exciting eye may improve the prognosis for the sympathizing eye[14,71]; however careful review of the data presented in these studies does not support this conclusion.[72] A review by Winter of 257 cases of histologically proven sympathetic ophthalmia indicated no benefit to the sympathizing eye from enucleation of the exciting eye, whether performed briefly before, concomitant with, or subsequent to the development of sympathetic ophthalmia at various elapsed intervals following injury.[13] This was also supported by the results of a prospective study.[6] Indeed, it is possible that the exciting eye may eventually provide the better visual acuity, and its enucleation would therefore deprive the patient of that visual potential.[72]

Another controversy is the possible role of evisceration versus enucleation. Even though evisceration may be technically easier and provides a faster recovery,[73] it seems not to protect against the development of sympathetic ophthalmia, probably because of retention of uveal remnants in the scleral shell.[74] Many cases of sympathetic ophthalmia following evisceration have been described in the older literature,[74,75] but it is not clear whether those larger rates were biased by the more limited resources for primary repair of those globes at the time of injury. Sympathetic ophthalmia after evisceration is probably rarer nowadays, but recent cases have been anecdotally reported.[76–79] Because this is far less common than in the past,[80,81] and management of sympathetic ophthalmia has significantly improved,[6,8,9] an issue raises whether evisceration should indeed be preferred to enucleation, particularly in blind eyes, after severe trauma and/or infection. This issue is not yet resolved,[73] especially considering the very low incidence of sympathetic ophthalmia and the changing trend from posttraumatic to postsurgical cases.[7,8] An additional complication to this controversy is the risk of inadvertently eviscerating occult tumors,[82] which may even outweigh the risk of sympathetic ophthalmia per se. It is advisable that patients with penetrating ocular injuries, as well as those undergoing intraocular surgeries with an increased risk of sympathetic ophthalmia (such as pars plana vitrectomy), are counseled about the possibility of developing the disease, early or even long after the traumatic or surgical insult.

PROGNOSIS

Before the use of corticosteroids, the visual prognosis of sympathetic ophthalmia was generally poor. However, after the advent of the corticosteroids and more recently of immunosuppressive agents, this prognosis dramatically improved.[8,9] Makley and Azar found that, in patients treated solely with systemic corticosteroids, a visual acuity of 20/60 or better was achieved in most of them, but relapses occurred in 60%, sometimes long after initial disease remission.[62] Chan et al. reported visual acuity of 20/40 or better in 50% of patients treated with steroids and immunosuppressive agents.[83] With prompt and aggressive corticosteroid therapy, and immunosuppressive agents, as needed, many eyes with sympathetic ophthalmia should retain reasonable vision.

In conclusion, sympathetic ophthalmia is a serious entity, often with many exacerbations and a relentlessly progressive course that may result in very poor vision. Cases associated with penetrating accidental trauma have been decreasing with improved repair of such globes, but, on the other hand, those following intraocular (particularly vitreoretinal) surgery are on the rise. Long-term follow-up of these patients is essential. It is hoped that, with the prompt and aggressive use of corticosteroids early in the course of the disease, and supplementation with immunosuppressive agents when indicated, the prognosis in these patients need not to be as grim as it had been in the past.

REFERENCES

1. Duke-Elder S. Sympathetic ophthalmitis. In: Duke-Elder S, editor. System of ophthalmology. vol 9. St Louis: Mosby; 1966. p. 558–93.
2. Goto H, Rao NA. Sympathetic ophthalmia and Vogt–Koyanagi–Harada syndrome. Int Ophthalmol Clin 1990;30:279–85.
3. Albert DM, Diaz-Rohena R. A historical review of sympathetic ophthalmia and its epidemiology. Surv Ophthalmol 1989;34:1–14.
4. Fuchs E. Über sympathisierende Entzündung (nebst Bemerkungen über seröse traumatische Iritis). Graefes Arch Ophthalmol 1905;61:365–456.
5. Liddy L, Stuart J. Sympathetic ophthalmia in Canada. Can J Ophthalmol 1972;7:157–9.
6. Kilmartin DJ, Dick AD, Forrester JV. Prospective surveillance of sympathetic ophthalmia in the UK and Republic of Ireland. Br J Ophthalmol 2000;84:259–63.
7. Sen HN, Nussenblatt RB. Sympathetic ophthalmia: what have we learned? Am J Ophthalmol 2009;148:632–3.
8. Vote BJ, Hall A, Cairns J, et al. Changing trends in sympathetic ophthalmia. Clin Experiment Ophthalmol 2004;32:542–5.
9. Castiblanco CP, Adelman RA. Sympathetic ophthalmia. Graefes Arch Clin Exp Ophthalmol 2009;247:289–302.
10. Gass JD. Sympathetic ophthalmia following vitrectomy. Am J Ophthalmol 1982;93:552–8.
11. Cha DM, Woo SJ, Ahn J, et al. A case of sympathetic ophthalmia presenting with extraocular symptoms and conjunctival pigmentation after repeated 23-gauge vitrectomy. Ocul Immunol Inflamm 2010;18:265–7.
12. Haruta M, Mukuno H, Nishijima K, et al. Sympathetic ophthalmia after 23-gauge transconjunctival sutureless vitrectomy. Clin Ophthalmol 2010;4:1347–9.
13. Winter FC. Sympathetic uveitis; a clinical and pathologic study of the visual result. Am J Ophthalmol 1955;39:340–7.
14. Lubin JR, Albert DM, Weinstein M. Sixty-five years of sympathetic ophthalmia. A clinicopathologic review of 105 cases (1913–1978). Ophthalmology 1980;87:109–21.
15. Buller AJ, Doris JP, Bonshek R, et al. Sympathetic ophthalmia following severe fungal keratitis. Eye 2006;20:1306–7.
16. Guerriero S, Montepara A, Ciraci L, et al. A case of sympathetic ophthalmia after a severe *Acanthamoeba* keratitis. Eye Contact Lens 2011;37:374–6.
17. Rathinam SR, Rao NA. Sympathetic ophthalmia following postoperative bacterial endophthalmitis: a clinicopathologic study. Am J Ophthalmol 2006;141:498–507.
18. Woods AC. Sympathetic ophthalmia: part 2. Am J Ophthalmol 1936;19:100–9.
19. Samuels B. Panophthalmitis and sympathetic ophthalmia. Arch Ophthalmol 1938;20:804–11.
20. Wong VG, Anderson R, O'Brien PJ. Sympathetic ophthalmia and lymphocyte transformation. Am J Ophthalmol 1971;72:960–6.
21. Rao NA, Robin J, Hartmann D, et al. The role of the penetrating wound in the development of sympathetic ophthalmia: experimental observations. Arch Ophthalmol 1983;101:102–4.
22. Sugita S, Sagawa K, Mochizuki M, et al. Melanocyte lysis by cytotoxic T lymphocytes recognizing the MART-1 melanoma antigen in HLA-A2 patients with Vogt–Koyanagi–Harada disease. Int Immunol 1996;8:799–803.
23. Hammer H. Cellular hypersensitivity to uveal pigment confirmed by leucocyte migration tests in sympathetic ophthalmitis and the Vogt–Koyanagi–Harada syndrome. Br J Ophthalmol 1974;58:773–6.
24. Rao NA, Wong VG. Aetiology of sympathetic ophthalmitis. Trans Ophthalmol Soc U K 1981;101:357–60.
25. Marak GE Jr. Recent advances in sympathetic ophthalmia. Surv Ophthalmol 1979;24:141–56.
26. Rao NA, Wacker WB, Marak GE Jr. Experimental allergic uveitis: clinicopathologic features associated with varying doses of S antigen. Arch Ophthalmol 1979;97:1954–8.
27. Rao NA. Mechanisms of inflammatory response in sympathetic ophthalmia and VKH syndrome. Eye 1997;11:213–6.
28. Yamaki K, Ohono S. Animal models of Vogt–Koyanagi–Harada disease (sympathetic ophthalmia). Ophthalmic Res 2008;40:129–35.

29. Yamaki K, Gocho K, Hayakawa K, et al. Tyrosinase family proteins are antigens specific to Vogt–Koyanagi–Harada disease. J Immunol 2000;165:7323–9.
30. Kawakami Y, Suzuki Y, Shofuda T, et al. T cell immune responses against melanoma and melanocytes in cancer and autoimmunity. Pigment Cell Res 2000;13(Suppl 8):163–9.
31. Reynard M, Shulman IA, Azen SP, et al. Histocompatibility antigens in sympathetic ophthalmia. Am J Ophthalmol 1983;95:216–21.
32. Azen SP, Marak GE Jr, Minckler DS, et al. Histocompatibility antigens in sympathetic ophthalmia. Am J Ophthalmol 1984;98:117–9.
33. Kilmartin DJ, Wilson D, Liversidge J, et al. Immunogenetics and clinical phenotype of sympathetic ophthalmia in British and Irish patients. Br J Ophthalmol 2001;85:281–6.
34. Shindo Y, Ohno S, Usui M, et al. Immunogenetic study of sympathetic ophthalmia. Tissue Antigens 1997;49:111–5.
35. Tiercy JM, Rathinam SR, Gex-Fabry M, et al. A shared HLA-DRB1 epitope in the DR beta first domain is associated with Vogt–Koyanagi–Harada syndrome in Indian patients. Mol Vis 2010;16:353–8.
36. Atan D, Turner SJ, Kilmartin DJ, et al. Cytokine gene polymorphism in sympathetic ophthalmia. Invest Ophthalmol Vis Sci 2005;46:4245–50.
37. Chan CC, Nussenblatt RB, Fujikawa LS, et al. Sympathetic ophthalmia. Immunopathological findings. Ophthalmology 1986;93:690–5.
38. Kuo PK, Lubin JR, Ni C, et al. Sympathetic ophthalmia: a comparison of the histopathological features from a Chinese and American series. Int Ophthalmol Clin 1982;22:125–39.
39. Croxatto JO, Rao NA, McLean IW, et al. Atypical histopathologic features in sympathetic ophthalmia. A study of a hundred cases. Int Ophthalmol 1982;4: 129–35.
40. Jakobiec FA, Marboe CC, Knowles DM 2nd, et al. Human sympathetic ophthalmia. An analysis of the inflammatory infiltrate by hybridoma-monoclonal antibodies, immunochemistry, and correlative electron microscopy. Ophthalmology 1983;90:76–95.
41. Shah DN, Piacentini MA, Burnier MN, et al. Inflammatory cellular kinetics in sympathetic ophthalmia a study of 29 traumatized (exciting) eyes. Ocular Immunol Inflamm 1993;1:255–62.
42. Abu El-Asrar AM, Struyf S, Van den Broeck C, et al. Expression of chemokines and gelatinase B in sympathetic ophthalmia. Eye (Lond) 2007;21:649–57.
43. Hooks JJ, Chan CC, Detrick B. Identification of the lymphokines, interferon-gamma and interleukin-2, in inflammatory eye diseases. Invest Ophthalmol Vis Sci 1988;29:1444–51.
44. Kuppner MC, Liversidge J, McKillop-Smith S, et al. Adhesion molecule expression in acute and fibrotic sympathetic ophthalmia. Curr Eye Res 1993;12: 923–34.
45. Jayaprakash Patil A, Edward DP, Wong M, et al. The role of perivascular melanophage infiltrates in the conjunctiva in sympathetic ophthalmia. Ocul Immunol Inflamm 2011;19:186–91.
46. Parikh JG, Saraswathy S, Rao NA. Photoreceptor oxidative damage in sympathetic ophthalmia. Am J Ophthalmol 2008;146:866–75 e2.
47. Zaharia MA, Lamarche J, Laurin M. Sympathetic uveitis 66 years after injury. Can J Ophthalmol 1984;19:240–3.
48. Galor A, Davis JL, Flynn HW Jr, et al. Sympathetic ophthalmia: incidence of ocular complications and vision loss in the sympathizing eye. Am J Ophthalmol 2009;148:704–10 e2.
49. Rao NA, Marak GE. Sympathetic ophthalmia simulating Vogt–Koyanagi–Harada's disease: a clinico-pathologic study of four cases. Jpn J Ophthalmol 1983;27:506–11.
50. Rao NA. Pathology of Vogt–Koyanagi–Harada disease. Int Ophthalmol 2007; 27:81–5.
51. Comer M, Taylor C, Chen S, et al. Sympathetic ophthalmia associated with high frequent deafness. Br J Ophthalmol 2001;85:496.
52. Read RW, Holland GN, Rao NA, et al. Revised diagnostic criteria for Vogt–Koyanagi–Harada disease: report of an international committee on nomenclature. Am J Ophthalmol 2001;131:647–52.
53. Dreyer WB, Jr., Zegarra H, Zakov ZN, et al. Sympathetic ophthalmia. Am J Ophthalmol 1981;92:816–23.
54. Sharp DC, Bell RA, Patterson E, et al. Sympathetic ophthalmia. Histopathologic and fluorescein angiographic correlation. Arch Ophthalmol 1984;102: 232–5.
55. Correnti AJ, Read RW, Kimble JA, et al. Imaging of Dalen–Fuchs nodules in a likely case of sympathetic ophthalmia by fluorescein angiography and OCT. Ophthalmic Surg Lasers Imaging 2010:1–3.
56. Bernasconi O, Auer C, Zografos L, et al. Indocyanine green angiographic findings in sympathetic ophthalmia. Graefes Arch Clin Exp Ophthalmol 1998; 236:635–8.
57. Saatci AO, Pasa E, Soylev MF, et al. Sympathetic ophthalmia and indocyanine green angiography. Arch Ophthalmol 2004;122:1568–9.
58. Moshfeghi AA, Harrison SA, Ferrone PJ. Indocyanine green angiography findings in sympathetic ophthalmia. Ophthalmic Surg Lasers Imaging 2005;36: 163–6.
59. Gallagher MJ, Yilmaz T, Cervantes-Castaneda RA, et al. The characteristic features of optical coherence tomography in posterior uveitis. Br J Ophthalmol 2007;91:1680–5.
60. Gupta V, Gupta A, Dogra MR, et al. Reversible retinal changes in the acute stage of sympathetic ophthalmia seen on spectral domain optical coherence tomography. Int Ophthalmol 2011;31:105–10.
61. Marak GE Jr. Phacoanaphylactic endophthalmitis. Surv Ophthalmol 1992;36: 325–39.
62. Makley TA Jr, Azar A. Sympathetic ophthalmia. A long-term follow-up. Arch Ophthalmol 1978;96:257–62.
63. Jabs DA, Rosenbaum JT, Foster CS, et al. Guidelines for the use of immunosuppressive drugs in patients with ocular inflammatory disorders: recommendations of an expert panel. Am J Ophthalmol 2000;130:492–513.
64. Tessler HH, Jennings T. High-dose short-term chlorambucil for intractable sympathetic ophthalmia and Behçet's disease. Br J Ophthalmol 1990;74: 353–7.
65. Gupta SR, Phan IT, Suhler EB. Successful treatment of refractory sympathetic ophthalmia in a child with infliximab. Arch Ophthalmol 2011;129:250–2.
66. Menghini M, Frimmel SA, Windisch R, et al. Efficacy of infliximab therapy in two patients with sympathetic ophthalmia. Klin Monbl Augenheilkd 2011; 228:362–3.
67. Keystone EC. Does anti-tumor necrosis factor-α therapy affect risk of serious infection and cancer in patients with rheumatoid arthritis? A review of long-term data. J Rheumatol 2011;38:1552–62.
68. Ozdemir H, Karacorlu M, Karacorlu S. Intravitreal triamcinolone acetonide in sympathetic ophthalmia. Graefes Arch Clin Exp Ophthalmol 2005;243:734–6.
69. Chan RV, Seiff BD, Lincoff HA, et al. Rapid recovery of sympathetic ophthalmia with treatment augmented by intravitreal steroids. Retina 2006;26: 243–7.
70. Mahajan VB, Gehrs KM, Goldstein DA, et al. Management of sympathetic ophthalmia with the fluocinolone acetonide implant. Ophthalmology 2009;116:552–7 e1.
71. Reynard M, Riffenburgh RS, Maes EF. Effect of corticosteroid treatment and enucleation on the visual prognosis of sympathetic ophthalmia. Am J Ophthalmol 1983;96:290–4.
72. Marak GE Jr. Sympathetic ophthalmia. Ophthalmology 1982;89:1291–2.
73. O'Donnell BA, Kersten R, McNab A, et al. Enucleation versus evisceration. Clin Exp Ophthalmol 2005;33:5–9.
74. Ruedemann AD. Sympathetic ophthalmia after evisceration. Trans Am Ophthalmol Soc 1963;61:274–314.
75. Green WR, Maumenee AE, Sanders TE, et al. Sympathetic uveitis following evisceration. Trans Am Acad Ophthalmol Otolaryngol 1972;76:625–44.
76. Griepentrog GJ, Lucarelli MJ, Albert DM, et al. Sympathetic ophthalmia following evisceration: a rare case. Ophthal Plast Reconstr Surg 2005;21: 316–8.
77. Androudi S, Theodoridou A, Praidou A, et al. Sympathetic ophthalmia following postoperative endophthalmitis and evisceration. Hippokratia 2010;14: 131–2.
78. Zhang Y, Zhang MN, Jiang CH, et al. Development of sympathetic ophthalmia following globe injury. Chin Med J 2009;122:2961–6.
79. Freidlin J, Pak J, Tessler HH, et al. Sympathetic ophthalmia after injury in the Iraq war. Ophthal Plast Reconstr Surg 2006;22:133–4.
80. du Toit N, Motala MI, Richards J, et al. The risk of sympathetic ophthalmia following evisceration for penetrating eye injuries at Groote Schuur Hospital. Br J Ophthalmol 2008;92:61–3.
81. Savar A, Andreoli MT, Kloek CE, et al. Enucleation for open globe injury. Am J Ophthalmol 2009;147:595–600 e1.
82. Eagle RC Jr, Grossniklaus HE, Syed N, et al. Inadvertent evisceration of eyes containing uveal melanoma. Arch Ophthalmol 2009;127:141–5.
83. Chan CC, Roberge RG, Whitcup SM, et al. 32 cases of sympathetic ophthalmia. A retrospective study at the National Eye Institute, Bethesda, Md., from 1982 to 1992. Arch Ophthalmol 1995;113:597–600.

Chapter 75

Vogt–Koyanagi–Harada Disease

Hiroshi Goto, P. Kumar Rao, Narsing A. Rao

INTRODUCTION AND HISTORICAL ASPECTS

Vogt–Koyanagi–Harada (VKH) disease is a bilateral granulomatous uveitis often associated with exudative retinal detachment and with extraocular manifestations, such as pleocytosis in the cerebrospinal fluid and, in some cases, vitiligo, poliosis, alopecia, and dysacusis.[1]

Poliosis associated with ocular inflammation was first described by Ali-ibn-Isa, an Arab physician who lived in the 1st century AD (cited by Pattison).[2] This association was reported by Schenkl in 1873,[3] by Hutchinson in 1892,[4] and by Vogt in 1906.[5] Harada described a primary posterior uveitis with exudative retinal detachments in association with cerebrospinal fluid pleocytosis.[6]

Three years later, in 1929, Koyanagi described six patients with bilateral chronic iridocyclitis, patchy depigmentation of the skin, patchy hair loss, and whitening of the hair, especially the eyelashes.[7] This constellation of findings was termed "uveitis with poliosis, vitiligo, alopecia, and dysacusis."[7] Babel in 1932[8] and Bruno and McPherson in 1945 combined the findings of Vogt, Koyanagi, and Harada and suggested that these processes represent a continuum of the same disease,[9] thereafter recognized as Vogt–Koyanagi–Harada syndrome.

When a patient presents with the ocular and the extraocular manifestations, the diagnosis of VKH is made with certainty. However, extraocular manifestations such as dysacusis and cutaneous changes are relatively rare, and the dermatologic changes mainly occur late in the course of the disease.[1,10] Because of the variation in clinical presentations of VKH, the American Uveitis Society (AUS) in 1978 recommended the following diagnostic criteria: (1) the absence of any history of ocular trauma or surgery; and (2) the presence of at least three of the following four signs: (a) bilateral chronic iridocyclitis; (b) posterior uveitis, including exudative retinal detachment, forme fruste of exudative retinal detachment, disc hyperemia or edema and "sunset glow" fundus; (c) neurologic signs of tinnitus, neck stiffness, cranial nerve, or central nervous system disorders, or cerebrospinal fluid pleocytosis; and (d) cutaneous findings of alopecia, poliosis, or vitiligo.[11]

Since VKH manifestations vary depending upon the clinical course, a given patient may not initially present with the features required for the diagnosis of VKH by AUS criteria. Read and Rao recently evaluated the utility of the existing AUS criteria in 71 consecutive patients with VKH who were diagnosed based on the clinical features and the course of the disease, combined with fluorescein angiography with or without utrasonography in selected cases.[12] The authors concluded that AUS criteria for diagnosis of VKH may not be adequate. Taking into account the multisystem nature of VKH and allowing for the different ocular findings present in the early and late stages of the disease, the First International Workshop on VKH proposed revised diagnostic criteria to include clinical manifestations at various stages of disease.[13] These revised diagnostic criteria are summarized in Box 75.1.

In the past, constellation of these ocular signs and symptoms warranted the term "syndrome," but in recent years the entity has been well characterized; thereafter the International Workshop on VKH adopted the term Vogt–Koyanagi–Harada disease.[13]

EPIDEMIOLOGY

The incidence of VKH is variable. It appears to be more common in Japan, where it accounts for 6.7% of all uveitis referrals.[14] In the USA it accounts for 1–4% of all uveitis clinic referrals.

VKH tends to affect more pigmented races, such as Asians, Hispanics, American Indians, and Asian Indians.[1,15] In the USA there appears to be variability in the racial distribution of patients with VKH disease.[1,11,16,17] In northern California VKH was seen mainly in Asians (41%), followed by whites (29%), Hispanics (16%), and blacks (14%).[17] In contrast, reports from southern California show that 78% of VKH patients were Hispanic while 3% were white, 10% were Asian, and 6% were black.[1] A series reported from the National Institutes of Health (NIH) showed that 50% of VKH patients were white, 35% were black, and 13% were Hispanic.[17] However, most of those patients reported in the NIH series had remote American Indian ancestry. Most studies report that women tend to be affected more frequently than men; however, Japanese investigators have not found such a female predilection.[15] Most patients are in their second to fifth decades of life, but children may also be affected.[1,18]

CLINICAL DESCRIPTION

Typical clinical features of VKH include bilateral panuveitis associated with exudative retinal detachment, meningism associated with headache and pleocytosis of cerebrospinal fluid, tinnitus or hearing loss, and cutaneous changes, such as alopecia, poliosis, and vitiligo. However, all of these extraocular features are rarely seen during the initial presentation, and the clinical features vary depending upon the stage of the disease as well as the effect of medical treatment. Presence of ocular and two or more extraocular features is considered as a complete form of VKH disease.[13] Incomplete VKH disease includes bilateral

Box 75.1 The revised diagnostic criteria proposed by the First International Workshop on Vogt–Koyanagi–Harada (VKH) disease*

A. Complete VKH disease
  1. Bilateral ocular involvement (a or b must be met, depending on the stage of disease when the patient is examined)
    a. Early manifestations of disease
      (1) There must be evidence of a diffuse choroiditis (with or without anterior uveitis, vitreous inflammatory reaction, or optic disc hyperemia), which may manifest as one of the following:
        (a) Focal areas of subretinal fluid, or
        (b) Bullous serous retinal detachments
      (2) With equivocal fundus findings, both of the following must be present as well:
        (a) Focal areas of delay in choroidal perfusion, multifocal areas of pinpoint leakage, large placoid areas of hyperfluorescence, pooling within subretinal fluid, and optic-nerve staining (listed in order of sequential appearance) by fluorescein angiography, and
        (b) Diffuse choroidal thickening, without evidence of posterior scleritis by ultrasonography
    b. Late manifestations of disease
      (1) History suggestive of prior presence of findings from la, and either both (2) and (3) below, or multiple signs from (3):
      (2) Ocular depigmentation (either of the following manifestations is sufficient):
        (a) Sunset glow fundus, or
        (b) Sugiura's sign
      (3) Other ocular signs:
        (a) Nummular chorioretinal depigmented scars, or
        (b) Retinal pigment epithelium clumping and/or migration, or
        (c) Recurrent or chronic anterior uveitis
  2. Neurological/auditory findings (may have resolved by time of examination)
    a. Meningismus (malaise, fever, headache, nausea, abdominal pain, stiffness of the neck and back, or a combination of these factors; headache alone is not sufficient to meet the definition of meningismus, however), or
    b. Tinnitus, or
    c. Cerebrospinal fluid pleoytosis
  3. Integumentary finding (not preceding onset of central nervous system or ocular disease)
    a. Alopecia, or
    b. Poliosis, or
    c. Vitiligo

B. Incomplete VKH disease (point 1 and either 2 or 3 must be present)
  1. Bilateral ocular involvement as defined for complete VKH disease
  2. Neurologic/auditory findings as defined for complete VKH disease above, or
  3. Integumentary findings as defined for complete VKH disease above.

C. Probable VKH disease
  1. Bilateral ocular involvement as defined for complete VKH disease above.

**In all cases there should not be a history of penetrating ocular injury or surgery preceding the initial onset of uveitis and no clinical or laboratory evidence suggestive of other ocular disease criteria.*

(Modified from Read RW, Holland GN, Rao NA et al. Revised diagnostic criteria for Vogt–Koyanagi–Harada disease: report of an international committee on nomenclature. Am J Ophthalmol 2001;131:647–52.[13])

typical ocular involvement plus either neurologic/auditory or cutaneous changes, whereas probable VKH disease is composed of just ocular manifestations.[13] However, some of these probable VKH patients can develop cutaneous manifestations during the chronic or chronic recurrent stage of the disease.

The prodromal stage

Initial manifestations of VKH disease may include non-specific viral-like illness, commonly referred to as a prodromal stage. This stage may last only a few days and may be limited to headaches, nausea, dizziness, fever, orbital pain, and meningism. Light sensitivity and tearing may occur 1–2 days following the above symptoms. These neurological signs include cranial nerve palsies and optic neuritis. Cerebrospinal fluid analysis usually reveals pleocytosis.

The acute uveitic stage

This stage follows the prodromal phase and presents with blurring of vision in both eyes. One eye may be affected first, followed a few days later by the second eye. Despite a delay in symptoms, careful examination will reveal bilateral posterior uveitis. This uveitis consists of thickening of the posterior choroid with elevation of the peripapillary retinochoroidal layer, multiple serous retinal detachments (Fig. 75.1), hyperemia and edema of the optic nerve head.

Rarely VKH disease can present with optic disc hyperemia and edema without serous retinal detachments (Fig. 75.2).

Thickened choroid can be detected by ultrasonography (Fig. 75.3). Alteration in the retinal pigment epithelium (RPE) associated with multifocal choroidal inflammation is easily observed with fluorescein angiography, which reveals hypofluorescent dots at the early phase followed by multiple focal areas of leakage and subretinal fluid accumulation at the late phase (Fig. 75.4).

Indocyanine green angiography (ICGA) (Fig. 75.5) could be useful to evaluate choroidal inflammatory changes such as early choroidal stromal vessel hyperfluorescence and leakage, and hypofluorescent dark dots at the level of the choroid.[19,20]

The inflammation eventually becomes diffuse, extending into the anterior segment and revealing the presence of flare and cells in the anterior chamber. Less commonly, mutton-fat keratic precipitates, small nodules on the iris surface and pupillary margin, may be observed;[1] however, these anterior inflammatory changes are more common in the recurrent phase. The inflammatory infiltrate in the ciliary body and choroid may cause forward displacement of the lens iris diaphragm (Fig. 75.6), leading to acute angle closure glaucoma or annular choroidal detachment.[21,22] These intraocular changes are typically bilateral; rarely, however, the process can be restricted to one eye.[23]

The chronic uveitic stage

The chronic or convalescent stage occurs several weeks after the acute uveitic stage and is characterized by development of vitiligo (Fig. 75.7), poliosis, and depigmentation of the choroids. Perilimbal vitiligo, also known as Sugiura's sign (Fig. 75.8), may develop at this stage among the patients who have melanosis at the palisade of Vogt, such as Japanese patients.[1,13]

Choroidal depigmentation occurs a few months after the uveitic phase. This leads to the characteristic pale disc with a bright red-orange choroid known as sunset glow fundus (Fig. 75.9). In Hispanics, the sunset glow fundus may show foci of RPE changes in the form of hyperpigmentation or hypopigmentation. The juxtapapillary area may show marked depigmentation. At this stage small, yellow, well-circumscribed areas of chorioretinal atrophy may appear, mainly in the inferior midperiphery of the fundus. This convalescent phase may last for several months.

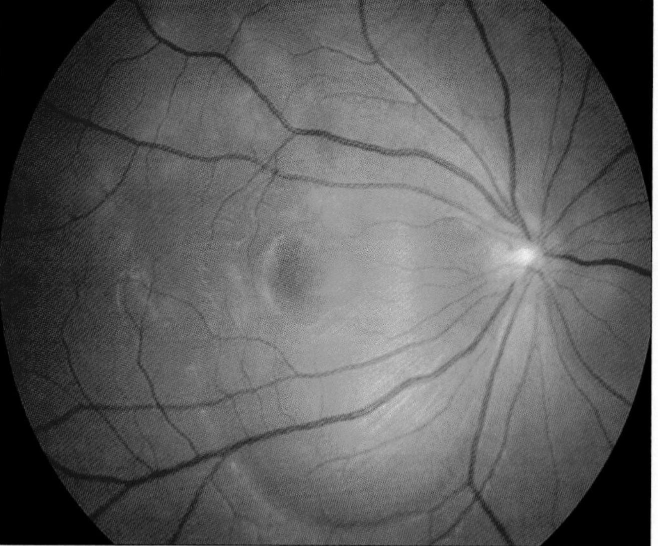
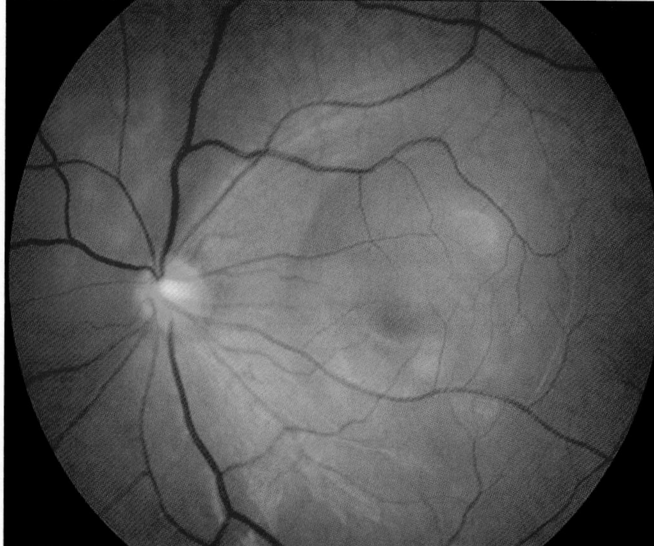

Fig. 75.1 Bilateral multiple serous retinal detachments at the acute uveitis stage of Vogt–Koyanagi–Harada disease.

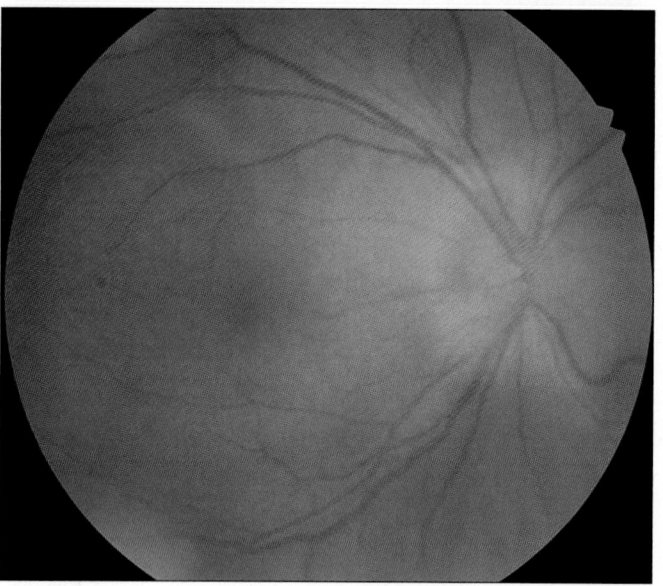
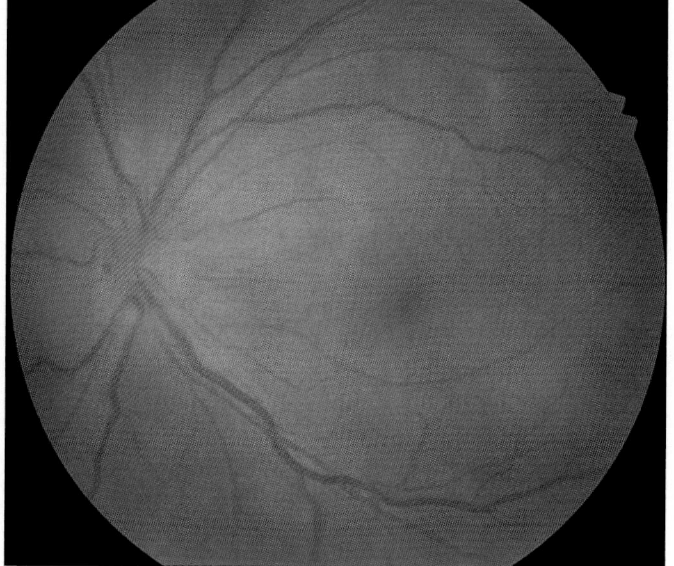

Fig. 75.2 Bilateral hyperemia and edema of the optic disc at the acute uveitis stage of Vogt–Koyanagi–Harada disease without serous retinal detachment.

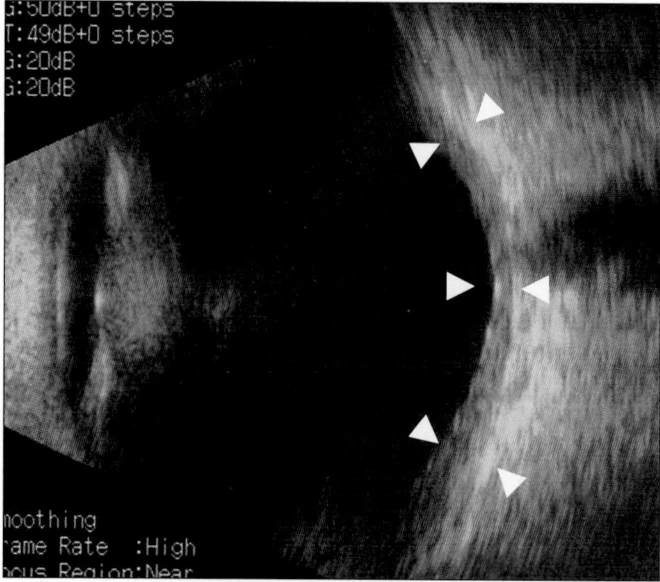

Fig. 75.3 Ultrasonography showing thickened choroid (arrowheads).

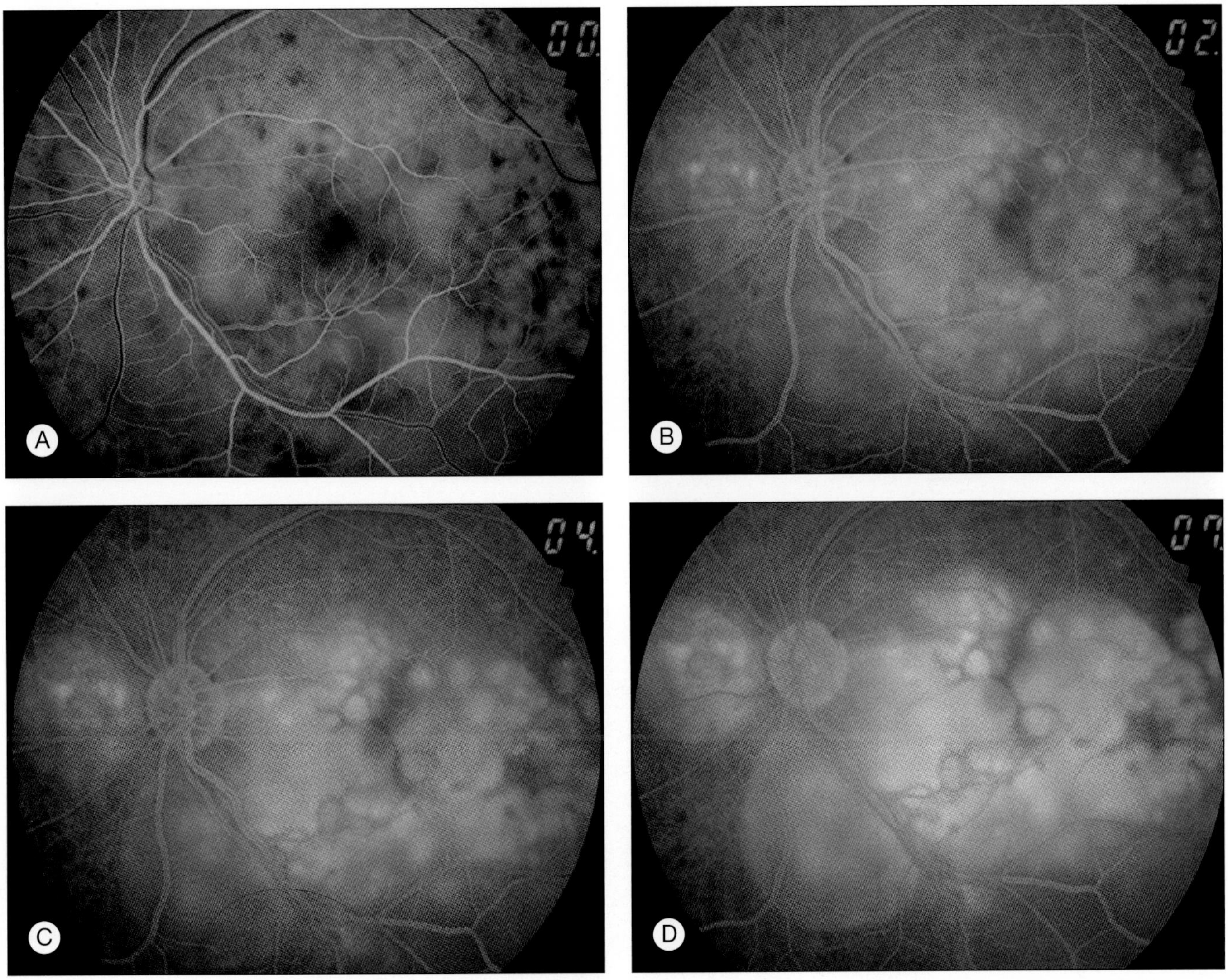

Fig. 75.4 (A) Early arteriovenous phase of fluorescein angiogram exhibiting multiple hypofluorescent dots with irregular hyperfluorescent background. (B) Subsequently, multiple hyperfluorescent dots at the retinal pigment epithelium level are noted. (C) Dye leakage during mid-phase of the angiogram. (D) Subretinal dye pooling at the area of serous retinal detachment during the late phase.

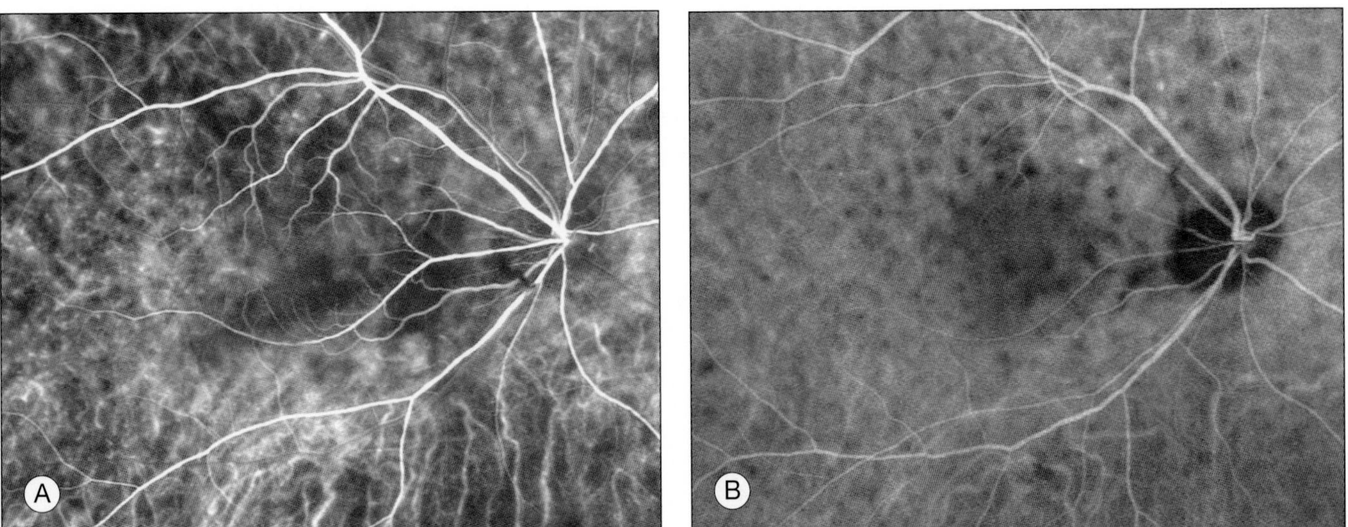

Fig. 75.5 (A) Early phase of the indocyanine green angiogram showing vascular leakage in the choroid. (B) Late phase of angiogram showing multiple hypofluorescent dots.

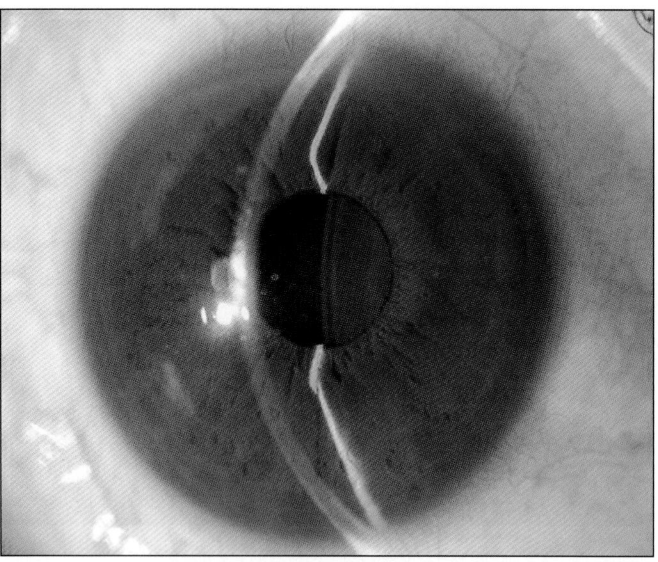

Fig. 75.6 Shallow anterior chamber caused by the anterior displacement of the lens associated with inflammatory infiltrates at the ciliary body.

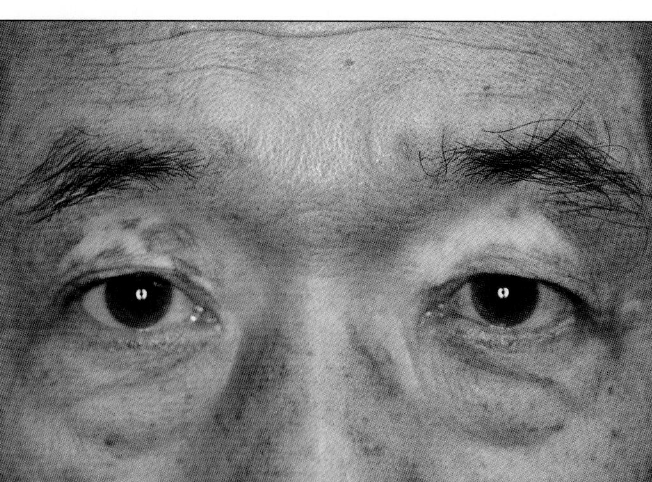

Fig. 75.7 Bilateral upper-eyelid vitiligo.

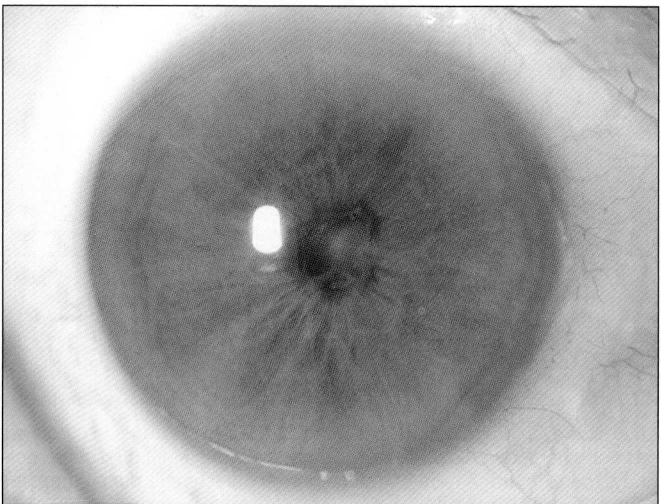

Fig. 75.8 Chronic stage of Vogt–Koyanagi–Harada disease showing extensive posterior synechiae and loss of pigment at the limbus (Sugiura's sign).

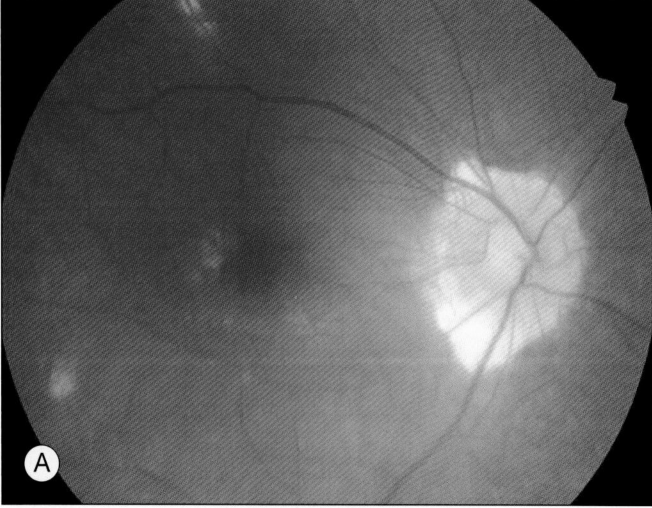

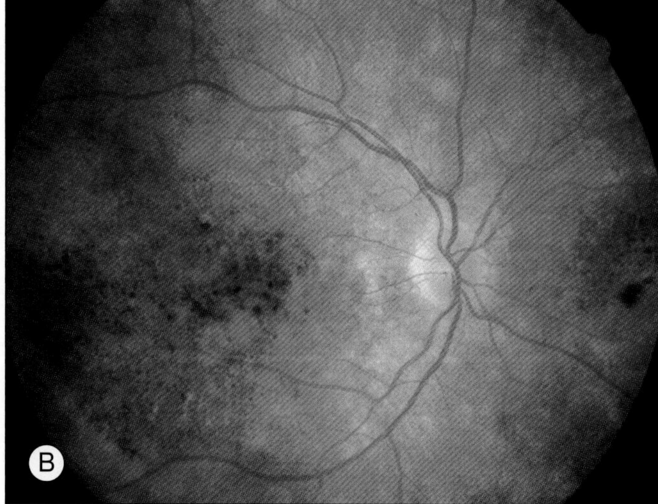

Fig. 75.9 Chronic stage of Vogt–Koyanagi–Harada disease revealing sunset glow fundus with juxtapapillary depigmentation and oval retinal pigment epithelium atrophic lesions in an Asian patient (A) and in a Hispanic patient (B).

The chronic recurrent stage

The chronic recurrent stage consists of a smoldering panuveitis with acute episodic exacerbations of granulomatous anterior uveitis. Recurrent posterior uveitis with exudative retinal detachment is uncommon. The anterior uveitis may be resistant to local and systemic corticosteroid therapy. Iris nodules may be seen during this phase (Fig. 75.10). The most visually debilitating complication of the chronic inflammation during this stage appears to be the development of subretinal neovascular membranes.[24] Posterior subcapsular cataract, as well as glaucoma, either angle closure or open angle, and posterior synechiae, may also be seen.[25,26] Recurrence of the intraocular inflammation may lead to extensive chorioretinal atrophy.

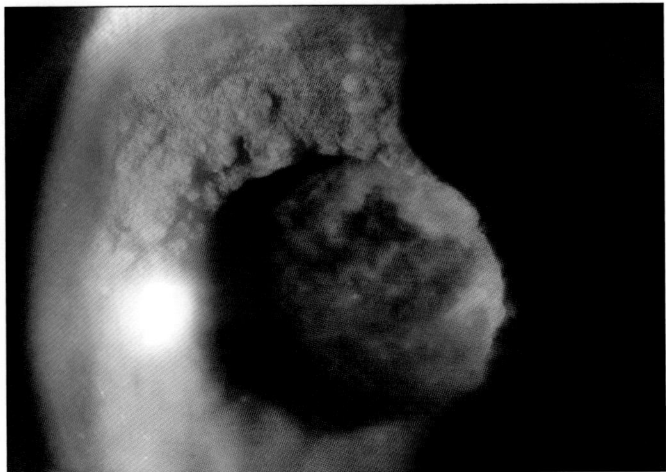

Fig. 75.10 Multiple iris nodules at the iris in chronic recurrent stage.

Frequency of distinguishing clinical features

Clinical features of ocular and extraocular manifestations of 180 patients with VKH disease and 967 patients with non-VKH disease analyzed by stepwise logistic regression models are listed in Table 75.1.[27] In the acute stage, exudative retinal detachment was most likely to be found, whereas in the chronic stage, sunset glow fundus was most common. Prevalence of sunset glow fundus can be low (67.5%) in patients treated with systemic corticosteroid from the initial acute uveitic stage.[28]

PATHOLOGY AND PATHOGENESIS

VKH is a non-necrotizing diffuse granulomatous inflammation involving the uvea. Although a granulomatous process is the primary feature of the disease, the histopathologic changes vary depending on the stage of the disease.[29] Uvea is thickened by diffuse infiltration of lymphocytes and macrophages, admixed with epithelioid cells and multinucleated giant cells containing melanin granules. The neural retina is detached from the RPE, and the subretinal space contains proteinaceous fluid exudates (Fig. 75.11). Dalen–Fuchs nodules, which

Table 75.1 Distinguishing clinical features of acute and chronic VKH disease[27]

Dependent variable = VKH	Odds ratio estimate (95% CI)	*P* value
Acute disease		
Exudative retinal detachment	>999 (48.02, >999)	<0.0001
Alopecia	81.23 (2.47, >999)	0.01
Disc hyperemia	5.28 (1.02, 27.42)	0.05
Asian	24.48 (2.38, 251.9)	0.007
Hispanic	59.76 (3.77, 948.2)	0.004
Chronic disease		
Sunset glow fundus	141.66 (54.65, 367.2)	<0.0001
Vitiligo	11.73 (3.59, 38.33)	<0.0001
Alopecia	3.20 (1.40,7.31)	0.0005
Nummular chorioretinal scars	2.83 (1.34, 5.98)	0.01
Vitreous cells	0.39 (0.18, 0.83)	0.02
Asian	3.48 (1.60, 7.60)	0.002
Hispanic	13.25 (4.63, 37.88)	0.0003

(Reproduced with permission from Rao NA, Gupta A, Dustin L, et al. Frequency of distinguishing clinical features in Vogt–Koyanagi–Harada disease. Ophthalmology 2010;117:591–9 [Table 8].)

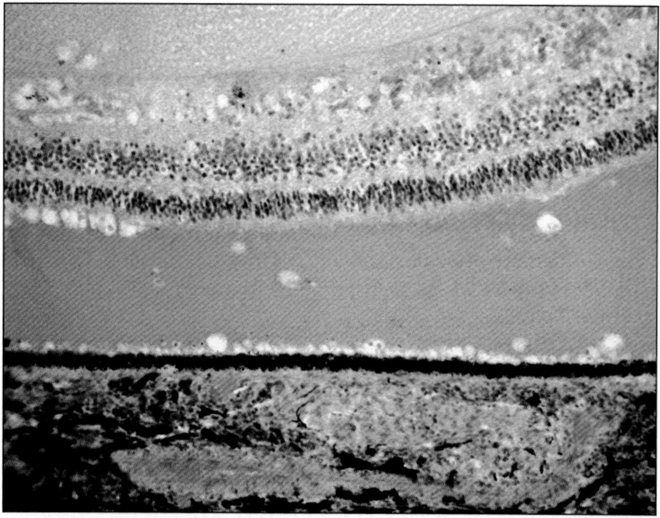

Fig. 75.11 Acute uveitic stage of Vogt–Koyanagi–Harada disease shows serous detachment of the retina, preservation of choriocapillaris from inflammatory cell infiltration, and thickening of choroid from granulomatous inflammatory cell infiltration (hematoxylin and eosin). (Courtesy of Professor H. Inomata.)

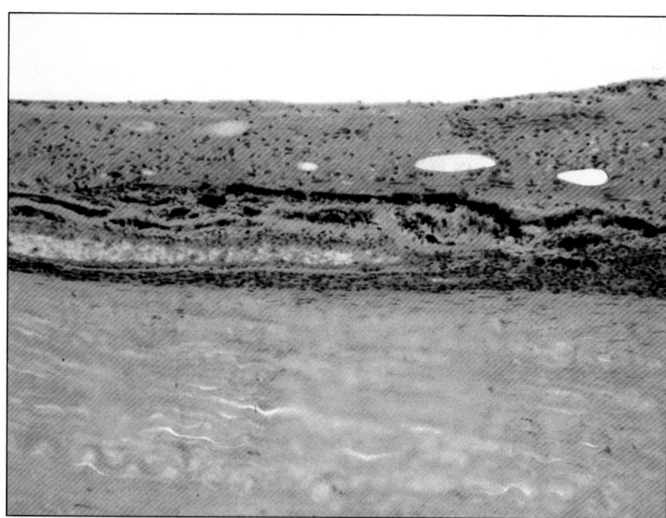

Fig. 75.13 Chronic recurrent stage of Vogt–Koyanagi–Harada disease shows choroidal inflammation, retinal pigment epithelium proliferation, and degeneration of overlying retina (hematoxylin and eosin). (Courtesy of Professor H. Inomata.)

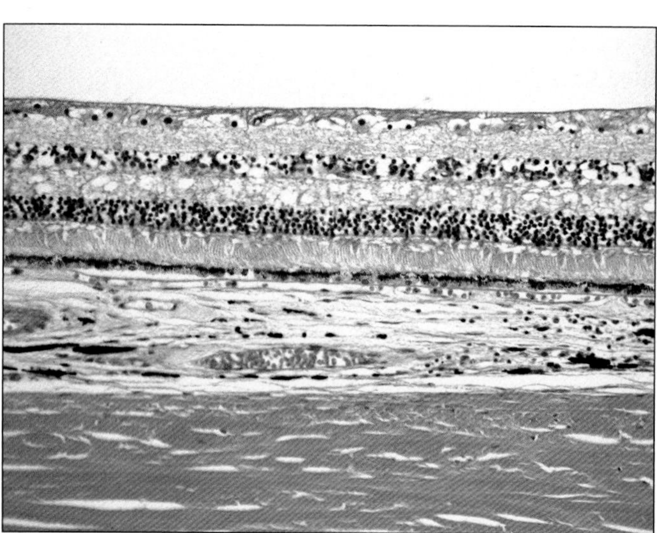

Fig. 75.12 Convalescent stage of Vogt–Koyanagi–Harada disease, exhibiting loss of choroidal melanocytes and infiltration of lymphocytes and plasma cells in the choroid. Note relatively intact retinal pigment epithelium and neurosensory retina (hematoxylin and eosin). (Courtesy of Professor H. Inomata.)

represent focal aggregates of epithelioid histiocytes admixed with RPE, are located between Bruch's membrane and the RPE.[29] In the convalescent stage, the choroidal melanocytes decrease in number and disappear (Fig. 75.12), resulting in the sunset glow appearance of the fundus.[29] During the chronic stage, the numerous focal yellowish oval or round lesions seen in the inferior peripheral fundus by ophthalmoscopy histologically display a focal loss of RPE cells and the formation of chorioretinal adhesions.[29] In the long-standing chronic recurrent stage, the RPE and neural retina show degenerative changes (Fig. 75.13). The RPE may reveal hyperplasia and fibrous metaplasia with or without associated subretinal neovascularization.[29]

Although the exact cause for the inflammation directed at the melanocytes remains unknown, current evidence suggests that it involves an autoimmune process driven by T lymphocytes against an as-yet unidentified antigen(s) associated with melanocytes.[1,30,31]

The antigenic peptides to induce autoimmune response in the uveal tract may include tyrosinase or tyrosinase-related proteins.[32,33] Experimental animal studies, as well as T-cell clones raised specific to tyrosinase family protein from the peripheral blood of patients with VKH, suggest that autoreactive T cells against tyrosinase and/or tyrosinase-related proteins may play a role in the development of VKH in a genetically susceptible individual.[33]

Cytokines are known to play an important role in the pathogenesis of VKH disease. Interleukin-21, a member of the IL-2 family exerting pleiotropic effects on the immune system, could be involved in the pathogenesis of VKH disease, possibly by promoting IL-17 secretion.[34]

$CD4^+CD25^{high}$ Treg cells have been shown to be involved in the pathogenesis of autoimmune diseases. Reduction of number or impaired function of $CD4^+CD25^{high}$ Treg cells has been reported in patients with VKH.[35]

There is a strong association with the human leukocyte antigen (HLA) DR4 in Japanese patients with VKH disease, and these patients and individuals from Korea showed predominant alleles of DRB1*0405 and HLA-DRB1 *0410.[36] Significant difference in the prevalence of HLA-DRB1 *0405 between the VKH patients and control subjects was also demonstrated in the Middle East.[37] However, in other racial groups, such as mixed Hispanic individuals from southern California, either HLA-DR1 or HLA-DR4 was found in 84% of patients with VKH disease.[38] Indeed, there was a higher relative risk with HLA-DR1 than HLA-DR4 (4.11 versus 1.96, respectively). Similar HLA-DR1 and HLA-DR4 subtypes were noted in 89% of mixed Mexican patients.[39] These studies indicate that specific HLA genes may confer risk for development of VKH disease.

INVESTIGATIONS

Imaging studies

In the vast majority of cases, the diagnosis of VKH disease is a clinical one when the patient presents with ocular and extraocular manifestations. However, when the disease presents without extraocular changes, fluorescein angiography is essential for the diagnosis. Indocyanine green angiography is also useful to evaluate choroidal inflammatory changes.

In patients with inadequate pupillary dilation caused by posterior synechiae or dense vitritis that obscures the view of the fundus, ultrasonography may help to establish the diagnosis.[40] Ultrasound biomicroscopic examination and other recent ophthalmic viewing system during the uveitic stage may reveal shallow anterior chamber, ciliochoroidal detachment, and thickened ciliary body.

In addition to angiography and ultrasonography, optical coherence tomography (OCT) and scanning laser ophthalmoscopy (SLO) have been found useful for substantiating the diagnosis. Serous retinal detachment can be clearly observed by OCT (Fig. 75.14). Thickened choroid can be demonstrated by OCT with enhanced depth imaging (Fig. 75.15). OCT has been used not only for diagnosis but for monitoring resolution of the serous retinal detachment[41,42] and choroidal thickness[43] with corticosteroid therapy. In the chronic stage, changes of the RPE can be clearly depicted as decreased fundus autofluorescence[44] (Fig. 75.16).

Lumbar puncture

Although lumbar puncture is not necessary for the diagnosis of VKH disease with typical ocular and extraocular manifestations, this procedure is a useful adjunctive test in cases with atypical features. Ohno et al. found that more than 80% of patients with VKH disease had cerebrospinal fluid pleocytosis, consisting mostly of lymphocytes.[17] In their study, the pleocytosis was present in 80% of patients within 1 week and in 97% of patients within 3 weeks of the onset of uveitis. The cerebrospinal fluid pleocytosis, however, is transient and resolves within 8 weeks

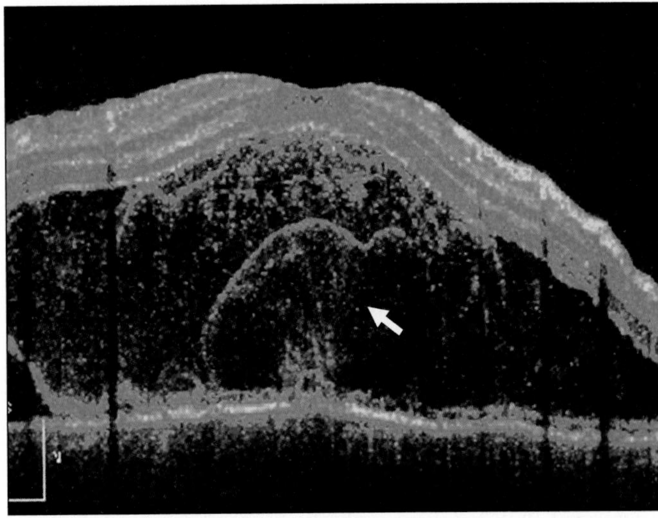

Fig. 75.14 Optical coherence tomography showing serous retinal detachment at the acute uveitic stage. Note the presence of fibrin in subretinal space (arrow).

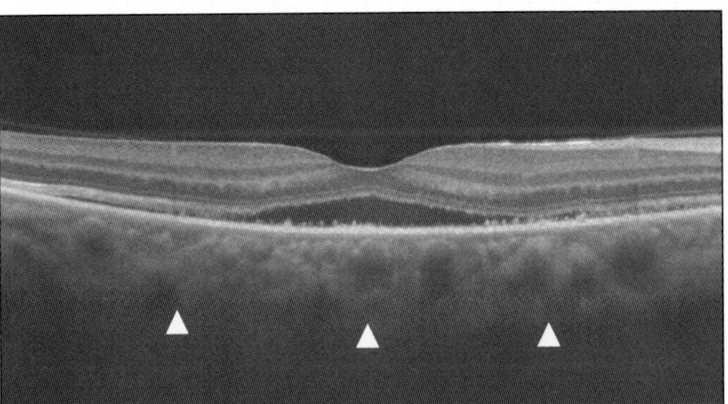

Fig. 75.15 Optical coherence tomography 9 days after systemic corticosteroid therapy showing thickened choroid at the macular area (arrowheads).

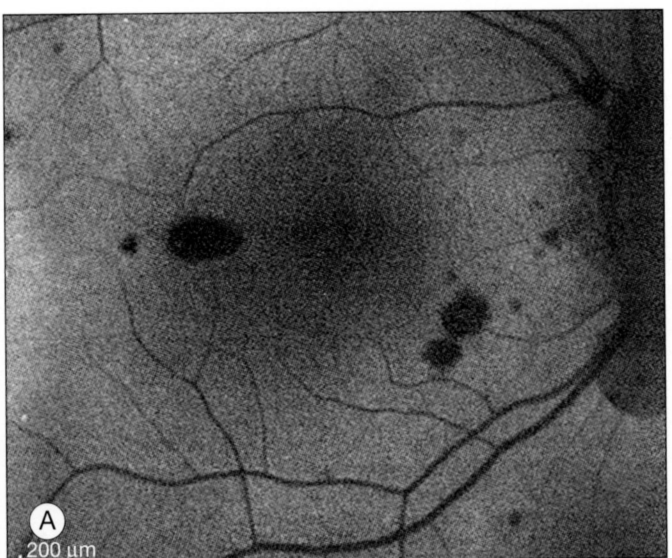

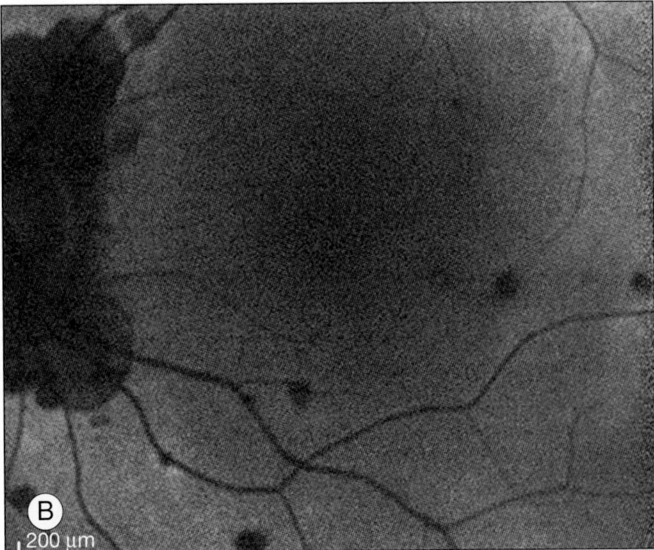

Fig. 75.16 Fundus autofluorescence imaging shows decreased autofluorescence at the atrophic nummular scars.

even in patients who develop recurrences of intraocular inflammation. Cytologic analysis may reveal melanin-containing histiocyte in patients with pleocytosis.[45]

DIFFERENTIAL DIAGNOSIS

The differential diagnosis of VKH disease includes sympathetic ophthalmia, uveal effusion syndrome, posterior scleritis, acute posterior multifocal placoid pigment epitheliopathy (APMPPE), and sarcoidosis.[1] Sympathetic ophthalmia can present with bilateral panuveitis associated with retinal detachment and meningism. However, a history of penetrating ocular injury is the rule in this disorder. Extraocular manifestations, such as dysacusis, vitiligo, poliosis, and alopecia, can occur in sympathetic ophthalmia, but they are rare.[46]

Uveal effusion syndrome may clinically mimic VKH disease. Angiographically, the effusion syndrome may reveal numerous fluorescent blotches in the subretinal space during the serous detachment phase. The syndrome can involve both eyes, although not simultaneously. Unlike VKH disease, the effusion syndrome lacks intraocular inflammation. Posterior scleritis affects predominantly women and is often bilateral. Patients may present with pain, photophobia, and loss of vision, and the vitreous often reveals cells. Exudative retinal detachment and choroidal folds may be noted. Ultrasonography can help to differentiate posterior scleritis from VKH disease. The former reveals flattening of the posterior aspect of the globe, thickening of the posterior coats of the eye, retrobulbar edema, and high internal reactivity of the thickened sclera. Other entities, such as sarcoidosis and APMPPE can be differentiated based on their clinical features, ultrasonography, and fluorescein angiography.

TREATMENT

Although data from randomized trials are lacking, early and aggressive use of systemic corticosteroids followed by slow tapering over 3–6 months is the acceptable treatment of choice to suppress the intraocular inflammation and to prevent the development of complications related to the ocular inflammation.[1] Such treatment may prevent progression of the disease to the chronic recurrent stage and may also reduce the incidence and/or severity of extraocular manifestations. If the ocular inflammation relapses after tapering of systemic corticosteroids, the relapse may reflect too-rapid tapering of the corticosteroids. Such recurrences become increasingly steroid-resistant, and cytotoxic or immunosuppressive agents are usually required to control the inflammation. Patients with inflammatory cell infiltration in the anterior chamber require topical corticosteroids and cycloplegics to reduce ciliary spasm and prevent posterior synechiae formation.

High-dose oral corticosteroids, 80–100 mg per day of prednisone or 200 mg of intravenous methylprednisolone for 3 days, followed by oral administration of high-dose corticosteroids with a slow taper, are the mainstay of therapy for VKH disease.[47,48] The use of intravenous corticosteroids, up to 1 g/day for 3 days, followed by a slow taper has been recommended by some. However, Sasamoto et al. found a similar beneficial effect of decreased intraocular inflammation with either 1 g or 200 mg per day of intravenous corticosteroids.[48] Of course, as is always the case when corticosteroids are prescribed, careful attention to possible risks and side-effects is warranted.

Box 75.2 Immunosuppressive/cytotoxic agents used in the treatment of Vogt–Koyanagi–Harada disease

- Corticosteroids[1,48,49]
- Oral prednisone 100–200 mg initially, followed by gradual taper over 3–6 months
- Pulse dose of methylprednisolone 1 g/day for 3 days, followed by gradual tapering of oral prednisone over 3–6 months
- Intravenous methylprednisolone 100–200 mg/day for 3 days, followed by gradual tapering of oral prednisone over 3–6 months
- Immunosuppressive agents[1]
- Cyclosporin 5 mg/kg per day
- FK506 0.1–0.15 mg/kg per day
- Cytotoxic agents[1]
- Azathioprine 1–2.5 mg/kg per day
- Mycophenolate mofetil 1–3 g/day
- Cyclophosphamide 1–2 mg/kg per day
- Chlorambucil 0.1 mg/kg per day; dose adjusted every 3 weeks to a maximum of 18 mg/day
- Biologics[50]
- Anti-TNF-α monoclonal antibody

Although the initial episode of uveitis can be managed successfully in the majority of cases with intravenous and/or oral corticosteroids, recurrences do not respond as well to systemic corticosteroid treatment.[1] Such patients may show some initial response to subtenon injections of triamcinolone acetonide, but they usually require immunosuppressive or cytotoxic agents, such as cyclosporine, azathioprine, cyclophosphamide, chlorambucil, mycophenolate mofetil (CellCept), and tacrolimus (FK506). Cyclosporine 5 mg/kg per day is generally preferred when the intraocular inflammation is corticosteroid-resistant or when the patient experiences intolerable side-effects from the long-term use of corticosteroids. Recently, a biologic agent, anti-TNF-α antibody, has been reported in the management of VKH disease.[49]

Administration of the immunosuppressives, cytotoxic agents, and biologics requires a careful pretreatment evaluation and careful subsequent evaluations during the follow-up examinations for any side-effects associated with the therapy. Various immunosuppressive and cytotoxic agents used in the treatment of VKH disease are summarized in Box 75.2.

COMPLICATIONS AND MANAGEMENT

A retrospective analysis of the records of 101 patients with VKH disease followed at the Doheny Eye Institute revealed the development of at least one complication in 51% of eyes.[50] Cataract occurred in 42%, glaucoma in 27%, choroidal neovascularization in 11% (Fig. 75.17), and subretinal fibrosis in 6% (Fig. 75.18). The patients who developed these complications had a significantly longer median duration of disease and significantly more recurrences than did those patients who developed no complications. Moreover, eyes possessing a better visual acuity at presentation had better visual acuity at final follow-up, and patients who developed VKH at a more advanced age had a worse visual acuity.[50]

There is general agreement that cataract surgery should be delayed until the intraocular inflammation has subsided, at which time safe cataract extraction with posterior-chamber intraocular lens implantation can be successfully accomplished. Occasionally, patients with significant vitreous opacities and debris may require a combined procedure of pars plana vitrectomy and lensectomy.[24]

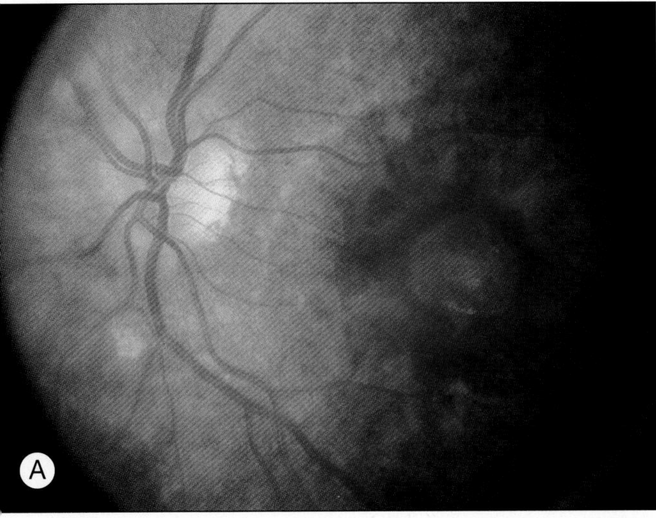

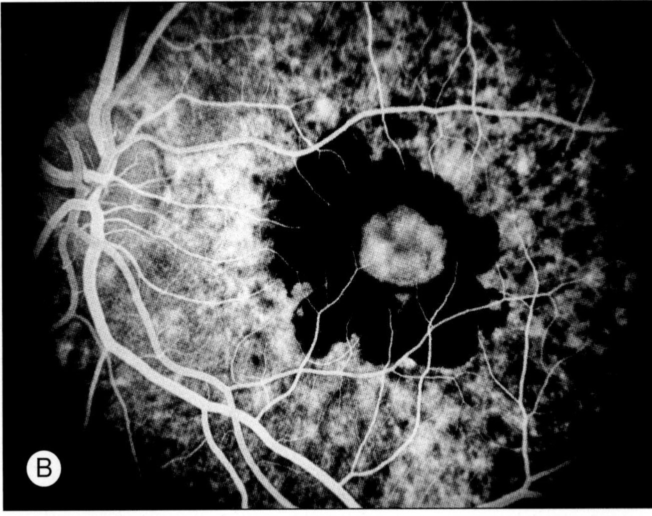

Fig. 75.17 Submacular choroidal neovascular membrane and hemorrhage during the chronic recurrent stage (A); the fluorescein angiogram shows a typical neovascular membrane (B).

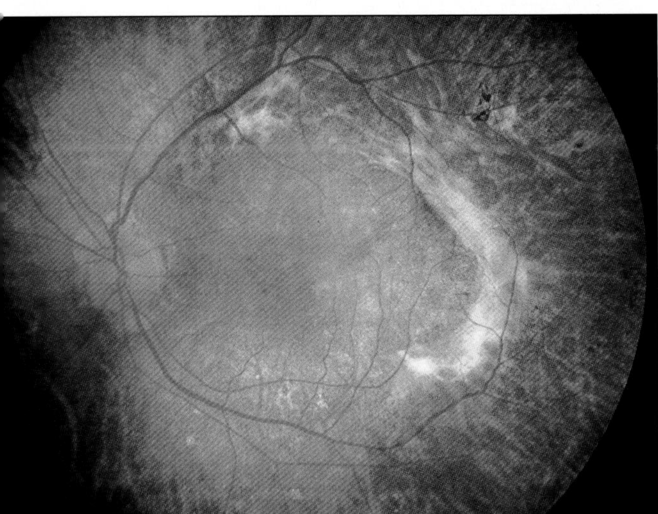

Fig. 75.18 Subretinal fibrosis in a patient with chronic recurrent stage of Vogt–Koyanagi–Harada disease.

Angle closure due to peripheral anterior synechiae and posterior synechiae may cause glaucoma.[25] Acute angle closure with elevated intraocular pressure has been reported as a presenting sign of VKH disease. Although sustained elevated intraocular pressure can be controlled by medical therapy alone, most patients require surgical intervention in the form of iridectomy, trabeculectomy with 5-fluorouracil or mitomycin C and tube-shunt surgery.

Chronic recurrent anterior uveitis and fundus pigmentary disturbances seem to predispose patients to the development of choroidal neovascularization[24] (Fig. 75.18). These subretinal membranes present with white gliotic raised masses, which may be associated with subretinal hemorrhage. ICG angiography is useful for detecting the membranes and photocoagulation may help with the management. Photodynamic therapy with verteporfin for subfoveal choroidal neovascularization has been attempted with some success.[51] Intravitreal injection of an anti-vascular endothelial growth factor (VEGF) may be an option to treat CNV in eyes with VKH syndrome.[52]

PROGNOSIS

In general, those VKH patients who are treated with initial high-dose systemic corticosteroids followed by gradual tapering will usually have a fair visual prognosis; nearly two-thirds of these patients retain 20/40 or better visual acuity.[1,48] On average, most patients require treatment for 6 months. The complications of chronic recurrent VKH disease include cataract, glaucoma, choroidal neovascularization, subretinal fibrosis, and optic atrophy.[1,50,53]

CONCLUSION

VKH is a bilateral granulomatous panuveitis that usually presents with serous retinal detachment, with signs of meningeal irritation, with or without extraocular manifestations such as poliosis, vitiligo, and auditory disturbances. In most cases the diagnosis is a clinical one, but the diagnosis of atypical cases may require the use of fluorescein angiography, lumbar puncture, and ultrasonography. VKH is treated initially with high-dose systemic corticosteroids. Successful outcome requires a gradual tapering of the corticosteroids over a 3–6 month period. Complications of this disease include cataract, glaucoma, choroidal neovascularization, and subretinal fibrosis. The overall prognosis for adequately managed cases is fair, with nearly 60–70% of patients retaining vision of 20/40 or better.

REFERENCES

1. Moorthy RS, lnomata H, Rao NA. Vogt–Koyanagi–Harada syndrome. Surv Ophthalmol 1995;39:265–92.
2. Pattison EM. Uveo-meningoencephalitic syndrome (Vogt–Koyanagi–Harada). Arch Neurol 1965;12:197–205.
3. Schenkl A. Ein Fall von plötzlich aufgetretener Poliosis circumscripta der Wimpern. Arch Dermatol Syph 1873;5:137–9.
4. Hutchinson J. A case of blanched eyelashes. Arch Surg 1892;4:357.
5. Vogt A. Frühzeitiges Ergrauen der Zilien und Bemerkungen über den sogenannten plötzlichen Eintritt dieser Veränderung. Klim Monatsbl Augenheilkd 1906;44:228–42.
6. Harada E. Beitrag zur klinischen Kenntnis von nichteitriger Choroiditis (choroiditis diffusa acuta). Acta Soc Ophthalmol Jpn 1926;30:356–78.
7. Koyanagi Y. Dysakusis, Alopecia und Poliosis bei schwerter Uveitis nichttraumatischen Ursprungs. Klin Monatsbl Augenheilkd 1929;82:194–211.

8. Babel J. Syndrome de Vogt–Koyanagi (Uveite bilaterale, poliosis, alopecie, vitiligo et dysacousie). Schweiz Med Wochenschr NR 1932;4:1136–40.
9. Bruno MG, McPherson Jr SD. Harada's disease. Am J 0phthalmol 1949;32: 513–22.
10. Beniz J, Forster DJ, Lean JS, et al. Variations in clinical features of the Vogt-Koyanagi–Harada syndrome. Retina 1991;11:275–80.
11. Snyder DA, Tessler HA. Vogt–Koyanagi–Harada syndrome. Am J Ophthalmol 1980;90:69–75.
12. Read RW, Rao NA. Utility of existing Vogt–Koyanagi–Harada syndrome diagnostic criteria at initial evaluation of the individual patient: a retrospective analysis. Ocul Immunol Inflamm 2000;8:227–34.
13. Read RW, Holland GN, Rao NA, et al. Revised diagnostic criteria for Vogt-Koyanagi–Harada disease: report of an international committee on nomenclature. Am J Ophthalmol 2001;131:647–52.
14. Goto H, Mochizuki M, Yamaki S, et al. Epidemiological survey of intraocular inflammation in Japan. Jpn J Ophthalmol 2007;51:41–4.
15. Shimizu K. Harada's, Behçet's, Vogt–Koyanagi syndromes: are they clinical entities? Trans Am Acad Ophthalmol Otolaryngol 1973;77:281–90.
16. Nussenblatt RB. Clinical studies of Vogt–Koyanagi–Harada's disease at the National Eye Institute, NIH, USA. Jpn J Ophthalmol 1988;32:330–3.
17. Ohno S, Char DH, Kimura SJ, et al. Vogt–Koyanagi–Harada syndrome. Am J Opthalmlol 1977;83:735–40.
18. Forster DJ, Green RL, Rao NA. Unilateral manifestation of the Vogt–Koyanagi–Harada syndrome in a 7-year-old child. Am J Ophthalmol 1991;111:380–2.
19. Herbort CP, Mantovani A, Bouchenaki N. Indocyanine green angiography in Vogt–Koyanagi–Harada disease: angiographic signs and utility in patient follow-up. Int Ophthalmol 2007;27:173–82.
20. Miyanaga M, Kawaguchi T, Miyata K, et al. Indocyanine green angiography findings in initial acute pretreatment Vogt–Koyanagi–Harada disease in Japanese patients. Jpn J Ophthalmol 2010;54:377–82.
21. Kawano Y, Tawara A, Nishioka Y, et al. Ultrasound biomicroscopic analysis of transient shallow anterior chamber in Vogt–Koyanagi–Harada syndrome. Am J Ophthalmol 1996;121:720–3.
22. Yamamoto N, Naito K. Annular choroidal detachment in patients with Vogt–Koyanagi–Harada disease. Graefes Arch Clin Exp Opthalmol 2004;242: 355–8.
23 Usui Y, Goto H, Sakai J, et al. Presumed Vogt–Koyanagi–Harada disease with unilateral ocular involvement: report of three cases. Graefes Arch Clin Exp Ophthalmol 2009;247:1127–32.
24. Moorthy RS, Chong LP, Smith RE, et al. Subretinal neovascular membranes in Vogt–Koyanagi–Harada syndrome. Am J Ophthalmol 1993;116:164–70.
25. Forster DJ, Rao NA, Hill RA, et al. Incidence and management of glaucoma in Vogt–Koyanagi–Harada syndrome. Ophthalmology 1993;100:613–8.
26. Moorthy RS, Rajeev B, Smith RE, et al. Incidence and management of cataracts in Vogt–Koyanagi–Harada syndrome. Am J Ophthalmol 1999;118: 197–204.
27. Rao NA,, Gupta A, Dustin L, et al. Frequency of distinguishing clinical features in Vogt–Koyanagi–Harada disease. Ophthalmology 2010;117:591–9.
28. Keino H, Goto H, Usui M. Sunset glow fundus in Vogt–Koyanagi–Harada disease with or without chronic ocular inflammation. Graefes Arch Clin Exp Ophthalmol 2002;240:878–82.
29. Inomata H, Rao NA. Depigmented atrophic lesions in sunset glow fundi of Vogt–Koyanagi–Harada disease. Am J Ophthalmol 2001;131:607–14.
30. Norose K, Yano A. Melanoma specific Th1 cytotoxic T lymphocyte lines in Vogt–Koyanagi–Harada disease. Br J Ophthalmol 1996;80:1002–8.
31. Sugita S, Sagawa K, Mochizuki M, et al. Melanocyte lysis by cytotoxic T lymphocytes recognizing the MART-1 melanoma antigen in HLA-A2 patients with Vogt–Koyanagi–Harada disease. Int Immunol 1996;8:799–803.
32. Gocho K, Kondo I, Yamaki K. Identificaiton of autoreactive T cells in Vogt–Koyanagi–Harada disease. Invest Ophthalmol Vis Sic 2001;42:2004–9.
33. Hayakawa K, Ishikawa M, Yamaki K. Ultrastructural changes in rat eyes with experimental Vogt–Koyanagi–Harada disease. Jpn J Ophthalmol 2004;48: 222–7.
34. Li F, Yang P, Liu X ,et al. Upregulation of interleukin 21 and promotion of interleukin 17 production in chronic or recurrent Vogt–Koyanagi–Harada disease. Arch Ophthalmol 2010:128:1449–54.
35. Chen L, Yang P, Zhou H, et al. Diminished frequency and function of $CD4^{+}CD25^{high}$ regulatory T cells associated with active uveitis in Vogt–Koyanagi–Harada syndrome. Invest Ophthalmol Vis Sci 2008;49:3475–82.
36. Shindo Y, Ohno S, Yamamoto T, et al. Complete association of the HLA-DRB1 04 and DQ1 04 alleles with Vogt–Koyanagi–Harada's disease. Hum Immunol 1994;39:169–76.
37. Iqniebi A, Gaafar A, Sheereen A, et al. HLA-DRB1among patients with Vogt–Koyanagi–Harada disease in Saudi Arabia. Mol Vis 2009;15:1876–80.
38. Weisz JM, Holland GN, Roer LN, et al. Association between Vogt–Koyanagi–Harada syndrome and HLA-DR1 and DR4 in Hispanic patients living in Southern California. Ophthalmology 1995;102:1012–5.
39. Arellanes-Garcia L, Bautista N, More P, et al. HLA-DR is strongly associated with Vogt–Koyanagi–Harada disease in Mexican Mestizo patients. Ocul Immunol Inflamm 1998;6:93–100.
40. Forster DJ, Cano MR, Green RL, et al. Echographic features of the Vogt–Koyanagi–Harada syndrome. Arch Ophthalmol 1990;108:1421–6.
41. Yamaguchi Y, Otani T, Kishi S. Tomographic features of serous retinal detachment with multilobular dye pooling in acute Vogt–Koyanagi–Harada disease. Am J Ophthalmol 2007;144:260–5.
42. Ishihara K, Hangai M, Kita M, et al. Acute Vogt–Koyanagi–Harada disease in enhanced spectral-domain optical coherence tomography. Ophthalmology 2009;116:1799–807.
43. Fong AH, Li KK, Wong D. Choroidal evaluation using enhanced depth imaging spectral domain optical coherence tomography in Vogt–Koyanagi–Harada disease. Retina 2011;31:502–99.
44. Vasconcelos-Santos DV, Sohn EH, Sadda S, et al. Retinal pigment epithelial changes in chronic Vogt–Koyanagi–Harada disease: fundus autofluorescence and spectral domain-optical coherence tomography findings. Retina. 2010;30: 33–41.
45. Tsai JH, Sukavatcharin S, Rao NA. Utility of lumbar puncture in diagnosis of Vogt–Koyanagi–Harada disease. Int Ophthalmol 2007;27:189–94.
46. Rao NA, Marak GE. Sympathetic ophthalmia simulating Vogt–Koyanagi–Harada's disease: a clinico-pathologic study of four cases. Jpn J Ophthalmol 1983;27:506–11.
47. Rubsamen PE, Gass JDM. Vogt–Koyanagi–Harada syndrome. Clinical course, therapy, and long-term visual outcome. Arch Ophthalmol 1991;109:682–7.
48. Sasamoto Y, Ohno S, Matsuda H. Studies on corticosteroid therapy in Vogt–Koyanagi–Harada disease. Ophthalmologica 1990;201:162–7.
49. Wang Y, Gaudio PA. Infliximab therapy for 2 patients with Vogt–Koyanagi–Harada syndrome. Ocul Immuno Inflamm 2008;16:167–71.
50. Read RW, Rechodouni A, Butani N, et al. Complications and prognostic factors in Vogt–Koyanagi–Harada disease. Am J Ophthalmol 2001;131:599–606.
51. Nowilaty SR, Bouhaimed M. Photodynamic Therapy Study Group. Photodynamic therapy for subfoveal choroidal neovascularisation in Vogt–Koyanagi–Harada disease. Br J Ophthalmol 2006;90:982–6.
52. Wu L, Evans T, Saravia M, et al. Intravitreal bevacizumab for choroidal neovascularization secondary to Vogt–Koyanagi–Harada syndrome. Jpn J Ophthalmol 2009;53:57–60.
53. Kuo IC, Rechdouni A, Rao NA, et al. Subretinal fibrosis in a patient with Vogt–Koyanagi–Harada syndrome. Ophthalmology 2000;107:1721–8.

White Spot Syndromes and Related Diseases

Chapter 76

Rukhsana G. Mirza, Lee M. Jampol

INTRODUCTION

The white spot syndromes (WSS) are a group of diseases characterized by inflammation and dysfunction of the outer retina, retinal pigment epithelium, choroid, or a combination of these. They often present a diagnostic and therapeutic challenge for clinicians and researchers. The etiologies of WSS remain unknown. This chapter discusses: birdshot chorioretinopathy (BCR), acute posterior multifocal placoid pigment epitheliopathy (APMPPE), serpiginous choroiditis, relentless placoid chorioretinitis, persistent placoid maculopathy, multifocal choroiditis and panuveitis (MFC), punctate inner choroidopathy (PIC), progressive subretinal fibrosis and uveitis syndrome (PSFU), multiple evanescent white dot syndrome (MEWDS), acute zonal occult outer retinopathy (AZOOR), acute idiopathic blind spot enlargement (AIBSE), and acute macular neuroretinopathy (AMN). Many entities are included in the differential diagnosis of these diseases. These include: granulomatous diseases, such as sarcoid, tuberculosis, sympathetic ophthalmia; masquerade syndromes like syphilis and intraocular lymphoma; infectious etiologies including toxoplasmosis, pneumocystis choroidopathy; and other entities such as presumed ocular histoplasmosis, and Behçet disease.[1] In addition, in some cases, degenerative processes such as drusen may appear similar to the whitish-yellow lesions of WSS.

The WSS each have distinct features, but do share some characteristics. Blurred vision, photopsias, visual field changes, floaters, and changes in contrast sensitivity can occur. Although these entities are thought to be inflammatory in nature, vitritis and iritis are not a necessary finding. The white spots themselves may be subtle or a prominent finding. Inflammatory multifocal chorioretinopathies may actually be a more descriptive term.

The white spot syndromes may present in one or both eyes. When bilateral, they may be asymmetric. The age of onset is generally greater than 50, but can range from the second to the sixth decade of life.

An autoimmune etiology has been hypothesized[2] and proposed specifically for birdshot chorioretinopathy, acute zonal occult outer retinopathy (AZOOR), and multiple evanescent white dot syndrome (MEWDS).[3] As yet, no characteristic pattern of antiretinal antibodies has been found. These entities need to be distinguished from entities with known neoplasias such as cancer-associated retinopathy (CAR) or melanoma-associated retinopathy (MAR). There are similar features including panretinal dysfunction, rapid progression, ERG changes, family history of autoimmune disease, retinal antibody activity on Western blot, and improvement in symptoms with immunosuppression. An increased prevalence of systemic autoimmunity in both patients with WSS and their first- as well as second-degree relatives, was found by Pearlman and colleagues.[4] This suggests that this group of diseases occurs in families with inherited immune dysregulation that predisposes to autoimmunity.

It has also been suggested that several of these entities may be "related" or even represent a spectrum of the same process. Multifocal choroiditis (MFC), punctate inner choroiditis (PIC), MEWDS, acute macular neuroretinopathy (AMN), and AZOOR share commonalities and Gass referred to them as the AZOOR complex.[5] These include female preponderance, zones of visual field loss that are usually contiguous to the blind spot, photopsias, and ERG changes such as reduced amplitudes. In addition, MFC and APMPPE have also been found in the same patient decades apart.[6] Other diseases that have been noted in the same patient include MEWDS and AZOOR as well as MFC and PIC. This overlap may give support to a common underlying genetic predisposition.[2]

BIRDSHOT CHORIORETINOPATHY

The term birdshot retinochoroidopathy was first used in 1980 by Ryan and Maumenee.[7] It was a descriptive term for patients with multiple small, cream-colored fundus findings. These lesions are scattered around the optic disc and radiate to the equator in a "shotgun" pattern. Other terms such as vitiliginous chorioretinitis have been used.[8] It has come to be known as birdshot chorioretinopathy (BCR) due to the histopathologic evidence that the primary lesions of the disease are in the choroid.[9] It is a bilateral, chronic process with vitritis, retinal vasculitis, and cystoid macular edema (CME). Furthermore, it demonstrates the strongest link between any disease and any HLA class I antigen.[10]

Clinical course

Clinical symptoms

Patients present with complaints of blurred vision, floaters, and photopsias. Most have vision of 20/40 or better.[9] The eye is generally not red or painful. Severe nyctalopia despite normal visual acuity may be a presenting symptom.[11] Individuals also may describe an alteration in color vision[12] or visual fields.[13] Although Gass described a few patients who concurrently had vitiligo of the skin,[8] BCR is thought to be a purely ocular disease.

Epidemiology

BCR is a rare chronic posterior uveitis. Shah and colleagues did an extensive review of English literature in 2005 and reported the following epidemiologic characteristics.[9] Birdshot chorioretinopathy accounts for 0.6–1.5% of patients referred to tertiary centers for uveitis, or 6–7.9% of patients with posterior uveitis. There is a slight female predominance in the literature, at 54.1%. The mean reported age at the onset of disease is 53 years. It is generally not a disease of children. The oldest reported age at onset was 79 years. Patients are predominantly white; there have only been two reported exceptions. Finally, the HLA-A29 allele (which is present in about 7% of Caucasians) is strongly associated with BCR.[14] The presence of this allele has been associated with a risk factor of 50–224 to develop BCR. Ninety percent or more of patients with BCR are HLA-A29-positive. Further sequencing of this allele has uncovered 11 subtypes. The HLA-A29*02 subtype is 20 times more prevalent in Caucasians than the HLA-A29*01 type, and the rest are exceedingly rare.[15] HLA-A29*02 subtype is most commonly associated with BCR.

Fundus findings

It is important to recognize that symptoms can precede the onset of the classic fundus findings by several years.[16] There is a range of presentations of the lesions associated with BCR. These birdshot lesions can be oval or round in shape, typically about ½ or ¼ disc diameter in size. They appear deep to the retina (Fig. 76.1). They can be subtle, and asymmetric between eyes. The lesions can be distinct or poorly defined and can occasionally coalesce. They tend to cluster near the nerve and most commonly nasal and inferior to the disc.[17,18] There is a pattern of linear radiation away from the nerve to the periphery[7] (Fig. 76.2). They may appear to follow choroidal blood vessels peripherally. There is no hyperpigmentation or clumping noted. The retinal pigment epithelium (RPE) and overlying retina appear intact. There has been a report of these choroidal lesions preceding symptom onset in BCR, but this is not the norm.[19]

Other ocular findings

The anterior segment generally has minimal inflammation without prominent keratic precipitates. Fine keratic precipitates have been described in some series.[18] Due to the mild nature of anterior segment inflammation, posterior synechiae do not occur. Signs of posterior inflammation include retinal vasculitis, optic disc edema, CME, and epiretinal membrane formation. Rhegmatogenous retinal detachment has been reported.[7,20,21] It is unclear if this is related to this disease entity or to an association with uveitis. Other common findings include diffuse narrowing of the retinal arterioles, perivascular nerve fiber layer hemorrhages, and tortuosity of retinal vessels. Choroidal neovascularization (CNV) can occur.[10,22,23] It has been postulated that this occurs due to the uveitic component causing CNV rather than ischemic factors.[24,25]

A consensus document on the diagnostic criteria for BCR was published in 2006.[26] Required characteristics include: bilateral disease, presence of at least three peripapillary lesions inferior or nasal to the optic nerve in at least one eye, low-grade anterior segment inflammation (less than or equal to 1+ cells), and low grade vitreous inflammation (less than or equal to 2+ vitreous haze). Supportive findings include: HLA-A29 positive, retinal vasculitis, and CME. Finally, exclusion criteria include: presence of significant keratic precipitates, posterior synechiae, or diagnosis of infectious, neoplastic, or inflammatory disease that may cause multifocal choroidal lesions.

Clinical course and prognosis

The disease is chronic in nature and apparently does not regress. Again, symptoms of blurred vision, color deficiency, contrast sensitivity issues, and visual field problems may be present for years prior to the onset of fundus lesions. Visual acuity may be normal despite these complaints. It remains a poorly understood disease and no consensus on management and treatment has been found. Many patients have a slow decline in vision, despite treatment.[9]A final visual acuity of 20/40 or better in the best-seeing eye was reported in 75.1% of patients. However, 9.8% of patients were legally blind at follow-up (in the review of literature by Shah and colleagues[9]). Generally, macular edema was the commonest cause of visual decline in 50.5%.[9] Choroidal neovascular membranes developed in 5% of eyes.[22,23] These occur near the optic disc and can be bilateral. Finally, optic disc edema leading to atrophy can also affect visual prognosis.

Imaging

Fluorescein angiography

The creamy white spots have variable appearance on fluorescein angiography (FA) and the disease may be more evident clinically than with this mode of imaging (Fig. 76.3). The lesions

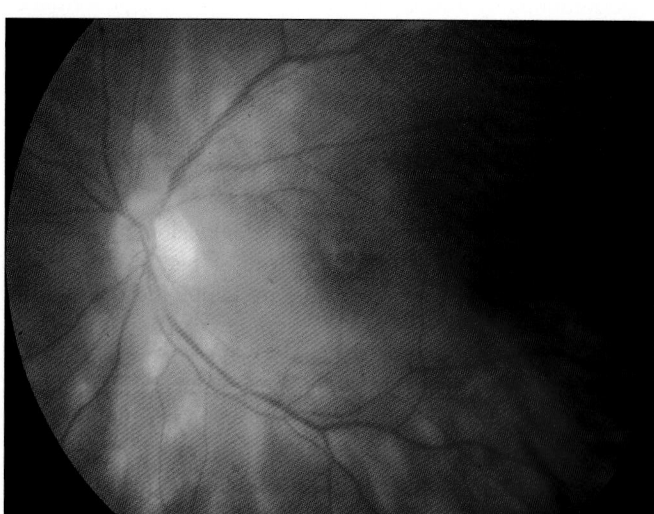

Fig. 76.1 Fundus photo of the left posterior pole showing a hazy view and the distribution of deep creamy oval lesions.

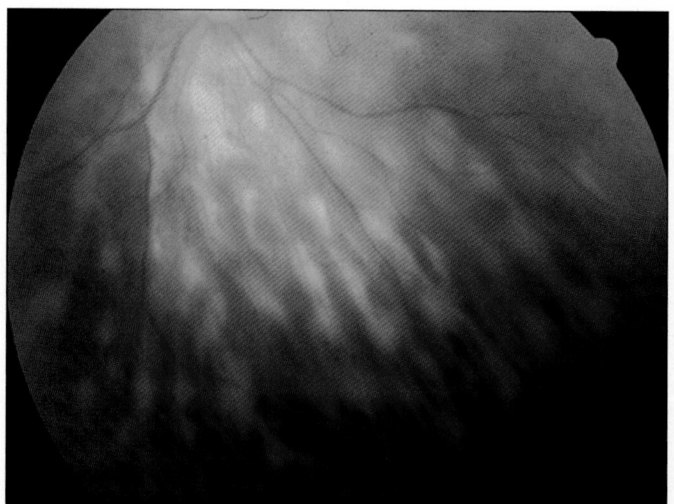

Fig. 76.2 Fundus photo showing the “birdshot” pattern extending linearly from the nerve to the periphery.

can hypofluoresce in the early phase and there can be diffuse hyperfluorescence in the late phases (Fig. 76.4). One theory suggests that the lesions are likely in the outer choroid and associated with large choroidal vessels, thus many of the lesions show neither hypofluorescence or hyperfluorescence in any phase. The diffuse hyperfluorescence seen may represent a deep inflammatory focus that accumulates fluorescein.[18] Angiographic findings may include increased transit time, leakage from retinal vasculature leading to CME, optic disc hyperfluorescence (Fig. 76.5), and disc or retinal neovascularization.[8,27,28]

Indocyanine green angiography

Indocyanine green angiography (ICGA) is an important diagnostic test. In the active disease,[28] the birdshot lesions appear hypofluorescent during the intermediate phase of angiography and appear to be bordered by medium-to-large vessels[28–30] (Fig. 76.6). The choroidal vessels appear indistinct. Late in the ICGA, there is diffuse choroidal hyperfluorescence. As with all the white spot syndromes, theories to explain this hypofluorescence include choroidal ischemia versus blockage from inflammatory infiltrates. However, in birdshot chorioretinopathy it is agreed upon that the site of the pathology is primarily the choroid. In the acute stages, the inflammatory infiltrates may be denser and block fluorescence. In late stages of the disease, it is thought that the lesions become more atrophic and choroidal vasculature may become more visible. The lesions can become more isofluorescent in this phase of the disease or they may remain hypofluorescent.[27,28]

Optical coherence tomography

This mode of imaging has primarily been used to follow CME, which is the most common cause of vision loss in BCR[31]

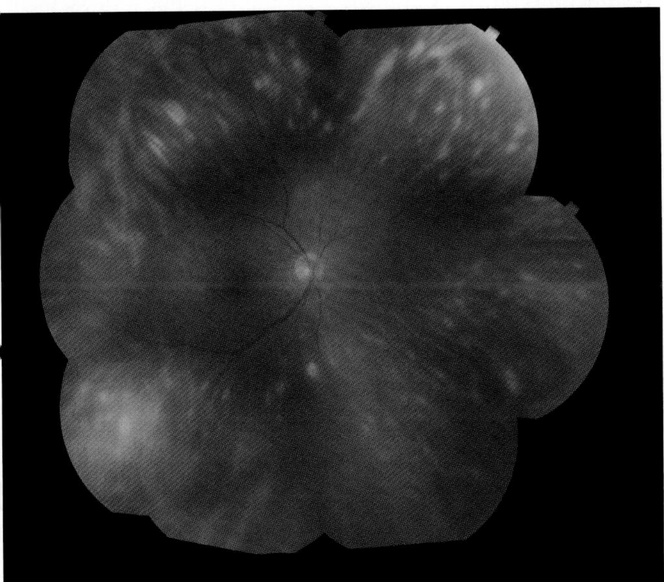

Fig. 76.3 Color montage of right eye showing the distribution of spots.

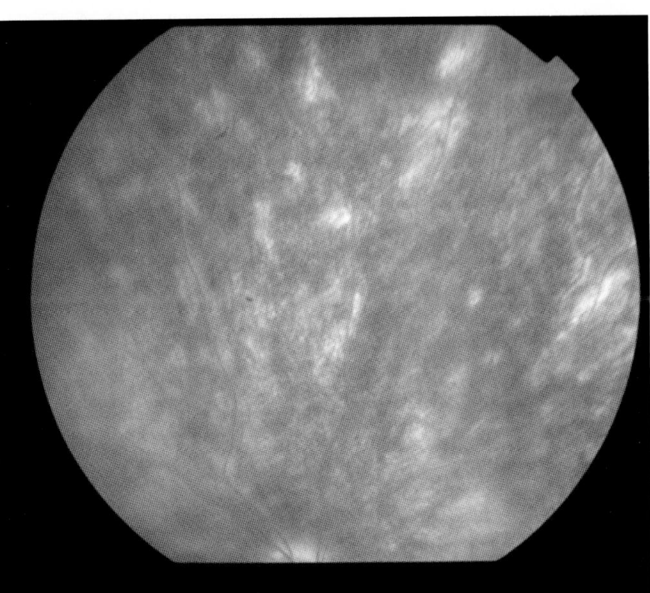

Fig. 76.4 FA of periphery showing hyperfluorescence of lesions.

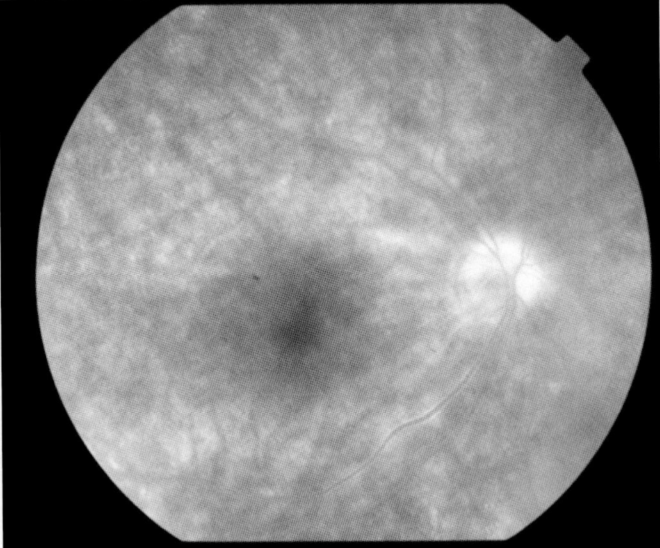

Fig. 76.5 FA showing hyperfluorescence of the optic nerve.

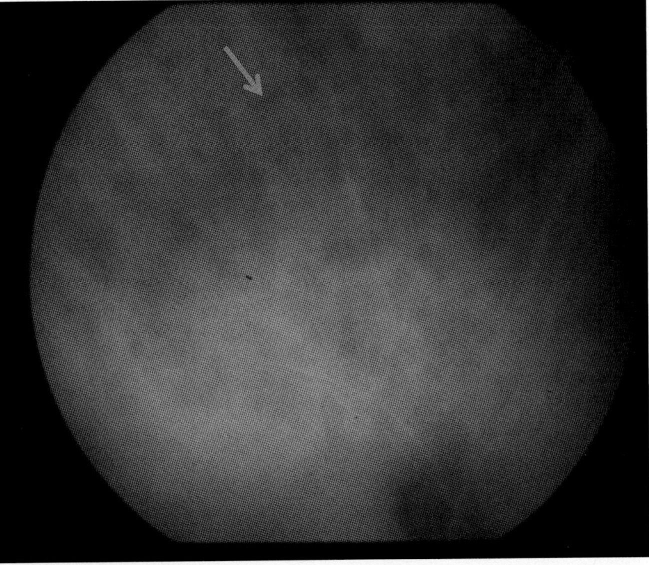

Fig. 76.6 ICG showing hypofluorescent lesions exceeding the number seen clinically.

(Fig. 76.7). Photoreceptor loss is not a prominent finding early on in the course.

Fundus autofluorescence

Giuliari and colleagues looked at fundus autofluorescence (FAF) of 18 eyes and found a spectrum of patterns.[31] They found that hypoautofluorescent lesions on FAF did not necessarily correspond to clinical birdshot lesions. Commonly (15/18 eyes) more FAF lesions denoting RPE defects were seen than clinical lesions. Koizumi and colleagues looked at 8 patients. They found that some of these hypofluorescent lesions could be placoid in nature and involve the macula.[32] In addition, a perivascular (retinal) linear hypofluorescent FAF pattern was noted by both groups of investigators.[31,32] It was postulated that this finding may suggest that the retinal vessels may play a role in inflammatory-driven damage of the RPE and serve as a conduit for inflammatory factors. The observation that the clinical choroidal lesions did not always correspond to the FAF defects suggests that the choroid and RPE may be affected independently.[32] Furthermore, RPE defects in the macula could also be another cause of vision loss in these individuals. FAF may be valuable in evaluating these patients as lesions may be clinically difficult to see.

Electrophysiology

Priem and coworkers also studied pattern-evoked cortical potentials and found abnormal findings in 53.3% of patients.[33]

Electroretinogram

Electroretinography (ERG) is an important test for following BCR. Abnormal electroretinograms (ERGs) were reported in 88.8% of patients.[9] There appear to be two groups of patients: those who develop abnormal ERG early in the disease process and those that develop abnormal results late in the course.[34] Early ERGs may demonstrate supernormal ERG amplitudes which may be related to retinal inflammation. In this stage, there may be a greater decrease in b-wave amplitude versus a-wave amplitude.[21,34] This is a negative ERG pattern, and is not pathognomonic to BCR. It suggests that the Müller and bipolar cells are more affected than the photoreceptor–retinal pigment epithelium complex. This has been seen in autoimmune retinopathy. Rod dysfunction may occur before cone dysfunction: the rod b-wave may be affected prior to photopic b-wave and flicker response in most patients. In late phases of the disease, there is a progressive decrease in a- and b-wave amplitudes. ERG findings have been noted to improve with treatment.[35] Some authors argue that the reversible nature of the ERG abnormalities suggest a non-ischemic etiology.[15] Inflammation of the retinal vasculature could lead to inner retinal dysfunction, while choroidal inflammation could be the cause of altered outer retinal function.

Electrooculogram

Shah and colleagues found that 66.5% of eyes reported in the literature with electrooculography (EOG) findings had abnormal results.[9] Decreased Arden ratios, representing RPE dysfunction, were reported.[34] These ratios further decline with disease progression.

Visual field testing

Visual field abnormalities are present in patients with BCR. These include: peripheral constriction, enlarged blind spot, central or paracentral scotomas, and generalized diminished sensitivity.[8,17,18,20,33] It is not certain whether these visual field defects occur due to ganglion cell, optic nerve, or outer retinal dysfunction, but it is unlikely that the birdshot lesions themselves cause blind spots.[9] Visual field abnormalities may be reversible with immunosuppression.[36]

Systemic associations

There are no definitive systemic associations. Shah and colleagues'[9] review of the literature revealed hearing loss in some patients.[8,37] As mentioned earlier, cutaneous vitiligo associated with BCR has also been reported in a few patients.[8,18] In addition, Priem and Oosterhuis reported an increased incidence of vascular disease in their series. Of 102 patients, 16 had hypertension, 5 had coronary artery disease, 2 had a history of cerebrovascular accident, and 2 had a central retinal vein occlusion.[18] These numbers are not impressive considering the age of the patients.

Pathogenesis

The pathogenesis of BCR is unknown. Inflammation appears to be a primary feature. The histopathological findings in a few eyes with BCR have been reported. These suggest that the spots may be related to accumulation of lymphocytes in the choroid at multiple levels, occasionally associated with hemorrhage.[38] Some of the foci were adjacent to the choroidal vessels. The RPE, ciliary body, and iris were not involved. Some lymphocytes were found around the retinal blood vessels and in the optic disc. The lymphocytes were primarily CD8+T-lymphocytes. Inflammation is strongly associated with HLA-A29, which suggests a genetic predisposition to this disease. However the fact that HLA-A29 is present in 7% of the white population, and BCR is so rare tells

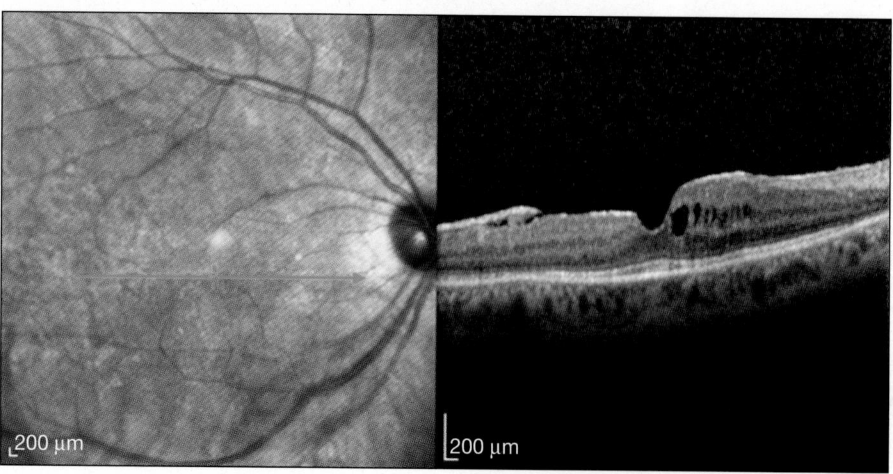

Fig. 76.7 Optical coherence tomography showing cystoid macular edema and epiretinal membrane seen here in a patient with birdshot chorioretinitis.

us other factors are at work. Other genes are highly suspected. The more recent discovery of HLA class I-specific killer cell immunoglobulin-like receptors (KIR) led to epidemiological studies implicating KIR-HLA gene combinations in disease.[39] The combination of KIR and HLA gene variants appears to increase the risk of developing BCR in HLA-A29-positive individuals. The presence of these in the absence of strong inhibition may activate natural killer cells and T cells against intraocular self-antigens thus inciting an autoimmune process. Familial history of autoimmunity is likely.[2]

Differential diagnosis

Birdshot chorioretinopathy can usually be distinguished from other disorders by history and physical findings. However, entities such as pars planitis, intraocular B-cell lymphoma, syphilitic chorioretinitis, sarcoidosis, sympathetic ophthalmia, and other white spot diseases, especially multifocal choroiditis and panuveitis syndrome, should be considered. Sarcoidosis (see Chapter 78, Sarcoidosis) and BCR may be the most difficult to distinguish from each other.[9]

Management/treatment

In the review of the literature by Shah and colleagues[9] most cases were treated; however, no definitive guidelines for the initiation of treatment were given. This chronic progressive disease may not be sight-threatening in the early course, but macular edema with retinal damage, photoreceptor dysfunction, RPE atrophy, and optic nerve damage are the end results. Corticosteroids have been the mainstay of treatment. Oral, sub-Tenon's, intraocular, and most recently sustained release fluocinolone acetonide[40] have been used. Corticosteroids can reduce CME,[7,21,41,42] inflammation,[21] and optic disc edema.[41] They have also been reported to decrease symptoms such as nyctalopia and issues with contrast sensitivity.[11] Systemic steroids carry their own risks. Local steroid injections increase the risk of cataract and cause glaucoma with repeated dosing. Implantation of a fluocinolone acetonide sustained-release device has been shown to eliminate the need for systemic therapy, however it also has a high risk of cataract progression and glaucoma.[40]

Immunosuppressive therapy

Steroid-sparing agents have been used for long-term management of refractory cases. The three classes of immunosuppressives have been used. Cyclosporine has been used as it inhibits T lymphocytes and prevents S-Ag-induced experimental uveitis.[10] Low-dose cyclosporine has proven to have positive visual effect in conjunction with steroids or alone.[43] Nephrotoxicity is the primary side-effect and hypertension can be a problem.[43] Antimetabolites such as azathioprine, mycophenolate mofetil, and methotrexate have been adjunctive or used in monotherapy. Side-effects of these drugs include bone-marrow suppression and hepatotoxicity.[44] The use of the alkylating agents cyclophosphamide and chlorambucil has also been reported. Side-effects such as bone-marrow suppression and development of malignancies must be weighed for this class. Daclizumab, a monoclonal antibody against the alpha-subunit of the IL-2 receptor of T cells, has recently been found to have value in treating BCR.[44,45] The long-term efficacy of these agents needs to be determined and weighed against potential side-effects.

Anti-VEGF therapy has been documented to be useful in treating CNV associated with inflammatory chorioretinal disorders.[46]

In following our patients, we recommend: ERG yearly, Goldmann visual field examination at least yearly, close monitoring of visual acuity, optical coherence tomography (OCT) to evaluate epiretinal membranes and CME, and FA to assess disc and retinal vascular leakage.

Summary

Birdshot chorioretinopathy is a bilateral, chronic progressive disease characterized by deep round lesions in a "birdshot" pattern. Symptoms including blurred vision, photopsias, scotomas, nyctalopia, and poor contrast sensitivity. These can develop years before the onset of fundus findings. The process is associated with a low-grade inflammation of the anterior and posterior segments. Visual prognosis is threatened by the ultimate development of CME, RPE atrophy, and optic nerve pallor. Chronic immune suppression is the mainstay of therapy.

PLACOID DISEASES

Acute posterior multifocal placoid pigment epitheliopathy (APMPPE), serpiginous choroiditis (SC), relentless placoid chorioretinitis (RPC), and persistent placoid maculopathy (PPM), are grouped together due to the "placoid" nature of the lesions that are associated with them. The etiology of these lesions is still poorly understood. They share similarities on fluorescein and indocyanine green angiography; there exists a debate regarding the nature of the hypofluorescence that is seen in these studies. Some argue that primary choroidal ischemia is the cause of the pathology, while others believe that this is blockage from swollen outer retina or RPE. In actuality, it may be a combination of these with newer OCT studies suggesting that the outer retinal layer may be the site of primary insult.

Acute posterior multifocal placoid pigment epitheliopathy

Acute posterior multifocal placoid pigment epitheliopathy (APMPPE) was first described in 1968 by Gass.[47] He presented 3 healthy young female patients who developed the acute onset of bilateral central vision loss associated with multifocal placoid (plate-like) lesions at the level of the outer retina and the RPE, although he had also considered a primary choroiditis. Discussion regarding the site and etiology of the lesions would continue as the disease was further described in later years.[48–57]

Clinical course

Clinical symptoms

Patients present with rapid onset of central vision loss that may be described as blurred vision, paracentral scotoma, metamorphopsia, "spots" in the vision, and photopsias.[58] Initial vision at presentation is 20/25 or worse in about 77% of eyes and 20/40 or worse in 58%.[58] Deficits can be unilateral or bilateral (more common 75%).[59] If unilateral, the second eye can become involved in a few days or weeks. Headaches, stiff neck, and malaise may accompany these ocular symptoms. A history of an antecedent viral syndrome or recent vaccination may be obtained.

Epidemiology

Males and females are equally affected and generally this occurs in young adults. Typically this presents between age 20 and 50 with the mean age of onset being 26.[58,59] Recently, Taich and Johnson describe a syndrome resembling APMPPE in older adults (over age 50).[60] These elderly individuals characteristically may have a worse outcome, with moderate or severe vision

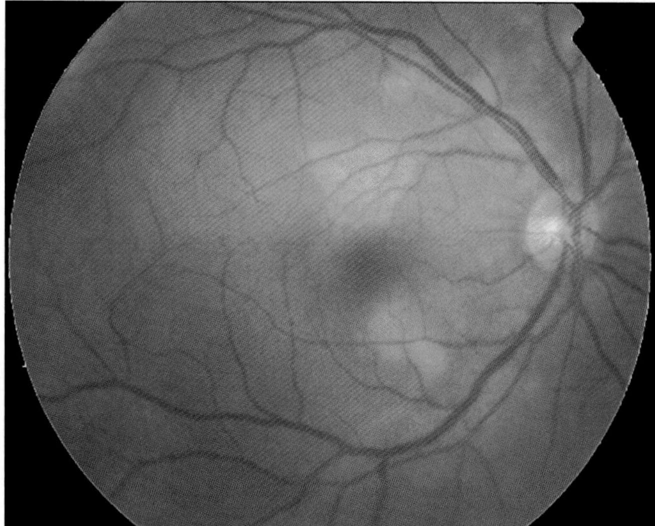

Fig. 76.8 Fundus photo of the right eye showing placoid opacification during the acute phase.

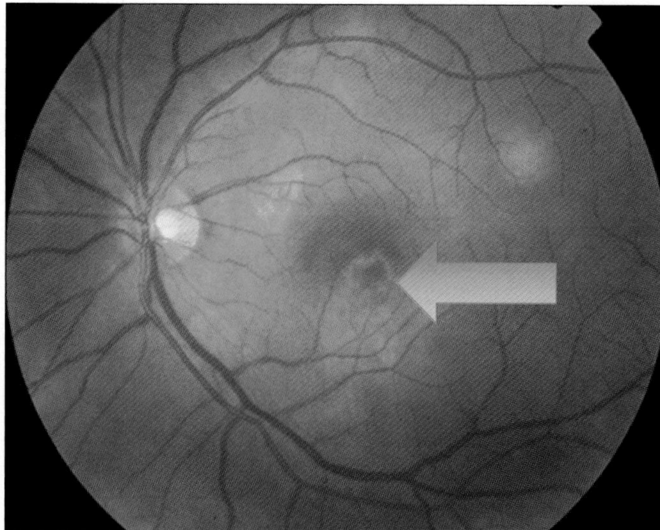

Fig. 76.9 Fundus photo of the left eye. Lesions of differing ages can be seen. Some mild pigment mottling can be seen (arrow).

loss due to the development of geographic atrophy and CNV. These patients resemble the entity persistent placoid maculopathy (see below) and may not have APMPPE.

Fundus findings

Gass described the presence of multiple round and confluent cream colored, flat lesions with indistinct margins scattered in the posterior pole. Lesions are not found anterior to the equator. The presence of these lesions is typically bilateral (Figs 76.8, 76.9). Fresh lesions can develop over the next few weeks, therefore lesions of differing ages can be visible. The placoid lesions tend to clear centrally initially leaving hypopigmentation. Later there is mild pigment mottling which develops into condensation of the pigment midperipherally, finally an increasing degree of coarse pigment clumping occurs (Fig. 76.10). These lesions can enlarge, but generally do not. In the original article, there was no description of serous macular detachment associated with APMPPE. However, later reports described localized serous retinal detachments over the lesions.[52,55,61–65] This feature occasionally makes it difficult to distinguish APMPPE from Harada's disease,[62,66,67] and some have thought that these entities may form a spectrum of disease.[68] It is more likely that there is an underlying common pathology that leads to the serous fluid.[69] Gass commented on how remarkably the choroid and retina remain relatively intact during the course of the disease. However, Spaide described choroidal infiltrations in the periphery[70] of a patient with acute APMPPE. In addition, multiple authors have described an association with retinal vasculitis[71,72] and retinal vein occlusion has also been seen.[71,72] Other findings can include subhyaloid hemorrhage[72] and rare CNV.[73] Case reports have also illustrated optic nerve involvement with disc edema.[71,74]

Other ocular findings

Although vitritis is not a significant component of APMPPE, the degree of ocular inflammation varies widely. An anterior uveitis[75] and granulomatous anterior uveitis[76] have been described. In addition, corneal stromal infiltrates[77] have been mentioned.

Clinical course and prognosis

Generally there is improvement of the visual symptoms within 2–4 weeks. APMPPE has a relatively good prognosis when compared with other placoid white spot syndromes. However Fiore and colleagues[58] reviewed the literature as well as a cohort from their own institution and showed that approximately 50% of patients have an incomplete recovery and 25% of patients have 20/40 vision or worse. Sixty percent of eyes have residual visual symptoms. Foveal involvement at presentation is an important prognosticator. Eighty-eight percent of eyes without foveal involvement proceed to full visual recovery in contrast to 53% of eyes that presented with foveal involvement. Unfortunately, approximately 70% of eyes present with foveal involvement. Photoreceptor involvement may ultimately limit visual prognosis. Progressive improvement of visual acuity usually follows the resolution of the lesions. Gass initially reported that visual recovery could continue on for months after the lesions resolved, even up to 6 months.[47] Most visual recovery occurs within 1 month.[49,51,52,55,58,61]

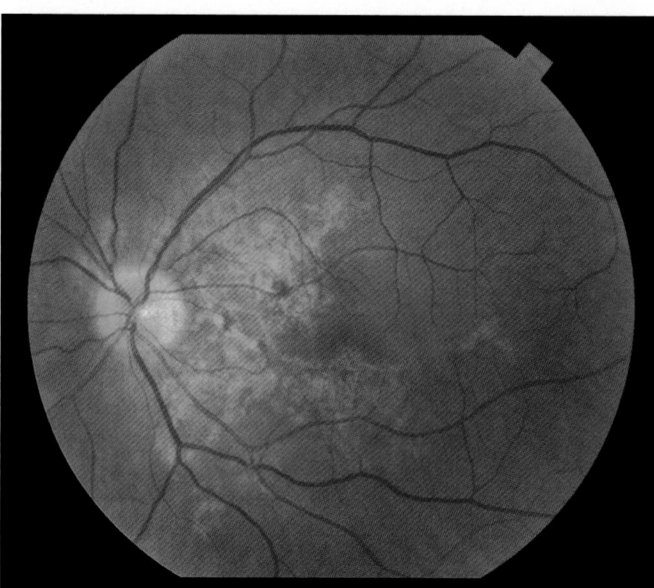

Fig. 76.10 Color fundus photo of healed acute posterior multifocal placoid pigment epitheliopathy.

Imaging

Fluorescein angiography

Gass[47] described the lesions in the early phase as nonfluorescent (Fig. 76.11) and that the choroidal fluorescence is obstructed.

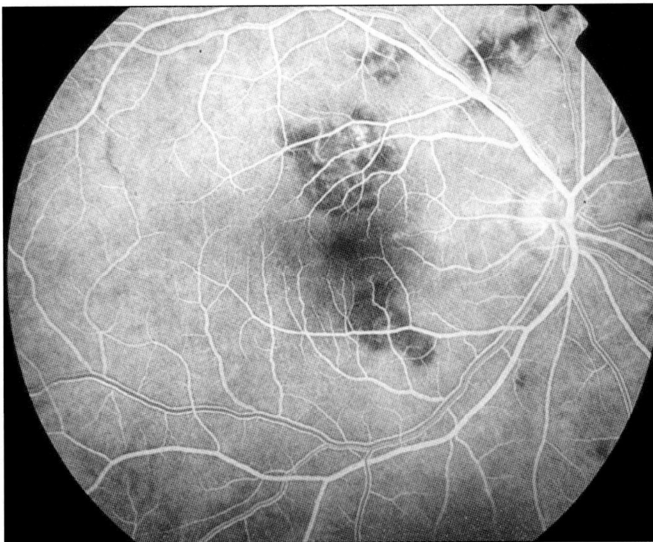
Fig. 76.11 FA shows early hypofluorescence of placoid areas.

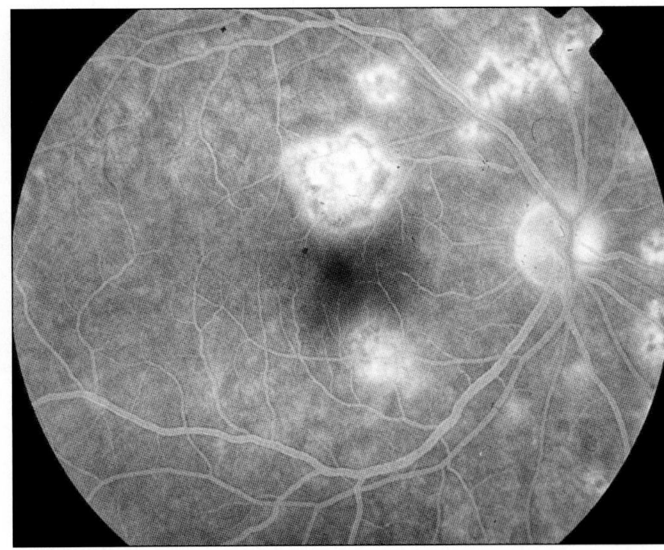
Fig. 76.12 FA in the late phases shows hyperfluorescence.

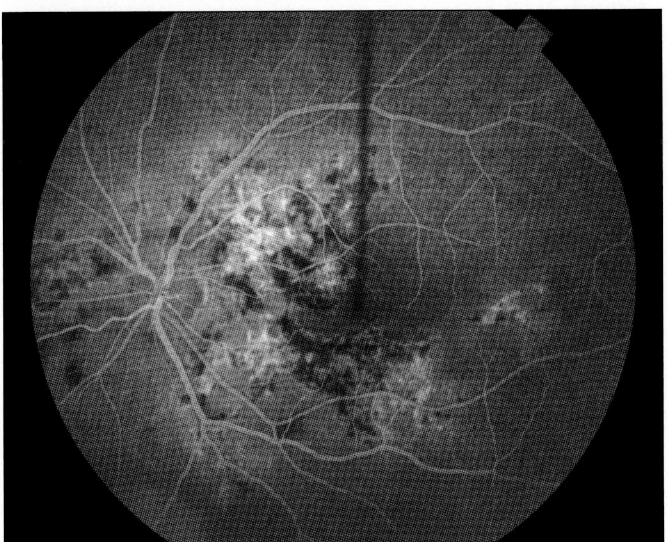
Fig. 76.13 Early FA. As the process becomes inactive, window defects develop. Pigment clumping is seen and blocks fluorescence as well.

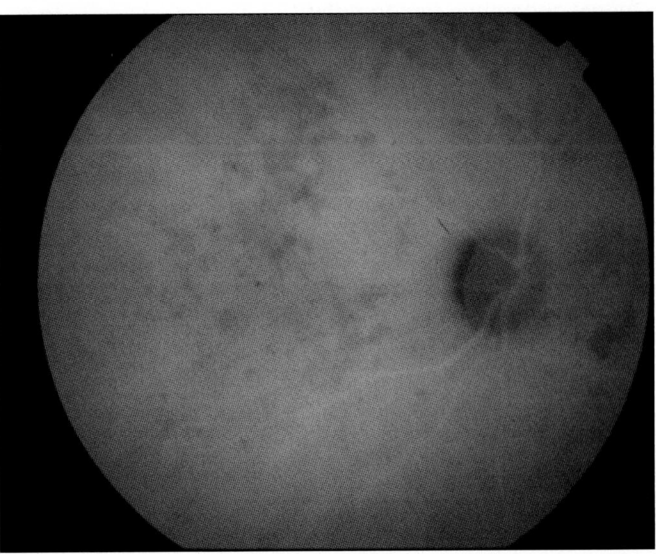
Fig. 76.14 ICG shows hypofluorescent areas.

Later in the angiogram there is a progressive, irregular staining of the lesions (Fig. 76.12). Ryan and Maumenee postulated that this could represent localization to the RPE or choriocapillaris rather than implying an infiltrate of the outer choroid.[48] Gass also stated that the underlying choroidal circulation appeared intact below the healing lesions.[47] However, later ICGA studies suggested that some choroidal hypoperfusion did exist.[78,79] This is discussed below. As the process becomes inactive, hyperfluorescence corresponding to window defects in the RPE develops and staining is no longer evident (Fig. 76.13). There is a clear visibility of the large choroidal vessels in areas of confluent atrophy. However, this does not exist in all areas, implying some RPE remains intact.[53] Either loss of the choriocapillaris or abnormal circulation in the confluent atrophied areas is suggested. In addition to these FA findings, there is also blocked fluorescence from pigment clumping.

The retinal vessels and optic nerve appeared normal[47,53] in original descriptions; however later reports described an association with retinal vasculitis, retinal vein occlusions, and disc edema.

Indocyanine green angiography

Since ICGA studies focus on the choroidal circulation, its findings in APMPPE have been important in developing theories of pathogenesis.[79–84] Acute lesions show early hypofluorescence (Fig. 76.14). In the late phases, these lesions become more defined in shape. These areas are more numerous than the placoid lesions seen clinically. As the disease heals, the hypofluorescence in the late phase becomes less defined and smaller. This lends some support to the theory of choroidal ischemia as an underlying factor in the pathogenesis of APMPPE. It is postulated that there is more hypofluorescence in the acute phase due to the additional presence of swollen outer retina or RPE cells in

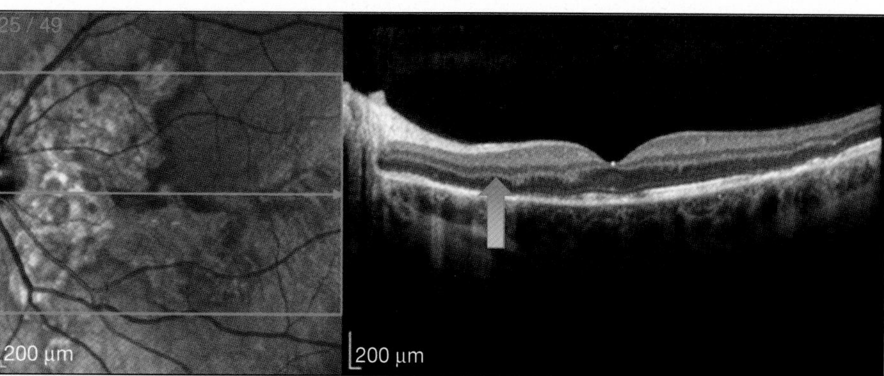

Fig. 76.15 OCT showing disruption of the outer retina.

response to choroidal ischemia (clinically presenting as placoid lesions). As these disappear, there is less blockage and thus less hypofluorescence. Photoreceptor damage may also play a role in this as well, as elucidated by OCT studies and discussed below. Studies show that the hypofluorescence in the late phases can also completely resolve,[78] suggesting that choroidal vasculopathy, if present, may be a transient process.

Optical coherence tomography

Many studies have described the OCT findings in APMPPE.[67,85–90] Garg and Jampol reported outer retinal abnormalities in APMPPE using time domain technology. A serous retinal detachment had reflective material within the subretinal fluid. It was postulated that this was either proteinaceous material or edematous RPE. There was rapid resolution of the serous detachment and the material disappeared.[64]

Lofoco and colleagues showed that in the acute phases the OCT revealed a mild hyperreflective area above the RPE in the photoreceptor layer corresponding to the placoid lesions. Later the OCT scan revealed a nodular hyperreflective lesion in the plane of the RPE with mild underlying backscattering. They theorized that the hyperreflective areas may indicate inflammatory tissue and inflammatory cells or the presence of ischemic edema in the outer retinal layers.[90] As ultra-high resolution (UHR)-OCT developed, Scheufele and colleagues show disruption of the outer retina early in the disease (Fig. 76.15). RPE disruption occurs as the lesions heal.[91] Backscatter of lesions was observed in the acute inflammatory phase in UHR as well. They found photoreceptor atrophy as the lesions began to heal and persistence of it post resolution. They suggested that the backscattering of acute lesions in the outer retina represents inflamed or damaged photoreceptor cell bodies. In addition to illustrating photoreceptor and RPE degeneration, spectral domain OCT has also shown that in some patients with fluid associated with the placoid lesions, that there may actually be accumulation of intraretinal fluid rather than an exudative retinal detachment.[64,85]

Fundus autofluorescence

FAF imaging is directed at the retinal pigment epithelial layer and is therefore especially useful in APMPPE. Several studies have described FAF findings[67,87,89,92,93] (Fig 76.16).

Spaide compared angiographic findings with autofluorescence. He noted that the early hypofluorescence seen on angiogram did not match up with observable changes of the RPE and he suggested this means there are choriocapillaris perfusion defects. In the late phase of the angiogram, there was staining of some of the lesions. These late-staining lesions matched the size and shape of lesions seen in fundus autofluorescence. As the

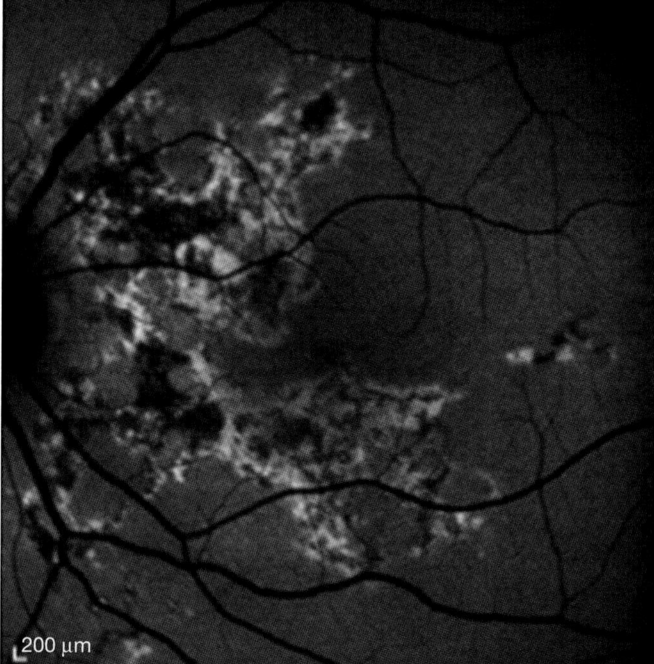

Fig. 76.16 FAF shows areas of hyper- and hypoautofluorescence corresponding to clinical changes in pigmentation.

lesions resolved clinically, they became pigmented centrally with a depigmented halo. On autofluorescence, centrally there was intense hyperautofluorescence, and the depigmented halo was hypoautofluorescent, implying atrophy. He postulated there was a centripetal contraction of the placoid lesions that produced this appearance. He notes the autofluorescence changes lagged behind the clinical appearance. In addition, he found that choroidal abnormalities seemed more numerous on fluorescein and indocyanine green angiography. He concluded the RPE abnormalities were a result of the choroidal abnormalities.[93]

Electrophysiology

Although these functional studies are not essential in the diagnosis of APMPPE, they do emphasize the role of RPE involvement as described by Fishman and colleagues. The electroretinogram is normal to minimally subnormal. However, abnormal light:dark ratios have been documented on EOG, suggesting a diffuse RPE problem. Furthermore, the ERG and EOG abnormalities can normalize, suggesting that this can be a transient RPE problem.[53]

Systemic associations

APMPPE has been linked to CNS manifestations[94–96] including cerebral vasculitis,[97–103] meningo-encephalitis[104] and stroke.[105–109] Cases of APMPPE associated with CN VI palsy[110] and transient hearing loss[111] have also been cited. Headaches are a common symptom and APMPPE has mimicked migraine with aura.[112] Although many patients give a history of viral illness, the symptoms of malaise and headaches may thus be more related to a widespread underlying vasculitis. Cerebrospinal fluid analysis has shown pleocytosis,[113] which lends credence to this. The CNS associations are not benign and death, though uncommon, is possible.

Systemic vasculitis[114] has been implicated in APMPPE and has been described in a P-ANCA-positive patient.[115,116] Other associations with erythema nodosum,[49,57] ulcerative colitis,[117] thyroiditis,[118] nephritis,[119,120] and juvenile rheumatoid arthritis[121] lead to an underlying immune mediated or inflammatory link. Other associations include granulomatous diseases such as: Wegener's granulomatosis (granulomatosis with polyangiitis),[122] pulmonary TB,[123] sarcoidosis.[97,124]

Pathogenesis

When Gass first described APMPPE, he believed that the abnormalities were primarily at the level of the RPE. He believed that there was blockage of fluorescence due to damaged RPE cells, and these cells stained in the late phases. He stated that the retinal and choroidal circulations looked remarkably intact.[47] Van Buskirk and coworkers first described an alternate theory that choroidal perfusion was the primary problem and that the hypofluorescence seen with angiography was due to lack of perfusion of the choriocapillaris.[57] ICG studies found that the choroid did appear hypoperfused as described above. However, Fishman and colleagues' study of ERG and EOG revealed that the ERG and thus the retina remained relatively intact compared to the EOG. Therefore, a diffuse RPE process was implicated in the acute phase of the disease. It also confirmed the transitory nature of this process as the EOG could normalize.[53] The fact that the ERG was generally normal, did not favor a primary widespread choriocapillaris defect.

Currently, some believe that there is a vascular insult affecting the choroid that may cause partial choroidal ischemia leading to RPE damage and ultimately affect photoreceptors. Imaging studies support this. In addition, the systemic associations of this disease point to an underlying vasculitis. It is still possible that a primary process involving the outer retina and RPE could secondarily cause choroidal abnormalities on angiography. It appears that there may be a trigger, either inflammatory or infectious in nature, that incites this process. Furthermore, an association with HLA-B7 and HLA-DR2[125] has been described and this suggests there are certain individuals who are more susceptible to this process.

Although exact etiology is unknown, there may be an association with viral illness;[126] specifically, mumps[127] and adenovirus have been mentioned.[128,129] In half of the cases presented by Ryan and Maumenee there was an overt viral illness prodrome.[48] In addition to viral infections, an association with bacterial infections has also been described. Two case reports implicate Lyme disease.[130,131] Another case report described APMPPE post acute bacterial infection with group A streptococcus.[132] APMPPE has also been found in cases post various vaccinations such as influenza,[133] varicella,[134] meningococcal C conjugate,[135] and hepatitis B.[136] Molecular mimicry has been implicated in the cases of post-vaccination APMPPE.[133] Sequence similarities between the introduced antigens and RPE could incite an immune reaction.

A delayed-type hypersensitivity (DTH) reaction may bring all these associations together.[82] In this process, there is an activation of sensitized T lymphocytes by various stimuli such as bacteria, viruses, and fungi. Previously primed T cells release lymphokines that then activate macrophages and cytotoxic T cells. Macrophages then give rise to epithelioid cells and giant cells that can lead to granulomas. The systemic associations such as CNS inflammation as mentioned above could be explained in this manner. The fluorescein and ICG findings could also be explained by a choroidal DTH reaction causing choroidal vascular occlusion.

A thrombotic process of the choroid has also been postulated. Elevated anticardiolipin antibodies were found in a patient with acute APMPPE. These levels were normal a year after resolution of the disease.[137] The association with retinal vein occlusion supports a thrombotic etiology. Furthermore, elevated anticardiolipin antibodies have been associated with a number of viral infections and in many cases also associated with thrombosis.[138]

Differential diagnosis

The diagnosis of APMPPE is made clinically based on examination, time course, and imaging characteristics. Other white spot diseases are in the differential diagnosis and should be considered. These include: serpiginous choroidopathy (which should be considered in recurrent, chronic cases), relentless placoid chorioretinitis, which should be thought of in severe, persistent, and recurrent cases, and multifocal evanescent white dot syndrome. Other considerations include: diffuse unilateral subacute neuroretinitis, Harada's disease,[62,66–68] TB, sarcoid, fungal disease, choroidal metastasis or lymphomatous infiltrate,[48] and syphilis.[139]

Management/treatment

Laboratory investigations are usually not necessary. Certain investigations may be useful in questionable cases. Spinal fluid analysis for pleocytosis,[114] anticardiolipin antibodies,[137] and association with HLA-B7 and HLA-DR2[125] are among them.

No therapy has been proven useful in the management of acute APMPPE. A review of the data from the literature on corticosteroids does not provide clear direction.[58] However, some make a case for intravenous steroids and immunosuppressive agents to be considered when there is central nervous system involvement.[140]

Rarely CNV can develop. Bruch's membrane appears less affected in APMPPE compared to serpiginous choroiditis, and therefore CNV is less prevalent. Anti-VEGF agents have been found to be useful in treating CNV.[141,142] Photodynamic therapy has been used as well; however, its use is cautioned as it can exacerbate inflammation and possible choroidal ischemia, which are present in the acute stages of APMPPE.[73]

Summary

APMPPE is a bilateral inflammatory process involving the RPE, the choriocapillaris, and outer retina. There is an equal incidence in males and females. A viral prodrome is often associated with this entity. There are characteristic findings on fluorescein angiography including early hypofluorescence with late staining in the acute phase. This process becomes inactive over the period of weeks without intervention and in comparison to other WSS it has a relatively good prognosis. The pathogenesis is controversial but choroidal hypoperfusion leading to RPE and photoreceptor damage may play a role or the outer retina and RPE may be the primary site of damage.

Serpiginous choroiditis

Serpiginous choroiditis (SC) also known as helicoid peripapillary chorioretinal degeneration,[143] geographic helicoid peripapillary choroidopathy,[144] and geographical choroidopathy[145] is a rare disease of unknown etiology. It is usually bilateral, chronic, and progressive. The lesions involve the outer retina, RPE, choriocapillaris, and large choroidal vessels.[146] Patients present with acute geographic or serpentine lesions that are gray or gray-yellow (due to disruption of the RPE or outer retina).

Clinical course

Clinical symptoms

Patients are often asymptomatic until the lesions affect the fovea. Blurred vision occurs at this point.[147,148] Although this is a bilateral disease, typically the patient becomes symptomatic unilaterally with foveal involvement. Small central or paracentral scotomas may be present. These are absolute in their acute stages, and become relative with healing.[148]

Epidemiology

SC is a disease of healthy individuals. The onset is usually between the ages of 30 and 70. However, cases of SC have been reported in younger individuals.[148] Most reports of SC involve Caucasians; however, SC has also been reported in Asians,[149] African Americans,[148] and Hispanics.[150] The literature reflects a slight predilection for males.[146] No family history is elicited. One study done in a Finnish population showed a higher prevalence of HLA-B7 in patients with SC.[151]

Fundus findings

Two variants of SC are seen. The classic appearance, seen in approximately 80% of cases,[146] starts with geographic patches of gray or creamy yellow placoid lesions in the peripapillary region. It generally progresses in a centrifugal manner with finger-like or serpentine projections. In one report, a centripetal direction was described.[147] The outer retina appears edematous, and serous retinal detachments may be seen.[152,153] As these active lesions resolve (with or without) treatment over the next several weeks, extensive RPE and choriocapillaris atrophy occurs (Fig. 76.17). SC has recurrences and therefore it is common to see lesions of different ages. Recurrences can occur at the edge of old scars (Fig. 76.18), but not always. As the disease becomes chronic, chorioretinal atrophy, subretinal fibrosis, and RPE clumping is seen.[146] Since most patients become symptomatic only when the fovea becomes involved, about two-thirds present with bilateral chorioretinal scarring.[154]

Macular serpiginous choroiditis[149,150] is the second variant (Figs 76.19–76.22). There is no difference in the lesions of macular serpiginous and peripapillary diseases except for location.[151] There is generally a poorer prognosis for the macular variant as the fovea is affected at the start. Vision loss may also be related to presence of CNV.[150] However, Sahu and coworkers, in a more recent report, did not observe CNV in their series.[155] Macular SC may be misdiagnosed as macular degeneration, macular dystrophies, or toxoplasmosis.[146]

Other ocular findings

Although serpiginous choroiditis is not usually associated with a marked inflammatory response, nongranulomatous anterior uveitis[156,157] has been seen. More commonly – estimated in about a third of patients – there are fine vitreous cells.[153] The eye is white. Additional retinal findings have been described. These include CNV, which affects 13–20% of eyes,[158–163] vein occlusions,[164,165] retinal vasculitis,[165] usually a periphlebitis, CME,[166] and bilateral full-thickness macular holes.[167] Optic nerve abnormalities such as optic disc edema[147] and disc neovascularization[162] can be seen at the active stage of serpiginous choroiditis.

Clinical course and prognosis

Serpiginous choroiditis is characterized by multiple recurrences at intervals of months to years. Healing of individual lesions takes place in 2[151] to 8 weeks,[146] but new lesions appear later.[147] Generally acute lesions are seen in one eye at a time.

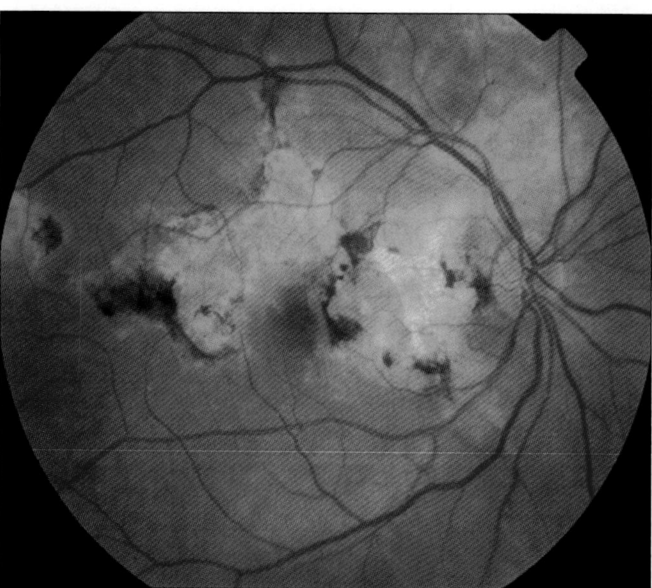

Fig. 76.17 Fundus photo showing the geographic projections in the inactive phase.

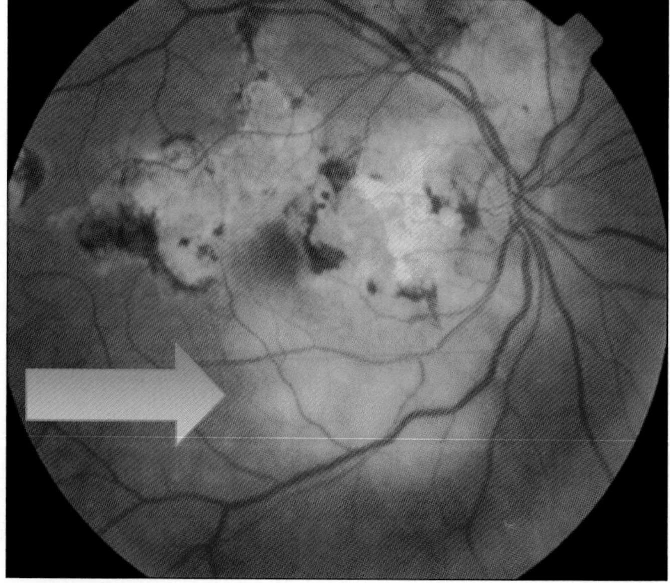

Fig. 76.18 Fundus photo showing recurrence of serpiginous choroiditis near the edge of a scar.

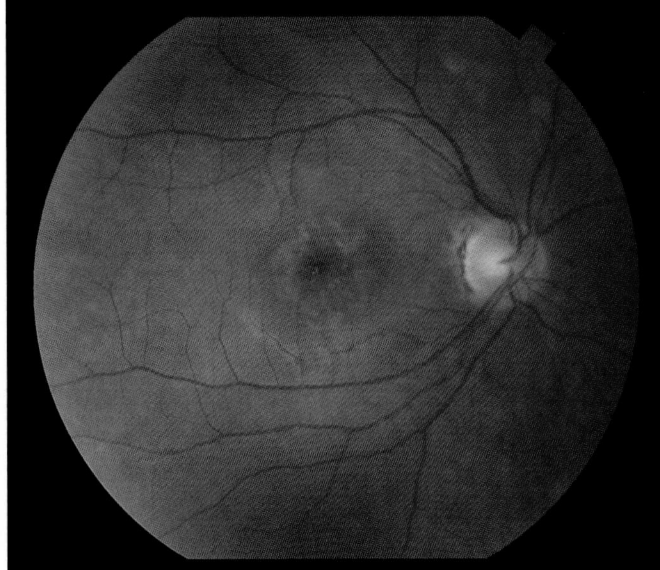

Fig. 76.19 Fundus photo of subacute macular serpiginous choroiditis.

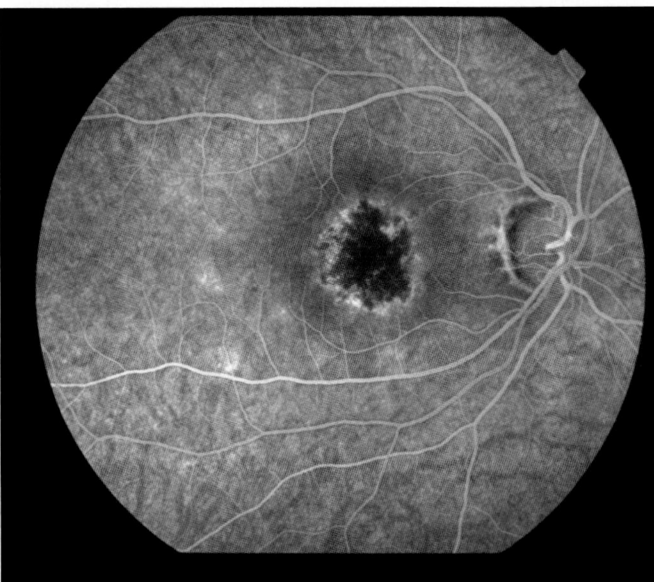

Fig. 76.20 Early FA shows hypofluorescence.

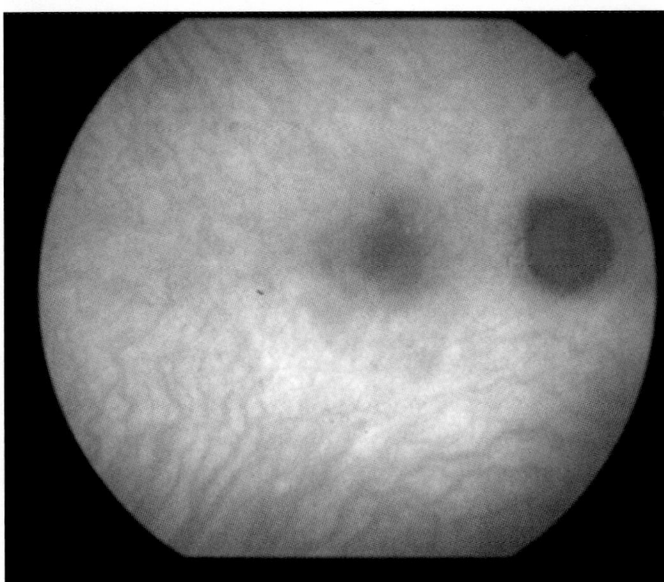

Fig. 76.21 ICG showing hypofluorescence centered in the macula.

Visual loss is correlated with proximity to the fovea. There can be some incomplete recovery, but due to the recurrences, 75% of patients develop central visual loss in one or both eyes. Final visual acuity is less than 20/200 in up to 25% of eyes regardless of treatment.[168]

Imaging

Fluorescein angiography

In the acute SC, the lesions show hypofluorescence during the early phase of the study[144] (Fig. 76.23). This is likely due to a combination of blockage by swollen outer retina and RPE and nonperfusion of the choriocapillaris. The borders of the lesion may be hyperfluorescent, representing intact choriocapillaris. As the study progresses, the previous hypofluorescent lesions become variably hyperfluorescent and this intensifies over time representing staining of the acute lesions (Fig. 76.24). Retinal vascular staining may be seen near active lesions. Pigmentary changes then develop and there is often pronounced atrophy. Angiography at this stage shows mottled hyperfluorescence with increased fluorescence in the late phases representing leakage of dye from the damaged choriocapillaris at the periphery of the lesion. CNV can occur and appears as late leakage, usually at the edge of a scar.

Indocyanine green angiography

ICGA[169–172] is useful in evaluating SC. Giovannini and colleagues describe how ICGA allows a greater understanding of the disease. In particular, ICGA allowed: (1) better staging of SC, revealing choroidal alterations when there was no clinical or FA evidence; (2) better identification of the active lesions, which appear to be larger at the choroidal level in comparison with the corresponding retinal lesions; and (3) persistence of choroidal activity even when the signs of retinal activity had disappeared.[171] The ICG pattern is characterized by hypofluorescent areas persisting from early to late phases (Fig. 76.25). The hypofluorescence has been reported to be less pronounced in later phases, which may represent delayed perfusion rather than nonperfusion.[173] The hypofluorescent lesions appear more extensive on ICGA in comparison to clinical examination and fluorescein angiography.

Optical coherence tomography

OCT findings have been described recently.[174–178] Spectral domain OCT illustrates retinal atrophy with disruption of the photoreceptor layers in affected areas. There is thinning of the RPE and intraretinal fluid including cystic changes can be seen.[174] There is increased reflectance of the choroid and the deeper retinal layers. Disruption of the photoreceptor inner/outer segments is seen in active and inactive lesions[175] (Fig. 76.26).

Fundus autofluorescence

As SC involves the RPE, FAF[175,178,179] images are helpful in demarcating this disease. New lesions appear hyperautofluorescent and old lesions are hypoautofluorescent (Fig. 76.27). Recurrences are characterized by hyperautofluorescent lesions at the borders

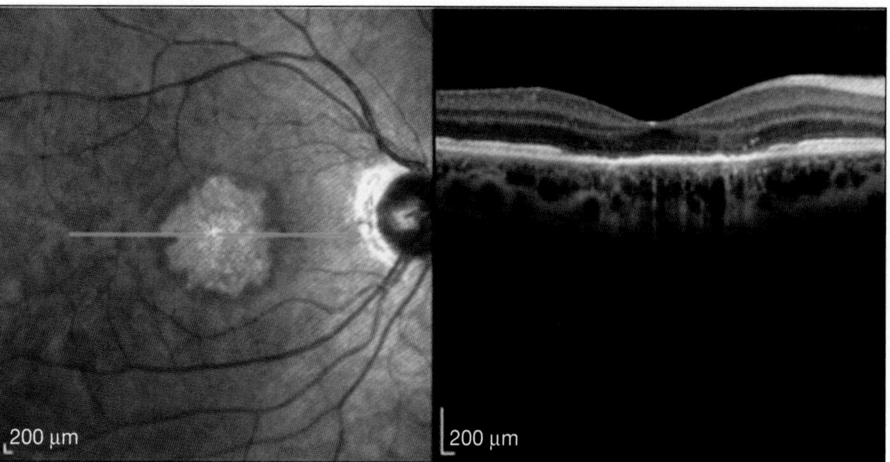

Fig. 76.22 OCT in macular serpiginous choroiditis shows outer retinal disruption.

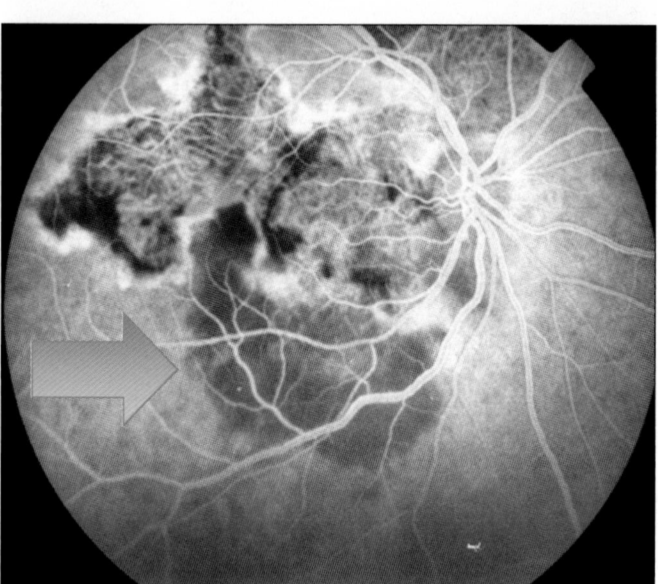

Fig. 76.23 FA shows hypofluorescence corresponding to the new lesion (arrow).

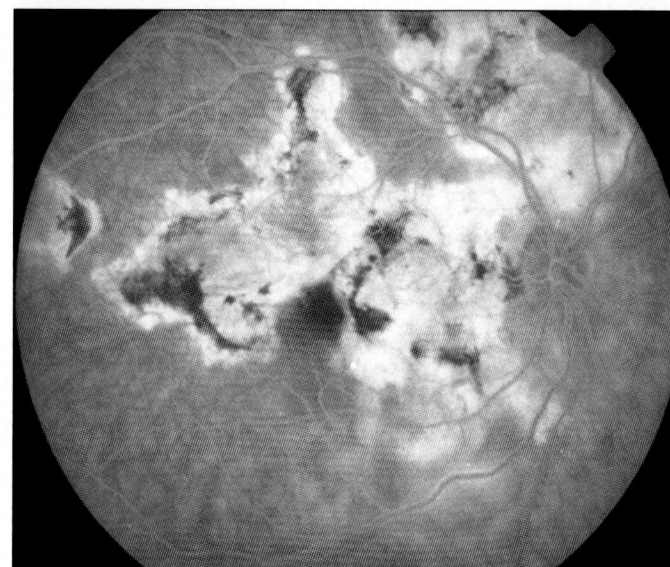

Fig. 76.24 FA in the late phases shows that previously hypofluorescent lesions become variably hyperfluorescent.

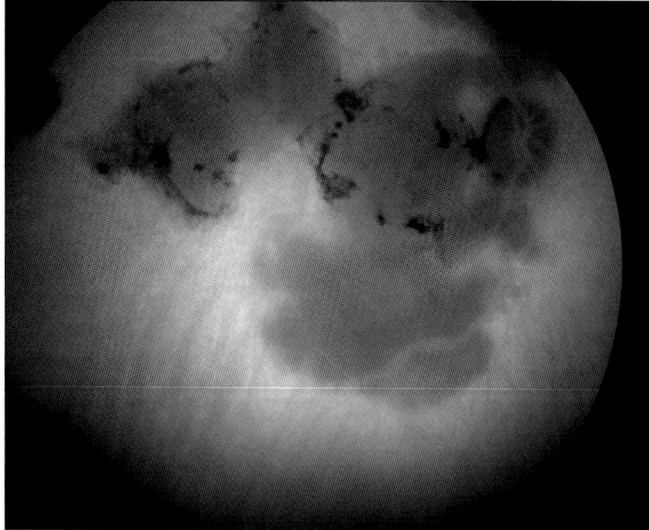

Fig. 76.25 ICG of this patient is characterized by persistent hypofluorescence.

of old hypoautofluorescent areas.[179] Hyperautofluorescence was detected 2–5 days after the appearance of acute lesions.[178] Piccolino and colleagues compared FAF to ICGA and OCT and found that the acute hyperautofluorescent areas were less extensive than the perfusion defect delineated by ICGA. When compared to OCT, there was increased reflectance of the photoreceptor layer corresponding to the area of hyperautofluorescence. As the disease progressed, the hyperautofluorescent area became hypoautofluorescent and the photoreceptor changes persisted.

In developing countries, especially India, individuals with evidence of tuberculosis may have serpiginous-like lesions. (See differential diagnosis section below and Chapter 82, Mycobacterial infections). FAF appears to distinguish the lesions of SC from TB-related disease. TB-related diseases have a stippled hypoautofluorescence corresponding to lesions, which is not as homogenous as SC.[179]

Electrophysiology

Results of ERG are normal,[148,153] and EOG is abnormal only when there is extensive disease.[153]

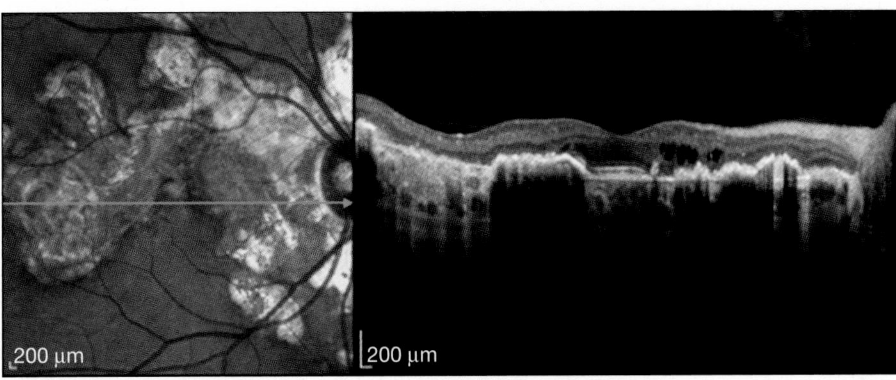

Fig. 76.26 OCT shows retinal atrophy and disruption of the photoreceptor layers. Cystic fluid is seen here as well. The fovea is spared.

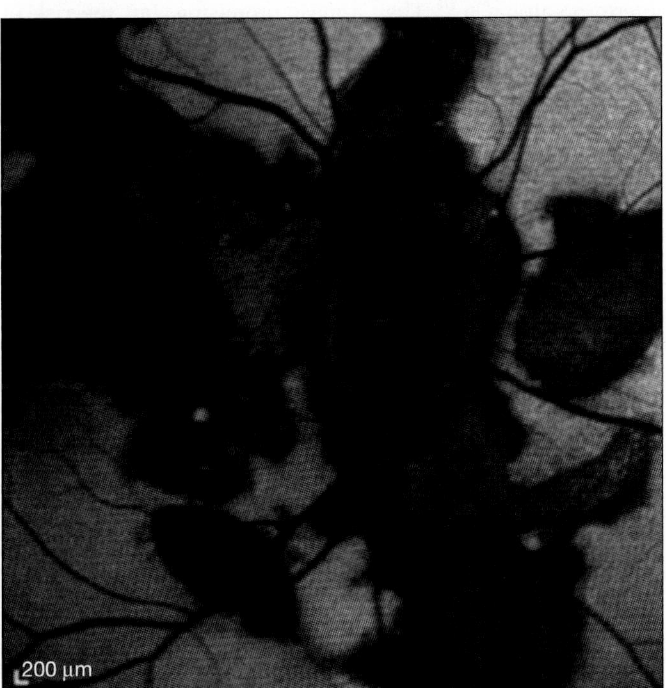

Fig. 76.27 FAF image shows hypoautofluorescent lesions corresponding to retinal pigment epithelium atrophy in projections surrounding the nerve.

Perimetry

Goldmann visual field examination shows that scotomas corresponding to an area of activity are not permanent.[148] Scotomas corresponding to fundus lesions are present, but are not absolute and usually are denser centrally and less peripherally. More recently microperimetry[180] studies confirm this finding.

Systemic associations

Reports have described SC in patients with various systemic diseases: Crohn's disease,[181] SLE,[182] celiac disease,[183] and extrapyramidal dystonia.[184] These are likely coincidental associations. Systemic vasculitides can cause choroidal ischemic syndromes, which may resemble SC.

Pathogenesis

The pathogenesis of serpiginous choroiditis remains unknown. Postulated etiologies have included autoimmune, infectious, vascular, and degenerative.[146]

The inflammatory nature of the disease is supported by histopathology with inflammatory lymphocytic infiltrate in the choroid (more prominent at the margin of the lesion).[161,185] Clinically, the presence of anterior uveitis, vitritis, and retinal vasculitis also points to an inflammatory etiology. Like APMPPE, the report of an association with HLA- B7 suggests some individuals are more susceptible to this process.[151] Broekhuyse found a sensitization to S-antigen in SC patients.[186] Acute SC lesions respond to steroids and immune modulating agents consistent with an immune-mediated process.

A microbial origin of SC has been suggested, but the evidence is not convincing. Herpes virus has been found in aqueous humor[187] and VZV and HSV DNA were detected in the aqueous of a subset of patients with serpiginous choroiditis, suggesting that these viruses may be involved. Conversely, Akpek and Chan described the lack of herpes virus DNA in choroidal tissues at autopsy of a patient with SC.[185] No viral DNA was amplified, including HSV, CMV, EBV, VZV, or HHV-8. Furthermore, there are reports of recurrences while on antiviral therapy.[168] Pisa and colleagues studied 5 patients with SC to assess the presence of fungal infection by the presence of antibodies in human serum samples.[188] Antibodies against *Candida* were apparent in 4 of the 5 patients.

Vasculopathy, either primary or secondary, has also been proposed.[146,173,189] The clinical presence of phlebitis and branch retinal vein occlusions supports this etiology. King and colleagues noted elevated factor VIII in association with SC.[190] This could lead to an occlusive vascular phenomenon due to vascular endothelial injury as seen in diseases such as scleroderma, Raynaud disease, polymyalgia rheumatica, and temporal arteritis. Fluorescein and ICGA also suggest vascular involvement. Hayreh's early work showed that closure of the cilioretinal vessels could produce lesions that look something like SC.[191] However, the lack of systemic vascular disease in SC does not support vasculopathy.

Finally, a degenerative etiology has been proposed. The nature of SC's chronic and progressive nature and later onset in life lends some support to this.[146] One case showed an association with unilateral extrapyramidal dystonia,[184] which could be supportive or coincidental. The presence of inflammation and lack of familial inheritance, the sporadic nature of SC, and occasional recovery of vision are not supportive of a degenerative condition.

Differential diagnosis

APMPPE must be considered. Patients with APMPPE are usually younger. The acute lesions are bilateral and scattered throughout the posterior pole. Recurrences are very rare. CNV is a rare complication in APMPPE compared to serpiginous choroiditis.

Visual prognosis is better with APMPPE. Persistent placoid maculopathy and relentless placoid chorioretinitis should also be considered and will be discussed later in this chapter. Other white spot syndromes such as birdshot choroidopathy and multifocal choroiditis and panuveitis syndrome as well as presumed ocular histoplasmosis may also be considerations.

Tuberculous serpiginous choroiditis (see Chapter 82, Mycobacterial infections) can resemble idiopathic serpiginous choroiditis. TB-related serpiginous choroiditis is associated with more vitritis compared to serpiginous choroiditis. In addition, patients with TB choroiditis have more multifocal lesions involving the periphery. SC has larger lesions compared to TB and is more likely to have lesions extending from the optic nerve head.[192] Fluorescein angiography does not distinguish between these two entities. Fundus autofluorescence may. Hypofluorescence corresponding to RPE loss in SC is more homogeneous compared to the variegated pattern and stippled hyperautofluorescence of tuberculous disease.[178]

Other diagnostic considerations include: sarcoidosis,[193] systemic non-Hodgkin lymphoma,[194] antiphospholipid antibody syndrome,[195] toxoplasmosis,[196] syphilis, and posterior scleritis.[197]

With macular SC, one must think about choroidal ischemia in the differential diagnosis.[150] This can occur with systemic vascular diseases such as systemic lupus erythematosus, toxemia of pregnancy, disseminated intravascular coagulation, thrombotic thrombocytopenic purpura, and malignant hypertension as an etiology for macular vision loss.

Management/treatment

Although the diagnosis is suspected by clinical history, examination, and imaging characteristics, a preliminary workup could include TB skin test, chest X-ray, quanterferon gold test if TB is strongly suggested,[198] ACE, VDRL, fluorescent treponemal antibody absorption test, toxoplasma titers, and a viral screen. Abrez and colleagues suggest an aqueous tap if anterior chamber cells are noted with an evaluation by PCR for viral etiology.[157]

As serpiginous choroiditis is a rare disease, controlled trials comparing treatments are not available. Much of what we know comes from small case series.[199] Due to the relapsing and progressive nature of SC, treatment should be aimed at both the acute inflammatory episode as well as preventing recurrences.

Steroids have been a mainstay of treatment and multiple routes of administration have been described. Oral prednisone,[152] sub-Tenon's triamcinolone, intravenous pulse methylprednisolone therapy,[200] intravitreal triamcinolone acetonide,[201–204] and intravitreous fluocinolone acetonide implant.[205] Systemic prednisone therapy of 60–80 mg/day is a commonly prescribed therapeutic regimen. Aggressive corticosteroid therapy is useful in treating acute attacks, but since the steroids are tapered, is not useful in preventing recurrences. Relapses are common when tapering the medication. A case report described using an intravitreous fluocinolone acetonide implant which resulted in ongoing control of the disease for 14 months postoperative follow-up.[205] This delivery route avoids the side-effects of systemic steroids. However, cataract and glaucoma from this route of administration are often seen.

Corticosteroids can be used alone, or in combination with other immunosuppressive therapy.[206,207] Antibiotics (cyclosporine),[208,209] antimetabolites (azathioprine),[210] alkylating agents (cyclophosphamide and chlorambucil)[211,212] have been used. Cyclosporine alone has been used with mixed results. Triple-agent immunosuppression with cyclosporine, azathioprine, and prednisone was described by Hooper and Kaplan.[213] They reported 5 patients with bilateral SC in whom visual recovery was promoted by this regimen. The therapy was given for 8 weeks prior to tapering. Two patients relapsed. Another study reported 4 patients maintained on a low dose of triple therapy for 12–69 months. Three of 4 patients did achieve remission off the drugs.[206] Alkylating agents have shown some promise, but side-effects including bone-marrow suppression, nausea, fatigue, as well as one case of development of transitional epithelial carcinoma of the bladder, did occur.[211] For this reason, these agents should probably be reserved for sight-threatening disease that has failed conventional immunosuppressive therapy.[146]

Other more recent therapies have included infliximab[214] and interferon-alpha-2a.[215] They appear promising, but the risk of systemic side-effects should be weighed. Patients receiving systemic management for SC are often jointly managed with a rheumatologist, internist, or oncologist.

Treatment is also aimed at managing complications of SC. These include CNV and CME. Reports have described the use of anti-VEGF agents for inflammatory chorioretinal disorders.[216–219] CNV in SC appears to be responsive to this treatment. Photodynamic therapy[220,221] has also been used with some success, however the clinician should be mindful that choroidal ischemia and inflammation is inherent in SC and could be exacerbated by this treatment. For extrafoveal CNV, thermal photocoagulation is possible.

Acetazolamide[222] may be useful in the management of CME related to SC. It is thought that CME develops due to RPE dysfunction. After 2 weeks of treatment, there was complete resolution of CME with improvement of visual acuity in one case report.

Follow-up can include Amsler grid use by the patient to monitor for relapses and foveal involvement.

Summary

Serpiginous choroiditis is a chronic, progressive, bilateral disease. The course of the disease includes destruction of the choriocapillaris, RPE, and atrophy of the overlying retina. Treatment is aimed at immune suppression, and carries significant side-effects. Visual prognosis is determined by the proximity of active disease to the fovea.

Relentless placoid chorioretinitis

Relentless placoid chorioretinitis (RPC) was described in 2000 by Jones and colleagues.[223] They reported 6 patients resembling both APMPPE and serpiginous choroiditis, but with an atypical time course and retinal distribution. The term ampiginous has been used to describe similar patients.[224] It is likely that some previous descriptions of multifocal serpiginous[225] and recurrent APMPPE represent this entity.[226]

Clinical course

Clinical symptoms

The commonest complaint is sudden painless blurring.[227] Patients also describe metamorphopsia, floaters, or can be asymptomatic.

Epidemiology

Patients were aged 17–51 in the report by Jones and colleagues.[223] There was no gender predilection. In a series by Jyotirmay and colleagues, a male preponderance was found with a mean age of 34.[227] The patients have no consistent medical disorder or viral prodrome.

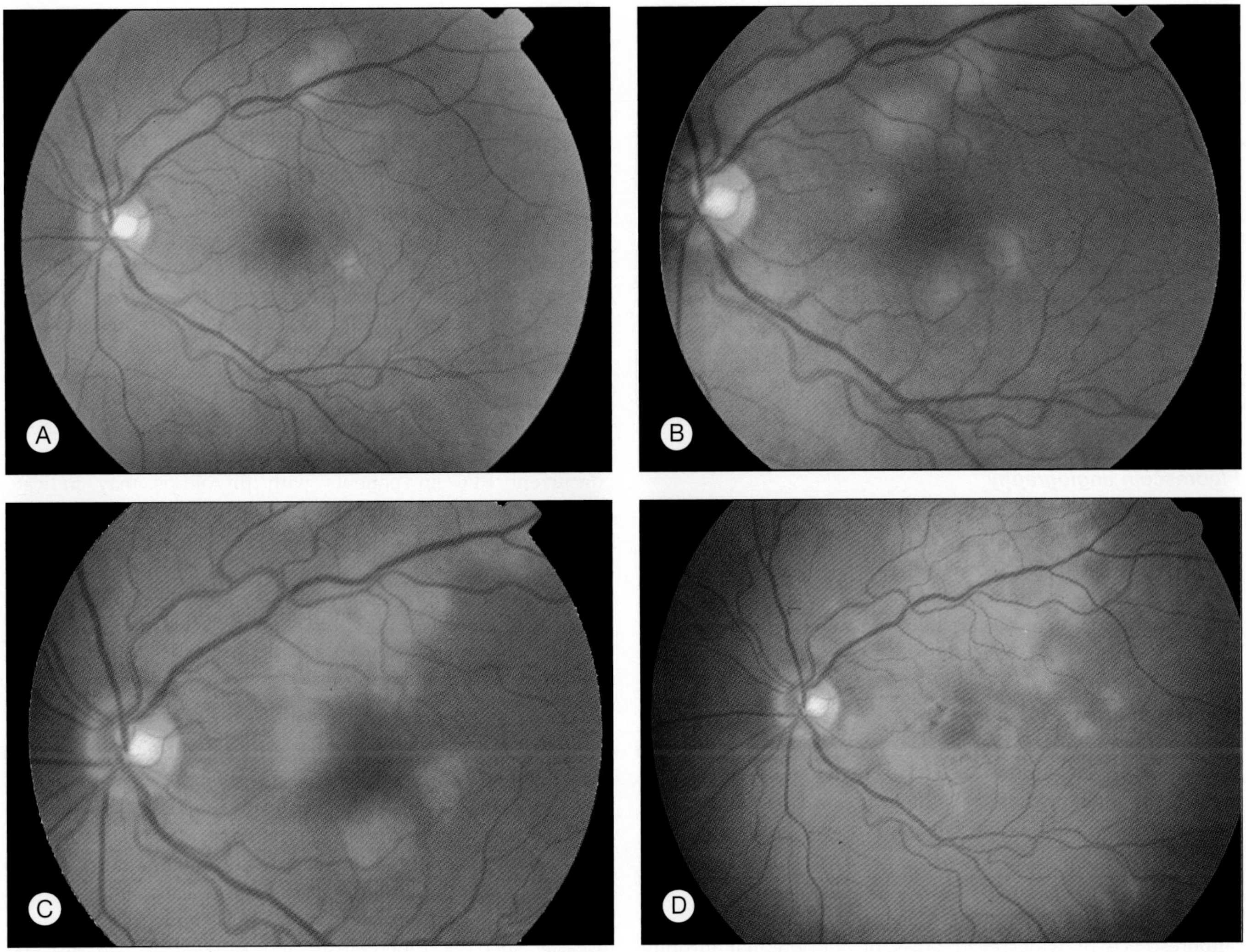

Fig. 76.28 (A–D) Fundus photos of a patient with relentless placoid chorioretinitis documenting progression of posterior creamy white lesions at the level of the RPE over the course of one month.

Fundus findings

In most cases, patients have bilateral posterior creamy-white lesions at the level of the RPE (Fig. 76.28). The lesions (in almost all cases) tend to be smaller than those of APMPPE (approximately ½ disc area)[227] (Fig. 76.29). Lesions can be active in both eyes simultaneously. As they heal, pigmented chorioretinal atrophy develops. Lesions can persist and grow. A hallmark of this disease is the eventual presence of numerous (>50 to hundreds) lesions with involvement anterior and posterior to the equator. This is in contrast to APMPPE which is limited to the posterior pole. One study found that lesions more commonly appear in the periphery first and in the posterior pole later.[227] The fovea is commonly involved.

Other findings have included a mild vitritis, occasional subretinal fluid, and disc swelling.[223] In their study of 26 eyes in 16 patients, Jyotirmay and colleagues found subretinal fibrosis, as well as epiretinal membranes as rare findings.[227] Interestingly, CNV was not described in either case series.[222,227,228]

Other ocular findings

Jones et al. described a patient with herpetic keratitis and corneal infiltrates in their series. Iritis with keratic precipitates as well as episcleritis can also occur.[223,228]

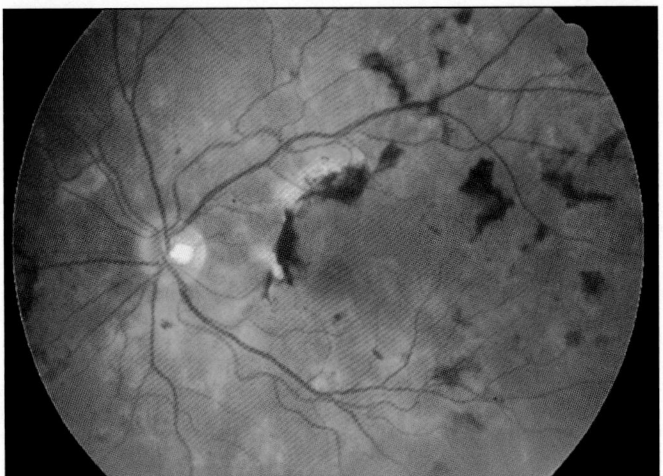

Fig. 76.29 Fundus photo of the same patient 2 years later. Healed lesions show pigmented chorioretinal atrophy. The fovea is spared.

Clinical course and prognosis

The clinical course is prolonged and relapsing. In 4 out of the original 6 patients, active lesions were seen bilaterally and concurrently. This is in contrast to serpiginous chorioretinitis in which usually only one eye is active at a time. Pigmented chorioretinal atrophy develops within weeks. Throughout the long clinical course, lesions persisted and grew. There was also the appearance of new lesions for 5–24 months despite therapy, and involved eyes developed 50 or more lesions. Some patients showed recurrences months to years after onset. These can occur after significant periods of inactivity.

Permanent vision loss is usually mild. However, central vision was affected in all untreated cases. Vision dropped as much as 6 lines in the acute stage in Jones et al.'s study.[223] Some patients showed improvement in vision. Patients who received prolonged systemic steroids seemed to have decreased activity and improved visual outcome. Only 2 out of 6 patients had a final vision worse than 20/40 in the original series. Jyotirmay and colleagues report a favorable visual outcome in over 96% of their patients.[227]

Imaging

Fluorescein angiography

Similar to APMPPE and SC, fluorescein studies reveal early hypofluoresence due to either blockage or choriocapillaris nonperfusion. Later phases show staining.

Indocyanine green angiography

ICGA shows hypofluorescence in the areas corresponding to the clinical lesions. This persists into the late phases. Again this shows similarity to APMPPE and SC.

Optical coherence tomography

There has been only one report. During the active stage of the disease with foveal lesions, the OCT showed subfoveal fluid.[229] In addition, a pigment epithelial detachment with hyperreflectivity of the inner and outer retinal layers was present. Further study is warranted.

Fundus autofluorescence

FAF of RPC has been reported in one patient. Marked hypoautofluorescence of widespread areas of chorioretinal atrophy was seen.[230]

Electrophysiology

A decrease in the electrooculogram and electroretinogram results (scotopic, photopic, and flicker) has been reported.[223] Other reports do not show this finding.[229]

Systemic associations

In Jones and colleagues' case series, one patient had Hashimoto thyroiditis and aseptic meningitis. Two other patients presented with nonspecific upper respiratory tract infections.[223] Jyotirmay et al.'s series reported 2 patients with Hashimoto thyoroiditis, and one patient with type 1 diabetes mellitus.[227] There has been a recent case report of RPC associated with central nervous system lesions in a 20-year-old male.[231]

Pathogenesis

The similarity to APMPPE and serpiginous choroiditis suggests that there is some common pathophysiology. The reports of concurrent RPC in patients with thyroiditis may indicate inflammatory or immune processes. The presence of uveitis, disc edema, and corneal infiltrates has also been described in APMPPE.

Choroidal ischemia either primary or secondary due to an inflammatory etiology is a consideration, as it is in APMPPE and SC. The presence of RPC in a patient with CNS lesions may indicate a small-vessel vasculitis.[231]

Differential diagnosis

APMPPE and serpiginous choroiditis are the main considerations (Table 76.1). Time course as well as the number and location of the lesions distinguish these diseases. There may be some resemblance to other white spot diseases including: multifocal choroiditis and birdshot chorioretinopathy. Other processes such as Harada's disease, neoplastic infiltration of the choroid, infections such as syphilis, and granulomatous diseases such as tuberculosis and sarcoidosis can also be considered.[223]

Table 76.1 Comparison of APMPPE, serpiginous choroiditis, and relentless placoid chorioretinitis

	APMPPE	Serpiginous choroiditis	Relentless placoid chorioretinitis
Age	Young	Young to middle-aged	Young to middle-aged
Course	Lesions heal over weeks	Lesions heal over weeks to months	Continued activity, growth of lesions, new lesions
Visual outcome	Good	Poor if fovea involved	Poor if fovea involved
Ocular involvement	Posterior pole	Posterior pole, usually peripapillary	Posterior pole and anterior to equator
Systemic involvement	Headaches, CNS signs	None	None
Recurrences	Usually uniphasic	Recurrences contiguous with old lesions	Noncontiguous recurrences
Treatment	Usually does well without treatment	Immunosuppression	Immunosuppression

Management/treatment

The best regimen is as yet unknown. Jones et al. described decreased activity and improved vision in patients who were treated with prolonged steroids versus patients who were untreated or treated less aggressively.[223] Antiviral therapy was not effective. Immunosuppression with cyclosporine was also described, but recurrence was noted when it was tapered. Mycophenolate mofetil with prednisone was used in one patient who also had CNS lesions.[232] Jyotirmay and colleagues used steroids (including sub-Tenon's) in combinations with azathioprine, or cyclophosphamide.

Summary

Relentless placoid chorioretinitis is a disease of unknown etiology that resembles APMPPE and serpiginous choroiditis. It has a prolonged and relapsing course. Many creamy lesions appear in the periphery, midperiphery, and macula. They grow in size, and eventually heal leaving pigmented chorioretinal atrophy. Commonly active lesions are found bilaterally. A hallmark of this disease is the eventual presence of 50 to hundreds of lesions that are seen throughout the fundus. Despite the vast distribution, including foveal involvement, visual prognosis is fairly good. Aggressive prolonged immunosuppressive therapy appears indicated.

Persistent placoid maculopathy

Persistent placoid maculopathy (PPM) was recently described by Golchet and colleagues. It superficially resembles macular serpiginous choroiditis but differs in its clinical course and visual prognosis.[233] CNV is a common feature of PPM, and usually the major cause of visual loss.

Clinical course

Clinical symptoms

Patients present with gradual, painless, decreased vision more commonly in one eye. Photopsias and decline in color vision can be seen.[233]

Epidemiology

In the original description there were 6 patients. Five patients were men and one was a woman. The range of ages was 50–68. All patients were Caucasian. There were no consistent systemic medical problems.[233]

Fundus findings

Patients have bilateral symmetric whitish plaque-like lesions at the level of the outer retina and RPE (Fig. 76.30). These lesions are centered in the fovea and not contiguous with the optic disc. There is a jigsaw pattern to margins of the lesions. During the course of the disease, there is very gradual fading of the whitish lesions in all patients.[233] This can take months to years. In addition to the central lesions, one patient had small white lesions nasal and superior to the disc at the time of presentation. Another patient developed a small lesion nasal to the disc in the course of follow-up. The central lesion grew in size in one of 6 patients in Golchet's series. RPE mottling and pigment clumping without CNV developed in 2 eyes. In all other eyes, no increase in pigmentation, atrophy, or scarring occurred until CNV developed.

Other ocular findings

No patients had any cells in the anterior chamber or vitritis.

Clinical course and prognosis

This macular disorder superficially resembles macular serpiginous. Vision is minimally affected, however, until the development of CNV or atrophy. The largest decrease in vision in eyes with no CNV was 4 Snellen lines to 20/60 in Golchet et al.'s series. This patient improved to 20/25 with corticosteroids.[233] Only one eye without CNV had a poor visual outcome. Nine of 12 eyes developed CNV and disciform scar formation.

Imaging

Fluorescein angiography

FA showed early hypofluorescence with partial filling in the late phase. No leakage or staining was seen, unless CNV was present (Figs 76.31, 76.32).

Indocyanine green angiography

ICGA revealed persistent hypofluorescence throughout the angiogram (Fig. 76.33). The large choroidal vessels in the affected areas were seen. In one case, the hypofluorescence showed partial resolution on follow-up.[233]

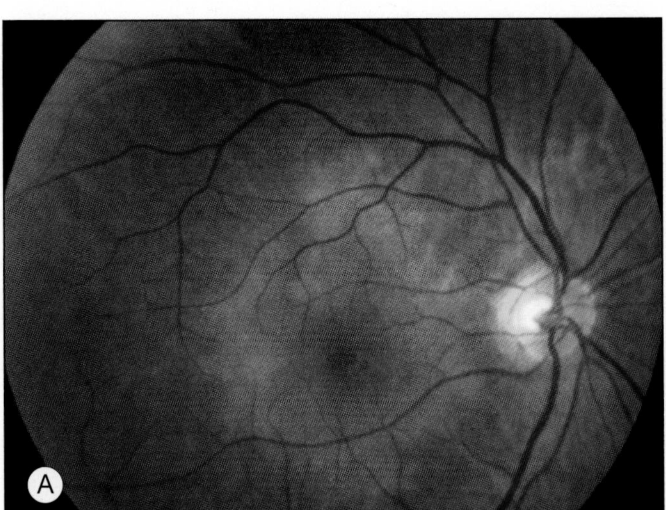

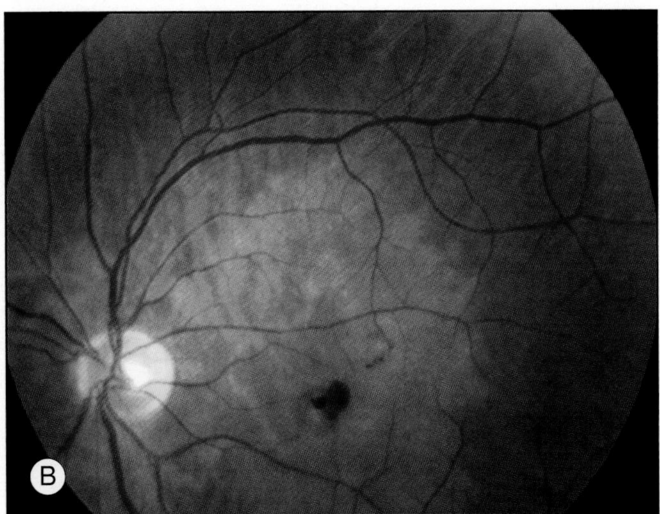

Fig. 76.30 Fundus photos of the right (A) and left (B) eye of a patient with persistent placoid maculopathy. Bilateral whitish plaques are seen. They are centered on the fovea. The left eye also shows a macular hemorrhage consistent with choroidal neovascularization.

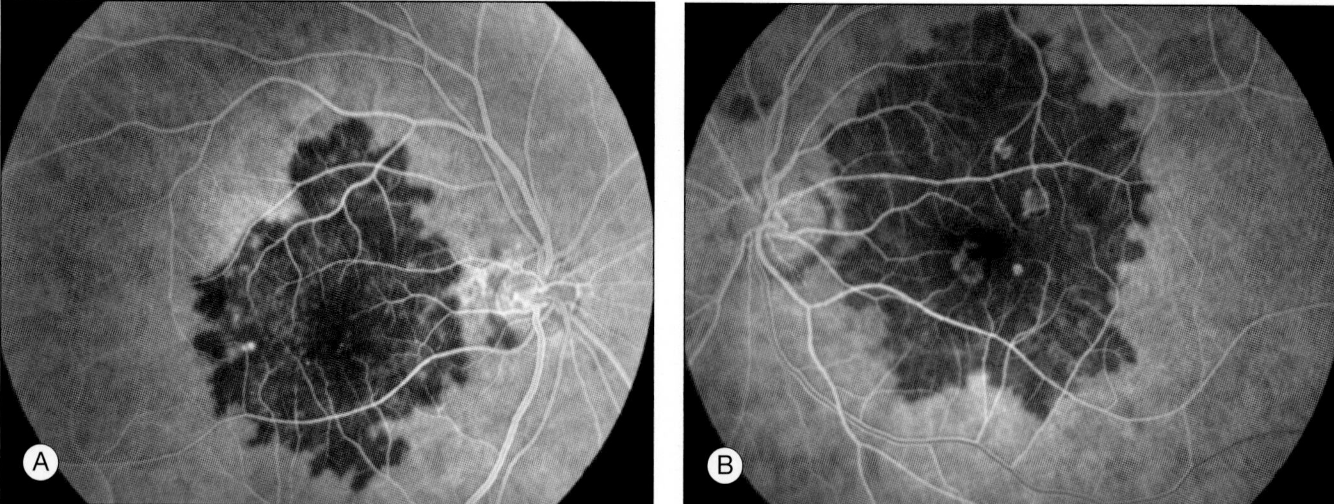

Fig. 76.31 Early FA of the right (A) and left (B) eye show hypofluorescence corresponding to the clinically seen macular lesions.

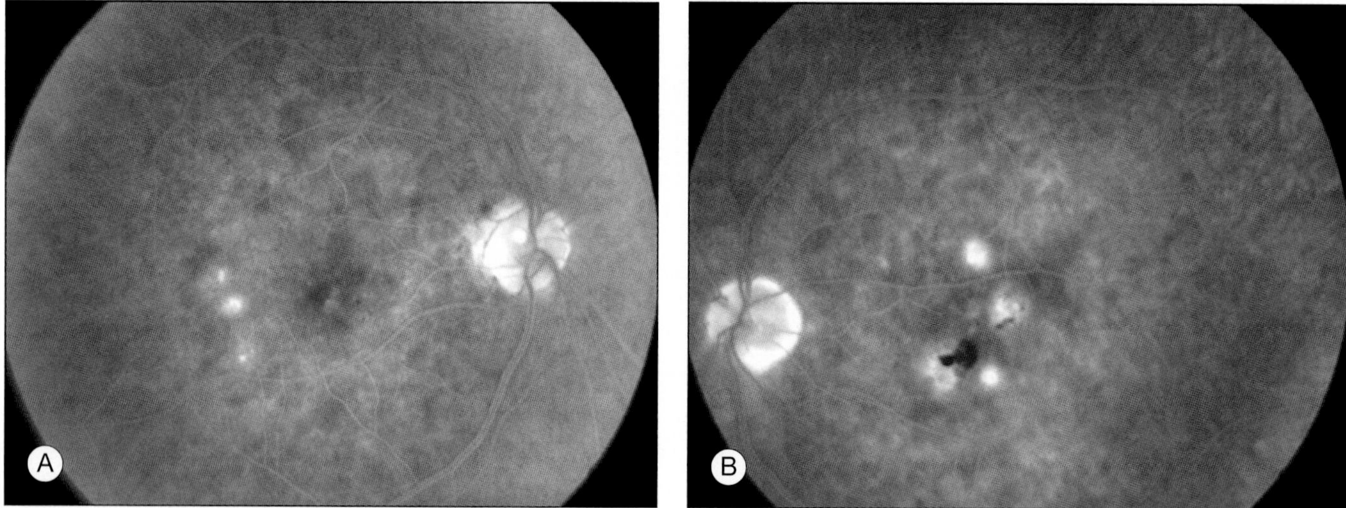

Fig. 76.32 Late FA of the right (A) and left (B) eye shows that there may be some slight hyperfluorescence corresponding to the lesion. There are some focal areas of hyperfluorescence that corresponds to choroidal neovascularization.

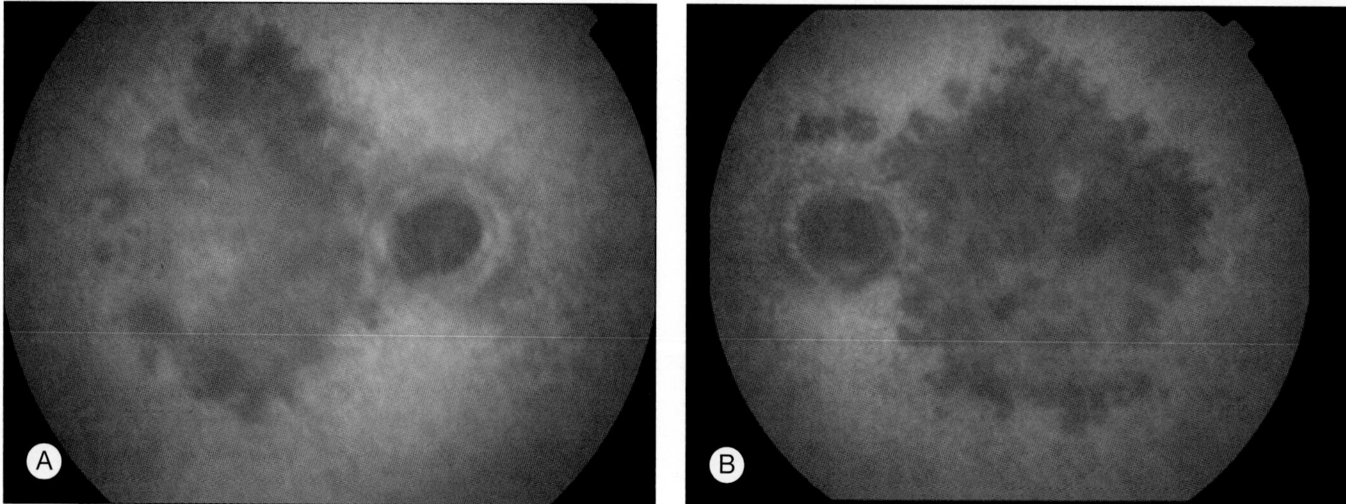

Fig. 76.33 ICGA shows persistent hypofluorescence.

Optical coherence tomography

There is a limited description of OCT findings in this rare entity. A mildly blunted fovea and normal RPE was seen in one patient.[233] Another case report described extensive RPE damage and CNV.[234]

Fundus autofluorescence

Hypofluorescence correlating to RPE damage would be expected and has been seen in one case.[234] This was noted in a patient with concurrent CNV. Further study is warranted.

Electrophysiology

One patient had a normal electroretinogram.[233]

Systemic associations

Three patients had vascular disease, including cardiac disease, myocardial infarction, hypertension, transient ischemic attack, and coronary artery disease. Two patients had type 2 diabetes. One patient had colon carcinoma and thrombocytopenia. Hyperthyroidism and cutaneous pemphigus were also reported by Golchet et al.[233]

Pathogenesis

There is similar speculation about pathology as with other placoid white spot entities. Choroidal hypoperfusion,[235] blockage by swollen RPE cells and inflammatory lesions in the outer retina, or a combination of these have been suggested to explain the hypofluorescence on ICG.[235] However, extensive choroidal hypoperfusion would not be expected in patients who maintain good vision.

Differential diagnosis

In addition to macular serpiginous choroiditis, other considerations include APMPPE, relentless placoid chorioretinitis, and syphilitic posterior placoid chorioretinitis[233] (Table 76.2). The visual outcome, number of lesions, and common association with CNV of this process distinguishes itself from the other white spot entities. The fluorescein angiogram in syphilis shows late staining unlike PPM, as well as clinical signs of inflammation due to the infectious etiology (see Chapter 84, Spirochetal infections).

Management/treatment

Oral or periocular corticosteroids have been used with subsequent improvement in vision. The role of steroids requires further investigation. Anti-VEGF agents have been used to treat CNV, with good results in one report.[236,237]

Summary

Persistent placoid maculopathy is a unique placoid white spot entity. Bilateral symmetric white lesions centered in the macula and not contiguous with the optic nerve are seen. These fade over months to years and are rarely associated with pigmentary changes and atrophy. Visual outcome is related to the development of CNV, which is very common.

MULTIFOCAL CHOROIDITIS AND PANUVEITIS, PUNCTATE INNER CHOROIDOPATHY, AND PROGRESSIVE SUBRETINAL FIBROSIS AND UVEITIS SYNDROME

Multifocal choroiditis and panuveitis (MFC), punctate inner choroidopathy (PIC), and progressive subretinal fibrosis and uveitis syndrome (PSFU) are conditions characterized by inflammation at the level of the RPE and outer retina. It does not appear to be a true choroiditis. Chorioretinal scars are left by the inflammation. The etiologies and pathogenesis of these entities are unclear. Jampol and Wiredu[238] have classified these entities as the same disease as their ophthalmosopic appearance and clinical courses are similar. MFC and PIC will be presented first, with a common differential and treatment. This section will end with a brief discussion of the rare PSFU.

Multifocal choroiditis and panuveitis

MFC was first described in 2 young patients in 1973 by Nozik and Dorsch.[239] They reported a chorioretinopathy that resembled presumed ocular histoplasmosis (POHS) but was associated with a bilateral anterior uveitis (see Chapter 70, Ocular histoplasmosis). Later, Dreyer and Gass[240] coined the term multifocal choroiditis and panuveitis, describing 28 patients with uveitis and lesions at the level of the RPE and choriocapillaris. Deutsch and Tessler[241] reported a series of 28 patients in 1984 with what they termed inflammatory pseudohistoplasmosis. Their series included patients with concurrent systemic diseases such as tuberculosis, sarcoidosis, and syphilis. Morgan and Schatz,[242] 2 years later, described 11 patients with a recurrent idiopathic multifocal choroiditis.

Clinical course

Clinical symptoms

Patients present with decreased central vision, photopsias, floaters, metamorphopsia, paracentral or temporal scotomas, ocular discomfort, and photophobia. Photopsias often correspond to lesions in the peripapillary area and indicate activity of the disease. Visual acuity can range from 20/20 to light perception. More than half present with vision less than 20/100 in the worse eye.[240,242]

Epidemiology

MFC occurs predominantly in Caucasian,[243] myopic women between the second and sixth decades of life.[240,242] Most affected patients are in their 30s. In addition, they have never lived in areas that are endemic for histoplasmosis.

Fundus findings

In the acute phase of MFC, yellow round or oval lesions, ranging in number from one to scores, are seen in the outer retina and RPE. They range in size from 50 to 1000 μm. They occur in the posterior pole, peripapillary region, and midperiphery. The nasal retina often shows clustering.[244] The lesions can also be arranged in linear scars parallel to the ora in the periphery[245] (Fig. 76.34). Previously, this linear appearance was thought to be pathognomonic for POHS.[246,247] Active lesions can be associated with subretinal fluid. As inflammation resolves, the lesions become atrophic with a variable amount of pigment ("punched out" appearance). They can also enlarge in size. There can be bridging subretinal scars between the disciform or atrophic scars.[248] Cantrill and Folk described 5 patients who developed sharply angulated subretinal scars as the lesions healed.[249] They noted broad scar formation in the macula as the lesions coalesced that could be related to serous and hemorrhagic macular detachment. During active phases, exudative retinal detachment may overlie areas of activity.

In recurrent episodes, new chorioretinal lesions may develop. Optic disc edema can be seen and atrophy may occur. Optic disc neovascularization can very rarely be seen.[241] The peripapillary region may have a characteristic subretinal fibrosis[250] that has

Table 76.2 Persistent placoid maculopathy compared with macular serpiginous choroditis

	Persistent placoid maculopathy	Macular serpiginous choroiditis*	Acute posterior multifocal placoid pigment epitheliopathy*
Lesion characteristics	Long-standing geographic central whitish plaques involving the fovea	Variable sizes and shapes, heal to scars and atrophy in weeks	Multiple postequatorial cream-colored placoid lesions of varying sizes; fade in 1–2 weeks
Visual acuity	Normal to mildly affected (20/20–20/60) with good prognosis for recovery unless complicated by CNV or atrophy	Rapid decrease in central vision to counting fingers with poor prognosis for recovery	Sudden onset of moderate vision loss, photopsia, and scotomas with excellent prognosis for recovery
Gender	Only 6 patients	Male = female	Male = female
Laterality	Bilateral, symmetric (6/6 patients)	Eventually all bilateral, usually asymmetric	Usually bilateral and symmetric
FA characteristics	Early hypofluorescence followed by partial filling-in in the late phase	Early hypofluorescence of the central portion of the lesion surrounded by progressive hyperfluorescence at the margins with eventual late staining	Early hypofluorescence followed by late hypofluorescence and staining; window defects appear in the quiescent stage
ICGA characteristics	Persistent hypofluorescence throughout the angiogram	Early hypofluorescence with some resolution in the late phase; no staining of lesion borders	Hypofluorescence of the active and healed lesions
Complications	CNV in 11/12 eyes, with 9 resulting in disciform macular scars so far; RPE mottling in 1/12 eyes. Atrophy.	CNV and disciform macular scars in up to 35%; RPE mottling and subretinal scar formation common; RPE detachments, vein and artery occlusions described	Most patients spontaneously recover; rare cases of permanent loss of vision secondary to RPE alterations or CNV; also, reports of CME, papillitis, bilateral central vein occlusions, and associated CNS vasculitis
Clinical course	Persistent lesions with mild decrease in VA unless complicated by CNV or RPE damage	Multiple discrete recurrences usually adjacent to old lesions, variably spaced over many years	Acute transients decrease in VA associated with a viral prodrome and rare recurrences

CME, cystoid macular edema; CNV, choroidal neovascularization; FA, fluorescein angiography; ICGA, indocyanine green angiography; RPE, retinal pigment epithelium; VA, visual acuity.
**For references, see original publication.*
(Reproduced with permission from Golchet PR, Jampol LM, Wilson D, et al. Persistent placoid maculopathy: a new clinical entity. Ophthalmology *2007;114(8):1530–40.).*

been described as a "napkin ring" configuration (Fig. 76.35). Retinal vessels may be narrowed. Periphlebitis may develop. Cystoid macular edema occurs in 10–20% of individuals. CNV develops in 25–30% of cases and can be the presenting sign.[240,242,243]

Other ocular findings

MFC may have a mild to moderate anterior uveitis. Nongranulomatous keratic precipitates and posterior synechiae can be present. Iris abnormalities, such as neovascularization or abnormal avascular areas on fluorescein angiography, have been

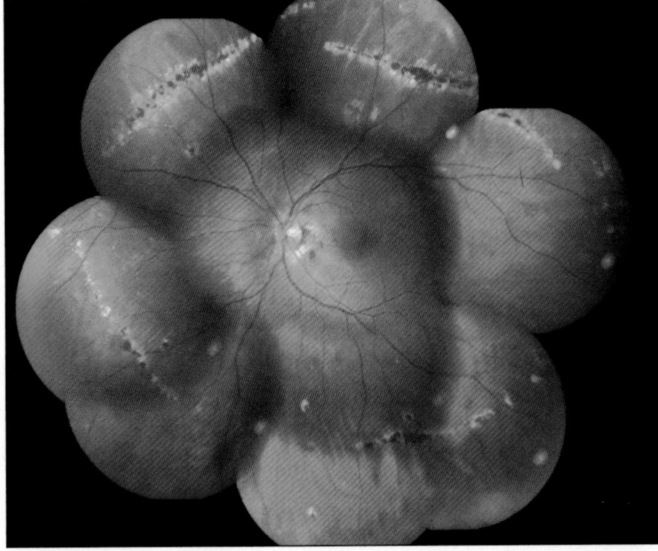

Fig. 76.34 Linear scars parallel to the ora are seen in the periphery. (Courtesy of Medical University of Innsbruck, Austria.)

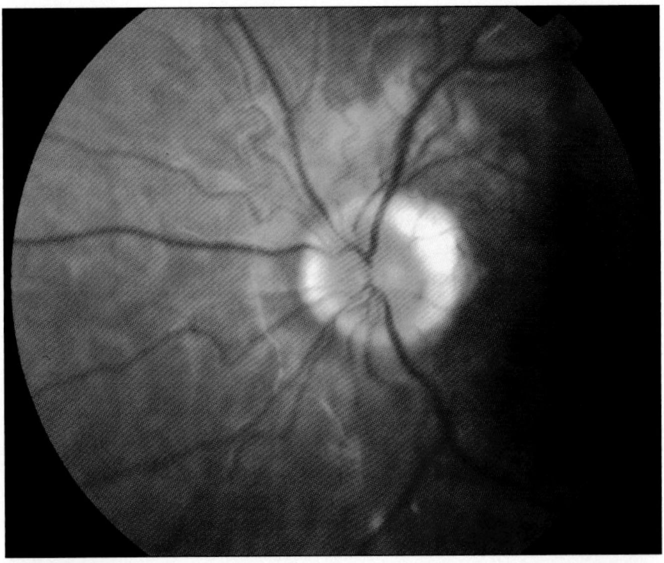

Fig. 76.35 Fundus photo showing a characteristic subretinal fibrosis ("napkin ring").

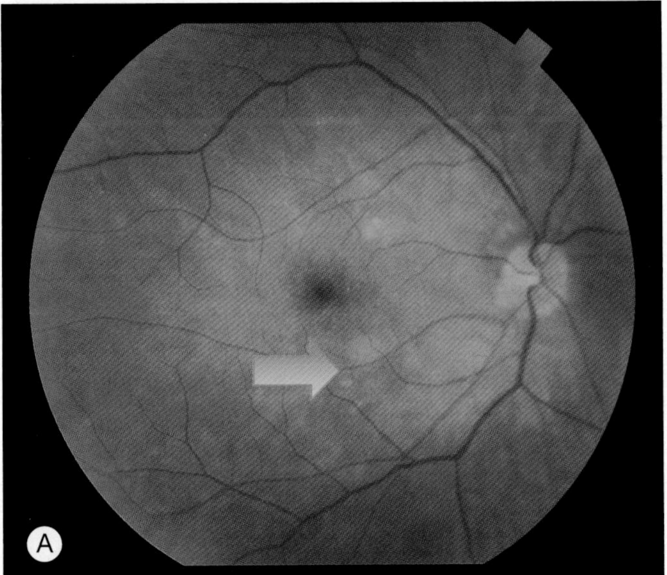

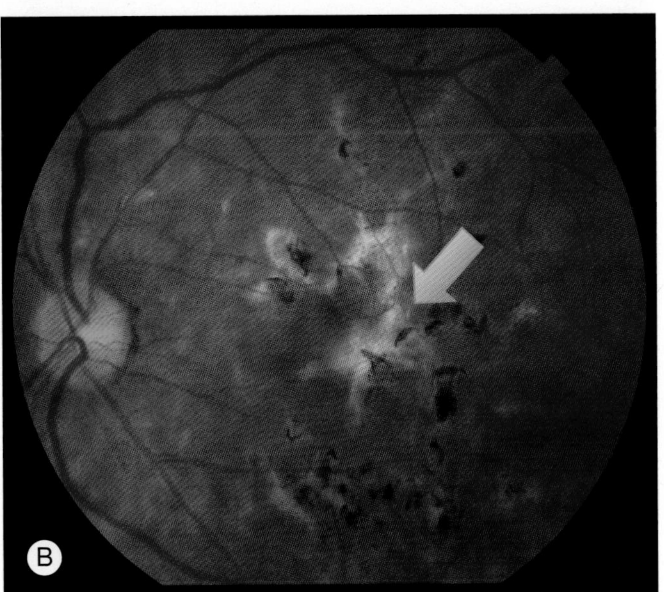

Fig. 76.36 Fundus photos of the right (A) and left (B) eyes. The right eye shows subtle acute lesions (arrow). The left eye shows chronic disease. Bridging fibrosis is seen between scars (thin arrow).

reported.[251] Vitritis, if present, is usually mild or moderate. Findings may be asymmetric.

Clinical course and prognosis

MFC waxes and wanes, but vision loss can occur. Most patients tend to have recurrent episodes that can involve the central or peripheral vision. These can resolve spontaneously or with the aid of immunosuppressants. Some patients retain excellent vision, but have persistent photopsias. About 25% of patients have a more chronic course that involves more inflammation, or CNV. Recurrent inflammation may cause CME, vitreous haze, and swelling around old scars (Fig. 76.36). New lesions that are not contiguous with old scars can develop. CNV is the most common cause of visual loss in MFC and can be seen with either inactive macular scars or recurrent inflammation. The long-term visual prognosis of MFC is variable. Brown and colleagues[244] followed 41 patients (68 eyes) for a mean of 39 months. They found that 66% of eyes ended up with 20/40 vision or better. Only 21% of eyes ended up 20/200 or worse. The majority of the cases with poor vision were due to CNV and less commonly CME. Foveal atrophy and uveitic neovascular glaucoma were other causes in their series. About one-third of patients developed CNV. Thorne and colleagues[252] studied 66 patients (122 eyes) and found that 55% of patients presented with vision worse than 20/50 and 38% presented with vision worse than 20/200. CNV was found in 22% of patients at presentation and was the most common cause of vision loss. Presence of epiretinal membrane and CME were other causes of vision loss. Use of immunosuppressive therapy was associated with an 83% reduction in the risk of posterior pole complications, including new or recurrent CNV.

Imaging

Fluorescein angiography

In the acute phase, the clinical lesions appear hypofluorescent on FA. Late in the angiogram, the lesions stain[242] (Figs 76.37, 76.38). CNV may be present in the peripapillary or macular areas. In the healed phase, the lesions become atrophic and show a window defect on angiography. A recent study of CNV in MFC revealed that most CNV is classic and clearly demonstrated unless blocked by subretinal blood.[253] The researchers further compared this with OCT (both stratus and spectralis), and found that CNV could be missed with this mode of imaging. They recommended FA be used in cases with suspected neovascularization.

Indocyanine green angiography

ICGA shows hypofluorescent round spots that may be far more numerous than seen on clinical examination and fluorescein angiography[254–256] (Fig. 76.39).

Optical coherence tomography

In the active phase, stratus OCT findings show an RPE irregularity corresponding to a clinical lesion. This RPE irregularity resolves with treatment.[257] In our experience with spectral domain OCT, the lesion disrupts the photoreceptor layer with potential normalization with treatment (Fig. 76.40). Retinal thinning may occur. Vance and colleagues describe SD-OCT imaging of acute lesions that showed drusen-like material between the

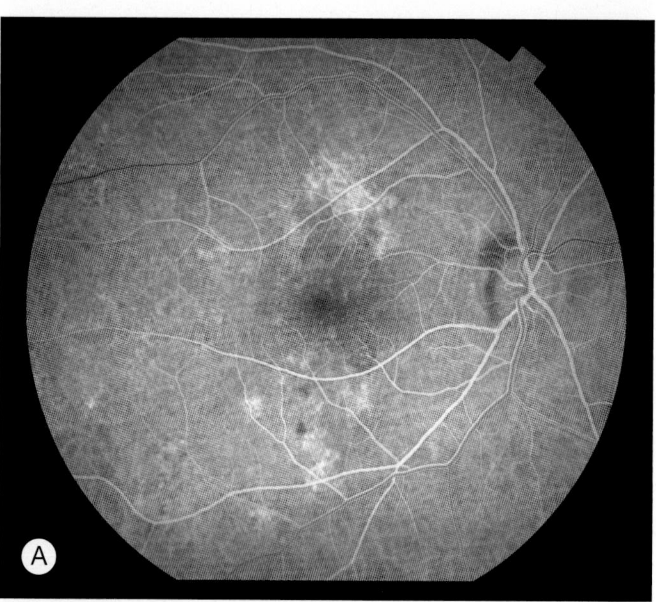

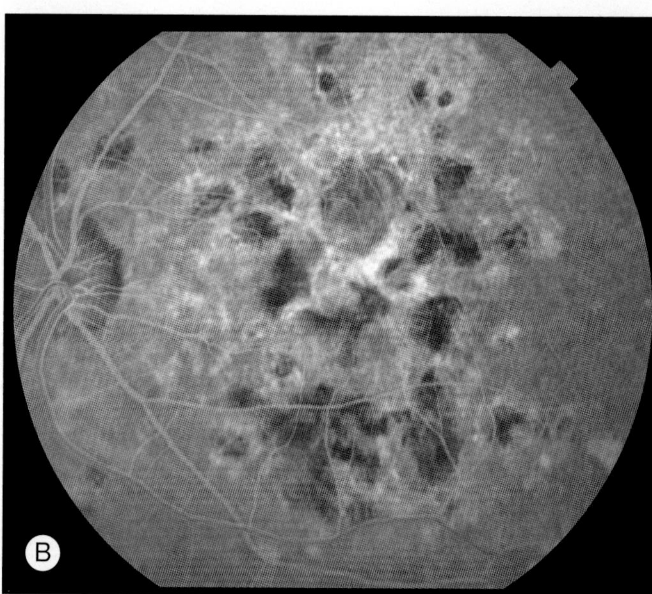

Fig. 76.37 Early FA of the right (A) and left (B) eye of a patient with new onset of symptoms in the right eye. The left eye has had poor vision for some time.

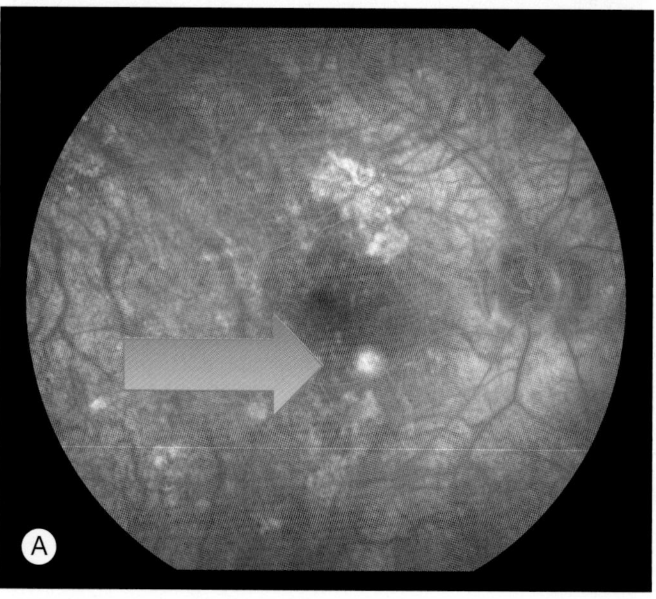

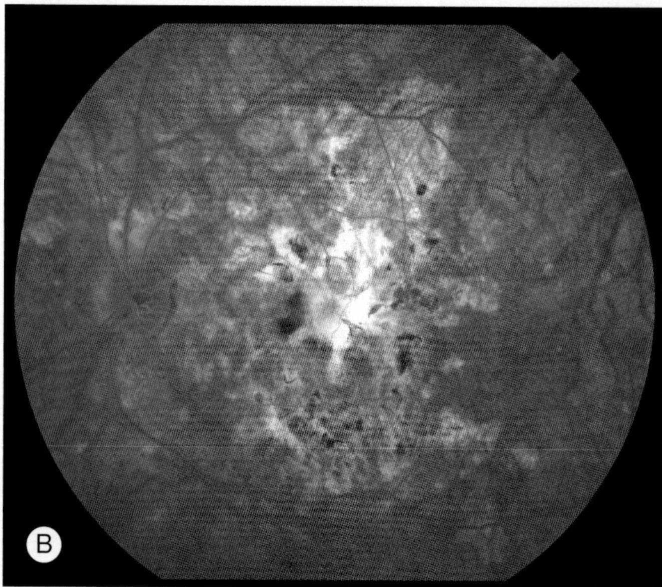

Fig. 76.38 Late FA of the right (A) and left (B) eye shows an acute hyperfluorescent lesion in the right (arrow). The left eye shows staining of the scars.

RPE and Bruch's membrane as well as a localized choroidal hyperreflectivity below the material.[258] These lesions disappear with treatment.

Fundus autofluorescence

Hyperautofluorescence was observed in the areas of fresh lesions. This resolved when immunosuppression was instituted. In the majority of patients, punctate hypoautofluorescent spots were seen on FAF corresponding to areas of chorioretinal atrophy (inactive lesions)[259] (Fig. 76.41).

Electrophysiology testing

Dreyer and Gass[240] reported ERGs on 29 eyes of 16 patients. They observed normal or borderline results in 41% of patients, moderately reduced results in 17%, and severely reduced results in 21% of eyes. Oh and colleagues used multifocal ERG (mfERG) to study pre- and post-treatment results; however, due to the sensitivity of this test, it becomes almost extinguished with active MFC.[260] Electrophysiologic tests are not used commonly in the management of MFC, as with other white spot diseases such as birdshot chorioretinopathy.

Visual field testing

Blind spot enlargement as a manifestation of multifocal choroiditis was described in 1991.[261] Enlarged blind spot in the setting of a normal optic nerve has been seen in acute idiopathic blind spot enlargement (AIBSE) and in patients with multiple evanescent white dot syndrome (MEWDS). The enlargement is thought to be due to peripapillary retinal dysfunction rather than an optic nerve problem. This is supported by the fact that color vision and pupillary responses have been reported to be normal in these patients. The enlarged blind spot can resolve with inactivity of disease. Photoreceptor outer segment abnormalities may be a cause of the blind spot enlargement.[262] Visual field testing may also demonstrate scotomas related to areas of chorioretinal scarring or serous detachments related to active lesions. Visual fields are an important way to monitor MFC.

Systemic associations

An association between MFC and Epstein–Barr Virus (EBV) has been suggested.[263] It was postulated that EBV triggers an immune response that starts a persistent intraocular inflammatory response. Immunoglobulin M antibodies directed against the viral capsid antigen or the Epstein–Barr early antigen were present in patients with MFC in one series with none in controls.[263,264] However, this could not be reproduced.[265] Some patients with MFC may also have or develop sarcoidosis. These individuals are often not distinguishable from those who have idiopathic MFC.

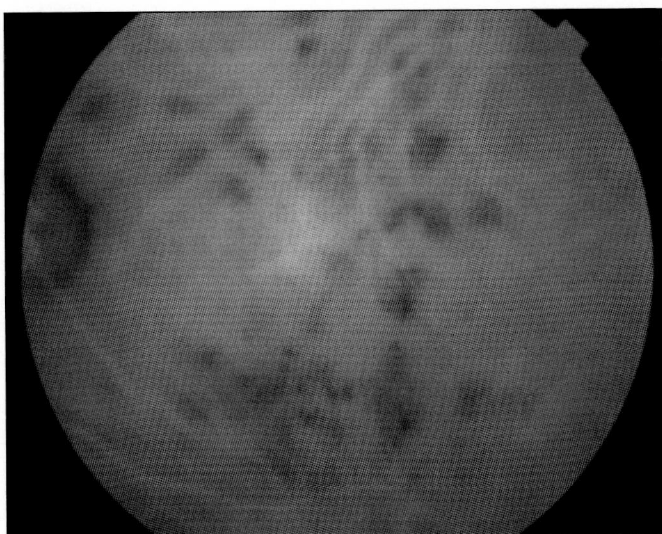

Fig. 76.39 ICG shows numerous hypofluorescent round spots.

Punctate inner choroidopathy

PIC was first described in 1984.[266] Watzke reported 10 myopic women with blurred vision, photopsias, or paracentral scotomas with small yellow–white lesions of the inner choroid and RPE. These lesions were associated with overlying subretinal fluid. Acute lesions healed to atrophic scars and developed more pigmentation with time. Choroidal neovascular membranes developed in more than half of these individuals.[267]

Clinical course

Clinical symptoms

In a survey of 77 people with PIC conducted by Gerstenblith and colleagues,[268] scotomas were the presenting complaint in 91% of patients, followed by blurred vision (86%), photopsias (73%), floaters (69%), metamorphopsia (65%), and decreased peripheral vision (26%). Most (85%) presented with unilateral symptoms.

Epidemiology

PIC is a disease of young, relatively healthy, myopic women. An estimation of a national incidence is approximately 100–200 cases

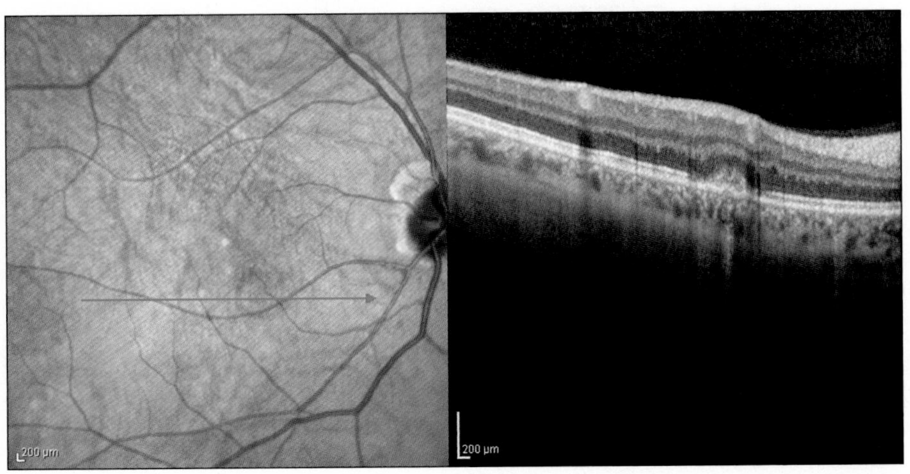

Fig. 76.40 OCT of the right eye shows a hyperreflective lesion in the outer retina corresponding to an acute lesion.

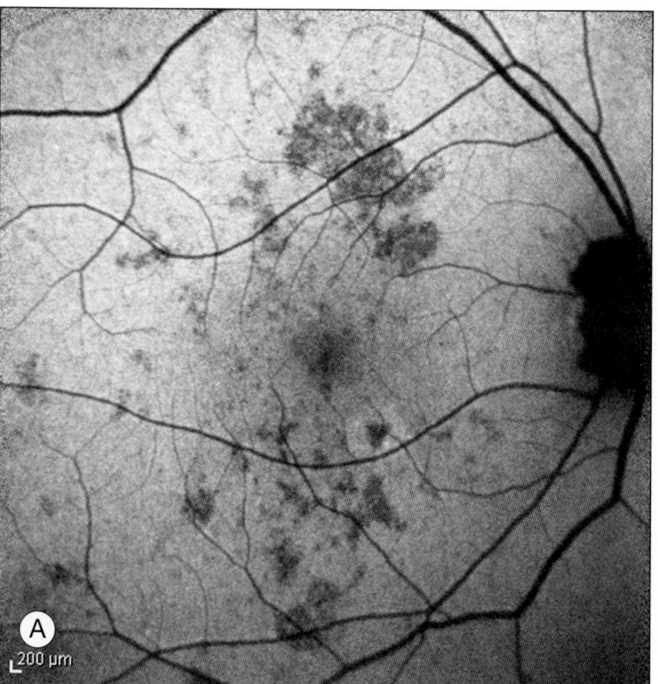

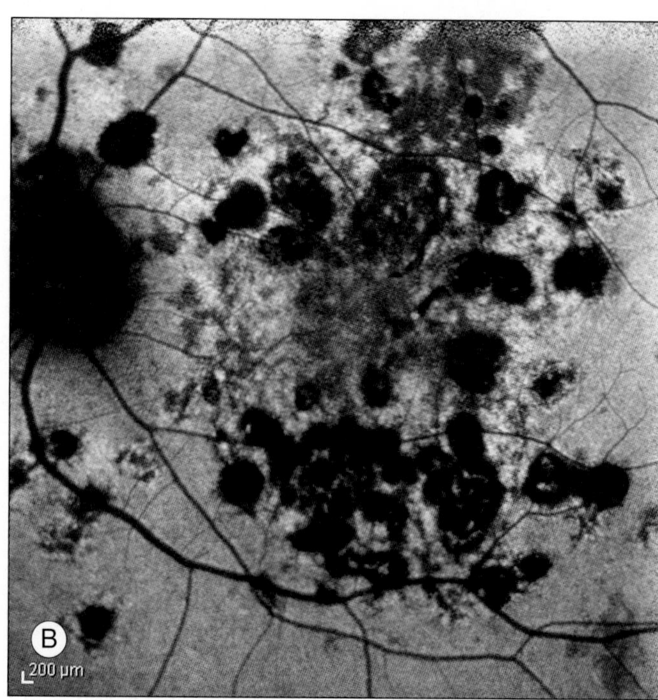

Fig. 76.41 (A,B) Fundus autofluorescence corresponding to inactive lesions that have developed chorioretinal scars.

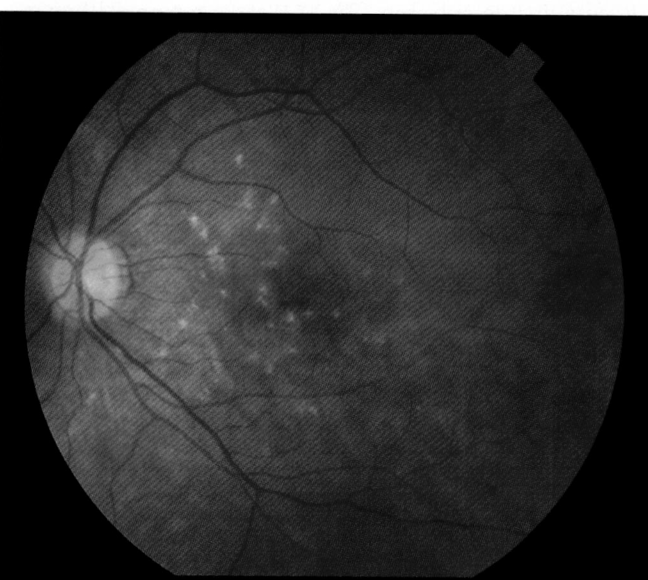

Fig. 76.42 Fundus photo of the posterior pole showing small round lesions that are characteristic.

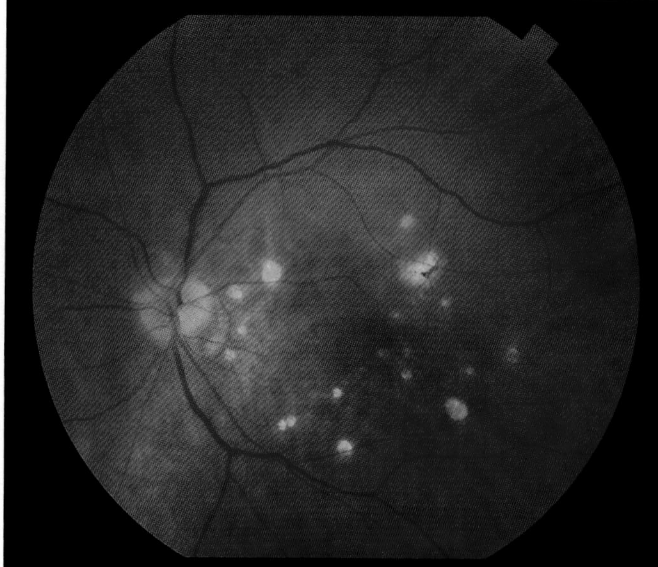

Fig. 76.43 Expansion of scars in the inactive phase is common.

per year.[269] This is probably an underestimation. Ninety percent of patients are women. Eighty-five percent of patients are myopic, and 97% are Caucasian.[268] The mean age at presentation is 30 years (range 15–55). Patel and colleagues[270] described the presentation and outcome of PIC patients at a tertiary referral center and found similar trends. Mean refraction is -4.6 diopters.[271]

Fundus findings

Multiple gray or yellow, small round lesions are seen scattered throughout the posterior pole.[268] (Fig. 76.42). Occasionally there is a linear pattern. The lesions are at the level of the outer retina, RPE, and inner choroid and a neurosensory detachment may be present. With time, these spots evolve into atrophic chorioretinal scars. After 2–3 years, they become more distinct, pigment, and appear similar to the punched out lesions of POHS (Fig. 76.43). Some lesions disappear without sequelae. CNV commonly develops.

Other ocular findings

Generally, PIC is not associated with anterior or posterior segment inflammation.

Clinical course and prognosis

Brown and colleagues reported that 88% of 16 patients had bilateral disease, despite its most commonly being a unilateral

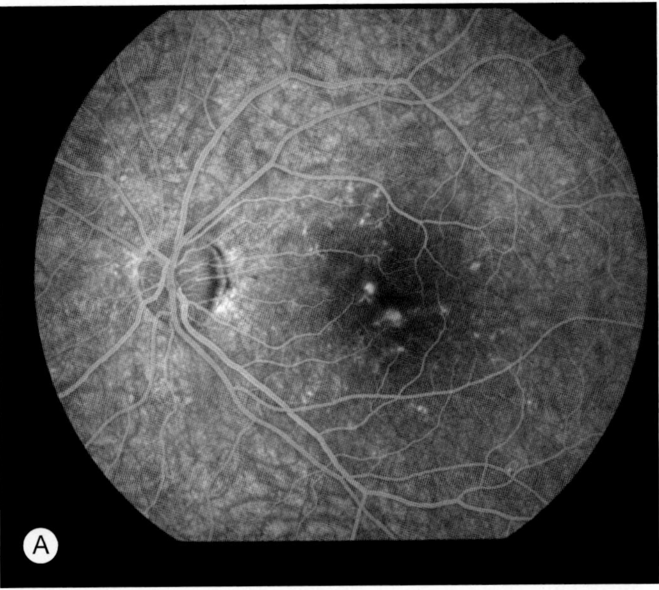

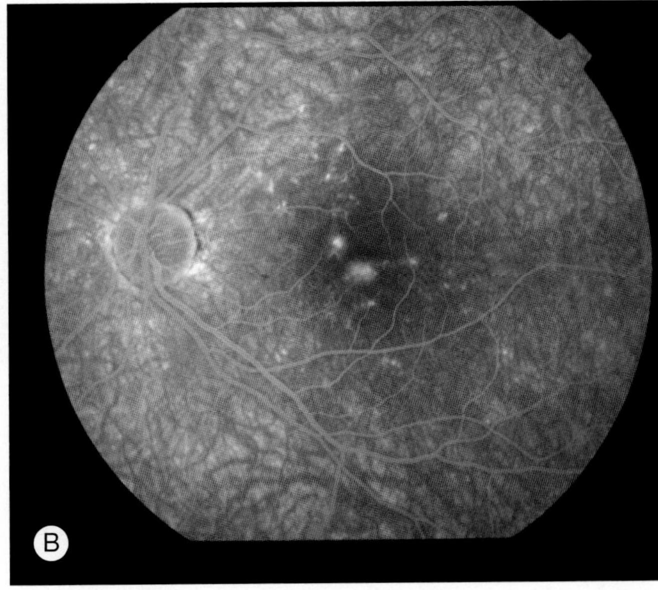

Fig. 76.44 (A,B) Fluorescein angiography shows increasing fluorescence (staining) and some slight leakage of lesions is seen.

complaint.[244] Patients generally become asymptomatic after one month. The scars continue to become atrophic and pigmented over the next 2–3 years. These scars appear to involve the RPE and choriocapillaris. Recurrences are common. Brown and colleagues followed patients for a mean length of 51 months.[244] They found that 77% of eyes had a final vision of 20/40 or better. Twenty-three percent had a vision of 20/50 or worse. Twenty percent had a vision of 20/200 or worse. The primary cause of this poor vision was CNV. Approximately 40% of eyes developed CNV and it generally appeared within one year of presentation. Smaller areas of CNV (<100 μm) were more likely to spontaneously resolve as compared with larger areas (>200 μm). Essex and colleagues[271] in a larger study recently reported the clinical features and outcome of 136 PIC patients (271 eyes) with a mean follow-up of 6.2 years. They found 63 fellow eyes that were normal at presentation. Of these, 56 (88%) remained unchanged. Only 3 (5%) developed PIC lesions and 4 (6%) developed CNV. In eyes with PIC lesions, 49 of 74 eyes (66%) remained unchanged. New PIC lesions developed in 9 eyes (12%) and CNV developed in 16 (22%).

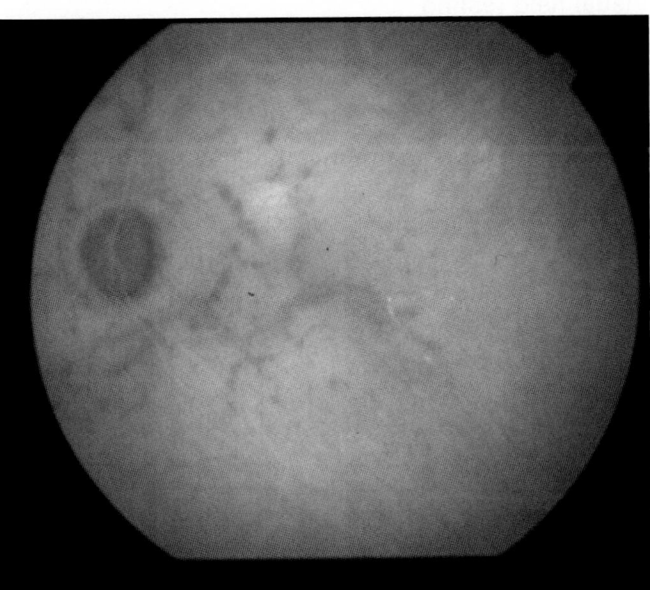

Fig. 76.45 ICG shows numerous hypofluorescent spots.

Imaging

Fluorescein angiography

PIC lesions can appear hyperfluorescent in the arterial phase or may appear as blocked fluorescence (Fig. 76.44A). In later phases, the lesions stain[266] (Fig. 76.44B). More lesions are seen on FA than are clinically visible. Tiny punctuate hyperfluorescent lesions may be seen scattered in the posterior pole. In later stages of disease, as the RPE atrophies, window defects are seen. Leakage of fluorescein into the subretinal space is also possible.

Olsen and colleagues described CNV in six patients with PIC.[272] They found that a fibrotic response followed the development of CVN and there was often a dumbbell-shaped pattern of subretinal fibrosis.

Indocyanine green angiography

As with other white spot diseases, the PIC lesions hypofluoresce in the early, middle, and late phases of ICGA[273,274] (Fig. 76.45). Many more lesions are seen on ICGA than are clinically visible or seen in FA.[275] Tiffin and colleagues described choroidal vascular abnormalities.[274] In addition to the hypofluorescent lesions that, in some cases, corresponded to clinically seen lesions, larger choroidal vessels were seen crossing these areas. Several choroidal vessels also showed hyperfluorescence of the vessel wall. They postulated focal choroidal ischemia in the areas of hypofluorescence and possibly a vasculitis in the area of hyperfluorescence of the vessel walls.

Optical coherence tomography

Stepien and Carroll[276] described spectral domain OCT findings in a patient with PIC with recurrent activity. In addition to seeing fluid associated with CNV, outer retinal irregularity was described. A homogenous thickening was seen overlying chorioretinal lesions (Fig. 76.46). This resolved with treatment. The pattern we see with SD-OCT is similar to MFC. There is sub-RPE solid looking material that pushes up the RPE and may extend into the retina.

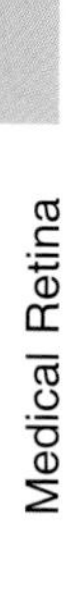

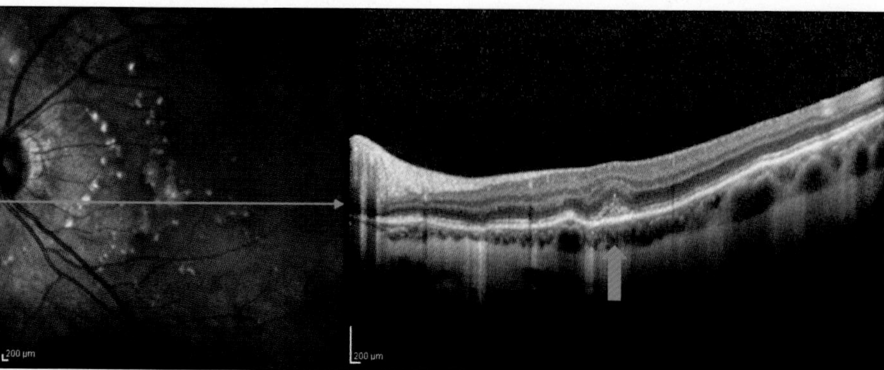

Fig. 76.46 OCT of an active lesion in punctate inner choroidopathy.

Electrophysiology

Reddy and colleagues found that 7 out of 16 patients with PIC had normal ERGs.[277] Three of the 7 patients had some asymmetry in b-wave amplitudes between the two eyes which correlated to the number of lesions in each eye.

Visual field testing

Reddy and colleagues also studied visual fields in 22 eyes of patients with PIC.[277] Ten eyes (45%) had normal visual fields. Nine eyes (41%) had enlargement of the blind spot, many of which extended toward the macula. Three eyes (14%) had central/paracentral scotomas. They postulated that this is related to the peripapillary clustering of lesions. The visual fields improved without treatment in most patients at follow-up. Photoreceptor outer segment abnormalities are the cause of the blind spot enlargement.[262]

Pathogenesis

The cause of MFC and PIC is not understood. It is uncertain if they are separate entities or on a spectrum of a single disease. They typically affect young, otherwise healthy women. There are yellow lesions at the level of the outer retina as seen by OCT and RPE, as well as evidence of some choroidal involvement. The lesions of MFC and PIC eventually atrophy and look similar to the punched out lesions of POHS. CNV can develop, leading to bridging scars and subretinal fibrosis. Patients can also develop blind spots and scotomas that can improve with or without treatment. These field defects can be associated with abnormalities of the outer retina as seen on ERG. MFC has been reported to occur in patients with other white spot syndromes such as APMPPE and MEWDS.[6,278] Becker and Jampol proposed a common genetic hypothesis for autoimmune involvement in these inflammatory processes.[2] The interplay of genetics, immune dysregulation, and environmental triggers may play a role in the different presentations of these clinical entities. Atan and colleagues[279] recently studied MFC and PIC and found similarities in the association with a IL-10 haplotype, and negative associations with a TNF haplotype. These genetic loci are known to be associated with noninfectious uveitis and autoimmunity. They state that definitive proof will necessitate genomewide sequence analysis. However, their data support the idea that genetic factors have a strong effect on clinical phenotype.

Differential diagnosis

The differential diagnosis for MFC and PIC includes: presumed ocular histoplasmosis syndrome, sarcoidosis, Vogt–Koyanagi–Haradas syndrome, sympathetic ophthalmia, myopic degeneration maculopathy, and other white spot syndromes such as serpiginous choroiditis, and birdshot chorioretinopathy.

Infectious etiologies may be considered given the patient's history and health status. These include viral (herpes simplex, herpes zoster, Epstein–Barr, cytomegalovirus, Coxsackie), bacterial (syphilis, tuberculosis, *Borrelia burgdorfori*, septic choroiditis, metastatic endophthalmitis), fungal (histoplasmosis, *Cryptococcus*, coccidioidomycosis, *Candida*), protozoal (toxoplasmosis, *Pneumocystis carinii*), and worms (diffuse unilateral subacute neuroretinitis).

Neoplastic masquerading diseases such as intraocular lymphoma can be considered as well.

Differentiation of MFC and POHS

Both entities may show punched out chorioretinal scars, peripapillary scarring, and CNV. Classically, the teaching is that the difference between these two entities is the presence of inflammation with MFC and absence with POHS. However, MFC can be present without signs of inflammation. Parnell and colleagues[248] differentiated MFC from POHS based on clinical features, morphology of photographed fundus lesions, and fluorescein angiography. Clinically, MFC patients may develop photopsias and visual field defects. Clinically, distinctive features of MFC include multiple small white lesions clustered in the macula, nasal retina, or equator, a mixture of acute and inactive lesions, progressive growth of lesions, and subretinal fibrous metaplasia with bridging tissue between scars. Other changes include hyperplastic changes around the nerve ("napkin ring"), myopic-appearing nerve, sheathing of vessels or narrowed vessels, and inflammation seen as CME, vitritis, or disc edema (see Chapter 70, Ocular histoplasmosis.)

Differentiation of MFC and PIC

Although we believe that these two entities are on the same spectrum of a single disease, there are a few studies that have proposed distinct features. Kedhar and colleagues[243] studied 66 patients (122 eyes) with MFC and 13 patients (22 eyes) with PIC. They found that the median range of age at presentation was less in PIC patients at 29 years compared with MFC at 45 years. Patients with MFC presented with a higher frequency of structural complications such as cataract, CME and ERM while PIC patients did not have these. They found that PIC patients were more likely to develop CNV (76.9%) versus those with MFC (27.7%). MFC patients were more likely to have complications from intraocular inflammation and bilateral visual impairment of 20/50 or worse. These differences are likely secondary to more widespread inflammatory disease with MFC.

Shimada and colleagues[280] looked at 14 eyes of 14 patients who were diagnosed with MFC (8 eyes) or PIC (6 eyes) that underwent surgical excision of a choroidal neovascular membrane. They found that CNV obtained from both types of patients expressed VEGF and CD68. In 3 of 8 MFC eyes, intraocular inflammatory findings were found clinically. In these eyes, immunohistochemistry showed that the CNV was infiltrated with CD20-positive B lymphocytes. No B lymphocytes were found in the PIC patients, or the 5 MFC patients without clinical inflammation. Therefore, the amount of inflammation in MFC may explain the differences.

Management/treatment

Treatment is aimed at inflammation and its sequelae (CME and CNV). Multifocal choroiditis and panuveitis may be associated with significant anterior and posterior inflammation. This can be managed with topical, periocular, intraocular, and systemic corticosteroids. Steroid-sparing agents are used when steroids are not tolerated or recurrence is frequent. Although PIC is not associated with significant visible inflammation, the lesions do respond to immunosuppressives. CNV can be managed with thermal laser if extrafoveal, photodynamic therapy,[281] steroids and/or anti-VEGF therapy. PDT can be in conjunction with systemic or local steroids as the etiology of the CNV is in part inflammatory in these entities and PDT can incite inflammation. This has been found to be effective.[282] Amer and Lois[267] in their extensive review of literature on PIC suggest that PDT may best achieve closure of already formed neovascularization, while immunosuppressive agents may be most effective in the early stages of development of CNV. Anti-VEGF therapy has been found to be promising in several studies of CNV caused by MFC[283–286] and PIC.[282,287,288] An additional complication in these patients due to the demographics (young females) is concomitant pregnancy. Steroid therapy is possible during pregnancy; other agents may affect fertility, however, and teratogenicity is unclear in humans.

Progressive subretinal fibrosis and uveitis syndrome

PSFU is a rare entity that was first described by Palestine and colleagues in 1984.[289] Three young women with intraocular inflammation and fibrotic subretinal lesions that progressively enlarged and coalesced were characterized. The patients also developed macular edema. Several authors have described progressive subretinal fibrosis in association with multifocal choroiditis.[240,249,290] This entity is also known as diffuse subretinal fibrosis syndrome.

Clinical course

Clinical symptoms

Patients, in the acute phase, present with unilateral decreased vision,[291] floaters, possibly photopsias, scotomas, and metamorphopsia.

Epidemiology

Kaiser and Gragoudas[291] reviewed the literature and found that patients are predominantly young, healthy, and myopic. Ages generally ranged from 20 to 40 years old. However, there may be a bimodal curve, as Gass described 3 elderly individuals (mean age 71) with biopsy-proved PSFU.[292]

Fundus findings

Numerous small (100–500 μm) yellow spots are seen at the level of the choriocapillaris, RPE, and deep retina.[291] There is clustering in the posterior pole, but there can be extension to the mid-periphery. The lesions can be associated with hazy yellow subretinal fluid. There is rapid development of subretinal scarring.

Other ocular findings

Anterior chamber reaction and vitritis is usually mild. Optic disc edema has been reported.[293] Other signs of inflammation such as posterior synechiae, keratic precipitates, and iris atrophy have been reported.[291]

Clinical course and prognosis

PSFU usually presents asymmetrically but is usually bilateral. Within a few days to weeks after development of the multifocal lesions, fluid starts to accumulate. Over the next several months, subretinal fibrosis develops. This further coalesces and forms sheets of fibrotic tissue under the retina. This is associated with marked decrease in vision. In Brown and colleagues' study, 7 of 10 eyes of patients with PSFU had vision worse than 20/200 after 2 years.[244] Only 2 of 10 eyes had vision of 20/40 or better. CNV and subretinal hemorrhages develop. The second eye can develop lesions within months of the first eye.[291]

Imaging

Fluorescein angiography

The lesions associated with PSFU are characterized by early hyperfluorescence followed by late leakage in the acute phase.[249,277,294] As fibrosis develops, there is staining in the late phases. CNV may be seen on FA but is uncommon and may be difficult to assess due to the fibrotic component.

Electrophysiology

Variable results have been seen in a few patients.[249,289,290]

Systemic associations

Case reports of PSFU in association with ectodermal dysplasia[295] and ulcerative colitis[296] have appeared. This may point to a genetic or inflammatory etiology, but due to the rarity of this disease, no conclusions can be reached.

Pathogenesis

Histopathology from a patient with PSFU showed a severely gliotic retina and thick subretinal fibrotic tissue. There was granulomatous lymphocytic infiltration in the choroid. The subretinal tissue was derived from retinal pigment epithelial cells. There was a predominance of B cells and plasma cells.[294]

Differential diagnosis

Considerations include other white spot syndromes, especially multifocal choroiditis and birdshot chorioretinopathy. Presumed ocular histoplasmosis syndrome, sarcoid panuveitis, tuberculosis, syphilis, Vogt–Koyanagi–Harada disease, and toxoplasmosis are other entities to rule out.

Management/treatment

Treatment is based on early diagnosis and aggressive management. Once severe subretinal fibrosis develops in the macula, treatment is of little benefit. High-dose systemic or intravitreal steroids have been used. However, these have generally been of little visual benefit.[249,289] Other immunosuppressives such as cyclosporine and azathioprine have been used with better results[244] and more recently a case report using infliximab improved vision.[297] Due to the rarity of this entity, however, a description of best treatment is not possible. Chronic therapy may be needed, and systemic glucocorticoids may be helpful in limiting damage to the fellow eye.

Summary

Multifocal choroiditis and panuveitis syndrome, punctate inner choroidopathy, and progressive subretinal fibrosis and uveitis syndrome are entities that present predominantly in young, healthy, myopic women. They present commonly unilaterally with lesions that are small and multifocal. With new imaging techniques, the outer retina is implicated as well as the RPE and choroid. They have varied outcomes; visual prognosis is generally dependent on the status of the macula and development of CNV or fibrosis. Treatments are aimed at reversing these processes. It is unclear if these are distinct entities, but likely they are on a spectrum of disease processes dependent on an interplay of genetic predisposition and environmental triggers.

MULTIPLE EVANESCENT WHITE DOT SYNDROME, ACUTE ZONAL OCCULT OUTER RETINOPATHY, ACUTE IDIOPATHIC BLIND SPOT ENLARGEMENT, AND ACUTE MACULAR NEURORETINOPATHY

Multiple evanescent white dot syndrome (MEWDS), acute zonal occult outer retinopathy (AZOOR), acute idiopathic blind spot enlargement (AIBSE), and acute macular neuroretinopathy (AMN) are presented together in this final section on WSS. These entities have shown an overlap with each other and on occasion with other WSS as discussed below.

Multiple evanescent white dot syndrome

Multiple evanescent white dot syndrome (MEWDS), originally described in 1984,[298] is an acute, multifocal, usually unilateral retinopathy affecting young adults. Multiple white dots are seen at the level of the outer retina or RPE.

Clinical course

Clinical symptoms

Patients usually present with acute onset of blurred vision in one eye. They also complain of a blind spot or "spots" in their periphery correlating to a temporal scotoma. Photopsias (especially temporally) are common. Patients also may relate flu-like symptoms.[298]

Epidemiology

No particular racial or regional predisposition for MEWDS has been reported. There is a strong female predominance (75%). Initial visual acuity ranges from 20/20 to 20/300 and, after an average duration of approximately 6 weeks, almost always returns to normal levels. Patients are young, and cases of MEWDS have been reported in children as young as 10 years old and in patients as old as 67 years old.[299,300] Most patients, however, cluster near the mean age of 27 years. Asano and colleagues report a high prevalence of myopes in their series.[301]

Fundus findings

Numerous, small (100–200 μμ) white spots are seen at the level of the RPE or deep retina (Fig. 76.47). The white dots are mostly concentrated in the paramacular area, usually sparing the fovea itself, and are less prominent and numerous beyond the vascular arcades.[298] Vitreal cells, retinal venous sheathing, and blurring of the disc margins are often present. The classic macular appearance is a granularity (Fig. 76.48). In atypical cases this may be the primary feature present.[302] The white spots disappear completely after a number of weeks or months. They may be replaced by mild pigment mottling, or rarely chorioretinal scarring resembling multifocal choroiditis. Recently, an appearance of transient brown areas has been described after the white spots resolve. These resemble the lesions of AMN, but are more numerous and widespread.[303] Rarely, a progressive geographic circumpapillary discoloration, appearing as a large white lesion, can be a presenting sign[304] and peripapillary scarring may be seen after the acute lesions have healed.[305]

Rare instances of late CNV have also been noted with MEWDS.[306,307] Some "idiopathic" cases of CNV could represent MEWDS with resolution of other ocular changes before presentation. In a patient with concurrent Best disease, there was

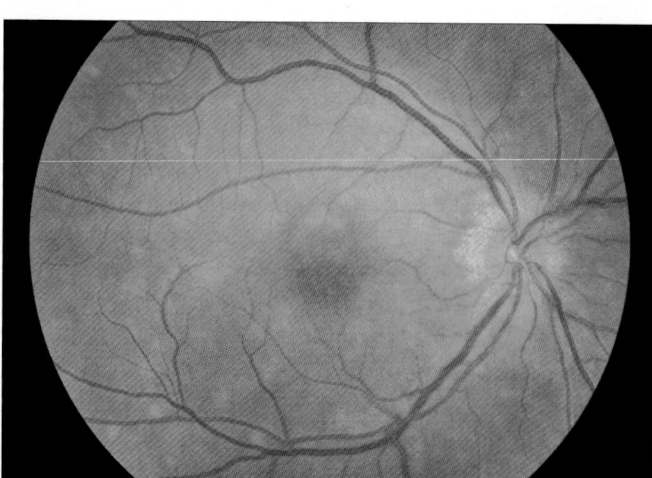

Fig. 76.47 Fundus photo showing subtle numerous white spots at the level of the RPE/deep retina. There are also blurred disc margins. There is foveal granularity.

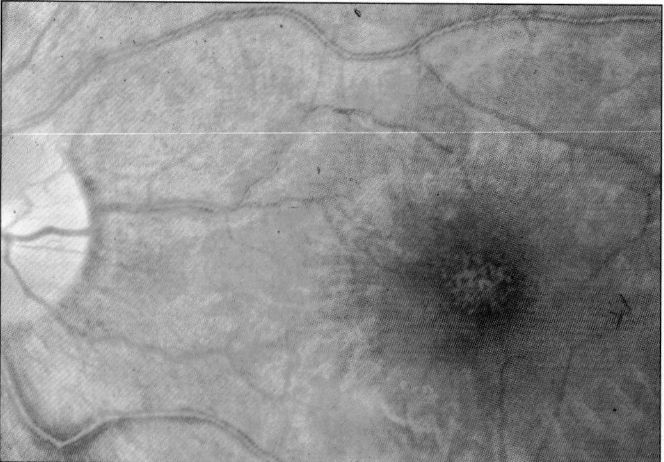

Fig. 76.48 Fundus photo showing granularity of the fovea. This may be the only presenting feature.

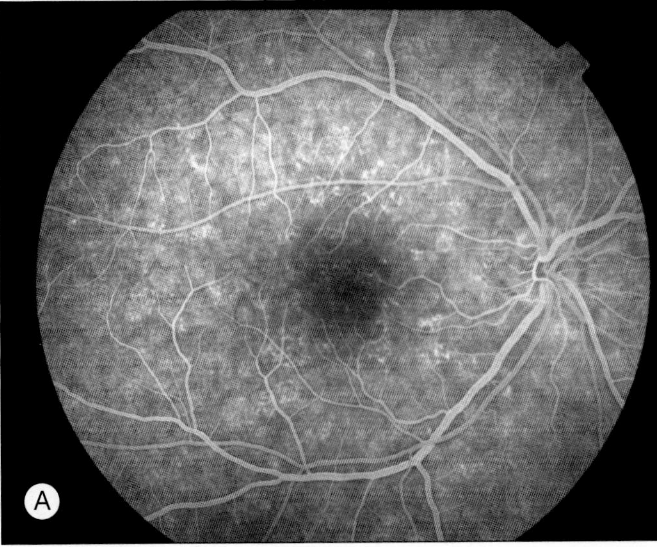
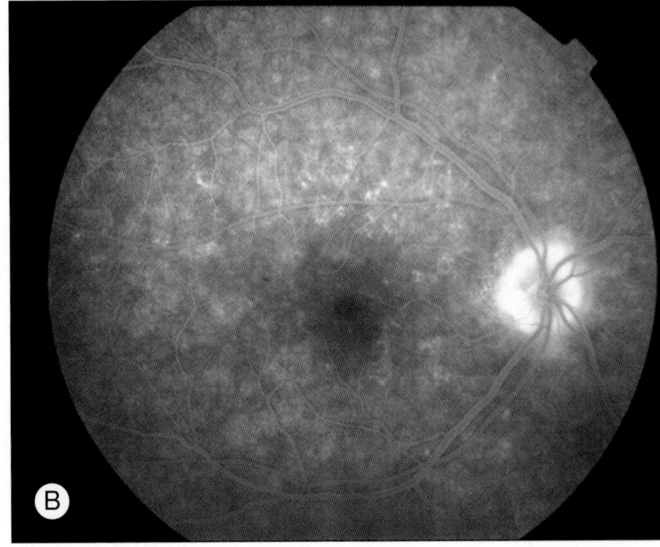

Fig. 76.49 FA of the right eye (A) early and (B) late. There is subtle early and late hyperfluorescence of the white dots in a wreath-like pattern.

a severity of visual symptoms that may have been due to the additive affect of the two RPE disorders.[308] More recently there have been reports that idiopathic CNV may actually present prior to the onset of other more typical clinical and angiographic features of MEWDS or other inflammatory chorioretinal diseases.[309,310]

There has been a single report of a retinal tear associated with acute MEWDS.[311]

Other ocular findings

Mild iritis may be present. Vitritis may be seen but is often absent.

Clinical course and prognosis

MEWDS is usually a self-limited disease, and recovery of visual function occurs over several weeks (3–10 weeks) with a concurrent dramatic improvement of the electroretinogram (ERG) and early receptor potential (ERP) amplitudes.[298,312] Some cases of recurrent MEWDS have been reported, but determinants predisposing toward recurrence have not been identified.[313] Although usually unilateral, bilateral MEWDS has been reported. Bilateral involvement can be either simultaneous or sequential (seen as recurrence of MEWDS in the opposite eye). Bilateral cases may show asymmetric involvement, with only one symptomatic eye, or simultaneous symptoms.[314] There is a chronic form of MEWDS with evidence of multiple recurrences over many years and involving both eyes.[315] Vision returns to baseline between recurrences in most patients. Some patients complain of visual field disturbances or photopsias even after vision has normalized. Fine and colleagues describe 3 cases of MEWDS going on to develop AZOOR.[316] This suggests that there may be a common pathogenetic factor in these diseases.

OCT has shown that the inflammatory lesions of MEWDS are likely at the level of the photoreceptors and RPE (see below). The change in the photoreceptor architecture noted acutely returns to normal.[317,318] The integrity of foveal cones specifically has been studied with OCT and foveal reflection analyzer, and also shows recovery.[319] The foveal granularity is associated with disruption of the IS–OS junction in the fovea with outer retinal swelling. This recovers partially. Although clinical lesions are usually present in one eye, photoreceptor dysfunction has been found to be bilateral in some cases.[318,320] Photoreceptor recovery supports the good prognosis associated with MEWDS. However, MEWDS can rarely be followed by a diagnosis of AZOOR with attenuation of the photoreceptors[316] (see AZOOR section). CNV is rare, but if present can affect visual prognosis.

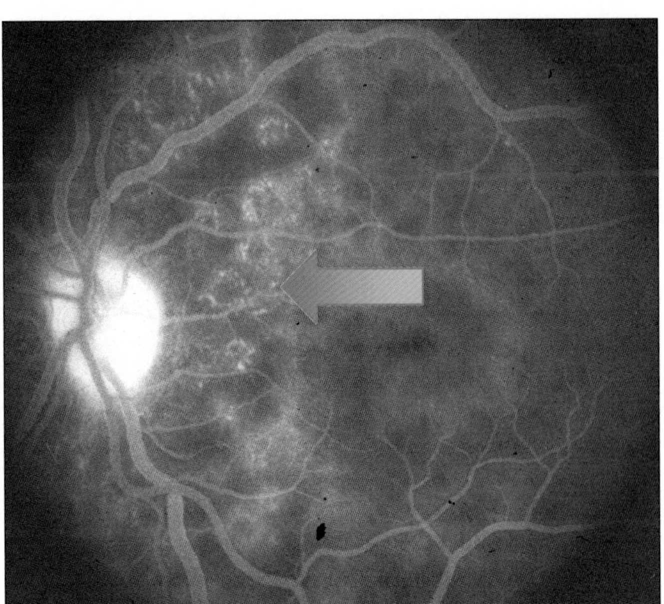

Fig. 76.50 Left eye FA close-up of wreath-like pattern (arrow); a diffuse, noncystoid leakage is seen in the outer retina in the macula.

Imaging

Fluorescein angiography

FA findings include early and late hyperfluorescence of the white dots in a wreath-like pattern; diffuse, but patchy, late staining at the level of the RPE and retina; and disc capillary leakage. A diffuse noncystoid leakage may be seen in the macula (Figs 76.49, 76.50). After resolution of the acute lesions, window defects may be noted in the macula corresponding to the clinical granularity seen and, less often, elsewhere. Chorioretinal scars with blockage and window defects may occasionally be seen. Of note, in the subacute phase, angiography can still show the lesions after they clinically have resolved.[303] Focal areas of vascular staining are sometimes noted.

Indocyanine green angiography

ICGA angiography in patients with MEWDS shows no abnormalities of large choroidal vessels in the early phase, but hypofluorescent lesions are evident in the late phase, corresponding to the white dots[321] (Fig. 76.51). These hypofluorescent spots are more numerous than those clinically seen. The hypofluorescence in the late phase suggests but does not prove that MEWDS may affect the choriocapillaris, as well as its well-known effect on the RPE and photoreceptors.[322,323] These lesions gradually disappear upon recovery,[323,324] but abnormalities on ICGA have been reported to be present up to 9 months after the initial presentation, even after clinical symptoms have resolved.[325] Since ICGA reveals lesions not seen clinically or by FA,[326] it has been recommended with some enthusiasm in the patients with MEWDS, mainly to help establish a diagnosis.[327] Signs are seen longer with ICG testing than with the clinical or fluorescein examination.[328] It has been suggested that the blind spot enlargement of MEWDS corresponds to multiple peripapillary lesions, sometimes only detected with ICGA. More recently, Gross and colleagues describe a new clinical variation in which small "dots" in the inner retina or at the level of the RPE are distinguished from larger "spots" which appear externally in the subpigment epithelial area. These lesions appear in late ICGA as small hypofluorescent lesions overlying larger hypofluorescent ones.[329] Dell'Omo and colleagues point out that the variations in angiographic and ICG studies could reflect that different anatomical structures are involved during the natural evolution of the disease.[330]

Optical coherence tomography

OCT findings were first described using STRATUS technology. A dome-shaped reflective lesion in the subretinal space was seen corresponding to a clinical white dot. An increased reflectivity in the choroid was seen below this lesion in the acute phase. In the recovery phase, there was a decrease in size of the subretinal material and less reflectivity in the choroid. Ultimately, deep retinal lesions disappeared, but reflectivity was seen in the choroid for several months after active disease.[331] High resolution OCT revealed disturbance in the photoreceptor inner/outer segment (IS–OS) junction[332–334] (Fig. 76.52). In cases of recurrent MEWDS, a thinning of the outer nuclear layer was seen. RPE disturbance was not a prominent feature.[334] Li and colleagues emphasized that the disruption of the photoreceptor outer segments can be restored anatomically. Functional studies also showed recovery.[318] In addition, although lesions typically occurred unilaterally, the photoreceptor dysfunction is bilateral in most cases.[318] Focal disruption of the IS–OS segment photoreceptor layer[302] is seen even in atypical cases where white spots are not present. Therefore, this study is of particular importance in making the diagnosis of MEWDS (Fig. 76.53).

Fundus autofluorescence

Dell'Omo and colleagues studied MEWDS in the acute and subacute phases and characterized specific FAF findings. Hypoautofluorescent areas were seen concentrated around the optic disc and posterior pole. Areas of hyperautofluorescence were seen as well, corresponding to the white dots.[335] Furino and colleagues described this as well.[336] In the recovery phase, many of the hypoautofluorescent lesions faded, while others persisted. The areas of hyperautofluorescence became smaller and more consolidated. They also retracted centripetally, becoming smaller with a ring of hypoautofluoresence around them, or became entirely hypoautofluorescent. In other cases, they disappeared altogether without becoming hypoautofluorescent.[335]

Electrophysiology

Electrophysiologic studies in patients with acute MEWDS[312] have found reduced ERG a-wave and reduced ERP amplitudes that would suggest a primary involvement of the outer segments of photoreceptors. Focal ERG studies reveal delayed recovery of oscillatory potential (OP), which implies some inner retinal involvement.[337] Studies[338] have used foveal densitometry and color matching to show that, even with normal ERG findings, abnormalities exist during the active stage of MEWDS at the level of the cone photoreceptor outer segments. A transient metabolic disturbance at the level of the pigment epithelium–photoreceptor complex has been suggested. Multifocal electroretinography (mfERG) shows areas of depression that correspond to scotomas while full-field ERG shows a general depression. These abnormalities resolve after 6 weeks.[339] In addition, mfERG shows supernormal amplitudes of the first-order kernel of N1- and P1-wave amplitudes at the beginning of the disease; these values decrease to normal or subnormal values by 2 weeks and may be helpful in detecting early stages of MEWDS or for follow-up.[340]

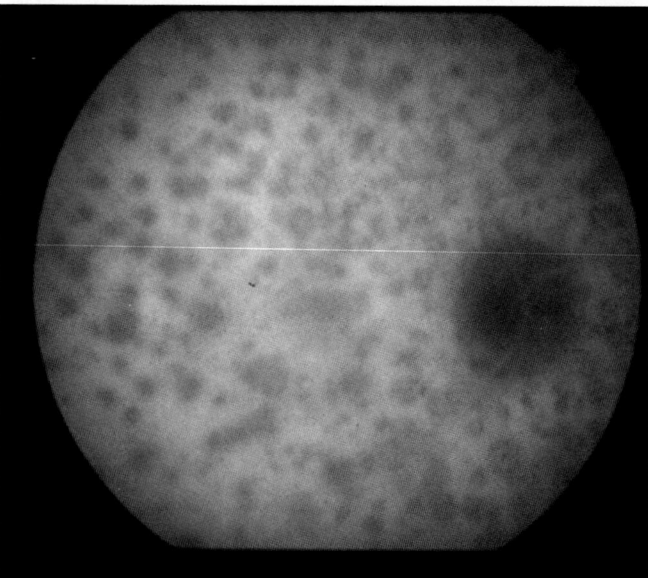

Fig. 76.51 ICG showing numerous hypofluorescent spots including confluent lesions around the disc.

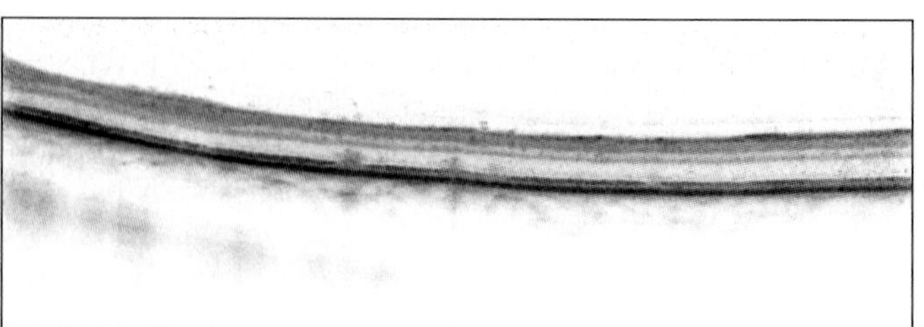

Fig. 76.52 OCT shows discontinuity of IS–OS line. (Courtesy of Medical University of Vienna.)

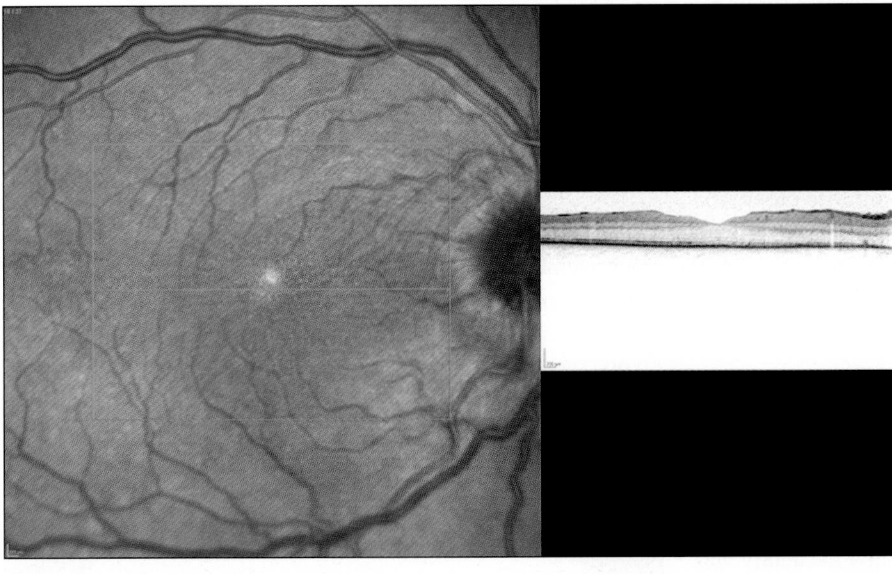

Fig. 76.53 OCT through the fovea shows swelling of the outer retinal layers and granules at the level of the RPE. (Courtesy of Medical University of Vienna.)

Visual field testing

Visual field testing can range from normal to a generalized depression to cecocentral or arcuate scotomas.[341] Visual field testing often shows an enlarged blind spot. Visual field abnormalities may persist for an extended period beyond the resolution of clinical lesions.[342] Newer microperimetry testing also shows enlarged blindspots.[343] In addition, microperimetry has shown decreased retinal sensitivity in areas of IS–OS abnormalities, when correlated with SD-OCT.[344]

Pathogenesis

The cause of MEWDS is unknown. Gass has used the term AZOOR (acute zonal occult outer retinopathy) complex to encompass the following entities: MEWDS, multifocal choroiditis, punctate inner choroidopathy (PIC), acute idiopathic blind-spot enlargement, acute macular neuroretinopathy, acute annular outer retinopathy, and AZOOR. Others have espoused similar opinions.[345,346] He suggested that these diseases represent parts of a spectrum of what is probably a single disease. Gass believed that these diseases may be of viral origin, with the virus entering the retina from the peripapillary area or at the ora serrata. He speculated that the virus gains access to the photoreceptor cells and spreads from cell to cell. He believed that the difference in clinical presentation results from genetic and immune system differences. In this case, a search for a virus or infectious agent as a trigger would be indicated.[5] To date, there is no direct evidence supporting this hypothesis; no virus has been reproducibly isolated in patients with these various diseases.

At the present time we do not have definite evidence for a viral or an immunologic cause for MEWDS. The response of a single patient with chronic relapsing MEWDS to cyclosporine therapy suggests an autoimmune component.[347] Laatikainen and Immonen[348] described an increased level of protein in the cerebrospinal fluid in MEWDS patients. The occurrence of MEWDS following varicella infection,[306] vaccination for hepatitis A[349] or hepatitis B,[350] or most recently reported in a young girl after vaccination for human papilloma virus and meningococcus[351] suggests environmental triggers. One case of MEWDS from China with no previous or concurrent illness exhibited increased serum immunoglobulin M (IgM) and IgG values.[352] Recovery of vision in 3 weeks was coincident with the return of the IgM value to normal values. Data from this case suggested that MEWDS might be associated with a viral syndrome, although tests for herpes zoster, herpes simplex, mumps, and measles were inconclusive. Any explanation of the etiology of MEWDS must explain the strong female predominance, the occurrence of occasional chronic relapsing cases, the occasional occurrence of MEWDS in patients with other white spot syndromes, and the excellent visual outcome in almost every case. The HLA locus may be important. A preliminary study found the frequency of HLA-B51 haplotype to be 3.7 times more common in patients with MEWDS than a normal control group.[353,354]

Our present suggestion is that a variety of relatively common susceptibility genes may be responsible for MEWDS. These predispose to immune dysregulation. Precipitated by environmental triggers, MEWDS may develop. If this theory is true, then patients with MEWDS may demonstrate a family or personal history of autoimmunity. In investigating this, we have found an increased prevalence of autoimmunity in patients with white spot syndromes and their families.[2,4] While the etiology of MEWDS is studied further, we believe that MEWDS is a distinct clinical entity that should not be confused with other WSS.

Differential diagnosis

The differential diagnosis of MEWDS includes other WSS: acute posterior multifocal placoid pigment epitheliopathy (APMPPE), birdshot chorioretinopathy, acute idiopathic blind spot syndrome, acute macular neuroretinopathy, and acute zonal occult outer retinopathy (discussed elsewhere in this chapter). Other chorioretinopathies such as sarcoidosis and diffuse unilateral subacute neuroretinitis must be considered. In older patients, ocular infiltration by lymphoma must be ruled out.

Patients with MEWDS often present with signs and symptoms suggesting primary optic nerve disease, including disc edema, visual loss, afferent pupillary defect, enlarged blind spot, and other optic nerve field defects. Dodwell et al.[355] reported 5 cases that were initially misdiagnosed as primary optic nerve disease, as the white spots were subtle findings. Optic nerve involvement in MEWDS could theoretically contribute to the central visual loss, visual field loss, afferent pupillary defect, and even dyschromatopsia. MEWDS should be considered in the differential diagnosis of young, healthy patients who present with unilateral or bilateral optic nerve dysfunction.[356,357]

The challenge of correctly diagnosing MEWDS lies in its variable, sometimes subtle, presentation and the rapid reversal of the visual loss with disappearance of the white dots. These factors may explain its recent discovery, and the scarcity of documented cases. MEWDS has shown overlapping with other WSS in the same patient. We believe that AIBSE may be a feature of MEWDS, MCP, and other WSS. In very rare cases, MEWDS can evolve into AZOOR.[316] Its uncertain association with other ophthalmic conditions such as AZOOR, AMN, and MFC requires further investigation.

Management/treatment

The natural course of MEWDS is excellent and often no intervention is required. There has been one case report that used steroid pulse therapy in an attempt to hasten recovery. The patient presented with 20/400 vision and a field defect and it is reported that immediately after the completion of therapy his acuity was 20/25 with full recovery of his visual field deficits.[358] However, the risk-to-benefit ratio should be evaluated in this type of treatment and further study is needed to validate this. Although CNV is not common in MEWDS, anti-VEGF therapy has been used with success in a few cases. This also warrants further study.[359,360]

Summary

MEWDS usually presents in young females who may describe a viral prodrome. Generally the retinopathy is unilateral, but studies have shown that this may be bilateral or asymmetric. White dots are the classic hallmark of this condition; however, atypical cases that present with a foveal granularity or CNV have also been described. The course is almost always good, and generally no intervention is required.

Acute zonal occult outer retinopathy

Acute zonal occult outer retinopathy (AZOOR) is linked to the white spot syndromes although it has no white spots. In the early 1990s, Dr Donald Gass[361] described 13 patients with what he called acute zonal occult outer retinopathy. These were, in general, young, healthy patients, who abruptly developed photopsias and the presence of a scotoma in a local area of the retina. Examination showed minimal fundus changes; however a dense scotoma could be plotted in the involved area. With the passage of time, these zones often developed pigment epithelial mottling, bone spicule pigmentation, and some choroidal atrophy (Fig. 76.54). The changes, when widespread, could resemble retinitis pigmentosa. The disease has been recently reviewed.[362]

Gass[5,363] also used the term AZOOR complex. Within the description he included MEWDS, AIBSE, AMN, PIC, and MFC. He felt that these diseases were somehow related; they demonstrated outer retinal dysfunction and usually occurred in young, healthy females.

Clinical course

Clinical symptoms

Patients with AZOOR have the abrupt onset of a scotoma related to outer retinal dysfunction. Most have photopsias. There may be recurrences, new scotomas or an increase in the size of the scotoma. The scotoma is often contiguous with the optic nerve. The disease may be unilateral initially but many progress to bilaterality.

Epidemiology

AZOOR is seen in all ethnic groups, although the literature shows a predominance of Caucasians. There is a marked predominance of women. Most patients are young, although occasionally elderly patients are involved. Some of the patients relate a preceding viral illness. There is no definite association with any systemic diseases.

Fundus findings

The fundus initially appears normal; subsequently the area of involvement will show retinal atrophy and mottling. The arterioles attenuate (Fig. 76.55). The area of involvement is often peripapillary but usually the central vision is good unless a scotoma extends to the fovea. The appearance may resemble

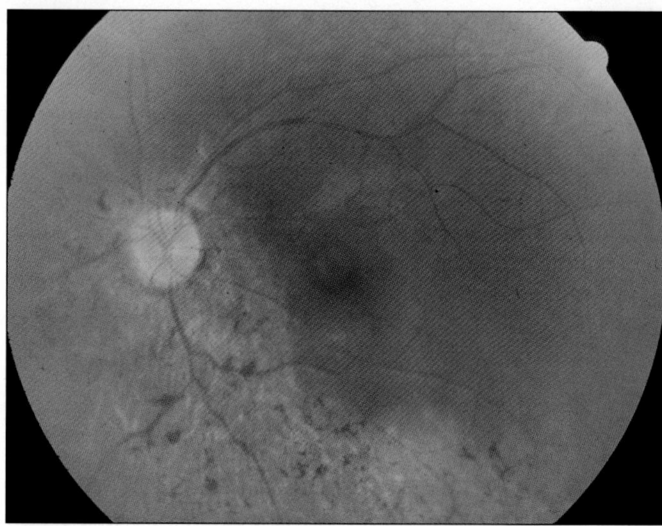

Fig. 76.54 Fundus photo of advanced acute zonal occult outer retinopathy. Pigment epithelial atrophy and bone spicule formation can be seen in continuity with the disc.

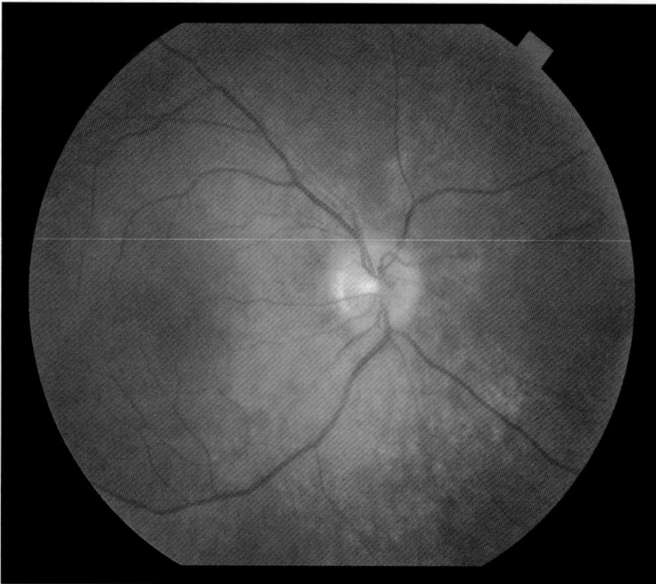

Fig. 76.55 Fundus photo. Subtle fundus changes are seen. Arteriolar attenuation is present.

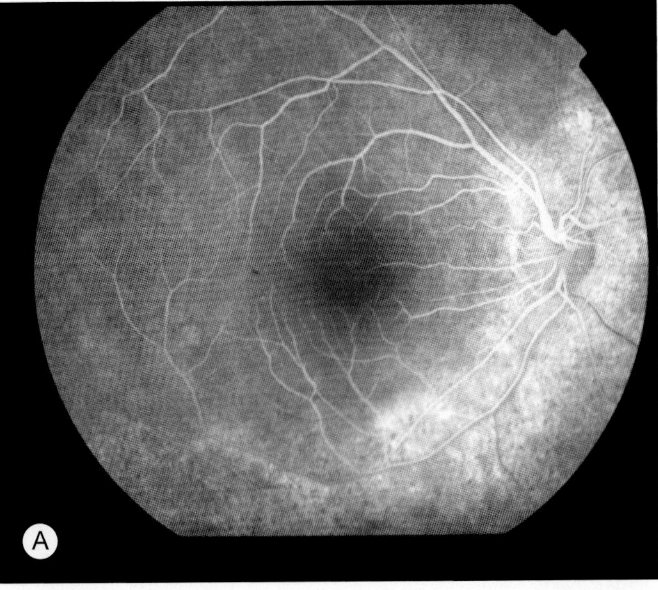

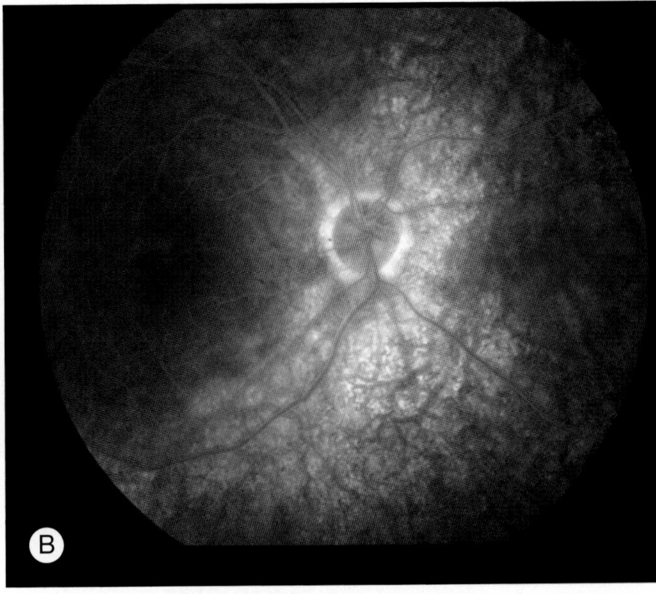

Fig. 76.56 (A,B) FA shows peripapillary zonal RPE abnormalities with window-type defects.

sectoral retinitis pigmentosa. The appearance can also resemble diffuse unilateral subacute neuroretinitis (DUSN). CNV is seen rarely.[364]

Other ocular findings

The eyes are quiet without evidence of anterior chamber reaction. There may be some vitreous cells; often these are minimal. Disc leakage, retinal vascular staining, and some CME may be seen.

Clinical course and prognosis

Patients may show progression, with new areas of retinal involvement. Occasionally there may also be some improvement in visual function in the involved areas. Gass[363] noted that most cases were active for about 6 months and then stabilized. We have, however, seen patients with persisting, advancing disease.

Imaging

Fluorescein angiography

Initially the fluorescein angiogram may be normal. Then window defects and abnormalities at the level of the pigment epithelium become apparent. Retinal arteriolar narrowing in the areas of involvement may be seen. Retinal vessel staining and leakage may be seen (Fig. 76.56).

Indocyanine green angiography

ICGA may be normal or may show hypofluorescence in the area of involvement.

Fundus autofluorescence

Spaide has demonstrated the value of autofluorescence in defining the area of retinal involvement.[365,366] Involved areas often show marked hypoautofluorescence. Peripapillary hypofluorescence may be present with a rim of surrounding hyperfluorescence (Fig. 76.57). Some cases may have a normal pattern, at least at the onset.

Optical coherence tomography

OCT evaluation, especially spectral domain OCT, demonstrates absence or irregularity of the IS–OS photoreceptor line in the areas of retinal involvement (Fig. 76.58).[366–368] With chronicity, atrophy of the RPE and thinning of the retina may be seen with the outer nuclear layer and then the inner nuclear layer thinning. Disruption may extend to the inner retina as well.

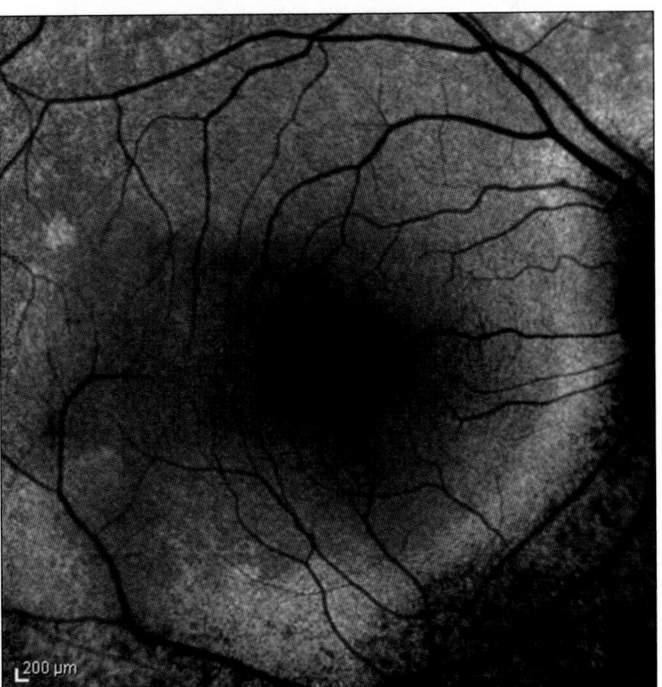

Fig. 76.57 FAF shows peripapillary hypofluorescence with a rim of surrounding hyperfluorescence.

Visual field testing

Scotomas (usually peripheral and temporal) develop often in continuity with the optic disc. These are usually dense. With healing, some improvement may occur, but the functional loss is often permanent (Fig. 76.59).

Electrophysiology

Focal ERG demonstrates abnormalities in the area of the scotoma. Full-field ERGs are almost always abnormal, if large enough

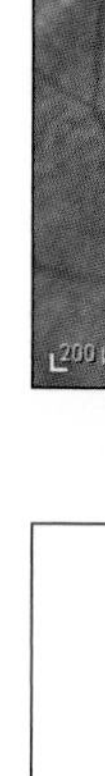

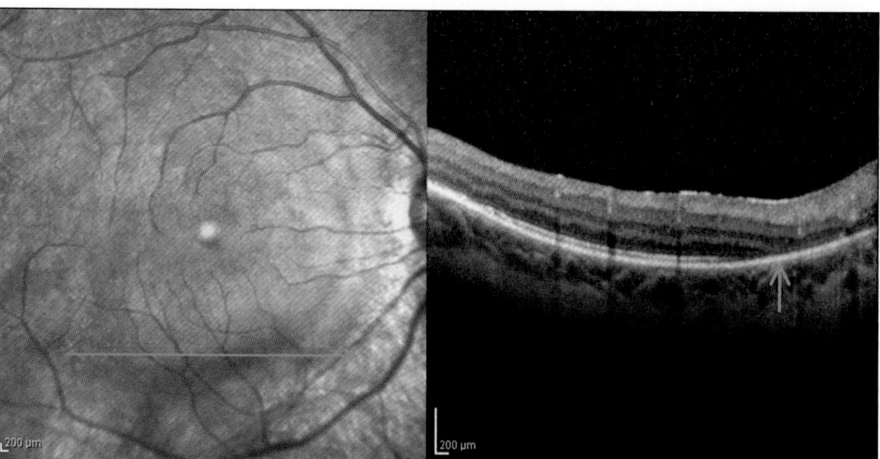

Fig. 76.58 OCT shows absence of the IS–OS photoreceptor line in the area of retinal involvement (arrow).

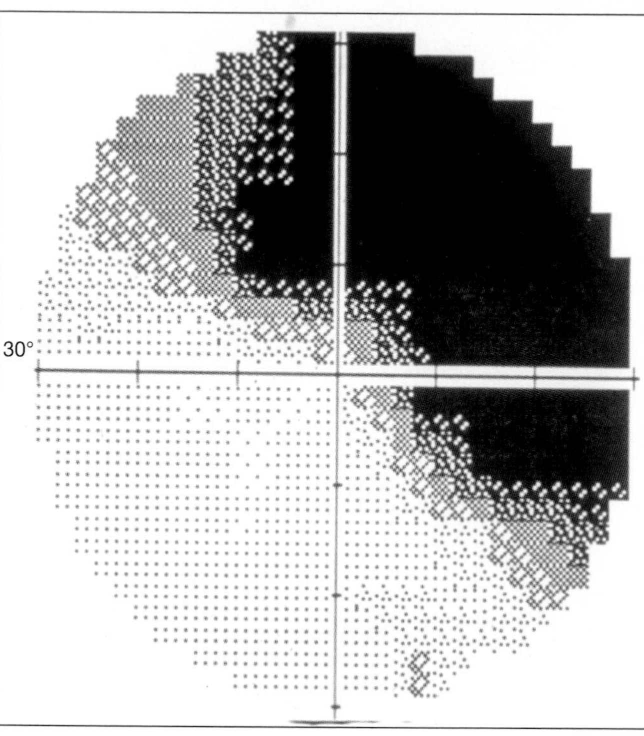

Fig. 76.59 Perimetry shows a dense zonal defect.

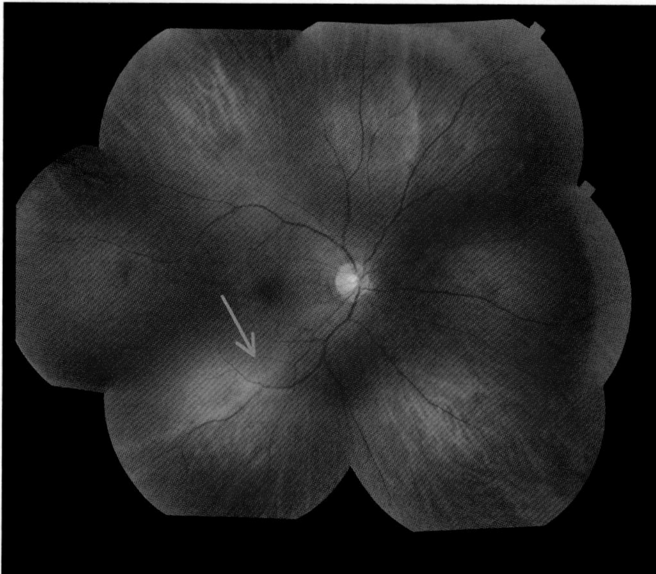

Fig. 76.60 Fundus photo of acute annular occult outer retinopathy. A grey-white line (arrow) is present between the normal retina to the right and involved retina to the left. (Courtesy of Manjot K. Gill, MD.)

areas of the retina are involved.[363] EOG testing is usually abnormal.

Association with ocular systemic diseases

There may be a relationship between AZOOR and other white spot syndromes. Some patients can begin with MEWDS and then subsequently show evidence of diffuse photoreceptor degeneration consistent with AZOOR.[369] Some patients that initially fit into the spectrum of punctate inner choroidopathy or multifocal choroiditis may develop severe widespread retinal dysfunction, again, consistent with AZOOR.[370] Thus there exist type 1 AZOOR (no other white spot syndrome) and type 2, which begins as another white spot syndrome. A few patients do not show any clinical retinal abnormalities (only photoreceptor dysfunction) – type 3.

Gass also described an entity that he called acute annular occult outer retinopathy:[371,372] Patients develop a scotoma with a grey–white line in the fundus between normal retina and involved retina (Figs 76.60 and 76.61). This line of activity fades. The areas of involvement subsequently may show evolution similar to AZOOR with RPE changes and retinal thinning. The relationship of this entity to classic AZOOR is uncertain.

Systemic autoimmune diseases have been noted in some patients with AZOOR.[362] An association with multiple sclerosis and pars planitis is possible.[373] Like other white spot syndromes, it may occur in patients with immune dysfunction.[2,4]

Pathogenesis

Mechanisms causing vision loss with the development of AZOOR remain obscure. Could this be an autoimmune attack on the retina? The possible association with systemic autoimmune disease suggests this.[4] No specific antiretinal antibodies have been identified and the presence of antibodies may be incidental or a secondary phenomenon (epiphenomenon) not related to the underlying disease process.

Gass suggested that AZOOR was possibly a viral infection, with the virus entering the eye from the optic disc and thus producing peripapillary lesions.[5] There is little evidence supporting an infectious etiology of AZOOR at this point.

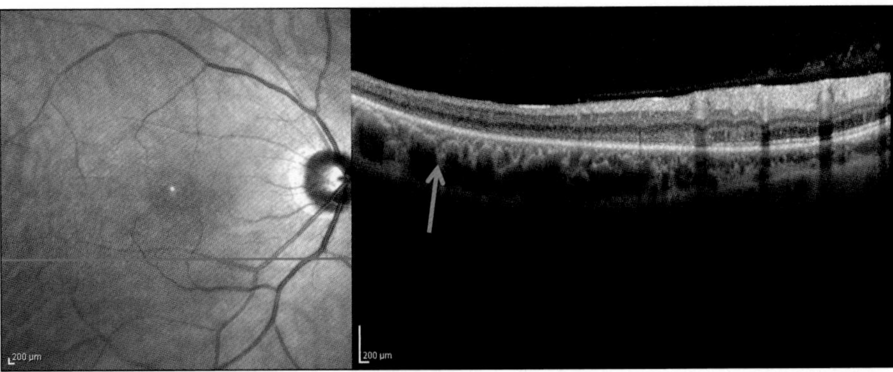

Fig. 76.61 OCT shows retinal thinning in the involved area. (Courtesy of Manjot K. Gill, MD.)

Differential diagnosis

The visual loss of AZOOR must be distinguished from optic neuropathies. OCT should show IS–OS junction abnormalities in the involved area. It may initially be difficult to distinguish AZOOR from other entities with outer retinal dysfunction. Patients with hereditary retinal diseases (e.g. retinitis pigmentosa) develop changes that can resemble AZOOR. These changes may be sectoral or asymmetric. Some of the patients with hereditary diseases have been shown to have antiretinal antibodies (the role these play in the pathophysiology of the diseases is unproven). Retinal dystrophies are usually bilateral, symmetric, and slowly progressive, distinguishing them from AZOOR. Patients with cancer-associated retinopathy (CAR) or melanoma-associated retinopathy (MAR) may show outer or inner retinal dysfunction with autoantibodies against the retina. These cases can resemble AZOOR. A less well-defined group of patients have been felt to have "autoimmune retinopathies" without cancer where antiretinal antibodies and perhaps even cell-mediated immunity may cause retinal dysfunction.[374] The clinical presentation of AZOOR – local and segmental, often peripapillary, or at least contiguous with the disc – helps in the diagnosis.

Management/treatment

No proven therapy exists. Systemic corticosteroids and other immunosuppressive drugs have been suggested to be beneficial.[306] Antiviral drugs and antibacterial drugs have also been tried. Recently Mahajan and Stone[375] reported the response of 3 patients to valacyclovir. Although these patients did show clinical improvement, they were early on in their course and their clinical appearances were not yet typical for AZOOR; thus the value of this drug for AZOOR remains uncertain.

Summary

AZOOR is a disease of sectoral or zonal outer retinal dysfunction, often adjacent to the optic nerve. Although the fundus initially appears normal, the development of retinitis pigmentosa-like changes occurs. Outer retinal and RPE changes are seen in most cases and some inflammation may be seen. At the present time there is no definitive evidence of an infectious cause of AZOOR. Autoimmune disease is suggested by the female predominance and possible response to immune suppressive therapy. Differentiating this condition from hereditary retinal degenerations, CAR, MAR, and autoimmune retinopathies is necessary. Some patients may initially present as another white spot syndrome and then show an evolution to a more diffuse photoreceptor degeneration consistent with AZOOR.

Acute idiopathic blind spot enlargement

Acute idiopathic blind spot enlargement (AIBSE) was first described by Fletcher and colleagues in 1988.[376] They reported 7 young patients with sudden onset of photopsias and a temporal scotoma involving the blind spot. A normal fundus was described in 5 patients, with 2 patients demonstrating peripapillary pigmentary changes. Enlarged blind spots have also been described in a variety of white spot syndromes such as MEWDS, MCP, PIC, AMN, and AZOOR. It is unclear if AIBSE is a distinct entity.

Clinical course

Clinical symptoms

The initial symptoms of 27 patients with AIBSE were described by Volpe and colleagues.[377] Loss of vision was the most common complaint, present in 25 patients. This was further described as blurring, awareness of a loss of part of their visual field, or "looking through a film." Positive visual phenomena were reported in 23 patients. These were described as photopsias, swirling movement within a scotoma, colored lights, or after "flash bulb" phenomena.

Epidemiology

AIBSE has been described in primarily young women.[377]

Fundus findings

Fletcher described a normal fundus and normal optic disc appearance.[376] However, ophthalmoscopic findings in Volpe and colleagues' study showed a normal exam in only 8 patients. Retinal findings such as pigmentary changes in the peripapillary region, periphery, or macula were seen. Other vitreoretinal abnormalities included white dots, macular edema, and vitritis. Optic disc swelling or hyperemia that was not commensurate with the blind spot size was present in 12 out of the 27 patients.

Ocular findings

Afferent pupillary defects and dyschromatopsia can be noted in patients.[377] Photostress recovery has been noted to be prolonged.[376] This has been related to photoreceptor dysfunction.

Clinical course and prognosis

In Volpe and colleagues' study, most (16 of 27) presented with 20/20 vision. Ten patients presented with 20/25 to 20/50, while only 1 had vision of 20/200. Watzke and Shults believed most cases of AIBSE are white spot syndromes.[378] They studied 21 patients with AIBSE and noted that unless examined within the first 2 weeks of onset, the underlying chorioretinal disease could be missed. The natural course of AIBSE is that the photopsias resolve with time, but persistent visual field defects remain. The course does not seem to demonstrate progressive worsening.[377,378]

Imaging

Fluorescein angiography

FA can be normal,[379] or show disc staining in the late phase.[377]

Indocyanine green angiography

Pece and colleagues[380] describe a case of AIBSE in which ICGA showed multiple hypofluorescent spots throughout the fundus that were not visible clinically. They reported that these abnormalities resolved over 4 weeks. This picture is consistent with MEWDS.

Optical coherence tomography

Spaide and colleagues[381] assessed visual field defects in diseases of the AZOOR-complex (MEWDS, MCP, AZOOR) and correlated them to spectral domain OCT scans. They found that there was a defect in boundary between the photoreceptor inner and outer segments. These IS–OS defects were found in the peripapillary region, chorioretinal scars, and CNV. In their study, there was no widespread dysfunction. Furthermore, there could be improvement in the IS–OS defects as well as visual fields with treatment. Sugahara and colleagues present a case of AIBSE in its convalescent stage.[382] In this stage, the IS–OS and external limiting membrane lines (ELM) were intact. However, Verhoeff's membrane, which is located at the cone outer segment tips (COSTs) was absent in the area of a persistent scotoma. This correlated to reduced responses on mfERG.

Electrophysiology

Full-field ERGs are generally normal in AIBSE; however, mfERG shows abnormalities coincident with areas of scotomas.[377,383]

Visual field testing

Goldmann and Humphrey visual field testing reveals an enlarged blind spot of varying sizes (Fig. 76.62). There is a common feature of steep margins.[377,384] Visual field recovery has been seen in other white spot diseases with enlarged blind spots; however, AIBSE has been noted to not recover entirely.[377] Blue-cone sensitivity has been shown to be decreased in AIBSE.[385] This can be elicited with blue-on-yellow perimetry.

Pathogenesis

The etiology is unknown, but AIBSE appears to be a result of photoreceptor outer segment dysfunction. The disease can rarely have recurrences but it does not appear to be progressive. It is therefore thought that an environmentally triggered factor is more plausible than an autoimmune condition.[377] Due to the female predilection, it has also been postulated that hormonal or genetic factors may be at play.[377] It seems like most if not all of these cases are subtle white spot syndromes.

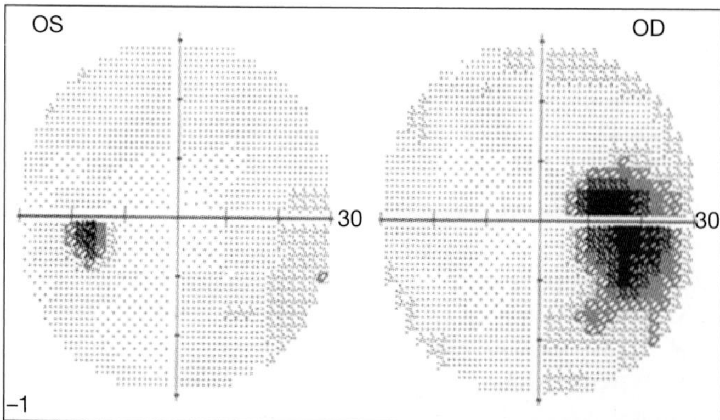

Fig. 76.62 Visual fields showing an enlarged blind spot. (Courtesy of Nicholas J. Volpe, MD and Alexander J. Brucker, MD.)

Differential diagnosis

Patients with AIBSE have been misdiagnosed with optic neuritis and migraines.[377] Other considerations include the white spot syndromes mentioned: AZOOR, MCP, PIC, AMN, and MEWDS.

Management/treatment

This is a self-limited and nonprogressive process.

Summary

AIBSE is a disease of predominantly young, healthy women. Patients present with scintillations in their temporal visual field associated with an enlarged blind spot. Classically, there are no significant optic disc or retinal findings. Visual fields improve, but may retain a persistent defect. Enlarged blind spots are also seen with MCP, MEWDS, PIC, and AZOOR. MEWDS can occur without white spots and it seems plausible that many cases of AIBSE represent subtle MEWDS or other white spot syndromes.

Acute macular neuroretinopathy

Acute macular neuroretinopathy (AMN) was first described in 1975 by Bos and Deutman.[386] It is a rare condition that causes acute transient or permanent visual changes.[387] The distinct macular lesions of AMN are reddish-brown in appearance and wedge-shaped or flower-like pointing to or encircling the fovea. The level of the retina involved has been controversial. Originally it was thought to be a disease of the inner retina. Newer imaging techniques have shown the outer retina is involved as well.[388-390] Fawzi and colleagues use multimodal imaging and find that the disease appears to start at the level of the outer plexiform layer and then rapidly involves the outer retina (paper in preparation).

Clinical course

Clinical symptoms

Patients complain of decreased vision and paracentral scotomas. A viral prodrome or drug use may be present.

Epidemiology

AMN occurs in young, healthy women in the second to fourth decades of life.[386] In a review of the literature, Turbeville reported that 83% of reported cases to 2002 were women with a mean age of 27 years.[391]

Fundus findings

One or several small lesions are seen surrounding the fovea at the level of the outer retina. These may be round, oval, or petaloid[386,391] (Fig. 76.63). They appear brown or dark red compared to the surrounding retina.[386,390] The lesions are best seen on red-free photography. Retinal hemorrhages have been reported.[391] No abnormality is seen in the retinal vessels or optic disc.

Clinical course and prognosis

The disease process may be unilateral or bilateral. Patients may present several days after the development of scotomas.[391] The lesions may develop rapidly or over the course of days to weeks. Turbeville and colleagues noted a different time course in those cases that were related to viral prodrome and those that developed in association with epinephrine (see below). Patients who reported an influenza-like illness had an onset of scotomas generally over days to weeks, though sudden onset was also possible. With time, the symptoms and lesions resolved, though patients remain mildly symptomatic. In contrast, all the epinephrine cases were sudden, bilateral, and did not seem to resolve with time. They postulated that this may represent different mechanisms.

Rarely, recurrences may occur in one or both eyes. The acute retinal lesions fade but generally do not disappear completely. Complete recovery has been reported in a few cases.[391] Newer imaging techniques as further discussed below suggest that there are persistent anatomical changes in the outer retina despite subjective or clinical improvement.[393]

Imaging

Fluorescein angiography

Usually FA results are normal. Sometimes there may be a slight hypofluorescence corresponding to blockage from the clinically seen lesions.[386,390,394]

Indocyanine green angiography

ICGA is normal.[395]

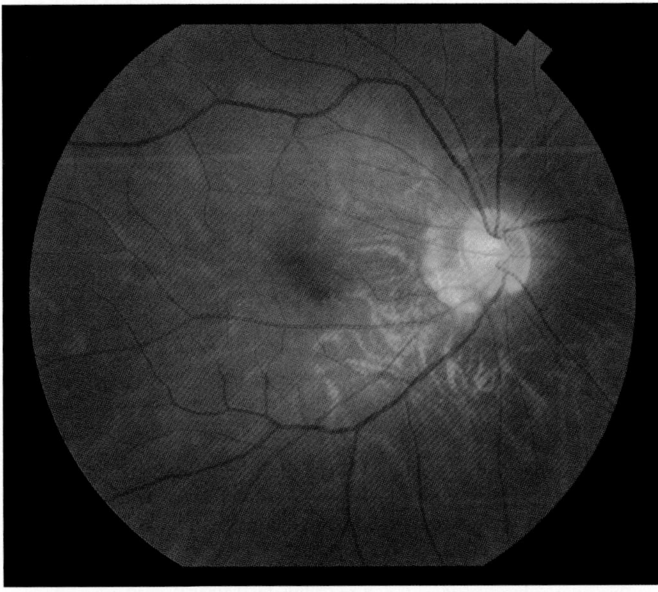

Fig. 76.63 Fundus photo of a patient with acute macular neuroretinopathy. Subtle macular reddish-brown lesions are seen.

Optical coherence tomography

Much of the recent literature on AMN is devoted to OCT findings.[387,389,392,395–400] Feigl and Haas[396] first described a high reflectivity band corresponding to the retinal pigment epithelium–choriocapillaris complex using time domain OCT. Others noted focal macular thinning likely corresponding to the recovery phase.[401] Spectral domain studies have shown distortion of the IS–OS junction and focal thinning of the outer retina.[398] The reddish-brown clinical lesions correspond to focal OS/RPE defects (Fig. 76.64). These usually persist; however, outer nuclear layer (ONL) thinning may be more prominent in larger lesions.[402] The infrared images seen with OCT highlight the lesions well. The findings on infrared reflectance and OCT change rapidly over time in the first few weeks, and may be the reason why the early inner retinal changes are missed. Very subtle pigmentary changes involving the RPE have been suggested to cause the reddish appearance (Fawzi, data in preparation).

Fundus autofluorescence

Subtle hypoautofluorescence corresponding to clinically seen lesions has been reported.[387]

Electrophysiology

Multifocal ERG has shown decreased foveal peaks in affected eyes.[388,400] Researchers using mfERG localize the lesion to the outer retina affecting the photoreceptor or bipolar cell layer, and changes may persist for longer durations.[403,404] ERG and EOG are generally normal.[405]

Visual fields

Paracentral scotomas are seen corresponding exactly to the shape and location of the clinical lesions. Patients can often draw their scotoma on an Amsler grid.[386] When defects are very small, microperimetry may be helpful.[406]

Systemic associations

Turbeville and colleagues summarized the reported associations.[391] Oral contraceptive use, flu-like syndrome, contrast media exposure, epinephrine use, trauma, history of headaches/migraines, postpartum hypotension, and hypotensive shock have all been described in patients who developed AMN.

Pathogenesis

The cause is unknown. Imaging shows involvement of the photoreceptors and the development of zones of outer retinal thinning. Turbeville and colleagues review theories of pathogenesis,

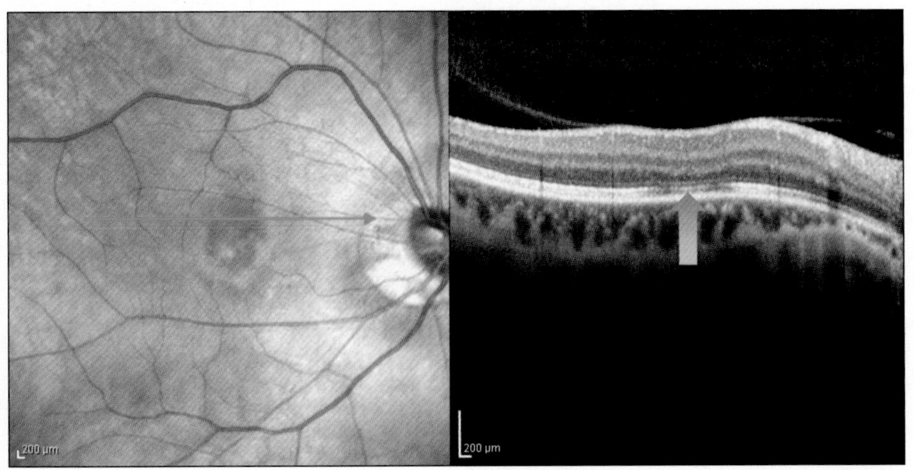

Fig. 76.64 OCT shows that the lesions correspond to focal OS/RPE defects (arrow).

which include hormonal predisposition, infectious processes (44% of reported cases to 2002 had a flu-like syndrome), decreased blood flow to the outer retina causing transient ischemia, and increased thoracic pressure causing a sudden increase in intravascular pressure damaging the blood-retina barrier.[391] The early involvement of the outer plexiform layer, as well as the vascular associations, suggest a vascular insult to the outer capillary network (Fawzi, data in preparation).

AMN-like lesions may be seen in patients with MEWDS[407] or AIBSE.[408]

Differential diagnosis

Other white spot diseases should be considered including MEWDS and AIBSE. Other entities included in the differential are central serous chorioretinopathy, old inner retinal infarcts, and optic neuritis.

Management/treatment

The disease is self-limited. Visual acuity and visual field defects improve over time, though subtle symptoms may persist. No treatment has been shown effective.

Summary

AMN is a rare condition, but should be considered in young, female patients with an acute onset of paracentral scotomas. A history of viral prodrome is common. The typical reddish-brown lesions are found in the macula and best seen with red-free light or infrared reflectance. This disease involves the outer retina as evidenced by OCT imaging. It is a self-limited process and no treatment has been proven effective.

Acknowledgment

Supported in part by a grant from Kevin Hitzeman and Mary Dempsey.

REFERENCES

1. Quillen DA, Davis JB, Gottlieb JL, et al. The white dot syndromes. Am J Ophthalmol 2004;137(3):538–50.
2. Jampol LM, Becker KG. White spot syndromes of the retina: a hypothesis based on the common genetic hypothesis of autoimmune/inflammatory disease. Am J Ophthalmol 2003;135(3):376–9.
3. Heckenlively JR, Ferreyra HA. Autoimmune retinopathy: a review and summary. Semin Immunopathol 2008;30(2):127–34.
4. Pearlman RB, Golchet PR, Feldmann MG, et al. Increased prevalence of autoimmunity in patients with white spot syndromes and their family members. Arch Ophthalmol 2009;127(7):869–74.
5. Gass JD. Are acute zonal occult outer retinopathy and the white spot syndromes (AZOOR complex) specific autoimmune diseases? Am J Ophthalmol 2003;135(3):380–1.
6. Mathura JR, Jampol LM, Daily MJ. Multifocal choroiditis and acute posterior multifocal placoid pigment epitheliopathy occurring in the same patient. Arch Ophthalmol 2004;122(12):1881–2.
7. Ryan SJ, Maumenee AE. Birdshot retinochoroidopathy. Am J Ophthalmol 1980;89(1):31–45.
8. Gass JD. Vitiliginous chorioretinitis. Arch Ophthalmol 1981;99(10):1778–87.
9. Shah KH, Levinson RD, Yu F, et al. Birdshot chorioretinopathy. Surv Ophthalmol 2005;50(6):519–41.
10. Nussenblatt RB, Mittal KK, Ryan S, et al. Birdshot retinochoroidopathy associated with HLA-A29 antigen and immune responsiveness to retinal S-antigen. Am J Ophthalmol 1982;94(2):147–58.
11. Ladas JG, Arnold AC, Holland GN. Control of visual symptoms in two men with birdshot retinochoroidopathy using low-dose oral corticosteroid therapy. Am J Ophthalmol 1999;128(1):116–8.
12. Holland GN, Shah KH, Monnet D, et al. Longitudinal cohort study of patients with birdshot chorioretinopathy II: color vision at baseline. Am J Ophthalmol 2006;142(6):1013–18.
13. Gordon LK, Monnet D, Holland GN, et al. Longitudinal cohort study of patients with birdshot chorioretinopathy. IV. Visual field results at baseline. Am J Ophthalmol 2007;144(6):829–37.
14. Priem HA, Kijlstra A, Noens L, et al. HLA typing in birdshot chorioretinopathy. Am J Ophthalmol 1988;105(2):182–5.
15. Monnet D, Brézin AP. Birdshot chorioretinopathy. Curr Opin Ophthalmol 2006;17(6):545–50.
16. Soubrane G, Bokobza R, Coscas G. Late developing lesions in birdshot retinochoroidopathy. Am J Ophthalmol 1990;109(2):204–10.
17. Gasch AT, Smith JA, Whitcup SM. Birdshot retinochoroidopathy. Br J Ophthalmol 1999;83(2):241–9.
18. Priem HA, Oosterhuis JA. Birdshot chorioretinopathy: clinical characteristics and evolution. Br J Ophthalmol 1988;72(9):646–59.
19. Lim L, Harper A, Guymer R. Choroidal lesions preceding symptom onset in birdshot chorioretinopathy. Arch Ophthalmol 2006;124(7):1057–8.
20. Fuerst DJ, Tessler HH, Fishman GA, et al. Birdshot retinochoroidopathy. Arch Ophthalmol 1984;102(2):214–9.
21. Kaplan HJ, Aaberg TM. Birdshot retinochoroidopathy. Am J Ophthalmol 1980;90(6):773–82.
22. Soubrane G, Coscas G, Binaghi M, et al. Birdshot retinochoroidopathy and subretinal new vessels. Br J Ophthalmol 1983;67(7):461–7.
23. Brucker AJ, Deglin EA, Bene C, et al. Subretinal choroidal neovascularization in birdshot retinochoroidopathy. Am J Ophthalmol 1985;99(1):40–4.
24. Felder KS, Brockhurst RJ. Neovascular fundus abnormalities in peripheral uveitis. Arch Ophthalmol 1982;100(5):750–4.
25. Henkind P. Ocular neovascularization. The Krill memorial lecture. Am J Ophthalmol 1978;85(3):287–301.
26. Levinson RD, Brezin A, Rothova A, et al. Research criteria for the diagnosis of birdshot chorioretinopathy: results of an international consensus conference. Am J Ophthalmol 2006;141(1):185–7.
27. Howe LJ, Woon H, Graham EM, et al. Choroidal hypoperfusion in acute posterior multifocal placoid pigment epitheliopathy. An indocyanine green angiography study. Ophthalmology 1995;102(5):790–8.
28. Fardeau C, Herbort CP, Kullmann N, et al. Indocyanine green angiography in birdshot chorioretinopathy. Ophthalmology 1999;106(10):1928–34.
29. Stanga PE, Lim JI, Hamilton P. Indocyanine green angiography in chorioretinal diseases: indications and interpretation: an evidence-based update. Ophthalmology 2003;110(1):15–21; quiz 22–3.
30. Howe LJ, Stanford MR, Graham EM, et al. Choroidal abnormalities in birdshot chorioretinopathy: an indocyanine green angiography study. Eye (Lond) 1997;11(Pt 4):554–9.
31. Giuliari G, Hinkle DM, Foster CS. The spectrum of fundus autofluorescence findings in birdshot chorioretinopathy. J Ophthalmol 2009; e-Pub doi: 10.1155/2009/567693.
32. Koizumi H, Pozzoni MC, Spaide RF. Fundus autofluorescence in birdshot chorioretinopathy. Ophthalmology 2008;115(5):e15–20.
33. Priem HA, De Rouck A, De Laey JJ, et al. Electrophysiologic studies in birdshot chorioretinopathy. Am J Ophthalmol 1988;106(4):430–6.
34. Hirose T, Katsumi O, Pruett RC, et al. Retinal function in birdshot retinochoroidopathy. Acta Ophthalmol (Copenh) 1991;69(3):327–37.
35. Holder GE, Robson AG, Pavesio C, et al. Electrophysiological characterisation and monitoring in the management of birdshot chorioretinopathy. Br J Ophthalmol 2005;89(6):709–18.
36. Thorne JE, Jabs DA, Kedhar SR, et al. Loss of visual field among patients with birdshot chorioretinopathy. Am J Ophthalmol 2008;145(1):23–8.
37. Heaton JM, Mills RP. Sensorineural hearing loss associated with birdshot retinochoroidopathy. Arch Otolaryngol Head Neck Surg 1993;119(6):680–1.
38. Gaudio PA, Kaye DB, Crawford JB. Histopathology of birdshot retinochoroidopathy. Br J Ophthalmol 2002;86(12):1439–41.
39. Levinson RD, Du Z, Luo L, et al. Combination of KIR and HLA gene variants augments the risk of developing birdshot chorioretinopathy in HLA-A*29-positive individuals. Genes Immun 2008;9(3):249–58.
40. Rush RB, Goldstein DA, Callanan DG, et al. Outcomes of birdshot chorioretinopathy treated with an intravitreal sustained-release fluocinolone acetonide-containing device. Am J Ophthalmol 2011;151(4):630–6.
41. Godel V, Baruch E, Lazar M. Late development of chorioretinal lesions in birdshot retinochoroidopathy. Ann Ophthalmol 1989;21(2):49–52.
42. Oh KT, Christmas NJ, Folk JC. Birdshot retinochoroiditis: long term follow-up of a chronically progressive disease. Am J Ophthalmol 2002;133(5):622–9.
43. Vitale AT, Rodriguez A, Foster CS. Low-dose cyclosporine therapy in the treatment of birdshot retinochoroidopathy. Ophthalmology 1994;101(5):822–31.
44. Jap A, Chee SP. Immunosuppressive therapy for ocular diseases. Curr Opin Ophthalmol 2008;19(6):535–40.
45. Sobrin L, Huang JJ, Christen W, et al. Daclizumab for treatment of birdshot chorioretinopathy. Arch Ophthalmol 2008;126(2):186–91.
46. Battaglia Parodi M, Iacono P, Verbraak FD, et al. Antivascular endothelial growth factors for inflammatory chorioretinal disorders. Dev Ophthalmol 2010;46:84–95.
47. Gass JD. Acute posterior multifocal placoid pigment epitheliopathy. Arch Ophthalmol 1968;80(2):177–85.
48. Ryan SJ, Maumenee AE. Acute posterior multifocal placoid pigment epitheliopathy. Am J Ophthalmol 1972;74(6):1066–74.
49. Deutman AF, Oosterhuis JA, Boen-Tan TN, et al. Acute posterior multifocal placoid pigment epitheliopathy. Pigment epitheliopathy of choriocapillaritis? Br J Ophthalmol 1972;56(12):863–74.
50. Deutman AF, Boen-Tan TN, Oosterhuis JA. Proceedings: Acute posterior multifocal placoid pigment epitheliopathy. Ophthalmologica 1973;167(5):368–72.
51. Fitzpatrick PJ, Robertson DM. Acute posterior multifocal placoid pigment epitheliopathy. Arch Ophthalmol 1973;89(5):373–6.
52. Savino PJ, Weinberg RJ, Yassin JG, et al. Diverse manifestations of acute posterior multifocal placoid pigment epitheliopathy. Am J Ophthalmol 1974;77(5):659–62.

53. Fishman GA, Rabb MF, Kaplan J. Acute posterior multifocal placoid pigment epitheliopathy. Arch Ophthalmol 1974;92(2):173–7.
54. Lewis RA. Acute posterior multifocal placoid pigment epitheliopathy. A recurrence. Arch Ophthalmol 1975;93(3):235–8.
55. Holt WS, Regan CD, Trempe C. Acute posterior multifocal placoid pigment epitheliopathy. Am J Ophthalmol 1976;81(4):403–12.
56. Scuderi G, Recupero SM, Valvo A. Acute posterior multifocal placoid pigment epitheliopathy. Ann Ophthalmol 1977;9(2):189–94.
57. Van Buskirk EM, Lessell S, Friedman E. Pigmentary epitheliopathy and erythema nodosum. Arch Ophthalmol 1971;85(3):369–72.
58. Fiore T, Iaccheri B, Androudi S, et al. Acute posterior multifocal placoid pigment epitheliopathy: outcome and visual prognosis. Retina 2009;29(7): 994–1001.
59. Jones NP. Acute posterior multifocal placoid pigment epitheliopathy. Br J Ophthalmol 1995;79(4):384–9.
60. Taich A, Johnson MW. A syndrome resembling acute posterior multifocal placoid pigment epitheliopathy in older adults. Trans Am Ophthalmol Soc 2008;106:56–62; discussion 62–3.
61. Bird AC, Hamilton AM. Placoid pigment epitheliopathy. Presenting with bilateral serous retinal detachment. Br J Ophthalmol 1972;56(12):881–6.
62. Kayazawa F, Takahashi H. Acute posterior multifocal placoid pigment epitheliopathy and Harada's disease. Ann Ophthalmol 1983;15(1):58–62.
63. Kremer I, Yassur Y. Unilateral atypical retinal pigment epitheliopathy associated with serous retinal detachment. Ann Ophthalmol 1992;24(2):75–7.
64. Garg S, Jampol LM. Macular serous detachment in acute posterior multifocal placoid pigment epitheliopathy. Retina 2004;24(4):650–1.
65. Birnbaum AD, Blair MP, Tessler HH, et al. Subretinal fluid in acute posterior multifocal placoid pigment epitheliopathy. Retina 2010;30(5):810–4.
66. Furusho F, Imaizumi H, Takeda M. One case of Harada disease complicated by acute posterior multifocal placoid pigment epitheliopathy-like recurrence in both eyes. Jpn J Ophthalmol 2001;45(1):117–8.
67. Lee GE, Lee BW, Rao NA, et al. Spectral domain optical coherence tomography and autofluorescence in a case of acute posterior multifocal placoid pigment epitheliopathy mimicking Vogt–Koyanagi–Harada disease: case report and review of literature. Ocul Immunol Inflamm 2011;19(1): 42–7.
68. Wright BE, Bird AC, Hamilton AM. Placoid pigment epitheliopathy and Harada's disease. Br J Ophthalmol 1978;62(9):609–21.
69. Williams DF, Mieler WF. Long-term follow-up of acute multifocal posterior placoid pigment epitheliopathy. Br J Ophthalmol 1989;73(12):985–90.
70. Spaide RF, Yannuzzi LA, Slakter J. Choroidal vasculitis in acute posterior multifocal placoid pigment epitheliopathy. Br J Ophthalmol 1991;75(11): 685–7.
71. Abu El-Asrar AM, Aljazairy AH. Acute posterior multifocal placoid pigment epitheliopathy with retinal vasculitis and papillitis. Eye (Lond) 2002;16(5): 642–4.
72. De Souza S, Aslanides IM, Altomare F. Acute posterior multifocal placoid pigment epitheliopathy associated with retinal vasculitis, neovascularization and subhyaloid hemorrhage. Can J Ophthalmol 1999;34(6):343–5.
73. Bowie EM, Sletten KR, Kayser DL, et al. Acute posterior multifocal placoid pigment epitheliopathy and choroidal neovascularization. Retina 2005;25(3): 362–4.
74. Frohman LP, Klug R, Bielory L, et al. Acute posterior multifocal placoid pigment epitheliopathy with unilateral retinal lesions and bilateral disk edema. Am J Ophthalmol 1987;104(5):548–50.
75. Lowes M. Placoid pigment epitheliopathy presenting as an anterior uveitis. A case report. Acta Ophthalmol (Copenh) 1977;55(5):800–6.
76. Alvi NP, Fishman GA. Granulomatous anterior uveitis presenting with acute posterior multifocal placoid pigment epitheliopathy. Doc Ophthalmol 1995;89(4):347–53.
77. Oh KT, Park DW. Acute posterior multifocal placoid pigment epitheliopathy with corneal stromal infiltrates. Am J Ophthalmol 1998;125(4):556–8.
78. Howe LJ, Woon H, Graham EM, et al. Choroidal hypoperfusion in acute posterior multifocal placoid pigment epitheliopathy. An indocyanine green angiography study. Ophthalmology 1995;102(5):790–8.
79. Dhaliwal RS, Maguire AM, Flower RW, et al. Acute posterior multifocal placoid pigment epitheliopathy. An indocyanine green angiographic study. Retina 1993;13(4):317–25.
80. Schneider U, Inhoffen W, Gelisken F. Indocyanine green angiography in a case of unilateral recurrent posterior acute multifocal placoid pigment epitheliopathy. Acta Ophthalmol Scand 2003;81(1):72–5.
81. Stanga PE, Lim JI, Hamilton P. Indocyanine green angiography in chorioretinal diseases: indications and interpretation: an evidence-based update. Ophthalmology 2003;110(1):15–21; quiz 22–3.
82. Park D, Schatz H, McDonald HR, et al. Acute multifocal posterior placoid pigment epitheliopathy: a theory of pathogenesis. Retina 1995;15(4):351–2.
83. Van Liefferinge T, Sallet G, De Laey JJ. Indocyanine green angiography in cases of inflammatory chorioretinopathy. Bull Soc Belge Ophtalmol 1995;257:73–81.
84. Yuzawa M, Kawamura A, Matsui M. Indocyanine green video angiographic findings in acute posterior multifocal placoid pigment epitheliopathy. Acta Ophthalmol (Copenh) 1994;72(1):128–33.
85. Montero JA, Ruiz-Moreno JM, Fernandez-Munoz M. Spectral domain optical coherence tomography findings in acute posterior multifocal placoid pigment epitheliopathy. Ocul Immunol Inflamm 2011;19(1):48–50.
86. Cheung CM, Yeo IY, Koh A. Photoreceptor changes in acute and resolved acute posterior multifocal placoid pigment epitheliopathy documented by spectral-domain optical coherence tomography. Arch Ophthalmol 2010; 128(5):644–6.
87. Batioglu F, Ozmert E, Kurt R. Fundus autofluorescence and spectral optical coherence tomography findings in a case with acute posterior multifocal placoid pigment epitheliopathy. Ann Ophthalmol (Skokie) 2008;40(3–4): 185–9.
88. Lim LL, Watzke RC, Lauer AK, et al. Ocular coherence tomography in acute posterior multifocal placoid pigment epitheliopathy. Clin Exp Ophthalmol 2006;34(8):810–2.
89. Souka AA, Hillenkamp J, Gora F, et al. Correlation between optical coherence tomography and autofluorescence in acute posterior multifocal placoid pigment epitheliopathy. Graefes Arch Clin Exp Ophthalmol 2006;244(10): 1219–23.
90. Lofoco G, Ciucci F, Bardocci A, et al. Optical coherence tomography findings in a case of acute multifocal posterior placoid pigment epitheliopathy (AMPPPE). Eur J Ophthalmol 2005;15(1):143–7.
91. Scheufele TA, Witkin AJ, Schocket LS, et al. Photoreceptor atrophy in acute posterior multifocal placoid pigment epitheliopathy demonstrated by optical coherence tomography. Retina 2005;25(8):1109–12.
92. Yeh S, Forooghian F, Wong WT, et al. Fundus autofluorescence imaging of the white dot syndromes. Arch Ophthalmol 2010;128(1):46–56.
93. Spaide RF. Autofluorescence imaging of acute posterior multifocal placoid pigment epitheliopathy. Retina 2006;26(4):479–82.
94. Pagnoux C, Thorne C, Mandelcorn ED, et al. CNS involvement in acute posterior multifocal placoid pigment epitheliopathy. Can J Neurol Sci 2011;38(3): 526–8.
95. Althaus C, Unsöld R, Figge C, et al. Cerebral complications in acute posterior multifocal placoid pigment epitheliopathy. Ger J Ophthalmol 1993;2(3): 150–4.
96. Stoll G, Reiners K, Schwartz A, et al. Acute posterior multifocal placoid pigment epitheliopathy with cerebral involvement. J Neurol Neurosurg Psychiatry 1991;54(1):77–9.
97. Prokosch V, Becker H, Thanos S, et al. Acute posterior multifocal placoid pigment epitheliopathy with concurrent cerebral vasculitis and sarcoidosis. Graefes Arch Clin Exp Ophthalmol 2010;248(1):151–2.
98. Massé H, Guyomard JL, Baudet D, et al. Mitoxantrone therapy for acute posterior multifocal placoid pigment epitheliopathy with cerebral vasculitis. Case Report Med 2009; e-Pub doi: 2009:481512.
99. de Vries JJ, den Dunnen WF, Timmerman EA, et al. Acute posterior multifocal placoid pigment epitheliopathy with cerebral vasculitis: a multisystem granulomatous disease. Arch Ophthalmol 2006;124(6):910–3.
100. Hsu CT, Harlan JB, Goldberg MF, et al. Acute posterior multifocal placoid pigment epitheliopathy associated with a systemic necrotizing vasculitis. Retina 2003;23(1):64–8.
101. Weinstein JM, Bresnick GH, Bell CL, et al. Acute posterior multifocal placoid pigment epitheliopathy associated with cerebral vasculitis. J Clin Neuroophthalmol Sep 1988;8(3):195–201.
102. Wilson CA, Choromokos EA, Sheppard R. Acute posterior multifocal placoid pigment epitheliopathy and cerebral vasculitis. Arch Ophthalmol 1988;106(6): 796–800.
103. Sigelman J, Behrens M, Hilal S. Acute posterior multifocal placoid pigment epitheliopathy associated with cerebral vasculitis and homonymous hemianopia. Am J Ophthalmol 1979;88(5):919–24.
104. Kersten DH, Lessell S, Carlow TJ. Acute posterior multifocal placoid pigment epitheliopathy and late-onset meningo-encephalitis. Ophthalmology 1987; 94(4):393–6.
105. Luneau K, Newman NJ, Srivastava S, et al. A case of acute posterior multifocal placoid pigment epitheliopathy with recurrent stroke. J Neuroophthalmol 2009;29(2):111–8.
106. Jaramillo A, Gaete G, Romero P, et al. Acute pontine infarct in a 16-year-old man with acute posterior multifocal placoid pigment epitheliopathy. A case report. J Stroke Cerebrovasc Dis 2009;18(2):164–6.
107. Bugnone AN, Hartker F, Shapiro M, et al. Acute and chronic brain infarcts on MR imaging in a 20-year-old woman with acute posterior multifocal placoid pigment epitheliopathy. AJNR Am J Neuroradiol 2006;27(1): 67–9.
108. Al Kawi A, Wang DZ, Kishore K, et al. A case of ischemic cerebral infarction associated with acute posterior multifocal placoid pigment epitheliopathy, CNS vasculitis, vitamin B(12) deficiency and homocysteinemia. Cerebrovasc Dis 2004;18(4):338–9.
109. Bewermeyer H, Nelles G, Huber M, et al. Pontine infarction in acute posterior multifocal placoid pigment epitheliopathy. J Neurol 1993;241(1):22–6.
110. Gibelalde A, Bidaguren A, Ostolaza JI, et al. [Pigmentary epitheliopathy multifocal acute placoid associated with paralysis of VI cranial par]. Arch Soc Esp Oftalmol 2009;84(3):159–62.
111. Clearkin LG, Hung SO. Acute posterior multifocal placoid pigment epitheliopathy associated with transient hearing loss. Trans Ophthalmol Soc UK 1983;103 (Pt 5):562–4.
112. Spencer BR, Kunimoto DY, Patel DR, et al. Acute multifocal posterior placoid pigment epitheliopathy (AMPPPE) mimicking migraine with aura. Cephalalgia 2009;29(6):694–8.
113. Fishman GA, Baskin M, Jednock N. Spinal fluid pleocytosis in acute posterior multifocal placoid pigment epitheliopathy. Ann Ophthalmol 1977; 9(1):36.
114. Hedges TR, Sinclair SH, Gragoudas ES. Evidence for vasculitis in acute posterior multifocal placoid pigment epitheliopathy. Ann Ophthalmol 1979;11(4):539–42.

115. Matsuo T, Horikoshi T, Nagai C. Acute posterior multifocal placoid pigment epitheliopathy and scleritis in a patient with pANCA-positive systemic vasculitis. Am J Ophthalmol 2002;133(4):566–8.
116. Matsuo T. Eye manifestations in patients with perinuclear antineutrophil cytoplasmic antibody-associated vasculitis: case series and literature review. Jpn J Ophthalmol 2007;51(2):131–8.
117. Di Crecchio L, Parodi MB, Saviano S, et al. Acute posterior multifocal placoid pigment epitheliopathy and ulcerative colitis: a possible association. Acta Ophthalmol Scand 2001;79(3):319–21.
118. Jacklin HN. Acute posterior multifocal placoid pigment epitheliopathy and thyroiditis. Arch Ophthalmol 1977;95(6):995–7.
119. Laatikainen LT, Immonen IJ. Acute posterior multifocal placoid pigment epitheliopathy in connection with acute nephritis. Retina 1988;8(2):122–4.
120. Priluck IA, Robertson DM, Buettner H. Acute posterior multifocal placoid pigment epitheliopathy. Urinary findings. Arch Ophthalmol 1981;99(9): 1560–2.
121. Bridges WJ, Saadeh C, Gerald R. Acute posterior multifocal placoid pigment epitheliopathy in a patient with systemic-onset juvenile rheumatoid arthritis: treatment with cyclosporin A and prednisone. Arthritis Rheum 1995;38(3): 446–7.
122. Chiquet C, Lumbroso L, Denis P, et al. Acute posterior multifocal placoid pigment epitheliopathy associated with Wegener's granulomatosis. Retina 1999;19(4):309–13.
123. Anderson K, Patel KR, Webb L, et al. Acute posterior multifocal placoid pigment epitheliopathy associated with pulmonary tuberculosis. Br J Ophthalmol 1996;80(2):186.
124. Dick DJ, Newman PK, Richardson J, et al. Acute posterior multifocal placoid pigment epitheliopathy and sarcoidosis. Br J Ophthalmol 1988;72(1):74–7.
125. Wolf MD, Folk JC, Panknen CA, et al. HLA-B7 and HLA-DR2 antigens and acute posterior multifocal placoid pigment epitheliopathy. Arch Ophthalmol 1990;108(5):698–700.
126. Nga AD, Ramli N, Mimiwati Z. Post viral acute multifocal posterior placoid pigment epithiopathy in a teenage child. Med J Malaysia 2009;64(2):176–8.
127. Borruat FX, Piguet B, Herbort CP. Acute posterior multifocal placoid pigment epitheliopathy following mumps. Ocul Immunol Inflamm 1998;6(3):189–93.
128. Thomson SP, Roxburgh ST. Acute posterior multifocal placoid pigment epitheliopathy associated with adenovirus infection. Eye (Lond) 2003;17(4): 542–4.
129. Azar P, Gohd RS, Waltman D, et al. Acute posterior multifocal placoid pigment epitheliopathy associated with an adenovirus type 5 infection. Am J Ophthalmol 1975;80(6):1003–5.
130. Augsten R, Pfister W, Königsdörffer E. [Acute posterior multifocal placoid pigment epitheliopathy (APMPPE) and borreliosis]. Klin Monbl Augenheilkd 2009;226(6):512–3.
131. Wolf MD, Folk JC, Nelson JA, et al. Acute, posterior, multifocal, placoid, pigment epitheliopathy and Lyme disease. Arch Ophthalmol 1992;110(6):750.
132. Lowder CY, Foster RE, Gordon SM, et al. Acute posterior multifocal placoid pigment epitheliopathy after acute group A streptococcal infection. Am J Ophthalmol 1996;122(1):115–7.
133. Mendrinos E, Baglivo E. Acute posterior multifocal placoid pigment epitheliopathy following influenza vaccination. Eye (Lond) 2010;24(1):180–1.
134. Fine HF, Kim E, Flynn TE, et al. Acute posterior multifocal placoid pigment epitheliopathy following varicella vaccination. Br J Ophthalmol 2010;94(3): 282–3, 363.
135. Yang DS, Hilford DJ, Conrad D. Acute posterior multifocal placoid pigment epitheliopathy after meningococcal C conjugate vaccine. Clin Exp Ophthalmol 2005;33(2):219–21.
136. Brézin AP, Massin-Korobelnik P, Boudin M, et al. Acute posterior multifocal placoid pigment epitheliopathy after hepatitis B vaccine. Arch Ophthalmol 1995;113(3):297–300.
137. Uthman I, Najjar DM, Kanj SS, et al. Anticardiolipin antibodies in acute multifocal posterior placoid pigment epitheliopathy. Ann Rheum Dis 2003;62(7): 687–8.
138. Uthman IW, Bizri AR, Gharavi AE. Infections and antiphospholipid antibodies. J Med Liban 2000;48(5):324–6.
139. Menon SR, Fleischhauer J, Jost K, et al. Clinical and electrophysiological course of acute syphilitic posterior placoid chorioretinitis. Klin Monbl Augenheilkd 2005;222(3):261–3.
140. O'Halloran HS, Berger JR, Lee WB, et al. Acute multifocal placoid pigment epitheliopathy and central nervous system involvement: nine new cases and a review of the literature. Ophthalmology 2001;108(5):861–8.
141. Mavrakanas N, Mendrinos E, Tabatabay C, et al. Intravitreal ranibizumab for choroidal neovascularization secondary to acute multifocal posterior placoid pigment epitheliopathy. Acta Ophthalmol 2010;88(2):e54–55.
142. Battaglia Parodi M, Iacono P, Verbraak FD, et al. Antivascular endothelial growth factors for inflammatory chorioretinal disorders. Dev Ophthalmol 2010;46:84–95.
143. Franceschetti A. A curious affection of the fundus oculi: helicoid peripapillar chorioretinal degeneration. Its relation to pigmentary paravenous chorioretinal degeneration. Doc Ophthalmol 1962;16:81–110.
144. Schatz HS, Maumenee AEM, Patz A. Geographic helicoid peripapillary choroiodopathy: clinical presentation and fluorescein angiographic findings. Trans Am Acad Ophthalmol Otolaryngol 1974;78:747–61.
145. Hamilton AM, Bird AC. Geographical choroidopathy. Br J Ophthalmol 1974;58(9):784–97.
146. Lim WK, Buggage RR, Nussenblatt RB. Serpiginous choroiditis. Surv Ophthalmol 2005;50(3):231–44.
147. Laatikainen L, Erkkilä H. Serpiginous choroiditis. Br J Ophthalmol 1974;58(9):777–83.
148. Weiss H, Annesley WH, Shields JA, et al. The clinical course of serpiginous choroidopathy. Am J Ophthalmol 1979;87(2):133–42.
149. Hardy RA, Schatz H. Macular geographic helicoid choroidopathy. Arch Ophthalmol 1987;105(9):1237–42.
150. Mansour AM, Jampol LM, Packo KH. Macular serpiginous choroiditis. Retina 1988;8(2):125–31.
151. Erkkilä H, Laatikainen L, Jokinen E. Immunological studies on serpiginous choroiditis. Graefes Arch Clin Exp Ophthalmol 1982;219(3):131–4.
152. Hoyng C, Tilanus M, Deutman A. Atypical central lesions in serpiginous choroiditis treated with oral prednisone. Graefes Arch Clin Exp Ophthalmol 1998;236(2):154–6.
153. Chisholm IH, Gass JD, Hutton WL. The late stage of serpiginous (geographic) choroiditis. Am J Ophthalmol 1976;82(3):343–51.
154. Laatikainen L, Erkkilä H. A follow-up study on serpiginous choroiditis. Acta Ophthalmol (Copenh) 1981;59(5):707–18.
155. Sahu DK, Rawoof A, Sujatha B. Macular serpiginous choroiditis. Indian J Ophthalmol 2002;50(3):189–96.
156. Masi RJ, O'Connor GR, Kimura SJ. Anterior uveitis in geographic or serpiginous choroiditis. Am J Ophthalmol 1978;86(2):228–32.
157. Abrez H, Biswas J, Sudharshan S. Clinical profile, treatment, and visual outcome of serpiginous choroiditis. Ocul Immunol Inflamm 2007;15(4): 325–35.
158. Baglivo E, Boudjema S, Pieh C, et al. Vascular occlusion in serpiginous choroidopathy. Br J Ophthalmol 2005;89(3):387–8.
159. Blumenkranz MS, Gass JD, Clarkson JG. Atypical serpiginous choroiditis. Arch Ophthalmol 1982;100(11):1773–5.
160. Lee DK, Suhler EB, Augustin W, et al. Serpiginous choroidopathy presenting as choroidal neovascularisation. Br J Ophthalmol 2003;87(9):1184–5.
161. Wu JS, Lewis H, Fine SL, et al. Clinicopathologic findings in a patient with serpiginous choroiditis and treated choroidal neovascularization. Retina 1989;9(4):292–301.
162. Laatikainen L, Erkkilä H. Subretinal and disc neovascularisation in serpiginous choroiditis. Br J Ophthalmol 1982;66(5):326–31.
163. Jampol LM, Orth D, Daily MJ, et al. Subretinal neovascularization with geographic (serpiginous) choroiditis. Am J Ophthalmol 1979;88(4):683–9.
164. Baglivo E, Safran AB, Borruat FX. Multiple evanescent white dot syndrome after hepatitis B vaccine. Am J Ophthalmol 1996;122(3):431–2.
165. Friberg TR. Serpiginous choroiditis with branch vein occlusion and bilateral periphlebitis. Case report. Arch Ophthalmol 1988;106(5):585–6.
166. Steinmetz RL, Fitzke FW, Bird AC. Treatment of cystoid macular edema with acetazolamide in a patient with serpiginous choroidopathy. Retina 1991;11(4): 412–5.
167. Gregory ME, Bhatt U, Benskin S, et al. Bilateral full thickness macular holes in association with serpiginous choroiditis. Ocul Immunol Inflamm 2009;17(5):328–9.
168. Christmas NJ, Oh KT, Oh DM, et al. Long-term follow-up of patients with serpinginous choroiditis. Retina 2002;22(5):550–6.
169. Squirrell DM, Bhola RM, Talbot JF. Indocyanine green angiographic findings in serpiginous choroidopathy: evidence of a widespread choriocapillaris defect of the peripapillary area and posterior pole. Eye (Lond) 2001; 15(Pt 3):336–8.
170. Salati C, Pantelis V, Lafaut BA, et al. A 8 months indocyanine angiographic follow-up of a patient with serpiginous choroidopathy. Bull Soc Belge Ophtalmol 1997;265:29–33.
171. Giovannini A, Mariotti C, Ripa E, et al. Indocyanine green angiographic findings in serpiginous choroidopathy. Br J Ophthalmol 1996;80(6):536–40.
172. Giovannini A, Ripa E, Scassellati-Sforzolini B, et al. Indocyanine green angiography in serpiginous choroidopathy. Eur J Ophthalmol 1996;6(3): 299–306.
173. Van Liefferinge T, Sallet G, De Laey JJ. Indocyanine green angiography in cases of inflammatory chorioretinopathy. Bull Soc Belge Ophtalmol 1995;257:73–81.
174. Punjabi OS, Rich R, Davis JL, et al. Imaging serpiginous choroidopathy with spectral domain optical coherence tomography. Ophthalmic Surg Lasers Imaging 2008;39(4 Suppl):S95–8.
175. Arantes TE, Matos K, Garcia CR, et al. Fundus autofluorescence and spectral domain optical coherence tomography in recurrent serpiginous choroiditis: case report. Ocul Immunol Inflamm 2011;19(1):39–41.
176. Gallagher MJ, Yilmaz T, Cervantes-Castañeda RA, et al. The characteristic features of optical coherence tomography in posterior uveitis. Br J Ophthalmol 2007;91(12):1680–5.
177. van Velthoven ME, Ongkosuwito JV, Verbraak FD, et al. Combined en-face optical coherence tomography and confocal ophthalmoscopy findings in active multifocal and serpiginous chorioretinitis. Am J Ophthalmol 2006; 141(5):972–5.
178. Cardillo Piccolino F, Grosso A, Savini E. Fundus autofluorescence in serpiginous choroiditis. Graefes Arch Clin Exp Ophthalmol 2009;247(2):179–85.
179. Yeh S, Forooghian F, Wong WT, et al. Fundus autofluorescence imaging of the white dot syndromes. Arch Ophthalmol 2010;128(1):46–56.
180. Pilotto E, Vujosevic S, Grgic VA, et al. Retinal function in patients with serpiginous choroiditis: a microperimetry study. Graefes Arch Clin Exp Ophthalmol 2010;248(9):1331–7.
181. Ugarte M, Wearne IM. Serpiginous choroidopathy: an unusual association with Crohn's disease. Clin Exp Ophthalmol 2002;30(6):437–9.
182. Fuentes-Paez G, Celis-Sanchez J, Torres J, et al. Serpiginous choroiditis in a patient with systemic lupus erythematosus. Lupus 2005;14(11):928–9.

183. Mulder CJ, Pena AS, Jansen J, et al. Celiac disease and geographic (serpiginous) choroidopathy with occurrence of thrombocytopenic purpura. Arch Intern Med 1983;143(4):842.
184. Richardson RR, Cooper IS, Smith JL. Serpiginous choroiditis and unilateral extrapyramidal dystonia. Ann Ophthalmol 1981;13(1):15–9.
185. Akpek EK, Chan CC, Shen D, et al. Lack of herpes virus DNA in choroidal tissues of a patient with serpiginous choroiditis. Ophthalmology 2004; 111(11):2071–5.
186. Broekhuyse RM, van Herck M, Pinckers AJ, et al. Immune responsiveness to retinal S-antigen and opsin in serpiginous choroiditis and other retinal diseases. Doc Ophthalmol 1988;69(1):83–93.
187. Madhavan HN, Priya K, Biswas J. Current perspectives of herpesviral retinitis and choroiditis. Indian J Pathol Microbiol 2004;47(4):453–68.
188. Pisa D, Ramos M, García P, et al. Fungal infection in patients with serpiginous choroiditis or acute zonal occult outer retinopathy. J Clin Microbiol 2008;46(1):130–5.
189. Babel J. [Geographic and helicoid choroidopathies. Clinical and angiographic study; attempted classification]. J Fr Ophtalmol 1983;6(12):981–93.
190. King DG, Grizzard WS, Sever RJ, et al. Serpiginous choroidopathy associated with elevated factor VIII–von Willebrand factor antigen. Retina 1990;10(2): 97–101.
191. Hayreh SS, Baines JA. Occlusion of the posterior ciliary artery. I. Effects on choroidal circulation. Br J Ophthalmol 1972;56(10):719–35.
192. Vasconcelos-Santos DV, Rao PK, Davies JB, et al. Clinical features of tuberculous serpiginous-like choroiditis in contrast to classic serpiginous choroiditis. Arch Ophthalmol 2010;128(7):853–8.
193. Edelsten C, Stanford MR, Graham EM. Serpiginous choroiditis: an unusual presentation of ocular sarcoidosis. Br J Ophthalmol 1994;78(1):70–1.
194. Rattray KM, Cole MD, Smith SR. Systemic non-Hodgkin's lymphoma presenting as a serpiginous choroidopathy: report of a case and review of the literature. Eye (Lond) 2000;14 (Pt 5):706–10.
195. Tang J, Fillmore G, Nussenblatt RB. Antiphospholipid antibody syndrome mimicking serpiginous choroidopathy. Ocul Immunol Inflamm 2009;17(4): 278–81.
196. Mahendradas P, Kamath G, Mahalakshmi B, et al. Serpiginous choroiditis-like picture due to ocular toxoplasmosis. Ocul Immunol Inflamm 2007;15(2): 127–30.
197. Sonika, Narang S, Kochhar S, et al. Posterior scleritis mimicking macular serpiginous choroiditis. Indian J Ophthalmol 2003;51(4):351–3.
198. Mackensen F, Becker MD, Wiehler U, et al. QuantiFERON TB-Gold - a new test strengthening long-suspected tuberculous involvement in serpiginous-like choroiditis. Am J Ophthalmol 2008;146(5):761–6.
199. Akpek EK, Ilhan-Sarac O. New treatments for serpiginous choroiditis. Curr Opin Ophthalmol 2003;14(3):128–31.
200. Markomichelakis NN, Halkiadakis I, Papaeythymiou-Orchan S, et al. Intravenous pulse methylprednisolone therapy for acute treatment of serpiginous choroiditis. Ocul Immunol Inflamm 2006;14(1):29–33.
201. Pathengay A. Intravitreal triamcinolone acetonide in serpiginous choroidopathy. Indian J Ophthalmol 2005;53(1):77–9.
202. Wadhwa N, Garg SP, Mehrotra A. Prospective evaluation of intravitreal triamcinolone acetonide in serpiginous choroiditis. Ophthalmologica 2010; 224(3):183–7.
203. Adigüzel U, Sari A, Ozmen C, et al. Intravitreal triamcinolone acetonide treatment for serpiginous choroiditis. Ocul Immunol Inflamm 2006;14(6):375–8.
204. Karacorlu S, Ozdemir H, Karacorlu M. Intravitreal triamcinolone acetonide in serpiginous choroiditis. Jpn J Ophthalmol 2006;50(3):290–1.
205. Seth RK, Gaudio PA. Treatment of serpiginous choroiditis with intravitreous fluocinolone acetonide implant. Ocul Immunol Inflamm 2008;16(3):103–5.
206. Akpek EK, Baltatzis S, Yang J, et al. Long-term immunosuppressive treatment of serpiginous choroiditis. Ocul Immunol Inflamm 2001;9(3):153–67.
207. Vonmoos F, Messerli J, Moser HR, et al. Immunosuppressive therapy in serpiginous choroiditis - case report and brief review of the literature. Klin Monbl Augenheilkd 2001;218(5):394–7.
208. Araujo AA, Wells AP, Dick AD, et al. Early treatment with cyclosporin in serpiginous choroidopathy maintains remission and good visual outcome. Br J Ophthalmol 2000;84(9):979–82.
209. Leznoff A, Shea M, Binkley KE, et al. Cyclosporine in the treatment of non-microbial inflammatory ophthalmic disease. Can J Ophthalmol 1992;27(6): 302–6.
210. Vianna RN, Ozdal PC, Deschênes J, et al. Combination of azathioprine and corticosteroids in the treatment of serpiginous choroiditis. Can J Ophthalmol 2006;41(2):183–9.
211. Akpek EK, Jabs DA, Tessler HH, et al. Successful treatment of serpiginous choroiditis with alkylating agents. Ophthalmology 2002;109(8):1506–13.
212. Sahin OG. Long-term cyclophosphamide treatment in a case with serpiginous choroiditis. Case Report Ophthalmol 2010;1(2):71–6.
213. Hooper PL, Kaplan HJ. Triple agent immunosuppression in serpiginous choroiditis. Ophthalmology 1991;98(6):944–51; discussion 951–2.
214. Seve P, Mennesson E, Grange JD, et al. Infliximab in serpiginous choroiditis. Acta Ophthalmol 2010;88(8):e342–343.
215. Sobaci G, Bayraktar Z, Bayer A. Interferon alpha-2a treatment for serpiginous choroiditis. Ocul Immunol Inflamm 2005;13(1):59–66.
216. Battaglia Parodi M, Iacono P, Verbraak FD, et al. Antivascular endothelial growth factors for inflammatory chorioretinal disorders. Dev Ophthalmol 2010;46:84–95.
217. Rouvas A, Petrou P, Douvali M, et al. Intravitreal ranibizumab for the treatment of inflammatory choroidal neovascularization. Retina 2011;31(5):871–5.
218. Song MH, Roh YJ. Intravitreal ranibizumab for choroidal neovascularisation in serpiginous choroiditis. Eye (Lond) 2009;23(9):1873–5.
219. Julián K, Terrada C, Fardeau C, et al. Intravitreal bevacizumab as first local treatment for uveitis-related choroidal neovascularization: long-term results. Acta Ophthalmol 2011;89(2):179–84.
220. Lim JI, Flaxel CJ, LaBree L. Photodynamic therapy for choroidal neovascularisation secondary to inflammatory chorioretinal disease. Ann Acad Med Singapore 2006;35(3):198–202.
221. Park SP, Ko DA, Chung H, et al. Photodynamic therapy with verteporfin for juxtafoveal choroidal neovascularization in serpiginous choroiditis. Ophthalmic Surg Lasers Imaging 2006;37(5):425–8.
222. Steinmetz RL, Fitzke FW, Bird AC. Treatment of cystoid macular edema with acetazolamide in a patient with serpiginous choroidopathy. Retina 1991; 11(4):412–5.
223. Jones BE, Jampol LM, Yannuzzi LA, et al. Relentless placoid chorioretinitis: A new entity or an unusual variant of serpiginous chorioretinitis? Arch Ophthalmol 2000;118(7):931–8.
224. Nussenblatt RB, Whitcup S, Palestine AG. Uveitis: Fundamentals and clinical practice. 2nd ed. St Louis: Mosby; 1996.
225 Arora SK, Gupta V, Gupta A, et al. Diagnostic efficacy of polymerase chain reaction in granulomatous uveitis. Tuber Lung Dis 1999;79(4):229–33.
226. Lyness AL, Bird AC. Recurrences of acute posterior multifocal placoid pigment epitheliopathy. Am J Ophthalmol 1984;98(2):203–7.
227. Jyotirmay B, Jafferji SS, Sudharshan S, et al. Clinical profile, treatment, and visual outcome of ampiginous choroiditis. Ocul Immunol Inflamm 2010;18(1):46–51.
228. Jones NP. Acute posterior multifocal placoid pigment epitheliopathy. Br J Ophthalmol 1995;79(4):384–9.
229. Amer R, Florescu T. Optical coherence tomography in relentless placoid chorioretinitis. Clin Exp Ophthalmol 2008;36(4):388–90.
230 Yeh S, Forooghian F, Wong WT, et al. Fundus autofluorescence imaging of the white dot syndromes. Arch Ophthalmol 2010;128(1):46–56.
231. Yeh S, Lew JC, Wong WT, et al. Relentless placoid chorioretinitis associated with central nervous system lesions treated with mycophenolate mofetil. Arch Ophthalmol 2009;127(3):341–3.
232. Chung YM, Yeh TS, Liu JH. Increased serum IgM and IgG in the multiple evanescent white-dot syndrome. Am J Ophthalmol 1987;104(2):187–8.
233. Golchet PR, Jampol LM, Wilson D, et al. Persistent placoid maculopathy: a new clinical entity. Trans Am Ophthalmol Soc 2006;104:108–20.
234. Kovach JL. Persistent placoid maculopathy imaged with spectral domain OCT and autofluorescence. Ophthalmic Surg Lasers Imaging 2010;41(Suppl): S101-103.
235. Khairallah M, Ben Yahia S. Persistent placoid maculopathy. Ophthalmology 2008;115(1):220–1.
236. Parodi MB, Iacono P, Bandello F. Juxtafoveal choroidal neovascularization secondary to persistent placoid maculopathy treated with intravitreal bevacizumab. Ocul Immunol Inflamm 2010;18(5):399–401.
237. Battaglia Parodi M, Iacono P, Verbraak FD, et al. Antivascular endothelial growth factors for inflammatory chorioretinal disorders. Dev Ophthalmol 2010;46:84–95.
238. Jampol LM, Wiredu A. MEWDS, MFC, PIC, AMN, AIBSE, and AZOOR: one disease or many? Retina 1995;15(5):373–8.
239. Nozik RA, Dorsch W. A new chorioretinopathy associated with anterior uveitis. Am J Ophthalmol 1973;76(5):758–62.
240. Dreyer RF, Gass DJ. Multifocal choroiditis and panuveitis. A syndrome that mimics ocular histoplasmosis. Arch Ophthalmol 1984;102(12):1776–84.
241. Deutsch TA, Tessler HH. Inflammatory pseudohistoplasmosis. Ann Ophthalmol 1985;17(8):461–5.
242. Morgan CM, Schatz H. Recurrent multifocal choroiditis. Ophthalmology 1986;93(9):1138–47.
243. Kedhar SR, Thorne JE, Wittenberg S, et al. Multifocal choroiditis with panuveitis and punctate inner choroidopathy: comparison of clinical characteristics at presentation. Retina 2007;27(9):1174–9.
244. Brown J, Folk JC, Reddy CV, et al. Visual prognosis of multifocal choroiditis, punctate inner choroidopathy, and the diffuse subretinal fibrosis syndrome. Ophthalmology 1996;103(7):1100–5.
245. Spaide RF, Yannuzzi LA, Freund KB. Linear streaks in multifocal choroiditis and panuveitis. Retina 1991;11(2):229–31.
246. Borodoker N, Cunningham ET, Yannuzzi LA, et al. Peripheral curvilinear pigmentary streak in multifocal choroiditis. Arch Ophthalmol 2002;120(4): 520–1.
247. Fonseca RA, Dantas MA, Kaga T, et al. Subretinal fibrosis and linear streaks in multifocal choroiditis. Arch Ophthalmol 2001;119(1):142.
248. Parnell JR, Jampol LM, Yannuzzi LA, et al. Differentiation between presumed ocular histoplasmosis syndrome and multifocal choroiditis with panuveitis based on morphology of photographed fundus lesions and fluorescein angiography. Arch Ophthalmol 2001;119(2):208–12.
249. Cantrill HL, Folk JC. Multifocal choroiditis associated with progressive subretinal fibrosis. Am J Ophthalmol 1986;101(2):170–80.
250. Buerk BM, Rabb MF, Jampol LM. Peripapillary subretinal fibrosis: a characteristic finding of multifocal choroiditis and panuveitis. Retina 2005;25(2): 228–9.
251. Wiechens B, Nölle B. Iris angiographic changes in multifocal chorioretinitis with panuveitis. Graefes Arch Clin Exp Ophthalmol 1999;237(11):902–7.
252. Thorne JE, Wittenberg S, Jabs DA, et al. Multifocal choroiditis with panuveitis: Incidence of ocular complications and of loss of visual acuity. Ophthalmology 2006;113(12):2310–16.

253. Kotsolis AI, Killian FA, Ladas ID, et al. Fluorescein angiography and optical coherence tomography concordance for choroidal neovascularisation in multifocal choroidtis. Br J Ophthalmol 2010;94(11):1506–8.
254. Slakter JS, Giovannini A, Yannuzzi LA, et al. Indocyanine green angiography of multifocal choroiditis. Ophthalmology 1997;104(11):1813–9.
255. Vadalà M, Lodato G, Cillino S. Multifocal choroiditis: indocyanine green angiographic features. Ophthalmologica 2001;215(1):16–21.
256. Cimino L, Auer C, Herbort CP. Sensitivity of indocyanine green angiography for the follow-up of active inflammatory choriocapillaropathies. Ocul Immunol Inflamm 2000;8(4):275–83.
257. Yeh S, Forooghian F, Wong WT, et al. Fundus autofluorescence imaging of the white dot syndromes. Arch Ophthalmol 2010;128(1):46–56.
258. Vance SK, Khan S, Klancnik JM, et al. Characteristic spectral-domain optical coherence tomography findings of multifocal choroiditis. Retina 2011;31(4):717–23.
259. Haen SP, Spaide RF. Fundus autofluorescence in multifocal choroiditis and panuveitis. Am J Ophthalmol 2008;145(5):847–53.
260. Oh KT, Folk JC, Maturi RK, et al. Multifocal electroretinography in multifocal choroiditis and the multiple evanescent white dot syndrome. Retina 2001;21(6):581–9.
261. Khorram KD, Jampol LM, Rosenberg MA. Blind spot enlargement as a manifestation of multifocal choroiditis. Arch Ophthalmol 1991;109(10):1403–7.
262. Spaide RF, Koizumi H, Freund KB. Photoreceptor outer segment abnormalities as a cause of blind spot enlargement in acute zonal occult outer retinopathy-complex diseases. Am J Ophthalmol 2008;146(1):111–20.
263. Tiedeman JS. Epstein–Barr viral antibodies in multifocal choroiditis and panuveitis. Am J Ophthalmol 1987;103(5):659–63.
264. Schenck F, Böke W. [Retinal vasculitis with multifocal chorioretinitis]. Klin Monbl Augenheilkd 1990;197(5):378–81.
265. Spaide RF, Sugin S, Yannuzzi LA, et al. Epstein–Barr virus antibodies in multifocal choroiditis and panuveitis. Am J Ophthalmol 1991;112(4):410–13.
266. Watzke RC, Packer AJ, Folk JC, et al. Punctate inner choroidopathy. Am J Ophthalmol 1984;98(5):572–84.
267. Amer R, Lois N. Punctate inner choroidopathy. Surv Ophthalmol 2011;56(1):36–53.
268. Gerstenblith AT, Thorne JE, Sobrin L, et al. Punctate inner choroidopathy: a survey analysis of 77 persons. Ophthalmology 2007;114(6):1201–4.
269. Brown J, Folk JC, Reddy CV, et al. Visual prognosis of multifocal choroiditis, punctate inner choroidopathy, and the diffuse subretinal fibrosis syndrome. Ophthalmology 1996;103(7):1100–5.
270. Patel KH, Birnbaum AD, Tessler HH, et al. Presentation and outcome of patients with punctate inner choroidopathy at a tertiary referral center. Retina 2011;31(7):1387–91.
271. Essex RW, Wong J, Fraser-Bell S, et al. Punctate inner choroidopathy: clinical features and outcomes. Arch Ophthalmol 2010;128(8):982–7.
272. Olsen TW, Capone A, Sternberg P, et al. Subfoveal choroidal neovascularization in punctate inner choroidopathy. Surgical management and pathologic findings. Ophthalmology 1996;103(12):2061–9.
273. Akman A, Kadayifçilar S, Aydin P. Indocyanine green angiographic findings in a case of punctate inner choroidopathy. Eur J Ophthalmol 1998;8(3):191–4.
274. Tiffin PA, Maini R, Roxburgh ST, et al. Indocyanine green angiography in a case of punctate inner choroidopathy. Br J Ophthalmol 1996;80(1):90–1.
275. Levy J, Shneck M, Klemperer I, et al. Punctate inner choroidopathy: resolution after oral steroid treatment and review of the literature. Can J Ophthalmol 2005;40(5):605–8.
276. Stepien KE, Carroll J. Using spectral-domain optical coherence tomography to follow outer retinal structure changes in a patient with recurrent punctate inner choroidopathy. J Ophthalmol ePub 2011, 753741; doi: 10.1155/2011/753741.
277. Reddy CV, Brown J, Folk JC, et al. Enlarged blind spots in chorioretinal inflammatory disorders. Ophthalmology 1996;103(4):606–17.
278. Bryan RG, Freund KB, Yannuzzi LA, et al. Multiple evanescent white dot syndrome in patients with multifocal choroiditis. Retina 2002;22(3):317–22.
279. Atan D, Fraser-Bell S, Plskova J, et al. Punctate inner choroidopathy and multifocal choroiditis with panuveitis share haplotypic associations with IL10 and TNF loci. Invest Ophthalmol Vis Sci 2011;52(6):3573–81.
280. Shimada H, Yuzawa M, Hirose T, et al. Pathological findings of multifocal choroiditis with panuveitis and punctate inner choroidopathy. Jpn J Ophthalmol 2008;52(4):282–8.
281. Spaide RF, Freund KB, Slakter J, et al. Treatment of subfoveal choroidal neovascularization associated with multifocal choroiditis and panuveitis with photodynamic therapy. Retina 2002;22(5):545–9.
282. Chan WM, Lai TY, Lau TT, et al. Combined photodynamic therapy and intravitreal triamcinolone for choroidal neovascularization secondary to punctate inner choroidopathy or of idiopathic origin: one-year results of a prospective series. Retina 2008;28(1):71–80.
283 Fine HF, Zhitomirsky I, Freund KB, et al. Bevacizumab (avastin) and ranibizumab (lucentis) for choroidal neovascularization in multifocal choroiditis. Retina 2009;29(1):8–12.
284. Parodi MB, Iacono P, Kontadakis DS, et al. Bevacizumab vs photodynamic therapy for choroidal neovascularization in multifocal choroiditis. Arch Ophthalmol 2010;128(9):1100–3.
285. Chang LK, Spaide RF, Brue C, et al. Bevacizumab treatment for subfoveal choroidal neovascularization from causes other than age-related macular degeneration. Arch Ophthalmol 2008;126(7):941–5.
286. Uparkar M, Borse N, Kaul S, et al. Photodynamic therapy following intravitreal bevacizumab in multifocal choroiditis. Int Ophthalmol 2008;28(5):375–7.
287. Vossmerbaeumer U, Spandau UH, von Baltz S, et al. Intravitreal bevacizumab for choroidal neovascularisation secondary to punctate inner choroidopathy. Clin Exp Ophthalmol 2008;36(3):292–4.
288. Rosen E, Rubowitz A, Ferencz JR. Exposure to verteporfin and bevacizumab therapy for choroidal neovascularization secondary to punctate inner choroidopathy during pregnancy. Eye (Lond) 2009;23(6):1479.
289. Palestine AG, Nussenblatt RB, Parver LM, et al. Progressive subretinal fibrosis and uveitis. Br J Ophthalmol 1984;68(9):667–73.
290. Salvador F, Garcia-Arumí J, Mateo C, et al. Multifocal choroiditis with progressive subretinal fibrosis. Report of two cases. Ophthalmologica 1994;208(3):163–7.
291. Kaiser PK, Gragoudas ES. The subretinal fibrosis and uveitis syndrome. Int Ophthalmol Clin 1996;36(1):145–52.
292. Gass JD, Margo CE, Levy MH. Progressive subretinal fibrosis and blindness in patients with multifocal granulomatous chorioretinitis. Am J Ophthalmol 1996;122(1):76–85.
293. Alves C, Meyer I, Toralles MB, et al. [Association of human histocompatibility antigens with ophthalmological disorders.] Arq Bras Oftalmol 2006;69(2):273–8.
294. Kim MK, Chan CC, Belfort R, et al. Histopathologic and immunohistopathologic features of subretinal fibrosis and uveitis syndrome. Am J Ophthalmol 1987;104(1):15–23.
295. Huffman RI, Huang JJ. Subretinal fibrosis and uveitis syndrome in a patient with ectodermal dysplasia. Ocul Immunol Inflamm 2009;17(5):348–50.
296. Fuentes-Páez G, Martínez-Osorio H, Herreras JM, et al. Subretinal fibrosis and uveitis syndrome associated with ulcerative colitis. Int J Colorectal Dis 2007;22(3):333–4.
297. Adán A, Sanmartí R, Burés A, et al. Successful treatment with infliximab in a patient with diffuse subretinal fibrosis syndrome. Am J Ophthalmol 2007;143(3):533–4.
298. Jampol LM, Sieving PA, Pugh D, et al. Multiple evanescent white dot syndrome. I. Clinical findings. Arch Ophthalmol 1984;102(5):671–4.
299. Olitsky SE. Multiple evanescent white-dot syndrome in a 10-year-old child. J Pediatr Ophthalmol Strabismus 1998;35(5):288–9.
300. Lim JI, Kokame GT, Douglas JP. Multiple evanescent white dot syndrome in older patients. Am J Ophthalmol 1999;127(6):725–8.
301. Asano T, Kondo M, Kondo N, et al. High prevalence of myopia in Japanese patients with multiple evanescent white dot syndrome. Jpn J Ophthalmol 2004;48(5):486–9.
302. Shelsta HN, Rao RR, Bhatt HK, et al. Atypical presentations of multiple evanescent white dot syndrome without white dots: a case series. Retina 2011;31(5):973–6.
303. Huang J, Spaide R. Appearance of brown areas after resolution of the acute phase of multiple evanescent white dot syndrome. Retina 2004;24(5):814–6.
304. Luttrull JK, Marmor MF, Nanda M. Progressive confluent circumpapillary multiple evanescent white-dot syndrome. Am J Ophthalmol 1999;128(3):378–80.
305. Daniele S, Daniele C, Ferri C. Association of peripapillary scars with lesions characteristic of multiple evanescent white-dot syndrome. Ophthalmologica 1995;209(4):217–9.
306. McCollum CJ, Kimble JA. Peripapillary subretinal neovascularization associated with multiple evanescent white-dot syndrome. Arch Ophthalmol 1992;110(1):13–4.
307. Wyhinny GJ, Jackson JL, Jampol LM, et al. Subretinal neovascularization following multiple evanescent white-dot syndrome. Arch Ophthalmol 1990;108(10):1384–5.
308. Park DW, Polk TD, Stone EM. Multiple evanescent white dot syndrome in a patient with Best disease. Arch Ophthalmol 1997;115(10):1342–3.
309. Papadia M, Herbort CP. Idiopathic choroidal neovascularisation as the inaugural sign of multiple evanescent white dot syndrome. Middle East Afr J Ophthalmol 2010;17(3):270–4.
310. Machida S, Fujiwara T, Murai K, et al. Idiopathic choroidal neovascularization as an early manifestation of inflammatory chorioretinal diseases. Retina 2008;28(5):703–10.
311. Ikeda N, Ikeda T, Nagata M, et al. Location of lesions in multiple evanescent white dot syndrome and the cause of the hypofluorescent spots observed by indocyanine green angiography. Graefes Arch Clin Exp Ophthalmol 2001;239(3):242–7.
312. Sieving PA, Fishman GA, Jampol LM, et al. Multiple evanescent white dot syndrome. II. Electrophysiology of the photoreceptors during retinal pigment epithelial disease. Arch Ophthalmol 1984;102(5):675–9.
313. Aaberg TM, Campo RV, Joffe L. Recurrences and bilaterality in the multiple evanescent white-dot syndrome. Am J Ophthalmol 1985;100(1):29–37.
314. Jost BF, Olk RJ, McGaughey A. Bilateral symptomatic multiple evanescent white-dot syndrome. Am J Ophthalmol 1986;101(4):489–90.
315. Tsai L, Jampol LM, Pollock SC, et al. Chronic recurrent multiple evanescent white dot syndrome. Retina 1994;14(2):160–3.
316. Fine HF, Spaide RF, Ryan EH, et al. Acute zonal occult outer retinopathy in patients with multiple evanescent white dot syndrome. Arch Ophthalmol 2009;127(1):66–70.
317. Forooghian F, Stetson PF, Gross NE, et al. Quantitative assessment of photoreceptor recovery in atypical multiple evanescent white dot syndrome. Ophthalmic Surg Lasers Imaging 2010;41(Suppl):S77–80.
318. Li D, Kishi S. Restored photoreceptor outer segment damage in multiple evanescent white dot syndrome. Ophthalmology 2009;116(4):762–70.
319. Kanis MJ, van Norren D. Integrity of foveal cones in multiple evanescent white dot syndrome assessed with OCT and foveal reflection analyser. Br J Ophthalmol 2006;90(6):795–6.

320. Li D, Kishi S. Loss of photoreceptor outer segment in acute zonal occult outer retinopathy. Arch Ophthalmol 2007;125(9):1194–200.
321. Ie D, Glaser BM, Murphy RP, et al. Indocyanine green angiography in multiple evanescent white-dot syndrome. Am J Ophthalmol 1994;117(1): 7–12.
322. Borruat FX, Auer C, Piguet B. Choroidopathy in multiple evanescent white dot syndrome. Arch Ophthalmol 1995;113(12):1569–71.
323. Obana A, Kusumi M, Miki T. Indocyanine green angiographic aspects of multiple evanescent white dot syndrome. Retina 1996;16(2):97–104.
324. Obana A, Kusumi M, Moriwaki M, et al. [Two cases of multiple evanescent white dot syndrome examined with indocyanine green angiography.] Nippon Ganka Gakkai Zasshi 1995;99(2):244–51.
325. Yen MT, Rosenfeld PJ. Persistent indocyanine green angiographic findings in multiple evanescent white dot syndrome. Ophthalmic Surg Lasers 2001;32(2):156–8.
326. Herbort CP, Borruat FX, de Courten C, et al. [Indocyanine green angiography in posterior uveitis]. Klin Monbl Augenheilkd 1996;208(5):321–6.
327. Stanga PE, Lim JI, Hamilton P. Indocyanine green angiography in chorioretinal diseases: indications and interpretation: an evidence-based update. Ophthalmology 2003;110(1):15–21; quiz 22–13.
328. Tsukamoto E, Yamada T, Kadoi C, et al. Hypofluorescent spots on indocyanine green angiography at the recovery stage in multiple evanescent white dot syndrome. Ophthalmologica 1999;213(5):336–8.
329. Gross NE, Yannuzzi LA, Freund KB, et al. Multiple evanescent white dot syndrome. Arch Ophthalmol 2006;124(4):493–500.
330. Dell'Omo R, Wong R, Marino M, et al. Relationship between different fluorescein and indocyanine green angiography features in multiple evanescent white dot syndrome. Br J Ophthalmol 2010;94(1):59–63.
331. Amin HI. Optical coherence tomography findings in multiple evanescent white dot syndrome. Retina 2006;26(4):483–4.
332. Gerstenblith AT, Thorne JE, Sobrin L, et al. Punctate inner choroidopathy: a survey analysis of 77 persons. Ophthalmology 2007;114(6):1201–4.
333. Sikorski BL, Wojtkowski M, Kaluzny JJ, et al. Correlation of spectral optical coherence tomography with fluorescein and indocyanine green angiography in multiple evanescent white dot syndrome. Br J Ophthalmol 2008;92(11): 1552–7.
334. Nguyen MH, Witkin AJ, Reichel E, et al. Microstructural abnormalities in MEWDS demonstrated by ultrahigh resolution optical coherence tomography. Retina 2007;27(4):414–18.
335. Dell'Omo R, Mantovani A, Wong R, et al. Natural evolution of fundus autofluorescence findings in multiple evanescent white dot syndrome: a long-term follow-up. Retina 2010;30(9):1479–87.
336. Furino C, Boscia F, Cardascia N, et al. Fundus autofluorescence and multiple evanescent white dot syndrome. Retina 2009;29(1):60–3.
337. Horiguchi M, Miyake Y, Nakamura M, et al. Focal electroretinogram and visual field defect in multiple evanescent white dot syndrome. Br J Ophthalmol 1993;77(7):452–5.
338. Keunen JE, van Norren D. Foveal densitometry in the multiple evanescent white-dot syndrome. Am J Ophthalmol 1988;105(5):561–2.
339. Chen D, Martidis A, Baumal CR. Transient multifocal electroretinogram dysfunction in multiple evanescent white dot syndrome. Ophthalmic Surg Lasers 2002;33(3):246–9.
340. Feigl B, Haas A, El-Shabrawi Y. Multifocal ERG in multiple evanescent white dot syndrome. Graefes Arch Clin Exp Ophthalmol 2002;240(8):615–21.
341. Nakao K, Isashiki M. Multiple evanescent white dot syndrome. Jpn J Ophthalmol 1986;30(4):376–84.
342. Hamed LM, Glaser JS, Gass JD, et al. Protracted enlargement of the blind spot in multiple evanescent white dot syndrome. Arch Ophthalmol 1989;107(2): 194–8.
343. Boscarino MA, Johnson TM. Microperimetry in multiple evanescent white dot syndrome. Can J Ophthalmol 2007;42(5):743–5.
344. Hangai M, Fujimoto M, Yoshimura N. Features and function of multiple evanescent white dot syndrome. Arch Ophthalmol 2009;127(10):1307–13.
345. Holz FG, Kim RY, Schwartz SD, et al. Acute zonal occult outer retinopathy (AZOOR) associated with multifocal choroidopathy. Eye (Lond) 1994; 8(Pt 1):77–83.
346. Jacobson SG, Morales DS, Sun XK, et al. Pattern of retinal dysfunction in acute zonal occult outer retinopathy. Ophthalmology 1995;102(8):1187–98.
347. Figueroa MS, Ciancas E, Mompean B, et al. Treatment of multiple evanescent white dot syndrome with cyclosporine. Eur J Ophthalmol 2001;11(1): 86–8.
348. Laatikainen L, Immonen I. Multiple evanescent white dot syndrome. Graefes Arch Clin Exp Ophthalmol 1988;226(1):37–40.
349. Fine L, Fine A, Cunningham ET. Multiple evanescent white dot syndrome following hepatitis a vaccination. Arch Ophthalmol 2001;119(12):1856–8.
350. Baglivo E, Safran AB, Borruat FX. Multiple evanescent white dot syndrome after hepatitis B vaccine. Am J Ophthalmol 1996;122(3):431–2.
351. Cohen SM. Multiple evanescent white dot syndrome after vaccination for human papilloma virus and meningococcus. J Pediatr Ophthalmol Strabismus. ePub 2009 Jun;25:1–3; doi: 10.3928/01913913-20090616-01.
352. Chung YM, Yeh TS, Liu JH. Increased serum IgM and IgG in the multiple evanescent white-dot syndrome. Am J Ophthalmol 1987;104(2):187–8.
353. Desarnaulds AB, Borruat FX, Herbort CP, et al. [Multiple evanescent white dot syndrome: a genetic predisposition?] Klin Monbl Augenheilkd 1996;208(5):301–2.
354. Borruat FX, Piguet B, Herbort CP. Acute posterior multifocal placoid pigment epitheliopathy following mumps. Ocul Immunol Inflamm 1998;6(3): 189–93.
355. Dodwell DG, Jampol LM, Rosenberg M, et al. Optic nerve involvement associated with the multiple evanescent white-dot syndrome. Ophthalmology 1990;97(7):862–8.
356. Fong KS, Fu ER. Multiple evanescent white dot syndrome–an uncommon cause for an enlarged blind spot. Ann Acad Med Singapore 1996;25(6): 866–8.
357. Reddy CV, Brown J, Folk JC, et al. Enlarged blind spots in chorioretinal inflammatory disorders. Ophthalmology 1996;103(4):606–17.
358. Takahashi Y, Ataka S, Wada S, et al. A case of multiple evanescent white dot syndrome treated by steroid pulse therapy. Osaka City Med J 2006;52(2): 83–6.
359. Battaglia Parodi M, Iacono P, Verbraak FD, et al. Antivascular endothelial growth factors for inflammatory chorioretinal disorders. Dev Ophthalmol 2010;46:84–95.
360. Rouvas AA, Ladas ID, Papakostas TD, et al. Intravitreal ranibizumab in a patient with choroidal neovascularization secondary to multiple evanescent white dot syndrome. Eur J Ophthalmol 2007;17(6):996–9.
361. Gass JD. Acute zonal occult outer retinopathy. Donders Lecture: The Netherlands Ophthalmological Society, Maastricht, Holland, June 19, 1992. J Clin Neuroophthalmol 1993;13(2):79–97.
362. Monson DM, Smith JR. Acute zonal occult outer retinopathy. Surv Ophthalmol 2011;56(1):23–35.
363. Gass JD, Agarwal A, Scott IU. Acute zonal occult outer retinopathy: a long-term follow-up study. Am J Ophthalmol 2002;134(3):329–39.
364. Cohen SYM, Jampol LMM. Choroidal neovascularization in peripapillary acute zonal occult outer retinopathy. Cases & Brief Reports 2007;1(4):220–2.
365. Spaide RF. Collateral damage in acute zonal occult outer retinopathy. Am J Ophthalmol 2004;138(5):887–9.
366. Fujiwara T, Imamura Y, Giovinazzo VJ, et al. Fundus autofluorescence and optical coherence tomographic findings in acute zonal occult outer retinopathy. Retina 2010;30(8):1206–16.
367. Li D, Kishi S. Loss of photoreceptor outer segment in acute zonal occult outer retinopathy. Arch Ophthalmol 2007;125(9):1194–200.
368. Spaide RF, Koizumi H, Freund KB. Photoreceptor outer segment abnormalities as a cause of blind spot enlargement in acute zonal occult outer retinopathy-complex diseases. Am J Ophthalmol 2008;146(1):111–20.
369. Fine HF, Spaide RF, Ryan EH, et al. Acute zonal occult outer retinopathy in patients with multiple evanescent white dot syndrome. Arch Ophthalmol 2009;127(1):66–70.
370. Zweifel SA, Kim E, Bailey Freund K. Simultaneous presentation of multifocal choroiditis and acute zonal occult outer retinopathy in one eye. Br J Ophthalmol 2011;95(2):288–97.
371. Gass JD, Stern C. Acute annular outer retinopathy as a variant of acute zonal occult outer retinopathy. Am J Ophthalmol 1995;119(3):330–4.
372. Fekrat S, Wilkinson CP, Chang B, et al. Acute annular outer retinopathy: report of four cases. Am J Ophthalmol 2000;130(5):636–44.
373. Sharma SM, Watzke RC, Weleber RG, et al. Acute zonal occult outer retinopathy (AZOOR) and pars planitis: a new association? Br J Ophthalmol 2008;92(4):583–4.
374. Heckenlively JR, Ferreyra HA. Autoimmune retinopathy: a review and summary. Semin Immunopathol 2008;30(2):127–34.
375 Mahajan VB, Stone EM. Patients with an acute zonal occult outer retinopathy-like illness rapidly improve with valacyclovir treatment. Am J Ophthalmol 2010;150(4):511–8.
376. Fletcher WA, Imes RK, Goodman D, et al. Acute idiopathic blind spot enlargement. A big blind spot syndrome without optic disc edema. Arch Ophthalmol 1988;106(1):44–9.
377. Volpe NJ, Rizzo JF, Lessell S. Acute idiopathic blind spot enlargement syndrome: a review of 27 new cases. Arch Ophthalmol 2001;119(1):59–63.
378. Watzke RC, Shults WT. Clinical features and natural history of the acute idiopathic enlarged blind spot syndrome. Ophthalmology 2002;109(7): 1326–35.
379. de Smet MD, Yamamoto JH, Mochizuki M, et al. Cellular immune responses of patients with uveitis to retinal antigens and their fragments. Am J Ophthalmol 1990;110(2):135–42.
380. Pece A, Sadun F, Trabucchi G, et al. Indocyanine green angiography in enlarged blind spot syndrome. Am J Ophthalmol 1998;126(4):604–7.
381. Spaide RF, Koizumi H, Freund KB. Photoreceptor outer segment abnormalities as a cause of blind spot enlargement in acute zonal occult outer retinopathy-complex diseases. Am J Ophthalmol 2008;146(1):111–20.
382. Sugahara M, Shinoda K, Matsumoto SC, et al. Outer retinal microstructure in a case of acute idiopathic blind spot enlargement syndrome. Case Report Ophthalmol 2011;2(1):116–22.
383. Kondo N, Kondo M, Miyake Y. Acute idiopathic blind spot enlargement syndrome: prolonged retinal dysfunction revealed by multifocal electroretinogram technique. Am J Ophthalmol 2001;132(1):126–8.
384. Singh K, de Frank MP, Shults WT, et al. Acute idiopathic blind spot enlargement. A spectrum of disease. Ophthalmology 1991;98(4):497–502.
385. Machida S, Haga-Sano M, Ishibe T, et al. Decrease of blue cone sensitivity in acute idiopathic blind spot enlargement syndrome. Am J Ophthalmol 2004;138(2):296–9.
386. Bos PJ, Deutman AF. Acute macular neuroretinopathy. Am J Ophthalmol 1975;80(4):573–84.
387. Yeh S, Hwang TS, Weleber RG, et al. Acute macular outer retinopathy (AMOR): A reappraisal of acute macular neuroretinopathy using multimodality diagnostic testing. Arch Ophthalmol 2011;129(3):365–8.
388. El-Dairi M, Bhatti MT, Vaphiades MS. A shot of adrenaline. Surv Ophthalmol 2009;54(5):618–24.

389. Vance SK, Spaide RF, Freund KB, et al. Outer retinal abnormalities in acute macular neuroretinopathy. Retina 2011;31(3):441–5.
390. Miller MH, Spalton DJ, Fitzke FW, et al. Acute macular neuroretinopathy. Ophthalmology 1989;96(2):265–9.
391. Turbeville SD, Cowan LD, Gass JD. Acute macular neuroretinopathy: a review of the literature. Surv Ophthalmol 2003;48(1):1–11.
392 Rush JA. Acute macular neuroretinopathy. Am J Ophthalmol 1977;83(4): 490–4.
393. Chan WM, Liu DT, Tong JP, et al. Longitudinal findings of acute macular neuroretinopathy with multifocal electroretinogram and optical coherence tomography. Clin Exp Ophthalmol 2005;33(4):439–42.
394. O'Brien DM, Farmer SG, Kalina RE, et al. Acute macular neuroretinopathy following intravenous sympathomimetics. Retina 1989;9(4):281–6.
395. Abu el-Asrar AM. Serpiginous (geographical) choroiditis. Int Ophthalmol Clin 1995;35(2):87–91.
396. Feigl B, Haas A. Optical coherence tomography (OCT) in acute macular neuroretinopathy. Acta Ophthalmol Scand 2000;78(6):714–6.
397. Mirshahi A, Scharioth GB, Klais CM, et al. Enhanced visualization of acute macular neuroretinopathy by Heidelberg retina tomography. Clin Exp Ophthalmol 2006;34(6):596–9.
398. Monson BK, Greenberg PB, Greenberg E, et al. High-speed, ultra-high-resolution optical coherence tomography of acute macular neuroretinopathy. Br J Ophthalmol 2007;91(1):119–20.
399. Hughes EH, Siow YC, Hunyor AP. Acute macular neuroretinopathy: anatomic localisation of the lesion with high-resolution OCT. Eye (Lond) 2009;23(11):2132–4.
400. Maschi C, Schneider-Lise B, Paoli V, et al. Acute macular neuroretinopathy: contribution of spectral-domain optical coherence tomography and multifocal ERG. Graefes Arch Clin Exp Ophthalmol 2011;249(6):827–31.
401. Kuznik-Borkowska A, Cohen SY, Broïdo-Hooreman O, et al. [Acute macular neuroretinopathy.] J Fr Ophtalmol 2006;29(3):319–22.
402. Vance SK, Khan S, Klancnik JM, et al. Characteristic spectral-domain optical coherence tomography findings of multifocal choroiditis. Retina. 2011.;31(4): 717–23.
403. Maturi RK, Yu M, Sprunger DT. Multifocal electroretinographic evaluation of acute macular neuroretinopathy. Arch Ophthalmol 2003;121(7):1068–9.
404. Browning AC, Gupta R, Barber C, et al. The multifocal electroretinogram in acute macular neuroretinopathy. Arch Ophthalmol 2003;121(10):1506–7.
405. Sieving PA, Fishman GA, Salzano T, et al. Acute macular neuroretinopathy: early receptor potential change suggests photoreceptor pathology. Br J Ophthalmol 1984;68(4):229–34.
406. Gómez-Torreiro M, Gómez-Ulla F, Bolívar Montesa P, et al. Scanning laser ophthalmoscope findings in acute macular neuroretinopathy. Retina 2002; 22(1):108–9.
407. Gass JD, Hamed LM. Acute macular neuroretinopathy and multiple evanescent white dot syndrome occurring in the same patients. Arch Ophthalmol 1989;107(2):189–93.
408. Singh K, de Frank MP, Shults WT, et al. Acute idiopathic blind spot enlargement. A spectrum of disease. Ophthalmology 1991;98(4):497–502.

Autoimmune Retinopathies

H. Nida Sen, Robert B. Nussenblatt

Chapter 77

INTRODUCTION

Autoimmune retinopathies (AIR) represent a group of inflammatory mediated retinopathies with otherwise unexplained vision loss associated with visual field deficits, photoreceptor dysfunction as evidenced on electroretinography (ERG), and the presence of circulating autoantibodies targeted against retinal antigens. Clinically, the fundus often appears normal, but some patients may show retinal vascular attenuation, diffuse retinal atrophy with or without pigmentary changes or waxy disc pallor. There are usually few or no intraocular inflammatory cells.[1,2]

AIR presumably results from an immunologic attack on the retina by antibodies directed against retinal antigens. The first case of vision loss and photoreceptor degeneration associated with cancer was described by Sawyer et al. in 1976.[3] Paraneoplastic retinopathy, as a term, was first used by Klingele and associates in 1984, and has become the more general term used for autoimmune retinopathies associated with systemic malignancy since then.[4] Several forms of autoantibody-mediated retinopathy are described: cancer-associated retinopathy (CAR) syndrome, melanoma-associated retinopathy (MAR) syndrome, or autoimmune retinopathy of other types.[3,5–11] AIR can be categorized in two groups: (i) autoimmune retinopathy associated with cancer or other malignancies (paraneoplastic retinopathy or paraneoplastic autoimmune retinopathy); (ii) autoimmune retinopathy without any evidence of malignancy (nonparaneoplastic autoimmune retinopathy). Cancer-associated retinopathy and other paraneoplastic retinopathies will be covered in Chapter 134 (Remote effects of cancer on the retina). Autoimmune retinopathy is the preferred term for an acquired, presumed immunologically mediated retinopathy caused by antiretinal autoantibodies in the absence of a malignancy. This chapter will emphasize the latter.

EPIDEMIOLOGY AND MECHANISMS

The prevalence of AIR is unknown, but the condition is believed to be rare. Clinical reports of nonparaneoplastic AIR consist only of case reports and a few small cohorts.[12,13] AIR remains an ill-defined disorder and the lack of standardized diagnostic criteria may be contributing to the underestimation of its prevalence. Though circulating autoantibodies to retinal antigens have been shown to be associated with retinal dysfunction, the mechanisms by which these antibodies cause dysfunction are not entirely understood.[14] Multiple retinal proteins have been found to be antigenic, including recoverin, carbonic anhydrase, α-enolase, arrestin, transducin-β, carbonic anhydrase II, TULP1, neurofilament protein, heat shock protein-70, photoreceptor-cell-specific nuclear receptor (PNR), Müller-cell-specific antigen, transient receptor potential cation channel, subfamily M, member 1 (TRPM1) and many other yet-unidentified antigens[15,16] (Table 77.1). Some of these antigens are retina-specific, such as recoverin and rhodopsin, while others can be found in nonretinal tissues as well, such as enolase. Among these, recoverin and enolase are the most extensively studied antigens in the context of AIR. Recoverin is a 23 kDa calcium-binding protein found in both rods and cones. Enolase is a 48 kDa glycolytic enzyme whose α- and β-isoforms are found in many tissues, and γ-isoform in neuronal tissues.[39] In a large series, more than 30% of patients with antiretinal antibodies tested positive for antienolase antibody.[40] Antibodies against α-enolase appear to be fairly ubiquitous; they are found in multiple autoimmune diseases and even in healthy subjects.[41–44] This has been, in part, attributed to the multifunctional nature of α-enolase.[14,25,45]

Table 77.1 Proteins targeted by antiretinal antibodies

Protein		
Recoverin (23 kD)		CAR, npAIR[6,17–24]
Alpha-enolase (46 kD)		CAR, npAIR [20,21,25–28]
Carbonic anhydrase II (CA II) (30 kD)		npAIR[20,21]
Tubby-like protein 1 (TULP-1) (65 kD)		CAR[29]
Heat shock protein 70 (HSC 70) (70 kD)		CAR[19]
Transducin (35 kD)		MAR[30]
Arrestin (S-Antigen) (48 kD)		MAR, npAIR[21,31]
Interphotoreceptor binding protein (IRBP) (141 kD)		npAIR[21]
Unknown proteins	22 kD, 34 kD, 35 kD, 37 kD, 40 kD, 68 kD	npAIR[32–34]
	34 kD, 40 kD, 46 kD, 60 kD, 70 kD	CAR [22,35–38]

Antibodies against the listed proteins were identified in the serum of patients with AIR or AIR-like clinical findings. CAR, cancer-associated retinopathy; MAR, melanoma-associated retinopathy; npAIR, non-paraneoplastic autoimmune retinopathy.

Of all these antigens, recoverin and CAR has the strongest association. Recoverin has been shown to be expressed by the tumor cells of patients with CAR.[46] While antirecoverin antibody is most specific to CAR, it has also been found in patients with nonparaneoplastic AIR, as well as patients with small-cell lung carcinoma without any retinopathy.[17,18,47] Recoverin and α-enolase have been shown to be highly expressed in cancer cells in patients with paraneoplastic AIR. It is plausible that the disease is triggered by molecular mimicry between retinal proteins and tumor antigens in cases of paraneoplastic AIR and presumed viral or bacterial proteins[26] in the case of nonparaneoplastic AIR.[26,48,49] Regardless of the presence or absence of malignancy, autoimmune retinopathies appear to share common clinical features.

Experimental studies have attempted to shed light on the pathogenic mechanisms of autoimmune retinopathy. *In vitro* studies have demonstrated that some of the antiretinal antibodies are, indeed, cytotoxic to retinal cells, and that the cellular internalization of the antibody leads to apoptosis.[19,25,27,50–52] This antibody-mediated apoptosis is independent of complement and involves caspase pathways and intracellular calcium influx. Similarly, *in vivo* studies showed that intravitreal injection of antirecoverin antibody causes apoptosis of retinal cells and a decrease in ERG responses.[19,53,54] Recoverin also acts as a uveitogenic antigen and can induce autoimmune retinopathy-like disease in animal models leading to reduced scotopic and photopic ERG responses.[55,56] Both *in vitro* and *in vivo* studies showed that antirecoverin antibody-triggered apoptosis occurs only in recoverin-positive cells.[57] Antirecoverin antibodies target photoreceptor cells and anti-α-enolase antibodies appear to target ganglion cells. Antibodies targeting retinal bipolar cells have been associated with MAR. Additionally, injection of immunoglobulins isolated from serum of patients with MAR into the vitreous of monkeys led to ERG changes similar to those observed in MAR, indicating the pathogenicity of the antiretinal antibodies.[58] Evidence from these studies suggests that antiretinal autoantibodies can target virtually any retinal cell type – photoreceptor cells, ganglion cells, bipolar cells – and cause retinal dysfunction.[20,50,59] It is still unclear, however, why some patients with antiretinal antibodies develop retinopathy while others do not.

CLINICAL FEATURES

Clinical features of AIR are quite variable. Serum antiretinal autoantibodies have been associated with loss of vision and visual field defects as well as electrophysiologic changes in patients with autoimmune retinopathy, but the exact mechanism has not been fully understood. In particular, the pathogenicity and specificity of these autoantibodies with respect to clinical findings have yet to be determined. Nevertheless, patients with AIR appear to share common clinical features despite the heterogeneity in the detectable circulating antiretinal antibodies.[12,20,60]

The clinical manifestations of nonparaneoplastic AIR is quite variable, there are no clear guidelines or consensus on the diagnosis of autoimmune retinopathy. Commonly recognized clinical manifestations include:[12,13]

1. Symptoms: acute, subacute or chronic onset of photopsia, dyschromatopsia, nyctalopia, photoaversion, scotomas, sometimes central vision loss.
2. Fundus findings: normal-appearing fundus, or waxy disc pallor, attenuated retinal vasculature and retinal pigment epithelial (RPE) atrophy or mottling. There are few or no intraocular inflammatory cells.
3. Psychophysical tests:
   Visual fields: constricted visual fields, central or paracentral scotomas.
   Electroretinogram (ERG): ERG can show abnormalities in rods, cones, Müller cells or bipolar cell responses or a combination of these.

Patients with nonparaneoplastic AIR present with subacute or chronic vision loss. Patients typically complain of color vision changes, photosensitivity or photoaversion, and varying degrees of nyctalopia. Other presenting symptoms include floaters, photopsias, scotomas, most commonly paracentral, and constricted visual fields. Of these, photosensitivity, photoaversion, difficulty seeing in bright light, reduced visual acuity, dyschromatopsia and central scotomas are suggestive of cone dysfunction, whereas nyctalopia (night blindness) and midperipheral scotomas are suggestive of rod dysfunction. Depending on the extent and the distinct retinal cell involvement, visual acuity, particularly in the earlier stages, may be deceivingly good. On presentation to a tertiary care center, most patients may have been diagnosed with nonspecific retinal degeneration or isolated cases of retinitis pigmentosa (RP). Fundus examination can be unremarkable or may show signs of retinal degeneration such as waxy disc pallor, attenuated retinal vasculature with or without pigmentary changes, or diffuse atrophy. There may be mild or no inflammatory cells in the anterior chamber or the vitreous[12,13,61] (Fig. 77.1).

Ancillary testing with fluorescein angiography (FA) or optical coherence tomography (OCT) may show mild retinal vascular staining or leakage, or cystoid macular edema (CME) in some cases.[12] Visual field testing may confirm scotomas and constricted visual fields. While static visual field testing may be better for demonstrating and following central and paracentral scotomas, kinetic visual fields are better for measuring peripheral field constriction. However, kinetic visual fields have the disadvantage of examiner dependence, the need for patient cooperation, inter-tester variability, and lack of standardization of parameters.[62,63] ERG may demonstrate abnormal rod, cone, Müller cell, and bipolar cell responses and delay in implicit times.[12,13,26,32] However, the majority of studies involving ERG findings in AIR come from paraneoplastic retinopathies (Fig. 77.2).

AIR is almost always bilateral, although involvement can be asymmetric. A family or a personal history of systemic autoimmune disease can be common among patients with nonparaneoplastic AIR.[12,33] There is a female preponderance (63–66%), and average age at diagnosis appears to range from 51 years to 56 years.[12,13,20] The typical patient would be a middle-aged or older adult in their fifth to sixth decades with no history of visual problems prior to the onset of photopsias, scotomas, and other symptoms consistent with AIR, and no family history of RP.

As might be expected for an entity with no consensus in diagnosis, retrospective studies in patients with nonparaneoplastic AIR showed that clinical features vary considerably. In one study, diffuse retinal atrophy was seen in the majority of patients (83%) and pigment deposits in only a small proportion (13%), macular edema was present in approximately half of the cases, while another study showed pigmentary changes in approximately half of the patients and macular edema in 24%. The most

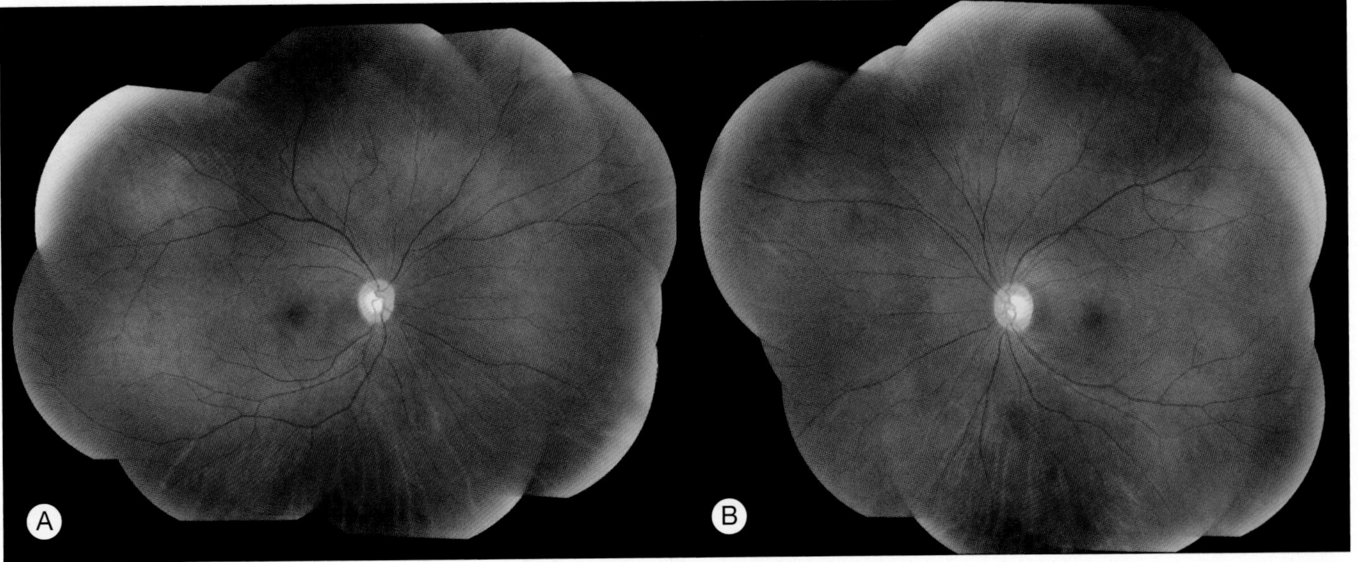

Fig. 77.1 (A,B) Fundus photo of a 57-year-old patient with systemic lupus erythematosus and autoimmune retinopathy. Note the mild attenuation of retinal vasculature and mild optic nerve pallor.

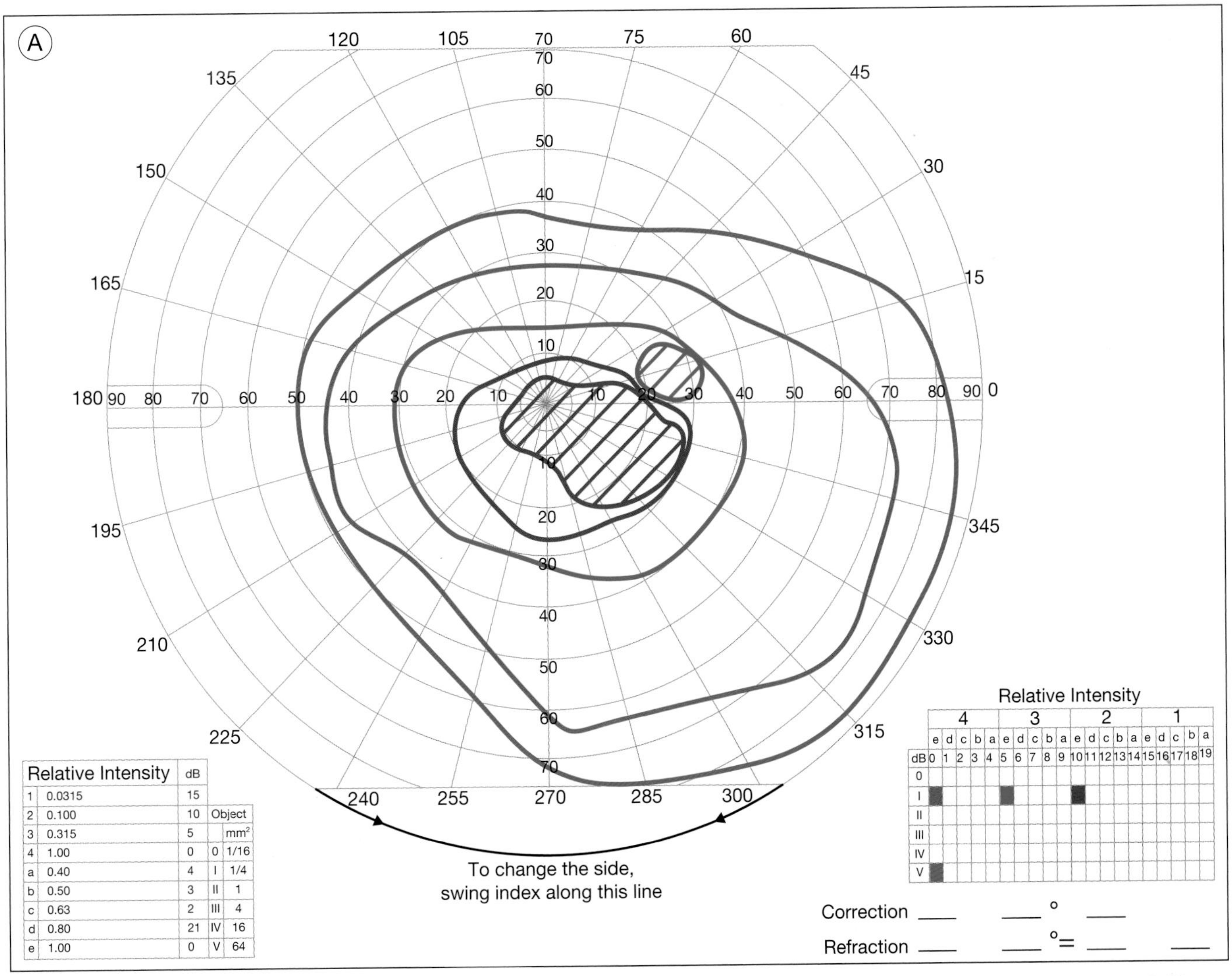

A

120 105 70 75 60
135 45
150 30
165 15
180 90 80 70 60 50 40 30 20 10 10 20 30 40 50 60 70 80 90 0
195 345
210 330
225 315
240 255 270 285 300

To change the side,
swing index along this line

Relative Intensity		dB	Object	
1	0.0315	15		
2	0.100	10	Object	
3	0.315	5		mm²
4	1.00	0	0	1/16
a	0.40	4	I	1/4
b	0.50	3	II	1
c	0.63	2	III	4
d	0.80	21	IV	16
e	1.00	0	V	64

Relative Intensity

	4					3					2					1				
	e	d	c	b	a	e	d	c	b	a	e	d	c	b	a	e	d	c	b	a
dB	0	1	2	3	4	5	6	7	8	9	10	11	12	13	14	15	16	17	18	19
0																				
I																				
II																				
III																				
IV																				
V																				

Correction ____ ____ ° ____

Refraction ____ ____ °= ____ ____

Fig. 77.2 (A,B,C) Goldman visual field of an autoimmune retinopathy patient shows central and paracentral scotoma in the right (A) and left (B) eye.

Continued

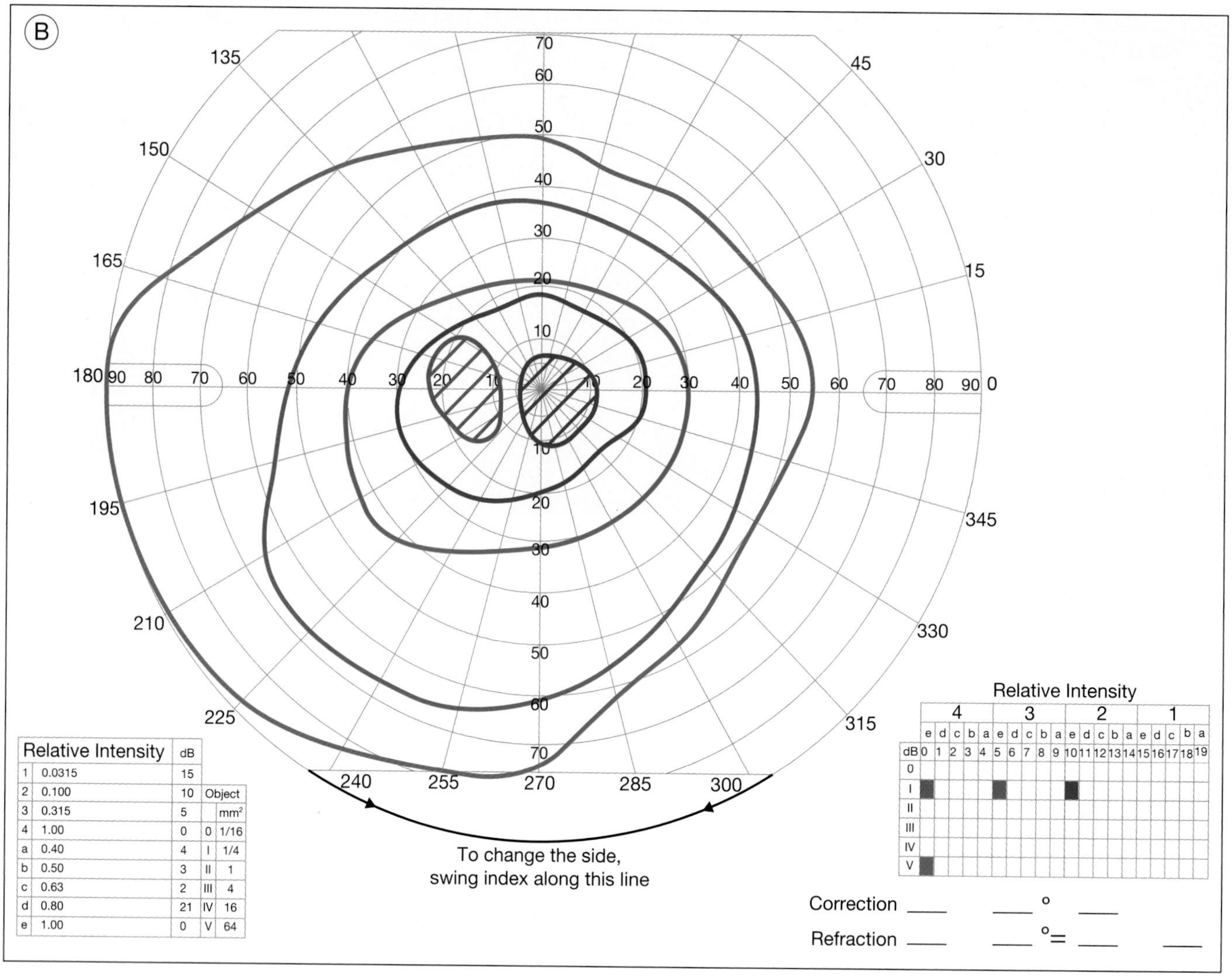

(B)

135 150 165 180 195 210 225 240 255 270 285 300 315 330 345 0 15 30 45

To change the side, swing index along this line

	Relative Intensity	dB		Object mm²
1	0.0315	15		
2	0.100	10		
3	0.315	5		
4	1.00	0	0	1/16
a	0.40	4	I	1/4
b	0.50	3	II	1
c	0.63	2	III	4
d	0.80	21	IV	16
e	1.00	0	V	64

Relative Intensity

	4					3					2					1				
	e	d	c	b	a	e	d	c	b	a	e	d	c	b	a	e	d	c	b	a
dB	0	1	2	3	4	5	6	7	8	9	10	11	12	13	14	15	16	17	18	19
0																				
I																				
II																				
III																				
IV																				
V																				

Correction ____ ____ ° ____

Refraction ____ ____ °= ____ ____

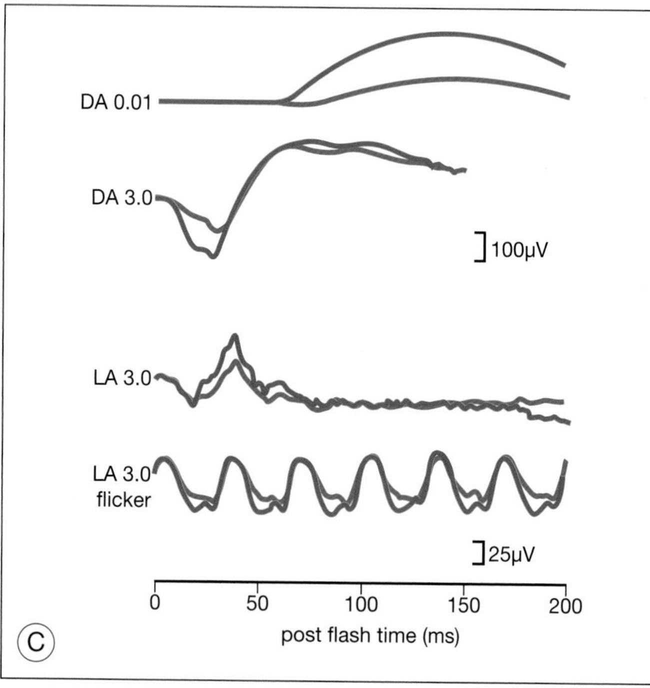

Fig. 77.2 Cont'd (C) ERG responses of the same patient shows reduced amplitudes for both rod- and cone-mediated responses. Blue traces indicate baseline ERG recordings; red traces were recorded 1 month after treatment with rituximab (Rituxan®, Genentech, Inc., CA), a chimeric anti-CD20 antibody. Note the improvement in rod-mediated responses. ERGs were recorded according to ISCEV standards. DA, dark adapted; LA, light adapted; number indicates flash intensity (cd-s/m²). Note different scales for DA and LA ERGs. (Courtesy of Brett Jeffrey, PhD.)

common symptoms at onset were subacute vision loss, photopsias, and nyctalopia. Similarly, in a series of 12 patients with antienolase-associated retinopathy, clinical characteristics included visual loss, normal-appearing fundus in most except for vascular attenuation, optic nerve head pallor in some, and mainly abnormal cone responses. In all of these studies, however, there was a female predominance and the age at onset was similar.[12,13,20,26,]

DIAGNOSIS

The diagnosis of AIR is difficult as there are no definitive or standardized tests. The presumptive diagnosis relies on the presence of the above clinical manifestations, usually more than one, along with demonstration of serum antiretinal antibodies. Most patients will have more than one antiretinal antibody. If the clinical features of autoimmune retinopathy and the circulating antiretinal antibodies are present, and if there is no malignancy at presentation or following a thorough investigation, a diagnosis of nonparaneoplastic AIR is made (Table 77.2).

In addition to an extensive review of systems and history to rule out any malignancy, a thorough physical exam and basic laboratory investigations accompanied by age- and gender-appropriate investigations are typically undertaken prior to starting treatment. These investigations are best performed or facilitated by an internist or the primary care physician. Because the diagnosis of AIR is presumptive, it is very important that a clear communication between the ophthalmologist and the primary medical team is established regarding the uncertainty of the diagnosis and the possible overlap with paraneoplastic retinopathy, so an appropriate investigation can be undertaken. Imaging with MRI or CT should be guided by the review of systems and patients' individual risk factors, and, as such, determined by the patient's primary medical team.

Demonstration of serum antiretinal antibodies can be done using various methods, including Western blot (WB), immunohistochemistry (IHC) or enzyme-linked immunosorbent assay (ELISA). Western blot is a protein immunoblot of patients' serum incubated with extracts of a normal donor human retina and shows antiretinal IgG bands. It identifies antibody activity based on size of the protein, and the interpretation relies on intensity of protein bands on a photographic film. The results may be affected by multiple technical factors and lack specificity. For example, a 23 kDa band on WB does not necessarily mean antibody against recoverin; there may be other antigens with the same size. The immunohistochemical detection of antiretinal antibodies, on the other hand, involves fixing patient serum against frozen donor human retina (or monkey or mouse retina) using immunohistochemical staining. Sections are then analyzed using light microscopy to determine which layers of the retina show binding of the antiretinal antibody. The advantage with IHC is the ability to localize the specific site of binding within the retina (Fig. 77.3). ELISA is similar, in principle, to WB and IHC and involves adding various dilutions of patient sera into wells coated with specific retinal proteins and binding is detected using secondary antibodies.[10,64] All of these techniques, however, lack standardization.[15] Moreover, it is important to remember that the mere presence of these autoantibodies does not warrant a diagnosis of AIR, nor does it mean they are pathogenic. Antiretinal antibodies have been detected in patients with other retinal diseases, uveitis, retinal degenerations including age-related macular degeneration, and even in normal controls.[21,65–68] Conversely, they can be negative in patients with clinical features of what would be considered AIR.[20] Despite the caveats, there are few centers in the United States that perform antiretinal antibody testing. One center provides these services commercially through a CLIA (clinical laboratory improvement amendments) certified laboratory.[69] WB and IHC are the more commonly performed techniques.

Autoimmune retinopathy, similar to paraneoplastic retinopathy, can be associated with various antiretinal antibodies. Initially detected autoantibodies in nonparaneoplastic AIR were antirecoverin antibodies.[17] Later, antibodies directed against the inner plexiform layer,[11] Müller cells (35 kDa) or other unidentified retinal proteins have been described.[32,64] One of the most commonly detected antibodies on WB in nonparaneoplastic AIR appears to be one with a molecular weight of about 35 kDa which was detected in about 25% of autoimmune retinopathies.[20]

Table 77.2 Diagnostic criteria for nonparaneoplastic AIR (proposed by the authors)

Must have all of the criteria	Must have ≥2 of the criteria
No evidence of malignancy	Symptoms: Photopsias or scotomas or dychromatopsia or nyctalopia or photoaversion
No family history of RP	Fundus changes*
(+) serum antiretinal antibodies	Visual field abnormality*
	ERG abnormality*

**Fundus changes, visual field or ERG abnormalities as described in clinical manifestations and diagnosis section (see text).*

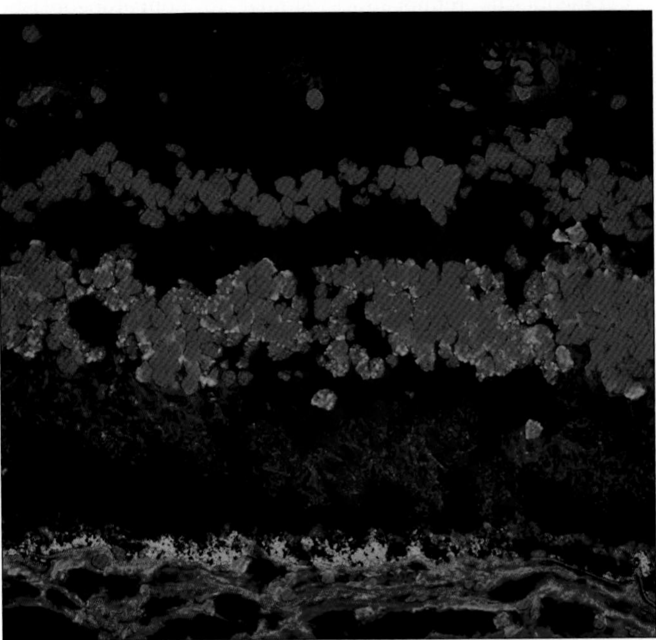

Fig. 77.3 Immunohistochemistry performed using serum of autoimmune retinopathy patient against fresh-frozen human donor retina shows staining at the photoreceptor inner and outer segments as well as outer nuclear layer. (Courtesy of Chi Chao Chan, MD.)

Autoimmune retinopathy can be associated with systemic autoimmune diseases, especially those that are autoantibody-mediated. In fact, cases of nonparaneoplastic AIR have been described in the setting of systemic lupus erythematosus.[12,70]

In a large cohort, only 47% of patients who presented with signs and symptoms compatible with AIR had any detectable antiretinal antibodies. Of these, patients with a history of cancer were more likely to have detectable antiretinal antibodies (63.5%) than those who did not (41.1%).[20] In the same study, the authors showed antirecoverin antibodies exclusively in the paraneoplastic AIR group, antibodies against 35 kDa protein were mostly found in nonparaneoplastic AIR patients' sera whereas anti-α-enolase was somewhat equally distributed in both groups. The fact that half of patients with symptoms and signs compatible with AIR tested negative for any antiretinal antibody with the techniques currently available, highlights the difficulty of diagnosis.

DIFFERENTIAL DIAGNOSIS

Since there are no standardized tests for nonparaneoplastic AIR, the differential diagnosis is as challenging as its diagnosis. A variety of retinopathies are associated with the detection of antiretinal antibodies in serum. In addition, the clinical features seen in autoimmune retinopathy are not specific or unique to AIR and can be seen in other forms of retinopathies.

The spectrum of disorders that may show clinical or laboratory similarities to AIR can be studied in four groups:

1. Paraneoplastic disorders (e.g., CAR, MAR)
2. White-dot syndrome spectrum disorders (e.g., acute zonal occult outer retinopathy)
3. Retinal degenerative disorders (e.g., retinitis pigmentosa, cone–rod dystrophy)
4. Non-infectious and infectious uveitis syndromes

Paraneoplastic retinopathies, similar to nonparaneoplastic AIR, are characterized by vision loss, photopsias, nyctalopia, and scotomas. Cancer-associated retinopathy is typically associated with antirecoverin antibody, and most commonly associated with small-cell carcinoma of the lung. It is important to remember that a non-neoplastic form of antirecoverin antibody-associated retinopathy has also been described.[6,7,17] MAR occurs in patients with cutaneous melanoma and is characterized by a negative waveform on standardized full-field ERG due to reduction in b-wave amplitudes. In addition to similar symptoms as in nonparaneoplastic AIR, patients tend to have diffuse fundus depigmentation. Paraneoplastic retinopathies typically have a more rapid decline; with rapid progression of vision and visual field loss, as well as ERG changes, spontaneous recovery has not been observed. Vision loss can precede the identification of malignancy.[60,61] It is important to differentiate paraneoplastic retinopathy from non-paraneoplastic AIR because of significant implications on treatment. The features of paraneoplastic retinopathy are covered in detail in Chapter 134 (Remote effects of cancer on the retina).

White-dot syndromes such as acute zonal occult outer retinopathy (AZOOR) or multiple evanescent white-dot syndrome (MEWDS) have been suggested to be associated with antiretinal antibodies.[64,71] AZOOR and MEWDS have overlapping features and cases of MEWDS evolving into AZOOR have been described.[72] However, immunohistochemical testing of sera of patients with AZOOR failed to show antiretinal antibodies.[73] AZOOR can present with similar symptoms, visual field, and ERG findings to nonparaneoplastic AIR; it is typically bilateral but asymmetric and majority of patients either stabilize or show partial recovery without treatment. MEWDS, despite having similar symptoms, is a unilateral retinopathy which is characterized by afferent pupillary defect, optic nerve swelling and spontaneous recovery, and hence is more readily differentiated from AIR. Both AZOOR and MEWDS may show enlarged blind spot on visual fields. In addition, the majority of eyes affected by AZOOR may show fundus autofluorescence abnormalities which has not been observed in AIR.[33,74,75]

Antiretinal antibodies have also been reported to occur in patients with RP, a hereditary retinal degeneration. However, up to 60% of patients with RP may lack a family history of retinal degeneration. Indeed, some patients who are eventually diagnosed as nonparaneoplastic AIR are initially diagnosed as isolated cases of RP. Approximately 10% to 37% of patients with RP may have circulating antiretinal antibodies.[10,76] Additionally, 90% of patients with RP and macular cysts have circulating antiretinal antibodies on WB, compared with 13% of patients with RP without macular cysts and 6% of controls.[21] Most commonly detected antibodies are targeted against carbonic anhydrase II and α-enolase.[18] In some cases of RP, rapid progression of visual field loss and CME appears to be associated with presence of antiretinal antibodies.[21,65] In retinal degenerations, whether the antibodies precede the onset of retinopathy or whether antiretinal autoantibodies are a consequence of retinal damage is unclear. Additionally, whether the presence of these autoantibodies has a significant impact on clinical course has yet to be determined.

Antiretinal antibodies have also been found in patients with retinal vasculitis, uveitis patients with Vogt–Koyanagi–Harada syndrome (VKH), Behçet disease, and sympathetic ophthalmia. In patients with VKH, antibody reactivity to photoreceptors correlated with disease activity. However, all these syndromes are characterized by significant intraocular inflammation in addition to their unique fundus findings, making the differentiation rather unproblematic. Other rare cases of retinopathies associated with antiretinal antibodies include onchocerciasis and ocular toxoplasmosis. Antibodies to retinal pigment epithelium (RPE), neural retina or photoreceptor layer has been described in these infectious retinopathies.[60,68,77] Typical fundus findings in these entities are helpful in differentiating them from nonparaneoplastic AIR. In all of the aforementioned diseases, it is unclear if the antibodies preceded the retinal disease or if the immune reactivity is simply a consequence of the retinal degenerative process.

TREATMENT AND PROGNOSIS

Various forms of immunomodulatory approaches have been tried in an attempt to treat autoimmune retinopathy. Theoretically, because of the presumed autoimmune nature of the disease, immunosuppression for nonparaneoplastic AIR is the most sensible treatment strategy. However, because of the ambiguity in diagnosis and lack of standardization in therapeutic outcomes, management of AIR poses an enormous challenge. The immunosuppressive therapy can be considered empiric at this time because of our lack of understanding of this condition. If undertaken, a long-term treatment is needed in most cases and therapy is not helpful once widespread retinal degeneration occurs. Most treatment-related case series are regarding paraneoplastic retinopathy and include chemotherapy, corticosteroids, intravenous immunoglobulin (IVIG), or plasmapheresis.[22] Recently, successful treatment of autoimmune retinopathy or associated cancer with more targeted biologic agents have also been reported.[35,78,79]

Immunosuppressive therapy should be administered by a rheumatologist, immunologist or a uveitis specialist well versed in the management of such therapy. Immunosuppressive agents such as mycophenolate mofetil, cyclosporine or corticosteroids may help improve visual function in some autoimmune retinopathy patients. In a cohort of 24 nonparaneoplastic AIR patients that received therapy with various combinations of prednisone, cyclosporine, azathioprine, mycophenolate mofetil, periocular or intravitreal steroid injections, 15 of the 24 showed varying degrees of improvement in visual acuity or visual field. CME improved in almost half of the patients, unfortunately, ERG was not routinely performed. Decrease in antiretinal antibodies following treatment may be seen in some cases,[12,22,60] however clinical significance of this finding is unclear.

In addition to systemic and local corticosteroids, most commonly used immunosuppressive agents in the treatment of AIR include intravenous immunoglobulin (IVIG), antimetabolites such as mycophenolate mofetil, azathioprine, and T-cell inhibitors such as cyclosporine.[12] IVIG has multiple mechanisms of action, some of which are not completely understood. When used in the treatment of autoimmune disorders, its effect is believed to be due to its interaction with Fc receptors on effector cells or by acting as anti-idiotypic antibodies directed against idiotypes on circulating autoantibodies. This mechanism may be at play in autoantibody-mediated diseases. Other mechanisms may involve clearance of immune complex deposits, presence of neutralizing antibodies in IVIG, its effect on the number of T-cell subsets, proinflammatory monocytes or regulatory T cells.[80] IVIG has been used in several uveitic syndromes refractive to conventional therapy. Its use is limited by cost and long infusions. Typical dose ranges between 1 and 2.5 g/kg each infusion, and the infusions can be administered every 4–8 weeks although different protocols have been used. Major side-effects include hypersensitivity and anaphylactic reactions and thrombotic events.[81] Similarly, plasmapheresis has also been used in paraneoplastic autoimmune retinopathy. Plasmapheresis, also known as therapeutic plasma exchange, involves extracorporeal elimination of large molecular weight plasma proteins from the blood. The regimen for plasmapheresis is determined according to the pathologic substance desired to be removed. To replace volume, albumin, albumin–saline combination or fresh-frozen plasma can be used, the latter is preferred to avoid depletion of coagulation factors and immunoglobulins. Its effect is believed to be due to removal of immune complexes and immune reactants. The effect may be rapid but is often short-lived, therefore, more sustainable immunomodulation is often required. Major side-effects include paresthesias, muscle cramps, urticarial and anaphylactic reactions.[22]

Less frequently, targeted B-cell therapy, such as anti-CD20 monoclonal antibody (Rituximab), has also been used in the treatment of AIR. Rituximab targets CD20 found on B cells which are the precursors of antibody-secreting plasma cells.[20,79] Although there is anecdotal evidence, the benefit of immunosuppressive therapy in AIR is also not definite. There are no clear guidelines on how to institute and manage immunosuppressives in patients with AIR, owing to the rarity and ambiguity surrounding this entity. Therefore, the treating physician typically extrapolates from guidelines that are established for other ocular inflammatory disorders.[82] These drugs can take several weeks to have an effect and it may take up to several months to observe a clinical effect in the form of improvement or stabilization on visual fields or ERG. More rapid improvement has been reported in CAR patients treated with IVIG.[22]

Adding to the challenges in the management is the lack of parameters to guide treatment. There have been no clear indicators for prognosis. Whether the autoantibodies would disappear in response to treatment, or whether their disappearance would be accompanied by clinical improvement is still unclear. Regardless, patients treated with immunosuppressives need to be closely monitored for side-effects. The most common side-effects with azathioprine and mycophenolate mofetil are gastrointestinal upset, nausea, and less commonly, vomiting. The most common severe side-effects are reversible bone marrow suppression and hepatotoxicity. The most serious side-effects of cyclosporine are nephrotoxocitiy, which occurs less commonly at lower doses (2–5 mg/kg/day), and hypertension. Regular complete blood count with differential, and chemistry panel including hepatic and renal function tests should be performed during therapy. Patients should be encouraged to report any side-effects as early intervention in the form of discontinuation or dose adjustments can be critical.

The response to treatment is very variable, with more favorable results achieved in paraneoplastic retinopathy, particularly CAR, with a combination of chemotherapy and immunomodulation. It has also been suggested that those with a family history of autoimmune disorders may be less likely to respond to immunosuppression.[12,83] Our experience indicates that with treatment only a minority of patients with AIR show improvement in visual function, and some remain stable. This may be due to late presentation to our center with significant loss seen on both ERG and visual fields at presentation. Whether an earlier attempt to treat with immunosuppressives would be more beneficial is not clear. Early treatment attempts would require establishing a clear diagnosis using sensitive and specific assays and more definitive clinical criteria. While most of the immunosuppressives used in the treatment of AIR can be instituted and managed safely, a better understanding of the disease is needed to justify more aggressive and potentially beneficial treatment approaches.

Despite evolving research, the relationship between antiretinal antibodies and retinal dysfunction is not fully understood. Limitations in diagnostic assays also limit therapeutic investigations. Regardless, until more is known the mainstay of treatment remains immunosuppression following a thorough investigation to rule out malignancy. Clearly, additional studies are needed to identify the specificity and pathogenicity of antiretinal antibodies and the appropriate treatment.

REFERENCES

1. Weinstein JM, Kelman SE, Bresnick GH, et al. Paraneoplastic retinopathy associated with antiretinal bipolar cell antibodies in cutaneous malignant melanoma. Ophthalmology 1994;101:1236–43.
2. Jacobson DM, Thirkill CE, Tipping SJ. A clinical triad to diagnose paraneoplastic retinopathy. Ann Neurol 1990;28:162–7.
3. Sawyer RA, Selhorst JB, Zimmerman LE, et al. Blindness caused by photoreceptor degeneration as a remote effect of cancer. Am J Ophthalmol 1976;81:606–13.
4. Klingele TG, Burde RM, Rappazzo JA, et al. Paraneoplastic retinopathy. J Clin Neuroophthalmol 1984;4:239–45.

5. Jacobson DM, Miller NR, Newman NJ, editors. Paraneoplastic diseases of neuro-ophthalmologic interest. In: Walsh & Hoyt's clinical neuro-ophthalmology. 5th ed. Baltimore, MD: Williams & Wilkins; 2008. p. 2497–551.
6. Thirkill CE, Roth AM, Keltner JL. Cancer-associated retinopathy. Arch Ophthalmol 1987;105:372–5.
7. Keltner JL, Thirkill CE. Cancer-associated retinopathy vs recoverin-associated retinopathy. Am J Ophthalmol 1998;126:296–302.
8. Vaphiades MS,Brown H, Whitcup SM. Node way out: Comments by Keltner JL, Thirkill CE. Surv Ophthalmol 2000;45:77–83.
9. Weinstein JM, Kelman SE, Bresnick GH. Paraneoplastic retinopathy associated with antiretinal bipolar cell antibodies in cutaneous malignant melanoma. Ophthalmology 1994;101:1236–43.
10. Potter MJ, Thirkill CE, Dam OM. Clinical and immunocytochemical findings in a case of melanoma-associated retinopathy. Ophthalmology 1999;106: 2121–5.
11. Mizener JB, Kimura AE, Adamus G. Autoimmune retinopathy in the absence of cancer. Am J Ophthalmol 1997;123:607–18.
12. Ferreyra HA, Jayasundera T, Khan NW, et al. Management of autoimmune retinopathies with immunosuppression. Arch Ophthalmol 2009; 127:390–7.
13. Larson TA, Gottlieb CC, Zein WM, et al. Autoimmune retinopathy: prognosis and treatment. Invest Ophthalmol Vis Sci 2010;51:E-Abstract 6375.
14. Adamus G. Autoantibody-induced apoptosis as a possible mechanism of autoimmune retinopathy. Autoimmunity Rev 2003;2:63–9.
15. Forooghian F, Macdonald IM, Heckenlively JR, et al. The need for standardization of antiretinal antibody detection and measurement. Am J Ophthalmol 2008;146(4):489–95.
16. Kondo M, Sanuki R, Ueno S, et al. Identification of autoantibodies against TRPM1 in patients with paraneoplastic retinopathy associated with ON bipolar cell dysfunction. PLoS One 2011;6(5):e19911.
17. Whitcup SM, Vistica BP, Milam AH, et al. Recoverin-associated retinopathy: a clinically and immunologically distinctive disease. Am J Ophthalmol 1998;126: 230–7.
18. Heckenlively JR, Fawzi AA, Oversier J, et al. Autoimmune retinopathy: patients with antirecoverin immunoreactivity and panretinal degeneration. Arch Ophthalmol 2000;118(11):1525–33.
19. Ohguro H, Ogawa K, Maeda T, et al. Cancer-associated retinopathy induced by both anti-recoverin and anti-hsc70 antibodies in vivo. Invest Ophthalmol Vis Sci 1999;40(13):3160–7.
20. Adamus G, Ren G, Weleber RG. Autoantibodies against retinal proteins in paraneoplastic and autoimmune retinopathy. BMC Ophthalmol 2004; 4:5.
21. Heckenlively JR, Jordan BL, Aptsiauri N. Association of antiretinal antibodies and cystoid macular edema in patients with retinitis pigmentosa. Am J Ophthalmol 1999;127:565–73.
22. Guy J, Aptsiauri N. Treatment of paraneoplastic visual loss with intravenous immunoglobulin: report of 3 cases. Arch Ophthalmol 1999;117:471–7.
23. Polans AS, Burton MD, Haley TL, et al. Recoverin, but not visinin, is an autoantigen in the human retina identified with a cancer-associated retinopathy. Invest Ophthalmol Vis Sci 1993;34:81–90.
24. Keltner JL, Thirkill CE, Tyler NK, et al. Management and monitoring of cancer-associated retinopathy. Arch Ophthalmol 1992;110:48–53.
25. Adamus G, Amundson D, Seigal GM, et al. Anti-enolase a autoantibodies in cancer-associated retinopathy: epitope mapping and cytoxicity on retinal cells. J Autoimmun 1998;11:671–7.
26. Weleber RG, Watzke RC, Shults WT, et al. Clinical and electrophysiologic characterization of paraneoplastic and autoimmune retinopathies associated with antienolase antibodies. Am J Ophthalmol 2005;139:780–94.
27. Ren G, Adamus G. Cellular targets of anti-alpha-enolase autoantibodies of patients with autoimmune retinopathy. J Autoimmun 2004;23:161–7.
28. Adamus G, Aptsiauri N, Guy J, et al. The occurrence of serum autoantibodies against enolase in cancer-associated retinopathy. Clin Immunol Immunopathol 1996;78:120–9.
29. Kikuchi T, Arai J, Shibuki H, et al. Tubby-like protein 1 as an autoantigen in cancer-associated retinopathy. J Neuroimmunol 2000;103:26–33.
30. Potter MJ, Adamus G, Szabo SM, et al. Autoantibodies to transducin in a patient with melanoma-associated retinopathy. Am J Ophthalmol 2002;134: 128–30.
31. Bazhin AV, Dalke C, Willner N, et al.Cancer-retina antigens as potential paraneoplastic antigens in melanoma-associated retinopathy. Int J Cancer 2009;124: 140–9.
32. Peek R, Verbraak F, Coevoet HM, et al. Muller cell-specific autoantibodies in a patient with progressive loss of vision. Invest Ophthalmol Vis Sci 1998;39: 1976–9.
33. Mantel I, Ramchand KV, Holder GE, et al. Macular and retinal dysfunction of unknown origin in adults with normal fundi: evidence for an autoimmune pathophysiology. Exp Mol Pathol 2008;84:90–101.
34. Keltner JL, Thirkill CE. The 22-kDa antigen in optic nerve and retinal diseases. J Neuroophthalmol 1999;19:71–83.
35. Espandar L, O'Brien S, Thirkill C, et al. Successful treatment of cancer-associated retinopathy with alemtuzumab. J Neurooncol 2007;83:295–302.
36. Ohkawa T, Kawashima H, Makino S, et al. Cancer-associated retinopathy in a patient with endometrial cancer. Am J Ophthalmol 1996;122:740–2.
37. Murphy MA, Thirkill CE, Hart Jr WM. Paraneoplastic retinopathy: a novel autoantibody reaction associated with small-cell lung carcinoma. J Neuroophthalmol 1997;17:77–83.
38. Masaoka N, Emoto Y, Sasaoka A, et al. Fluorescein angiographic findings in a case of cancer-associated retinopathy. Retina 1999;19:462–4.
39. McAleese SM, Dunbar B, Fothergill JE, et al. Complete amino acid sequence of the neurone-specific gamma isozyme of enolase (NSE) from human brain and comparison with the non-neuronal alpha form (NNE). Eur J Biochem 1988;178:413–7.
40. Adamus G, Wilson DJ. The need for standardization of antiretinal antibody detection and measurement. Am J Ophthalmol 2009;147(3):557, author reply 557–8.
41. Shin SJ, Kim BC, Kim TI, et al. Anti-alpha-enolase antibody as a serologic marker and its correlation with disease severity in intestinal Behçet's disease. Dig Dis Sci 2011;56(3):812–18.
42. Lee JH, Cho SB, Bang D, et al. Human anti-alpha-enolase antibody in sera from patients with Behçet's disease and rheumatologic disorders. Clin Exp Rheumatol 2009;27(2 Suppl 53):S63–6.
43. Forooghian F, Adamus G, Sproule M, et al. Enolase autoantibodies and retinal function in multiple sclerosis patients. Graefes Arch Clin Exp Ophthalmol 2007;245(8):1077–84.
44. Vermeulen N, Arijs I, Joossens S, et al. Anti-alpha-enolase antibodies in patients with inflammatory bowel disease. Clin Chem 2008;54:534–41.
45. Pancholi V. Multifunctional a-enolase: its role in diseases. Cell Mol Life Sci 2001;58:902–20.
46. Thirkill CE, Tait RC, Tyler NK, et al. Intraperitoneal cultivation of small-cell carcinoma induces expression of the retinal cancer-associated retinopathy antigen. Arch Ophthalmol 1993;111:974–8.
47. Bazhin AV, Shifrina ON, Savchenko MS, et al. Low titre autoantibodies against recoverin in sera of patients with small cell lung cancer but without a loss of vision. Lung Cancer 2001;34:99–104.
48. Polans A, Witkowska D, Haley T, et al. Recoverin, a photoreceptor-specific calcium-binding protein, is expressed by the tumor of a patient with cancer-associated retinopathy. Proc Natl Acad Sci U S A 1995;92:9176–80.
49. Matsubara S, Yamaji Y, Soto M, et al. Expression of a photoreceptor protein, recoverin, as a cancer-associated retinopathy autoantigen in human lung cancer cell lines. Br J Cancer 1996;74:1419–22.
50. Adamus G. Autoantibody-induced apoptosis as a possible mechanism of autoimmune retinopathy. Autoimmun Rev 2003;2(2):63–8.
51. Chen W, Elias RV, Cao W, et al. Anti-recoverin antibodies cause the apoptotic death of mammalian photoreceptor cells in vitro. J Neurosci Res 1999;57: 706–18.
52. Adamus G, Webb S, Shiraga S, et al. Anti-recoverin antibodies induce an increase in intracellular calcium, leading to apoptosis in retinal cells. J Autoimmun 2006;26:146–53.
53. Adamus G, Machnicki M, Elerding H, et al. Antibodies to recoverin induce apoptosis of photoreceptor and bipolar cells in vivo. J Autoimmun 1998;11: 523–33.
54. Adamus G, Machnicki M, Seigel GM. Apoptotic retinal cell death induced by antirecoverin autoantibodies of cancer-associated retinopathy. Invest Ophthalmol Vis Sci 1997;38:283–91.
55. Gery I, Chanaud 3rd NP, Anglade E. Recoverin is highly uveitogenic in Lewis rats. Invest Ophthalmol Vis Sci 1994;35:3342–5.
56. Lu Y, He S, Jia L, et al. Two mouse models for recoverin-associated autoimmune retinopathy. Mol Vis 2010;16:1936–48.
57. Williams RC, Peen E. Apoptosis and cell penetration by autoantibody may represent linked processes. Clin. Exp. Rheumatol 1999; 17:643–7.
58. Lei B, Bush RA, Milam AH, et al. Human melanoma-associated retinopathy (MAR) antibodies alter the retinal ON-response of the monkey ERG in vivo. Invest Ophthalmol Vis Sci 2000;41:262–6.
59. Adamus G, Chan CC. Experimental autoimmune uveitides: multiple antigens, diverse diseases. Int Rev Immunol 2002;21(2–3):209–29.
60. Hooks JJ, Tso MO, Detrick B. Retinopathies associated with antiretinal antibodies. Clin Diagn Lab Immunol 2001;8:853–8.
61. Chan JW. Paraneoplastic retinopathies and optic neuropathies. Surv Ophthalmol 2003;48:12–38.
62. Shapiro LR, Johnson CA. Quantitative evaluation of manual kinetic perimetry using computer simulation. Appl Opt 1990;29:1445–50.
63. Keltner JL, Johnson CA, Spurr JO, et al. Comparison of central and peripheral visual field properties in the optic neuritis treatment trial. Am J Ophthalmol 1999;128:543–53.
64. Heckenlively JR, Ferreyra HA. Autoimmune retinopathy: a review and summary. Semin Immunopathol 2008;30:127–34.
65. Heckenlively JR, Aptsiauri N, Nusinowitz S, et al. Investigations of antiretinal antibodies in pigmentary retinopathy and other retinal degenerations. Trans Am Ophthalmol Soc 1996;94:179–200.
66. Cherepanoff S, Mitchell P, Wang JJ, et al. Retinal autoantibody profile in early age-related macular degeneration: preliminary findings from the Blue Mountains Eye Study. Clin Experiment Ophthalmol 2006;34:590–5.
67. Joachim SC, Bruns K, Lackner KJ, et al. Analysis of IgG antibody patterns against retinal antigens and antibodies to alpha-crystallin, GFAP, and alpha-enolase in sera of patients with "wet" age-related macular degeneration. Graefes Arch Clin Exp Ophthalmol 2007;245:619–26.
68. Ko AC, Brinton JP, Mahajan VB, et al. Seroreactivity against aqueous-soluble and detergent-soluble retinal proteins in posterior uveitis. Arch Ophthalmol 2011;129:415–20.
69. Ocular Immunology Laboratory, Oregon Health & Science University [homepage on the Internet]. Portland, OR: OHS; no date [cited 2012 Feb]. http//www.ohsu.edu/xd/health/services/casey-eye/clinical-services/diagnostic-services/upload/Ocular-Immunology-Web-2.pdf.
70. Cao X, Bishop RJ, Forooghian F, et al. Autoimmune retinopathy in systemic lupus erythematosus: histopathologic features. Open Ophthalmol J 2009;28;3: 20–5.

71. Brown Jr J, Folk JC. Current controversies in the white dot syndromes. Multifocal choroiditis, punctate inner choroidopathy, and the diffuse subretinal fibrosis syndrome. Ocul Immunol Inflamm 1998;6(2):125–7.
72. Fine HF, Spaide RF, Ryan Jr EH, et al. Acute zonal occult outer retinopathy in patients with multiple evanescent white dot syndrome. Arch Ophthalmol 2009;127(1):66–70.
73. Jacobson SG, Morales DS, Sun XK, et al. Pattern of retinal dysfunction in acute zonal occult outer retinopathy. Ophthalmology 1995;102:1187–98.
74. Fujiwara T, Imamura Y, Giovinazzo VJ, et al. Fundus autofluorescence and optical coherence tomographic findings in acute zonal occult outer retinopathy. Retina 2010;30:1206–16.
75. Yeh S, Forooghian F, Wong WT, et al. Fundus autofluorescence imaging of the white dot syndromes. Arch Ophthalmol 2010;128:46–56.
76. Galbraith, GM, Emerson D, Fudenberg HH, et al. Antibodies to neurofilament protein in retinitis pigmentosa. J. Clin. Invest 1986;78:865–9.
77. Chan, CC, Nussenblatt RB, Kim MK, et al. Immunopathology of ocular onchocerciasis. 2. Antiretinal autoantibodies in serum and ocular fluids. Ophthalmology 1987;94:439–43.
78. Sen HN, Chan CC, Caruso RC, et al. Waldenström's macroglobulinemia-associated retinopathy. Ophthalmology 2004;111:535–9.
79. Mahdi N, Faia LJ, Goodwin J, et al. A case of autoimmune retinopathy associated with thyroid carcinoma. Ocul Immunol Inflamm 2010;18:322–3.
80. Kaveri SV, Lacroix-Desmazes S, Bayry J. The antiinflammatory IgG. N Engl J Med 2008;17;359:307–9.
81. Le Hoang P, Cassoux N, George F, et al. Intravenous immunoglobulin (IVIg) for the treatment of birdshot retinochoroidopathy. Ocul Immunol Inflamm 2000;8:49–57.
82. Jabs DA, Rosenbaum JT, Foster CS, et al. Guidelines for the use of immunosuppressive drugs in patients with ocular inflammatory disorders: recommendations of an expert panel. Am J Ophthalmol 2000;130:492–513.
83. Jacobson DM, Thirkill CE, Tipping SJ. A clinical triad to diagnose paraneoplastic retinopathy. Ann Neurol 1990;28(2):162–7. Ophthalmol 1998;126:230–7.

Chapter 78

Sarcoidosis

Yasir Jamal Sepah, Douglas A. Jabs, Quan Dong Nguyen

Sarcoidosis is a multisystem granulomatous disorder of unknown etiology characterized by intrathoracic involvement. The disease was first described as early as 1869, but its protean presentation and clinical course still make sarcoidosis a diagnostic and therapeutic challenge for modern-day physicians. Ocular involvement is common and has been previously reported to occur in approximately 15–25% of patients with sarcoidosis.[1,2] However, some series have reported higher rates. Posterior-segment manifestations may account for up to 28% of the lesions seen in patients with ocular sarcoid. Most large case series of patients with uveitis report that approximately 5% of patients with uveitis have biopsy-confirmed systemic sarcoidosis.[3–6]

GENERAL CONSIDERATIONS

Epidemiology

Sarcoidosis is worldwide in its distribution, but it is most frequently recognized in developed countries where adequate diagnostic facilities are available. Although all races are affected, series in the USA generally show that the disease is more prevalent in blacks than in whites. It has also been noted that the prevalence of sarcoidosis in black populations of Africa and South America is less than what has been observed in the African American population.[7–9] Both sexes are affected, with the overall frequency showing a very slight excess of females (approximately 60%). Sarcoidosis is a disease of young adults, with almost three-fourths of cases occurring in those younger than 40 years of age. Children may be affected, but this is uncommon.[6–10] The clinical course of childhood sarcoidosis is often atypical; that is, there is less frequent pulmonary involvement and more frequent extrathoracic disease.[11,12] A recent study of 46 caucasian children from Denmark reported the four most frequent presenting symptoms to be erythema nodosum (22%), iridocyclitis (22%), peripheral lymphadenopathy (15%), and cutaneous sarcoidosis (7%). Overall, a good prognosis was observed. Moreover, erythema nodosum was generally associated with good outcomes while central nervous system (CNS) involvement was associated with a poor prognosis.[13] These children must be differentiated from children with juvenile rheumatoid arthritis and those with familial juvenile systemic granulomatosis[14–17] because of the similarity of ocular and articular involvement. Many cases of familial juvenile systemic granulomatosis are misdiagnosed as childhood sarcoidosis.[18]

Etiology and pathogenesis

The etiology of sarcoidosis is unknown. Multiple etiologies have been proposed, including a variety of infectious agents, allergy to pine pollen and peanut dust, chewing pine pitch, and hypersensitivity to chemicals such as beryllium or zirconium. To date, there is no conclusive evidence to implicate any of these as an etiologic agent. Familial studies and human leukocyte antigen (HLA) typing have suggested a possible genetic predisposition, but these studies are far from conclusive.[19] A cooperative multicenter study, A Case Control Etiologic Study of Sarcoidosis (ACCESS), enrolled 736 biopsy-confirmed cases from 10 centers in the USA and suggested a genetic predisposition for sarcoidosis, presenting evidence for the allelic variation at the HLA-DRB1 locus as a contributing factor to the disease. The most significant finding was the relationship between *DRB1*0401* and eye involvement ($P \leq 0.0008$; odds ratio (OR) 3.49) in the study population. Although only 2% of blacks had a *DRB1*0401* allele, a similar OR was present in both blacks and whites.[19]

Patients with sarcoidosis are characterized by depression of delayed-type hypersensitivity, reflected by T-cell anergy, and skin tests that are often negative. Peripheral blood lymphocytes from patients with sarcoidosis show diminished responses to mitogens.

Bronchoalveolar lavage has enabled investigators to determine the immunologic events at the area of active disease in the lungs. These studies have shown entirely different results from peripheral blood lymphocytes. In the lungs, there is an excess of helper T lymphocytes (CD4+). These activated helper T cells spontaneously secrete lymphokines, including interleukin-2 (IL-2), and will polyclonally activate B cells to produce immunoglobulins. These studies have been interpreted to show that an active T-cell-driven immunologic response occurs at the target organ site and eventually leads to granuloma formation.[21,22] Studies of bronchoalveolar lavage fluids have suggested that macrophages may also play a role in the pathogenesis of pulmonary sarcoidosis by inducing changes in the pulmonary microvasculature.[23]

Immunohistologic studies of biopsy tissue from patients with sarcoidosis have demonstrated the presence of cells of macrophage lineage and activated T cells in the granuloma. The vast majority of lymphocytes are T cells of the helper subset (CD4+) and express activation markers, including class II antigens and the IL-2 receptor.[24–26]

Clinical features

The organs most frequently involved in sarcoidosis are the lungs, lymph nodes and spleen, skin, eyes, nervous system, and bones and joints[1,19,27–29] (Table 78.1).

Intrathoracic sarcoidosis

Several series have demonstrated that intrathoracic involvement is the most common manifestation of sarcoidosis and occurs in 90% of patients. An abnormality on chest radiograph examination is evident at the onset of sarcoidosis in almost all patients. Chest radiograph abnormalities have been classified according to a simple staging system, which closely correlates with the eventual outcome. Stage 0 is characterized by a normal chest radiograph; stage 1 is characterized by bilateral hilar lymphadenopathy without pulmonary infiltration and is seen in 65% of patients with pulmonary sarcoidosis; stage 2 is characterized by hilar lymphadenopathy associated with pulmonary infiltration and is seen in 22% of patients with sarcoid; stage 3 sarcoid is characterized by pulmonary infiltration with fibrosis but without bilateral hilar adenopathy and occurs in 13% of patients. The overall rates of radiographic resolution are 59%, 39%, and 38% for stage 1, 2, and 3 disease, respectively.[1]

Extrapulmonary lesions

Involvement of the reticuloendothelial system, particularly the extrapulmonary lymph nodes or spleen, or both, is common and occurs in 23–37% of patients with sarcoidosis. Biopsy of a palpable lymph node is often used for histologic confirmation of the diagnosis of sarcoidosis (see below). Skin lesions occur frequently in sarcoidosis and include erythema nodosum, lupus pernio, maculopapular rashes, cutaneous plaques, and subcutaneous nodules. Lupus pernio (dusky-purple infiltration of the skin of the nose) and sarcoid plaques are typically associated with chronic disease, whereas erythema nodosum (especially in the presence of polyarthritis) is typically associated with acute sarcoid or Lofgren syndrome.[30] Neurosarcoidosis occurs in 2–7% of patients with sarcoid. Facial palsy is the most frequent manifestation of neurosarcoidosis. Other presentations include other cranial nerve palsies, papilledema, peripheral neuropathy, meningitis, space-occupying cerebral lesions, cavernous sinus syndrome,[31] and endocrine disorders such as hypopituitarism or diabetes insipidus resulting from space-occupying lesions. Musculoskeletal involvement includes bone cysts in patients with chronic sarcoid, polyarthralgias, and periarthritis in patients with acute sarcoid, and, less commonly, myopathy from granulomatous lesions within muscles.[1,19,29,31–35]

Table 78.1 Organ system involvement in sarcoidosis

Organ system	Frequency (%)
Intrathoracic	84–93
Hilar nodes	60–77
Lung parenchyma	40–56
Lymph nodes	23–37
Eyes	11–32
Skin	12–27
Erythema nodosum	4–31
Spleen	1–18
Bones	2–9
Parotid	5–8
Central nervous system	2–7

Investigations

Radiological evaluation

Chest X-ray

The single best test for the evaluation of patients with suspected sarcoidosis is the chest film, since it is abnormal in approximately 90% of patients with sarcoid. Although the chest film is the best test for detecting the presence of sarcoidosis, it does not unequivocally establish the diagnosis, though neither does a negative chest X-ray rule out the disease.

High-resolution computed tomography (CT)

The CT findings in sarcoidosis can be divided into three main categories:

1. Parenchymal findings
2. Large and small airway findings
3. Mediastinal findings.

The presence of diffuse nodular opacities (1–5 mm) with irregular borders in the perilymphatic distribution typically in the upper and middle lung zones is the most common and almost universal finding in the lung parenchyma.[36] The presence of architectural distortion is also exclusive to sarcoidosis as opposed to other diseases with perilymphatic distribution.[37] "Sarcoid galaxy sign," which is a collection of multiple granulomas and gives the impression of an opacity, is present in 10–20% of patients with pulmonary sarcoidosis.[38] Extensive fibrosis, mostly distributed in the upper and middle zones associated with architectural distortion, is also seen in 20–25% of cases. The presence of air trapping at end expiration has been reported frequently. Terasaki et al.[39] reported air trapping on expiration in 45 (98%) of their study patients. Devies et al.[40] demonstrated that the extent of air trapping on expiration was correlated with the pulmonary function of the patient.

Large-airway involvement is seen in 1–3% of patients with pulmonary sarcoidosis. This typically presents with tracheal stenosis due to granuloma formation within the tracheal mucosa or submucosa or secondary to lymph node compression from the outside. More than 60% of patients with sarcoidosis are reported to have smooth thickening of the smaller airways.[36]

The classic radiologic finding in the mediastinum of a sarcoid patient is symmetric bilateral hilar adenopathy with some form of paratracheal adenopathy. Symmetry is an important diagnostic feature of the sarcoid hilar adenopathy as it is uncommon in the major diagnostic alternatives, including tuberculosis and lymphoma.[36]

Gallium scan

Gallium-67 is a radioactive isotope with a half-life of 78 hours and is administered intravenously to patients as Ga-citrate. In the vascular system, the half-life of Ga drops to 12 hours. Ga is taken up by activated macrophages in the epithelioid cell granulomas. Such uptake is detected by gamma cameras 48 hours after injection and is assessed in the liver, spleen, thorax, eyes, and lacrimal and salivary glands. Scanning has also been suggested as a useful diagnostic test for sarcoidosis. The test is again nonspecific, and gallium uptake is seen in other diseases, including Sjögren syndrome, tuberculosis, radiation therapy, and lymphoma. It has been proposed that the combination of gallium scanning and an elevated angiotensin-converting enzyme (ACE) level is highly specific for sarcoidosis, but these studies have employed patients specifically chosen for very active sarcoid.[41] As such, these tests may be of less utility in a patient with presumed sarcoid uveitis and no obvious evidence of systemic sarcoidosis. The best use of these tests may be in following patients with active disease.[42,43]

In a study of 22 patients with sarcoid uveitis compared to 70 patients with uveitis secondary to other disorders, Power et al.[44] reported that the sensitivity and specificity of an elevated ACE alone in diagnosing sarcoidosis were 73% and 83%, respectively, and that the sensitivity and specificity of the gallium scan alone were 91% and 84%, respectively. Using the combination of a gallium scan and an elevated serum ACE, the specificity for diagnosing sarcoidosis was 100% and the sensitivity was 73%. The authors concluded that the combination of serum ACE level and whole-body gallium scan might be useful for diagnosing sarcoidosis in patients with uveitis. However, because of the study design inherent in investigating the values of these tests, their actual utility in patients with normal chest radiographs and without clinical evidence of sarcoid remains uncertain. Furthermore, because the reported prevalence of sarcoid uveitis is approximately 5% among patients with biopsy-confirmed systemic sarcoidosis,[3–6] routine screening of all patients with uveitis by both ACE levels and gallium scan may have a low positive predictive value and, therefore, may be misleading. Nevertheless, in selected patients in whom sarcoidosis is highly likely, these tests may be useful.

Magnetic resonance imaging (MRI) and positive emission tomography scan (PET)

Fluorodeoxyglucose PET (^{18}F-FDG PET) scanning has become of great importance in the study and follow-up of patients with cancer. However, in recent years, its role in the diagnosis and management of other conditions such as sarcoidosis has been explored. Although the sensitivity of a whole-body PET scan to detect sarcoid lesions is 80–100%, the findings are nonspecific and histology is required to confirm or rule out sarcoidosis. MRI has been successfully used in the evaluation of organ-specific damage in patients with sarcoidosis, especially cardiac and musculoskeletal tissue.[41,44–48]

Histology

Histologic confirmation (Table 78.2) is generally required to establish the diagnosis of sarcoid. The only clinical situation when diagnosis of sarcoidosis can be strongly considered reliably without biopsy is Löfgren syndrome (see below). Otherwise, biopsy should be done. Sites most often biopsied include the lungs, mediastinal lymph nodes, skin, peripheral lymph nodes, liver, and conjunctiva. Biopsy of clinically evident skin lesions or palpable lymph nodes is frequently performed because of the high yield and low morbidity. Fiberoptic bronchoscopy with transbronchial lung biopsy is positive in 80% of patients with intrapulmonary sarcoidosis. This procedure is routinely performed by pulmonary physicians and has a relatively low morbidity. The next step in such a scenario is cervical mediastinoscopy, which is both highly invasive and an expensive procedure. The requirement of general anesthesia further increases the chances of complications from the procedure. From the patient's perspective it is important that further possibilities of minimally invasive techniques for the diagnosis of sarcoidosis are explored. Development of linear echoendoscopes and subsequent procedures (endoscopic ultrasound-guided fine-needle aspiration (EUS-FNA) and endobronchial ultrasound-guided transbronchial needle aspiration (EBUS-TBNA)) has opened new diagnostic possibilities for sarcoidosis. Both techniques allow real-time monitoring of the needle. Several investigators have reported a high sensitivity of 72–85% for EBUS-TBNA and minimal complications. In a randomized control trial (RCT) Tremblay et al.[49] have shown that the diagnostic yield of EBUS-guided TBNA (95.8%) versus the conventional TBNA (73.1%) was 22.7% greater. Sensitivity and specificity were 60.9% and 100%, respectively, in the standard TBNA group, and 83.3% and 100%, respectively, in the EBUS-guided TBNA group (absolute increase in sensitivity of 22.5%). EUS-FNA was used for diagnosis of sarcoidosis and had a yield of 82% and sensitivity of 89–94% by assessing noncaseating granulomas in mediastinal nodes.[50] The liver biopsy is often positive in patients with sarcoidosis, but the finding of granulomatous lesions on liver biopsy must be interpreted with caution, as they can be produced by other disorders. Other potential biopsy sites include peripheral lymph nodes and minor salivary glands.

Conjunctival biopsies are positive in 25–57% of patients with histologically documented sarcoidosis. Variations in these reports are the result of whether clinically evident lesions are biopsied or whether a "blind" conjunctival biopsy is performed. However, the yield can be increased by techniques such as bilateral conjunctival biopsies and serial sectioning of the specimens, and careful inspection of the conjunctiva for any visibly evident nodules which can be biopsied. Transconjunctival lacrimal gland biopsy can also be used for histologic diagnosis, but the procedure is not performed routinely.[42,51]

Immunology

The Kveim skin test was a simple, specific, outpatient skin test using human sarcoid tissue. It was positive in 78% of patients with sarcoidosis and was helpful in delineating multisystemic sarcoidosis from other granulomatous disorders. The antigen was a saline suspension of human sarcoid tissue prepared from the spleen of a patient suffering from active sarcoidosis. This material was injected intradermally, and the site inspected for nodule formation after 3–6 weeks. A palpable nodule was biopsied, and the finding of noncaseating granulomas on biopsy established the diagnosis of sarcoid.[19,52,53] Concerns about the injection of human tissue, with its potential for disease transmission, have essentially eliminated the use of the Kveim test.

Noninvasive tests

Multiple attempts have been made to find noninvasive tests that could be both sensitive and specific in the diagnosis of sarcoidosis. These have included measurement of serum calcium, urinary calcium, serum lysozyme, and serum immunoglobulins. Although all these may be abnormal in patients with sarcoid, they are nonspecific and nondiagnostic. The serum ACE level has been touted as a useful measurement in the diagnosis of sarcoidosis. The ACE level is frequently abnormal in patients

Table 78.2 Yield of different biopsy sites in the diagnosis of sarcoidosis

Technique	Study	Positive/total	(%)
Liver biopsy	Branson and Park (1954)[103]	48/63	76
	Israel and Sones (1964)[52]	22/24	92
	Klatskin (1976)[104]	17/23	94
Scalene lymph node biopsy	Beahrs et al. (1957)[105]	20/34	59
	Rochlin and Enterline (1958)[106]	27/34	79
	Williams and Webb (1962)[107]	32/39	82
Scalene fat pad biopsy	Romer et al. (1973)[108]	115/142	81
	Rasmussen and Neukirch (1976)[109]	41/99	52
Mediastinoscopy	Carlens (1964)[110]	118/123	96
	Palva (1964)[111]	27/28	96
	Romer et al. (1973)[108]	47/48	98
Lung biopsy, transbronchial	Koerner et al. (1975)[112]	21/23	91
Bronchoscope	Koontz (1978)[113]	74/104	71
Conjunctival biopsy	Crick et al. (1961)[114]	20/79	25
	Bornstein et al. (1962)[115]	16/64	25
	Kahn et al. (1977)[116]	20/60	33
	Solomon et al. (1978)[117]	8/15	57
	Garver (unpublished, 1980)	10/21	48
	Nichols et al. (1980)[118]	30/55	55
	Karcioglu and Brear (1985)[119]	14/28	50
Minor salivary gland biopsy	Nessan and Jacoway (1979)[120]	44/75	58

(Modified from Green WR. Inflammatory diseases and conditions of the eye. In: Spencer WH, editor. Ophthalmic pathology: an atlas and textbook, vol. 3. Philadelphia, PA: WB Saunders; 1986.)

with active sarcoidosis and appears to reflect the total-body granuloma content in such patients. As such, it may be useful in following patients with active sarcoid.[43,52,54] However, it is not diagnostic of sarcoidosis and appears to be of limited utility in the diagnostic dilemma of patients with possible sarcoid uveitis but a normal chest film.

For following patients with active intrapulmonary sarcoid, pulmonary function tests, particularly forced vital capacity, forced expiratory volume, and diffusing capacity, are far more useful. Changes in pulmonary function tests are often used to follow patients with sarcoidosis and to adjust the corticosteroid dosage.[27]

Jabs and Johns[55] reported that over 80% of patients with ocular sarcoid had their ocular lesions at the time of diagnosis of sarcoidosis, and Hunter and Foster[48] reported that 3% of patients with uveitis were diagnosed as having sarcoid after the initial evaluation for a systemic disease revealed no diagnosable systemic disorder. Although patients who present with uveitis should be evaluated for sarcoid, repetitive workups appear to have limited value unless new symptoms arise.

COURSE AND PROGNOSIS

There appear to be two distinct paradigms of sarcoidosis, acute and chronic, with differences in onset, natural history, course, prognosis, and response to treatment. Acute sarcoidosis tends to have an abrupt, explosive onset in young patients and to go into spontaneous remission within 2 years of onset. Acute iritis is often seen in acute sarcoidosis. The response to systemic corticosteroids is generally quite good, and the long-term complications are minimal. Löfgren's syndrome comprises erythema nodosum, bilateral hilar adenopathy, and acute iritis; it generally has a good long-term prognosis.[1,19,29]

Chronic sarcoidosis is defined as disease persistence of greater than 2 years. The disease may have a more insidious onset and generally has intrapulmonary involvement with chronic pulmonary disease as a major source of morbidity. Corticosteroid therapy is generally required and may be prolonged. Chronic ocular disease, particularly chronic uveitis, may be a feature of chronic sarcoidosis.[1,19,27,29,55]

The overall mortality from sarcoidosis is 3–5%, but neurosarcoid is associated with a mortality of 10%.[47] Corticosteroids are the mainstay of treatment, although antimalarial agents can be used for patients with mucocutaneous lesions. Patients with hilar adenopathy without abnormalities of pulmonary function and without intrapulmonary infiltration may not need systemic corticosteroid treatment.

OCULAR MANIFESTATIONS

Multiple studies have documented the common occurrence of ocular involvement in sarcoidosis and the various ocular manifestations of sarcoid. Frequency estimates vary and have ranged as high as 50%.[47] However, most series report rates that are generally closer to 15–28%.[1,19,29,32,55,56] These differences undoubtedly relate to case ascertainment methods, the patient population studied, definitions of ophthalmic involvement, and the nature of the evaluation conducted. Racial differences influence not only the mode of presentation for ocular sarcoidosis but also the frequency of patients with ocular involvement. When the same diagnostic criteria were applied, Japanese patients with sarcoidosis were found to have ocular disease six times more frequently than Finnish patients, and they were also more likely to present with ocular symptoms of sarcoidosis. In the USA, the African American population is twice as likely to have ocular disease as opposed to caucasian patients. Furthermore, high frequencies of ocular involvement are reported when keratoconjunctivitis sicca is sought carefully and included as evidence of lacrimal involvement in sarcoidosis.[47]

Sarcoidosis may affect most of the ocular structures, as well as the orbit and adnexa. Ocular lesions described in sarcoidosis include: anterior uveitis, iris nodules, conjunctival nodules, scleral nodule,[57] and corneal disease with either band keratopathy or interstitial keratitis; posterior segment disease, including chorioretinitis, periphlebitis, chorioretinal nodules, vitreous inflammation, and retinal neovascularization; and orbital disease, including involvement of the lacrimal gland, nasolacrimal duct, optic nerve, and orbital granulomas. The various ocular lesions along with the prevalence estimates are outlined in Table 78.3.

Table 78.3 Ocular manifestations of sarcoidosis

Ocular manifestations	Frequency in patients with ocular sarcoid (%)
Anterior segment disease	
Anterior uveitis	66–70
Acute	15–32
Chronic	39–53
Iris nodules	11–16
Conjunctival lesions	7–47
Cornea	
Band keratopathy	5–14
Interstitial keratitis	1
Posterior segment disease	
Vitritis	3–25
Periphlebitis	10–17
Chorioretinitis	11
Choroidal nodules	4–5
Retinal neovascularization	1–5
Orbital and other disease	26
Lacrimal gland	7–60
Keratoconjunctivitis sicca	5–60
Enlargement	7–28
Orbital granuloma	1
Optic nerve granuloma	<1–7

Anterior uveitis is the most common ocular manifestation and occurs in approximately two-thirds of patients with ocular sarcoid. The uveitis may be an acute iridocyclitis or a chronic granulomatous uveitis. Acute iridocyclitis is most often seen in patients with acute sarcoid but can be seen in those with chronic sarcoid as well. The prognosis is worse for those with chronic disease, who may develop complications such as secondary glaucoma, band keratopathy, cataracts, macular edema, and visual loss. Iris nodules are occasionally seen in association with anterior uveitis in patients with sarcoidosis.

Conjunctival and corneal lesions in patients with sarcoidosis are less common. These are generally described as conjunctival nodules, which on biopsy reveal the characteristic granuloma formation of sarcoidosis. Occasionally a nonspecific or phlyctenular keratoconjunctivitis is described in association with other mucocutaneous lesions of sarcoidosis. The cornea is infrequently involved but may develop band keratopathy either because of chronic uveitis or because of hypercalcemia. In addition, occasional cases of interstitial keratitis in association with sarcoidosis have been described.

The frequency of orbital, and particularly lacrimal gland, lesions varies widely among series and depends on the patient selection and investigations used. Clinical enlargement is present in less than one-third of patients with ocular sarcoid, but when sought, keratoconjunctivitis sicca may be present in a greater percentage.[29,32,47,55-57] Orbital granuloma, independent of the lacrimal gland, occurs infrequently.[58-60] Massive lacrimal gland enlargement simulating a lacrimal gland tumor may occur and require biopsy.

POSTERIOR SEGMENT DISEASE

Posterior segment lesions are reported to occur in approximately 14–28% of patients with ocular sarcoid.[6,13,29,32,46,47,55,56,61,62] The actual frequency may be higher, since most patients with posterior segment disease also have anterior uveitis. Posterior lesions include vitritis, chorioretinitis, periphlebitis, vascular occlusion, retinal neovascularization, and optic nerve head granulomas.

Vitreous infiltration in patients with sarcoidosis can appear as cellular infiltration, often as a nonspecific vitritis. More classically, however, the lesions demonstrate clumping and an accumulation of vitreous debris, called either "snowballs" or a "string of pearls" (Fig. 78.1). These lesions may be somewhat similar in appearance to those seen in pars planitis, although snowball formation is generally not seen in sarcoid uveitis. Sarcoid granulomata can also present in the optic nerve, peripheral retina, pars plana, and anterior choroid, and can be imaged by high-resolution ultrasound biomicroscopy as different forms of uveal thickening.[63]

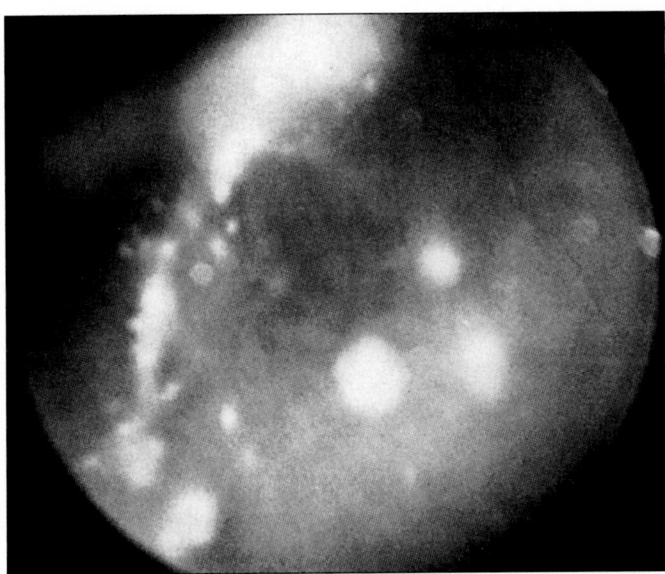

Fig. 78.1 Vitreous inflammation in a patient with sarcoidosis.

Perivascular sheathing is the second most common finding and occurs in 10–17% of patients with ocular sarcoid. It is generally a midperipheral periphlebitis without significant vascular occlusion (Figs 78.2 and 78.3). However, several series have documented the occasional occurrence of occlusive retinal vascular disease, particularly branch retinal vein occlusion (Fig. 78.4). Central retinal vein occlusion is less common. Histologic studies have demonstrated vascular compromise by the granulomatous inflammatory material.[64,65] More severe forms of periphlebitis have been called "candle-wax drippings." Sanders and Shilling[66] have described an "acute retinopathy of sarcoidosis" with extensive perivascular sheathing, vascular occlusion, and intraretinal hemorrhages. These cases were complicated by subsequent retinal neovascularization.

Deeper chorioretinal lesions have also been reported. These can vary in size from small "Dalen–Fuchs-like" granulomas to large choroidal nodules simulating a metastatic tumor. If located in the macular region, these lesions can cause severe visual loss. Corticosteroid therapy has been able to shrink these lesions. Exudative retinal detachments are rarely seen in patients with sarcoid uveitis but do occur in those patients with large nodular chorioretinal granulomas. These detachments appear to be an overlying detachment of the neurosensory retina and may resolve with oral corticosteroid therapy.[5,67]

Visual loss can occur from epiretinal membrane formation and cystoid macular edema in patients with sarcoidosis. Once the inflammation has been controlled, pars plana vitrectomy with membrane peeling may have a beneficial effect on restoring vision, although development of cataract and membrane recurrence may require additional surgeries.[68,69] In one small uncontrolled case series, triamcinolone acetonide was injected into the vitreous cavity to assist the visualization of the vitreous for the vitrectomy,[70] but the role of this approach is uncertain.

Peripheral retinal neovascularization or neovascularization of the optic nerve head is present in less than 5% of patients with

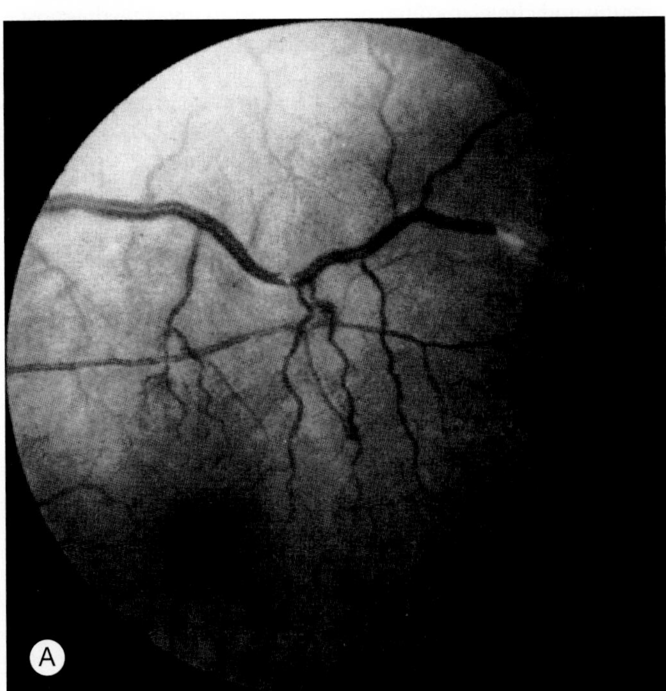

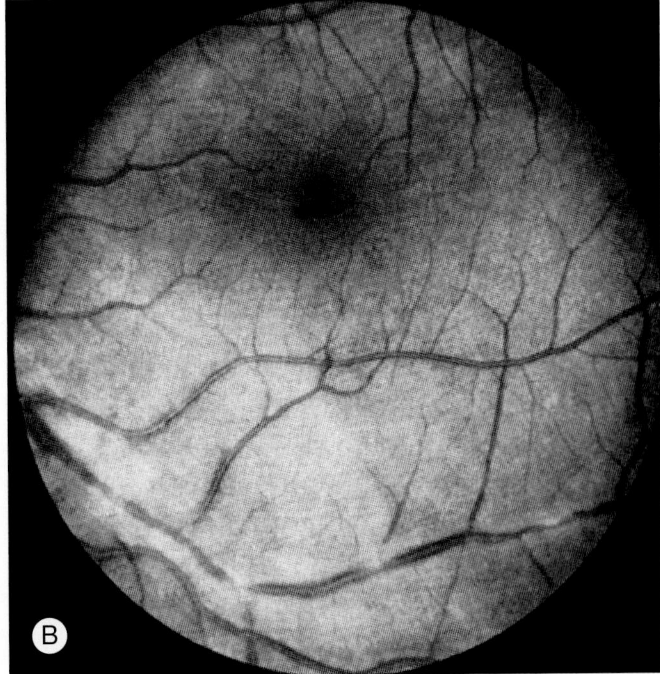

Fig. 78.2 (A and B) Perivascular sheathing in a patient with sarcoidosis. (Reproduced with permission from Green WR. Inflammatory diseases and conditions of the eye. In: Spencer WH, editor. Ophthalmic pathology: an atlas and textbook, vol. 3. Philadelphia, PA: WB Saunders; 1986.)

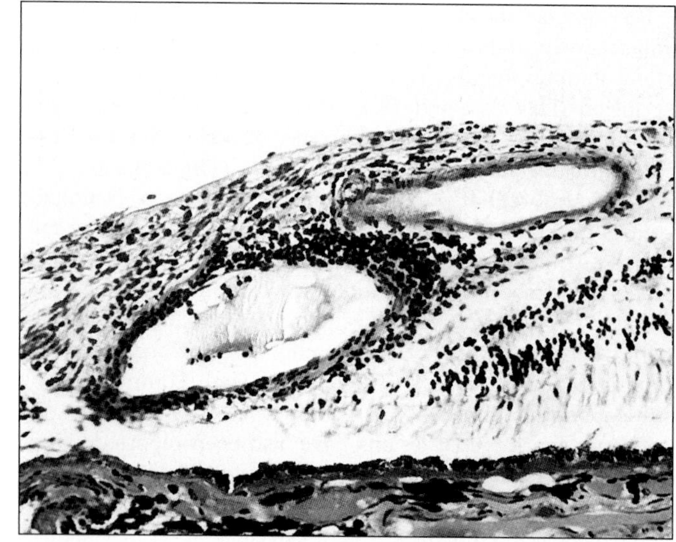

Fig. 78.3 Histopathology of periphlebitis in a patient with sarcoidosis (periodic acid–Schiff reaction; ×225). (Reproduced with permission from Green WR. Inflammatory diseases and conditions of the eye. In: Spencer WH, editor. Ophthalmic pathology: an atlas and textbook, vol. 3. Philadelphia, PA: WB Saunders; 1986.)

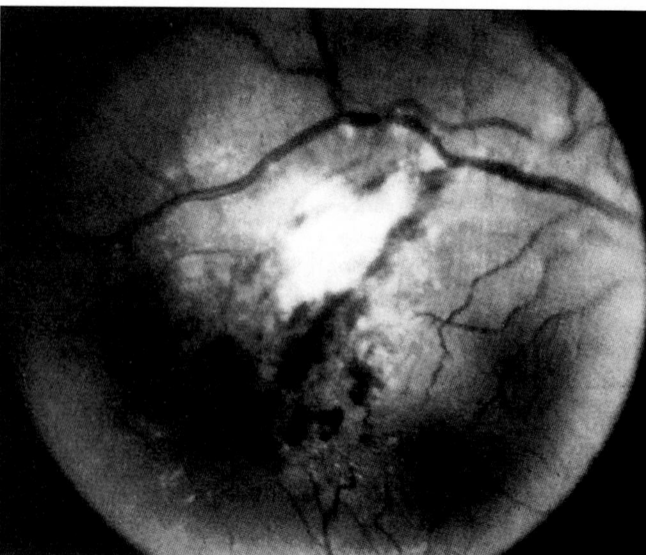

Fig. 78.4 Perifoveal branch vein occlusion in a patient with sarcoidosis.

ocular sarcoid, but can be associated with significant visual loss due to vitreous hemorrhage. Peripheral retinal neovascularization is generally seen in patients with a defined vaso-occlusive disorder such as a branch retinal vein occlusion. The peripheral neovascular lesions may even simulate a sea fan, similar to that seen in sickle-cell disease. Neovascularization of the disc may also develop after a branch or central vein occlusion. The rare occurrence of peripapillary choroidal neovascularization in the absence of uveitis or optic nerve disease has been reported, and described to be responsive to oral corticosteroids.[70] Doxanas and coworkers[71] described a patient with sarcoidosis and a steroid-responsive neovascularization of the optic nerve head without retinal nonperfusion (Fig. 78.5). Hoogstede and Copper[65] described one case of subretinal neovascularization, which they attributed to sarcoid uveitis. Duker et al.[72] reported the clinical features of proliferative sarcoid retinopathy in 11 eyes of seven patients. In these cases the new retinal vessels were associated with concomitant peripheral retinal capillary nonperfusion. The authors suggested that in these patients capillary nonperfusion secondary to microvascular shutdown, rather than a direct effect of inflammation, was the stimulus for the formation of retinal neovascularization.

It has been reported that when posterior-segment involvement is seen in patients with sarcoid uveitis, there is an increased frequency of CNS involvement. In a retrospective review of the literature, Gould and Kaufman[73] suggested that the prevalence of CNS involvement increased from 2% to 30% when fundus lesions were found. However, Spalton and Sanders[74] found no such association, thus leaving the association not well confirmed.

Optic nerve involvement, particularly multiple granulomas of the optic nerve head, occur in 0.5–7.0% of patients with ocular sarcoid[29,32,53,55,74] (Fig. 78.6). Histologic descriptions have shown granuloma formation[53,75] (Fig. 78.7). Optic disc edema without granulomatous invasion of the optic nerve head may be seen in patients either with chronic uveitis or with papilledema[34] from CNS sarcoid. Occasionally, isolated sarcoid optic neuropathy (optic atrophy, optic neuritis, optic disc edema) may occur and may be the first manifestation of neurosarcoidosis.[76–78]

In addition to these conventionally observable lesions, Mizuno and Takahashi[79] have used cycloscopy to document the common occurrence of lesions in the ciliary processes of patients with intraocular sarcoidosis. In their series, nodules of the ciliary processes were seen in 41% of eyes, waxy exudates in 24%, and cyclitic membrane-like exudates in 3%. Only 20% of eyes with intraocular sarcoid had no observable lesions.

DIAGNOSIS

Ocular sarcoidosis can present as a myraid of signs and symptoms. Such variability in presentation makes the diagnosis challenging and clinicians often need to resort to invasive diagnostic techniques in order to rule out or establish the diagnosis. In 2006 the scientific community came together at the first International Workshop on Ocular Sarcoidosis (IWOS) in Tokyo, Japan and established criteria for the diagnosis of ocular sarcoidosis when ocular changes are present in the presence or absence of clinical signs of systemic disease. The IWOS diagnostic criteria consist of seven clinical and five laboratory investigations. The IWOS diagnostic criteria allow ophthalmologists to arrive at one of the following four conclusions with a minimally invasive approach: (1) definite; (2) presumed; (3) probable; and (4) possible ocular sarcoidosis. A summary of the IWOS diagnostic criteria and laboratory investigation is given in Table 78.4. A proposed outline to the approach in evaluating a patient for possible ocular sarcoid is shown in Fig. 78.8.

One concern that ophthalmologists may have using the IWOS criteria would be that it was developed based on the information available from the Japanese population and the criteria may not be valid in other ethnicities. However, results from a recent survey of 24 uveitis specialists from around the world suggest that a significant number of ophthalmologists use the IWOS criteria to establish a diagnosis of ocular sarcoidosis.[80] Employing the IWOS diagnostic criteria allows for diagnosis in the absence of a biopsy, provides information for both the clinician and patient with regard to prognosis, and encourages

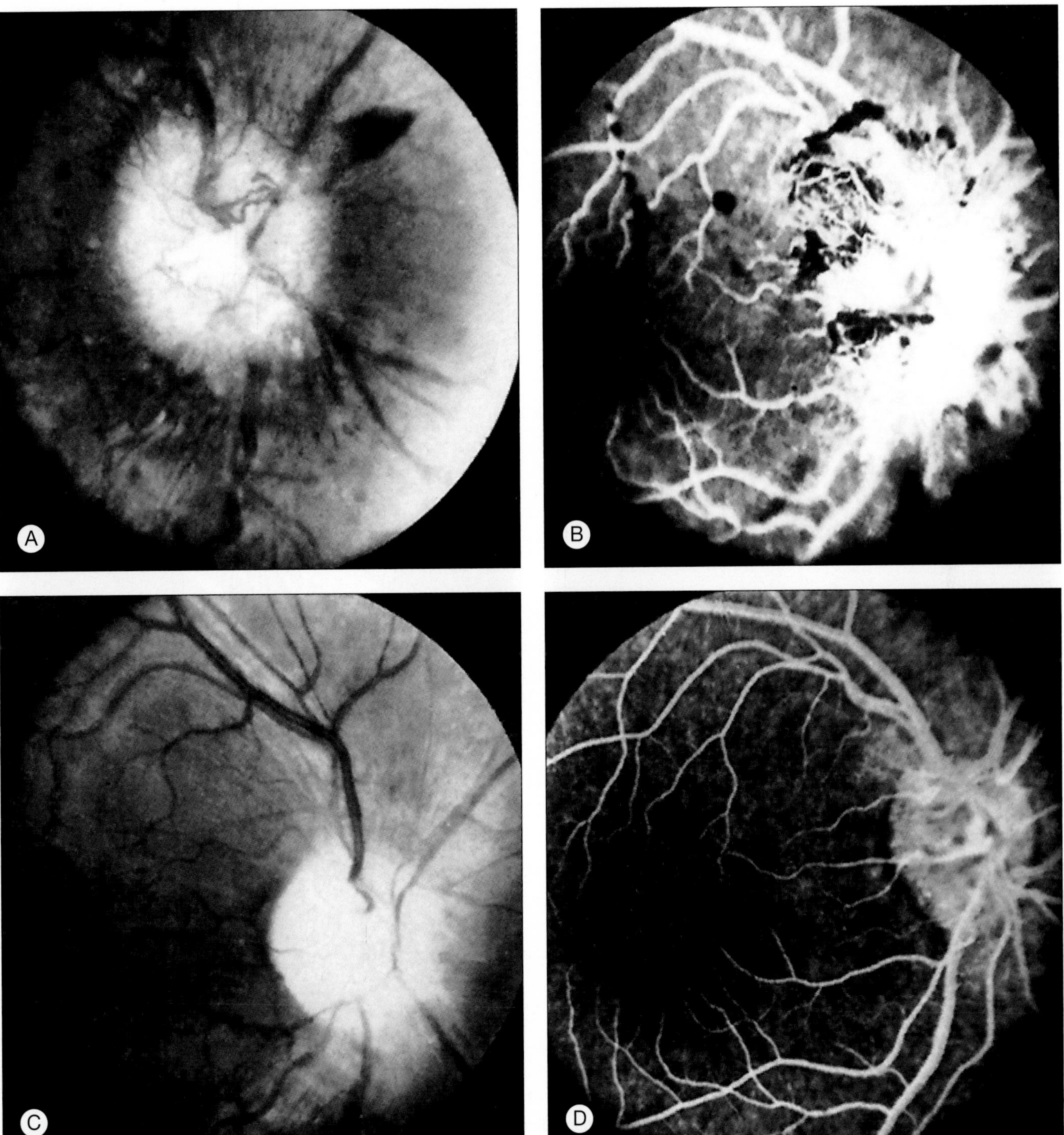

Fig. 78.5 Neovascularization of the optic nerve in a patient with sarcoidosis. Fundus photography (A), and fluorescein angiogram (B), right eye, and fundus photograph (E) and fluorescein angiogram (F), left eye, before steroid treatment. Fundus photograph (C) and fluorescein angiogram (D), right eye, and fundus photograph (G).

Continued

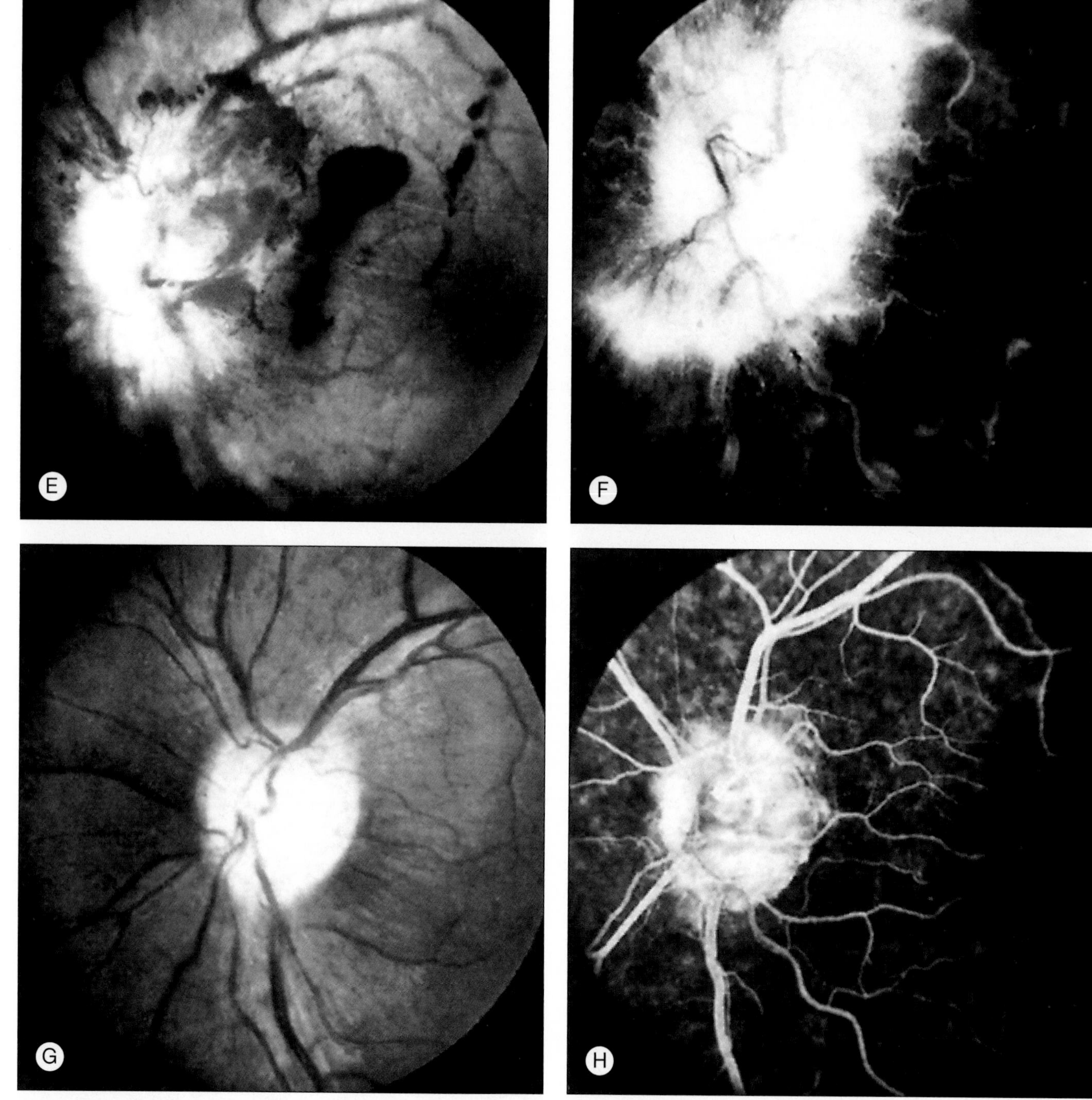

Fig. 78.5 Cont'd Fluorescein angiogram (H), left eye, after treatment, demonstrating resolution of disc neovascularization. (Reproduced with permission from Doxanas MT, Kelley JS, Prout TE. Sarcoidosis with neovascularization of the optic nerve head. Am J Ophthalmol 1980;90: 347–51.)

nonspecialists to consider sarcoidosis as a putative diagnosis. Although there are limitations of the IWOS diagnostic criteria, they certainly help to limit the investigations that a patient with suspected sarcoidosis may have to undergo and help the caregiver to formulate a standardized approach towards establishing the diagnosis.

As is the case in any other form of uveitis, there needs to be a systematic approach to establishing a diagnosis of ocular sarcoidosis and ruling out its major differentials. Patients may present with no systemic disease. Once the clinician suspects any form of uveitis, it is extremely important to differentiate whether it is of infectious or noninfectious etiology, as the management will be different in each case. After carefully ruling out the possibility of an infectious cause of the uveitis, ophthalmologists may follow the IWOS criteria for diagnosis. However, if the clinical and ancillary evidence is not enough to commit to a diagnosis or rule out the possibility in patients with ocular sarcoidosis, a biopsy may be performed. It is important for the ophthalmologist to consider referring patients with suspected sarcoidosis to an internist whenever there is evidence of

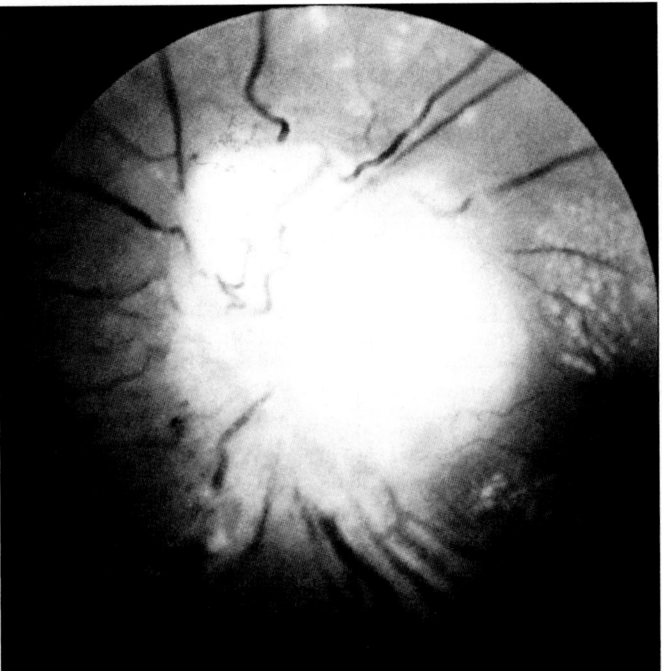

Fig. 78.6 Optic nerve mass in a patient with sarcoidosis. (Courtesy of Robert Nussenblatt.)

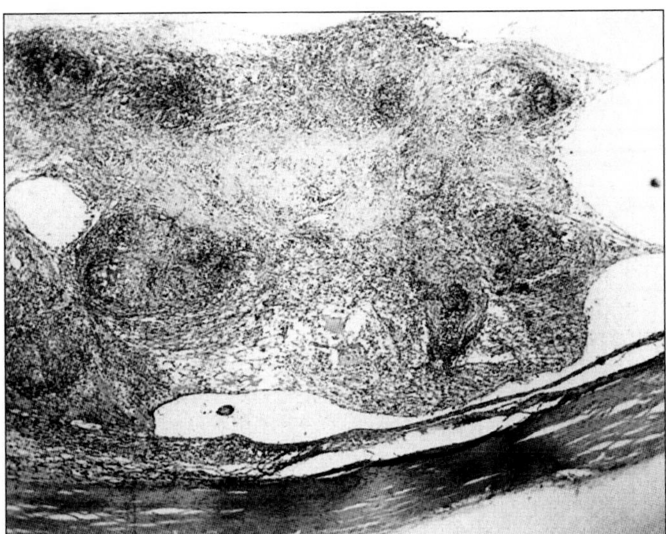

Fig. 78.7 Granulomatous inflammatory mass coming from the optic nerve head in a patient with sarcoidosis (hematoxylin & eosin; ×35). (Reproduced with permission from Green WR. Inflammatory diseases and conditions of the eye. In: Spencer WH, editor. Ophthalmic pathology: an atlas and textbook, vol. 3. Philadelphia, PA: WB Saunders; 1986.)

Table 78.4 Clinical signs, laboratory investigations, and diagnostic criteria proposed by the International Workshop on Ocular Sarcoidosis

Clinical signs suggestive of ocular sarcoidosis
1. Mutton-fat KPs (large and small) and/or iris nodules at pupillary margin (Koeppe) or in stroma (Bussacca) 2. Trabecular meshwork (TM) nodules and/or tent-shaped peripheral anterior synechiae (PAS) 3. Snowballs/string-of-pearl vitreous opacities. 4. Multiple chorioretinal peripheral lesions (active and atrophic) 5. Nodular and/or segmental periphlebitis (± candle-wax drippings) and/or macroaneurysm in an inflamed eye 6. Optic disc nodule(s)/granuloma(s) and/or solitary choroidal nodule 7. Bilaterality (assessed by clinical examination or investigational tests showing subclinical inflammation)
Laboratory investigations in suspected ocular sarcoidosis
1. Negative tuberculin test in a BCG-vaccinated patient or having had a positive PPD (or Mantoux) skin test previously 2. Elevated serum angiotensin-converting enzyme (ACE) and/or elevated serum lysozyme 3. Chest X-ray; look for bilateral hilar lymphadenopathy 4. Abnormal liver enzyme tests (any two of alkaline phosphatase, ASAT. ALAT, LDH or γ-GT) 5. Chest CT scan in patients with negative chest X-ray
Diagnostic criteria for ocular sarcoidosis (Fig. 78.8)
All other possible causes of uveitis, in particular tuberculous uveitis, have to be ruled out.
1. Biopsy supported diagnosis with a compatible uveitis → Definite ocular sarcoidosis 2. Biopsy not done; presence of bilateral hilar lymphadenopathy with a compatible uveitis → Presumed ocular sarcoidosis 3. Biopsy not done and bilateral hilar lymphadenopathy-negative; presence of three of the suggestive intraocular signs and two positive investigational tests → Probable ocular sarcoidosis 4. Biopsy negative, four of the suggestive intraocular signs and two of the investigations are positive → Possible ocular sarcoidosis

BCG, bacille Calmette-Guérin; PPD, purified protein derivative; ASAT, aspartate aminotransferase; ALAT, alanine aminotranseferase; LDH, lactate dehydrogenase; γ-GT, glutamyl transferase.

extrapulmonary involvement or the diagnosis of systemic disease needs to be confirmed.

COURSE AND PROGNOSIS

Karma and coworkers[56] classified the course of ocular sarcoidosis as monophasic, relapsing, or chronic. The three different courses of uveitis correlated with visual outcome. Patients with monophasic uveitis retained 20/30 or better visual acuity in 88% of eyes, with relapsing uveitis in 72% of eyes, and with chronic uveitis in none of the six eyes. Similarly, those with monophasic uveitis had a visual acuity of 20/70 or worse in 12% of eyes, with relapsing uveitis in 28% of eyes, and chronic uveitis in 67% of eyes. Hence the course of uveitis appears to correlate with the long-term visual outcome.

The development of secondary glaucoma in association with sarcoid uveitis appears to be a poor prognostic sign and is associated with severe visual loss. In one series,[55] most of these patients had a panuveitis with both anterior- and posterior-segment involvement associated with the development of secondary glaucoma, suggesting a more severe ocular disease. Treatment should be directed towards promptly suppressing the inflammation and minimizing any potential ocular complications.

In a retrospective study of 60 patients with sarcoid-associated uveitis who were followed at a subspecialty eye care and referral center, Dana et al.[81] identified prognostic factors for visual outcomes in sarcoid uveitis. The factors most strongly associated with both a lack of visual acuity improvement and a final visual acuity worse than 20/40 were: (1) delay in presentation to a uveitis subspecialist of greater than 1 year; (2) development of glaucoma; and (3) presence of intermediate or posterior uveitis.

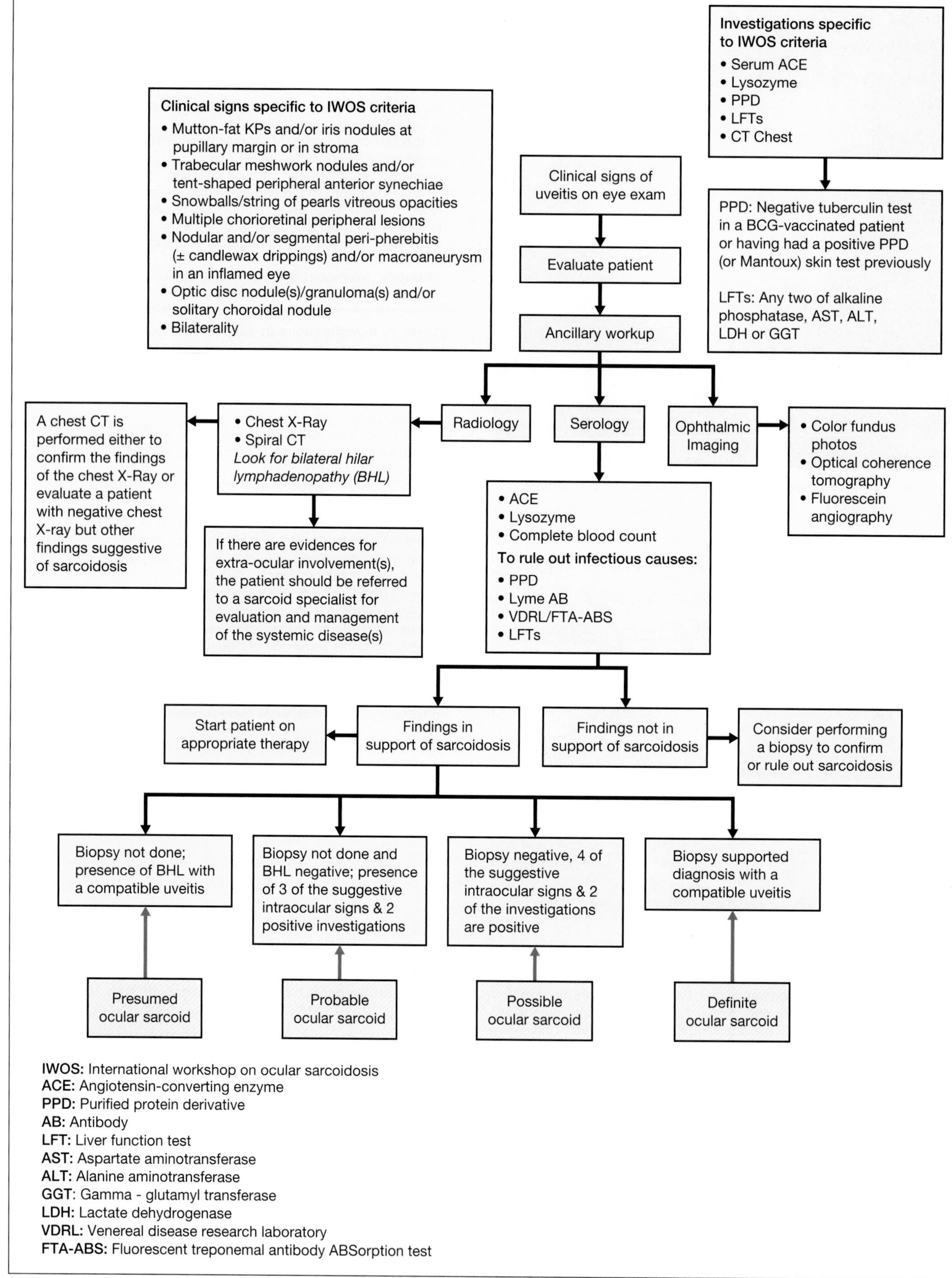

Fig. 78.8 Schematic outline for the evaluation of patients with suspected sarcoidosis.

There was a substantial increase in the relative odds of both visual improvement and the likelihood of achieving a visual acuity of at least 20/40 among patients in whom systemic corticosteroids were used for treatment. Because patients with more severe disease are more likely to receive systemic corticosteroid therapy, this result strongly supports the use of systemic corticosteroids for selected patients with sarcoid uveitis. Miserocchi et al. evaluated the risk factors for visual outcomes in 44 patients retrospectively and their multivariate results suggest that only the presence of cystoid macular edema was significantly associated with worse visual outcome.[82]

THERAPY

Treatment of any form of uveitis depends upon the initial presentation of the patient, severity of the disease, and accompanied complications. Nonetheless, the goals of therapy remain the same and include preservation of visual acuity, prompt identification of all sources of inflammation, zero tolerance toward any degree of inflammation, and proper management of complications such as macular edema, cataract, and glaucoma. The management of uveitis can be quite complex and may involve employment of multiple therapeutic options, some of which do have potential significant and serious side-effects. Timely referral to uveitis specialists is of the utmost priority and importance to allow correct diagnosis, and prompt and aggressive treatment with appropriate therapeutic agents, which may help to preserve vision and reduce the risks of irreversible ocular injury secondary to cumulative damage in patients with uveitis. A proposed outline for the management of ocular sarcoidosis is shown in Fig. 78.9. However, it is of the utmost importance to recognize that the approach to the management of each patient should be individualized. The proposed scheme only serves as a generalized recommendation. If there are any concerns regarding the

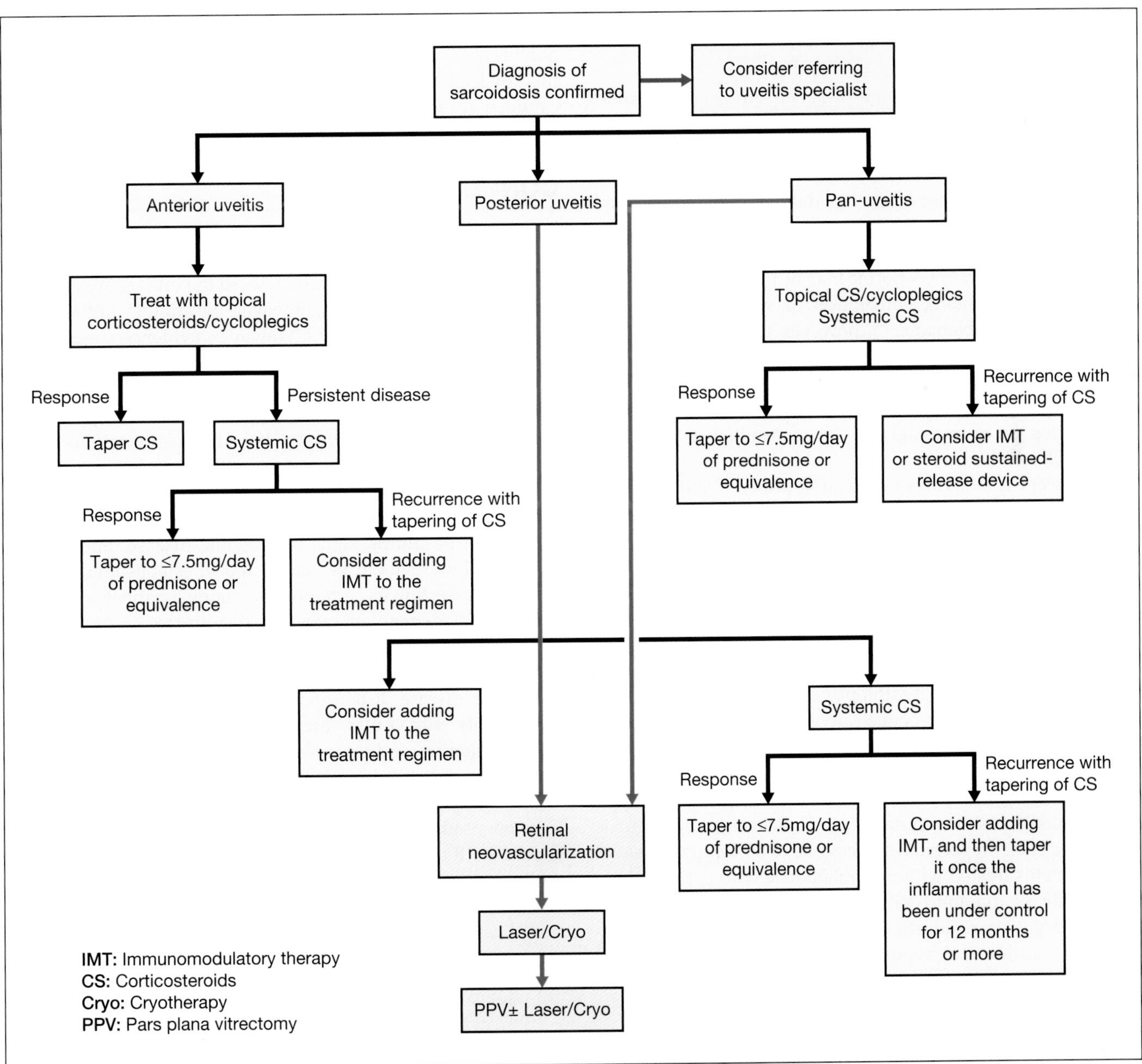

Fig. 78.9 Proposed treatment algorithm for patients with ocular sarcoidosis.

diagnosis and management of a patient with ocular sarcoidosis, it may be beneficial for the patient if he/she can be referred to a uveitis specialist who is experienced in managing the disease.

Established therapy

Treatment of the anterior uveitis associated with sarcoidosis is generally achieved with intensive topical corticosteroids, which may require several months to reach quiescence. In some patients with refractory anterior uveitis, the judicious use of oral corticosteroids may be necessary to suppress the inflammation. Patients with sarcoidosis generally respond to corticosteroid therapy, but chronic therapy may be necessary. Posterior-segment lesions in sarcoidosis generally require the use of systemic corticosteroids. Dosages are often in the range of prednisone 40–80 mg/day initially. Maintenance therapy with systemic corticosteroids should be less than 7.5 mg/day of prednisone or equivalence. Posterior-segment lesions such as perivascular sheathing and peripheral chorioretinal nodules that are not associated with visual loss may not mandate oral corticosteroid therapy. However, vascular occlusion, neovascularization, macular mass lesions, and optic disc lesions may produce profound visual loss and most likely require corticosteroid therapy.

Although corticosteroids are very effective in controlling inflammation initially, their long-term use is often associated with significant complications and side-effects. The use of steroid-sparing agents is indicated if chronic steroid usage (≥7.5 mg of prednisone or equivalent daily) is required to control the inflammation. Occasionally, corticosteroid-sparing agents such as hydroxychloroquine, methotrexate, azathioprine, mycophenolate mofetil, or cyclosporine may be useful in patients with corticosteroid-dependent sarcoidosis in whom corticosteroid side-effects are problematic;[83–86] however, their usages may not be without risk. Patients being treated with these agents, including corticosteroids, require very thorough and experienced clinical oversight by specialists (such as uveitis specialists, rheumatologists, or oncologists) who are familiar with employing such classes of drugs.

More recently, methotrexate,[87] azathioprine,[88,89] and mycophenolate[90] have been widely employed as steroid-sparing agents in the management of chronic uveitis. In a retrospective series of 386 patients, methotrexate was found to control uveitis in 66% of patients.[91] However, in 16% of patients, toxicity and adverse events secondary to the drug led to its discontinuation. A delay of up to 6 months in response to therapy with methotrexate has also been reported, which has prompted the use of intraocular injections of the drug.[88] Azathioprine has been reported to be beneficial in patients with ocular sarcoidosis who do not respond to methotrexate. However, in a retrospective study of patients with intermediate uveitis, a 25% rate of discontinuation was noted within the first year of therapy due to toxicity. Mycophenolate mofetil has shown promising results in terms of low toxicity. Deuter et al.[90] reported a success rate of 86% in patients with chronic uveitis treated with mycophenolate with a discontinuation of only 5% due to toxicity. A small series of seven patients diagnosed with sarcoidosis has also reported the drug to be beneficial.[92] Galor et al. reported a response rate of 70%, 42%, and 58% at 6 months for mycophenolate mofetil, methotrexate, and azathioprine, respectively, in 321 patients with nonspecific ocular inflammation.[93] Although the time to response for azathioprine and mycophenolate was similar, the former had more toxicity-related events reported.

Other immunomodulatory therapeutic agents have been employed in the management of sarcoidosis. Baughman and Lower reported a 58% complete and 28% partial improvement in patients with ocular sarcoidosis when treated with leflunomide. Only two of the 28 patients discontinued therapy due to toxicity in this study.[94]

Biologics

Biologics, antagonists of tumor necrosis factor (TNF) such as adalimumab (humanized monoclonal antibody), infliximab (chimeric monoclonoal antibody), and etanercept (soluble TNF receptor antagonist) have been reported in small studies to benefit patients with chronic uveitis.[95–99] However, there is a lack of evidence from RCTs supporting the use of adalimumab and infliximab, while it has been shown in a double-masked RCT that etanercept is no better than placebo when treating chronic uveitis.[61,62] Several groups have also reported the development of uveitis in patients receiving anti-TNF therapy,[98,100,101] at a significantly higher rate, with etanercept followed by infliximab and adalimumab.[102] Although the mechanism of this phenomenon is not yet fully understood, several reports of anti-TNF therapy leading to a sarcoidosis-like reaction suggest that a very cautious approach should be taken when using these agents to treat ocular sarcoidosis.

CONCLUSION

Sarcoidosis is a multiorgan disease with protean manifestations, including ocular involvement. Throughout the years, significant advancements have been made toward the understanding of the pathogenesis of sarcoidosis; however, the etiology of the disease is not completely elucidated. However, evidence suggests that the pathophysiology most likely involves T cells. Sarcoid is one of the most common causes of uveitis of all types - anterior, intermediate, and/or posterior. Therefore, it is important for ophthalmologists to recognize that ocular manifestations may be the initial presentation of a patient with sarcoidosis.

The IWOS has established criteria for the diagnosis of ocular sarcoidosis when ocular changes are present in the presence or absence of clinical signs of systemic disease. Such criteria are helpful and should be considered in establishing the diagnosis and asserting its certainty. Managing a patient with ocular sarcoid will depend on whether the disease is unilateral or bilateral, whether there is presence or absence of systemic involvement, and how such involvements are at the time of the ocular disease. It is important for ophthalmologists caring for patients with ocular sarcoid to collaborate with internists, pulmolnologists, and sarcoid specialists to provide patients with comprehensive and complete care.

There are existing therapeutic options and approaches that may be used in bringing the disease into quiescence, which should be the goals for both ocular and systemic diseases. In addition, potential new drugs are currently in development that may lead to disease quiescence with fewer side-effects and complications in the future.

REFERENCES

1. James DG, Neville E, Siltzbach LE. A worldwide review of sarcoidosis. Ann NY Acad Sci 1976;278:321–34.
2. James DG. Sarcoidosis. In: Wyngaarden JB, Smith LH Jr, editors. Cecil textbook of medicine. 17th ed. Philadelphia: WB Saunders; 1985.
3. Henderly DE, Genstler AJ, Smith RE, et al. Changing patterns of uveitis. Am J Ophthalmol 1987;103:131–6.

4. Karma A. Ophthalmic changes in sarcoidosis. Acta Ophthalmol Suppl 1979: 1–94.
5. Perkins ES, Folk J. Uveitis in London and Iowa. Ophthalmologica 1984; 189:36–40.
6. Rosenbaum JT. Uveitis. An internist's view. Arch Intern Med 1989; 149:1173–6.
7. Statement on sarcoidosis. Joint statement of the American Thoracic Society (ATS), the European Respiratory Society (ERS) and the World Association of Sarcoidosis and Other Granulomatous Disorders (WASOG) adopted by the ATS Board of Directors and by the ERS Executive Committee, February 1999. Am J Respir Crit Care Med 1999;160:736–55.
8. Rybicki BA, Major M, Popovich J Jr, et al. Racial differences in sarcoidosis incidence: a 5-year study in a health maintenance organization. Am J Epidemiol 1997;145:234–41.
9. Lazarus A. Sarcoidosis: epidemiology, etiology, pathogenesis, and genetics. Dis Mon 2009;55:649–60.
10. James DG, Neville E, Siltzbach LE. A worldwide review of sarcoidosis. Ann NY Acad Sci 1976;278:321–34.
11. Rosenberg AM, Yee EH, Mackenzie JW. Arthritis in childhood sarcoidosis. J Rheumatol 1983;10:987–90.
12. Seamone CD, Nozik RA. Sarcoidosis and the eye. Ophthalmol Clin North Am 1992;5:567–76.
13. Milman N, Hoffmann AL. Childhood sarcoidosis: long-term follow-up. Eur Respire J 2008;31:592–8.
14. Blain JG, Riley W, Logothetis J. Optic nerve manifestations of sarcoidosis. Arch Neurol 1965;13:307–9.
15. Jabs DA, Houk JL, Bias WB, et al. Familial granulomatous synovitis, uveitis, and cranial neuropathies. Am J Med 1985;78:801–4.
16. Rose CD, Eichenfield AH, Goldsmith DP, et al. Early onset sarcoidosis with aortitis – "juvenile systemic granulomatosis?" J Rheumatol 1990;17:102–6.
17. Scerri L, Cook LJ, Jenkins EA, et al. Familial juvenile systemic granulomatosis (Blau's syndrome). Clin Exp Dermatol 1996;21:445–8.
18. Latkany PA, Jabs DA, Smith Justine R, et al. Multifocal choroiditis in patients with familial juvenile systemic granulomatosis. Am J Ophthalmol 2002;134: 897–904.
19. James DG. Sarcoidosis. In: Wyngaarden JB, Smith LH Jr, editors. Cecil textbook of medicine. 17th ed. Philadelphia: WB Saunders; 1985.
20. Rossman MD, Thompson B, Frederick M, et al. HLA-DRB1*1101: a significant risk factor for sarcoidosis in blacks and whites. Am J Hum Genet 2003;73: 720–35.
21. Crystal RG, Roberts WC, Hunninghake GW, et al. NIH conference. Pulmonary sarcoidosis: a disease characterized and perpetuated by activated lung T-lymphocytes. Ann Intern Med 1981;94:73–94.
22. Hunninghake GW, Crystal RG. Pulmonary sarcoidosis: a disorder mediated by excess helper T-lymphocyte activity at sites of disease activity. N Engl J Med 1981;305:429–34.
23. Meyer KC, Kaminski MJ, Calhoun WJ, et al. Studies of bronchoalveolar lavage cells and fluids in pulmonary sarcoidosis. I. Enhanced capacity of bronchoalveolar lavage cells from patients with pulmonary sarcoidosis to induce angiogenesis in vivo. Am Rev Respir Dis 1989;140:1446–9.
24. Buechner SA, Winkelmann RK, Banks PM. T-cell subsets in cutaneous sarcoidosis. Arch Dermatol 1983;119:728–32.
25. Chan CC, Wetzig RP, Palestine AG, et al. Immunohistopathology of ocular sarcoidosis. Report of a case and discussion of immunopathogenesis. Arch Ophthalmol 1987;105:1398–402.
26. Semenzato G, Agostini C, Zambello R, et al. Activated T-cells with immunoregulatory functions at different sites of involvement in sarcoidosis – phenotypic and functional evaluations. Ann NY Acad Sci 1986;465:56–73.
27. Johns CJ, Schonfeld SA, Scott PP, et al. Longitudinal study of chronic sarcoidosis with low-dose maintenance corticosteroid therapy. Outcome and complications. Ann NY Acad Sci 1986;465:702–12.
28. Mayock RL, Bertrand P, Morrison CE, et al. Manifestations of sarcoidosis. Analysis of 145 patients, with a review of nine series selected from the literature. Am J Med 1963;35:67–89.
29. James DG. Ocular sarcoidosis. Ann NY Acad Sci 1986;465:551–63.
30. Mana J, Marcoval J, Graells J, et al. Cutaneous involvement in sarcoidosis. Relationship to systemic disease. Arch Dermatol 1997;133:882–8.
31. Zarei M, Anderson JR, Higgins JN, et al. Cavernous sinus syndrome as the only manifestation of sarcoidosis. J Postgrad Med 2002;48:119–21.
32. Obenauf CD, Shaw HE, Sydnor CF, et al. Sarcoidosis and its ophthalmic manifestations. Am J Ophthalmol 1978;86:648–55.
33. Delaney P. Neurologic manifestations in sarcoidosis: review of the literature, with a report of 23 cases. Ann Intern Med 1977;87:336–45.
34. James DG, Zatouroff MA, Trowell J, et al. Papilloedema in sarcoidosis. Br J Ophthalmol 1967;51:526–9.
35. Sugo A, Seyama K, Yaguchi T, et al. [Cardiac sarcoidosis with myopathy and advanced A-V nodal block in a woman with a previous diagnosis of sarcoidosis.] Nihon Kyobu Shikkan Gakkai Zasshi 1995;33:1111–8.
36. Wilson AG, Hansell DM. Immunologic diseases of the lung. In: Armstrong P, Wilson AG, Hansell DM, editors. Imaging of the diseases of the chest. London: Mosby; 2000. p. 637–88.
37. Nishino M, Lee KS, Itoh H, et al. The spectrum of pulmonary sarcoidosis: variations of high-resolution CT findings and clues for specific diagnosis. Eur J Radiol 2010;73:66–73.
38. Nakatsu M, Hatabu H, Morikawa K, et al. Large coalescent parenchymal nodules in pulmonary sarcoidosis: "sarcoid galaxy" sign. AJR Am J Roentgenol 2002;178(6):1389–93.
39. Terasaki H, Fujimoto K, Muller NL, et al. Pulmonary sarcoidosis: comparison of findings of inspiratory and expiratory high-resolution CT and pulmonary function tests between smokers and nonsmokers. AJR Am J Roentgenol 2005;185:333–8.
40. Davies CW, Tasker AD, Padley SP, et al. Air trapping in sarcoidosis on computed tomography: correlation with lung function. Clin Radiol 2000;55: 217–21.
41. Nosal A, Schleissner LA, Mishkin FS, et al. Angiotensin-I-converting enzyme and gallium scan in noninvasive evaluation of sarcoidosis. Ann Intern Med 1979;90:328–31.
42. Weinreb RN. Diagnosing sarcoidosis by transconjunctival biopsy of the lacrimal gland. Am J Ophthalmol 1984;97:573–6.
43. Rohatgi PK, Ryan JW, Lindeman P. Value of serial measurement of serum angiotensin converting enzyme in the management of sarcoidosis. Am J Med 1981;70:44–50.
44. Power WJ, Neves RA, Rodriguez A, et al. The value of combined serum angiotensin-converting enzyme and gallium scan in diagnosing ocular sarcoidosis. Ophthalmology 1995;102:2007–11.
45. Akbar JJ, Meyer CA, Shipley RT, et al. Cardiopulmonary imaging in sarcoidosis. Clin chest med 2008;29:429–43, viii.
46. Mana J. Magnetic resonance imaging and nuclear imaging in sarcoidosis. Curr Opin Pulm Med 2002;8:457–63.
47. Crick RP, Hoyle C, Smellie H. The eyes in sarcoidosis. Br j ophthalmol 1961;45:461–81.
48. Hunter DG, Foster CS. Isolated ocular sarcoidosis – late development of systemic manifestations in uveitis patients. Invest Ophthalmol Vis Sci 1991;32: 681–681.
49. Tremblay A, Stather DR, Maceachern P, et al. A randomized controlled trial of standard vs endobronchial ultrasonography-guided transbronchial needle aspiration in patients with suspected sarcoidosis. Chest 2009;136:340–6.
50. Annema JT, Veselic M, Rabe KF. Endoscopic ultrasound-guided fine-needle aspiration for the diagnosis of sarcoidosis. Eur Respir J 2005;25:405–9.
51. Weinreb RN, Tessler H. Laboratory diagnosis of ophthalmic sarcoidosis. Surv Ophthalmol 1984;28:653–64.
52. Israel HL, Sones M. Selection of biopsy procedures for sarcoidosis diagnosis. Arch Intern Med 1964;113:255–60.
53. Green WR. Inflammatory disease and conditions of the eye. In: Spencer WH, editor. Ophthalmic pathology: an atlas and textbook. Philadelphia, PA: WB Saunders, 1986.
54. Baarsma GS, La Hey E, Glasius E, et al. The predictive value of serum angiotensin converting enzyme and lysozyme levels in the diagnosis of ocular sarcoidosis. Am J Ophthalmol 1987;104:211–7.
55. Jabs DA, Johns CJ. Ocular involvement in chronic sarcoidosis. Am J Ophthalmol 1986;102:297–301.
56. Karma A, Huhti E, Poukkula A. Course and outcome of ocular sarcoidosis. Am J Ophthalmol 1988;106:467–72.
57. Qazi FA, Thorne JE, Jabs DA. Scleral nodule associated with sarcoidosis. Am J Ophthalmol 2003;136:752–4.
58. Khan JA, Hoover DL, Giangiacomo J, et al. Orbital and childhood sarcoidosis. J Pediatr Ophthalmol Strabismus 1986;23:190–4.
59. Collison JM, Miller NR, Green WR. Involvement of orbital tissues by sarcoid. Am J Ophthalmol 1986;102:302–7.
60. Faller M, Purohit A, Kennel N, et al. Systemic sarcoidosis initially presenting as an orbital tumour. Eur Respir J 1996:474–6.
61. Foster CS, Tufail F, Waheed NK, et al. Efficacy of etanercept in preventing relapse of uveitis controlled by methotrexate. Arch Ophthalmol 2003;121: 437–40.
62. Smith JA, Thompson DJ, Whitcup SM, et al. A randomized, placebo-controlled, double-masked clinical trial of etanercept for the treatment of uveitis associated with juvenile idiopathic arthritis. Arthritis Rheum 2005;53:18–23.
63. Gentile RC, Berinstein DM, Liebmann J, et al. High-resolution ultrasound biomicroscopy of the pars plana and peripheral retina. Ophthalmology 1998;105:478–84.
64. Gass JD, Olson CL. Sarcoidosis with optic nerve and retinal involvement. Arch Ophthalmol 1976;94:945–50.
65. Hoogstede HA, Copper AC. A case of macular subretinal neovascularisation in chronic uveitis probably caused by sarcoidosis. Br J Ophthalmol 1982; 66:530–5.
66. Sanders MD, Shilling JS. Retinal, choroidal, and optic disc involvement in sarcoidosis. Trans Ophthalmol Soc UK 1976;96:140–4.
67. Letocha CE, Shields JA, Goldberg RE. Retinal changes in sarcoidosis. Can J Ophthalmol 1975;10:184–92.
68. Kiryu J, Kita M, Tanabe T, et al. Pars plana vitrectomy for cystoid macular edema secondary to sarcoid uveitis. Ophthalmology 2001;108:1140–4.
69. Kiryu J, Kita M, Tanabe T, et al. Pars plana vitrectomy for epiretinal membrane associated with sarcoidosis. Jpn J ophthalmol 2003;47:479–83.
70. Sonoda KH, Enaida H, Ueno A, et al. Pars plana vitrectomy assisted by triamcinolone acetonide for refractory uveitis: a case series study. Br J Ophthalmol 2003;87:1010–4.
71. Doxanas MT, Kelley JS, Prout TE. Sarcoidosis with neovascularization of the optic nerve head. Am J Ophthalmol 1980;90:347–51.
72. Duker JS, Brown GC, McNamara JA. Proliferative sarcoid retinopathy. Ophthalmology 1988;95:1680–6.
73. Gould H, Kaufman HE. Sarcoid of the fundus. Arch Ophthalmol 1961;65: 453–6.
74. Spalton DJ, Sanders MD. Fundus changes in histologically confirmed sarcoidosis. Br J ophthalmol 1981;65:348–58.

75. Kelley JS, Green WR. Sarcoidosis involving the optic nerve head. Arch Ophthalmol 1973;89:486–8.
76. Ing EB, Garrity JA, Cross SA, et al. Sarcoid masquerading as optic nerve sheath meningioma. Mayo Clin Proc 1997;72:38–43.
77. Katz B. Disc edema, transient obscurations of vision, and a temporal fossa mass. Surv ophthalmol 1991;36:133–9.
78. Mansour AM. Sarcoid optic disc edema and optociliary shunts. J Clin Neuro-Ophthalmol 1986;6:47–52.
79. Mizuno K, Takahashi J. Sarcoid cyclitis. Ophthalmology 1986;93:511–7.
80. Wakefield D, Zierhut M. Controversy: ocular sarcoidosis. Ocul Immunol Inflamm 2010;18:5–9.
81. Dana MR, Merayo-Lloves J, Schaumberg DA, et al. Prognosticators for visual outcome in sarcoid uveitis. Ophthalmology 1996;103:1846–53.
82. Miserocchi E, Modorati G, Di Matteo F, et al. Visual outcome in ocular sarcoidosis: retrospective evaluation of risk factors. Available online at: www.ncbi.nlm.nih.gov/pubmed/21374555 (accessed 03/03/2011).
83. Gedalia A, Molina JF, Ellis GS, et al. Low-dose methotrexate therapy for childhood sarcoidosis. J pediatr 1997;130:25–9.
84. Kaye O, Palazzo E, Grossin M, et al. Low-dose methotrexate: an effective corticosteroid-sparing agent in the musculoskeletal manifestations of sarcoidosis. Br J Rheumatol 1995;34:642–4.
85. Lower EE, Baughman RP. Prolonged use of methotrexate for sarcoidosis. Arch Intern Med 1995;155:846–51.
86. Mathur A, Kremer JM. Immunopathology, rheumatic features, and therapy of sarcoidosis. Curr Opin Rheumatol 1992;4:76–80.
87. Samson CM, Waheed N, Baltatzis S, et al. Methotrexate therapy for chronic noninfectious uveitis: analysis of a case series of 160 patients. Ophthalmology 2001;108:1134–9.
88. Taylor SR, Habot-Wilner Z, Pacheco P, et al. Intraocular methotrexate in the treatment of uveitis and uveitic cystoid macular edema. Ophthalmology 2009;116:797–801.
89. Muller-Quernheim J, Kienast K, Held M, et al. Treatment of chronic sarcoidosis with an azathioprine/prednisolone regimen. Eur Respir J 1999;14:1117–22.
90. Deuter CME, Doycheva D, Stuebiger N, et al. Mycophenolate sodium for immunosuppressive treatment in uveitis. Ocular Immunol Inflamm 2009;17:415–9.
91. Kempen JH, Altaweel MM, Holbrook JT, et al. The multicenter uveitis steroid treatment trial: rationale, design, and baseline characteristics. Am J Ophthalmol 2010;149:550–61 e10.
92. Bhat P, Cervantes-Castaneda RA, Doctor PP, et al. Mycophenolate mofetil therapy for sarcoidosis-associated uveitis. Ocul Immunol Inflamm 2009;17:185–90.
93. Galor A, Perez VL, Hammel JP, et al. Comparison of antimetabolite drugs as corticosteroid-sparing therapy for noninfectious ocular inflammation. Ophthalmology 2008;115:1826–32.
94. Baughman RP, Lower EE. Leflunomide for chronic sarcoidosis. Sarcoidosis Vasculitis Diffuse Lung Dis 2004;21:43–8.
95. Reiff A, Takei S, Sadeghi S, et al. Etanercept therapy in children with treatment-resistant uveitis. Arthritis Rheum 2001;44:1411–5.
96. Baughman RP, Bradley DA, Lower EE. Infliximab in chronic ocular inflammation. Int J Clin Pharmacol Ther 2005;43:7–11.
97. Galor A, Perez VL, Hammel JP, et al. Differential effectiveness of etanercept and infliximab in the treatment of ocular inflammation. Ophthalmology 2006;113:2317–23.
98. Tynjala P, Lindahl P, Honkanen V, et al. Infliximab and etanercept in the treatment of chronic uveitis associated with refractory juvenile idiopathic arthritis. Ann Rheum Dis 2007;66:548–50.
99. Diaz-Llopis M, Garcia-Delpech S, Salom D, et al. Adalimumab therapy for refractory uveitis: a pilot study. J Ocul Pharmacol Ther 2008;24:351–61.
100. Schmeling H, Horneff G. Etanercept and uveitis in patients with juvenile idiopathic arthritis. Rheumatol (Oxf) 2005;44:1008–11.
101. Hashkes PJ, Shajrawi I. Sarcoid-related uveitis occurring during etanercept therapy. Clin Exp Rheumatol 2003;21:645–6.
102. Lim LL, Fraunfelder FW, Rosenbaum JT. Do tumor necrosis factor inhibitors cause uveitis? A registry-based study. Arthritis Rheum 2007;56:3248–52.
103. Branson JH, Park JH. Sarcoidosishepatic involvement: presentation of a case with fatal liver involvement; including autopsy findings and review of the evidence for sarcoid involvement of the liver as found in the literature. Ann Intern Med 1954;40:111–45.
104. Klatskin G. Hepatic granulomata: problems in interpretation. Ann NY Acad Sci 1976;278:427–32.
105. Beahrs OH, Woolner LB, Kirklin JW, et al. Carcinomatous transformation of mixed tumors of the parotid gland. AMA Arch Surg 1957;75:605–13; discussion 604–13.
106. Rochlin DB, Enterline HT. Prescalene lymph node biopsies; a report of 142 cases. Am J Surg 1958;96:372–8.
107. Williams TK, Webb WR. Prescalene node biopsy. An evaluation. Arch Surg 1962;84:261–4.
108. Romer F, Paulsen S, Antonius V, et al. Sarcoidosis in a Danish "amt". A retrospective epidemiologic study of sarcoidosis in Ringkobing Amt from 1960 to 1969. Dan Med Bull 1973;20:112–20.
109. Rasmussen SM, Neukirch F. Sarcoidosis. A clinical study with special reference to the choice of biopsy procedure. Acta Med Scand 1976;199:209–16.
110. Carlens E. Biopsies in connection with bronchoscopy and mediastinoscopy in sarcoidosis; a comparison. Acta Med Scand Suppl 1964;425:237–8.
111. Palva T. Mediastinal sarcoidosis. Acta Otolaryngol Suppl 1964;188:258.
112. Koerner SK, Sakowitz AJ, Appelman RI, et al. Transbronchinal lung biopsy for the diagnosis of sarcoidosis. N Engl J Med 1975;293:268–70.
113. Koontz CH. Lung biopsy in sarcoidosis. Chest 1978;74:120–1.
114. Crick RP, Hoyle C, Smellie H. The eyes in sarcoidosis. Br J Ophthalmol 1961;45:461–81.
115. Bornstein JS, Frank MI, Radner DB. Conjunctival biopsy in the diagnosis of sarcoidosis. N Engl J Med 1962;267:60–4.
116. Khan F, Wessely Z, Chazin SR, et al. Conjunctival biopsy in sarcoidosis: A simple, safe, and specific diagnostic procedure. Ann Ophthalmol 1977;9:671–6.
117. Solomon DA, Horn BR, Byrd RB, et al. The diagnosis of sarcoidosis by conjunctival biopsy. Chest 1978;74:271–3.
118. Nichols CW, Eagle RC Jr, Yanoff M, et al. Conjunctival biopsy as an aid in the evaluation of the patient with suspected sarcoidosis. Ophthalmology 1980;87:287–91.
119. Karcioglu ZA, Brear R. Conjunctival biopsy in sarcoidosis. Am J Ophthalmol 1985;99:68–73.
120. Nessan VJ, Jacoway JR. Biopsy of minor salivary glands in the diagnosis of sarcoidosis. N Engl J Med 1979;301:922–4.

Intermediate Uveitis

Chapter 79

Phoebe Lin, Glenn J. Jaffe

INTRODUCTION

Intermediate uveitis is defined anatomically, according to the Standardized Uveitis Nomenclature working group, as intraocular inflammation in which the primary site is the vitreous, but it commonly involves the peripheral retina as well.[1] The origin of the inflammatory cells includes the ciliary body pars plana, the peripheral retinal vessels, and the peripheral choroid. Previously used terminology for this entity includes pars planitis, peripheral uveitis, peripheral cyclitis, hyalitis, and vitritis. The term "pars planitis" now specifically refers to a subcategory of idiopathic intermediate uveitis characterized by the presence of snowbanks and snowballs, which will be described in more detail below.

EPIDEMIOLOGY AND DEMOGRAPHICS

Because the currently used nomenclature for uveitis was agreed upon in 2005, current prevalence and incidence figures for this anatomic category of uveitis are sparse. Although various groups have reported the frequency of intermediate uveitis in their uveitis practices, ranging from 4 to 15.4%, these figures are subject to referral bias since the reports originate from tertiary care referral clinics.[2–6] In pediatric uveitis, it accounts for up to 25% of cases.[7,8] The overall population prevalence of different types of uveitis based on anatomic location including intermediate uveitis has been investigated in several population studies since 2005. Gritz and Wong found a prevalence ratio for intermediate uveitis of 4.0 per 100 000 persons in a cross-sectional retrospective study using a database of individuals in northern California receiving care through a single large health maintenance organization.[9] The incidence was 1.5 per 100 000 person-years. These figures were reported with the stipulation that the prevalence may have been underestimated because a significant proportion of included patients did not have dilated fundus examinations, and the anatomic uveitis location was, therefore, unknown. Another study utilizing the Veterans Affairs database in the Pacific Northwest region found that the prevalence of intermediate uveitis was approximately 3.3 per 100 000 persons.[10] The annual incidence of pars planitis in Olmstead County, Minnesota, was 2.08 per 100 000 persons.[11]

Although intermediate uveitis can occur at any age, it tends to occur in a younger age range. Average age of onset was 31 years (range 8–64 years) in one study,[12] and 30 years (range 6–76 years) in another.[13] There appears to be no gender predilection for this anatomic subtype of uveitis, although certain entities that can cause intermediate uveitis, such as sarcoidosis, have a strong female bias.[14] In certain uveitis practices, such as that reported by Thorne and colleagues, intermediate uveitis appears to be slightly more common in women (66.4%).[13] Racial predilection likely depends on the etiology, but there appears to be no race preference in pars planitis.

PRESENTATION AND CLINICAL FINDINGS

The most common symptoms of intermediate uveitis include blurry vision and floaters, whereas pain, redness, and photophobia are less common than in other types of uveitis. Although typically bilateral over time (74.5–80% bilateral),[3,12,13,15] it is frequently asymmetric and may begin unilaterally. Findings on clinical examination at onset include anterior vitreous cells or diffuse vitreous haze, and, to a lesser extent, anterior chamber involvement. Vitreous haze is graded on a scale of 0–4+ based on the level of optic nerve and retinal vessel obscuration.[16] Snowballs (see below for discussion on histopathology) are whitish inflammatory vitreous opacities in clusters frequently found in the inferior vitreous cavity (Fig. 79.1). Snowbanks are identified as whitish gray confluent preretinal membranes most commonly seen along the inferior pars plana, and peripheral retina (Fig. 79.2A). Over time, these may develop into organized fibrovascular membranes that are prone to vitreous hemorrhage and retinal detachment. The vascular component of this snowbank is continuous with the retinal vessels (Fig. 79.2B). Commonly, a

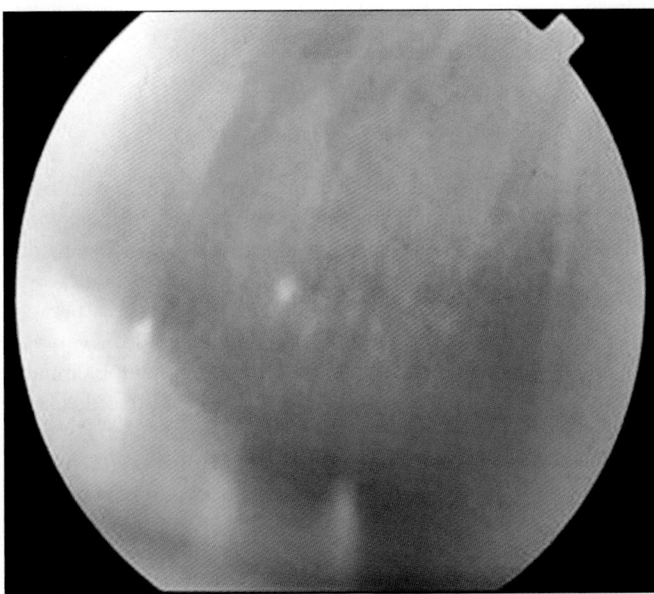

Fig. 79.1 Snowballs seen in the inferior vitreous cavity in a patient with pars planitis.

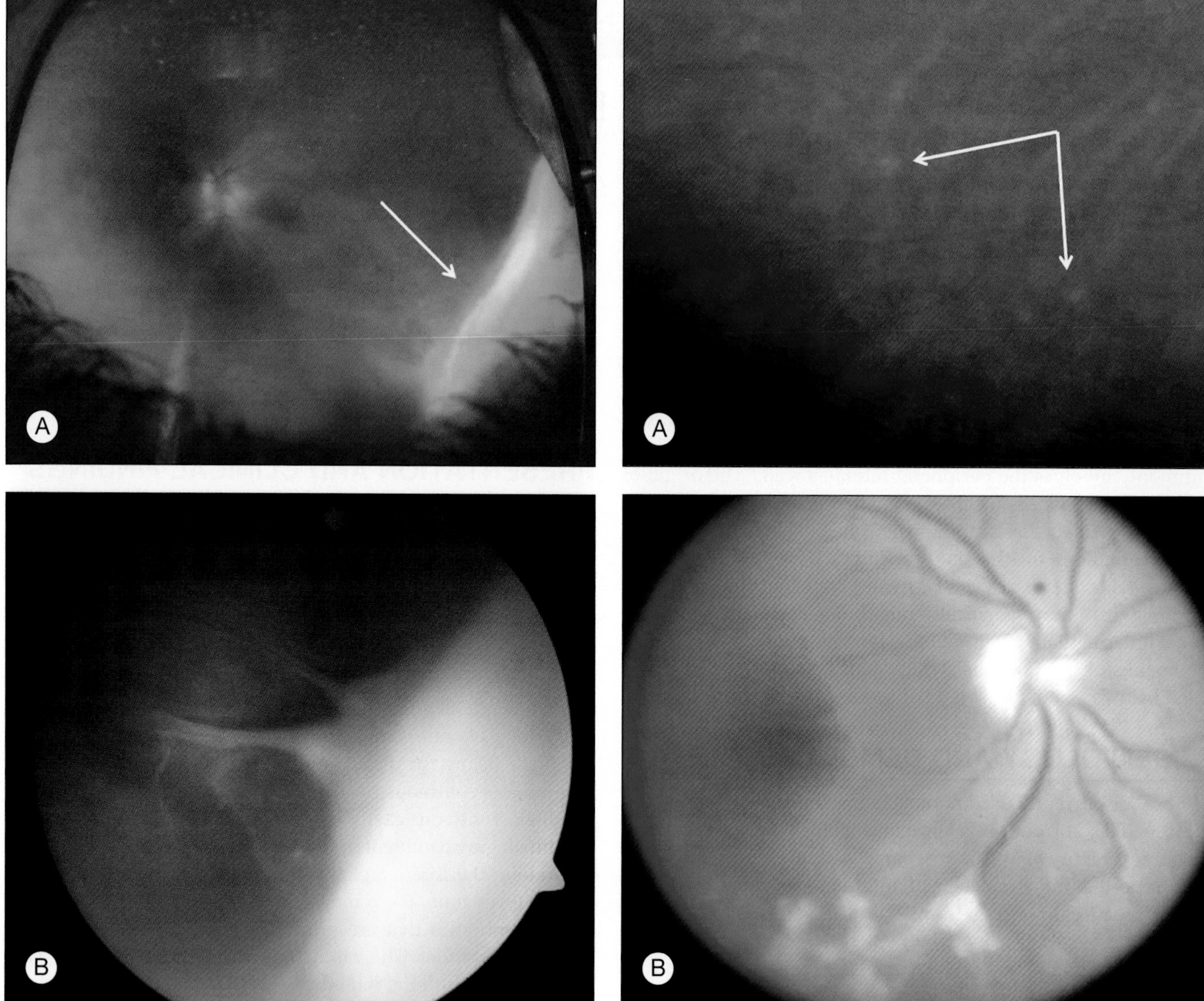

Fig. 79.2 Inferotemporal pars plana snowbank in a patient with idiopathic unilateral pars planitis. (A) Wide-field view. Snowbank noted by arrow. (B) Retinal vessel incorporated into snowbank in magnified view of A.

Fig. 79.3 (A) Focal periphlebitis (designated by arrows) in a patient with sarcoid intermediate uveitis. (B) Granulomatous exudative periphlebitis (candle-wax drippings or taches de bougie).

peripheral vasculitis manifested by perivascular sheathing is seen in intermediate uveitis, and may indicate an increased probability of associated systemic disease.[12] According to one study, periphlebitis in the setting of intermediate uveitis was associated with an increased rate of multiple sclerosis (MS) or optic neuritis.[17] It is important to note that sarcoidosis can also present as an isolated periphlebitis or as granulomatous inflammation in the form of snowballs. Periphlebitis in sarcoidosis can present with a wide spectrum of appearances, from scant focal periphlebitis to exudative candle-wax drippings (taches de bougie) (Fig. 79.3). Yellowish peripheral punched-out chorioretinal lesions that might represent active or old choroidal granulomata are highly suspicious for sarcoidosis, although once these are present, the anatomic designation is panuveitis rather than intermediate uveitis. Obliterative peripheral vasculitis may result in peripheral neovascularization and resultant vitreous hemorrhage (Fig. 79.4). Cystoid macular edema (CME) is a common finding, occurring in over 40% of individuals at diagnosis of intermediate uveitis (Fig. 79.5).[13] Clinically apparent optic nerve edema also occurs in a small percentage of patients with intermediate uveitis.

Imaging

Although the majority of cases of intermediate uveitis are diagnosed by clinical examination, various imaging modalities give useful adjunctive information to guide diagnosis and management. For instance, in the setting of media opacity from cataract, ultrasound biomicroscopy (UBM) can be used to detect pars plana exudates. Identification of cyclitic membranes by UBM can be of great value in preoperative planning. B-scan ultrasonography can be used to diagnose and measure macular thickening with a great degree of accuracy, sensitivity, and

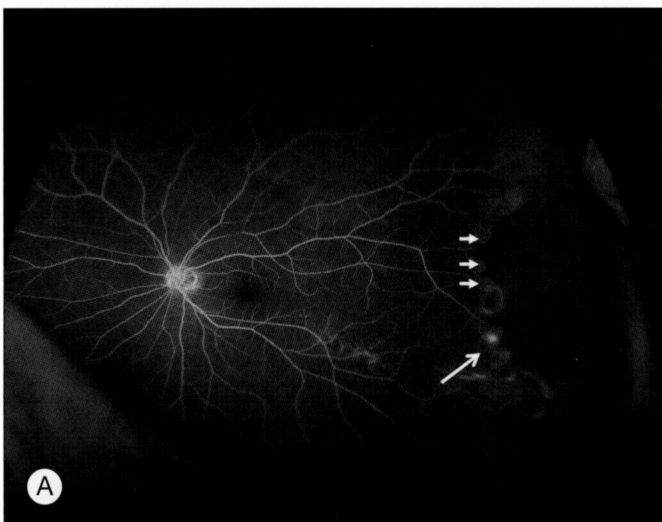

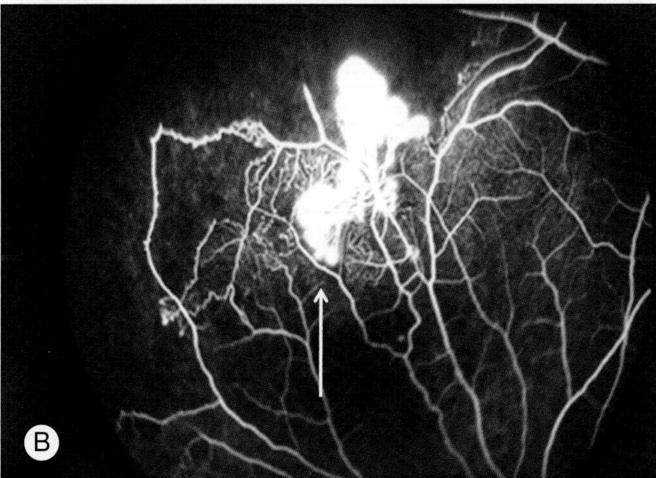

Fig. 79.4 Peripheral nonperfusion and neovascularization (NV) in 2 patients with sarcoidosis-associated intermediate uveitis. (A) Wide-field fluorescein angiography showing severe peripheral nonperfusion (short arrows) and an early neovascular tuft (long arrow). (B) Advanced peripheral NV (arrow).

specificity in the setting of media opacity or intolerance to fluorescein angiography and optical coherence tomography (OCT).[18] Fluorescein angiography is useful to detect CME, vasculitis, peripheral nonperfusion, and peripheral neovascularization. OCT is important to identify and follow CME as a gauge of disease activity in intermediate uveitis.[19] In some cases, concentric macular retinal thickening without frank CME, as determined by OCT, can be used to monitor response to treatment.[20]

DIFFERENTIAL DIAGNOSIS AND WORKUP

The cause of intermediate uveitis can be determined by investigating the presence of systemic findings or historical clues. Although the vast majority of cases are idiopathic (nearly 70%),[21] the most common known inflammatory etiologies include sarcoidosis and MS, whereas infectious causes can include syphilis, Lyme disease, and tuberculosis (Table 79.1). Pars planitis is, by definition, idiopathic intermediate uveitis characterized by the presence of snowbanks and snowballs. Thorne et al. found that 36% of their intermediate uveitis patients had pars planitis.[13] In one study by Rodriguez et al., 22.2% of cases of intermediate uveitis at a referral center were due to sarcoidosis, whereas 8.0% were due to MS.[21] One out of 112 cases at this center was due to Lyme disease. In two other studies, 14.8 and 16.2% had MS, respectively.[17,22]

Tests that warrant investigation on all patients with intermediate uveitis include rapid plasma reagin and fluorescent treponemal antibody absorption test to test for syphilis, chest X-ray, angiotensin-converting enzyme (ACE), and tuberculin skin test with anergy panel, to evaluate sarcoidosis and tuberculosis. If clinical suspicion is high for sarcoidosis in the setting of a negative ACE and chest X-ray, one should consider a gallium scan, pulmonary function tests, or a chest computed tomography scan. A careful review of systems should be performed to determine if there are risks associated with MS, including urinary retention, neurologic weakness or symptoms, or evidence of previous optic neuritis (Table 79.2).[23] In a significant number of patients, as is the case in our experience, pars planitis can be the first manifestation of a central nervous system demyelinating process, so it is important to elicit the appropriate history and keep a low threshold for the diagnosis of MS. Because there is growing evidence that early treatment of MS with systemic interferon therapy may reduce long-term disability, it is important to consider this systemic association seriously upon initial presentation.[24–26] Evaluation by a neurologist, magnetic resonance imaging (MRI) of the brain, and cerebrospinal fluid studies should be considered in new-onset intermediate uveitis, even without the above symptoms, given that early disease can by asymptomatic.

If there is a history of exposure to deer or ticks, especially if the patient lives or travels in an endemic area, and there is an associated history of a target lesion, or systemic flu-like symptoms, then *Borrelia burgdorferi* antibody should be tested. Exposure to cats might prompt serum antibody testing for *Bartonella*.[27] In the elderly population, intraocular lymphoma should be suspected and there should be a lower threshold to perform diagnostic vitrectomy, especially if there is limited response to corticosteroids.[28,29] If intraocular lymphoma is highly suspected, a lumbar puncture for cytological evaluation of the cerebrospinal fluid and neuroimaging are adjunctive diagnostic tests to consider. Bilateral pars planitis has been found in patients who have human T-cell lymphotropic virus type 1 (HTLV-1) infection, which is endemic in Japan, the Caribbean islands, parts of Central Africa, and South America.[30] The latter can be diagnosed with serological testing for antibodies against HTLV-1. Gastrointestinal disturbances associated with a pars planitis-like clinical presentation should prompt referral to a gastroenterologist since it has been reported in association with inflammatory bowel disease and Whipple's disease.[31,32] Other masquerade syndromes, such as intermediate uveitis secondary to tumor necrosis from retinoblastoma or uveal melanoma or even metastasis from other types of systemic cancer, must be evaluated in the appropriate clinical settings.[33] Finally, mild vitritis and CME in the setting of recent cataract surgery should prompt consideration of pseudophakic CME. One should consider indolent endogenous or exogenous endophthalmitis as a possibility if there is a poor response or worsening with corticosteroids in the setting of the appropriate risk factors, such as immunocompromised state or recent intraocular surgery.

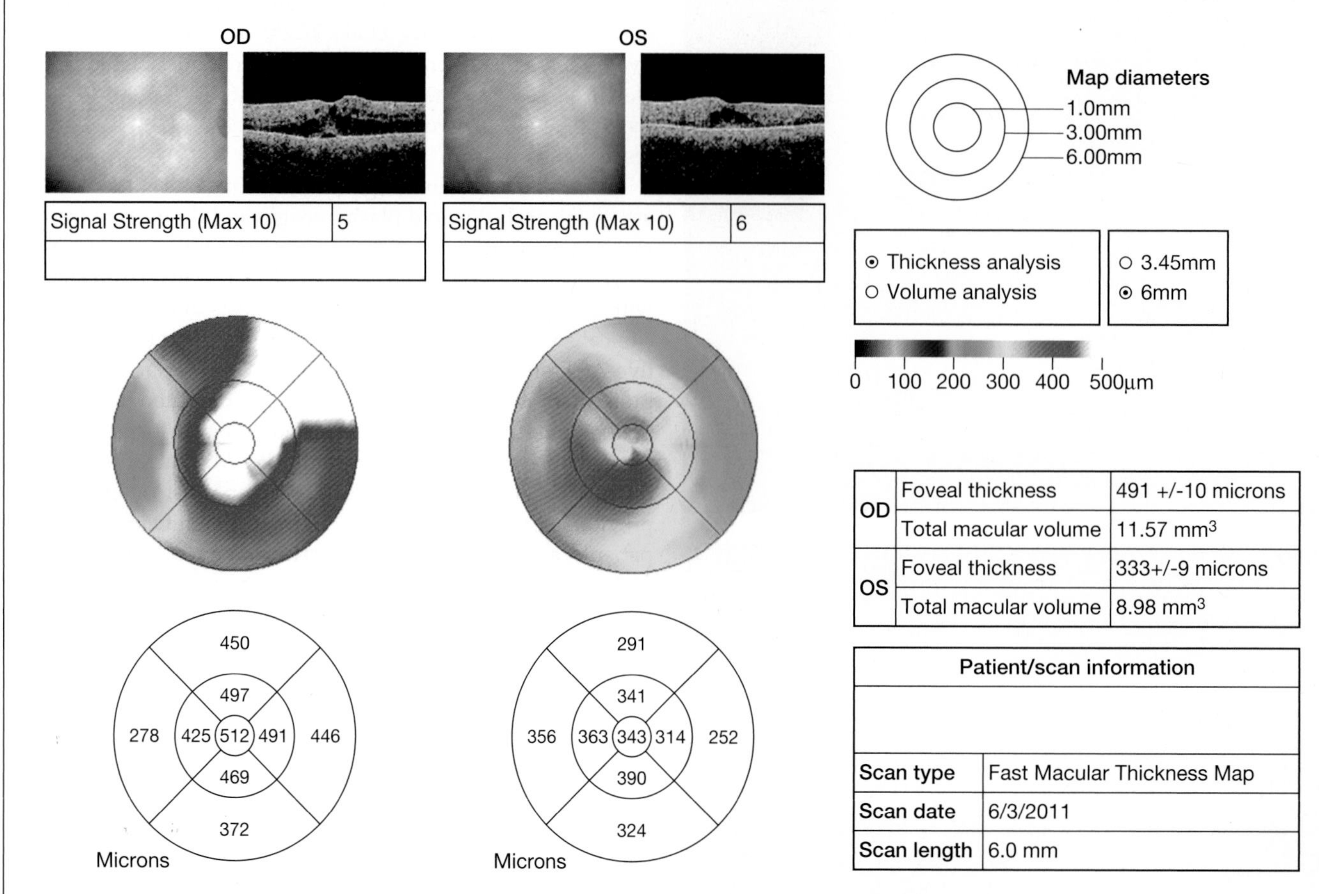

Fig. 79.5 Bilateral cystoid macular edema in a patient with otherwise quiescent intermediate uveitis.

Table 79.1 Differential diagnosis of intermediate uveitis

Infectious
Lyme disease (*Borrelia burgdorferi*) Syphilis (*Treponema pallidum*) Toxocariasis (*Toxocara canis*) Toxoplasmosis (*Toxoplasma gondii*) Tuberculosis (*Mycobacterium tuberculosis*) Cat-scratch disease (*Bartonella, Rochalimaea*) Whipple's disease (*Tropherema whipelli*) HTLV-1 Hepatitis C Epstein–Barr virus Endophthalmitis (*Propionibacterium acnes*, indolent fungal infection)
Immune
Sarcoidosis Multiple sclerosis Inflammatory bowel disease Behçet's disease Idiopathic Pars planitis
Masquerade
Lymphoma (usually B-cell, NHL) Leukemia Amyloidosis Other neoplasms: retinoblastoma, uveal melanoma Irvine–Gass syndrome (CME with subtle inflammation)

HTLV-1, human T-lymphotropic virus-1; NHL, non-Hodgkin's lymphoma; CME, cystoid macular edema.

HISTOPATHOLOGY AND PATHOPHYSIOLOGY

On histopathologic examination, snowballs are isolated vitreous granulomas consisting of lymphocytes, macrophages, epithelioid cells, and multinucleated giant cells.[34] Snowbanks consist of collapsed vitreous collagen, membranous fibroglial cells, blood vessels, and lymphocytes as well as hyperplastic pars plana nonpigmented epithelium.[35] Periphlebitis is denoted by lymphocytic infiltration and cuffing of the peripheral retinal venules.[34] Because the term "intermediate uveitis" is an anatomic designation, one should avoid assigning a single etiologic or pathophysiologic process to it given that various systemic diseases and infectious processes can result in inflammation in this anatomic location. The pathogenesis of the autoimmune causes of intermediate uveitis involves overlapping principles as well as some distinguishing characteristics, and will be discussed here for pars planitis and sarcoidosis.

Pars planitis

Although it is thought that noninfectious intermediate uveitis arises from an autoimmune response, the antigenic stimulus has not yet been clearly identified. Bora et al. described a novel 36 kDa nucleopore complex protein that was found to be six to eight times higher in the sera of 81% of active pars planitis patients compared with controls ($P < 0.05$).[36] The exact function of this protein and its role in the pathogenesis of pars planitis are unknown, although there are indications that other nucleopore complex proteins may be involved in myeloid

Table 79.2 Systemic symptoms and signs of multiple sclerosis by site

Anatomic location	Symptoms	Signs
Cerebrum	Cognitive impairment	Deficits in attention, reasoning, and executive function; dementia (late)
	Depression	Flat affect
	Hemisensory and motor	Upper motor neuron signs
Optic nerve	Unilateral vision loss	rAPD, Uthoff phenomenon (exacerbation in hot temperatures), Pulfrich effect (difficulty judging path of oncoming cars)
Cerebellum	Tremor	Action tremor
	Clumsiness and poor balance	Gait ataxia
Brainstem	Diplopia, oscillopsia	INO, nystagmus
	Vertigo	
	Impaired swallowing	
	Impaired speech	
Spinal cord	Weakness	
	Stiffness and painful spasms	Spasticity, Lhermitte's sign (painful electric-shock sensation down spine upon neck flexion)
	Bladder dysfunction	
	Retention	
	Frequency, urgency	
Other	Pain	
	Fatigue	
	Temperature sensitivity and exercise intolerance	

rAPD, relative afferent papillary defect; INO, internuclear ophthalmoplegia. (Modified from Compston A, Coles A. Multiple sclerosis. Lancet 2008;372: 1502–17.)

leukemogenesis and autoantibody formation.[37,38] Wetzig et al. found that endstage idiopathic intermediate uveitis in a familial case of bilateral intermediate uveitis was characterized immunopathologically by a predominance of CD4+ T lymphocytes and overwhelming predominance of glial cells in the pars plana snowbank; the latter is a characteristic unique to this type of uveitis.[39] It has been proposed that pars planitis represents a similar pathoetiological entity as MS, although with expression either isolated to the eye or starting in the eye.[40] Indeed, patients with MS have increased circulating CD54+ lymphocytes and antibodies that recognize glial proteins.[41] Raja et al.[22] discovered that a human leukocyte antigen (HLA)-DR15 allele, which is known to be associated with MS, was significantly associated with pars planitis compared with controls (odds ratio, 2.86; $P = 0.004$). Although no specific autoantigen has been clearly determined, components of vitreous, in addition to the glial elements mentioned above, have been implicated. Circulating lymphocytes isolated from pars planitis patients appear to proliferate in response to type II collagen.[35] Furthermore, Hultsch produced a clinical entity similar to pars planitis by giving owl monkeys multiple intravitreal injections of hyaluronic acid.[42]

Interleukin-8 (IL-8), a cytokine that is involved in neutrophil and T-lymphocyte recruitment, and soluble intercellular adhesion molecule 1 (sICAM-1), which is expressed at sites of inflammation to aid in leukocyte adhesion and migration, were elevated in the blood of patients with intermediate uveitis compared to controls. Furthermore, elevated sICAM-1 and IL-8 were associated with development of systemic disease. Elevated IL-8 was associated with signs of inflammatory activity such as periphlebitis and the presence of vitreous exudates. Rather than explaining the pathogenesis of this ocular condition, these markers may be indicators of systemic disease or activity, even in the absence of systemic symptoms.[43,44]

Sarcoidosis

Sarcoidosis is also thought to be a CD4 T-lymphocyte-mediated process in the eye and in other actively affected tissues. Efforts to elucidate an infectious cause for sarcoidosis have met with little success. Patients with active sarcoidosis have a predominantly Th1 cytokine profile with elevated levels of IL-2 and interferon-gamma, and diminished levels of IL-4. Despite the predominance of CD4+ T cells in ocular tissues affected by the disease, elevated peripheral levels of immunoglobulin, B-cell hyperactivity in the peripheral blood, and a loss of delayed-type hypersensitivity to the tuberculin skin test (anergy) argues for an unusual partitioning of the immune response.[41,45] We have found that approximately 50% of patients with sarcoid-associated uveitis are anergic to delayed-type hypersensitivity testing.[46] The latter observations underline the importance of an anergy panel to accompany a tuberculin skin test in the initial workup of intermediate uveitis. HLA associations in sarcoidosis also differ from pars planitis and have not been clearly elucidated. In one study by Rossman et al., ocular sarcoidosis was associated with the HLA-DRB1*0401 allele in both blacks and whites.[47]

TREATMENT

Unilateral disease

Once an infectious cause has been ruled out, the primary treatment of choice is corticosteroids. If an underlying systemic condition is suspected, then systemic treatment with appropriate referral to a rheumatologist or infectious disease specialist is warranted. For unilateral noninfectious intermediate uveitis in the absence of systemic disease, periocular corticosteroids are initiated (Fig. 79.6), although some clinicians utilize systemic steroids. In our practice, posterior subtenon Kenalog is given at 40 mg/mL, 1 mL total. If there is little to no response in 3–4 weeks, a second injection can be given, or alternatively, if the patient is pseudophakic and does not have glaucoma, an intravitreal injection of preservative-free triamcinolone acetonide can be offered. If smoldering uveitic CME is present without other

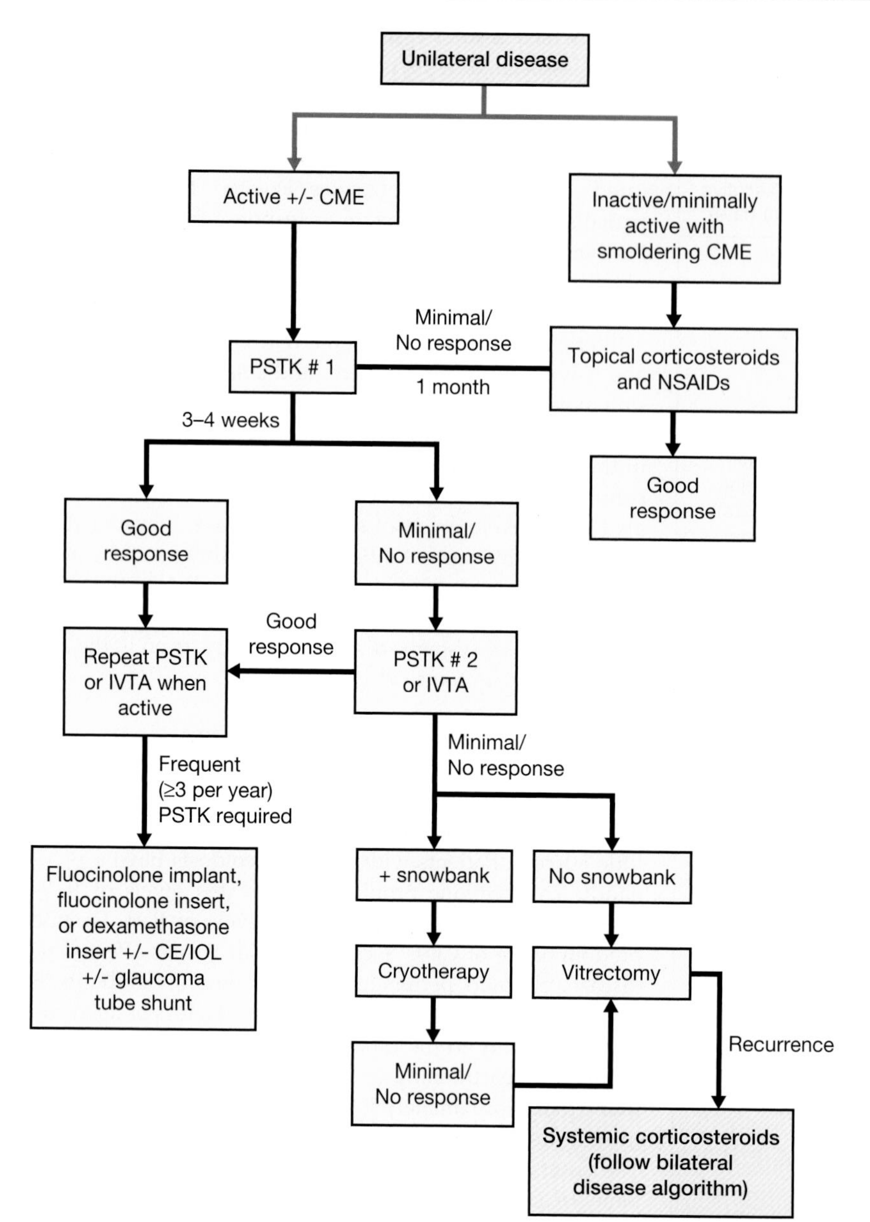

Fig. 79.6 Treatment algorithm for unilateral disease. CME, cystoid macular edema; PSTK, posterior subtenon Kenalog; IVTA, intravitreal triamcinolone acetonide; CE/IOL, cataract extraction with intraocular lens implant; NSAIDs, nonsteroidal anti-inflammatory drugs.

evidence of active inflammatory disease, a trial of topical corticosteroids in combination with nonsteroidal anti-inflammatory drops can be applied prior to considering either periocular or intravitreal corticosteroids.[48] Alternatively, bevacizumab has been investigated for its efficacy in treating uveitic CME. In a study comparing intravitreal bevacizumab with intravitreal triamcinolone acetonide for uveitic CME, after removing the effect on cataract formation the triamcinolone group appeared to have significantly better visual acuity outcomes. Triamcinolone was also more effective in reducing macular thickness than bevacizumab.[49]

If the patient has benefited from periocular or intraocular corticosteroid, but has documented recurrence when the corticosteroids have waned, then a corticosteroid intravitreal implant can be considered, especially if the patient is already pseudophakic (Fig. 79.7). If the patient is phakic, combined lens extraction, intraocular lens implantation, and insertion of a fluocinolone acetonide sustained drug delivery system (Retisert)

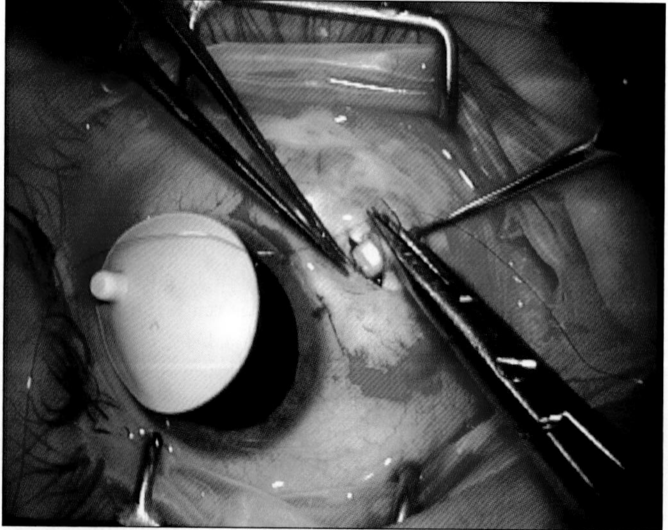

Fig. 79.7 Fluocinolone acetonide implant placement.

can be performed.[50] If the patient has known glaucoma, then combined glaucoma tube shunt and fluocinolone implant surgery should be considered and has been found to be effective.[51] In young patients, combined surgery should proceed only after achieving relative quiescence given the robust inflammatory response after incisional surgery and careful consideration of the loss of accommodation that will occur after removing the crystalline lens. Alternatively, a dexamethasone intravitreal insert (Ozurdex)[52] can be applied to circumvent the need for incisional surgery. If there is little to no response after two corticosteroid injections (either posterior subtenon or intravitreal), then therapeutic/diagnostic vitrectomy can be considered. If a snowbank is present, cryotherapy can be applied.[53] Peripheral laser photocoagulation has also been used to treat pars planitis, resulting in a decrease in the amount of corticosteroid needed and in decreased vitritis, although the rate of epiretinal membrane increased.[54] If peripheral neovascularization occurs, then peripheral laser is indicated. Finally, oral prednisone can be used, applying the algorithm for bilateral disease below.

Bilateral disease

Bilateral disease usually warrants treatment with systemic corticosteroids, starting at 1 mg/kg/day tapered to the lowest levels required to achieve quiescence over a 2-month period. If greater than 10 mg of oral prednisone is required for longer than 4 months, or when treating children, in whom long-term corticosteroids can cause growth retardation, steroid-sparing immunosuppressives should be initiated (Fig. 79.8). If one is not aware of the systemic risks or does not choose to monitor appropriately for systemic risks referral to or co-management with an internist or rheumatologist is highly recommended.

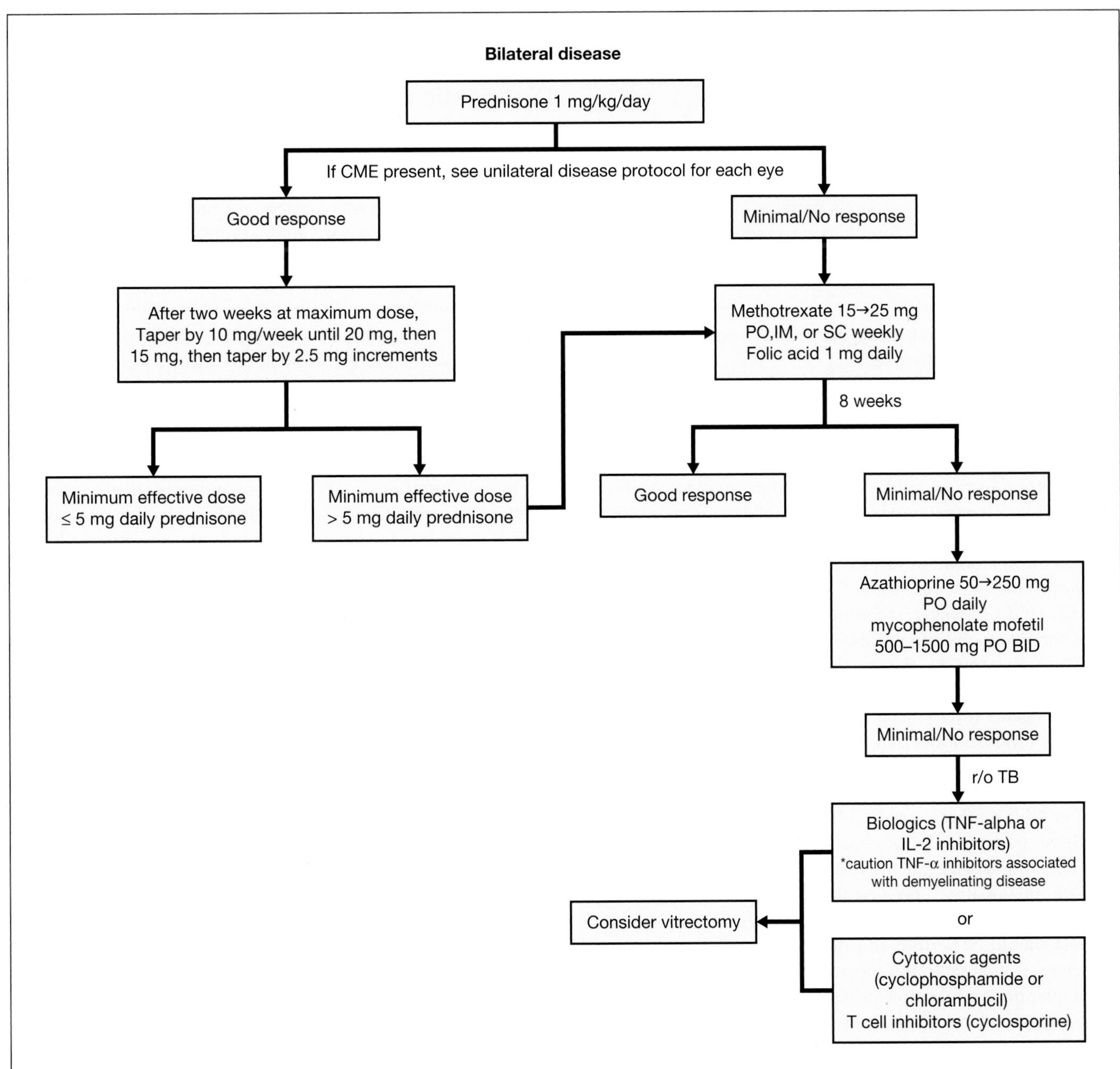

Fig. 79.8 Treatment algorithm for bilateral disease.

We have had good success treating sarcoidosis-associated intermediate and panuveitis with methotrexate starting at 12.5–15 mg PO weekly and escalating to 25 mg PO weekly, along with folic acid, 1 mg/day. Dosage is based on treatment response and tolerability. Because of its relative safety in children, methotrexate is often used as a first-line agent with a short course of bridging corticosteroids. It should be noted that methotrexate should not be used in pregnancy given its teratogenicity and fetal abortive effects. Common side-effects of methotrexate include nausea, vomiting, and oral stomatitis. If gastrointestinal side-effects prevent oral dosing, intramuscular or subcutaneous injections can be administered instead. Hepatotoxicity, cytopenia, and interstitial pneumonitis can also occur with methotrexate use. Liver function tests and complete blood counts are evaluated before initiation of therapy and should be monitored every 8–12 weeks thereafter. The dose of methotrexate should be reduced if the aspartate aminotransferase or alanine aminotransferase level is more than twice normal on two separate occasions, but any elevation may warrant at least dose reduction. In the first study on the use of methotrexate in ocular sarcoidosis, 100% of 11 patients decreased their dosage of corticosteroids, 86% successfully discontinued prednisone, and 90% had preserved or improved visual acuity, although all patients in this study had panuveitis rather than isolated intermediate uveitis.[55] In a multicentered retrospective study in which methotrexate was used to treat noninfectious uveitis patients of all anatomic subtypes, methotrexate was found to be moderately effective in controlling inflammation, although the side-effect profile was beneficial.[56] Information regarding the effectiveness of methotrexate on the intermediate uveitis subgroup in the latter study was difficult to interpret given that 76.2% were inactive at the time of starting methotrexate.

In patients unable to tolerate methotrexate or who fail to achieve treatment success on this agent, other antimetabolites, including azathioprine or mycophenolate mofetil, can be initiated. Galor et al. compared the three antimetabolites in the treatment of noninfectious ocular inflammation in a retrospective cohort study. They suggested that mycophenolate mofetil controlled inflammation more rapidly than methotrexate, when "control of inflammation" was defined by quiescent inflammation on ≤10 mg oral prednisone.[57] There were several caveats in the latter study, however, including significantly younger age in the methotrexate group, and the use of prior immunosuppressive drug therapy in the azathioprine and mycophenolate groups. If antimetabolites are minimally effective, a course of cytotoxic agents (cyclophosphamide or chlorambucil) or T-cell inhibitors (cyclosporine) can be given with close attention to toxic side-effects. Alternatively, the tumor necrosis alpha (TNF-α) inhibitors adalimumab or infliximab can be initiated in combination with methotrexate,[58] although it is important to note that there are a number of reports of these biologics causing demyelinating disease such as MS and progressive multifocal leukoencephalopathy.[59] Because they have also been implicated in the reactivation of latent tuberculosis,[60] an updated tuberculin skin test should be performed prior to initiating these drugs. If the patient is anergic to the tuberculin skin test due to sarcoidosis, a quantiferon tuberculosis test can be performed.[61]

The biologics daclizumab and infliximab have both been used to treat ocular sarcoidosis with success.[62,63] Etanercept is a TNF-α inhibitor that is no longer used as often in the treatment of uveitis since it has been associated with increased inflammation or lack of ocular inflammation control. In one study of 22 uveitis patients who received anti-TNF-α therapy, infliximab was more effective than etanercept in controlling ocular inflammation.[64] Referral to a rheumatologist is typically sought once the patient requires immunosuppressive medication stronger than the antimetabolites.

Recently, the results of the Multicenter Uveitis Steroid Treatment trial were published, comparing systemic anti-inflammatory therapy with the fluocinolone acetonide implant for intermediate, posterior, and panuveitis.[65] The study demonstrated no significant difference in visual acuity outcome at 24 months, but improved control of uveitis activity, vitreous haze, and a trend towards better control of CME in the implant group by 24 months. The rate of ocular complications, such as elevated intraocular pressure requiring glaucoma surgery or cataracts, was significantly higher in the implant group, as expected, whereas adverse systemic events, while infrequent in both groups, were slightly lower in the implant group, although the risk of hospitalization did not differ between the two groups.[65]

Diagnostic and therapeutic vitrectomy

Diagnostic and therapeutic vitrectomy is considered in patients who are not responsive to the above treatment regimens or if intraocular lymphoma is highly suspected. In a prospective randomized study, Tranos et al. demonstrated better visual acuity and improved fluorescein angiographic CME characteristics after vitrectomy, compared with standard medical therapy consisting of systemic corticosteroids and immunosuppressives. However, this study was underpowered to achieve statistical significance.[66] A number of other studies also appear to show a moderate level of success in treating CME with pars plana vitrectomy, which is thought to be effective by debulking soluble and cellular vitreous inflammatory mediators, and by allowing easier access to the vitreous cavity of aqueous inhibitory molecules such as transforming growth factor-ß and alpha-melanocyte stimulating hormone.[67–69] We perform a diagnostic vitrectomy if an infectious source such as herpetic viral infection or toxoplasmosis is suspected but cannot be confirmed using other methods, or if intraocular lymphoma is suspected, in which case the specimen is sent for cytopathological evaluation and/or flow cytometry. If intraocular lymphoma is diagnosed, a neurologic workup and MRI may be necessary to determine if there is central nervous system disease. If isolated to the eye or in the setting of central nervous system lymphoma with a recurrence restricted to the eye, orbital irradiation or intravitreal rituximab alone or in combination with methotrexate can be administered with success.[70–72]

CLINICAL COURSE AND COMPLICATIONS

Clinical course

Patients with inflammatory intermediate uveitis often have a favorable visual acuity outcome. In one study of patients with pars planitis, mean visual acuity after 10 years of follow-up was 20/30, 75% maintained a visual acuity of 20/40 or better, and one-third maintained normal visual acuity without treatment.[11] In a study by Kalinina Ayuso and colleagues, younger age at onset decreased the visual prognosis and increased the rates of complications;[73] however, another study showed higher rates of remission in patients who presented at a younger age. Mean time to remission in the latter study, which occurred at a rate of 34%, was 8.6 years.[12]

Complications

Causes of vision loss in intermediate uveitis include CME, uveitic glaucoma, retinal detachment, vitreous hemorrhage, cataracts, and epiretinal membranes. Band keratopathy, especially prominent in children with chronic intermediate uveitis, can also cause vision loss. Chronic CME accounts for most cases of permanent visual loss, and occurred at a rate of 41.2% over 15 years according to one large retrospective cohort study, and at a rate of 45.7% in a separate study.[11,13] Concentric retinal macular thickening can also be seen in patients with intermediate uveitis, although it does not necessarily need to be treated.[20] The 15-year rates of cataract and epiretinal membranes were 34.2% and 44.4%, respectively, in the report by Donaldson et al.[11] An increased rate of CME appears to be associated with cigarette smoking. In one large case-control study, the odds ratio of a smoker (versus a nonsmoker) having intermediate uveitis with CME was 8.4 compared with an odds ratio of 1.5 in intermediate uveitis without CME.[4] In the report from Thorne et al., the odds ratio of having CME at presentation was 3.9 compared with a reference group of patients who had never smoked.[13]

In the late stages of intermediate uveitis peripheral neovascular and fibrous membranes can extend on to the ciliary body to form cyclitic and/or retrolenticular membranes, resulting in ciliary body detachment and hypotony. Prevention of progression to this stage is the mainstay of management. Once this develops, surgical intervention can be attempted to remove the cyclitic membrane and reverse hypotony to prevent phthisis, but success in improving visual outcome is poor.[74] Retinal detachment in the setting of active inflammatory disease should be repaired after relative quiescence is achieved, if possible. Combined surgery with fluocinolone implant and placement of silicone oil can be considered given the lipophilic nature of fluocinolone and its ability to be dispersed throughout the silicone oil.[75]

REFERENCES

1. Jabs DA, Nussenblatt RB, Rosenbaum JT. Standardization of uveitis nomenclature for reporting clinical data. Results of the First International Workshop. Am J Ophthalmol 2005;140:509–16.
2. Bonfioli AA, Damico FM, Curi AL, et al. Intermediate uveitis. Semin Ophthalmol 2005;20:147–54.
3. Lai WW, Pulido JS. Intermediate uveitis. Ophthalmol Clin North Am 2002;15:309–17.
4. Lin P, Loh AR, Margolis TP, et al. Cigarette smoking as a risk factor for uveitis. Ophthalmology 2010;117:585–90.
5. Lin P, Tessler HH, Goldstein DA. Family history of inflammatory bowel disease in patients with idiopathic ocular inflammation. Am J Ophthalmol 2006;141:1097–104.
6. Henderly DE, Genstler AJ, Smith RE, et al. Changing patterns of uveitis. Am J Ophthalmol 1987;103:131–6.
7. Kump LI, Cervantes-Castaneda RA, Androudi SN, et al. Analysis of pediatric uveitis cases at a tertiary referral center. Ophthalmology 2005;112:1287–92.
8. Tugal-Tutkun I, Havrlikova K, Power WJ, et al. Changing patterns in uveitis of childhood. Ophthalmology 1996;103:375–83.
9. Gritz DC, Wong IG. Incidence and prevalence of uveitis in Northern California; the Northern California Epidemiology of Uveitis Study. Ophthalmology 2004; 111:491–500; discussion
10. Suhler EB, Lloyd MJ, Choi D, et al. Incidence and prevalence of uveitis in Veterans Affairs Medical Centers of the Pacific Northwest. Am J Ophthalmol 2008;146:890–6 e8.
11. Donaldson MJ, Pulido JS, Herman DC, et al. Pars planitis: a 20-year study of incidence, clinical features, and outcomes. Am J Ophthalmol 2007;144:812–7.
12. Vidovic-Valentincic N, Kraut A, Hawlina M, et al. Intermediate uveitis: long-term course and visual outcome. Br J Ophthalmol 2009;93:477–80.
13. Thorne JE, Daniel E, Jabs DA, et al. Smoking as a risk factor for cystoid macular edema complicating intermediate uveitis. Am J Ophthalmol 2008;145:841–6.
14. Tugal-Tutkun I, Aydin-Akova Y, Guney-Tefekli E, et al. Referral patterns, demographic and clinical features, and visual prognosis of Turkish patients with sarcoid uveitis. Ocul Immunol Inflamm 2007;15:337–43.
15. Althaus C, Sundmacher R. Intermediate uveitis: epidemiology, age and sex distribution. Dev Ophthalmol 1992;23:9–14.
16. Madow B, Galor A, Feuer WJ, et al. Validation of a photographic vitreous haze grading technique for clinical trials in uveitis. Am J Ophthalmol 2011;152: 170–6.
17. Malinowski SM, Pulido JS, Folk JC. Long-term visual outcome and complications associated with pars planitis. Ophthalmology 1993;100:818–24; discussion 25.
18. Lai JC, Stinnett SS, Jaffe GJ. B-scan ultrasonography for the detection of macular thickening. Am J Ophthalmol 2003;136:55–61.
19. de Smet MD, Okada AA. Cystoid macular edema in uveitis. Dev Ophthalmol 2010;47:136–47.
20. Castellano CG, Stinnett SS, Mettu PS, et al. Retinal thickening in iridocyclitis. Am J Ophthalmol 2009;148:341–9.
21. Rodriguez A, Calonge M, Pedroza-Seres M, et al. Referral patterns of uveitis in a tertiary eye care center. Arch Ophthalmol 1996;114:593–9.
22. Raja SC, Jabs DA, Dunn JP, et al. Pars planitis: clinical features and class II HLA associations. Ophthalmology 1999;106:594–9.
23. Compston A, Coles A. Multiple sclerosis. Lancet 2008;372:1502–17.
24. Curkendall SM, Wang C, Johnson BH, et al. Potential health care cost savings associated with early treatment of multiple sclerosis using disease-modifying therapy. Clin Ther 2011;33:914–25.
25. Jacobs LD, Beck RW, Simon JH, et al. Intramuscular interferon beta-1a therapy initiated during a first demyelinating event in multiple sclerosis. CHAMPS Study Group. N Engl J Med 2000;343:898–904.
26. Comi G, Filippi M, Barkhof F, et al. Effect of early interferon treatment on conversion to definite multiple sclerosis: a randomised study. Lancet 2001;357: 1576–82.
27. Ormerod LD, Dailey JP. Ocular manifestations of cat-scratch disease. Curr Opin Ophthalmol 1999;10:209–16.
28. Sabet-Peyman EJ, Eberhart CG, Janjua K, et al. Persistent intermediate uveitis associated with latent manifestation of facial large B-cell non-Hodgkin lymphoma. Ocul Immunol Inflamm 2009;17:322–4.
29. Mruthyunjaya P, Jumper JM, McCallum R, et al. Diagnostic yield of vitrectomy in eyes with suspected posterior segment infection or malignancy. Ophthalmology 2002;109:1123–9.
30. Buggage RR. Ocular manifestations of human T-cell lymphotropic virus type 1 infection. Curr Opin Ophthalmol 2003;14:420–5.
31. Boskovich SA, Lowder CY, Meisler DM, et al. Systemic diseases associated with intermediate uveitis. Cleve Clin J Med 1993;60:460–5.
32. Thaler S, Grisanti S, Klingel K, et al. Intermediate uveitis and arthralgia as early symptoms in Whipple's disease. Int J Infect Dis 2010;14(Suppl 3):e388–9.
33. Soheilian M, Mirbabai F, Shahsavari M, et al. Metastatic cutaneous melanoma to the vitreous cavity masquerading as intermediate uveitis. Eur J Ophthalmol 2002;12:324–7.
34. Eichenbaum JW, Friedman AH, Mamelok AE. A clinical and histopathological review of intermediate uveitis ("pars planitis"). Bull N Y Acad Med 1988;64: 164–74.
35. Pederson JE, Kenyon KR, Green WR, et al. Pathology of pars planitis. Am J Ophthalmol 1978;86:762–74.
36. Bora NS, Bora PS, Tandhasetti MT, et al. Molecular cloning, sequencing, and expression of the 36 kDa protein present in pars planitis. Sequence homology with yeast nucleopore complex protein. Invest Ophthalmol Vis Sci 1996; 37:1877–83.
37. Courvalin JC, Lassoued K, Bartnik E, et al. The 210-kD nuclear envelope polypeptide recognized by human autoantibodies in primary biliary cirrhosis is the major glycoprotein of the nuclear pore. J Clin Invest 1990;86:279–85.
38. Kraemer D, Wozniak RW, Blobel G, et al. The human CAN protein, a putative oncogene product associated with myeloid leukemogenesis, is a nuclear pore complex protein that faces the cytoplasm. Proc Natl Acad Sci U S A 1994;91: 1519–23.
39. Wetzig RP, Chan CC, Nussenblatt RB, et al. Clinical and immunopathological studies of pars planitis in a family. Br J Ophthalmol 1988;72:5–10.
40. Nissenblatt MJ, Masciulli L, Yarian DL, et al. Pars planitis – a demyelinating disease? Arch Ophthalmol 1981;99:697.
41. Boyd SR, Young S, Lightman S. Immunopathology of the noninfectious posterior and intermediate uveitides. Surv Ophthalmol 2001;46:209–33.
42. Hultsch E. Peripheral uveitis in the owl monkey. Experimental model. Mod Probl Ophthalmol 1977;18:247–51.
43. Klok AM, Luyendijk L, Zaal MJ, et al. Elevated serum IL-8 levels are associated with disease activity in idiopathic intermediate uveitis. Br J Ophthalmol 1998;82:871–4.
44. Klok AM, Luyendijk L, Zaal MJ, et al. Soluble ICAM-1 serum levels in patients with intermediate uveitis. Br J Ophthalmol 1999;83:847–51.
45. Bianco A, Spiteri MA. Peripheral anergy and local immune hyperactivation in sarcoidosis: a paradox or birds of a feather. Clin Exp Immunol 1997;110:1–3.
46. Chow JH, Mettu PS, Srivastava SK, et al. PPD and positive skin test controls in the evaluation of anergy in uveitis patients. ARVO Meeting Abstracts April 11, 2008.
47. Rossman MD, Thompson B, Frederick M, et al. HLA-DRB1*1101: a significant risk factor for sarcoidosis in blacks and whites. Am J Hum Genet 2003;73: 720–35.
48. Hogewind BF, Zijlstra C, Klevering BJ, et al. Intravitreal triamcinolone for the treatment of refractory macular edema in idiopathic intermediate or posterior uveitis. Eur J Ophthalmol 2008;18:429–34.
49. Soheilian M, Rabbanikhah Z, Ramezani A, et al. Intravitreal bevacizumab versus triamcinolone acetonide for refractory uveitic cystoid macular edema: a randomized pilot study. J Ocul Pharmacol Ther 2010;26:199–206.

50. Chieh JJ, Carlson AN, Jaffe GJ. Combined fluocinolone acetonide intraocular delivery system insertion, phacoemulsification, and intraocular lens implantation for severe uveitis. Am J Ophthalmol 2008;146:589–94.
51. Malone PE, Herndon LW, Muir KW, et al. Combined fluocinolone acetonide intravitreal insertion and glaucoma drainage device placement for chronic uveitis and glaucoma. Am J Ophthalmol 2010;149:800–6 e1.
52. Ghosn CR, Li Y, Orilla WC, et al. Treatment of experimental anterior and intermediate uveitis by a dexamethasone intravitreal implant. Invest Ophthalmol Vis Sci 2011;52:2917–23.
53. Okinami S, Sunakawa M, Arai I, et al. Treatment of pars planitis with cryotherapy. Ophthalmologica 1991;202:180–6.
54. Pulido JS, Mieler WF, Walton D, et al. Results of peripheral laser photocoagulation in pars planitis. Trans Am Ophthalmol Soc 1998;96:127–37; discussion 37–41.
55. Dev S, McCallum RM, Jaffe GJ. Methotrexate treatment for sarcoid-associated panuveitis. Ophthalmology 1999;106:111–8.
56. Gangaputra S, Newcomb CW, Liesegang TL, et al. Methotrexate for ocular inflammatory diseases. Ophthalmology 2009;116:2188–98 e1.
57. Galor A, Jabs DA, Leder HA, et al. Comparison of antimetabolite drugs as corticosteroid-sparing therapy for noninfectious ocular inflammation. Ophthalmology 2008;115:1826–32.
58. Neri P, Zucchi M, Allegri P, et al. Adalimumab (Humira): a promising monoclonal anti-tumor necrosis factor alpha in ophthalmology. Int Ophthalmol 2011;31:165–73.
59. Li SY, Birnbaum AD, Goldstein DA. Optic neuritis associated with adalimumab in the treatment of uveitis. Ocul Immunol Inflamm 2010;18:475–81.
60. Salgado E, Gomez-Reino JJ. The risk of tuberculosis in patients treated with TNF antagonists. Expert Rev Clin Immunol 2011;7:329–40.
61. Milman N, Soborg B, Bo Svendsen C, et al. Quantiferon test for tuberculosis screening in sarcoidosis patients. Scand J Infect Dis 2011.
62. Gallagher M, Quinones K, Cervantes-Castaneda RA, et al. Biological response modifier therapy for refractory childhood uveitis. Br J Ophthalmol 2007; 91:1341–4.
63. Lindstedt EW, Baarsma GS, Kuijpers RW, et al. Anti-TNF-alpha therapy for sight threatening uveitis. Br J Ophthalmol 2005;89:533–6.
64. Galor A, Perez VL, Hammel JP, et al. Differential effectiveness of etanercept and infliximab in the treatment of ocular inflammation. Ophthalmology 2006;113:2317–23.
65. Kempen JH, Altaweel MM, Holbrook JT, et al. Randomized comparison of systemic anti-inflammatory therapy versus fluocinolone acetonide implant for intermediate, posterior, and panuveitis: the Multicenter Uveitis Steroid Treatment Trial. Ophthalmology 2011;118:1916–26.
66. Tranos P, Scott R, Zambarakji H, et al. The effect of pars plana vitrectomy on cystoid macular oedema associated with chronic uveitis: a randomised, controlled pilot study. Br J Ophthalmol 2006;90:1107–10.
67. Becker M, Davis J. Vitrectomy in the treatment of uveitis. Am J Ophthalmol 2005;140:1096–105.
68. Dugel PU, Rao NA, Ozler S, et al. Pars plana vitrectomy for intraocular inflammation-related cystoid macular edema unresponsive to corticosteroids. A preliminary study. Ophthalmology 1992;99:1535–41.
69. Verbraeken H. Therapeutic pars plana vitrectomy for chronic uveitis: a retrospective study of the long-term results. Graefes Arch Clin Exp Ophthalmol 1996;234:288–93.
70. Levy-Clarke GA, Chan CC, Nussenblatt RB. Diagnosis and management of primary intraocular lymphoma. Hematol Oncol Clin North Am 2005;19:739–49, viii.
71. Pe'er J, Hochberg FH, Foster CS. Clinical review: treatment of vitreoretinal lymphoma. Ocul Immunol Inflamm 2009;17:299–306.
72. Smith JR, Rosenbaum JT, Wilson DJ, et al. Role of intravitreal methotrexate in the management of primary central nervous system lymphoma with ocular involvement. Ophthalmology 2002;109:1709–16.
73. Kalinina Ayuso V, ten Cate HA, van den Does P, et al. Young age as a risk factor for complicated course and visual outcome in intermediate uveitis in children. Br J Ophthalmol 2011;95:646–51.
74. Yu EN, Paredes I, Foster CS. Surgery for hypotony in patients with juvenile idiopathic arthritis-associated uveitis. Ocul Immunol Inflamm 2007;15: 11–7.
75. Dayani PN, Chow J, Stinnett SS, et al. Pars plana vitrectomy, fluocinolone acetonide implantation, and silicone oil infusion for the treatment of chronic, refractory uveitic hypotony. Am J Ophthalmol 2011;152:849–56 e1.

Chapter 80

Rheumatic Disease

Alastair K. Denniston, Mary Gayed, David Carruthers, Caroline Gordon, Philip I. Murray

INTRODUCTION

Many rheumatic diseases have ocular and adnexal complications. These range from relatively mild ocular surface problems to potentially blinding intraocular and orbital disease. It is important to know which ophthalmic conditions can be associated with rheumatic disease, and to have a greater understanding of those diseases. Close collaboration with a rheumatologist is often essential, particularly in the management of these patients.

The aims of this chapter are to provide: (1) an overview of the ophthalmic conditions commonly associated with rheumatic disease; (2) a detailed disease-specific section on the systemic and ocular manifestations and management of various rheumatic diseases, including the systemic vasculitides, paying particular attention to posterior segment disease; and (3) a knowledge of the potential ocular complications of the treatment of rheumatic disease.

AN APPROACH TO THE ASSESSMENT OF THE PATIENT WITH POSSIBLE RHEUMATIC DISEASE

Patients may present to the ophthalmologist with a known rheumatic disease and it may be assumed that the ophthalmic problem is a manifestation of their rheumatic disease. Alternatively, patients may present who do not have a known diagnosis of rheumatic disease. In this group it is important to know which ophthalmic conditions are associated with rheumatic disease, and to be aware that some are common to many rheumatic diseases, such as keratoconjunctivitis sicca, and scleritis. Therefore, one must have knowledge of those diseases and how to differentiate between them. This will involve taking a full ophthalmic and medical history, performing a detailed examination, and ordering appropriate investigations.

Common ocular presentations of rheumatic disease

Keratoconjunctivitis sicca and other corneal presentations

Keratoconjunctivitis sicca (KCS, or "dry eye syndrome") is a common ocular manifestation of a number of rheumatic diseases including rheumatoid arthritis (RA), systemic lupus erythematosus (SLE), scleroderma, and relapsing polychondritis. Symptoms vary from slight irritation and burning in mild disease to severe pain and blurred vision arising from increasing corneal involvement. Clinical examination using slit-lamp biomicroscopy reveals a small or absent tear meniscus with a tear film break-up time of less than 10 seconds. Corneal abnormalities, which may be highlighted with fluorescein drops and a cobalt blue light, include punctate epitheliopathy, mucus filaments, strands, and plaques. Additional staining with Rose Bengal or Lissamine Green drops reveals a characteristic interpalpebral pattern, with greatest staining nasal and temporal to the corneal limbus. Tear production, as measured by Schirmer's test, is reduced. Wetting of the test strip by less than 5 mm after 5 minutes in the un-anesthetized eye indicates severe tear deficiency. It should be noted that the correlation of dry eye symptoms with observed disease is poor. Many more patients report "dry eyes" than have visible disease, and many asymptomatic patients do have some degree of keratoconjunctivitis sicca.[1]

Other less common corneal presentations of rheumatic disease include the sight-threatening peripheral ulcerative keratitis (PUK). The etiology is uncertain but it has been suggested that immune complex deposition at the corneal limbus results in an obliterative vasculitis and stromal melt. It is most commonly associated with RA or systemic vasculitis, in particular granulomatosis with polyangiitis (previously known as Wegener's granulomatosis).[2,3] Clinical features include variable pain and redness and reduced vision, uni/bilateral peripheral corneal ulceration with epithelial defect and stromal thinning, associated limbal inflammation, and scleritis.

Scleritis/episcleritis

Scleritis

Inflammation of the sclera is an extremely painful, potentially blinding condition. It may be classified according to location (anterior – 90%, or posterior – 10%), distribution (diffuse or nodular), and destruction (necrotizing or non-necrotizing). The majority of anterior scleritis is non-necrotizing (diffuse or nodular) and necrotizing disease may occur with and without inflammation.

Scleritis is associated with systemic disease in around 40–50% of patients, of which most are cases of a rheumatic disease, such as RA, granulomatosis with polyangiitis, relapsing polychondritis, SLE, sarcoidosis, polyarteritis nodosa, inflammatory bowel disease, psoriatic arthritis, ankylosing spondylitis, and gout.[4] It is commonest in middle-aged women. Scleritis is bilateral in 50% of cases, but both eyes may not be affected at the same time.[5] The pain (constant/deep/boring) can be so severe that it may wake the patient at night. The eye has an intense red/dark red appearance. The globe may be very tender to touch. A bluish hue implies scleral thinning from previous active scleritis due to the underlying blue/black uveal tissue showing through the translucent sclera. Scleral thinning can eventually result in high degrees of astigmatism. The degree of redness and scleral thinning is more easily seen under room light or in daylight than by the slit lamp. Topical phenylephrine 2.5% causes blanching of the more superficial episcleral vessels but does not change the engorgement of deeper scleral vessels and can often help differentiate between scleritis and episcleritis. The most severe type is necrotizing anterior scleritis with inflammation. Apart from the severe pain and redness, there may be tearing and photophobia. White avascular areas surrounded by injected edematous sclera are present that may lead to scleral necrosis. An associated anterior uveitis suggests advanced disease. Complications of scleritis include peripheral ulcerative keratitis, acute stromal keratitis, sclerosing keratitis, uveitis, cataract, astigmatism, glaucoma, and globe perforation.

Posterior scleritis is uncommon but is probably underdiagnosed. It is a potentially sight-threatening condition. It may be overlooked on account of more obvious anterior scleral inflammation or because there is isolated posterior disease and thus the eye appears white and quiet (often despite severe symptoms). It is associated with systemic disease (usually RA or systemic vasculitis) in up to one-third of cases. There is mild–severe deep pain (may be referred to brow or jaw), reduced vision, diplopia, and hypermetropic shift. The eye is white (unless anterior involvement) but may be associated with lid edema, proptosis, lid retraction, restricted motility, shallow anterior chamber, choroidal folds, annular choroidal detachment, exudative retinal detachments, macular edema, and optic disc edema. Diagnosis (and response to therapy) may be assisted by B-scan ultrasonography with measurement of scleral thickening and fluid in Tenon's space (T-sign).

Episcleritis

This common condition is a benign, recurrent inflammation of the episclera. Being superficial it is easily distinguished from deeper scleral inflammation, in that it is less painful and the involved vessels blanch on instillation of topical phenylephrine 2.5%. It is more common in young women, often self-limiting, and may require little or no treatment. It is not usually associated with any systemic disease, although around 10% may have an underlying rheumatic disease.[6]

Uveitis

Acute anterior uveitis

In acute anterior uveitis (AAU) patients typically present with pain, photophobia, redness, and blurred vision. Examination findings are of anterior segment inflammation including circumlimbal injection, keratic precipitates (especially inferior), anterior chamber (AC) flare, cells, and fibrin (fibrin is a key feature in HLA-B27-associated uveitis). A hypopyon is suggestive of HLA-B27-associated disease, Behçet disease, or severe intraocular infection.[7] Posterior synechiae are common in both idiopathic and HLA-B27-associated AAU and every effort should be made to break them at time of presentation. Vitreous cells may be seen as "spill-over" inflammation, but vitritis is not a dominant feature. Occasionally cystoid macular edema (CME) may be seen (especially in HLA-B27 disease), but this is more commonly a feature of intermediate, posterior or pan-uveitis. It is estimated that up to one-third of patients with AAU have ankylosing spondylitis (AS).[8] Treatment is with intensive topical corticosteroid and mydriatic. If severe, subconjunctival corticosteroid and mydriatic, oral corticosteroid or even intravenous corticosteroid may be given. Recurrent disease (especially if frequent or severe) may be an indication for maintenance systemic treatment.

Chronic anterior uveitis

In chronic anterior uveitis (CAU) patients are typically asymptomatic, so the condition may be picked up on routine optometric review or in screening in the context of juvenile idiopathic arthritis (JIA). Anterior chamber cells and flare are noted and with time posterior synechiae, cataract, band keratopathy, and secondary glaucoma are common.

Intermediate uveitis

This is defined anatomically as the predominant amount of inflammation being in the vitreous. Patients typically present with floaters but may have reduced vision in the context of associated CME. Examination findings include vitritis, retinal periphlebitis, snowball vitreous opacities, and snowbanks at the vitreous base. It is commonly idiopathic (pars planitis type) but may be associated with systemic disease; the main rheumatic disease association is with sarcoidosis, but multiple sclerosis is also a recognized cause.

Posterior uveitis

Patients typically present with visual symptoms, arising from retinal and/or choroidal inflammation; an associated retinal vasculitis may be seen. A number of rheumatic diseases may be associated with posterior uveitis, including Behçet disease and sarcoidosis.

Panuveitis

In panuveitis (inflammation involving anterior chamber, vitreous, and retina/choroid) the presentation is usually with visual problems (reduced acuity, floaters) with redness, photophobia, and pain being a more minor feature.

Other retinal presentations

Retinal vasculitis may be associated with Behçet disease, sarcoidosis, systemic vasculitis, and SLE, but may also be associated with infections (herpesviruses, toxoplasma) and nonrheumatic systemic diseases (such as multiple sclerosis).

Orbital presentations

Rheumatic diseases – notably ANCA-associated vasculitis (ANCA = antineutrophil cytoplasmic antibodies) and SLE – may be associated with orbital inflammation or periorbital edema. Orbital inflammation may present with reduced vision, acute proptosis, lid edema, conjunctival injection and chemosis, reduced ocular motility, and raised intraocular pressure. It may be misdiagnosed as orbital cellulitis, thyroid-associated ophthalmopathy, or another form of orbital inflammation. Inflammation sometimes includes a myositis that may be demonstrated by imaging using CT and B-scan ultrasound (enlargement of extraocular muscles).

Neuro-ophthalmic presentations

Neuro-ophthalmic complications of rheumatic disease are most commonly seen in the systemic vasculitides and include optic neuropathy, ocular motility abnormalities, and retrochiasmal lesions. They are discussed in more detail under the specific rheumatic diseases (see below).

Investigations

The investigations ordered will depend on the history and examination findings. A baseline set of tests might include: full blood count, erythrocyte sedimentation rate, C-reactive protein, urea and electrolytes, liver function tests, rheumatoid factor, antinuclear antibody, antineutrophil cytoplasmic antibody, angiotensin-converting enzyme, uric acid, syphilis serology, chest X-ray, and urinalysis.

Therapeutic considerations

Many patients will require systemic treatment, such as corticosteroids, immunosuppressants (methotrexate, azathioprine, mycophenolate mofetil, cyclosporine), and biologics (anti-TNF, rituximab - anti-CD20) for their rheumatic and ophthalmic disease. Where possible this should be undertaken in conjunction with a rheumatologist who has an expertise in this type of therapy. Ophthalmologists should only prescribe these drugs if they have a detailed knowledge of their action, route of administration, side-effects, and how to monitor for them, as the treatments themselves have potentially serious complications. Most patients with sight-threatening disease are likely to be prescribed oral corticosteroid, and these have numerous, well-recognized side-effects, including glucocorticoid-induced bone disease.[9] Fortunately, in patients with ocular inflammation the commonly used immunosuppressants do not appear to increase overall or cancer mortality.[10]

DISEASE-SPECIFIC SECTION

Rheumatoid arthritis

General considerations

Rheumatoid arthritis (RA) is a deforming peripheral arthritis that is classically symmetrical with a predilection for the small joints of the hands and feet and may be associated with sight-threatening ocular disease.

Epidemiology

RA is the commonest of the inflammatory arthritides, with an incidence of around 3 in 10000 per annum and a prevalence of 1% among adults in industrialized nations.[11-13] Epidemiological risk factors include age (increases with age), female gender (3–5 times greater risk than male),[13] and smoking.[14]

Articular and systemic disease

Typical features of the arthritis of RA are its symmetrical small joint distribution and its deforming nature, giving rise to the classic appearance of ulnar deviation ("rheumatoid hands"). All synovial joints may be affected, including the metacarpophalangeal joints (MCP), proximal interphalangeal joints (PIP), the interphalangeal joint of the thumb, metatarsophalangeal joints, wrist, elbows, hip joints, knees, and the atlanto-axial joint.[15] Degenerative changes of the atlanto-axial joint may make intubation hazardous and should be considered when planning anesthesia. In contrast to noninflammatory degenerative arthritis such as osteoarthritis, patients commonly complain of morning stiffness that improves with exercise.[15]

Extra-articular features are common and affect many systems.[16] One-quarter of patients with RA develop solid lesions within the subcutaneous tissues of extensor surfaces known as rheumatoid nodules. Cardiac complications includes accelerated atherosclerotic coronary artery disease, pericarditis, heart block or valvular dysfunction.[17] Respiratory complications include pleural effusions, nodules of the pleura or lung tissue, and interstitial fibrosis; a severe variant of interstitial fibrosis associated with RA and coal-miners' pneumoconiosis is known as Caplan syndrome.[18] Other systemic complications include renal amyloidosis and a chronic anemia and/or leucopenia. The combination of RA, splenomegaly, and leucopenia is known as Felty syndrome.[19]

Box 80.1 The 2010 American College of Rheumatology (ACR)/ European League Against Rheumatism (EULAR) classification criteria for rheumatoid arthritis[21]

The criteria are aimed at classification of newly presenting patients. In addition, patients with erosive disease typical of rheumatoid arthritis (RA) with a history compatible with prior fulfillment of the 2010 criteria should be classified as having RA.

Target population (Who should be tested?)

1. Patients that have at least 1 joint with definite clinical synovitis (swelling)

2. Patients with the synovitis not better explained by another disease

Classification criteria for RA
(score-based algorithm: add score of categories A–D; a score of >6/10 is needed for classification of a patient as having definite RA)

	Score
A. Joint involvement	
1 large joint	0
2–10 large joints	1
1–3 small joints (with or without involvement of large joints)	2
4–10 small joints (with or without involvement of large joints)	3
>10 joints (at least 1 small joint)	5
B. Serology (at least 1 test result is needed for classification)	
Negative RF *and* negative ACPA	0
Low-positive RF *or* low-positive ACPA	2
High-positive RF *or* high-positive ACPA	3
C. Acute-phase reactants (at least 1 test result is needed for classification)	
Normal CRP *and* normal ESR	0
Abnormal CRP *or* abnormal ESR	1
D. Duration of symptoms	
<6 weeks	0
≥6 weeks	1

(Adapted from Aletaha D, Neogi T, Silman AJ, et al. 2010 Rheumatoid Arthritis Classification Criteria: an American College of Rheumatology/European League Against Rheumatism collaborative initiative. Arthritis Rheum 2010;62:2569–81.)

Vasculitis is a rare but important complication of RA which ranges in severity from nail-fold infarcts to severe life-threatening systemic vasculitis.[20]

In addition to clinical assessment, the diagnosis may be supported by systemic investigations such as the measurement of inflammatory markers, rheumatoid factor, and anticitrullinated protein antibodies (ACPA) (Box 80.1).[21]

Ocular disease

In RA, anterior segment disease is more common than posterior segment disease. Common anterior segment disease includes keratoconjunctivitis sicca, Sjögren syndrome, episcleritis, scleritis, and various forms of keratitis.

Scleritis occurs in 1–6% of patients with RA, and in up to 14% of patients with rheumatoid vasculitis.[2,4,5] Scleritis in the context of RA may present with severe pain and may be diffuse or nodular, anterior or posterior, and necrotizing or non-necrotizing in pattern.[6] Of greatest concern is scleromalacia perforans, in which scleral destruction is not typically painful and not associated with visible signs of inflammation.[2,6] Episcleritis may also be seen in the context of RA.[6,22]

Corneal complications of RA are wide-ranging with varying risk of perforation. Marginal keratitis without apparent inflammation may result in peripheral thinning giving rise to the appearance of "contact lens cornea". More significant are peripheral ulcerative keratitis and keratolysis ("corneal melt") both of which have a high risk of perforation.[2] Necrotizing keratitis or scleritis in the context of RA are associated with increased mortality.[23]

Posterior segment lesions in RA include posterior scleritis and rarely a retinal vasculitis. Retinal vasculitis is probably underdiagnosed. In one study of 60 patients with RA the rate of retinal vasculitis was 18% even in the absence of clinical features of retinal vasculitis.[24] This study is supported by a number of case reports describing typical retinal vasculitis associated with fluorescein angiographic evidence of leakage and a single case of retinal exudation in the context of scleritis that the authors attribute to vasculitis.[25,26]

Treatment-related ocular complications of RA include cataract (corticosteroid), elevated intraocular pressure (corticosteroid), and retinopathy (chloroquine and to a lesser extent hydroxychloroquine).

Treatment

Treatment of systemic disease

The goals of treatment in RA are to alleviate symptoms and to prevent tissue destruction (usually of joints) and loss of function. Permanent damage to the joints may occur early in the disease and thus best practice is now to treat early and aggressively. The 2008 recommendations of the American College of Rheumatology (ACR) advise a hierarchical approach based on disease activity (low, moderate or high) and duration of disease (<6 months, 6–24 months, and 24 months).[27] In addition to appropriate anti-inflammatory pharmacological interventions (such as NSAIDs, intra-articular and oral corticosteroids), disease-modifying anti-rheumatic drugs (DMARDs) such as methotrexate and leflunomide are recommended first-line and may be used in combination according to activity and duration of disease. The ACR recommendations for use of biologics (such as anti-TNF therapies) include high disease activity, poor prognostic features (such as the presence of rheumatoid nodules, secondary Sjögren syndrome, rheumatoid vasculitis, longer duration of disease, and failure of DMARDs).[27] Anti-TNF therapy may also be used with methotrexate. Other biologic therapies include rituximab (anti-CD20) and abatacept (fusion protein of CTLA-4 and IgG).[28]

Treatment of ocular disease

Mild superficial ocular disease (such as mild keratoconjunctivitis sicca or episcleritis) may be adequately controlled with topical therapies such as artificial tear substitutes.[29] Non-necrotizing anterior scleritis may be managed with oral NSAIDs, but necrotizing disease frequently requires systemic corticosteroid. Uncontrolled ocular inflammation warrants escalation of systemic treatment that should be coordinated with a rheumatologist. In addition, sight-threatening inflammation such as necrotizing scleritis or corneal melt requires urgent rescue therapy such as pulsed intravenous methylprednisolone.[2] In our practice we administer up to three pulses of 500–1000 mg methylprednisolone on consecutive days that is usually followed by commencing or increasing a course of oral corticosteroid (in addition to DMARD/biologic therapy).

Seronegative spondyloarthropathies

General considerations

Spondyloarthropathy is a term used to describe a group of interrelated inflammatory arthropathies affecting the synovium and extra-articular sites (Box 80.2).[30] The spondylarthropathies include the following conditions: ankylosing spondylitis, reactive arthritis, inflammatory bowel disease-related arthritis, juvenile spondyloarthropathies, and psoriatic arthritis. Clinical manifestations include inflammatory back pain, enthesitis (inflammation of the entheses, where tendons or ligaments insert into the bone), dactylitis (inflammation of an entire digit), uveitis, and usually an asymmetrical arthritis that affects lower limbs. There is a strong association with the class I MHC molecule HLA-B27. Based on a systematic review, which included nearly 30000 patients, the mean prevalence of uveitis in spondylarthropathies has been estimated at 33% overall, with acute anterior uveitis being the most common type seen.[31]

Box 80.2 The European Spondyloarthropathy Study Group (ESSG) spondyloarthropathy classification criteria

Presence of
Inflammatory spinal pain
Or
Synovitis – asymmetrical or predominantly in the lower limbs and one or more of the following
And
One or more of the following:
Family history – first- or second-degree relative with AS, psoriasis, acute iritis, reactive arthritis or inflammatory bowel disease
Inflammatory bowel disease
Past or present alternating buttock pain
Past or present spontaneous pain or tenderness on examination of the site of insertion of the Achilles tendon or plantar fascia (enthesitis)
Episode of diarrhea occurring <1 month before the onset of arthritis
Non-gonococcal urethritis or cervicitis occurring <1 month before the onset of arthritis

(Reproduced with permission from Dougados M, van der Linden S, Juhlin R, et al. The European Spondylarthropathy Study Group preliminary criteria for the classification of spondylarthropathy. Arthritis Rheum 1991;34:1218–27.)

Epidemiology

Spondyloarthropathies occur particularly in individuals who are positive for HLA-B27 but additional environmental factors are also thought to play a role. It can be difficult to differentiate these disorders, because their clinical features may overlap and undifferentiated forms of spondyloarthropathy are well recognized.[32] Spondyloarthropathies as a whole have a prevalence of 0.5–1.9% of the population.

Ankylosing spondylitis

General considerations

Ankylosing spondylitis (AS) is an HLA-B27-associated chronic inflammatory axial arthritis typically presenting in young men with a strong association with anterior uveitis.

Epidemiology

AS is the commonest of the spondyloarthropathies. Its prevalence varies between 0.1 and 0.4% of the population, depending on the frequency of HLA-B27 in that population. This results in significant geographic variation with extremely low rates of AS in South Africa, low rates in Japan, higher rates in Germany compared to other European countries and very high rates in the natives of Eurasia and the North American circumpolar/sub-Arctic areas.[33] AS is commoner in males, with a male: female ratio of 2–3:1, although it has been suggested that it may be underdiagnosed in females due to them having milder disease.[34]

Articular and systemic disease

The hallmark of AS is inflammatory back pain presenting with buttock pain, early morning stiffness (minimum 30 minutes), relieved by exercise and NSAIDs, worse with rest, and night pain.[35] The shoulders and hips are regarded as axial joints and are affected in up to 50% of patients.[36] In AS an asymmetrical oligoarthritis is uncommon, but may be a predictor of more severe disease if it presents early in the disease course.[36]

Enthesitis is a characteristic feature of AS and may occur at any enthesis, but is most commonly seen in the foot at the insertion of the Achilles tendon and of the plantar fascia onto the calcaneus. The classic cardiac abnormalities in AS are aortitis, aortic regurgitation, and conduction abnormalities, which are seen in up to 9% of long-term follow-up patients.[37]

Disease is monitored using a combination of instruments, including BASDAI (Bath Ankylosing Spondylitis Assessment Index), BASFI (Bath Ankylosing Spondylitis Function Index), inflammatory markers (CRP/ESR), Visual Analogue Scale, swollen joint count, and X-rays of spine and pelvis.

Ocular disease

The commonest ocular complication of AS is recurrent AAU. It is almost always unilateral but may affect both eyes sequentially (described as "flip-flop" pattern). Rarely the anterior uveitis may become persistent. The presentation is of typical AAU but inflammation is classically more severe (often with fibrin in the anterior chamber) and recurrences more frequent than in idiopathic AAU.[38–40] Hyopyon may also be present in severe cases. AAU may lead to sight loss via recurrent or persistent CME, secondary glaucoma, and cataract.[38–40] Treatment-related ocular complications of AS include cataract and elevated intraocular pressure (secondary to corticosteroid usage).

Treatment

Treatment of systemic disease

The goal of treatment in AS is to restore and maintain posture and movement to as near normal as possible, which is achieved through lifelong physical therapy, and medical and surgical treatment. NSAIDs (non-steroidal anti-inflammatory drugs) are the basis of treating AS. They reduce pain and stiffness within 48–72 hours in several studies; a good response may also be used to support the diagnosis.[41,42] Unlike many inflammatory rheumatic diseases, systemic corticosteroids do not have a major part in the treatment of AS although peripheral arthritis often responds to steroid treatment.[41]

DMARDs (disease-modifying antirheumatic drugs), such as sulfasalazine and methotrexate, are effective for the peripheral manifestations of AS, but there is limited efficacy for treating axial manifestations.[43,44] Anti-TNF agents, such as etanercept, infliximab, and adalimumab are recommended as treatment options for patients with AS if disease is not sufficiently controlled after treatment with two or more DMARDs.

Treatment of ocular disease

The mainstay of treatment for AS-associated AAU is intensive topical corticosteroids and a mydriatic (as for idiopathic AAU), but it should be noted that subconjunctival treatment and oral corticosteroids are more commonly required to adequately control inflammation in HLA-B27-associated versus idiopathic AAU. Anti-TNF agents, such as infliximab, etanercept, and adalimumab, as part of studies for the treatment of the underlying AS can also reduce the frequency of AAU recurrences.[45,46]

Reactive arthritis (previously known as Reiter syndrome)

General considerations

Reactive arthritis (ReA) is a sterile inflammation of the joints triggered by an infection, associated with frequently occurring extra-articular symptoms.

Epidemiology

There are a few population-based studies which have estimated the incidence to be between 10 and 30 per 100 000 per annum.[47] HLA-B27 is positive in 60–80% of patients with reactive arthritis. The most commonly associated infections are urogenital (*Chlamydia trachomatis*) or gastrointestinal (*Yersinia*, *Salmonella*, *Shigella* and *Campylobacter*).[48–50]

Articular and systemic disease

Characteristically patients will have an asymmetric oligoarthritis of the large lower limb joints, but the upper limbs and small joints (usually PIP joints rather than MCP joints) are affected. Other features include inflammatory lower back pain similar to AS, dactylitis, enthesitis, erythema nodosum, and keratoderma blenorrhagica (pustular skin lesions on the soles of feet), indistinguishable from pustular psoriasis.[48]

Ocular disease

The commonest ocular complications of ReA are anterior segment disease. Conjunctivitis forms part of the classical triad of ReA, but is usually only seen at first presentation and early in the disease . Of more consequence is recurrent AAU that may occur in up to 50% of patients, although in only up to 20% patients at the initial attack.[40,48] As described for other forms of AAU, these attacks may be associated with spillover vitreous cells and CME, and very rarely optic disc edema.

Rarely ReA may be associated with panuveitis or multifocal choroiditis;[51,52] the rarity of such cases is underlined by many series of ReA patients in which no cases of panuveitis or posterior uveitis were identified.[48,53]

Treatment

Treatment of systemic disease

The underlying infection should be treated as appropriate.[54] Acute arthritis can be treated with NSAIDs and intra-articular corticosteroids. DMARDs such as sulphasalazine or methotrexate should be considered in patients with a prolonged disease course.[54]

Treatment of ocular disease

ReA-associated AAU is treated as for idiopathic AAU with intensive topical corticosteroids and a mydriatic. As noted previously for other HLA-B27-associated AAU, subconjunctival treatment and oral corticosteroids may be required to adequately control inflammation. Rare cases of posterior segment inflammation are likely to require systemic immunosuppression.

Inflammatory bowel disease

General considerations

Peripheral and axial arthritis are associated with inflammatory bowel disease (IBD), especially Crohn's disease and ulcerative colitis.

Epidemiology

The incidence of peripheral arthritis is reported to be between 5% and 10% in ulcerative colitis and 10% and 20% in Crohn's disease, respectively.[55] Men and women are affected equally.

Spondylitis occurs in 1–26% of patients with IBD and males are more often affected than females. In addition, the prevalence of AS in IBD (1–6%) is higher than in the general population.[55]

Articular and systemic disease

IBD-related arthritis is often a clinical diagnosis as radiology is often normal with no joint erosion or deformity. Two distinct types of arthritis have been described: type 1 (pauciarticular) and type 2 (polyarticular).[55,56]

Ocular disease

Ophthalmic complications are estimated to occur in 3.5–12% of patients with IBD, occurring more commonly earlier in the disease.[57] The commonest ocular complications of IBD are uveitis, episcleritis, and scleritis.

Uveitis is usually of recurrent AAU type, occurring in around 5% of IBD patients, but in up to 50% of IBD patients who are also positive for HLA-B27.[58] Less commonly, a chronic bilateral anterior uveitis may be seen, which has a female gender preponderance.[59] Scleritis is a well-recognized feature of IBD and has been reported to parallel the activity of the bowel disease. Scleritis is usually anterior but may be posterior; it may be non-necrotizing or necrotizing, leading to a risk of scleromalacia perforans.[60] Retinal artery occlusions and ischemic optic neuropathy are reported and may reflect the prothrombotic tendency seen in some patients with IBD. Other reported associations with IBD include keratitis, retinal vasculitis, posterior uveitis, cystoid macular edema, optic neuritis, neuroretinitis, Brown's syndrome and orbital myositis.[60] A recent community survey also suggested that there is a high prevalence of "dry eye" (up to 42%), which was associated with 5-aminosalicylate use, although it was not clear if this was causative or a surrogate marker of disease activity.[61] Interestingly, a family history of IBD has been proposed as an independent risk factor for the development of idiopathic ocular inflammation, including uveitis.[62]

Treatment

Treatment of systemic disease

Treatment depends on the severity of symptoms. Patients with mild oligoarthritis usually respond to relative rest, physiotherapy, and intra-articular corticosteroid injections.[55,56] Most of the patients respond to NSAIDs because they control the symptoms and joint and enthesis inflammation, but they do not stop joint destruction, and they may have significant side-effects including exacerbation of IBD and produce small intestine and colon ulcers. Hence, they are recommended for patients with mild exacerbations, to control symptoms in arthritis flares, but their use must be limited to the minimal effective dose and time.[55,56]

Type 1 arthritis is related to disease activity and therefore therapy of the underlying IBD is the treatment of choice. Treatment of type 2 IBD arthritis and axial arthropathies generally requires long-term treatment with a DMARD, such as sulfasalazine or methotrexate. In addition treatment with systemic on intra-articular corticosteroids can be used.[55] A number of IBD patients will also be using anti-TNF agents to control their bowel symptoms.

Treatment of ocular disease

IBD-associated AAU is treated as for idiopathic AAU with intensive topical corticosteroids and a mydriatic; it should be noted that the more chronic form of anterior uveitis may require more prolonged treatment.[63] The treatment of scleritis will depend on the pattern and severity of disease seen, but will often require immunosuppression.[63]

Psoriatic arthritis

General considerations

Psoriatic arthritis (PsA) is the combination of an inflammatory arthritis (peripheral arthritis and/or sacroiliitis or spondylitis), psoriasis, and the absence of serological tests for rheumatoid factor.[30] In 2006, however, the CASPAR (ClASsification Criteria for Psoriatic ARthritis) was developed (Box 80.3). This has been demonstrated to have high sensitivity and specificity for the diagnosis of PsA (see below).[30,64]

Epidemiology

Psoriatic arthritis (PsA), can occur at any age but is commonest between 30 and 50 years of age. It affects male and females equally.[30,65] The exact prevalence of PsA is unknown, but it is estimated to effect 0.3–1% of the US population and 7–42% of patients with psoriasis.[30,65,66]

Articular and systemic disease

PsA can cause a variety of articular symptoms, varying from an isolated monoarthritis to an extensive destructive arthritis. Articular involvement can be divided into five subtypes: DIP (distal interphalangeal) joint involvement, mono/oligoarticular, symmetrical polyarthritis, arthritis mutilans, and spondylarthropathy. It is important that patients with longstanding PsA have cervical spine X-rays before a general anesthetic, as there can be a clinically silent erosive/inflammatory arthritis causing atlantoaxial or subaxial instability, as in RA.[67] Dactylitis or "sausage digit" occurs in 30–40% of patients with PsA. In addition 20–40% of patients have symptomatic enthesitis generally affecting the foot at the insertion of the Achilles tendon and of the plantar fascia onto the calcaneus.[64,68] There appears no correlation between the severity of skin psoriasis and joint involvement, but skin symptoms do tend to precede joint symptoms. Psoriasis can be assessed using a variety of tools including: PASI (Psoriasis Area and Severity Index), health assessment questionnaires, and Psoriatic Arthritis Response Criteria (PsARC).

Ocular disease

Ophthalmic complications are estimated to occur in 10% of patients with psoriasis,[69] and 31% of patients with PsA.[70] The most common presentations are conjunctivitis (up to 20%) or uveitis (7%).[70] Paiva and coworkers compared the nature of uveitis in PsA to that seen with a previous cohort of

Box 80.3 The CASPAR criteria for psoriatic arthritis

Presence of
Inflammatory articular disease (joint, spine or enthesis)
And
At least 3 points scored from the following
- Current psoriasis (2 points), a personal history of psoriasis (1 point) or a family history of psoriasis (1 point)
- Typical psoriatic nail dystrophy (1 point); this includes onycholysis, pitting, hyperkeratosis
- Dactylitis (1 point): current or previous episode noticed by rheumatologist
- Juxta-articular new bone formation (1 point): hand or foot X-rays
- Rheumatoid factor-negative (1 point): preferably by enzyme-linked immunosorbent assay

(Adapted with permission from Taylor W, Gladman D, Helliwell P, et al. Classification criteria for psoriatic arthritis: development of new criteria from a large international study. Arthritis Rheum 2006;54:2665–73.)

spondylarthropathy patients. Interestingly this suggested that PsA-associated uveitis was more likely to be insidious in onset (19% versus 3%), bilateral (38% versus 7%), chronic in duration (31% versus 6%) or posterior (44% versus 17%).[71] Episcleritis, scleritis, keratoconjunctivitis sicca, and keratitis are also reported.[69,70]

Treatment

Treatment of systemic disease

NSAIDs are normally used for musculoskeletal symptoms, based on the evidence from other rheumatic diseases.[72] Intra-articular corticosteroid can be used, but oral corticosteroids should be used cautiously as they can be associated with a "post-steroid psoriasis flare." Methotrexate can be used for both skin psoriasis and PsA, but care must be taken as the risk of hepatotoxicity seems to be higher in patients with psoriasis, possibly due to a higher tendency of non-alcoholic steatohepatitis (NASH). Sulfasalazine can be used for articular symptoms; there is no benefit for the skin psoriasis. Leflunomide has demonstrated to be effective at treating PsA.[72] Cyclosporine can achieve rapid improvement of the skin lesions of psoriasis, but there is little evidence regarding its effectiveness in PsA. There are concerns regarding possibly causing hypertension and renal insufficiency, so the dose needs to be kept as low as possible and careful monitoring is indicated as these reversible events are reversible if picked up soon after onset.[72]

Anti-TNF agents (etanercept/infliximab/adalimumab) are generally reserved for severe disease. They have been shown to be effective at treating peripheral arthritis, psoriasis, enthesitis, and dactylitis.[73] Further work is currently being undertaken to look at other possible biologic targets including: alefacept, which is a fully human fusion protein that blocks interaction between LFA-3 on the antigen-presenting cell; rituximab, an anti-CD20 agent; and ustekinumab, an IL-12/IL-23 inhibitor.[73]

Treatment of ocular disease

PsA-associated AAU is treated as for idiopathic AAU with intensive topical corticosteroids and a mydriatic, but more persistent anterior uveitis may require prolonged treatment. Cataract, which may be associated with chronic intraocular inflammation, corticosteroid usage, and possibly P-UVA treatment,[74] requires surgical treatment with appropriate immunosuppressive perioperative care.

Juvenile idiopathic arthritis

General considerations

Juvenile idiopathic arthritis (JIA) is the most common rheumatic disease occurring in childhood. It is characterized by persistent inflammation of the joints, with onset prior to age 16 years.

Epidemiology

The reported incidence of JIA varies between 0.8 to 23 per 100 000 per annum, with a prevalence rate between 7 and 400 per 100 000 children. There are reported differences between different ethnic groups: JIA is more frequent in children of European descent than in children of African, Asian or East Indian origin.[75]

Articular and systemic disease

JIA is classified using the ILAR (International League of Associations of Rheumatologists) classification (Box 80.4). The main clinical feature of JIA is defined as: "swelling within a joint or limitation in range of movement with joint pain or tenderness, which persists for a minimum of 6 weeks, observed by a

Box 80.4 The International League of Associations of Rheumatologists (ILAR) classification of juvenile idiopathic arthritis

Systemic arthritis
Definition: Arthritis in one or more joints with or preceded by fever of at least 2 weeks' duration that is documented to be daily ("quotidian") for at least 3 days, and accompanied by one or more of the following:
1. Evanescent (nonfixed) erythematous rash
2. Generalized lymph node enlargement
3. Hepatomegaly and/or splenomegaly
4. Serositis

Exclusions (below): a, b, c, d

Oligoarthritis
Definition: Arthritis affecting 1–4 joints during the first 6 months of disease. Two subcategories are recognized:
1. Persistent oligoarthritis: Affecting not more than 4 joints throughout the disease course
2. Extended oligoarthritis: Affecting a total of more than 4 joints after the first 6 months of disease

Exclusions (below): a, b, c, d, e

Polyarthritis (rheumatoid factor negative)
Definition: Arthritis affecting 5 or more joints during the first 6 months of disease; a test for RF is negative.
Exclusions (below): a, b, c, d, e

Polyarthritis (rheumatoid factor positive)
Definition: Arthritis affecting 5 or more joints during the first 6 months of disease; two or more tests for RF at least 3 months apart during the first 6 months of disease are positive.
Exclusions (below): a, b, c, e

Psoriatic arthritis
Definition: Arthritis and psoriasis, or arthritis and at least two of the following:
1. Dactylitis
2. Nail pitting or onycholysis
3. Psoriasis in a first-degree relative

Exclusions (below): b, c, d, e

Enthesitis-related arthritis
Definition: Arthritis and enthesitis, or arthritis or enthesitis, with at least two of the following:
1. The presence of or a history of sacroiliac joint tenderness and/or inflammatory lumbosacral pain
2. The presence of HLA-B27 antigen
3. Onset of arthritis in a male over 6 years of age
4. Acute (symptomatic) anterior uveitis
5. History of ankylosing spondylitis, enthesitis-related arthritis, sacroiliitis with inflammatory bowel disease, Reiter syndrome, or acute anterior uveitis in a first-degree relative

Exclusions (below): a, d, e.

Undifferentiated arthritis
Definition: Arthritis that fulfils criteria in no category or in two or more of the above categories.

Exclusions
The principle of this classification is that all categories of JIA are mutually exclusive. This principle is reflected in the list of possible exclusions for each category:
a. Psoriasis or a history of psoriasis in the patient or first-degree relative
b. Arthritis in an HLA-B27-positive male beginning after the 6th birthday
c. Ankylosing spondylitis, enthesitis-related arthritis, sacroiliitis with inflammatory bowel disease, Reiter syndrome, or acute anterior uveitis, or a history of one of these disorders in a first-degree relative
d. The presence of IgM rheumatoid factor on at least two occasions at least 3 months apart
e. The presence of systemic JIA in the patient

The application of exclusions is indicated under each category, and may change as new data become available.

(Reproduced with permission from Petty RE, Southwood TR, Manners P, et al. International League of Associations for Rheumatology classification of juvenile idiopathic arthritis: second revision, Edmonton, 2001. J Rheumatol 2004;31:390–2.)

physician and which is not due to primary mechanical disorders or to other identifiable causes."[76]

Ocular disease

The major ocular manifestation of JIA is uveitis. Uveitis is present in around 10% of JIA patients at presentation but may occur in up to one-third of patients at some point during their disease although the exact estimate depends on the type of population sampled.[77–81] Inflammation is typically a chronic anterior uveitis with a white eye, which is usually bilateral (70%) but may initially present with unilateral disease. Recurrent acute anterior uveitis is less commonly seen and when it does occur is usually in the context of HLA-B27.

The risk of developing uveitis in association with JIA has been stratified according to age of onset, type of arthritis, and the presence of ANA, with uveitis occurring in up to half of the highest-risk group (oligoarticular – persistent and extended, ANA-positive disease). Interestingly, a recent study has suggested that age and ANA status may be less useful in predicting risk in boys (versus girls).[82] It should be noted that the gold standard for determining ANA is via immunofluorescence on HEp-2 cells; ELISA-determined ANA was not found to be predictive.[83] Antihistone antibodies are also associated with risk of uveitis but are less widely used in clinical practice.[83] Since the chronic anterior uveitis has minimal if any of the symptoms commonly associated with inflammation, screening is recommended. The recommendations of the American Academy of Pediatrics are summarized in Table 80.1.[84]

JIA-associated uveitis is more commonly seen in girls,[81] but male gender is a risk factor for worse disease, with significantly higher rates of CME by 5 years of follow-up (50% versus 4%) and need for cataract surgery (59% versus 32%). Other reported predictors of worse outcome are uveitis present at time of diagnosis[85,86] and elevated laser flare values.[87]

The key sight-threatening complications of JIA-associated uveitis are band keratopathy (60%), cataract (40%), glaucoma (10–25%), and CME (10%). Posterior synechiae are present in most cases.[77,88,89] Less commonly, vitritis and a peripheral retinal vasculitis are reported.[77,80,88,89]

Treatment

Treatment of systemic disease

The management of JIA is based on a combination of medical treatment, physical and occupational therapy, and surgical management. NSAIDs can be used for all types of mild JIA, to treat pain and stiffness. Oral corticosteroids must be used minimally in children because of the effects on bone and growth, the main indications are severe fever, serositis and macrophage activation syndrome. Intra-articular corticosteroids can be used, and encouraging results have been reported in children with monoarthritis.[90] Methotrexate is used for patients with polyarthritis, other DMARDs that have been shown to be effective include sulfasalazine and leflunomide. Etanercept can be used in patients who fail to respond to methotrexate therapy and has been demonstrated to be effective both in the short and long term management of JIA.[91–93] Infliximab, was not shown to be superior to placebo in polyarticular JIA.[94] Adalimumab is licensed for use in JIA, and was found to be effective in children with polyarticular JIA.[95] Abatacept is an alternative biological agent which is a selective T-cell co-stimulator inhibitor. In randomized controlled trials (RCTs) abatacept was superior to placebo in children with polyarticular arthritis, including those who were anti-TNF treatment failures.[96,97] There is some concern regarding the potential increased risk of cancers in children using anti-TNF agents.[98] Further studies are being undertaken to investigate the potential future role of other biologics, including rituximab, IL(interleukin)-1 and IL-6 antagonists.

Table 80.1 American Academy of Pediatrics guidelines on frequency of ophthalmologic examination in patients with juvenile idiopathic arthritis

Type	ANA	Age at onset (yr)	Duration of disease (yr)	Risk category	Eye examination frequency (mth)
Oligoarthritis or polyarthritis	+	≤6	≤4	High	3
	+	≤6	>4	Moderate	6
	+	≤6	>7	Low	12
	+	>6	≤4	Moderate	6
	+	>6	>4	Low	12
	–	≤6	≤4	Moderate	6
	–	≤6	>4	Low	12
	–	>6	NA	Low	12
Systemic disease (fever, rash)	NA	NA	NA	Low	12

Recommendations for follow-up continue through childhood and adolescence.
ANA, antinuclear antibodies; NA, not applicable; mth, month; yr, year.
(Reproduced with permission from Cassidy J, Kivlin J, Lindsley C, Nocton J. Ophthalmologic examinations in children with juvenile rheumatoid arthritis. Pediatrics 2006;117:1843–5.)

Treatment of ocular disease

Systemic immunosuppression is usually required to control both the systemic disease and its ocular manifestations, although some children may only require topical corticosteroid and a mydriatic. What constitutes a "safe" level of topical corticosteroid usage in children is controversial. In a recent retrospective study by Thorne and coworkers topical corticosteroid use was associated with development of cataract and this was independent of active uveitis or presence of posterior synechiae.[99] Importantly, there appeared to be no significant increase of cataract when chronic administration was no more than twice daily.[99] The need for frequent topical corticosteroid to control the uveitis usually requires the introduction of methotrexate often given by the subcutaneous route weekly rather than orally. If methotrexate cannot adequately control the inflammation then it requires the addition of an anti-TNF agent; adalimumab appears to be the drug of choice, with effective control of the uveitis in 16/18 children in one study.[100] There are some reports of uveitis occurring in association with etanercept.[101]

Cataract surgery is challenging and requires very careful preparation, perioperative care and intensive postoperative management. It is vital that the patient's carers are fully aware of the importance of adherence to prescribed therapy and follow-up visits. Traditionally cataract removal for these patients was by pars plana vitrectomy/lensectomy followed by aphakia, but it is now more common to use intraocular lenses at the time of surgery.[102–104] Postoperative posterior synechiae and intraocular lens deposits are common, but overall visual improvement is encouraging, with a recent series of 17 eyes reporting an improvement in visual acuity of 2 lines or more in all patients with no increase of CME, glaucoma or hypotony,[103] but it should be noted that other studies do report significant rates of secondary glaucoma and CME.[104]

Systemic lupus erythematosus

General considerations

Systemic lupus erythematosus (SLE) is a multisystem autoimmune disease predominantly affecting women of childbearing age. The classification criteria for SLE are summarized in Box 80.5.[105]

Epidemiology

SLE has a prevalence of around 28 cases per 100 000,[106] predominantly affecting women of child-bearing age (15–45 years); the female: male ratio peak is 12:1. SLE is more common in non-Caucasians, in whom it is both more severe and earlier in onset.[107]

Articular and systemic disease

SLE is a systemic disease that can cause constitutional or organ-specific symptoms. The skin, mucous membranes, joints, kidney, brain, serous membranes, lung, heart, and occasionally the gastrointestinal tract may all be involved.[105,106] Arthritis in SLE can divided into a deforming and nondeforming arthropathy. Constitutional symptoms consist of fever, malaise, fatigue, weight loss, lymphadenopathy, and anorexia.[106] There are multiple cutaneous manifestations of lupus: commonly these include photosensitivity (>50% of patients), butterfly/malar rash, painful/painless oral ulcers, diffuse alopecia, and livedo reticularis.[106]

Renal disease is one of the most serious SLE manifestations and a prognostic indicator of disease severity. Renal biopsy is used to determine the class of nephropathy as classified by the International Society of Nephrology (ISN)/Renal Pathology Society (RPS) guidelines.[108]

Neuropsychiatric SLE (NPSLE) is a major diagnostic and treatment problem. The ACR has provided classification criteria, describing central and peripheral types of neurological involvement that may be found in lupus patients.[106]

Box 80.5 The 1997 updated American College of Rheumatology criteria for systemic lupus erythematosus

For the purposes of clinical trials, a diagnosis of SLE is made on the presence of at least four out of 11 criteria being present simultaneously or sequentially.

1. **Malar rash**
   Fixed erythema, flat or raised, over the malar eminences, tending to spare the nasolabial folds
2. **Discoid rash**
   Erythematous raised patches with adherent keratotic scaling and follicular plugging; atrophic scarring may occur in older lesions
3. **Photosensitivity**
   Skin rash as a result of unusual reaction to sunlight, by patient history or physician observation
4. **Oral ulcers**
   Oral or nasopharyngeal ulceration, usually painless, observed by physician
5. **Nonerosive arthritis**
   Involving 2 or more peripheral joints, characterized by tenderness, swelling, or effusion
6. **Pleuritis or pericarditis**
   (a) Pleuritis: convincing history of pleuritic pain or rubbing heard by a physician or evidence of pleural effusion
   OR
   (b) Pericarditis: documented by electrocardiogram or rub or evidence of pericardial effusion
7. **Renal disorder**
   (a) Persistent proteinuria > 0.5 g per day or > than 3+ if quantitation not performed
   OR
   (b) Cellular casts: may be red cell, hemoglobin, granular, tubular, or mixed
8. **Neurological disorder**
   (a) Seizures: in the absence of offending drugs or known metabolic derangements, e.g., uremia, ketoacidosis, or electrolyte imbalance
   OR
   (b) Psychosis: in the absence of offending drugs or known metabolic derangements, e.g., uremia, ketoacidosis, or electrolyte imbalance
9. **Hematological disorder**
   At least one of the following:
   (a) Hemolytic anemia – with reticulocytosis
   (b) Leucopenia < 4000/mm^3 on ≥ 2 occasions
   (c) Lymphopenia < 1500/mm^3 on ≥ 2 occasions
   (d) Thrombocytopenia < 100 000/mm^3 in the absence of offending drugs
10. **Immunologic disorder**
   At least one of the following:
   (a) Anti-DNA: antibody to native DNA in abnormal titer
   (b) Anti-Sm: presence of antibody to Sm nuclear antigen
   (c) Positive finding of antiphospholipid antibodies on:
      1. An abnormal serum level of IgG or IgM anticardiolipin antibodies
      2. A positive test result for lupus anticoagulant using a standard method, *or*
      3. A false-positive test result for at least 6 months confirmed by *Treponema pallidum* immobilization or fluorescent treponemal antibody absorption test
11. **Positive antinuclear antibody**
   An abnormal titer of antinuclear antibody by immunofluorescence or an equivalent assay at any point in time and in the absence of potential drug causes

(Modified from Hochberg MC. Updating the American College of Rheumatology revised criteria for the classification of systemic lupus erythematosus. Arthritis Rheum 1997;40:1725.)

Pulmonary features of SLE include pleurisy, pneumonitis, pulmonary hemorrhage, pulmonary embolism, pulmonary hypertension, and diaphragmatic weakness causing shrinking lungs. Pericarditis is the most common cardiological manifestation; others include myocarditis, endocarditis, accelerated atherosclerosis, and, rarely, pericardial tamponade.[106]

Abdominal pain, nausea, vomiting, and diarrhea occur in up to 50% of SLE patients. Gastrointestinal involvement includes mesenteric vasculitis (high risk of death), aseptic peritonitis (with or without ascites), subacute bowel obstruction, hepatitis, sclerosing cholangitis, protein-losing enteropathy, pancreatitis, and ascites.[109]

Cytopenias, including anemia, leucopenia or thrombocytopenia, are commonly associated with SLE; they may be immune-mediated or due to other factors, e.g. menstrual losses. Antiphospholipid antibodies and lupus anticoagulant are found in about 30–40% of patients, associated with venous and arterial thrombosis, recurrent fetal loss, pre-eclampsia, headache, and epilepsy.[106]

A firm diagnosis of lupus is made based on appropriate clinical findings and the measurement of at least one antibody. There are a number of antibodies associated with SLE, the most common being ANA (antinuclear antibody). Other associated autoantibodies include anti-dsDNA (double stranded DNA) in approximately 60% of patients, the highly specific anti-Sm antibody (Smith proteins) in 10–30% of patients, and anti-RNP (ribonucleoprotein) also in 10–30% of patients.[105,106]

Ocular disease

Ophthalmic complications are common in SLE, affecting up to one-third of patients. The commonest complication is keratoconjunctivitis sicca but sight-threatening posterior segment and neuro-ophthalmic disease is also seen (reviewed by Sivaraj and coworkers).[110]

Common ocular surface diseases related to SLE include KCS (25% of SLE patients).[111,112] Peripheral ulcerative keratitis is a rare but serious complication requiring urgent immunosuppression.[2]

Episcleritis is observed in 1–2% and scleritis in 1% of patients with SLE.[6,113] Scleritis may be anterior or posterior, necrotizing or non-necrotizing, and may indicate activity of the underlying disease.

Occasionally SLE may cause orbital inflammation and present with acute proptosis, lid edema, conjunctival injection and chemosis, reduced ocular motility and elevated intraocular pressure, with myositis and panniculitis also reported.[114,115] Orbital inflammation may also be associated with posterior scleritis.

Lupus retinopathy was first described by Bergmeister in 1929. Its prevalence is estimated at around 10%, although this is variable depending on the population studied.[116] The classic clinical picture is of cotton-wool spots, retinal hemorrhages, and vascular abnormalities (arterial narrowing with capillary dilation, and venous dilation and tortuosity) (Figs 80.1–80.3). Additional features may include retinal edema, hard exudates, and microaneurysms. Retinopathy is usually bilateral but may be asymmetric.[117]

Severe vaso-occlusive retinopathy is much less common but potentially devastating. Whereas mild retinopathy may be picked up as an incidental finding, vaso-occlusive retinopathy usually presents with visual symptoms such as reduced acuity, visual field loss, and distortion. In addition it is strongly associated with the life-threatening complication of CNS lupus.[118] The clinical appearance is of widespread arteriolar occlusion and capillary nonperfusion. Subsequently neovascularization is common (up to 72% cases) (Figs 80.4, 80.5),[118] and may be complicated by vitreous hemorrhage (up to 63%), retinal traction, and detachment (up to 27%).[118] The occurrence of vaso-occlusive disease is strongly associated with the presence of antiphospholipid antibodies (up to fourfold increased risk).[119] Primary antiphospholipid syndrome (i.e. antiphospholipid antibodies in the absence of SLE or any other systemic disease) may be associated with a similar severe vaso-occlusive retinopathy but with cotton-wool spots being less common. The severe vaso-occlusive retinopathy is sometimes described as a retinal vasculitis, but this is not generally supported by histological examination.[120]

Occlusion of the larger retinal vessels may occur and again is associated with the presence of antiphospholipid antibodies. Manifestations include branch retinal arteriolar or central retinal artery occlusion (B/CRAO) (Fig. 80.6), branch or central retinal vein occlusion (B/CRVO), and combined retinal arterial and venous occlusions.[118,120]

Other retinal manifestations of SLE include an unusual bilateral pigmentary retinopathy that may resemble retinitis pigmentosa but is proposed to be ischemic in origin.[121] Coexisting systemic hypertension may result in features of hypertensive retinopathy. Choroidal involvement in SLE (lupus choroidopathy) may also cause significant visual morbidity. Choroidopathy results in single or multifocal serous detachments of the retina and retinal pigment epithelium (RPE), which may mimic idiopathic central serous chorioretinopathy (CSC).[122] The degree of visual symptoms depends on the anatomical location of the detachment(s). These serous detachments may become extensive over time but conversely may reverse with control of the underlying systemic disease.[122] Fluorescein angiography (and indocyanine green angiography) is helpful as it not only demonstrates typical CSC-like leakage from the choroid into the subretinal and sub-RPE spaces but also demonstrates the degree of choroidal ischemia.

Optic nerve disease is uncommon (about 1% patients with SLE). The spectrum of disease described includes anterior and posterior ischemic optic neuropathy, and acute optic neuritis (which is also thought to be ischemic in origin).[123] Bilateral optic disc swelling in SLE may arise due to either idiopathic

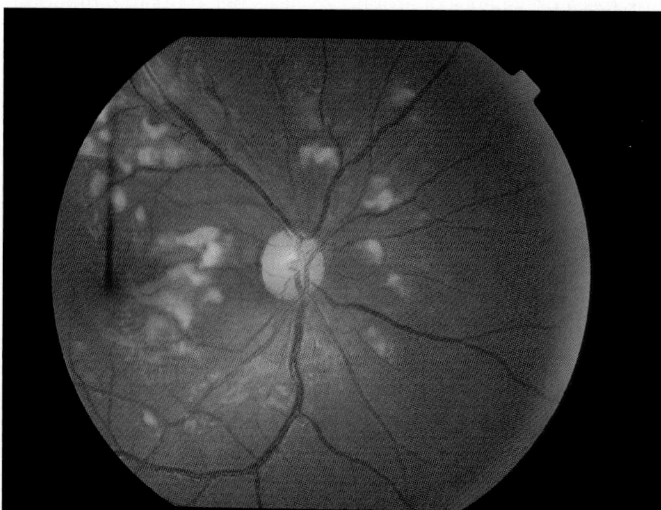

Fig. 80.1 Acute lupus retinopathy with cotton-wool spots, arterial narrowing, venous dilation, and tortuosity.

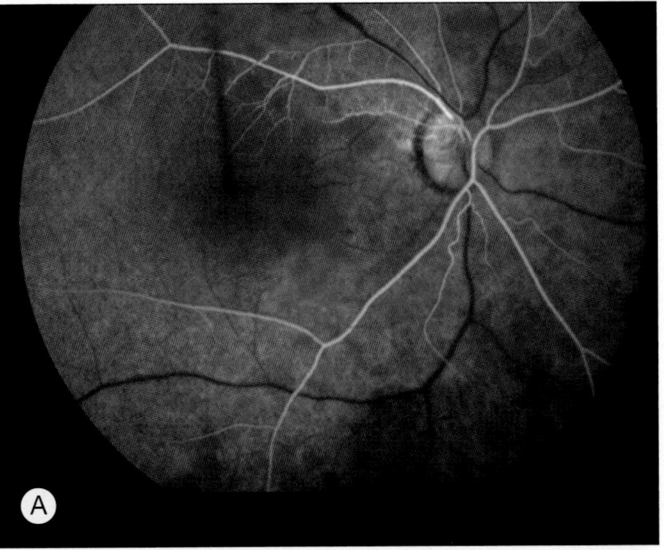

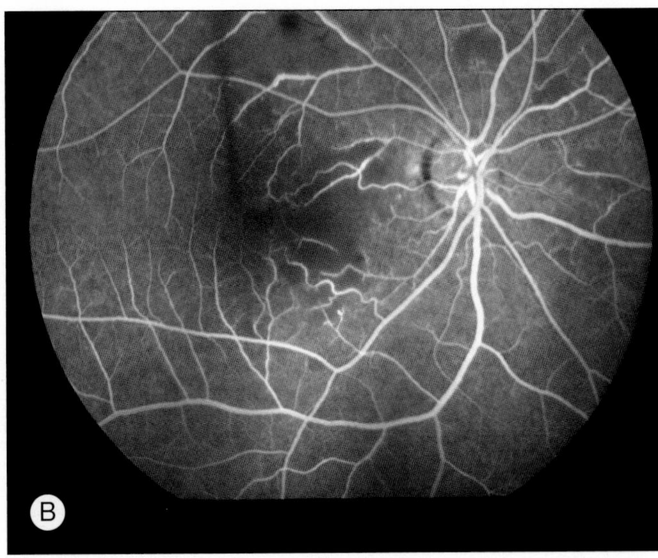

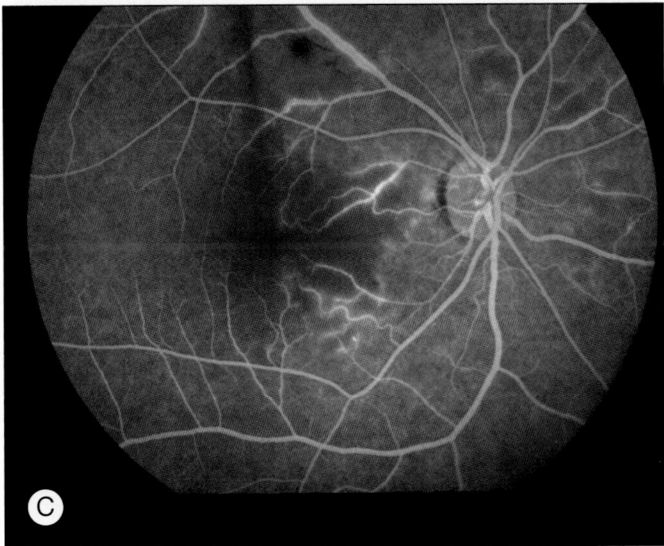

Fig. 80.2 Fundus fluorescein angiography of the same patient: (A) early, (B) arteriovenous, and (C) late phases demonstrating capillary "dropout," vessel wall staining, and leakage.

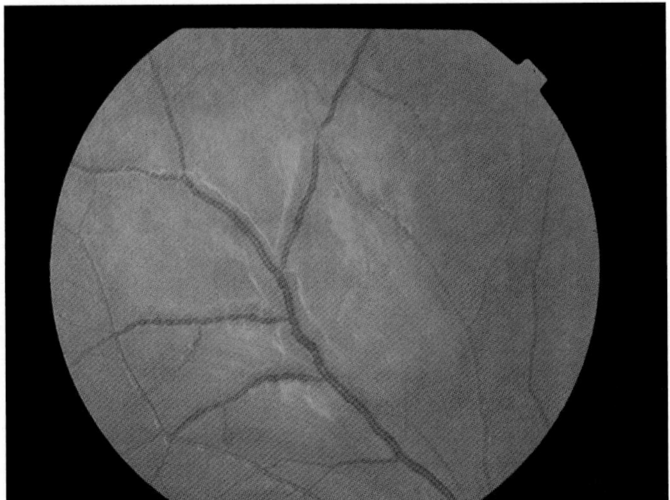

Fig. 80.3 Detail of the same patient showing venous beading.

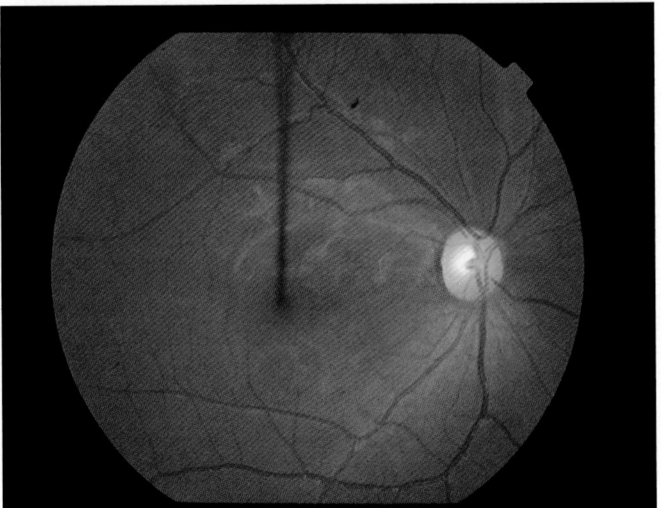

Fig. 80.4 The same patient one year later, showing resolution of cotton-wool spots. Careful examination, however, reveals two areas of abnormal neovascularization.

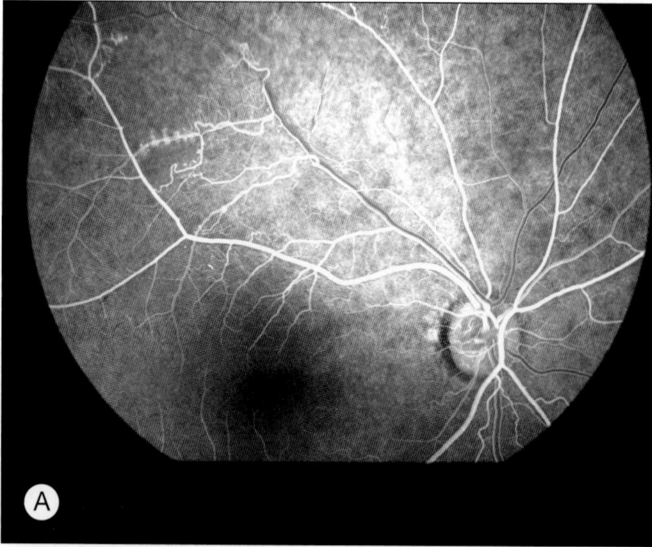

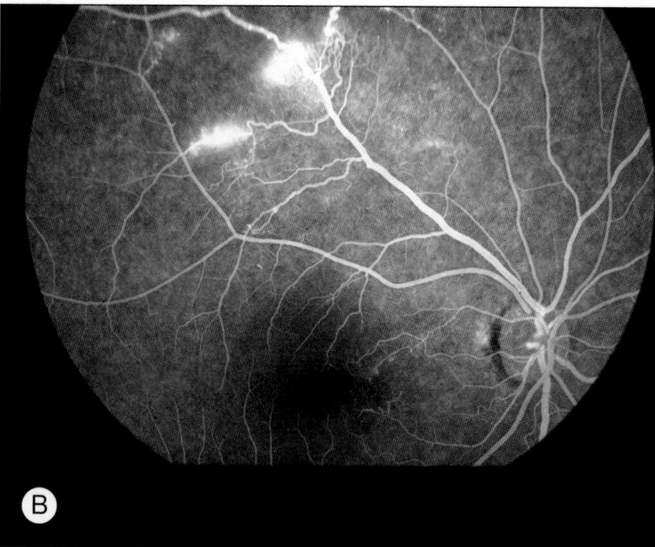

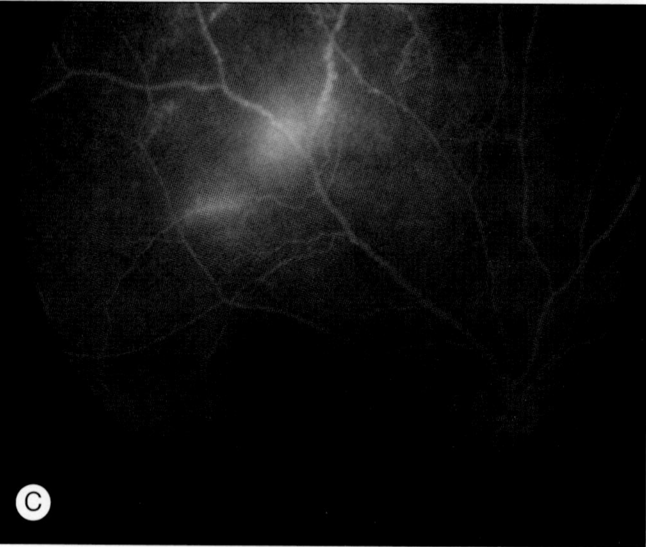

Fig. 80.5 Fundus fluorescein angiography of the same patient: (A) early, (B) arteriovenous, and (C) late phases demonstrating the presence of active new vessels. These did not resolve with immunosuppression and required sectoral laser photocoagulation.

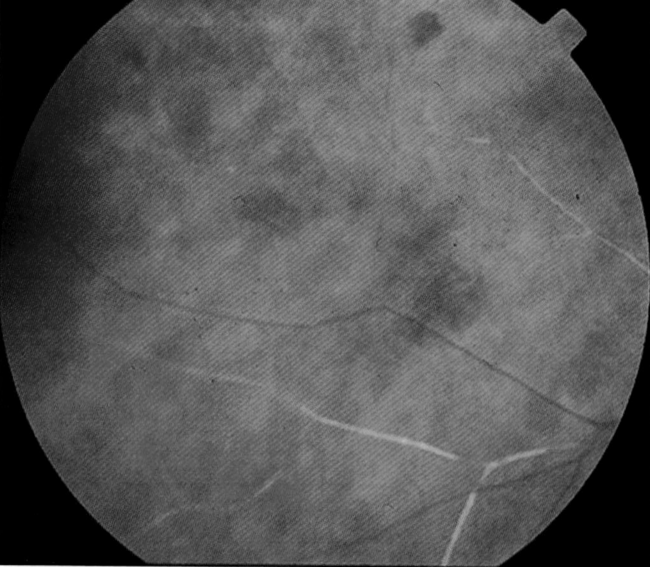

Fig. 80.6 Branch retinal arteriole occlusion in a patient with systemic lupus erythematosus and antiphospholipid syndrome.

intracranial hypertension or accelerated systemic hypertension, both of which are more common in SLE.

Other neuro-ophthalmic complications of SLE include ocular motility abnormalities (causes include brain stem infarcts, cranial neuropathies, tenosynovitis, myositis and Miller–Fisher syndrome), nystagmus, ptosis, and migraine.[110]

Finally, it should be noted that patients with SLE are immunosuppressed (both due to disease and treatment) and may present with severe intraocular infections. Retinal necrosis due to herpes simplex virus, varicella zoster virus, and cytomegalovirus have been reported. Other ocular infections include tuberculous choroidal abscess, and nocardia endophthalmitis.[124,125]

Treatment

Treatment of systemic disease

The treatment of SLE is tailored to the severity of disease. General lifestyle advice includes avoidance of sunlight and use of sun block. Patients should have regular disease assessments, and be screened for SLE complications, such as infection, diabetes, hyperlipidemia, and hypertension. Women of childbearing age should be advised regarding the importance of good disease control before conception, the need for close monitoring during pregnancy, and the risk of postpartum disease flare.

Mild cases with intermittent rashes, arthritis, and other mucocutaneous features can usually be treated with corticosteroid creams, short courses of NSAIDs, and hydroxychloroquine (<6.5 mg/kg/day). More severe cases of SLE usually require oral corticosteroids. Patients who need 10 mg/day of prednisone or more despite hydroxychloroquine, or those who present with more severe manifestations (such as nephritis, gastrointestinal vasculitis or central nervous system disease) that need higher initial doses of prednisone (0.5–1 mg/kg/day) are likely to need azathioprine, methotrexate, mycophenolate mofetil or cyclophosphamide as steroid-sparing immunosuppressive agents. If conservative treatment and traditional DMARDs fail then biologics should be considered.

Rituximab is a monoclonal antibody against the B-lymphocyte marker CD20 expressed on B cells, it has been used in SLE patients since 2002, and observational studies have suggested that rituximab is effective in treating active SLE refractory to standard immunosuppressant.[126] Recent data have demonstrated that repeated treatment with rituximab is effective in treating refractory SLE and has a favorable safety profile.[127] Lightstone and coworkers are currently investigating the possibility of corticosteroid avoidance regimes.[128]

Treatment of ocular disease

In SLE, control of the systemic disease often improves the ophthalmic disease. The presence of severe ophthalmic disease should prompt the rheumatologist to look for evidence of systemic activity, and warrants escalation of systemic therapy. Additional local and regional treatments may also be indicated depending on the type of ocular complication. For example, KCS may benefit from a range of treatments, including tear replacement therapy (preservative-free preparations preferred), punctal occlusion, lid hygiene, topical corticosteroids or cyclosporine, and environmental measures.[110]

Mild anterior segment inflammation may respond to topical corticosteroids (keratitis or anterior uveitis), or topical NSAIDs (episcleritis). In more severe anterior segment inflammation, such as scleritis or disease affecting the posterior segment or orbit, systemic treatment is required. Non-necrotizing scleritis may respond to oral NSAIDs, but most severe inflammatory disease will require high-dose systemic corticosteroid often in combination with the immunosuppressive agents listed above. Significant retinal vascular occlusions associated with antiphospholipid antibodies may be treated with warfarin or low-dose acetylsalicylic acid (in addition to immunosuppression). Retinal neovascularization usually requires panretinal photocoagulation. Persistent vitreous hemorrhage or tractional retinal detachment may require vitreoretinal surgery.[110,118]

Sjögren syndrome

General considerations

Sjögren syndrome is a slowly progressive, inflammatory autoimmune disease primarily affecting the exocrine glands.

Epidemiology

Sjögren syndrome predominantly affects females in the fourth to fifth decade of life. The female: male ratio is 9:1. In a population-based study in Minnesota, incidence of Sjögren syndrome was estimated to be 3.9 per 100 000 per year.[129]

Articular and systemic disease

Sjögren syndrome is clinically characterized by sicca symptoms: dry eyes and mouth due to failure of the salivary and mucosal glands. Sjögren syndrome may be primary or secondary to a pre-existing disorder such as SLE, rheumatoid arthritis, systemic sclerosis, vasculitis, autoimmune thyroid disease or primary biliary cirrhosis.[130,131]

The primary syndrome is associated with hypergammaglobulinemia with very high total IgG levels and strongly positive antinuclear antibody, rheumatoid factor, and anti-Ro and anti-La antibody levels. The extraglandular manifestations include arthralgia, Raynaud phenomenon, peripheral neuropathy, myositis, liver and interstitial nephritis or renal tubular acidosis. Immune complex deposition resulting from ongoing B-cell hyperactivity is associated with increased morbidity and lymphoma risk.[130]

Ocular disease

The cardinal ocular sign of Sjögren syndrome is keratoconjunctivitis sicca (KCS), which may range from mild irritation in its early stage to severe tear deficiency with ocular surface inflammation and damage resulting in severe visual loss.[1] Assessment of tear production, tear stability, and careful examination of the ocular surface are key.[1] Posterior segment disease is rare. Rosenbaum and Bennett described a series of eight patients with Sjögren syndrome and uveitis, reporting that in all cases the disease was bilateral and chronic; in their report they describe anterior and posterior disease (but no chorioretinitis) with posterior synechiae, cataract, and pars plana exudation being common.[132]

Treatment

Treatment of systemic disease

Sjögren syndrome is a chronic disease with a wide clinical spectrum, making it necessary for regular follow-up. Treatment of sicca symptoms is essential, and includes general measures such as avoidance of dry atmospheres, humidification of rooms, and chewing sugarless chewing gum.[131] Hydroxychloroquine can be effective for treating the subgroup of Sjögren sufferers who have inflammatory myalgias and arthralgias. Anti-TNF-α agents have not shown clinical efficacy, and larger controlled trials are needed to establish the efficacy of rituximab.[131,133]

Treatment of ocular disease

The treatment of KCS is predominantly with frequent use of preservative-free tear substitutes, with a range of viscosities to suit the patient, their visual needs, and even the time of day. RCTs have shown topical 0.05% cyclosporine to be beneficial for patients with moderate to severe dry eye disease.[134,135] In the presence of associated inflammation of the ocular surface, topical glucocorticoids may be required.[29]

Sarcoidosis

This is dealt with separately in Chapter 78 (Sarcoidosis).

Familial juvenile systemic granulomatosis (Blau syndrome)

General considerations

Familial juvenile systemic granulomatosis (Blau syndrome or Jabs syndrome) is a rare autosomal dominant disorder, associated with mutations in the NOD2/CARD 15 gene.[136–139] It was described by Blau in 1990, as a triad of polyarthritis, iritis, and granulomatous papulosquamous rash. There may also be an environmental role, with one series finding Mycobacterium avium ss. paratuberculosis DNA to be present in Blau syndrome tissue in all cases (n = 5).[140]

Epidemiology

Little is known about the epidemiology of familial juvenile systemic granulomatosis. It is thought to occur worldwide, with equal gender and race distribution.[138] In a study looking at the experience of two centers (four families), all affected members carried a NOD2/CARD 15 mutation while it was absent in all the unaffected members.[138] The disease is autosomal dominant in nature, with an observed element of "anticipation" (worsening of symptoms in succeeding generations).[138]

Articular and systemic disease

Familial juvenile systemic granulomatosis presents with a polyarticular arthritis, associated with synovial and tenosynovial cysts, resulting in swelling of the affected joints and tendons.[138] Campylodactyly (multidigit contracture of the interphalangeal joints) can occur secondary to inflammation.[138]

Familial juvenile systemic granulomatosis can be distinguished from childhood sarcoidosis by the absence of pulmonary involvement.[138,141] The rash is described as papulo-erythematous, and usually affects the trunk and extremities.[138] In addition, familial juvenile systemic granulomatosis can be associated with a large vessel vasculitis, and cranial nerve palsies;[138] Crohn's disease is reported to occur in 30% of patients.[142]

Ocular disease

The cardinal ocular sign of familial juvenile systemic granulomatosis is a chronic anterior uveitis or panuveitis with multifocal choroiditis.[143] Complications of uveitis are common including cataract, glaucoma, band keratopathy, and CME. Also reported are subepithelial corneal infiltrates, optic disc edema, ischemic optic neuropathy, and retinal vasculopathy.[143,144]

Treatment

Treatment of systemic disease

Treatment for familial juvenile systemic granulomatosis is largely empirical. Prednisone can be used (dose will be dependent on the severity of disease).[138,139] Immunosuppressive agents, such as methotrexate and azathioprine, have been used with little effect.[138,139] There are also isolated reports of benefit from infliximab and anakinra (IL-1 receptor antagonist) in refractory cases.[138,139]

Treatment of ocular disease

Due to the chronicity of disease, long-term immunosuppression is generally required[144] that may be supplemented with topical and local treatment (as described previously) when needed for flares of ocular disease.

Scleroderma

General considerations

Scleroderma (also called systemic sclerosis) is a multisystem disease of unknown etiology characterized by tissue thickening and fibrosis, often with involvement of internal organs. Scleroderma is usually divided into two forms: a localized form confined to the skin and subcutaneous tissues, and systemic sclerosis that effects both the skin and internal organs.

Epidemiology

The precise estimate for the incidence and prevalence of scleroderma are unknown. This is likely due to a combination of true variation over different populations and differences in case ascertainment and disease classification.[145] Reported prevalence estimates in North America have varied from 13.8 cases per 100 000 from 1950 to 1979 to 28.6 cases per 100 000 in 1985.[146] A Canadian study estimated the prevalence in Quebec in 2003 to be 44.3 cases per 100 000.[145,147] Scleroderma is more common in women, with a female : male ratio of 4–6 : 1. Multiple studies have demonstrated increased incidence and severity of scleroderma in people of African descent.

Articular and systemic disease

Cutaneous manifestations may initially present with inflammation, edema, and reduced sweat and oil production. The characteristic cutaneous features include scleroderma (symmetrical skin thickening proximal to MCP joints), Raynaud phenomenon, Barnett's sign (vertical striation on neck extension), telangiectasia, calcinosis, "mauskopf" facies (caused by tightening of skin and a reduced oral aperture. Gastrointestinal effects include esophageal dysmotility, gastro-esophageal reflux disease (GORD), and intestinal dysmotility.[148]

Pulmonary disease is the leading cause of mortality in scleroderma, manifestations include interstitial lung disease, and/or pulmonary hypertension.

Scleroderma patients will for the most part have a positive ANA (85–90%), in addition 60–70% will be positive for one of the scleroderma-exclusive antibodies (anticentromere, Scl-70 and anti-RNA polymerase III).

Ocular disease

Ocular involvement is common, particularly of the eyelids and anterior segment. Lid involvement occurs in up to two-thirds of patients, resulting in progressive skin tightness, blepharophimosis, and occasionally lagophthalmos. Small lid telangiectasia occurs in up to 21% of patients.[149,150] Ocular surface disease is also very common, with KCS affecting up to 79% patients. KCS may occur as part of secondary Sjögren syndrome. It should be noted when interpreting IOP measurements in scleroderma that central corneal thickness increases during the first eight years of disease and may affect IOP readings.[151,152]

Although retinopathy may be seen in patients with scleroderma it is usually in the context of secondary hypertension, and is of a clinical appearance typical of hypertensive retinopathy (cotton-wool spots, exudation, neuroretinal edema, hemorrhages). Milder retinal changes may also occur in normotensive patients with scleroderma, as shown by Ushiyama et al. where 34% of normotensive scleroderma patients (versus 8% controls) had retinal findings such as hard exudates and vascular tortuosity.[116] Other reported retinal features include combined CRVO and CRAO, bilateral CRVO, BRVO and parafoveal telangiectasia. Interestingly, fundus fluorescein angiography (FFA) studies suggest that abnormality of the choroidal vasculature occurs in around one-third of patients, with hyperfluorescence in the late phase corresponding with areas of hypopigmentation.[153] Other reported ocular complications include cranial nerve palsies, Brown syndrome, and ophthalmoplegia.[154]

Treatment of systemic disease

Scleroderma is a heterogeneous condition, with multiple degrees of severity, so optimal management involves an individual patient approach: assessing current organ involvement, assessing potential problems, and aggressive treatment of more serious organ involvement.[155] Optimal management of blood pressure is a key aspect for managing these patients. Corticosteroids are commonly used at low doses for inflammatory arthritis, but there is no convincing RCT evidence. Cyclophosphamide has been demonstrated in two recent RCTs to be beneficial in scleroderma-associated lung fibrosis and skin disease. Methotrexate has been demonstrated to be effective for skin manifestations in early disease. Mycophenolate mofetil has been demonstrated to be effective for skin, lung, and survival in open-label trials, but work is being undertaken to assess this further.[156] At present there is some evidence that anti-TNF agents may improve inflammatory arthritis, disability, and possibly skin manifestations.[157] In patients with severe diffuse cutaneous scleroderma autologous hematopoietic stem cell transplantation results in sustained improvement of skin thickening and stabilization of organ function. There are two large RCTs currently under way in Europe and the United States to investigate this further.[158]

Treatment of ocular disease

Keratoconjunctivitis sicca may usually be controlled with topical therapy as previously described.[29] In addition to systemic immunosuppression, treatment of blood pressure is an important factor in preventing or treating retinopathy.

Polymyositis and dermatomyositis

General considerations

Myositis is a collective term used to describe polymyositis and dermatomyositis, which are due to chronic inflammation of striated muscle, associated with elevated muscle enzymes. Myositis may present with or without cutaneous and systemic features.

Epidemiology

Several classification criteria have been proposed, the most frequent are the Bohan and Peter criteria (Box 80.6).[159] The precise incidence of myositis is unknown, but is estimated to be between 2 and 10 new cases per million persons at risk per year.[160,161] The reported female: male incidence ratio is 2.5:1.[161] Similar to SLE and systemic sclerosis, there is a higher incidence in people of African descent, with a younger age of onset.

Box 80.6. The Bohan and Peter criteria for the diagnosis of polymyositis and dermatomyositis

Individual criteria
1. Symmetric proximal muscle weakness
2. Muscle biopsy evidence of myositis
3. Increase in serum skeletal muscle enzymes
4. Characteristic electromyography pattern
5. Typical rash of dermatomyositis

Diagnostic criteria
Polymyositis:
Definite: all of 1–4
Probable: any three of 1–4
Possible: any two of 1–4
Dermatomyositis:
Definite: 5 plus any three of 1–4
Probable: 5 plus any two of 1–4
Possible: 5 plus any one of 1–4

(Modified from Bohan A, Peter JB. Polymyositis and dermatomyositis (first of two parts). N Engl J Med 1975;292:344–7.)

Myositis can be associated with other autoimmune conditions, particularly scleroderma and mixed connective tissue disease, and occasionally in SLE, RA, and Sjögren syndrome.[162] There is an increased risk of malignancy in both polymyositis and dermatomyositis. The greatest risk is in dermatomyositis (standardized incidence ratio (SIR): 3.0) which is associated with ovarian, lung, pancreatic, stomach, colorectal and non-Hodgkin lymphoma. Polymyositis is associated with a significant but lower increased risk (SIR: 1.2–1.5), of malignancy particularly non-Hodgkin lymphoma, and lung and bladder cancer.[163]

Articular and systemic disease

Myositis often presents as a subtle, progressive, painless symmetrical weakness over 3–6 months, affecting proximal more than distal muscles.[161] Dermatomyositis is characteristically associated with a heliotrope rash (purplish rash over the periorbital area) and Gottron papules (scaly or erythematous papules and plaques over bony prominences, particularly elbows and knees). Subcutaneous calcinosis (nodules or plaques of calcification over the elbows, forearms, knuckles, axillae, or buttocks), occurs particularly in juvenile dermatomyositis, but occasionally also in adult cases.[161]

Arthralgias and synovitis of small or large joints may occur in patients with myositis, even without an associated connective tissue disease. A deforming arthropathy of the proximal and distal interphalangeal joints occurs typically in patients with inflammatory myopathy and antisynthetase antibodies.[161,162] Interstitial lung disease is also more likely to develop in DM or PM patients with anti-Jo-1 or other antisynthetase antibodies. Subclinical cardiac involvement including myocarditis, pericarditis, arrhythmias, and congestive cardiac failure have been reported. Gastrointestinal tract musculature involvement may occur, causing dysphonia, dysphagia, pseudo-obstruction or malabsorption.[161,162]

Ocular disease

The classic heliotrope eyelid eruption of dermatomyositis is a familiar periocular sign of disease. Actual ocular involvement with myositis of the extraocular muscles is rare.[164] A retinopathy with cotton-wool spots is described in both these conditions, most commonly seen in children and usually (but not exclusively) in the context of systemic vasculitis. Retinopathy is usually mild, but in its severe retinal vasculitis form may lead to permanent visual loss.[165,166] Conjunctivitis, anterior uveitis, and episcleritis are also reported.[166,167]

Treatment

Treatment of systemic disease

There are no large RCTs exploring the treatment of myositis, so treatment is based on case series, open-label trials, and small RCTs. General measures for treating are rehabilitation, avoidance of aspiration, and sun protection. Primary initial therapy is oral corticosteroid.[162,168] Initially patients should be treated with prednisone 1 mg/kg, daily for 4–6 weeks before tapering the dose, but in more severe disease IV methylprednisolone up to 1 g/day for three consecutive days is recommended. Immunosuppressant therapy at an early stage may be required to facilitate corticosteroid reduction and side-effects from corticosteroids, and the first choice agents are methotrexate and azathioprine. In severe cases, in particular those associated with vasculitis or interstitial lung disease, cyclophosphamide has been recommended.[162,168] Intravenous immunoglobulin has been proposed in patients with rapidly progressing disease, and alternative agents include cyclosporine, mycophenolate mofetil, possibly rituximab (ongoing phase II clinical trials), and anti-TNF agents (although studies have found an increased risk of disease flare).[169]

Treatment of ocular disease

Systemic immunosuppression is required to control both the systemic disease and its ocular manifestations. Vasculitis regimens such as intravenous cyclophosphamide and methylprednisolone are commonly used.[167]

Relapsing polychondritis

General considerations

Relapsing polychondritis is a rare autoimmune disease of unknown etiology, primarily effecting cartilaginous structures throughout the body.

Epidemiology

Relapsing polychondritis has an estimated incidence rate of 3.5 per million per annum; the peak onset is between 40 and 60 years. Equal frequency has been reported in both genders and all racial groups. Over 30% of cases are associated with existing autoimmune and hematological conditions, including RA, SLE, Sjögren syndrome, AS, lymphoma, and IBD.[170]

Articular and systemic disease

Relapsing polychondritis is a multisystem disease that can affect the cartilaginous structures in the eyes, ears, nose, laryngotracheobronchial, and costal cartilages (Table 80.2). It causes inflammation of hyaline cartilage with a predilection for ear cartilage.[171] Involvement of the parasternal joints, including the sternoclavicular, costochondral, and manubriosternal articulations, is typical for this condition. Peripheral joint disease is reported in 70% of patients, and is usually nonerosive and asymmetric.[171]

Ocular disease

Ophthalmic disease occurs in around half of patients with relapsing polychondritis. In a series of 112 patients, Isaak and coworkers reported that 19% patients had ocular symptoms at the onset of disease, with 51% developing ocular symptoms during the course of disease. Episcleritis (39%) and scleritis (14%) are common.[172] Anterior uveitis was reported as just 9% in the Isaak series but has been reported to be as prevalent as 30% in other series.[173] Other anterior segment findings include KCS and peripheral ulcerative keratitis.[174] The commonest posterior segment presentation is posterior scleritis, which may be severe and be associated with serous retinal detachments and frank proptosis.[175–177] Retinopathy consisting of cotton-wool spots and intraretinal hemorrhages is reported to occur in up to 9% of patients. Other posterior segment features are branch or central retinal vein occlusions and ischemic optic neuropathy.[172] Cranial neuropathies may also be seen.

Table 80.2 Systemic features of relapsing polychondritis

Organ involvement	Clinical manifestation
Ear	External inflammation, loss of hearing, tinnitus, vertigo
Eye	Episcleritis, scleritis, ulcerative keratitis, uveitis, proptosis
Nose	Crusting, rhinorrhea, epistaxis, saddle nose
Large airways	Hoarseness, aphonia, wheezing, inspiratory stridor, nonproductive cough, dyspnea
Joints	Parasternal joints, peripheral joints (mono- or oligoarticular)
Heart	Aortic and mitral valvular disease
Skin	Aphthous ulcers, purpura, papules, nodules or ulcerations

(Reproduced with permission from Lahmer T, Treiber M, von Werder A, et al. Relapsing polychondritis: an autoimmune disease with many faces. Autoimmun Rev 2010;9:540–6.)

Treatment

Treatment of systemic disease

First-line therapy for relapsing polychondritis is corticosteroid, initially started at 1 mg/kg prednisone daily; if necessary three pulses IV methylprednisolone can be administered. Immunosuppressives should be used for severe disease causing organ compromise or where corticosteroids have not provided a satisfactory response within a few weeks. The choice of immunosuppressant is empirical; the most commonly used agents are cyclophosphamide, azathioprine, cyclosporine, and methotrexate.[170] There are case reports reporting success with anti-TNF agents (etanercept/infliximab/adalimumab), anakinra, and rituximab.[178]

Treatment of ocular disease

Systemic immunosuppression is required to control both the systemic disease and its severe ocular manifestations. Vasculitis regimens may be required. Anterior uveitis, episcleritis, and KCS may be additionally controlled with topical therapy as previously described.

Primary systemic vasculitis

The vasculitides are a heterogeneous group of diseases involving inflammation of blood vessels with subsequent tissue destruction and/or organ damage. The vasculitides can be considered to be primary or secondary (commonly associated with another connective tissue disease or infection). They are predominantly arterial in nature, though capillaries and less commonly veins are involved. Local tissue disruption is caused by inflammatory cell infiltrate in the vessel wall and subsequent tissue ischemia from vessel occlusion. The primary systemic vasculitides are an uncommon group of diseases (combined annual incidence >100 new cases per million).[179] Classification is usually based on the predominantly affected vessel (Box 80.7). Recently the term ANCA-associated vasculitis (AAV) has been used to describe those small vessel conditions where there are similar immunopathological tissue mechanism: granulomatosis with polyangiitis (GPA, Wegener's granulomatosis), microscopic polyangiitis (MPA), and Churg–Strauss syndrome (CSS).[180,181]

In parallel with advances in our understanding of the immunobiology of the vasculitides, it is becoming increasingly recognized that therapy for vasculitis needs to be tailored to the specific diagnosis and the phase of disease in that individual. An understanding of the natural history of the specific conditions and assessment to identify the extent and activity of disease is required to achieve this.

Box 80.7 Classification of vasculitides according to the Chapel Hill consensus

Primary vasculitides
Large artery
Giant cell arteritis
Takayasu arteritis
Medium artery
Polyarteritis nodosa
Kawasaki disease
Small artery and vein
Granulomatosis with polyangiitis (Wegener's granulomatosis)*
Microscopic polyangiitis*
Churg–Strauss syndrome*
Henoch–Schonlein purpura
Leukocytoclastic vasculitis
Essential cryoglobulinemic vasculitis
Other
Behçet disease
Cogan syndrome
Secondary vasculitides
Connective tissue disease
Hepatitis B/C
HIV

These vasculitides are associated with ANCA.
Recently Watts et al. have suggested a possible fourth category, no predominant vessel size, to describe Behçet disease, primary central nervous system (CNS) vasculitis and Cogan syndrome.[180]
(Modified from Jennette JC, Falk RJ, Andrassy K, et al. Nomenclature of systemic vasculitides. Proposal of an international consensus conference. Arthritis Rheum 1994;37:187–92.)

Progression and prognosis of primary systemic necrotizing vasculitis

Classification of the vasculitides is most often based on the size of vessel involved (Box 80.7).[182] The initial and predominant inflammatory process is granulomatous in some cases, with the vasculitic phase of the illness only presenting later. This is typical of GPA, where constitutional and upper respiratory symptoms may be present for several years prior to diagnosis, thus delaying the commencement of appropriate therapy and adding to the morbidity and mortality of the condition.

Though the vasculitides are characteristically relapsing diseases, the frequency of relapse depends on the specific underlying diagnosis. In polyarteritis nodosa (PAN) the risk is low, which contrasts with ANCA-associated vasculitides where relapse is as high as 50%.[183] Prior to the introduction of effective therapy, the 5-year survival of systemic necrotizing vasculitis (SNV) was only 15%; corticosteroids improved this figure to 48%, while the combination corticosteroids and cyclophosphamide (CP) gave a significant improvement, with 5-year survival reaching 80%. However, this improved survival came at a cost with recurrent flares of disease activity leading to the accumulation of organ damage, with appreciable morbidity also related to drug toxicity.

Aims of therapy

The aim of therapy in SNV must be to suppress disease activity so that organ damage is limited.

Clinical tools to assess disease activity and damage are used to aid in assessment and management of these complex diseases. These scoring systems have predictive value for severe disease where patients are at higher risk of mortality, thus supporting a more aggressive approach to therapy. The Birmingham Vasculitis Activity Score (BVAS) provides a weighted numerical score based on the specific organ involved and the severity of that involvement. A high score reflects either critical organ involvement or multisystem disease and predicts a higher mortality.[184] The Vasculitis Damage Index (VDI) is a cumulative score where items of organ damage must be present for a period of at least 3 months and be attributable to effects of the disease, its therapy or other undefined causes. A high VDI score identifies a subgroup of patients with more severe or fatal disease.[185]

Thorough clinical assessment to differentiate vasculitis localized to a single organ (such as ocular vasculitis) from more systemic disease is important, as the former group may not require systemic immunosuppression. Use of a systematic approach in clinical assessment, such as that provided on the BVAS form, can help clinicians identify previously unsuspected disease symptoms or signs, such as purpura or vascular bruits. Urinalysis is a simple critical investigation to identify renal involvement. Laboratory tests may provide supportive evidence of active systemic disease. A rise in C-reactive protein indicates active inflammation in the absence of infection. The presence of ANCA supports a diagnosis of one of the AAV but should not on its own prompt introduction of immunosuppressive therapy without appropriate clinical features. MPO-ANCA is seen in MPA and CSS, while PR3-ANCA is most commonly seen in GPA. Tissue samples for histopathological examination may be needed to confirm a diagnosis and exclude alternatives such as infection or malignancy. Therefore, a combination of clinical tools and laboratory investigations can help support a diagnosis of SNV and help differentiate disease activity, where immunosuppressive therapy may be required, from irreversible organ damage, where more therapy may be potentially harmful.

A diagnosis of vasculitis is not an indication to commence aggressive therapy in every patient. Some small vessel disease, such as Henoch–Schonlein purpura (HSP) or isolated leukocytoclastic vasculitis (LCV), where an initiating event is identified, may be self-limiting and need no therapy. Corticosteroids alone may be enough for the large vessel vasculitides. It is the AAV and PAN where a more aggressive approach is indicated to minimize organ damage. The approach outlined below can also be applied to other vasculitides where there is critical organ-threatening disease (such as sight-threatening scleritis in rheumatoid vasculitis).

Induction stage

Cyclophosphamide in combination with corticosteroids are the drugs of choice for remission induction. Continuous oral cyclophosphamide (2 mg/kg/day) in conjunction with oral prednisone (1 mg/kg reducing to 10 mg daily by 3 months) induces remission in most by 3 months.[186] Remission induction takes longer in some patients, increasing the risk of drug-related toxicity. A safer and equally effective approach is to use intermittent pulses of intravenous cyclophosphamide.[187] The pulse interval is an important factor and a suggested induction regimen has been provided (Table 80.3).

Maintenance stage

AT six months, cyclophosphamide should be switched to milder maintenance therapy, such as azathioprine (2 mg/kg/day) or methotrexate. Co-trimoxazole has also been shown to reduce the relapse rate in GPA, possibly by eliminating nasal carriage of Staphylococcus aureus. Other maintenance agents that have been used in small series include cyclosporine, leflunomide, and

Table 80.3 Pulse cyclophosphamide induction regimen

Drug doses	Methylprednisolone 10 mg/kg plus Cyclophosphamide 15 mg/kg
Dose interval	0, 2 ,4, 7, 10, 13 weeks Switch after six pulses to consolidation phase with monthly infusions ×3. If in remission, maintenance treatment with methotrexate or azathioprine can be commenced
Dose reductions	Age (>70 yr), renal impairment, infection, neutropenia
Toxicity	Nausea, alopecia, neutropenia, infertility, hemorrhagic cystitis

Box 80.8 The American College of Rheumatology 1990 criteria for the classification of giant cell arteritis

The presence of *three or more* of the following five criteria is associated with 93.5% sensitivity and 91.2% sensitivity for GCA.

1. Age ≥50 years at disease onset
2. New onset of localized headache
3. Temporal artery tenderness or decreased pulse
4. ESR ≥50 mm/h
5. Arterial biopsy with necrotizing arteritis with a predominance of mononuclear cell infiltrates or granulomatous process with multinucleate giant cells

(Reproduced with permission from Hunder GG, Bloch DA, Michel BA, et al. The American College of Rheumatology 1990 criteria for the classification of giant cell arteritis. Arthritis Rheum 1990;33:1122–8.)

mycophenolate mofetil. The duration that maintenance therapy should be continued is not clear, but in diseases where the relapse rate is high (e.g. AAV) therapy should probably be continued for 3–5 years.

Adjuvant therapy

Where disease control is proving difficult and in the presence of severe organ involvement, pulses of methylprednisolone (1 g on three consecutive days) may be used but should not delay the commencement of cyclophosphamide. Plasma exchange and intravenous immunoglobulin are other potential treatment modalities.

Treatment of relapse

Fewer items of damage accumulate after relapse than at first presentation,[185] but for major relapses a short course of cyclophosphamide (six pulses) with an early transfer to maintenance methotrexate, azathioprine or cyclosporine is one approach. Patients with recurrent relapses may be exposed to several courses of cyclophosphamide, increasing the risk of drug-related toxicity (bladder cancer, infertility, myelodysplasia). Methotrexate may be used as an alternative to cyclophosphamide for less severe relapse.

Alternative approaches to therapy

A number of alternative therapies have been trialed. A short course of higher-dose pulsed cyclophosphamide may induce an early remission, but has an increased risk of neutropenia and infection. Autologous stem cell transplantation after intensive immunosuppression has been successfully carried out in a few patients with severe unremitting disease. Anti-T cell monoclonal antibodies (Campath-1H and anti-CD4) have produced dramatic responses in some patients. Anti-TNF agents have not shown any benefit over standard therapy,[188] although several case reports suggest a benefit in some cases of treatment-resistant vasculitis. More promising results have been shown using the B-cell depleting anti-CD20 antibody rituximab.[189]

Large vessel vasculitides

Giant cell arteritis

General considerations

Giant cell arteritis (GCA) or temporal arteritis is a vasculitis that typically effects elderly patients, and is highly corticosteroid-responsive. Symptoms tend to begin insidiously, most commonly headaches, scalp tenderness, myalgias, fever, anorexia, and weight loss.[190] In some cases, however, disease can present abruptly with a major complication such as loss of vision.[191]

Epidemiology

GCA is predominantly a disease of the elderly. It rarely affects those under 50 years, with a mean age of presentation of 70–75 years. There is a 2:1 female:male ratio. It is estimated to affect approximately 220 patients per million per year.[180,192,193]

Articular and systemic disease

GCA targets branches of the external carotid artery; patient symptoms include headaches, scalp tenderness, jaw and tongue claudication. There is an increased risk of transient ischemic attack (TIA) or stroke, as a result of arteritis of the vertebral and basilar arteries. Systemic features of GCA, such as fever, malaise, fatigue, weakness, anorexia, weight loss, and depression are present in 40–50% of patients. The arteritic process can involve other large vessels and subclavian or brachial arteries presenting with upper limb claudication or an aortitis (thoracic > abdominal) is well recognized in 10–20% of patients. There is thought to be an association with polymyalgia rheumatica.[194]

Ocular disease

Many patients present with temporal headache but no visual loss, but anterior ischemic optic neuropathy (AION) due to arteritis of the short posterior ciliary arteries is the major complication of GCA, and typically presents as acute painless loss of vision. The diagnosis is straightforward when seen with devastating loss of vision (often perception of light), a relative afferent pupillary defect, and typical optic disc edema in the context of systemic features typical of the disease. With time optic atrophy ensues with complete loss of vision. Nevertheless in some patients it is difficult to distinguish between an arteritic and nonarteritic cause of AION. Failure to differentiate these two can be catastrophic as involvement of the second eye in arteritic AION ranges from 10% if treated to 95% if untreated. A detailed ocular and general history is essential and examination reveals a tender, thickened, nonpulsatile superficial temporal artery. Characteristically there is an elevated erythrocyte sedimentation rate (ESR) and C-reactive protein (CRP). A definitive diagnosis is made on temporal artery biopsy (TAB) but a positive biopsy is not always required to make a diagnosis (American College of Rheumatology classification criteria for GCA – Box 80.8).[195] Nevertheless all patients with a clinical and/or laboratory diagnosis, or where the diagnosis is in doubt should have therapy instigated and a TAB performed. A TAB is normally performed within 48–72 hours of commencing corticosteroid therapy. A recent study has shown that on 459 cases of biopsy-proven GCA the odds of a positive biopsy were 1.5 times greater with an ESR of 47–107 mm/hr, 5.3 times greater with a CRP >2.45 mg/dl, and 4.2 times greater with platelets >400/μL.[196]

More problematic are those presenting with posterior ischemic optic neuropathy (with an apparently normal optic disc in the acute phase) and who may not report typical features; in the series by Hayreh, around 10% of the IONs seen were posterior ischemic optic neuropathy (PION).[191] The estimates of visual loss from GCA vary widely from 13% to 70%, with lower estimates being seen in a recent series that may reflect improved diagnosis and earlier treatment. The visual loss is usually severe (<20/200), and visual recovery is uncommon despite appropriate therapy.[197] Visual field loss may be complete, altitudinal or occasionally an arcuate (Bjerrum-type) scotoma. Amaurosis fugax may be a warning of impending ION or other serious ischemic pathology. An ischemic retinopathy with cotton-wool spots (and sometimes retinal hemorrhages) may be seen and can precede optic nerve involvement.[198,199] Other ophthalmic complications of biopsy-proven GCA include cilioretinal artery occlusion (CRAO), and ocular ischemic syndrome occurring in about 14%, 20%, and 1% respectively of patients. Occasionally there is extraocular muscle dysfunction with symptoms of transient or permanent diplopia.[191]

Treatment

Corticosteroids are the mainstay of treatment, with almost all patients who present to a rheumatologist responding to 40–60 mg oral prednisone. Those patients presenting to an ophthalmologist with or without vision loss should have three IV pulses of methylprednisolone 1 g for 3 days, then oral prednisone 1 mg/kg/day. Corticosteroid taper can occur after 4 weeks with resolution of symptoms and a fall in inflammatory markers.[200] It is reasonable to aim for a dose of 15 mg by 3 months of therapy. In addition, low-dose aspirin (to reduce the risk of arterial thrombus and visual loss) and bone protection (bisphosphonates and calcium and vitamin D supplementation) with or without a proton pump inhibitor could be considered.[200] On average 18 months of corticosteroid treatment is required, but up to 40% may need long-term therapy due to relapsing disease. A corticosteroid sparing agent may need to be introduced, such as methotrexate, azathioprine, and leflunomide. The role of biological agents in treatment is not currently established. There is no evidence that they are beneficial when used at disease onset but may be helpful in relapsing disease to minimize corticosteroid dose and thus side-effects. Recently encouraging results have been demonstrated with the biologics infliximab, etanercept, rituximab, and tociluzimab.[201–203]

Takayasu's arteritis

General considerations

Takayasu's arteritis is a rare inflammatory disease of unknown etiology, characterized by granulomatous vasculitis affecting large arteries, in particular the aorta and its main branches.

Epidemiology

Takayasu's arteritis is very rare, with an annual incidence of 2.6 per million in North America and 1.2 per million in Japan. It is classically described in women of childbearing age of Southeast Asian, South African, and Latin American background[204–206] (see Box 80.9[207]).

Box 80.9 The American College of Rheumatology criteria for the classification of Takayasu arteritis

For purposes of classification, a patient is said to have Takayasu arteritis if *at least three* of these six criteria are present. The presence of any three or more criteria yields a sensitivity of 90.5% and a specificity of 97.8%

1. Age at disease onset < 40 years
   Development of symptoms or findings related to Takayasu arteritis at age under 40 years
2. Claudication of extremities
   Development and worsening of fatigue and discomfort in muscles of one or more extremities while in use, especially the upper extremities
3. Decreased brachial artery pulse
   Decreased pulsation of one or both brachial arteries
4. BP difference >10 mmHg
   Difference of >10 mmHg in systolic blood pressure between arms
5. Bruit over subclavian arteries or aorta
   Bruit audible on auscultation over one or both subclavian arteries or abdominal aorta
6. Arteriogram abnormality
   Arteriographic narrowing or occlusion of the entire aorta, its primary branches, or large arteries in the proximal upper or lower extremities, not due to arteriosclerosis, fibromuscular dysplasia, or similar causes; changes usually focal or segmental

(Reproduced with permission from Arend WP, Michel BA, Bloch DA, et al. The American College of Rheumatology 1990 criteria for the classification of Takayasu arteritis. Arthritis Rheum 1990;33:1129–34.)

Articular and systemic disease

At the time of diagnosis, 10–20% of patients are clinically asymptomatic and the disease is diagnosed incidentally on vascular examination. The most common findings on examination are hypertension, bruits, diminished or absent pulses, and asymmetric blood pressure readings in the extremities. Of symptomatic patients, 80–90% can present with either systemic or vascular symptoms, or a combination of both. Systemic features include fever, malaise, weight loss, arthralgia, and night sweats.[204–206]

Vascular symptoms are more common and are as a result of active vasculitis or vascular damage from previous inflammation resulting in stenosis or aneurysm formation. Involvement of the carotid and vertebral arteries can lead to central nervous system involvement. Clinically patients may be asymptomatic, or have symptoms including transient ischemic attacks, stroke, dizziness, syncope, headache or visual changes. Mesenteric involvement is common. The most common cardiac manifestation is aortic regurgitation. Cutaneous manifestations such as erythema nodosum and pyroderma granulosum have been observed in 3–28% of patients.[204–206]

Ocular disease

Ophthalmic disease occurs in around one-third of patients with Takayasu arteritis. The most common ocular complication is hypertensive retinopathy (16–30%), followed by Takayasu retinopathy (13–15%), and ocular ischemic syndrome (around 4%).[208,209] Takayasu retinopathy may progress from small vessel dilation (stage 1), to microaneurysms (stage 2), arteriovenous anastomoses (stage 3), and finally additional complications, such as retinal neovascularization and vitreous hemorrhage (stage 4).[208] Other recognized complications include AION, PION, and neovascular glaucoma. The presence of ischemic ocular complications is associated with non-recordable right upper limb blood pressure.[209]

Treatment

Corticosteroids are the mainstay of treatment. Initially it is recommended that prednisone is started at 1 mg/kg/day (maximum 60 mg/day), for a month then tapered gradually.[210,211] If patients have severe disease or refractory disease, steroid-sparing agents need to be considered.

Corticosteroid-sparing agents that can be considered are azathioprine (2 mg/kg/day), and methotrexate (20–25 mg/week).[210,212] Other agents with limited data available include cyclophosphamide, mycophenolate mofetil, leflunomide and minocycline, and the biological agents infliximab, tocliziumab, and abatacept.[210,212]

Non-medical interventions such as angioplasty, stent insertion, arterial reconstruction, and bypass grafting may also be required.[210,211]

Medium vessel vasculitides

Polyarteritis nodosa

General considerations

Polyarteritis nodosa (PAN) is a necrotizing inflammation of medium vessels with or without glomerulonephritis, which can be secondary to hepatitis B, and is ANCA-negative.

Epidemiology

PAN is a very uncommon disease, being estimated to occur at less than 1 per million per year (United Kingdom data). The major environmental risk factor is hepatitis B; other associated viruses are HIV and parvovirus B19.[193]

Articular and systemic disease

PAN has a wide spectrum of disease, ranging from very mild limited disease to life threatening organ involvement. Arthralgia or arthritis may be present in up to 50% of patients. An intermittent, asymmetrical, predominantly lower limb, nondeforming arthritis may occur in up to 20% of cases. Myalgias may occur in up to 50% of patients.[213,214]

Cutaneous features are seen in 25–60%: these include infarctions, ulcerations, livedo reticularis, subcutaneous nodules, and ischemic changes of distal digits.[215] Peripheral neuropathy or mononeuritis multiplex may be seen. CNS involvement with headaches, seizures, cranial nerve dysfunction, stroke, and cerebral hemorrhage are less common. Renal involvement can result in hypertension as a result of renal artery stenosis or renal impairment/failure due to multiple microaneurysms and infarcts as a consequence of vascular occlusion. Abdominal pain, which can occur in up to 70% of patients as a result of gastrointestinal involvement, can be severe, with bowel ischemia occurring.[213,214]

Ocular disease

Ophthalmic disease occurs in around 10–20% of patients with PAN, and may reflect direct ocular involvement or be secondary to its systemic effects (notably hypertension from renal disease). Retinal disease includes retinal vasculitis and hypertensive retinopathy. Other ophthalmic complications include peripheral ulcerative keratitis, episcleritis, scleritis (both anterior and posterior), serous retinal detachments, ischemic optic neuropathy, cranial neuropathies, and cerebral disease resulting in visual field defects.[216–218]

Treatment

Pulsed IV cyclophosphamide and corticosteroids has been found to achieve better disease control and sustained remission compared to corticosteroids alone, but the long-term survival remains unchanged.[219,220] Patients with hepatitis-associated PAN are recommended to have high-dose corticosteroid therapy tapered over 2 weeks followed by antiviral agents, and plasma exchange.[219,220]

Kawasaki disease

General considerations

Kawasaki disease predominantly affects young children and is the most common cause of acquired heart disease in the United States and Japan. It is the second commonest vasculitis of childhood after Henoch–Schonlein purpura.

Epidemiology

The highest incidence rate is in Japan – 216 cases per 100 000 per year in children under 5 years of age – with a peak incidence at between 9 and 11 months of age.[221] There are possible familial and infectious links.[193]

Articular and systemic disease

Kawasaki disease is usually defined as a persistent fever for a minimum of 5 days with a minimum of four out of the following: (1) polymorphous rash; (2) bilateral conjunctival injection without exudates; (3) oropharyngeal involvement, including red fissured lips, strawberry tongue, and red pharynx without exudates; (4) peripheral changes including edema of extremities, sole erythema, and periungual desquamation; and (5) cervical lymphadenopathy. Arthritis of the small joints is common, and is associated with a bluish discoloration over the PIPs. Axial arthropathy and effusions can also occur, but the articular symptoms will usually resolve after the acute phase.[222,223]

The most serious manifestation is that of the cardiovascular system, which can result in aneurysms (especially the coronary arteries), myocarditis, and congestive cardiac failure. Other clinical manifestations include gastrointestinal manifestations, urethritis, facial nerve palsy (rare), and sensorineural hearing loss.[222,223]

Ocular disease

Bilateral conjunctival injection without purulent discharge is one of the hallmarks of Kawasaki disease. Additionally, bilateral anterior uveitis is common in the first week of illness.[224] Rare ocular manifestations include optic neuritis and ophthalmic artery obstruction.[225]

Treatment

Kawasaki disease is treated with a single IV dose of immunoglobulin and high-dose aspirin. The aspirin dose can be reduced once the fever finishes. If patients fail to respond to the first dose of IV immunoglobulin, treatment options include a repeat infusion, infliximab, IV methylprednisolone, and plasmapheresis.[226–229]

Small vessel vasculitides

Granulomatosis with polyangiitis (Wegener's granulomatosis)

General considerations

Granulomatosis with polyangiitis (GPA) is a multisystem disease of unknown etiology, characterized by granulomatous inflammation, tissue necrosis, and varying degrees of vasculitis. It can affect any organ, but has a predilection for the upper respiratory tract, lungs, and kidneys.

Epidemiology

GPA has a slight male predominance, which is more marked in Caucasians. GPA is a rare disease, with a prevalence ranging from 3 per 100 000 in the United States to up to 16 per 100 000 in Northern Europe.[230,231] GPA predominantly affects older individuals, but 15% of cases have been reported in childhood.[232] GPA is highly associated with PR3 (proteinase 3) ANCA.[233]

Articular and systemic disease

Musculoskeletal symptoms can occur in up to 60% of patients. Commonly a migratory polyarthritis affecting the large joints or a polyarthritis can occur.

Presenting symptoms in up to 75% of patients will be of upper respiratory tract disease (nasal, sinus, tracheal and/or ear abnormalities). The "saddle nose deformity" results from nasal bridge collapse, and other nasal manifestations include nasal pain, stuffiness, crusts, epistaxis, mucosal erosion, and septal perforation. A characteristic feature of mouth involvement is "strawberry gums," an intense gingivitis that responds to systemic treatment. A serious complication is subglottic stenosis secondary to tracheal inflammation and scarring, as this may require a tracheostomy.[3] Nonspecific systemic features may occur, particularly during active disease, which include fever, malaise, arthralgias, anorexia, and weight loss.[3]

Pulmonary involvement may present as cough, hemoptysis, dyspnea, or pleuritic or other forms of chest pain; however one-third of patients with pulmonary lesions have asymptomatic disease. Renal involvement occurs in about 80% of GPA patients.

Ocular disease

Ophthalmic disease occurs in around 50% of patients in this condition and is an important cause of morbidity and blindness, with vision loss occurring in around 8%.[3] Although orbital disease is the most common ocular complication of the disease, almost any part of the ophthalmic system may be affected.

Orbital disease occurs in up to 20% of patients with GPA. It may present with acute or subacute proptosis, and may be associated with ocular motility disturbance (resulting in diplopia), and optic nerve compression or infiltration potentially leading to blindness. Severe proptosis may also lead to sight-threatening exposure keratopathy. It should be noted that although proptosis is common in these patients, chronic orbital inflammation may lead to orbital socket contraction with enophthalmos, restrictive ophthalmopathy, and chronic pain.[234]

Important nonorbital presentations of GPA include scleritis (7–10% of patients), peripheral ulcerative keratitis, and an ulcerative conjunctivitis with a chronic cicatrizing course.[235] The scleritis may be anterior or posterior; necrotizing scleritis is often associated with corneal disease (marginal corneal ulcer/PUK). Uveitis is uncommon (around 3%). Anterior, posterior and panuveitis have all been described in this context and may be isolated or associated with scleritis.[236,237] Retinal vasculitis may occur and ranges in severity from cotton-wool spots to severe vaso-occlusive disease, with neovascularization and related consequences. Neuro-ophthalmic consequences most commonly occur secondary to orbital involvement, but may also arise due to vasculitis causing ischemic optic neuropathy. In a study of 59 patients with ANCA-associated vasculitis and ocular inflammation, 75% had scleritis, and with time these patients had a 2.75-fold higher mortality than other patients with inflammatory eye disease.[238]

Treatment

Like other vasculitides, the suggested treatment to induce remission is pulsed IV cyclophosphamide with oral steroids.[219,239] Corticosteroid-sparing agents that can be substituted for cyclophosphamide once remission has been achieved are methotrexate or azathioprine. If disease is limited then methotrexate in combination with oral corticosteroid can be used rather than cyclophosphamide.[219] Biologics are now increasingly used in the management, initially infliximab and more recently rituximab.[240] Rituximab has been used in clinical trials to induce remission in GPA, with favorable results compared to cyclophosphamide, and in sight-threatening ocular and orbital disease.[189,241] Treatment is primarily directed against the systemic disease, although it should be noted that the severity of ophthalmic involvement may be an important factor in escalating therapy.

Microscopic polyangiitis

General considerations

Microscopic polyangiitis (MPA) is a necrotizing vasculitis, predominantly affecting small vessels, associated with MPO (myeloperoxidase) ANCA.

Epidemiology

MPA has an incidence of 5 per million per year, with a peak age of onset of between 65 and 75 years; it is more common in men.[231]

Articular and systemic disease

Renal involvement is very common, affecting up to 90% of patients. Rapidly progressive glomerulonephritis may occur, resulting in acute renal failure necessitating renal dialysis. Varying degrees of pulmonary involvement can occur; these can range from mild dyspnea to life-threatening pulmonary hemorrhage. Involvement of both the central and peripheral nervous system is described, and includes peripheral neuropathy, mononeuritis multiplex, cerebral hemorrhage/infarction, seizures or headache. Other systemic manifestations include cardiac, gastrointestinal, otorhinolaryngeal, and venous thromboembolism.[215,242,243]

Ocular disease

Ophthalmic disease is rare in MPA, with one series noting ocular involvement in only 1 of 85 patients with MPA.[242] In small case series and isolated reports the following ophthalmic complications have been noted: scleritis, anterior uveitis with hypopyon, retinal vasculitis (ranging from cotton-wool spots to neovascularization and vitreous hemorrhage) and peripheral nonulcerative keratitis.[244,245]

Treatment

Recommended treatment for severe MPA is oral corticosteroid with pulsed IV cyclophosphamide to induce remission.[219,239] In milder active disease (no threatened vital organ disease or damage), methotrexate or azathioprine and oral corticosteroid can be used, but there is a higher risk of relapse.[239] If patients have failed to achieve remission and have persistent low activity, IV immunoglobulin can be used to achieve remission.[219] There is sparse data in the literature regarding the use of biologics, mainly infliximab and rituximab.[246]

Churg–Strauss syndrome

General considerations

Churg–Strauss syndrome (CSS) is a primary, multisystem, eosinophilic vasculitis associated with upper and lower respiratory tract disease and ANCA.

Epidemiology

CSS is estimated to have a prevalence of 10 to 15 per million. The mean age of diagnosis is 55 years. It has equal gender incidence.[247]

Articular and systemic disease

Churg–Strauss syndrome can affect virtually any organ system in the body. Systemic symptoms include fever, weight loss, arthralgias, and, rarely, arthritis.[247]

Pulmonary involvement is nearly universal in CSS, with 96–100% having asthma. Other pulmonary manifestations include pulmonary infiltrates, pulmonary hemorrhage, and pleural effusions.

Peripheral neuropathy occurs commonly (65–75%), usually with mononeuritis multiplex. CNS involvement may include cranial nerve palsies, ischemic optic neuropathy, cerebral hemorrhage or infarction, convulsions, coma, and psychosis.

Abdominal pain is the most common gastrointestinal symptom. Cardiac involvement includes eosinophilic endomyocarditis, coronary vasculitis, valvular heart disease, congestive heart failure, hypertension, and pericarditis. Skin lesions are common and typically include nonthrombocytopenic palpable purpura, with erythematous, maculopapular, or pustular lesions being reported. Renal involvement is fairly typical, but unlike other necrotizing vasculitides such as GPA or microscopic polyangiitis, renal failure is rare.[247–249]

Ocular disease

Ophthalmic disease may arise from two processes: vasculitis and granuloma formation. Clinical presentations include conjunctival nodules,[250] peripheral ulcerative keratitis, episcleritis, scleritis, uveitis (rare), retinal vasculitis,[251] retinal artery occlusion, ischemic optic neuropathy, cranial neuropathies[252] and orbital disease (presenting with an orbital inflammatory syndrome).[251]

Treatment

As with other ANCA-positive vasculitides, remission induction is normally achieved with oral corticosteroids and cyclophosphamide or with a DMARD such as methotrexate or azathioprine in less severe disease.[219,239] Rituximab is currently undergoing clinical trials, but there have been promising results published.[253]

OCULAR COMPLICATIONS OF RHEUMATOLOGICAL THERAPIES

General

Ocular complications of rheumatological therapies may relate to (1) direct drug-specific toxic effects, such as chloroquine retinopathy, (2) indirect drug-specific side-effects, such as corticosteroid-induced ocular hypertension resulting in secondary glaucoma, and (3) drug non-specific complications relating to immunosuppression, such as opportunistic infections.

Corticosteroids

Most treatment-related visual morbidity is associated with corticosteroid treatment. The association between posterior subcapsular cataract and exogenous corticosteroids is well established.[254] Cataract surgery in patients with rheumatic diseases is generally successful, although there must be strict control of any intraocular inflammation prior to surgery and in the postoperative phase. Prognosis will be worse if there is visually significant posterior segment disease. Increased intraocular pressure due to exogenous corticosteroids may occur in up to 30% of the normal population, with 5% experiencing an increase of more than 15 mmHg (reviewed by Clark[255]). Corticosteroid-induced ocular hypertension must be monitored and treated where there is a risk of progression to secondary glaucoma.

Antimalarials

The aminoquinolones chloroquine and hydroxychloroquine have been widely used in the treatment of SLE. These drugs can cause a reversible, visually insignificant keratopathy (cornea verticillata) and, more importantly, an irreversible sight-threatening maculopathy. Clinical progression is of loss of the foveal reflex followed by a fine granular appearance of the macula and finally a "bull's eye" maculopathy presenting as a central scotoma. Endstage disease includes generalized atrophy, peripheral pigmentation, arteriolar attenuation, and optic atrophy.[256]

Retinopathy is rare with hydroxychloroquine when used at currently recommended doses (<6.5 mg/kg/d), but increases markedly towards 1% after 5–7 years of usage or a cumulative dose of 1000 g of hydroxychloroquine.[257,258] The risk with chloroquine is thought to be significantly greater, with an increased risk at over 460 g chloroquine. In both cases, risk increases with increasing dose, increasing duration, and reduced renal function. The American Academy of Ophthalmology (AAO) 2011 guidelines recommend screening for all patients at baseline or within first year of use, and to start annual screening after 5 years of use (or earlier if additional risk factors).[258] Assessments should include dilated retinal examinations, and white 10–2 automated visual field testing which should be interpreted with a low threshold for abnormality and with retesting if abnormalities are seen. Additionally, they recommend that one or more of the following should be performed where available: spectral domain optical coherence tomography, multifocal electroretinography or fundus autofluorescence.[258] High-risk patients include those on a dose of >6.5 mg/kg, with a duration of >5 years, obese patients, those with renal or hepatic disease, those with pre-existing retinal disease or those over the age of 60 years.[258] Amsler grid testing is no longer recommended. Although fundus examinations are advised for documentation, the aim is to detect changes before visible maculopathy. The AAO authors stress the importance of counseling patients regarding the risk of toxicity and the rationale for screening.

REFERENCES

1. The definition and classification of dry eye disease: report of the Definition and Classification Subcommittee of the International Dry Eye WorkShop (2007). Ocul Surf 2007;5:75–92.
2. Galor A, Thorne JE. Scleritis and peripheral ulcerative keratitis. Rheum Dis Clin North Am 2007;33:835–54, vii.
3. Tarabishy AB, Schulte M, Papaliodis GN, et al. Wegener's granulomatosis: clinical manifestations, differential diagnosis, and management of ocular and systemic disease. Surv Ophthalmol 2010;55:429–44.
4. Akpek EK, Thorne JE, Qazi FA, et al. Evaluation of patients with scleritis for systemic disease. Ophthalmology 2004;111:501–16.
5. Galor A, Thorne JE, Jabs DA. Rheumatic disease and scleritis. Ophthalmology 2007;114:1232.
6. Watson PG, Hayreh SS. Scleritis and episcleritis. Br J Ophthalmol 1976;60:163–91.
7. Zaidi AA, Ying GS, Daniel E, et al. Hypopyon in patients with uveitis. Ophthalmology 2010;117:366–72.
8. Rothova A, van Veenedaal WG, Linssen A, et al. Clinical features of acute anterior uveitis. Am J Ophthalmol 1987;103:137–45.
9. Weinstein RS. Clinical practice. Glucocorticoid-induced bone disease. N Engl J Med 2011;365:62–70.
10. Kempen JH, Daniel E, Dunn JP, et al. Overall and cancer related mortality among patients with ocular inflammation treated with immunosuppressive drugs: retrospective cohort study. BMJ 2009;339:b2480.
11. Symmons D, Turner G, Webb R, et al. The prevalence of rheumatoid arthritis in the United Kingdom: new estimates for a new century. Rheumatology (Oxford) 2002;41:793–800.

12. Gabriel SE, Crowson CS, O'Fallon WM. The epidemiology of rheumatoid arthritis in Rochester, Minnesota, 1955–1985. Arthritis Rheum 1999;42: 415–20.
13. Gabriel SE. The epidemiology of rheumatoid arthritis. Rheum Dis Clin North Am 2001;27:269–81.
14. Sugiyama D, Nishimura K, Tamaki K, et al. Impact of smoking as a risk factor for developing rheumatoid arthritis: a meta-analysis of observational studies. Ann Rheum Dis 2010;69:70–81.
15. Majithia V, Geraci SA. Rheumatoid arthritis: diagnosis and management. Am J Med 2007;120:936–9.
16. Turesson C, O'Fallon WM, Crowson CS, et al. Extra-articular disease manifestations in rheumatoid arthritis: incidence trends and risk factors over 46 years. Ann Rheum Dis 2003;62:722–7.
17. Avina-Zubieta JA, Choi HK, Sadatsafavi M, et al. Risk of cardiovascular mortality in patients with rheumatoid arthritis: a meta-analysis of observational studies. Arthritis Rheum 2008;59:1690–7.
18. Schreiber J, Koschel D, Kekow J, et al. Rheumatoid pneumoconiosis (Caplan's syndrome). Eur J Intern Med 2010;21:168–72.
19. Balint GP, Balint PV. Felty's syndrome. Best Pract Res Clin Rheumatol 2004;18:631–45.
20. Bartels CM, Bridges AJ. Rheumatoid vasculitis: vanishing menace or target for new treatments? Curr Rheumatol Rep 2010;12:414–19.
21. Aletaha D, Neogi T, Silman AJ, et al. 2010 Rheumatoid arthritis classification criteria: an American College of Rheumatology/European League Against Rheumatism collaborative initiative. Arthritis Rheum 2010;62:2569–81.
22. Akpek EK, Uy HS, Christen W, et al. Severity of episcleritis and systemic disease association. Ophthalmology 1999;106:729–31.
23. Foster CS, Forstot SL, Wilson LA. Mortality rate in rheumatoid arthritis patients developing necrotizing scleritis or peripheral ulcerative keratitis. Effects of systemic immunosuppression. Ophthalmology 1984;91:1253–63.
24. Giordano N, D'Ettorre M, Biasi G, et al. Retinal vasculitis in rheumatoid arthritis: an angiographic study. Clin Exp Rheumatol 1990;8:121–5.
25. Martin MF, Scott DG, Gilbert C, et al. Retinal vasculitis in rheumatoid arthritis. Br Med J Clin Res Ed 1981;282:1745–6.
26. Matsuo T, Koyama T, Morimoto N, et al. Retinal vasculitis as a complication of rheumatoid arthritis. Ophthalmologica 1990;201:196–200.
27. Saag KG, Teng GG, Patkar NM, et al. American College of Rheumatology 2008 recommendations for the use of nonbiologic and biologic disease-modifying antirheumatic drugs in rheumatoid arthritis. Arthritis Rheum 2008;59: 762–84.
28. Maxwell L, Singh JA. Abatacept for rheumatoid arthritis. Cochrane Database Syst Rev 2009;CD007277.
29. Management and therapy of dry eye disease: report of the Management and Therapy Subcommittee of the International Dry Eye WorkShop (2007). Ocul Surf 2007;5:163–78.
30. Dougados M, van der Linden S, Juhlin R, et al. The European Spondylarthropathy Study Group preliminary criteria for the classification of spondylarthropathy. Arthritis Rheum 1991;34:1218–27.
31. Zeboulon N, Dougados M, Gossec L. Prevalence and characteristics of uveitis in the spondyloarthropathies: a systematic literature review. Ann Rheum Dis 2008;67:955–9.
32. Rudwaleit M, Taylor WJ. Classification criteria for psoriatic arthritis and ankylosing spondylitis/axial spondyloarthritis. Best Pract Res Clin Rheumatol 2010;24:589–604.
33. Gabriel SE, Michaud K. Epidemiological studies in incidence, prevalence, mortality, and comorbidity of the rheumatic diseases. Arthritis Res Ther 2009;11:229.
34. Lee W, Reveille JD, Davis Jr JC, et al. Are there gender differences in severity of ankylosing spondylitis? Results from the PSOAS cohort. Ann Rheum Dis 2007;66:633–8.
35. van der Heijde D, Lie E, Kvien TK, et al. ASDAS, a highly discriminatory ASAS-endorsed disease activity score in patients with ankylosing spondylitis. Ann Rheum Dis 2009;68:1811–18.
36. Zochling J, van der Heijde D, Burgos-Vargas R, et al. ASAS/EULAR recommendations for the management of ankylosing spondylitis. Ann Rheum Dis 2006;65:442–52.
37. Amor B, Dougados M, Listrat V, et al. Are classification criteria for spondylarthropathy useful as diagnostic criteria? Rev Rhum Engl Ed 1995;62: 10–5.
38. Rosenbaum JT. Acute anterior uveitis and spondyloarthropathies. Rheum Dis Clin North Am 1992;18:143–51.
39. Linssen A, Dekker-Saeys AJ, Dijkstra PF, et al. The use of HLA-B27 as a diagnostic and prognostic aid in acute anterior uveitis AAU in The Netherlands. Doc Ophthalmol 1986;64:217–23.
40. Tay-Kearney ML, Schwam BL, Lowder C, et al. Clinical features and associated systemic diseases of HLA-B27 uveitis. Am J Ophthalmol 1996;121: 47–56.
41. Dougados M, Dijkmans B, Khan M, et al. Conventional treatments for ankylosing spondylitis. Ann Rheum Dis 2002;61(Suppl 3):iii40–50.
42. van der Heijde D, Baraf HS, Ramos-Remus C, et al. Evaluation of the efficacy of etoricoxib in ankylosing spondylitis: results of a fifty-two-week, randomized, controlled study. Arthritis Rheum 2005;52:1205–15.
43. Clegg DO, Reda DJ, Abdellatif M. Comparison of sulfasalazine and placebo for the treatment of axial and peripheral articular manifestations of the seronegative spondylarthropathies: a Department of Veterans Affairs cooperative study. Arthritis Rheum 1999;42:2325–9.
44. Roychowdhury B, Bintley-Bagot S, Bulgen DY, et al. Is methotrexate effective in ankylosing spondylitis? Rheumatology (Oxford) 2002;41:1330–2.
45. Rudwaleit M, Rodevand E, Holck P, et al. Adalimumab effectively reduces the rate of anterior uveitis flares in patients with active ankylosing spondylitis: results of a prospective open-label study. Ann Rheum Dis 2009;68:696–701.
46. Braun J, Baraliakos X, Listing J, Sieper J. Decreased incidence of anterior uveitis in patients with ankylosing spondylitis treated with the anti-tumor necrosis factor agents infliximab and etanercept. Arthritis Rheum 2005;52: 2447–51.
47. Soderlin MK, Kautiainen H, Puolakkainen M, et al. Infections preceding early arthritis in southern Sweden: a prospective population-based study. J Rheumatol 2003;30:459–64.
48. Lee DA, Barker SM, Su WP, et al. The clinical diagnosis of Reiter's syndrome. Ophthalmic and nonophthalmic aspects. Ophthalmology 1986;93:350–6.
49. Saari KM, Kauranen O. Ocular inflammation in Reiter's syndrome associated with *Campylobacter jejuni* enteritis. Am J Ophthalmol 1980;90:572–3.
50. Saari KM, Vilppula A, Lassus A, et al. Ocular inflammation in Reiter's disease after *Salmonella* enteritis. Am J Ophthalmol 1980;90:63–8.
51. Needham AD, Harding SP, Carey P. Bilateral multifocal choroiditis in Reiter syndrome. Arch Ophthalmol 1997;115:684–5.
52. Conway RM, Graham SL, Lassere M. Incomplete Reiter's syndrome with focal involvement of the posterior segment. Aust N Z J Ophthalmol 1995;23:63–6.
53. Rosenbaum JT. Characterization of uveitis associated with spondyloarthritis. J Rheumatol 1989;16:792–6.
54. Leirisalo-Repo M. Reactive arthritis. Scand J Rheumatol 2005;34:251–9.
55. Rothfuss KS, Stange EF, Herrlinger KR. Extraintestinal manifestations and complications in inflammatory bowel diseases. World J Gastroenterol 2006; 12:4819–31.
56. Rodriguez-Reyna TS, Martinez-Reyes C, Yamamoto-Furusho JK. Rheumatic manifestations of inflammatory bowel disease. World J Gastroenterol 2009;15:5517–24.
57. Hopkins DJ, Horan E, Burton IL, et al. Ocular disorders in a series of 332 patients with Crohn's disease. Br J Ophthalmol 1974;58:732–7.
58. Greenstein AJ, Janowitz HD, Sachar DB. The extra-intestinal complications of Crohn's disease and ulcerative colitis: a study of 700 patients. Medicine (Baltimore) 1976;55:401–12.
59. Lyons JL, Rosenbaum JT. Uveitis associated with inflammatory bowel disease compared with uveitis associated with spondyloarthropathy. Arch Ophthalmol 1997;115:61–4.
60. Ghanchi FD, Rembacken BJ. Inflammatory bowel disease and the eye. Surv Ophthalmol 2003;48:663–76.
61. Cury DB, Moss AC. Ocular manifestations in a community-based cohort of patients with inflammatory bowel disease. Inflamm Bowel Dis 2010;16: 1393–6.
62. Lin P, Tessler HH, Goldstein DA. Family history of inflammatory bowel disease in patients with idiopathic ocular inflammation. Am J Ophthalmol 2006;141:1097–104.
63. Soukiasian SH, Foster CS, Raizman MB. Treatment strategies for scleritis and uveitis associated with inflammatory bowel disease. Am J Ophthalmol 1994;118:601–11.
64. Taylor W, Gladman D, Helliwell P, et al. Classification criteria for psoriatic arthritis: development of new criteria from a large international study. Arthritis Rheum 2006;54:2665–73.
65. Shbeeb M, Uramoto KM, Gibson LE, et al. The epidemiology of psoriatic arthritis in Olmsted County, Minnesota, USA, 1982–1991. J Rheumatol 2000;27:1247–50.
66. Ibrahim G, Waxman R, Helliwell PS. The prevalence of psoriatic arthritis in people with psoriasis. Arthritis Rheum 2009;61:1373–8.
67. Jenkinson T, Armas J, Evison G, et al. The cervical spine in psoriatic arthritis: a clinical and radiological study. Br J Rheumatol 1994;33:255–9.
68. van Romunde LK, Cats A, Hermans J, et al. Psoriasis and arthritis. II. A cross-sectional comparative study of patients with "psoriatic arthritis" and seronegative and seropositive polyarthritis: clinical aspects. Rheumatol Int 1984;4: 61–5.
69. Rehal B, Modjtahedi BS, Morse LS, et al. Ocular psoriasis. J Am Acad Dermatol 2011;65:1202–12.
70. Lambert JR, Wright V. Eye inflammation in psoriatic arthritis. Ann Rheum Dis 1976;35:354–6.
71. Paiva ES, Macaluso DC, Edwards A, et al. Characterisation of uveitis in patients with psoriatic arthritis. Ann Rheum Dis 2000;59:67–70.
72. Nash P, Clegg DO. Psoriatic arthritis therapy: NSAIDs and traditional DMARDs. Ann Rheum Dis 2005;64(Suppl 2):ii74–7.
73. Mease PJ. Psoriatic arthritis: update on pathophysiology, assessment and management. Ann Rheum Dis 2011;70(Suppl 1):i77–i84.
74. Current status of oral PUVA therapy for psoriasis. Eye protection revisions. J Am Acad Dermatol 1982;6:851–5.
75. Saurenmann RK, Rose JB, Tyrrell P, et al. Epidemiology of juvenile idiopathic arthritis in a multiethnic cohort: ethnicity as a risk factor. Arthritis Rheum 2007;56:1974–84.
76. Petty RE, Southwood TR, Manners P, et al. International League of Associations for Rheumatology classification of juvenile idiopathic arthritis: second revision, Edmonton, 2001. J Rheumatol 2004;31:390–2.
77. BenEzra D, Cohen E, Behar-Cohen F. Uveitis and juvenile idiopathic arthritis: a cohort study. Clin Ophthalmol 2007;1:513–18.
78. Berk AT, Kocak N, Unsal E. Uveitis in juvenile arthritis. Ocul Immunol Inflamm 2001;9:243–51.
79. Boone MI, Moore TL, Cruz OA. Screening for uveitis in juvenile rheumatoid arthritis. J Pediatr Ophthalmol Strabismus 1998;35:41–3.
80. Chylack Jr LT. The ocular manifestations of juvenile rheumatoid arthritis. Arthritis Rheum 1977;20:217–23.

81. Saurenmann RK, Levin AV, Feldman BM, et al. Prevalence, risk factors, and outcome of uveitis in juvenile idiopathic arthritis: a long-term followup study. Arthritis Rheum 2007;56:647–57.
82. Saurenmann RK, Levin AV, Feldman BM, et al. Risk factors for development of uveitis differ between girls and boys with juvenile idiopathic arthritis. Arthritis Rheum 2010;62:1824–8.
83. Nordal EB, Songstad NT, Berntson L, et al. Biomarkers of chronic uveitis in juvenile idiopathic arthritis: predictive value of antihistone antibodies and antinuclear antibodies. J Rheumatol 2009;36:1737–43.
84. Cassidy J, Kivlin J, Lindsley C, et al. Ophthalmologic examinations in children with juvenile rheumatoid arthritis. Pediatrics 2006;117:1843–5.
85. Ayuso VK, Ten Cate HA, van der Does P, et al. Male gender and poor visual outcome in uveitis associated with juvenile idiopathic arthritis. Am J Ophthalmol 2010;149:987–93.
86. Kalinina AV, Ten Cate HA, van der Does P, et al. Male gender as a risk factor for complications in uveitis associated with juvenile idiopathic arthritis. Am J Ophthalmol 2010;149:994–9.
87. Christoph T, Carsten H, Martin R, et al. Elevated laser flare values correlate with complicated course of anterior uveitis in patients with juvenile idiopathic arthritis. Acta Ophthalmol 2011;896:e521–e527.
88. Key III SN, Kimura SJ. Iridocyclitis associated with juvenile rheumatoid arthritis. Am J Ophthalmol 1975;80:425–9.
89. Rosenberg AM, Oen KG. The relationship between ocular and articular disease activity in children with juvenile rheumatoid arthritis and associated uveitis. Arthritis Rheum 1986;29:797–800.
90. Beukelman T, Guevara JP, Albert DA. Optimal treatment of knee monarthritis in juvenile idiopathic arthritis: a decision analysis. Arthritis Rheum 2008; 59:1580–8.
91. Prakken B, Albani S, Martini A. Juvenile idiopathic arthritis. Lancet 2011;377:2138–49.
92. Giannini EH, Ilowite NT, Lovell DJ, et al. Long-term safety and effectiveness of etanercept in children with selected categories of juvenile idiopathic arthritis. Arthritis Rheum 2009;60:2794–804.
93. Lovell DJ, Giannini EH, Reiff A, et al. Etanercept in children with polyarticular juvenile rheumatoid arthritis. Pediatric Rheumatology Collaborative Study Group. N Engl J Med 2000;342:763–9.
94. Ruperto N, Lovell DJ, Cuttica R, et al. A randomized, placebo-controlled trial of infliximab plus methotrexate for the treatment of polyarticular-course juvenile rheumatoid arthritis. Arthritis Rheum 2007;56:3096–106.
95. Lovell DJ, Ruperto N, Goodman S, et al. Adalimumab with or without methotrexate in juvenile rheumatoid arthritis. N Engl J Med 2008;359:810–20.
96. Ruperto N, Lovell DJ, Quartier P, et al. Long-term safety and efficacy of abatacept in children with juvenile idiopathic arthritis. Arthritis Rheum 2010;62:1792–802.
97. Ruperto N, Lovell DJ, Quartier P, et al. Abatacept in children with juvenile idiopathic arthritis: a randomised, double-blind, placebo-controlled withdrawal trial. Lancet 2008;372:383–91.
98. Diak P, Siegel J, La GL, et al. Tumor necrosis factor alpha blockers and malignancy in children: forty-eight cases reported to the Food and Drug Administration. Arthritis Rheum 2010;62:2517–24.
99. Thorne JE, Woreta FA, Dunn JP, et al. Risk of cataract development among children with juvenile idiopathic arthritis-related uveitis treated with topical corticosteroids. Ophthalmology 2010;117:1436–41.
100. Biester S, Deuter C, Michels H, et al. Adalimumab in the therapy of uveitis in childhood. Br J Ophthalmol 2007;91:319–24.
101. Lim LL, Fraunfelder FW, Rosenbaum JT. Do tumor necrosis factor inhibitors cause uveitis? A registry-based study. Arthritis Rheum 2007;56:3248–52.
102. Quinones K, Cervantes-Castaneda RA, Hynes AY, et al. Outcomes of cataract surgery in children with chronic uveitis. J Cataract Refract Surg 2009;35: 725–31.
103. Grajewski RS, Zurek-Imhoff B, Roesel M, et al. Favourable outcome after cataract surgery with IOL implantation in uveitis associated with juvenile idiopathic arthritis. Acta Ophthalmol ePub 11 February, 2011;doi: 10.1111/j. 1755-3768.2011.02110.x.
104. Kotaniemi K, Penttila H. Intraocular lens implantation in patients with juvenile idiopathic arthritis-associated uveitis. Ophthalmic Res 2006;38:318–23.
105. Hochberg MC. Updating the American College of Rheumatology revised criteria for the classification of systemic lupus erythematosus. Arthritis Rheum 1997;40:1725.
106. Smith PP, Gordon C. Systemic lupus erythematosus: clinical presentations. Autoimmun Rev 2010;10:43–5.
107. Alarcon GS, Friedman AW, Straaton KV, et al. Systemic lupus erythematosus in three ethnic groups: III. A comparison of characteristics early in the natural history of the LUMINA cohort. LUpus in MInority populations: NAture vs Nurture. Lupus 1999;8:197–209.
108. Weening JJ, D'Agati VD, Schwartz MM, et al. The classification of glomerulonephritis in systemic lupus erythematosus revisited. Kidney Int 2004;65: 521–30.
109. Sultan SM, Ioannou Y, Isenberg DA. A review of gastrointestinal manifestations of systemic lupus erythematosus. Rheumatology (Oxford) 1999;38: 917–32.
110. Sivaraj RR, Durrani OM, Denniston AK, et al. Ocular manifestations of systemic lupus erythematosus. Rheumatology (Oxford) 2007;46:1757–62.
111. Jensen JL, Bergem HO, Gilboe IM, et al. Oral and ocular sicca symptoms and findings are prevalent in systemic lupus erythematosus. J Oral Pathol Med 1999;28:317–22.
112. Read RW. Clinical mini-review: systemic lupus erythematosus and the eye. Ocul Immunol Inflamm 2004;12:87–99.
113. Lachmann SM, Hazleman BL, Watson PG. Scleritis and associated disease. Br Med J 1978;1:88–90.
114. Stavrou P, Murray PI, Batta K, et al. Acute ocular ischaemia and orbital inflammation associated with systemic lupus erythematosus. Br J Ophthalmol 2002;86:474–5.
115. Grimson BS, Simons KB. Orbital inflammation, myositis, and systemic lupus erythematosus. Arch Ophthalmol 1983;101:736–8.
116. Ushiyama O, Ushiyama K, Koarada S, et al. Retinal disease in patients with systemic lupus erythematosus. Ann Rheum Dis 2000;59:705–8.
117. Coppeto JR. Retinopathy and systemic lupus erythematosus. Arch Ophthalmol 1984;102:1748–9.
118. Jabs DA, Fine SL, Hochberg MC, et al. Severe retinal vaso-occlusive disease in systemic lupus erythematous. Arch Ophthalmol 1986;104:558–63.
119. Asherson RA, Merry P, Acheson JF, et al. Antiphospholipid antibodies: a risk factor for occlusive ocular vascular disease in systemic lupus erythematosus and the "primary" antiphospholipid syndrome. Ann Rheum Dis 1989;48: 358–61.
120. Graham EM, Spalton DJ, Barnard RO, et al. Cerebral and retinal vascular changes in systemic lupus erythematosus. Ophthalmology 1985;92:444–8.
121. Sekimoto M, Hayasaka S, Noda S, et al. Pseudoretinitis pigmentosa in patients with systemic lupus erythematosus. Ann Ophthalmol 1993;25:264–6.
122. Jabs DA, Hanneken AM, Schachat AP, et al. Choroidopathy in systemic lupus erythematosus. Arch Ophthalmol 1988;106:230–4.
123. Jabs DA, Miller NR, Newman SA, et al. Optic neuropathy in systemic lupus erythematosus. Arch Ophthalmol 1986;104:564–8.
124. Wang JC, Chuah GC, Yap EY. Tuberculous choroidal granulomas in a patient with systemic lupus erythematosus. A case report. Int Ophthalmol 2001;24: 107–9.
125. Ishibashi Y, Watanabe R, Hommura S, et al. Endogenous *Nocardia asteroides* endophthalmitis in a patient with systemic lupus erythematosus. Br J Ophthalmol 1990;74:433–6.
126. Favas C, Isenberg DA. B-cell-depletion therapy in SLE – what are the current prospects for its acceptance? Nat Rev Rheumatol 2009;5:711–16.
127. Turner-Stokes T, Lu TY, Ehrenstein MR, et al. The efficacy of repeated treatment with B-cell depletion therapy in systemic lupus erythematosus: an evaluation. Rheumatology (Oxford) 2011.
128. Lightstone L. Lupus nephritis: where are we now? Curr Opin Rheumatol 2010;22:252–6.
129. Pillemer SR, Matteson EL, Jacobsson LT, et al. Incidence of physician-diagnosed primary Sjögren syndrome in residents of Olmsted County, Minnesota. Mayo Clin Proc 2001;76:593–9.
130. Fox RI. Sjögren's syndrome. Lancet 2005;366:321–31.
131. Mavragani CP, Moutsopoulos NM, Moutsopoulos HM. The management of Sjögren's syndrome. Nat Clin Pract Rheumatol 2006;2:252–61.
132. Rosenbaum JT, Bennett RM. Chronic anterior and posterior uveitis and primary Sjogren's syndrome. Am J Ophthalmol 1987;104:346–52.
133. Ramos-Casals M, Tzioufas AG, Stone JH, et al. Treatment of primary Sjögren syndrome: a systematic review. JAMA 2010;304:452–60.
134. Sall K, Stevenson OD, Mundorf TK, et al. Two multicenter, randomized studies of the efficacy and safety of cyclosporine ophthalmic emulsion in moderate to severe dry eye disease. CsA Phase 3 Study Group. Ophthalmology 2000;107:631–9.
135. Barber LD, Pflugfelder SC, Tauber J, et al. Phase III safety evaluation of cyclosporine 0.1% ophthalmic emulsion administered twice daily to dry eye disease patients for up to 3 years. Ophthalmology 2005;112:1790–4.
136. Rothova A. Ocular involvement in sarcoidosis. Br J Ophthalmol 2000;84: 110–16.
137. Fretzayas A, Moustaki M, Vougiouka O. The puzzling clinical spectrum and course of juvenile sarcoidosis. World J Pediatr 2011;7:103–10.
138. Becker ML, Rose CD. Blau syndrome and related genetic disorders causing childhood arthritis. Curr Rheumatol Rep 2005;7:427–33.
139. Punzi L, Furlan A, Podswiadek M, et al. Clinical and genetic aspects of Blau syndrome: a 25-year follow-up of one family and a literature review. Autoimmun Rev 2009;8:228–32.
140. Dow CT, Ellingson JL. Detection of *Mycobacterium avium ss. paratuberculosis* in Blau syndrome tissues. Autoimmune Dis 2011;2011:127692.
141. James DG. A comparison of Blau's syndrome and sarcoidosis. Sarcoidosis 1994;11:100–1.
142. Geha RS, Notarangelo LD, Casanova JL, et al. Primary immunodeficiency diseases: an update from the International Union of Immunological Societies Primary Immunodeficiency Diseases Classification Committee. J Allergy Clin Immunol 2007;120:776–94.
143. Latkany PA, Jabs DA, Smith JR, et al. Multifocal choroiditis in patients with familial juvenile systemic granulomatosis. Am J Ophthalmol 2002;134: 897–904.
144. Latkany P. Blau syndrome. Ophthalmology 2004;111:853–4.
145. Bernatsky S, Joseph L, Pineau CA, et al. Scleroderma prevalence: demographic variations in a population-based sample. Arthritis Rheum 2009;61:400–4.
146. Mayes MD, Lacey Jr JV, Beebe-Dimmer J, et al. Prevalence, incidence, survival, and disease characteristics of systemic sclerosis in a large US population. Arthritis Rheum 2003;48:2246–55.
147. Chifflot H, Fautrel B, Sordet C, et al. Incidence and prevalence of systemic sclerosis: a systematic literature review. Semin Arthritis Rheum 2008;37: 223–35.
148. Ebert EC. Esophageal disease in progressive systemic sclerosis. Curr Treat Options Gastroenterol 2008;11:64–9.
149. West RH, Barnett AJ. Ocular involvement in scleroderma. Br J Ophthalmol 1979;63:845–7.

150. Horan EC. Ophthalmic manifestations of progressive systemic sclerosis. Br J Ophthalmol 1969;53:388–92.
151. Emre S, Kayikcioglu O, Ates H, et al. Corneal hysteresis, corneal resistance factor, and intraocular pressure measurement in patients with scleroderma using the Reichert ocular response analyzer. Cornea 2010;29:628–31.
152. Serup J, Serup L. Increased central cornea thickness in localized scleroderma morphoea. Metab Pediatr Syst Ophthalmol 1985;8:11–4.
153. Serup L, Serup J, Hagdrup H. Fundus fluorescein angiography in generalized scleroderma. Ophthalmic Res 1987;19:303–8.
154. Tailor R, Gupta A, Herrick A, et al. Ocular manifestations of scleroderma. Surv Ophthalmol 2009;54:292–304.
155. Kowal-Bielecka O, Landewe R, Avouac J, et al. EULAR recommendations for the treatment of systemic sclerosis: a report from the EULAR Scleroderma Trials and Research group EUSTAR. Ann Rheum Dis 2009;68:620–8.
156. Le EN, Wigley FM, Shah AA, et al. Long-term experience of mycophenolate mofetil for treatment of diffuse cutaneous systemic sclerosis. Ann Rheum Dis 2011;70:1104–7.
157. Phumethum V, Jamal S, Johnson SR. Biologic therapy for systemic sclerosis: a systematic review. J Rheumatol 2011;38:289–96.
158. Vonk MC, Marjanovic Z, van den Hoogen FH, et al. Long-term follow-up results after autologous haematopoietic stem cell transplantation for severe systemic sclerosis. Ann Rheum Dis 2008;67:98–104.
159. Bohan A, Peter JB. Polymyositis and dermatomyositis first of two parts. N Engl J Med 1975;292:344–7.
160. Patrick M, Buchbinder R, Jolley D, et al. Incidence of inflammatory myopathies in Victoria, Australia, and evidence of spatial clustering. J Rheumatol 1999;26:1094–100.
161. Mastaglia FL, Phillips BA. Idiopathic inflammatory myopathies: epidemiology, classification, and diagnostic criteria. Rheum Dis Clin North Am 2002;28:723–41.
162. Mastaglia FL, Garlepp MJ, Phillips BA, et al. Inflammatory myopathies: clinical, diagnostic and therapeutic aspects. Muscle Nerve 2003;27:407–25.
163. Hill CL, Zhang Y, Sigurgeirsson B, et al. Frequency of specific cancer types in dermatomyositis and polymyositis: a population-based study. Lancet 2001; 357:96–100.
164. Susac JO, Garcia-Mullin R, Glaser JS. Ophthalmoplegia in dermatomyositis. Neurology 1973;23:305–10.
165. Yeo LM, Swaby DS, Situnayake RD, et al. Irreversible visual loss in dermatomyositis. Br J Rheumatol 1995;34:1179–81.
166. Cohen BH, Sedwick LA, Burde RM. Retinopathy of dermatomyositis. J Clin Neuroophthalmol 1985;5:177–9.
167. Backhouse O, Griffiths B, Henderson T, et al. Ophthalmic manifestations of dermatomyositis. Ann Rheum Dis 1998;57:447–9.
168. McHugh N. Disease management dermatomyositis/polymyositis. Rheumatology (Oxford) 2011;50:12–4.
169. Dalakas MC, Hohlfeld R. Polymyositis and dermatomyositis. Lancet 2003; 362:971–82.
170. Lahmer T, Treiber M, von Werder A, et al. Relapsing polychondritis: an autoimmune disease with many faces. Autoimmun Rev 2010;9:540–6.
171. Balsa A, Expinosa A, Cuesta M, et al. Joint symptoms in relapsing polychondritis. Clin Exp Rheumatol 1995;13:425–30.
172. Isaak BL, Liesegang TJ, Michet Jr CJ. Ocular and systemic findings in relapsing polychondritis. Ophthalmology 1986;93:681–9.
173. Matas BR. Iridocyclitis associated with relapsing polychondritis. Arch Ophthalmol 1970;84:474–6.
174. Messmer EM, Foster CS. Vasculitic peripheral ulcerative keratitis. Surv Ophthalmol 1999;43:379–96.
175. Magargal LE, Donoso LA, Goldberg RE, et al. Ocular manifestations of relapsing polychondritis. Retina 1981;1:96–9.
176. Anderson Sr B. Ocular lesions in relapsing polychondritis and other rheumatoid syndromes. The Edward Jackson memorial lecture. Am J Ophthalmol 1967;64:35–50.
177. McKay DA, Watson PG, Lyne AJ. Relapsing polychondritis and eye disease. Br J Ophthalmol 1974;58:600–5.
178. McCarthy EM, Cunnane G. Treatment of relapsing polychondritis in the era of biological agents. Rheumatol Int 2010;30:827–8.
179. Basu N, Watts R, Bajema I, et al. EULAR points to consider in the development of classification and diagnostic criteria in systemic vasculitis. Ann Rheum Dis 2010;69:1744–50.
180. Watts RA, Suppiah R, Merkel PA, et al. Systemic vasculitis – is it time to reclassify? Rheumatology (Oxford) 2011;50:643–5.
181. Falk RJ, Gross WL, Guillevin L, et al. Granulomatosis with polyangiitis Wegener's: an alternative name for Wegener's granulomatosis. Arthritis Rheum 2011;63:863–4.
182. Jennette JC, Falk RJ, Andrassy K, et al. Nomenclature of systemic vasculitides. Proposal of an international consensus conference. Arthritis Rheum 1994; 37:187–92.
183. Gordon M, Luqmani RA, Adu D, et al. Relapses in patients with a systemic vasculitis. Q J Med 1993;86:779–89.
184. Luqmani RA, Bacon PA, Moots RJ, et al. Birmingham Vasculitis Activity Score (BVAS) in systemic necrotizing vasculitis. QJM 1994;87:671–8.
185. Exley AR, Carruthers DM, Luqmani RA, et al. Damage occurs early in systemic vasculitis and is an index of outcome. QJM 1997;90:391–9.
186. Langford CA, Talar-Williams C, Barron KS, et al. Use of a cyclophosphamide-induction methotrexate-maintenance regimen for the treatment of Wegener's granulomatosis: extended follow-up and rate of relapse. Am J Med 2003;114: 463–9.
187. Adu D, Pall A, Luqmani RA, et al. Controlled trial of pulse versus continuous prednisolone and cyclophosphamide in the treatment of systemic vasculitis. QJM 1997;90:401–9.
188. Morgan MD, Drayson MT, Savage CO, et al. Addition of infliximab to standard therapy for ANCA-associated vasculitis. Nephron Clin Pract 2011;117: c89–c97.
189. Stone JH, Merkel PA, Spiera R, et al. Rituximab versus cyclophosphamide for ANCA-associated vasculitis. N Engl J Med 2010;363:221–32.
190. Hunder GG. Clinical features of GCA/PMR. Clin Exp Rheumatol 2000;18:S6–8.
191. Hayreh SS, Podhajsky PA, Zimmerman B. Ocular manifestations of giant cell arteritis. Am J Ophthalmol 1998;125:509–20.
192. Direskeneli H, Aydin SZ, Kermani, et al. Development of outcome measures for large-vessel vasculitis for use in clinical trials: opportunities, challenges, and research agenda. J Rheumatol 2011;38:1471–9.
193. Watts RA, Scott DG. Epidemiology of the vasculitides. Semin Respir Crit Care Med 2004;25:455–64.
194. Cantini F, Niccoli L, Storri L, et al. Are polymyalgia rheumatica and giant cell arteritis the same disease? Semin Arthritis Rheum 2004;33:294–301.
195. Hunder GG, Bloch DA, Michel BA, et al. The American College of Rheumatology 1990 criteria for the classification of giant cell arteritis. Arthritis Rheum 1990;33:1122–8.
196. Walvick MD, Walvick MP. Giant cell arteritis: laboratory predictors of a positive temporal artery biopsy. Ophthalmology 2011;118:1201–4.
197. Danesh-Meyer H, Savino PJ, Gamble GG. Poor prognosis of visual outcome after visual loss from giant cell arteritis. Ophthalmology 2005;112: 1098–103.
198. Melberg NS, Grand MG, Dieckert JP, et al. Cotton-wool spots and the early diagnosis of giant cell arteritis. Ophthalmology 1995;102:1611–14.
199. Johnson MC, Lee AG. Giant cell arteritis presenting with cotton wool spots. Semin Ophthalmol 2008;23:141–2.
200. Ghosh P, Borg FA, Dasgupta B. Current understanding and management of giant cell arteritis and polymyalgia rheumatica. Expert Rev Clin Immunol 2010;6:913–28.
201. Hoffman GS, Cid MC, Rendt-Zagar KE, et al. Infliximab for maintenance of glucocorticosteroid-induced remission of giant cell arteritis: a randomized trial. Ann Intern Med 2007;146:621–30.
202. Martinez-Taboada VM, Rodriguez-Valverde V, Carreno L, et al. A double-blind placebo controlled trial of etanercept in patients with giant cell arteritis and corticosteroid side effects. Ann Rheum Dis 2008;67:625–30.
203. Bhatia A, Ell PJ, Edwards JC. Anti-CD20 monoclonal antibody (rituximab) as an adjunct in the treatment of giant cell arteritis. Ann Rheum Dis 2005;64: 1099–100.
204. Cong XL, Dai SM, Feng X, et al. Takayasu's arteritis: clinical features and outcomes of 125 patients in China. Clin Rheumatol 2010;29:973–81.
205. Hall S, Barr W, Lie JT, et al. Takayasu arteritis. A study of 32 North American patients. Medicine (Baltimore) 1985;64:89–99.
206. Nasu T. Takayasu's truncoarteritis in Japan. A statistical observation of 76 autopsy cases. Pathol Microbiol (Basel) 1975;43:140–6.
207. Arend WP, Michel BA, Bloch DA, et al. The American College of Rheumatology 1990 criteria for the classification of Takayasu arteritis. Arthritis Rheum 1990;33:1129–34.
208. Chun YS, Park SJ, Park IK, et al. The clinical and ocular manifestations of Takayasu arteritis. Retina 2001;21:132–40.
209. Peter J, David S, Danda D, et al. Ocular manifestations of Takayasu arteritis: a cross-sectional study. Retina 2011;31:1170–8.
210. Mukhtyar C, Guillevin L, Cid MC, et al. EULAR recommendations for the management of large vessel vasculitis. Ann Rheum Dis 2009;68:318–23.
211. Park MC, Lee SW, Park YB, et al. Clinical characteristics and outcomes of Takayasu's arteritis: analysis of 108 patients using standardized criteria for diagnosis, activity assessment, and angiographic classification. Scand J Rheumatol 2005;34:284–92.
212. Valsakumar AK, Valappil UC, Jorapur V, et al. Role of immunosuppressive therapy on clinical, immunological, and angiographic outcome in active Takayasu's arteritis. J Rheumatol 2003;30:1793–8.
213. Pettigrew HD, Teuber SS, Gershwin ME. Polyarteritis nodosa. Compr Ther 2007;33:144–9.
214. Dillon MJ, Eleftheriou D, Brogan PA. Medium-size-vessel vasculitis. Pediatr Nephrol 2010;25:1641–52.
215. Kluger N, Pagnoux C, Guillevin L, et al. Comparison of cutaneous manifestations in systemic polyarteritis nodosa and microscopic polyangiitis. Br J Dermatol 2008;159:615–20.
216. Blodi FC, Sullivan PB. Involvement of the eyes in periarteritis nodosa. Trans Am Acad Ophthalmol Otolaryngol 1959;63:161–5.
217. Moore JG, Sevel D. Corneo-scleral ulceration in periarteritis nodosa. Br J Ophthalmol 1966;50:651–5.
218. Yamamoto S, Takeuchi S. Episcleritis as the primary clinical manifestation in a patient with polyarteritis nodosa. Jpn J Ophthalmol 2000;44:151–3.
219. Mukhtyar C, Guillevin L, Cid MC, et al. EULAR recommendations for the management of primary small and medium vessel vasculitis. Ann Rheum Dis 2009;68:310–7.
220. Gayraud M, Guillevin L, le TP, et al. Long-term followup of polyarteritis nodosa, microscopic polyangiitis, and Churg–Strauss syndrome: analysis of four prospective trials including 278 patients. Arthritis Rheum 2001;44: 666–75.
221. Nakamura Y, Yashiro M, Uehara R, et al. Epidemiologic features of Kawasaki disease in Japan: results of the 2007–2008 nationwide survey. J Epidemiol 2010;20:302–7.

222. Gedalia A, Cuchacovich R. Systemic vasculitis in childhood. Curr Rheumatol Rep 2009;11:402–9.
223. Gedalia A. Kawasaki disease: an update. Curr Rheumatol Rep 2002;4:25–9.
224. Ohno S, Miyajima T, Higuchi M, et al. Ocular manifestations of Kawasaki's disease (mucocutaneous lymph node syndrome). Am J Ophthalmol 1982; 93:713–17.
225. Farvardin M, Kashef S, Aleyasin S, et al. Sudden unilateral blindness in a girl with Kawasaki disease. J Pediatr Ophthalmol Strabismus 2007;44:303–4.
226. Ogata S, Bando Y, Kimura S, et al. The strategy of immune globulin resistant Kawasaki disease: a comparative study of additional immune globulin and steroid pulse therapy. J Cardiol 2009;53:15–9.
227. Imagawa T, Mori M, Miyamae T, et al. Plasma exchange for refractory Kawasaki disease. Eur J Pediatr 2004;163:263–4.
228. Sundel RP, Burns JC, Baker A, et al. Gamma globulin re-treatment in Kawasaki disease. J Pediatr 1993;123:657–9.
229. Sundel RP, Baker AL, Fulton DR, et al. Corticosteroids in the initial treatment of Kawasaki disease: report of a randomized trial. J Pediatr 2003;142:611–16.
230. Schilder AM. Wegener's granulomatosis vasculitis and granuloma. Autoimmun Rev 2010;9:483–7.
231. Ntatsaki E, Watts RA, Scott DG. Epidemiology of ANCA-associated vasculitis. Rheum Dis Clin North Am 2010;36:447–61.
232. Mahr AD, Neogi T, Merkel PA. Epidemiology of Wegener's granulomatosis: lessons from descriptive studies and analyses of genetic and environmental risk determinants. Clin Exp Rheumatol 2006;24:S82–91.
233. Rao NV, Wehner NG, Marshall BC, et al. Characterization of proteinase-3 PR-3, a neutrophil serine proteinase. Structural and functional properties. J Biol Chem 1991;266:9540–8.
234. Talar-Williams C, Sneller MC, Langford CA, et al. Orbital socket contracture: a complication of inflammatory orbital disease in patients with Wegener's granulomatosis. Br J Ophthalmol 2005;89:493–7.
235. Robinson MR, Lee SS, Sneller MC, et al. Tarsal-conjunctival disease associated with Wegener's granulomatosis. Ophthalmology 2003;110:1770–80.
236. Tanihara H, Nakayama Y, Honda Y. Wegener's granulomatosis with rapidly progressive retinitis and anterior uveitis. Acta Ophthalmol (Copenh) 1993; 71:853–5.
237. Huong du LT, Tran TH, Piette JC. Granulomatous uveitis revealing Wegener's granulomatosis. J Rheumatol 2006;33:1209–10.
238. Watkins AS, Kempen JH, Choi D, et al. Ocular disease in patients with ANCA-positive vasculitis. J Ocul Biol Dis Infor 2009;3:12–9.
239. Lapraik C, Watts R, Bacon P, et al. BSR and BHPR guidelines for the management of adults with ANCA associated vasculitis. Rheumatology (Oxford) 2007;46:1615–16.
240. Booth A, Harper L, Hammad T, et al. Prospective study of TNFalpha blockade with infliximab in anti-neutrophil cytoplasmic antibody-associated systemic vasculitis. J Am Soc Nephrol 2004;15:717–21.
241. Taylor SR, Salama AD, Joshi L, et al. Rituximab is effective in the treatment of refractory ophthalmic Wegener's granulomatosis. Arthritis Rheum 2009; 60:1540–7.
242. Guillevin L, Durand-Gasselin B, Cevallos R, et al. Microscopic polyangiitis: clinical and laboratory findings in eighty-five patients. Arthritis Rheum 1999;42:421–30.
243. Lhote F, Cohen P, Genereau T, et al. Microscopic polyangiitis: clinical aspects and treatment. Ann Med Interne (Paris) 1996;147:165–77.
244. Hara A, Ohta S, Takata M, et al. Microscopic polyangiitis with ocular manifestations as the initial presenting sign. Am J Med Sci 2007;334: 308–10.
245. Gallagher MJ, Ooi KG, Thomas M, et al. ANCA associated pauci-immune retinal vasculitis. Br J Ophthalmol 2005;89:608–11.
246. Walsh M, Jayne D. Rituximab in the treatment of anti-neutrophil cytoplasm antibody associated vasculitis and systemic lupus erythematosus: past, present and future. Kidney Int 2007;72:676–82.
247. Noth I, Strek ME, Leff AR. Churg–Strauss syndrome. Lancet 2003;361: 587–94.
248. Guillevin L, Cohen P, Gayraud M, et al. Churg–Strauss syndrome. Clinical study and long-term follow-up of 96 patients. Medicine (Baltimore) 1999;78: 26–37.
249. Masi AT, Hunder GG, Lie JT, et al. The American College of Rheumatology 1990 criteria for the classification of Churg–Strauss syndrome (allergic granulomatosis and angiitis). Arthritis Rheum 1990;33:1094–100.
250. Margolis R, Kosmorsky GS, Lowder CY, et al. Conjunctival involvement in Churg–Strauss syndrome. Ocul Immunol Inflamm 2007;15:113–5.
251. Takanashi T, Uchida S, Arita M, et al. Orbital inflammatory pseudotumor and ischemic vasculitis in Churg–Strauss syndrome: report of two cases and review of the literature. Ophthalmology 2001;108:1129–33.
252. Weinstein JM, Chui H, Lane S, et al. Churg–Strauss syndrome (allergic granulomatous angiitis). Neuro-ophthalmologic manifestations. Arch Ophthalmol 1983;101:1217–20.
253. Pepper RJ, Fabre MA, Pavesio C, et al. Rituximab is effective in the treatment of refractory Churg–Strauss syndrome and is associated with diminished T-cell interleukin-5 production. Rheumatology (Oxford) 2008;47:1104–5.
254. West SK, Valmadrid CT. Epidemiology of risk factors for age-related cataract. Surv Ophthalmol 1995;39:323–34.
255. Clark AF, Wordinger RJ. The role of steroids in outflow resistance. Exp Eye Res 2009;88:752–9.
256. Hobbs HE, Sorsby A, Freedman A. Retinopathy following chloroquine therapy. Lancet 1959;2:478–80.
257. Lee AG. Hydroxychloroquine screening. Br J Ophthalmol 2005;89:521–2.
258. Marmor MF, Kellner U, Lai TY, et al. Revised recommendations on screening for chloroquine and hydroxychloroquine retinopathy. Ophthalmology 2011; 118:415–22.

Chapter 81

HIV-Associated Infections

Igor Kozak, J. Allen McCutchan, William R. Freeman

Acquired immunodeficiency syndrome (AIDS) is a potentially fatal multisystem syndrome characterized by profound disruption of the immune system and a propensity for various opportunistic infections and neoplasms. AIDS is caused by either of two human immunodeficiency viruses (HIV-1 [formerly HTLV-3] or HIV-2).[1–3] HIV-1 entered humans from chimpanzees nearly a century ago and, after passing unrecognized among West Africans,[4,5] came to the United States via Haiti in the 1970s. AIDS was recognized first in 1981 as outbreaks of usual opportunistic infections (OIs) in homosexual men in three American cities.

Ocular involvement occurs in up to 73% of AIDS patients,[6,7] with the most common lesions being a retinal vasculopathy consisting of cotton-wool spots, retinal hemorrhages, and infectious retinopathy such as cytomegalovirus (CMV), herpetic, toxoplasmic, or luetic retinitis.

EPIDEMIOLOGY OF HIV INFECTION AND AIDS

By 2010 an estimated 1.1 million people were living with HIV in the United States, approximately 56 000 new HIV infections have occurred annually for more than a decade, and about 15 000 patients die annually. This difference between incidence and mortality increases the prevalence of HIV infection by about 40 000 persons annually. Since 1996 AIDS has been converted from an inevitably progressive and fatal disease into a manageable chronic condition by three-drug regimens referred to as highly active or combination antiretroviral therapy (HAART or CART). HIV is spread by homo- and heterosexual intercourse, blood exposures through shared needles among intravenous drug users, or peripartum or by breast feeding of infants.[8–11]

OCCUPATIONAL EXPOSURE TO HIV

The average risk of HIV transmission in healthcare workers after percutaneous exposure to HIV-infected blood is approximately 0.3% without treatment.[12,13] This risk is further lowered by double-gloving and is probably much lower in the ophthalmic setting.[14] Postexposure prophylaxis (PEP) with two or three antiretroviral drugs appears likely to dramatically reduce the transmission of HIV even after high-risk injuries.[15] Because PEP should be started as soon as possible after injury, healthcare institutions should have well-developed procedures that provide for expert consultation and ready access to a combination of drugs for persons at high risk of injuries, such as surgeons, invasive proceduralists, and phlebotomists.

Currently, for percutaneous injuries, the US Public Health Service recommends 4 weeks of treatment with a two-drug regimen if the exposure is less severe (solid needle and superficial injury) and the source patient has asymptomatic HIV infection or known low viral load (<1500 RNA copies/ml) [class I patient]. An expanded three-drug regimen is recommended if the exposure is severe (large-bore hollow needle, deep puncture, visible blood on device, or needle used in patient's artery or vein) or if the source patient has symptomatic HIV infection, AIDS, acute seroconversion, or known high viral load [class II patient]. The recommended two-drug regimens for HIV/PEP are: (a) tenofavir plus emtricitabine or (b) zidovudine plus lamivudine. Tenofovir is generally better tolerated, but should not be used in persons with renal insufficiency. Three-drug regimens involve adding ritonavir-boosted (/r) lopinavir/r or darunavir/r. Alternatives for constructing an expanded regimen in cases of resistance, drug interactions, or intolerance include darunavir/r, atazanavir/r, or raltegravir. For mucous membrane or nonintact skin exposures, the two-drug regimen is recommended for all small volume exposures (a few drops) and large volume (major blood splash) exposure in a class I patient, with three-drug expanded regimens recommended for large volume exposure in a class II patient.[13]

HIV VIROLOGY AND PATHOGENESIS

HIV infection usually gradually depletes CD4 lymphocytes, resulting in decreased blood levels of this crucial subset of "helper" T cells.[16] AIDS patients typically become ill only after CD4+ helper T cells reach less than 200/ml, a level that no longer supports cell-mediated immunity at levels needed to contain infections by select opportunistic viral, bacterial, or fungal pathogens.

Understanding of HIV infection was revolutionized by the development in the mid-1990s of assays that measured the levels of HIV in the blood. All stages of HIV infection were seen to be characterized by a high rate of viral replication in most patients. Levels of plasma HIV-1 RNA predict the rate of clinical progression in HIV patients.[17–23] Both high replication and an error-prone reverse transcription process promote frequent mutations in the HIV genome that result in the emergence of variants that can better resist either control by the hosts antibody and cell-mediated immune responses or by antiretroviral drugs, if drugs are present in insufficient numbers or at low blood levels that fail to fully suppress HIV replication. Under selective pressure from antiretroviral agents, mutations that confer a decreased sensitivity to individual drugs are selected and stored in latent cells where they last for decades.[24–27]

THERAPY OF HIV INFECTIONS

Treatment of HIV has evolved rapidly over the past 25 years (1986–2011) with the development of more than 30 drugs that fall into at least four classes based on which of the steps in HIV replication they inhibit. These steps include: (a) binding to receptors and entry into the host cell; (b) reverse transcription of HIV RNA to proviral DNA; (c) integration of proviral DNA into the host cell genome; and (d) maturation of HIV after budding by the action of HIV protease.[28] Coadministration of drugs from several of the classes delays or prevents the emergence of drug-resistant HIV by minimizing viral replication. However, HIV may develop resistance to all available therapy because (a) patients have difficulty maintaining high levels of adherence over long periods and (b) cross-resistance is common to drugs within a class.[29-32] After failure of a regimen, the next combination of drugs is less likely to be successful in fully suppressing HIV replication which is the necessary condition for prolonged success. For details of recent expert guidelines on HIV therapy consult Guidelines for the Use of Antiretroviral Agents in HIV-1-Infected Adults and Adolescents, which is constantly updated and available at this NIH website: http://www.aidsinfo.nih.gov/ContentFiles/AdultandAdolescentGL.pdf (cited February 2012).

CLINCIAL SPECTRUM OF HIV

HIV infection and disease is highly variable in presentation and includes asymptomatic, various chronic or recurring constitutional signs and symptoms, and a plethora of opportunistic conditions. The "acute retroviral syndrome," that is, early or primary infection with HIV, is characterized by fever, pharyngitis, skin rash, arthralgias, malaise, mucosal ulcerations, and neurologic manifestations such as aseptic meningitis.[33]

Patients chronically infected with HIV may present with a prodrome of generalized, nontender lymph node enlargement, fevers and night sweats, weight loss, and diarrhea for weeks or months, formerly termed AIDS-related complex (ARC). Nearly all HIV-seropositive patients will progress to AIDS, but a small minority, called "long-term nonprogressors" or "elite controllers," suppress their infections naturally (without treatment) to the point of very low or undetectable levels of plasma HIV. Although highly active antiretroviral therapy (HAART) often reduces plasma viremia of HIV-1 to undetectable levels, latent viral reservoirs of resting CD4 lymphocytes persist for years and reappear in the blood if therapy is stopped.[34]

Opportunistic infections are responsible for the deaths of most AIDS patients, but consequences of coinfections with hepatitis C and B, such as hepatic insufficiency or hepatocellular carcinoma, have become increasingly important, in part because HIV promotes progression of these infections.[35] The most common pathogens encountered in AIDS patients are cytomegalovirus (CMV), *Candida albicans*, *Pneumocystis jiroveci* (formerly *carinii*), *Mycobacterium tuberculosis* and *M. avium-intracellulare*, *Cryptococcus neoformans*, herpes simplex virus (HSV), *Cryptosporidium* spp., *Toxoplasma gondii*, and varicella zoster virus (VZV).[3,36] CMV retinitis can be the initial sign of tissue-invasive systemic CMV infection in these patients, although it is restricted to patients with advanced immunosuppression (CD4+ count less than 50). CMV may present also in the gastrointestinal tract, brain and spinal cord, or other organs.[37]

INFECTION CONTROL RELATED TO HIV

The US Centers for Disease Control and Prevention (CDC) recommendations for universal precautions to prevent the occupational transmission of HIV and other bloodborne viruses in the healthcare setting were provided in 1988 and have not been amended.[38]

The CDC provided specific guidelines for ophthalmologic examinations in addition to the general recommendations. The use of gloves (especially if the skin of the examiner is compromised in any way) and good handwashing technique after procedures or examinations involving the eye are recommended because HIV may be present in tears.

Sterilization of all instruments and equipment that come into contact with the eye in all patients is necessary using gas or steam autoclaving or a 5- to 10-minute soak in one of the following solutions: 3% hydrogen peroxide solution, 10% solution of sodium hypochlorite (common household bleach), or 70% ethanol or isopropanol. Instruments disinfected in this manner should be rinsed in water and dried before reuse.[39,40] Damage to tonometer tips has been reported with the use of 70% isopropanol; thus a 5- to 10-minute soak in 3% H_2O_2 or 1:10 dilution of household bleach may be preferable.[41] It should be noted that there is no evidence of HIV transmission through contact with tears or instruments used to examine these patients.[39]

Contact lenses used in trial fittings on all patients should be disinfected by use of any commercially available cleaning method or solution.[42] Inactivation of HIV by various disinfectants on surfaces has been reviewed.[43] Guidelines for preventing transmission of HIV through transplantation of human tissue and organs (including corneal transplants) have been set forth.[44] Specific recommendations for postexposure management of needle-stick injuries or mucosal membrane exposures to secretions from patients with HIV infection have been published.[45]

OCULAR FINDINGS IN AIDS: AN OVERVIEW

HIV has been detected in the cornea,[46] conjunctival epithelium,[47] and in tears,[46] but at very low titers. Ocular manifestations of AIDS may be seen in up to 100% of patients. They are less common, but may be seen in patients with earlier, symptomatic HIV infection.[48] Most common are cotton-wool spots and other noninfectious retinopathies,[49] CMV retinitis, and conjunctival Kaposi sarcoma, followed less frequently by herpes zoster ophthalmicus,[50,51] retinal toxoplasmosis, choroidal *P. carinii* infection, herpes simplex and herpes zoster retinitis (acute retinal necrosis [ARN]), and cryptococcal choroiditis.[6,52-59]

Iritis may occur in association with viral retinitis but especially with CMV; it is mild. Acute iritis may be associated with the use of oral rifabutin (used for the treatment and prophylaxis of mycobacterial infections) or intravenous cidofovir used for CMV retinitis.[60]

Choroidal infection with *Cryptococcus*, *Pneumocystis*, *M. tuberculosis*, *Aspergillus*, *Toxoplasma*, *Histoplasma*, and *M. avium-intracellulare* usually is associated with systemic infection.[61,62] *Histoplasma capsulatum* chorioretinitis and endophthalmitis,[63] *Paracoccidioidomycosis brasiliensis* chorioretinitis,[64] keratitis sicca, cranial nerve paralysis, Roth's spots, papilledema, perivasculitis, and fungal corneal ulcers are rare but have been reported.[65]

NONINFECTIOUS RETINOPATHY

Noninfectious retinopathy refers to cotton-wool spots, retinal hemorrhages, and microvascular abnormalities that do not progress, enlarge, or cause visual symptoms. No infectious cause of these lesions has been demonstrated, and they appear to represent nonspecific retinal microvascular disease. A correlation between the number of cotton-wool spots and decreased cerebral blood flow (as shown by technetium 99^{m} hexamethylpropyleneamine oxime single photon emission computed tomography) was shown in 25 patients with AIDS or symptomatic HIV infection.[66]

Cotton-wool spots are the most common ocular lesion seen in AIDS, occurring in 25–50% of patients[6,67] and in up to 75% of cases by autopsy examination.[57] In one study, up to 92% of AIDS patients were found to have evidence of retinovascular disease when examined using fluorescein angiography.[67]

Cotton-wool spots seen by ophthalmoscopy are a result of microinfarction of the nerve fiber layer of the retina. In AIDS these lesions usually are confined to the posterior pole near the optic disc[67] (Fig. 81.1). Histopathologic study of retinal cotton-wool spots in AIDS patients has demonstrated that these lesions have pathologic features identical to those seen in cotton-wool spots of other cause. Similar to the cotton-wool spots seen in other systemic diseases, this lesion in AIDS demonstrates no associated inflammation, no cells in the vitreous, and no vascular leakage on fluorescein angiography (Fig. 81.2). Attempts to isolate organisms from cotton-wool spots in the hope of explaining their cause in AIDS as infectious have been unsuccessful, and the cause of this lesion in AIDS remains elusive.[6,57,68,69]

Cotton-wool spots have been speculated to be harbingers of CMV retinitis or perhaps sites of susceptibility to CMV infection, but substantiation of these ideas is lacking. Histopathologic studies of eyes at autopsy have failed to show clear evidence of a viral cause of cotton-wool spots.[70–72]

We have reported that noninfectious retinopathy is not seen in HIV-seronegative men and is rare in ARC, but it is very common in patients with AIDS even in the absence of active opportunistic ophthalmic infection.[48] It is striking that this lesion may be seen in 50–75% of AIDS patients, and studies using multiple examinations indicate that the more frequently these patients are examined, the higher the incidence may be.[6,49] Cotton-wool spots probably are ophthalmoscopically visible for 6–12 weeks, and owing to the transient nature of the lesion and its apparent noninfectious cause, treatment is not indicated at this time.[73]

In a cross-sectional study, the median CD4 count (per microliter [μl]) in patients with cotton-wool spots was 14 cells (range 0–160) and was 8 cells (range 0–42) in patients with CMV retinitis.[74] In the absence of other systemic vascular disease, such as hypertension or diabetes mellitus, AIDS must be considered in the differential diagnosis of cotton-wool spots owing to their very high prevalence in these patients. Whether these lesions are an early manifestation of AIDS remains to be elucidated, but they may be apparent in HIV-infected persons before the onset of opportunistic infections.[48]

Morphologic studies have shown that the number of retrobulbar optic nerve fibers in patients with AIDS is decreased compared with the number of optic nerve fibers in normal control eyes as a result of axonal degeneration and an associated decrease in the number of optic nerve axons.[75–77] Infarctions of the nerve fiber layer develop in most patients with AIDS, and the number of such infarctions increases over time.[6,49] Visual dysfunction associated with multiple nerve fiber layer infarctions may be manifested by defects in color-vision and contrast-sensitivity testing in patients with AIDS.[78] Interestingly, in vivo studies of the retinal nerve fiber layer have shown both broad and slit-like defects, suggesting that retinal nerve fiber loss and optic nerve fiber loss are related to subclinical vision loss in HIV patients without infectious retinitis.[79] Electroretinographic studies of HIV patients without retinitis also have shown retinal dysfunction.[80,81]

Retinal hemorrhages are seen in AIDS in association with CMV retinitis, cotton-wool spots, and as an isolated finding. These lesions have been reported in up to 30%[52,67,82] of AIDS patients, and autopsy evidence of retinal hemorrhages has been reported to be as high as 40%. Retinal hemorrhages usually take the form of flame-shaped lesions in the posterior pole, dot-blot hemorrhages, or as punctate intraretinal hemorrhages peripherally (Fig. 81.3). Occasionally the hemorrhage is manifested as Roth's spots (hemorrhage with a white central area).[52,67] The pattern of retinal hemorrhages changes over time. The hemorrhages do not appear to be related to a bleeding diathesis or coagulopathy, but rather seem to be a manifestation of AIDS itself.[6] Vision loss from retinal hemorrhage has not been described, and treatment is conservative if the lesions are not associated with CMV retinitis or septicemia.

Microvascular pathologic findings in AIDS, as demonstrated by fluorescein angiography, include microaneurysms, telangiectasias, focal areas of nonperfusion, and capillary loss.[67] These

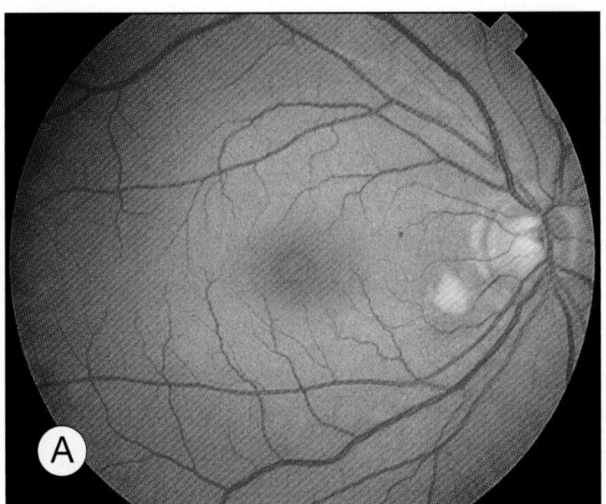

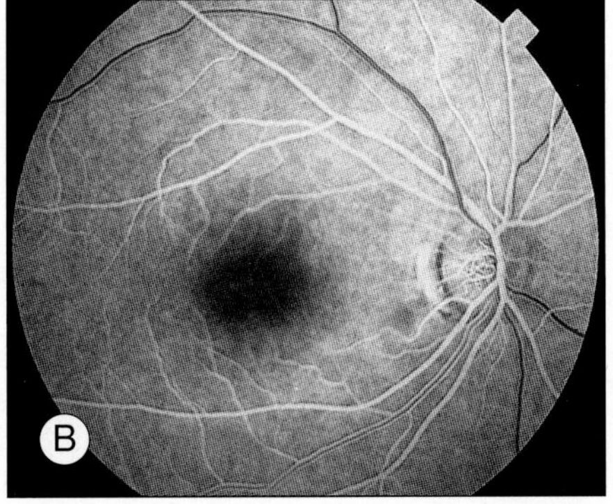

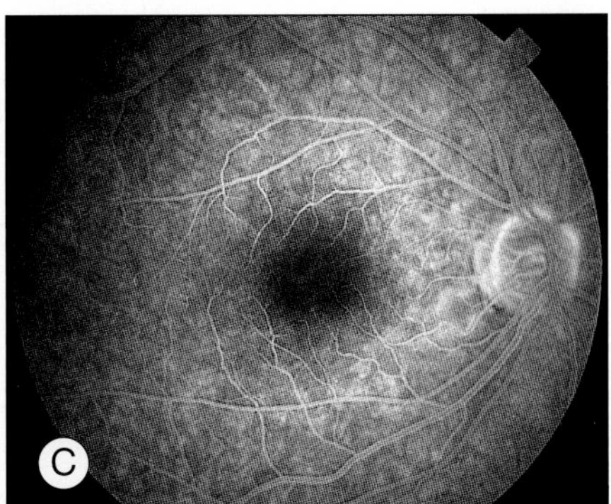

Fig. 81.1 (A) Retinal cotton-wool spot seen inferotemporal to the disc. (B) Early fluorescein angiogram shows blockage and possible nonperfusion. (C) Late angiogram shows staining, presumably from damaged retinal microvasculature.

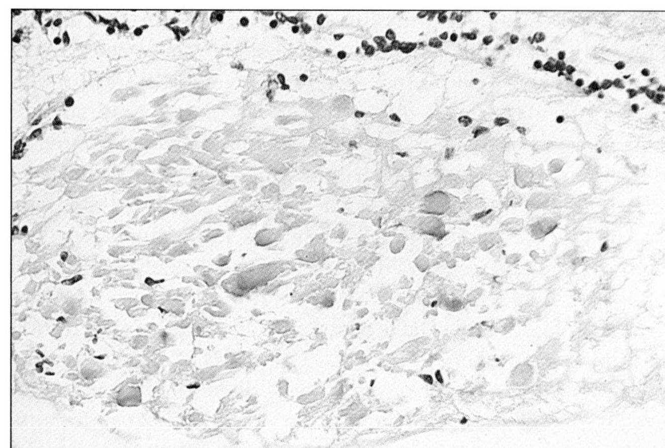
Fig. 81.2 Photomicrograph of retinal cotton-wool spot shows cytoid bodies and swelling of the nerve fiber layer of the retina. Retinal cellular elements are seen at the top of the photograph.

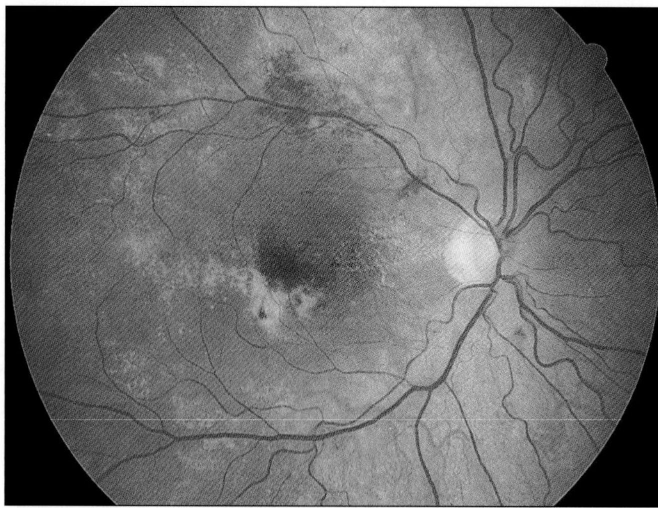
Fig. 81.4 CMV retinitis with hemorrhagic areas are seen superior to the fovea and a more dense area just below the fovea. Borders are opaque and associated with variable amounts of hemorrhage.

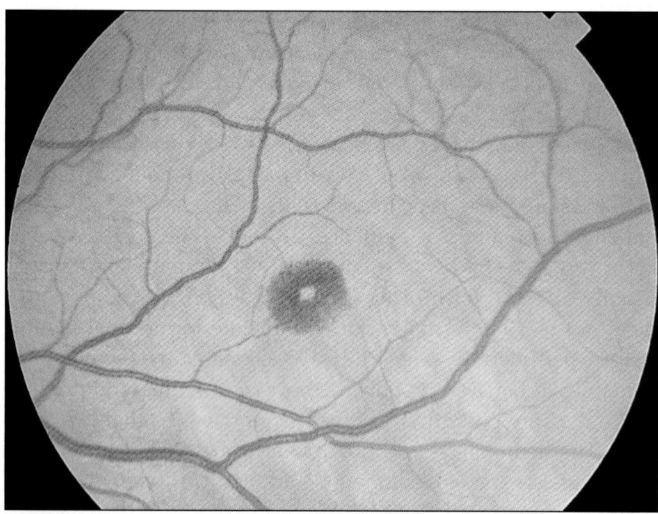
Fig. 81.3 White, centered retinal hemorrhage (Roth's spot) seen in an HIV-infected patient. These lesions do not progress.

changes are similar to the changes seen in diabetes mellitus. The histologic findings of periodic acid–Schiff (PAS)-positive thickening of blood vessels and precapillary arteriolar closure also correlate with the findings in diabetes mellitus.

Branch or central retinal vein occlusion, branch retinal artery occlusion, and ischemic maculopathy have been reported in HIV patients without infectious retinitis. The incidence is unknown. It is possible that the cause may be related to lupus anticoagulant and other clotting abnormalities seen in HIV-infected patients.[83,84] Abnormalities of retinal blood flow have also been reported in HIV patients and may contribute to the pathogenesis of microvascular abnormalities.[85–88]

INFECTIOUS RETINOPATHY

Cytomegalovirus retinitis

Pathogenesis, diagnosis, and clinical manifestations

Cytomegalovirus (CMV) infection is a major cause of morbidity and mortality in AIDS. CMV retinitis has been reported to occur in 15–40% of AIDS patients with the rate declining since the arrival of HAART.[37,52,89,90] In contrast to the noninfectious lesions of AIDS, CMV retinitis demands aggressive treatment to prevent severe visual loss.[6,91,92] Patients with active CMV disease may have systemic symptoms of fever, arthralgia, and pneumonitis, or leukopenia, retinitis, or hepatitis; blood cultures and urine specimens may be positive for CMV. CMV retinitis often is the presenting sign of systemic CMV infection, and all patients should be thoroughly evaluated for systemic disease.

The clinical presentation of CMV retinitis in AIDS is similar in many respects to CMV retinitis found in iatrogenically immunosuppressed patients and infants with cytomegalic inclusion disease.[93,94] Correlation of the clinical and typical pathologic findings at autopsy has been demonstrated.[95] Specifically, it is known that CMV is a neurotropic virus with a tendency to infect neural tissues and the retina. Necrosis of the retina in AIDS-associated CMV retinitis is typical, with pathognomonic cytomegaly and minimal inflammatory cells present in the lesions. Choroidal involvement is rare, and whether vascular endothelium is involved is unclear. These lesions also may appear as noncontiguous patches rather than the more commonly seen contiguous spreading lesion. Antigens to CMV have been found by immunofluorescence, immunoperoxidase staining, and DNA hybridization techniques.[96,97] The most distinctive anterior segment finding is the presence of fine stellate keratic precipitates on the corneal endothelium.[98] Retinal vascular nonperfusion and retinal neovascularization resulting from CMV retinitis and choroiditis also have been reported.[99]

CMV is a slowly progressive necrotizing retinitis that may affect the posterior pole, the periphery, or both, and may be unilateral or bilateral. Involved retinal areas appear as white intraretinal lesions, areas of infiltrate, and often necrosis along the vascular arcades in the posterior pole. In addition, prominent retinal hemorrhages often are present within the necrotic area or along its leading edge (Fig. 81.4). Peripherally, CMV retinitis occurs commonly; it tends to have a less intense white appearance, with areas of granular, white retinitis that may or may not demonstrate associated retinal hemorrhage (Fig. 81.5). As the

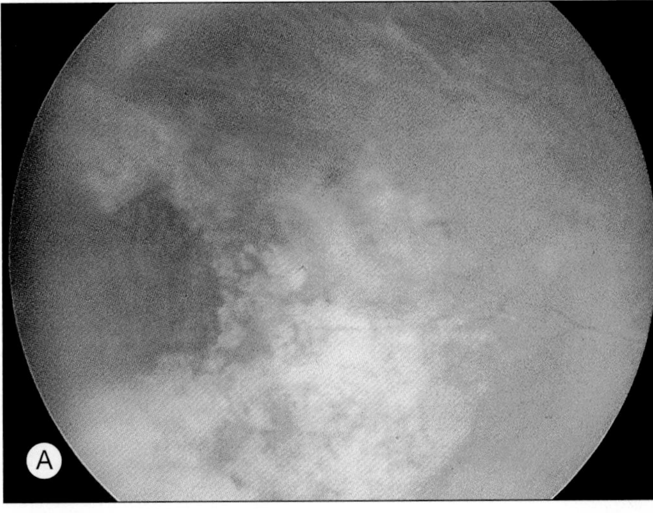

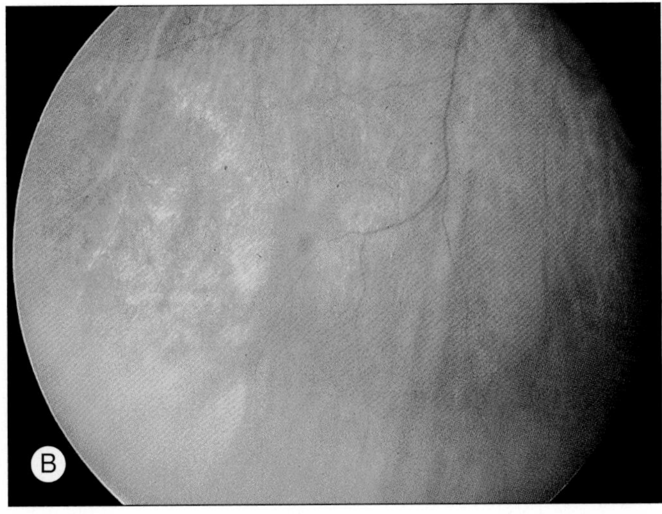

Fig. 81.5 (A) Peripheral CMV retinitis without retinal hemorrhage is characterized by white areas of retinal necrosis. (B) After healing, CMV retinitis leaves behind a glial scar without opacification (not same eye as in panel A). Often only minimal pigmentary changes are seen.

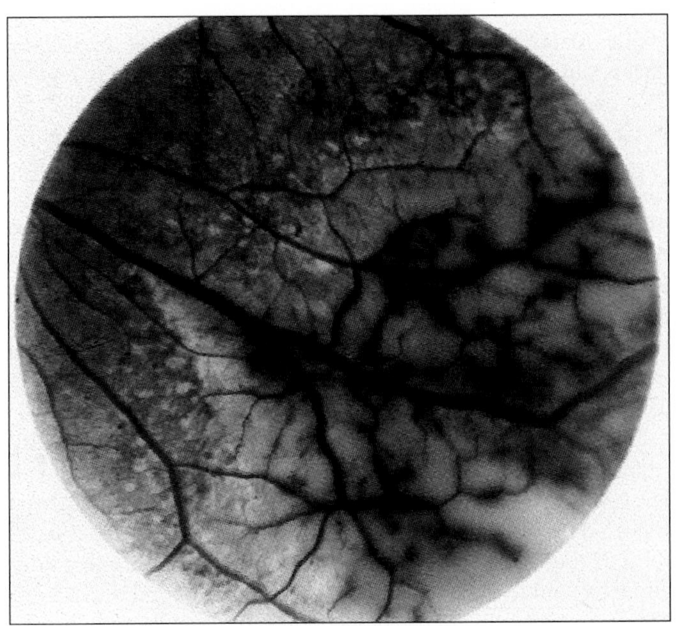

Fig. 81.6 Fluorescein angiogram of CMV retinitis lesion shows lack of perfusion and blockage, as well as staining and leakage of fluorescein from damaged retinal vessels.

retinitis progresses, an area of atrophic, avascular retina may remain with underlying retinal pigment epithelial atrophy or hyperplasia.[6,37,100] Peripheral CMV retinitis is common in AIDS patients who initially may report only floaters with or without a visual field deficit. Wide-angle fundus photography and fluorescein angiography may be of benefit if the diagnosis is uncertain. These techniques may be used to document progression of retinitis, and fluorescein leakage in areas of retinitis may be helpful in confirming the diagnosis (Fig. 81.6).

Reactivation of CMV retinitis is characterized by reopacification of the border of the lesion followed by advancement. Smoldering retinitis (Fig. 81.7) and subtle reactivation may be difficult to recognize without prior fundus photographs. Several studies have shown that wide-angle fundus photographs are a more sensitive indicator of retinitis progression than is clinical examination by indirect ophthalmoscopy.[101,102]

Several investigators have shown that untreated CMV retinitis is inexorably progressive in AIDS patients.[6,52,94,96,102,103] As in our experience, untreated CMV becomes bilateral in the vast majority of patients. In an observational study of 26 patients treated for CMV retinitis, vision scores decreased with greater abnormalities found on ophthalmologic examination. Visual symptoms were most strongly related to findings in the worse eye. Patients reported considerable impairment, including blurred vision (42%), difficulty reading (40%), difficulty driving (44%), treatment interference with social activities (40%), and substantial trouble with vision (50%).[104] Treatment of AIDS-related CMV retinitis minimizes loss of vision and may protect previously uninfected eyes, prolonging visual independence.[105]

Recurrent CMV retinitis exhibiting a foveal-sparing pattern within 1500 mm of the foveola has been described and occurs primarily in patients with recurrent CMV retinitis resistant to treatment ("clinically resistant"), particularly that which has arisen temporally. Despite its foveolar proximity and ultimate significant loss of function, the pattern of progression allows for preservation of useful foveal vision for longer periods than would have been expected.[106]

Other manifestations of CMV retinitis include retinal edema, attenuated vessels, perivascular sheathing, and exudative retinal detachment[107] (Fig. 81.8). In addition, vitritis and anterior uveitis are often seen, and optic atrophy may occur as a late manifestation resulting from widespread retinal destruction. CMV occasionally may be demonstrated in vitreous biopsy specimens in these patients.[95] The yield may be higher in the presence of marked vitritis because CMV is a cell-associated virus. Other causes of retinitis, including herpes simplex retinitis,[93,108] toxoplasmosis,[62] candidal infection, Behçet disease, syphilis, acute retinal necrosis,[109,110] and subacute sclerosing panencephalitis, usually can be distinguished from CMV on clinical grounds, although this may not be the case in retinitis caused by other members of the herpesvirus family.[109] CMV has a very characteristic clinical appearance, but the lesions in CMV retinitis vary from patient to patient, and it is important to maintain a high index of suspicion for the above infections, especially in light

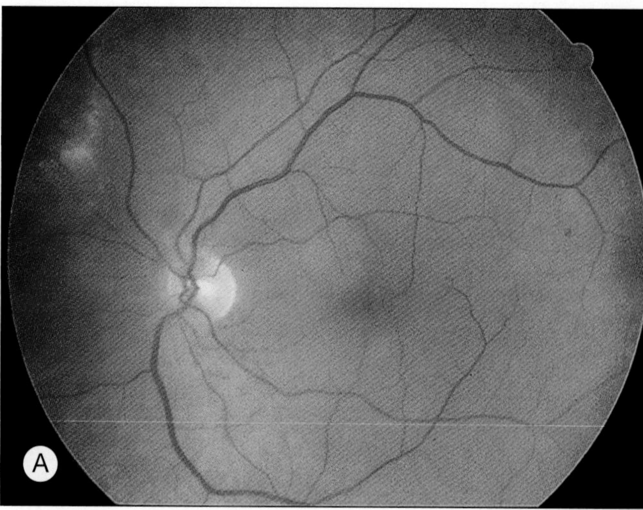

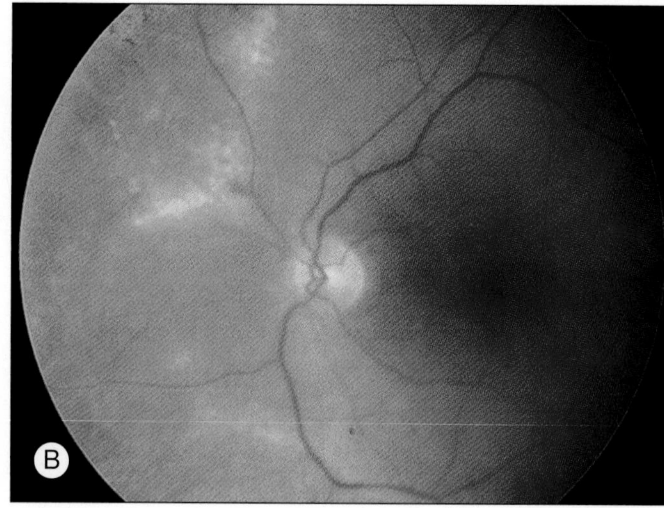

Fig. 81.7 Smoldering CMV retinitis is a low grade of retinitis border activity that is associated with slow progression of retinitis. It may be difficult to diagnose without fundus photographs. (A) Low grade CMV lesion. (B) Lesion has progressed slowly over 2 months.

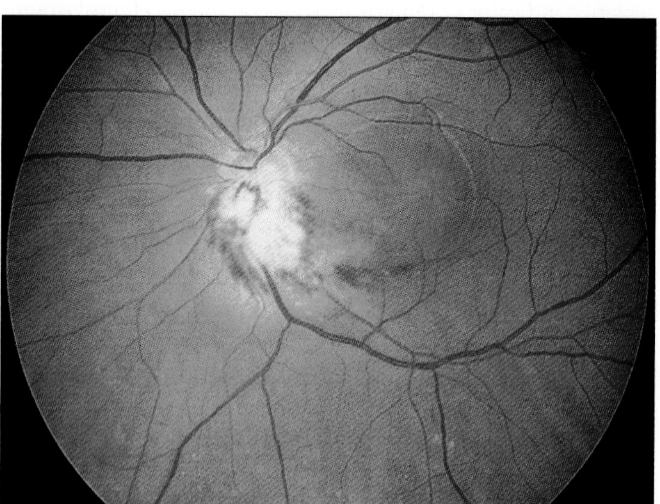

Fig. 81.8 CMV affecting the perifoveal area or the optic nerve can result in an exudative retinal detachment often involving the macula. If there has not been actual involvement of a vital structure, treatment may result in improvement of central vision.

of frequent superinfection of AIDS patients with multiple organisms.[6,82,83]

CMV retinitis is a reflection of underlying active systemic CMV infection. In almost all cases it is a blinding disease if not controlled. Thus, in the face of changing mental status, development of focal signs on neurologic examination, or other symptoms consistent with subacute encephalitis in AIDS patients, a comprehensive ophthalmologic examination is indicated, and an increased index of suspicion of CMV infection of the CNS and possible CMV retinitis is warranted. There is also evidence that patients with CMV retinitis, especially peripapillary disease, have a much higher incidence of CMV encephalitis. CMV infection of the brain, optic nerves, and retinas from 47 consecutive autopsies of patients with AIDS was examined.[111] Immunocytochemistry demonstrated CMV infection in 11 (23%) brains, 2 (2%) of 94 optic nerves, and 38 (40%) of 94 retinas. Ten (91%) of 11 patients with CMV encephalitis had concurrent retinitis. While 10 (42%) of 24 patients with CMV retinitis had CMV encephalitis, when the retinitis included the peripapillary region, 75% had encephalitis. The optic nerve parenchyma usually was not infected histologically despite extensive peripapillary retinitis. The strength of these associations suggests that CMV retinitis defines a group of patients with AIDS at risk for development of CMV encephalitis (relative risk, 9.5%), especially when the retinitis involves the peripapillary region (relative risk, 13%). Furthermore, in patients with AIDS without CMV retinitis, central nervous system symptoms are unlikely to be attributable to CMV encephalitis.[111] The pathologic correlation between ocular and cerebral lesions in patients with AIDS has been reviewed.[112]

CMV retinitis is less frequent in children with AIDS, with reported rates of approximately 5–6%, though rates of extraocular CMV are higher than in adults. CMV retinitis has been reported in young children with high absolute CD4 counts, though these counts are low relative to the child's age. Older children tend to have low absolute CD4 counts similar to adults. There is a higher incidence of bilateral and posterior pole disease in children, however this is likely due in part to delays in diagnosis in children from lack of subjective vision complaints.[113–115]

Screening techniques for retinal and systemic CMV infection

Screening for CMV retinitis is a difficult problem. Many patients who are CMV-viremic or -viruric may not have end-organ disease, and studies employing quantitative CMV polymerase chain reaction (PCR) in plasma or CMV antigenemia have not been able to definitively predict the development of CMV retinitis.[116] Currently no laboratory marker exists that reliably predicts the occurrence of clinical CMV retinitis.

Urine is culture-positive for CMV in more than 50% of homosexual men and the majority of AIDS patients; thus urine culture may not be of diagnostic value. Serology in AIDS patients is nonspecific, and documentation of rising CMV titers is unusual.[6,96] Studies of newly diagnosed CMV retinitis patients indicate that many are CMV culture-negative in the blood. Positive blood cultures for CMV, fever, and weight loss are associated with more extensive CMV retinitis at the time of diagnosis.[117] The results of virologic blood assays for CMV also have been associated with clinical outcome in patients with CMV retinitis.[118] Thus assays for the detection of CMV antigenemia may be a simple and rapid means of identifying those patients with unilateral retinitis at highest risk of developing CMV retinitis of the fellow eye or of visceral CMV disease if intravitreal injections or implants are used as the sole treatment for CMV retinitis.[119]

A positive PCR result supports the clinical diagnosis and may be useful for monitoring response to antiviral treatment. By prospective monitoring for increases in plasma CMV DNA copy number, it may be possible to identify HIV-seropositive patients who are at imminent risk for development of symptomatic CMV retinitis.[120]

It is also reasonable and practical to use the CD4 cell count as a threshold below which to screen patients, since the risk of CMV retinitis increases at CD4 cell counts below 50/mm^3.[74] The incidence and prevalence of CMV retinitis in a cohort study of patients with CD4 cell counts below 0.10×10^9/L (100/μl) revealed a 25% chance for the development of CMV retinitis by 4 years of follow-up. Among those subjects in whom CMV retinitis developed, about 19% had retinitis before a CD4 cell count of less than 0.05×10^9/L (<50/μl) was observed, and 81% had CMV retinitis after the CD4 cell count reached this threshold.[121] In the HAART era, some patients may develop CMV retinitis with CD4 counts above 100/ml, probably because of incomplete restoration of the immune repertoire against CMV.[122]

A technique for screening for central CMV retinitis, entoptic perimetry, employs patient visualization of moving particles on a computer monitor, appears to have a very high sensitivity and specificity (over 90%) in detecting CMV retinitis within the central 30-degrees radius of fixation[79] (Fig. 81.9).

Techniques for detection of CMV DNA based on PCR are increasingly being applied to ocular fluids; however, the clinical significance of such findings can sometimes be unclear. The application of PCR-based methods to ocular fluids made a useful contribution to the treatment of the patients.[123]

This appears to be a sensitive and specific diagnostic assay that could assist in the diagnosis of CMV retinitis.[124] PCR detection of CMV DNA has been reported to be a more sensitive method than analysis of locally produced antibodies by calculating a Goldman–Witmer coefficient to determine local ocular antibody production. There is also an immune predisposition to the development of CMV retinitis in patients with AIDS.[125,126]

Treatment of CMV retinitis

The treatment of CMV retinitis has been reviewed.[127,128] Treatment may be systemic, local, or a combination of the two. There are currently five medications approved by the US Food and Drug Administration (FDA) for the treatment of CMV retinitis: ganciclovir, valganciclovir, cidofovir, foscarnet. Fomivirsen, the first antisense drug with a relatively long duration of action, is no longer available in the United States.

Systemic therapy of CMV retinitis

CMV retinitis may be treated systemically or intravitreally. However, systemic treatment is associated with less spread of CMV retinitis from one eye to the other.[128] In addition, local treatment including the sustained release ganciclovir implant has been shown to be associated with higher risk of the development of systemic CMV.[129,130]

Systemic CMV may cause gastrointestinal disease, with colitis being the most common manifestation as well as esophagitis. Systemic CMV diagnosis may be difficult and usually requires histopathologic evidence of CMV infection. The cumulative incidence of systemic CMV disease that becomes clinically apparent is approximately 25%.[131] Therefore, although systemic CMV disease may not be clinically apparent at the time of diagnosis of CMV retinitis, some experts believe that initial systemic therapy may be warranted despite the inconvenience, expense, and potential toxicities.

Intravenous ganciclovir

Ganciclovir is a nucleoside analog of 2-deoxyguanosine, similar to acyclovir.[132] Despite its structural similarities with acyclovir, ganciclovir is much more active in vitro against CMV than acyclovir.[133] Ganciclovir inhibits all herpesviruses, including CMV, by preventing DNA elongation. CMV lacks the virally specified thymidine kinase (TK) that converts ganciclovir (or acyclovir) to its monophosphate form.[134] TK-altered strains resistant to acyclovir are as sensitive to ganciclovir as the unaltered parent strains. Thus ganciclovir is phosphorylated to its triphosphate form much more efficiently than acyclovir, which accounts for the greater activity of ganciclovir against CMV.[135]

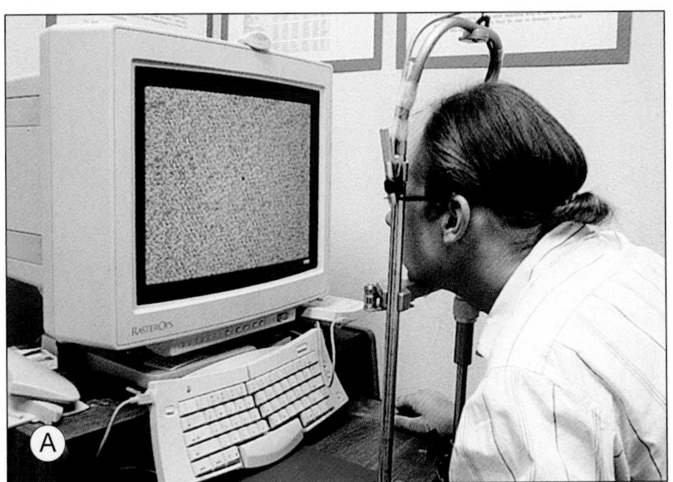

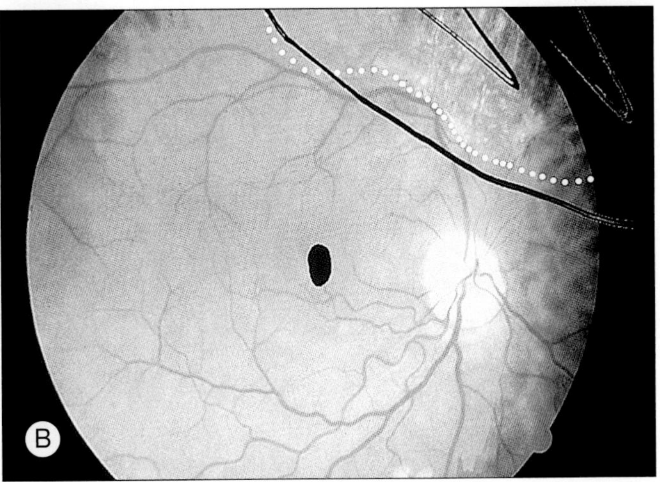

Fig. 81.9 Entoptic perimetry can allow detection of CMV retinitis lesions. (A) The patient is asked to view particle motion programmed on a monitor. (B) An overlay of the CMV lesion (dotted white border) and the patient's own sketch of the scotoma seen (black line).

The majority of AIDS patients treated with ganciclovir respond within 2–4 weeks with decreased retinal opacification and stabilization of the retinitis[89] (Fig. 81.10). Ganciclovir is commercially available as an intravenous and oral formulation (and also is included in an intraocular device), and indefinite maintenance therapy is necessary as long as the patient remains in immune failure with a CD4 count below 50/µl. An intravenous loading dose of 5 mg/kg every 12 hours for 14–21 days should be followed by maintenance doses of 5 mg/kg/day. If the drug is discontinued, retinitis often recurs within 10–21 days, continuing its progression at the borders of healed areas.[89] Recurrences have been common, even during maintenance therapy, being reported 3 weeks to 5 months after institution of therapy and occurring in 30–40% of patients.[89] Many investigators have found that discontinuation or delay of ganciclovir therapy results in nearly 100% recurrence of retinitis, at which time reinstitution of the loading dose regimen often is necessary.[134,136,137] Multiple series in patients with AIDS and CMV retinitis have shown response rates of 80–100%, with 60–80% of patients achieving a remission with ganciclovir therapy.[37,137–141]

The treatment of CMV retinitis usually includes an induction phase followed by a maintenance phase to prevent relapse. Before the advent of HAART, relapse occurred almost universally, given a sufficiently long period after induction courses of ganciclovir. Therapy therefore continued for a lifetime. The median time to relapse in patients treated with just an induction dose is 3–4 weeks.[137]

Most clinicians use a 14-day induction course of intravenous ganciclovir consisting of 5 mg/kg/day every 12 hours and indefinite maintenance of 5 mg/kg/day. Lower doses and every-other-day dosing schedules have been associated with high rates of early relapse. Since treatment may be lifelong if the patient's CD4 count cannot be elevated with anti-HIV therapy, usually a permanent or semipermanent indwelling venous catheter is placed at the onset of therapy if intravenous therapy is chosen as maintenance therapy. Ganciclovir requires modification of dosing in the presence of renal insufficiency.

Side-effects of ganciclovir include granulocytopenia, neurologic dysfunction, abnormal liver function tests, and rarely, thrombocytopenia. The most serious toxicity is granulocytopenia, which may occur in up to one-third of patients when defined as less than 500 neutrophils per microliter.[137] Granulocytopenia is generally reversible, and this adverse effect is exacerbated when used with AZT.[142] The use of colony-stimulating factors rGM-CSF (recombinant granulocyte–macrophage colony-stimulating factor) and rG-CSF (recombinant granulocyte colony-stimulating factor) for reversing or preventing neutropenia may be useful.

The prevalence of CMV resistance to ganciclovir is unknown, but ever-increasing induction regimens may be necessary to control CMV retinitis. Strains of CMV that develop resistance to ganciclovir may remain susceptible to foscarnet. Because of the question of ganciclovir resistance, a trial of combined vs alternating foscarnet–ganciclovir maintenance therapy has been reported to be effective.[143]

Visual acuity depends on the location of the involved retina, and involvement of the fovea or optic nerve may result in decreased visual acuity even if there has been a response to therapy. Ganciclovir has been shown to be effective in preserving visual acuity. For example, 73% of eyes maintained a visual acuity of 20/40 or better when treated with ganciclovir.[144]

Oral ganciclovir

Oral ganciclovir (FDA approved, 1994) can be used for maintenance therapy of CMV retinitis after it has been healed with intravenous ganciclovir therapy. Studies using this drug regimen have shown efficacy, but it is clear that oral ganciclovir is less effective than intravenous ganciclovir for many patients.

Perhaps the most common use of oral ganciclovir is in patients being treated with intravitreal therapy (injections of cidofovir or ganciclovir implant) to prevent systemic CMV disease. Such use of oral ganciclovir also may reduce the incidence of CMV in the fellow eye if it is not involved.[145,146] Oral ganciclovir for prophylaxis or treatment of CMV retinitis has been replaced by oral valganciclovir, which provides much higher blood levels.

Valganciclovir

Valganciclovir, the valine ester of ganciclovir, is an orally administered formulation of ganciclovir. The valine ester confers

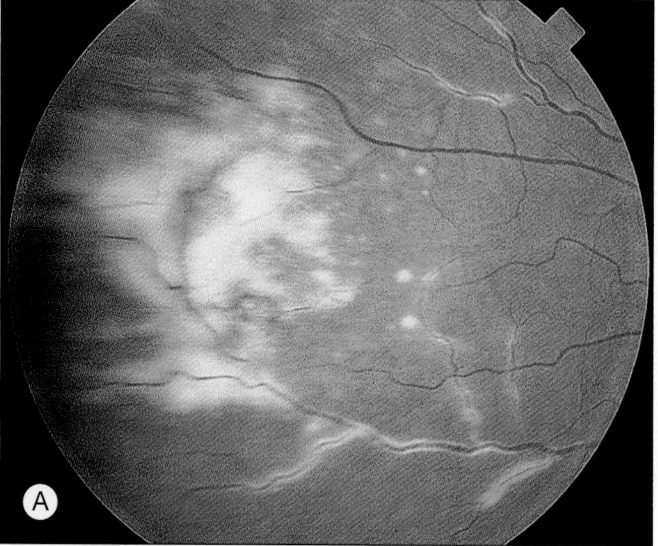

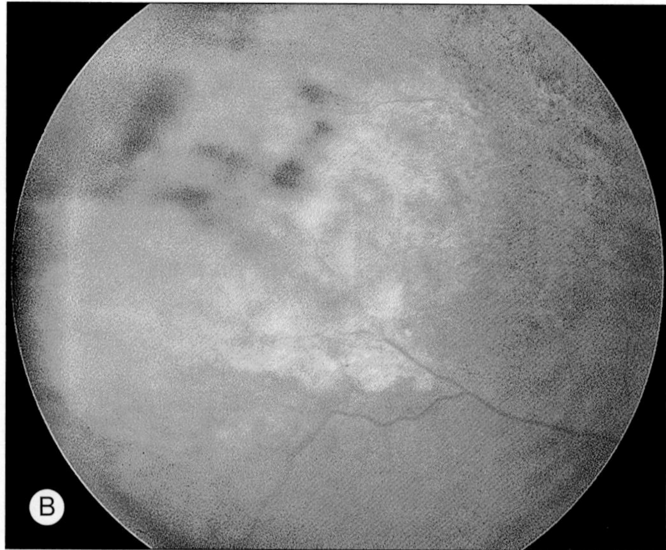

Fig. 81.10 (A) Active peripheral CMV retinitis with secondary retinal vasculitis. (B) The area is healed after intravenous ganciclovir therapy. Note absence of border opacification. Also seen are pigmentary changes characteristic of healed CMV.

enhanced permeability and absorption of the molecule through the cell membranes of the gut. Once in the bloodstream, the valine ester is cleaved from the molecule by esterases, rendering plasma levels of ganciclovir comparable to those achieved with intravenous ganciclovir administration. A single-dose randomized crossover pharmacokinetic study reported the absolute ganciclovir bioavailability after oral valganciclovir administration is 60.9% compared to 5.6% bioavailability of oral ganciclovir.[147] A randomized crossover dose-ranging study determined that plasma levels of ganciclovir after an 875 mg dose of valganciclovir are similar to the plasma levels achieved with a dose of 5 mg/kg of intravenous ganciclovir (AUC 24.8 mg/ml per h vs 26 mg/ml per h). The authors suggested the 900 mg dose of valganciclovir would approximate the AUC value of the 5 mg/kg dose of IV ganciclovir.[148]

Valganciclovir has been studied for induction therapy for CMV retinitis. Martin et al. (Valganciclovir Study Group) reported a multicenter randomized, controlled clinical trial comparing oral valganciclovir 900 mg twice a day for 3 weeks' induction therapy followed by 900 mg daily for 1 week maintenance therapy with intravenous ganciclovir 5 mg/kg twice a day for 3 weeks' induction therapy followed by 5 mg/kg once daily for one week of maintenance therapy. After 4 weeks both groups received continued maintenance therapy with 900 mg valganciclovir daily. Eighty patients with newly diagnosed CMV retinitis were randomized to each group in a 1:1 ratio. Primary endpoint was photographically determined progression of CMV retinitis within 4 weeks after the initiation of treatment. In the valganciclovir group, 9.9% of patients had progression of CMV retinitis within the first 4 weeks compared to 10.0% of patients assigned to IV ganciclovir. This 0.1 percentage point difference was not significant (95% CI –9.7 to 10.0). Secondary endpoints included the achievement of a prospectively defined successful response to induction therapy and the time to progression of CMV retinitis. Seventy-seven percent of patients receiving IV ganciclovir and 71.9% of patients receiving oral valganciclovir achieved a satisfactory response to induction therapy. This 5.2 percentage point difference was not significant (95% CI –20.4 to 10.1). The median times to progression of retinitis were 125 days in the IV ganciclovir group and 160 days in the oral valganciclovir group. The relative risk of progression of retinitis in the valganciclovir group compared to the ganciclovir group was 0.90 (95 CI 0.58–1.38). Diarrhea was the most common adverse effect during the study and occurred more frequently in the valganciclovir group compared to the ganciclovir group (19% vs 10%, P = 0.11). Neutropenia occurred with similar frequency in each group. Catheter-related side-effects were seen more frequently in the IV ganciclovir group than in the valganciclovir group.[149] No clinical trials have been published specifically comparing efficacy of valganciclovir for maintenance therapy of CMV retinitis.

Lalezari et al. (Roche Valganciclovir Study Group) reported a large safety study of valganciclovir. The adverse event profile was similar to that reported from previous studies of intravenous and oral ganciclovir. Adverse events of note were diarrhea (38%), nausea (23%), fever (18%), neutropenia (absolute neutrophil count <500 cells/mm^3) (10%), and anemia (hemoglobin <8.0 g/dl) (12%), thrombocytopenia (platelet count <25 000 cells/mm^3) (2%).[150]

In summary, oral valganciclovir offers the obvious advantage of extreme effectiveness against CMV retinitis without the difficulties and inconveniences of intravenous administration. Furthermore, because valganciclovir is converted to ganciclovir in the bloodstream, its pharmacologic safety profile, including side-effects, is no different than that of intravenously administered ganciclovir. Thus oral valganciclovir is an effective and safe alternative to intravenous ganciclovir for the treatment of CMV retinitis. Oral ganciclovir has become unavailable but is now supplanted by valganciclovir.

Foscarnet

The second drug for the treatment of CMV retinitis in patients with AIDS was licensed by the FDA in 1993. Foscarnet is a pyrophosphate analog with broad antiviral activity via inhibition of viral polymerases, such inhibition not being dependent on activation or phosphorylation by viral or cellular enzymes. Foscarnet inhibits DNA chain elongation by preventing pyrophosphate exchange.[151]

Foscarnet inhibits the DNA polymerase of CMV and other herpesviruses (HSV-1, HSV-2, VZV, and Epstein–Barr virus [EBV]) and the replication of HIV in vitro and in vivo.[152] Both herpesvirus and HIV replication may be inhibited by therapeutically achievable concentrations of foscarnet. Since the drug is not metabolized and is excreted by the kidney, the dosage must be adjusted for renal insufficiency. Foscarnet also has been used successfully to treat HIV-infected patients with acyclovir-resistant HSV and VZV infections, in addition to CMV retinitis. Foscarnet acts directly on the viral polymerase of all herpesviruses and on the reverse transcriptase of HIV-1. Resistance of CMV to foscarnet is associated with mutations in the genes of these polymerases. Cross-resistance to antiviral drugs is likely to be an increasing problem, since patients with AIDS are living longer as a result of HAART and of the drugs used in the prophylaxis of various opportunistic infections, as well as because of the experience gained in the management of HIV-related problems.

Foscarnet has been shown to be useful against ganciclovir-resistant herpesviruses, such as CMV, because a mutation in a DNA polymerase gene conferring resistance to ganciclovir and acyclovir differs from the region conferring resistance to foscarnet.[153] Foscarnet also is an effective inhibitor of the HIV reverse transcriptase enzyme and acts in a dose-dependent manner. AZT and foscarnet have synergistic activity in vitro against HIV, and in vivo, foscarnet has activity against HIV as measured by surrogate markers.[154]

The use of foscarnet salvage therapy in patients with CMV retinitis who are intolerant of or resistant to ganciclovir was studied in AIDS patients with CMV retinitis who had documented hematologic intolerance or resistance to ganciclovir therapy. This study showed that in patients intolerant of ganciclovir, salvage foscarnet therapy resulted in a longer time to retinitis progression than reported previously in historic controls who terminated ganciclovir therapy. In patients who exhibited clinical resistance to ganciclovir, foscarnet appeared to have efficacy in controlling retinitis. No significant differences in either efficacy or toxicity were observed in the range of foscarnet maintenance doses studied.[155]

A large, randomized, multicenter, blinded clinical trial (the Foscarnet–Ganciclovir Cytomegalovirus Retinitis Trial) compared ganciclovir with foscarnet in the treatment of CMV retinitis in patients with AIDS. No difference was reported between the treatment groups in the rate of progression of retinitis;

however, the median survival was 8.5 months in the ganciclovir group and 12.6 months in the foscarnet group. Excess mortality was reported in a subset of patients in the foscarnet group whose renal function was compromised at entry. Differences in mortality could not be explained entirely on the basis of less antiretroviral therapy in the ganciclovir group, which suggests beneficial interactions between foscarnet and antiretroviral nucleosides. These results indicate that, for patients with AIDS and CMV retinitis, treatment with foscarnet initially offers a survival advantage over treatment with ganciclovir, although foscarnet was not as well tolerated as ganciclovir.[156]

A marginally prolonged survival seen in patients treated with foscarnet compared with those treated with ganciclovir may have been due to a direct effect on HIV replication. Both drugs had a suppressive effect on circulating p24 antigen, which was predictive of improved survival. The inhibitory effect on CMV replication also may have a beneficial effect on limiting HIV replication.[157]

A randomized, controlled, comparative trial of foscarnet and ganciclovir demonstrated that they equally controlled CMV retinitis but that foscarnet was associated with a longer survival. However, foscarnet was less well tolerated than ganciclovir, primarily because of the nature of its side-effects. Since foscarnet and ganciclovir have different side-effects, initial treatment of CMV retinitis should be individualized.[158]

The most frequently reported major adverse effect associated with foscarnet administration is nephrotoxicity, with dose-limiting toxicity occurring frequently and cases of acute renal failure having been observed. Symptomatic hypocalcemia has been reported and may be responsible for arrhythmias and seizures, and the risk is increased by concurrent administration of intravenous pentamidine. Bone marrow suppression with neutropenia, anemia, and thrombocytopenia can be seen with foscarnet administration. Neutropenia was reported to be less common with foscarnet than with ganciclovir (14% vs 34%).[156]

Practical guidelines for the use of foscarnet include administration through an infusion pump to avoid the potential consequences of overdose or too rapid infusion, adequate hydration of patients with saline loading[159] to reduce the risk of nephrotoxicity, avoidance of administration of other potentially nephrotoxic agents, and monitoring of renal function two or three times per week during induction therapy and once per week during maintenance therapy, with the dosage being recalculated on the basis of patient weight and serum creatinine. Studies of foscarnet doses have suggested that patients receiving high maintenance doses (120 mg/kg/day) have slower rates of retinitis progression.[160,161]

Foscarnet is active against HIV, and studies have shown that it raises the CD4 count transiently and decreases viral antigenemia (p24 antigen). Because of its efficacy against CMV and HIV, it would appear to be a potentially effective agent for treating HIV-infected patients; however, it is currently only available for intravenous administration, and its use is associated with substantial toxicity (see above).[154,162]

Cidofovir

Cidofovir, (S)-1-[3-hydroxy-2-(phosphonylmethoxy)propyl]cytosine, formerly known as HPMPC, was the first antiviral nucleotide analog available for the treatment of CMV retinitis. Cidofovir is active in uninfected cells, may act preemptively, and may retain activity against ganciclovir-resistant strains. Preclinical studies showed the major toxicity of cidofovir to be dose-, schedule-, and species-dependent nephrotoxicity. The concomitant administration of probenecid protects animal models against cidofovir-induced nephrotoxicity. Four treatment modifications are indicated clinically to reduce the incidence of cidofovir-related nephrotoxicity: dose reduction or interruption for changes in renal function; concomitant administration of probenecid; administration of 1 liter of normal saline 1 hour before infusion; and extension of the dosing interval.[163]

The treatment of CMV retinitis with intravenous cidofovir was demonstrated to be effective in slowing the progression of peripheral CMV retinitis in patients with previously untreated CMV retinitis and AIDS. Intravenous cidofovir also has been used for long-term suppression of CMV retinitis. Biweekly therapy (after induction therapy) was reported to have a time to progression of CMV retinitis of 120 days in one randomized, controlled trial[164] and 2.5 months in another randomized, controlled trial.[165,166] Treatment and subsequent maintenance of CMV retinitis with 20 μg of intravitreously injected cidofovir, given at 5- to 6-week intervals, also is safe and highly effective.[167]

Treatment with parenteral cidofovir is complicated by nephrotoxicity, which can be reduced with saline hydration and concomitant administration of probenecid. Despite these additional treatments, the long-term reports from the HPMPC Peripheral Cytomegalovirus Retinitis Trial showed a rate of proteinuria of 1.22 per patient-year and a rate of elevated serum creatinine of 0.41 per patient-year. Thus many patients may have difficulty tolerating cidofovir for a prolonged time. Neutropenia has also been reported with cidofovir.

Unfortunately parenteral cidofovir has also been found to have ocular toxicity, including a high incidence of iritis (up to 50%), including recurrent iritis, and a risk of profound ocular hypotony with vision loss, similar to the iritis and hypotony seen with intravitreal injections of cidofovir.[168–170] It has been estimated in one study that cidofovir-related iritis developed in half of patients within approximately 4 months. The long-term reports from the HPMPC Peripheral Cytomegalovirus Retinitis Trial showed a rate of cidofovir-associated uveitis of 0.20 per person-year and a rate of significant ocular hypotony of 0.16 per patient-year.[166] Thus in the setting of iritis in HIV-infected patients, use of systemic cidofovir or rifabutin should be considered potential causes of iritis, and these drugs may need to be discontinued.

Nephrotoxicity may be cumulative in some patients and appears to be related to toxicity in the proximal tubule. This "secretory toxicity" also may be responsible for the hypotony and iritis that the drug causes when given intravenously or intravitreously. The ciliary body and the proximal tubule of the kidney have many similarities in terms of the mechanism involved in the secretion of fluids across epithelia. Oral administration of probenecid before and after the intravenous infusion appears to help ameliorate the nephrotoxicity of the drug, but the ocular side-effects of iritis and hypotony occur despite concomitant probenecid administration.

CMV resistance

Many patients taking chronic maintenance therapy for CMV retinitis develop resistant virus. Development of in vitro resistance of CMV to ganciclovir and foscarnet and disease progression has been shown in several small studies,[171,172] and mechanisms of resistance to ganciclovir have been described.[173] In one prospective, randomized study of 207 patients with newly diagnosed CMV retinitis, drug-resistant CMV occurred in four of nine ganciclovir-treated patients and in none of five foscarnet-treated patients.[118] In patients with CMV retinitis and AIDS treated with either oral or intravenous ganciclovir, isolates of CMV after a median exposure of 75 and 165 days, respectively, showed increasing resistance in vitro.[174] Jabs et al. reported that the cumulative incidence of ganciclovir resistance at 9 months was 27.5%.[172] Similar incidence rates of resistance occur for foscarnet and cidofovir.[175] In addition, the incidence of resistance to valganciclovir appears to be similar to that for ganciclovir.[176]

Resistance to an anti-CMV drug can be described as phenotypic, expressed as an inhibitory concentration 50% greater than a certain threshold (IC50). This is determined typically via plaque reduction assays, DNA hybridization assays, or antigen-reduction assays that require large amounts of viable virus often requiring culturing.[174,177–179] Genotypic resistance is defined by the presence of a mutation in the CMV genome conferring resistance to a particular drug. PCR amplification techniques allow fast detection of resistance-conferring mutations in the viral genome, requiring only small amounts of viral nucleic acids and can use nonviable virus.[180–182] Low-level ganciclovir resistance is typically associated with mutations in the CMV *UL97* gene. *UL97* codes for a phosphotransferase that catalyzes the first step of ganciclovir activation to the triphosphate form. High-level ganciclovir resistance is typically caused by mutations in both the CMV *UL97* and *UL54* genes. *UL54* codes for the cytomegalovirus DNA polymerase.[173] Mutations in the *UL54* gene are also responsible for foscarnet and cidofovir resistance.[173,183–186] *UL54* mutations responsible for foscarnet resistance are usually distinct from those causing ganciclovir–cidofovir resistance. However, low-grade ganciclovir–foscarnet cross-resistance has been reported, plus Chou et al. reported a DNA polymerase mutation causing resistance to ganciclovir, cidofovir, and foscarnet.[172,173,182–184]

Treatment strategies in resistant CMV

When clinically resistant retinitis appears, many clinicians employ an alternative antiviral agent systemically; intravenous cidofovir or foscarnet are alternatives. Unfortunately, as mentioned above, there can be cross-resistance between CMV isolates resistant to ganciclovir and resistant to cidofovir and/or foscarnet; this must be borne in mind in such patients. The probability of developing foscarnet or cidofovir resistance while taking these drugs appears similar to the rates of development of resistance to ganciclovir.[175] For this reason, clinicians often employ intravitreal therapies including the ganciclovir intraocular device when systemic therapy begins to fail. Intravitreal therapies appear to be more effective in such circumstances, largely because they deliver higher doses of anti-CMV medication to the retina.[187] In such circumstances, it is recommended to continue to treat the patient with some form of systemic therapy, often oral valganciclovir, to help prevent systemic CMV infection or infection of the fellow eye. Studies have shown that treatment with the ganciclovir implant alone is associated with a higher risk of contralateral CMV retinitis and extraocular CMV.[188,189]

Combination therapies: ganciclovir–foscarnet

Several studies have shown that combinations of foscarnet and ganciclovir are more effective in the treatment of recurrent or resistant retinitis than is continued monotherapy.[91,189] Such combination intravenous therapy also has been shown to be safe and effective in children with CMV retinitis.[190] Unfortunately, combination intravenous therapy with these two drugs necessitates multiple intravenous infusions daily and has a marked negative effect on patients' lifestyle. Combination of IV foscarnet and oral valganciclovir has supplanted this combination intravenous therapy.

The combination of foscarnet and ganciclovir in patients with AIDS and CMV retinitis who have relapsed has been shown to be more effective than either agent given alone;[143] however, combination therapy was associated with the greatest negative impact of treatment on quality-of-life measures.

To determine the best therapeutic systemic regimen for treatment of relapsed CMV retinitis, a multicenter randomized controlled clinical trial of 279 patients with AIDS and either persistently active or relapsed CMV retinitis was reported. Patients were randomized to one of three therapeutic regimens: induction with foscarnet sodium at 90 mg/kg intravenously every 12 hours for 2 weeks, followed by maintenance at a dosage of 120 mg/kg per day (foscarnet group); induction with ganciclovir sodium at 5 mg/kg intravenously every 12 hours for 2 weeks followed by maintenance at 10 mg/kg per day (ganciclovir group); or continuation of previous maintenance therapy plus induction with the other drug (either ganciclovir or foscarnet) for 2 weeks followed by maintenance therapy with both drugs, ganciclovir sodium at 5 mg/kg per day and foscarnet sodium at 90 mg/kg per day (combination therapy group). The mortality rate was similar among the three groups. Median survival times were as follows: foscarnet group, 8.4 months; ganciclovir group, 9.0 months; and combination therapy group, 8.6 months (P = 0.89). Comparison of retinitis progression revealed that combination therapy was the most effective regimen for controlling the retinitis. The median times to retinitis progression were as follows: foscarnet group, 1.3 months; ganciclovir group, 2.0 months; and combination therapy group, 4.3 months (P = 0.001). Although no difference could be detected in visual acuity outcomes, visual field loss and retinal area involvement on fundus photographs both paralleled the progression results, with the most favorable results in the combination therapy group. The rates of visual field loss were as follows: foscarnet group, 28 degrees per month; ganciclovir group, 18 degrees per month; combination therapy group, 16 degrees per month (P = 0.009). The rates of increase of retinal area involved by CMV were as follows: foscarnet group, 2.47% per month; ganciclovir group, 1.40% per month; and combination therapy group, 1.19% per month (P = 0.04). Although side-effects were similar among the three treatment groups, combination therapy was associated with the greatest negative impact of treatment on quality-of-life measures. This study suggests that for patients with AIDS and CMV retinitis whose retinitis has relapsed and who can tolerate both drugs, combination therapy appears to be the most effective therapy for controlling CMV retinitis.[143] Small series suggest that combined intravitreal injections of ganciclovir and foscarnet may be effective in treating CMV retinitis when the infection is clinically resistant to either intravitreal drug alone.[191]

Summary of initial systemic CMV retinitis treatment

The initial treatment of CMV retinitis is usually oral valganciclovir 900 mg twice a day for induction therapy of approximately 3 weeks followed by 900 mg daily for maintenance therapy. Intravenous ganciclovir can be used if a patient has a contraindication to oral treatment such as malabsorption. The dose for intravenous ganciclovir is 5 mg/kg twice a day for induction therapy for 2–3 weeks followed by maintenance therapy at 5 mg/kg daily or 6 mg/kg 5 days/week. Induction therapy with intravenous foscarnet is dosed at 90 mg/kg twice a day for approximately 2 weeks followed by maintenance therapy at 120 mg/kg daily. Intravenous cidofovir for induction therapy is dosed at 5 mg/kg weekly for approximately 3 weeks followed by maintenance therapy dosed at 3–5 mg/kg every 2 weeks.

Intraocular therapy of viral retinitis

Ganciclovir

Because of the difficulties associated with systemic ganciclovir, foscarnet, and cidofovir, interest in local administration has increased. Obviously, intraocular (or periocular) treatment will not affect the systemic CMV infection, but in some patients, especially those with systemic toxicity resulting from the drug, local administration may have certain advantages.

In 40 patients with primary CMV retinitis involving 57 eyes, all had received one 14-day course of intravenous ganciclovir and all were free of other end-organ CMV disease. All affected eyes received weekly intravitreal injections of 400 mg of ganciclovir for maintenance therapy. Median survival of patients was at least 13 months. Fifteen patients had 19 new opportunistic infections during the observation period, but none developed new nonocular CMV disease. Active retinitis recurred in 68.4% of the eyes while receiving maintenance therapy, with a median time to progression of 14.7 weeks. CMV retinitis occurred in 30.4% of the previously uninvolved eyes (follow-up 3.1 years). Bacterial endophthalmitis complicated treatment in one eye, and retinal detachment developed in five eyes. Thus the long-term treatment of CMV retinitis with weekly intraocular injections of ganciclovir was associated with survival and ocular outcomes similar to those reported with systemic ganciclovir.[192]

Intravitreal ganciclovir also was shown to be an effective alternative to systemic ganciclovir in patients with severe neutropenia and in patients who chose to continue receiving systemic zidovudine or didanosine.[193] Injections of high-dose intravitreal ganciclovir using a 2 mg dose revealed that weekly 2 mg injections appear to offer superior control of retinitis for periods of months or longer.[194] Highly concentrated ganciclovir solution for intravitreal injection also reduced repeated amaurosis and ocular pain and was reported by patients to have improved their comfort and quality of life, thus increasing their compliance to treatment and reducing side-effects, as compared with usual protocols.[195]

Foscarnet

Intravitreal foscarnet at a dose of 2.4 mg per injection given one or two times weekly also appears to be a safe and effective treatment method for CMV retinitis. Resistance to this treatment regimen may develop, however.[196] High-dose intravitreal foscarnet for CMV retinitis was shown to be a safe, effective, and useful alternative in patients with intolerance to intravenous therapy.[197]

Ganciclovir intraocular device

An intraocular sustained-release ganciclovir delivery implant that releases drug into the vitreous is commercially available.[198] These surgically implanted, time-release implants have been shown to be more effective than intravenous ganciclovir alone in delaying the progression of CMV retinitis.[129,199,200]

Insertion of the device requires a pars plana incision and a partial vitrectomy. The implant is sewn into the pars plana behind the lens.[198] Insertion of the ganciclovir intraocular device (GIOD) requires trimming the strut of the device so that it is nearly flush with the drug pellet. A 5.5 mm incision can be made 4 mm posterior to the limbus with a microvitreoretinal blade or similar instrument (Fig. 81.11). A unimanual bipolar intraocular cautery can be used to coagulate bleeding choroid. It is important to ensure that the incision is full-thickness, since the device can be inserted inadvertently under the pars plana. A suture is placed through the preplaced hole (the surgeon must make the hole) in the strut of the device; 8–0 Prolene can be used. The device is anchored in the middle of the wound, and running or interrupted sutures can be used to close the wound. Astigmatism can result from overzealous wound closure; this is usually transient. This procedure can be performed in an outpatient setting under local anesthesia.

Despite the relative ease of insertion, it has become clear that the risk of retinal detachment in the first 2 months after insertion is substantially higher than if other methods are used to control retinitis, though in the long term there is no statistical difference in retinal detachment rate.[198,201–203] In addition, the risk of postoperative endophthalmitis appears to be a real one, with incidences on the order of 1% or sometimes higher.[204] The intravitreal levels attained by this drug are over twice those after intravenous administration, and this appears to be associated with a

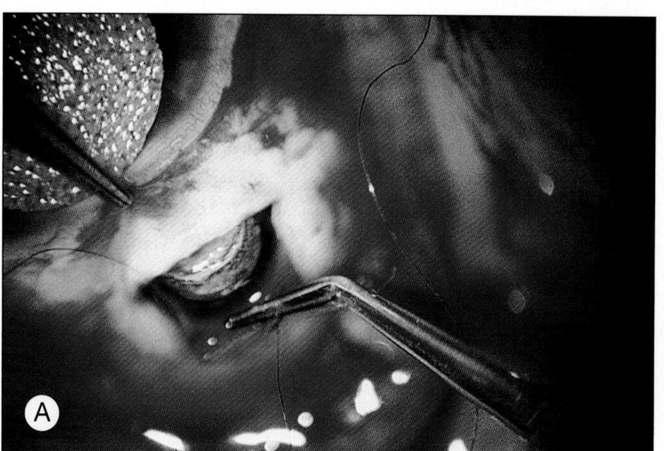

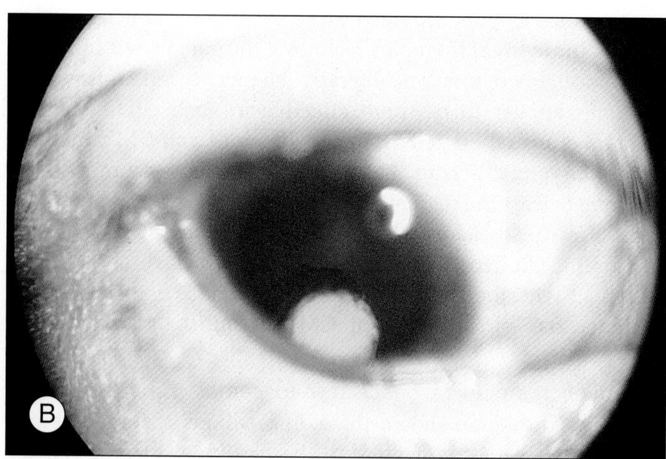

Fig. 81.11 (A) Insertion of ganciclovir intraocular device. (B) The device can be seen inferotemporally through a dilated pupil.

lower incidence of resistance and progression of retinitis. This is particularly true in newly diagnosed cases, but failure can occur in up to 25% of such cases within the first 2 months. In a study of 91 implants in 70 eyes, GIOD was effective as an adjunct to continued systemic therapy in those patients with recurrent CMV retinitis.[200] Intraocular sustained-release implants have been used to treat acute CMV disease and to prevent recurrence. Pathology studies of eyes having undergone implantation with the GIOD have shown no evidence of intraocular toxicity.[136] It is not certain whether implants should be exchanged at the 7-month time period or whether retinitis should be allowed to reactivate before replacing the implant.

Intravitreal cidofovir

Another form of intraocular therapy is intravitreal cidofovir (HPMPC), which is injected every 6 weeks. This work was initiated after discovery of long-acting properties of the drug in the eye. The safety and efficacy of intravitreal cidofovir for CMV retinitis in humans were reported in a phase I/II unmasked, consecutive case series in a single-center institutional referral practice. Eligible patients with AIDS had active CMV retinitis in at least one eye, despite adequate intravenous therapy with ganciclovir or foscarnet, were intolerant to intravenous therapy, were noncompliant with intravenous therapy, or refused intravenous therapy. In a preliminary safety study (group 1), 10 eyes of nine patients received 14 injections of cidofovir while being treated concurrently with intravenous ganciclovir. In a dose-escalating efficacy study (group 2), eight eyes of seven patients received 11 injections of cidofovir as sole treatment for CMV retinitis. The primary outcome was time to retinitis progression. In group 1 eyes receiving 20 μg of cidofovir, the median time to retinitis progression was between 49 and 92 days (mean, 78 days). In group 2 eyes treated with 20 μg of cidofovir with probenecid, the median time to retinitis progression was 64 days (mean 63 days). Hypotony occurred in the two eyes treated with a 100 μg dose of cidofovir and in one of three eyes receiving a 40 μg dose. No adverse effects resulted from the remaining 20 μg cidofovir injections. Cidofovir was found to be safe and effective for the local treatment of CMV retinitis, providing a long duration of antiviral effect (Fig. 81.12).[205]

It was then shown that injections of 20 μg of intravitreal HPMPC resulted in complete suppression of CMV replication with no advancement of retinitis borders when given every 6 weeks.[170,205–209] This medication must be given with oral probenecid. Probenecid 2 g is given orally 2 hours before, and 1 g 2 hours and 8 hours after injection.

Two types of adverse events may occur after intravitreal cidofovir injection: iritis and hypotony. The incidence of these is not dissimilar to what is seen after intravenous administration. The incidence of iritis can be reduced from 70% to 18% if oral probenecid is used, and it is now recommended universally. Iritis can be managed with topical steroids and cycloplegia; however, it may lead to cataract and synechiae in the long term. A mild, asymptomatic 20% reduction in intraocular pressure (IOP) is seen almost universally after cidofovir injection, and this appears to be of no concern. The mechanism of this has been defined by ultrasound biomicroscopy, which has disclosed that severe hypotony after cidofovir injections is associated with ciliary body atrophy.[206] Reduction in aqueous flow has been demonstrated by aqueous fluorophotometry. This effect on secretory epithelia also is probably responsible for the nephrotoxicity of the drug when given intravenously. Indeed, probenecid also is given before and after each intravenous infusion to prevent uptake by the proximal tubule of the kidney and associated nephrotoxicity. Profound hypotony with vision loss occurs in approximately 1% of injections.

A retrospective, cohort study described iritis and hypotony after treatment with intravenous cidofovir for CMV retinitis in association with intraocular inflammation.[168] Eleven cases of iritis (26%) occurred among 43 patients. In six cases the iritis was bilateral. Patients who experienced iritis were more likely to have been previously treated for CMV retinitis (P = 0.03), to be diabetic (P = 0.05), or to be receiving protease inhibitors (P = 0.001). The onset of iritis occurred at a mean (±SD) of 4.9 ± 1.8 days after a cidofovir dose and after a mean (±SD) of 4.2 ± 1.6 doses of cidofovir. Six eyes of four patients had hypotony. Five eyes of five patients had a persistent decrease in visual acuity of at least 2 Snellen lines. Acute intraocular inflammation may occur with or without hypotony after intravenous cidofovir therapy, similar to the reactions seen after intravitreous

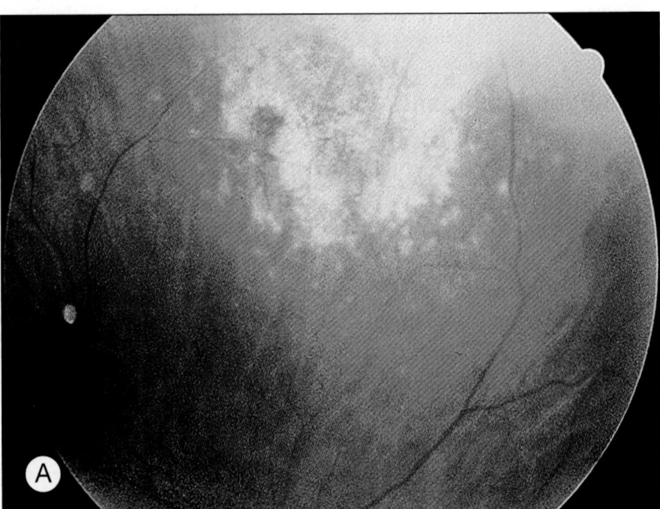

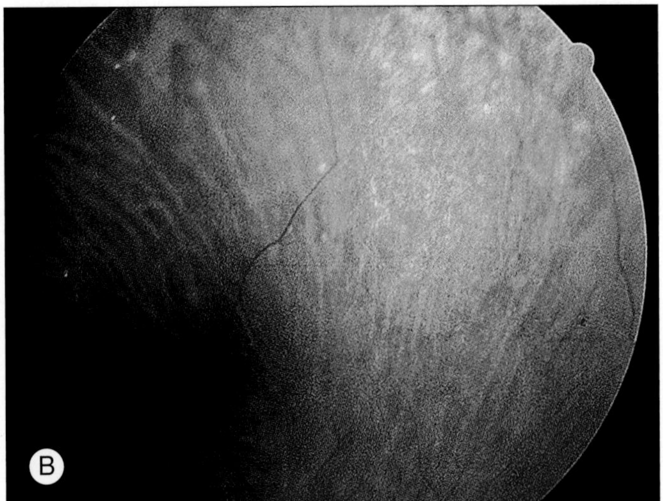

Fig. 81.12 (A) Active CMV retinitis with no systemic treatment. The eye was injected with a single injection of cidofovir 20 μg via the pars plana. (B) The retinitis remains healed 53 days later, with no other therapy.

administration. Cidofovir therapy can be continued in some patients if medical necessity warrants, but inflammation may recur or permanent hypotony develop.

A lower cidofovir dose (10 µg) has been used to investigate methods of reducing the toxicity of intravitreal cidofovir. This dose is effective in healing retinitis in 75% of patients, but the response in 25% is inadequate. The 10 µg dose, however, is not associated with a significant incidence of iritis or IOP lowering. Cidofovir should be diluted in a sterile manner by a pharmacist. It can be diluted in normal saline and frozen for extended periods in single-dose vials.

The efficacy and safety of multiple intravitreal cidofovir (HPMPC) injections given every 5–6 weeks for the maintenance treatment of CMV retinitis with 20 µg intravitreally injected was shown to be highly effective, with only rare episodes of reactivation and progression.[170]

A correlation between IOP and CD4 T-lymphocyte counts in patients with HIV with and without CMV retinitis has been described.[210] IOP was measured with calibrated Goldmann applanation tonometers in two groups of patients. Group A included 84 HIV patients (120 eyes) with CMV retinitis, and group B included 110 HIV patients (183 eyes) without CMV retinitis; 33 patients without HIV (66 eyes) were included as a control group. Step-wise regression analysis of IOP included correlation with CMV retinitis (presence, extent, and activity), CD4 T-lymphocyte count, age, and gender. The mean IOP was 9.8 mmHg in group A, 12.6 mmHg in group B, and 16.1 mmHg in the control group. All three groups were statistically different from each other when intraocular pressure was compared ($P < 0.0001$). Step-wise regression showed that low CD4 T-lymphocyte count and extent of CMV retinitis both correlated to low IOP. These results demonstrate that IOP is lower than normal in patients with HIV and that decreased CD4 T-lymphocyte count is the major factor associated with low IOP, accounting for 20% of the effect. The extent of CMV retinitis accounts for 8% of the effect.

Fomivirsen

Fomivirsen, formerly called ISIS 2922, was approved by the FDA in August 1998 for the treatment of CMV retinitis in AIDS patients intolerant of or who have a contraindication to other CMV regimens or who were insufficiently responsive to previous treatments for CMV retinitis. Fomivirsen is the first of a class of antisense oligonucleotides. This compound possesses potent anti-CMV activity, but does not target the CMV viral DNA polymerase. Fomivirsen is a 21-base synthetic phosphorothioate oligonucleotide designed to be complementary to CMV mRNA that encodes for the major immediate early region (IE2) proteins of CMV. Binding to this location results in specific inhibition of gene expression that is critical to production of essential viral proteins.[211–213]

Following intravitreal administration, the rate of vitreous clearance of fomivirsen is first-order with a half-life of approximately 55 hours in humans. Measurable concentrations of drug are not detected in the systemic circulation after intravitreal injection making the interaction of fomivirsen with systemic drugs unlikely. Preclinical studies of fomivirsen by Freeman and associates suggested that this type of antiviral antisense compound does inhibit viral replication; however, it did cause changes in the RPE and intraocular inflammation at doses only moderately higher than the dose needed to treat retinitis by the intravitreal route.[214]

The Vitravene Study Group published the data from the clinical trials involving fomivirsen. Two prospective randomized open-label controlled clinical trials (USA/Brazilian and EuroCanadian Studies) compared two fomivirsen regimens for the treatment of reactivated CMV retinitis or CMV retinitis that was persistently active despite other anti-CMV treatments. The more intense schedule (regimen A) included 61 patients (67 eyes) and consisted of three weekly 330 µg (0.05 ml) intravitreal injections for induction, then 330 µg every 2 weeks for maintenance therapy. The less intense schedule (regimen B) included 32 patients (39 eyes) and utilized a 330 µg injection for induction on day 1 and day 15, then 330 µg injections every 4 weeks for maintenance therapy. The study endpoint was time to progression based on masked evaluation of serial fundus photos. Eligibility criteria included AIDS patients with active CMV retinitis who had failed prior treatment with ganciclovir, foscarnet, or cidofovir.[215]

In the USA/Brazilian study, median time to progression was 106 days (interpolated median 88.6 days) for regimen A; 267 days (interpolated median 111.3 days) for regimen B ($P = 0.2179$ Wilcoxon rank sum test; 0.2950 log rank). In the EuroCanadian study the median time to progression was not determinable for regimen A; only four patients progressed (25th percentile 91 days). The median time to progression for regimen B was 403 days (interpolated median 182 days).[216]

The safety and toxicity of fomivirsen was also reported by the Vitravene study group. The most often reported adverse events were anterior chamber inflammation and increased IOP. Retinal pigment epitheliopathy occurred in 5/10 patients in the trial for newly diagnosed CMV retinitis with the 330 µg dose; this prompted a change to the reported 165 µg dose used for the remainder of the study. No episodes of retinal pigment epitheliopathy were reported with the 165 µ dose. No patients developed retinal pigment epitheliopathy in the 330 µg less intense regimen.

Independent of the randomized clinical trials, there have been reports of Vitravene-induced peripheral retinal toxicity and serious inflammation with vision loss. In clinical practice fomivirsen has been used as a fourth-line drug for CMV retinitis resistant to other therapy. The approved dose of fomivirsen is 330 µg intravitreally every 2 weeks for induction therapy for two doses followed by 330 µg intravitreally every month for maintenance therapy. Fomivirsen is no longer available in the United States.[217]

Investigational agents for CMV retinitis

Maribavir

Maribavir (1263W94), which completed phase II trials but failed to achieve study goals in a phase III trial in 2009, is a benzimidazole compound with in vitro activity against CMV. It does not require intracellular activation and has demonstrated activity against clinical isolates resistant to ganciclovir or foscarnet. The mechanism of action of maribavir is mediated through inhibition of the CMV *UL97* gene product. The drug inhibits viral DNA synthesis through blocking of terminal DNA processing. UL97 is involved in the monophosphorylation of ganciclovir and is essential for viral growth. Maribavir has no effect on the metabolism of HIV protease inhibitors. *UL97* mutants that are compromised in their ability to phosphorylate ganciclovir are fully susceptible to maribavir. In vitro IC50 of maribavir was 0.12 mM compared to ganciclovir at 0.53 mM.[218,219]

Tomeglovir

Tomeglovir is a 4-sulphonamide substituted naphthalene derivative with good activity in vitro against laboratory-adapted and clinical strains of CMV (IC50 1.17 μM vs 5.77 μM ganciclovir). Tomeglovir is also active against ganciclovir-resistant strains. Preclinical studies showed a significant decrease in mortality at all dosages in CMV-infected immunodeficient mice treated with tomeglovir. Metabolism occurs via the CYP3A4 system, although the effects of tomeglovir on the metabolism of HIV protease inhibitors has not been formally reported. Drug-resistant strains of CMV generated by in vitro passage in the presence of tomeglovir contained mutations in the *UL89* and *UL104* genes, suggesting that this novel non-nucleoside class of compounds inhibits CMV by preventing cleavage of the polygenic concatameric viral DNA into unit-length genomes. Safety and tolerability studies of single oral doses (up to 2000 mg) of tomeglovir in healthy male volunteers have been performed without significant adverse events being observed.[220,221]

Rhegmatogenous retinal detachment in CMV retinitis

Retinal detachment is a common cause of vision loss in patients with CMV retinitis. In the pre-HAART era, the incidence rate of retinal detachment in patients with CMV retinitis was approximately 33% per eye per year.[137,144,203,222–224] The incidence of retinal detachment in immunosuppressed patients with CMV retinitis was believed to be higher in patients treated with anti-CMV therapies, specifically ganciclovir.[225–227] These retinal detachments were characterized by multiple peripheral breaks in areas of healed atrophic retinitis; and in some patients severe proliferative vitreoretinopathy resulted (Fig. 81.13).[228] Detachment occurred from weeks to months after institution of intravenous ganciclovir therapy and was frequently bilateral. Retinal detachment may also complicate the course of CMV retinitis.

However, it now appears that rhegmatogenous retinal detachment is associated with healed or active CMV retinitis due to breaks in the necrotic retina.[229] Results of a multicenter, prospective, randomized, controlled clinical trial analyzing incidence and risk factors for rhegmatogenous retinal detachment in a population of patients with newly diagnosed CMV retinitis treated with foscarnet vs ganciclovir revealed that retinal detachment in patients with CMV retinitis is unrelated to the type of intravenous therapy used or to refractive error. The median time to retinal detachment in an involved eye with CMV retinitis and free of retinal detachment at baseline was 18.2 months.[223]

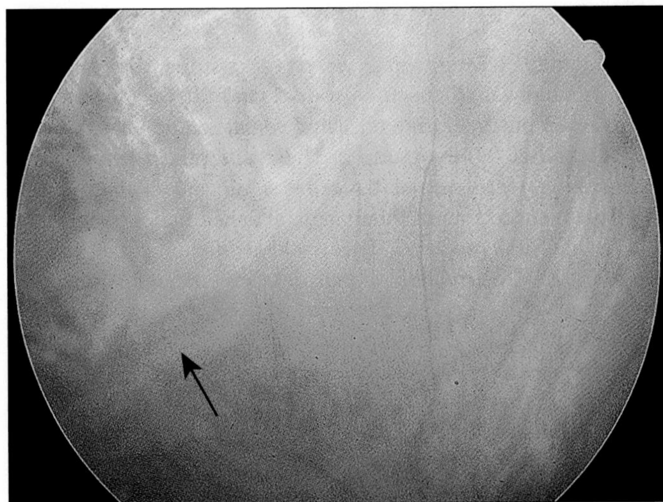

Fig. 81.13 Retinal breaks are seen just peripheral to the area of border opacification; the retina is detached.

Studies have confirmed that the risk factors for retinal detachment in eyes with CMV retinitis include the extent of peripheral CMV disease, as well as retinitis activity and involvement of the anterior retina near the vitreous base.[203,223,230] This is logical, considering that in most cases the causative retinal breaks are within or at the border of healed CMV retinitis lesions. In addition, any intervention that violates the vitreous (e.g. vitreous biopsy or insertion of the ganciclovir implant) would be expected to accelerate the development of vitreous detachment or liquefaction, which would increase the risk of retinal detachment.[199,201,203]

With the advent of HAART therapy the incidence of CMV retinitis-related retinal detachment has decreased by 60%. The success of HAART in the reduction of retinal detachment risk may be related to the improved immune control over CMV replication, thus protecting against progression of disease to larger lesion sizes. The altered pattern of inflammation with HAART-mediated immune improvement may also change the course of vitreous detachment, a key step in the development of CMV-related detachments, thus altering the retinal detachment risk.[199,203,231]

Patients with AIDS and CMV retinitis are surviving longer as a result of the use of HAART and improved treatment of opportunistic infections. As a result, though the incidence rate of retinal detachment is lower, the overall prevalence of retinal detachment may become an increasingly common cause of visual morbidity in these patients. In the pre-HAART era, the incidence and outcome of retinal detachment complicating CMV retinitis were studied at two London AIDS centers. Patients with CMV retinitis were identified prospectively and underwent standard treatment. Retinal detachments were diagnosed during regular follow-up. If retinal reattachment surgery was performed, a standard procedure of vitrectomy and internal tamponade with silicone oil was employed. Of 147 patients with CMV retinitis, 41 (28%) developed retinal detachments (47 eyes); 43 detachments were rhegmatogenous and four were exudative. At the last clinic visit, eight eyes (53%) maintained a visual acuity of 6/60 or better. The visual results of surgery are good in selected patients, bearing in mind the progressive nature of the underlying disease and poor life expectancy.[232]

Vitrectomy with silicone oil tamponade also was studied in eyes with retinal detachments related to CMV retinitis or acute retinal necrosis.[233] Anatomic reattachment was achieved in all eyes, and preservation of ambulatory vision was achieved in most eyes. Visual acuity was limited by concomitant optic nerve disease in some eyes. The authors noted that surgical repair employing silicone oil produces excellent results and that prognosis for vision is strongly related to preoperative visual acuity.

Treatment of retinal detachment consists of vitrectomy, posterior hyaloid removal, and intraocular tamponade with silicone oil or long-acting gas.[234] Retinal reattachment surgery in 29 eyes of 24 patients with AIDS and retinal detachment associated with CMV retinitis was described by Freeman et al.[229] In this study the total retinal reattachment rate was 76%, and the macular attachment rate was 90% after one operation. The mean postoperative visual acuity (best corrected) was 20/60, but in some patients visual acuity decreased because of progressive CMV retinitis. Prophylactic laser photocoagulation of fellow eyes did not appear to prevent retinal detachment (Fig. 81.14).

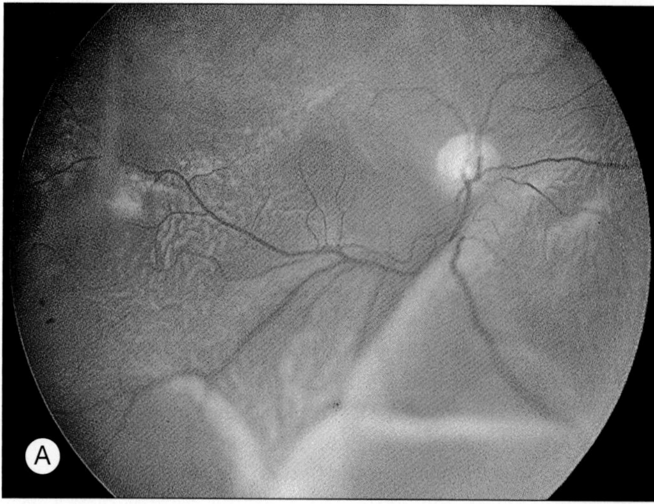

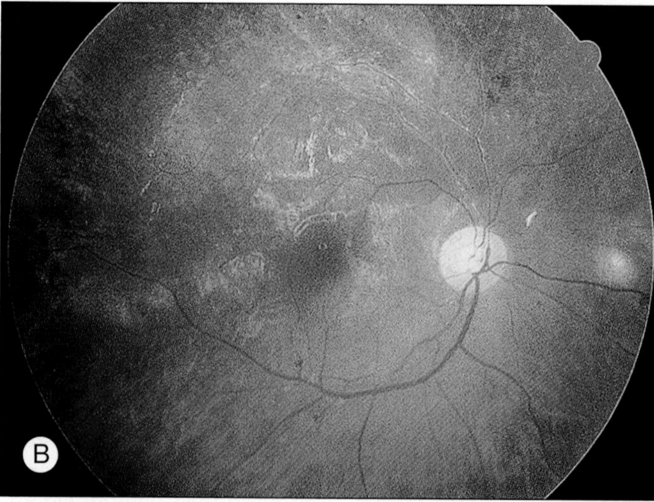

Fig. 81.14 (A) Preoperatively the macula has been shallowly detached, associated with a rhegmatogenous CMV-related retinal detachment. (B) Postoperatively the retina is reattached; silicone oil is in place, and the visual acuity is 20/40. Good visual recovery may be possible even with macula-off detachments because the detachment may be shallow as the vitreous is well formed; the retina may not be completely detached from the macula, and the macular detachments may be shallow.

The repair of retinal detachment in eyes with viral retinitis is complex and is performed using a combination of pars plana vitrectomy, internal tamponade (usually with silicone oil or a long-acting gas such as perfluoropropane), and endolaser often combined with scleral buckling.[229] Pneumatic retinopexy can cause retinal traction and seldom is useful in these eyes. The most common causes of rhegmatogenous retinal detachment in AIDS patients with viral retinitis are acute retinal necrosis syndrome and previously treated CMV retinitis. In these eyes proliferative vitreoretinopathy occasionally is established at the time of detachment or has the potential to occur as a result of multiple retinal breaks and necrosis combined with intraocular inflammation. Scleral buckling alone often is unsuccessful in these cases because of the numerous areas of retinal necrosis and break formation. Retinal breaks are often not apparent until the time of vitrectomy, and the configurations of the retinal detachments are atypical because of peripheral retinal scarring and adhesion to the pigment epithelium and choroid. Thus in these eyes rhegmatogenous retinal detachments may not extend to the ora serrata. In eyes with CMV retinitis, we have favored an approach using complete delamination of the posterior hyaloid combined with endodrainage and permanent tamponade with silicone oil, although we have had good success with intraocular long-acting gases in cases of more limited retinitis and retinal detachment. We have had a very high surgical success rate with this approach. Patients with AIDS and CMV retinitis appear to be surviving longer, and survival after retinal reattachment surgery has been increased to between 6 months and 2 years.[229]

To determine if scleral buckling is of any benefit in surgical repair of CMV-associated retinal detachment if combined with vitrectomy, silicone oil, and inferior midperipheral endolaser, 22 consecutive eyes with CMV-associated retinal detachments were repaired with vitrectomy and endolaser to all breaks and to the inferior midperipheral retina using silicone oil without scleral buckling. Results were compared with another series of 56 consecutive eyes undergoing vitrectomy, silicone oil injection, endolaser to all breaks, and 360 degrees encircling scleral buckling. Total retinal reattachment rates were 84% for group 1 and 86% for group 2. Rates of macular reattachment were 91% for group 1 and 91% for group 2. Mean best postoperative refracted visual acuity was 20/66 for group 1 and 20/67 for group 2. Median best postoperative refracted visual acuity was 20/74 for group 1 and 20/80 for group 2. These differences between the two groups were not statistically significant. Patients who underwent surgery with the macula attached had a better postoperative visual outcome. Thus, scleral buckling may not be necessary in CMV-related retinal detachment if repaired with vitrectomy, silicone oil, and inferior midperipheral endolaser.[235] Elimination of scleral buckling may reduce intraoperative time, patient morbidity, and the risk of an accidental needle-stick. Patients with macula-on-retinal detachments also should be considered for surgery before macular detachment occurs.[236]

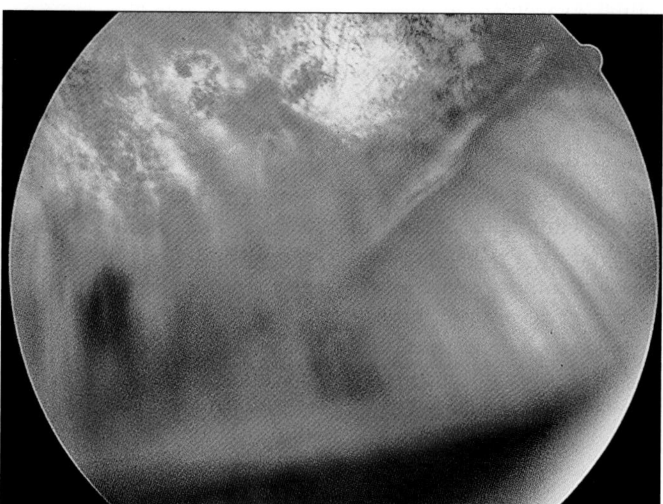

Fig. 81.15 Postoperatively, inferior retinal redetachment posterior to scleral buckle with use of silicone oil. The detachment has been walled off by laser that was applied intraoperatively. Inferior laser photocoagulation may obviate the need for encircling scleral buckling in CMV-related retinal detachments.

The long-term visual results of CMV retinal detachment surgery are still in question, however, and visual acuity may be limited by factors such as refractive problems resulting from silicone oil and cataract[228,237–241] (Fig. 81.15). In addition, posterior capsule fibrosis is very common if subsequent cataract surgery is performed in the presence of silicone oil. Methods to reduce visual acuity loss from cataract include judicious use of gas tamponade with scleral buckling instead of silicone oil, and removal of silicone oil prior to or at the time of cataract surgery. Posterior capsule fibrosis can be treated with Nd:YAG capsulotomy, though success is higher if the silicone oil has been previously removed.[238]

The general operative approach to these eyes is by pars plana vitrectomy, and the surgeon should leave the lens intact whenever possible. After the vitreous gel is removed, all epiretinal membranes are segmented and traction is removed, allowing the retina to become mobile. In some cases the peripheral vitreous gel is adherent to the necrotic peripheral retina and cannot be removed without causing further retinal damage. The use of a soft-tipped extrusion needle may allow the surgeon to remove the posterior hyaloid over broad areas of the retina. A posterior retinotomy is made, and, if an endoretinal biopsy is to be performed, it is done at the location of the posterior retinotomy that will be used for internal drainage.[229,234] A pneumohydraulic exchange is made through the retinotomy site, attaching the retina and filling the eye with air using a constant-pressure, sterile, air-delivery pump. Retinopexy is placed around all breaks in eyes to be treated with a long-acting gas. The peripheral retina may be encircled with either a small buckle or a band to relieve vitreous base traction, which may become a problem later in these inflamed eyes. In eyes with widespread retinal necrosis, most surgeons use silicone oil because it permanently tamponades all retinal breaks, including future sites of retinal necrosis and break formation.

In the HAART era, PVR may be seen in CMV detachment. This may be due to immune recovery uveitis causing a propensity to intraocular inflammation.[242] The management of CMV-related rhegmatogenous retinal detachments has been reviewed.[243] Certainly, it may be useful in acute retinal necrosis (ARN) because rhegmatogenous retinal detachment develops in a large number of patients with ARN. Similar considerations apply in bilateral healed CMV retinitis. The difficulty in both diseases is that all areas of retinal involvement must be surrounded with three rows of argon laser treatment. It is often impossible to carry out treatment to the ora serrata, however, and fluid may leak anteriorly and cause retinal detachment despite treatment. The widespread availability of the indirect laser ophthalmoscopic delivery system should solve this problem. In addition, subretinal fluid may break through a wall of laser treatment if the mass of detached retina and subretinal fluid is relatively large. For this reason most surgeons advocate placement of a panretinal type of pattern within the area of healing retinitis as well.[244–247]

HIV disease/CMV retinitis in the HAART era

Since the advent of HAART many patient have had dramatic restoration of immune system function. This also may be associated with a sustained drop in the plasma HIV viral load to low or undetectable levels. This suppression of plasma viremia may be prolonged; however, the HIV genome may still be found.[37,248] As mentioned earlier, with the prevalent use of HAART, the incidence of CMV retinitis has decreased approximately 75%.[249–252] For patients with CMV retinitis on HAART the risk of vision loss is lower,[249] the risk of retinal detachment is approximately 60% less, and long term survival is much higher.[203,249]

In fact, for patients who have healed CMV retinitis and respond to HAART, discontinuation of maintenance therapy for CMV disease has been shown to be safe in a subset of patients.[249,253–257] We have found that some of these patients may discontinue anti-CMV therapy without reactivation of retinitis (Fig. 81.16). These data suggest that HAART therapy also is permitting at least partial immune reconstitution in some patients. Thus a trial of withdrawal of CMV therapy may be indicated in some patients with good response to HAART therapy and well-healed CMV retinitis. Patients should have a sustained CD4 count elevation of over 100 cells/mm^3 for at least 3–6 months before discontinuing anti-CMV treatment and should be carefully monitored for reactivation. Reactivation of CMV retinitis may occur after successful HAART therapy when the CD4 count diminishes.[258] In addition, some patients may develop CMV retinitis on HAART with CD4 counts above 100/μl, probably because of incomplete restoration of the immune repertoire against CMV.[122]

The effects of HAART on the natural history of other AIDS-related opportunistic disorders have been summarized[259,260] and reflect the improvement or resolution of changes in the natural history of these disorders with inflammatory syndromes. The development of CMV retinitis relatively soon after initiation of HAART has been described.[261]

Immune recovery uveitis

In conjunction with the dramatic improvements in the immune system reported in some patients on HAART therapy, inflammation at sites of OIs is common, and related to recovery of immunity with effective antiretroviral therapy.[262] The syndrome

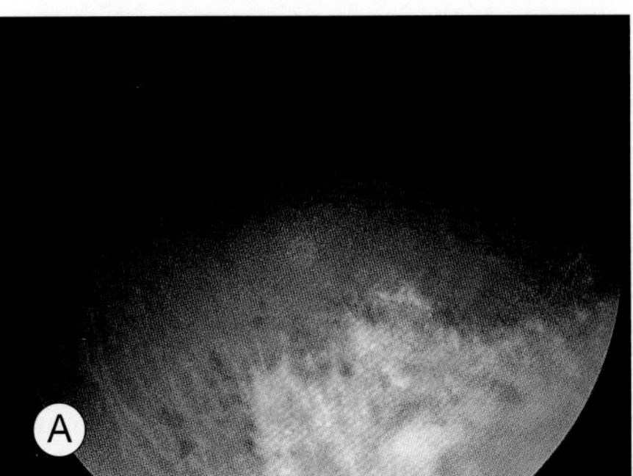

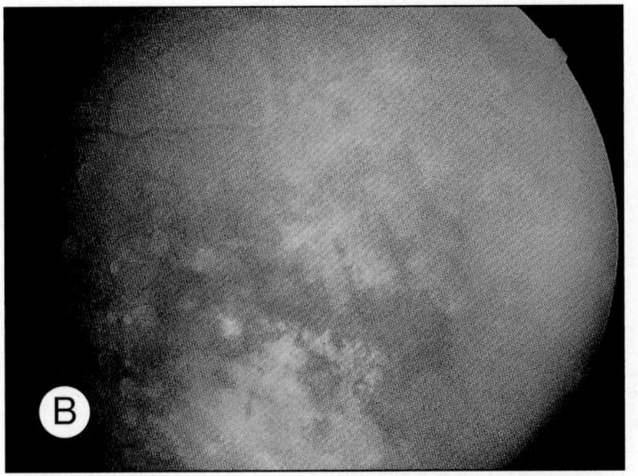

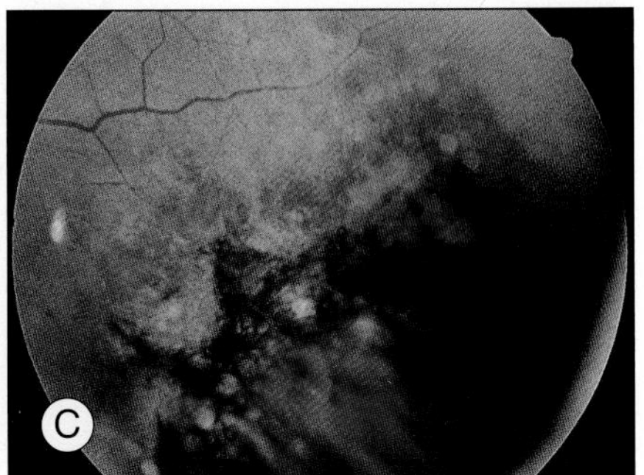

Fig. 81.16 (A) Active CMV retinitis required treatment with systemic ganciclovir. (B) The patient was subsequently treated with highly active antiretroviral therapy, with increase in CD4+ cell count to over 100 cells/ml. The retinitis had remained healed. (C) The patient's systemic anti-CMV therapy was withdrawn, and the retinitis has remained healed for over 6 months. The CD4+ cell count remains over 100.

has been described in the eye as "immune recovery vitritis" or "immune recovery uveitis" (IRU).[263–269]

Immune recovery uveitis appears to occur in eyes with healed CMV lesions in patients with immune reconstitution on HAART. The incidence rate of this phenomenon has varied, with reports from 0.11 to 0.83 per person-year in HAART responders with CMV retinitis.[268,269] Jabs et al. reported the frequency of IRU at 15.5% of 200 prevalent cases of CMV retinitis.[270] Arevalo et al. reported IRU in 37.5% of 32 patients.[271] Eyes in which CMV retinitis lesions involve large surface areas of retina seem to be at higher risk for the development of IRU.[272] Previous treatment with cidofovir may also be a risk factor.[273] Patients with IRU exhibit signs of inflammation such as iritis, vitritis, macular edema, and epiretinal membrane formation (Fig. 81.17).[274–277] Cataract, vitreomacular traction, proliferative vitreoretinopathy, optic disc and retinal neovascularization, panuveitis with hypopyon, and uveitic angle closure glaucoma with posterior synechia have also been reported in IRU.[278–284] Vision loss from these inflammatory sequelae may range from mild to moderate and is usually associated with macular edema and associated macular surface changes or cataract in most cases.

The pathophysiology of IRU is not well understood. One hypothesis is that once the CMV retinitis is healed and the immune system is reconstituted, the patient can mount an inflammatory response to residual CMV antigens in retinal glial cells in or adjacent to the necrotic CMV lesion. Another hypothesis is that control of CMV retinitis is incomplete in certain individuals with continued subclinical virus or viral protein production that stimulates the immune system. It has been reported that CMV antigens persist in cells of all retinal layers at the borders of clinically healed CMV lesions and in CMV infected retinal glial cells after treatment with ganciclovir.[283–285]

Periocular steroids may be used successfully to treat this disorder, but ophthalmologists should be aware of CD4 cell counts. It appears that if the CD4 cell count is elevated above 60/mm^3, treatment of immune recovery vitritis can be carried out without reactivation of retinitis (Fig. 81.13).[262,278] Recently, one case of reactivated CMV retinitis has been reported after treatment of IRU with periocular steroids.[286] Intravitreal triamcinolone is also effective in reducing macular edema, however, caution is needed not to reactivate retinitis.[287,288]

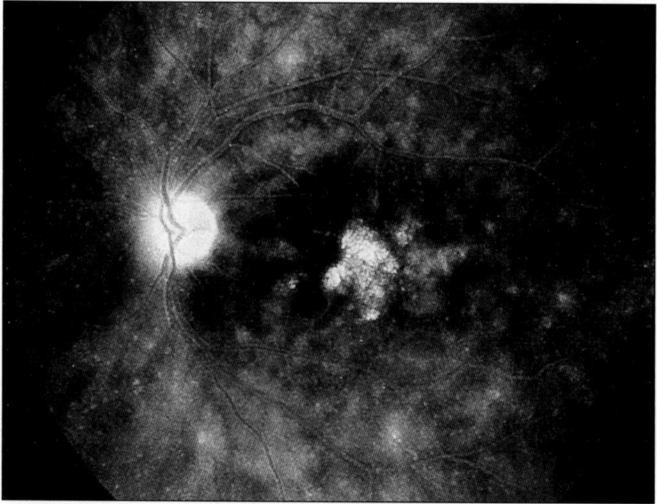

Fig. 81.17 Macular edema in a patient with immune recovery uveitis.

Other complications of CMV retinitis

Central visual loss in AIDS patients with CMV retinitis occurs in two forms: direct macular tissue destruction and secondary involvement as part of rhegmatogenous retinal detachment. We treated 32 patients (35 eyes) with macular exudation that caused reversible visual loss and initially manifested as neurosensory retinal detachment and lipid exudates. Of 35 eyes, 25 showed papillary or peripapillary active retinitis and 10 showed retinitis 1500–3000 μm from the fovea. Of 23 eyes with reduced vision that were followed up until healing of the retinitis and resolution of subretinal fluid and lipid exudates, 22 (96%) showed visual improvement with anti-CMV treatment. Our findings suggest that macular exudation is a reversible cause of visual loss in patients with CMV retinitis.[107]

Cystoid macular edema can occur in the setting of resolving CMV retinitis in patients with immunodeficiency other than AIDS. This entity is distinct from serous macular exudation, which can occur in patients with AIDS with active CMV retinitis involving the posterior pole.[289]

Herpetic retinitis

Acute retinal necrosis in HIV patients

Acute retinal necrosis (ARN) has been reported in AIDS patients.[290] It is a devastating disease characterized by the acute onset of a fulminant panuveitis with confluent, well-demarcated areas of retinitis, plus prominent anterior uveitis, occlusive retinal and choroidal vasculitis, vitritis, and papillitis.[54,109,291,292] In most cases the cause of the clinical syndrome of ARN is varicella zoster but HSV can also cause ARN. The retinitis is characterized by deep retinal whitening, minimal hemorrhage, and a rapid progression. In some cases, ARN in AIDS patients may be preceded by VZV optic neuropathy.[293] A history of preceding cutaneous zoster infection may be helpful in making the diagnosis in such cases.[294,295] In addition, the CD4 count is usually above 60/ml.[292] The diagnosis of ARN is clinical based on criteria established by the American Uveitis Society that do not include immune status of the patient.[296]

No evidence of retinal vascular abnormalities may be present either clinically or angiographically early in the course of ARN. Retinal detachment is a common sequela, with multiple retinal breaks evident within areas of retinal necrosis. Retinal atrophy, often accompanied by proliferative vitreoretinopathy, is a common endstage finding, and there may be associated anterior uveitis, scleritis, and ocular hypotension.[109]

Large numbers of herpesvirus particles in retinal tissue affected with ARN have been demonstrated by electron microscopy using endoretinal biopsy techniques. Virus may be detectable only during the acute phase of the disease.[109] Necrotic retinal tissue or retina reduced to thin glial remnants may not demonstrate virus. The difficulty in growing virus from these specimens is consistent with the hypothesis of VZV as the causative agent, since VZV is difficult to isolate and grow in vitro. CMV initially was believed to be the presumed infectious agent of ARN, but subsequent studies have not confirmed this.[297]

Studies employing endoretinal biopsy and PCR techniques have enabled definitive identification and culture of the causative virus, which has important diagnostic and therapeutic implications. Recent studies have suggested that combination antiviral therapy given intravenously (usually acyclovir or ganciclovir in combination with foscarnet), if given promptly, can arrest the disease and salvage vision.[189] Retinal detachment in VZV retinitis is common (up to two-thirds of patients) and may be associated with PVR or retinal shortening. Repair with vitrectomy and silicone oil after relief of traction with membrane segmentation and sometimes retinotomy may result in useful vision.[189,298] Prophylactic barrier laser around lesions should be considered to lower the risk of retinal detachment in ARN.

Ganciclovir has good efficacy against all herpesviruses but has a lower therapeutic index and must be given indefinitely because it acts as a virostatic agent. Determination of a specific viral cause early in the course of the disease when large numbers of viral particles are present is therefore imperative. Both HSV and VZV may be sensitive to acyclovir. However, VZV requires higher serum concentrations than HSV. Treatment for ARN in AIDS patients is usually based on established treatment for non-HIV-infected patients. Acyclovir IV 500 mg/m^2 or 10 mg/kg every 8 hours is effective followed by oral famciclovir 500 mg TID, acyclovir 800 mg five times a day or valacyclovir 1000 mg TID for maintenance therapy.[85] Duration of maintenance therapy is controversial, with reports of contralateral ARN infection decades later.[299] This may support lifetime maintenance therapy, especially in immunosuppressed AIDS patients. Valacyclovir 1000 mg TID has been reported effective for initial treatment of ARN in a small series of immunocompetent individuals.[300] Intravenous foscarnet may be used in acyclovir resistant cases.[301,302] Corticosteroids have been used to decrease vitritis in immunocompetent patients with ARN, but steroids are usually contraindicated in HIV patients with advanced immunosuppression.[85,294]

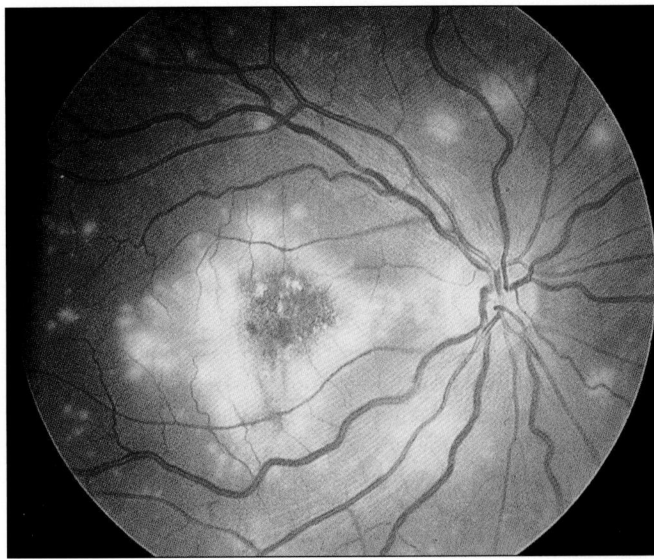

Fig. 81.18 Deep, round retinal lesions seen superior to the optic disc are characteristic of varicella zoster retinitis in AIDS patients, also termed progressive outer retinal necrosis (PORN) syndrome.

Progressive outer retinal necrosis

Progressive outer retinal necrosis (PORN) is another variant of herpetic retinitis in AIDS patients and is nearly always caused by VZV. The incidence of PORN has decreased during the HAART era.[303] It has been described in association with VZV as the onset of retinitis either succeeded by or coincident with an eruption of dermatomal zoster.[304] Most patients with this syndrome have had low CD4 cell counts (i.e., below 50/ml). PORN syndrome is an extremely rapid progressive necrotizing retinitis characterized by early patchy multifocal deep outer retinal lesions (Fig. 81.18) with late diffuse thickening of the retina, absence of vascular inflammation and minimal to no vitreous inflammation.[305] Severe vision loss develops as a result of a widespread retinal necrosis and from retinal detachment, the latter reported in up to 70% of patients in early studies.[305-312] Perivascular clearing of the retinal opacification is characteristic of PORN syndrome (Fig. 81.19).[305]

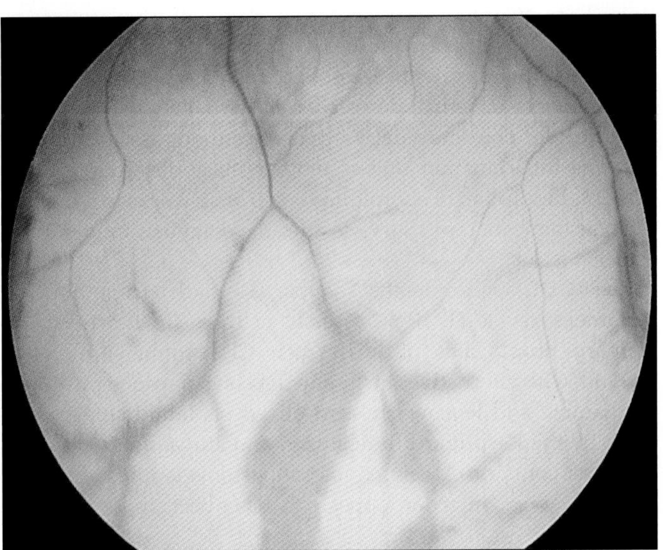

Fig. 81.19 Varicella zoster retinitis in an HIV patient shows retinal opacification and perivascular "clearing." The perivascular edema and necrosis is cleared first; the tissue is not spared.

Therapy of PORN often requires immediate high-dose anti-zoster or -HSV therapy. The earliest reports of treatment of PORN with single intravenous antivirals, primarily acyclovir, showed poor visual results. Engstrom et al. reported final vision of no light perception (NLP) in 67% of 63 eyes within 4 weeks.[305] Poor outcomes with IV acyclovir were possibly due to development of HSV or VZV resistance to acyclovir in patients who developed PORN while on prophylactic anti-HSV therapy with acyclovir. Recent studies have shown improved visual outcomes employing combination intravenous and intravitreal antiviral treatment. Scott et al. reported final vision of 20/80 or better in 5 of 11 eyes (45%) with only two of 11 eyes (18%) progressing to NLP vision utilizing a regimen of intravitreal ganciclovir and foscarnet plus IV foscarnet and IV ganciclovir or oral valganciclovir. In addition, the authors' data suggested that laser demarcation may be beneficial to decrease the rate of retinal detachment.[306] Combination of antiviral drugs and HAART preserved vision in a report by Kim et al.[312]

Nonviral intraocular infections in AIDS patients

Nonviral intraocular infections have been reported in AIDS patients. Autopsy studies have documented numerous infections. Many of the opportunistic infections seen in patients with AIDS can be prevented with appropriate prophylactic agents.[313]

Pneumocystis carinii choroidopathy

In 1987 Macher and associates[314] described a patient with AIDS with disseminated pneumocystosis, and choroidal *P. carinii* was found at autopsy; no clinical correlation was reported. In 1989 Rao and colleagues[58] reported the histopathologic findings in an autopsy series of three patients with AIDS who clinically demonstrated yellow choroidal infiltrates while receiving aerosolized pentamidine for *P. carinii* pneumonia (PCP) prophylaxis. In two cases a presumptive diagnosis of disseminated pneumocystosis was made by ophthalmologic examination. Histopathologically, the choroidal infiltrates were eosinophilic, acellular, vacuolated, and frothy, with the infiltrates within the choroidal vessels and choriocapillaris. Both Gomori's methenamine-silver stain and electron microscopy demonstrated organisms.

In 1989 Freeman et al. described a woman with AIDS with multifocal, slowly enlarging, round-to-oval lesions in the choroid.[315] Fluorescein angiography revealed early hypofluorescence with late staining of the lesions, which appeared deep to the retinal circulation, without evidence of retinal involvement or inflammation (Fig. 81.20). A transscleral choroidal biopsy revealed, by electron microscopy, cystic structures characteristic of *P. carinii* within necrotic choroid.

A multicenter study of pneumocystis choroidopathy in 1991 reported 21 patients with AIDS and presumed *P. carinii* choroidopathy.[316] The lesions were characteristically yellow to pale yellow, appeared in the choroid, and were found in the posterior pole. They enlarged slowly before systemic anti-pneumocystis therapy and eventually resolved. Of 21 patients, 18 were receiving topical therapy with aerosolized pentamidine. There was little evidence of retinal destruction by visual acuity and visual field testing. The choroidal infiltrates were not associated with vitreous inflammation unless another infectious retinitis was present. Resolution of choroiditis took from 6 weeks to 4 months after systemic therapy. Survival after the diagnosis ranged from 2 to 36 weeks.

The CDC recommends double strength trimethoprim-sulfamethoxazole (TMP-SMX) daily or three times weekly for primary prophylaxis of PCP when CD4 counts are below 200/ml, with alternatives including dapsone, dapsone plus pyrimethamine and leucovorin, aerosolized pentamidine administered by the Respirgard II nebulizer, and atovaquone.[313] PCP is the most common AIDS-defining opportunistic infection. Choroidal *P. carinii* infection appears to have been more common when the prophylactic use of nonsystemically absorbed aerosolized pentamidine for PCP was widespread. The choroidal lesions of *P. carinii* appear as pale, cream- or orange-colored, space-occupying lesions from several hundred to several thousand microns in size and they rarely are symptomatic or lead to a decrease in visual acuity. The lesions may be unilateral or bilateral.[58,315,317–319] *P. carinii* choroidopathy appears to be a marker for disseminated pneumocystosis and should be treated systemically. The need for maintenance systemic therapy for choroidopathy has not been established.

Although the diagnosis of disseminated pneumocystosis may be suggested by the characteristic appearance of *P. carinii* choroidopathy, isolated retinal disease may rarely be the earliest clinical manifestation of disseminated pneumocystosis. The incidence of *P. carinii* choroiditis has decreased, probably because of more widespread use of systemic PCP prophylaxis such as trimethoprim–sulfamethoxazole, immune restoration from HAART, and decreased use of aerosolized pentamidine for prophylaxis and therapy.[320]

Ocular toxoplasmosis

Toxoplasmosis is a common CNS opportunistic infection in patients with AIDS. Ocular toxoplasmosis is much less common,[62,321,322] with reported incidence of 3% in HIV-infected patients in France.[323] US incidence is decreased in the HAART era by immune restoration and primary toxoplasmosis prophylaxis with TMP-SMX for those with CD4 counts less than 200/ml.[85] Eight patients with presumed ocular toxoplasmic retinochoroiditis were described in 1988 by Holland et al.[62] In two cases the diagnosis was confirmed histologically. Lesions were usually bilateral (5/8) and multifocal, with vitreous inflammation noted clinically. Therapy resulted in remission, but reactivation and disease progression followed in two of three patients when therapy was stopped. Three patients had retinal tears or detachment as a result of severe retinal necrosis. The ocular lesions were the first manifestation of toxoplasmosis in four of five patients with disseminated disease, although all patients had pre-existing HIV infection, and in four the diagnosis of AIDS had not been made. In four of five patients with no evidence of nonocular infection, evidence of *Toxoplasma* was demonstrated

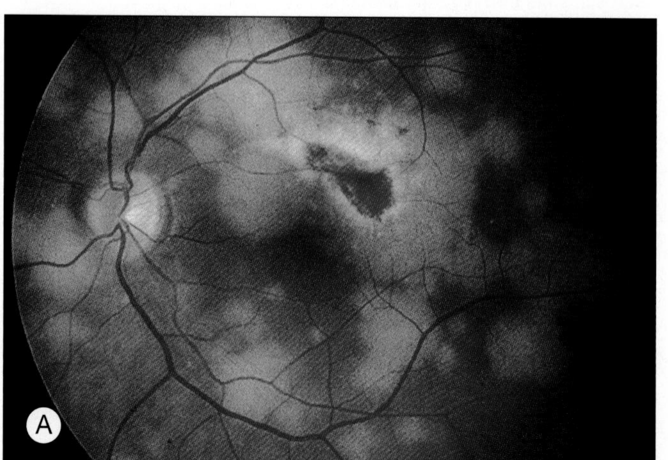

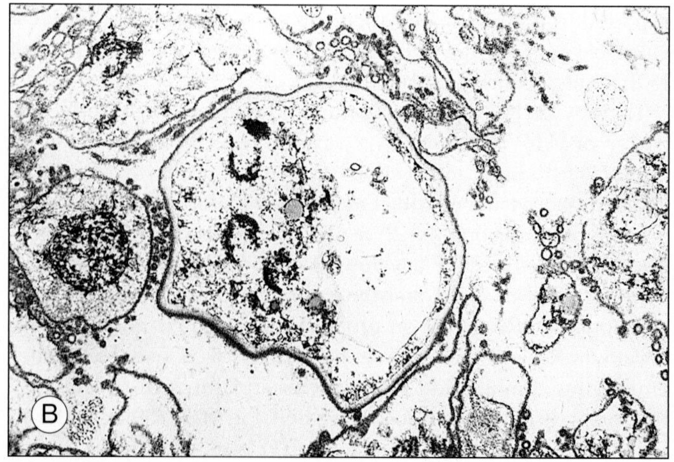

Fig. 81.20 (A) Pneumocystis choroiditis. The round lesions are associated with minimal inflammation. Overlying the lesions in the superior portion of the macula is a typical CMV retinitis lesion. (B) Electron micrograph of *Pneumocystis carinii* organisms seen after choroidal biopsy.

in the CNS (encephalitis or brain abscess). No patient had evidence of pre-existing chorioretinal scars, and all had IgG antibodies to *T. gondii* at the time of diagnosis. Ocular disease was believed to be secondary to reactivation of *Toxoplasma* or to newly acquired or newly disseminated disease to the eye from nonocular sites of disease (Fig. 81.21).

Retinal toxoplasmosis in HIV infection may present as a focal necrotizing nonhemorrhagic retinitis that does not heal spontaneously and may simulate ARN, CMV, or luetic retinitis.[85,324] Prominent vitreous and anterior chamber reaction, relative absence of retinal hemorrhage, and thick, densely opaque yellow-white lesions with smooth nongranular borders suggest toxoplasmosis. Endoretinal biopsy or PCR techniques may be useful if diagnosis is difficult.[85,325,326]

Ocular toxoplasmosis often presents differently in AIDS compared to immunocompetent individuals, spreading as a contiguous or multifocal retinitis. AIDS patients more often have extensive areas of retinal necrosis plus multiple areas of active infection.[327,328] Histopathologic studies show absent to scant inflammatory cells in the infected retina of immunocompromised patients. AIDS patients can develop ocular toxoplasmosis in the absence of preexisting chorioretinal scars. This pattern combined with frequent systemic toxoplasmosis at diagnosis suggests that acquired disease is more common than reactivation of congenital disease.[85,329] For immunocompetent individuals, current evidence also suggests that most patients with ocular toxoplasmosis were infected postnatally, even though the risk of ocular toxoplasmosis is higher from congenital infection[330] (Fig. 81.21). Ocular toxoplasmosis in AIDS patients has also been reported to cause miliary disease, optic neuritis, panophthalmitis, and acute unilateral iridocyclitis without retinal lesions.[331,332] Ocular toxoplasmosis is diagnosed clinically and using PCR from a vitreous fluid sample.

Ocular, as well as disseminated, toxoplasmosis in patients with AIDS is treated with standard antitoxoplasma regimens used in immunocompetent patients such as sulfadiazine (4–6 g/day) or clindamycin in sulfa allergic patients plus pyrimethamine/leucovorin, with apparent response rates of 80%.[333] TMP-SMX was reported in a small (77 patients) randomized trial to be effective and better tolerated than pyrimethamine–sulfadiazine.[334] Other treatments for patients unable to tolerate sulfa drugs such as azithromycin or atovaquone have been primarily studied for CNS toxoplasmosis in AIDS patients and ocular toxoplasmosis in immunocompetent patients.[335–337] Atovaquone was originally synthesized as an antimalarial and has been shown to have activity against both *P. carinii* and *T. gondii*. Ocular toxoplasmosis in patients with AIDS frequently recurs when medical therapy is terminated so maintenance therapy generally is given. Corticosteroids may be given as adjunctive therapy for intracranial toxoplasmosis to reduce cerebral edema, although this is unproved; systemic corticosteroids are sometimes given to reduce inflammation in ocular disease, although these should be administered cautiously in HIV-infected patients. In addition, resolution of ocular toxoplasmosis in AIDS patients has been seen without corticosteroid therapy.[62]

Toxoplasma retinitis is decreasing because of more widespread use of HAART and of prophylaxis, such as TMP-SMX.[320] Currently the CDC recommends consideration of discontinuing maintenance therapy (sulfadiazine plus pyrimethamine/leucovorin with clindamycin used in sulfa-allergic patients) for toxoplasma encephalitis if a patient maintains a CD4 count above 200/ml for greater than 6 months.

Fungal diseases

Candida albicans

Since HIV can be a consequence of intravenous drug use, which is also associated with candidemia, it is surprising that candida endophthalmitis is not seen more frequently in HIV patients. Focal retinal and chorioretinal lesions and endophthalmitis from *Candida* spp. have been described in patients with AIDS.[55,338] Traditional therapy for candida endophthalmitis has been systemic amphotericin B. However, limited vitreous penetration has resulted in treatment failures, plus adverse effects including nephrotoxicity discourage its use.[339] Trials comparing oral fluconazole to IV amphotericin B for systemic candidemia in immunocompetent patients suggested equivalent efficacy with

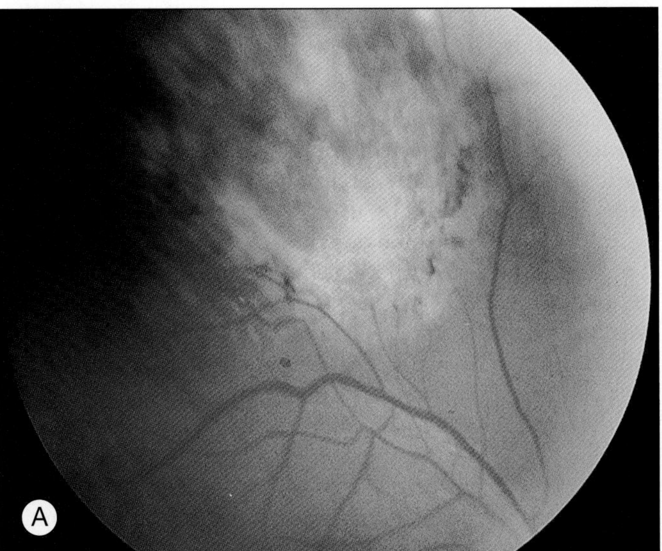

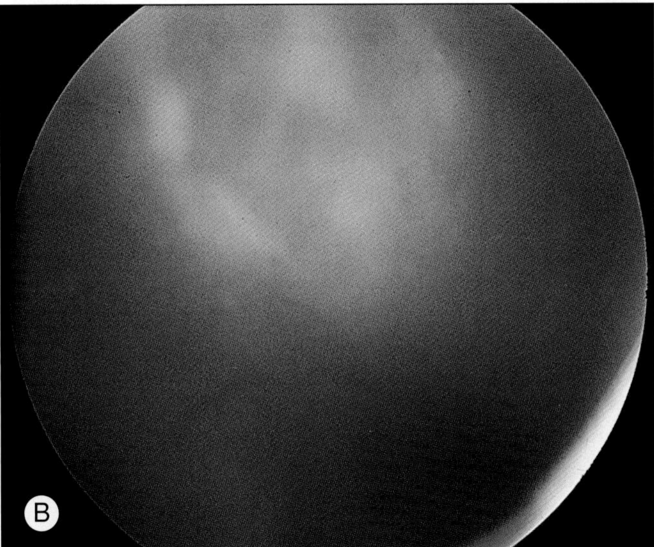

Fig. 81.21 (A) Toxoplasmosis retinitis in an HIV patient who was healed after antitoxoplasmosis therapy with clindamycin. (B) Systemic treatment for toxoplasmosis was withdrawn 6 months later, and the retinitis reactivated.

fluconazole being the less toxic.[340] Vitrectomy and intravitreal amphotericin B can be helpful in cases failing systemic therapy.

Cryptococcus neoformans

Cryptococcal infections may occur in 5–10% of patients with AIDS[341] and are associated with both direct and indirect ocular complications. Cryptococcal infection is a common occurrence in AIDS, resulting in meningitis and secondary ocular involvement. Chorioretinitis, endophthalmitis, or both, caused by direct intraocular invasion of the organism, have been described in immunosuppressed patients.[342,343] Visual loss caused by cryptococcal infection has been demonstrated to result from invasion of the visual pathways, including the optic nerve, tract, and chiasm.

The treatment of cryptococcal disease in patients with AIDS usually consists of an "induction" phase of about 2 weeks followed by a "consolidation" phase of about 8 weeks. Amphotericin B (>7 mg/kg/day) is most commonly used for induction, if possible combined with 5-flucytosine 100 mg/kg daily in four divided doses. If necessary because of toxicity, amphotericin can be replaced by fluconazole (800–1200 mg/day); a third phase of prolonged maintenance therapy with oral fluconazole (200 mg/day) is continued unless CD4 counts are above 200/ml. Ophthalmologic complications of cryptococcal meningitis were seen infrequently before the description of AIDS .

Histoplasmosis

Histoplasmosis was initially reported in patients with AIDS in 1982, and in the next eight years more than 100 systemic cases were reported,[344] mostly disseminated disease that presents as fevers without localized symptoms. The treatment of histoplasmosis in patients with AIDS usually consists of an induction phase with amphotericin B followed by a lifelong maintenance phase with either amphotericin B or itraconazole.[345]

Gonzales et al. reported bilateral endogenous endophthalmitis in an HIV-positive patient presenting with severe subretinal exudation, choroidal granulomas, and intraretinal hemorrhage leading to bilateral exudative retinal detachments. Vitreous cultures grew *H. capsulatum* var. capsulatum. Treatment involved systemic and bilateral intravitreal amphotericin B plus vitrectomy/scleral buckle in one eye.[346] Ala-Kauhaluoma et al. reported a case of panuveitis in disseminated histoplasmosis in an HIV patient treated with liposomal amphotericin B, HAART, and topical steroids that ended up with anterior segment scarring.[347]

Aspergillosis

Endogenous endophthalmitis caused by *Aspergillus fumigatus* rarely has been described in AIDS and can arrive in the eye hematogenously or through extension to the orbit from adjacent sinuses. One case of disseminated, invasive aspergillosis with ocular involvement noted at autopsy was described in 13 patients with pulmonary aspergillosis; no clinical correlation of ocular findings was reported.[348] Whereas four cases of orbital aspergillosis in HIV were reported, ocular aspergillosis is very rare in the HIV population.[349]

Coccidioidomycosis

To our knowledge, no cases of ocular coccidioidomycosis have been described in patients with AIDS. In a retrospective review of 77 patients with HIV infection and coccidioidomycosis, no case of endogenous endophthalmitis secondary to coccidioidomycosis was described, although disseminated disease (including meningitis) was described in a majority of patients.[350] Other unusual mycotic infections causing endophthalmitis, some in association with chorioretinitis, but not necessarily HIV-seropositive patients, are reviewed by McDonnell and Green.[351]

Paracoccidioidomycosis

Severe CNS plus ocular infection with *Paracoccidioides brasiliensis* that simulated CNS and ocular toxoplasmosis has been reported in a pregnant HIV-positive patient. The infection caused severe iridocyclitis, vitritis, plus a granulomatous chorioretinal lesion also involving the optic nerve that ultimately progressed to retinal detachment, NLP vision, and enucleation despite treatment.[352]

Advances in antifungal therapy

Fungal endophthalmitis traditionally has been treated with intravenous amphotericin B. Limitation of vitreous penetration plus systemic toxicity limit its effectiveness.[353] Flucytosine and fluconazole have higher vitreous penetration but are limited by lack of broad coverage against many of the organisms typically seen in fungal endophthalmitis. As a result, vitrectomy and intravitreal amphotericin B is usually recommended in serious fungal endophthalmitis or cases unresponsive to systemic therapy.[354]

The triazole antifungal medications fluconazole, itraconazole, voriconazole, posaconazole, and ravuconazole are orally available and are less toxic drugs that can treat a variety of fungal organisms.[355]

Older drugs such fluconazole, which treats candida, and cryptococci and itraconazole, which treat histoplamosis and aspergillus, remain valuable. Voriconazole has been shown to have mean aqueous and vitreous minimum inhibitory concentrations for 90% of isolates (MIC90) for a wide spectrum of yeast and molds, including *Candida* and *Aspergillus* spp. after oral administration. Voriconazole and posaconazole have also been reported to successfully treat fungal endophthalmitis that was unresponsive to traditional antifungal agents.[356,357] Voriconazole and posaconazole have been shown to have efficacy against *Candida albicans* isolates from HIV patients.[358]

Bacterial retinitis

Syphilis

Concurrent ocular syphilis appears to be more common in HIV-infected than in uninfected persons.[359] Ophthalmic manifestations of syphilis usually occur during or shortly after the secondary stage. Syphilitic uveitis and chorioretinitis in HIV-infected patients have been described. Nine patients with ocular syphilis and concurrent HIV infection were described by McLeish and colleagues in 1990.[360] They found iridocyclitis in three of 15 eyes, vitritis in one eye, retinitis or neuroretinitis in five eyes, papillitis in two eyes, optic perineuritis in two eyes, and retrobulbar neuritis in two eyes. The three of nine patients with AIDS had the worst initial visual acuities. Six of nine had concomitant neurosyphilis. Benzathine benzylpenicillin, the only treatment in three of the patients, led to relapses in all three. Seven of nine patients treated with high-dose intravenous penicillin responded dramatically to therapy with no evidence of relapse.[360]

Concurrent ocular syphilis and neurosyphilis reported in two patients with HIV infection, in addition to a review of 13 other

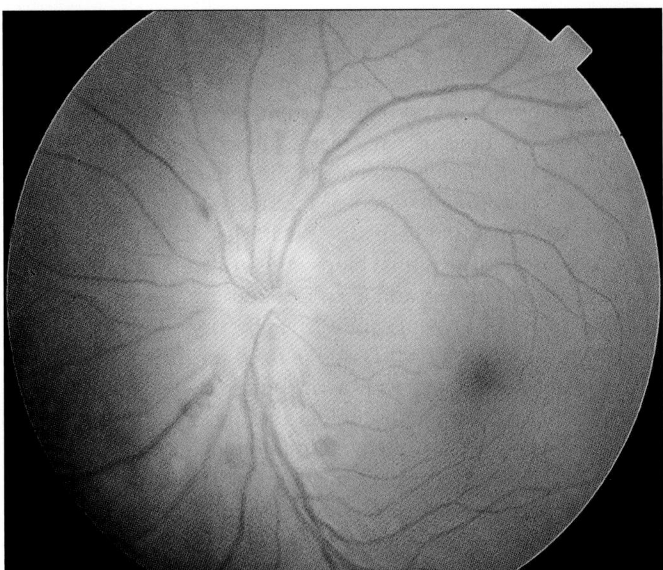

Fig. 81.22 Papillitis and vitritis from syphilis in an HIV-positive patient. Intravenous penicillin resolved the findings.

HIV-infected patients with ocular syphilis, revealed that 11 of the 13 HIV-infected patients with ocular syphilis had neurosyphilis.[361] The authors stress that neuro-ophthalmic syphilis may be the presenting feature of HIV infection and that ocular syphilis is strongly associated with concurrent neurosyphilis in patients that are HIV-seropositive (Fig. 81.22).

Necrotizing retinitis has been reported in a patient with HIV and syphilis. In some cases the appearance of luetic retinitis as a focal expanding white lesion may simulate CMV retinitis, ARN, or toxoplasmic retinitis. Marked inflammation of the vitreous and anterior chamber usually accompanies syphilitic retinal disease with posterior synechiae and keratic precipitates.[82,362]

Standard treatment of primary and secondary syphilis with 2.4 MU of intramuscular benzathine penicillin in patients with and without HIV infection produce similar excellent clinical responses. Serolological responses to therapy (reducing non-treponemal antibody to unreactive levels), the primary method for ascertaining adequate treatment, are less certain in HIV patients.[363]

For retinitis, treatment for neurosyphilis with intravenous penicillin should be used and ceftriaxone may be used when penicillin is contraindicated. With regard to diagnosis, false-negative serum rapid plasma reagin (RPR) and Venereal Disease Research Laboratories (VDRL) may occur uncommonly with HIV-infection. Thus additional, more specific tests are recommended in this population (i.e. fluorescent treponemal antibody, absorbed [FTA-ABS]).[363]

INVASIVE DIAGNOSTIC TECHNIQUES FOR RETINAL DISEASE

In difficult cases, biopsy of the vitreous, choroid, or retina may allow for diagnosis of retinal disease. Vitreous biopsy may yield a diagnosis if a moderate to heavy cellular infiltrate is present. Most modern vitrectomy machines use sterile, disposable tubing and cassettes so that vitreous washings obtained are sterile. These washings may be filtered or centrifuged for appropriate stains, cultures, and cytologic study.

An alternative method may be used to obtain undiluted vitreous at the time of pars plana vitrectomy. After the infusion cannula can be visualized within the eye, the cannula is connected to a sterile, constant-air infusion pump, and a vitrectomy is carried out under air. In phakic eyes, a minus-power contact lens is used to visualize the retina under air. In this way the entire volume of the vitreous cavity may be removed in an undiluted form for study.

Appropriate processing of vitreous obtained as part of a diagnosis is mandatory, and the testing performed should reflect the differential diagnosis. Where infection is suspect, plating of undiluted vitreous on appropriate culture media for aerobic bacteria (chocolate and blood agar, brain–heart media), anaerobic bacteria (thioglycolate media and cooked meat broth), media for acid-fast bacilli, and fungal culture media is imperative and should be done in the operating room. Smears of the undiluted gel should be stained for these etiologic agents, and cytologic smears also should be obtained. In addition, histopathologic stains are useful in ruling out intraocular neoplasms, particularly intraocular lymphoma. Other important diagnostic aids include the use of cytospin preparations that concentrate the cells in vitreous washings, and the use of cell blocks, should enough cellular material be present in a vitreous specimen. The choice of fixatives should be considered carefully. In general, the use of electron microscopic fixatives such as glutaraldehyde may destroy the antigenicity of proteins, rendering immunostaining impossible. Buffered paraformaldehyde will preserve many antigens, although in some cases, frozen, nonfixed tissue is required. In situ hybridization may work on fixed or fresh tissue and can be valuable in determining the presence of pathogenic DNA.[364]

PCR techniques also may be useful in analyzing aqueous or vitreous specimens in difficult cases. Nonfixed fluids are best; they can be frozen for later evaluation or processed fresh. In cases of active retinitis, the test is very sensitive, although it may be somewhat nonspecific because it may detect CMV in the blood in the absence of retinal infection. Choroidal biopsies may be indicated when infiltrative processes of the choroid are seen clinically. Fungal, bacterial, protozoal, or parasitic disease may cause metastatic focal or diffuse infiltrative lesions in the choroid.[365] Tuberculous disease and neoplastic disorders, including lymphoma, also may produce such lesions. All such diseases respond temporarily, if at all, to steroid therapy, and in many cases the diagnosis cannot be made by study of vitreous cells. Before undertaking this diagnostic procedure, prior arrangements for appropriate histologic examination of all materials obtained must be made, since the amount of material that can be obtained is usually small. Any cultures to be taken should be performed by direct plating of the tissue onto the appropriate media in the operating room, as outlined above.

Thorough preoperative examination of the posterior segment is necessary. The choroidal lesion to be biopsied must be well localized. Echography can be used to gain further information regarding the consistency of the lesion and the presence of subretinal or suprachoroidal fluid. It can also be useful in determining if an intraocular lesion has extraocular extension. It is best to select a site distant from the macular area; a nasal area of involvement is best.

In the operating room, the conjunctiva is removed from the limbus 360 degrees, and all four rectus muscles are isolated. Tenon's capsule is cleaned from the quadrant to be biopsied, and the margins of the lesion are marked. It is advantageous to choose a site where a serous or exudative retinal detachment is present overlying the lesion in question because this provides an added margin of safety. A half-thickness scleral dissection is performed 5–10 mm^2 and fashioned into a "trap door." Preplaced 5-0 polyester sutures can be used to allow the trap door to be closed quickly. A smaller area of underlying sclera is closed by diathermy to prevent bleeding, and then an area 3–4 mm on each side is resected. Care is taken to remove choroid and not retina. The trap door is then closed with 5-0 polyester sutures, and the area of resection is examined with the indirect ophthalmoscope. Some sclera should be visible if a full-thickness choroidal biopsy was performed. Retinal incarceration in the biopsy site is a potential source of problems and may have to be addressed using internal pars plana surgical techniques. Vitreous in the biopsy implies retinal incarceration or a retinal break that must be repaired using pars plana vitrectomy techniques. Using this technique, embolic bacterial endophthalmitis, pneumocystis choroidopathy, and other pathologic entities may be diagnosed. Because of the potential to damage the retina or perforate the eye, in some cases it may be preferable to perform a pars plana vitrectomy before choroidal biopsy. This will allow maintenance of intraocular pressure, as well as rapid internal access to the retina should complications arise.

Endoretinal biopsy has been reported to be of value in the diagnosis of viral retinitis. Freeman et al.[109] first reported this technique in 1986. We pursued this technique in patients with CMV retinitis (Fig. 81.23). After healing of retinitis with ganciclovir, rhegmatogenous retinal detachment developed in a large number of these patients as a result of numerous breaks in areas of necrotic and healed retina. We showed in several eyes that persistent infection was present, as viral particles were seen. At this time we do not recommend endoretinal biopsy for all cases of viral retinitis. Rather, we treat such cases with the appropriate antiviral drug and await a response. Response may not indicate a specific viral cause, however, because some drugs treat multiple viruses. In certain cases it is helpful to obtain an etiologic diagnosis. As new antiviral and immunostimulating drugs become available, viral retinitis may not take on the so-called classic clinical appearance, and aggressive diagnostic techniques may become more important. Currently we obtain endoretinal biopsies at the time of pars plana vitrectomy to repair rhegmatogenous retinal detachments in these patients. During these procedures, undiluted vitreous specimens are taken for viral cultures, and in some cases in situ nucleic acid hybridization studies are done. The retinal biopsy (described below) is divided into three small pieces, and each is placed on a small wedge of sterile paper or on an agar sandwich in the operating room using the operating microscope. Tissue is fixed in glutaraldehyde for electron microscopy, as well as in buffered formalin for light microscopy and some immunologic studies. The third piece of tissue may be frozen for further immunologic studies or cultured for virus. It is important to remember that the choice of fixative and tissue preparation technique is critically important; if an incorrect choice is made, it may not be possible to arrive at a diagnosis. Even when obtaining an endoretinal biopsy, the vitreous should also be examined because vitreous biopsy in cases of infectious retinitis may be positive for the causative organism. One can also perform endoretinal biopsy in nondetached retinas. The preliminary results in animals have been encouraging, and refinement of these techniques in the future may shed light on a variety of retinal disorders.

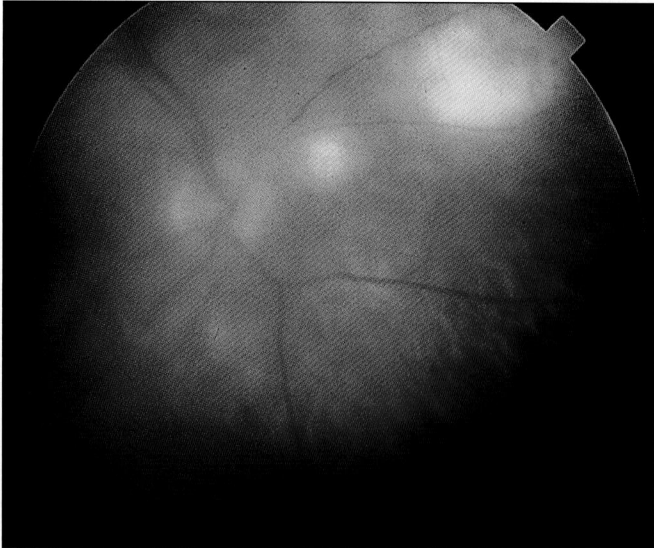

Fig. 81.23 Retinal lymphoma in an HIV-positive patient can present as an atypical retinitis. Diagnosis was made by endoretinal biopsy.

In eyes undergoing endoretinal biopsy a pars plana vitrectomy with complete removal of the hyaloid is performed. The biopsy site also is used for internal drainage. To determine the etiologic diagnosis, it is important to make this location at the junction of healed and normal or active retinitis. Vessels are cauterized only posterior to the biopsy site. We prefer to use the pointed 20-gauge intraocular unimanual bipolar cautery. Low power must be used, and major vessels posterior to the biopsy site are cauterized. Using motorized vertical cutting scissors, a rectangular strip of retina is excised, which crosses the site of active retinitis or the leading border. The strip may be 2 mm wide and 3–5 mm long. It is chosen from an area of necrotic or gliotic nonfunctional retina so that no visual loss occurs. Removal of the tissue from the eye through the 20-gauge sclerotomy with a forceps may crush and mutilate the tissue, so, instead, we prefer to guide the tissue toward the sclerotomy with a pick or pick forceps. The tissue is released, and the instrument is then removed from the eye while the infusion bottle is elevated to the high position. In this way the tissue is hydraulically directed into the sclerotomy site and plugs it. The tissue is gently teased out of the sclerotomy with a 0.12 mm forceps and spread over the cornea, removing all folds.

Any ocular tissue, but particularly small endoretinal biopsy specimens, must be processed with care. The surgeon must decide in advance on the location of the area to be biopsied and the fixatives and numbers of specimens to be processed. We have developed a mount that allows more facile mounting of retinal biopsy specimens.[366] The agar–albumin sandwich technique allows the small piece of retinal tissue to be floated onto a slab of clear agar and then "glued" to it with liquid agar that has been warmed in a microwave oven. When the tissue is draped on the agar, it can be readily identified and not lost during processing. Multiple sections of the tissue can then be cut for processing and immunostaining. The technique also works well for electron microscopy and other morphologic studies.

ANTIRETROVIRAL THERAPY

Expert guidelines for use of these drugs are continuously updated.[367] Many other antiretroviral agents are undergoing preclinical and clinical studies. Currently available drugs do not eradicate latent HIV infection which returns when drugs are stopped (Table 81.1). When used in combination, they usually decrease viral replication, improve immunologic status, reduce risk of infectious complications, and prolong life. Drugs active against the patient's HIV strain should always be used in combination for full potency and prevention of resistance.

SYNOPSIS

The common retinal manifestations of AIDS include noninfectious and infectious retinopathy. Chemotherapeutic agents have been developed to treat all known causes of infectious retinopathy and have been shown to be successful in clinical trials, although they are not without complications. The results of treatment of CMV retinitis with foscarnet, ganciclovir, valganciclovir, or cidofovir are very encouraging, but systemic toxicity and the availability of only one convenient oral preparation, valganciclovir, are serious problems, as is the development of

Table 81.1 Currently licensed antiretroviral drugs in the United States in 2011 by class

Brand name	Generic name	Manufacturer name
Multi-class combination products		
Atripla	efavirenz, emtricitabine and tenofovir disoproxil fumarate	Bristol–Myers Squibb and Gilead Sciences
Nucleoside reverse transcriptase inhibitors (NRTIs)		
Combivir	lamivudine and zidovudine	GlaxoSmithKline
Emtriva	emtricitabine, FTC	Gilead Sciences
Epivir	lamivudine, 3TC	GlaxoSmithKline
Epzicom	abacavir and lamivudine	GlaxoSmithKline
Retrovir	zidovudine, azidothymidine, AZT, ZDV	GlaxoSmithKline
Trizivir	abacavir, zidovudine, and lamivudine	GlaxoSmithKline
Truvada	tenofovir disoproxil fumarate and emtricitabine	Gilead Sciences, Inc.
Videx EC	enteric coated didanosine, ddI EC	Bristol–Myers Squibb
Videx	didanosine, dideoxyinosine, ddI	Bristol–Myers Squibb
Viread	tenofovir disoproxil fumarate, TDF	Gilead
Zerit	stavudine, d4T	Bristol–Myers Squibb
Ziagen	abacavir sulfate, ABC	GlaxoSmithKline
Nonnucleoside reverse transcriptase inhibitors (NNRTIs)		
Edurant	rilpivirine	Tibotec Therapeutics
Intelence	etravirine	Tibotec Therapeutics
Rescriptor	delavirdine, DLV	Pfizer
Sustiva	efavirenz, EFV	Bristol–Myers Squibb
Nonnucleoside reverse transcriptase inhibitors (NNRTIs)		
Viramune (immediate release)	nevirapine, NVP	Boehringer Ingelheim
Viramune XR (extended release)	nevirapine, NVP	Boehringer Ingelheim
Protease inhibitors (PIs)		
Agenerase	amprenavir, APV	GlaxoSmithKline
Aptivus	tipranavir, TPV	Boehringer Ingelheim
Crixivan	indinavir, IDV,	Merck
Fortovase	saquinavir (no longer marketed)	Hoffmann–La Roche
Invirase	saquinavir mesylate, SQV	Hoffmann–La Roche
Kaletra	lopinavir and ritonavir, LPV/RTV	Abbott Laboratories
Lexiva	fosamprenavir calcium, FOS-APV	GlaxoSmithKline
Norvir	ritonavir, RTV	Abbott Laboratories
Prezista	darunavir	Tibotec, Inc.
Reyataz	atazanavir sulfate, ATV	Bristol–Myers Squibb
Viracept	nelfinavir mesylate, NFV	Agouron Pharmaceuticals
Fusion inhibitors		
Fuzeon	enfuvirtide, T-20	Hoffmann–La Roche & Trimeris
Entry inhibitors – CCR5 co-receptor antagonist		
Selzentry	maraviroc	Pfizer
HIV integrase strand transfer inhibitors		
Isentress	raltegravir	Merck & Co., Inc.

rhegmatogenous retinal detachment after healing of retinitis. The vitreoretinal surgeon is commonly involved with AIDS patients in two scenarios. Retinal detachment can now be successfully repaired in a high percentage of cases of CMV retinitis eyes with a good visual outcome. Second, in some cases a tissue diagnosis is required because of the possibility of other forms of viral retinitis; this should be kept in mind when treating these patients, as well as the possibility of endogenous bacterial or fungal endophthalmitis. Implantation of ganciclovir implants can successfully control retinitis but may be associated with retinal detachment, endophthalmitis, and vitreous hemorrhage. Noninfectious, AIDS-associated retinopathy, manifested by retinal cotton-wool spots and hemorrhage, is extremely common. The presence of these lesions may suggest the diagnosis of AIDS in the appropriate clinical setting. Although the pathogenesis of these lesions remains obscure, the lesions do not cause visual loss and should not be confused with infectious retinitis. The advent of highly active antiretroviral therapy has changed the short-term natural history of opportunistic infections of patients infected with HIV and is associated with a new ocular inflammatory syndrome, immune recovery uveitis.

REFERENCES

1. Review of draft for revision of HIV infection classification system and expansion of AIDS surveillance case definition. MMWR Morb Mortal Wkly Rep 1991;40:787.
2. Revision of the CDC surveillance case definition for acquired immunodeficiency syndrome. Council of State and Territorial Epidemiologists; AIDS Program, Center for Infectious Diseases. MMWR Morb Mortal Wkly Rep 1987;36(Suppl 1):1S–15S.
3. CDC. HIV prevalence estimates. MMWR Morb Mortal Wkly Rep 2008;57 (39):1073–6.
4. Deeks SG, Smith M, Holodniy M, et al. HIV-1 protease inhibitors: a review for clinicians. JAMA 1997;277:145–53.
5. Zhu T, Korber BT, Nahmias AJ, et al. An African HIV-1 sequence from 1959 and implications for the origin of the epidemic. Nature 1998;391: 594–7.
6. Freeman WR, Lerner CW, Mines JA, et al. A prospective study of the ophthalmologic findings in the acquired immune deficiency syndrome. Am J Ophthalmol 1984;97:133–42.
7. Jabs DA, Green R, Fox R, et al. Ocular manifestations of acquired immune deficiency syndrome. Ophthalmology 1989;96:1092–9.
8. Centers for Disease Control and Prevention [Internet]. Atlanta, GA: CDC; 2002 [cited 2010 Jan 26]. Cases of HIV infection and AIDS in the United States, 2002, HIV/AIDS surveillance report, Vol. 14. Available from: http://www.cdc.gov/hiv/surveillance/resources/reports/2002report/.
9. Hogg RS, Health KV, Yi B, et al. Improved survival among HIV-infected individuals following initiation of antiretroviral therapy. JAMA 1998;279: 450–4.
10. Palella FJ, Delaney KM, Moorman AC, et al. Declining morbidity and mortality among patients with advanced human immunodeficiency virus infection. N Engl J Med 1998;338:853–60.
11. Padian NS, Shiboski SC, Jewell NP. Female-to-male transmission of human immunodeficiency virus. JAMA 1991;266:1664–7.
12. Centers for Disease Control and Prevention [Internet]. Atlanta, GA: CDC; 2002 [cited 2012 Jan 26]. Surveillance of healthcare personnel with HIV/AIDS, as of December 2002. Available from: http://www.cdc.gov/ncidod/hip/BLOOD/hivpersonnel.htm.
13. US Public Health Service. Updated US public health service guidelines for the management of occupational exposures to HBV, HCV, and HIV and recommendations for postexposure prophylaxis. MMWR Recomm Rep 2005; 541–7.
14. Marcus R. Surveillance of health care workers exposed to blood from patients infected with the human immunodeficiency virus. N Engl J Med 1988;319:1118–23.
15. Cardo DM, Culver DH, Ciesielski CA, et al. A case-control study of HIV seroconversion in health care workers after percutaneous exposure. N Engl J Med 1997;137:1485–90.
16. Fauci AS. Immunopathogenic mechanisms of HIV infection. Ann Intern Med 1996;124:654–63.
17. Coombs RW, Welles SL, Hooper C, et al. Association of plasma human immunodeficiency virus type 1 RNA level with risk of clinical progression in patients with advanced infection. J Infect Dis 1996;174:704–12.
18. Hughes MD, Johnson VA, Hirsch MS. Monitoring plasma HIV-1RNA levels in addition to CD4 lymphocyte count improves assessment of antiretroviral therapeutic response. Ann Intern Med 1997;127:929–38.
19. Mellors JW, Kingsley LA, Rinaldo Jr CR, et al. Quantitation of HIV-1 RNA in plasma predicts outcome after seroconversion. Ann Intern Med 1995;122: 573–9.
20. Mellors JW, Rinaldo Jr CR, Gupta P, et al. Prognosis in HIV-1 infection predicted by the quantity of virus in plasma. Science 1996;272:1167–70.
21. Mellors JW, Munoz A, Giorgi JV, et al. Plasma viral load and CD4 lymphocytes as prognostic markers of HIV-1 infection. Ann Intern Med 1997;126: 946–54.
22. O'Brien WA, Hartigan PM, Martin D, et al. Changes in plasma HIV-1 RNA and CD4 lymphocyte counts and the risk of progression to AIDS. N Engl J Med 1996;334:426–31.
23. Welles SL, Jackson JB, Yen-Lieberman B, et al. Prognostic value of plasma human immunodeficiency virus type 1 (HIV-1) RNA levels in patients with advanced HIV-1 disease and with little or no zidovudine therapy. J Infect Dis 1996;174:696–703.
24. Feinberg MB. Changing the natural history of HIV disease. Lancet 1996; 348:239–46.
25. Havlir DV, Richman DD. Viral dynamics of HIV: implications for drug development and therapeutic strategies. Ann Intern Med 1996;124:984–94.
26. Ho DD, Neumann AU, Perelson AS, et al. Rapid turnover of plasma virions and CD4 lymphocytes in HIV-1 infection. Nature 1995;373:123–6.
27. Perelson AS, Newmann AU, Markowitz M, et al. HIV-1 dynamics in vivo: virion clearance rate, infected cell life-span, and viral generation time. Science 1996;271:1582–6.
28. McDonald CK, Kuritzkes DR. Human immunodeficiency virus type 1 protease inhibitors. Arch Intern Med 1997;157:951–9.
29. Gulick RM, Mellor JW, Havlir D, et al. Treatment with indinavir, zidovudine, and lamivudine in adults with human immunodeficiency virus infection and prior antiretroviral therapy. N Engl J Med 1997;337:734–9.
30. Hammer SM, Squires KE, Hughes MD, et al. A controlled trial of two nucleoside analogues plus indinavir in persons with human immunodeficiency virus infection and CD4 cell counts of 200 per cubic millimeter or less. N Engl J Med 1997;337:725–33.
31. Ledergerber B, Egger M, Opravil M, et al. Clinical progression and virological failure on highly active antiretroviral therapy in HIV-1 patients: a prospective cohort study. Swiss HIV Cohort Study. Lancet 1999;353:863–81.
32. Cervia JS, Smith MA. Enfuvirtide (T-20): a novel human immunodeficiency virus type 1 fusion inhibitor. Clin Infect Dis 2003;37:1102–6.
33. Pedersen C, Lindhardt BO, Jensen BL, et al. Clinical course of primary HIV infection: consequences for subsequent course of infection. Br Med J 1989; 299:154–7.
34. Chun T, Stuyver L, Mezell S, et al. Presence of an inducible HIV-1 latent reservoir during highly active antiretroviral therapy. Proc Natl Acad Sci U S A 1997;94:13193–7.
35. Joshi D, O'Grady J, Dietrich D, et al. Increasing burden of liver disease in patients with HIV infection. Lancet 2011;377(9772):1198–209.
36. Update: Acquired Immunodeficiency Syndrome – United States. MMWR Morb Mortal Wkly Rep 1986;35:757–66.
37. Henderly DE, Freeman WR, Smith RE, et al. Cytomegalovirus retinitis as the initial manifestation of the acquired immune deficiency syndrome. Am J Ophthalmol 1987;103:316–20.
38. Update: Universal precautions for prevention of transmission of human immunodeficiency virus, hepatitis B virus, and other bloodborne pathogens in health-care settings. MMWR Morb Mortal Wkly Rep 1988;37:377–88.
39. Leads from the MMWR. Recommendations for preventing possible HTLV-III/LAV virus from tears. JAMA 1985;254:1429.
40. Update: Acquired Immunodeficiency Syndrome – United States. MMWR Morb Mortal Wkly Rep 1985;35:17–21.
41. Key CB, Whitman J. Alcohol soaking damages applanation tonometer heads. Arch Ophthalmol 1986;104:800.
42. Vogt M, Ho DD, Bakar S, et al. Safe disinfection of contact lenses after contamination with HTLV-III. Ophthalmology 1986;93:771–4.
43. Sattar SA. Springthorpe vs Survival and disinfectant inactivation of the human immunodeficiency virus: a critical review. Rev Infect Dis 1991;13: 430–47.
44. Centers for Disease Control and Prevention, Department of Health and Human Services. Guidelines for preventing transmission of human immunodeficiency virus through transplantation of human tissue and organs. MMWR Morb Mortal Wkly Rep 1994;43:1–17.
45. Centers for Disease Control and Prevention. Update: provisional Public Health Service recommendations for chemoprophylaxis after occupational exposure to HIV. MMWR Morb Mortal Wkly Rep 1996;45:468–72.
46. Ablashi DV, Sturzenegger S, Hunter EA, et al. Presence of HTLV-III in tears and cells from the eyes of AIDS patients. J Exp Pathol 1987;3:693–703.
47. Fujikawa LS, Salahuddin SZ, Ablashi D, et al. Human T-cell leukemia/ lymphotropic virus type III in the conjunctival epithelium of a patient with AIDS. Am J Ophthalmol 1985;100:507–9.
48. Freeman WR, Chen A, Henderly D, et al. Prognostic and systemic significance of non-infectious AIDS associated retinopathy. Invest Ophthalmol Vis Sci 1987;28(suppl):9.
49. Freeman WR, Chen A, Henderly DE, et al. Prevalence and significance of acquired immunodeficiency syndrome-related retinal microvasculopathy. Am J Ophthalmol 1989;107:229–35.
50. Cole EL, Meisler DM, Calabrese LH, et al. Herpes zoster ophthalmicus and acquired immune deficiency syndrome. Arch Ophthalmol 1984;102:1027–9.
51. Sandor EV, Millman A, Croxson TS, et al. Herpes zoster ophthalmicus in patients at risk for the acquired immune deficiency syndrome (AIDS). Am J Ophthalmol 1986;101:153–5.

52. Holland GN, Pepose JS, Pettit TH, et al. Acquired immune deficiency syndrome, ocular manifestations. Ophthalmology 1983;90:859–73.
53. Kestelyn P, Van de Perre P, Rouvroy D, et al. A prospective study of the ophthalmologic findings in the acquired immune deficiency syndrome in Africa. Am J Ophthalmol 1985;100:230–8.
54. Lipson BK, Freeman WR, Beniz J, et al. Optic neuropathy associated with cryptococcal arachnoiditis in AIDS patients. Am J Ophthalmol 1989;107: 523–7.
55. Morinelli EN, Dugel PU, Riffenburgh R, et al. Infectious multifocal choroiditis in patients with acquired immune deficiency syndrome. Ophthalmology 1993;100:1014–21.
56. Pepose JS, Hilborne LH, Cancilla PA, et al. Concurrent herpes simplex and cytomegalovirus retinitis and encephalitis in the acquired immune deficiency syndrome (AIDS). Ophthalmology 1984;91:1669–77.
57. Pepose JS, Nestor MS, Holland GN, et al. An analysis of retinal cotton-wool spots and cytomegalovirus retinitis in the acquired immunodeficiency syndrome. Am J Ophthalmol 1983;95:118–9.
58. Rao NA, Zimmerman PL, Boyer D, et al. A clinical, histopathologic, and electron microscopic study of *Pneumocystis carinii* choroiditis. Am J Ophthalmol 1989;107:218–28.
59. Weiss A, Margo CE, Ledord DK, et al. Toxoplasmic retinochoroiditis as an initial manifestation of the acquired immune deficiency syndrome. Am J Ophthalmol 1986;101:248–9.
60. Arevalo JF, Russack V, Freeman WR. New ophthalmic manifestations of presumed rifabutin-related uveitis. Ophthalmic Surg Lasers 1997;28:321–4.
61. Glasgow BJ, Engstrom Jr RE, Holland GN, et al. Bilateral endogenous fusarium endophthalmitis associated with acquired immunodeficiency syndrome. Arch Ophthalmol 1996;114:873–7.
62. Holland GN, Engstrom RE, Glasgow BJ, et al. Ocular toxoplasmosis in patients with the acquired immunodeficiency syndrome. Am J Ophthalmol 1988;106:653–67.
63. Gonzales CA, Scott IU, Chaudhry NA, et al. Endogenous endophthalmitis caused by *Histoplasma capsulatum* var. capsulatum: a case report and literature review. Ophthalmology 2000;107:725–9.
64. Finamor LP, Muccioli C, Martins MC, et al. Ocular and central nervous system paracoccidioidomycosis in a pregnant woman with acquired immunodeficiency syndrome. Am J Ophthalmol 2002;134:456–9.
65. Santos C, Parker J, Dawson C, et al. Bilateral fungal corneal ulcers in a patient with AIDS-related complex. Am J Ophthalmol 1985;102:118–9.
66. Geier SA, Schielke E, Klauss V, et al. Retinal microvasculopathy and reduced cerebral blood flow in patients with acquired immunodeficiency syndrome. Am J Ophthalmol 1992;113:100–1.
67. Newsome DA, Green W, Miller ED, et al. Microvascular aspects of acquired immune deficiency syndrome retinopathy. Am J Ophthalmol 1984;98: 590–601.
68. Freeman WR, O'Connor GR. Acquired immune deficiency syndrome retinopathy, pneumocystis, and cotton-wool spots. Am J Ophthalmol 1984;98: 235–7.
69. Kwok S, O'Donnell JJ, Wood IS. Retinal cotton-wool spots in a patient with *Pneumocystis carinii* infection. N Engl J Med 1982;307:184–5.
70. Faber DW, Wiley CA, Bergeron-Lynn G, et al. Role of human immunodeficiency virus and cytomegalovirus in the pathogenesis of retinitis and retinal vasculopathy in AIDS patients. Invest Ophthalmol Vis Sci 1992;33: 2345–53.
71. Gonzalez CR, Wiley CA, Arevalo JF, et al. Polymerase chain reaction detection of cytomegalovirus and human immunodeficiency virus-1 in the retina of patients with acquired immune deficiency syndrome with and without cotton-wool spots. Retina 1996;16:305–11.
72. Honrubia FM, Ferrer E, Torron C, et al. Study of the retinal fiber layer in patients with acquired immunodeficiency syndrome. Ger J Ophthalmol 1994;3:1–4.
73. Mansour AM, Rodenko G, Dutt R. Half-life of cotton wool spots in the acquired immunodeficiency syndrome. Int J STD AIDS 1990;1:132–3.
74. Kuppermann BD, Petty JG, Richman DD, et al. Cross-sectional prevalence of CMV retinitis in AIDS patients: correlation with CD4 counts. Invest Ophthalmol Vis Sci 1992;33:750.
75. Sadun AA, Pepose JS, Madigan MC, et al. AIDS-related optic neuropathy: a histological, virological and ultrastructural study. Graefes Arch Clin Exp Ophthalmol 1995;233:387–98.
76. Sadun AA, Tenhula WN, Heller KB. Optic nerve pathology associated with AIDS: ultrastructural changes. [ARVO Abstract] Invest Ophthalmol Vis Sci (Suppl). 1990.
77. Tenhula WN, Sadun AA, Heller KB, et al. Optic nerve axon losses in AIDS. Morphometric comparisons. [ARVO Abstract]. Invest Ophthalmol Vis Sci (Suppl). 1990;31:1793.
78. Quiceno JI, Capparelli E, Sadun AA, et al. Visual dysfunction without retinitis in patients with acquired immunodeficiency syndrome. Am J Ophthalmol 1992;113:8–13.
79. Plummer DJ, Arevalo JF, Fram N, et al. Effectiveness of entoptic perimetry for locating peripheral scotomas caused by cytomegalovirus retinitis. Arch Ophthalmol 1996;114:828–31.
80. Latkany PA, Holopigian K, Lorenzo-Latkany M, et al. Electroretinographic and psychophysical findings during early and late stages of human immunodeficiency virus infection and cytomegalovirus retinitis. Ophthalmology 1997;104:445–53.
81. Falkenstein IA, Bartsch DU, Azen SP, et al. Multifocal electroretinography in HIV-positive patients without infectious retinitis. Am J Ophthalmol 2008; 146(4):579–88.
82. Holland GN, Gottlieb MS, Foos RY. Retinal cotton-wool patches in acquired immunodeficiency syndrome. N Engl J Med 1982;307:1702.
83. Conway MD, Tong P, Olk RJ. Branch retinal artery occlusion (BRAO) combined with branch retinal vein occlusion (BRVO) and optic disc neovascularization associated with HIV and CMV retinitis. Int Ophthalmol 1995–1996; 19:249–52.
84. Cunningham Jr ET, Levinson RD, Jampol LM, et al. Ischemic maculopathy in patients with acquired immunodeficiency syndrome. Am J Ophthalmol 2001;132:727–33.
85. Levinson RD, Dunn JP, Holland GN. Ophthalmic disorders associated with selected primary and acquired immunodeficiency diseases. In: Duane's clinical ophthalmology. CD-ROM. Hagerstown: Harper and Row; 2004. ch. 40.
86. Dejaco-Ruhswurm I, Kiss B, Rainer G, et al. Ocular blood flow in patients infected with human immunodeficiency virus. Am J Ophthalmol 2001; 132:719–25.
87. Lim MC, Cumberland WG, Minassian SL, et al. Decreased macular leukocyte velocity in HIV-infected individuals. Am J Ophthalmol 2001;132:710–8.
88. Dadgostar H, Holland GN, Huang X, et al. Hemorheologic abnormalities associated with HIV infection: in vivo assessment of retinal microvascular blood flow. Invest Ophthalmol Vis Sci 2006;47(9):3933–8.
89. Henderly DE, Freeman WR, Causey DM, et al. Cytomegalovirus retinitis and response to therapy with ganciclovir. Ophthalmology 1987;94:425–34.
90. Jabs DA, Bartlett JG. AIDS and ophthalmology: a period of transition. Am J Ophthalmol 1997;124:227–33.
91. Studies of Ocular Complications of AIDS Research Group in collaboration with the AIDS Clinical Trials Group. Foscarnet–ganciclovir cytomegalovirus retinitis trial 4 - visual outcomes. Ophthalmology 1994;101:1250–61.
92. Collaborative DHPG Treatment Study Group. Treatment of serious cytomegalovirus infections with 9-(1,3-dihydroxy-2-propoxymethyl) guanine in patients with AIDS and other immunodeficiencies. N Engl J Med 1986;314: 801–5.
93. Cogan DG. Immunosuppression and eye disease. Am J Ophthalmol 1977;83: 777–88.
94. Egbert PR, Pollard RB, Gallagher JG, et al. Cytomegalovirus retinitis in immunosuppressed hosts. II. Ocular manifestations. Ann Intern Med 1980;93:664.
95. DeVenecia G, Zu Rhein GM, Pratt MV, et al. Cytomegalic inclusion retinitis in an adult, a clinical, histopathologic, and ultrastructural study. Arch Ophthalmol 1971;86:44.
96. Friedman AH, Orellana J, Freeman WR, et al. Cytomegalovirus retinitis: a manifestation of the acquired immune deficiency syndrome (AIDS). Br J Ophthalmol 1983;67:372–80.
97. Kennedy PGE, Newsome DA, Hess J, et al. Cytomegalovirus but not human T lymphotropic virus type III/lymphadenopathy associated virus detected by in-situ hybridization in retinal lesions in patients with the acquired immune deficiency syndrome. Br Med J 1986;293:162–4.
98. Brody JM, Butrus SI, Laby DM, et al. Anterior segment findings in AIDS patients with cytomegalovirus retinitis. Graefes Arch Clin Exp Ophthalmol 1995;233:374–6.
99. Saran BR, Pomilla PV. Retinal vascular nonperfusion and retinal neovascularization as a consequence of cytomegalovirus retinitis and cryptococcal choroiditis. Retina 1996;16:510–2.
100. Palestine AG, Stevens G, Lane HC, et al. Treatment of cytomegalovirus retinitis with dihydroxy propoxymethyl guanine. Am J Ophthalmol 1986;101: 95–101.
101. Studies of Ocular Complications of AIDS Research Group in collaboration with the AIDS Clinical Trials Group. Assessment of cytomegalovirus retinitis – clinical evaluation vs centralized grading of fundus photographs. Arch Ophthalmol 1996;114:791–805.
102. Studies of Ocular Complications of AIDS Research Group in collaboration with the AIDS Clinical Trials Group. Clinical vs photographic assessment of treatment of cytomegalovirus retinitis. Foscarnet–ganciclovir cytomegalovirus retinitis trial report 8. Arch Ophthalmol 1996;114:848–55.
103. Roarty JD, Fisher EJ, Nussbaum JJ. Long-term visual morbidity of cytomegalovirus retinitis in patients with acquired immune deficiency syndrome. Ophthalmology 1993;100:1685–8.
104. Wu AW, Coleson LC, Holbrook J, et al, for Studies of Ocular Complications of AIDS Research Group. Measuring visual function and quality of life in patients with cytomegalovirus retinitis: development of a questionnaire. Arch Ophthalmol 1996;114:841–7.
105. Bloom PA, Sandy CJ, Migdal CS, et al. Visual prognosis of AIDS patients with cytomegalovirus retinitis. Eye 1995;9:697–702.
106. Luckie AP, Ai E. A foveal-sparing pattern of cytomegalovirus retinitis in the acquired immunodeficiency syndrome. Aust NZ J Ophthalmol 1996;24: 53–9.
107. Gangan PA, Besen G, Munguia D, et al. Macular serous exudation in patients with acquired immunodeficiency syndrome and cytomegalovirus retinitis. Am J Ophthalmol 1994;118:212–9.
108. Minkler DS, Mcleon EB, Shaw CM, et al. Herpes virus hominis encephalitis and retinitis. Arch Ophthalmol 1976;94:89–95.
109. Freeman WR, Thomas EL, Rao NA, et al. Demonstration of herpes group virus in the acute retinal necrosis syndrome. Am J Ophthalmol 1986;102:701–9.
110. Young SJ, Bird AC. Bilateral acute retinal necrosis. Br J Ophthalmol 1978;62:581–90.
111. Bylsma SS, Achim CL, Wiley CA, et al. The predictive value of cytomegalovirus retinitis for cytomegalovirus encephalitis in acquired immunodeficiency syndrome. Arch Ophthalmol 1995;113:89–95.
112. Leger F, Vital C, Vital A, et al. Pathologic correlations between ocular and cerebral lesions in 36 AIDS patients. Clin Neuropathol 1997;16:45–8.

113. Livingston PG, Kerr NC, Sullivan JL. Ocular disease in children with vertically acquired human immunodeficiency virus infection. J AAPOS 1998;2:177–81.
114. Du LT, Coats DK, Kline MW, et al. Incidence of presumed cytomegalovirus in HIV-infected pediatric patients. J AAPOS 1999;3:245–9.
115. Baumal CR, Levin AV, Read SE. Cytomegalovirus retinitis in immunosuppressed children. Am J Ophthalmol 1999;127:550–8.
116. Rasmussen L, Zipeto D, Wolitz RA, et al. Risk for retinitis in patients with AIDS can be assessed by quantitation of threshold levels of cytomegalovirus DNA burden in blood. J Infect Dis 1997;176:1146–55.
117. Studies of Ocular Complications of AIDS Research Group in collaboration with the AIDS Clinical Trials Group. Foscarnet–ganciclovir cytomegalovirus retinitis trial 5 – clinical features of cytomegalovirus retinitis at diagnosis. Am J Ophthalmol 1997;124:141–57.
118. Studies of Ocular Complications of AIDS Research Group in collaboration with the AIDS Clinical Trials Group. Cytomegalovirus (CMV) culture results, drug resistance, and clinical outcome in patients with AIDS and CMV retinitis treated with foscarnet or ganciclovir. J Infect Dis 1997;176:50–8.
119. Pannuti CS, Kallas EG, Muccioli C, et al. Cytomegalovirus antigenemia in acquired immunodeficiency syndrome patients with untreated cytomegalovirus retinitis. Am J Ophthalmol 1996;122:847–52.
120. Rasmussen L, Morris S, Zipeto D, et al. Quantitation of human cytomegalovirus DNA from peripheral blood cells of human immunodeficiency virus-infected patients could predict cytomegalovirus retinitis. J Infect Dis 1995;171:177–82.
121. Hoover DR, Peng Y, Saah A, et al. Occurrence of cytomegalovirus retinitis after human immunodeficiency virus immunosuppression. Arch Ophthalmol 1996;114:821–7.
122. Song MK, Schrier RD, Smith IL. Paradoxical activity of CMV retinitis in patients receiving highly active antiretroviral therapy. Retina 2002;22:262–7.
123. Mitchell SM, Fox JD. Aqueous and vitreous humor samples for the diagnosis of cytomegalovirus retinitis. Am J Ophthalmol 1995;120:252–3.
124. McCann JD, Margolis TP, Wong MG, et al. A sensitive and specific polymerase chain reaction-based assay for the diagnosis of cytomegalovirus retinitis. Am J Ophthalmol 1995;120:219–26.
125. Schrier RD, Freeman WR, Wiley CA, et al. Immune predispositions for cytomegalovirus retinitis in AIDS. The HNRC Group. J Clin Invest 1995;95:1741–6.
126. Dunn JP, Martin DF [Internet]. Medscape from WebMD Ophthalmology; 2003 Sep 30 [cited 2012 Jan 26]. Treatment of cytomegalovirus (CMV) retinitis in the era of highly active antiretroviral therapy. Available (with account) from: http://medscape.com/viewprogram/663.
127. See RF, Rao NA. Cytomegalovirus retinitis in the era of combined highly active antiretroviral therapy. Ophthalmol Clin North Am 2002;15:529–36, viii.
128. Stalder N, Sudre P, Olmari M, et al. Cytomegalovirus retinitis: decreased risk of bilaterality with increased use of systemic treatment. Swiss HIV Cohort Study Group. Clin Infect Dis 1997;24:620–4.
129. Martin DF, Kuppermann BD, Wolitz RA, et al. Oral ganciclovir for patients with cytomegalovirus retinitis treated with a ganciclovir implant. Roche Ganciclovir Study Group. N Engl J Med 1999;340:1063–70.
130. Jabs DA, Martin BK, Forman MS. Cytomegalovirus resistance to ganciclovir and clinical outcomes of patients with cytomegalovirus retinitis. Ophthalmol 2003;135:26–34.
131. Chiron Ganciclovir Implant Study Group. A randomized, controlled, multicenter clinical trial of sustained-release intraocular ganciclovir implant in AIDS patients with CMV retinitis (abstract 1215). Program and abstracts of the Thirty-fifth Interscience Conference on Antimicrobial Agents and Chemotherapy (San Francisco). Washington, DC: American Society for Microbiology; 1995.
132. Bach MC, Bagwell SP, Knapp NP, et al. 9-(1,3-dihydroxy-2-propoxymethyl) guanine for cytomegalovirus infections in patients with the acquired immunodeficiency syndrome. Ann Intern Med 1985;103:381.
133. Sha BE, Benson CA, Deutsch TA, et al. Suppression of cytomegalovirus retinitis in persons with AIDS with high-dose intravenous acyclovir. J Infect Dis 1991;164:777–80.
134. Biron KK, Stanat SC, Sorrell JB, et al. Metabolic activation of the nucleoside analog 9-[[2-hydroxy-1-(hydroxymethyl) ethoxy]methyl] guanine in human diploid fibroblasts infected with human cytomegalovirus. Proc Natl Acad Sci U S A 1985;82:2473–7.
135. Field AK, Daview ME, Dewitt C, et al. 9-[[2-hydroxy-1-(hydroxymethyl) ethoxy]methyl] guanine: a selective inhibitor of herpes group virus replication. Proc Natl Acad Sci U S A 1983;80:4139–43.
136. Anand R, Font RL, Fish RH, et al. Pathology of cytomegalovirus retinitis treated with sustained release intravitreal ganciclovir. Ophthalmology 1993;100:1032–9.
137. Jabs DA, Enger C, Bartlett JG. Cytomegalovirus retinitis and acquired immunodeficiency syndrome. Arch Ophthalmol 1989;107:75–80.
138. Holland GN, Sidikaro Y, Kreiger AE, et al. Treatment of cytomegalovirus retinopathy with ganciclovir. Ophthalmology 1987;94:815–23.
139. Jacobson MA, O'Donnell JJ, Porteous D, et al. Retinal and gastrointestinal disease due to cytomegalovirus in patients with the acquired immune deficiency syndrome: prevalence, natural history, and response to ganciclovir therapy. Q J Med 1988;67:473–86.
140. Orellana J, Teich SA, Friedman AH, et al. Combined short- and long-term therapy for the treatment of cytomegalovirus retinitis using ganciclovir (BW B759U). Ophthalmology 1987;94:831–8.
141. Studies of Ocular Complications of AIDS Research Group in collaboration with the AIDS Clinical Trials Group. Mortality in patients with the acquired immunodeficiency syndrome treated with either foscarnet or ganciclovir for cytomegalovirus retinitis. N Engl J Med 1992;326:213–20.
142. Hoechst H, Dieterich D, Bozzette S, et al. Toxicity of combined ganciclovir and zidovudine for cytomegalovirus disease associated with AIDS. Ann Intern Med 1990;113:111–7.
143. Studies of Ocular Complications of AIDS Research Group in collaboration with the AIDS Clinical Trials Group. Combination foscarnet and ganciclovir therapy vs monotherapy for the treatment of relapsed cytomegalovirus retinitis in patients with AIDS: the cytomegalovirus retreatment trial. Arch Ophthalmol 1996;114:23–33.
144. Gross JG, Bozzette SA, Mathews WC, et al. Longitudinal study of cytomegalovirus retinitis in acquired immune deficiency syndrome. Ophthalmology 1990;97:681–6.
145. Spector SA, McKinley GF, Lalezari JP, et al. Oral ganciclovir for the prevention of cytomegalovirus disease in persons with AIDS. N Engl J Med 1996;334:1491–7.
146. Oral Ganciclovir European and Australian Cooperative Study Group. Intravenous vs oral ganciclovir: European/Australian comparative study of efficacy and safety in the prevention of cytomegalovirus retinitis recurrence in patients with AIDS. The Oral Ganciclovir European and Australian Cooperative Study Group. AIDS 1995;9:471–7.
147. Jung D, Dorr A. Single-dose pharmacokinetics of valganciclovir in HIV- and CMV-seropositive subjects. J Clin Pharmacol 1999;39:800–4.
148. Brown F, Banken L, Saywell K, et al. Pharmacokinetics of valganciclovir and ganciclovir following multiple oral dosages of valganciclovir in HIV- and CMV-seropositive volunteers. Clin Pharmacokinet 1999;37:167–76.
149. Martin DF, Sierra-Madero J, Walmsley S, et al. A controlled trial of valganciclovir as induction therapy for cytomegalovirus retinitis. N Engl J Med 2002;346:1119–26.
150. Lalezari J, Lindley J, Walmsley S, et al. A safety study of oral valganciclovir maintenance treatment of cytomegalovirus retinitis. J Acquir Immune Defic Syndr 2002;30:392–400.
151. Crumpacker CS. Mechanism of action of foscarnet against viral polymerases. Am J Med 1992;92(Suppl 2A):3–7.
152. Bergdahl S, Sonnerbor A, Larsson A, et al. Declining levels of HIV p24 antigen in serum during treatment with foscarnet. Lancet 1988;1:1052.
153. Crumpacker CS, Kowalsky PN, Oliver SA, et al. Resistance of herpes simplex virus to 9-[[2-(hydroxymethyl) ethoxy]methyl] guanine (2-NDG); physical mapping of drug synergism within the viral DNA polymerase locus. Proc Natl Acad Sci U S A 1984;81:1556–60.
154. Jacobson MA, Crowe S, Levy J, et al. Effect of foscarnet therapy on infection with human immunodeficiency virus in patients with AIDS. J Infect Dis 1988;158:862–5.
155. Jacobson MA, Wulfsohn M, Feinberg JE, et al. Phase II dose-ranging trial of foscarnet salvage therapy for cytomegalovirus retinitis in AIDS patients intolerant of or resistant to ganciclovir (ACTG protocol 093). AIDS Clinical Trials Group of the National Institute of Allergy and Infectious Diseases. AIDS 1994;8:451–9.
156. Studies of Ocular Complications of AIDS Research Group in collaboration with the AIDS Clinical Trials Group. Morbidity and toxic effects associated with ganciclovir or foscarnet therapy in a randomized cytomegalovirus retinitis trial. Arch Intern Med 1995;155:65–74.
157. Studies of Ocular Complications of AIDS Research Group in collaboration with AIDS Clinical Trials Group. Antiviral effects of foscarnet and ganciclovir therapy on human immunodeficiency virus p24 antigen in patients with AIDS and cytomegalovirus retinitis. J Infect Dis 1995;172:613–21.
158. Jabs DA. Controversies in the treatment of cytomegalovirus retinitis: foscarnet vs ganciclovir. Infect Agents Dis 1995;4:131–42.
159. Deray G, Martinez F, Katlama C, et al. Foscarnet nephrotoxicity: mechanism, incidence, and prevention. Am J Nephrol 1989;9:316–21.
160. Holland GN, Levinson RD, Jacobson MA. Dose-related difference in progression rates of cytomegalovirus retinopathy during foscarnet maintenance therapy. AIDS Clinical Trials Group Protocol 915 Team. Am J Ophthalmol 1995;119:576–86.
161. Berthe P, Baudouin C, Garraffo R, et al. Toxicologic and pharmacokinetic analysis of intravitreal injections of foscarnet, either alone or in combination with ganciclovir. Invest Ophthalmol Vis Sci 1994;35:1038–45.
162. Palestine AG, Polis MA, De Smet MD, et al. A randomized controlled trial of foscarnet in the treatment of cytomegalovirus retinitis in patients with AIDS. Ann Intern Med 1991;115:665–73.
163. Lalezari JP. Cidofovir: a new therapy for cytomegalovirus retinitis. J Acquir Immune Defic Syndr 1997;14 (Suppl 1):22–6.
164. Lalezari JP, Stagg RJ, Kuppermann BD, et al. Intravenous cidofovir for peripheral cytomegalovirus retinitis in patients with AIDS: a randomized, controlled trial. Ann Intern Med 1997;126:257–63.
165. Studies of Ocular Complications of AIDS Research Group in collaboration with the AIDS Clinical Trials Group. Long-term follow-up of patients with AIDS treated with parenteral cidofovir for cytomegalovirus: the HPMPC Peripheral Cytomegalovirus Retinitis Trial. AIDS 2000;14:1571–81.
166. Studies of Ocular Complications of AIDS Research Group in collaboration with the AIDS Clinical Trials Group. Parenteral cidofovir for cytomegalovirus retinitis in patients with AIDS: the HPMPC peripheral cytomegalovirus retinitis trial – a randomized, controlled trial. Ann Intern Med 1997;126:264–74.
167. Rahhal FM, Arevalo JF, Chavez de la Paz E, et al. Treatment of cytomegalovirus retinitis with intravitreous cidofovir in patients with AIDS: a preliminary report. Ann Intern Med 1996;125:98–103.

168. Davis JL, Taskintuna I, Freeman WR, et al. Iritis and hypotony after treatment with intravenous cidofovir for cytomegalovirus retinitis. Arch Ophthalmol 1997;115:733–7.
169. Kirsch LS, Arevalo JF, Chavez de la Paz E, et al. Intravitreal cidofovir (HPMPC) treatment of cytomegalovirus retinitis in patients with acquired immune deficiency syndrome. Ophthalmology 1995;102:533–43.
170. Rahhal FM, Arevalo JF, Munguia D, et al. Intravitreal cidofovir for the maintenance treatment of cytomegalovirus retinitis. Ophthalmology 1996;103: 1078–83.
171. Jabs DA, Dunn JP, Enger C, et al. Cytomegalovirus retinitis and viral resistance: prevalence of resistance at diagnosis, 1994. Cytomegalovirus Retinitis and Viral Resistance Study Group. Arch Ophthalmol 1996;114:809–14.
172. Jabs DA, Enger C, Dunn JP, et al. Cytomegalovirus retinitis and viral resistance: 4. Ganciclovir resistance. J Infect Dis 1998;177:770–3.
173. Smith KL, Cherrington JM, Jiles RE, et al. High-level resistance of cytomegalovirus to ganciclovir is associated with alterations in both the UL97 and DNA polymerase genes. J Infect Dis 1997;176:69–77.
174. Drew WL, Stempton MJ, Andrews J, et al. Cytomegalovirus (CMV) resistance in patients with CMV retinitis and AIDS treated with oral or intravenous ganciclovir. J Infect Dis 1999;179:1352–5.
175. Jabs DA, Enger C, Forman M, et al. Incidence of foscarnet resistance and cidofovir resistance in patients treated for cytomegalovirus retinitis. The Cytomegalovirus Retinitis and Viral Resistance Study Group. Antimicrob Agents Chemother 1998;42:2240–1.
176. Boivin G, Gilbert C, Gaudreau A, et al. Rate of emergence of cytomegalovirus (CMV) mutations in leukocytes of patients with acquired immunodeficiency syndrome who are receiving valganciclovir as induction and maintenance therapy for CMV retinitis. J Infect Dis 2001;184:1598–602.
177. Drew WL, Miner RC, Saleh E, et al. Antiviral susceptibility of cytomegalovirus: criteria for detecting resistance to antivirals. Clin Diagn Virol 1993;1: 179–85.
178. Landry ML, Stanat S, Biron K, et al. A standardized plaque reduction assay for determination of drug susceptibilities of cytomegalovirus clinical isolates. Antimicrob Agents Chemother 2000;44:688–92.
179. Cihlar T, Fuller MD, Cherrington JM. Characterization of drug resistance-associated mutations in the human cytomegalovirus DNA polymerase gene by using recombinant mutant viruses generated from overlapping DNA fragments. J Virol 1998;72:5927–36.
180. Weinberg A, Jabs DA, Chou S, et al. Mutations conferring foscarnet resistance in a cohort of patients with acquired immunodeficiency syndrome and cytomegalovirus retinitis. J Infect Dis 2003;187:777–84.
181. Spector SA, Hsia K, Wolf D, et al. Molecular detection of human cytomegalovirus and determination of genotypic ganciclovir resistance in clinical specimens. Clin Infect Dis 1995;21 (Suppl 2):S170–3.
182. Erice A. Resistance of human cytomegalovirus to antiviral drugs. Clin Microbiol Rev 1999;12:286–97.
183. Chou S, Lurain NS, Weinberg A, et al. Interstrain variation in the human cytomegalovirus DNA polymerase sequence and its effect on the genotypic diagnosis of antiviral drug resistance. Antimicrob Agents Chemother 1999;43:1500–2.
184. Chou S, Marousek G, Parenti DM, et al. Mutation in region III of the DNA polymerase gene conferring foscarnet resistance in cytomegalovirus isolates from 3 subjects receiving prolonged antiviral therapy. J Infect Dis 1998;178:526–30.
185. Gilbert C, Bestman-Smith J, Boivin G. Resistance of herpesvirus to antiviral drugs: clinical impacts and molecular mechanisms. Drug Resist Update 2002;5:88–114.
186. Hu H, Jabs DA, Forman MS, et al. Comparison of cytomegalovirus (CMV) UL97 gene sequences in the blood and vitreous of patients with acquired immunodeficiency syndrome and CMV retinitis. J Infect Dis 2002;185:861–7.
187. Arevalo JF, Gonzalez C, Capparelli EV, et al. Intravitreous and plasma concentrations of ganciclovir and foscarnet after intravenous therapy in patients with AIDS and cytomegalovirus. J Infect Dis 1995;172:951–6.
188. Jabs DA, Martin BK, Forman MS, et al. Cytomegalovirus resistance to ganciclovir and clinical outcomes of patients with cytomegalovirus retinitis. Am J Ophthalmol 2003;135:26–34.
189. Kuppermann BD, Flores-Aguilar M, Quiceno J, et al. Combination ganciclovir and foscarnet therapy in the treatment of clinically resistant cytomegalovirus retinitis in patients with the acquired immune deficiency syndrome. Am J Ophthalmol 1993;111:1359–66.
190. Walton RC, Whitcup SM, Mueller BU, et al. Combined intravenous ganciclovir and foscarnet for children with recurrent cytomegalovirus retinitis. Ophthalmology 1995;102:1865–70.
191. Desatnik HR, Foster RE, Lowder CY. Treatment of clinically resistant cytomegalovirus retinitis with combined intravitreal injections of ganciclovir and foscarnet. Am J Ophthalmol 1996;122:121–3.
192. Hodge WG, Lalonde RG, Sampalis J, et al. Once-weekly intraocular injections of ganciclovir for maintenance therapy of cytomegalovirus retinitis: clinical and ocular outcome. J Infect Dis 1996;174:393–6.
193. Montero MC, Pastor M, Buenestado C, et al. Intravitreal ganciclovir for cytomegalovirus retinitis in patients with AIDS. Ann Pharmacother 1996;30: 717–23.
194. Young S, Morlet N, Besen G, et al. High-dose (2000-microgram) intravitreous ganciclovir in the treatment of cytomegalovirus retinitis. Ophthalmology 1998;105:1404–10.
195. Baudouin C, Chassain C, Caujolle C, et al. Treatment of cytomegalovirus retinitis in AIDS patients using intravitreal injections of highly concentrated ganciclovir. Ophthalmologica 1996;210:329–35.
196. Tognon MS, Turrini B, Masiero G, et al. Intravitreal and systemic foscarnet in the treatment of AIDS-related CMV retinitis. Eur J Ophthalmol 1996;6: 179–82.
197. Diaz-Llopis M, Espana E, Munoz G, et al. High dose intravitreal foscarnet in the treatment of cytomegalovirus retinitis in AIDS. Br J Ophthalmol 1994;78:120–4.
198. Sandorn GE, Anand R, Torti RE, et al. Sustained-release ganciclovir therapy for treatment of cytomegalovirus retinitis: use of an intravitreal device. Arch Ophthalmol 1992;110:188–95.
199. Martin DF, Parks DJ, Mellow SD, et al. Treatment of cytomegalovirus retinitis with an intraocular sustained-release ganciclovir implant: a randomized controlled clinical trial [see comments]. Arch Ophthalmol 1994;112:1531–9.
200. Marx JL, Kapusta MA, Patel SS, et al. Use of the ganciclovir implant in the treatment of recurrent cytomegalovirus retinitis. Arch Ophthalmol 1996; 114:815–20.
201. Martin DF, Ferris FL, Brothers RJ, et al. Retinal detachment in eyes treated with a ganciclovir implant [Letter]. Arch Ophthalmol 1995;113:1355.
202. Martin DF, Dunn JP, Davis JL, et al. Use of the ganciclovir implant for the treatment of cytomegalovirus retinitis in the era of potent antiretroviral therapy: recommendations of the International AIDS Society – USA panel. Am J Ophthalmol 1999;127:329–39.
203. Kempen JH, Jabs DA, Dunn JP, et al. Retinal detachment risk in cytomegalovirus retinitis related to the acquired immunodeficiency syndrome. Arch Ophthalmol 2001;119:33–40.
204. Shane TS, Martin DF. Endophthalmitis after ganciclovir implant in patients with AIDS and cytomegalovirus retinitis. Am J Ophthalmol 2003;136: 649–54.
205. Kirsch LS, Arevalo JF, De Clercq E, et al. Phase I/II study of intravitreal cidofovir for the treatment of cytomegalovirus retinitis in patients with the acquired immunodeficiency syndrome. Am J Ophthalmol 1995;119:466–76.
206. Banker AS, Arevalo JF, Munguia D, et al. Intraocular pressure and aqueous humor dynamics in patients with AIDS treated with intravitreal cidofovir (HPMPC) for cytomegalovirus retinitis. Am J Ophthalmol 1997;124:168–80.
207. Besen B, Flores-Aguilar M, Assil KK, et al. Long-term therapy for herpes retinitis in an animal model with high-concentrated liposome-encapsulated HPMPC. Arch Ophthalmol 1995;113:661–8.
208. Kirsch LS, Arevalo JF, Chavez de la Paz E, et al. Intravitreal cidofovir (HPMPC) treatment of cytomegalovirus retinitis in patients with acquired immune deficiency syndrome [published erratum appears in Ophthalmology 102:702, 1995]. Ophthalmology 1995;102:533–42; discussion 542–3.
209. Taskintuna I, Rahhal FM, Arevalo JF, et al. Low-dose intravitreal cidofovir (HPMPC) therapy of cytomegalovirus retinitis in patients with acquired immune deficiency syndrome. Ophthalmology 1997;104:1049–57.
210. Arevalo JF, Munguia D, Faber D, et al. Correlation between intraocular pressure and CD4 T-lymphocyte counts in patients with human immunodeficiency virus with and without cytomegalovirus retinitis. Am J Ophthalmol 1996;122:91–6.
211. Azad RF, Driver VB, Tanaka K, et al. Antiviral activity of a phosphorothioate oligonucleotide complementary to RNA of the human cytomegalovirus major immediate-early region. Antimicrob Agents Chemother 1993;37:1945–54.
212. Anderson KP, Fox MC, Brown-Driver V, et al. Inhibition of human cytomegalovirus immediate-early gene expression by an antisense oligonucleotide complementary to immediate-early RNA. Antimicrob Agents Chemother 1996;40:2004–11.
213. The Vitravene Study Group. A randomized controlled clinical trial of intravitreous fomivirsen for treatment of newly diagnosed peripheral cytomegalovirus retinitis in patients with AIDS. Am J Ophthalmol 2002;133:467–74.
214. Freeman WR. Retinal toxic effects associated with intravitreal fomivirsen. Arch Ophthalmol 2001;119:458.
215. The Vitravene Study Group. Randomized dose-comparison studies of intravitreous fomivirsen for treatment of cytomegalovirus retinitis that has reactivated or is persistently active despite other therapies in patients with AIDS. Am J Ophthalmol 2002;133:475–83.
216. The Vitravene Study Group. Safety of intravitreous fomivirsen for treatment of cytomegalovirus retinitis patients with AIDS. Am J Ophthalmol 2002;133: 484–98.
217. Jabs DA, Griffiths PD. Fomivirsen for the treatment of cytomegalovirus retinitis. Am J Ophthalmol 2002;133:552–6.
218. Biron KK, Harvey RG, Chamberlain SS. Potent and selective inhibition of human cytomegalovirus replication by 1263W94, a benzimidazole L-riboside with a unique mode of action. Antimicrob Agents Chemother 2002;46: 2365–72.
219. Koszalka GW, Johnson NW, Good SS, et al. Preclinical and toxicology studies of 1263W94, a potent and selective inhibitor of human cytomegalovirus replication. Antimicrob Agents Chemother 2002;46:2373–80.
220. Wang LH, Peck RW, Yin Y, et al. Phase I safety and pharmacokinetic trials of 1263W94, a novel oral anti-human cytomegalovirus agent, in healthy and human immunodeficiency virus-infected subjects. Antimicrob Agents Chemother 2003;47:1334–42.
221. Lalezari JP, Aberg JA, Wang LH, et al. Phase I dose escalation trial evaluating the pharmacokinetics, anti-human cytomegalovirus (HCMV) activity, and safety of 1263W94 in human immunodeficiency virus-infected men with asymptomatic HCMV shedding. Antimicrob Agents Chemother 2002;46: 2969–76.
222. Kempen JH, Jabs DA, Wilson LA, et al. Risk of vision loss in patients with cytomegalovirus retinitis and the acquired immunodeficiency syndrome. Arch Ophthalmol 2003;121:466–76.

223. Freeman WR, Friedberg DN, Berry C, et al. Risk factors for development of rhegmatogenous retinal detachment in patients with cytomegalovirus retinitis. Am J Ophthalmol 1993;116:713–20.
224. Studies of Ocular Complications of AIDS (SOCA) Research Group in Collaboration with the AIDS Clinical Trials Group (ACTG). Rhegmatogenous retinal detachment in patients with cytomegalovirus retinitis. Foscarnet–Ganciclovir Cytomegalovirus Retinitis Trial. Am J Ophthalmol 1997;124:61–70.
225. Broughton WL, Cupples HP, Parver LM. Bilateral retinal detachment following cytomegalovirus retinitis. Arch Ophthalmol 1978;96:618–24.
226. Freeman WR, Henderly DE, Wan WL. Rhegmatogenous retinal detachment in treated cytomegalovirus retinitis: prevalence, pathophysiology, and treatment. Am J Ophthalmol 1987;103:527–36.
227. Sidikaro Y, Silver L, Holland GN, et al. Rhegmatogenous retinal detachments in patients with AIDS and necrotizing retinal infections. Ophthalmology 1991;98:129–35.
228. Irvine AR. Treatment of retinal detachment due to cytomegalovirus retinitis in patients with AIDS. Trans Am Ophthalmol Soc 1991;89:349–63.
229. Freeman WR, Quiceno JI, Crapotta JA, et al. Surgical repair of rhegmatogenous retinal detachment in immunosuppressed patients with cytomegalovirus retinitis. Ophthalmology 1992;99:466–74.
230. Holland GN, Buhles WC, Mastre B, et al. A controlled retrospective study of ganciclovir treatment for cytomegalovirus retinopathy: use of a standardized system for the assessment of disease outcome. Arch Ophthalmol 1989;107: 1759–66.
231. Freeman WR. Retinal detachment in cytomegalovirus retinitis: should our approach be changed? Retina 1999;19:27–33.
232. Sandy CJ, Bloom PA, Graham EM, et al. Retinal detachment in AIDS-related cytomegalovirus retinitis. Eye 1995;9:277–81.
233. Regillo CD, Vander JF, Duker JS, et al. Repair of retinitis-related retinal detachments with silicone oil in patients with acquired immunodeficiency syndrome. Am J Ophthalmol 1992;113:21–7.
234. Freeman WR. Application of vitreoretinal surgery to inflammatory and infectious diseases of the posterior segment. Int Ophthalmol Clin 1992;32: 15–33.
235. Nasemann JE, Mutsch A, Wiltfang R, et al. Early pars plana vitrectomy without buckling procedure in cytomegalovirus retinitis-induced retinal detachment. Retina 1995;15:111–6.
236. Garcia RF, Flores-Aguilar M, Quiceno JI, et al. Results of rhegmatogenous retinal detachment repair in cytomegalovirus retinitis with and without scleral buckling. Ophthalmology 1995;102:236–45.
237. Davis JL, Chuang EL. Management of retinal detachment associated with CMV retinitis in AIDS patients. Eye 1992;6:28–34.
238. Tanna AP, Kempen JH, Dunn JP. Incidence and management of cataract after retinal detachment repair with silicone oil in immune compromised patients with cytomegalovirus retinitis. Am J Ophthalmol 2003;136:1009–15.
239. Irvine AR, Lonn L, Schwartz D, et al. Retinal detachment in AIDS: long-term results after repair with silicone oil. Br J Ophthalmol 1997;81:180–3.
240. Meldrum ML, Aaberg TM, Patel A, et al. Cataract extraction after silicone oil repair of retinal detachments due to necrotizing retinitis. Arch Ophthalmol 1996;114:885–92.
241. Azen SP, Scott IU, Flynn Jr HW, et al. Silicone oil in the repair of complex retinal detachments. A prospective observational multicenter study. Ophthalmology 1998;105:1587–97.
242. Karavellas MP, Song M, MacDonald JC, et al. Long-term posterior and anterior segment complications of immune recovery uveitis associated with cytomegalovirus retinitis. Am J Ophthalmol 2000;130:57–64.
243. Baumal CR, Reichel E. Management of cytomegalovirus-related rhegmatogenous retinal detachments. Ophthalmic Surg Lasers 1998;29:916–25.
244. Althaus C, Loeffler KU, Schimkat M, et al. Prophylactic argon laser coagulation for rhegmatogenous retinal detachment in AIDS patients with cytomegalovirus retinitis. Graefes Arch Clin Exp Ophthalmol 1998;236:359–64.
245. Davis JL, Hummer J, Feuer WJ. Laser photocoagulation for retinal detachment and retinal tears in cytomegalovirus retinitis. Ophthalmology 1997;104:2053–2060; discussion 2060–1.
246. McCluskey P, Grigg J, Playfair TJ. Retinal detachments in patients with AIDS and CMV retinopathy: a role for laser photocoagulation. Br J Ophthalmol 1995;79:153–6.
247. Meffert SA, Ai E. Laser photocoagulation prophylaxis for CMV retinal detachments. Ophthalmology 1998;105:1353–5.
248. Finzi D, Hermankova M, Pierson T, et al. Identification of a reservoir for HIV-1 in patients on highly active antiretroviral therapy. Science 1997;278: 1295–300.
249. Kempen JH, Martin BK, Wu AW, et al. The effect of cytomegalovirus retinitis on the quality of life of patients with AIDS in the era of highly active antiretroviral therapy. Ophthalmology 2003;110:987–95.
250. Palella Jr FJ, Delaney KM, Moorman AC, et al. Declining morbidity and mortality among patients with advanced human immunodeficiency virus infection. HIV Outpatient Study Investigators. N Engl J Med 1998;338:853–60.
251. Varani S, Spezzacatena P, Manfredi R, et al. The incidence of cytomegalovirus (CMV) antigenemia and CMV disease is reduced by highly active antiretroviral therapy. Eur J Epidemiol 2000;16:433–7.
252. Deayton JR, Wilson P, Sabin CA, et al. Changes in the natural history of cytomegalovirus retinitis following the introduction of highly active antiretroviral therapy. AIDS 2000;14:1163–70.
253. MacDonald JC, Torriani FJ, Morse LS, et al. Lack of reactivation of cytomegalovirus (CMV) retinitis after stopping CMV maintenance therapy in AIDS patients with sustained elevations in CD4 T cells in response to highly active antiretroviral therapy. J Infect Dis 1998;177:1182–7.
254. Jabs DA, Bolton SG, Dunn JP, et al. Discontinuing anticytomegalovirus therapy in patients with immune reconstitution after combination antiretroviral therapy. Am J Ophthalmol 1998;126:817–22.
255. MacDonald JC, Karavellas MP, Torriani FJ, et al. Highly active antiretroviral therapy-related immune recovery in AIDS patients with cytomegalovirus retinitis. Ophthalmology 2000;107:877–81.
256. Curi AL, Muralha A, Muralha L, et al. Suspension of anticytomegalovirus maintenance therapy following immune recovery due to highly active antiretroviral therapy. Br J Ophthalmol 2001;85:471–3.
257. Whitcup SM, Fortin E, Lindblad AS, et al. Discontinuation of anticytomegalovirus therapy in patients with HIV infection cytomegalovirus. JAMA 1999;282:1633–71.
258. Vrabec TR, Baldassano VF, Whitcup SM. Discontinuation of maintenance therapy in patients with quiescent cytomegalovirus retinitis and elevated CD4 counts. Ophthalmology 1998;105:1259–64.
259. Sepkowitz KA. Effect of HAART on natural history of AIDS-related opportunistic disorders. Lancet 1998;351:228–30.
260. Michelet C, Arvieux C, Francois C, et al. Opportunistic infections occurring during highly active antiretroviral treatment. AIDS 1998;12:1815–22.
261. Jacobson MA, Zegans M, Pavan PR, et al. Cytomegalovirus retinitis after initiation of highly active antiretroviral therapy. Lancet 1997;349:1443–5.
262. Elston JW, Thaker H. Immune reconstitution inflammatory syndrome. Int J STD AIDS 2009;23:221–4.
263. Karavellas MP, Lower CY, Macdonald JC, et al. Immune recovery vitreitis associated with inactive cytomegalovirus retinitis: a new syndrome. Arch Ophthalmol 1998;116:169–75.
264. Otiti-Sengeri J, Meenken C, van den Horn GJ, et al. Ocular immune reconstitution inflammatory syndromes. Curr Opin HIV AIDS 2008;3:432–7.
265. Holland GN. Pieces of a puzzle: toward better understanding of intraocular inflammation associated with human immunodeficiency virus infection. Am J Ophthalmol 1998;125:383–5.
266. Zegans ME, Walton RC, Holland GN, et al. Transient vitreous inflammatory reactions associated with combination antiretroviral therapy in patients with AIDS and cytomegalovirus retinitis. Am J Ophthalmol 1998;125:292–300.
267. Holland GN. Immune recovery uveitis. Ocul Immunol Inflamm 1999;7: 215–21.
268. Karavellas MP, Plummer DJ, Macdonald JC, et al. Incidence of immune recovery vitreitis in cytomegalovirus retinitis patients following institution of successful highly active antiretroviral therapy. J Infect Dis 1999;179:697–700.
269. Nguyen QD, Kempen JH, Bolton SG, et al. Immune recovery uveitis in patients with AIDS and cytomegalovirus retinitis after highly active antiretroviral therapy. Am J Ophthalmol 2000;129:634–9.
270. Jabs DA, Van Natta ML, Kempen JH, et al. Characteristics of patients with cytomegalovirus retinitis in the era of highly active antiretroviral therapy. Am J Ophthalmol 2002;133:48–61.
271. Arevalo JF, Mendoza AJ, Ferretti Y. Immune recovery uveitis in AIDS patients with cytomegalovirus retinitis treated with highly active antiretroviral therapy in Venezuela. Retina 2003;23:495–502.
272. Karavellas MP, Azen SP, Macdonald JC, et al. Immune recovery vitreitis in AIDS: clinical predictors, sequella, and treatment outcomes. Retina 2001;21: 1–9.
273. Song M, Azen SP, Buley A, et al. Effect of anti-cytomegalovirus therapy on the incidence of immune recovery uveitis in AIDS patients with healed cytomegalovirus retinitis. Am J Ophthalmol 2003;136:696–702.
274. Newsome R, Casswell T, O'Moore E, et al. Cystoid macular oedema in patients with AIDS and cytomegalovirus retinitis on highly active antiretroviral therapy. Br J Ophthalmol 1998;82:456–7.
275. Silverstein BE, Smith JH, Sykes SO, et al. Cystoid macular edema associated with cytomegalovirus retinitis in patients with acquired immunodeficiency syndrome. Am J Ophthalmol 1998;125:412–5.
276. Whitcup SM. Cytomegalovirus retinitis in the era of highly active antiretroviral therapy. JAMA 2000;283:653–7.
277. Karavellas MP, Song MK, Macdonald JC, et al. Long-term posterior and anterior segment complications of immune recovery uveitis associated with cytomegalovirus retinitis. Am J Ophthalmol 2000;130:57–64.
278. Sanislo SR, Lowder CY, Kaiser PK. Optic nerve head neovascularization in a patient with inactive cytomegalovirus retinitis and immune recovery. Am J Ophthalmol 1998;126:318–20.
279. Canzano JC, Reed JB, Morse LS. Vitreomacular traction syndrome following highly active antiretroviral therapy in AIDS patients with cytomegalovirus retinitis. Retina 1998;18:443–7.
280. Robinson MR, Csasky KG, Lee SS, et al. Fibrovascular changes misdiagnosed as cytomegalovirus retinitis reactivation in a patient with immune recovery. Clin Infect Dis 2004;38:139–41.
281. Biswas J, Choudhry S, Kumarasamy, et al. Immune recovery vitreitis presenting as panuveitis following therapy with protease inhibitors. Indian J Ophthalmol 2000;48:313–5.
282. Goldberg DE, Freeman WR. Uveitic angle closure glaucoma in a patient with inactive cytomegalovirus and immune recovery uveitis. Ophthalmic Surg Lasers 2002;33:421–5.
283. Goldberg DE, Wang H, Azen SP, et al. Long term visual outcome of patients with cytomegalovirus retinitis treated with highly active antiretroviral therapy. Br J Ophthalmol 2003;87:853–5.
284. Kuppermann BD, Holland GN. Immune recovery uveitis. Am J Ophthalmol 2000;130:103–6.
285. Pepose JS, Newman C, Bach MC, et al. Pathologic features of cytomegalovirus retinopathy after treatment with the antiviral agent ganciclovir. Ophthalmology 1987;94:414–24.

286. D'Alessandro L, Bottaro E. Reactivation of CMV retinitis after treatment with subtenon corticosteroids for immune recovery uveitis in patients with AIDS. Scand J Infect Dis 2002;34:780–2.
287. Morrison VL, Kozak I, LaBree LD, et al. Intravitreal triamcinolone acetate for the treatment of immune recovery uveitis macular edema. Ophthalmology 2007;114(2):334–9.
288. Shah AM, Oster SF, Freeman WR. Viral retinitis after intravitreal triamcinolone injection in patients with predisposing medical comorbidities. Am J Ophthalmol 2010;149(3):433–40.
289. Maguire AM, Nichols CW, Crooks GW. Visual loss in cytomegalovirus retinitis caused by cystoid macular edema in patients without the acquired immune deficiency. Ophthalmology 1996;103:601–5.
290. Omerod LD, Larkin JA, Margo CA, et al. Rapidly progressive herpetic retinal necrosis: a blinding disease characteristic of advanced AIDS. [see commentary by C.L. Lowder, pp. 46–47]. Clin Infect Dis 1998;26:34–5.
291. Forster DJ, Dugel PU, Frangieh GT, et al. Rapidly progressive outer retinal necrosis in the acquired immunodeficiency syndrome. Am J Ophthalmol 1990;110:341–8.
292. Duker JS, Blumenkranz MS. Diagnosis and management of the acute retinal necrosis (ARN) syndrome. Surv Ophthalmol 1991;35:327–43.
293. Friedlander S, Rahhal FM, Ericson L, et al. Optic neuropathy preceding acute retinal necrosis in acquired immunodeficiency syndrome. Arch Ophthalmol 1996;114:1481–5.
294. Culbertson WW, Atherton SS. Acute retinal necrosis and similar retinitis syndromes. Int Ophthalmol Clin 1993;33:129–43.
295. Sellitti TP, Huang AJ, Schiffman J, et al. Association of herpes zoster ophthalmicus with acquired immunodeficiency syndrome and acute retinal necrosis. Am J Ophthalmol 1993;116:297–301.
296. Holland GN. Standard diagnostic criteria for the acute retinal necrosis syndrome. Executive Committee of the American Uveitis Society. Am J Ophthalmol 1994;117:663–7.
297. Abe T, Tsuchida K, Tamai M. A comparative study of the polymerase chain reaction and local antibody production in acute retinal necrosis syndrome and cytomegalovirus retinitis. Graefes Arch Clin Exp Ophthalmol 1996;234: 419–24.
298. Weinberg DV, Lyon AT. Repair of retinal detachments due to herpes varicella-zoster virus retinitis in patients with acquired immune deficiency syndrome. Ophthalmology 1997;104:279–82.
299. Schlingemann RO, Bruinenberg M, Wertheim-Van Dillen P, et al. Twenty years' delay of fellow eye involvement in herpes simplex virus type 2-associated bilateral acute retinal necrosis syndrome. Am J Ophthalmol 1996;122:891–2.
300. Aslanides IM, De Souza S, Wong DTW, et al. Oral valacyclovir in the treatment of acute retinal necrosis syndrome. Retina 2002;22:352–4.
301. Chatis PA, Miller CH, Schrager LE, et al. Successful treatment with foscarnet of an acyclovir-resistant mucocutaneous infection with herpes simplex virus in a patient with the acquired immunodeficiency syndrome. N Engl J Med 1989;320:297–300.
302. Safrin S, Berger TG, Gilson I, et al. Foscarnet therapy in five patients with AIDS and acyclovir-resistant varicella-zoster virus infection. Ann Intern Med 1991;115:19–21.
303. Dunn JP. Viral retinitis. Ophthalmol Clin North Am 1999;12:109.
304. Pavesio CE, Mitchell SM, Barton K, et al. Progressive outer retinal necrosis (PORN) in AIDS patients: a different appearance of varicella-zoster retinitis. Eye 1995;9:271–6.
305. Engstrom RJ, Holland GN, Margolis TP, et al. The progressive outer retinal necrosis syndrome. A variant of necrotizing herpetic retinopathy in patients with AIDS. Ophthalmology 1994;101:1488–502.
306. Scott IU, Luu KM, Davis JL. Intravitreal antivirals in the management of patients with acquired immunodeficiency syndrome with progressive outer retinal necrosis. Arch Ophthalmol 2002;120:1219–22.
307. Ciulla TA, Rutledge BK, Morley MG, et al. The progressive outer retinal necrosis syndrome: successful treatment with combination antiviral therapy. Ophthalmic Surg Lasers 1998;29:198–206.
308. Margolis TP, Lowder CY, Holland GN, et al. Varicella-zoster virus retinitis in patients with the acquired immunodeficiency syndrome. Am J Ophthalmol 1991;112:119–31.
309. Spaide RF, Martin DF, Teich SA, et al. Successful treatment of progressive outer retinal necrosis syndrome. Retina 1996;16:479–87.
310. Meffert SA, Kertes PJ, Lim P, et al. Successful treatment of progressive outer retinal necrosis using high-dose intravitreal ganciclovir. Retina 1997;17: 560–2.
311. Perez-Blasquez E, Traspas R, Marin IM, et al. Intravitreal ganciclovir treatment in progressive outer retinal necrosis. Am J Ophthalmol 1997;124: 418–21.
312. Kim SJ, Equi R, Belair ML, et al. Long-term preservation of vision in progressive outer retinal necrosis treated with combination antiviral drugs and highly active antiretroviral therapy. Ocul Immun Inflamm 2007;15: 425–7.
313. Kaplan JE, Benson, C, Holmes KK, et al. Guidelines for Prevention and Treatment of Opportunistic Infections in HIV-Infected Adults and Recommendations of the U.S. Public Health Service and the Infectious Disease Society of America. MMWR Recomm Rep 2009;58(RR04):1–198.
314. Macher AM, Bardenstein DS, Zimmerman LE. Pneumocystis carinii choroiditis in a male homosexual with AIDS and disseminated pulmonary and extrapulmonary *P. carinii* infection. N Engl J Med 1987;236:1092.
315. Freeman WR, Gross JG, Labelle J, et al. Pneumocystis carinii choroidopathy: a new clinical entity. Arch Ophthalmol 1989;107:863–7.
316. Shami MJ, Freeman WR, Friedberg D, et al. A multicenter study of pneumocystis choroidopathy. Am J Ophthalmol 1991;112:15–22.
317. Dugel PU, Rao NA, Forster DJ, et al. *Pneumocystis carinii* choroiditis after long-term aerosolized pentamidine therapy. Am J Ophthalmol 1990;110: 113–7.
318. Foster RE, Lowder CY, Meisler DM, et al. Presumed *Pneumocystis carinii* choroiditis: unifocal presentation, regression with intravenous pentamidine, and choroiditis recurrence. Ophthalmology 1991;98:1360–5.
319. Sneed SR, Blodi CF, Berger BB, et al. *Pneumocystis carinii* choroiditis in patients receiving inhaled pentamidine. N Engl J Med 1989;322:936–7.
320. Centers for Disease Control and Prevention. HIV/AIDS surveillance report 1999;11:2–38.
321. Parke II DW, Font RL. Diffuse toxoplasmic retinochoroiditis in a patient with AIDS. Arch Ophthalmol 1986;104:571–5.
322. Heinemann MH, Gold JMW, Maisel J. Bilateral toxoplasma retinochoroiditis in a patient with acquired immune deficiency syndrome. Retina 1986;6:224.
323. Cochereau-Massin I, LeHoang P, Lautier-Frau M, et al. Ocular toxoplasmosis in human immunodeficiency virus-infected patients. Am J Ophthalmol 1992;114:130–5.
324. Elkins BS, Holland GN, Opremcak EM, et al. Ocular toxoplasmosis misdiagnosed as cytomegalovirus retinopathy in immunocompromised patients. Ophthalmology 1994;101:499–507.
325. Berger BB, Egwuagu CE, Freeman WR, et al. Miliary toxoplasmic retinitis in acquired immunodeficiency syndrome. Arch Ophthalmol 1993;111:373–6.
326. Cano-Parra JL, Diaz-Llopis ML, Cordoba JL, et al. Acute iridocyclitis in a patient with AIDS diagnosed as toxoplasmosis by PCR. Ocul Immunol Inflamm 2000;8:127–30.
327. Moshfeghi DM, Dodds EM, Couto CA, et al. Diagnostic approaches to severe, atypical toxoplasmosis mimicking acute retinal necrosis. Ophthalmology 2004;111:716–25.
328. Moorthy RS, Smith RE, Rao NA. Progressive ocular toxoplasmosis in patients with acquired immunodeficiency syndrome. Am J Ophthalmol 1993;115: 742–7.
329. Holland GN. Ocular toxoplasmosis: a global reassessment. Part II: Disease manifestations and management. Am J Ophthalmol 2004;137:1–17.
330. Holland GN. Ocular toxoplasmosis: a global reassessment. Part I: Epidemiology and course of disease. Am J Ophthalmol 2003;136:973–88.
331. Grossniklaus HE, Specht CS, Allaire G, et al. Toxoplasma gondii retinochoroiditis and optic neuritis in acquired immune deficiency syndrome. Report of a case. Ophthalmology 1990;97:1342–6.
332. Rehder JR, Burnier MBJ, Pavesio CE, et al. Acute unilateral toxoplasmic iridocyclitis in an AIDS patient. Am J Ophthalmol 1988;106:740–1.
333. Tate Jr GW, Martin RG. Clindamycin in the treatment of human ocular toxoplasmosis. Can J Ophthalmol 1977;12:188–95.
334 Torre D, Casari S, Speranza F, et al. Randomized trial of trimethoprim-sulfamethoxazole versus pyrimethamine-sulfadiazine for therapy of toxoplasmic encephalitis in patients with AIDS. Antimicrob Agents Chemother 1998;2: 1346–9.
335. Jacobson JM, Hafner R, Remington J, et al. Dose-escalation, phase I/II study of azithromycin and pyrimethamine for the treatment of toxoplasmic encephalitis in AIDS. AIDS 2001;15:583–9.
336. Bosch-Driessen LH, Verbraak FD, Suttorp-Schulten MSA, et al. A prospective, randomized trial of pyrimethamine and azithromycin vs pyrimethamine and sulfadiazine for the treatment of ocular toxoplasmosis. Am J Ophthalmol 2002;134:34–40.
337. Pearson PA, Piracha AR, Sen H, et al. Atovaquone for the treatment of toxoplasma retinochoroiditis in immunocompetent patients. Ophthalmology 1999;106:148–53.
338. Friedman AH. The retinal lesions of the acquired immune deficiency syndrome. Trans Am Ophthalmol Soc 1984;82:447–91.
339. Edwards JE, Foos RY, Montomerie JZ, et al. Ocular manifestations of candida septicemia: review of seventy-six cases of hematogenous candida endophthalmitis. Medicine (Baltimore) 1974;53:47–75.
340. Rex JH, Bennet JE, Sugar AM, et al. A randomized trial comparing fluconazole with amphoteracin B for the treatment of candidemia in patients without neutropenia. N Engl J Med 1994;331:1325–30.
341. Panther LA, Sande MA. Cryptococcal meningitis in AIDS. In: Sande MA, Volberding PA, editors. The medical management of AIDS, 2nd ed. Philadelphia: WB Saunders; 1997.
342. Shields JA, Wright DM, Augsburger JJ, et al. Cryptococcal chorioretinitis. Am J Ophthalmol 1980;89:210.
343. Wykoff CA, Albini TA, Couvillion SS, et al. Intraocular Cryptococcoma. Arch Ophthalmol 2009;127(5):700–2.
344. Wheat LJ, Connolly-Stringfield PA, Baker RL, et al. Disseminated histoplasmosis in the acquired immune deficiency syndrome: clinical findings, diagnosis and treatment, and review of the literature. Medicine (Baltimore) 1990;69:361–74.
345. Wheat J, Hafner R, Wulfsohn M, et al. Prevention of relapse of histoplasmosis with itraconazole in patients with the acquired immunodeficiency syndrome. Ann Intern Med 1993;118:610–6.
346. Gonzales CA, Scott IU, Chaudhry NA, et al. Endogenous endophthalmitis caused by *Histoplasma capsulatum* var. capsulatum: a case report and literature review. Ophthalmology 2000;107:725–9.
347. Ala-Kauhaluoma M, Aho I, Ristola M, et al. Involvement of intraocular structures in disseminated histoplasmosis. Acta Ophthalmol 2010;88(4): 493–6.
348. Denning DW, Follansbee SE, Scolaro M, et al. Pulmonary aspergillosis in the acquired immunodeficiency syndrome. N Engl J Med 1991;324:654–62.

349. Kronish JW, Johnson TE, Gilberg SM, et al. Orbital infections in patients with human immunodeficiency virus infection. Ophthalmology 1996;103(9): 1483–92.
350. Fish DG, Ampel NM, Galgiani JN, et al. Coccidioidomycosis during human immunodeficiency virus infection: a review of 77 patients. Medicine (Baltimore) 1990;69:384–91.
351. McDonnell PJ, Green WR, Endophthalmitis. In: Mandell GL, Gordon RG, Bennett JE, editors. Principles and practice of infectious diseases, 4th ed. New York: Churchill Livingstone; 1995.
352. Finamor LP, Muccioli C, Martins MC, et al. Ocular and central nervous system paracoccidioidomycosis in a pregnant woman with acquired immunodeficiency syndrome. Am J Ophthalmol 2002;134:456–9.
353. Hariprasad SM, Mieler WF, Holz ER, et al. Determination of vitreous, aqueous, and plasma concentration of orally administered voriconazole in humans. Arch Ophthalmol 2004;122:42–7.
354. Brod RD, Flynn HW, Miller D. Endogenous fungal endophthalmitis. In: Duane's clinical ophthalmology. Hagerstown: Harper and Row; 2004. CD-ROM. ch 11.
355. Riddell 4th J, Comer GM, Kauffman CA. Treatment of endogenous fungal endophthalmitis: focus on new antifungal agents. Clin Infect Dis 2011;52: 648–53.
356. Garbino J, Ondrusova A, Baligvo E, et al. Successful treatment of *Paecilomyces lilacinus* endophthalmitis with voriconazole [published correction appears in Scand J Infect Dis 2003; 35:79]. Scand J Infect Dis 2002;34:701–3.
357. Kim JE, Perkins SL, Harris GJ. Voriconazole treatment of fungal scleritis and epibulbar abscess resulting from scleral buckle infection. Arch Ophthalmol 2003;121:735–7.
358. Ruhnke M, Schmidt-Westhausen A, Trautmann M. In vitro activities of voriconazole (UK-109,496) against fluconazole-susceptible and -resistant *Candida albicans* isolates from oral cavities of patients with human immunodeficiency virus infection. Antimicrob Agents Chemother 1997;41:575–7.
359. Tucker JD, Li JZ, Robbins GK, et al. Ocular syphilis among HIV-infected patients: a systematic analysis of the literature. Sex Transm Infect 2011;87: 4–8.
360. McLeish WM, Pulido JS, Holland S, et al. The ocular manifestations of syphilis in the human immunodeficiency virus type 1-infected host. Ophthalmology 1990;97:196–203.
361. Levy JH, Liss RA, Maguire AM. Neurosyphilis and ocular syphilis in patients with concurrent human immunodeficiency virus infection. Retina 1989;9: 175–80.
362. Gass JDM, Braunstein RA, Chenoweth RG. Acute syphilitic posterior placoid chorioretinitis. Ophthalmology 1990;97:1288–97.
363. Farhi D, Benhaddou N, Grange P, et al. Clinical and serologic baseline and follow-up features of syphilis according to HIV status in the post-HAART era. Medicine (Baltimore) 2009;88:331–40.
364. Freeman WR, Wiley CA. In situ nucleic acid hybridization. Surv Ophthalmol 1988;34:187–92.
365. de Smet MD. Differential diagnosis of retinitis and choroiditis in patients with acquired immunodeficiency syndrome. Am J Med 1992;92:17S–21S.
366. Schneiderman TE, Faber DW, Gross JG, et al. The agar–albumin sandwich technique for processing retinal biopsy specimens. Am J Ophthalmol 1989;108:567–71.
367. HHS Panel on Antiretroviral Guidelines for Adults and Adolescents [Internet]. Department of Health and Human Services; 2011 Oct 14 [cited 2012 Jan 26]. Guidelines for the use of antiretroviral agents in HIV-1-infected adults and adolescents. Available from: http://www.aidsinfo.nih.gov/ContentFiles/AdultandAdolescentGL.pdf.

Mycobacterial Infections

Chapter 82

Perumalsamy Namperumalsamy, Sivakumar R. Rathinam

INTRODUCTION

Ocular mycobacterial infection represents an important form of extra pulmonary infection which encompasses tubercular (TB) as well as nontubercular mycobacterial (NTM) diseases in and around the eye. It presents with diverse clinical manifestations because of a number of factors that are related to the microbe and the host. In spite of recent revolutionary advances in diagnostic technologies, establishing the diagnosis as well as treating the disease are clinical challenges. Mycobacterial disease is known to have affected humans for more than a century and still it continues to be a global health concern. There are several challenges as far as TB is concerned. To list a few, TB stands as the most common opportunistic infection in HIV-positive patients in many developing countries. In 2009, 1.7 million people died from TB, including 380 000 people with concomitant HIV infection, which equates to about 4700 deaths a day.[1] Yet another global threat is the emergence of multidrug-resistant (MDR-TB) and extensively drug-resistant strains of tuberculosis (XDR-TB). The World Health Organization has estimated there are 11.1 million patients with tuberculosis worldwide, of which 440 000 cases are due to MDR-TB. XDR-TB cases have been confirmed in 58 countries.[1] A second important concern is the emergence of NTM infections, both in immune-competent and immune-compromised individuals in previously unrecognized settings and with new clinical manifestations.[2] Clinical manifestations of NTM simulate typical tuberculosis. Lack of better laboratory tools for differentiation, lack of treatment guidelines, and resistance to routine antitubercular treatment challenge the early management of mycobacterial infections.

PULMONARY AND EXTRAPULMONARY TUBERCULOSIS

Tuberculosis is an infection caused by a rod-shaped, non-spore-forming, aerobic bacterium, *Mycobacterium tuberculosis*. Bacilli spread by small airborne droplets from infected patients. Once the droplet nuclei are inhaled, the bacilli settle in the airways. If the infection is not contained by the immune system, in around 3–8 weeks, local spread and spread to regional lymph nodes in the lungs occur. Subsequent spread to other organs results in extrapulmonary tuberculosis (EPTB). EPTB is reported to be increasing over the last several years.[3] Organs affected in EPTB include lymph nodes, pleura, central nervous system, eyes, musculoskeletal system, genitourinary tract and gastrointestinal tract. Symptoms and clinical presentations of EPTB are variable and depend on the organ involved. Unlike pulmonary TB patients, EPTB patients are less likely to present with cough, dyspnea, hemoptysis, abnormal chest X-ray, night sweats, weight loss, anorexia or fatigue. They may present with higher rates of abdominal pain, diarrhea, infertility, monoarticular joint pain or adenopathy depending upon the organ involved. Ocular tuberculosis represents an extrapulmonary dissemination of the bacilli primarily from lungs. However patients with ocular TB may have normal chest X-ray and negative chest complaints; alternatively they may have evidence of other forms of EPTB such as tubercular lymphadenitis. Ophthalmologists have to include appropriate questions in the history and consider extra-ocular systems whenever a tubercular etiology is suspected. It is essential to rule out EPTB and involvement of other systems in patients who may appear only to harbor pulmonary tuberculosis.

OCULAR TUBERCULOSIS

Tuberculosis is one of the most common infectious uveitis in tropical countries.[4–6] It is either unilateral or asymmetrically bilateral, characterized by a chronic and insidious course. Anatomically, tubercular uveitis may present as anterior, intermediate, posterior or pan-uveitis; it more often presents as granulomatous than nongranulomatous uveitis.

Three classic forms of ocular tuberculosis have been described. Direct ocular infection from an exogenous source may involve ocular adnexa, conjunctiva, sclera or cornea. The second form results from a hypersensitivity reaction to distant foci of infection causing episcleritis, phlyctenulosis, and occlusive retinal vasculitis of the type observed in Eales disease. The third form relates to the hematogenous spread of *M. tuberculosis* from pulmonary or extrapulmonary sites. The manifestations of this form of ocular tuberculosis are numerous (Figs 82.1 to 82.5), including lupus vulgaris, episcleritis, scleritis, necrotizing scleritis, posterior scleritis, interstitial keratitis, subretinal abscess, optic disc granuloma (Fig. 82.2), choroiditis, chorioretinitis, and choroidal granuloma (Fig. 82.3). Fundus fluorescein angiography may show a well-demarcated choroidal tubercle with initial hypo- and then late hyperfluorescence in such patients. Vessel wall staining, vascular leakage, disc staining and pooling of dye in the area of exudative detachment are other signs commonly seen in fluorescein angiography (Fig. 82.4B,C). Multifocal chorioretinitis with pigmented scars often indicates a tubercular etiology.[4] Exudative retinal hemorrhagic periphlebitis (Fig. 82.2) in a patient with uveitis is highly suggestive of tubercular etiology. Healed periphlebitis results in sclerosed venules. Presence of perivascular healed chorioretinal scars in such patients would also suggest tubercular cause. Serpiginous-like choroiditis (SLC) of presumed tubercular etiology closely mimics classic

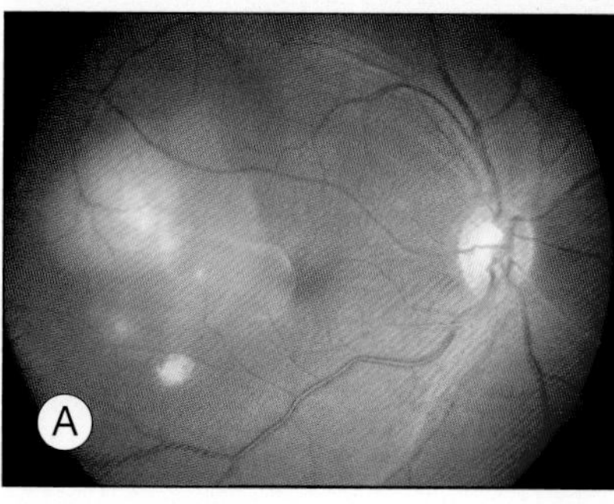

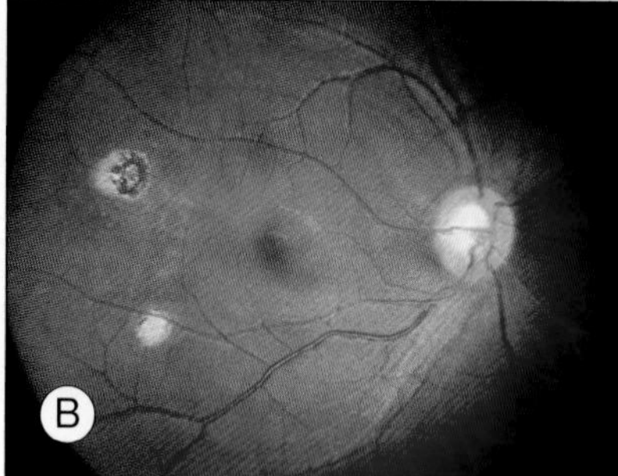

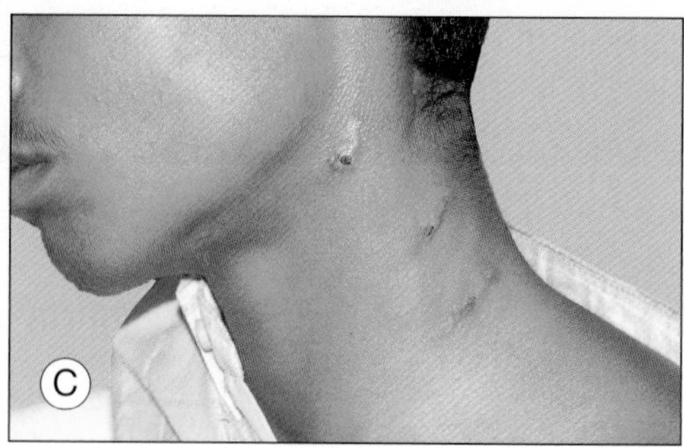

Fig. 82.1 (Patient 1) (A) Pretreatment fundus photograph of right eye showing a choroidal tubercle with adjoining exudative detachment. A healed scar is below the active lesion. (B) Fundus photograph of the right eye after antitubercular treatment showing healed scars with resolution of exudative detachment. (C) Multiple tubercular cervical sinuses in the neck of the same patient.

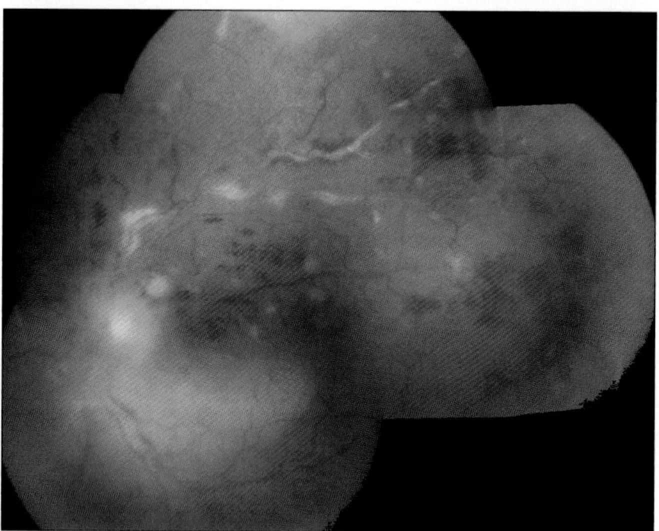

Fig. 82.2 (Patient 2) Fundus photograph showing tubercular disc granuloma, vasculitis, and multifocal retinitis in a smear positive pulmonary tuberculosis patient.

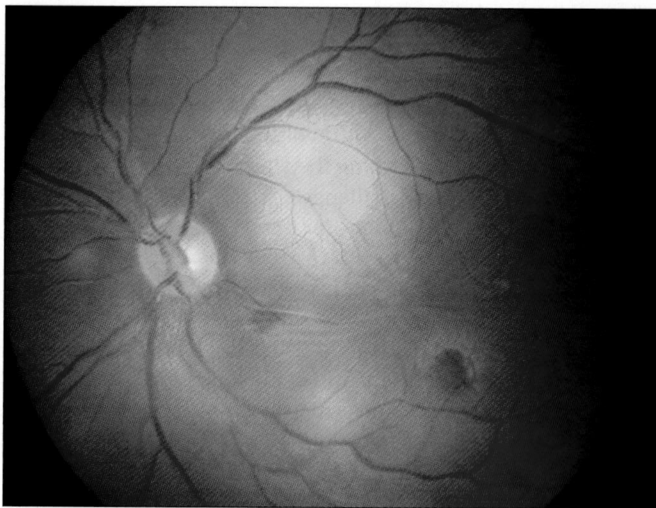

Fig. 82.3 (Patient 3) Fundus photograph showing old healed choroiditis as well as active recurrent lesions with varying chronology of choroidal lesions in the right eye. Mantoux skin test was necrotic and chest X-ray showed calcified lymph nodes.

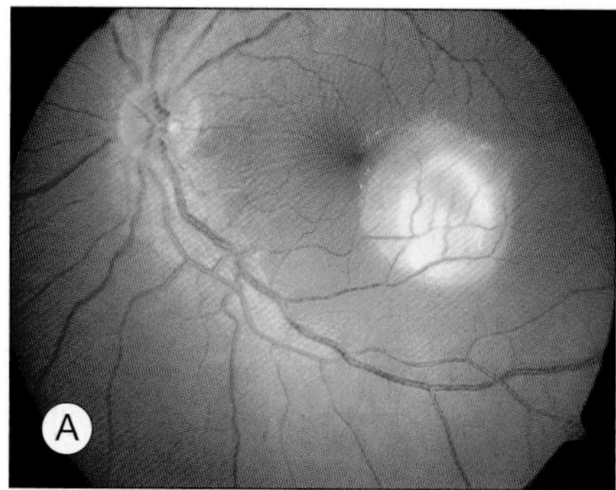

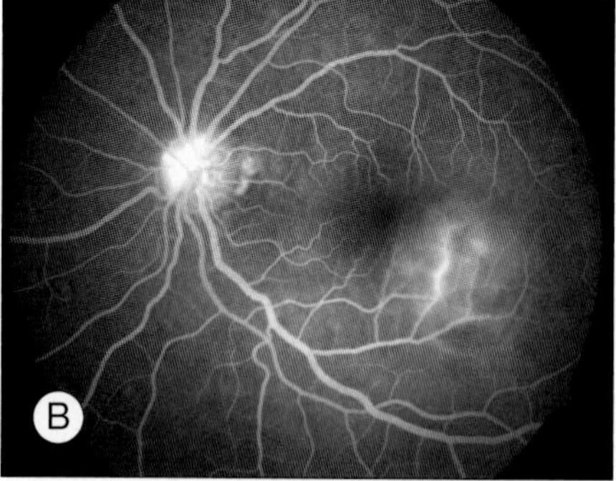

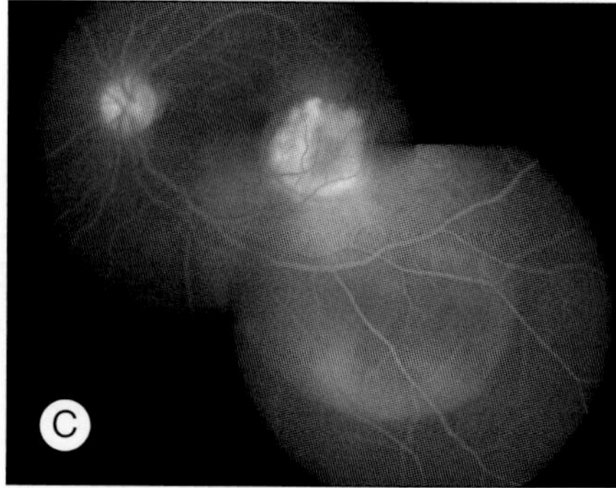

Fig. 82.4 (Patient 4) (A) Choroidal tubercle with choroidal folds, with shallow serous retinal detachment. (B) Fundus fluorescein angiogram shows vascular staining and perivascular leakage overlying the lesion suggestive of active retinal vasculitis. (C) Fundus fluorescein angiogram shows a well-demarcated choroidal tubercle showing increasing hyperfluorescence with pooling of dye in the area of neurosensory detachment in the late phase extending beyond the tubercle with late disc staining.

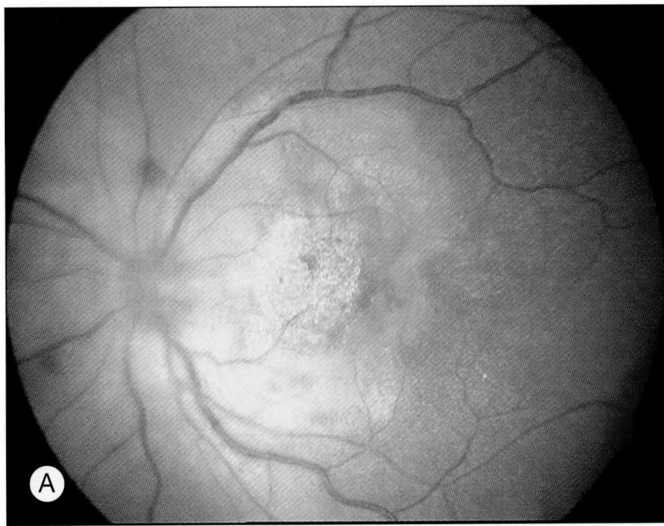

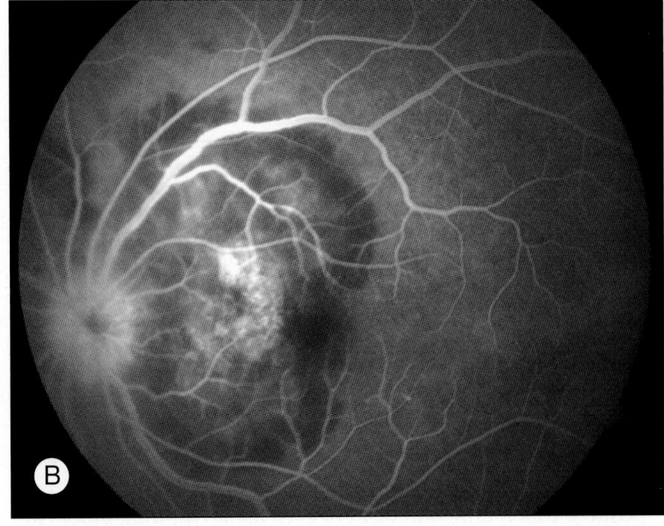

Fig. 82.5 (Patient 5) (A) Pretreatment fundus photograph of the left eye showing serpiginous-like choroiditis partly healed in the center with an active peripheral lesion, disc hyperemia with vitreous reaction. Vitreous was positive for real-time PCR for *M. tuberculosis.* (B) Fundus fluorescein angiogram of the same patient showing hyperfluorescence in the older central lesion and hypofluorescence in the active peripheral lesion, vessel wall staining, and disc staining.

serpiginous choroidopathy (SC) (Fig. 82.5A,B). Patients with SLC, however, are more likely to have multifocal scattered highly pigmented lesions with vitreous cells in contrast to classic SC, which is characteristically seen in the peripapillary area.[4,5]

Thus tubercular uveitis has a variable presentation, making the clinical diagnosis challenging. To help the clinician, a diagnostic criterion has been recommended. Diagnosis is considered as definitive TB only when the bacilli are isolated from the ocular tissues. The criterion for presumed tuberculous uveitis is reported to be presence of any one of the following clinical signs, such as choroidal granuloma, broad-based posterior synechiae, retinal vasculitis with or without choroiditis, or serpiginous-like choroiditis with a positive tuberculin skin test or QuantiFERON-TB Gold test, or any other relevant tests, such as chest radiograph and computed tomography.[4] Good response to anti tubercular treatment and absence of recurrence further supports the diagnosis of presumed ocular tuberculosis.

Differential diagnosis

Granulomatous uveitis may also be seen in patients with herpes simplex or varicella zoster infection, phacoantigenic uveitis, sarcoidosis, syphilis, leprosy, Vogt–Koyanagi–Harada disease and sympathetic ophthalmia. Other causes of choroidal granulomas include syphilis, sarcoidosis, and fungal lesions.[4,5]

Pathogenesis

Tissue damage in ocular tuberculosis is not only a direct consequence of infection but it is also due to non-resolving inflammation that results from a sensitive balance between protective immunity and destructive pathology.[7] Molecular studies and sequencing of the *M. tuberculosis* genome have identified specific and highly immunogenic antigens. These are the so-called 6 kDa early secretory antigenic target (ESAT-6) and the 10 kDa culture filtrate protein (CFP-10). They are capable of eliciting vigorous helper T-cell responses with resultant cytotoxicity in cellular models. They cause cell lysis and may enable the bacteria to invade and spread within the alveolar epithelium. Recent studies indicate ESAT-6 may also stimulate the trafficking of infected macrophages into the granulomas, to utilize the granulomas as foci of macrophage recruitment, infection, and subsequent bacterial dissemination.

Host genetic factors appear to play a role in disease severity. Abnormalities in the genes encoding the interferon-gamma receptor chain and genes encoding interleukin-12 are important in determining the susceptibility to disseminated mycobacterial disease.[8] Pulmonary alveolar macrophages express complement and toll-like receptors and destroy the bacteria when they fuse with lysosomes. However, the mycobacteria can inhibit fusion with lysosomes, and may then thrive in the phagosome. Retinal pigment epithelium (RPE) shares several functions with the macrophages, including expression of toll-like receptors, complement, and phagocytosis of bacteria. Clinicopathologic study combined with molecular analysis revealed distribution of the mycobacteria in the RPE even though the retina and uvea were involved with the inflammatory process. The authors suggest a possibility of reactivation of sequestered organisms in cases of recurrent inflammation.[9]

NONTUBERCULOUS MYCOBACTERIAL INFECTIONS

More recently, nontuberculous mycobacterial (NTM) disease appears to be increasing.[10] The genus *Mycobacterium* contains more than 125 species; these saprophytic mycobacteria are ubiquitous in the environment, and may be present in soil, water, and dust particles. Both rapid and slow-growing NTM have been implicated in ocular infection, *M. chelonae* and *M. abscessus* are often reported to result in severe and progressive endophthalmitis. NTM endophthalmitis has been reported after uncomplicated phacoemulsification and intraocular lens implantation, laser in situ keratomileusis, endothelial keratoplasty, scleral buckling, and intravitreal injections.[11] Difficulty in management is mainly due to delay in the diagnosis and varying sensitivity to antibiotics. In many studies, initial cultures took variable periods to demonstrate growth or failed entirely to show the causative organism. Etiologies were often misdiagnosed as *Propionibacterium* acnes, nocardial or fungal endophthalmitis.[11] NTM are resistant to most conventional antimycobacterial drugs but are sensitive to a variety of other antibiotics. Amikacin, moxifloxacin, and to a lesser extent levofloxacin and ciprofloxacin demonstrate significant effectiveness against NTM.[12] Biofilm-forming, nonpigmented, rapidly growing mycobacteria have also been shown to result in endophthalmitis. These organisms show resistance to eradication strategies, resistance to innate host immune responses, and to antibiotics.[13] Large gaps still exist in our knowledge on ocular NTM infection. Accurate biomarkers to predict exposure, latency, relapse, and resistant diseases are being investigated and are not yet available for clinical use.

LATENT TUBERCULOSIS

Latent tuberculosis infection (LTBI) is diagnosed when there is a positive tuberculin skin test (TST) in an asymptomatic person with no clinical or radiographic signs of active tuberculosis. The clinical relevance of this condition is that the patient may progress to active tuberculosis. After entry into the human system, organisms can either begin to proliferate immediately, causing primary TB, or be cleared by the immune system. Alternatively, by slowing their metabolism or becoming dormant, they adapt to stressful conditions generated by the infected host and remain silent to the immune system. When the environmental conditions are favorable, activation may result in clinically apparent disease.

LABORATORY EVALUATION

A complete systemic history and examination are fundamental steps in the evaluation of all patients with ocular tuberculosis and may reveal evidence of pulmonary and other extrapulmonary tuberculosis. Recent advances in diagnostic tools for tuberculous infection, including molecular biology techniques, IFN-γ release assays, and radiodiagnostics have improved the specificity of the diagnosis. However, all these investigations have their own strengths and limitations.[14] The suboptimal specificity and sensitivity of existing diagnostic tools delay the diagnosis and treatment of active ocular infection. Clear understanding of their principles and proper test selection are needed to obtain relevant clinical support.

Positive reaction after Mantoux or TST intradermal injection of tuberculin purified protein derivative (PPD) indicate a successful cellular immune response by the patient. The antigen used in TST is a mixture of more than 200 proteins derived from *M. tuberculosis*. They can cross-react with BCG and NTM antigens, undermining the specificity of the test. Hence TST has limited specificity and a positive result may not confirm disease. The American Thoracic Society and the United States Centers for Disease Control (CDC) consider reactions of 5 mm or more to be positive in very high-risk individuals (e.g., abnormal chest X-ray, HIV patients), 10 mm or more in high-risk patients (e.g., patients from endemic areas), and 15 mm or more in patients with no identified risk factors. In addition, a negative test does not rule out TB. In a study on patients with histopathologically proven ocular tuberculosis, 40% had negative TST results.[15]

To study the immune response of the patient, novel in vitro tests have been developed using ESAT-6 and CFP-10 proteins (see pathogenesis). Commercially available QuantiFERON (QFT) and TSPOT.TB are commonly known as interferon-gamma release assays (IGRA). T cells, collected from the patient are exposed to these specific tubercular antigens. The assay measures the interferon-γ (IFN-γ) released by sensitized T cells of the patient. The CDC guidelines state that IGRAs can be used in all situations in which the TST is currently used. Canada and United Kingdom national guidelines suggest using IGRAs only to confirm a positive TST.[16] Although these tests were originally designed to screen for latent tuberculosis, they have been tested in active systemic and ocular tuberculosis cohorts as well. A meta-analysis on IGRA concludes that the diagnostic sensitivities of both IGRAs are higher than that of tuberculin skin tests and the specificity, lower.[17] TST and QFT were found equally predictive of progression to TB disease; QFT was not found superior to TST in a cohort of adolescents in a high systemic TB burden population from South Africa,[18] as well as in uveitis.[19] The QFT result together with the TST may increase the sensitivity.[20] Positive and negative predictive values of IGRA depend on prevalence of TB in that population. As far as systemic TB is concerned, there is increasing evidence that IGRAs perform differently in high burden compared to low burden countries. Because of the low prevalence of TB in the United States, the low pretest probability and low positive predictive value, IGRAs may not be useful as a standard part of the uveitis workup.[21] The lack of a gold standard for diagnosis of TB infection prevents an effective and interpretable comparison of the IGRAs and the TST in ocular tuberculosis.[21]

Radiologic examination of the chest may reveal infiltrations, cavitation, hilar adenopathy, pleural effusion, or fibrotic or calcific lesions in some patients. The predominant route of infection to ocular tissues is by hematogenous spread from the lungs; however, the pulmonary focus may not be evident clinically or radiographically in all patients. In a cohort of histopathologically proven ocular TB patients, 57% of patients had negative chest radiograph results.[15] Hence an initial negative workup does not rule out the infection, and repeat workup may be needed. More recently, high resolution computed tomography of the chest was found to be a useful tool in the diagnosis of granulomatous uveitis. Some centers further recommend use of positron emission tomography/CT-guided lymph node identification for biopsy to aid the diagnosis of tuberculosis-associated uveitis.[22]

Isolation of *M. tuberculosis* by culture remains the cornerstone for diagnosis; however, isolation from inflamed ocular tissue is not always possible. Whenever it is possible, the specimen is often too small for all procedures, such as Ziehl Neelsen staining, inoculation in liquid and solid media, species identification, and drug susceptibility testing. Biopsy specimens may be obtained for histopathological analysis from either the iris or by retinochoroidal biopsy. The absence of acid-fast bacilli or of caseating necrosis in the biopsy specimen does not rule out tuberculosis. In such circumstances, tests based on nucleic acid amplification are rapid and more specific for *M. tuberculosis*. Diagnosis based on detection of mycobacterial DNA through PCR and real time PCR is becoming the method of choice because of rapid test results and the ability to test in a very small sample.[15]

Resistance to anti-TB drugs may be caused by chromosomal mutations in genes encoding drug targets resulting in MDR-TB. Proper management of MDR-TB relies on early recognition of drug resistance. Clinical diagnosis of drug resistance is checked by drug susceptibility testing. It is performed on all positive mycobacterial cultures on Middlebrook 7H10 agar, with 1%

proportional method for isoniazid, rifampicin, ethambutol, streptomycin, ciprofloxacin, and kanamycin. Drug susceptibility testing by conventional mycobacterial culture is slow and elaborate, requiring sequential procedures for the diagnosis. Several molecular diagnostic tests, such as the Sanger-based DNA sequencing methods, are expected to lead to faster identification of MDR and XDR strains.[23]

TREATMENT

Antitubercular therapy is highly effective in reducing the recurrences of uveitis in patients with manifest TB. The systemic management of TB is complex and requires the input of infectious disease experts. The WHO recommends new patients with both pulmonary TB and extrapulmonary TB to be treated with a four-drug regimen (isoniazid 5 mg/kg/day, rifampicin 10 mg/kg/day, ethambutol 15 mg/kg/day, and pyrazinamide 20–25 mg/kg/day). Ethambutol and pyrazinamide are stopped after 2 months and isoniazid and rifampicin are continued for 4–6 months. Corticosteroids seem to have a potential benefit in patients with tubercular pericarditis and meningitis.[24] Similarly, steroids are used in ocular TB as well. More evidence is required on the dose and duration of corticosteroid treatment in ocular infections. In patients with coexisting HIV and systemic tuberculosis, initiation of concomitant antitubercular and antiretroviral therapy may result in exacerbation of inflammation and clinical deterioration.[25] Either addition of corticosteroids or delaying the administration of highly active antiretroviral therapy (HAART) for the first 2 months of antituberculosis treatment is advised. Hepatotoxic effects are seen with all first-line antituberculosis therapies and usually present as nausea, vomiting, and abdominal pain in the right upper quadrant. In most patients, even if hepatotoxic effects develop, severe liver injury can be avoided and antituberculosis therapy can be completed by following a comprehensive management algorithm.[26] Drug dosage and adverse reactions are summarized in Table 82.1.

Table 82.1 Five groups of antituberculosis drugs[26,30]

Drug	Dose	Adverse reaction	Additional information
GROUP 1 Four first-line oral antituberculosis drugs			
Isoniazid	4–6 mg/kg (up to 300 mg)	Transient increase in hepatic enzyme Peripheral neuropathy	Use during pregnancy is considered safe Crosses the blood–brain barrier
Rifampicin	8–12 mg/kg	Hepatotoxicity Thrombocytopenia	Safe during pregnancy
Ethambutol	15–20 mg/kg	Reversible dose-related retrobulbar neuritis, typically begins 3–6 months after the start of therapy Hepatotoxicity	Crosses placental barrier, but considered safe in pregnancy Better ocular penetration Does not cross meninges
Pyrazinamide	20–25 mg/kg	Pruritus Hepatotoxicity	Safe during pregnancy Crosses the blood–brain barrier
GROUP 2* Fluoroquinolones*	**GROUP 3** Injectable drugs**	**GROUP 4†**	**GROUP 5‡**
Ofloxacin (15 mg/kg)	Capreomycin (15 mg/kg)	Ethionamide/prothionamide (15 mg/kg)	Clofazimine (100 mg)
Levofloxacin (15 mg/kg)	Kanamycin (15 mg/kg)	Cycloserine/terizidone (15 mg/kg)	Amoxicillin with clavulanate (875/125 mg every 12 h)
Moxifloxacin (7·5–10 mg/kg)	Amikacin (15 mg/kg)	P-aminosalicylic acid (acid salt) 150 mg/kg	Linezolid (600 mg)
	Streptomycin (15 mg/kg)		Imipenem§ (500–1000 mg every 6 h) Clarithromycin‡ (500 mg/12 h) Thioacetazone (150 mg)

**A fluoroquinolone should always be included in the treatment of MDR and XDR tuberculosis.*
***There should always be one injectable drug in the treatment of MDR and XDR tuberculosis. Preference to the following sequence: capreomycin, kanamycin, followed by amikacin.*
†Group 4 Use all the necessary drugs to make up at least four active basic drugs; start with ethionamide, cycloserine, finally aminosalicylic acid, rarely streptomycin.
‡Group 5 Less-effective drugs or drugs on which clinical data are sparse. Preference to the following order: clofazimine, amoxicillin-clavulanate, linezolid, imipenem or meropenem, clarithromycin, and thioacetazone.
§Except imipenem and clarithromycin all other drugs are given as single dose per day.
MDR, multidrug-resistant tuberculosis; XDR, extensively drug-resistant tuberculosis.

Drug-resistant tuberculosis

MDR tuberculosis is defined as the disease caused by organisms that are resistant to isoniazid and rifampicin, which are two first-line anti-TB drugs. XDR-TB is defined as tuberculosis that is caused by organisms resistant to isoniazid and rifampicin and to any one of the fluoroquinolones and at least one of the injectable second-line drugs. MDR and XDR tuberculosis are generally thought to have high morbidity and mortality rates and drug-resistant strains have evolved mainly due to incomplete or improper treatment of TB patients. MDR and XDR-TB are now global threats.[1] In the vast majority of clinical settings in the developing world, culture and drug-susceptibility testing are not available. Most cases likely go undetected due to insufficient laboratory infrastructure for diagnosis.[27,28] At present, MDR-TB is treated by a combination of 8–10 drugs with therapies lasting up to 18–24 months; only four of these drugs were actually developed to treat TB. Such suboptimal therapy leads to almost 30% of MDR-TB patients experiencing treatment failure. The current situation necessitates the immediate identification of new and more potent drugs.[29] A better prognosis can be obtained, however, with the right combination and rational use of drugs chosen in a stepwise selection process through five groups on the basis of efficacy, safety, and cost.[30]

Detection of drug resistance is possible only in culture isolates, because of challenges in isolating the organisms from the eye; drug susceptibility testing is difficult in ocular TB. This has serious implications, specifically in uveitis. When a trial of antitubercular treatment fails in presumed ocular TB, there is a very high possibility for the uveitis specialist to assume a nontubercular etiology and to start corticosteroids or immunosuppressive treatment to control inflammation.[28] In such situations, molecular diagnostic studies may be of help.

The WHO has developed a new six-point Stop TB Strategy addressing the key challenges facing TB control.[1] Its goal is to dramatically reduce the global burden of tuberculosis by 2015 by ensuring all TB patients, including those co-infected with HIV and those with drug-resistant TB, benefit from universal access to high-quality diagnosis and patient-centered treatment. The strategy also supports the development of new and effective tools to prevent, detect, and treat TB. If success is achieved and quality care is provided as per the International Standard of TB Care, it is anticipated the incidence of extrapulmonary tuberculosis, including ocular TB, will decline.

REFERENCES

1. World Health Organization. Global tuberculosis control 2010. World Health Organization. Available at www.who.int/tb/publications/global_report; accessed June 6, 2011.
2. Griffith DE, Aksamit T, Brown-Elliott BA, et al. An official ATS/IDSA statement: diagnosis, treatment, and prevention of nontuberculous mycobacterial diseases. Am J Respir Crit Care Med 2007;15:367–416.
3. Gonzalez OY, Adams G, Teeter LD, et al. Extra-pulmonary manifestations in a large metropolitan area with a low incidence of tuberculosis. Int J Tuberc Lung Dis 2003;7:1178–85.
4. Gupta A, Bansal R, Gupta V, et al. Ocular signs predictive of tubercular uveitis. Am J Ophthalmol 2010;149:562–70.
5. Vasconcelos-Santos DV, Rao PK, Davies JB, et al. Clinical features of tuberculous serpiginouslike choroiditis in contrast to classic serpiginous choroiditis. Arch Ophthalmol 2010;128:853–8.
6. Rathinam SR, Namperumalsamy P. Global variation and pattern changes in epidemiology of uveitis. Indian J Ophthalmol 2007;55:173–83.
7. Dorhoi A, Reece ST, Kaufmann SHE. For better or for worse: the immune response against *Mycobacterium tuberculosis* balances pathology and protection. Immunol Rev 2011;240:235–51.
8. Krishnan N, Robertson BD, Thwaites G. The mechanisms and consequences of the extra-pulmonary dissemination of *Mycobacterium tuberculosis*. Tuberculosis (Edinb) 2010;90:361–6.
9. Rao NA, Saraswathy S, Smith RE. Tuberculous uveitis: distribution of *Mycobacterium tuberculosis* in the retinal pigment epithelium. Arch Ophthalmol 2006;124:1777–9.
10. Shenai S, Rodrigues C, Mehta A. Time to identify and define non-tuberculous mycobacteria in a tuberculosis-endemic region. Int J Tuberc Lung Dis 2010; 14:1001–8.
11. Matieli LCV, De Freitas D, Sampaio J, et al. Mycobacterium abscessus endophthalmitis: treatment dilemma and review of the literature. Retina (Philadelphia, Pa) 2006;26:826–9.
12. Caballero AR, Marquart ME, O'Callaghan RJ, et al. Effectiveness of fluoroquinolones against *Mycobacterium abscessus* in vivo. Curr Eye Res 2006;31: 23–9.
13. Holland SP, Pulido JS, Miller D, et al. Biofilm and scleral buckle-associated infections. A mechanism for persistence. Ophthalmology 1991;98:933–8.
14. Vasconcelos-Santos DV, Zierhut M, Rao NA. Strengths and weaknesses of diagnostic tools for tuberculous uveitis. Ocul Immunol Inflamm 2009;17: 351–5.
15. Wroblewski KJ, Hidayat AA, Neafie RC, et al. Ocular tuberculosis: a clinicopathologic and molecular study. Ophthalmology 2011;118:772–7.
16. Schluger NW, Burzynski J. Recent advances in testing for latent TB. Chest 2010;138:1456–63.
17. Sester M, Sotgiu G, Lange C, et al. Interferon-γ release assays for the diagnosis of active tuberculosis: a systematic review and meta-analysis. Eur Respir J 2011;37:100–11.
18. Mahomed H, Hawkridge T, Verver S, et al. The tuberculin skin test versus QuantiFERON TB GoldH in predicting tuberculosis disease in an adolescent cohort study in South Africa. PLoS ONE 2011;6(3):e17984. doi:10.1371/journal.pone.0017984.
19. Babu K, Satish V, Satish S, et al. Utility of QuantiFERON TB gold test in a south Indian patient population of ocular inflammation. Indian J Ophthalmol 2009; 57:427–30.
20. Marcus A, Hla MH, Soon-Phaik C. Diagnosis of tuberculous uveitis: clinical application of an interferon-gamma release assay. Ophthalmology 2009;116: 1391–6.
21. Albini TA, Karakousis PC, Rao NA. Interferon-gamma release assays in the diagnosis of tuberculous uveitis. Am J Ophthalmol 2008;146:486–8.
22. Doycheva D, Deuter C, Hetzel J, et al. The use of positron emission tomography/CT in the diagnosis of tuberculosis-associated uveitis. Br J Ophthalmol [Internet] Oct 8, 2010 [cited 2011 May 11]. Available from: http://www.ncbi.nlm.nih.gov/pubmed/20935307.
23. Campbell PJ, Morlock GP, Sikes RD, et al. Molecular detection of mutations associated with first- and second-line drug resistance compared with conventional drug susceptibility testing of *Mycobacterium tuberculosis*. Antimicrob Agents Chemother 2011;55: 2032–41.
24. Kadhiravan T, Deepanjali S. Role of corticosteroids in the treatment of tuberculosis: an evidence-based update. Indian J Chest Dis Allied Sci 2010;52: 153–8.
25. Rathinam SR, Lalitha P. Paradoxical worsening of ocular tuberculosis in HIV patients after antiretroviral therapy. Eye (Lond) 2007;21:667–8.
26. Senousy BE, Belal SI, Draganov PV. Hepatotoxic effects of therapies for tuberculosis. Nat Rev Gastroenterol Hepatol 2010;7:543–56.
27. Koul A, Arnoult E, Lounis N, et al. The challenge of new drug discovery for tuberculosis. Nature 2011;469:483–90.
28. Rathinam SR. Treating uveitis in the developing world setting. Int Ophthalmol Clin 2010;50:219–28.
29. Rao NA, Irfan M, Soomro MM, et al. Drug resistance pattern in multidrug resistance pulmonary tuberculosis patients. J Coll Physicians Surg Pak 2010 Apr;20(4):262–5.
30. Caminero JA, Sotgiu G, Zumla A, et al. Best drug treatment for multidrug-resistant and extensively drug-resistant tuberculosis. Lancet Infect Dis 2010;10: 621–9.

Eales Disease

Perumalsamy Namperumalsamy, Dhananjay Shukla

Chapter 83

INTRODUCTION

Eales disease is an idiopathic, occlusive perivasculitis affecting peripheral retina in young men, leading to retinal nonperfusion, new vessel formation, and recurrent vitreous hemorrhages. Eales disease was reported from the UK, USA, and Canada in the latter half of the 19th century and early 20th century.[1,2] The eponym originated from the first description of a syndrome of recurrent vitreous hemorrhage in young men with epistaxis and constipation by Henry Eales.[3] Most cases in the last decade have been reported from the Indian subcontinent, with a few reports from Turkey, Saudi Arabia, and Iran.[4–13] However, the incidence of Eales disease appears to have declined globally, due probably to improved general health and living standards and reduced incidence of tuberculosis (TB),[1,2,10] as well as to improved etiologic diagnosis in a heterogeneous group of allegedly primary vasculitides, previously amalgamated as presumed Eales disease.[14] Most patients are healthy young men, aged 20–40 years; the mean age of onset is generally earlier in Asians than in Caucasians.[2,15–17]

CLINICAL FEATURES AND NATURAL HISTORY

Three sequential vascular responses which determine the natural course of Eales disease are inflammation, occlusion, and neovascularization.[1,2,10,15] Most patients are asymptomatic at the stages of inflammation and occlusion. The disease starts quietly as multiple, peripheral inflammatory branch retinal vein occlusions: fine, solid white lines representing venous sheathing are the commonest clinical presentation (Fig. 83.1).[1,2] As active vasculitis slowly resolves, the fuzzy vascular sheathing, with indistinct margins, becomes well defined and distinct. Retinal arteries may be involved later, but their involvement is not central to the disease presentation,[1] and is generally suggestive of other conditions like systemic vasculitides.[11,18] Other clinical features which suggest alternative inflammatory etiologies are exudative or focal vasculitis, cotton-wool spots,[11,18] and central retinal involvement including macular and optic disc edema, choroiditis, anterior uveitis, and vitritis.[2,14]

As the occlusions are primarily venous, they occur gradually, allowing development of compensatory phenomena like collaterals, microaneurysms, capillary telangiectasia, corkscrew vessels, and venous beading; some of these changes may be observed by careful examination of the apparently uninvolved fellow eye of a patient with unilateral involvement. Prolonged and extensive retinal nonperfusion eventually leads to peripheral neovascularization in up to 80% of eyes; disc neovascularization is rare.[2,4,15] New vessels bleed into vitreous, resulting in the classic presentation of Eales disease: a sudden, unilateral blurring of vision or floaters[15,17] (Fig. 83.2). Vision often improves, but recurrences are common. The second eye is ultimately affected in 50–90% of cases, after a gap of 3–10 years.[2,4,14,15] Isolated episodes of vitreous hemorrhage usually settle down without visual deficit; recurrent bleeds lead to progressive contraction of vitreous cortex, resulting in tractional retinal detachments, secondary retinal tears, and epimacular membranes.[1] Though anterior-segment neovascularization occurs in a small fraction of eyes, the prognosis is better than what is typically associated with iris neovascularization.[4]

Charamis graded the evolution of Eales disease into four stages. Stage I was characterized by mild peripheral perivasculitis; stage II by extensive inflammation involving larger vessels; neovascularization and vitreous hemorrhage heralded stage III; and tractional complications marked stage IV.[19] A system for grading Eales disease on the basis of the degree and extent of retinal vasculopathy, neovascular proliferations, and vitreous hemorrhage has also been proposed.[20] However, the course of the disease is variable, and a fixed sequence of stages may not be followed consistently.[1,2]

PATHOLOGY AND PATHOGENESIS

The classic histopathological connotation of the term "vasculitis" is a type III hypersensitivity reaction with deposition of immune complexes in the vessel wall.[21] This definition is not applicable to retinal vasculitis in general, and Eales disease in particular, which represents perivascular cuffing with inflammatory cells, graded by clinical appearance rather than vascular caliber or type of immune response.[11,21] Most authors have therefore used the terms "vasculitis" and "perivasculitis" interchangeably in the context of Eales disease.

Central to the visually debilitating complications of Eales disease is retinal hypoxia. Inflammation causes hypoxia by an increase in the metabolic demands of cells and a reduction in metabolic substrates caused by inflammatory vascular occlusion. Hypoxia in turn triggers further inflammation, setting up a vicious cycle.[22] This sequence suggest a pathogenetic role for both angiogenic factors and inflammatory cytokines in Eales disease, in a manner similar to noninflammatory vascular diseases like diabetic retinopathy. A simultaneous upregulation of vascular endothelial growth factor (VEGF), and interleukins (IL-6 and IL-9) has indeed been observed during the proliferative phases of both diabetic retinopathy and Eales disease.[7] Other biochemical analyses have also implicated retinal autoimmunity, angiogenic growth

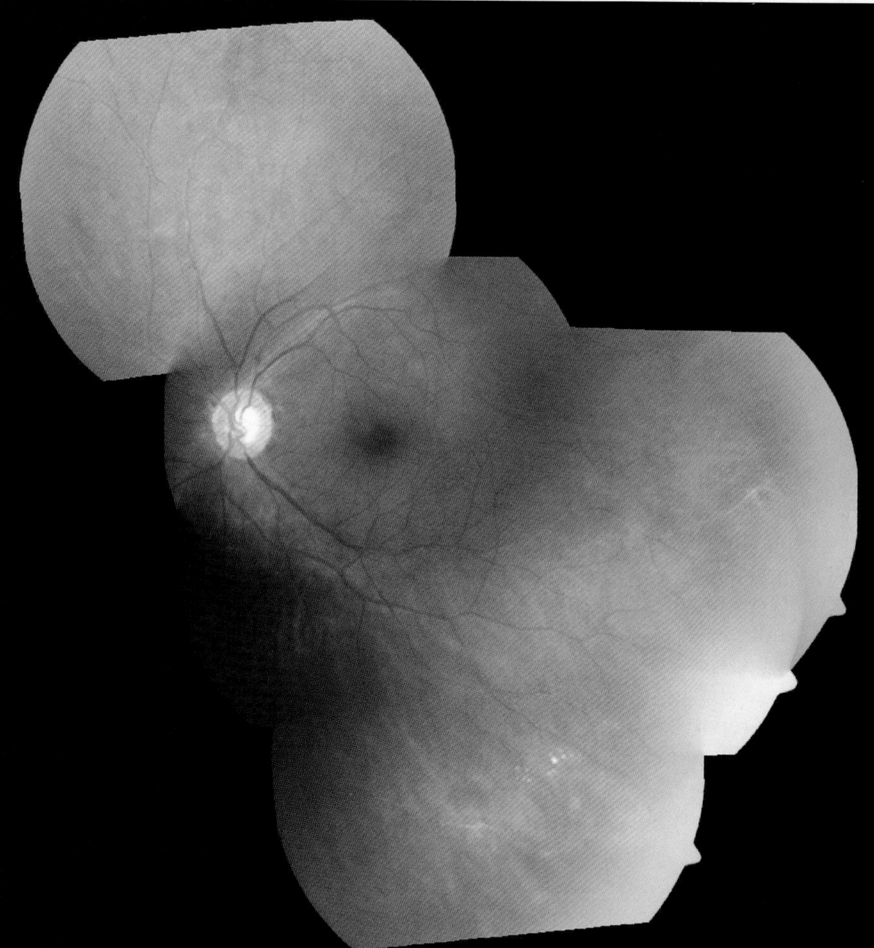

Fig. 83.1 The most common presentation of Eales disease is solid columns of sheathing in peripheral veins, as seen here in superior, inferior, and inferotemporal periphery. A few hard exudates inferiorly suggest resolved retinal edema. The posterior pole and visual acuity are unaffected.

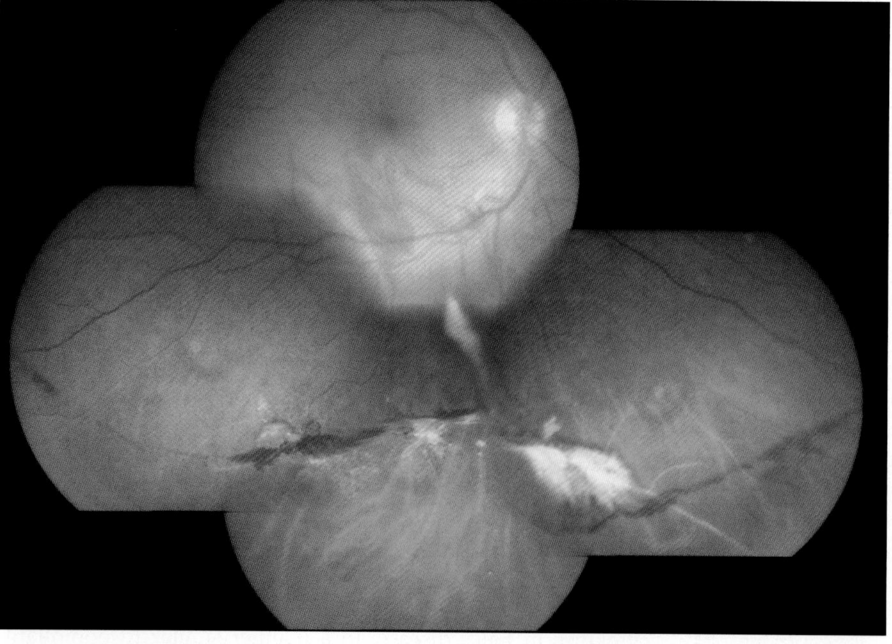

Fig. 83.2 Classic presentation of Eales disease is floaters or blurring of vision due to vitreous hemorrhage from peripheral new vessels. Recurrent bleeds lead to epiretinal membrane formation, which is beginning at the posterior pole. Note the linear, extensive sheathing of the peripheral retinal vessels.

factors, and oxidative stress in causing inflammation and neovascularization in Eales disease.[2] Recent serologic and genetic studies have reinforced the role of cell-mediated immunity in Eales disease, particularly interleukins and tumor necrosis factor-alpha.[9,12]

The pathogenesis of inflammatory vascular occlusions in Eales disease remains unclear. Systemic association with neurological, vestibuloauditory, hematological, and parasitic diseases and infections have been proposed but never proven.[2,15] The most frequently reported association is with systemic TB. While viable organisms have not been demonstrated from the eyes with Eales disease, polymerase chain reaction-based studies have identified mycobacterial DNA in vitreous and epiretinal tissue.[23,24] These findings make the case for hypersensitivity to tuberculoprotein; the case is reinforced by the presence of Mantoux tuberculin skin test positivity in the majority of patients.[2] This concept continues to be popular among current researchers.[11] Several other studies have however disputed this notion by demonstrating Mantoux positivity in healthy controls, as well as Mantoux negativity among Eales patients.[2,15,25]

DIFFERENTIAL DIAGNOSIS

Eales disease is a diagnosis of exclusion (see Fig. 83.3). Several ocular and systemic inflammatory and noninflammatory diseases cause retinal vascular sheathing or occlusion, which may closely resemble Eales disease. However, a battery of investigations is not necessary for every patient. A detailed history and a thorough systemic examination rule out most of the mimicking diseases; only a few tailored investigations are required to clinch the diagnosis.

Among noninflammatory vascular occlusions, primary branch retinal vein occlusion mimics Eales most closely. The former occurs at an arteriovenous crossing; the crossing artery is frequently sclerosed. The occlusions are not multiple and peripheral like Eales, and affect older age groups. Proliferative diabetic retinopathy may also exhibit sheathing of vessels during active stage (as part of the appearance labeled "featureless retina") or at involutional stage. Central retinal vein occlusion in a young adult should be investigated for inflammatory etiology (see diagnostic workup, below) because it represents a rare presentation of Eales.[1] Coats disease, familial exudative vitreoretinopathy (FEVR) and sickle-cell disease also show similar peripheral nonperfusion and should be ruled out. Though Coats disease also occurs in male patients, they are typically younger and have unilateral disease with prominent telangiectasia, more exudation, and less neovascularization or vitreous hemorrhage. FEVR and sickle-cell retinopathy have distinctive clinical and angiographic features, as well as familial and systemic associations respectively, to distinguish them from Eales disease.

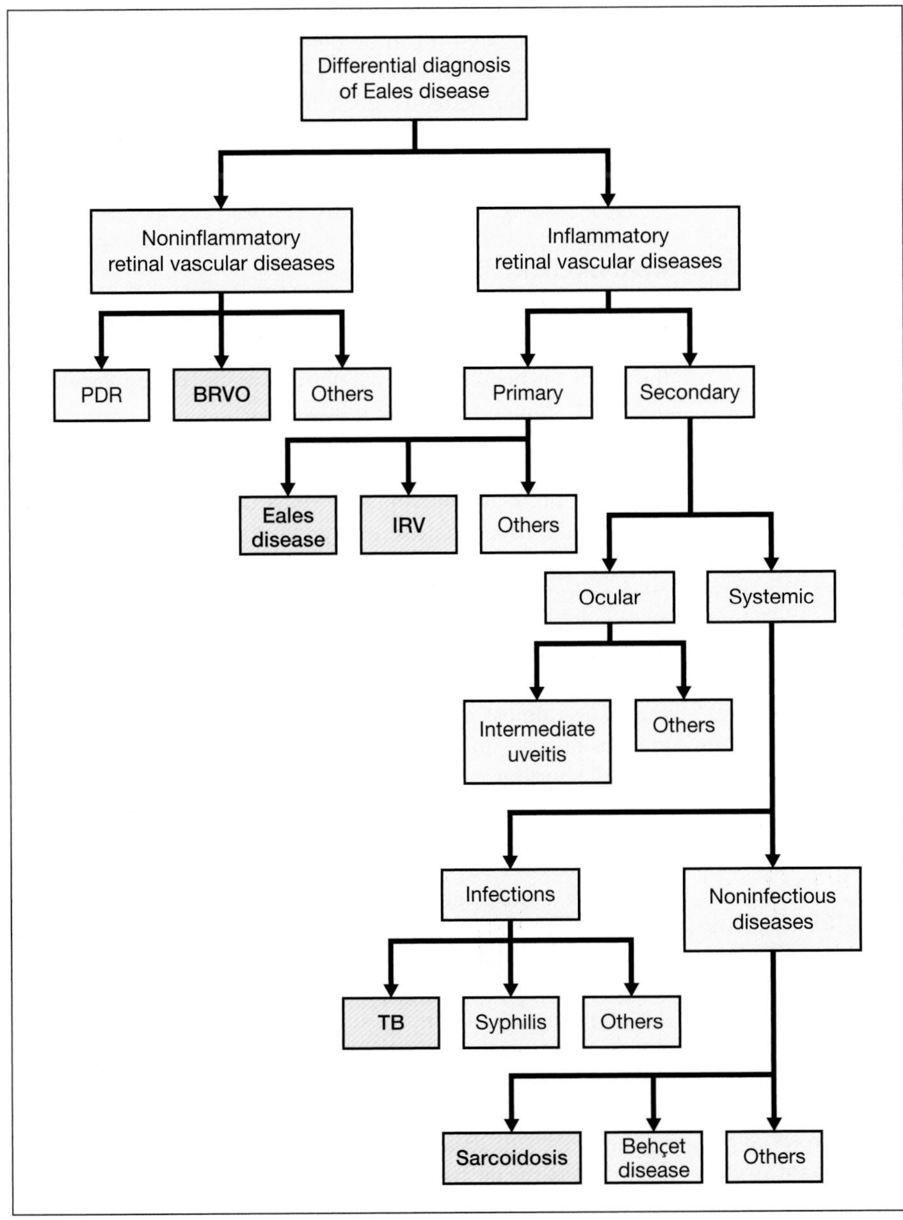

Fig. 83.3 Differential diagnosis of Eales disease. PDR, proliferative diabetic retinopathy; BRVO, branch retinal vein occlusion; IRV, idiopathic retinal vasculitis; TB, tuberculosis.

Ocular inflammatory conditions like intermediate uveitis, endophthalmitis, multifocal choroiditis, and birdshot retinopathy may have associated retinal vasculitis, but primary lesions are generally prominent and unmistakable. Systemic TB should be ruled out in every case of retinal vasculitis because of its endemic presence, especially in the Indian subcontinent.[26] However, TB typically causes anterior and/or posterior uveitis along with retinal vasculitis, which is generally florid and associated with vitritis and choroiditis.[26] Syphilis, like TB, needs to be screened by default because of its recent re-emergence with human immunodeficiency virus (HIV), as well as its protean and nonpathognomonic presentations, though uveitis is most frequent.[27] Retinal periphlebitis occurs in about half the cases of leptospirosis, the most widespread zoonosis globally. Nongranulomatous uveitis, vitritis, and papillitis help in differentiation.[28] Retinal vasculitis can also occur along with necrotizing retinitis, though arteries are involved more commonly.[11]

Like TB and syphilis, sarcoidosis also has no pathognomonic signs, and needs to be ruled out in most ocular inflammations. Vasculitis is typically segmental and nodular, with snowball vitreous exudates and granulomatous uveitis. Diagnosis is based on key ophthalmic signs and laboratory investigations.[29] Although uncommon, Behçet disease is the classic presentation of occlusive retinal vasculitis along the Silk Route. It involves both arteries and veins, and is accompanied by severe uveitis, vitritis, and retinal infiltrates; orogenital aphthoses are diagnostic.[30] Systemic vasculitides primarily cause retinal arterial occlusions rather than vasculitis: only small-vessel vasculitis, specifically systemic lupus erythematosus (SLE), is worth a mention in the differential diagnosis of Eales disease. SLE manifests more like hypertensive retinopathy than vasculitis, presenting typically with cotton-wool spots and retinal hemorrhages, and sometimes, choroidopathy.[31]

Primary retinal vasculitis

Once the diseases causing secondary vasculitis are ruled out, the two main conditions which remain in the picture are Eales disease and idiopathic retinal vasculitis. When the vasculitis is more posterior, sectorial and exudative; neovascularization, vitreous hemorrhage, and recurrences are uncommon; and presentation is gender-neutral, some authorities prefer the term "idiopathic retinal vasculitis" rather than Eales disease.[2] Though the differentiation is rather semantic as workup remains the same (see below), Eales disease has the unusual combination of minimal peripheral vascular inflammation but extensive vascular occlusions and neovascularization leading to recurrent vitreous hemorrhages, justifying the continued use of the eponym.[2]

DIAGNOSTIC WORKUP FOR EALES DISEASE

The purpose of the workup is to search for a cause for vasculitis and to rule out infections. This is best done by meticulous history-taking and systemic examination; laboratory investigations should be tailored to the positive findings from history and examination.[32]

After considering the age and sex of the patient, one should elicit information about residence, occupation, eating habits, and travel, which may help with the diagnosis of leptospirosis, syphilis, and toxoplasmosis. Similarly, cough, fever, and night sweats (TB or sarcoidosis), joint pain and swelling (SLE, Behçet disease), orogenital ulcerations (Behçet disease, syphilis), recurrent abortions and sexually transmitted disease (syphilis, HIV), skin rashes, nodules, or vesicles (SLE, Behcet disease, sarcoidosis), and neurological symptoms (sarcoidosis, multiple sclerosis) reveal underlying diseases which should be investigated further.

A detailed examination for systemic disease, especially for skin and mucosa, joints, respiratory and central nervous systems by an internist rules out important systemic associations, some of which may be life-threatening. Only a few basic screening investigations are universally required in retinal vasculitis which the ophthalmologist should order before referral to the internist: a complete hemogram, peripheral smear, erythrocyte sedimentation rate, tuberculin skin test, chest X-ray, rapid plasma reagin (RPR for syphilis), enzyme-linked immunosorbent assay for HIV, and urinanalysis are sufficient to screen for most common diseases causing vasculitis; further investigations are required only when history, examination, and/or aforementioned investigations point towards a specific disease.[11,32]

Fluorescein angiography helps mainly to identify peripheral new vessels and the extent of retinal nonperfusion, bordered by compensatory phenomena like collaterals and microaneurysms (Fig. 83.4). Active vasculitis appears as leakage from the stained vessel walls, though it can be detected clinically. B-scan ultrasound is a key presurgical investigation to assess the retinal status, posterior vitreous detachment (PVD), and tractional membranes obscured by vitreous hemorrhage. While assessing PVD, one must beware of vitreoschisis and an anomalous PVD, both common in Eales disease.[33]

MANAGEMENT

Patients with resolved vasculitis and clear media should be followed up at 6–12-month intervals. When the vision is good and the macula is healthy, minimal peripheral vasculitis may also be observed, though with close follow-up.[2,32]

Once systemic and ocular infections have been ruled out by history, examination, and investigations, corticosteroids are the mainstay of treatment for active vasculitis. Periocular depot steroids like triamcinolone acetonide, 40 mg/mL, are effective in most cases with unilateral disease.[34] When the vasculitis is bilateral or severe, or when there is inadequate response to periocular injections, systemic corticosteroids (typically, oral prednisolone, 1 mg/kg body weight/day) should be considered.[34] In the authors' experience, corticosteroids by these two routes are almost always enough to control the inflammation in Eales disease; immunosuppressive agents are rarely required. A small short-term case series reported successful resolution of active vasculitis in Eales disease with intravitreal injection of triamcinolone acetonide, 4 mg/mL.[5] The rationale of choosing intravitreal over sub-Tenon's route and the potential predicament of bilateral treatment were not explained. In the presence of a positive tuberculin test, some investigators recommend antitubercular therapy.[1,15] However, its role in the treatment of Eales disease is unproven and controversial, and should be decided by an internist.[2]

Peripheral scatter photocoagulation in the areas with new vessels, preferably guided by angiographic retinal nonperfusion, is the treatment of choice once the proliferative stage is reached.[1,2,4,10,14,15] Treatment should be extended posteriorly according to the posterior spread of the retinal nonperfusion and the presence of posterior or disc neovascularization.[2] Scatter photocoagulation is not recommended for peripheral retinal nonperfusion in the absence of neovascularization: peripheral nonperfusion is nearly universal in eyes with Eales disease.[20] Photocoagulation is also contraindicated in the presence of active vasculitis, which is likely to flare up and release more angiogenic factors, aggravating neovascularization (Fig. 83.5).[2] Pretreatment with corticosteroids sometimes mitigates the need for subsequent photocoagulation as well.

Persistent vitreous hemorrhage is the most frequent indication for vitrectomy. Early intervention (within 3–6 months) begets

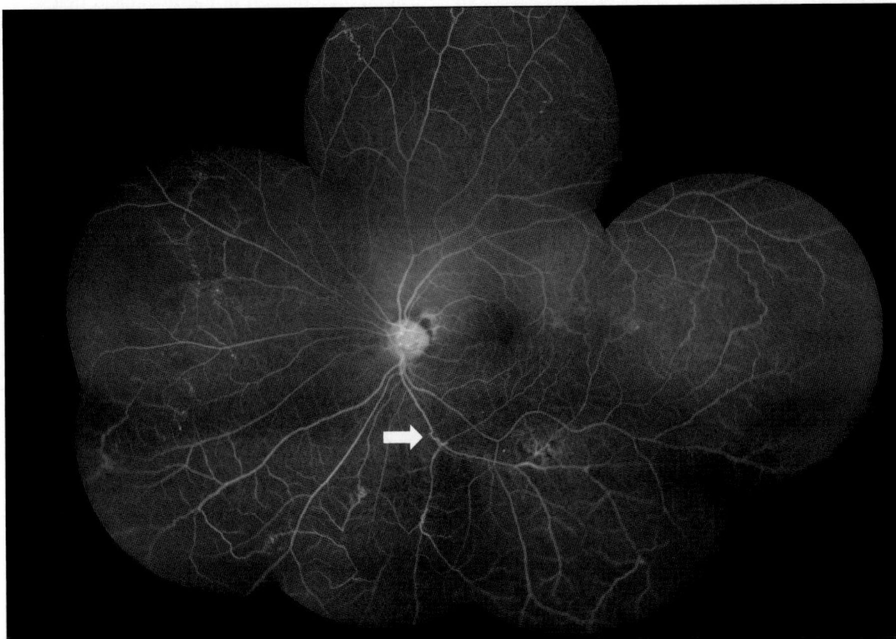

Fig. 83.4 Midphase angiogram of a patient with Eales disease showing scattered peripheral areas of capillary microaneurysms, telangiectasia, collateral formation, and retinal nonperfusion, most prominent at 3:00 and 9:00 meridians. The posterior pole is largely unaffected. The inflammatory sheathing of inferotemporal retinal vein from the first branching downwards (arrow) is not apparent due to resolution of active vasculitis.

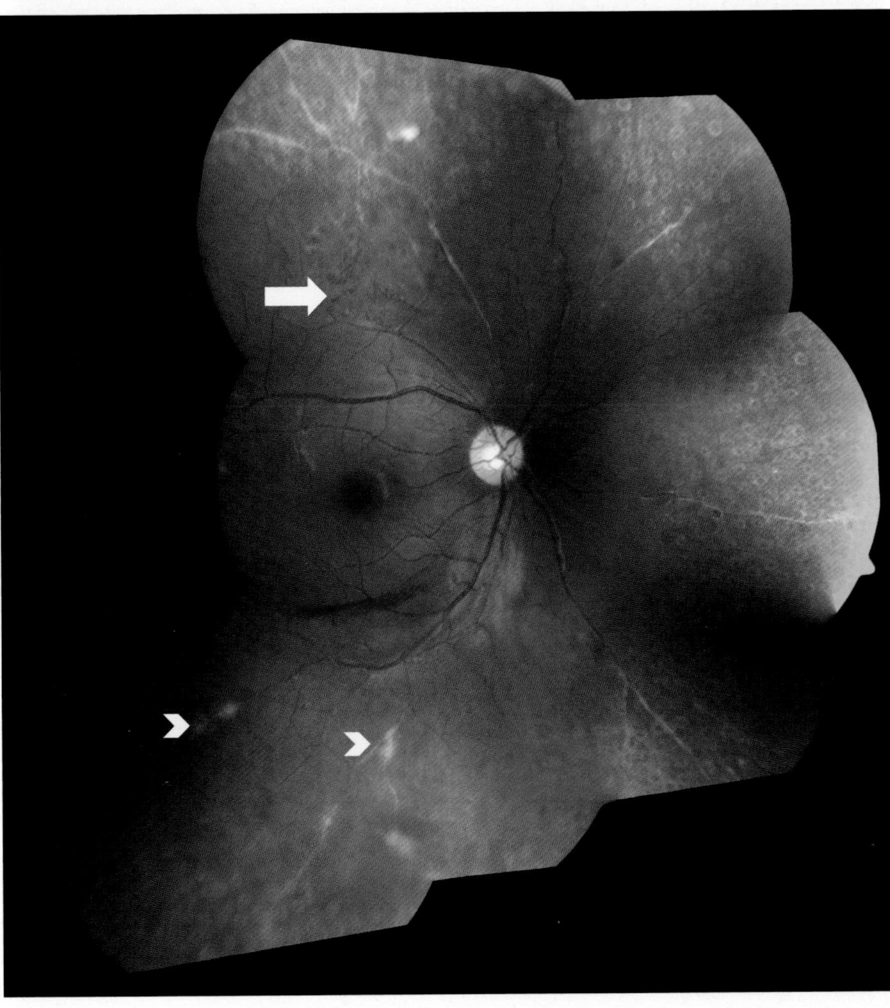

Fig. 83.5 This patient underwent peripheral scatter photocoagulation for postinflammatory neovascularization in Eales disease. The picture shows a simultaneous recurrence of neovascularization (arrow) and vascular inflammation (arrowheads): the inflammation was treated before neovascularization. Note the lack of involvement of the posterior pole.

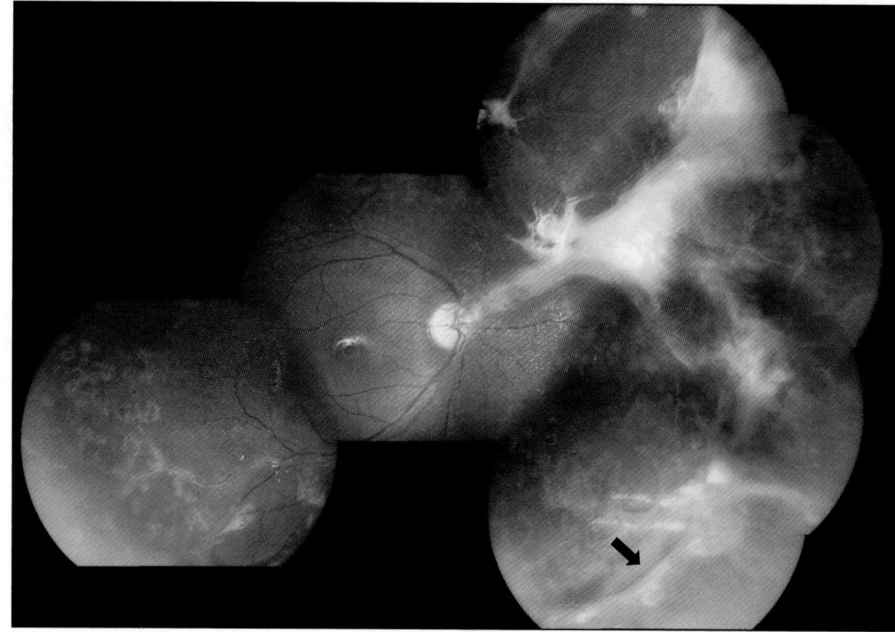

Fig. 83.6 Postvitrectomy view of an eye with persistent vitreous hemorrhage and membranes due to Eales disease: Note the relatively spared macula in spite of a large nasal residual tractional band with multiple attachments. Peripheral scatter photocoagulation marks are visible all around; indentation of the encircling belt buckle is seen inferonasally (arrow). (Reproduced with permission from Shukla D, Kanungo S, Prasad NM, et al. Surgical outcomes for vitrectomy in Eales' disease. Eye 2008;22:900–4.)

better visual outcomes;[35] epimacular membranes or extramacular retinal detachment warrant consideration of early vitrectomy; and macular detachment mandates immediate vitrectomy. Results of vitrectomy in Eales disease have been reported for about three decades; however, there is marked discrepancy in the reported outcomes due to variability in case selection, mainly PVD status and retinal detachment.[4,8,33,35] With modern surgical instrumentation, good surgical outcomes are possible in spite of incomplete or anomalous PVD and tractional sequelae (Fig. 83.6).[8] Encircling belt buckles may help improve the anatomical outcomes of vitrectomy in the presence of peripheral tractional membranes.[8] Recently, anti-VEGF drugs like bevacizumab and ranibizumab have been used as adjuvants to scatter photocoagulation and vitrectomy. While bevacizumab probably has merit in treating neovascularization refractory to scatter photocoagulation[6] and as an adjuvant to vitrectomy, it cannot substitute vitrectomy for vitreous hemorrhage in Eales disease, and can precipitate tractional complications.[13] The patient should therefore be cautioned about the need for vitrectomy prior to anti-VEGF injection.

SUMMARY

Though numerous ocular and systemic diseases cause retinal vasculitis, isolated retinal vasculitis, as seen in Eales disease, has few systemic associations.[36] A detailed history and clinical examination, and specific investigations as indicated by the positive findings are cost-effective and sufficient. Once the diagnosis of Eales disease is established, most cases are usually observed;[14] corticosteroids are required when vasculitis is significant. Peripheral scatter photocoagulation is effective in the proliferative disease, but should be delayed in favor of corticosteroids in the presence of active inflammation. Recurrent vitreous hemorrhage and tractional complications require consideration of early vitrectomy. With judicious use of medical and surgical treatment options, visual prognosis is good in most cases. While corticosteroids and scatter photocoagulation remain the standard of care, pharmacotherapy using antiangiogenic molecules, antioxidants, and antibodies against specific inflammatory cytokines may play a larger role in the future treatment of this enigmatic disease.[2,7,9,12]

REFERENCES

1. Patnaik B, Nagpal PN, Namperumalsamy P, et al. Eales disease: clinical features, pathophysiology, etiopathogenesis. Ophthalmol Clin North Am 1998;11:601–18.
2. Biswas J, Sharma T, Gopal L, et al. Eales disease – an update. Surv Ophthalmol 2002;47:197–214.
3. Eales H. Retinal haemorrhages associated with epistaxis and constipation. Brim Med Rev 1880;9:262.
4. Atmaca LS, Batioglu F, Atmaca Sonmez P. A long-term follow-up of Eales' disease. Ocul Immunol Inflamm 2002;10:213–21.
5. Ishaq M, Feroze AH, Shahid M, et al. Intravitreal steroids may facilitate treatment of Eales' disease (idiopathic retinal vasculitis): an interventional case series. Eye 2007;21:1403–5.
6. Kumar A, Sinha S. Rapid regression of disc and retinal neovascularization in a case of Eales disease after intravitreal bevacizumab. Can J Ophthalmol 2007 ;42:335–6.
7. Murugeswari P, Shukla D, Rajendran A, et al. Proinflammatory cytokines and angiogenic and anti-angiogenic factors in vitreous of patients with proliferative diabetic retinopathy and Eales' disease. Retina 2008;28:817–24.
8. Shukla D, Kanungo S, Prasad NM, et al. Surgical outcomes for vitrectomy in Eales' disease. Eye 2008;22:900–4.
9. Saxena S, Pant AB, Khanna VK, et al. Interleukin-1 and tumor necrosis factor-alpha: novel targets for immunotherapy in Eales disease. Ocul Immunol Inflamm 2009;17:201–6.
10. Das T, Pathengay A, Hussain N, et al. Eales' disease: diagnosis and management. Eye 2010;24:472–82.
11. El-Asrar AMA, Herbort CP, Tabbara KF. A clinical approach to the diagnosis of retinal vasculitis. Int Ophthalmol 2010;30:149–73.
12. Sen A, Paine SK, Chowdhury IH, et al. Association of interferon-gamma, interleukin-10, and tumor necrosis factor-alpha gene polymorphisms with occurrence and severity of Eales' disease. Invest Ophthalmol Vis Sci 2011; 52:171–8.
13. Patwardhan SD, Azad R, Shah BM, et al. Role of intravitreal bevacizumab. In: Eales disease with dense vitreous hemorrhage: a prospective randomized control study. Retina 2011;31:866–70.
14. Schubert HD. Eales' disease. In: Guyer DR, Yannuzzi LA, Chang S, et al. editors. Retina – vitreous – macula. Philadelphia: W.B. Saunders; 1999. p. 415–20.
15. Das T, Biswas J, Kumar A, et al. Eales' disease study. Indian J Ophthalmol 1994;42:3–18.
16. Elliot AJ. Recurrent intraocular hemorrhage in young adults (Eales's disease); a report of 31 cases. Trans Am Ophthalmol Soc 1954;52:811–75.
17. Spitznas M, Meyer-Schwicherath G, Stephan B. The clinical picture of Eales' disease. Graefes Arch Klin Exp Ophthalmol 1975;73–85.
18. Stanford MR, Verity DH. Diagnostic and therapeutic approach to patients with retinal vasculitis. Int Ophthalmol Clin 2000;40:69–83.
19. Charamis J. On the classification and management of the evolutionary course of Eales' disease. Trans Ophthalmol Soc UK 1965;85:157–60.

20. Das TP, Namperumalsamy P. Photocoagulation in Eales' disease. Results of prospective randomised clinical study. Presented in XXVI Int Cong Ophthalmol, Singapore, 1990.
21. Graham EM, Stanford MR, Whitcup SM. Retinal vasculitis. In: Pepose, JS, Holland GN, Wilhelmus, KR, editors. Ocular infection and immunity. St. Louis: Mosby; 1996. p.538–51.
22. Eltzschig HK, Carmeliet P. Hypoxia and inflammation. N Engl J Med 2011;17;656–65.
23. Biswas J, Therese L, Madhavan HN. Use of polymerase chain reaction in detection of *Mycobacterium tuberculosis* complex DNA from vitreous sample of Eales' disease. Br J Ophthalmol 1999;83:994.
24. Madhavan HN, Therese KL, Gunisha P, et al. Polymerase chain reaction for detection of Mycobacterium tuberculosis in epiretinal membrane in Eales' disease. Invest Ophthalmol Vis Sci 2000;41:822–5.
25. Muthukkaruppan V, Rengarajan K, Chakkalath HR, et al. Immunological status of patients of Eales' disease. Indian J Med Res 1989;90:351–9.
26. Bansal R, Gupta A, Gupta V, et al. Role of anti-tubercular therapy in uveitis with latent/manifest tuberculosis. Am J Ophthalmol 2008;146:772–9.
27. Chao JR, Khurana RN, Fawzi AA, et al. Syphilis: reemergence of an old adversary. Ophthalmology 2006;113:2074–9.
28. Shukla D, Rathinam SR, Cunningham Jr ET. Leptospiral uveitis in the developing world. Int Ophthalmol Clin 2010;50:113–24.
29. Herbort CP, Rao NA, Mochizuki M. International criteria for the diagnosis of ocular sarcoidosis: results of the first international workshop on ocular sarcoidosis (IWOS). Ocul Immunol Inflamm 2009;17:160–9.
30. Davatchi F, Shahram F, Chams-Davatchi C, et al. Behçet's disease in Iran: analysis of 6500 cases. Int J Rheum Dis 2010;13:367–73.
31. Aristodemou P, Stanford M. Therapy insight: the recognition and treatment of retinal manifestations of systemic vasculitis. Nat Clin Pract Rheumatol 2006;2:443–51.
32. George RK, Walton RC, Whitcup SM, et al. Primary retinal vasculitis. Systemic associations and diagnostic evaluation. Ophthalmology 1996;103:384–9.
33. Badrinath SS, Gopal L, Sharma T, et al. Vitreoschisis in Eales' disease: pathogenic role and significance in surgery. Retina 1999;19:51–4.
34. George RK, Nussenblatt RB. Treatment of retinal vasculitis. Ophthalmol Clin North Am 1998;11:673–80.
35. Kumar A, Kumar A, Tiwari HK, et al. Comparative evaluation of early vs. deferred vitrectomy in Eales' disease. Acta Ophthalmol Scand 2000;78:77–8.
36. Saurabh K, Das R, Biswas J, et al. Profile of retinal vasculitis in a tertiary eye care center in Eastern India. Indian J Ophthalmol 2011;59:297–301.

Chapter 84

Spirochetal Infections

Julie H. Tsai, Narsing A. Rao

INTRODUCTION

The history of spirochetal infections in the eye extends back to the first reported observations of spirochetes isolated from the nervous system.[1] Today, the most common organisms encountered in the tissues of the eye and ocular adnexae are *Treponema pallidum*, the infectious entity causing syphilis; *Borrelia burgdorferi*, the organism responsible for Lyme disease; and *Leptospira* species, which upon infection produces a host of local and systemic findings typical of leptospirosis. While the majority of these diseases can be treated effectively in the early stages, recognition of the constellation of symptoms often requires a high degree of clinical suspicion.

SYPHILITIC UVEITIS

Infection with the spirochete *T. pallidum* results in the constellation of ocular and systemic findings associated with syphilis. Sexual transmission is the most common means of inoculation, though direct contact with an active lesion or spread via transfusion are also potential routes of infection. Prior to the advent of penicillin, the disease was associated with high morbidity and mortality; however, as the antibiotic became widely available, the incidence of syphilitic disease dropped steeply. In recent years, changing socioeconomic factors and increases in high-risk sexual behavior, infection with human immunodeficiency virus (HIV), and antibiotic resistance have all contributed to resurgence of the disease. Worldwide, there are an estimated 12 million new cases annually, with 90% found in developing nations, and increases in reported cases are seen most commonly in cases of men having sex with men and those who are coinfected with HIV.[2,3]

While uncommon, ocular manifestations are typically associated with neurosyphilis, which can occur early or late in the course of infection.[4] Symptoms can be seen roughly 2–6 months after initial infection.[5] The most common ocular finding is uveitis, occurring in 2.5–5% of patients with tertiary syphilis. Clinical signs are protean and can include iritis, chorioretinitis, panuveitis, vitritis, and placoid chorioretinitis.[6,7]

Epidemiology and pathogenesis

The only known reservoir for syphilis is in the human, and historically, infection had been limited to populations with poor hygiene, limited access to healthcare, and low socioeconomic status. Worldwide, syphilis cases have increased in the past 10 years, up 33.5% between 2000 and 2004 in the USA and 41.5% between 1999 and 2001 in the UK.[3,5] The most current surveillance in the USA indicates that the number of reported cases is rising each year, up 39% since 2006 in the USA. Specifically, the rates are rising sharply among young black men between the ages of 15 and 24, with 58.2 cases per 100 000 compared to 19.3 in 2005.[3]

The local and systemic response to *T. pallidum* is complex, and is initiated as the bacteria enter the body through intact mucosa. Local invasion of the tissues ensues, and dissemination occurs via blood and the lymphatic system. On the microscopic level, lymphocytic infiltration is seen, either diffuse or focal, surrounding the blood vessels of affected organs. In the eye, this can be found in the iris, ciliary body, and choroid, along with chronic granulomatous inflammation, including epithelioid histiocytes and multinucleated giant cells. Mononuclear cells, sensitized T lymphocytes, macrophages, and plasma cells can also be seen. This inflammation and the resulting adaptive immune response cause the tissue destruction characteristic of syphilis as the bacteria do not produce an intrinsic toxin.

Local antibodies are also produced against the lipid, protein, and lipoprotein components of *T. pallidum*. The majority of bacteria are eradicated by opsonization and engulfed by macrophages. Those organisms that are resistant to phagocytosis may persist locally at the site of inoculation. Dissemination can occur despite the development of the humoral and cellular response, and without treatment, the bacteria can persist in the human host for decades, resulting in continued transmission and end-organ damage.[8]

Ocular manifestations

Uveitis is the most common ocular finding, occurring in 2.5–5% of patients with tertiary disease.[6] Findings can include keratic precipitates and iritis in the anterior segment of the eye. The iritis and iridocyclitis may manifest as either granulomatous or nongranulomatous inflammation. Dilated iris capillaries may also be noted (roseola), and these dilated and tortuous vessels may be a result of obliterative endarteritis. Chorioretinitis is also common and can present in a variety of ways. Vitritis, vasculitis, papillitis, periphlebitis, exudative retinal detachment, uveal effusion, central retinal vein occlusion, subretinal neovascular membrane formation, retinal necrosis, and neuroretinitis have all been described.[9–13] Yellow or gray placoid lesions can often be seen in the macula or juxtapapillary locations. This condition is also termed acute syphilitic posterior placoid chorioretinitis.[7,14] The lesions often have atrophic centers and are flat, with no evidence of fluid or hemorrhage. Fluorescein angiography reveals early hypofluorescence and late stain of the lesion with distinctive "leopard spot" hypofluorescence (Fig. 84.1). In patients with HIV, posterior uveitis is more common. A dense vitritis can also

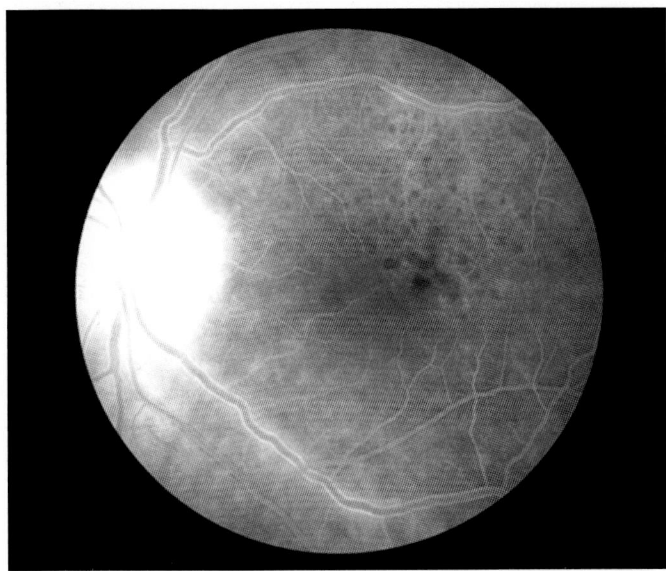

Fig. 84.1 Late fluorescein angiographic image of the left eye in a patient with ocular syphilis with focal hypofluorescence, leakage of the optic disc, and staining of the retinal veins. (Reproduced with permission from Chao JR, Khurana RN, Fawzi AA, et al. Syphilis: reemergence of an old enemy. Ophthalmology 2006;113:2074–9.)

be the only presenting sign of syphilitic uveitis in HIV-positive patients.[9,15,16] Recently, a more defined presentation of diffuse, creamy retinitis with overlying punctuate retinal precipitates has been described in HIV-positive patients diagnosed with syphilitic uveitis.[17–19]

Other ocular findings include interstitial keratitis of the cornea; chancre and nonspecific papillary reaction of the conjunctiva; episcleral and scleral inflammation, most commonly associated with conjunctival involvement; and inflammation of the optic nerve presenting as optic neuritis. Cataract can also be seen, both in congenital as well as acquired disease. Glaucoma in syphilis is often due to uveitis, though it may occur in either congenital or acquired infection. Lastly, the classic pupillary finding in syphilis is the Argyll Robertson pupil, which is seen in late syphilis or early neurosyphilis, manifesting with anisocoria and light-near dissociation upon clinical testing.

Findings in neurosyphilis are variable and dependent on the stage of disease. These may include stroke-like symptoms due to vasculitis and vascular compromise in early neurosyphilis, which may affect the cranial nerve nuclei as well as the centers for saccadic and smooth pursuit. Focal intracranial gummas may cause visual field deficits and superior orbital fissure syndrome, depending on the location of origination. Horner syndrome and internuclear ophthalmoplegia may also be observed in these patients. Late neurosyphilis may result in general paresis and tabes dorsalis.

Diagnosis

A high level of clinical suspicion is required for the appropriate diagnosis of syphilitic uveitis, due to its variable clinical presentation. In HIV-infected individuals, the presentation of syphilitic uveitis may be atypical; thus a strong clinical suspicion is especially important in evaluating those patients. Appropriate laboratory studies can aid in confirming the diagnosis and rule out other disease entities. Visualization of the organism in lesion exudates or tissue via dark-field microscopy with immunofluorescent staining is considered the gold standard and the quickest and most direct approach for establishing the diagnosis; however, the availability of such facilities limits its utility in clinical practice.[20] In addition, these tests are highly specific, but not very sensitive for widespread detection of infection.

Serologic testing with nontreponemal and treponemal tests is most commonly used in ophthalmic clinical practice. Nontreponemal tests detect the antibody to cardiolipin cholesterol antigen, and most clinicians are familiar with the Venereal Disease Research Laboratory (VDRL) and rapid plasma reagin (RPR) tests. These tests are best suited for general screening in a population with a low prevalence of syphilis, as well as for monitoring treatment efficacy as the titers decrease with appropriate therapy.

Treponemal tests, such as the fluorescent treponemal antibody absorption tests (FTA-ABS) and the microhemagglutinin assay for *T. pallidum* (MHA-TP), are more specific than the nontreponemal tests and may be just as sensitive. However, they are more expensive and a proportionate increase in false positives can occur if they are applied to a low-risk population. Thus, they may be used initially in patients who have a high probability of infection. Generally, once these tests are positive, the patient remains positive for life.

The use of a singular type of serologic test is insufficient for diagnosis, as each has its limitations, specifically the false-positive test results in patients without syphilis. False-positive test results may be associated with certain infections (e.g., Lyme disease, leptospirosis, malaria) and medical conditions (e.g., autoimmune disorders, intravenous drug use, pregnancy). A good rule of thumb in the evaluation of the patient with suspected syphilitic infection is to obtain a nontreponemal test and, if the initial study is reactive, confirm the diagnosis with a treponemal test. For those individuals with a positive treponemal screening test, a standard nontreponemal test with titer should be ordered to guide therapeutic decisions. If the nontreponemal test is negative, a different treponemal study should be ordered to confirm the results of the initial test. If the second treponemal test is positive, treatment should be initiated; alternatively, those patients with a history of prior therapy should be followed by observation unless a review of their sexual history indicates a likelihood of re-exposure.[21,22]

Newer testing, which may not always be available to the clinician, includes polymerase chain reaction (PCR) assays and rapid specific treponemal tests. PCR assays, if available, should be conducted on frozen specimens (shipped according to the laboratory specifications), but cannot discern between live or dead organisms. The rapid tests, which may use as little as 10–50 μL of sample, are considered to be equivalent to the older specific treponemal antibody tests, and have similar limitations in terms of distinguishing active versus inactive infection.[23,24]

For HIV-infected individuals, these serologic tests are often accurate and reliable for diagnosis as well as following the response to therapy. Atypical results (i.e., unusually high/low/fluctuating titers) without corresponding clinical findings suggestive of early syphilis should prompt the clinician to investigate further and consider other tests to confirm the diagnosis.[21] False-negative tests may occur due to insufficient production of antibody to the bacterial proteins, or an overall lack of immunoreactivity.

Consideration of further testing is warranted in all patients with neurosyphilis, as no single test can be used to diagnose this presentation in all instances. Cerebrospinal fluid (CSF) analysis, along with VDRL and FTA-ABS tests, may need to be considered in confirming the diagnosis of neurosyphilis.[4] CSF FTA-ABS is often too sensitive and thus the role of this test is still controversial. CSF VDRL does have the advantage over CSF FTA-ABS in cases requiring differentiation of current active infection from past infection. Leukocytosis and elevated protein concentrations can be seen in the CSF and these findings are often present for more than 1 year in those individuals with neurologic symptoms. This is consistent with neurosyphilis and warrants treatment even if test results are negative.

In summary, the reagin tests (VDRL, RPR) are used in screening for early syphilis infection. The treponemal tests (FTA-ABS, MHA-TP) can be used to confirm the diagnosis and guide management. The nontreponemal tests with titer (VDRL, RPR) can be used to follow therapeutic adequacy. Lastly, further investigation should be considered in patients with HIV, or in cases of neurosyphilis.

Differential diagnoses

The clinical findings and possible differential diagnoses for syphilitic uveitis are listed in Table 84.1. The most critical diagnosis to make may be acute syphilitic posterior chorioretinitis, and one must rule out acute posterior multifocal placoid pigment epitheliopathy and atypical serpiginous choroidopathy. In these instances, the use of intravitreal steroid or systemic immunosuppressive therapy for treatment of these conditions may unmask an underlying infection.[14] It is important to emphasize that a high degree of clinical suspicion is vital in order to make the diagnosis, and that serologic confirmation is required.

Treatment

The clinician who diagnoses syphilitic infection in a patient has two responsibilities: to report the case to the state Department of Health;[25] and to determine if he or she is comfortable in managing and following the therapeutic regimen for the patient. A survey of infectious disease practitioners conducted in 2008 found variation in the management of syphilis among the experts, particularly in cases where patients were coinfected with HIV.[20] It is the recommendation of the authors that the ophthalmologist treat the patient in consultation with an infectious disease specialist.

Penicillin G is the preferred treatment for all stages of syphilis (Table 84.2). The dose, route of administration, and duration of therapy are determined by the stage and clinical findings. Sexual partners of the infected individual also need to be evaluated and treated.[21] For patients with a penicillin allergy, alternative antibiotics may be used; however, as the other medications are not as effective as penicillin, skin testing and desensitization are recommended, especially in those patients who are coinfected with HIV. As for patients diagnosed with congenital syphilis, treatment with aqueous penicillin G or procaine penicillin G via intravenous administration is recommended. Other antibiotics such as ceftriaxone and ampicillin have been used, but there is no optimal therapy for congenital syphilis noted at this time.

Syphilitic uveitis or other ocular manifestations associated with neurosyphilis should be treated according to the

Table 84.1 Differential diagnosis of ocular syphilis with laboratory workup

Disease/disorder	Possible serologic/laboratory testing
Toxoplasmosis	IgM-ELISA, IgG-ELISA for antibodies to *Treponema gondii*
Rubella	IgM-ELISA, IgG-ELISA for rubella; rubella titer
Cytomegalovirus (CMV)	CMV DNA PCR
Human immunodeficiency virus (HIV)	ELISA
Herpes simplex virus (HSV)	Diagnostic viral culture, HSV-1/HSV-2 serologic assays
Varicella-zoster virus (VZV)	Diagnostic viral culture, antibody assays
HLA-B27-related uveitis	HLA-B27 genetic testing
Primary intraocular lymphoma	Cytology on vitreous or aqueous humor; neuroradiologic and CSF studies
Sarcoidosis	Angiotensin-converting enzyme (ACE) level
Tuberculosis	PPD, QuantiFERON gold testing
Idiopathic uveitis	Diagnosis of exclusion after testing for other uveitic entities

IgM/IgG, immunoglobulin M/G; ELISA, enzyme-linked immunoabsorbent assay; PCR, polymerase chain reaction; HLA, human leukocyte antigen; CSF, cerebrospinal fluid; PPD, purified protein derivative.

Table 84.2 Recommended treatment of syphilis

Stage of disease	Preferred treatment	Alternative treatment
Primary, secondary, or early latent	Benzathine penicillin G 2.4 million units IM, single dose	Doxycycline 100 mg po BID ×2 weeks or tetracycline 500 mg po QID ×2 weeks
Late latent, latent syphilis of unknown duration, tertiary stage, or those who fail primary therapy	Benzathine penicillin G 2.4 million units IM, administered weekly ×3 weeks	Doxycycline 100 mg po BID ×4 weeks or tetracycline 500 mg po QID ×4 weeks
Neurosyphilis	Aqueous penicillin G 3–4 million units IV every 4 hours ×10–14 days	Procaine penicillin 2.4 million units IM daily ×10–14 days and probenecid 500 mg po QID ×10–14 days

Notes: (1) Human immunodeficiency virus-positive patients should be treated with penicillin at all stages of infection, and those allergic to penicillin should be desensitized and then treated with the full regimen. (2) All patients with tertiary syphilis should have a cerebrospinal fluid analysis and be evaluated for neurosyphilis.

(Adapted from Centers for Disease Control and Prevention. Sexually transmitted diseases treatment guidelines, 2010. MMWR 2010;59:26–40.)

recommendations for neurosyphilis.[4] A CSF examination is recommended for all patients with syphilitic eye disease to guide therapy. The recommended regimen is aqueous crystalline penicillin G delivered intravenously, as no alternative has been proven scientifically effective. In those patients who have failed primary therapy and show evidence of tertiary syphilis, asymptomatic neurosyphilis may be present and may warrant evaluation of the CSF.[21] With regard to neurosyphilis in the HIV-positive patient, treatment with intravenous penicillin utilizing the neurosyphilis recommendations results in rapid resolution of findings.[19] It is important to note that therapy must be of a duration and dose sufficient to cure neurosyphilis, regardless of CSF findings.[26]

Success with therapy may be evaluated by improvement in clinical findings and seroconversion or low titers upon nontreponemal testing. The published criteria for treatment of early syphilis describe four- to eightfold decreases in nontreponemal titers that should occur by 3–6 months, respectively. It is important to realize that these criteria cannot be used in monitoring treatment efficacy in HIV-positive patients. In these individuals, serologic testing may be inaccurate, and this often justifies the aggressive treatment regimen in this population.

Once the infection has been appropriately treated, adjunctive therapy with corticosteroids may be applied for any residual ocular inflammation related to syphilis. Topical corticosteroids are beneficial for anterior uveitis and interstitial keratitis, whereas systemic corticosteroid therapy may be required in order to resolve symptoms of residual scleritis, posterior uveitis, or optic neuritis. Corticosteroid regimens should always be administered concurrently with antibiotic therapy.

Course and outcome

Outcomes of syphilitic uveitis and systemic disease are dependent on early diagnosis and appropriate antibiotic therapy. These cases often result in full visual recovery and improvement in other systemic findings. Untreated cases of syphilitic uveitis often lead to worsening of intraocular inflammation, development of glaucoma secondary to chronic uveitis, and retinal necrosis. Chronic vitritis and optic atrophy may also occur. Treatment in HIV-positive individuals should be initiated early and aggressively, utilizing the regimen recommended for neurosyphilis.

UVEITIS ASSOCIATED WITH LYME DISEASE

Lyme disease is a multisystem disorder found in North America, Europe, and Asia. In the USA, the manifestations are caused by infection with *Borrelia burgdorferi*, a spirochete transmitted by the *Ixodes* tick species. The disease can be broken down into stages: stage 1, which often begins days to weeks after the tick bite and is denoted by the pathognomonic finding of erythema migrans in conjunction with fever, malaise, and arthralgias; stage 2, which is the phase of dissemination of the spirochete to multiple organs in the days, weeks, or months after infection; and stage 3, which often occurs after a disease-free period lasting months to years.

In all cases, a history of tick bite may be absent in 50% of individuals.[27] The dissemination to multiple organ systems, particularly the skin, heart, joints, and nervous system, along with neurological manifestations (e.g., cranial and peripheral neuropathies and meningoencephalitis), is the hallmark of stage 2 disease.[28] Chronic arthritis and conduction defects may also develop.[29] The lymphocytoma, another skin lesion, may develop, especially on the earlobe or breast, and the initial erythema migrans fades and reappears.[28] These findings may take days, weeks, or even months to manifest clinically.

The third or late stage of disease often occurs after a disease-free period lasting months to years, and may occur despite adequate antibiotic therapy.[30] Chronic symptoms mark this phase of infection, and common conditions include chronic relapsing arthritis of the knee; acrodermatitis chronica atrophicans, a rash that results in atrophy of the skin and underlying structures; and late neurologic manifestations (e.g., encephalopathy, demyelination, and dementia).[28,29,31,32]

Ocular disease associated with Lyme borreliosis can manifest at any stage of infection. Though well documented, the majority of cases persist in case reports and case series, with few definitive, large-scale studies in the scientific literature.

Epidemiology and pathogenesis

In the USA, the endemic areas are clustered around three regions: (1) the northeast, down as far south to Virginia, with hyperendemic regions in Connecticut and New York; (2) the Midwest, in the states of Michigan, Wisconsin, and Minnesota; and (3) the west, primarily in northern California. Certain areas of Europe and Asia are also affected, particularly in regions with a temperate climate. It is unclear why there is a preponderance of cases localized to the northeastern USA.[30]

The pathogenesis of the disease is similar to that induced by the spirochete *T. pallidum*, and follows in three distinct stages. The first stage, or early infection, is believed to be due to spirochetemia. After an incubation period of 3–32 days, the spirochete multiplies and induces proinflammatory responses in both the innate and adaptive immune systems. This is clinically observed as the characteristic skin rash, erythema migrans, at the site of the tick bite.[33] Within days to weeks, *B. burgdorferi* can be recovered from many areas of the body. All affected tissues show some infiltration of lymphocytes and plasma cells, along with vascular damage (e.g., mild vasculitis or hypervascular occlusion).

The immunological response of the host to parasitic invasion is the likely etiology for the manifestations of stage 2 and 3 disease.[34] The specific immunoglobulin M (IgM) response provides for polyclonal B-cell activation and increased levels of circulating immune complexes, while the specific IgG response develops over weeks in response to spirochetal polypeptides and nonprotein antigens.[30] Spirochetal killing is primarily due to bactericidal B-cell responses and utilizes the complement pathway. For the majority of cases, the innate and adaptive response is capable of controlling widespread dissemination of the disease without antibiotic therapy; however, without appropriate therapy, *B. burgdorferi* can survive for several years in particular loci, such as joints, skin, and nervous system.[29]

Ocular manifestations

Ocular findings in Lyme disease are less prominent compared to the significant systemic manifestations and can appear at any stage of disease. Conjunctivitis is the most common finding, present in 11% of patients with early-stage Lyme disease.[35] Ophthalmologists are generally not consulted as the nonspecific findings of conjunctival and periorbital inflammation are mild in nature and self-limiting. Neuro-ophthalmic complications are associated with the neurologic involvement in stage 2 disease and commonly manifest as ocular motility problems due to cranial nerve palsies, optic neuritis, papilledema, and pseudotumor cerebri in the setting of meningoencephalitis.[31,36,37] Stromal keratitis, episcleritis, and symblepharon formation have been reported in stage 3 disease.[38]

Intraocular inflammation often presents as chorioretinitis and vitreous inflammation, though there have been a variety of clinical presentations associated with Lyme disease.[35,39,40] Vitreous involvement may be nonspecific, with or without associated retinal pathology, such as retinal vasculitis.[40] Clinically, the presence of disc edema in the setting of posterior-segment inflammation may be related to chronic posterior-segment inflammation rather than the neurologic involvement from borreliosis (Fig. 84.2). Appropriate neuro-ophthalmic testing should be undertaken to evaluate the potential of other central nervous system complications.

Diagnosis

The clinical diagnosis of Lyme disease is dependent on the following: appearance of the pathognomonic skin rash (erythema migrans) in a patient with a history of tick bite and/or residence in an endemic region; or the appearance of the skin lesion in addition to involvement of two organ systems in those patients without a history of a tick bite or residence in a nonendemic region. The diagnostic criteria for Lyme disease as recommended by the Centers for Disease Control and Prevention (CDC) are listed in Table 84.3.[41,42]

Culture of *B. burgdorferi* from peripheral blood, areas of skin rash, and CSF provides for definitive diagnosis.[43,44] However, positive cultures are often difficult to obtain as they mainly occur early on in the disease process. In these cases, sensitivity is highest in tissue culture, with the positive rates of culture dropping significantly for plasma and CSF.[30] For ocular disease, serological testing is often more helpful in diagnosis as these manifestations can occur several years after initial inoculation. These results, along with a clinical history suggestive of infection, provide the basis for diagnosis of Lyme disease.

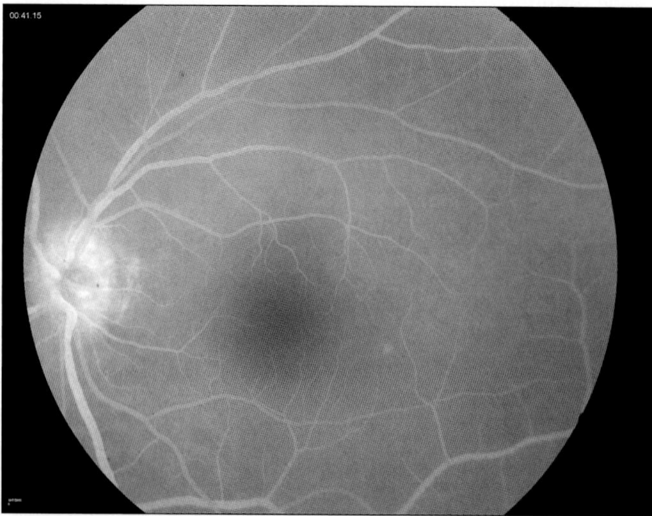

Fig. 84.2 Fluorescein angiogram depicting disc edema and mild vitritis in a 44-year-old Caucasian male with positive serology for Lyme borreliosis. There is a nonspecific window defect temporal to the fovea. (Courtesy of Thomas J. Federici, MD.)

The CDC recommends a two-step approach in which serologic samples are tested: first, an enzyme-linked immunosorbent assay (ELISA) is performed to detect the presence of IgG and IgM specific for *B. burgdorferi*. Equivocal results are then tested by Western blotting. According to CDC criteria, the IgM Western blot is considered positive if two of the following three bands are present: the 23, 39, and 41 kDa, though the combination of the 23 and 41 kDa bands may still be considered a false-positive result. The IgG Western blot may be considered to be positive if five of the following 10 bands are present: 18, 23, 28, 30, 39, 41, 45, 58, 66, and 93 kDa.[41] The results still need to be interpreted with care, as a portion of the normal population has IgG reactivity to the 41-kDa flagellar antigen of the spirochete and thus the presence of the band alone cannot be utilized in serologic diagnosis.[30]

As a final note of caution, these tests, though commonly used, can be insensitive during the first few weeks of infection, prior to the development of host antibody response. Actively infected individuals will have a positive IgG response. For those patients with active disease lasting more than 4–8 weeks, an elevated IgM response is likely to be a false positive, and thus an IgM response should not be used to support the diagnosis of an infection after that time period.[30] In instances where the disease course is much more aggressive and severe than initially anticipated, coinfection with *Babesia microti* or *Ehrlichia phagocytophilia* (causing human babesiosis and granulocytic anaplasmosis, respectively) should be considered.[45–47]

Differential diagnoses

Given the various ocular manifestations of Lyme disease, the clinician needs to rule out both infectious and noninfectious etiologies with similar clinical presentations. In terms of other infectious etiologies, findings on the clinical examination as well as appropriate serologic/diagnostic tests should be undertaken to rule out syphilis, tuberculosis, viral meningitis/encephalitis, viral keratitis, infectious arthritis and mononucleosis, and mumps. Examination should also incorporate the following noninfectious etiologies in the differential diagnosis: sarcoidosis, collagen vascular diseases, vasculitis, Vogt–Koyanagi–Harada syndrome, and multiple sclerosis.

Treatment

Therapy for Lyme borreliosis consists of antibiotic treatment for the systemic infection, though preventive measures (i.e., protective clothing, repellents, and acaricides), landscape

Table 84.3 Criteria for diagnosis of Lyme disease

Presence of any one of the following criteria satisfies the diagnosis of Lyme disease.

1. Development of erythema migrans (EM) within 30 days of exposure in an endemic area; size of lesion should be at least 5 cm
2. In the absence of EM, history of exposure to endemic area, with signs involving one organ system and positive laboratory test
3. No history of exposure to endemic area, but with EM as well as involvement of two organ systems
4. No history of exposure to endemic area, but with EM and a positive serology

(Adapted from Case definitions for public health surveillance. MMWR Morb Mortal Wkly Rep 1997;46(RR-10):1–55 and Recommendations for public health surveillance. MMWR Morb Mortal Wkly Rep 1995;44:590–1.)

modifications, and tick checks are often the best defense against infection as they reduce exposure. Vaccination was once offered to individuals between the ages of 15 and 70 years who may travel to or live in endemic regions;[48] however, the vaccine is no longer available, as the manufacturer has discontinued production, citing low demand. Currently, a single dose of doxycycline (200 mg) can be prescribed for individuals as a preventive measure within 72 hours of a documented tick bite.[49]

With regard to management of ocular findings, the most effective treatment strategy is still unclear.[35] Systemic therapy should be initiated in consultation with an infectious disease specialist (Table 84.4). Diplopia secondary to cranial nerve palsies should be addressed according to the severity of patient symptoms. Adjunct corticosteroids have been beneficial in treating the specific ocular manifestations: topical applications for anterior-segment manifestations (e.g., keratitis and episcleritis), and intravitreous injections for macular edema.[38,50–52] Systemic corticosteroids have been utilized in more severe cases of ocular inflammation, such as vision-threatening uveitis, scleritis, or optic neuritis; however, the use may be controversial, as a higher incidence of relapses has been observed.[31] Inadequate treatment in the early stages may lead to relapses and development of late-stage manifestations.[31] Treatment of concomitant infections should also be addressed if the clinical findings persist despite prolonged antibiotic therapy.

Table 84.4 Treatment of Lyme disease

Early infection – local or disseminated	
Adults	Doxycycline 100 mg orally twice daily for 14–21 days
	Amoxicillin 500 mg orally three times a day for 14–21 days
In case of doxycycline/amoxicillin allergy:	
	Cefuroxime 500 mg orally twice daily for 14–21 days
	Erythromycin 250 mg orally four times daily for 14–21 days
Children	Amoxicillin 50 mg/kg body weight per day in three divided doses for 14–21 days
In case of penicillin allergy:	
	Cefuroxime 30 mg/kg per day in two divided doses for 14–21 days
Neurological and/or ocular abnormalities (early or late)	
Adults	Ceftriaxone 2 g IV once a day for 14–28 days
	Cefotaxime 2 g IV every 8 hours for 14–28 days
In case of ceftriaxone or penicillin allergy:	
	Doxycycline 100 mg orally 3 times a day for 30 days
Children	Ceftriaxone 75–100 mg/kg per day (maximum 2 g) IV once a day for 14–28 days
	Cefotaxime 150 mg/kg per day in three to four divided doses (maximum 6 g) for 14–28 days

Notes: (1) Avoid doxycycline in pregnant women. (2) Chronic Lyme disease symptoms seen in late disease may require long-term antibiotic therapy (2 or more months of oral antibiotics, or 1 or more months of IV antibiotics). (Adapted from Steere AC. Lyme disease. N Engl J Med 2001;345:115–25.)

Disease course and outcome

The majority of patients respond well to systemic antibiotic therapy; however, posterior uveitis, stromal keratitis, and neurotrophic keratitis can be slow to respond to treatment. Untreated disease can have a relapsing course for several years, though the number of patients with chronic symptoms, most notably arthritis, decreases 10–20% each year, with few individuals having symptoms beyond 5 years.[30]

OCULAR LEPTOSPIROSIS

Leptospirosis is a zoonotic infection with a worldwide distribution, with higher incidence in tropical and subtropical climates. Initially described by Weil in 1886, infection causes a severe condition characterized by acute fever, malaise, and uveitis. Most human infection may be asymptomatic, and there is a wide spectrum of disease presentation which ranges from nonspecific febrile illness to multiorgan involvement associated with high mortality rates.

Systemic disease often begins with nonspecific symptoms of headache, fevers, myalgias, malaise, and conjunctival chemosis with or without subconjunctival hemorrhage. The fevers may be mild, moderate, or severe. Anicteric disease affects 80–90% of patients, but 10–15% go on to develop severe systemic septicemia or multiorgan failure (icteric leptospirosis, or Weil disease). Mortality ranges from less than 5–30%, but those figures are unreliable.[53,54] Poor prognostic factors include involvement of the liver, renal failure, rhabdomyolysis, and altered sensorium.[55]

Leptospirosis is rapidly becoming a major public health problem in several countries, both in the developing world as well as in urban areas. Diagnosis is difficult and requires a high level of suspicion, as the manifestations vary by the affected organ system. It is often misdiagnosed as aseptic meningitis, encephalitis, influenza, dengue fever, hepatitis, gastroenteritis, typhoid, or malaria.[56] Often, the immunologic symptoms (e.g., uveitis) occur after an asymptomatic period, which may last anywhere from 2 months to 2 years, making clinical assessment difficult, and laboratory testing near impossible in these patients.

Epidemiology and pathogenesis

The genus *Leptospira* consists of two strains: *L. interrogans*, which causes the infectious disease in humans, and *L. biflexia*, which is a saprophytic strain. The natural reservoir for *Leptospira* is wild animals, particularly rodents, but dogs and other domestic livestock may also be affected. The spirochete colonizes the renal tubules of the animal host, and survives excretion in the urine. It also survives as a free-living organism in contaminated soil or water. Individuals at high risk for infection include abattoir workers, farmers, veterinarians, miners, and sewer workers who contract the disease via direct contact with diseased animals. Indirect contact is more common after exposure to wet soil or water through occupational exposure or recreational exposures (e.g., water sports in either fresh or sea water, ecotourism in endemic regions) as the spirochete has the ability to enter the human body through intact mucosa or abraded epidermis. The appearance of this rural tropical disease in urban centers of developing regions is often secondary to a lack of sanitation in areas of rapid expansion and growth. Sporadic outbreaks have also been reported in developed countries.[57,58]

Hematogenous dissemination allows the organisms to invade the central nervous system as well as the aqueous humor of the eye; transendothelial migration occurs via systemic vasculitis, resulting in a broad spectrum of presentations, including pulmonary hemorrhage, damage to the renal tubule structures, and hepatic cell destruction.[59] It is unclear which mechanism allows for *Leptospira* to cause infection: innate bacterial virulence factors, direct tissue damage secondary to hemolytic toxins, or innate host immune responses.

In the eye, the mechanisms surrounding leptospiral uveitis remain unclear. Invasion of the vitreous by neutrophils, macrophages, lymphocytes, and plasma cells can be seen within 10 days of infection in a rabbit model.[60] Antibodies to *Leptospira* in the aqueous coincided with the intraocular appearance of plasma cells. Extensive veterinary studies on equine recurrent uveitis (ERU) suggest that it is an organ-specific, autoimmune disorder, and that leptospiral uveitis in horses is a separate and distinct subset of ERU.[61] Molecular studies on human eyes are not currently available.

Ocular manifestations

In the acute phase of infection, the incidence of ocular signs ranges from 2 to 90% of cases, suggesting that the majority of findings may be nonspecific and diagnosed only when there is a high index of suspicion. Conjunctival hyperemia, chemosis, and subconjunctival hemorrhage are most commonly seen in these cases. Changes in the retinal vasculature and the presence of retinal hemorrhages have been reported, along with disc hyperemia and retinal vasculitis.[57]

After the initial septicemic phase, a period of relative quiescence precedes the development of ocular symptoms. These can range from a localized anterior uveitis to diffuse panuveitis. Findings are generally nongranulomatous, though granulomatous reactions may be seen in rare cases. Anterior-segment findings can include hypopyon in 12% of cases, and a fibrinous reaction may be present. Cataract can also be present, and, in rare cases, spontaneous absorption of the lens opacity has been reported. The symptoms of photophobia, blurred vision, and pain are generally self-limited.[62]

In the posterior segment, vitritis is common, and the presentation of vitreous strands, or veil opacities that attach to the optic disc, can often be seen. There may be other vitreous precipitates in the posterior vitreous, and snowbanking may be seen. Nonocclusive vasculitis, periphlebitis, choroiditis, and papillitis have also been described.[57]

Diagnosis

Clinical diagnosis of systemic leptospirosis is difficult given the nonspecific symptoms and variable presentations reported in the literature. The diagnostic dilemma extends to the ocular manifestations, where the differential diagnosis for leptospiral uveitis includes such entities as human leukocyte antigen (HLA)-B27-associated uveitis, Behçet disease, and sarcoidosis (Table 84.5). The clinician cannot rely on the examination alone; rather, a high index of suspicion in an endemic region, or in individuals who may have exposure due to socioeconomic or recreational factors, needs to be taken into account. The ophthalmologist faced with a potential diagnosis of leptospirosis will also need to look toward laboratory testing to confirm the clinical suspicion.

Table 84.5 Differential diagnosis of leptospirosis

HLA-B27-related uveitis	Sarcoidosis
Behçet disease	Syphilis
Eales disease	Toxoplasmosis
Endophthalmitis	Leprosy
Tuberculosis	

HLA, human leukocyte antigen.

The gold standard for laboratory testing is the microscopic agglutination test (MAT), which is comprised of the agglutination of live leptospires by titrated amounts of patient serum.[53,56] Generally, 12–16 of the known serovars of any given geographic region are used in the test with the endpoint read using dark-field microscopy. A fourfold change in the titer or seroconversion is considered positive, with a compatible clinical presentation. Of note, false negatives can occur if the infection is due to a serovar not present in the testing panel, and false positives can also occur if there are any residual antibodies to a prior exposure in an endemic area. In chronic cases, a titer of 1:100 is considered a positive test. The main difficulty in obtaining MAT testing lies in that large numbers of leptospiral cultures need to be maintained; thus, only large reference laboratories are able to conduct this laboratory test. Other diagnostic procedures, including a *Leptospira* dipstick test, ELISA, and microscopic slide agglutination tests, may be more widely available. Newer laboratory techniques, including PCR for the detection of leptospiral DNA, are currently in development.[63]

Treatment

Antibiotic therapy for systemic disease is extremely effective. Supportive care, when required, should be initiated for those individuals suffering from multiorgan involvement. Intravenous penicillin G has been effective for severe systemic infection, but for less severe presentations, doxycycline given 100 mg twice daily for 1 week was shown to be effective in eradicating leptospires from all target organs within 3 days.[64] Azithromycin has been studied for the treatment of leptospirosis in those individuals unable to take or tolerate doxycycline; further clinical trials are warranted to determine whether this could be considered a reasonable alternative.[65]

Treatment for leptospiral uveitis includes local administration of corticosteroids, as they are the mainstay for therapy for ocular inflammation. Dose and route of delivery are dependent on the location, laterality, and severity of the symptoms. It is unclear if systemic antibiotic therapy during the early phase of infection provides any protective role in the prevention of immunologic sequelae such as uveitis, though a recent study suggests that those treated in the septicemic phase developed only mild disease.[66]

Disease course and outcome

Visual recovery and potential are generally good, with one large series reporting that more than 50% of patients regained 20/20 vision.[62] Most patients have mild disease (anicteric) and recover within 1–2 weeks. For systemic disease, mortality varies from less than 1% to more than 20%, and is dependent on the severity of disease and involvement of multiple organ systems.[53]

REFERENCES

1. Nichols HJ. Observations on a strain of *Spirochaeta pallida* isolated from the nervous system. J Exp Med 1914;19:362–71.
2. Puech C, Gennai S, Pavese P, et al. Ocular manifestations of syphilis: recent cases over a 2.5-year period. Graefes Arch Clin Exp Ophthalmol 2010;248: 1623–9.
3. Centers for Disease Control and Prevention. Sexually transmitted disease surveillance 2009. Atlanta: U.S. Department of Health and Human Services; 2010.
4. Marra CM. Update on neurosyphilis. Curr Infect Dis Rep 2009;11:127–34.
5. Durnian JM, Naylor G, Saeed AM. Ocular syphilis: the return of an old acquaintance. Eye (Lond) 2004;18:440–2.
6. Aldave AJ, King JA, Cunningham ET, Jr. Ocular syphilis. Curr Opin Ophthalmol 2001;12:433–41.
7. Gass JD, Braunstein RA, Chenoweth RG. Acute syphilitic posterior placoid chorioretinitis. Ophthalmology 1990;97:1288–97.
8. Peeling RW, Hook EW, 3rd. The pathogenesis of syphilis: the great mimicker, revisited. J Pathol 2006;208:224–32.
9. Kuo IC, Kapusta MA, Rao NA. Vitritis as the primary manifestation of ocular syphilis in patients with HIV infection. Am J Ophthalmol 1998;125:306–11.
10. Levy JH, Liss RA, Maguire AM. Neurosyphilis and ocular syphilis in patients with concurrent human immunodeficiency virus infection. Retina 1989;9: 175–80.
11. Fu EX, Geraets RL, Dodds EM, et al. Superficial retinal precipitates in patients with syphilitic retinitis. Retina 2010;30:1135–43.
12. Pillai S, DiPaolo F. Bilateral panuveitis, sebopsoriasis, and secondary syphilis in a patient with acquired immunodeficiency syndrome. Am J Ophthalmol 1992;114:773–5.
13. Passo MS, Rosenbaum JT. Ocular syphilis in patients with human immunodeficiency virus infection. Am J Ophthalmol 1988;106:1–6.
14. Song JH, Hong YT, Kwon OW. Acute syphilitic posterior placoid chorioretinitis following intravitreal triamcinolone acetonide injection. Graefes Arch Clin Exp Ophthalmol 2008;246:1775–8.
15. Browning DJ. Posterior segment manifestations of active ocular syphilis, their response to a neurosyphilis regimen of penicillin therapy, and the influence of human immunodeficiency virus status on response. Ophthalmology 2000;107: 2015–23.
16. Villanueva AV, Sahouri MJ, Ormerod LD, et al. Posterior uveitis in patients with positive serology for syphilis. Clin Infect Dis 2000;30:479–85.
17. Wickremasinghe S, Ling C, Stawell R, et al. Syphilitic punctate inner retinitis in immunocompetent gay men. Ophthalmology 2009;116:1195–200.
18. Tran TH, Cassoux N, Bodaghi B, et al. Syphilitic uveitis in patients infected with human immunodeficiency virus. Graefes Arch Clin Exp Ophthalmol 2005;243:863–9.
19. Hughes EH, Guzowski M, Simunovic MP, et al. Syphilitic retinitis and uveitis in HIV-positive adults. Clin Exp Ophthalmol 2010;38:851–6.
20. Dowell D, Polgreen PM, Beekmann SE, et al. Dilemmas in the management of syphilis: a survey of infectious diseases experts. Clin Infect Dis 2009;49: 1526–9.
21. Workowski KA, Berman S. Sexually transmitted diseases treatment guidelines, 2010. MMWR Recomm Rep 2010;59:1–110.
22. Tramont EC. *Treponema pallidum* (syphilis). In: Mandell GL, Bennett J, Dolin R, editors. Mandell, Douglas and Bennett's principles and practice of infectious disease, 7th ed. Philadelphia: Churchill-Livingstone; 2010. p. 3035–53.
23. Behrhof W, Springer E, Brauninger W, et al. PCR testing for *Treponema pallidum* in paraffin-embedded skin biopsy specimens: test design and impact on the diagnosis of syphilis. J Clin Pathol 2008;61:390–5.
24. Borelli S, Monn A, Meyer J, et al. Evaluation of a particle gel immunoassay as a screening test for syphilis. Infection 2009;37:26–8.
25. Chorba TL, Berkelman RL, Safford SK, et al. Mandatory reporting of infectious diseases by clinicians. JAMA 1989;262:3018–26.
26. Gordon SM, Eaton ME, George R, et al. The response of symptomatic neurosyphilis to high-dose intravenous penicillin G in patients with human immunodeficiency virus infection. N Engl J Med 1994;331:1469–73.
27. Reik L, Jr, Burgdorfer W, Donaldson JO. Neurologic abnormalities in Lyme disease without erythema chronicum migrans. Am J Med 1986;81:73–8.
28. Duray PH, Steere AC. Clinical pathologic correlations of Lyme disease by stage. Ann N Y Acad Sci 1988;539:65–79.
29. Steere AC. Lyme disease. N Engl J Med 2001;345:115–25.
30. Steere AC. *Borrelia burgdorferi* (Lyme disease, Lyme borreliosis). In: Mandell GL, Bennett JE, Dolin R, editors. Mandell, Douglas and Bennett's principles and practice of infectious disease. Philadelphia: Churchill-Livingstone; 2009. p. 3071–81.
31. Winterkorn JM. Lyme disease: neurologic and ophthalmic manifestations. Surv Ophthalmol 1990;35:191–204.
32. Rahn DW. Lyme disease: clinical manifestations, diagnosis, and treatment. Semin Arthritis Rheum 1991;20:201–18.
33. Glickstein L, Moore B, Bledsoe T, et al. Inflammatory cytokine production predominates in early Lyme disease in patients with erythema migrans. Infect Immun 2003;71:6051–3.
34. Lesser RL, Kornmehl EW, Pachner AR, et al. Neuro-ophthalmologic manifestations of Lyme disease. Ophthalmology 1990;97:699–706.
35. Zaidman GW. The ocular manifestations of Lyme disease. Int Ophthalmol Clin 1997;37:13–28.
36. Karma A, Seppala I, Mikkila H, et al. Diagnosis and clinical characteristics of ocular Lyme borreliosis. Am J Ophthalmol 1995;119:127–35.
37. Jacobson DM, Frens DB. Pseudotumor cerebri syndrome associated with Lyme disease. Am J Ophthalmol 1989;107:81–2.
38. Zaidman GW. Episcleritis and symblepharon associated with Lyme keratitis. Am J Ophthalmol 1990;109:487–8.
39. Rothova A, Kuiper H, Spanjaard L, et al. Spiderweb vitritis in Lyme borreliosis. Lancet 1991;337:490–1.
40. Mikkila HO, Seppala IJ, Viljanen MK, et al. The expanding clinical spectrum of ocular Lyme borreliosis. Ophthalmology 2000;107:581–7.
41. Recommendations for test performance and interpretation from the Second National Conference on Serologic Diagnosis of Lyme Disease. MMWR Recomm Rep 1995;44:590–1.
42. Case definitions for infectious conditions under public health surveillance. Centers for Disease Control and Prevention. MMWR Recomm Rep 1997;46: 1–55.
43. Wormser GP, Bittker S, Cooper D, et al. Comparison of the yields of blood cultures using serum or plasma from patients with early Lyme disease. J Clin Microbiol 2000;38:1648–50.
44. Berger BW, Johnson RC, Kodner C, et al. Cultivation of *Borrelia burgdorferi* from erythema migrans lesions and perilesional skin. J Clin Microbiol 1992;30: 359–61.
45. Krause PJ, Telford SR, 3rd, Spielman A, et al. Concurrent Lyme disease and babesiosis. Evidence for increased severity and duration of illness. JAMA 1996;275:1657–60.
46. Krause PJ, McKay K, Thompson CA, et al. Disease-specific diagnosis of coinfecting tickborne zoonoses: babesiosis, human granulocytic ehrlichiosis, and Lyme disease. Clin Infect Dis 2002;34:1184–91.
47. Wormser GP, Dattwyler RJ, Shapiro ED, et al. The clinical assessment, treatment, and prevention of Lyme disease, human granulocytic anaplasmosis, and babesiosis: clinical practice guidelines by the Infectious Diseases Society of America. Clin Infect Dis 2006;43:1089–134.
48. Recommendations for the use of Lyme disease vaccine. Recommendations of the Advisory Committee on Immunization Practices (ACIP). MMWR Recomm Rep 1999;48:1–17, 21–5.
49. Nadelman RB, Nowakowski J, Fish D, et al. Prophylaxis with single-dose doxycycline for the prevention of Lyme disease after an *Ixodes scapularis* tick bite. N Engl J Med 2001;345:79–84.
50. Orlin SE, Lauffer JL. Lyme disease keratitis. Am J Ophthalmol 1989;107: 678–80.
51. Flach AJ, Lavoie PE. Episcleritis, conjunctivitis, and keratitis as ocular manifestations of Lyme disease. Ophthalmology 1990;97:973–5.
52. Reibaldi M, Faro S, Motta L, et al. Intravitreal triamcinolone for macular edema in Lyme disease. Graefes Arch Clin Exp Ophthalmol 2008;246:457–8.
53. Leptospirosis: an emerging public health problem. Wkly Epidemiol Rec 2011; 86:45–50.
54. Martins MG, Matos KT, da Silva MV, et al. Ocular manifestations in the acute phase of leptospirosis. Ocul Immunol Inflamm 1998;6:75–9.
55. Dupont H, Dupont-Perdrizet D, Perie JL, et al. Leptospirosis: prognostic factors associated with mortality. Clin Infect Dis 1997;25:720–4.
56. Vinetz JM. Leptospirosis. Curr Opin Infect Dis 2001;14:527–38.
57. Rathinam SR. Ocular manifestations of leptospirosis. J Postgrad Med 2005;51:189–94.
58. Update: leptospirosis and unexplained acute febrile illness among athletes participating in triathlons – Illinois and Wisconsin, 1998. MMWR Recomm Rep 1998;47:673–6.
59. Levett PN, Haake DA. Leptospirosis. In: Mandell GL, Bennett JE, Dolin R, editors. Mandell, Douglas and Bennett's principles and practices of infectious diseases. 7th ed. Philadelphia: Churchill-Livingstone; 2009. p. 3059–65.
60. Witmer RH. Experimental leptospiral uveitis in rabbits. AMA Arch Ophthalmol 1954;53:547–59.
61. Kalsow CM, Dwyer AE. Retinal immunopathology in horses with uveitis. Ocul Immunol Inflamm 1998;6:239–51.
62. Rathinam SR, Rathnam S, Selvaraj S, et al. Uveitis associated with an epidemic outbreak of leptospirosis. Am J Ophthalmol 1997;124:71–9.
63. Rathinam SR, Namperumalsamy P. Leptospirosis. Ocul Immunol Inflamm 1999;7:109–18.
64. Truccolo J, Charavay F, Merien F, et al. Quantitative PCR assay to evaluate ampicillin, ofloxacin, and doxycycline for treatment of experimental leptospirosis. Antimicrob Agents Chemother 2002;46:848–53.
65. Hospenthal DR, Murray CK. In vitro susceptibilities of seven Leptospira species to traditional and newer antibiotics. Antimicrob Agents Chemother 2003;47:2646–8.
66. Pappachan JM, Mathew S, Thomas B, et al. The incidence and clinical characteristics of the immune phase eye disease in treated cases of human leptospirosis. Indian J Med Sci 2007;61:441–7.

Chapter 85

Ocular Toxoplasmosis

Rubens Belfort Jr, Claudio Silveira, Cristina Muccioli

INTRODUCTION

Toxoplasmosis is a common zoonosis caused by the infection with *Toxoplasma gondii,* and it is also the most important and frequent cause of infectious retinal disease and posterior uveitis. Toxoplasmosis can cause severe, life-threatening disease, specially in newborns and immunosuppressed patients but the majority of *T. gondii* infections in immunocompetent patients remain asymptomatic.[1,2]

In the eye it can cause blindness secondary to the retinitis present in the posterior pole of the eye or vitreoretinal complications in the acute or recurrent form of the disease.[3] Ocular toxoplasmosis (OT) represents 50–85% of the posterior uveitis cases in Brazil and about 25% of cases in the United States.[4] The prevalence of OT in the United States is not well determined but it ranges from 0.6 to 2% according to published reports and in Brazil, the prevalence ranges from 10 to 17.7%.[5]

Ocular toxoplasmosis may occur either in a congenital or a postnatal acquired form, and in both the eye may be affected during the acute phase of the infection or, more commonly, many months to years later.[6] Many concepts related to OT have changed in the last years and are presented in Box 85.1.

Beef probably is not an important source of transmission; undercooked lamb, pork, and chicken are the common culprits as well as food and environment contaminated by the feces of infected cats. Transmission can also occur via organ transplantation and blood transfusion.[7] Recently, water has been associated with the transmission of ocular toxoplasmosis on different continents.[8]

Fetal toxoplasmosis tends to occur only when the woman acquires the infection during or months before the pregnancy. The infection may be severe and is a frequent cause of abortion in the first months of pregnancy. When the fetus is infected, OT may become clinically apparent decades later and when it does, it presents bilaterally 85% of the time.[9] Even women with IgG serum antibodies against toxoplasma may not be always protected against transmitting congenital toxoplasmosis to the fetus.[10]

Box 85.1 Wrong concepts in ocular toxoplasmosis

- All cases congenital
- Must present as a “retinochoroiditis”
- Vertical transmission (pregnancy) only once in life
- Cats and meat are the only source
- No treatment to avoid recurrences
- All patients need antitoxoplasmic drugs for 4–6 weeks
- Recurrences are related only to local factors

BIOLOGY, LIFE CYCLE, AND TRANSMISSION

Toxoplasma gondii is an obligate, intracellular protozoan parasite that undergoes a life cycle which includes both sexual and asexual reproduction. The sexual cycle occurs exclusively in felines, which shed a large number of infectious oocysts in their feces once in life, usually for a few weeks. Members of the cat family are its definitive hosts (hosts in which the parasite reproduces sexually), but hundreds of other species, including mammals, birds, and reptiles, may serve as intermediate hosts.[11] The parasite can be found in the host's tissues, such as muscles, retina, nervous system, and body fluids (saliva, milk, semen, urine, and peritoneal fluid).[12]

T. gondii exists in three forms: the oocyst, the tachyzoite, and the bradyzoite (also called the tissue cyst). Once the cyst is ingested by the intermediate hosts it causes disease with the production of tachyzoites. Under the pressure of the immune response the bradyzoites are formed. They are very resistant and may remain in the retina as well as the central nerve system and different muscles such as the tongue and heart for many years.[13] The bradyzoites can remain dormant in the host for years without tissue damage and, for unknown causes, may rupture, causing reactivation of the ocular acute and recurrent disease.[14]

Strains/clonal populations: haplogroups genetics

The ability to identify parasite types may provide new insights into the pathogenesis of this disease, and genotyping ultimately may become an important diagnostic and prognostic tool.[15]

The majority of strains identified in Europe and North America are classified into three distinct genotypes (types I, II, and III). Type I strains are very virulent and types II and III strains are less virulent. All of them can cause disease in humans. Type I strains are considered to be more often associated with postnatal acquired ocular infections, and type II strains are more associated with congenital infections and toxoplasmic encephalitis.[16] Atypical strains as well as mixed infections have been identified in many parts of the world and these atypical strains seem to be common in Brazil.[17] The genetic make up of *T. gondii* is more complex than previously recognized and unique or divergent genotypes may contribute to different clinical outcomes of toxoplasmosis in different localities.[18]

Atypical toxoplasmic retinochoroiditis as well as variations in the clinical presentation and severity of disease have been attributed to several factors, including the genetic heterogeneity of the host and the genotype of the parasite responsible for infection.[19]

PATHOGENESIS

Serologic evidence of previous toxoplasma infection is present in 20–70% of individuals in different countries, depending on a variety of factors including climate, hygiene, and dietary habits. There is no consistent correlation between the prevalence of serum antibodies and the frequency of ocular disease.[20] Different factors, such as the pathogenicity of the toxoplasmosis strains, may play an important role.[21]

Ocular toxoplasmosis in immunocompetent patients is characterized histologically by foci of granulomatous chorioretinal inflammation and coagulative necrosis of the retina with sharply demarcated borders. Inflammatory changes can be widespread in the eye and involve choroid, iris, and trabecular meshwork. Immunosuppressed patients with ocular toxoplasmosis have both tachyzoites and tissue cysts in areas of retinal necrosis and within retinal pigment epithelial cells.[22] Parasites can occasionally be found in the iris, choroid, vitreous, and optic nerve. The lesions tend to be diffuse and often are active in both eyes.[23,24]

OCULAR DISEASE

The retina is the primary site of *T. gondii* infection in the eye and the hallmark is a necrotizing retinochoroiditis satellite lesion adjacent to old hyperpigmented scars accompanied by vitreous inflammation and anterior uveitis. Retinal vasculitis is also present (Fig. 85.1). OT is characterized by recurrent episodes of necrotizing retinochoroiditis thought to be caused by the proliferation of live organisms that emerge from tissue cysts and/or an inflammatory reaction triggered by autoimmune mechanisms.[25]

The most common clinical signs of active ocular toxoplasmosis are blurring or loss of vision and floaters. Depending on the location of the lesions and the anterior chamber and vitreous inflammation patients can be more or less symptomatic.[26]

The diagnosis is clinical and suspected based on the ocular examination, the exclusion of the differential diagnostic entities (see below), and the presence of circulating antibodies for toxoplasmosis. It is important to perform both biomicroscopy and indirect ophthalmoscopy in both eyes. In special cases other procedures such as optical coherence tomography or fluorescein angiography may be necessary to diagnose and manage complications like macular edema and vasculitis.[27] Toxoplasmic retinochoroiditis can be associated with severe morbidity if disease extends to structures critical for vision, including the macula and optic nerve, if there is damage to the eye from inflammation or if there are complications such as retinal detachment due to necrotic hole formation or tractional changes or neovascularization.[28]

Recurrence frequency varies between individuals and is unpredictable, not only with respect to frequency but also regarding the retina site and its clinical presentation[29] (Fig. 85.2).

Toxoplasmic retinochoroiditis lesions have the same fundus characteristics, whether they result from congenital or acquired infections (Fig. 85.3). Acute and new lesions are usually intensely white, focal lesions with overlying vitreous inflammatory haze. Active lesions that are accompanied by a severe vitreous inflammatory reaction will have the classic "headlight in the fog" appearance. Anterior uveitis is characterized by inflammatory cells in the aqueous, medium-sized keratic precipitates, and posterior synechiae.[30]

Eyes with active toxoplasmic retinochoroiditis will occasionally develop retinal vasculitis with vascular sheathing and hemorrhages in response to reactions between circulating antibodies and local *T. gondii* antigens.[31] Typically, hyperpigmented scars of old and inactive lesions are present, and recurrent lesions occur at the border of healed scar as a satellite lesion.[32]

In most cases toxoplasmic retinochoroiditis is a self-limited disease. Untreated lesions generally begin to heal after 1 or 2 months, although the time course is variable, and in some cases active disease may persist for months.[33] HIV-infected patients have a tendency to present with diffuse retinitis with less vitreous involvement since they do not generate a vigorous inflammatory response. A high number of recurrences may be seen (Figs 85.4 and 85.5).

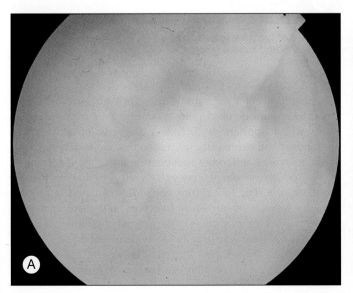

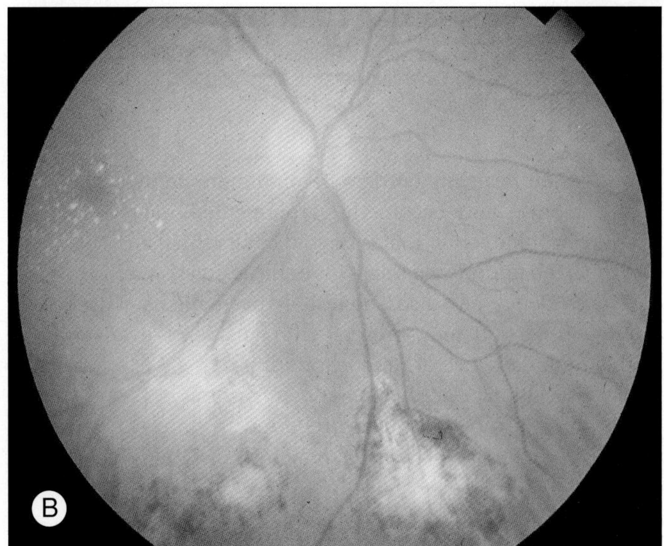

Fig. 85.1 (A) Acute necrotizing toxoplasmic retinochoroiditis with vasculitis and vitritis. (B) Macular star with healed lesion 6 months later.

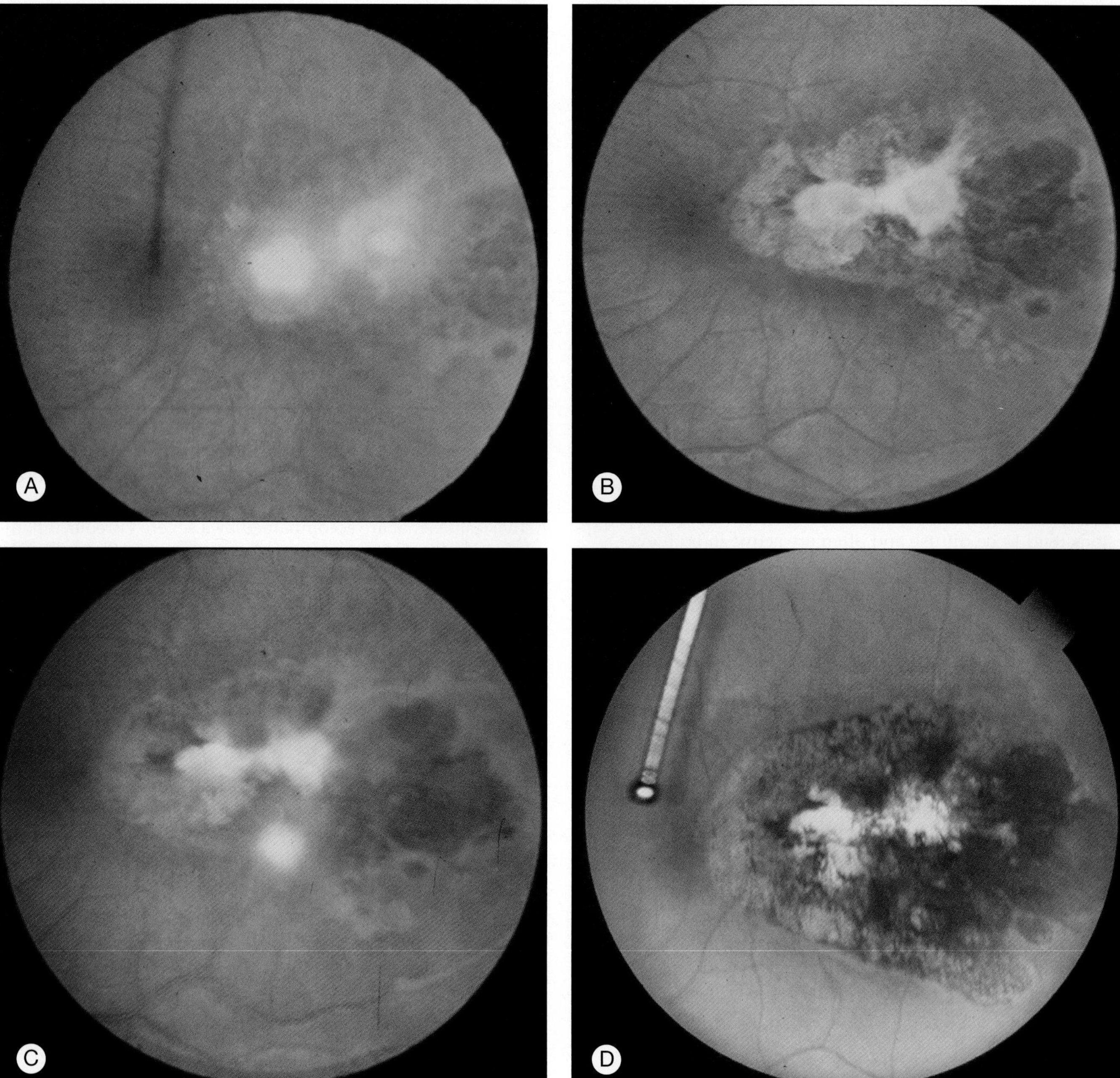

Fig. 85.2 Recurrent toxoplasmosis followed for 10 years. (A) Active lesion contiguous to recurrent scars showing different degrees of hyperpigmentation. (B) One year later, lesions healed. (C) Another recurrence 3 years later; small asymptomatic new lesion. (D) Follow-up 10 years after the first picture.

As a lesion heals, its borders become more defined and after several months may become hyperpigmented. Large scars will have an atrophic center that is devoid of all retinal and choroidal elements; the underlying sclera gives the lesion its white center.[34] Recent evidence has also suggested that patients with recent acquired infection may present with vitritis or even anterior uveitis in the absence of retinochoroiditis.[35]

The association between Fuchs heterochromic iridocyclitis and ocular toxoplasmosis has been reported in different countries and the pathologic mechanisms remain unknown.[36]

LABORATORY TECHNIQUES

Parasites are found rarely in intraocular fluids, and invasive diagnostic tests such as retinal biopsy are associated with serious risks that prevent their routine use. Different serologic tests exist and should be used only to confirm past exposure to *T. gondii;* it is inappropriate to base a diagnosis of ocular toxoplasmosis on the presence of antibodies alone. There is no minimal level of antibodies necessary to make the diagnosis of OT; any positive serology is enough therefore to diagnose ocular toxoplasmosis. The IgG serum antibodies can persist at high titers for years after an acute infection, and there is a high prevalence of such antibodies in the general population. Because active retinal lesions are usually foci of recurrent disease, serum IgG titers may be low and IgM may be absent. The serologic determination of IgA antibodies may help to determine the time of the primary infection since they last for less time in the serum.[37]

The development of molecular biology techniques has allowed the identification of *T. gondii* DNA in the aqueous humor and the vitreous, as well as ocular tissue sections of patients with presumed toxoplasmic retinochoroiditis, by polymerase chain reaction (PCR) techniques even when organisms are not identified on histopathologic examination.[38,39]

The differential diagnoses comprise infectious diseases such as rubella, cytomegalovirus, syphilis, herpes simplex, tuberculosis, and toxocariasis. Noninfectious conditions like retinal and choroidal coloboma, retinoblastoma, retinopathy of prematurity, gyrate atrophy, retinal vascular membrane, and serpiginous choroidopathy among others have to be excluded in some presentations.[40]

OUTCOMES AND COMPLICATIONS

Toxoplasmic retinochoroiditis can result in permanent loss of vision because of retinal necrosis, uveitis, and its complications. Central vision will be lost if lesions affect the fovea, maculopapillary bundle, or optic disc. Other reported complications include macular edema, retinal neovascularization, vascular occlusion and vitreoretinal lesions such as vitreous hemorrhage and epiretinal membranes. Subretinal neovascular membranes may be a cause of sudden loss of vision. Rhegmatogenous and tractional retinal detachments may occur as well as secondary glaucoma and cataracts.[41]

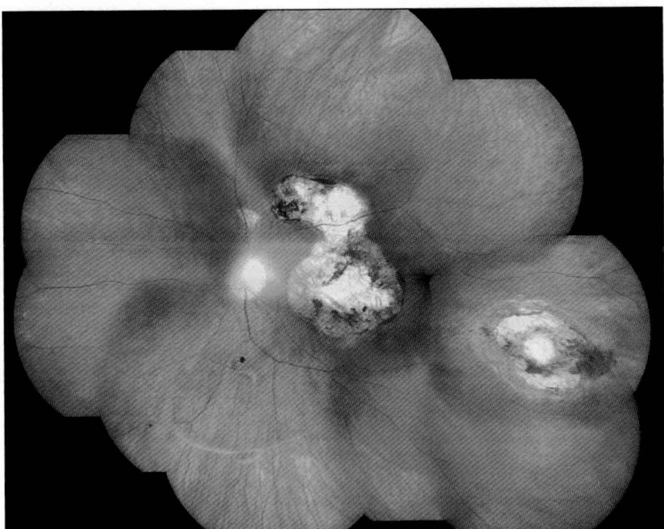

Fig. 85.3 Multiple toxoplasmic scars in a patient with congenital toxoplasmosis.

TREATMENT AND PREVENTION

There are many questions surrounding the treatment of ocular toxoplasmosis. Available drugs do not eliminate tissue cysts and cannot prevent chronic infection. No treatment has proven to be superior or even more effective than no treatment. It is accepted that steroids decrease the inflammation and therefore can lead to better vision function but should not be used without antitoxoplasmic drugs in order to avoid the worsening of the infection.[42] But the efficacy of the antitoxoplasmic agents and systemic steroids have never been studied in large clinical trials. There is no cure for toxoplasmosis since the tissue cysts are resistant to the available drugs and remain viable for many years.[43]

The combination of pyrimethamine, sulfadiazine, and corticosteroids, which is considered the "classic" therapy for ocular toxoplasmosis (Box 85.2), is the most common drug combination used and considered by many experts to be the best option.[44] Therapy with trimethoprim and sulfamethoxazole probably is equally effective and has fewer side-effects and better patient compliance. It may be considered, however, as having a higher risk to cause severe allergic reactions because of the long life of sulfamethoxazole.[45] Other drugs, such as systemic or intraocular clindamycin, have also been used.[46,47]

The duration of treatment depends on the individual clinical picture. Steroid treatment is often administered systemically and, as noted above, always associated with antitoxoplasmic drugs. Local drops are used when anterior uveitis is present.[48]

Traditional short-term treatments of active toxoplasmic retinochoroiditis lesions do not prevent subsequent recurrences. There

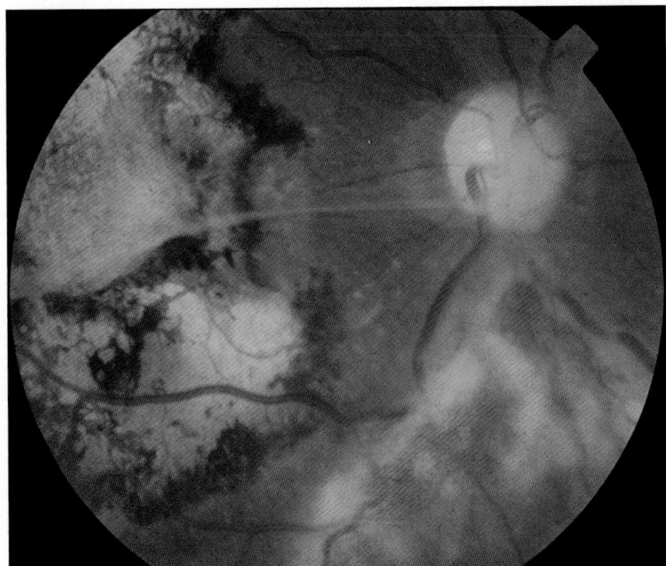

Fig. 85.4 Active CMV retinitis and old toxoplasmic scar in an AIDS patient.

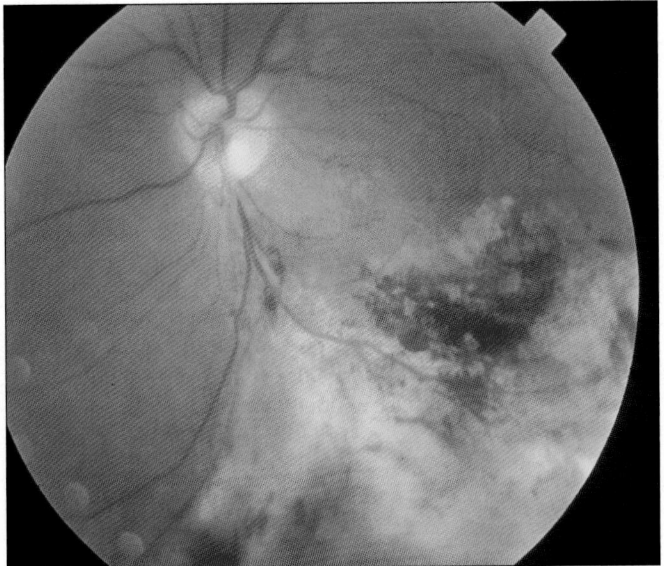

Fig. 85.5 Diffuse toxoplasmic retinitis in an HIV-infected patient.

Box 85.2 Classic therapy for ocular toxoplasmosis

- Pyrimethamine: 75–100 mg loading dose given over 24 hours, followed by 25–50 mg daily for 4–6 weeks depending on clinical response
- Sulfadizine: 2.0–4.0 g loading dose initially, followed by 1.0 g given 4 times daily for 4–6 weeks, depending or clinical response
- Prednisone: 40–60 mg daily for 2 to many weeks depending on clinical response; taper off before discontinuing pyrimethamine/ sulfadiazine
- Folinic acid: 5.0 mg tablet, 2–3 times weekly during pyrimethamine therapy

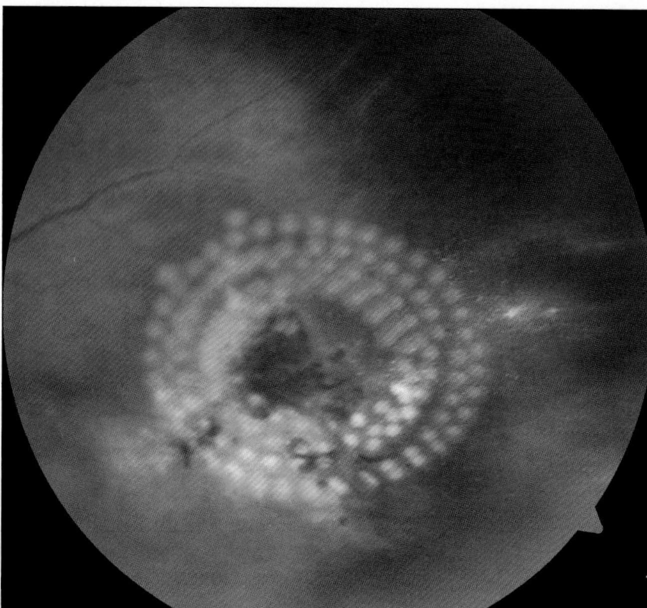

Fig. 85.6 Photocoagulated retinal hole adjacent to a peripheral toxoplasmic scar.

is no cure for OT since none of the available drugs penetrates the cyst.[49]

The combination of trimethoprim/sulfamethoxazole given for many months may decrease the number of recurrences and should be considered in higher-risk patients.[50] Periodical evaluation of the retina is mandatory in order to diagnose and treat potential sight-threatening complications such as retinal holes and retinal detachments (Fig. 85.6).

Classically, toxoplasmosis was considered as a self-limiting benign infection in the normal host, with treatment not necessary. Prevention of ocular toxoplasmosis in all patients with the acute form of systemic infection is debatable. Opinion is divided whether treatment should be offered in cases of recent acquired toxoplasmosis to decrease the population of tissue by cysts, thereby avoiding or decreasing later ocular involvement,[51] since its effectiveness has never been demonstrated.

When indicated, cataract surgery should be performed to restore vision and to allow the fundus examination in order to identify new lesions as well as retinal complications secondary to the uveitis. As a rule, patients with cataract secondary to ocular toxoplasmosis are operated on, typically with IOL (intraocular lens) implantation with good results, after at least 3 months of the uveitis being inactive.[52]

REFERENCES

1. Weiss LM, Dubey JP. Toxoplasmosis: A history of clinical observations. Int J Parasitol 2009;39(8):895–901. Review.
2. Commodaro AG, Belfort RN, Rizzo LV, et al. Ocular toxoplasmosis: an update and review of the literature. Mem Inst Oswaldo Cruz 2009;104(2):345–50. Review.
3. Nussenblatt RB. Ocular toxoplasmosis. In: Nussenblatt RB, Whitcup SM, Palestine AG. Uveitis: fundamentals and clinical practice, 2nd ed. St Louis: Mosby–Year Book; 1996. p. 211–28.
4. Jones JL, Kruszon-Moran D, Wilson M, et al. Toxoplasma gondii infection in the United States: seroprevalence and risk factors. Am J Epidemiol 2001;154:357–65.
5. Holland GN. Ocular toxoplasmosis: a global reassessment. Part I: epidemiology and course of disease. Am J Ophthalmol 2003;136(6):973–88.
6. Holland GN, O'Connor GR, Belfort R, et al. Toxoplasmosis. In: Pepose JS, Holland GN, Wilhelmus KR, editors. Ocular infection and immunity. St Louis: Mosby–Year Book; 1996. p. 1183–223.
7. Montoya JG, Liesenfeld O. Toxoplasmosis. Lancet 2004;363:1965–76. Review.
8. Bowie WR, King AS. Outbreak of toxoplasmosis associated with municipal drinking water. Lancet 1997;350:173–8.
9. Garza-Leon M, Muccioli C, Arellanes-Garcia L. Toxoplasmosis in pediatric patients. Int Ophthalmol Clin 2008;48:75–85.
10. Silveira C, Ferreira R, Muccioli C, et al.. Toxoplasmosis transmitted to a newborn from the mother infected 20 years earlier. Am J Ophthalmol 2003 Aug;136(2):370–1.
11. Remington JS, McLeod R, Thulliez P, et al. Toxoplasmosis. In: Remington JS, Klein J, editors. Infectious diseases of the fetus and newborn infant, 5th edn. Philadelphia: WB Saunders. 2001. p. 205–346.
12. Belfort Jr R, Muccioli C. Toxoplasmosis ocular. In: Fernando Arévalo J, Graue-Wiechers F, Quiroz-Mercado H, et al., editors. Uveítis y Tumores Intraoculares Temas Selectos. Venezuela: AMOLCA; 2008. vol. 1, p. 81–8.
13. Tenter AM, Heckeroth AR, Weiss LM. Toxoplasma gondii: from animals to humans. Int J Parasitol 2000;30(12–13):1217–58.
14. Silveira C, Vallochi AL, Rodrigues da Silva U, et al. *Toxoplasma gondii* in the peripheral blood of patients with acute and chronic toxoplasmosis. Br J Ophthalmol 2011;95(3):396–400.
15. Howe DK, Honoré S, Derouin F, Sibley LD. Determination of genotypes of *Toxoplasma gondii* strains isolated from patients with toxoplasmosis. J Clin Microbiol 1997;35(6):1411–4.
16. Vallochi AL, Muccioli C, Martins MC, et al. The genotype of *Toxoplasma gondii* strains causing ocular toxoplasmosis in humans in Brazil. Am J Ophthalmol 2005;139(2):350–1.
17. Vaudaux JD, Muccioli C, James ER, et al. Identification of an atypical strain of toxoplasma gondii as the cause of a waterborne outbreak of toxoplasmosis in Santa Isabel do Ivai, Brazil. J Infect Dis 2010;202(8): 1226–33.
18. Grigg ME, Ganatra J, Boothroyd JC, et al. Unusual abundance of atypical strains associated with human ocular toxoplasmosis. J Infect Dis 2001; 184(5):633–9.
19. Bottós J, Miller RH, Belfort RN, et al. UNIFESP Toxoplasmosis Group. Bilateral retinochoroiditis caused by an atypical strain of *Toxoplasma gondii*. Br J Ophthalmol 2009;93(11):1546–50.
20. Talabani H, Asseraf M, Yera H, et al. Contributions of immunoblotting, real-time PCR, and the Goldmann–Witmer coefficient to diagnosis of atypical toxoplasmic retinochoroiditis. J Clin Microbiol 2009;47(7):2131–5.
21. Saeij JP, Boyle JP, Boothroyd JC. Differences among the three major strains of *Toxoplasma gondii* and their specific interactions with the infected host. Trends Parasitol 2005;21:476–81.
22. Holland GN. Ocular toxoplasmosis: a global reassessment. Part II: disease manifestations and management. Am J Ophthalmol 2004;137:1–17.
23. Holland GN, Engstrom Jr RE, Glasgow BJ, et al. Ocular toxoplasmosis in patients with the acquired immunodeficiency syndrome. Am J Ophthalmol 1988;106(6):653–67.
24. Rehder JR, Burnier Jr MB, Pavesio CE, et al. Acute unilateral toxoplasmic iridocyclitis in an AIDS patient. Am J Ophthalmol 1988;106(6):740–1.
25. Arevalo JF, Belfort Jr R, Muccioli C, et al. Ocular toxoplasmosis in the developing world. Int Ophthalmol Clin 2010;50(2):57–69. Review.
26. Bonfioli AA, Orefice F. Toxoplasmosis. Semin Ophthalmol 2005;20(3):129–41. Review.
27. Pereira A, Orefice F. Toxoplasmosis. In: Foster CS, Vitale AT, editors. Diagnosis and treatment of uveitis. Philadelphia, PA: W.B. Saunders; 2001. p. 385–410.
28. Bosch-Driessen LH, Karimi S, Stilma JS, et al. Retinal detachment in ocular toxoplasmosis. Ophthalmology 2000;107(1):36–40.
29. Holland GN, Crespi CM, ten Dam-van Loon N, et al. Analysis of recurrence patterns associated with toxoplasmic retinochoroiditis. Am J Ophthalmol 2008;145(6):1007–13.
30. Rothova A. Ocular manifestations of toxoplasmosis. Curr Opin Ophthalmol 2003;14(6):384–8. Review.
31. Smith JR, Cunningham Jr ET. Atypical presentations of ocular toxoplasmosis. Curr Opin Ophthalmol 2002;13(6):387–92. Review.
32. Hovakimyan A, Cunningham Jr ET. Ocular toxoplasmosis. Ophthalmol Clin North Am 2002;15(3):327–32. Review.
33. Tabbara KF. Ocular toxoplasmosis. Int Ophthalmol 1990;14(5–6):349–51. Review.
34. Pleyer U, Torun N, Liesenfeld O. [Ocular toxoplasmosis.] Ophthalmologe 2007;104(7):603–15, quiz 616. Review

35. Holland GN, Muccioli C, Silveira C, et al. Intraocular inflammatory reactions without focal necrotizing retinochoroiditis in patients with acquired systemic toxoplasmosis. Am J Ophthalmol 1999;128(4):413–20.
36. Toledo de Abreu M, Belfort Jr R, Hirata PS. Fuchs' heterochromic cyclitis and ocular toxoplasmosis. Am J Ophthalmol 1982;93(6):739–44.
37. Vallochi AL, Nakamura MV, Schlesinger D, et al. Ocular toxoplasmosis: more than just what meets the eye. Scand J Immunol 2002;55:324–8.
38. Matos K, Muccioli C, Belfort Jr R, et al. Correlation between clinical diagnosis and PCR analysis of serum, aqueous, and vitreous samples in patients with inflammatory eye disease. Arq Bras Oftalmol 2007;70:109–14.
39. Fekkar A, Bodaghi B, Touafek F, et al. Comparison of immunoblotting, calculation of the Goldmann–Witmer coefficient, and real-time PCR using aqueous humor samples for diagnosis of ocular toxoplasmosis. J Clin Microbiol 2008;46(6):1965–7.
40. Vasconcelos-Santos DV, Dodds EM, Oréfice F. Review for disease of the year: differential diagnosis of ocular toxoplasmosis. Ocul Immunol Inflamm 2011;19(3):171–9.
41. London NJ, Hovakimyan A, Cubillan LD, et al. Prevalence, clinical characteristics, and causes of vision loss in patients with ocular toxoplasmosis. Eur J Ophthalmol 2011;21(6):811–19.
42. Stanford MR, Gilbert RE. Treating ocular toxoplasmosis: current evidence. Mem Inst Oswaldo Cruz 2009;104(2):312–5. Review.
43. Stanford MR, See SE, Jones LV, et al. Antibiotics for toxoplasmic retinochoroiditis: an evidence-based systematic review. Ophthalmology 2003;110:926–31; quiz 931–2. Review.
44. Rothova A, Meenken C, Buitenhuis HJ, et al. Therapy for ocular toxoplasmosis. Am J Ophthalmol 1993;115:517–23.
45. Soheilian M, Sadoughi MM, Ghajarnia M, et al. Prospective randomized trial of trimethoprim/sulfamethoxazole versus pyrimethamine and sulfadiazine in the treatment of ocular toxoplasmosis. Ophthalmology 2005;112(11):1876–82.
46. Soheilian M, Ramezani A, Azimzadeh A, et al. Randomized trial of intravitreal clindamycin and dexamethasone versus pyrimethamine, sulfadiazine, and prednisolone in treatment of ocular toxoplasmosis. Ophthalmology 2011;118(1):134–41.
47. Lasave AF, Díaz-Llopis M, Muccioli C, et al. Intravitreal clindamycin and dexamethasone for zone 1 toxoplasmic retinochoroiditis at twenty-four months. Ophthalmology 2010;117(9):1831–8.
48. Bosch-Driessen EH, Rothova A. Sense and nonsense of corticosteroid administration in the treatment of ocular toxoplasmosis. Br J Ophthalmol 1998;82:858–60.
49. Holland GN, Crespi CM, ten Dam-van Loon N, et al. Analysis of recurrence patterns associated with toxoplasmic retinochoroiditis. Am J Ophthalmol 2008;145(6):1007–13.
50. Silveira C, Belfort Jr R, Muccioli C, et al. The effect of long-term intermittent trimethoprim/sulfamethoxazole treatment on recurrences of toxoplasmic retinochoroiditis. Am J Ophthalmol 2002;134:41–6.
51. McLeod R, Kieffer F, Sautter M, et al. Why prevent, diagnose and treat congenital toxoplasmosis? Mem Inst Oswaldo Cruz 2009;104(2):320–44.
52. Van Gelder RN, Leveque TK. Cataract surgery in the setting of uveitis. Curr Opin Ophthalmol 2009;20(1):42–5.

Chapter 86

Helminthic Disease

Marcos Ávila, David Isaac

INTRODUCTION

Helminths have plagued mankind since before the era of our earliest recorded history.[1] It is possible to recognize features of helminthic infections from the ancient writings of Hippocrates, Egyptian medical papyri, and the Bible.[2] Nematode worms or roundworms are one of the two major phyla of the Helminths and include the major intestinal human worms (e.g., *Ascaris lumbricoides, Trichuris trichiura, Necator americanus, Ancylostoma duodenale, Strongyloides stercoralis*), animal worms (e.g., *Toxocara canis, Toxocara cati, Ancylosoma caninum, Baylìascaris procyonis*), and the filarial worms that can cause lymphatic filariasis (e.g., *Wuchereria bancrofti, Brugia malayi*) or onchocerciasis (*Onchocerca volvulus*).[1] The other phylum of the Helminths is called Platyhelminths, which is divided into trematodes (e.g., *Schistosoma mansoni*) and cestodes (e.g., *Taenia solium, Taenia saginata*). Many kinds of adult worms cannot develop on their own and parasitize human intestine; some in their larval stage can infect humans directly, causing tissue damage that includes the eye.[3] It is estimated that almost 1 billion people worldwide, especially in tropical areas and developing countries, are infected with one or more helminths.[4] This chapter discusses the most common helminthic diseases that affect the posterior segment of the eye: ocular toxocariasis, diffuse unilateral subacute neuroretinitis (DUSN), ocular onchocerciasis, and cysticercosis.

OCULAR TOXOCARIASIS

Toxocariasis is a infection caused by the nematode *T. canis* and less frequently by other roundworms such as *T. cati.*[3,5,6] Systemic effects of *Toxocara* infestation in the human are termed visceral larval migrans (VLM). VLM is usually a self-limited disease and typically affects young children from 6 months to 4 years of age.[5] Findings associated with the disorder range from a mild to moderate eosinophilia in an asymptomatic patient, fever, pallor, anorexia, malaise, hepatomegaly, and transient infiltrates of the lungs in symptomatic VLM to, more infrequently, a fulminating and fatal disease associated with pneumonia, congestive heart failure, or convulsions.[3,5,7] Ocular toxocariasis is unusual in adults but is an important cause of visual impairment during childhood, accounting for approximately 1% of all cases of uveitis among all ages in referral centers in the United States and Japan[8,9] and 3% of panuveitis in Switzerland.[10] Exact correlation between VLM and ocular toxocariasis is not well determined but patients with systemic disease rarely present with ocular involvement. In one study of 245 cases of VLM, only 5% had any indication of ocular disease.[11]

History

In 1907 Leiper first described the infestation of humans with canine nematodes.[12] Later, Wilder, in 1950, described nematode ocular infection.[13] In her study, Wilder reviewed the histopathology of 46 eyes primarily enucleated for suspicion of intraocular malignancy and nematode larvae were found in 24 eyes. Two years later Beaver and coworkers identified a *Toxocara* species larva in a liver biopsy from a child with visceral lesions and eosinophilia, identifying the etiological agent with this previously reported syndrome in children.[14] Nichols, in 1956, reported identifying *T. canis* (Toxocaridae family) in specimens originally studied by Wilder who first thought the worm to be part of Ancylostomidae family.[15] These studies demonstrated a common etiology for systemic and ocular diseases. In 1959 Irvine and Irvine[16] described histologic findings in a 4-year-old child presenting with strabismus, decreased vision, and retinal detachment. The eye was enucleated for suspicion of a tumor but an eosinophilic abscess with *Toxocara canis* larva on the pars plana region was demonstrated. This patient differed from cases reported by Wilder since the patient presented with clear media and the retina could be examined.[13] In 1960 Ashton[17] described four histopathologically proven cases of *Toxocara* endophthalmitis that presented with a posterior pole granuloma in a distinct fashion that represented a third classic form of this disorder. Duguid, in 1961,[18] described a case series of ocular toxocariasis and emphasized the difference between the posterior pole granuloma and diffuse chronic endophthalmitis, suggesting that clinical diagnosis could be perfomed in certain cases. In 1971 Wilkinson and Welch[19] reported 41 cases of proven or presumed ocular toxocariasis. Eyes with chronic endophthalmitis and leukocoria were much more likely to have been enucleated, whereas eyes with the posterior or peripheral isolated and visible granulomas were usually diagnosed clinically, and enucleation was not performed to confirm the diagnosis. Since then, several other relatively unusual forms of ocular *Toxocara* have been described and these are briefly discussed later. Association of *T. canis* and diffuse unilateral subacute neuroretinitis will be discussed separately in this chapter.

Parasitology

The *Toxocara* genus comprises 21 species including *T. canis* which is the most common cause of toxocariasis.[3,5,6,20] *T. canis* is a natural parasite of dogs and occasionally can infest human and other paratenic hosts such as rodents and rabbits.[21] Adult worms are cylindrical and long, measuring from 75 to 120 mm. Male worms are longer than female and in their development find five different stages from larvae to adult parasite.[20] Adult forms are found only on small intestine of puppies until 6 months of age (definitive host) and pregnant and lactating bitches. In older dogs and humans the cycle is not complete and because of this only the definitive host where worms reach sexual maturation can shed eggs in feces. To understand the pathogenesis of *T. canis* and the development of VLM and ocular toxocariasis it is necessary to understand the parasite life cycle.

Eggs lacking an embryo are shed in the feces of the definitive host (puppies). The eggs then develop an embryo and become infective in the environment in 2–6 weeks. Following ingestion by dogs or other parasite hosts, the infective eggs hatch and larvae penetrate the intestine wall and are carried by the circulation to a wide variety of tissues (liver, heart, lungs, brain, muscle, eyes). In the human and in adult dogs, this completes the life cycle, and the parasites are usually enclosed by an inflammatory granulomatous response that is primarily eosinophilic, although the larvae may remain viable for years under such conditions.[3,5,22,23] During pregnancy, the host response in the infected bitch is altered, and previously encysted larvae may resume migration,[23] crossing the placenta and affecting the canine fetus. In puppies, larvae reaching the lungs are coughed up and swallowed and, reaching the small intestine, they quickly mature into adult worms that produce infectious ova that are passed in fecal material. Prenatal infection is the primary route of transmission to puppies, however they can become infected after birth by ingestion of milk or feces from an infected nursing bitch.[6,22] The infection rate in puppies may approach 100%[24,25] and they start to shed over 200 000 eggs per day in feces from 3 to 6 weeks after initial infestation and may shed eggs until they are about 6 months old when the mature worms die[20] (Fig. 86.1).

Pathophysiology

Humans can be infested by ingestion of embryonated eggs or larvae. Eggs can be ingested accidentally after contact with

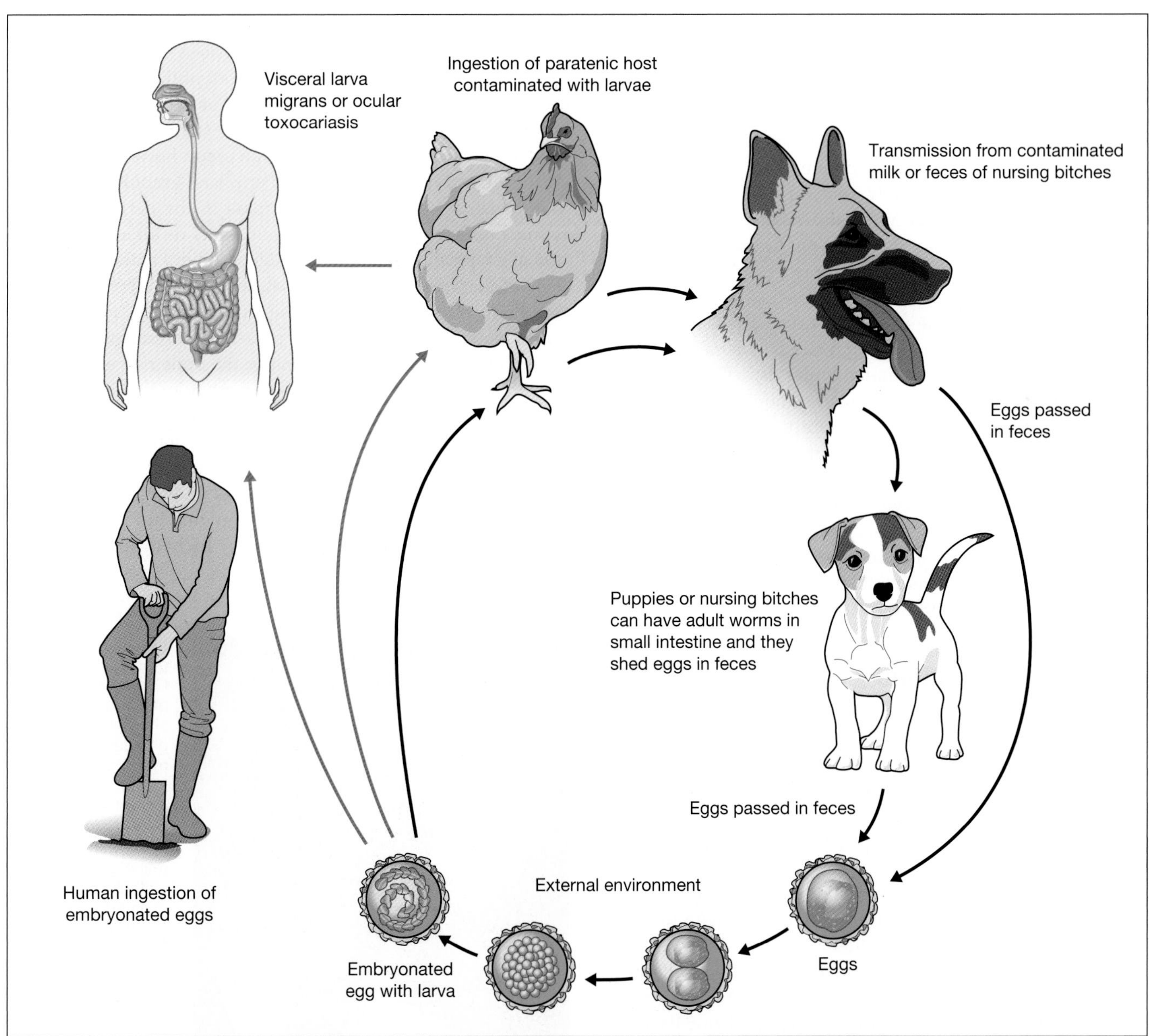

Fig. 86.1 Life cycle of *Toxocara canis*. Parasites mature and complete their cycle of life in puppies and pregnant bitches. Embryonated eggs are shed in feces and they mature in the external enviroment. Humans become infested by ingestion of embryonated eggs from contamined soil or larvae from paratenic hosts. Larvae are disseminate to organs originating visceral larva migrans or ocular toxocariasis.

puppies or by geophagia of soil containing embryonated eggs.[26–28] Outdoor parks and playgrounds (sandboxes) can be highly contaminated with embryonated eggs of *Toxocara*, since in this environment people routinely walk their pets.[29–33] Under optimal conditions embryonated eggs may remain viable for years.[34] Direct contact with untreated puppies is also an important form of transmission. Amaral et al. have shown that perianal hair from stray as well as owned dogs had embryonated eggs in 24% of cases and 99% of the total number of eggs were found in puppies.[25] A less frequent method of transmission is the ingestion of larvae from contamined meat. Several studies described infection by eating raw meat or liver from animals such as cows, chicken, and ducks.[35,36,37]

After ingesting embryonated ova, the parasites mature in the small intestine and transform to second stage larvae which penetrate the intestine wall, enter the lymphatic and portal circulation, and are disseminated to liver and lungs. Then the larvae reach the heart and are disseminated to other organs such as brain, kidney, heart, muscle, and eyes.[20] In human beings the parasites are enclosed by an inflammatory granulomatous reaction and the parasites do not evolve further.[22] The eosinophilic granuloma comprise the larva enveloped by a central core of eosinophils surrounded by mononuclear cells, histiocytes, epithelioid cells and giant cells. Because of the inability of the parasite to mature into an adult form in humans, a search for *T. canis* ova in human feces is inevitably unrewarding.[38]

T. canis can cause either VLM and ocular toxocariasis and the clinical manifestation depends on factors such as host immunological condition, inflammatory response, number of eggs/larvae ingested, frequency of ingestion, and localization of the second stage larvae in human tissues.[20] A large amount of ingested embryonated eggs may lead to a rapid increase in eosinophilia and rising antibody levels.[20] One study has shown that the degree of systemic eosinophilia in VLM has been correlated with level of exposure to *Toxocara* larvae.[39] A lower exposure to embryonated eggs may produce lower levels of antibodies and eosinophilia and may permit wider larval migration, reaching the eye.[20] Intraocular involvement by *T. canis* tends to occur in young patients, but in individuals who have developed ocular toxocariasis the age of onset is usually older than patients with VLM.[7,13,22,40] Mean age of presentation for systemic VLM is 2 years[5] versus 7.5 years for ocular toxocariasis.[11]

Clinical presentations

Although the average age of presentation is around 8 years for ocular toxocariasis,[5,11] the age at presentation may range from 2 to 30 years[11,41] and individual cases have been reported in adults with age up to 62 years.[41,42] Toxocara canis infection in adults and very young children is rare, probably because of better hygiene habits of adults and less contact with puppies, sandboxes, and geophagia.

The ocular involvement is typically unilateral, and bilateral disease is quite rare.[20,43] Patients usually present with unilateral visual impairment, leukokoria, and or strabismus in a relatively quiet eye. Careful slit-lamp examination can show cells in the anterior chamber (73%) and vitreous (100%),[44] and vitritis causing decrease in visual acuity was reported in 53% in one series.[9]

Based on ophthalmoscopic findings, ocular toxocariasis can be classified into these categories: peripheral granuloma; posterior pole granuloma; chronic endophthalmitis; or atypical presentations.

The presence of a retinal granuloma is the most common finding in ocular toxocariasis. Wilkinson and Welch,[19] in a study with 41 eyes diagnosed with the disease, reported that a peripheral granulomatous mass with relatively clear media was the most common form of presentation, being seen in 18 of 41 (44%) cases.[19] Stewart et al.,[9] in 2005, described 22 cases of ocular toxocariasis and in 50% of them peripheral granuloma was diagnosed. However, an isolated posterior pole inflammatory mass was the most common form of presentation in a series of 100 cases reported by Hagler et al.[45] and in 53% of 30 cases published by Oréfice and coworkers.[44]

Shields,[7] in a review in 1984, divided ocular toxocariasis into nine different categories, including DUSN.[7] Despite *T. canis* being described as one of the possible nematodes to cause DUSN, other roundworms are also causes of DUSN and therefore the disorder will be discussed separately in this chapter.

Peripheral granuloma

The peripheral granuloma, also described as the peripheral inflammatory mass form of *Toxocara* endophthalmitis, is usually seen in a quiet eye with varying levels of decreased vision and strabismus.[19] The vitreous and anterior chamber show mild to moderate reaction. Intense vitritis can occur, however at diagnosis the vitreous is generally clear. Peripheral granuloma presents as a dense, white inflammatory mass in the periphery of the retina. Localized traction on the retina may result in the production of a typical retinal fold from the periphery to the optic nerve (Fig. 86.2). This mass may be quite localized, spherical, and similar to those observed in the posterior pole. Fibrocellular bands may be observed running from a peripheral inflammatory mass to the more posterior retina or the optic nerve (Fig. 86.3). The prognosis in eyes with peripheral granulomatous inflammation is usually relatively good and visual acuity can be preserved. By the time this diagnosis is made, active inflammation is usually not progressive.[19] Ultrasound biomicroscopy study of 15 eyes with peripheral toxocariasis has shown alterations such as vitreous membranes in 86.6%, granuloma in 73.3%, pseudocysts in 53.3%, and thickening of ciliary body in 40% of studied

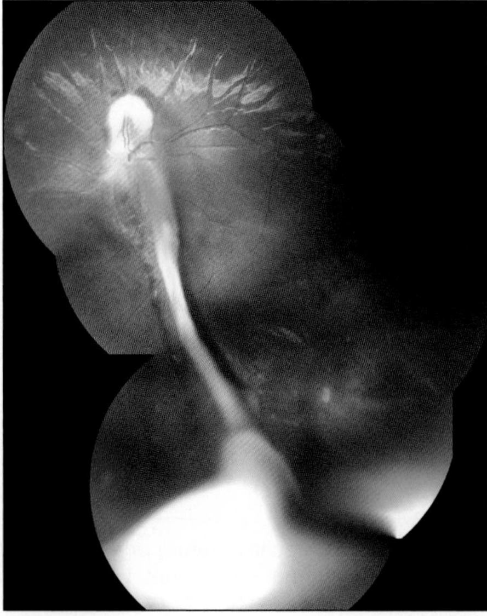

Fig. 86.2 Peripheral granuloma. Composite fundus photography showing peripheral granuloma (white mass) and retinal fold towards optic nerve head. There is hyperpigmentation of surrounding retinal pigmented epithelium and macular displacement inferiorly.

eyes.[46] Intra- and epiretinal traction bands can lead to production of both traction and rhegmatogenous retinal detachments, macular displacement and distortion, and optic nerve dysfunction.

Posterior pole granuloma

Posterior pole granuloma presents as white or gray spherical intraretinal or subretinal granuloma affecting the posterior pole. Most of the time it is diagnosed in a cicatricial stage when the lesion appears as a well-defined subretinal mass, measuring from 500 to 3000 μm, with no hemorrhage or exudates. Traction bands running from the mass to the surrounding retina may be observed. With cicatricial granulomas, there is very mild or no anterior chamber reaction and a low amount of cells in the vitreous cavity. Perilesional retina can show hyperpigmentation of retinal pigmented epithelium (RPE) and wrinkling of internal limiting membrane (Fig. 86.4). An optical coherence tomography case report has shown that the granuloma presents as a well-defined subretinal mass above the RPE (Fig. 86.5).[47] Active disease can show different stages of severity from mild anterior chamber and vitreous reaction to a very intense vitritis as seen in the chronic endophthalmitis form of the disease. During the active phase the posterior pole granuloma is observed as an ill-defined hazy mass surrounded by retinal exudates or hemorrhages.[19,20] A granuloma is usually seen in the posterior pole temporal to the optic nerve head; however, the occurrence of optic nerve granuloma has been described.[48] Due to posterior pole involvement, patients present with central visual impairment and can have strabismus and leukokoria. Macular lesions may be observed in association with peripheral inflammatory masses and choroidal neovascularization may occur as a late complication.[45,49,50]

Chronic endophthalmitis

Patients with chronic endophthalmitis are typically younger than those with more localized granulomatous forms of the disease. There is usually relatively clear media.[19] Localized granulomatous forms may be a late presentation of an acute form of the disease that had healed without development of retinal detachment or phthisis bulbi. As the vitreous clears it is possible to visualize the retinal lesions.[19] The history is usually negative for trauma, intraocular surgery, or bacterial and fungal endophthalmitis. However, a history of playing in sandboxes in public places and geophagia may be obtained.[19,27,28] External inspection usually reveals a quiet eye but severe intraocular

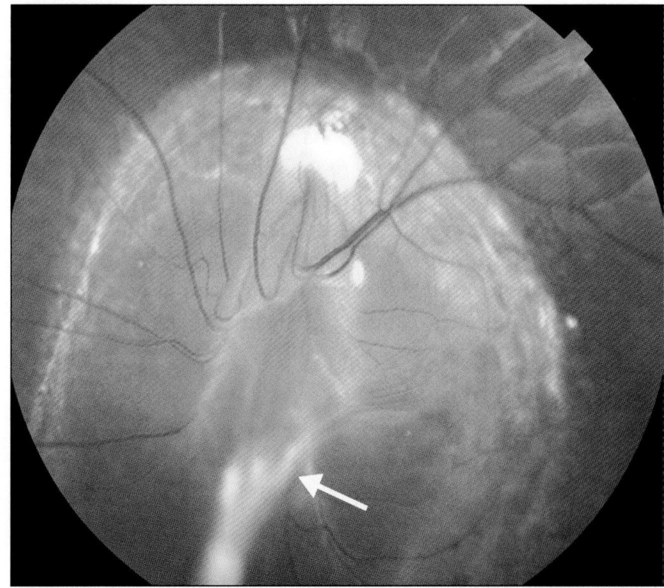

Fig. 86.3 Fibrocellular bands running from a peripheral granuloma to the optic nerve head (arrow).

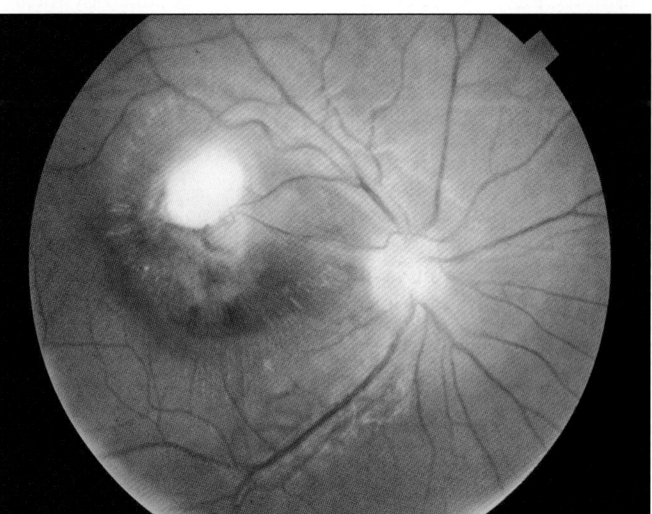

Fig. 86.4 Posterior pole granuloma. A posterior pole granuloma with surrounding retinal pigmented epithelium changes and internal retina wrinkling. (Courtesy of Fernando Oréfice, MD, and Editora Cultura Médica.)

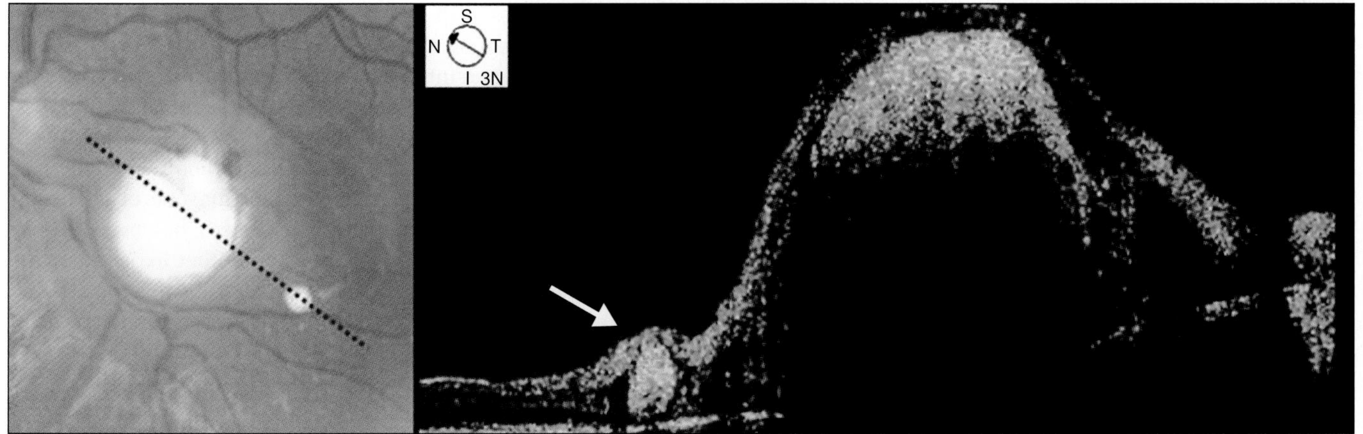

Fig. 86.5 Optical coherence tomography of a posterior pole granuloma showing its subretinal location. (Courtesy of Aline do Lago Coutinho, MD.)

inflammation can be present. In such cases leukokoria may be seen. Patients present with anterior chamber reaction that can vary from moderate to intense granulomatous reaction and can lead to hypopyon and posterior synechiae. The vitreous shows dense cellular infiltration with hazy media that can clear or develop cyclitic membranes, retinal traction and detachment that can be diagnosed ultrasonographically.[51] If vitreous clears, a localized granuloma can be seen. The prognosis in this form of endophthalmitis depends primarily on the degree of intravitreal organization and the development of complications such as retrolental membranes, cataract, glaucoma, retinal detachment, and phthisis bulbi.

Atypical presentations

Atypical forms of ocular toxocariasis have been reported. Most of them had a presumed diagnosis. These include: optic nerve granuloma and optic neuritis;[48] motile subretinal nematode,[52] which more recently many consider to be an early phase of DUSN; diffuse chorioretinitis;[7] conjunctivitis; keratitis; and lens involvement, including motile intralenticular larva and cataract.[7,22]

Diagnosis

Definitive diagnosis of ocular toxocariasis is obtained by means of histological demonstration of the larva or fragments of it in affected tissues. This evaluation is rarely performed and clinical signs; epidemiology (age, geophagia, contact with puppies, playing in sandboxes); imaging and serological tests are sufficient to permit the diagnosis despite the fact they do not confirm the presence of the parasite. Clinical presentation of localized granuloma in the periphery and posterior pole are very typical in many cases and a presumed diagnosis is made. In cases of chronic endophthalmitis when fundus examination is not possible due to media opacification specific ancillary tests such as ultrasonography or CT scan can help in establishing the differential diagnosis.

The enzyme-linked immunosorbent assay (ELISA) is the current serum test of choice to detect exposure to *T. canis*.[7] Intraocular fluids (aqueous humor, vitreous) can also be used to detect antibodies in a suspected case of ocular toxocariasis with a negative serum ELISA test.[7,41,53] The ELISA test employs antigens secreted by the second-stage larva and recombinant antigens have been produced from them that add even greater specificity to an already-reliable test (approximately 92%). The ELISA has a reasonably high degree of sensitivity as well (approximately 78%), at a titer greater than 1:32.[54] The immunodiagnostic tests used for VLM are not as reliable for ocular toxocariasis, and eosinophil count is not usually increased in these patients. Centers for Disease Control and Prevention consider serum ELISA titers less than 1:32 to be insignificant in the diagnosis of systemic toxocariasis[55] but others have stated that a serum titer of 1:8 is sufficient to support a diagnosis of ocular toxocariasis if the patient has signs and symptoms compatible with that disorder.[45] A positive test may represent a previous contact with the parasite and it does not necessarily mean that the patient suffers from either VLM or ocular toxocariasis. Ellis and coworkers have shown that 23% of 333 kindergarten children in rural North Carolina without signs of ocular toxocariasis exhibited a serum titer ≥1:32, and 32% had a titer ≥1:16.[55] Prestes-Carneiro and coworkers have shown that 14% of 182 ramdomly studied patients in rural Sao Paulo, Brazil, presented positive ELISA tests for *T. canis*.[56] Thus a positive serum titer cannot be used to confirm absolutely a diagnosis of ocular toxocariasis, although the absence of any serologic evidence of *Toxocara* infestation does not exclude the diagnosis but may assist in reducing the odds of this organism being the cause of ocular disease. Oréfice and coworkers studying 30 cases of presumed ocular toxocariasis found a positive ELISA test in 88% of them.[44] Another study has shown that only 45% of patients with clinically diagnosed ocular toxocariasis had titers higher than 1:32.[54]

Cytologic study of aqueous humor or vitrectomy samples may also be helpful in confirming the diagnosis of ocular toxocariasis. The presence of eosinophils in intraocular fluids is consistent with intraocular *Toxocara*. Remnants of *Toxocara* organisms have occasionally been recovered from vitrectomy specimens obtained at surgery.[57]

Differential diagnosis

Differential diagnosis of ocular toxocariasis includes: retinoblastoma, toxoplasmosis, other causes of endophthalmitis and uveitis, retinopahy of prematurity, Coats disease, persistent hyperplastic primary vitreous, and familial exudative vitreoretinopathy. In localized granulomas with clear media diagnosis can be determined by clinical evaluation (indirect binocular ophthalmoscope). In eyes with severe vitreous opacification, it may be impossible to make the appropriate diagnosis on the basis of morphologic features alone and considering the differential diagnosis is important.

Retinoblastoma

Retinoblastoma is the most common intraocular malignancy of childhood and also the most important entity frequently confused with ocular toxocariasis.[7] The first report of nematode intraocular endophthalmitis by Wilder[13] included enucleated eyes for suspicion of intraocular retinoblastoma. Shields and coworkers[58] reported that among 500 consecutive patients referred to them with leukokoria 42% had pseudoretinoblastoma and among them 15.6% had a final diagnosis of ocular toxocariasis. Patients with retinoblastoma are usually diagnosed before 2 years of age, being younger than a typical child with ocular toxocariasis. Sporadic retinoblastomas are more frequently confused with ocular toxocariasis since most of them are unilateral, and lack a family history of the malignancy. On ophthalmic evaluation, retinoblastoma usually does not present signs of intraocular inflammation, with clear vitreous and lack of posterior synechiae, cataract or cyclitic membranes, and the tumor presents a growing pattern that does not occur in toxocara granulomas.[7] In cases with opaque media the differential diagnosis is harder. Ultrasonography and CT scan may be very valuable in demonstrating an intraocular mass and calcifications of a retinoblastoma, or vitreous organization and tractional membranes, which is more frequently observed in ocular toxocariasis. In cases where the differential diagnosis is difficult, evaluation of intraocular fluids by ELISA or cytology may be of particular importance. If retinoblastoma is suspected, however, biopsy should be avoided and consultation with other experts may be a better path to reliable diagnosis. Risks and concerns relating to sampling retinoblastoma tissue are discussed in the oncology section of this book.

Toxoplasmosis

The typical lesion seen with protozoal *Toxoplama gondii* infection is focal granulomatous and necrotizing retinochoroiditis. It appears as a whitish or yellowish lesion, slightly elevated and with poorly defined limits.[20] During active disease, severe vitritis frequently occurs and in this case a differential diagnosis with chronic endophthalmitis caused by *Toxocara* can be very difficult. Ultrasonographic study can show vitreous membranes and an elevated mass that are more common in toxocariasis. Serological studies of antibodies to both parasites can be helpful in establishing differential diagnosis.

Other forms of endophthalmitis and uveitis

Bacterial endophthalmitis is frequently related to a recent history of trauma or intraocular surgery. These acute infections produce much more intraocular inflammation than a typical toxocariasis case. Endogenous endophthalmitis is rare, but an indolent infection may be nearly impossible to distinguish from nematode endophthalmitis. In such cases, laboratory diagnostic methods may be of value in determining the etiology. Pars planitis or chronic cyclitis is a condition that typically occurs in an older age group than that in which ocular toxocariasis occurs. Hogan and coworkers[59] described a case of pars planitis in which subsequent histologic examination demonstrated that the etiology was *T. canis*.

Retinopathy of prematurity

Patients with retinopathy of prematurity (ROP) have a positive history of prematurity and low birth weight, which is not common in ocular toxocariasis. ROP is usually diagnosed soon after birth and nontreated patients can develop cicatricial signs such as high myopia, temporal macular dragging, peripheral retinal folds and, in more severe disease, ROP stage V (retrolental fibroplasia). ROP affects both eyes while ocular toxocariasis is almost always unilateral. Morphologic features of ROP may be very similar to those of peripheral cicatricial ocular toxocariasis. In both conditions a peripheral white retinal mass may be associated with a fold of retina extending from the posterior pole to the granuloma.

Coats disease

Coats disease is a unilateral condition that affects predominantly young males in the same age group as does toxocariasis. Ophthalmoscopic and fluorescein angiographic evaluation show classic intraretinal telangiectatic vessels with association with yellow intraretinal and subretinal exudates. In later stages retinal detachment may be present and the differential diagnosis with ocular toxocariasis may be more difficult. In Coats disease vitreous shows no signs of marked inflammation and epiretinal membrane formation is not seen.

Persistent hyperplastic primary vitreous

Persistent hyperplastic primary vitreous (PHPV) is a congenital condition usually diagnosed within the first few weeks of life and presents itself almost always unilaterally. PHPV presents frequently with a retrolental fibrovascular mass that may be confused with toxocariasis. The involved eye is typically microphthalmic and this feature is not common in ocular toxocariasis.

Familial exudative vitreoretinopathy

Familial exudative vitreoretinopathy is an inherited disorder with typically bilateral occurrence. This disorder is associated with peripheral vascular abnormalities, pronounced exudation, vitreoretinal traction, and folds of retina extending from the posterior pole to a peripheral type of mass.

Treatment

Most ocular toxocariasis cases are diagnosed when there is a focal granuloma but no longer vitreous or surrounding active inflammation. In such cases treatment with anthelmintics or corticosteroids is not helpful and surgical treatment is considered when there is clinical cataract, vitreous membranes or opacification, or in cases of retinal detachment.

Medical therapy should be considered in cases of active inflammation. Topical and systemic corticosteroids are useful in managing acute inflammatory reaction and may reduce vitreous opacification and reduce or prevent membrane formation.[7,19,48,60,61] Topical mydriatics may prevent posterior synechia and secondary angle closure secondary to seclusio pupillae.[20] The exact role of anthelmintic therapy in ocular toxocariasis remains unclear and it is not proven that the use of this therapy can kill intraocular larva.[7] Despite this, the use of anthelmintic drugs or combination of them with corticosteroids has been reported with favorable results.[52] Anthelmintic drugs such as thiabendazole and diethylcarbamazine have been recommended in selected cases of VLM[60] and nowadays albendazole is the current drug of choice in the treatment of VLM,[30] showing its superiority over thiabendazole.[62] For the treatment of VLM currently recommended therapy is albendazole 400 mg twice a day for 5 days.[63] Treatment of ocular disease was described as a dose of 200 mg albendazole twice a day for one month.[20] If a subretinal larva is observed it can be destroyed with photocoagulation.[7] Intravitreal ranibizumab has been described to treat choroidal neovascularization secondary to ocular toxocariasis.[64]

Ocular surgery is indicated mainly in cases of ocular toxocariasis with retinal detachment[43,65,66] and pars plana vitrectomy is the preferred technique, allowing release of membrane traction and retinal reattachment in more than 70% of cases in some series.[45,66,67] Other indications for surgery include management of vitreous opacification, cataract, and glaucoma. Hagler and coworkers[45] reported 17 consecutive cases of retinal detachment secondary to ocular toxocariasis. In this report the retina was successfully reattached in 12 (71%) cases, and vision remained stable or improved in 15 (88%) of the 17 eyes. Small et al.[66] reported 12 cases of retinal detachment with a postoperative reattachment after vitreous surgery in 10 (83%), and visual acuity improved in 7 (70%) of the anatomic successes. Recently Giuliari and coworkers[67] presented 45 cases treated surgically for complicated ocular toxocariasis. Pars plana vitrectomy was the technique of choice in 58% of the cases, 38% had peripheral granuloma and postoperative visual acuity was equal or better than 20/300 in 60% of the eyes studied.

The most important approach to the management of ocular toxocariasis and VLM is prevention, decreasing the risk of ingestion of *T. canis* embryonated eggs or larvae. Effective measures include anthelmintic treatment of newborn puppies, nursing and lactating bitches after each pregnancy; hygienic disposal of dog feces; avoiding contact of children at risk with potentially contamined animals; avoiding eating raw meat of possible hosts; stopping children from playing in sandboxes in places where people walk their dogs; and improving hygiene habits in children, among others.

DIFFUSE UNILATERAL SUBACUTE NEURORETINITIS

Diffuse unilateral subacute neuroretinitis (DUSN) is an ocular disease caused by the presence of a nematode worm in the subretinal space. The disease affects predominantly children and young adults and often causes unilateral severe visual loss. In the acute stage it presents with an appearance of subacute retinitis, optic disc swelling, and mild to moderate vitritis while in late stages there is retinal and optic disc atrophy, retinal vessel narrowing, and severe visual impairment.

History and etiology

In 1978 Gass and Scelfo first described a clinical syndrome in which only one eye of a healthy child or young adult was affected.[68] Features of the syndrome include: insidious, usually severe loss of peripheral and central vision; vitritis; diffuse and focal pigment epithelial derangement with relative sparing of the macula; narrowing of the retinal vessels; optic atrophy; increased retinal circulation time; and subnormal electroretinographic findings.[68] Initially the syndrome was termed "unilateral retinal wipeout syndrome." Later, after recognition of signs of acute stages of the disease, the syndrome was named diffuse unilateral subacute neuroretinitis. The nematodal etiology of the syndrome was not yet clear, but from 36 patients reported, two revealed the presence of a subretinal worm at fundus examination, and both larvae were suspected to be from the *Toxocara* genus.[68,69] Later, in 1983, Gass and Braunstein described two different-sized nematodes causing the disease and postulated that the cause was probably not *T. canis*. The geographic distribution of both was different and the smaller worm (from 400 to 1000 μm in length) was proposed to be a larva of *Ancylostoma caninum*, while the larger one (from 1500 to 2000 μm in length) remained uncertain.[70] One year later, Kazacos and coworkers suggested that the larger larva previously described[70] was *Bayliascaris procyonis*, an intestinal nematode of raccoons and squirrels associated with central nervous system infections.[71,72] Association of DUSN and neural larva migrans has been reported and indirect immunofluorescence assays on serum and cerebrospinal fluid of one patient were positive for B. procyonis.[73] Other case reports of DUSN with confirmed serological evidence of *B. procyonis* infestation were reported and support its etiology as the larger nematode to cause DUSN.[74,75]

The exact etiology of the smaller larva remains unclear. Despite the first impression of the larvae being Toxocara,[69] later Gass and Braunstein[70] opined that *T. canis* might not be the cause of DUSN due to lack of consistent serologic evidence, the length of second-stage larva of *T. canis* being smaller than the small worm described, the clinical features being different than other forms of ocular toxocariasis, and the worldwide prevalence of *T. canis* did not fit with the limited distribution of DUSN. Gass theorized that *A. caninum*, a common parasite of dogs, could be the causative agent because it is a frequent cause of cutaneous larval migrans in the southeastern United States, its infective third-stage larva measures approximately 650 μm, it can survive in host tissues for months to years without changing size or shape, and cutaneous larval migrans had immediately preceded the onset of DUSN in some patients.[76] Casella and coworkers[77] also described cases of DUSN and cutaneous larva migrans, reinforcing that *A. caninum* could be a probable cause of the disease in Brazil. Cunha de Sousa and Nakashima[78] successfully extracted a subretinal worm in a 9-year-old Brazilian boy through a retinotomy after pars plana vitrectomy. This larva was morphologically similar to third-stage *T. canis* based on length of body and esophagus, tapered tail, and mouth shape. *Toxocara canis* causes visceral larva migrans and *A. caninum* causes cutaneous larva migrans, and there is evidence that both can be related to DUSN; thus confirmation of one as causative agent does not necessarily exclude the other as a possible cause. Cases of DUSN caused by non-nematode worm were reported by McDonald and coworkers. In such cases the larva related to DUSN was *Alaria mesocercaria*, a trematode worm.[79] Despite this report, nematodes are described as the main etiologic factors in DUSN. Among them, some filariae such as *Dirofilaria*,[80–82] have been proposed to cause the disease but *B. procyonis* as the large worm, *A. caninum* and/or *T. canis* as the small worms are the most probably etiologic factors.

Epidemiology

DUSN is an endemic disease in the southeasthern United States where the smaller worm (400–1000 μm) is most often seen and in the northern-midwestern part of the country where the larger worm (1500–2000 μm) is mostly related to the disease.[70,76] Its occurrence has been described also in the Caribbean,[9] Canada,[83] Germany,[84] Spain,[85] China,[86] and India.[81,82,87] It is endemic in South America, with most cases described in Brazil[77,88–91] and Venezuela.[92] In South America, DUSN is caused by a smaller worm, although in one case report a larger worm was found as the etiologic factor (Fig. 86.6).[93]

DUSN typically affects healthy patients in the second and third decades of life,[68,70] with a higher incidence in the male gender. In the typical disease only one eye is affected and a single motile subretinal nematode can be identified. Cases of nematodes infesting both eyes[89] or two nematodes infesting the same eye[85] are less frequently reported.

Pathophysiology

The complete pathophysiology of DUSN is not clearly determined but it is presumed that DUSN develops as a local reaction of outer retina to toxic products released by subretinal worm.[68] These products would also produce a toxic reaction to inner retina. Through the years there is a progressive loss of ganglion cells, secondary arterial narrowing, and optic atrophy.[76] Gass and Scelfo[68] reported histopathological findings from one eye of a patient with clinical evidence of DUSN. Histopathological analysis has shown a nongranulomatous vitritis, retinitis, and retinal and optic nerve perivasculitis. An extensive degeneration of the peripheral retina, mild degeneration of the posterior retina, retinal pigmented epithelium (RPE), choroiditis, and mild optic nerve atrophy were also observed. There was no eosinophilic reaction as usually seen in the typical granuloma of ocular toxocariasis. Histopathologic data were not sufficient to explain severe visual loss in this case (light perception), which contributed to speculation about the role of functional mechanisms in causing visual damage such as an inflammatory and/or toxic aggression towards retinal bipolar cells.[94] Recently Gomes and coworkers[95] and Casella and coworkers[96] described two case series of patients with DUSN studied by means of time domain optical coherence tomography (OCT). In both series the OCT main finding was diffuse atrophy of the retinal nerve fiber layer. The variability of the inflammatory signs and tissue damage seen in patients with the disease may reflect differences in host

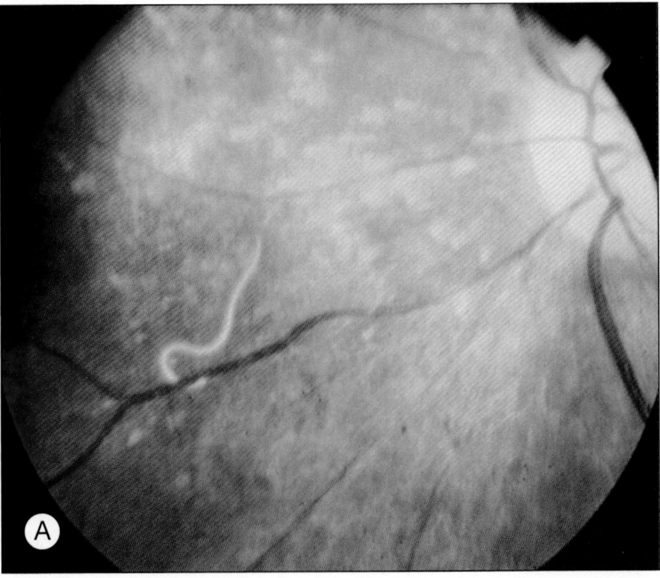

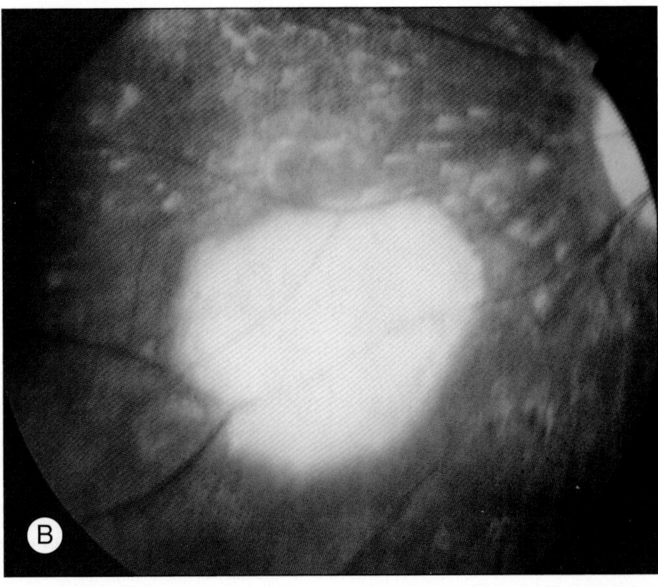

Fig. 86.6 Subretinal large nematode (A). Retinal aspect after photocoagulation of the nematode (B). (Reproduced with permission from Cialdini AP, de Souza EC, Avila MP. The first South American case of diffuse unilateral subacute neuroretinitis caused by a large nematode. Arch Ophthalmol. 1999;117:1431–2. Copyright © 1996 American Medical Association. All rights reserved.)

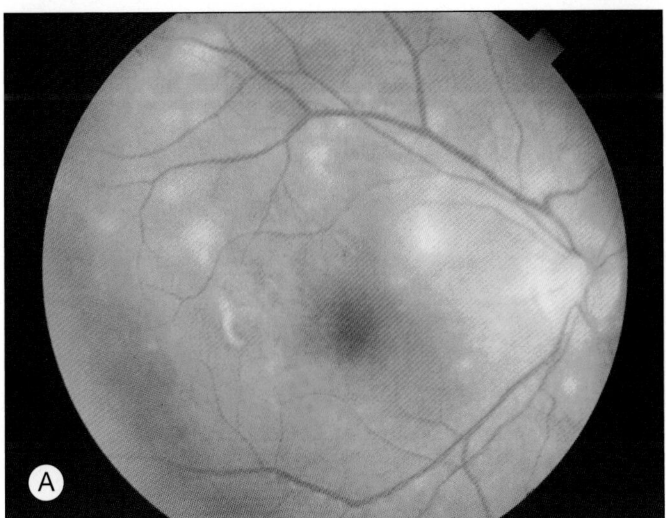

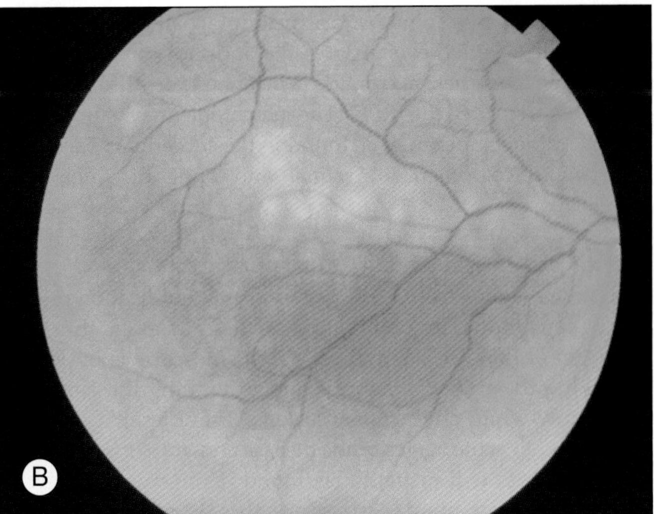

Fig. 86.7 Early stage presumed DUSN. Fundus photographs showing typical retinal finding: Crops of multifocal, gray-white or yellow lesions at the level of the outer retina. (Courtesy of Fernando Oréfice, MD and Editora Cultura Médica.)

immune response to the organism or the characteristics of the nematode itself.[97]

Clinical presentation

Clinical features of DUSN can be divided into early and late stages.

Early stage

Most patients with DUSN are asymptomatic or have mild symptoms in this stage of the disease.[90] Main symptoms include central or paracentral scotoma, floaters, mild to moderate visual loss, and ocular discomfort.[69] Signs include: afferent pupillary defect; mild to moderate vitritis; optic disc swelling; vasculitis and/or narrowing of retinal vessels. Less frequently, posterior segment signs include retinal and subretinal hemorrhages, serous exudation, and choroidal neovascularization.[69] The anterior segment is typically calm, although occasionally anterior uveitis may be present. The most characteristic retinal finding is the presence of recurrent crops of evanescent, multifocal, gray-white or yellow lesions at the level of the outer retina (Fig. 86.7). These active lesions are typically clustered in posterior pole, and the larva may be found in the surrounding area.[76] These lesions disappear in 1–2 weeks as the worm moves to other retinal area. Less than 1% of the lesions can lead to a focal chorioretinal scar that simulates that seen in the presumed ocular histoplasmosis syndrome.[97]

Late stage

Frequently in children, visual loss is insidious, and the patient comes to medical attention during the late stages of the disease.[97] If the nematode is not recognized and the condition is not treated, the disease evolves to its late stage. Main symptoms

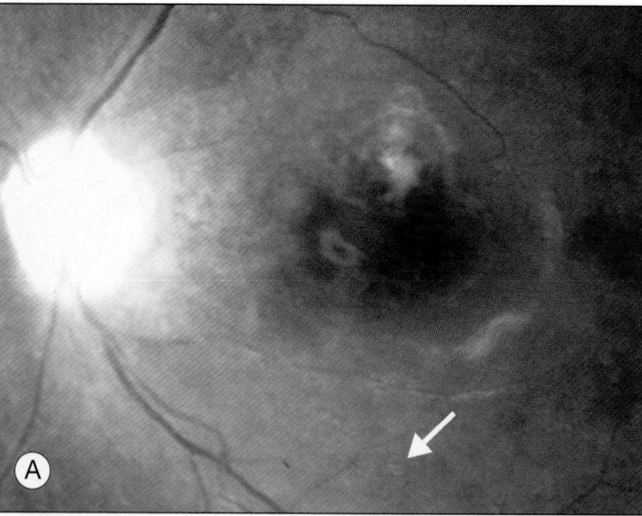

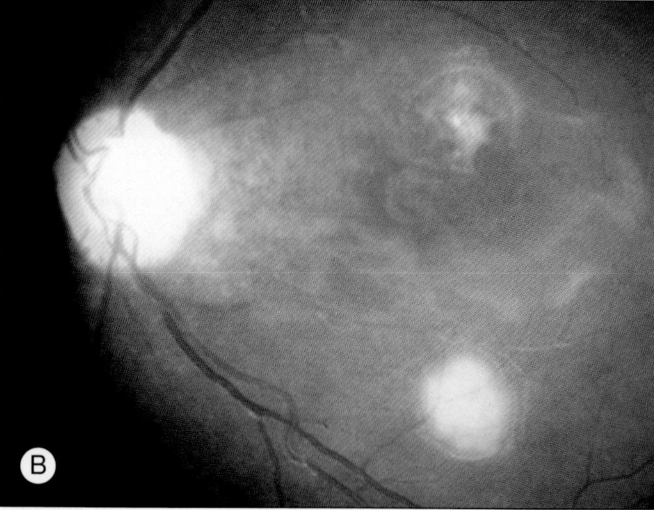

Fig. 86.8 (A) Arrow indicates the location of a subretinal nematode in the macular region. This case represents a late stage of DUSN with optic disc pallor, retinal pigmented epithelium changes and vascular narrowing. (B) Same eye after photocoagulation of the nematode. (Courtesy of Arnaldo Cialdini, MD.)

include a dense central or paracentral scotoma and severe permanent visual loss, while signs include an afferent pupillary defect in the affected eye, progressive optic atrophy, narrowing of the retinal arteries, and marked focal and/or diffuse degenerative changes in the RPE. The nematode may survive for 4 years or longer and may be found in the subretinal space even after the development of retinal and optic disc changes[97] (Fig. 86.8).

Diagnosis

Definitive diagnosis of DUSN is based on identification of subretinal nematode after observation of clinical aspects that raise suspicion of the disease. Indirect ophthalmoscopy is important in making the correct diagnosis and in locating the cluster of active gray-white outer retinal lesions. These lesions are typically found in acute stages of the disease and, if they are present, the nematode will usually be found biomicroscopically in their vicinity.[97] If theses lesions are absent, a detailed search of the entire fundus using a contact lens may locate the worm (Fig. 86.9). The rates of nematode identification in previous studies has varied from 33 to 52%.[92,95,98] A case report has shown that scanning laser ophthalmoscopy enhances contrast between the nematode and the ocular fundus and improves visualization and location of a moving worm.[99] In cases in which nematode is not located on fundus examination, a presumed diagnosis is established based on clinical findings, epidemiology, and ancillary exams.

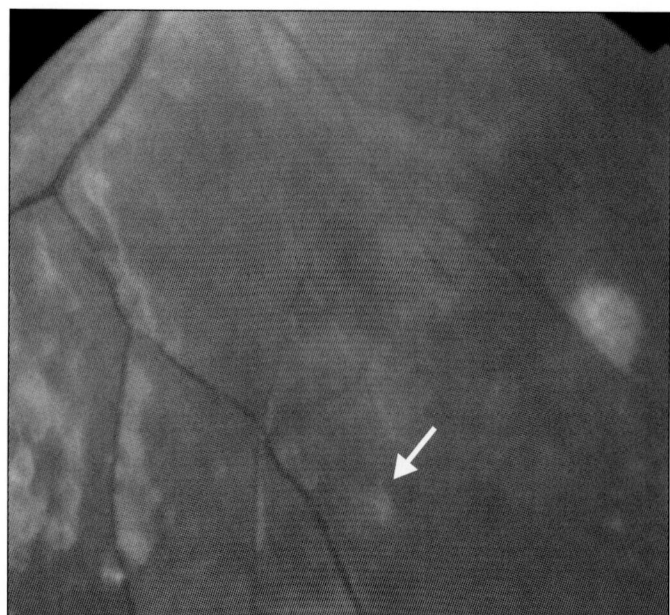

Fig. 86.9 Red-free retinography showing subretinal nematode (arrow) located on nasal-inferior retina.

Fluorescein angiography (FA) findings are different in acute and late stages of DUSN. During the early stages of the disease FA shows leakage of dye from the optic nerve head and perivenous phlebitis.[69] The active gray-white lesions exhibit early hypofluorescence and hyperfluorescence with staining in late phases of the angiogram. The aspect of the lesions on FA is very similar to the fluorescein pattern found in other white-dot syndromes, however in multiple evanescent white-dot syndrome (MEWDS) the lesions are hyperfluorescent on early angiogram. In early stages of the disease there are also minimal changes in RPE and cystoid macular edema may occur. In late stages of DUSN, FA shows diffuse hyperfluorescence from RPE window defects and delay in retinal perfusion (Fig. 86.10). Indocyanine green angiography (ICG) shows multiple small round hypofluorescent lesions that persist during all angiograms. Their aspect is similar to lesions found in birdshot chorioretinopathy.[100]

The electroretinogram (ERG) may be normal in the very early stage of the disease, however it typically varies from subnormal to severe decreased as the retinopathy progress. During all stages of the disease the b-wave is more affected than a-wave, possibly due to a toxic effect of the nematode and its products to retinal bipolar cells.[94] Rarely the ERG is extinguished[69,70] and the unaffected eye presents normal ERG. Eradication of the nematode in one case resulted in improvement in multifocal ERG amplitudes.[101]

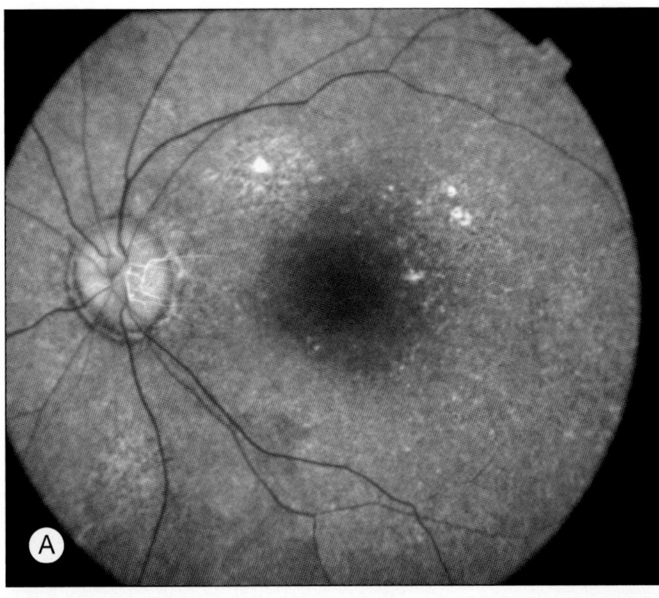

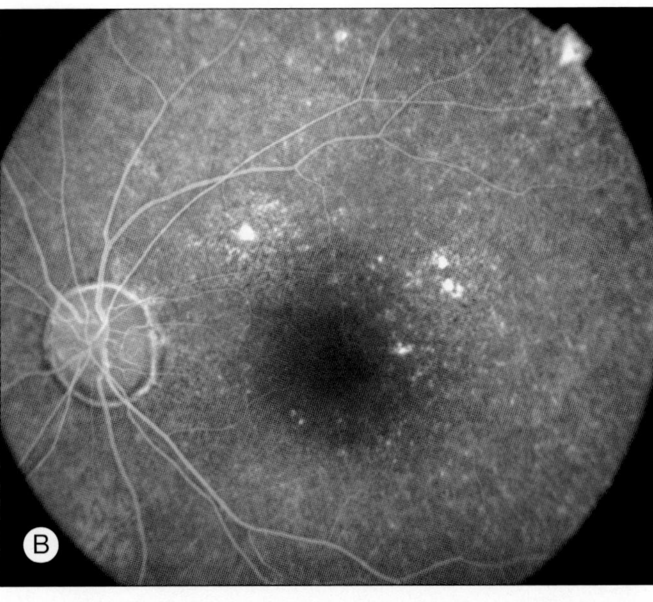

Fig. 86.10 Fluorescein angiography performed in a late stage of DUSN, showing diffuse hyperfluorescence from retinal pigmented epithelium window defects and delay in retinal perfusion.

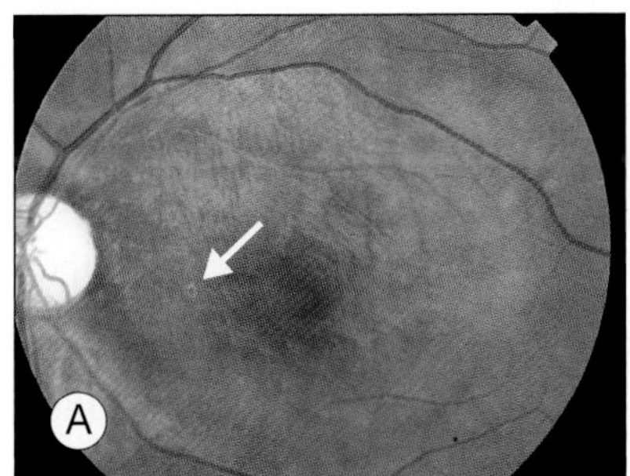

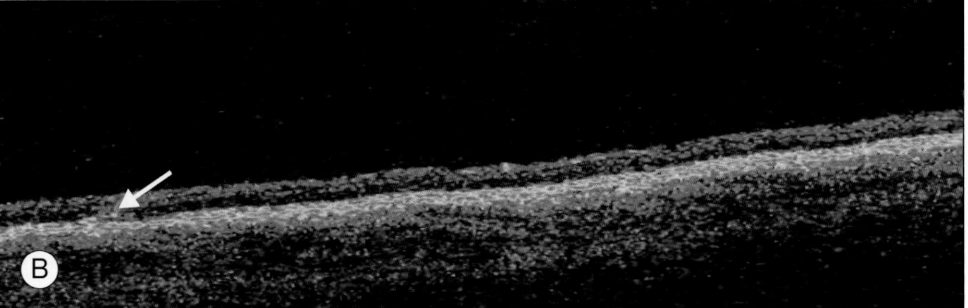

Fig. 86.11 (A) Color fundus photograph showing subretinal nematode (arrow). (B) Optical coherence tomography showing retinal atrophy and nematode in subretinal space (arrow). (Images courtesy of Antônio Marcelo Casella, MD.)

Optical coherence tomography (OCT) shows diffuse retinal thinning and diffuse retinal nerve layer atrophy.[95,96] Casella and coworkers also described focal retinal edema in areas affected by the worm and have shown the topography of subretinal worm by means of OCT[96] (Fig. 86.11). Gomes et al., studying 38 patients with DUSN, described statistical significance between retinal nerve fiber thickness and worse visual acuity.[95]

Serologic studies, stool examinations, and peripheral blood smears are of little value in making the diagnosis of DUSN.[69] Toxocaral and *B. procyonis* antibody titers have been suggested as diagnostic tools to try to characterize which nematode is producing the disease.[71] Recent study showed that ELISA cross-reactivity between them may be present and suggests a Western blot analysis to complete serological differentiation between *Toxocara* and *Baylisacaris* as cause of larva migrans.[102] ELISA test has been also used for serological characterization of cutaneous larva migrans caused by *A. caninum*.[103]

Differential diagnosis

DUSN can mimic several other chorioretinal diseases.[76] The disease presents differently in early and late stages and the differential diagnosis will be described separately for better comprehension.

In the early stages of DUSN, the typically seen gray-white lesions can mimic many other infectious and inflammatory conditions (Fig. 86.7). In DUSN, typical lesions occur in outer retina and after healing they normally present few or no RPE scars. In other infections such as toxoplasmosis, cytomegalovirus, and bacterial or fungal retinitis generally the inner retina is affected and there is prominent chorioretinal scarring left in the area of the retinitis. DUSN may also mimic white-dot syndromes such as acute posterior multifocal placoid pigment epitheliopathy (APMPPE), serpiginous choroiditis, multiple evanescent white-dot syndrome (MEWDS), multifocal choroiditis with panuveitis (MFC), and birdshot chorioretinopathy.[100] These entities are discussed in other chapters in more detail. Briefly, unlike DUSN, the active lesions in APMPPE and serpiginous choroiditis are accompanied by loss of visual acuity only when the lesions involve the center of the fovea, and they always cause permanent visible alterations in the pigment epithelium. APMPPE and serpiginous choroiditis occur in adults and are generally bilateral. In APMPPE, the electrooculogram may be abnormal but the ERG is normal, and visual prognosis is good. Serpiginous choroiditis has a worse prognosis than APMPPE and electrophysiologic tests are normal. MEWDS occurs in young adults, it is more frequent in women and may be distinguished from DUSN

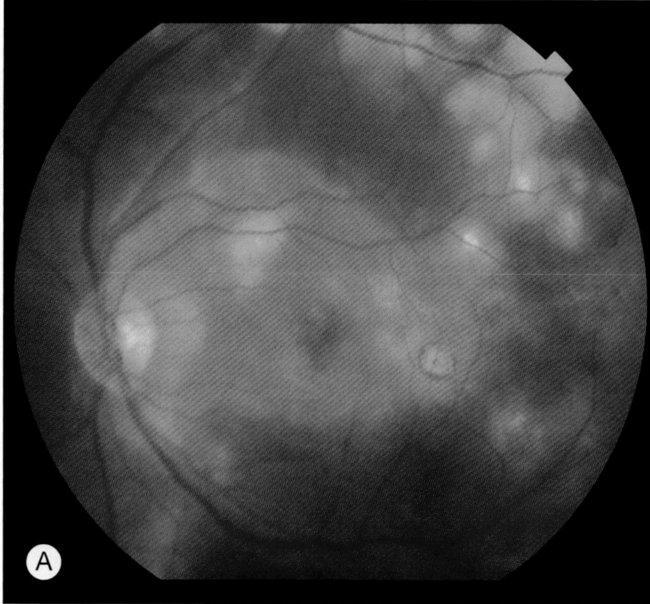

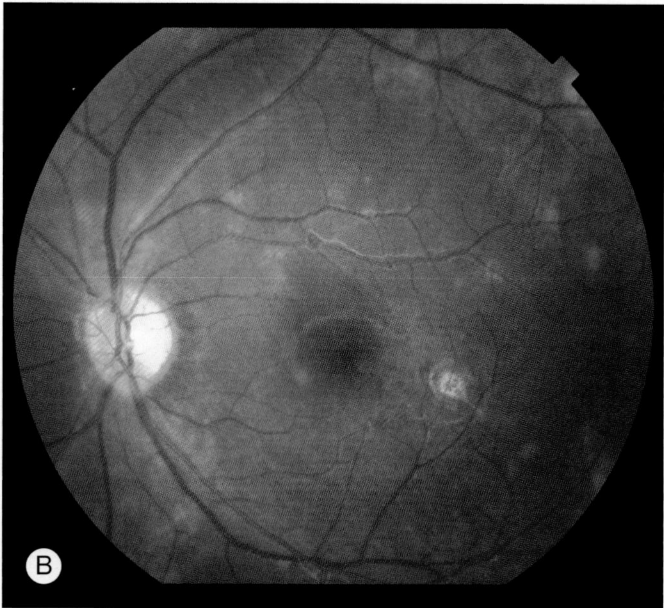

Fig. 86.12 (A) Color fundus photograph of a 9-year-old boy with unilateral multifocal retinitis diagnosed as presumed early stage of DUSN. (B) Appearance after 45 days. The patient was treated with albendazole 400 mg/day twice a day for 30 days. Visual acuity improved from 20/200 (A) to 20/70 (B).

by a frequent history of an antecedent flu-like illness and photopsia, widely scattered gray-white outer retinal lesions, an enlarged blind spot, hyperfluorescent dots seen from the early phases of fluorescein angiography (in DUSN lesions are initially hypofluorescent), a decrease in the ERG a-wave that normalizes as symptoms fade, and return of the fundus and visual function to normal in most patients within several months.[97] Birdshot chorioretinopathy often occurs in middle-aged women, is bilateral, and frequently associated with positive HLA-A29. Fundus changes include moderate vitritis, multiple scattered yellowish rounded lesions that may resemble DUSN lesions. Fluorescein angiography shows hypofluorescent lesions and may demonstrate active retinovascular leakage along the large retinal vessels, small vessel leakage, and cystoid or diffuse macular edema. Circulation times are often delayed and the vessels empty much more rapidly than in a normal eye.[100] Other uveitis can mimic DUSN. In Behçet disease, the white lesions involve the inner retina and the patient usually has other systemic manifestations of the disorder, including oral and/or genital ulcers, arthritis, and erythema nodosum. Patients with DUSN occasionally may demonstrate perivenous candle-wax-dripping exudate or subretinal exudate similar to that seen in patients with sarcoidosis.[76]

In late stage of the disease after fading of gray-white lesions and development of scattered focal chorioretinal scars, the fundus of patients with DUSN may be mistaken for the presumed ocular histoplasmosis syndrome (POHS). POHS is frequently bilateral, shows normal RPE between the focal scars, presents clear vitreous without inflammatory cells, and the lack of optic atrophy and retinal vessel narrowing. Retinitis pigmentosa (RP) is another important differential diagnostic entity. The presence of bone-spicule RPE hyperpigmentation, bilaterality, and posterior subcapsular cataract are common in RP but rare in DUSN.[97] Other causes of optic atrophy may mimic DUSN, such as trauma, retrobulbar or intracranial tumors, and sustained occlusion of ophthalmic artery.

Treatment

Prompt identification of the early signs of the disease allows treatment that can prevent late manifestations and encourage visual recovery/preservation. Treatment of DUSN can be performed with either photocoagulation of the nematode when it is identified during fundus examination (careful searching often with a contact lens is needed) or systemic anthelmintic drugs when the diagnosis is presumed. Photocoagulation of the subretinal worm is the current treatment of choice (Fig 86.6 and 86.8). It causes minimal or no post-treatment exacerbation of inflammation and is successful in causing prompt and permanent inactivation of the disease. Visual acuity improvement depends on the stage of the diagnosis.

Initially the use of oral anthelmintic was considered ineffective[70] but further studies have shown that thiabendazole is effective in the treatment of patients with a moderate degree of vitritis associated with a breakdown in the blood–retinal barrier.[104–106] Subsequently, ivermectin has been tried as a less toxic alternative to thiabendazole.[107] However, Casella and coworkers reported that ivermectin failed to kill a nematode that was subsequently identified and destroyed with laser photocoagulation.[108] Recent studies report case series of successful treatment of DUSN with albendazole[98,109] (Fig. 86.12). Cunha-de-Souza and coworkers[98] and Malaguido and coworkers[109] report the use of albendazole 400 mg/daily for 30 days with fading of active lesions and visual recovery. In patients with late-stage DUSN some degree of improvement of vision was observed. No adverse side-effects were observed in both studies, and this therapy has been advocated in cases of presumed DUSN where the nematode is not located.[90]

ONCHOCERCIASIS

Onchocerciasis (river blindness) is caused by the microfilarial stage of the nematode *Oncocerca volvulus* and is endemic in West Africa, but also in Yemen and in six countries of the Americas

(Brazil, Colombia, Ecuador, Guatemala, Mexico, and Venezuela).[91,110] According to the World Health Organization, onchocerciasis is the world's second leading cause of preventable blindness and its prevalence is estimated at 37 million individuals worldwide, most of them living on the African continent.[111] The filariae cause dermatitis, subcutaneous nodules due to encapsulation of parasites in fibrous tissue and eye disease. The disease is transmitted by an insect of the genus *Simulium* (Blackflies) which breed in fast-flowing rivers and streams, lending the name "river blindness." The vector ingests microfilariae during a blood-meal from a sick human. Then the parasites develop into infectious stages and are transmitted to other persons on subsequent bites. Humans are the only definitive host known.[110]

Clinical presentation

Ocular onchocerciasis can involve any part of the eye and disease manifestations are characterized either as posterior or anterior eye disease.[112]

Anterior eye disease prevalence has been described ranging from 43 to 48% of affected individuals in studied populations. The most frequently diagnosed anterior eye disease is the presence of microfilariae in the anterior chamber associated or not with iridocyclitis, followed by punctate epithelial keratitis, corneal microfilariae, sclerosing keratitis, and neovascularization leading to visual impairment and blindness in one or both eyes in 2–4% of patients.[113,114]

Posterior eye disease prevalence ranges from 34 to 75% of affected patients.[113,114] Posterior segment lesions include atrophy of RPE and choroid mainly in the posterior pole, hyperpigmentation clumping of RPE, white and shiny intraretinal deposits, retinitis, subretinal fibrosis, neuritis and optic nerve atrophy.[113–116] Patients may present with visual field loss and poor night vision and in patients with hyperpigmentation of RPE a differential diagnosis with retinitis pigmentosa is important. Another important differential diagnostic consideration is hypovitaminosis A, which can cause also night blindness and intraretinal white spots.

Treatment and prevention

Through the years the prevalence of ocular onchocerciasis is falling in endemic areas. This fact is due to several task forces of the World Health Organization in Africa and the Americas to reduce vector breeding and also to the treatment of patients with the disease, preventing blindness in affected and contamination of healthy individuals.

Ivermectin is a safe and effective microfilaricidal drug which has been donated by Merck and Company since 1987 to be delivered through mass drug administration programs to control onchocerciasis. Ivermectin rapidly kills the microfilariae and reduces the lifespan of adult worms. This therapeutic scheme is administered twice each year and the goal of these programs is to treat during the years at least 85% of the population at risk and completely eliminate transmission of the parasite in Africa and America by the year 2012.[110]

CYSTICERCOSIS

Cysticercosis is the infestation of human tissues by *Cysticercus cellulosae*, the larval form of *Taenia solium*, a common pork parasite that can cause taeniasis in man. The ingestion of contaminated and uncooked meat containing cysticerci leads to development of taeniasis, the infestation of human small intestine by the adult tapeworm of *T. solium* (definitive host). Cysticercosis occurs when the intermediate host (e.g., pork, man) ingests eggs of *T. solium* from contaminated food or water, or by autoinfection of the definitive host when there is accidental ingestion of eggs shed in the host feces.[117,118] The ingested eggs develop into larvae, which penetrate the small intestine wall reaching lymphatics and vascular system. The larvae then spread to highly vascularized organs such as brain, heart, muscles, and eyes, where they become a cystic structure containing the scolex named cysticercus (metacestode).[119] Cysticerci may remain viable in the ocular and central nervous system for years and ocular manifestations can be devastating as the cysticercus increases in size or dies releasing toxic products leading to a profound inflammatory reaction, causing blindness in 3–5 years.[120]

Clinical presentation

The central nervous system is the most affected system and neurocysticercosis is the most commonly diagnosed form of cysticercosis.[121] Neurocysticercosis is the main cause of acquired seizures worldwide. The disease can also lead to encephalopathy, meningeal signs, obstructive hydrocephalus, and other neurological abnormalities.[122] Cysticerci appear as cystic lesions on computed tomography (CT) or magnetic resonance imaging (MRI), and when calcified appear as hyperdense spots on radiographs.

Eyes and adnexial tissues are affected in 13–46% of infected individuals.[117] Cysticerci may be present in virtually all ocular and adnexial structures such as in the eyelids, orbit, extraocular muscles, subconjuntival space, anterior chamber, vitreous and subretinal space.[118,121,123–125] Vitreous and subretinal locations are the most often diagnosed locations of ocular cysticercosis, ranging from 68 to 74% of studied cases and 41% occured either subretinally or intraretinally in one series.[117,121] The parasite reaches the eye through posterior cilliary arteries to the subretinal space. A subretinal cysticercus is seen ophthalmoscopically as a cyst in subretinal space containing one scolex that usually presents as a white spot inside the cyst (Fig. 86.13). Associated findings may be observed, such as retinal pigmented epithelium hyperpigmentation, serous retinal detachment, retinal edema and/or hemorrhages, and severe uveitis in later stages (Fig. 86.14). Intravitreous cysticercus presents as a well-defined translucent floating cyst that can produce undulating movement, especially when stimulated by light. Epiretinal membranes or RPE changes in the spot where the parasites traverse the retina may be observed (Fig. 86.15).[119,123,126,127] Ultrasonography may be used to confirm the cystic nature of the parasite and MRI has been suggested to confirm ultrasonographic findings as well as determine the presence of possible other cysts in orbit or brain.[125]

Treatment

Intraocular cysticercosis is treated with surgical removal.[126–128] Treatment with systemic drugs has not been succesful[129] and killing the cyst without removing it might produce severe uveitis. An intravitreal cysticercus can be removed by pars plana vitrectomy and the subretinal cyst removal can be performed by either vitrectomy or transcleral removal.[126] The cysticercus should be removed unharmed, avoiding its rupture and release of intracystic material in the vitreous cavity, however there are reports of successful suction of the cyst during vitrectomy with

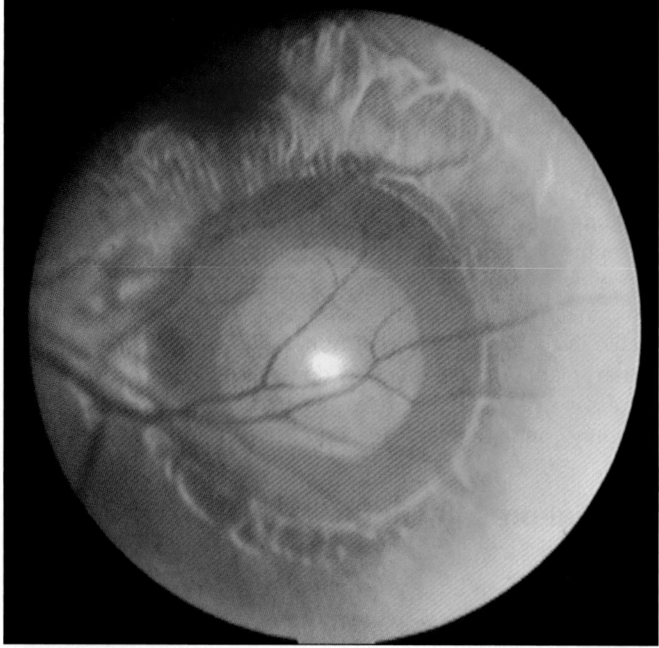

Fig. 86.13 Subretinal cysticercus in the posterior pole surrounded by hemorrhage.

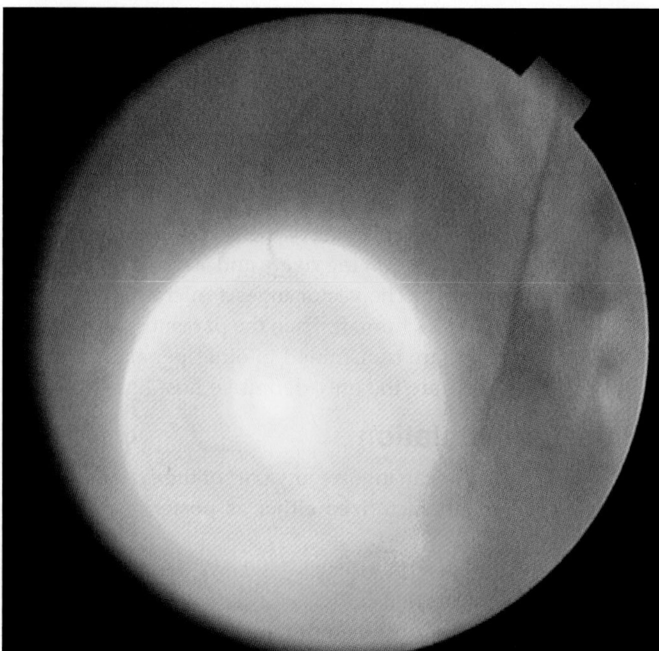

Fig. 86.14 Subretinal cysticercus located in the inferior retina.

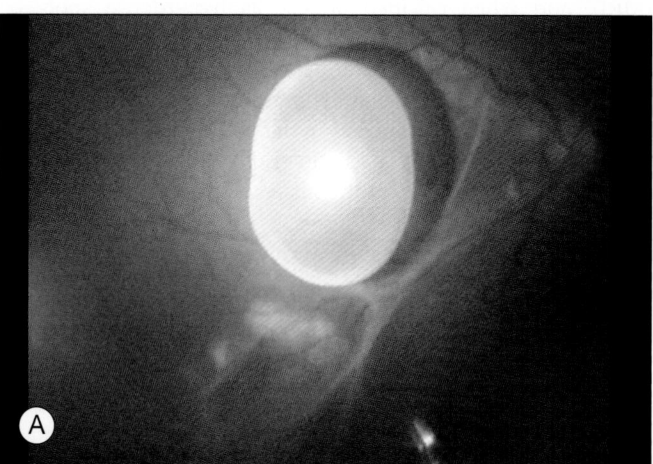

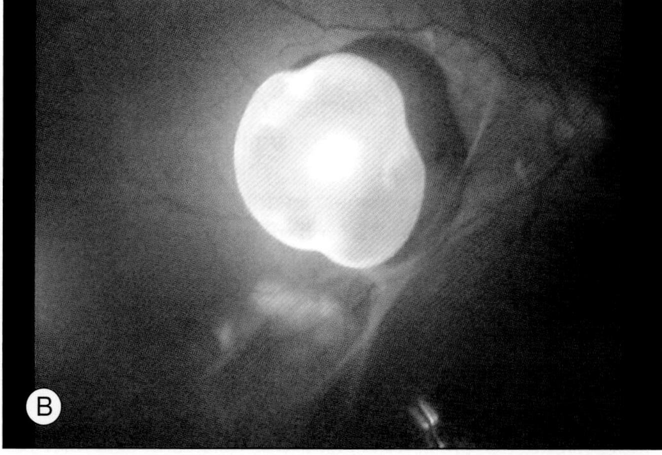

Fig. 86.15 Intravitreal cysticercus. It is possible to see an epiretinal membrane and pigmented epithelium changes inferiorly. This is the possible site from where the parasite passed from the subretinal space to the vitreous cavity. During vitrectomy it was possible to detect cyst movements as the light pipe was directed to it.

the vitreous cutter,[126,127] and rupture of intravitreal or partial removal of the subretinal cyst during vitrectomy followed by administration of intravitreous and systemic cortisteroids without postoperative significant inflammation.[119,128]

REFERENCES

1. Hotez PJ, Brindley PJ, Bethony JM, et al. Helminth infections: the great neglected tropical diseases. J Clin Invest 2008;118:1311–21.
2. Cox FEG. History of human parasitology. Clin Microbiol Rev 2002;15: 595–612.
3. Glickman LT, Magnaval J. Zoonotic roundworm infections. Infect Dis Clin North Am 1993;7:717–32.
4. Hotez PJ, Molyneux DH, Fenwick A, et al. Control of neglected tropical diseases. N Engl J Med 2007;357:1018–27.
5. Zinkham WH. Systemic visceral larval migrans. In Ryan SJ, Smith RE, editors. Selected topics on the eye in systemic disease. New York: Grune & Stratton; 1979. p. 167–75.
6. Schantz PM. Of worms, dogs, and human hosts: continuing challenges for veterinarians in prevention of human diseases. J Am Vet Med Assoc 1994;204: 1023–8.
7. Shields JA. Ocular toxocariasis: a review. Surv Ophthalmol 1984;28:361–81.
8. Goto H, Mochizuki M, Yamaki K, et al. Epidemiological survey of intraocular inflammation in Japan. Jpn J Ophthalmol 2007;51:41–4.
9. Stewart JM, Cubillan LD, Cunningham ET Jr. Prevalence, clinical features, and causes of vision loss among patients with ocular toxocariasis. Retina 2005;25:1005–13.
10. Tran VT, Auer C, Guex-Crosier Y, et al. Epidemiological characteristics of uveitis in Switzerland. Int Ophthalmol 1994–1995;18:293–8.
11. Brown DH. Ocular toxocara canis II. Clinical review. J Pediatr Ophthalmol 1970;7:182–91.
12. Leiper RT. Two new genera of nematodes occasionally parasitic in man. Br Med J 1907;1: 1296–8.
13. Wilder HC. Nematode endophthalmitis. Trans Am Acad Ophthalmol Otolaryngol 1950;55:99–109.
14. Beaver PC, Snyder CH, Carrera GM, et al. Chronic eosinophilia due to visceral larva migrans. Pediatrics 1952;9:7–19.
15. Nichols RL. The etiology of visceral larva migrans. I. Diagnostic morphology of infective second-stage *Toxocara* larvae. J Parasitol 1956;42:349–62.
16. Irvine WC, Irvine AR Jr. Nematode endophthalmitis: *Toxocara canis* – report of one case. Am J Ophthalmol 1959;47:185–91.
17. Ashton N. Larval granulomatosis of the retina due to *Toxocara*. Br J Ophthalmol 1960;44:129–48.

18. Duguid IM. Features of ocular infestation by *Toxocara*. Br J Ophthalmol 1961;45:789–96.
19. Wilkinson CP, Welch RB. Intraocular *Toxocara*. Am J Ophthalmol 1971; 71:921–30.
20. Rocha IML, Oréfice F, Soares IP, et al. Toxocaríase. In: Oréfice F, editor. Uveíte clínica e cirúrgica. 2nd ed. Rio de Janeiro: Cultura Médica; 2005.
21. Chieffi PP, Santos SV, Queiroz ML, et al. Human toxocariasis: contribution by Brazilian researchers. Rev Inst Med Trop S Paulo 2009;51:301–8.
22. Molk R. Ocular toxocariasis: a review of the literature. Ann Ophthalmol 1983;15:216–31.
23. Ottesen EA. Visceral larval migrans and other unusual helminth infections. In: Mandell GL, Douglas RG, Bennett JE, editors. Principles and practice of infectious diseases. 2nd ed. New York: John Wiley; 1979.
24. Mok CH. Visceral larva migrans: a discussion based in review of literature. Clin Pediatr 1968;7:565–73.
25. Amaral HL, Rassier GL, Pepe MS, et al. Presence of *Toxocara canis* eggs on the hair of dogs: a risk factor for visceral larva migrans. Vet Parasitol 2010; 174:115–8.
26. Marmor M, Glickman L, Shofer F, et al. *Toxocara canis* infection of children: epidemiological and neuropsychological findings. Am J Public Health 1987;77:554–9.
27. Schantz PM, Meyer D, Glickman LT. Clinical, serologic, and epidemiologic characteristics of ocular toxocariasis. Am J Trop Med Hyg 1979;28:24–8.
28. Schantz PM, Weis PE, Pollard ZF, et al. Risk factors for toxocaral ocular larva migrans: a case–control study. Am J Public Health 1980;70:1269–72.
29. Queiroz ML, Simonsen M, Paschoalotti MA, et al. Frequency of soil contamination by *Toxocara canis* eggs in the south region of São Paulo municipality (SP, Brazil) in a 18 month period. Rev Inst Med Trop Sao Paulo 2006;48: 317–9.
30. Despommier D. Toxocariasis: clinical aspects, epidemiology, medical ecology, and molecular aspects. Clin Microbiol Rev 2003;16:265–72.
31. Castillo D, Paredes C, Zanartu C. Environmental contamination with *Toxocara* spp. eggs in public squares and parks from Santiago, Chile, 1999. Bol Chil Parasitol 2000;55:86–91.
32. Giacometti A, Cirioni O, Fortuna M. Environmental and serological evidence for the presence of toxocariasis in the urban area of Ancona, Italy. Eur J Epidemiol 2000;16:1023–26.
33. Akdemir C. Visceral larva migrans among children in Kütahya (Turkey) and an evaluation of playgrounds for *T. canis* eggs. Turk J Pediatr 2010;52:158–62.
34. Borg OA, Woodruff AW. Prevalence of ova of *Toxocara* species in public places. Br Med J 1973;4:470–2.
35. Yoshikawa M, Nishiofuku M, Moriya K, et al. A familial case of visceral toxocariasis due to consumption of raw bovine liver. Parasitol Int 2008;57:525–9.
36. Hoffmeister B, Glaeser S, Flick H, et al. Cerebral toxocariasis after consumption of raw duck liver. Am J Trop Med Hyg 2007;76:600–2.
37. Morimatsu Y, Akao N, Akiyoshi H, et al. A familial case of visceral larva migrans after ingestion of raw chicken livers: appearance of specific antibody in bronchoalveolar lavage fluid of the patients. Am J Trop Med Hyg 2006;75:303–6.
38. Wilkinson CP. Ocular toxocariasis. In: Ryan SJ, editor. Retina. 4th ed. London: Elsevier; 2005.
39. Glickman LT, Schantz PM. Epidemiology and pathogenesis of zoonotic toxocariasis. Epidemiol Rev 1981;3:230–50.
40. Bass JL, Mehta KA, Glickman LT, et al. Clinically inapparent *Toxocara* infection in children. N Engl J Med 1983;308:723–4.
41. Alabiad CR, Albini TA, Santos CI, et al. Ocular toxocariasis in a seronegative adult. Ophthalmic Surg Lasers Imaging 2010;2:1–3.
42. Raistrick ER, Hart JC. Ocular toxocariasis in adults. Br J Ophthalmol 1976;60:365–70.
43. Benitez-del Castillo JM, Herreros G, Guillen JL, et al. Bilateral ocular toxocariasis demonstrated by aqueous humor enzyme-linked immunosorbent assay. Am J Ophthalmol 1995;119:514–6.
44. Oréfice F, Boratto LM, Silva HF. Presumível toxocaríase ocular – revisão de 30 casos (1978–1989) – Relato de dois casos atípicos. Rev Bras Oftalmol 1991;50:92–101.
45. Hagler WS, Pollard ZF, Jarrett WH, et al. Results of surgery for ocular *Toxocara canis*. Ophthalmology 1981;88:1081–6.
46. Cella W, Ferreira E, Torigoe AM, et al. Ultrasound biomicroscopy findings in peripheral vitreoretinal toxocariasis. Eur J Ophthalmol 2004;14(2):132–6.
47. do Lago A, Andrade R, Muccioli C, et al. Optical coherence tomography in presumed subretinal toxocara granuloma: case report. Arq Bras Oftalmol 2006;69:403–5.
48. Bird AC, Smith JL, Curtin VT. Nematode optic neuritis. Am J Ophthalmol 1970;69:72–7.
49. Gass JDM. Stereoscopic atlas of macular diseases. 4th ed. St Louis: Mosby; 1997.
50. Monshizadeh R, Ashrafzadeh MT, Rumelt S. Choroidal neovascular membrane: a late complication of inactive toxocara chorioretinitis. Retina 2000; 20:219–20.
51. Wan WL, Cano MR, Pince KJ, et al. Echographic characteristics of ocular toxocariasis. Ophthalmology 1991;98:28–32.
52. Rubin ML, Kaufman HE, Tierney JP, et al. An intraretinal nematode (a case report). Trans Am Acad Ophthalmol Otolaryngol 1968;72:855–66.
53. Sharkey JA, McKay PS. Ocular toxocariasis in a patient with repeatedly negative ELISA titers to *Toxocara canis*. Br J Ophthalmol 1993;77:253–4.
54. Schantz PM. Toxocara larva migrans now. Am J Trop Med Hyg 1989;41: 21–34.
55. Ellis GS Jr, Pakalnis VA, Worley G, et al. *Toxocara canis* infestation: clinical and epidemiological associations with seropositivity in kindergarten children. Ophthalmology 1986;93:1032–7.
56. Prestes-Carneiro LE, Souza DH, Moreno GC, et al. Toxocariasis/cysticercosis seroprevalence in a long-term rural settlement, São Paulo, Brazil. Parasitology 2009;136:681–9.
57. Maguire AM, Green WR, Michels RG, et al. Recovery of intraocular *Toxocara canis* by pars plana vitrectomy. Ophthalmology 1990;97:675–80.
58. Shields JA. Differential diagnosis of retinoblastoma. In: Guyer DR, Yannuzzi LA, Chang S, et al. editors. Retina–vitreous–macula. Philadelphia: W.B. Saunders; 1999.
59. Hogan MJ, Kimura SJ, Spencer WH. Visceral larval migrans and peripheral retinitis. JAMA 1965;194:1345–7.
60. O'Connor GR. Chemotherapy of toxoplasmosis and toxocariasis. In: Srinivasan BD, editor. Ocular therapeutics. New York: Masson; 1980.
61. Barisan-Asenbauer T, Maca SM, Hauff W, et al. Treatment of ocular toxocariasis with albendazole. J Ocul Pharm Therapeut 2001;17:287–94.
62. Sturchler D, Schubarth P, Gualzata M, et al. Thiabendazole vs albendazole in treatment of toxocariasis: a clinical trial. Ann Trop Med Parasitol 1989;83: 473–8.
63. Hotez PJ. Toxocara canis. In: Burg FD, Wald ER, Ingelfinger JR, et al. editors. Gellis and Kaganís current pediatric therapy. 15th ed. Philadelphia: W.B. Saunders; 1995. p. 683–4.
64. Lyall DA, Hutchison BM, Gaskell A, et al. Intravitreal ranibizumab in the treatment of choroidal neovascularisation secondary to ocular toxocariasis in a 13-year-old boy. Eye 2010;24:1730–1.
65. Amin HI, McDonald HR, Han DP, et al. Vitrectomy update for macular traction in ocular toxocariasis. Retina 2000;20:80–5.
66. Small KW, McCuen BW, de Juan E, et al. Surgical management of retinal traction caused by ocular toxocariasis. Am J Ophthalmol 1989;108:10–4.
67. Giuliari GP, Ramirez G, Cortez RT. Surgical treatment of ocular toxocariasis: anatomic and functional results in 45 patients. Eur J Ophthalmol 2011; 21(4):490–4.
68. Gass JDM, Scelfo R. Diffuse unilateral subacute neuroretinitis. J R Soc Med 1978;71:95–111.
69. Gass JD, Gilbert WR Jr, Guerry RK, et al. Diffuse unilateral subacute neuroretinitis. Ophthalmology 1978;85:521–45.
70. Gass JD, Braunstein RA. Further observations concerning the diffuse unilateral subacute neuroretinitis syndrome. Arch Ophthalmol 1983;101:1689–97.
71. Kazacos KR, Raymond LA, Kazacos EA, et al. The raccoon ascarid. A probable cause of human ocular larva migrans. Ophthalmology 1985;92:1735–44.
72. Kazacos KR, Vestre WA, Kazacos EA, et al. Diffuse unilateral subacute neuroretinitis syndrome: probable cause. Arch Ophthalmol 1984;102: 967–8.
73. Mets MB, Noble AG, Basti S, et al. Eye findings of diffuse unilateral subacute neuroretinitis and multiple choroidal infiltrates associated with neural larva migrans due to *Baylisascaris procyonis*. Am J Ophthalmol 2003;135:888–90.
74. Goldberg MA, Kazacos KR, Boyce WM, et al. Diffuse unilateral subacute neuroretinitis. Morphometric, serologic and epidemiologic support for *Baylisascaris* as a causative agent. Ophthalmology 1993;100:1695–701.
75. Brasil OF, Lewis H, Lowder CY. Migration of *Baylisascaris procyonis* into the vitreous. Br J Ophthalmol 2006;90:1203–4.
76. Gass JDM. Stereoscopic atlas of macular diseases: diagnosis and treatment, vol. 4. St Louis: Mosby; 1997. p. 622–8.
77. Casella AMB, Machado RA, Tsuro A, et al. Would *Ancylostoma caninum* be one of the agents of diffuse unilateral subacute neuroretinitis (D.U.S.N) in Brazil? Arq Bras Oftalmol 2001;64:473–6.
78. Cunha de Souza E, Nakashima Y. Diffuse unilateral subacute neuroretinitis. Report of transvitreal surgical removal of a subretinal nematode. Ophthalmology 1995;102:1183–6.
79. McDonald HR, Kazacos KR, Schatz H, et al. Two cases of intraocular infection with *Alaria mesocercaria* (Trematoda). Am J Ophthalmol 1994;117:447–55.
80. Parsons HE. Nematode chorioretinitis: report of a case, with photographs of a viable worm. Arch Ophthalmol 1952;47:799–800.
81. Nath R, Gogoi R, Bordoloi N, et al. Ocular dirofilariasis. Indian J Pathol Microbiol 2010;53:157–9.
82. Myint K, Sahay R, Mon S, et al. "Worm in the eye": the rationale for treatment of DUSN in south India. Br J Ophthalmol 2006;90(9):1125–7.
83. Yuen VH, Chang TS, Hooper PL. Diffuse unilateral subacute neuroretinitis syndrome in Canada. Arch Ophthalmol 1996;114:1279–82.
84. Kuchle M, Knorr HL, Medenblik-Frysch S, et al. Diffuse unilateral subacute neuroretinitis syndrome in a German most likely caused by the raccoon roundworm, *Baylisascaris procyonis*. Graefes Arch Clin Exp Ophthalmol 1993; 231:48–51.
85. Harto MA, Rodriguez-Salvador V, Avino JA, et al. Diffuse unilateral subacute neuroretinitis in Europe. Eur J Ophthalmol 1999;9:58–62.
86. Cai J, Wei R, Zhu L, et al. Diffuse unilateral subacute neuroretinitis in China. Arch Ophthalmol 2000;118:721–2.
87. Natesh S, Harsha K, Nair U, et al. Subretinal worm and repeat laser photocoagulation. Middle East Afr J Ophthalmol 2010;17:183–5
88. de Souza EC, da Cunha SL, Gass JD. Diffuse unilateral subacute neuroretinitis in South America. Arch Ophthalmol 1992;110:1261–3.
89. de Souza EC, Abujamra S, Nakashima Y, et al. Diffuse bilateral subacute neuroretinitis: first patient with documented nematodes in both eyes. Arch Ophthalmol 1999;117:1349–51.
90. Oréfice F, Garcia CAA, Paranhos FRL, et al. Neuroretinite subaguda unilateral difusa (DUSN). In: Oréfice F, editor. Uveíte clínica e cirúrgica. 2nd ed. Rio de Janeiro: Cultura Médica; 2005.

91. Sabrosa NA, Zajdenweber M. Nematode infections of the eye: toxocariasis, onchocerciasis, diffuse unilateral subacute neuroretinitis, and cysticercosis. Ophthalmol Clin North Am 2002;15:351–6.
92. Cortez R, Denny JP, Muci-Mendoza R, et al. Diffuse unilateral subacute neuroretinitis in Venezuela. Ophthalmology 2005;112(12):2110–4.
93. Cialdini AP, de Souza EC, Avila MP. The first South American case of diffuse unilateral subacute neuroretinitis caused by a large nematode. Arch Ophthalmol 1999;117:1431–2.
94. Oréfice F, Gonçalves ER, Siqueira RC, et al. Estudo de 21 casos de neuroretinite subaguda unilateral difusa (DUSN): dois casos com larva móvel subretiniana. Rev Bras Oftalmol 1994;53:23–45.
95. Gomes AH, Garcia CA, Segundo P de S, et al. Optic coherence tomography in a patient with diffuse unilateral subacute neuroretinitis. Arq Bras Oftalmol 2009;72:185–8.
96. Casella AM, Farah ME, Souza EC, et al. Retinal nerve fiber layer atrophy as relevant feature for diffuse unilateral subacute neuroretinitis (DUSN): case series. Arq Bras Oftalmol 2010;73:182–5.
97. Davis JL, Gass JDM, Olsen KR. Diffuse unilateral subacute neuroretinitis. In: Ryan SJ. editor. Retina. 4th ed. London: Elsevier; 2005.
98. Souza EC, Casella AM, Nakashima Y, et al. Clinical features and outcomes of patients with diffuse unilateral subacute neuroretinitis treated with oral albendazole. Am J Ophthalmol 2005;140:437–45.
99. Moraes LR, Cialdini AP, Avila MP, et al. Identifying live nematodes in diffuse unilateral subacute neuroretinitis by using the scanning laser ophthalmoscope. Arch Ophthalmol 2002;120:135–8.
100. Quillen DA, Davis JB, Gottlieb JL, et al. The white dot syndromes. Am J Ophthalmol 2004;137:538–50.
101. Martidis A, Greenberg PB, Rogers AH, et al. Multifocal electroretinography response after laser photocoagulation of a subretinal nematode. Am J Ophthalmol 2002;133:417–9.
102. Dangoudoubiyam S, Kazacos KR. Differentiation of larva migrans caused by *Baylisascaris procyonis* and *Toxocara* species by Western blotting. Clin Vaccine Immunol 2009;16:1563–8.
103. Kwon IH, Kim HS, Lee JH, et al. A serologically diagnosed human case of cutaneous larva migrans caused by *Ancylostoma caninum*. Korean J Parasitol 2003;41:233–7.
104. Gass JD, Callanan DG, Bowman CB. Successful oral therapy for diffuse unilateral subacute neuroretinitis. Trans Am Ophthalmol Soc 1991;89: 97–112.
105. Maguire AM, Zarbin MA, Conner TB, et al. Ocular penetration of thiabendazole. Arch Ophthalmol 1952;108:1675.
106. Gass JDM, Callanan DG, Bowman CB. Oral therapy in diffuse unilateral subacute neuroretinitis. Arch Ophthalmol 1992;110:675–80.
107. Callanan DG, Davis JL, Cohen SM, et al. The use of ivermectin in diffuse unilateral subacute neuroretinitis. Ophthalmology 1993;100(9 Suppl): 114–5.
108. Casella AM, Farah ME, Belfort R, Jr. Anthelmintic drugs in diffuse unilateral subacute neuroretinitis. Am J Ophthalmol 1998;125:109–11.
109. Malaguido MR, Casella AM, Malaguido DR. [Clinical treatment of diffuse unilateral subacute neuroretinitis with albendazole.] Arq Bras Oftalmol 2007;70:814–22.
110. Report from the 2009 Inter-American Conference on Onchocerciasis: progress towards eliminating river blindness in the Region of the Americas. Wkly Epidemiol Rec 2010;85(33):321–6.
111. Reddy M, Gill SS, Kalkar SR, et al. Oral drug therapy for multiple neglected tropical diseases: a systematic review. JAMA 2007;298:1911–24.
112. Hall LR, Pearlman E. Pathogenesis of onchocercal keratitis (river blindness). Clin Microbiol Rev 1999;12:445–53.
113. Newland HS, White AT, Greene BM, et al. Ocular manifestations of onchocerciasis in a rain forest area of west Africa. Br J Ophthalmol 1991;75:163–9.
114. Kayembe DL, Kasonga DL, Kayembe PK, et al. Profile of eye lesions and vision loss: a cross-sectional study in Lusambo, a forest-savanna area hyperendemic for onchocerciasis in the Democratic Republic of Congo. Trop Med Int Health 2003;8:83–9.
115. Semba RD, Murphy RP, Newland HS, et al. Longitudinal study of lesions of the posterior segment in onchocerciasis. Ophthalmology 1990;97:1334–41.
116. Bird AC, Anderson J, Fuglsang H. Morphology of posterior segment lesions of the eye in patients with onchocerciasis. Br J Ophthalmol 1976;60:2–20.
117. Duke-Elders S, Perkins ES. System of ophthalmology. Inflammations of the uveal tract: uveitis. St Louis: Mosby; 1966. ch. 3, v. 9, p. 478–87.
118. Orefice F. editor. Uveíte clínica e cirúrgica: texto e atlas. Rio de Janeiro: Cultura Médica; 2000. ch. 40. v. 2. p. 705–13.
119. Pantaleão GR, Borges de Souza AD, Rodrigues EB, et al. [The use of systemic and intravitreous steroid in inflammation secondary to intraocular cysticercosis: case report.] Arq Bras Oftalmol 2007;70:1006–9.
120. Junior L. Ocular cysticercosis. Am J Ophthalmol 1949;32: 523–48.
121. Wittig EO. Ocular cysticercosis: an epidemiological study. Arq Neuropsiquiatr 2001;59:693–701.
122. Shandera WX, Kass JS. Neurocysticercosis: current knowledge and advances. Curr Neurol Neurosci Rep 2006;6:453–9.
123. Kruger-Leite E, Jalkh AE, Quiroz H, et al. Intraocular cysticercosis. Am J Ophthalmol 1985;99:252–7.
124. Rath S, Honavar SG, Naik M, et al. Orbital cysticercosis: clinical manifestations, diagnosis, management, and outcome. Ophthalmology 2010;117:600–5.
125. Chung GW, Lai WW, Thulborn KR, et al. Magnetic resonance imaging in the diagnosis of subretinal cysticercosis. Am J Ophthalmol 2002;134:931–2.
126. Sharma T, Sinha S, Shah N, et al. Intraocular cysticercosis: clinical characteristics and visual outcome after vitreoretinal surgery. Ophthalmology 2003;110:996–1004.
127. Avila MP, Cialdini AP, Pereira AE, et al. Live cysticercus/Giant intraocular foreign bodies. Best of Show Video Awards. Annual Meeting, American Academy of Ophthalmology – Final Program 2003: 301.
128. Passos E, Frasson MC, Nehemy MB. Vitrectomia para o tratamento de cisticerco intrarretiniano. Rev Bras Oftalmol 1996;55:841–5.
129. Santos R, Chavarria M, Aguirre AE. Failure of medical treatment in two cases of intraocular cysticercosis. Am J Ophthalmol 1984;97:249–50.

Chapter 87

Endogenous Endophthalmitis: Bacterial and Fungal

Stephen G. Schwartz, Janet L. Davis, Harry W. Flynn Jr

EPIDEMIOLOGY AND RISK FACTORS

Endogenous endophthalmitis remains an uncommon but serious cause of intraocular inflammation.[1] The incidence may be increasing, due to several factors. An increasing number of immunocompromised patients are receiving antineoplastic agents, immunomodulating agents, and newer broad-spectrum antimicrobial agents, all of which may reduce normal flora.[2,3] Low-birthweight premature infants and patients with a history of intravenous substance abuse are at increased risk for endogenous endophthalmitis.[4] Other reported risk factors include long-term intravenous line placement, peripheral hyperalimentation, systemic corticosteroids, abdominal surgery, hemodialysis, HIV infection, systemic malignancy, diabetes mellitus, pregnancy or postpartum state,[5] massive systemic trauma, alcoholism, hepatic insufficiency, and genitourinary manipulation.[6]

One recent series of 64 cases over 10 years reported a culture positivity rate of 64%. Of culture-positive cases, fungi (predominantly *Candida* spp.) were isolated in 66%, Gram-negative bacteria in 19%, and Gram-positive bacteria in 15%. Fungal cases were associated with better visual outcomes.[7]

CLINICAL ASSESSMENT OF THE PATIENT

Infectious endophthalmitis may be categorized by the cause of the infection and by the characteristic timing of clinical signs and symptoms. One proposed categorization scheme is presented in Box 87.1.[8] In general, endogenous endophthalmitis is suspected in a patient without risk factors for exogenous endophthalmitis, such as prior surgery, trauma, or keratitis. Patients with endogenous endophthalmitis may present with varying degrees of pain, inflammation, and visual loss. In the anterior chamber, cell and flare, fibrin, posterior synechiae, and hypopyon may occur. In the posterior segment, findings may include vitreous opacification and chorioretinitis, including hemorrhage, cotton-wool spots, retinal opacification, and vasculitis. An insidious onset, focal vitreous opacities, and chorioretinal infiltrates suggest fungal etiology. Relatively more rapid progression and more severe intraocular inflammation suggest bacterial etiology.

Endogenous endophthalmitis may present as a relatively mild and nonspecific anterior uveitis.[9] Early in the clinical course, the clinical features may be subtle, making the diagnosis difficult. The rate of initial misdiagnosis has been reported as high as 63% in one large series.[10] A differential diagnosis of endogenous endophthalmitis is presented in Box 87.2.

Cases may be classified according to several criteria. One published classification scheme for endogenous bacterial endophthalmitis used zones of anatomic involvement (Box 87.3).[11]

Box 87.1 Classification of endophthalmitis and common causative organisms

- Acute-onset postoperative endophthalmitis
  - Coagulase-negative staphylococci
  - *Staphylococcus aureus*
  - *Streptococcus* spp.
- Chronic (delayed-onset) postoperative endophthalmitis
  - *Propionibacterium acnes*
  - *Candida parapsilosis*
  - Coagulase-negative staphylococci
- Filtering bleb-associated endophthalmitis
  - *Streptococcus* spp.
  - *Staphylococcus* spp.
  - *Haemophilus influenza*
- Post-traumatic endophthalmitis
  - *Staphylococcus* spp.
  - *Bacillus cereus*
- Endogenous endophthalmitis
  - *Candida albicans*
  - *Aspergillus* spp.
  - *Staphylococcus aureus*
  - Gram-negative organisms
- Endophthalmitis associated with microbial keratitis
  - Gram-negative organisms
  - *Staphylococcus aureus*
  - *Fusarium* spp.
- Endophthalmitis associated with intravitreal injection
  - Coagulase-negative staphylococci
  - *Streptococcus* spp.

(Adapted from Schwartz SG, Flynn HW Jr, Scott IU. Endophthalmitis: classification and current management. Expert Rev Ophthalmol 2007;2:385–96.)

Box 87.2 Differential diagnosis of endogenous endophthalmitis

- Uveitis
  - Anterior/intermediate
    - Pars planitis
  - Posterior
    - Vogt–Koyanagi–Harada disease
    - Posterior scleritis
    - Sarcoidosis
    - Syphilis
    - Tuberculosis
    - Sympathetic ophthalmia
    - Intraocular lymphoma
    - Lyme disease
- Tumor necrosis with inflammation
  - Retinoblastoma
- Disseminated toxoplasmosis
- Disseminated viral retinitis
- Vitreous metastases
- Occlusive diseases of the choriocapillaris
  - Disseminated intravascular coagulation
  - Thrombotic thrombocytopenic purpura
- Asteroid hyalosis

Another scheme, designed for endogenous fungal endophthalmitis, also used anatomic criteria (Box 87.4); in this series, the stage at initial diagnosis was statistically correlated to the final visual acuity.[12]

MEDICAL EVALUATION OF THE PATIENT

In contrast to patients with postoperative or post-traumatic endophthalmitis, nearly all patients with endogenous endophthalmitis have an identifiable systemic infection and require at least some degree of systemic evaluation. Generally, the medical evaluation is performed in consultation with an infectious disease specialist or other medical specialist. A high index of suspicion should be maintained, because both the ophthalmic and systemic symptoms are quite variable. In one series, 43% of patients with endogenous endophthalmitis had no nonocular symptoms.[13] Endogenous endophthalmitis may present prior to the onset of systemic symptoms,[14] or may occur in patients later found to have no other systemic infection.[15] In one series, the rate of negative systemic workup was over 40%.[16] In a patient not known to have systemic infection, intraocular cultures (aqueous, vitreous, or both) may be necessary to confirm the diagnosis. Intraocular cultures are also important in patients who progress despite treatment with empiric antimicrobial therapy.

Obtaining cultures from multiple sites may be necessary to make a specific diagnosis. In one series of patients with endogenous bacterial endophthalmitis, the rate of diagnostic cultures was 74% for vitreous, 72% for blood, and 96% overall.[17] The rates of positive cultures are lower in patients with endogenous fungal endophthalmitis. Rates of positive cultures have been reported in the range of 44–70%,[18] and as low as 18% in one prior series.[19]

Box 87. 3 Anatomic classification of endogenous bacterial endophthalmitis

Focal: One or a few discrete foci in the iris, ciliary body, retina, or choroid
Anterior diffuse: Severe generalized signs of inflammation in the anterior segment
Posterior diffuse: Intense inflammatory reaction in vitreous, obscuring the fundus
Panophthalmitis: Severe involvement of anterior segment, posterior segment, and orbital structures

(Adapted from Greenwald MJ, Wohl LG, Sell CH. Metastatic bacterial endophthalmitis: a contemporary reappraisal. Surv Ophthalmol 1986;31:81–101.)

Box 87.4 Classification of endogenous fungal endophthalmitis

Stage I: Chorioretinal changes without extension into the vitreous cavity
Stage II: Fungal mass penetrating through the inner limiting membrane and budding into the vitreous cavity
Stage III: Vitreous opacity resulting in a blurred fundus
Stage IV: Vitreous opacity plus retinal detachment

(Adapted from Takebayashi H, Mizota A, Tanaka M. Relation between stage of endogenous fungal endophthalmitis and prognosis. Graefes Arch Clin Exp Ophthalmol 2006;244:816–20.)

ENDOGENOUS BACTERIAL ENDOPHTHALMITIS

Endogenous bacterial endophthalmitis is reported to comprise between 2% and 8% of all cases of infectious endophthalmitis (Fig. 87.1).[20] Many bacteria have been reported to cause endogenous endophthalmitis. Gram-positive agents associated with bacterial endogenous endophthalmitis include *Staphylococcus areus*,[21] group B *Streptococcus*,[22] *Streptococcus pneumoniae*,[23] *Streptococcus bovis*,[24] *Propionibacterium acnes*,[25] *Listeria monocytogenes*,[26] *Bacillus* spp.,[27] *Nocardia* spp.,[28] and others. Gram-negative agents associated with bacterial endogenous endophthalmitis include *Klebsiella pneumoniae*,[29] *Pseudomonas aeruginosa*,[30] *Escherichia coli*,[31] *Enterococcus faecalis*,[32] *Neisseria meningitidis*,[33] *Proteus* spp.,[34] and others.

ENDOGENOUS FUNGAL ENDOPHTHALMITIS

Over 50 000 species of fungi have been reported, yet fewer than 200 of these are associated with clinical disease in humans and even fewer have been reported to cause endogenous endophthalmitis (Box 87.5). Fungi may be differentiated using several criteria, but are commonly divided between unicellular yeasts and multicellular molds. Molds contain tubular structures (hyphae). Some fungi may grow with both yeast-like and mold-like morphology in tissues or culture. Fungi may also be classified by pigmentation (moniliaceous versus dermatiaceous), virulence (pathogenic versus opportunistic), or clinical presentation (cutaneous, subcutaneous, or systemic).

Candida albicans is the most common yeast isolate and the most common overall fungal isolate in patients with endogenous fungal endophthalmitis.[35,36] *C. albicans* may be found as a

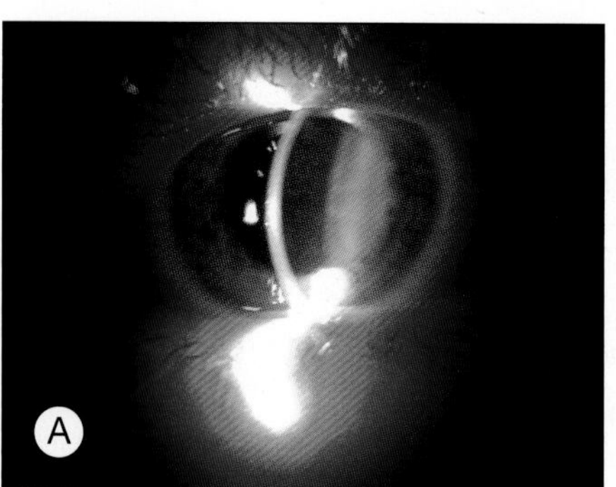

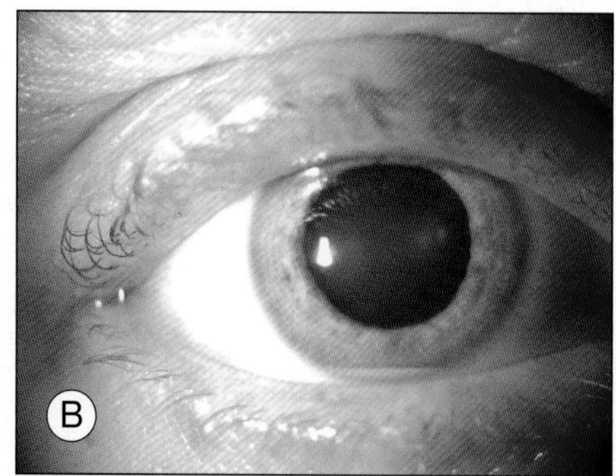

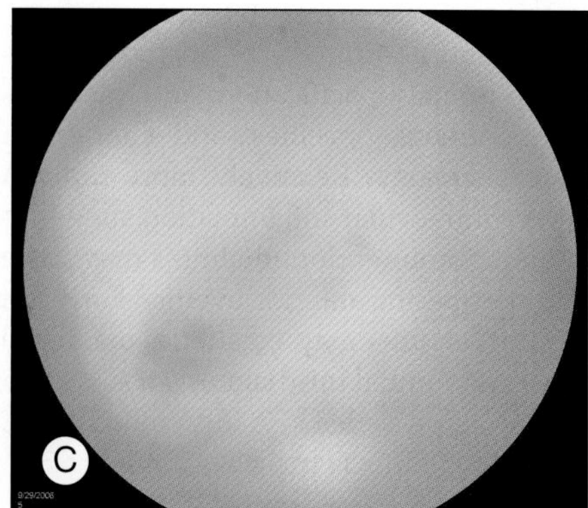

Fig. 87.1 Endogenous *Klebsiella pneumonia* endophthalmitis. (A) Note anterior chamber cell and flare. (B) Note hypopyon. (C) Note vitreous opacification overlying macular chorioretinitis and associated hemorrhage. (Case courtesy of Lisa C. Olmos, MD, MBA.)

Box 87.5 Fungal isolates

- Yeasts and yeast-like isolates
  - *Candida* species
    - *C. albicans*
    - *C. parapsilosis*
    - *C. tropicalis*
    - *C. glabrata*
  - *Cryptococcus neoformans*
  - *Trichosporon beigelii*
  - *Sporobolomyces salmonicolor*
- Hyaline molds – septate (colorless hyphae)
  - *Aspergillus* spp.
    - *A. fumigatus*
    - *A. niger*
    - *A. glaucus*
    - *A. flavus*
  - *Pseudoallescheria boydii*
  - *Fusarium* spp.
    - *F. solani*
    - *F. oxysporum*
  - *Bipolaris hawaiiensis*
  - *Paecilomyces* spp.
  - *Penicillium spp.*
- Hyaline molds – aseptate (colorless hyphae)
  - *Mucor* spp.
  - *Absidia* spp.
  - *Rhizopus* spp.
- Dermatiaceous molds (colored hyphae)
  - *Scedosporium* spp.
    - *S. apiopsermum*
    - *S. prolificans*
  - *Cladophialophora bantiana*
  - *Phialemoniunm curvatum*
- Dimorphic molds
  - *Blastomyces dermatitidis*
  - *Histoplasma capsulatum*
  - *Sporothrix schenckii*
  - *Coccidioides immitis*

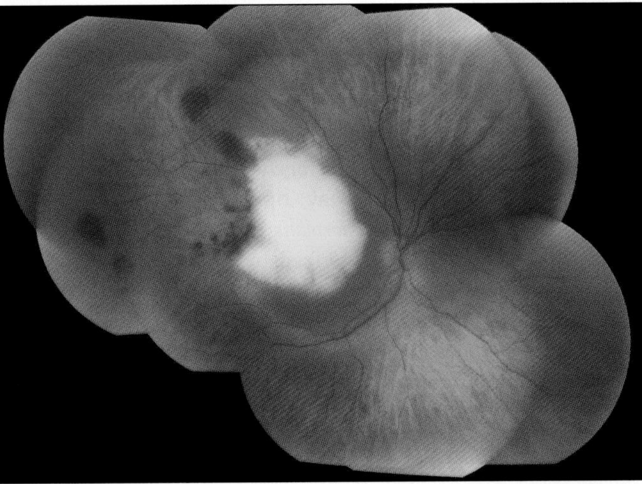

Fig. 87.2 Endogenous *Candida* endophthalmitis. Note creamy white chorioretinal lesion, with associated retinal hemorrhage and evidence of vasculitis.

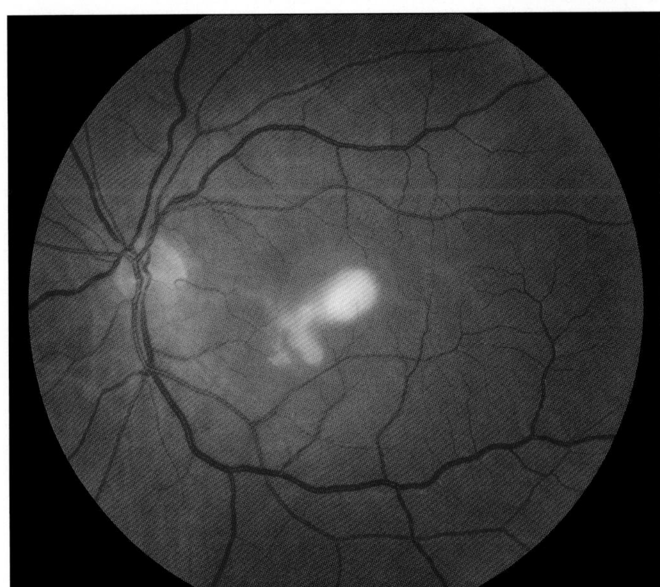

Fig. 87.3 Macular chorioretinitis, clinically suspected endogenous *Candida* endophthalmitis. This patient was an intravenous drug abuser and improved with empiric oral fluconazole. (Case courtesy of Jeffrey K. Moore, MD.)

commensal organism in the gastrointestinal tract and mucous membranes of healthy individuals.[37]Although the organism is of low virulence to healthy individuals, candidemia is associated with relatively high rates of morbidity and mortality.[38] In one series, the mortality rate among patients with candidemia and endogenous *Candida* endophthalmitis was reported as 77%.[39] *Candida* endophthalmitis is strongly associated with intravenous drug abuse.[40] Other *Candida* species reported to cause endophthalmitis include *C. tropicalis, C. parapsilosis, C. glabrata, C. guilliermondii,* and *C. krusei*. Among patients with diagnosed candidemia, reported rates of endogenous endophthalmitis range from less than 3%[41] to 44%.[42] The prevalence of *Candida* endophthalmitis may be decreasing, as systemic antifungals are now more commonly prescribed for patients with positive blood cultures.[43] The most characteristic clinical sign of *Candida* endophthlamitis is one or more creamy white, well-circumscribed chorioretinal lesion, less than 1 mm in diameter, most commonly in the posterior pole, with an overlying haze of vitreous inflammatory cells (Figs 87.2, 87.3). Yellow or fluffy-white vitreous opacities, sometimes connected by strands of inflammatory material ("string of pearls" configuration), may be noted. Recently, a subretinal abscess was reported in a patient with endogenous *C. albicans* endopthalmitis.[44] The initial misdiagnosis rate may be high; one series reported this rate to approach 50%.[45]

Aspergillus is the most common mold isolate and the second most common overall fungal isolate in patients with endogenous fungal endophthalmitis.[46] Reported risk factors include chronic pulmonary disease, liver transplantation,[47] and treatment with systemic corticosteroids, but rare cases are reported in apparently immunocompetent individuals.[48] Endogenous *Aspergillus* endophthalmitis is associated with a characteristic central macular chorioretinal inflammatory lesion.[49] A gravitational layering (pseudohypopyon) of inflammatory exudates in either the preretinal (subhyaloid) or subretinal space may be noted with the macular lesion. Additionally, *Aspergillus* endophthalmitis may be associated with retinal vascular occlusion, choroidal vascular occlusion, and exudative retinal detachment.[50] For these reasons, *Aspergillus* endophthalmitis generally has a poorer prognosis than *Candida* endophthalmitis. A case report documented a poor visual outcome, and eventual mortality, in a patient with acute myelogenous leukemia and bilateral endogenous *Aspergillus fumigatus* endophthalmitis despite prophylaxis with oral fluconazole. The intial ophthalmologic presentation was notable for diffuse hemorrhagic retinal necrosis, and the initial diagnosis was cytomegalovirus retinitis.[51]

Cryptococcus neoformans is associated with meningitis and visual loss through a variety of mechanisms, including cryptococcomas in the visual pathway, optic neuritis, and elevated intracranial pressure.[52] *C. neoformans* may cause endophthalmitis, which is typically characterized by nonspecific intraocular inflammation, making initial misdiagnosis relatively common. The most common presentation is a multifocal chorioretinitis.[53] Successful outcomes have been reported with a combination of systemic amphotericin B and fluconazole with intravitreal amphotericin B.[54]

Coccidioides immitis endophthalmitis is associated with chronic pulmonary or disseminated coccidioidomycosis.[55] Endogenous endophthalmitis is infrequently reported.[56] Asymptomatic patients with systemic coccidioidomycosis may have inactive chorioretinal scars, suggesting prior intraocular involvement.[57] Alternatively, a case of ocular coccidiomycosis has been reported 22 years following treatment of systemic disease.[58]

Rare causes of endogenous fungal endophthalmitis include *Histoplasma capsulatum*,[59] *Sporothrix schenckii*,[60] and others.

TREATMENT STRATEGIES

Although successful treatment of chorioretinitis in a patient with systemic candidiasis has been reported after simply removing an infected catheter,[61] most patients with endogenous endophthamitis require treatment with systemic antimicrobial agents. The choroid and retina are highly vascular structures, which suggests that systemic pharmacotherapy may be sufficient to treat infections confined to these structures, while severe intravitreal involvement may require intravitreal agents.[62] In patients not responding to systemic therapy, intravitreal therapy should be considered. There is no current consensus regarding the precise role of surgical techniques, such as pars plana vitrectomy (PPV). The Endophthalmitis Vitrectomy Study (EVS) did not enroll patients with endogenous endophthalmitis and therefore its results are not directly applicable to these patients.[63]

Systemic pharmacotherapies

Although the EVS reported no additional benefit using systemic amikacin and ceftazidime, patients with endogenous bacterial endophthalmitis are generally treated with systemic antimicrobials in order to manage systemic infections. The selection of systemic pharmacotherapies is frequently made in consultation with an infectious disease or other medical specialist. The management is typically individualized based on the severity of the ocular and sytemic infections.

Systemic antimicrobials are associated with variable intravitreal penetration. For example, in a prospective study, intravenous teicoplanin was reported to have poor intravitreal penetration.[64]A more recent series of patients with postoperative endophthalmitis reported that systemic meropenem and linezolid offered no additional benefits.[65]

Alternatively, both systemic gatifloxacin[66] and moxifloxacin[67] have been reported to reach potentially therapeutic intraocular drug levels in the noninflamed eye, but their specific benefit in the treatment of endogenous bacterial endophthalmitis remains unproven. Systemic gatifloxacin is no longer commercially available, due to an associated dysglycemia in some patients.[68] Additionally, systemic fluoroquinolones are associated with other serious adverse events, including tendinopathy, especially in the elderly and in patients taking systemic corticosteroids.[69]

A case report demonstrated that after a single dose of intravenous daptomycin, intravitreal concentrations of daptomycin were approximately 28% of the serum concentration, suggesting a potential role for this drug in the treatement of endogenous bacterial endophthalmitis.[70]

Systemic antibiotics may not prevent the onset of endogenous bacterial endophthalmitis. One case report documented that *Pseudomonas aeruginosa* endophthalmitis involved the second eye despite initation of intravenous ceftazidime.[71]

Commonly used systemic antifungals are reviewed in Box 87.6.

Amphotericin B has been widely used in the treatment of various fungal infections. An alternative liposomal formulation is also available,[72] but experience with this formulation in the treatment of endogenous fungal endophthalmitis is limited at this time.[73,74] Amphotericin B is administered intravenously, and is generally effective in the treatment of infections due to *Candida*,[75] *Aspergillus*,[76] *Blastomyces*,[77] *Coccidioides*,[78] and other fungi. The use of amphotericin B is limited by multiple toxic effects, including renal failure, chills, fever, vomiting, nausea, diarrhea, dyspnea, malaise, anemia, arrythmia, hypokalemia, and hearing loss.[79] The intravitreal penetration of systemic amphotericin B is relatively poor, and although successful treatment of *Candida* endophthalmitis has been reported using systemic amphotericin B alone,[80] this approach has a high rate of treatment failure.[81] Either a systemic agent with better intraocular penetration, or combined systemic and intravitreal treatment, is generally selected.

Azoles collectively represent an alternative antifungal drug class. The imidazoles (miconazole and ketoconazole) were used historically, but largely have been replaced by the newer triazoles (fluconazole, itraconazole, voriconazole, and posiconazole), although a case report documented a good outcome in endogenous *Aspergillus terreus* endophthalmitis using intravitreal amphotericin B, oral ketoconazole, and topical natamycin.[82]

Fluconazole has excellent gastrointestinal absorption and may be used orally or intravenously.[83] Intraocular penetration from the systemic circulation is generally excellent.[84] A case report documented good outcomes in a patient with bilateral endogenous *C. albicans* endophthalmitis using intravenous fluconazole and pars plana vitrectomy (PPV) in one eye only.[85] Fluconazole (with or without PPV) has also been reported to successfully

Box 87.6 Systemic antifungal agents

Amphotericin B 0.6–1 mg/kg/day IV
Azole compounds
- Fluconazole 400–1600 mg/day oral or IV
- Itraconazole 400–800 mg/day oral or IV
- Voriconazole 6 mg/kg/day oral or IV
- Posaconazole 400–800 mg/day oral or IV

Echinocandins
- Caspofungin 70 mg loading dose, then 50 mg/day IV
- Micafungin 50–150 mg/day IV
- Anidulafungin 50–100 mg/day

treat endophthalmitis caused by *C. tropicalis*,[86] *Coccidioides immitis*,[87] and *Cryptococcus neoformans*.[88] Fluconazole is generally well tolerated, with gastrointestinal disturbance as the major reported toxicity.[89] Oral fluconazole may be an appropriate antifungal choice in patients with chorioretinitis outside the posterior pole,[90] in patients who have been initially treated with intravenous amphotericin B,[91] and in patients at risk for toxicity.

Itraconazole also may be prescribed orally, but is used infrequently in the treatment of endogenous endophthalmitis.[92] It has relatively more effectiveness against *Aspergillus* than the other azoles,[93] but intraocular penetration is relatively poor.

Voriconazole is a synthetic second-generation azole derived from fluconazole. It may be used orally or intravenously. Voriconazole is generally effective against most *Candida* species (including those resistant to fluconazole, such as *C. krusei* and *C. glabrata*),[94] as well as *Aspergillus* and *Cryptococcus*.[95] Voriconazole has excellent intravitreal penetration from the systemic circulation.[96] Oral voriconazole alone has been reported to successfully manage a patient with presumed endogenous *Candida* endophthalmitis.[97]

Posaconazole is a newer azole with efficacy against *Candida*, *Aspergillus*, and *Zygomycetes*.[98] Relatively little is known about its intraocular penetration. Successful treatment of refractory *Fusarium* deep keratitis or endophthalmitis has been reported with oral (or oral plus topical) posaconazole.[99,100]

Commonly used echinochandins include caspofungin, micafungin, and anidulafungin. These are newer agents and, compared with amphotericin B and the azoles, relatively little has been reported about their use in endogenous endophthalmitis. Caspofungin may be effective against *C. albicans* resistant to azoles.[101] One case report documented successful treatment of *C. glabrata* endophthalmitis using only systemic caspofungin.[102] A second report documented treatment of *A. fumigatus* endophthalmitis resistant to intravitreal amphotericin and systemic voriconazole with systemic caspofungin.[103]

Intravitreal pharmacotherapies

In endogenous endophthalmitis, intravitreal pharmacotherapies may be used as adjunctive therapies to systemic medications.

The Endophthalmitis Vitrectomy Study (EVS) did not enroll patients with endogenous endophthalmitis and therefore its results are not applicable to these patients.[63] However, many of the principles of the EVS apply to patients with endogenous endophthalmitis. The EVS used intravitreal vancomycin and amikacin, which achieved broad-spectrum coverage of both Gram-positive and Gram-negative organisms. In a patient with bacteremia due to a known organism, targeted pharmacotherapy may be considered in patients with suspected ocular involvement. To reduce the risk of aminoglycoside toxicity, ceftazidime or ceftriaxone may be considered as an alternative to amikacin. Ceftazidime may precipitate when mixed with vancomycin, but this does not appear to affect its clinical efficacy.[104] Injecting antibiotics through separate syringes is generally recommended.

Intravitreal antifungals are listed in Box 87.7. Animal studies have suggested that intravitreal amphotericin B, 5–10 µg, is generally nontoxic.[105] A case series of patients inadvertently treated with very high doses reported severe noninfectious panophthalmitis, but ultimately good visual outcomes, following treatment with doses as high as 500 µg.[106] Intravitreal amphotericin B alone, without systemic therapy, has been reported to successfully treat endogenous *Candida* endopthalmitis.[107] A case report documented good outcomes using PPV, intravitreal liposomal amphotericin B, and systemic fluconazole in a patient with bilateral endogenous *C. albicans* endophthalmitis.[108]

Box 87.7 Intravitreal antifungal agents

Amphotericin B 0.005–0.01 mg/0.1 ml
Voriconazole 0.1 mg/0.2 ml
Caspofungin 0.1 mg/0.1 ml
Fluconazole (experimental)
Flucytosine (experimental)

Intravitreal fluconazole has been tested in animal models,[109,110] but does not appear to be any more effective than intravitreal amphotericin B and is thus rarely used clinically.[111] Intravitreal ketoconazole has been reported safe in a rabbit model,[112] but its use has not been reported in humans.

Based on animal models, intravitreal voriconazole appears to be nontoxic up to doses of 100 µg, and may be less toxic to the retina than intravitreal amphotericin B.[113] Intravitreal voriconazole, combined with PPV, has been reported to successfully treat a patient with endogenous *A. terreus* endophthalmitis resistant to PPV with repeated injections of intravitreal amphotericin B and systemic voriconazole.[114]

Intravitreal corticosteroids (e.g., dexamethasone 400 µg) may be a helpful adjunct in some patients with bacterial or fungal endophthalmitis, by reducing inflammation.[115] Generally, corticosteroids should be withheld until proper antimicrobials have been initiated, especially in patients with suspected fungal disease.

Surgical treatments

Although there is no general agreement on exactly which patients will benefit from PPV,[116] surgical treatments are typically reserved for patients with established vitreous involvement.[117] PPV offers the advantages of removing infectious organisms from the vitreous cavity and providing ample material for cultures. Disadvantages of PPV include surgical risks, such as retinal detachment, choroidal detachment, or sclerotomy site leakage. One large series reported improved outcomes in patients treated with PPV.[118] In patients with endogenous fungal endophthalmitis treated with PPV and systemic antifungals, adjunctive intravitreal antifungals were not used in one series of *Candida* cases.[119] In phakic patients with an uninvolved crystalline lens, lensectomy is not required at the time of vitreous surgery.[120]

Vitreous needle tap may be useful in hospitalized patients who are poor surgical candidates or in facilities where access to PPV instrumentation and support staff is limited (Fig. 87.4). Patients who fail to respond to tap and inject should be considered for PPV during subsequent follow-up.

SUGGESTED MANAGEMENT

In patients with clinically suspected endogenous endophthalmitis, the history, physical findings, and blood cultures may be useful to determine an etiology. Because of the relative infrequency of these cases (especially bacterial cases), there are no generally established treatment guidelines.[121]

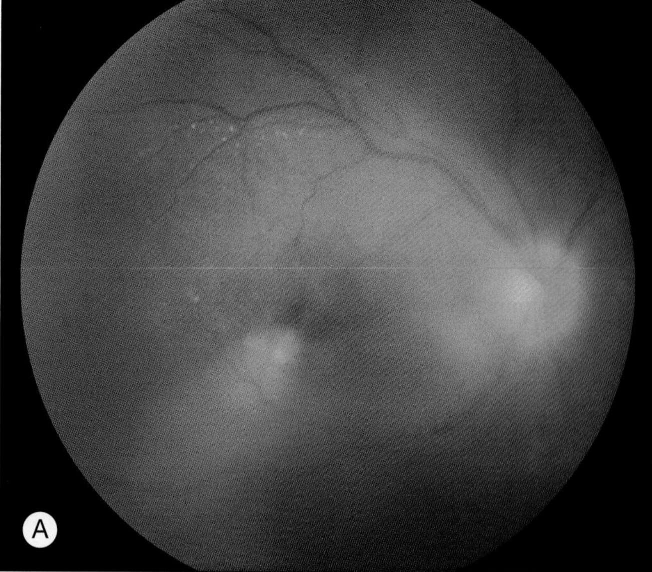

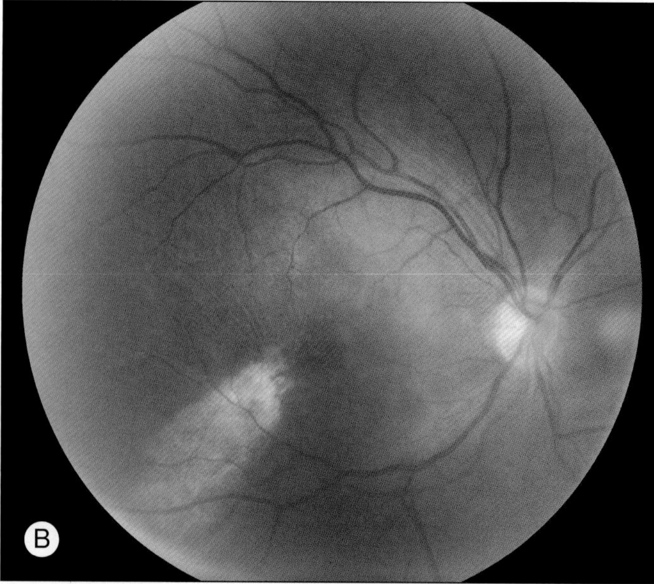

Fig. 87.4 (A) Endogenous methicillin-resistant *Staphylococcus aureus* endophthalmitis. Note white subretinal lesion with overlying vitritis. (B) Four months after treatment with intravitreal vancomycin and ceftazidime, as well as systemic vancomycin, the patient improved. Note clear vitreous and subretinal scar.

An insidious onset, diffuse vitreous opacities, and chorioretinal infiltrates suggest fungal etiology. Rapid progression and more severe intraocular inflammation suggest bacterial etiology. Other causes of vitreous cellular inflammation should be considered, including toxoplasmosis, sarcoidosis, syphillis, neoplastic etiologies, pars planitis, and dehemoglobinized vitreous hemorrhage.

In patients with clinically suspected endogenous endophthalmitis, consultation with an infectious disease or other medical specialist should be considered to search for evidence of bacteremia/fungemia or other organ involvement. Patients with chorioretinal infiltrates with no or minimal vitreous cells may be initially managed with systemic antimicrobials and close observation. Patients with moderate or severe vitreous inflammation, or patients with milder disease who progress despite systemic therapy, may be treated with systemic antimicrobials as well as PPV with intravitreal antimicrobials.

Using a high index of suspicion and these treatment suggestions, many patients will achieve good anatomic and visual outcomes. Unfortunately, some patients with endogenous endophthalmitis will lose vision despite prompt and appropriate therapy.

REFERENCES

1. Smith SR, Kroll AJ, Lou PL, et al. Endogenous bacterial and fungal endophthalmitis. Int Ophthalmol Clin 2007;47:173–83.
2. Essman TF, Flynn HW Jr, Smiddy WE, et al. Treatment outcomes in a 10-year study of endogenous fungal endophthalmitis. Ophthalmic Surg Lasers 1997;28:185–94.
3. Chakrabarti A, Shivaprakash MR, Singh R, et al. Fungal endophthalmitis: fourteen years' experience from a center in India. Retina 2008;28:1400–7.
4. Schiedler V, Scott IU, Flynn HW Jr, et al. Culture-proven endogenous endophthalmitis: clinical features and visual acuity outcomes. Am J Ophthalmol 2004;137:725–31.
5. Rahman W, Hanson R, Westcott M. A rare case of peripartum endogenous bacterial endophthalmitis. Int Ophthalmol 2011;31:113–5.
6. Smith SR, Kroll AJ, Lou PL, et al. Endogenous bacterial and fungal endophthalmitis. Int Ophthalmol Clin 2007;47:173–83.
7. Connell PP, O'Neill EC, Fabinyi D, et al. Endogenous endophthalmitis: 10-year experience at a tertiary referral centre. Eye 2011;25:66–72.
8. Schwartz SG, Flynn HW Jr, Scott IU. Endophthalmitis: classification and current management. Expert Rev Ophthalmol 2007;2:385–96.
9. Chhabra MS, Noble AG, Kumar AV, et al. *Neisseria meningitidis* endogenous endophthalmitis presenting as anterior uveitis. J Pediatr Ophthalmol Strabismus 2007;44:309–10.
10. Jackson TL, Eykyn SJ, Graham EM, et al. Endogenous bacterial endophthalmitis: a 17-year prospective series and review of 267 reported cases. Surv Ophthalmol 2003;48:403–23.
11. Greenwald MJ, Wohl LG, Sell CH. Metastatic bacterial endophthalmitis: a contemporary reappraisal. Surv Ophthalmol 1986;31:81–101.
12. Takebayashi H, Mizota A, Tanaka M. Relation between stage of endogenous fungal endophthalmitis and prognosis. Graefes Arch Clin Exp Ophthalmol 2006;244:816–20.
13. Khan A, Okhravi N, Lightman S. The eye in systemic sepsis. Clin Med 2002;2:444–8.
14. Kim SJ, Seo SW, Park JM, et al. Bilateral endophthalmitis as the initial presentation of bacterial meningitis. Korean J Ophthalmol 2009;23:321–4.
15. Shankar K, Gyanendra L, Hari S, et al. Culture proven endogenous bacterial endophthalmitis in apparently healthy individuals. Ocul Immunol Inflamm 2009;17:396–9.
16. Binder MI, Chua J, Kaiser PK, et al. Endogenous endophthalmitis: an 18-year review of culture-positive cases at a tertiary care center. Medicine 2003;82: 97–105.
17. Okada AA, Johnson RP, Liles WC, et al. Endogenous bacterial endophthalmitis: report of a ten-year retrospective study. Ophthalmology 1994;101: 832–8.
18. Anand AR, Madhavan HN, Neelam V, et al. Use of polymerase chain reaction in the diagnosis of fungal endophthalmitis. Ophthalmology 2001;108: 326–30.
19. McDonnell PJ, McDonnell JM, Brown RH, et al. Ocular involvement in patients with fungal infections. Ophthalmology 1985;92:706–9.
20. Okada AA, Johnson RP, Liles WC, et al. Endogenous bacterial endophthalmitis: report of a ten-year retrospective study. Ophthalmology 1994;101: 832–8.
21. Major JC Jr, Engelbert M, Flynn HW Jr, et al. *Staphylococcus aureus* endophthalmitis: antibiotic susceptibilities, methicillin resistance, and clinical outcomes. Am J Ophthalmol 2010;149:278–83.
22. Sparks JR, Recchia FM, Weitkamp JH. Endogenous group B streptococcal endophthalmitis in a preterm infant. J Perinatol 2007;27:392–4.
23. Torii H, Miyata H, Sugisaka E, et al. Bilateral endophthlamitis in a patient with bacterial meningitis caused by *Streptococcus pneumoniae*. Ophthalmologica 2008;222:357–9.
24. Hayasaka K, Nakamura H, Hayakawa K, et al. A case of endogenous bacterial endophthlamitis caused by *Streptococcus bovis*. Int Ophthalmol 2008;28: 55–7.
25. Montero JA, Ruiz-Moreno JM, Rodriguez AE, et al. Endogenous endophthalmitis by *Propionobacterium acnes* associated with leflunomide and adalimumab therapy. Eur J Ophthalmol 2006;16:343–5.
26. Augsten R, Konigsdorffer E, Dawczynski J, et al. [Listeria monocytogenes endophthalmitis.] Klin Monbl Augenheilkd 2004;221:1054–6.
27. Miller JJ, Scott IU, Flynn HW Jr, et al. Endophthalmitis caused by *Bacillus* species. Am J Ophthalmol 2008;145:883–8.
28. Kawakami H, Sawada A, Mochizuki K, et al. Endogenous *Nocardia farcinica* endophthalmitis. Jpn J Ophthalmol 2010;54:164–6.
29. Ang M, Jap A, Chee SP. Prognostic factors and outcomes in endogenous *Klebsiella pneumoniae* endophthalmitis. Am J Ophthalmol 2011;151(2):338–44.

30. Motley WW 3rd, Augsburger JJ, Hutchins RK, et al. *Pseudomonas aeruginosa* endogenous endophthalmitis with choroidal abscess in a patient with cystic fibrosis. Retina 2005;25:202–7.
31. Tseng CY, Liu PY, Shi ZY, et al. Endogenous endophthalmitis due to *Escherichia coli*: case report and review. Clin Infect Dis 1996;22:1107–8.
32. Rishi E, Rishi P, Nandi K, et al. Endophthalmitis caused by *Enterococcus faecalis*: a case series. Retina 2009;29:214–7.
33. Balaskas K, Potamitou D. Endogenous endophthalmitis secondary to bacterial meningitis from *Neisseria meningitidis*: a case report and review of the literature. Cases J 2009;2:149.
34. Leng T, Flynn HW Jr, Miller D, et al. Endophthalmitis caused by Proteus species: antibiotic sensitivities and visual acuity outcomes. Retina 2009; 29:1019–24.
35. Ness T, Pelz K, Hansen LL. Endogenous endophthalmitis: microorganisms, disposition, and prognosis. Acta Ophthalmol Scand 2007;85:852–6.
36. Lingappan A, Wykoff CC, Albini TA, et al. Endogenous fungal endophthalmitis: causative organisms, management strategies, and visual acuity outcomes. Am J Ophthalmol 2012;153:162–6.
37. Walsh TJ. Emerging fungal pathogens: evolving challenges to immunocompromised patients. In Scheld WM, Armstrong D, Hughes JM, editors. Emerging infections. Washington, DC: ASM Press; 1998. ch. 15.
38. Pappas PG, Rex JH, Lee J, et al. A prospective observational study of candidemia: epidemiology, therapy, and influences on mortality in hospitalized adult and pediatric patients. Clin Infect Dis 2003;37:634–43.
39. Menezes AV, Sigesmund DA, Demajo WA, et al. Mortality of hospitalized patients with *Candida* endopthalmitis. Arch Intern Med 1994;154:2093–7.
40. Connell PP, O'Neill EC, Amirul Islam FM, et al. Endogenous endophthalmitis associated with intravenous drug abuse: seven-year experience at a tertiary referral center. Retina 2010;30:1721–5.
41. Scherer WJ, Lee K. Implications of early systemic therapy on the incidence of endogenous fungal endophthalmitis. Ophthalmology 1997;104:1593–8.
42. Bross J, Talbot GH, Maislin G, et al. Risk factors for nosocomial candidemia: a case–control study in adults without leukemia. Am J Med 1989;87:614–20.
43. Donahue SP, Hein E, Sinatra RB. Ocular involvement in children with candidemia. Am J Ophthalmol 2003;135:886–7.
44. Kaburaki T, Takamoto M, Araki F, et al. Endogenous *Candida albicans* infection causing subretinal abscess. Int Ophthalmol 2010;30:203–6.
45. Schiedler V, Scott IU, Flynn HW Jr, et al. Culture-proven endogenous endophthalmitis: clinical features and visual acuity outcomes. Am J Ophthalmol 2004;137:725–31.
46. Ness T, Pelz K, Hansen LL. Endogenous endophthalmitis: microorganisms, disposition, and prognosis. Acta Ophthalmol Scand 2007;85:852–6.
47. Hashemi SB, Shishegar M, Nikeghbalian S, et al. Endogenous *Aspergillus* endophthalmitis occurring after liver transplantation: a case report. Transplant Proc 2009;41:2933–5.
48. Logan S, Rajan M, Graham E, et al. A case of aspergillus endophthalmitis in an immunocompetent woman: intra-ocular penetration of oral voriconazole: a case report. Cases J 2010;3:31.
49. Weishaar PD, Flynn HW Jr, Murray TG, et al. Endogenous *Aspergillus* endophthalmitis: clinical features and treatment outcomes. Ophthalmology 1998; 105:57–65.
50. Jampol LM, Dyckman S, Maniates V, et al. Retinal and choroidal infarction from *Aspergillus*: clinical diagnosis and clinicopathologic correlations. Trans Am Ophthalmol Soc 1988;86:422–40.
51. Georgala A, Layeux B, Kwan J, et al. Inaugural bilateral aspergillus endophthalmitis in a seriously immunocompromised patient. Mycoses 2011;54(5): 371–465.
52. Rex JH, Larsen RA, Dismukes WE, et al. Catastrophic visual loss due to *Cryptococcus neoformans* meningitis. Medicine 1993;72:207–24.
53. Henderly DE, Liggett PE, Rao NA. Cryptococcal chorioretinitis and endophthalmitis. Retina 1987;7:75–9.
54. Sheu SJ, Chen YC, Kuo NW, et al. Endogenous cryptococcal endophthalmitis. Ophthalmology 1998;105:377–81.
55. Zakka KA, Foos RY, Brown WJ. Intraocular coccidiomycosis. Surv Ophthalmol 1978;22:313–21.
56. Blumenkranz MS, Stevens DA. Endogenous coccidiodal endophthalmitis. Ophthalmology 1980;87:974–84.
57. Rodenbiker HT, Ganley JP, Galgiani JN, et al. Prevalence of chorioretinal scars associated with coccidiomycosis. Arch Ophthalmol 1981;99:71–5.
58. Stone JL, Kalina RE. Ocular coccidioidomycosis. Am J Ophthalmol 1993;116: 249–50.
59. Gonzales CA, Scott IU, Chaudhry NA, et al. Endogenous endophthalmitis caused by *Histoplasma capsulatum var. capsulatum*: a case report and literature review. Ophthalmology 2000;107:725–9.
60. Cartwright MJ, Promersberger M, Stevens GA. *Sporothrix schenckii* endophthalmitis presenting as granulomatous uveitis. Br J Ophthalmol 1993;77: 61–2.
61. Dellon AL, Stark WJ, Chretien PB. Spontaneous resolution of endogenous *Candida* endophthalmitis complicating intravenous hyperalimentation. Am J Ophthalmol 1975;79:648–54.
62. Riddell JIV, Comer GM, Kauffman CA. Treatment of endogenous fungal endophthalmitis: focus on new antifungal agents. Clin Infect Dis 2011;52: 648–53.
63. Endophthalmitis Vitrectomy Study Group. Results of the Endophthalmitis Vitrectomy Study: a randomized trial of immediate vitrectomy and of intravenous antibiotics for the treatment of postoperative bacterial endophthalmitis: Endophthalmitis Vitrectomy Study Group. Arch Ophthalmol 1995;113: 1479–96.
64. Briggs MC, McDonald P, Bourke R, et al. Intravitreal penetration of teicoplanin. Eye 1998;12:252–5.
65. Tappeiner C, Schuerch K, Goldblum D, et al. Combined meropenem and linezolid as a systemic treatment for postoperative endophthalmitis. Klin Monbl Augenheilkd 2010;227:257–61.
66. Hariprasad SM, Mieler WF, Holz ER. Vitreous and aqueous penetration of orally administered gatifloxacin in humans. Arch Ophthalmol 2004;121: 345–50.
67. Hariprasad SM, Shah GK, Mieler WF, et al. Vitreous and aqueous penetration of orally administered moxifloxacin in humans. Arch Ophthalmol 2006;124: 178–82.
68. Park-Wyllie LY, Juurlink DN, Kopp A, et al. Outpatient gatifloxacin therapy and dysglycemia in older adults. N Engl J Med 2006;354:1352–61.
69. Mehlhorn AJ, Brown DA. Safety concerns with fluoroquinolones. Ann Pharmacother 2007;41:1859–66.
70. Sheridan KR, Potoski BA, Shields RK, et al. Presence of adequate intravitreal concentrations of daptomycin after systemic intravenous administration in a patient with endogenous endophthalmitis. Pharmacotherapy 2010;30: 1247–51.
71. Chan WM, Liu DT, Fan DS, et al. Failure of systemic antibiotic in preventing sequential endogenous endophthalmitis of a bronchiectasis patient. Am J Ophthalmol 2005;139:549–50.
72. Rex JH, Walsh TJ, Sobel JD, et al. Practice guidelines for the treatment of candidiasis: Infectious Diseases Society of America. Clin Infect Dis 2000; 30:662–78.
73. Darling K, Singh J, Wilks D. Successful treatment of *Candida glabrata* endophthalmitis with amphotericin B lipid complex (ABLC). J Infect 2000;40: 92–4.
74. Virata SR, Kylstra JA, Brown JC, et al. Worsening of endogenous *Candida albicans* endophthalmitis during therapy with intravenous lipid complex amphotericin B. Clin Infect Dis 1999;28:1177–8.
75. Griffin JR, Pettit TH, Fishman LS, et al. Blood-borne *Candida* endophthalmitis. A clinical and pathologic study of 21 cases. Arch Ophthalmol 1973; 89:450–6.
76. Roney P, Barr CC, Chun CH, et al. Endogenous *Aspergillus* endophthalmitis. Rev Infect Dis 1986;8:955–8.
77. Lewis H, Aaberg TM, Fary DR, et al. Latent disseminated blastomycosis with choroidal involvement. Arch Ophthalmol 1988;106:527–30.
78. Blumenkranz MS, Stevens DA. Endogenous coccidiodal endophthalmitis. Ophthalmology 1980;87:974–84.
79. Lemke A, Kiderlen AF, Kayser O, et al. Appl Microbiol Biotechnol 2005; 68:151–62.
80. Kinyoun JL. Treatment of *Candida* endophthalmitis. Retina 1982;2:215–22.
81. Green WR, Bennett JE, Goos RD. Ocular penetration of amphotericin B: a report of laboratory studies and a case report of post surgical *Cephalosporium* endophthalmitis. Arch Ophthalmol 1965;73:769–75.
82. Dave VP, Majji AB, Suma N, et al. A rare case of *Aspergillus terreus* endogenous endophthalmitis in a patient of acute lymphoid leukemia with good clinical outcome. Eye 2011;25(8):1094–6.
83. Humphrey MJ, Jevons S, Tarbit MH. Pharmacokinetic evaluation of UK-49,858, a metabolically stable triazole antifungal drug, in animals and humans. Antimicrob Agents Chemother 1985;28:648–53.
84. Savani DJ, Perfect JR, Cobo LM, et al. Penetration of new azole compounds into the eye and efficacy in experimental *Candida* endophthalmitis. Antimicrob Agents Chemother 1987;31:6–10.
85. Annamalai T, Fong KC, Choo MM. Intravenous fluconazole for bilateral endogenous Candida endophthalmitis. J Ocul Pharmacol Ther 2011;27:105–7.
86. Christmas NJ, Smiddy WE. Vitrectomy and systemic fluconazole for treatment of endogenous fungal endophthalmitis. Ophthalm Surg Lasers 1996;27:1012–8.
87. Luttrull JK, Wan WL, Kubak BM, et al. Treatment of ocular fungal infections with oral fluconazole. Am J Ophthalmol 1995;119:477–81.
88. Urbak SF, Degn T. Fluconazole in the management of fungal ocular infections. Ophthalmologica 1994;208:147–56.
89. Como JA, Dismukes WE. Oral azole drugs as systemic antifungal therapy. N Engl J Med 1994;330:263–72.
90. Edwards JE Jr, Bodey GP, Bowden RA, et al. International conference for the development of a consensus on the management and prevention of severe candidal infections. Clin Infect Dis 1997;25:43–59.
91. Ackler ME, Vellend H, McNeely DM, et al. Use of fluconazole in the treatment of candidal endophthalmitis. Clin Infect Dis 1995;20:657–64.
92. van't Wout JW, Novakova I, Verhagen CA, et al. The efficacy of itraconazole against fungal infections in neutropenic patients: a randomized comparative study with amphotericin B. J Infect 1991;22:45–52.
93. Como JA, Dismukes WE. Oral azole drugs as systemic antifungal therapy. N Engl J Med 1994;330:263–72.
94. Pappas PG, Rex JH, Sobel JD, et al. Guidelines for treatment of candidiasis. Clin Infect Dis 2004;38:161–89.
95. Scott LJ, Simpson D. Voriconazole: a review of its use in the management of invasive fungal infections. Drugs 2007;67:269–98.
96. Hariprasad SM, Mieler WF, Holz ER, et al. Determination of vitreous, aqueous, and plasma concentrations of orally administered voriconazole in humans. Arch Ophthalmol 2004;122:42–7.
97. Biju R, Sushil D, Georgy NK. Successful management of presumed Candida endogenous endophthalmitis with oral voriconazole. Indian J Ophthalmol 2009;57:306–8.
98. Morris MI. Posaconazole: a new antifungal agent with expanded spectrum of activity. Am J Health Syst Pharm 2009;66:225–36.

99. Sponsel WE, Graybill JR, Nevarez HL, et al. Ocular and systemic posaconazole (SCH-56592) treatment of invasive *Fusarium solani* keratitis and endophthalmitis. Br J Ophthalmol 2002;86:829–30.
100. Tu EY, McCartney DL, Beatty RF, et al. Successful treatment of resistant ocular fusariosis with posaconazole (SCH-56592) . Am J Ophthalmol 2007;143: 222–7.
101. Bennett JE. Antimicrobial agents (continued): Antifungal Agents. In: Hardman JG, Limbird LE, editors. Goodman and Gilman's The pharmacological basis of therapeutics, 10th ed. New York: McGraw–Hill; 2001. p. 1295–312.
102. Sarria JC, Bradely JC, Habash R, et al. *Candida glabrata* endophthalmitis treated successfully with caspofungin. Clin Infect Dis 2005;40:46–8.
103. Durand ML, Kim IK, D'Amico DJ, et al. Successful treatment of *Fusarium* endophthalmitis with voriconazole and *Aspergillus* endophthalmitis with voriconazole plus caspofungin. Am J Ophthalmol 2005;140:552–4.
104. Kwok AK, Hui M, Panc CP, et al. An in vitro study of ceftazidime and vancomycin concentrations in various fluid media: implications for use in treating endophthalmitis. Invest Ophthalmol Vis Sci 2002;43:1182–8.
105. Axelrod AJ, Peyman GA, Apple DJ. Toxicity of intravitreal injection of amphotericin B. Am J Ophthalmol 1973;76:578–83.
106. Payne JF, Keenum DG, Sternberg P Jr, et al. Concentrated intravitreal amphotericin B in fungal endophthalmitis. Arch Ophthalmol 2010;128:1546–50.
107. Brod RD, Flynn HW Jr, Clarkson JG, et al. Endogenous *Candida* endophthalmitis: management without intravenous amphotericin B. Ophthalmology 1990;97:666–72.
108. Koc A, Onal S, Yenice O, et al. Pars plana vitrectomy and intravitreal liposomal amphotericin B in the treatment of Candida endophthalmitis. Ophthalmic Surg Lasers Imaging 2010 Mar;9:1–3. Epub ahead of print doi: 10.3928/15428877-20100215-35.
109. Schulman JA, Peyman G, Fiscella R, et al. Toxicity of intravitreal injection of fluconazole in the rabbit. Can J Ophthalmol 1987;22:304–6.
110. Velpandian T, Narayanan K, Nag TC, et al. Retinal toxicity of intravitreally injected plain and liposome formulation of fluconazole in rabbit eye. Indian J Ophthalmol 2006;54:237–40.
111. Urbak SF, Degn T. Fluconazole in the management of fungal ocular infections. Ophthalmologica 1994;208:147–56.
112. Yoshizumi MO, Banihashemi AR. Experimental intravitreal ketoconazole in DMSO. Retina 1988;8:210–5.
113. Gao H, Pennesi ME, Shah K, et al. Intravitreal voriconazole: an electroretinographic and histopathologic study. Arch Ophthalmol 2004;122:1687–92.
114. Kramer M, Kramer MR, Blau H, et al. Intravitreal voriconazole for the treatment of endogenous *Aspergillus* endophthalmitis. Ophthalmology 2006;113: 1184–6.
115. Schulman JA, Peyman GA. Intravitreal corticosteroids as an adjunct in the treatment of bacterial and fungal endophthalmitis: a review. Retina 1992;12: 336–40.
116. Kinyoun JL. Treatment of Candida endophthalmitis. Retina 1982;2:215–22.
117. Snip RC, Michels RG. Pars plana vitrectomy in the management of endogenous Candida endophthalmitis. Am J Ophthalmol 1976;82:699–704.
118. Jackson TL, Eykyn SJ, Graham EM, et al. Endogenous bacterial endophthalmitis: a 17-year prospective series and review of 267 reported cases. Surv Ophthalmol 2003;48:403–23.
119. Christmas NJ, Smiddy WE. Vitrectomy and systemic fluconazole for treatment of endogenous fungal endophthalmitis. Ophthalmic Surg Lasers 1996; 27:1012–8.
120. Huang SS, Brod RD, Flynn HW Jr. Management of endophthalmitis while preserving the uninvolved crystalline lens. Am J Ophthalmol 1991;112: 695–701.
121. Jackson TL, Eykyn SJ, Graham EM, et al. Endogenous bacterial endophthalmitis: a 17-year prospective series and review of 267 reported cases. Surv Ophthalmol 2003;48:403–23.

Chapter 88

Acute Retinal Necrosis Syndrome

G. Atma Vemulakonda, Jay S. Pepose, Russell N. Van Gelder

DEFINITION

In 1971 Urayama and coworkers[1] first reported six cases of an apparently new syndrome characterized by acute necrotizing retinitis, vitritis, retinal arteritis, choroiditis, and late-onset rhegmatogenous retinal detachment. Young and Bird[2] described two similar cases in 1978 and gave the syndrome the acronym BARN (bilateral acute necrosis syndrome). With the subsequent recognition of unilateral and asynchronous bilateral cases, the disease has been termed simply acute retinal necrosis syndrome, or ARN syndrome. Acute retinal necrosis syndrome is characterized by the initial onset of episcleritis or scleritis, periorbital pain, and anterior uveitis, which may be granulomatous or stellate in appearance. This is followed by decreased vision resulting from vitreous opacification, necrotizing retinitis, and, in some cases, optic neuritis or neuropathy. The retinitis appears as deep, multifocal, yellow-white patches, typically beginning in the peripheral fundus (Figs 88.1, 88.2) and then becoming concentrically confluent and spreading toward the posterior pole (Figs 88.3–88.5); the macula frequently is spared. An active vasculitis is present, with perivascular hemorrhages, sheathing, and terminal obliteration of arterioles by thrombi. The phase of active retinitis usually lasts 4–6 weeks.[3-8]

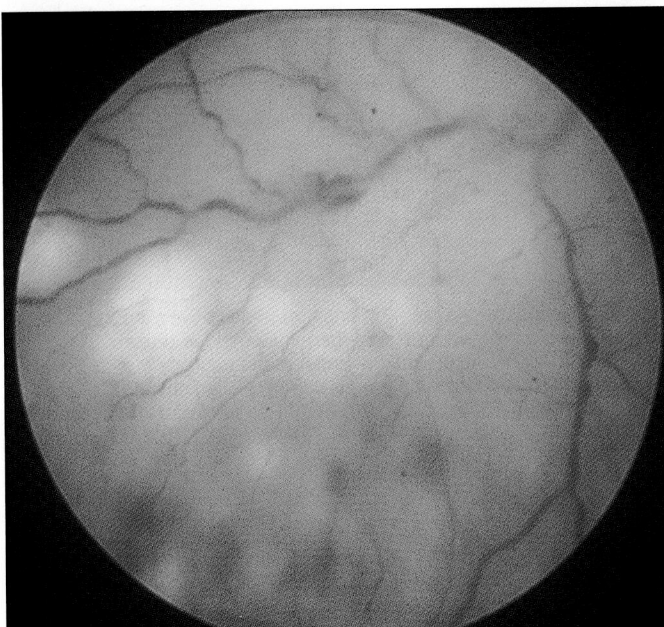

Fig. 88.1 Typical fundus appearance of early acute retinal necrosis syndrome demonstrating necrotizing peripheral retinitis, intraretinal hemorrhage, and vitritis.

With resolution, pigmentation of the peripheral lesions begins at their posterior margins, leaving a scalloped appearance (Fig. 88.6), frequently accompanied by retinal breaks at the junction of normal and necrotic retina. Giant retinal pigment epithelial tears may develop.[9] A rhegmatogenous retinal detachment has been observed in approximately 75% of untreated eyes, generally within 1–2 months after the onset of the disease. Earlier

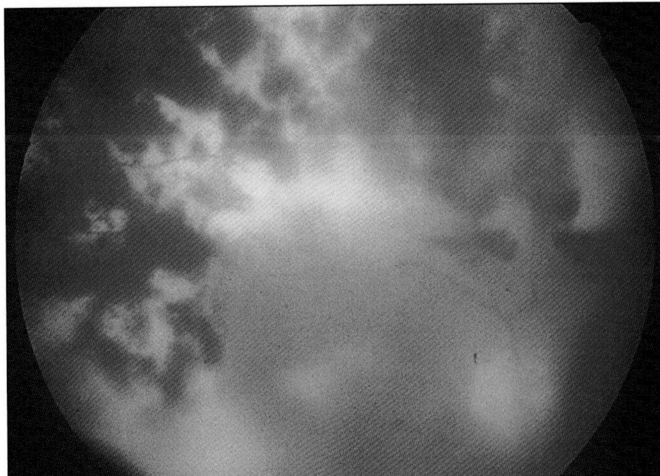

Fig. 88.2 White patches of retinal necrosis are seen in the periphery with isolated areas of necrosis more posterior early in the course of acute retinal necrosis.

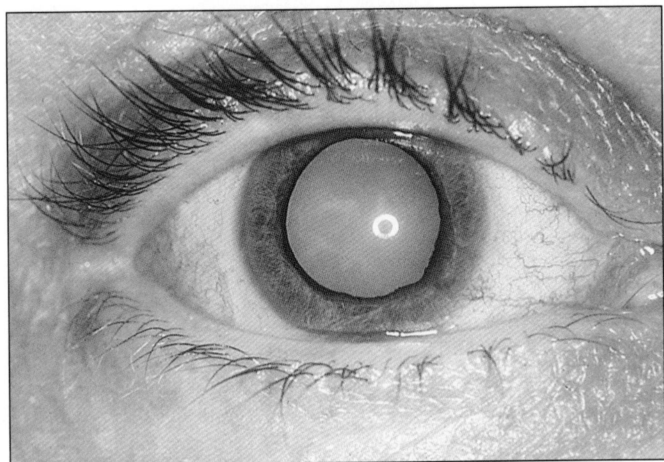

Fig. 88.3 Marked vitritis associated with acute retinal necrosis syndrome. Episcleritis and keratic precipitates are also often seen early in the syndrome.

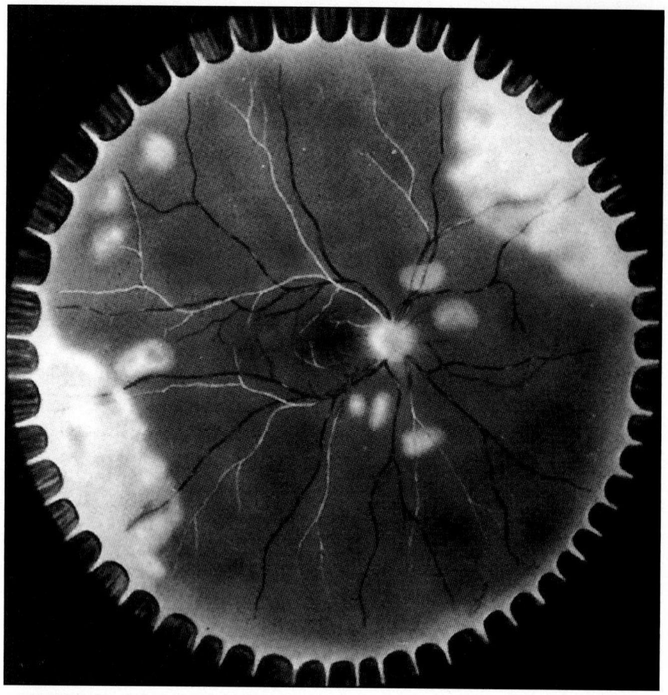

Fig. 88.4 Fundus appearance late in acute retinal necrosis syndrome. Dense vitritis, confluent retinal necrosis, and intraretinal hemorrhage are encroaching on the posterior pole.

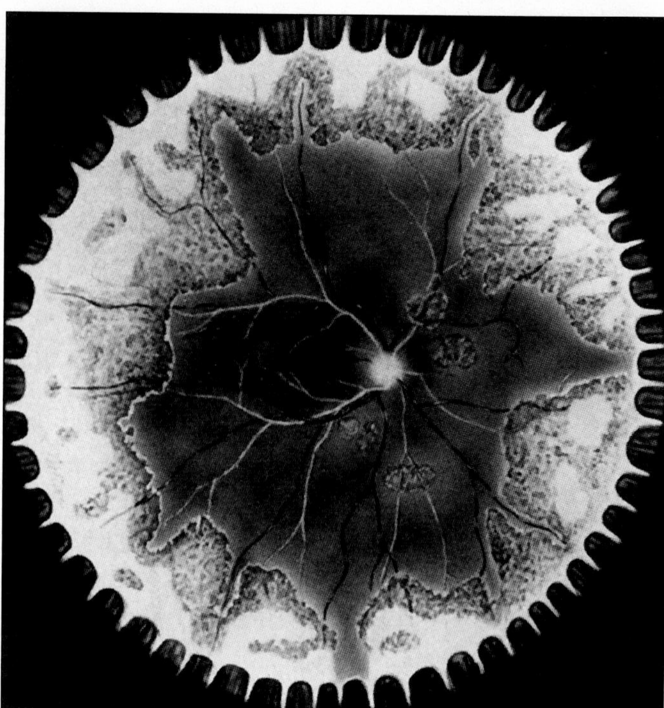

Fig. 88.6 During the resolution of active retinitis, the lesions become pigmented starting at their posterior margins, leaving a scalloped border between necrotic and normal-appearing retina.

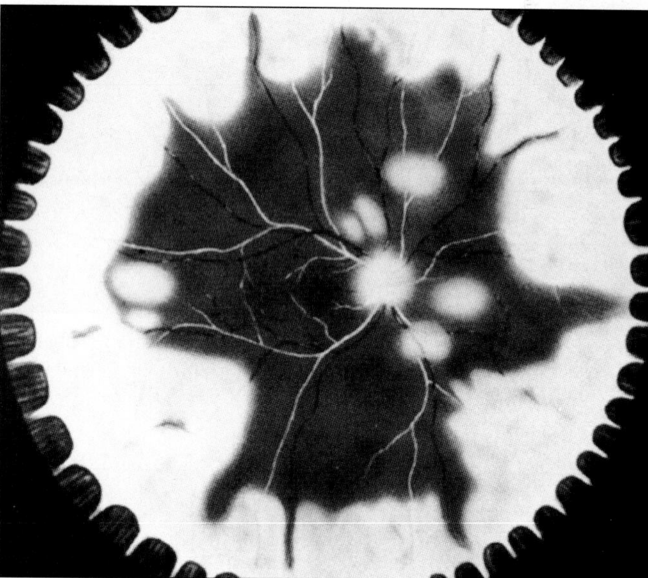

Fig. 88.5 The peripheral retinitis becomes confluent for 360 degrees and is accompanied by an obliterative vasculitis and papillitis.

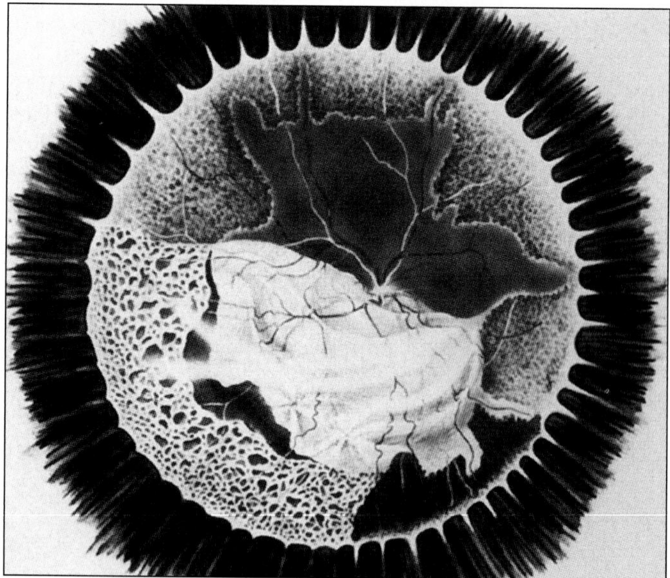

Fig. 88.7 Retinal breaks and the onset of proliferative vitreoretinopathy can lead to a combined tractional-rhegematogenous retinal detachment 1–2 months after the onset of the acute retinal necrosis syndrome. (Reproduced with permission from Clarkson JG, Blumenkranz MS, Culbertson WW, et al. Retinal detachment following the acute retinal necrosis syndrome. Ophthalmology 1984;91:1665–8.)

exudative and rhegmatogenous detachments have been noted, particularly in cases associated with herpes simplex virus (HSV).[3,6,8,10] Vitreous inflammation may lead to organization and proliferative vitreoretinopathy,[11] adding a traction component to the retinal detachment (Fig. 88.7). Vision may suddenly decrease as a result of anterior ischemic optic neuropathy. Macular pucker also may occur.

Computed tomography[12–14] and ultrasonography[14] have revealed enlargement of the optic nerve sheath in ARN cases associated with prominent optic disc edema. Since ARN patients can develop meningoencephalitis, it is helpful to keep this possibility in mind, look for symptoms and signs of neurologic disease, and refer the patient for further investigation as appropriate.[15] Even in ARN patients who are not immunocompromised and who have no clinical evidence of encephalitis, magnetic resonance imaging of selected cases has shown lesions of the lateral geniculate, optic tracts, and chiasm,[16] suggesting viral spread through the central nervous system by axoplasmic transport from retinal ganglion cells. An explanation for this has been shown in mouse models, where there is evidence to show that HSV1 infection may progress through the optic chiasm from one eye to the other and along the visual pathways leading to meningoencephalitis.[17]

The contralateral eye is involved in approximately one-third of untreated ARN cases, usually within 6 weeks of the onset of disease in the first eye.[9,18] However, the second eye can be affected as late as 34 years after involvement of the first eye,[19] and the fellow eye has become involved even after acyclovir treatment for ARN in the first eye.[20] Mild forms of ARN syndrome, characterized by patchy, peripheral retinal opacification, recently have been reported. These mild cases did not become rapidly confluent or lead to detachment.[21] It is unclear whether this atypical presentation is a result of intense acyclovir and corticosteroid therapy or a reflection of a wide range of disease severity. In addition, less involved forms of ARN have been reported after primary varicella, without concomitant therapy.[22]

PATIENT POPULATION

ARN syndrome occurs most commonly in otherwise healthy patients of either sex and of any age; in general, patients are not immunocompromised or systemically ill. However, ARN patients may demonstrate subclinical immune dysfunction. In one review of 216 patients with ARN, impaired cellular immunity was noted in 16%.[23] Skin testing of patients with ARN revealed anergy in five of seven tested cases and abnormal lymphocyte proliferative indices in one-third.[24] The significance of cutaneous anergy is unclear, however, since patients with zoster infections frequently demonstrate anergy.[25] Specific HLA haplotypes may increase the relative risk of developing ARN syndrome, such as the HLA-DQw7 antigen and phenotype Bw62, DR4 in white patients in the United States[26] and HLA-Aw33, B44, and DRw6 in Japanese patients.[27] Pleocytosis of the cerebrospinal fluid frequently accompanies the syndrome,[9,13,28] and intrathecal production of antibodies against herpesviruses has been demonstrated in selected cases.[4] Some patients present with ARN before, after, or at the same time as they show skin manifestations of varicella zoster infection[29,30] (e.g., primary varicella, herpes zoster ophthalmicus, or Ramsay Hunt syndrome). Unilateral ARN also has been noted after herpes simplex keratitis.[31] Diffuse cerebral atrophy and labyrinthine deafness have been reported following ARN,[32] and some investigators have suggested that ARN be considered as one of the uveomeningeal syndromes.[14]

With the increase in intravitreal steroid injections for a variety of retinal diseases, there have been reports of ARN occurring in immunocompetent patients and other patients who have medical comorbidities. As a result, this increased risk has led some to increase their vigilance for the development of viral retinitis following intravitreal injection [33–35]

Acute necrotizing retinitis that is clinically identical to ARN or shares many features with ARN has been reported in immunocompromised patients. ARN was first described in immunocompromised patients in 1985;[36] a recent case series described 26 cases of ARN in AIDS patients, noting a generally fulminant course.[37] The cause of the retinitis in these immunocompromised patients may be particularly diverse or multifactorial. For example, an AIDS patient died after an ARN-like syndrome with concurrent encephalitis, and herpes simplex viral antigens were localized in the central nervous system at postmortem examination.[38] In contrast, several immunocompromised patients have presented with ARN in association with skin manifestations of zoster.[39] Although ARN syndrome initially was defined as manifesting in otherwise healthy patients, many authorities have broadened the diagnostic criteria to include immunocompromised hosts.[39–42] It is the evolution of clinical signs and symptoms, and not the specific pathogen or immune status of the patient, that serves as the sole basis by which ARN syndrome has been defined (see Differential Diagnosis, below).

ETIOLOGY

Considerable evidence points to multiple members of the herpesvirus family in the etiology of ARN syndrome. In numerous studies, varicella zoster virus (VZV) has been the most frequent virus isolated,[43] sometimes in up to two-thirds of patients.[44] VZV was isolated in tissue culture from the vitreous of a blind eye enucleated early in the course of the disease, and specific varicella zoster antigens were identified in retinal tissue by immunocytologic staining[45] (Fig. 88.8). VZV was identified by electron microscopy in necrotic retinal tissue (Fig. 88.9) in two other cases

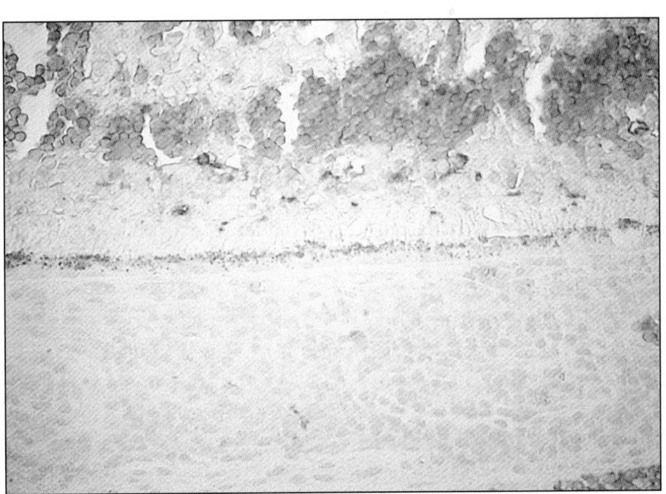

Fig. 88.8 Varicella zoster antigens (brown) are seen in cells scattered in all layers of a necrotic retina.

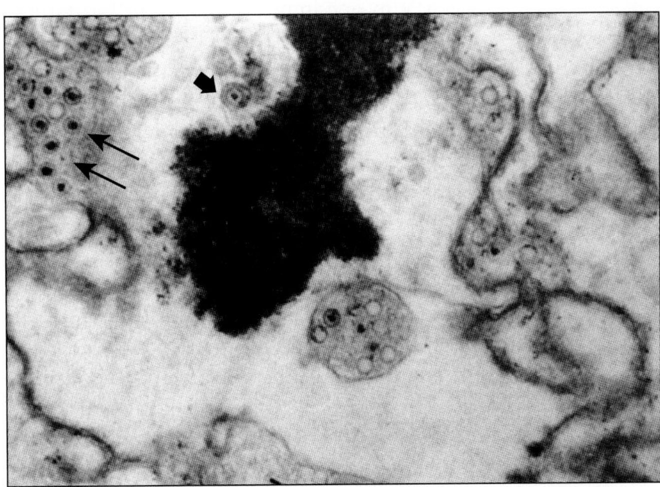

Fig. 88.9 Ultrastructural studies of necrotic retina reveal multiple 100 nm nucleocapsids (double arrows) and enveloped virions typical of a herpes-type virus. (Courtesy of M.S. Blumenkranz.)

of ARN.[46] Varicella zoster DNA in intraocular fluids of ARN cases has been confirmed by polymerase chain reaction (PCR),[47] and Witmer quotients of paired serum to intraocular fluid antibody levels have been diagnostic of varicella zoster in numerous cases.[48,49] Varicella zoster antigens have been demonstrated in vitreous aspirates of patients with ARN syndrome.[50]

Restriction endonuclease patterns of the ARN virus isolate were similar to those of typical varicella zoster strains and showed similar sensitivities to a panel of antiviral drugs.[51] Although strain heterogeneity has been observed in the varicella zoster viruses associated with ARN syndrome,[52] these data thus do not support the notion that the ARN virus represents a mutant strain of VZV with significant alterations in either the viral thymidine kinase or DNA polymerase genes. It therefore remains enigmatic why an "old virus" should give rise to a "new" syndrome.

Some reports have suggested that other members of the herpesvirus family may cause ARN, in about 20% of cases according to one study.[44] A number of studies have implicated HSV because of concurrent herpes simplex skin lesions,[53] the detection of herpes simplex antigens on vitreous cells,[7] the presence of immune complexes containing herpes simplex antigens in aqueous or serum,[54] the documentation of intraocular antibody synthesis directed against HSV,[49] diagnostic changes in serum antibody levels to herpes simplex, polymerase chain reaction detection of herpes simplex,[55] or the culture of herpes simplex from vitreous humor.[3,8,45] Several cases have been described of ARN caused by reactivation of HSV type 2.[47,55,56] Interestingly, patients with herpes simplex type 2 appear to be much younger (mean 21 years) than those with either herpes simplex type 1 or varicella zoster (mean age 40 years).[49,57,58] The proportion of ARN syndrome patients with disease caused by HSV-2 may be higher in Japan than in the United States, perhaps coincident with changing epidemiologic distributions of HSV-1 versus HSV-2 in this population.[59,60] Patients with ARN syndrome caused by herpes simplex type 1 appear to have a higher risk of encephalitis or meningitis than those with disease caused by VZV.[57,61–65]

In one study of a case of ARN,[66] cytomegalovirus (CMV) was cultured and CMV antigens were demonstrated in retinal tissue, but megalic cells or electron-dense cytoplasmic inclusions, which have uniformly typified CMV infection of the retina, were not identified. In another case the polymerase chain reaction yielded positive results for CMV in one immunocompetent individual, whose vitreous was negative for VZV and HSV types 1 and 2.[67] Epstein–Barr virus has also been postulated in some cases of ARN syndrome,[68,69] but definitive linkage of this nearly ubiquitous virus to disease remains problematic. Indeed, EBV has been found in 20% of normal cadaveric eyes,[70] and while one study found EBV by PCR in about one-sixth of their ARN cases, each case was also positive for VZV by PCR.[44]

PATHOLOGIC FEATURES

Studies of blind eyes enucleated early in the course of ARN have demonstrated retinal necrosis, hemorrhage, and considerable vitreous debris. The retinal necrosis is full-thickness, and an underlying choroiditis is present that may be granulomatous (Fig. 88.10). VZV DNA and antigens have been identified in lymphoid cells within choroidal infiltrates in an eye enucleated in the late stage of disease.[71] Eosinophilic intranuclear inclusions within cells of all layers of retina and retinal pigment epithelium were the first clues suggesting a possible viral etiology by a member of the herpes group.[46] There is histologic evidence of retinal arteritis (Fig. 88.11), although no virus particles have been detected in vascular endothelium. Deposits of immune complexes containing varicella zoster viral antigens have been demonstrated in retinal vessel walls by immunocytologic methods and may play a role in the vasculitis seen during active stages. The perivasculitis is not restricted to retinal vessels alone and can involve the extraocular muscles (Fig. 88.12). Immune complexes with herpes simplex also have been identified in intraocular fluids in ARN cases.

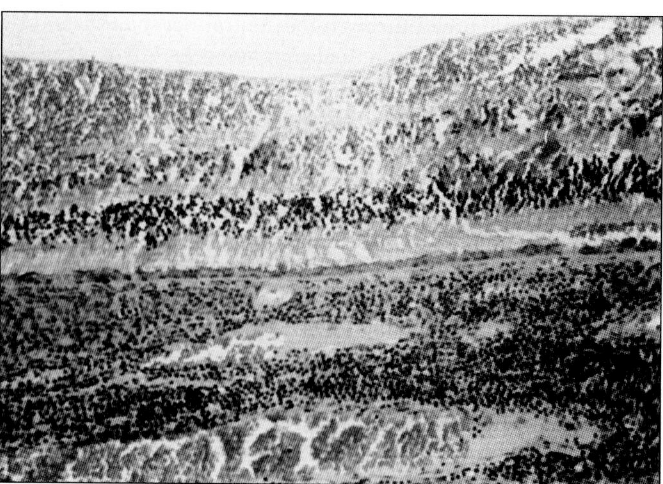

Fig. 88.10 Photomicrograph of a case of acute retinal necrosis shows full-thickness retinal necrosis with an underlying granulomatous choroiditis. (Courtesy of Robert Y. Foos.)

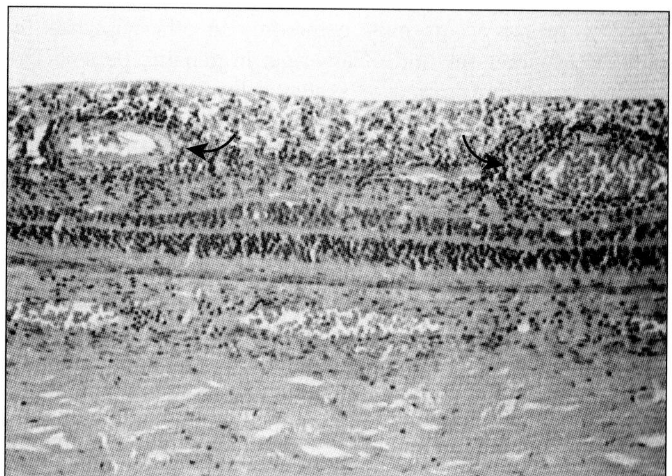

Fig. 88.11 Histologic evidence of retinal vasculitis (arrows) in acute retinal necrosis. (Courtesy of Robert Y. Foos.)

Ultrastructural studies of retinal tissue have revealed 180 nanometer virions containing icosahedral capsids, consistent with particles of the herpes group[46] (see Fig. 88.8). The optic nerve may be largely necrotic and heavily infiltrated with plasma cells, but no virus particles or antigens have been seen in the optic nerve. It is possible that the absence of viral antigens or particles reflects more the time point in the course of the disease when enucleation was performed in these rare cases than conclusive evidence regarding acute optic nerve infection. The

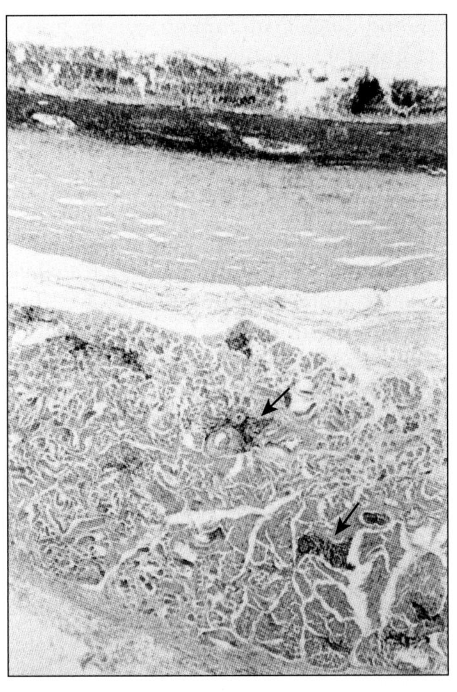

Fig. 88.12 Foci of perivascular inflammation (arrows) are seen in the inferior oblique muscle in a case of acute retinal necrosis. (Courtesy of Robert Y. Foos.)

multifocal, deep retinitis observed early in the course of ARN is compatible with either blood-borne spread of virus or transmission to the eye through a bilateral nerve pathway. An animal model of ARN using herpes simplex virus suggests that spread to the contralateral eye occurs by retrograde axonal transport between the suprachiasmatic nucleus of the hypothalamus and the contralateral retina.[72]

Retinal necrosis in ARN probably is the result of multiple factors, including a direct lytic viral infection of retina, immune complex disease mediating an obliterative arteritis, choroidal inflammation and occlusion, T-cell-mediated inflammation, and vitreous inflammation. All these elements contribute and lead to a combined traction-rhegmatogenous retinal detachment.

DIFFERENTIAL DIAGNOSIS

The American Uveitis Society released its criteria for diagnosis of acute retinal necrosis syndrome in 1994.[42] Under this definition, diagnosis of ARN syndrome is dependent solely on the observed clinical findings and their progression. Neither the identification of an etiologic agent nor knowledge of the patient's immune status is required to render a diagnosis of ARN syndrome. The diagnostic criteria are divided into mandatory and supporting categories and are summarized in Table 88.1. By this definition, retinal lesions presumptively caused by herpesviruses (but not part of other well-recognized syndromes such as CMV retinitis or progressive outer retinal necrosis [see below]) are covered under the umbrella term *necrotizing herpetic retinopathy*.

The differential diagnosis of ARN includes CMV retinopathy, syphilitic retinitis, toxoplasmosis (particularly in immunocompromised hosts), large cell lymphoma, and acute multifocal hemorrhagic retinal vasculitis. A more extensive differential diagnosis includes toxocariasis, fungal or bacterial retinitis, pars planitis, Behçet disease, sarcoidosis, commotio retinae, central retinal artery or ophthalmic artery occlusion, ocular ischemic syndrome, collagen-vascular disease, intraocular leukemia/lymphoma (including T-cell-mediated[73]) and retinoblastoma.

Table 88.1 American Uveitis Society criteria for diagnosis of acute retinal necrosis syndrome

Required clinical criteria	Supporting clinical criteria
One or more foci of retinal necrosis with discrete borders, located in peripheral retina	Optic neuropathy/atrophy
Rapid progression of disease in the absence of therapy	Scleritis
Circumferential spread of disease	Pain
Evidence of occlusive vasculopathy and arteriolar involvement	
A prominent inflammatory reaction in the vitreous and anterior chamber	

The syndrome of ARN is readily distinguished from a separate form of varicella zoster retinitis reported in human immunodeficiency virus (HIV)-infected patients, sometimes referred to as "progressive outer retinal necrosis syndrome" or PORN.[54,74] This latter entity shares an etiologic agent with some cases of ARN but is otherwise completely distinct. It is characterized by multifocal, patchy choroidal, and deep posterior retinal opacification that initially may be parafoveal. Additional features differentiating this syndrome from ARN include the absence of vitreous or anterior chamber inflammation or signs of active vasculitis. PORN progresses rapidly from the posterior pole to involve the entire retina, resulting in widespread retinal necrosis and atrophy. Despite a common etiologic agent, varicella zoster retinitis should not be referred to as the syndrome of ARN. Indeed, the two diseases may even affect different eyes of the same patient.[75]

Although the syndrome of ARN is a clinical diagnosis established on the basis of a constellation of evolving signs and symptoms, which may be pathognomonic in many cases, in atypical or difficult diagnostic cases ancillary clinical history or laboratory tests can support the diagnosis. It is important to assess the patient's level of immunocompetence, since knowledge of seropositivity to HIV and syphilis may help to establish the appropriate specific diagnosis. Diagnostic vitrectomy is appropriate in cases of uncertain diagnosis. The most sensitive and specific method for the detection of herpes viruses in vitreous specimens is the polymerase chain reaction (PCR). PCR assays are capable of detecting a single varicella zoster virion from vitreous biopsy.[76] Simultaneous PCR for multiple herpesviruses has been used to screen for an etiologic agent in atypical cases of ARN and has implicated both CMV[76] and HSV[47] as potentially causative. PCR can be performed in multiplex for VZV, HSV, CMV, and toxoplasmosis.[77] Sensitivity for each, even in multiplex testing, is at least 10 genomes per microliter. With application of quantitative PCR (qPCR), accurate estimates of pathogen load can be achieved.[78,79] These data suggest significant heterogeneity in the pathogen load among individual cases of disease. The great sensitivity of PCR can be problematic, however; assays that yield false-positive results, likely through amplification of latent virus in host tissue, have been reported.[76] False-negative results can also occur. Consensus has not yet been reached regarding the negative predictive value of a negative PCR test for viral DNA.

PCR requires meticulous technical performance and confirmation by probe hybridization to avoid specificity problems and is best performed by a laboratory with considerable experience with this method. In many cases, aqueous and/or vitreous sampling for PCR is becoming the diagnostic test of choice when faced with viral retinitis.[44,80]

In cases in which PCR is negative but clinical suspicion is high, endoretinal biopsy may be appropriate. Taking the biopsy from the transition zone between normal and necrotic retina during the acute phase of the disease greatly increases its diagnostic yield. In the past, obtaining paired serum and intraocular fluid specimens and applying a modified Witmer quotient was performed for diagnostic value even in the early stages of ARN syndrome. It also seemed to develop increasing sensitivity with time.[48,81] With the increased use of PCR, Witmer quotient appears to be used less frequently.[44,79,80] Quantitative antiviral antibody levels in acute and chronic sera from ARN patients are consistent with a specific etiologic diagnosis in a minority of cases and have been falsely negative in cases in which vitreous cultures were positive for herpesviruses.

TREATMENT AND PROGNOSIS

Treatment of ARN syndrome is complex and must be individualized in response to the many pathogenic and temporal facets of the disorder, as well as to the specific vitreoretinal pathologic findings at hand. Cases of ARN associated with mild or minimal inflammation have been reported in which ARN did not progress to extensive retinal necrosis, traction, or detachment.[21,22] Controlled, randomized, prospective treatment studies on ARN have not been conducted given the relative rarity of this disease, so current recommendations are based solely on anecdotal data and case series. Early studies indicated that the natural history of classic ARN syndrome carries a generally poor prognosis in untreated eyes,[9] with only 28% of affected eyes obtaining a final vision better than 20/200 because of rhegmatogenous retinal detachment (75% of affected eyes), optic nerve dysfunction, or macular abnormality. The advent of antiviral therapy and vitrectomy techniques[82] has decreased this level of vision loss to less than one-third of cases in recent years.[12] In one series of cases that were detected early and treated aggressively with acyclovir and laser photocoagulation, outcome for 13 eyes of 12 patients showed 20/40 or better vision in 46% of eyes and 20/400 or better in 92%.[83] However, the use of prophylactic laser photocoagulation has become more controversial than it was in the past.[84]

In light of the characterization and the determination of antiviral sensitivities of the varicella zoster isolate, acyclovir has been used in an effort to limit the direct cytopathic effect of virus on retinal tissue. Based on the dose required for a 50% reduction of virus plaques in tissue culture (ED_{50}), oral administration of acyclovir results in subtherapeutic serum levels; in contrast, intravenous acyclovir (13 mg/kg every 8 hours) results in an intravitreal acyclovir level[4] over three times the ARN ED_{50}. After intravenous administration of acyclovir to ARN patients (1500 mg/m^2/day in three divided doses), retinal lesions were first noted to regress 3.9 days after the beginning of therapy; new lesions did not develop, and existing lesions did not progress.[20] Historically, intravenous therapy for 5–10 days was followed by oral acyclovir at the zoster dosage (800 mg orally five times daily, assuming normal renal function) for up to 6 weeks after the onset of infection, and longer in immunocompromised patients. Valacyclovir (1 g orally three times daily) or famciclovir[85,86] (500 mg orally three times daily) may also be used following intravenous acyclovir administration. Side-effects of acyclovir include decreased renal function, gastrointestinal irritation, phlebitis, central nervous system dysfunction, and hypersensitivity reactions. Acyclovir has potent antiviral action against VZV, HSV types 1 and 2 (both of which have been implicated in ARN), and Epstein–Barr virus, but it has low activity against CMV. Valganciclovir is active against VZV, HSV, and CMV, but is FDA approved at present only for CMV retinitis.

In recent years many clinicians have moved to outpatient use of oral antivirals for treatment induction of ARN.[87–89] Prodrugs such as valacyclovir and famciclovir have high systemic absorption, are active against VZV and HSV, and may be used for prophylaxis against involvement of the second eye.[3,90] Valganciclovir, another prodrug, has been used in other cases.[91] Treatment algorithms have used oral valacyclovir 1 g 3 times daily, oral famciclovir 500 mg 3 times daily, or valganciclovir 450–900 mg 2 times daily until complete resolution of retinitis was observed. Some clinicians have used higher doses of valacyclovir 2 g 3–4 times daily to achieve resolution.[92] These medications are then generally slowly tapered over 1.5–75.7 months.[84,93] Recent studies have not found a significant superiority of intravenous to oral treatment induction, but these studies have been retrospective and limited by the relative rarity of this disease. Given the risk of encephalitis, particularly in patients with HSV-1-associated disease, close monitoring of patient mental status is warranted.

Recent studies have suggested an adjunctive role for intravitreal antiviral medication in the treatment of ARN syndrome. In one small series, three patients treated with intravitreal ganciclovir as well as intravenous foscarnet, ganciclovir, or acyclovir led to excellent outcomes,[94] while another three patients responded to intravitreal antiviral treatment despite progression on intravenous acyclovir.[95] A similar approach has been employed for progressive outer retinal necrosis.[96,97] Early administration of intravitreal antivirals also provides an opportunity for vitreous sampling (akin to the "tap and inject" for endophthalmitis), allowing for PCR-based identification of causative virus.

Acute decreases in vision in ARN patients can result from ischemic optic neuropathy and have led to trials of anticoagulants such as aspirin, along with high-dose oral steroids early after initiation of antiviral therapy. Systemic corticosteroids also may limit intraocular inflammation and the vitreous reaction, but are generally begun only after 24–48 hours of intravenous acyclovir. Virus particles or antigens have not been observed in the optic nerve in ARN, and it appears that the optic nerve dysfunction is caused by ischemia from swollen vascular endothelial cells, thrombotic arteriolar occlusion, and infiltration of the optic nerve by inflammatory cells. Hyperaggregation of platelets has been reported in six of seven patients with bilateral ARN studied, as determined by adenosine 5-diphosphate aggregation testing and partial prothrombin times.[98] Optic nerve dysfunction has been reported in ARN patients despite anticoagulation therapy or antiplatelet therapy. Studies have employed optic nerve sheath fenestration in conjunction with acyclovir therapy in a small group of ARN patients with optic neuropathy and disc edema, with reported improvement in final vision in six of eight eyes.[14] Better results were obtained in the subgroup that underwent decompression within 12 days of the onset of the optic neuropathy.

In early studies prior to current antiviral management techniques, the second eye became involved in 36% of ARN patients, usually within 6 weeks of the first eye's involvement.[20] More recent studies have suggested a fellow-eye involvement rate of ~3% with appropriate antiviral treatment.[84] The duration of systemic treatment to prevent fellow-eye involvement is not well established but generally risk is felt to be decreased in 6–12 weeks. However, bilateral ARN has been reported up to 34 years after the first eye was affected,[19] raising a question as to utility of very long-term or life-long prophylaxis in patients who have lost vision in one eye from ARN syndrome. Risk of second-eye involvement may also be dependent on the etiologic agent causing disease. Additionally, rare cases of reactivation in the originally affected eye have been reported.[99]

Retinal tears at the junction of normal and necrotic retina, as well as subsequent proliferative retinopathy creating a complicated combined traction-rhegmatogenous retinal detachment, pose a difficult problem in the management of ARN. Whereas Peyman et al.[7,18] obtained good results in selected patients with intravenous and intravitreal acyclovir in conjunction with prophylactic vitrectomy and scleral buckles in an uncontrolled study of active ARN cases that had not yet developed detachment, others have not been able to prevent retinal detachment by similar management,[100] while still others have found decreased incidence of secondary detachment, but no improvement in final mean visual acuity.[101] In a study of 13 eyes of 12 ARN patients, the incidence of retinal detachment despite intravenous acyclovir therapy was 84%, suggesting that antiviral therapy alone does not effectively preclude retinal detachment.

The use of prophylactic laser has been an issue of great debate in recent years. Several studies have demonstrated the benefit of prophylactic laser photocoagulation posterior to areas of active retinitis,[28,46,83,102] while others have found no decrease in the risk of retinal detachment.[103,104] One reason for this variability may be the small sample sizes used in these studies. Investigators have also postulated that generally the eyes receiving prophylactic photocoagulation have less vitritis, which allows for treatment. It is thought that vitritis over necrotic retina increases the risk of retinal detachment. They further reason that the eyes unable to receive prophylactic photocoagulation because of media opacity are at higher risk for retinal detachment than those with less vitritis and subsequently clearer media.[84] Without prospective randomized controlled studies, this question may not be definitively answered. Unfortunately, given the infrequency of this disease, it may be difficult to perform such a study.

One study found that retinal detachments appear to happen anywhere from 9 to 148 days from the onset of symptoms, so these eyes should be carefully examined at each office visit.[44] With the use of modern microsurgical techniques, including intravitreal silicone oil, air–fluid exchange, demarcating laser photocoagulation, and a long-acting gas tamponade, a high percentage of retinas can be anatomically reattached. However, it must be kept in mind that patients with minimal vision secondary to optic atrophy, macular pucker, or retinal dysfunction before detachment are unlikely to obtain improved visual function despite anatomically successful retinal reattachment.

As ARN syndrome appears to be due to reactivation of preexisting herpes viral infection with VZV or HSV, it is logical to ask whether vaccination might reduce the incidence of ARN syndrome. Zostavax® is an attenuated live herpes zoster virus vaccine that carries indication for reduction of incidence of shingles in individuals over age 60. In a large study of over 38 000 individuals, the vaccine reduced the incidence of shingles episodes by approximately 50%, with greater effect seen in the cohort of 60–70-year-olds than in those over age 80.[105] However, as this population is older than the typical ARN syndrome population, it is unclear whether use of this vaccine will impact rates of disease. Of greater interest is the question of whether childhood chickenpox vaccination with attenuated live virus will impact development of ARN syndrome. Reactivation of attenuated vaccine resulting in herpetic meningitis has been described[106] but to date no cases of ARN syndrome associated with vaccine reactivation have been reported. Similar questions will continue to arise with development of vaccines against HSV-1 and HSV-2.[107]

The syndrome of ARN remains a relatively recently described, potentially visually devastating disorder with multifactorial pathogenesis. Its successful management appears to depend on further advances in antiviral chemotherapy, control of the ischemic vasculopathy, and prevention of proliferative vitreoretinopathy.

REFERENCES

1. Urayama A, Yamada N, Sasaki T, et al. Unilateral acute uveitis with retinal periarteritis and detachment. Jpn J Clin Ophthalmol 1971;25:607–19.
2. Young NJ, Bird AC. Bilateral acute retinal necrosis. Br J Ophthalmol 1978;62(9):581–90.
3. Duker JS, Nielsen JC, Eagle Jr RC, et al. Rapidly progressive acute retinal necrosis secondary to herpes simplex virus, type 1. Ophthalmology 1990;97(12):1638–43.
4. el Azazi M, Samuelsson A, Linde A, et al. Intrathecal antibody production against viruses of the herpesvirus family in acute retinal necrosis syndrome. Am J Ophthalmol 1991;112(1):76–82.
5. Lewis ML, Culbertson WW, Post JD, et al. Herpes simplex virus type 1. A cause of the acute retinal necrosis syndrome. Ophthalmology 1989;96(6): 875–8.
6. Margolis T, Irvine AR, Hoyt WF, et al. Acute retinal necrosis syndrome presenting with papillitis and arcuate neuroretinitis. Ophthalmology 1988;95(7): 937–40.
7. Peyman GA, Goldberg MF, Uninsky E, et al. Vitrectomy and intravitreal antiviral drug therapy in acute retinal necrosis syndrome. Report of two cases. Arch Ophthalmol 1984;102(11):1618–21.
8. Watanabe J, Ashida M, Funaki A, et al. [A case of acute retinal necrosis syndrome caused by herpes simplex virus type 1.] Nippon Ganka Gakkai Zasshi 1989;93(1):65–71.
9. Fox GM, Blumenkranz M. Giant retinal pigment epithelial tears in acute retinal necrosis. Am J Ophthalmol 1993;116(3):302–6.
10. Matsuo T, Date S, Tsuji T, et al. Immune complex containing herpesvirus antigen in a patient with acute retinal necrosis. Am J Ophthalmol 1986;101(3): 368–71.
11. Ahmadieh H, Soheilian M, Azarmina M, et al. Surgical management of retinal detachment secondary to acute retinal necrosis: clinical features, surgical techniques, and long-term results. Jpn J Ophthalmol 2003;47(5):484–91.
12. Litoff D, Catalano RA. Herpes zoster optic neuritis in human immunodeficiency virus infection. Arch Ophthalmol 1990;108(6):782–3.
13. Sergott RC, Anand R, Belmont JB, et al. Acute retinal necrosis neuropathy. Clinical profile and surgical therapy. Arch Ophthalmol 1989;107(5):692–6.
14. Sergott RC, Belmont JB, Savino PJ, et al. Optic nerve involvement in the acute retinal necrosis syndrome. Arch Ophthalmol 1985;103(8):1160–2.
15. Cardine S, Chaze PA, Bourcier F, et al. [Bilateral acute retinal necrosis syndrome associated with meningoencephalitis caused by herpes simplex virus 2. A case report.] J Fr Ophtalmol 2004;27(7):795–800.
16. Farrell TA, Wolf MD, Folk JC, et al. Magnetic resonance imaging in a patient with herpes zoster keratouveitis and contralateral acute retinal necrosis. Am J Ophthalmol 1991;112(6):735–6.
17. Labetoulle M, Kucera P, Ugolini G, et al. Neuronal pathways for the propagation of herpes simplex virus type 1 from one retina to the other in a murine model. J Gen Virol 2000;81(Pt 5):1201–10.
18. Carney MD, Peyman GA, Goldberg MF, et al. Acute retinal necrosis. Retina 1986;6(2):85–94.
19. Falcone PM, Brockhurst RJ. Delayed onset of bilateral acute retinal necrosis syndrome: a 34-year interval. Ann Ophthalmol 1993;25(10):373–4.
20. Blumenkranz MS, Culbertson WW, Clarkson JG, et al. Treatment of the acute retinal necrosis syndrome with intravenous acyclovir. Ophthalmology 1986;93(3):296–300.

21. Matsuo T, Nakayama T, Koyama T, et al. A proposed mild type of acute retinal necrosis syndrome. Am J Ophthalmol 1988;105(6):579–83.
22. Kelly SP, Rosenthal AR. Chickenpox chorioretinitis. Br J Ophthalmol 1990; 74(11):698–9.
23. Rochat C, Herbort CP. [Acute retinal necrosis syndrome. Lausanne cases, review of the literature and new physiopathogenetic hypothesis.] Klin Monatsbl Augenheilkd 1994;204(5):440–9.
24. Rochat C, Polla BS, Herbort CP. Immunological profiles in patients with acute retinal necrosis. Graefes Arch Clin Exp Ophthalmol 1996;234(9):547–52.
25. Pepose JS. Skin test with varicella-zoster virus antigen for ophthalmic herpes zoster. Am J Ophthalmol 1984;98(6):825–7.
26. Holland GN, Cornell PJ, Park MS, et al. An association between acute retinal necrosis syndrome and HLA-DQw7 and phenotype Bw62, DR4. Am J Ophthalmol 1989;108(4):370–4.
27. Ichikaw T, Sakai J, Usui M. HLA antigens of patients with Kirisawa's uveitis and herpetic keratitis. Atarashii Ganka. 1989;6:107–14.
28. Sternberg Jr P, Han DP, Yeo JH, et al. Photocoagulation to prevent retinal detachment in acute retinal necrosis. Ophthalmology 1988;95(10):1389–93.
29. Browning DJ, Blumenkranz MS, Culbertson WW, et al. Association of varicella zoster dermatitis with acute retinal necrosis syndrome. Ophthalmology 1987;94(6):602–6.
30. Yeo JH, Pepose JS, Stewart JA, et al. Acute retinal necrosis syndrome following herpes zoster dermatitis. Ophthalmology 1986;93(11):1418–22.
31. Sado K, Kimura T, Hotta Y, et al. Acute retinal necrosis syndrome associated with herpes simplex keratitis. Retina 1994;14(3):260–3.
32. Severin M, Neubauer H. Bilateral acute vascular retinal necrosis. Ophthalmologica 1981;182(4):199–203.
33. Shah AM, Oster SF, Freeman WR. Viral retinitis after intravitreal triamcinolone injection in patients with predisposing medical comorbidities. Am J Ophthalmol 2010;149(3):433–40.
34. Aggermann T, Stolba U, Brunner S, et al. Endophthalmitis with retinal necrosis following intravitreal triamcinolone acetonide injection. Ophthalmologica 2006;220(2):131–3.
35. Toh T, Borthwick JH. Acute retinal necrosis post intravitreal injection of triamcinolone acetonide. Clin Experiment Ophthalmol 2006;34(4):380–2.
36. Neetens A, Stevens W, Taelman R, et al. Immune deficiency and necrotising retinopathy. Bull Soc Belge Ophtalmol 1985;215:73–86.
37. Batisse D, Eliaszewicz M, Zazoun L, et al. Acute retinal necrosis in the course of AIDS: study of 26 cases. AIDS 1996;10(1):55–60.
38. Freeman WR, Thomas EL, Rao NA, et al. Demonstration of herpes group virus in acute retinal necrosis syndrome. Am J Ophthalmol 1986;102(6):701–9.
39. Jabs DA, Schachat AP, Liss R, et al. Presumed varicella zoster retinitis in immunocompromised patients. Retina 1987;7(1):9–13.
40. Chambers RB, Derick RJ, Davidorf FH, et al. Varicella-zoster retinitis in human immunodeficiency virus infection. Case report. Arch Ophthalmol 1989;107(7):960–1.
41. Freeman WR, Wiley CA, Gross JG, et al. Endoretinal biopsy in immunosuppressed and healthy patients with retinitis. Indications, utility, and techniques. Ophthalmology 1989;96(10):1559–65.
42. Holland GN. Standard diagnostic criteria for the acute retinal necrosis syndrome. Executive Committee of the American Uveitis Society. Am J Ophthalmol 1994;117(5):663–7.
43. Muthiah MN, Michaelides M, Child CS, et al. Acute retinal necrosis: a national population-based study to assess the incidence, methods of diagnosis, treatment strategies and outcomes in the UK. Br J Ophthalmol 2007;91(11): 1452–5.
44. Lau CH, Missotten T, Salzmann J, et al. Acute retinal necrosis features, management, and outcomes. Ophthalmology 2007;114(4):756–62.
45. Culbertson WW, Blumenkranz MS, Pepose JS, et al. Varicella zoster virus is a cause of the acute retinal necrosis syndrome. Ophthalmology 1986;93(5): 559–69.
46. Culbertson WW, Blumenkranz MS, Haines H, et al. The acute retinal necrosis syndrome. Part 2: Histopathology and etiology. Ophthalmology 1982;89(12): 1317–25.
47. Cunningham Jr ET, Short GA, Irvine AR, et al. Acquired immunodeficiency syndrome: associated herpes simplex virus retinitis. Clinical description and use of a polymerase chain reaction-based assay as a diagnostic tool. Arch Ophthalmol 1996;114(7):834–40.
48. Pepose JS, Flowers B, Stewart JA, et al. Herpesvirus antibody levels in the etiologic diagnosis of the acute retinal necrosis syndrome. Am J Ophthalmol 1992;113(3):248–56.
49. Van Gelder RN, Willig JL, Holland GN, et al. Herpes simplex virus type 2 as a cause of acute retinal necrosis syndrome in young patients. Ophthalmology 2001;108(5):869–76.
50. Soushi S, Ozawa H, Matsuhashi M, et al. Demonstration of varicella-zoster virus antigens in the vitreous aspirates of patients with acute retinal necrosis syndrome. Ophthalmology 1988;95(10):1394–8.
51. Pepose JS, Biron K. Antiviral sensitivities of the acute retinal necrosis syndrome virus. Curr Eye Res 1987;6(1):201–5.
52. Abe T, Sato M, Tamai M. Variable R1 region in varicella zoster virus in fulminant type of acute retinal necrosis syndrome. Br J Ophthalmol 2000;84(2): 193–8.
53. Ludwig IH, Zegarra H, Zakov ZN. The acute retinal necrosis syndrome. Possible herpes simplex retinitis. Ophthalmology 1984;91(12):1659–64.
54. Margolis TP, Lowder CY, Holland GN, et al. Varicella-zoster virus retinitis in patients with the acquired immunodeficiency syndrome. Am J Ophthalmol 1991;112(2):119–31.
55. Rahhal FM, Siegel LM, Russak V, et al. Clinicopathologic correlations in acute retinal necrosis caused by herpes simplex virus type 2. Arch Ophthalmol 1996;114(11):1416–9.
56. Thompson WS, Culbertson WW, Smiddy WE, et al. Acute retinal necrosis caused by reactivation of herpes simplex virus type 2. Am J Ophthalmol 1994;118(2):205–11.
57. Ganatra JB, Chandler D, Santos C, et al. Viral causes of the acute retinal necrosis syndrome. Am J Ophthalmol 2000;129(2):166–72.
58. Tan JCH, Byles D, Stanford MR, et al. Acute retinal necrosis in children caused by herpes simplex virus. Retina 2001;21(4):344–7.
59. Hashido M, Lee FK, Nahmias AJ, et al. An epidemiologic study of herpes simplex virus type 1 and 2 infection in Japan based on type-specific serological assays. Epidemiol Infect 1998;120(2):179–86.
60. Itoh N, Matsumura N, Ogi A, et al. High prevalence of herpes simplex virus type 2 in acute retinal necrosis syndrome associated with herpes simplex virus in Japan. Am J Ophthalmol 2000;129(3):404–5.
61. Gain P, Chiquet C, Thuret G, et al. Herpes simplex virus type 1 encephalitis associated with acute retinal necrosis syndrome in an immunocompetent patient. Acta Ophthalmol Scand 2002;80(5):546–9.
62. Gaynor BD, Wade NK, Cunningham Jr ET. Herpes simplex virus type 1 associated acute retinal necrosis following encephalitis. Retina 2001;21(6):688–90.
63. Kim C, Yoon YH. Unilateral acute retinal necrosis occurring 2 years after herpes simplex type 1 encephalitis. Ophthalmic Surg Lasers 2002;33(3): 250–2.
64. Tada Y, Negoro K, Morimatsu M, et al. Findings in a patient with herpes simplex viral meningitis associated with acute retinal necrosis syndrome. AJNR Am J Neuroradiol 2001;22(7):1300–2.
65. Maertzdorf J, Van der Lelij A, Baarsma GS, et al. Herpes simplex virus type 1 (HSV-1)-induced retinitis following herpes simplex encephalitis: indications for brain-to-eye transmission of HSV-1. Ann Neurol 2000;48(6):936–9.
66. Rungger-Brandle E, Roux L, Leuenberger PM. Bilateral acute retinal necrosis (BARN). Identification of the presumed infectious agent. Ophthalmology 1984;91(12):1648–58.
67. Silverstein BE, Conrad D, Margolis TP, et al. Cytomegalovirus-associated acute retinal necrosis syndrome. Am J Ophthalmol 1997;123(2):257–8.
68. Kramer S, Brummer C, Zierhut M. Epstein–Barr virus associated acute retinal necrosis. Br J Ophthalmol 2001;85(1):114.
69. Gallego-Pinazo R, Harto M, Garcia-Medina JJ, et al. Epstein–Barr virus and acute retinal necrosis in a 5-year-old immunocompetent child. Clin Ophthalmol 2008;2(2):451–5.
70. Chodosh J, Gan YJ, Sixbey JW. Detection of Epstein–Barr virus genome in ocular tissues. Ophthalmology 1996;103(4):687–90.
71. Rummelt V, Wenkel H, Rummelt C, et al. Detection of varicella zoster virus DNA and viral antigen in the late stage of bilateral acute retinal necrosis syndrome. Arch Ophthalmol 1992;110(8):1132–6.
72. Vann VR, Atherton SS. Neural spread of herpes simplex virus after anterior chamber inoculation. Invest Ophthalmol Vis Sci 1991;32(9):2462–72.
73. Levy-Clarke GA, Buggage RR, Shen D, et al. Human T-cell lymphotropic virus type-1 associated t-cell leukemia/lymphoma masquerading as necrotizing retinal vasculitis. Ophthalmology 2002;109(9):1717–22.
74. Forster DJ, Dugel PU, Frangieh GT, et al. Rapidly progressive outer retinal necrosis in the acquired immunodeficiency syndrome. Am J Ophthalmol 1990;110(4):341–8.
75. Gariano RF, Berreen JP, Cooney EL. Progressive outer retinal necrosis and acute retinal necrosis in fellow eyes of a patient with acquired immunodeficiency syndrome. Am J Ophthalmol 2001;132(3):421–3.
76. Short GA, Margolis TP, Kuppermann BD, et al. A polymerase chain reaction-based assay for diagnosing varicella-zoster virus retinitis in patients with acquired immunodeficiency syndrome. Am J Ophthalmol 1997;123(2): 157–64.
77. Dabil H, Boley ML, Schmitz TM, et al. Validation of a diagnostic multiplex polymerase chain reaction assay for infectious posterior uveitis. Arch Ophthalmol 2001;119(9):1315–22.
78. Dworkin LL, Gibler TM, Van Gelder RN. Real-time quantitative polymerase chain reaction diagnosis of infectious posterior uveitis. Arch Ophthalmol 2002;120(11):1534–9.
79. Asano S, Yoshikawa T, Kimura H, et al. Monitoring herpesvirus DNA in three cases of acute retinal necrosis by real-time PCR. J Clin Virol 2004;29(3): 206–9.
80. Cottet L, Kaiser L, Hirsch HH, et al. HSV2 acute retinal necrosis: diagnosis and monitoring with quantitative polymerase chain reaction. Int Ophthalmol 2009;29(3):199–201.
81. Luyendijk L, vd Horn GJ, Visser OH, et al. Detection of locally produced antibodies to herpes viruses in the aqueous of patients with acquired immune deficiency syndrome (AIDS) or acute retinal necrosis syndrome (ARN). Curr Eye Res 1990;9(Suppl):7–11.
82. Blumenkranz M, Clarkson J, Culbertson WW, et al. Vitrectomy for retinal detachment associated with acute retinal necrosis. Am J Ophthalmol 1988;106(4):426–9.
83. Crapotta JA, Freeman WR, Feldman RM, et al. Visual outcome in acute retinal necrosis. Retina 1993;13(3):208–13.
84. Tibbetts MD, Shah CP, Young LH, et al. Treatment of acute retinal necrosis. Ophthalmology 2010;117(4):818–24.
85. Figueroa MS, Garabito I, Gutierrez C, et al. Famciclovir for the treatment of acute retinal necrosis (ARN) syndrome. Am J Ophthalmol 1997;123(2):255–7.
86. Klein JL, Sandy C, Migdal CS, et al. Famciclovir in AIDS-related acute retinal necrosis. AIDS 1996;10(11):1300–1.

87. Figueroa MS, Garabito I, Gutierrez C, et al. Famciclovir for the treatment of acute retinal necrosis (ARN) syndrome. Am J Ophthalmol 1997;123(2):255–7.
88. Aslanides IM, De Souza S, Wong DT, et al. Oral valacyclovir in the treatment of acute retinal necrosis syndrome. Retina 2002;22(3):352–4.
89. Emerson GG, Smith JR, Wilson DJ, et al. Primary treatment of acute retinal necrosis with oral antiviral therapy. Ophthalmology 2006;113(12):2259–61.
90. Pepose JS. The potential impact of the varicella vaccine and new antivirals on ocular disease related to varicella-zoster virus. Am J Ophthalmol 1997;123(2): 243–51.
91. Savant V, Saeed T, Denniston A, et al. Oral valganciclovir treatment of varicella zoster virus acute retinal necrosis. Eye (Lond) 2004;18(5):544–5.
92. Guex-Crosier Y, Meylan PR. High dosage of oral valaciclovir as an alternative treatment of varicella zoster acute retinal necrosis syndrome. Eye (Lond). 2006;20(2):247.
93. Aizman A, Johnson MW, Elner SG. Treatment of acute retinal necrosis syndrome with oral antiviral medications. Ophthalmology 2007;114(2): 307–12.
94. Chau Tran TH, Cassoux N, Bodaghi B, et al. Successful treatment with combination of systemic antiviral drugs and intravitreal ganciclovir injections in the management of severe necrotizing herpetic retinitis. Ocul Immunol Inflamm 2003;11(2):141–4.
95. Luu KK, Scott IU, Chaudhry NA, et al. Intravitreal antiviral injections as adjunctive therapy in the management of immunocompetent patients with necrotizing herpetic retinopathy. Am J Ophthalmol 2000;129(6):811–3.
96. Scott IU, Luu KM, Davis JL. Intravitreal antivirals in the management of patients with acquired immunodeficiency syndrome with progressive outer retinal necrosis. Arch Ophthalmol 2002;120(9):1219–22.
97. Roig-Melo EA, Macky TA, Heredia-Elizondo ML, et al. Progressive outer retinal necrosis syndrome: successful treatment with a new combination of antiviral drugs. Eur J Ophthalmol 2001;11(2):200–2.
98. Ando F, Kato M, Goto S, et al. Platelet function in bilateral acute retinal necrosis. Am J Ophthalmol 1983;96(1):27–32.
99. Matsuo T, Nakayama T, Baba T. Same eye recurrence of acute retinal necrosis syndrome. Am J Ophthalmol 2001;131(5):659–61.
100. Blumenkranz M, Clarkson J, Culbertson WW, et al. Visual results and complications after retinal reattachment in the acute retinal necrosis syndrome. The influence of operative technique. Retina 1989;9(3):170–4.
101. Hillenkamp J, N'lle B, Bruns C, et al. Acute retinal necrosis: clinical features, early vitrectomy, and outcomes. Ophthalmology 2009;116(10):1971–5.
102. Han DP, Lewis H, Williams GA, et al. Laser photocoagulation in the acute retinal necrosis syndrome. Arch Ophthalmol 1987;105(8):1051–4.
103. McDonald HR, Lewis H, Kreiger AE, et al. Surgical management of retinal detachment associated with the acute retinal necrosis syndrome. Br J Ophthalmol 1991;75(8):455–8.
104. Tibbetts MD, Shah CP, Young LH, et al. Treatment of acute retinal necrosis. Ophthalmology 2010;117(4):818–24.
105. Oxman M. A vaccine to prevent herpes zoster and postherpetic neuralgia in older adults. N Engl J Med 2005;352(22):2271–84.
106. Han J, Hanson D, Way S. Herpes zoster and meningitis due to reactivation of varicella vaccine virus in an immunocompetent child. Pediatr Infect Dis J 2011;30(3):266–8.
107. Pepose J, Keadle T, Morrison L. Ocular herpes simplex: changing epidemiology, emerging disease patterns, and the potential of vaccine prevention and therapy. Am J Ophthalmol 2006;141(3):547–57.

Chapter 89

Drug Toxicity of the Posterior Segment

Robert A. Mittra, William F. Mieler

A variety of systemic medications can generate retinal toxicity. Fortunately, in the majority of cases the loss of visual function is minimal or reversible following discontinuation of the inciting drug. Nevertheless, permanent or progressive visual loss may occur in some instances. We present those medications known to produce a well-described anomaly and have omitted others that have not been definitively proven to cause retinal abnormalities. The medications are grouped according to the type of retinal toxicity they produce, summarized in Box 89.1.

Box 89.1 Patterns of retinal toxicity

Disruption of the retina and retinal pigment epithelium
Phenothiazines
Thioridazine
Chlorpromazine
Chloroquine derivatives
Chloroquine
Hydroxychloroquine
Quinine sulfate
Clofazimine
Deferoxamine
Corticosteroid preparations
Cisplatin and BCNU (carmustine)

Vascular damage
Quinine sulfate
Cisplatin and BCN
Talc
Oral contraceptives
Aminoglycoside antibiotics
Interferon (carmustine)
Ergot alkaloids
Phenylpropanolamine

Cystoid macular edema
Epinephrine
Latanoprost
Nicotinic acid
Paclitaxel/docetaxel

Retinal folds
Acetazolamide
Chlorthalidone
Ethoxyzolamide
Hydrochlorothiazide
Metronidazole
Sulfa antibiotics
Triamterene

Crystalline retinopathy
Tamoxifen
Canthaxanthine
Methoxyflurane
Talc
Nitrofurantoin

Uveitis
Rifabutin
Cidofovir

Miscellaneous
Digoxin
Methanol

DISRUPTION OF THE RETINA AND RETINAL PIGMENT EPITHELIUM

Phenothiazines

Thioridazine

Blurred vision, dyschromatopsia (reddish or brownish discoloration of vision), and nyctalopia characterize acute toxicity with thioridazine.[1] In the earliest stages the fundus appearance may be normal or display only mild granular pigment stippling (Fig. 89.1). An intermediate stage is characterized by circumscribed nummular areas of retinal pigment epithelial (RPE) loss from the posterior pole to the midperiphery[2] (Fig. 89.2A). Fluorescein angiography (FA) reveals disruption of the choriocapillaris in these zones of pigment rarefaction (Fig. 89.2B). In late stages of thioridazine toxicity, widespread areas of depigmentation alternating with hyperpigmented plaques, vascular attenuation, and optic atrophy are seen[3] (Fig. 89.3).

Retinal toxicity from thioridazine is dependent more on the total daily dose than on the cumulative amount of drug received.[4]

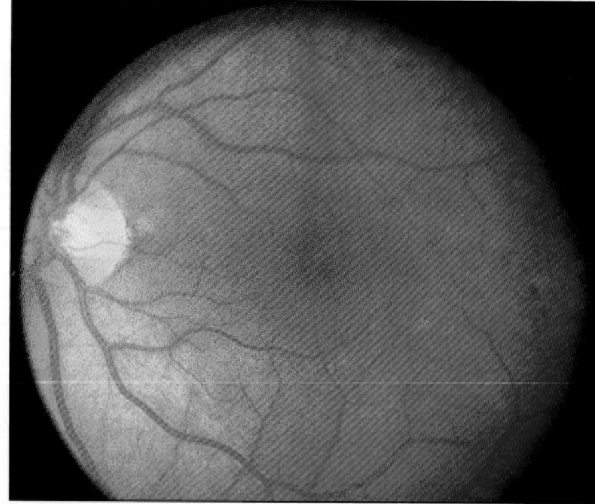

Fig. 89.1 Early thioridazine toxicity. Photograph shows mild granular pigment stippling temporal to the macular region.

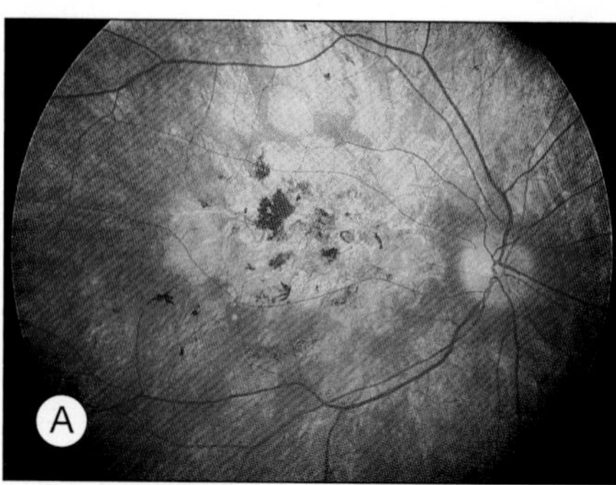

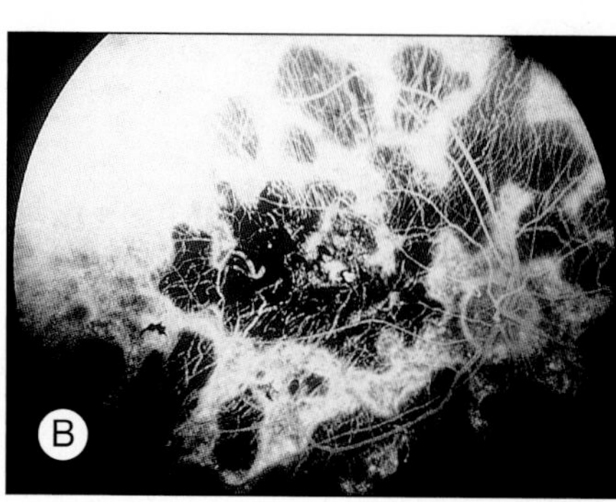

Fig. 89.2 Intermediate thioridazine toxicity. Photograph (A) and fluorescein angiogram (B) show central and peripheral nummular pigmentary changes with corresponding atrophy of the choriocapillaris.

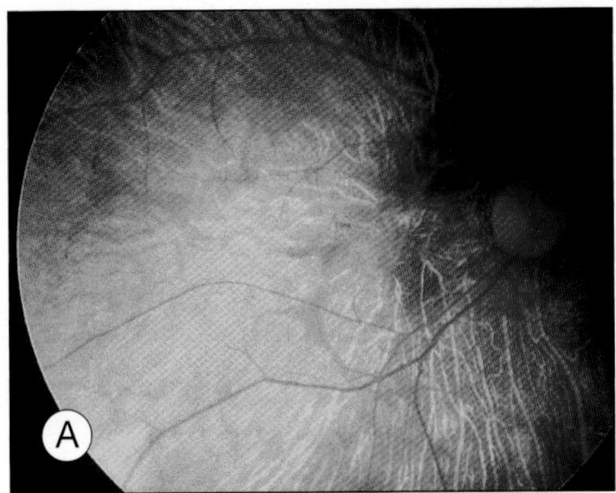

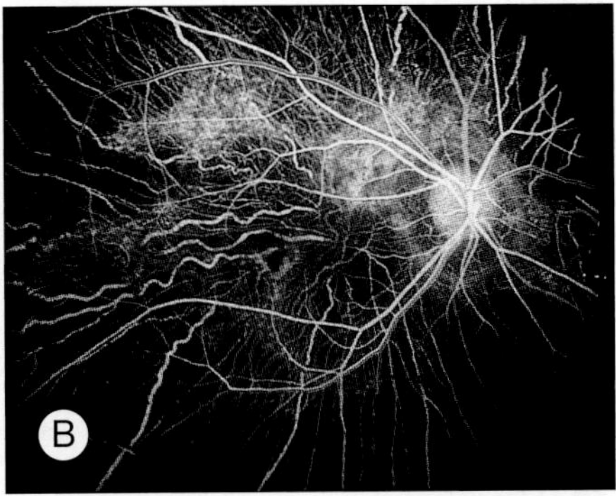

Fig. 89.3 Endstage thioridazine toxicity. Photograph (A) and fluorescein angiogram (B) show diffuse pigmentary and choriocapillaris atrophy, optic atrophy, and vascular attenuation. This severe endstage disease resembles choroideremia.

With higher daily doses, toxicity can occur rapidly, even within the first two weeks of therapy.[5] Toxicity is rare at dosages less than 800 mg/day. Nonetheless, a few cases have been reported with lower doses given over several years.[6-10] As a result, many now suggest that any patient taking thioridazine, regardless of the daily dose, should be monitored for the development of visual symptoms or fundus changes.

In the initial stages of toxicity, visual field testing can reveal mild constriction, paracentral scotomas, or ring scotomas. Electroretinography (ERG) is either normal or shows decreased oscillatory potentials. In the later stages, both the rod and cone functions of the ERG, as well as electrooculography (EOG), are markedly abnormal.[11] If the drug is stopped early, ERG testing often improves over the first year.[12] Histologic studies demonstrate that atrophy and disorganization of photoreceptor outer segments occurs primarily, with a secondary loss of the RPE and choriocapillaris.[3]

The early fundus changes associated with thioridazine often progress despite discontinuation of therapy.[2] It is unclear whether this degeneration represents continued toxicity of the drug or a delayed expansion of chorioretinal scarring to areas of subclinical, preexisting damage.[12] Visual function, in contrast to fundus appearance, usually improves over the first year after a toxic reaction, but there has been one report of severe progressive decline in vision after cessation of the drug.[13]

The mechanism of thioridazine-mediated toxicity remains unknown. Many phenothiazines bind melanin granules of the RPE and uveal tissue, but not all commonly instigate retinal toxicity.[14-16] The compound NP-207 (piperidylchlorophenothiazine hydrochloride) has a remarkably similar chemical structure to thioridazine, including the same piperidyl side chain. NP-207 was never marketed because of the pronounced pigmentary retinopathy that developed during early clinical trials.[17] This piperidyl side chain is not present in other phenothiazines such as chlorpromazine, which exhibit much less retinal toxicity. Experimental studies demonstrate that phenothiazines both alter enzyme kinetics and inhibit oxidative phosphorylation with subsequent abnormalities in rhodopsin synthesis.[18-20] Other studies postulate that phenothiazine toxicity is due to the drug's effect on the dopamine receptors in the retina.[21] Further study is necessary to determine whether these observed effects are involved in the pathogenesis of thioridazine toxicity.

A review of the daily and cumulative drug dosage is essential in patients taking thioridazine. Baseline fundus photography and possibly ERG testing may be helpful if future toxicity develops. Given the many antipsychotic medications available today, consideration of alternative agents may be discussed with the patient's psychiatrist. At the earliest sign of toxicity, thioridazine should be discontinued.

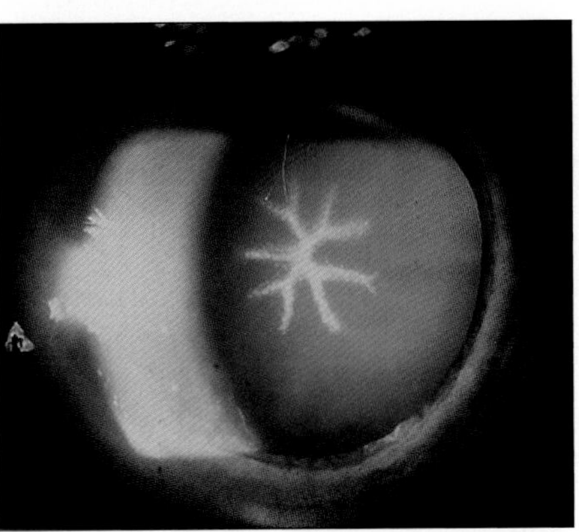

Fig. 89.4 Typical chlorpromazine-induced anterior stellate lens opacities. These findings are generally not felt to be of visual significance.

Chlorpromazine

Chlorpromazine is a piperazine similar to thioridazine but lacks the piperidyl side chain mentioned above. The compound binds strongly to melanin and can cause hyperpigmentation in the skin, conjunctiva, cornea, lens, and retina[22-28] (Fig. 89.4). Other ocular effects include oculogyric crisis, miosis, and blurred vision caused by paralysis of accommodation. Usual doses range from 40 to 75 mg/day, but dosages up to 800 mg/day are not uncommon.

Retinal toxicity from chlorpromazine is rare. When massive doses are given (e.g., 2400 mg/day for 12 months), pigmentary changes may occur in the retina with attenuation of retinal vessels and optic nerve pallor[25] (Fig. 89.5). Similar to thioridazine, the development and extent of toxicity are more closely related to daily dosage than total amount of drug taken.

Chloroquine derivatives

Chloroquine

Chloroquine was first used as an antimalarial drug in World War II. Currently it is prescribed for treatment of amebiasis, rheumatoid arthritis, and systemic lupus erythematosus in countries primarily outside the United States, and for prophylaxis against malaria. Retinal toxicity with degeneration of the RPE and neurosensory retina as a result of long-term daily use of chloroquine has been well described.[29-35] However, most cases of retinopathy have developed when a higher than currently recommended (3 mg/kg/day using lean body weight) dose was used.[36]A daily

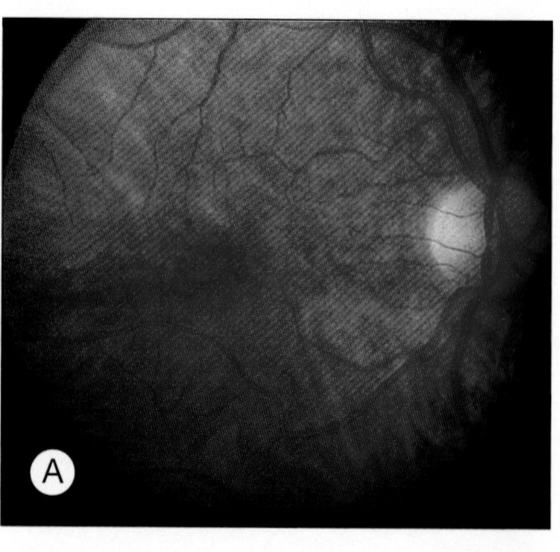

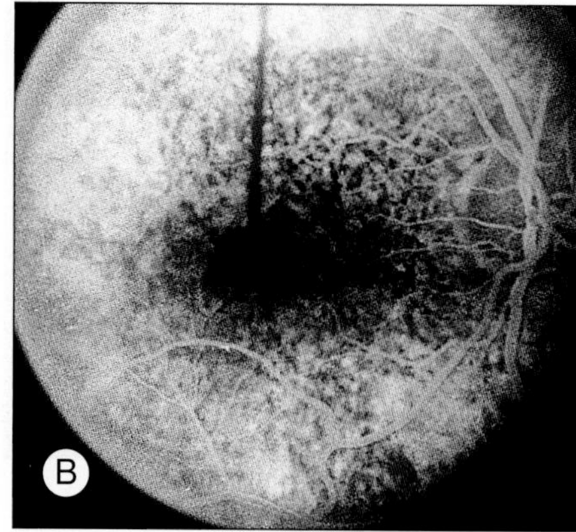

Fig. 89.5 Chlorpromazine toxicity. Photograph (A) and fluorescein angiogram (B) show granular pigmentary changes, though less severe than those generally seen with thioridazine.

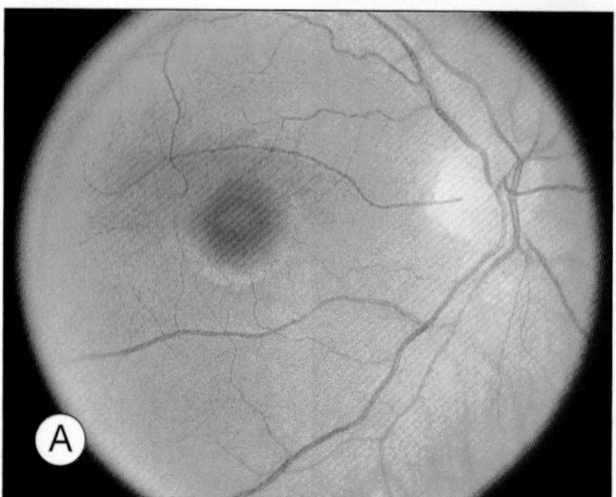

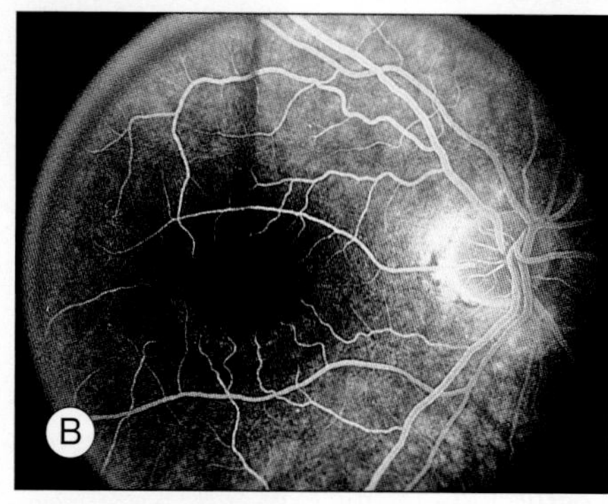

Fig. 89.6 Early chloroquine toxicity. Photograph (A) and fluorescein angiogram (B) show early perifoveal pigmentary changes. (Reproduced with permission from Mieler WF. Focal points. American Academy of Ophthalmology, December 1997.)

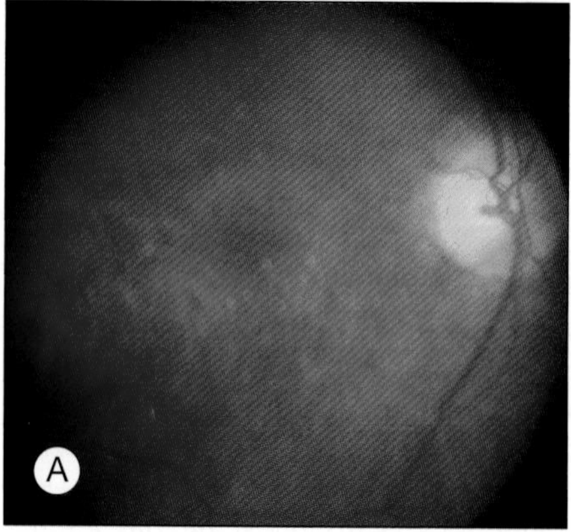

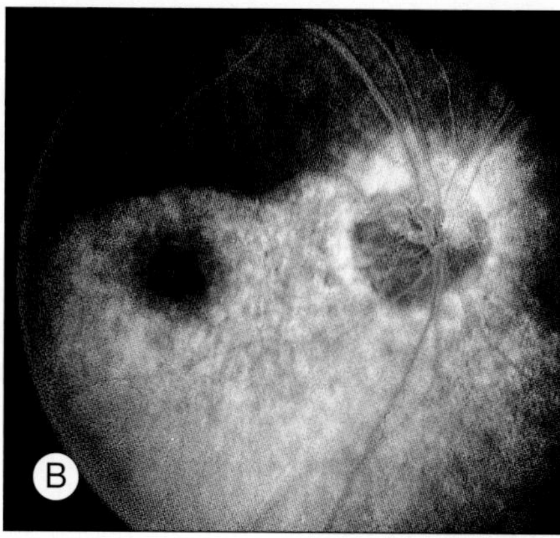

Fig. 89.7 Advanced chloroquine toxicity. Later photograph (A) and fluorescein angiogram (B) from the patient in Fig. 89.6 show marked progression with advanced widespread pigmentary changes. (Reproduced with permission from Mieler WF. Focal points. American Academy of Ophthalmology, December 1997.)

dose exceeding 250 mg with a total cumulative dose between 100 and 300 g is customarily needed to produce toxicity.[37] One study showed a 19% incidence of chloroquine retinopathy in patients taking a mean daily dose of 329 mg.[38] Conversely, with strict adherence to a low dose per diem, the incidence of retinal abnormalities is minimal even when cumulative doses reach over 1000 g.[39]

A paracentral scotoma may be the earliest manifestation of retinal toxicity and can precede the development of any ophthalmoscopic or ERG abnormality.[40] Subtle macular pigment stippling with a loss of the foveal light reflex (Fig. 89.6) usually appears on fundus examination before the development of a classic bull's-eye maculopathy, in which a ring of depigmentation surrounded by an area of hyperpigmentation is seen centered on the fovea (Fig. 89.7). Visual acuity decreases when the RPE abnormalities involve the center of the fovea. The peripheral retina can display pigment mottling, which may, in severe cases, develop into the appearance of primary tapetoretinal degeneration with narrowed retinal vessels, optic disc pallor, and eventual blindness (Fig. 89.8).

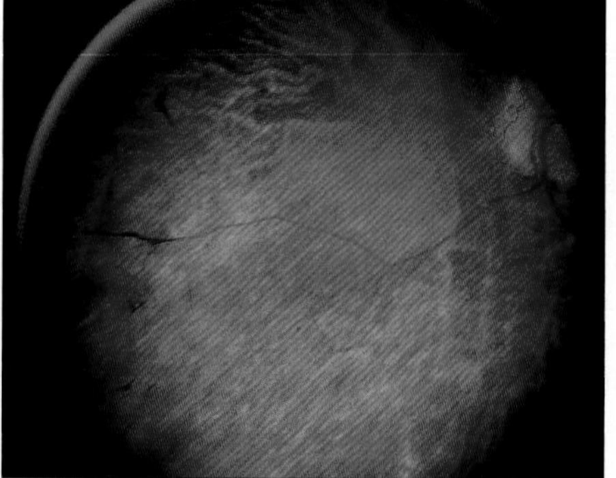

Fig. 89.8 Chloroquine retinopathy. Photograph shows bone-spicule pigmentary changes that can develop in advanced cases. The appearance is similar to endstage retinitis pigmentosa.

After the cessation of chloroquine treatment, early subtle macular changes can revert to normal. Although far advanced cases may progress despite discontinuation of the drug, most patients remain stable with long-term follow-up.[41,42] Chloroquine, however, is very slowly excreted from the body. It has been detected in the plasma, red blood cells, and urine of patients 5 years after their last known ingestion.[43] This prolonged presence may account for the rare cases of delayed onset of chloroquine retinopathy seen up to 7 years or longer after discontinuation.[44,45]

Fluorescein angiography can be helpful in the early demonstration of pigment abnormalities in the macula (see Figs 89.6, 89.7). There is minimal evidence of damage to the choriocapillaris on FA in the areas of pigment disturbance. The ERG and EOG may be abnormal early, although the EOG is sometimes supernormal initially and is not as helpful diagnostically.[46] Histopathologic sections demonstrate loss of RPE pigmentation with an accumulation of pigment-laden cells in the outer retinal layers with damage and reduction of photoreceptors.[47] Electron microscopic studies reveal more widespread damage to the retina, especially the ganglion cell layer.[48] The retinal nerve fiber layer thickness has been shown to be significantly decreased compared to normal in patients on chloroquine therapy and is correlated to the daily dose taken.[49] Fundus autofluorescence (FAF) and optical coherence tomography (OCT) findings suggest that the ganglion cell layer is affected by toxicity initially, especially surrounding the retinal vasculature.[50]

Like the phenothiazines, chloroquine is bound by melanin and concentrated in the RPE and uveal tissues.[51] It appears that chloroquine toxicity may be mediated by disruption of lysosomal function in the RPE and neural retina and by inhibition of critical enzymes and interference with their metabolic function.[44,52,53]

With the availability of hydroxychloroquine, a less toxic but similar medication, use of chloroquine has steadily waned. Screening for toxicity has been more fully evaluated recently for hydroxychloroquine (see below), and similar testing is likely appropriate for chloroquine as well. Color vision can be abnormal in early toxicity and use of the Standard Pseudoisochromatic Plates Part 2 (SPP-2) or the American Optical Hardy Rand Rittler (AO-HRR) color vision plates provides adequate sensitivity and specificity for detection of abnormalities.[54,55] Multifocal ERG testing may be abnormal in early toxicity even when other tests such as visual field and full-field ERG are normal.[56,57]

Hydroxychloroquine

Given the incidence of toxicity with chloroquine, most rheumatologists prefer hydroxychloroquine for the treatment of rheumatoid arthritis and systemic lupus erythematosus. Although it can produce a retinopathy identical to chloroquine, its occurrence is much less common.[58–61] Toxicity involving decreased visual acuity, paracentral scotoma, and a bull's-eye maculopathy has been documented[62–67] (Figs 89.9, 89.10). Many of these patients received above the recommended daily dosage of 6.5 mg/kg/day, but the classic fundus findings have been reported at lower doses as well.[62,64,67–69] Screening for toxicity becomes more important the longer the patient has been taking the drug as toxicity approaches 1% after 5–7 years of therapy and/or a cumulative dose of 1000 g.[70–72]

Several authors have questioned the utility of screening given the low yield, high cost, and the difficulty in diagnosing the condition early enough to prevent damage.[73–76] Nevertheless, if retinal and functional changes are detected early, severe visual impairment can be averted.[69,77]

The revised American Academy of Ophthalmology guidelines for screening include a baseline examination performed at the commencement of therapy.[78] Screening exams during the first five years of therapy can be performed during routine ophthalmic examination (interval to be determined by the age of the patient and the presence or absence of retinal or macular disease). Earlier recommendations emphasized dosing by weight. As most patients are given 400 mg/day of hydroxychloroquine, this dose is acceptable for all except for those with short stature (generally 5 feet 2 inches or less in height). These patients should be given a dose based on their ideal body weight, otherwise overdosage may occur.[79] Furthermore, the dosage may need to be altered if the patient has renal or liver dysfunction.

After five years of therapy, screening should be performed at least annually.[71] Current guidelines are centered around tests found to detect early toxicity often prior to any appreciable fundus findings. Patients should have a Humphrey 10–2 automated visual field test with a white test object and in addition should have one of three objective tests at each screening: multifocal electroretinogram (mfERG),[70,80–84] spectral domain OCT,[85–87] and/or FAF[88] (Fig. 89.11). Any abnormalities of the

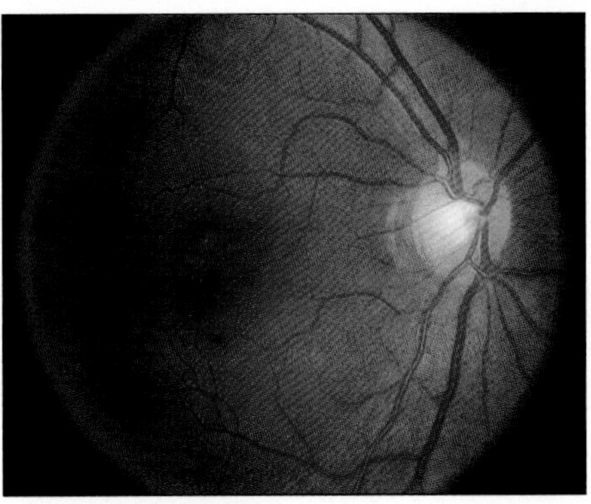

Fig. 89.9 Hydroxychloroquine toxicity. Photograph displays nonspecific pigmentary changes in the central macula.

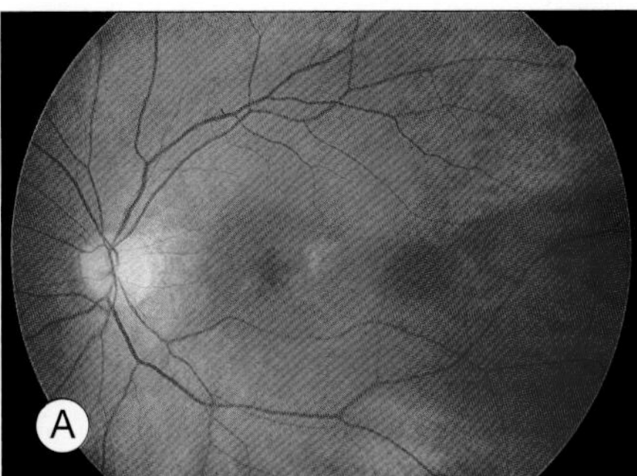

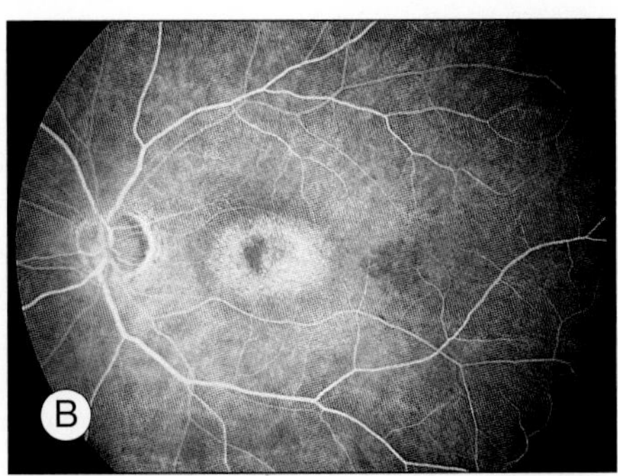

Fig. 89.10 Hydroxychloroquine toxicity. Photograph (A) and fluorescein angiogram (B) show a marked bull's-eye maculopathy, virtually identical to what has been described in association with chloroquine maculopathy. The patient was of short stature.

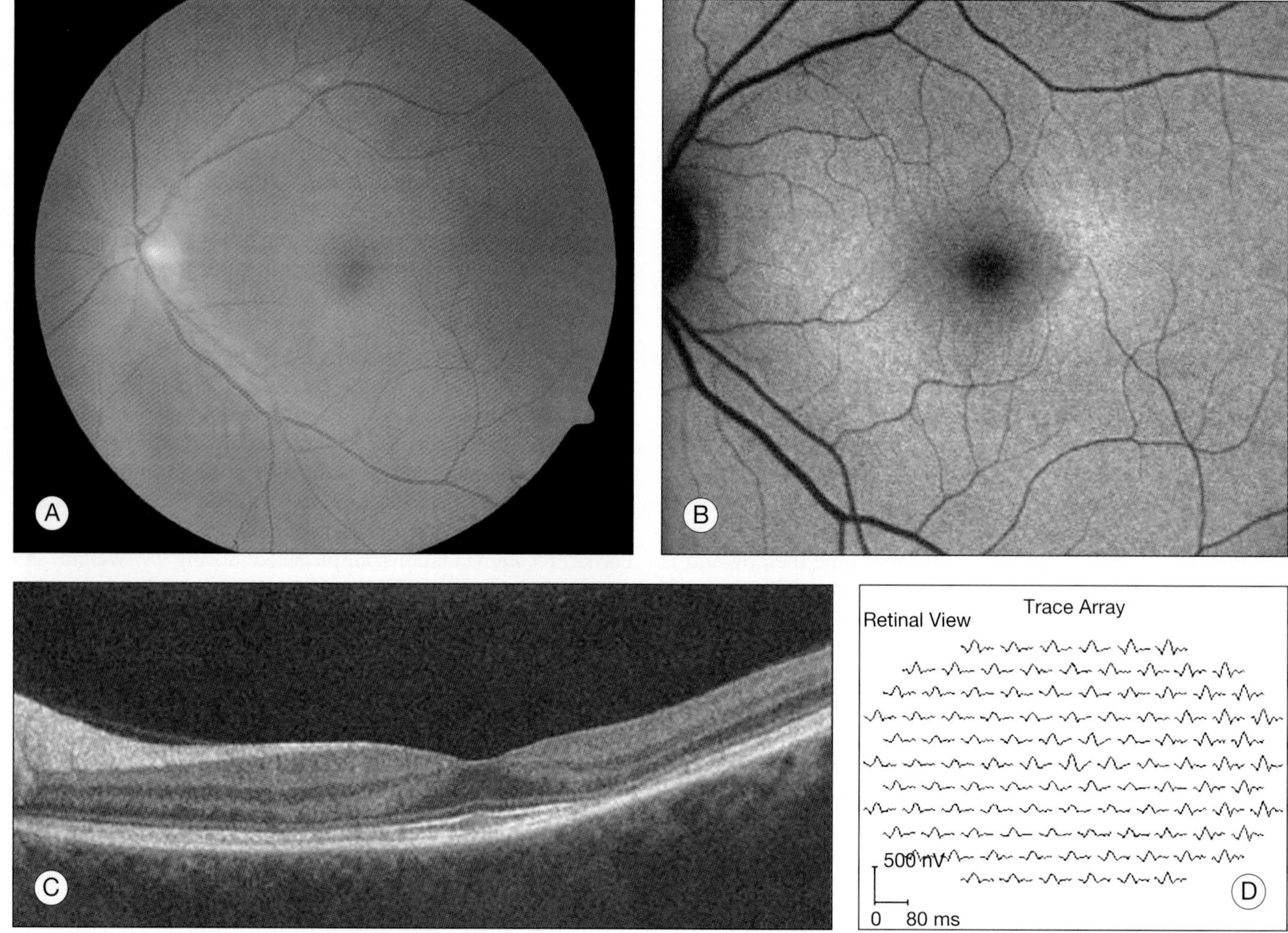

Fig. 89.11 Screening tests for hydroxychloroquine toxicity. Color photograph (A) showing very minimal macular pigment mottling in a patient on hydroxychloroquine for five years. Fundus autofluorescence (B) shows a minimal degree of abnormality in the macular region. Spectral domain optical coherence tomography (C) shows minimal disruption of the inner segment/outer segment junction. Multifocal electroretinogram (D) shows normal waveforms. (Courtesy of Michael Marmor, MD, Stanford, CA.)

pattern deviation on the Humphrey 10–2 visual fields should be taken seriously and the test repeated to confirm its reproducibility. In most situations, and since SD-OCT testing is so readily available, SD-OCT should also be obtained. While abnormalities on FAF are generally associated with concerns for active disease, the test has not yet been shown to be reliably predictable as a screening tool for future toxicity.

As noted in the preceding paragraph, it is imperative to discuss the risk of toxicity with patients and the rationale for screening (to detect, but not necessarily prevent visual loss).[78] If ocular toxicity occurs,[63,65,66,89] and is recognized at an early stage, efforts should be made to communicate this directly to the prescribing physician so that alternative treatment options can be discussed with the patient. In almost all cases, cessation of the drug should be suggested.

Quinine sulfate

Quinine sulfate was first used for the treatment of malaria in World War II, but it currently is prescribed for the management of nocturnal muscle cramps or "restless leg syndrome". The recommended daily dose is less than 2 g. Signs of systemic toxicity occur with doses greater than 4 g, and the fatal oral dose is 8 g. Ocular toxicity with quinine develops after an overdose, either by accidental ingestion or by attempted abortion or suicide. Rarely, chronic ingestion at low levels can result in ocular toxicity as well.[90] With an overdose, a syndrome known as *cinchonism* is rapidly produced, consisting of nausea, vomiting, headache, tremor, and sometimes hypotension and loss of consciousness. When patients awake they often are completely blind and have dilated, unreactive pupils.[91] In the acute stages of toxicity, fundus examination reveals mild venous dilation with minimal retinal edema and normal arterial caliber. The FA displays minimal abnormalities. ERG testing shows an acute slowing of the *a*-wave with increased depth, loss of oscillatory potentials, and a decreased *b*-wave.[92] EOG and visual-evoked potential (VEP) testing are also abnormal.

Over the next few days visual acuity returns, but the patient is left with a small central island of vision. There is a progressive attenuation of the retinal arterioles with the development of optic disc pallor over the next few weeks to months and iris depigmentation can occur[93] (Fig. 89.12). Early investigators believed the mechanism of quinine toxicity to be vascular in origin. This was based primarily on the fundus appearance several weeks after ingestion, which showed marked arteriolar attenuation and optic disc pallor.[91,94] More recent experimental and clinical studies have demonstrated minimal involvement of the retinal vasculature in the early stages of quinine toxicity.[91,94,95] Furthermore, ERG and histologic studies show that the site of toxicity is likely the retinal ganglion, bipolar, and photoreceptor cells.[91,95] The exact mechanism of quinine toxicity is unidentified, but some have suggested that it may act as an acetylcholine antagonist and disrupt cholinergic transmission in the retina.[96]

Clofazimine

Clofazimine is a red phenazine dye that has been used to treat dapsone-resistant leprosy, psoriasis, pyoderma gangrenosum, discoid lupus, and more recently, *Mycobacterium avium*-complex infections in AIDS patients. With treatment over several months, clofazimine crystals may accumulate in the cornea. Two cases of bull's-eye maculopathy with pigmentary retinopathy (Fig. 89.13) have been reported in AIDS patients with doses of 200 to 300 mg/day (total dose, 40–48 g).[97,98] Visual acuity was mildly affected, with reduced scotopic, photopic, and flicker ERG amplitudes. Cessation of treatment may result in the clearance of the corneal deposits but does not appear to affect the retinopathy.

Dideoxyinosine (DDI)

A midperipheral pigmentary retinopathy has been noted in three children with AIDS receiving high-dose therapy with the antiviral 2′, 3′-dideoxyinosine.[99] The cases were associated with ERG and EOG changes. The retinal toxicity stabilized after discontinuation of the medication. Several cases have now been described involving adult patients as well. A very similar midperipheral pattern of RPE abnormality has been noted (Fig. 89.14).

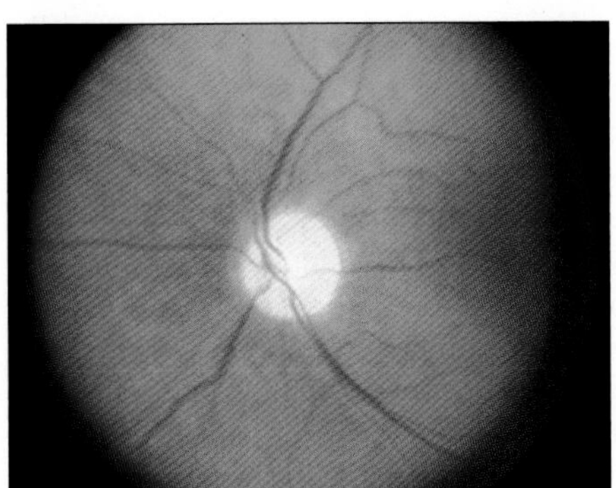

Fig. 89.12 Quinine toxicity. Photograph illustrates the characteristic optic nerve head pallor with diffuse arteriolar attenuation approximately two months after an intentional overdose of the medication.

Deferoxamine

Intravenous (IV) and subcutaneous (SQ) administration of deferoxamine has been used to treat patients who require repeated blood transfusions and subsequently develop complications of iron overload. High-dose IV and SQ therapy has produced visual loss, nyctalopia, peripheral and central field loss, and reduced ERG amplitudes and EOG ratios.[100,101] The fundus examination can be normal initially, or there may be a faint graying of the macula.[102] Pigmentary changes in the macula and periphery develop within a few weeks and are particularly highlighted by fluorescein angiography[103] (Fig. 89.15). Return of visual function occurs with cessation of therapy. Deferoxamine chelates many metals other than iron, and it is possible that the mechanism of toxicity may involve the removal of copper from the RPE.[100] Histopathologic changes occur primarily in the RPE and include loss of microvilli from the apical surface, patchy depigmentation, vacuolation of the cytoplasm, swelling and calcification of mitochondria, and disorganization of the plasma membrane.[104]

Corticosteroid preparations

The vehicles of several common corticosteroid preparations have been shown to cause retinal necrosis when inadvertently injected into the eye[105,106] (Fig. 89.16). The corticosteroids themselves probably have a minimal toxic effect on the retina.[107] Celestone Soluspan, with its vehicle benzalkonium chloride, and Depo-Medrol, with myristyl gamma-picolinium chloride, caused the most extensive retinal damage in an experimental study comparing several depot steroids.[108] If one of these agents is inadvertently injected, immediate surgical removal should be instituted.

Cisplatin and BCNU (carmustine)

Cisplatin and BCNU are used for the treatment of malignant gliomas and metastatic breast cancer. Three different types of retinal toxicity have been reported with these agents. One type of change consists of a pigmentary retinopathy of the macula with markedly decreased visual acuity and frequently abnormal electrophysiologic testing. This pigmentary change has been reported after administration of combined intra-arterial cisplatin and BCNU and with cisplatin alone for malignant glioma.[109,110]

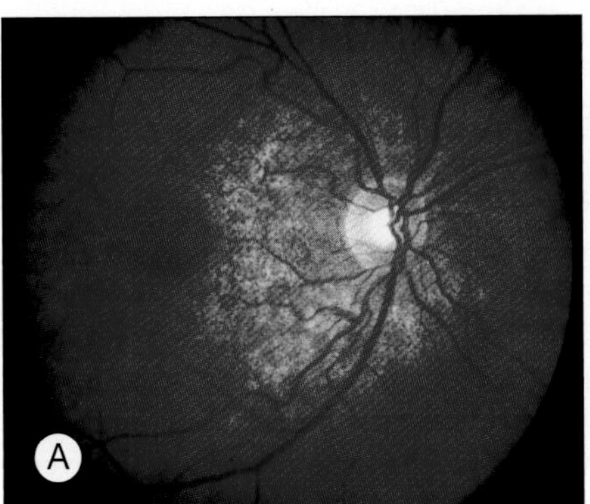

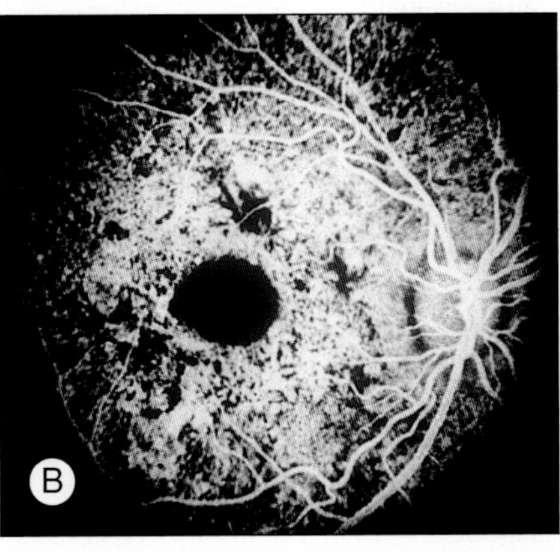

Fig. 89.13 Clofazimine toxicity. Photograph (A) and fluorescein angiogram (B) show moderate macular pigmentary changes in a bull's-eye pattern.

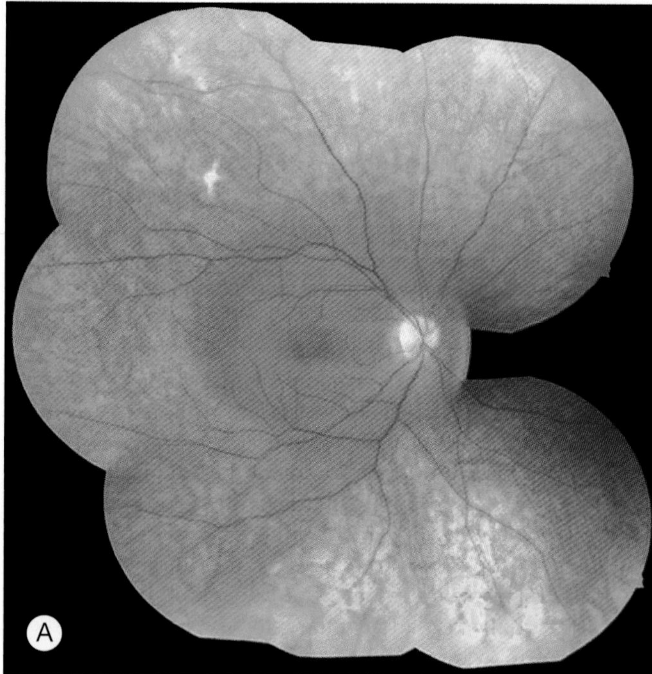

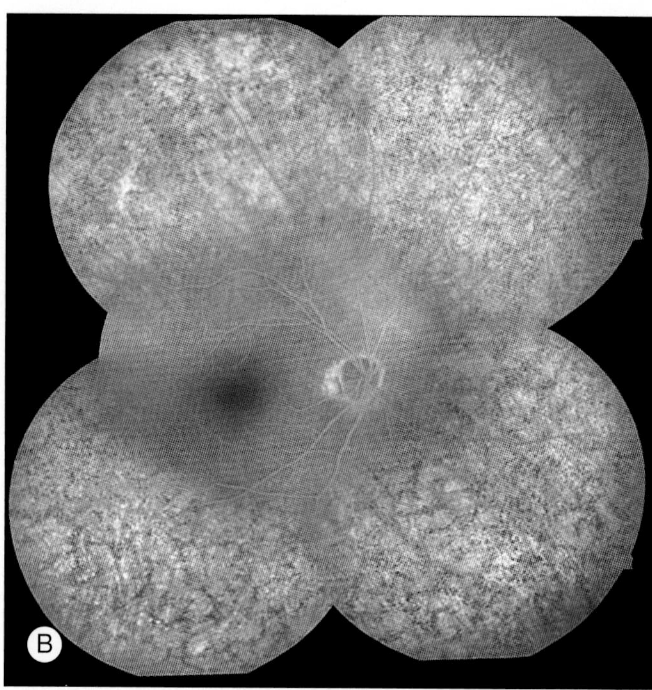

Fig. 89.14 Dideoxyinosine (DDI) toxicity. Photograph (A) showing severe midperipheral retinal pigmentary mottling in an adult having been exposed to DDI in the past. Fluorescein angiogram (B) highlights the RPE changes (Courtesy of David Sarraf, MD, Los Angeles, CA.)

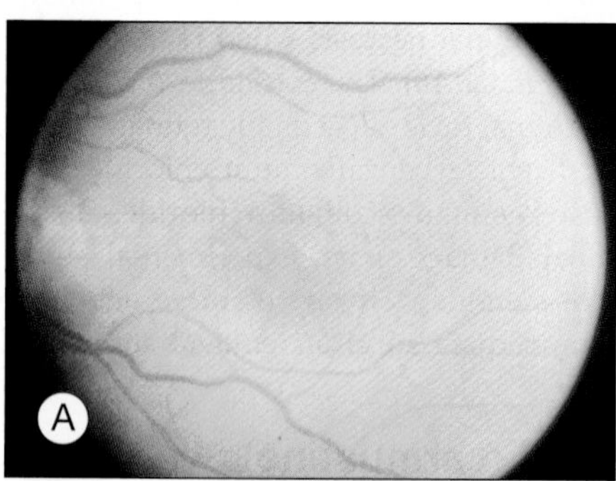

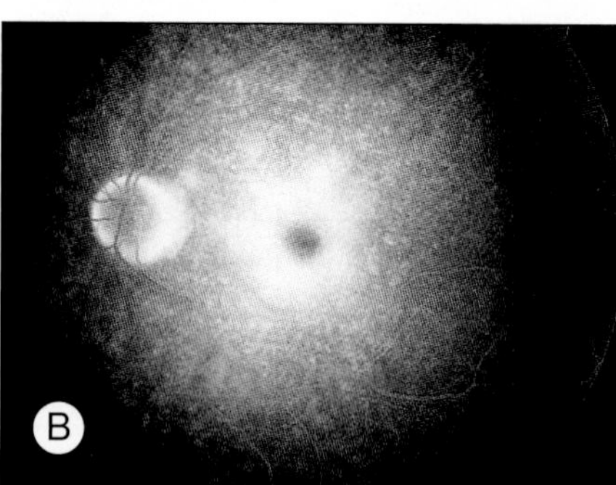

Fig. 89.15 Deferoxamine toxicity. Photograph (A) and fluorescein angiogram (B) show a diffuse pigmentary retinopathy with macular and retinal edema.

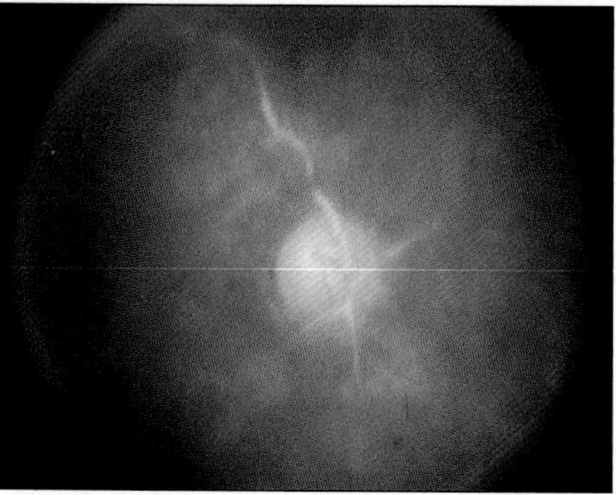

Fig. 89.16 Inadvertent intraocular corticosteroid injection. Photograph shows endstage retinopathy, with sclerotic vessels and diffuse pigmentary changes, after an inadvertent intraocular injection of corticosteroid.

These findings probably are the result of platinum toxicity of the retina. Severe bilateral visual loss was reported after intravenous cisplatin in a patient that received four times the intended dose for treatment of lymphoma.[111] Later histology showed a splitting of the outer plexiform layer.

A second type of retinopathy has been described and consists of cotton-wool spots, intraretinal hemorrhages, macular exudate, and optic neuropathy with disc swelling. This was reported in the setting of high-dose chemotherapy with cisplatin, cyclophosphamide, carmustine, and autologous bone-marrow transplantation for metastatic breast cancer.[112] The third type of change involves a vascular retinopathy or optic neuropathy, which can include arterial occlusion, vasculitis, and papillitis. This has been seen in approximately 65% of patients receiving intra-arterial BCNU alone or combined with cisplatin for malignant glioma.[110] These fundus changes are associated with a profound visual loss that begins about 6 weeks after the start of therapy. Other ocular effects may include orbital pain, chemosis, secondary glaucoma, internal ophthalmoplegia, and cavernous sinus syndrome. Injection of medication above the ophthalmic artery can still result in toxicity.[113] The visual loss usually is progressive, and no treatment is known.

Miscellaneous agents

Overdose of potassium iodate, an iodized salt used for iodine supplementation in areas endemic for goiter, has been shown to cause profound visual loss and extensive fundus pigmentary abnormalities.[114] Fluorescein angiography reveals RPE window defects and ERG and VEP testing shows marked impairment of retinal function. Visual acuity may improve slowly over several months. There have been two cases of pigmentary retinopathy with diminished ERG amplitudes reported after administration of denileuken diftitox.[115]

VASCULAR DAMAGE

Quinine sulfate

See above, Disruption of the retina and retinal pigment epithelium.

Cisplatin and BCNU (carmustine)

See above, Disruption of the retina and retinal pigment epithelium.

Talc

A characteristic retinopathy consisting of small, white, glistening crystals concentrated in the end arterioles of the posterior pole has been described in intravenous (IV) drug abusers[116–118] (Fig. 89.17). These addicts crush oral medications such as methylphenidate hydrochloride (Ritalin) or methadone HCl and then create an aqueous suspension by adding water and heating the mixture. The solution is subsequently drawn up into a syringe, with occasional attempts at filtering the mixture with cotton fibers, gauze, or cigarette filters. These oral medications contain talc (hydrous magnesium silicate) as inert filler material; after IV administration, talc particles embolize to the pulmonary vasculature, where the larger particles are trapped. After repeated injections over months to years, collateral vasculature develops, allowing the particles to enter the systemic circulation and embolize to other organs, including the eye. Even before shunt development, particles smaller than 7 μm can traverse the pulmonary capillary bed and enter the retinal circulation.[119]

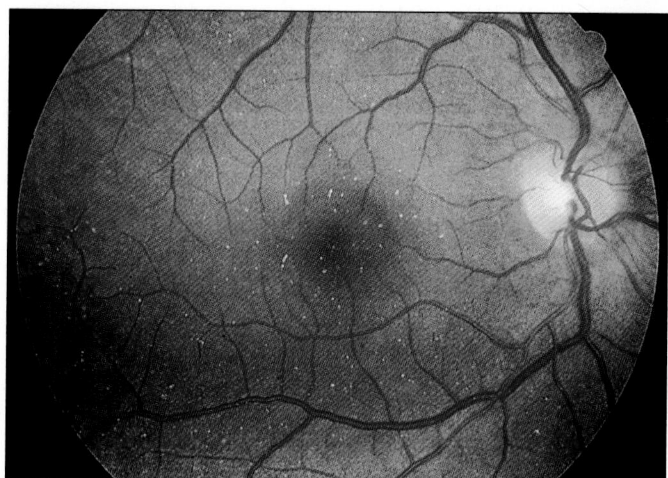

Fig. 89.17 Talc retinopathy. Characteristic perifoveal yellow-white glistening crystals.

Once a large number of talc particles lodge in the small arterioles of the retinal vasculature, a characteristic picture of an ischemic retinopathy begins to develop. Capillary nonperfusion, microaneurysm formation, cotton-wool spots, and venous loops can all be seen.[120] In severe cases optic disc and peripheral neovascularization and vitreous hemorrhage can develop[121,122] (Fig. 89.18). An experimental model of talc retinopathy in monkeys has demonstrated with light and electron microscopic techniques that the vascular abnormalities induced are very similar to other ischemic retinopathies seen in humans, such as sickle cell and hypertensive retinopathy.[123–125]

Once talc retinopathy is diagnosed, an attempt at educating the patient as to the cause of the disorder is indicated. Treatment of neovascularization and vitreous hemorrhage should be undertaken using laser photocoagulation and pars plana vitrectomy if necessary in a manner similar to that used for sickle cell or proliferative diabetic retinopathy.

Oral contraceptives

Oral contraceptives have been implicated in some cases of central retinal vein occlusion (CRV), retinal and cilioretinal artery obstruction, and retinal edema occurring in young women.[126–132] The synthetic estrogen and progesterone contained in contraceptive pills are thought to adversely effect coagulation factors and induce a hypercoagulable state leading to thromboembolic complications. Most of the studies reporting ocular complications are from the 1960s and 1970s, when the estrogen concentrations used in "the pill" were much higher (Fig. 89.19). Some recent prospective studies have failed to show an increased incidence of ocular complications with the drug, though one large study showed an increase in "retinal vascular findings".[133–135]

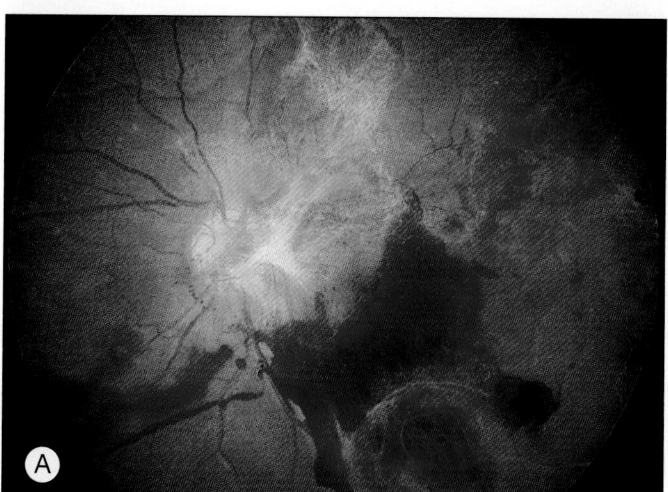

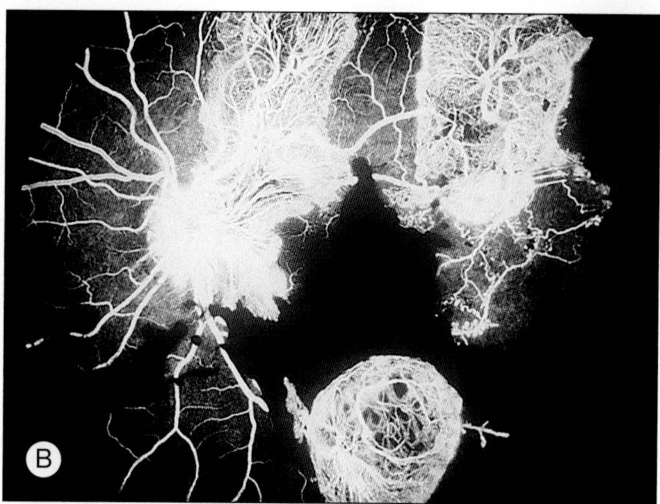

Fig. 89.18 Ischemic talc retinopathy. Photograph (A) and fluorescein angiogram (B) show widespread capillary dropout, neovascularization, and preretinal hemorrhage.

Aminoglycoside antibiotics

Retinal toxicity from aminoglycoside antibiotics has been reported after inadvertent intraocular injection of massive doses, intravitreal injection for bacterial endophthalmitis, prophylactic intravitreal injection after pars plana vitrectomy, prophylactic subconjunctival injections after routine ocular surgery, and with the use of small amounts in the infusion fluid during cataract extraction.[136–139] Gentamicin is the most toxic antibiotic in the aminoglycoside family, followed by tobramycin and amikacin.[140] Massive doses result in early superficial and intraretinal hemorrhages, retinal edema, cotton-wool patches, arteriolar narrowing, and venous beading[139] (Fig. 89.20). Fluorescein angiography reveals severe vascular nonperfusion in the acute stages. Visual loss is profound, and late rubeosis iridis, neovascular glaucoma, pigmentary retinopathy, and optic atrophy are common. Intravitreal injection of smaller doses thought to be safe for the eye (100–400 μg) can still cause toxicity with less severe fundus changes.[137–139] The major preservatives found in injectable gentamicin (methylparaben, propylparaben, sodium bisulfite, and edetate disodium) likely play an additive role in its ocular toxicity.

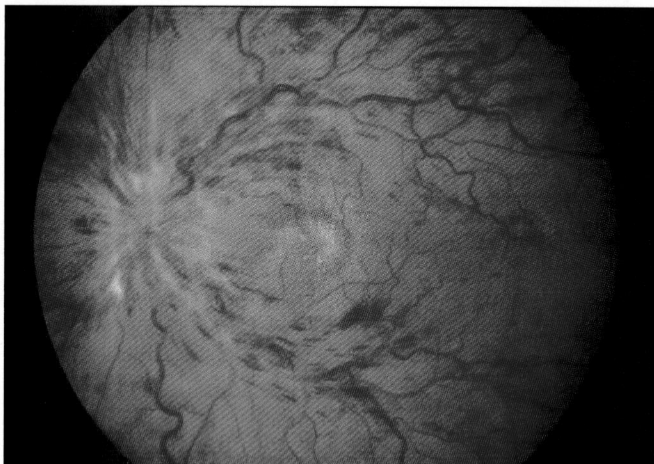

Fig. 89.19 Nonischemic central retinal vein occlusion (CRVO) in a 40-year-old hypertensive female on oral contraceptives. Upon stopping the oral contraceptives, the CRVO resolved without treatment.

A number of factors appear to affect the extent of toxicity observed with similar doses of these medications. Peyman found that retinal toxicity could be enhanced with an intravitreal injection directed at the posterior pole with the bevel of the needle pointed toward the retina, and Zachary and Forster demonstrated that an increased rate of injection during intraocular administration could also increase the retinal toxicity observed.[141,142] One investigator stated that eyes that have undergone a previous pars plana vitrectomy are at greater risk for gentamicin toxicity, but an experimental model has shown no difference between eyes that had cataract extraction alone compared with those that underwent lensectomy and vitrectomy.[143,144] Finally, increased ocular pigmentation protects the rabbit retina from aminoglycoside toxicity and may explain some of the wide variability seen with intraocular exposure in humans.[145,146]

Although clinical aminoglycoside toxicity appears to affect the retinal vasculature primarily, pathologic studies have revealed that gentamicin in small doses causes the formation of abnormal lamellar lysosomal inclusions in the RPE, and larger doses cause increasing amounts of retinal necrosis, first of the outer then inner segments.[147–150] Histologically, vessel closure appears to result from granulocytic plugging.

Prevention of aminoglycoside toxicity can be accomplished by abandoning the use of these medications as routine prophylaxis following intraocular surgery, eliminating them from intraocular infusion fluids used in vitrectomy and cataract surgery, and using alternative medications for the treatment of bacterial endophthalmitis. Animal studies have demonstrated that thinned sclera alone without perforation can result in markedly elevated intraocular gentamicin levels after subconjunctival injection.[151] If inadvertent intraocular injection does occur, immediate pars plana vitrectomy with posterior segment lavage should be performed.[152,153] Since there is some evidence that gravity plays a role in the predilection of gentamicin-induced toxicity for the macula, the patient should be placed upright as soon as possible after surgery.[154]

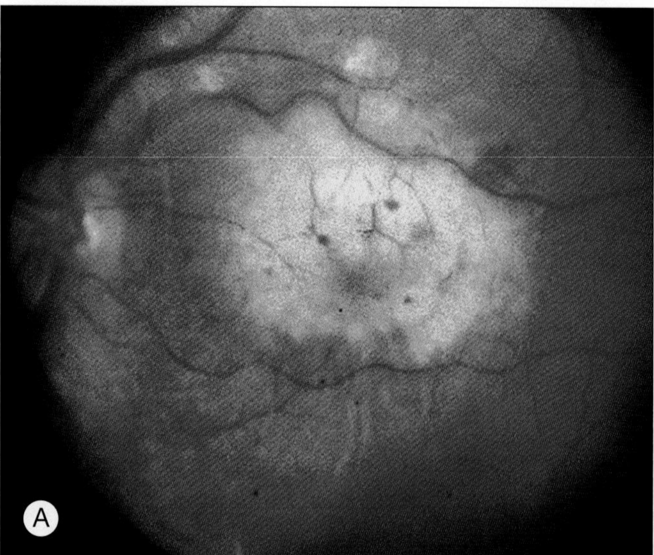

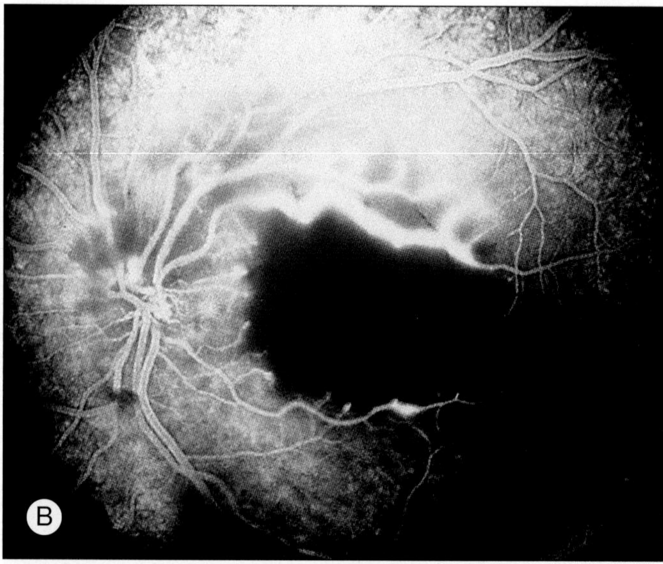

Fig. 89.20 Intraocular gentamicin injection. Photograph (A) and fluorescein angiogram (B) show acute macular necrosis, with virtually complete cessation of blood flow where presumably the medication came in contact with the retina while the patient was in a supine position during the early postoperative timeframe.

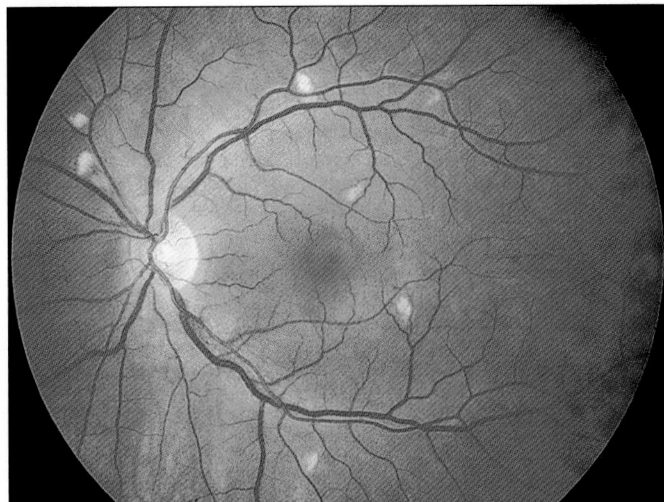

Fig. 89.21 Interferon retinopathy, consisting primarily of multiple cotton-wool spots dispersed throughout the posterior pole. The findings resolved following cessation of therapy.

Interferon

Interferon-α is used to treat Kaposi's sarcoma, hemangiomas of infancy, chronic hepatitis C, melanoma, renal cell carcinoma and in chemotherapy protocols for leukemia, lymphoma, and hemangiomatosis. Interferon therapy has been associated with the development of multiple cotton-wool spots associated with retinal hemorrhages[155–157] (Fig. 89.21). Optic disc edema, branch arterial and venous occlusion, central retinal venous obstruction, anterior ischemic optic neuropathy and CME have been reported with the more severe findings observed in patients receiving high dose therapy.[158–162] Visual acuity usually is not affected if the fundus findings are limited to cotton-wool spots and intraretinal hemorrhage. Changes are noted within the first 4–8 weeks of therapy and are seen more frequently in diabetic and hypertensive patients[163] (Fig. 89.22).

Intravitreal injection of interferon-α-2b is well tolerated in the rabbit eye up to dosages of 1 million units; 2 million units causes a vitreous haze and intraretinal hemorrhages.[164] Interferon toxicity may be caused by an increase in immune complex deposition and activated complement C5a with leukocyte infiltration. EOG testing may become abnormal in early toxicity.[165]

Miscellaneous agents

Ergot alkaloids in higher than recommended doses have been reported to cause retinal vasoconstriction,[166,167] and over-the-counter phenylpropanolamine used in appetite suppressants and decongestants has been implicated in one case of central retinal vein occlusion.[168] Gemcitabine is a chemotherapeutic agent used for non-small-cell lung carcinoma, breast, ovarian and pancreatic cancers. It has been associated with one case of Purtscher-like retinopathy[169] (Fig. 89.23).

CYSTOID MACULAR EDEMA

Epinephrine

The use of epinephrine compounds in glaucoma has decreased with the advent of newer, more efficacious agents. Topical epinephrine can cause macular edema in aphakic eyes, indistinguishable clinically and angiographically from postoperative aphakic cystoid macular edema (CME). In the largest controlled study, 28% of aphakic eyes treated with epinephrine and 13% of untreated aphakic eyes had macular edema, a difference that was statistically significant.[170] Most cases of CME resolve with cessation of epinephrine usage. This medication should be avoided in the treatment of the glaucomatous aphakic and pseudophakic eyes.

Nicotinic acid

High doses of niacin have been used to reduce serum lipid and cholesterol levels. Better-tolerated HMG-CoA reductase inhibitor agents have curtailed their utilization, though there has been a recent resurgence in their use in both monotherapy and combination therapy with statins. At doses greater than 1.5 g/day, a minority of patients will report blurred central vision, sometimes associated with a paracentral scotoma or metamorphopsia.[171] Fluorescein angiography fails to demonstrate vascular leakage despite the typical clinical appearance of CME[172,173] (Fig. 89.24). This has led to speculation of a direct toxic effect on Müller cells, resulting in intracellular edema.[174] Optical coherence tomography reveals cystoid spaces in the inner nuclear and outer plexiform layers.[175,176] With cessation of treatment, the CME resolves, and vision generally returns to normal. Given the rarity of this condition, only patients who are taking high-dose niacin and who have visual symptoms should be evaluated.

Latanoprost

Latanoprost is a prostaglandin analogue that is used for the control of a variety of forms of glaucoma. Although initial human and animal studies did not show an association between latanoprost and CME, recent case reports and studies have documented that approximately 2–5% of susceptible patients with glaucoma may develop CME and anterior uveitis, which resolves after discontinuation of the drug[177–185] (Fig. 89.25). This may be caused by the preservative used in the drug formulation.[186] Patients with CME who are taking latanoprost should undergo a trial off the medication before initiating further therapy for the edema. High-risk CME patients, such as those with a history of recent surgery or uveitis, should be managed with other agents.

Paclitaxel/docetaxel

Paclitaxel and docetaxel are similar antimicrotubule agents that are used for treatment of breast, lung, and prostate cancer. They have both been associated with angiographically negative CME (Fig. 89.26). The edema appears to respond to treatment with topical or systemic acetazolamide, and/or intravitreal anti-VEGF therapy.[187,188]

RETINAL FOLDS

Sulfa antibiotics, acetazolamide, chlorthalidone, disothiazide, ethoxyzolamide, hydrochlorothiazide, metronidazole, sulphonamide, topiramate, triamterene

Several medications, most with a structure similar to sulfanilamide, as those above, can cause a syndrome of transient acute myopia and anterior chamber shallowing. This is thought to occur as a result of ciliary body swelling, choroidal effusion, or

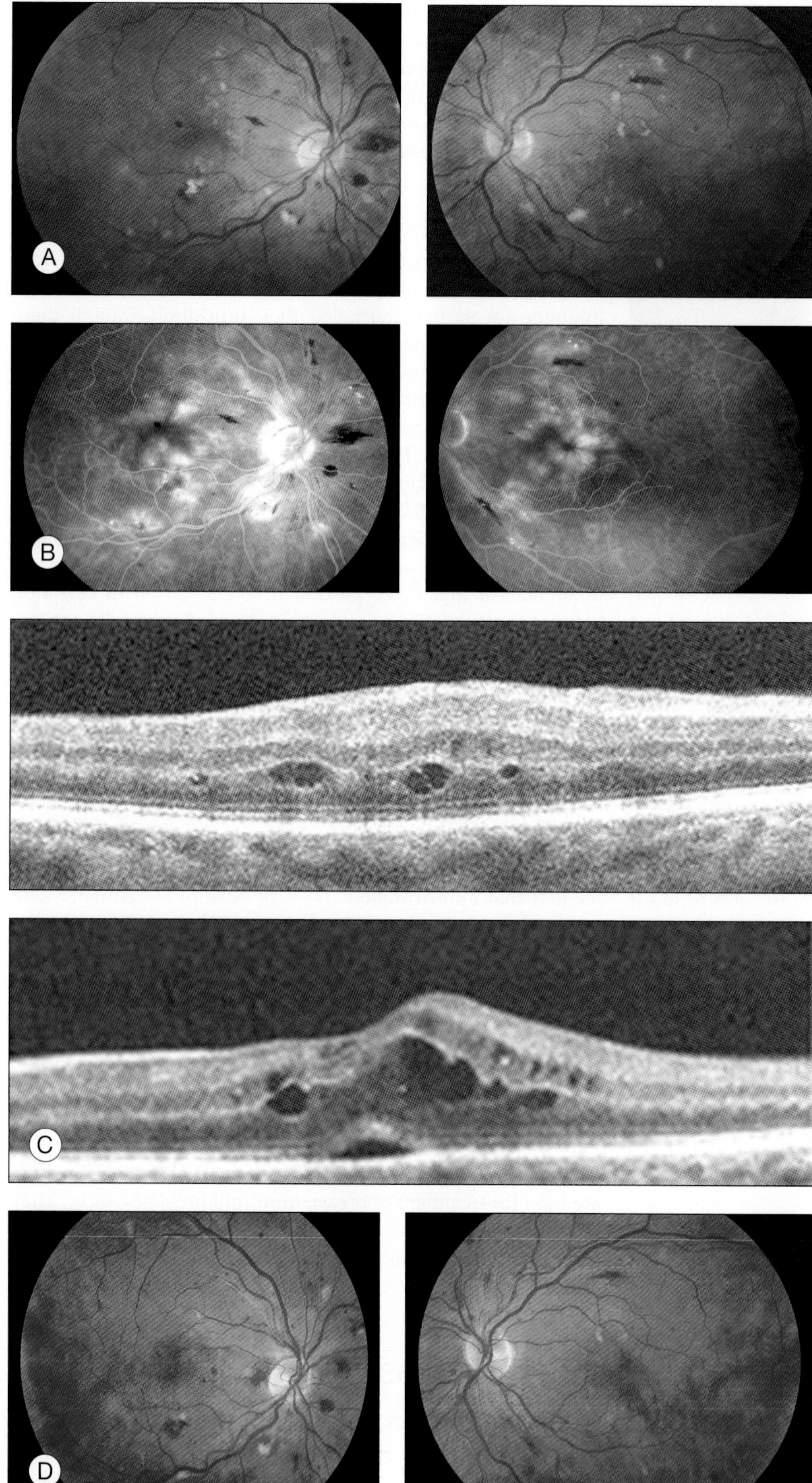

Fig. 89.22 Interferon microangiopathy. Photograph (A) and fluorescein angiogram (B) showing multiple cotton-wool spots and microangiopathy in a patient being treated for hepatitis C. Spectral domain optical coherence tomography (C) documents mild cystoid macular edema. Once the interferon was discontinued, photograph (D), taken one month later, documents significant resolution of the cotton-wool spots.

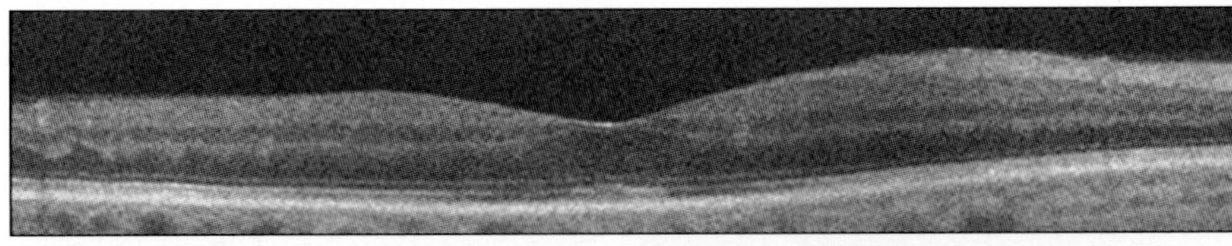

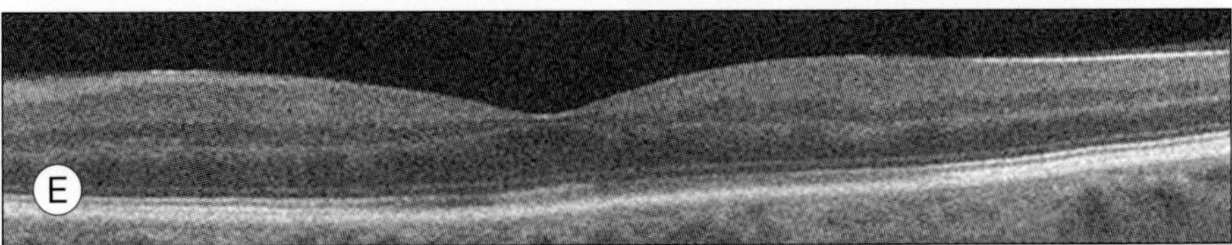

Fig. 89.22 Cont'd Spectral domain optical coherence tomography (E) shows resolution of the cystoid macular edema. (Courtesy of Joseph Maguire, MD, Philadelphia, PA.)

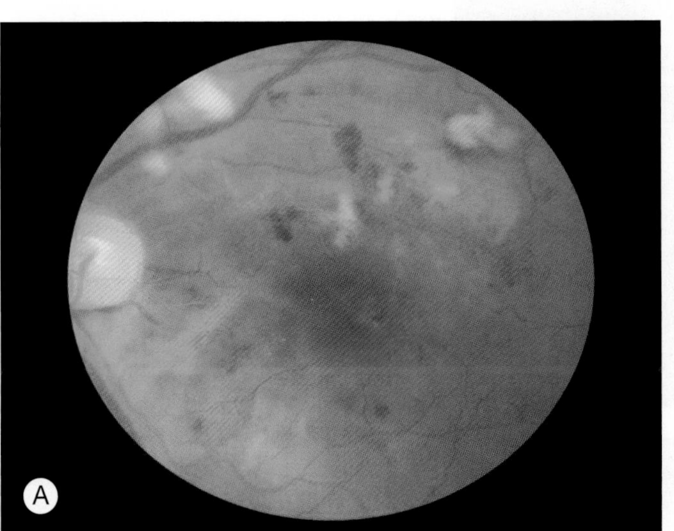

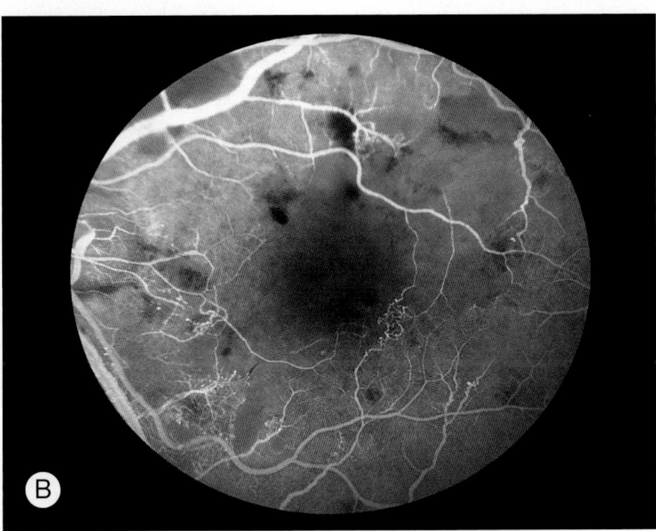

Fig. 89.23 Gemcitadine toxicity. Photograph (A) documents multiple cotton-wool spots, while the fluorescein angiogram (B) shows extensive capillary nonperfusion in a patient being treated for lung carcinoma.

both, or with swelling of the lens itself with subsequent forward rotation of the lens–iris diaphragm.[189–198] Retinal folds in the macula are seen in young patients with this syndrome, but FA does not reveal retinal leakage (Fig. 89.27). The folds presumably develop as a result of vitreous traction on the macula that is caused by the forward shift of the lens and iris.

CRYSTALLINE RETINOPATHY

Tamoxifen

Tamoxifen is an antiestrogen agent used in the treatment of estrogen-receptor-positive tumors such as advanced breast carcinoma (and in some estrogen-receptor-negative tumors such as hepatocellular carcinoma) and as adjuvant therapy after surgical resection of early disease. Retinal toxicity consisting of decreased visual acuity and color vision with white intraretinal crystalline deposits, macular edema, and punctate retinal pigmentary changes can occur.[199] The intraretinal deposits appear to reside in the inner retina and are most numerous in paramacular areas (Fig. 89.28). Early reports involved patients who had received high doses (60–100 mg/day, total dosage >100 g) of the drug over 1 year.[200] More recent studies have demonstrated that chronic low-dose administration (10–20 mg/day) with as little as 7.7 g total, also can cause ocular toxicity.[201–205] Even asymptomatic patients may exhibit intraretinal crystalline formation.[206] Visual function and edema improve after discontinuation of the drug, but the refractile deposits remain.

There has been a recent upturn in cases of tamoxifen-induced retinal crystals, as patients with aggressive glioblastoma are now being treated with 100–200 mg of tamoxifen on a daily basis (Fig. 89.29). Concurrent cystoid macular edema may be treated with intravitreal anti-VEGF therapy.

Fluorescein angiography demonstrates late focal staining in the macula consistent with CME. Decreased photopic and scotopic a- and b-wave amplitude is noted on ERG testing.[207] Light microscopy reveals lesions confined to the nerve fiber and inner plexiform layers, which stain positive for glycosaminoglycans. Small (3–10 μm) intracellular and large (30–35 μm) extracellular lesions within axons are noted on electron microscopy.[208] The lesions appear to represent products of axonal degeneration similar to corpora amylacea. Experimentally, tamoxifen inhibits glutamate uptake by RPE cells.[209] OCT findings in lower-dose therapy interestingly do not show an increase in macular edema, but rather a foveal cyst with disruption of the photoreceptor line, while high-dose therapy can show CME.[210–212]

Decreased vision with bilateral optic disc swelling and retinal hemorrhages has been reported in a patient just 3 weeks after

Text continues on page 1548

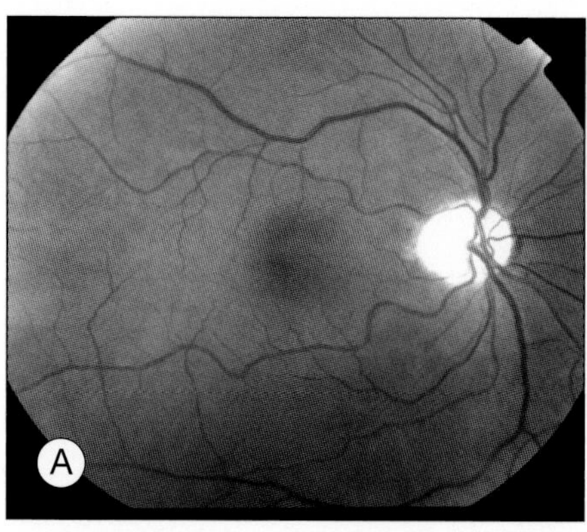

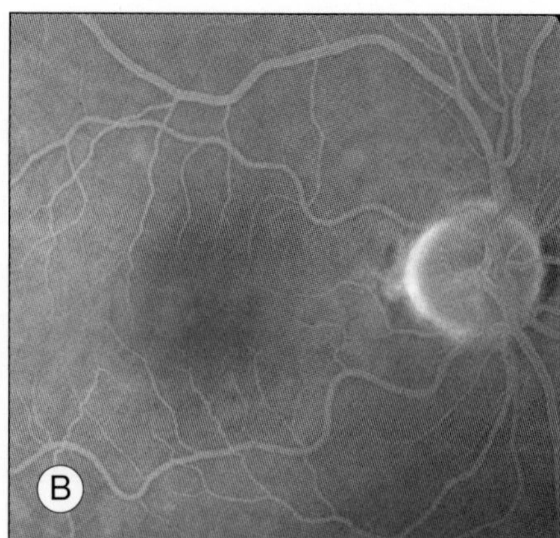

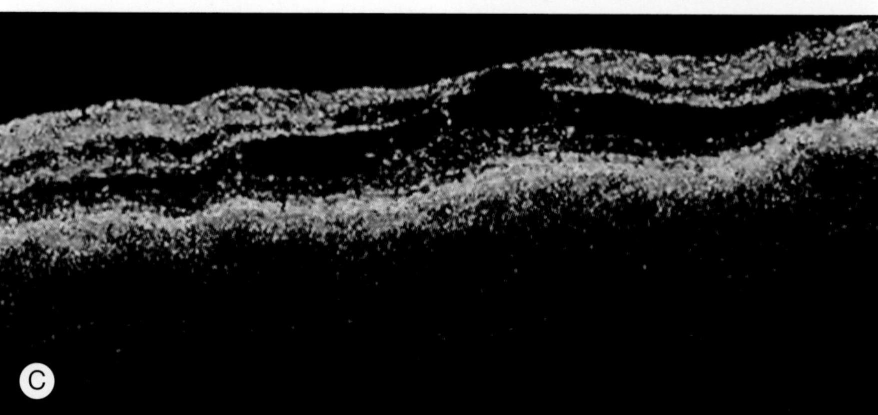

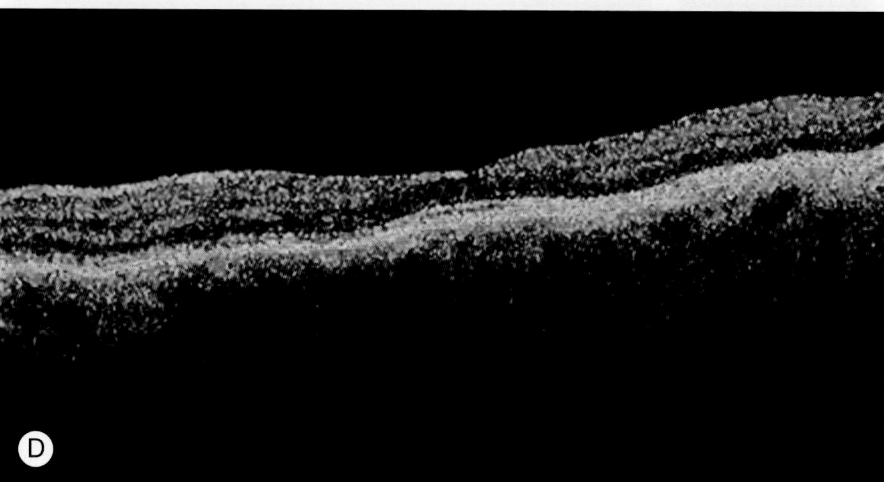

Fig. 89.24 Nicotinic acid maculopathy. Red free photograph (A) shows blunted foveal reflex, while the fluorescein angiogram (B) shows minimal late leakage. A time domain OCT (C) shows mild macular edema. The nicotinic acid was discontinued, and two weeks later, the OCT (D) returned to normal. The findings were bilateral. (Courtesy of Lawrence A Yannuzzi, MD, New York City, NY.)

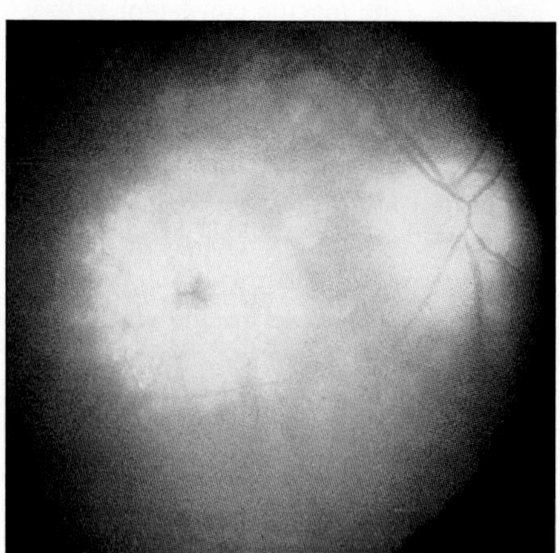

Fig. 89.25 Latanaprost-associated cystoid macular edema. Angiogram shows characteristic fluorescein filling of the cystic spaces.

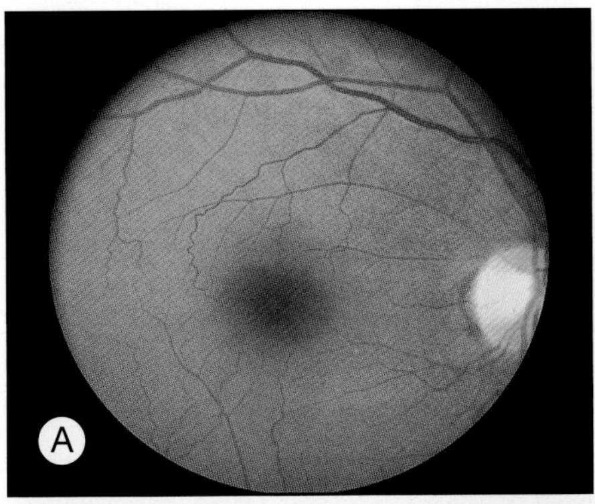
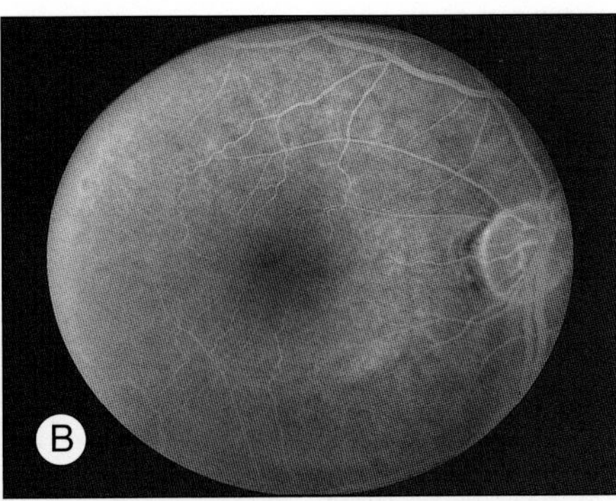
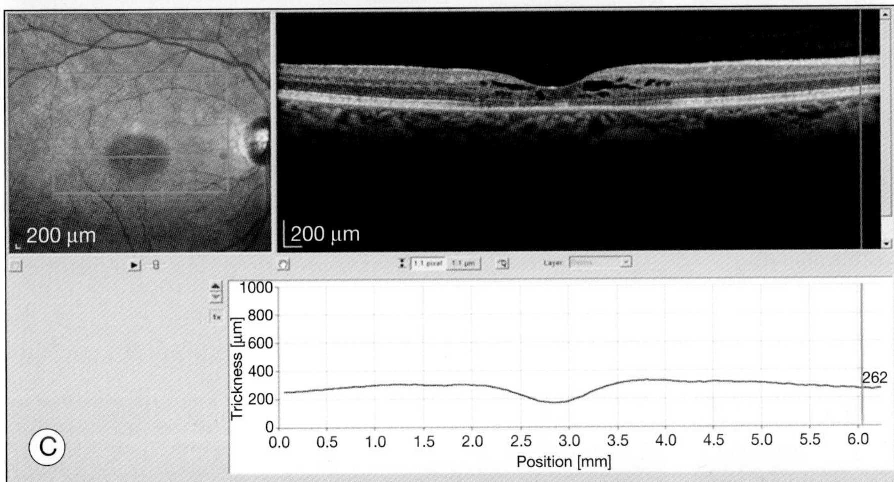

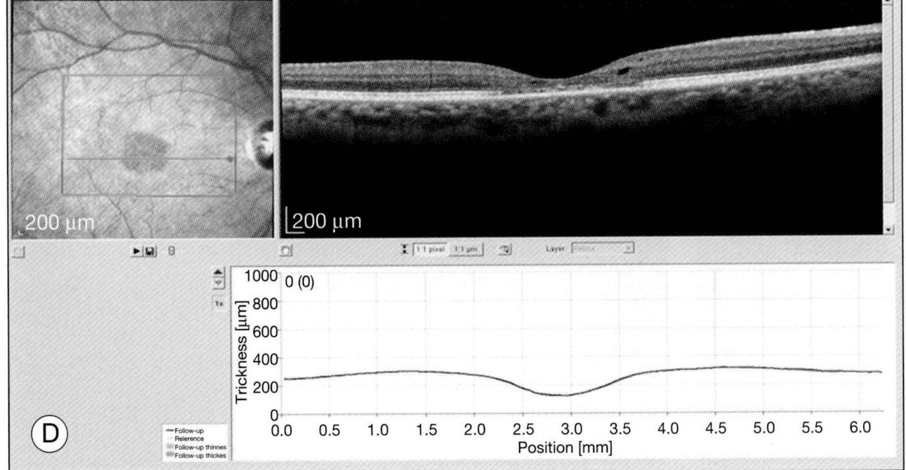

Fig. 89.26 Paclitaxel maculopathy. Photograph (A) showing a blunted foveal reflex in a patient on paclitaxel for treatment of metastatic breast carcinoma. The fluorescein angiogram (B) shows minimal late leakage of dye, though spectral domain optical coherence tomography (SD-OCT) (C) shows intraretinal cystic spaces. Upon treatment with topical carbonic anhydrase inhibitors, the cystic spaces on SD-OCT (D) gradually resolved. The findings were bilateral.

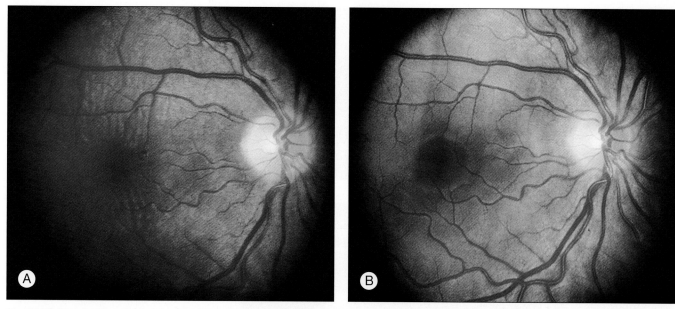

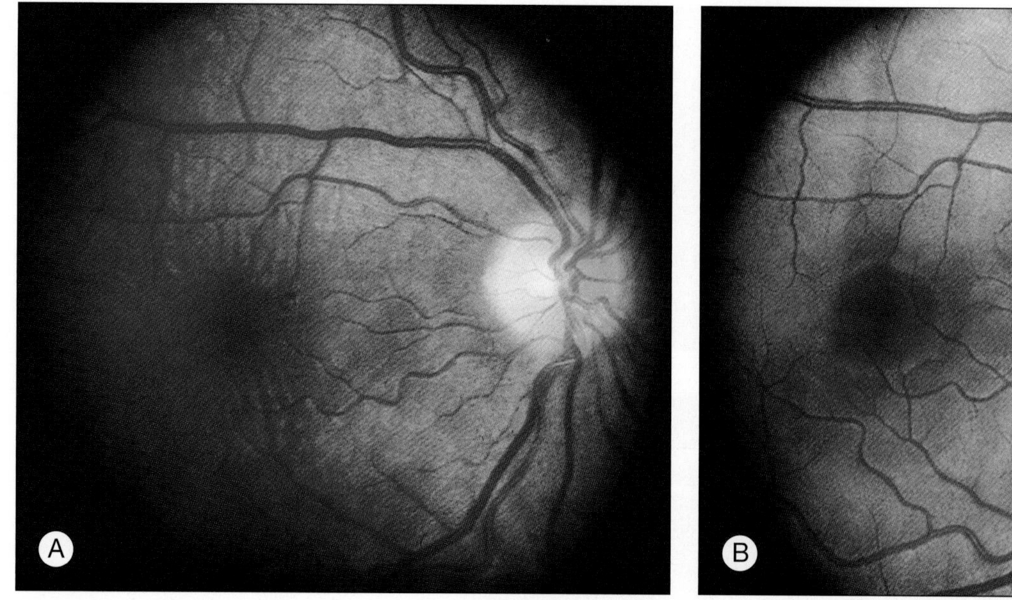

Fig. 89.27 Chlorthalidone-induced retinal folds. Photograph (A) shows perifoveal retinal folds associated with chlorthalidone therapy, which resolve within two weeks following discontinuation of the drug (B).

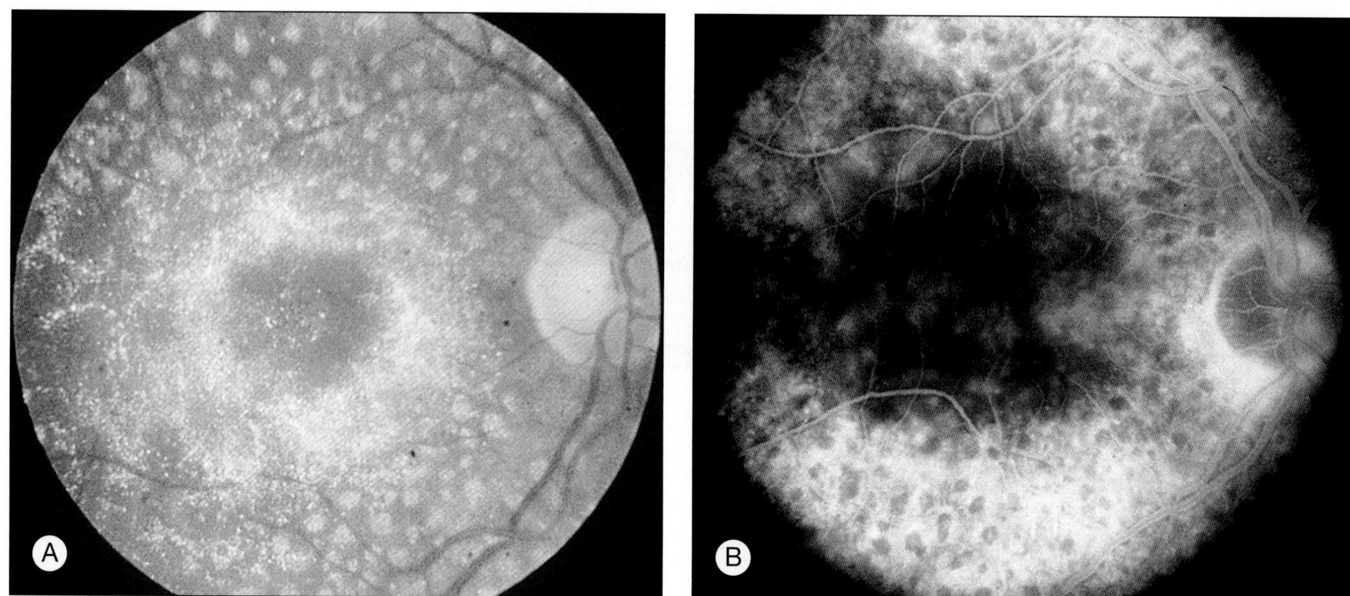

Fig. 89.28 Tamoxifen crystalline retinopathy. Characteristic yellow-white macular crystals are seen in a perifoveal distribution. The crystals were not felt to be of visual significance.

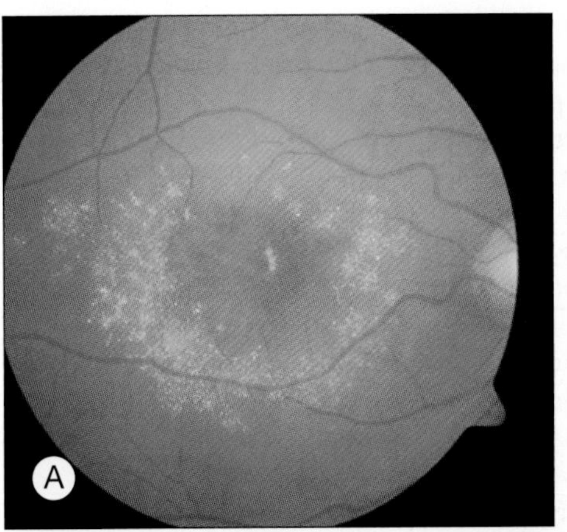

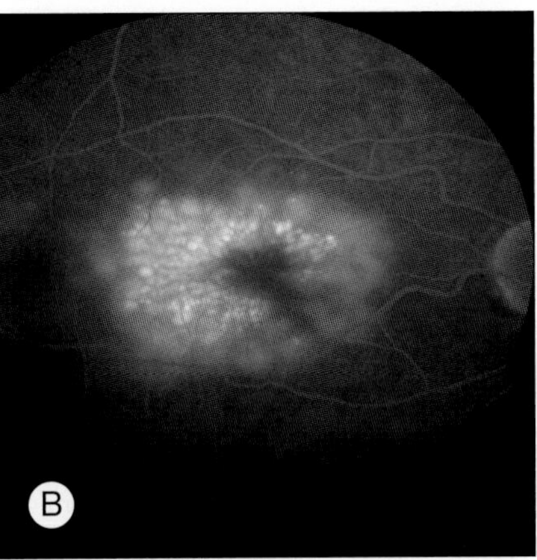

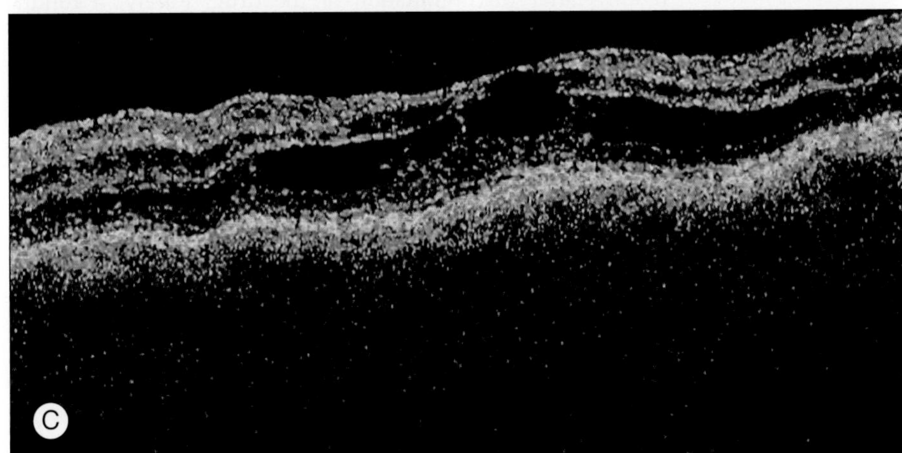

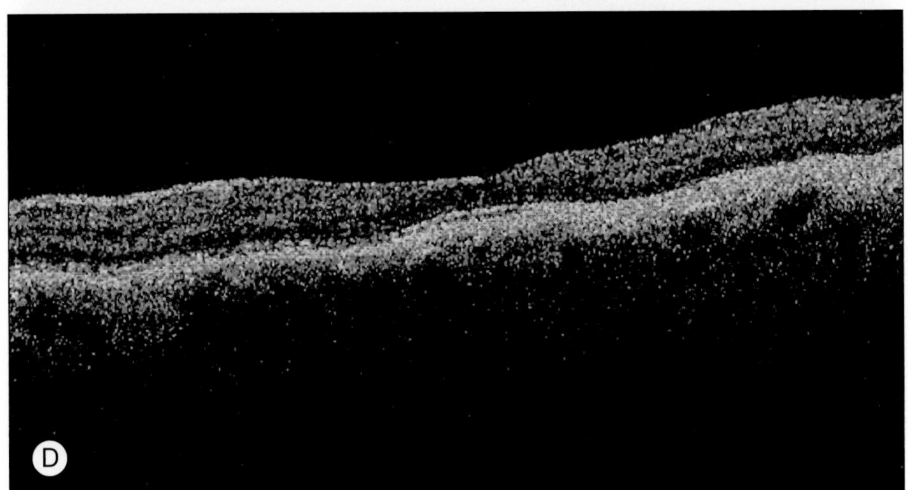

Fig. 89.29 Tamoxifen crystalline retinopathy in a patient with advanced glioblastoma being treated with high-dose tamoxifen. Photograph (A) shows perifoveal crystals, while the fluorescein angiogram (B) shows diffuse cystoid macular edema (CME). A time domain OCT (C) confirms the findings of diffuse CME. A follow-up OCT (D) several months later, following administration of intravitreal bevacizumab, shows resolution of the CME. The findings were bilateral. (Courtesy of David Sarraf, MD, Los Angeles, CA.)

commencement of therapy with tamoxifen. These findings resolved completely after the drug was stopped.[213] It is unclear whether the findings in this patient were related to the more commonly seen toxic effects. Optic neuropathy with tamoxifen has been reported as well.[214] With current low-dose therapy (10–20 mg/day), retinal lesions are rare, and routine examination of asymptomatic patients is not indicated.[206,215] If a patient taking tamoxifen is noted to have intraretinal crystals, FA should be performed, primarily to rule out juxtafoveal telangiectasis, which can have similar-appearing lesions.[216] With confirmed evidence of toxicity causing a visual disturbance, the medication should be stopped. For persistent macular edema, which has been noted after prolonged high-dose therapy after cessation of the drug, antivascular endothelial growth factor injection may be beneficial.[217]

Canthaxanthine

Canthaxanthine is a naturally occurring carotenoid. It is used as a food-coloring agent, for skin pigmentation in the treatment of vitiligo, and for the treatment of photosensitivity disorders such as erythropoietic protoporphyria, psoriasis, and photosensitive eczema. It also has been used over-the-counter in high doses as an oral tanning agent. Many reports have described a characteristic ring-shaped deposition of yellow-orange crystals in the superficial retina with high doses (usually a total dose greater than 19 g over 2 years)[218–220] (Fig. 89.30). The crystals appear more prominently in eyes with preexisting retinal disease and with concurrent use of beta-carotene.[218,221]

Patients usually are asymptomatic, and FA usually is normal. There have been published reports of both normal and abnormal ERG, EOG, dark adaptation, and static threshold perimetry.[222–225] Although only clinically evident in the macula, the lipid-soluble crystals are found pathologically in the entire inner retina and ciliary body.[226] The crystals are, as would be expected, larger and more numerous surrounding the fovea. Canthaxanthine crystals are localized to the spongy degeneration of the inner neuropil and are associated with atrophy of the Müller cells. Interestingly, a single case report showed OCT localization of crystals to the outer plexiform layer.[227] An experimental model of canthaxanthine-induced retinopathy also has demonstrated RPE cell vacuolization and disruption of phagolysosomes.[228]

With discontinuation of treatment, deposits may slowly clear over many years.[229,230] This slow reversal correlates with the detection of high plasma levels of canthaxanthine many months after discontinuation of the drug. Rarely, a fundus picture identical to canthaxanthine maculopathy can be seen in patients who have no known history of extradietary canthaxanthine.[231] A high dietary intake concurrent with preexisting retinal disease is thought to partially explain this phenomenon.

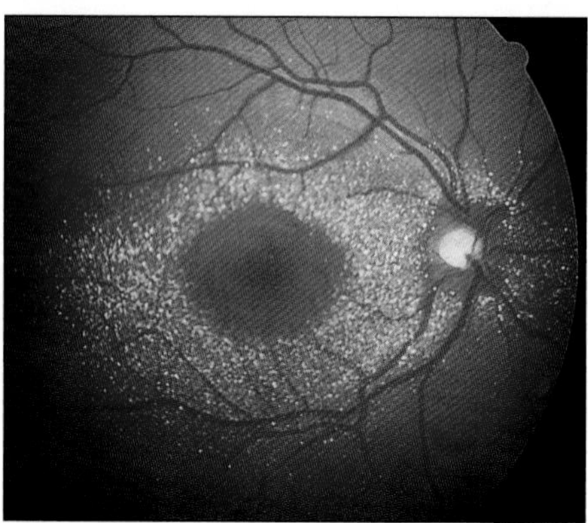

Fig. 89.30 Canthaxanthine retinopathy. Prominent perifoveal punctate yellow deposits in a doughnut-shaped ring surrounding the macula.

Methoxyflurane

Methoxyflurane is an inhalational anesthetic, which, if used for extended periods, especially in patients with renal insufficiency, causes irreversible renal failure as a result of deposition of calcium oxalate crystals in the kidney. These crystals are also deposited elsewhere throughout the body. Fundus examination of these patients reveals numerous yellow-white punctate lesions in the posterior pole and periarterially[232,233] (Fig. 89.31). The deposits are located histologically in both the RPE and inner retina.[234,235]

Talc

See Vascular damage above.

Miscellaneous agents

A single case of crystalline retinopathy following 19 years of nitrofurantoin (Macrodantin) use has been reported.[236] Three cases of rapid visual loss with fludarabine phosphate, a nucleoside analog, during treatment for SLE or metastatic melanoma were reported, with two of the cases exhibiting deep yellow retinal flecks.[237] Three patients receiving long-term ritonavir therapy as part of a highly active antiretroviral therapy regimen were reported to have a retinal pigment epitheliopathy, parafoveal telangiectasis, and intraretinal crystal deposits.[238]

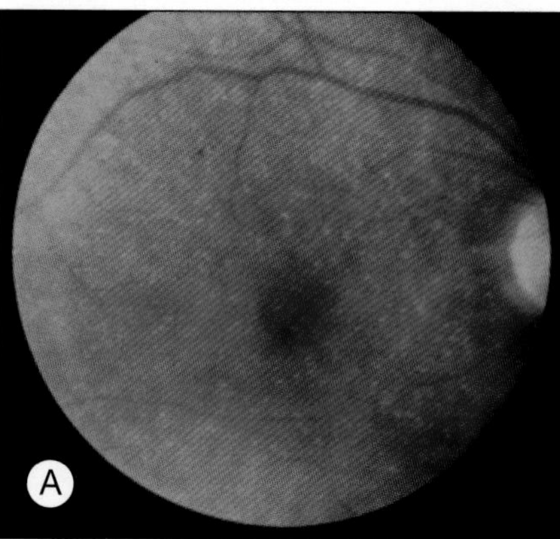

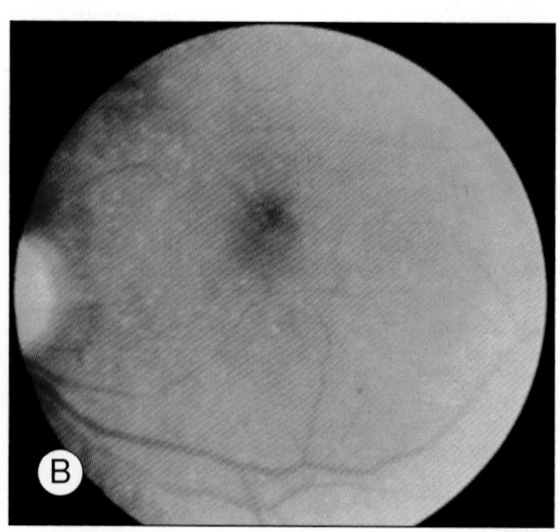

Fig. 89.31 Methoxyflurane crystals. (A,B) Photographs document intraretinal crystals dispersed throughout the posterior pole in a patient subjected to methoxyflurane anesthesia, who developed postoperative renal failure.

UVEITIS

Rifabutin

Rifabutin is a semisynthetic rifamycin antibiotic that is used for the treatment and prevention of disseminated *Mycobacterium avium*-complex (MAC) infection in patients with and without AIDS.[239–247] A small percentage of patients treated with higher doses of rifabutin (>450 mg/day) for systemic MAC infection, or lower doses (300 mg/day) for prophylaxis against MAC, can develop uveitis.[248] The uveitis usually is bilateral and can be severe enough to cause a hypopyon that simulates infectious endophthalmitis.[249] It can occur from 2 weeks to 14 months after initiation of the drug.[247] Concomitant use of clarithromycin and/or fluconazole (or itraconazole), especially when lower doses of rifabutin are used, greatly increases the chance of a uveitic episode.[250] Both systemic fluconazole and clarithromycin elevate rifabutin levels by inhibiting metabolism of the drug via the hepatic microsomal cytochrome P-450.[245] Although most cases have reported mainly an anterior uveitis and corneal endothelial deposits, posterior vitritis and retinal vasculitis have been described as well.[239,251]

Rifabutin-associated uveitis can be treated successfully with topical corticosteroids or by decreasing or discontinuing the medication. Long-term use may result in ERG abnormalities.[252] Patients without systemic MAC infection who are taking rifabutin for prophylaxis and also are taking fluconazole or clarithromycin should be warned about the potential for uveitis and counseled as to its signs and symptoms.

Cidofovir

Cidofovir, also known as HPMPC, is a nucleotide analogue that inhibits viral DNA polymerase and is used for the treatment of cytomegalovirus (CMV) retinitis.[253–262] Cidofovir therapy, with both intravenous and intravitreous (20 μg) routes of administration, has been associated with an anterior uveitis, hypotony, and visual loss.[263] These complications can be treated and sometimes prevented with the use of topical corticosteroids, cycloplegics, and oral probenecid. Cidofovir has been shown experimentally and clinically to cause a direct toxic effect to the ciliary body, with a resulting iritis and intraocular pressure decrease.[253,261] Although a 10 μg intravitreous dose had fewer side effects, it is also much less effective against CMV retinitis.[262] Investigations continue to try to determine the optimal dose and route of administration of cidofovir.

Latanoprost

See the drugs listed under Cystoid macular edema.

MISCELLANEOUS

Cardiac glycosides

Cardiac glycosides such as digoxin are used in the treatment of chronic heart failure and as antiarrhythmic agents. Although these drugs do not cause a characteristic fundus abnormality, ocular symptoms including blurred vision, scintillating scotomas, and xanthopsia (yellowing of vision) are common.[264,265] These changes probably are caused by direct toxicity to the photoreceptors. The visual symptoms are reversible with discontinuation of the drug.

Methanol

Methanol occasionally is ingested by alcoholics. Visual blurring and field deficits are seen within 18 hours. Early fundus findings include optic nerve hyperemia and retinal edema, and late findings include optic atrophy[8,266–273] (Fig. 89.32). OCT findings have shown the optic nerve head swelling with adjacent edema of the retinal nerve fiber layer.[274] Optic nerve toxicity is mediated by formic acid, a breakdown product of methanol, which directly affects the inner retina and optic nerve. The degree of systemic acidosis correlates well with the extent of visual dysfunction. Early hemodialysis is effective in removing methanol from the body, but if visual recovery is not evident by 6 days, it often remains permanently decreased.

Vigabatrin

Vigabatrin is used for treatment of epilepsy, and has been associated with optic atrophy and visual field defects.[275,276]

Sildenafil, tadalafil, vardenafil

Sildenafil, tadalafil, and vardenafil are a class of drugs that are potent inhibitors of phosophodiesterase-5 (PDE-5) and are used for the treatment of erectile dysfunction. Sildenafil also blocks PDE-6, though with only about 1/10 of its effect on PDE-5. PDE-6 is a key enzyme in the phototransduction cascade, and sildenafil modifies this cascade in photoreceptor outer segments causing a rise in cyclic guanosine monophosphate (cGMP). Commonly, patients notice a bluish dyschromotopsia (dose dependent) 1–2 hours after ingestion and this has been associated with a significant transient depression in the ERG in at least one study, though others have shown minimal to no effect on the ERG.[277–286] There appears to be no appreciable effect to slight increase in choroidal circulation with use of sildenafil on the ocular circulation and no adverse effects on those with early age-related macular degeneration.[287–292] There have been reported cases of nonarteritic ischemic optic neuropathy, central serous

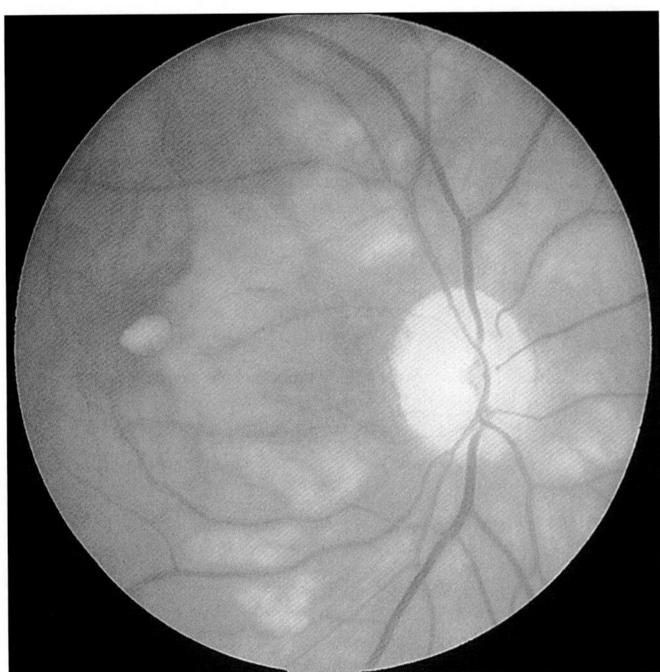

Fig. 89.32 Methanol poisoning. Acute changes revealing peripapillary retinal whitening and edema.

retinopathy, and cilioretinal artery obstruction with use of sildenafil and tadalafil.[293-305]

SUMMARY

Although there are thousands of systemic medications, only a small number of these agents produce retinal changes. Retinal toxicity can occur when agents are used at standard therapeutic levels, and when they are used for nonapproved indications. The mechanism by which toxicity develops is unknown in many cases. With numerous new medications reaching the market annually, ophthalmologists need to maintain a high index of suspicion that patients' symptoms and clinical findings may be related to one or more of their medications.

REFERENCES

1. Weekley RD, Potts AM, Reboton J, et al. Pigmentary retinopathy in patients receiving high doses of a new phenothiazine. Arch Ophthalmol 1960;64:65–76.
2. Meredith TA, Aaberg TM, Willerson D. Progressive chorioretinopathy after receiving thioridazine. Arch Ophthalmol 1978;96:1172–6.
3. Miller III FS, Bunt-Milam AH, Kalina RE. Clinical-ultrastructural study of thioridazine retinopathy. Ophthalmology 1982;89:1478–88.
4. Connell MM, Poley BJ, McFarlane JR. Chorioretinopathy associated with thioridazine therapy. Arch Ophthalmol 1964;71:816–21.
5. Hagopian V, Stratton DB, Busick RD. Five cases of pigmentary retinopathy associated with thioridazine administration. Am J Psychiatr 1966;123:97–100.
6. Hamilton D. Thioridazine retinopathy within the upper dosage limit [letter]. Psychosomatics 1985;26:823–4.
7. Heshe J, Engelstoft FH, Kirk L. Retinal injury developing under thioridazine treatment. Nord Psykiat T 1961;15:442–7.
8. Lam RW, Remick RA. Pigmentary retinopathy associated with low-dose thioridazine treatment. Can Med Assoc J 1985;132:737.
9. Neves MS, Jordan K, Dragt H. Extensive chorioretinopathy associated with very low dose thioridazine [letter]. Eye 1990;4:767–70.
10. Tekell JI, Silva JA, Maas JA, et al. Thioridazine-induced retinopathy. Am J Psychiatry 1996;153:1234–5.
11. Miyata, M, Imai, H, Ishikawa, S, et al. Changes in human electroretinography associated with thioridazine administration. Ophthalmologica 1980;181:175–80.
12. Marmor, MF. Is thioridazine retinopathy progressive? Relationship of pigmentary changes to visual function. Br J Ophthalmol 1990;74:739–42.
13. Chaudhry TA, Shamsi FA, Weitzman ML. Progressive severe visual loss after long-term withdrawal from thioridazine treatment. Eur J Ophthalmol 2006;16:651–3.
14. Potts AM. Further studies concerning accumulation of polycyclic compounds on uveal melanin. Invest Ophthalmol Vis Sci 1964;3:399–404.
15. Potts AM. The concentration of phenothiazines in the eye of experimental animals. Invest Ophthalmol Vis Sci 1962;1:522–30.
16. Potts AM. The reaction of uveal pigment in vitro with polycyclic compounds. Invest Ophthalmol Vis Sci 1964;3:405–16.
17. Kinross-Wright, JT. Clinical trial of a new phenothiazine compound NP-207. Psychiatr Res Rep Am Psychiatr Assoc 1956;4:89–94.
18. Bonting SL, Caravaggio LL, Canady MR. Studies on sodium potassium-activated adenosine triphosphatase. X. Occurrence in retinal rods and relation to rhodopsin. Exp Eye Res 1964;3:47–56.
19. Cerletti A, Meier-Ruge W. Toxicological studies on phenothiazine-induced retinopathy. Excerpts Medica International Congress Series 1968;145:170–88.
20. Muirhead JF. Drug effects on retinal oxidation: retinal alcohol: NAD+ oxido-reductase. Invest Ophthalmol Vis Sci 1967;6:635–41.
21. Fornaro P, Calabria G, Corallo G, et al. Pathogenesis of degenerative retinopathies induced by thioridazine and other antipsychotics: a dopamine hypothesis. Doc Ophthalmol 2002;105:41–9.
22. DeLong SL, Poley BJ, McFarlane JR. Ocular changes associated with long-term chlorpromazine therapy. Arch Ophthalmol 1965;73:611–7.
23. Mathalone MBR. Eye and skin changes in psychiatric patients treated with chlorpromazine. Br J Ophthalmol 1967;51:86–93.
24. Oshika T. Ocular adverse effects of neuropsychiatric agents: incidence and management. Drug Safety 1995;12:256–63.
25. Siddal JR. The ocular toxic findings with prolonged and high dosage chlorpromazine intake. Arch Ophthalmol 1965;74:460–4.
26. Wolf ME, Richer S, Berk MA, et al. Cutaneous and ocular changes associated with the use of chlorpromazine. Int J Clin Pharmacol Ther Toxicol 1993;31:365–7.
27. Webber SK, Domniz Y, Sutton GL, et al. Corneal deposition after high-dose chlorpromazine hydrochloride therapy. Cornea 2001;20:217–9.
28. Razeghinejad MR, Nowroozzadeh MH, Zamani M, et al. In vivo observations of chlorpromazine ocular deposits in a pt on long-term chlorpromazine therapy. Clin Exp Ophthalmol 2008;36:560–3.
29. Cambiaggi A. Unusual ocular lesions in a case of systemic lupus erythematosus. Arch Ophthalmol 1957;57:451–3.
30. Henkind P, Rothfield NF. Ocular abnormalities in patients treated with synthetic antimalarial drugs. N Engl J Med 1963;269:433–9.
31. Hobbs HE, Edeadie SP, Sommervile F. Ocular lesions after treatment with chloroquine. Br J Ophthalmol 1961;45:284–97.
32. Hobbs HE, Sorsby A, Freedman A. Retinopathy following chloroquine therapy. Lancet 1959;2:478–80.
33. Marks JS. Chloroquine retinopathy: is there a safe daily dose? Ann Rheum Dis 1982;41:52–8.
34. Nylander U. Ocular damage in chloroquine therapy. Acta Ophthalmol 1967;92:5–71.
35. Okun E, Gouras P, Bernstein H, et al. Chloroquine retinopathy. Arch Ophthalmol 1963;69:59–71.
36. Ochsendorf FR, Runne U. Chloroquine: consideration of maximum daily dose (3.5 mg/kg ideal weight) prevents retinopathy. Dermatology 1996;192:382–3.
37. Tobin DR, Krohel GB, Rynes RL. Hydroxychloroquine: seven-year experience. Arch Ophthalmol 1982;100:81–3.
38. Finbloom DS, Silver K, Newsome DA, et al. Comparison of hydroxychloroquine and chloroquine use and the development of retinal toxicity. J Rheumatol 1985;12:692–4.
39. Mackenzie AH, Scherbel AL. A decade of chloroquine maintenance therapy: rate of administration governs incidence of retinotoxicity. Arthritis Rheum 1968;11:496.
40. Hart WM, Burde RM, Johnston GP, et al. Static perimetry in chloroquine retinopathy: perifoveal patterns of visual field depression. Arch Ophthalmol 1984;102:377–80.
41. Brinkley JR, Dubois EL, Ryan SJ. Long-term course of chloroquine retinopathy after cessation of medication. Am J Ophthalmol 1979;88:1–11.
42. Carr RE, Henkind P, Rothfield N, et al. Ocular toxicity of antimalarial drugs. Am J Ophthalmol 1968;66:738.
43. Rubin M, Bernstein HN, Zvaifler NJ. Studies on the pharmacology of chloroquine. Arch Ophthalmol 1963;70:80–7.
44. Ehrenfeld M, Nesher R, Merin S. Delayed-onset chloroquine retinopathy. Br J Ophthalmol 1986;70:281–3.
45. Sassani JW, Brucker AJ, Cobbs W, et al. Progressive chloroquine retinopathy. Ann Ophthalmol 1983;15:19–22.
46. Heckenlively JR, Matin D, Levy J. Chloroquine retinopathy. Am J Ophthalmol 1980;89:150.
47. Wetterholm DH, Winter FC. Histopathology of chloroquine retinal toxicity. Arch Ophthalmol 1964;71:82–7.
48. Ramsey MS, Fine BS. Chloroquine toxicity in the human eye: histopathologic observation by electron microscopy. Am J Ophthalmol 1972;73:229–35.
49. Bonanomi MT, Dantas NC, Medeiros FA. Retinal nerve fiber layer thickness measurements in patients using chloroquine. Clin Experiment Ophthalmol 2006;34:130–6.
50. Kellner U, Kellner S, Weinitz S. Chloroquine retinopathy: lipofuscin- and melanin-related fundus autofluorescence, optical coherence tomography and multifocal electroretinography. Doc Ophthalmol 2008;116:119–27.
51. Bernstein H, Zvaifler N, Rubin M, et al. The ocular deposition of chloroquine. Invest Ophthalmol 1963;2:384–92.
52. Mahon GJ, Anderson HR, Gardiner TA, et al. Chloroquine causes lysosomal dysfunction in neural retina and implications for retinopathy. Curr Eye Res 2003;28:277–84.
53. Ivanina TA, Zueva MY, Lebedeva MM, et al. Ultrastructural alterations in rat and cat retina and pigment epithelium induced by chloroquine. Graefes Arch Clin Exp Ophthalmol 1983;22:32–8.
54. Vu BL, Easterbrook M, Hovis JK. Detection of color vision defects in chloroquine retinopathy. Ophthalmol 1999;106:1799–803.
55. Neubauer AS, Samari-Kermani K, Schaller U, et al. Detecting chloroquine retinopathy: electro-oculogram versus colour vision. Br J Ophthalmol 2002;87:902–8.
56. Kellner U, Kraus H, Forester MH. Multifocal ERG in chloroquine retinopathy: regional variance of retinal dysfunction. Graefes Arch Clin Exp Ophthalmol 2000;238:94–7.
57. Tzekov R. Ocular toxicity due to chloroquine and hydroxychloroquine. Doc Ophthalmol 2005;110:111–20.
58. Grierson DJ. Hydroxychloroquine and visual screening in a rheumatology outpatient clinic. Ann Rheum Dis 1997;56:188–90.
59. Levy GD, Munz SJ, Paschal J, et al. Incidence of hydroxychloroquine retinopathy in 1207 patients in a large multicenter outpatient practice. Arthritis Rheum 1997;40:1482–6.
60. Rynes RI. Ophthalmologic considerations in using antimalarials in the United States. Lupus 1996;5:73–4.
61. Coyle JT. Hydroxychloroquine retinopathy. Ophthalmol 108:243–4. 2001
62. Falcone PM, Paolini L, Lou PL. Hydroxychloroquine toxicity despite normal dose therapy. Ann Ophthalmol 1993;25:385–8.
63. Johnson MW, Vine AK. Hydroxychloroquine therapy in massive total doses without retinal toxicity. Am J Ophthalmol 1987;104:139–44.
64. Mavrikakis M, Papazoglou S, Sfikakis PP, et al. Retinal toxicity in long-term hydroxychloroquine treatment. Ann Rheum Dis 1996;55:187–9.
65. Shearer RV, Dubois EL. Ocular changes induced by long-term hydroxychloroquine therapy. Am J Ophthalmol 1967;64:245–52.
66. Weiner A, Sandberg MA, Gaudio AR, et al. Hydroxychloroquine retinopathy. Am J Ophthalmol 1991;112:528–34.
67. Weiser A, Sandberg MA, Gaadio AR, et al. Hydroxychloroquine retinopathy. Am J Ophthalmol 1991;121:582–4.

68. Bienfang D, Coblyn JS, Liang MH, et al. Hydroxychloroquine retinopathy despite regular ophthalmologic evaluaton: A consecutive case series. J Rheumatol 2000;27:2703–6.
69. Browning DJ. Hydroxychloroquine and chloroquine retinopathy: screening for drug toxicity. Am J Ophthalmol 2002;133:649–56.
70. Lyons JS, Severns ML. Detection of early hydroxychloroquine retinal toxicity enhanced by ring ratio analysis of multifocal electroretinography. Am J Ophthalmol 2007;143:801–9.
71. Mavrikakis I, Sfikakis PP, Mavrikakis E, et al. The incidence of irreversible retinal toxicity in patients treated with hydroxychloroquine: a reappraisal. Ophthalmol 2003;110:1321–6.
72. Wolfe F, Marmor MF. Rates and predictors of hydroxychloroquine retinal toxicity in patients with rheumatoid arthritis and systemic lupus erythematosus. Arthritis Care Res 2010;62:775–84.
73. Easterbrook M, Bernstein H. Ophthalmic monitoring of patients taking antimalarials: preferred practice patterns. J Rheumatol 1997;24:1390–2.
74. Morsman CDG, Livesey SJ, Richards IM, et al. Screening for hydroxychloroquine retinal toxicity: is it necessary? Eye 1990;4:572–6.
75. Shipley M, Silman A. Should patients on hydroxychloroquine have their eyes examined regularly? Br J Rheumatol 1997;30:514–5.
76. Silman A, Shipley M. Ophthalmological monitoring for hydroxy-chloroquine toxicity: a scientific review of available data. Br J Rheumatol 1997;36: 599–601.
77. Easterbrook M. Hydroxychloroquine retinopathy. Ophthalmol 2001;108: 2158–9.
78. Marmor MF, Kellner U, Lai TYY, et al. Recommendations on screening for chloroquine and hydroxychloroquine retinopathy. Ophthalmol 2011;118: 415–22.
79. Michaelides M, Stover N, Francis P, et al. Retinal toxicity associated with hydroxychloroquine and chloroquine. Arch Ophthalmol 2011;129:30–9.
80. Maturi RK, Yu M, Weleber RG. Multifocal electroretinographic evaluation of long-term hydroxychloroquine users. Arch Ophthalmol 2003;122: 973–81.
81. Penrose PF, Tzekov RT, Sutter EE, et al. Multifocal electroretinography evaluation for early detection of retinal dysfunction in patients taking hydroxychloroquine. Retina 2003;23:503–12.
82. Moschos MN, Moschos MM, Apostolopoulos M, et al. Assessing hydroxychloroquine toxicity by the multifocal ERG. Doc Ophthalmol 2004;108: 47–53.
83. Lai TY, Chan WM, Li H, et al. Multifocal electroretinographic changes in patients receiving hydroxychloroquine therapy. Am J Ophthalmol 2005;140: 794–807.
84. Lai TY, Ngai JW, Chan WM, et al. Visual field and multifocal electroretinography and their correlations in patients on hydroxychloroquine therapy. Doc Ophthalmol 2006;112:177–87.
85. Rodriguez-Padrilla JA, Hedges 3rd TR, Monson B, et al. High-speed ultra-high resolution optical coherence tomography findings in hydroxychloroquine retinopathy. Arch Ophthalmol 2007;125:775–80.
86. Stepien KE, Han DP, Schell J, et al. Spectral-domain optical coherence tomography and adaptive optics may detect hydroxychloroquine retinal toxicity before symptomatic visual loss. Trans Am Ophthalmol Soc 2009;107: 28–33.
87. Pasadhika S, Fishman GA, Choi D, et al. Selective thinning of the perifoveal inner retina as an early sign of hydroxychloroquine retinal toxicity. Eye 2010;24:75–762.
88. Kellner U, Renner AB, Tillack H. Fundus autofluorescence and mfERG for the early detection of retinal alterations in patients using chloroquine/ hydroxychloroquine. Invest Ophthalmol Vis Sci 2006;47:3531–8.
89. Maturi RK, Folk JC, Nichols B, et al. Hydroxychloroquine retinopathy. Arch Ophthalmol 1999;117:1262–2.
90. Horgan SE, Williams RW. Chronic retinal toxicity due to quinine in Indian tonic water. Eye 1995;9:637–63.
91. Brinton GS, Nortona EWD, Zahn JR, et al. Ocular quinine toxicity. Am J Ophthalmol 1980;90:403–10.
92. Lochhead J, Movaffaghy A, Falsini B, et al. The effect of quinine on the electroretinogram of children with pediatric cerebral malaria. J Infect Dis 2003;187:1342–5.
93. Traill A, Patmaraj R, Zamir E. Quinine iris toxicity. Arch Ophthalmol 2007;125:430.
94. Bacon P, Spalton DJ, Smith SE. Blindness from quinine toxicity. Br J Ophthalmol 1988;72:219–24.
95. Buchanan TAS, Lyness RW, Collins AD, et al. An experimental study of quinine blindness. Eye 1987;1:522–4.
96. Canning CR, Hague S. Ocular quinine toxicity. Br J Ophthalmol 1988;72: 23–6.
97. Craythorn JM, Swartz M, Creel DJ. Clofazimine-induced bull's-eye retinopathy. Retina 1986;6:50–2.
98. Cunningham CA, Friedberg DN, Carr RE. Clofazimine-induced generalized retinal degeneration. Retina 1990;10:131–4.
99. Whitcup SM, Butler KM, Caruso R, et al. Retinal toxicity in human immunodeficiency virus-infected children treated with 2',3'-dideoxyinosine. Am J Ophthalmol 1992;113:1–7.
100. Davies SC, Hungerford JL, Arden GB, et al. Ocular toxicity of high-dose intravenous desferrioxamine. Lancet 1983;2:181–4.
101. Mehta AM, Engstrom RE, Kreiger AE. Deferoxamine-associated retinopathy after subcutaneous injection. Am J Ophthalmol 1994;118:260–2.
102. Gass JDM. Stereoscopic atlas of macular diseases: diagnosis and treatment. 4th ed. St Louis: Mosby; 1997.
103. Haimovici R, D'Amico DJ, Gragoudas ES, et al. Deferoxamine Retinopathy Study Group: The expanded clinical spectrum of deferoxamine retinopathy. Ophthalmol 2002;109:164–71.
104. Rahl AHS, Hungerford JL, Ahmed AI. Ocular toxicity of desferrioxamine: light microscopic histochemical and ultrastructural findings. Br J Ophthalmol 1986;70:373–81.
105. Hida T, Chandler D, Arena JE, et al. Experimental and clinical observations of the intraocular toxicity of commercial corticosteroid preparations. Am J Ophthalmol 1986;101:190–5.
106. Pendergast SD, Eliott D, Machemer R. Retinal toxic effects following inadvertent intraocular injection of celestone soluspan. Arch Ophthalmol 1995;113: 1230–1.
107. McCuen II BW, Bessler M, Tano Y, et al. The lack of toxicity of intravitreally administered triamcinolone acetonide. Am J Ophthalmol 1981;91:785–8.
108. Piccolino FC, Pandolfo A, Polizzi A, et al. Retinal toxicity from accidental intraocular injection of depomedrol. Retina 2002;22:117–9.
109. Kupersmith MJ, Seiple WH, Holopigian K, et al. Maculopathy caused by intra-arterially administered cisplatin and intravenously administered carmustine. Am J Ophthalmol 1992;113:435–8.
110. Miller DF, Bay JW, Lederman RJ, et al. Ocular and orbital toxicity following intracarotid injection of BCNU (carmustine) and cisplatinum for malignant gliomas. Ophthalmology 1985;92:402–6.
111. Katz BJ, Ward JH, Digre KB, et al. Persistent severe visual and electroretinographic abnormalities after intravenous Cisplatin therapy. J Neruoophthalmol 2003;23:132–5.
112. Khawly JA, Rubin P, Petros W, et al. Retinopathy and optic neuropathy in bone marrow transplantation for breast cancer. Ophthalmology 1996;103: 87–95.
113. Margo CE, Murtagh FR. Ocular and orbital toxicity after intra-carotid cisplatin therapy. Am J Ophthalmol 1993;116:508–9.
114. Singalavaniga A, Ruangvaravate N, Dulayajinda D. Potassium iodate toxic retinopathy: a report of five cases. Retina 2000;20:378–83.
115. Ruddle JB, Harper CA, Honemann D, et al. A denileukin diftitox (Ontak) associated retinopathy? Br J Ophthalmol 2006;90:1070–1.
116. AtLee WE. Talc and cornstarch emboli in eyes of drug users. JAMA 1972;219:49.
117. Murphy SB, Jackson WB, Pare JAP. Talc retinopathy. Can J Ophthalmol 1978;13:152–6.
118. Tse DT, Ober RR. Talc retinopathy. Am J Ophthalmol 1980;90:624–40.
119. Schatz H, Drake M. Self-injected retinal emboli. Ophthalmology 1979;86:468.
120. Friberg TR, Gragoudas ES, Regan CDJ. Talc emboli and macular ischemia in intravenous drug abuse. Arch Ophthalmol 1979;97:1089.
121. Brucker AJ. Disk and peripheral retinal neovascularization secondary to talc and cornstarch emboli. Am J Ophthalmol 1979;88:864.
122. Kresca LJ, Goldberg MF, Jampol LM. Talc emboli and retinal neovascularization in a drug abuser. Am J Ophthalmol 1979;87:334.
123. Jampol LM, Setogawa T, Rednam KRV, et al. Talc retinopathy in primates: a model of ischemic retinopathy. I. Clinical studies. Arch Ophthalmol 1981; 99:1273–80.
124. Kaga N, Tso MOM, Jampol LM, et al. Talc retinopathy in primates: a model of ischemic retinopathy. II. A histopathologic study. Arch Ophthalmol 1982; 100:1644–8.
125. Kaga N, Tso MOM, Jampol LM. Talc retinopathy in primates: a model of ischemic retinopathy. III. An electron microscopic study. Arch Ophthalmol 1982;100:1649–57.
126. Gombos GM, Moreno DH, Bedrossian PB. Retinal vascular occlusion induced by oral contraceptives. Ann Ophthalmol 1975;7:215–7.
127. Goren GB. Retinal edema secondary to oral contraceptives. Am J Ophthalmol 1967;64:447–9.
128. Lyle TK, Wybar K. Retinal vasculitis. Br J Ophthalmol 1961;45:778–88.
129. Perry HD, Mallen FJ. Cilioretinal artery occlusion associated with oral contraceptives. Am J Ophthalmol 1977;84:56–8.
130. Stowe GC, Jakov AN, Albert DM. Central retinal vascular occlusion associated with oral contraceptives. Am J Ophthalmol 1978;86:798–801.
131. Varga M. Recent experiences on the ophthalmological complications of oral contraceptives. Ann Ophthalmol 1976;8:925–34.
132. Walsh FB, Clark DB, Thompson RS, et al. Oral contraceptives and neuro-ophthalmologic interest. Arch Ophthalmol 1965;74:628–40.
133. Garg SK, Chase P, Marshall G, et al. Oral contraceptives and renal and retinal complications in young women with insulin-dependent diabetes mellitus. JAMA 1994;271:1099–102.
134. Petersson GJ, Fraunfelder FT, Meyer SM. Oral contraceptives. Ophthalmology 1981;88:368–71.
135. Vessey MP, Hannaford P, Mant J, et al. Oral contraception and eye disease: findings in two large cohort studies. Br J Ophthalmol 1998;82:538–42.
136. Balian JV. Accidental intraocular tobramycin injection: a case report. Ophthalmic Surg 1983;14:353–4.
137. Campochiaro PA, Conway BP. Aminoglycoside toxicity – a survey of retinal specialists: implications for ocular use. Arch Ophthalmol 1991;109:946–50.
138. Campochiaro PA, Lim JI. Aminoglycoside toxicity in the treatment of endophthalmitis. Arch Ophthalmol 1994;112:48–53.
139. McDonald HR, Schatz H, Allen AW, et al. Retinal toxicity secondary to intraocular gentamicin. Ophthalmology 1986;93:871–7.
140. D'Amico DJ, Caspers-Velu L, Libert J, et al. Comparative toxicity of intravitreal aminoglycoside antibiotics. Am J Ophthalmol 1985;100:264–75.
141. Peyman GA, Vastine DW, Crouch ER, et al. Clinical use of intravitreal antibiotics to treat bacterial endophthalmitis. Trans Am Acad Ophthalmol Otolaryngol 1974;78:862–75.

142. Zachary IG, Forster RK. Experimental intravitreal gentamicin. Am J Ophthalmol 1976;82:604–11.
143. Rosenbaum JD, Krumholz DM, Metz DM. Gentamicin retinal toxicity after cataract surgery in an eye that underwent vitrectomy. Ophthalmic Surg Laser 1997;28:236–8.
144. Talamo JH, D'Amico DJ, Hanninen LA, et al. The influence of aphakia and vitrectomy on experimental retinal toxicity of aminoglycoside antibiotics. Am J Ophthalmol 1985;100:840–7.
145. Kane A, Barza M, Baum J. Intravitreal injection of gentamicin in rabbits: effect of inflammation and pigmentation on half-life and ocular distribution. Invest Ophthalmol Vis Sci 1981;20:593–7.
146. Zemel E, Loewenstein A, Lei B, et al. Ocular pigmentation protects the rabbit retina from gentamicin-induced toxicity. Invest Ophthalmol Vis Sci 1995;36: 1875–84.
147. Brown GC, Eagle RC, Shakin EP, et al. Retinal toxicity of intravitreal gentamicin. Arch Ophthalmol 1990;108:1740–4.
148. D'Amico DJ, Libert J, Kenyon KR, et al. Retinal toxicity of intravitreal gentamicin: an electron microscopic study. Invest Ophthalmol Vis Sci 1984;25: 564–72.
149. Hines J, Vinores SA, Campochiaro PA. Evolution of morphologic changes after intravitreous injection of gentamicin. Curr Eye Res 1993;12:521–9.
150. Conway BP, Tabatabay CA, Campochiaro PA, et al. Gentamicin toxicity in the primate retina. Arch Ophthalmol 1989;107:107–12.
151. Loewenstein A, Zemel E, Vered Y, et al. Retinal toxicity of gentamicin after subconjunctival injection performed adjacent to thinned sclera. Ophthalmol 2001;108:759–54.
152. Chu TG, Ferreira M, Ober RR. Immediate pars plana vitrectomy in the management of inadvertent intracameral injection of gentamicin: a rabbit experimental model. Retina 1994;14:59–64.
153. Burgansky Z, Rock T, Bartov E. Inadvertent intravitreal gentamicin injection. Eur J Ophthalmol 2002;12:138–40.
154. Lim JI, Anderson CT, Hutchinson A, et al. The role of gravity in gentamicin-induced toxic effects in a rabbit model. Arch Ophthalmol 1994;112: 1363–7.
155. Guyer DR, Tiedeman J, Yannuzzi LA, et al. Interferon-associated retinopathy. Arch Ophthalmol 1993;111:350–6.
156. Kawano T, Shegehira M, Uto H, et al. Retinal complications during interferon therapy for chronic hepatitis C. Am J Gastroenterol 1996;91:309–13.
157. Schulman JA, Liang C, Kooragayala LM, et al. Posterior segment complications in patients with hepatitis C treated with interferon and ribavirin. Ophthalmol 2003;110:437–42.
158. Kiratli H, Irkee M. Presumed interferon-associated bilateral macular arterial branch obstruction. Eye 2000;14:920–2.
159. Tokai R, Ikeda T, Miyaura T, et al. Interferon-associated retinopathy and cystoid macular edema. Arch Ophthalmol 2001;119:1077–9.
160. Hejny C, Sternberg P, Lawson DH, et al. Retinopathy associated with high-dose interferon alfa-2b therapy. Am J Ophthalmol 2001;131:782–7.
161. Fraunfelder FW, Fraunfelder FT. Interferon alfa-associated anterior ischemic optic neuropathy. Ophthalmology 2011;118:408–11.
162. Rubio JE, Charles S. Interferon-associated combined branch retinal artery and central retinal vein obstruction. Retina 2003;23:546–8.
163. Wilson RL, Ross RD, Wilson LM, et al. Interferon-associated retinopathy in a young, insulin-dependent diabetic patient. Retina 2000;20:413–5.
164. Kertes PJ, Britton WA, Addison DJ, et al. Toxicity of intravitreal interferon alpha-2b in the rabbit. Can J Ophthalmol 30:355–9.1995.
165. Crochet M, Ingster-Moati I, Even G, et al. Retinography caused by interferon alpha associated ribavirin therapy and the importance of the electro-oculogram: a case report. J Fr Ophthalmol 2004;27:257–62.
166. Gupta DR, Strobos RJ. Bilateral papillitis associated with Cafergot therapy. Neurology 1972;22:793.
167. Mindel JS, Rubenstein AE, Franklin B. Ocular ergotamine tartrate toxicity during treatment of Vacor-induced orthostatic hypotension. Am J Ophthalmol 1981;92:492–6.
168. Gilmer G, Swartz M, Teske M, et al. Over-the-counter phenylpropanolamine: a possible cause of central retinal vein occlusion. Arch Ophthalmol 1986;104:642.
169. Banach MJ, Williams GA. Purtscher retinopathy and necrotizing vasculitis with gemcitabine therapy. Arch Ophthalmol 2000;118:726–272.
170. Thomas JV, Gragoudas ES, Blair NP, et al. Correlation of epinephrine use and macular edema in aphakic glaucomatous eyes. Arch Ophthalmol 1978;96: 625–8.
171. Fraunfelder FW, Fraunfelder FT, Illingworth DR. Adverse ocular effects associated with niacin therapy. Br J Ophthalmol 1995;79:54–6.
172. Gass JDM. Nicotinic acid maculopathy. Am J Ophthalmol 1973;76:500–10.
173. Millay RH, Klein ML, Illingworth DR. Niacin maculopathy. Ophthalmology 1988;95:930–6.
174. Jampol LM. Niacin maculopathy. Ophthalmology 1988;95:1704–5.
175. Spirn MJ, Warren FA, Guyer DR, et al. Optical coherence tomography findings in nicotinic acid maculopathy. Am J Ophthalmol 2003;135:913–4.
176. Dajani HM, Lauer AK. Optical coherence tomography findings in niacin maculopathy. Can J Ophthalmol 2006;41:197–200.
177. Hoyng PFJ, Rulo AH, Greve EL, et al. Fluorescein angiographic evaluation of the effect of latanoprost treatment on blood–retinal barrier integrity: a review of studies conducted on pseudophakic glaucoma patients and on phakic and aphakic monkeys. Surv Ophthalmol 1997;41(Suppl 2):83–8.
178. Moroi S, Gottfredsdottir MS, Johnson MW, et al. Anterior uveitis and cystoid macular edema associated with latanoprost. Am Acad Ophthalmol Abstracts 1997;172.
179. Rowe JA, Hattenhauer MG, Herman DC. Adverse side effects associated with latanoprost. Am J Ophthalmol 1997;124:683–5.
180. Warwar RE, Bullock JD, Ballal D. Cystoid macular edema and anterior uveitis associated with latanoprost use. Ophthalmology 1998;105:263–8.
181. Halpern DL, Pasquale LR. Cystoid macular edema in aphakia and pseudophakia after use of prostaglandin analogs. Semin Ophthalmol 2002;17: 181–6.
182. Wand M, Gaudio AR, Shields MB. Latanoprost and cystoid macular edema in high-risk aphakic or pseudophakic eyes. J Cataract Refract Surg 2001;27: 1397–401.
183. Furuichi M, Chiba T, Abe K, et al. Cystioid macular edema associated with topical latanaprost in glaucomatous eyes with a normally functioning blood–ocular barrier. J Glaucoma 2001;10:233–6.
184. Lima MC, Paranhos Jr A, Salim S, et al. Visually significant cystoid macular edema in pseudophakic and aphakic patients with glaucoma receiving latanaprost. J Glaucoma 2000;9:317–21.
185. Schumer RA, Camras CB, Mandahl AK. Latanoprost and cystoid macular edema: is there a causal relation? Curr Opin Ophthalmol 2000;11: 94–100.
186. Miyake K, Ibaraki N. Prostaglandins and cystoid macular edema. Surv Ophthalmol 2002;47(Suppl1):S203–18.
187. Joshi MM, Garretson B. Paclitaxel retinopathy. Arch Ophthalmol 2007;125: 709–10.
188. Telender DG, Sarraf D. Cystoid macular edema with Docetaxel chemotherapy and the fluid retention syndrome. Semin Ophthalmol 2007;22:151–3.
189. Grinbaum A, Ashkenazi I, Avni I, et al. Transient myopia following metronidazole treatment for trichomonas vaginalis. JAMA 1992;267:511–2.
190. Ryan EH, Jampol LM. Drug-induced acute transient myopia with retinal folds. Retina 1986;6:220–3.
191. Soylev MF, Green RL, Feldon SE. Choroidal effusion as a mechanism for transient myopia induced by hydrochlorothiazide and triamterene. Am J Ophthalmol 1995;120:395–7.
192. Sen HA, O'Halloran HS, Lee WB. Case reports and small case series: topiramate-induced acute myopia and retinal striae. Arch Ophthalmol 2001;119:775–7.
193. Rhee DJ, Goldberg MJ, Parrish RK. Bilateral angle-closure glaucoma and ciliary body swelling from topiramate. Arch Ophthalmol 2001;119:1721–3.
194. Sankar PS, Pasquale LR, Grosskreutz CL. Uveal effusion and secondary angle-closure glaucoma associated with topiramate use. Arch Ophthalmol 2001;119: 1210–1.
195. Medeiros FA, Zhang XY, Bernd AS, et al. Angle-closure glaucoma associated with ciliary body detachment in patients using topiramate. Arch Ophthalmol 2003;121:282–5.
196. Fraunfelder FW, Fraunfelder FT, Keates EU. Topiramate-associated acute, bilateral, secondary angle-closure glaucoma. Ophthalmol 2004;111:109–11.
197. Craig JE, Ong TJ, Louis DL, et al. Mechanism of topiramate-induced acute-onset myopia and angle closure glaucoma. Am J Ophthalmol 2004;137: 193–5.
198. Mahesh G, Giridhar A, Saikumar SJ, et al. Drug-induced acute myopia following chlorthalidone treatment. Indian J Ophthalmol 2007;55:386–8.
199. Alwitry A, Gardner I. Tamoxifen maculopathy. Arch Ophthalmol 2002;120: 1402.
200. Kaiser-Kupfer MI, Kupfer C, Rodrigues MM. Tamoxifen retinopathy. Cancer Treat Rep 1978;62:315–20.
201. Chang T, Gonder JR, Ventresca MR. Low-dose tamoxifen retinopathy. Can J Ophthalmol 1992;27:148–9.
202. Griffiths MFP. Tamoxifen retinopathy at low dosage. Am J Ophthalmol 1987;104:185–6.
203. Pavlidis NA, Petris C, Briassoulis E, et al. Clear evidence that long-term, low-dose tamoxifen treatment can induce ocular toxicity. Cancer 1992;69: 2961–4.
204. Noureddin BN, Seoud M, Bashshur Z. et al. Ocular toxicity in low-dose tamoxifen: a prospective study. Eye 1999;13:729–33.
205. Yanyali AC, Freund KB, Sorenson JA, et al. Tamoxifen retinopathy in a male patient. Am J Ophthalmol 2001;131:386–7.
206. Heier JS, Dragoo RA, Enzenauer RW, et al. Screening for ocular toxicity in asymptomatic patients treated with tamoxifen. Am J Ophthalmol 1994;117: 772–5.
207. McKeown CA, Swartz M, Blom J, et al. Tamoxifen retinopathy. Br J Ophthalmol 1981;65:177–9.
208. Kaiser-Kupfer MI, Kupfer C, Rodrigues MM. Tamoxifen retinopathy: a clinicopathologic report. Ophthalmology 1981;88:89–93.
209. Maenpaa H, Mannerstrom M, Toimela T, et al. Glutamate uptake is inhibited by tamoxifen and toremifene in cultured retinal pigment epithelial cells. Pharmacol Toxicol 2002;91:116–22.
210. Gualino V, Cohen SY, Delyfer MN, et al. Optical coherence tomography findings in tamoxifen retinopathy. Am J Ophthalmol 2005;140:757–68.
211. Park SS, Zawadzki RJ, Truong SN, et al. Microcystoid maculopathy associated with tamoxifen use diagnoses by high-resolution fourier-domain optical coherence tomography. Retin Cases Brief Rep 2009;3:33–5.
212. Bourla DH, Sarraf D, Schwartz SD. Peripheral retinopathy and maculopathy in high-dose tamoxifen therapy. Am J Ophthalmol 2007;144:126–8.
213. Ashford AR, Donev I, Tiwari RP, et al. Reversible ocular toxicity related to tamoxifen therapy. Cancer 1988;61:33–5.
214. Colley SM, Elston JS. Tamoxifen optic neuropathy. Clin Exp Ophthalmol 2004;32:105–6.
215. Nayfield SG, Gorin MB. Tamoxifen-associated eye disease: a review. J Clin Oncol 1996;14:1018–26.

216. Kalina RE, Wells CG. Screening for ocular toxicity in asymptomatic patients with tamoxifen [letter]. Am J Ophthalmol 1995;119:112–3.
217. Bourla DH, Gonzales CR, Mango CW, et al. Intravitreous vascular endothelial growth factor (VEGF) inhibitor therapy for tamoxifen induced macular edema. Semin Ophthalmol 2007;22:87–8.
218. Chang TS, Aylward W, Clarkson JG, et al. Asymmetric canthaxanthine retinopathy. Am J Ophthalmol 1995;119:801–2.
219. Lonn LI. Canthaxanthine retinopathy. Arch Ophthalmol 1987;105:1590–1.
220. Espaillat A, Aiello LP, Arrigg PG, et al. Canthaxanthine retinopathy. Arch Ophthalmol 1999;117:412–3.
221. Cortin P, Boudreault G, Rousseau AP, et al. La retinopathie a la canthaxanthine. II. Facteurs predisposants. Can J Ophthalmol 1984;19:215–9.
222. Boudreault G, Cortin P, Corriveau LA, et al. La retinopathie a la canthaxanthine. I. Etude clinique de 51 consommateurs. Can J Ophthalmol 1983;18: 325–8.
223. Harnois C, Cortin P, Samson J, et al. Static perimetry in canthaxanthine maculopathy. Arch Ophthalmol 1988;106:58–60.
224. Metge P, Mandirac-Bonnefoy C, Bellaube P. Thesaurismose retinienne à la canthaxanthine. Bull Mem Soc Fr Ophtalmol 1984;95:547–9.
225. Weber U, Goerz G, Hennekes R. Carotenoid retinopathie. I. Morphologische und funktionell befunde. Klin Monatsbl Augenheilkd 1985;186:351–4.
226. Daicker B, Schiedt K, Adnet JJ, et al. Canthaxanthin retinopathy: an investigation by light and electron microscopy and physiochemical analysis. Graefes Arch Clin Exp Ophthalmol 1987;225:189–97.
227. Chan A, Duker JS. Ultrahigh-resolution optical coherence tomography of canthaxanthin retinal crystals. Ophthalmic Surg Lasers Imaging 2006;37: 138–9.
228. Scallon LJ, Burke JM, Mieler WF, et al. Canthaxanthine-induced retinal pigment epithelial changes in the cat. Curr Eye Res 1988;7:687–93.
229. Harnois C, Samson J, Malenfant M, et al. Canthaxanthine retinopathy: anatomic and functional reversibility. Arch Ophthalmol 1989;107:538–40.
230. Leyon H, Ros A, Nyberg S, et al. Reversibility of canthaxanthin deposits within the retina. Acta Ophthalmol 1990;68:607–11.
231. Oosterhuis JA, Remky H, Nijman NM, et al. Canthaxanthine-retinopathie ohne canthaxanthine-einnahime. Klin Monatsbl Augenheilkd 1989;194: 110–6.
232. Bullock JD, Albert DM. Fleck retina: appearance secondary to oxalate crystals from methoxyflurane anesthesia. Arch Ophthalmol 1975;93:26–31.
233. Novak MA, Roth AS, Levine MR. Calcium oxalate retinopathy associated with methoxyflurane abuse. Retina 1988;8:230–6.
234. Albert DM, Bullock JD, Lahav M, et al. Flecked retina secondary to oxalate crystals from methoxyflurane anesthesia: clinical and experimental studies. Trans Am Acad Ophthalmol Otolaryngol 1975;79:817–26.
235. Wells CG, Johnson RJ, Qingli L, et al. Retinal oxalosis: a clinicopathological report. Arch Ophthalmol 1989;107:1638–43.
236. Ibanez HE, Williams DF, Boniuk I. Crystalline retinopathy associated with long-term nitrofurantoin therapy. Arch Ophthalmol 1994;112:304–5.
237. Bishop R, Ding X, Heller C, et al. Rapid vision loss associated with fludarabine administration. Retina 2010;30:1272–7.
238. Roe RH, Jumper JM, Gualino V, et al. Retinal pigment epitheliopathy, macular telangiectasis, intraretinal crystal deposits in HIV-positive patients receiving ritonavir. Retina 2011;31:559–65.
239. Arevalo JF, Russack V, Freeman WR. New ophthalmic manifestations of presumed rifabutin-related uveitis. Ophthalmic Surg Laser 1997;28: 321–4.
240. Becker K, Schimkat M, Jablonowski H, et al. Anterior uveitis associated with rifabutin medication in AIDS patients. Infection 1996;24:36–8.
241. Jacobs DS, Piliero PJ, Kuperwaser MG, et al. Acute uveitis associated with rifabutin use in patients with human immunodeficiency virus infection. Am J Ophthalmol 1994;118:716–22.
242. Karbassi M, Nikou S. Acute uveitis in patients with acquired immunodeficiency syndrome receiving prophylactic rifabutin. Arch Ophthalmol 1995; 113:699–701.
243. Kelleher P, Helbert M, Sweeney J, et al. Uveitis associated with rifabutin and macrolide therapy for *Mycobacterium avium-intracellulare* infection in AIDS patients. Genitourin Med 1996;72:419–21.
244. Nichols CW. *Mycobacterium avium* complex infection, rifabutin, uveitis: is there a connection? Clin Infect Dis 1996;22:43–9.
245. Rifai A, Peyman GA, Daun M, et al. Rifabutin-associated uveitis during prophylaxis for *Mycobacterium avium* complex infection. Arch Ophthalmol 1995;113:707.
246. Saran BR, Maguire AM, Nichols C, et al. Hypopyon uveitis in patients with acquired immunodeficiency syndrome: treatment for systemic *Mycobacterium avium* complex infection with rifabutin. Arch Ophthalmol 1994;112: 1159–65.
247. Tseng AL, Walmsley SL. Rifabutin-associated uveitis. Ann Pharmacother 1995;29:1149–55.
248. Bhagat N, Read RW, Rao NA, et al. Rifabutin-associated hypopyon uveitis in human immunodeficiency virus-negative immunocompetent individuals. Ophthalmol 2001;108:750–2.
249. Khan MA, Singh J, Dhillon B. Rifabutin-induced uveitis with inflammatory vitreous infiltrate. Eye 2000;14:344–6.
250. Saha N, Bansal S, Bishop F, et al. Bilateral hypopyon and vitritis associated with rifabutin therapy in an immunocompetent patient taking itraconazole. Eye 2009;23(6):1481.
251. Chaknis MJ, Brooks SE, Mitchell KT, et al. Inflammatory opacities of the vitreous in rifabutin-associated uveitis. Am J Ophthalmol 1996;122: 580–2.
252. Ponjavic V, Granse L, Bengtsson Stigmar E,et al. Retinal dysfunction and anterior sefment depostits in a patient treated with rifabutin. Acta Ophthalmol Scand 2002;80:553–6.
253. Banker AS, Arevalo JF, Munguia D, et al. Intraocular pressure and aqueous humor dynamics in patients with AIDS treated with intravitreal cidofovir (HPMPC) for cytomegalovirus retinitis. Am J Ophthalmol 1997;124:168–80.
254. Davis JL, Taskintuna I, Freeman WR, et al. Iritis and hypotony after treatment with intravenous cidofovir for cytomegalovirus retinitis. Arch Ophthalmol 1997;115:733–7.
255. Friedberg DN. Hypotony and visual loss with intravenous cidofovir treatment of cytomegalovirus retinitis. Arch Ophthalmol 1997;115:801–2.
256. Jabs DA. Cidofovir. Arch Ophthalmol 1997;115:785–6.
257. Kirsch LS, Arevalo JF, De Clercq E, et al. Phase I/II study of intra-vitreal cidofovir for the treatment of cytomegalovirus retinitis in patients with the acquired immunodeficiency syndrome. Am J Ophthalmol 1995;119: 466–76.
258. Kirsch LS, Arevalo JF, de la Paz EC. Intravitreal cidofovir (HPMPC) treatment of cytomegalovirus retinitis in patients with acquired immune deficiency syndrome. Ophthalmology 1995;102:533–43.
259. Lea AP, Bryson HM. Cidofovir. Drugs 1996;52:225–30.
260. Rahal FM, Arevalo JF, Munguia D, et al. Intravitreal cidofovir for the maintenance treatment of cytomegalovirus retinitis. Ophthalmology 1996;103: 1078–83.
261. Taskintuna, I, Banker, AS, Rao, NA, et al. An animal model for cidofovir (HPMPC) toxicity: intraocular pressure and histopathologic effects. Exp Eye Res 1997;64:795–806.
262. Taskintuna I, Rahhal FM, Arevalo F, et al. Low-dose intravitreal cidofovir (HPMPC) therapy of cytomegalovirus retinitis in patients with acquired immune deficiency syndrome. Ophthalmology 1997;104:1049–57.
263. Wang L, Damji KF, Chialant D, et al. Hypotony after intravenous cidofovir therapy for the treatment of cytomegalovirus retinitis. Can J Ophthalmol 2002;37:419–22.
264. Blair JR, Mieler WF. Retinal toxicity associated with commonly encountered systemic agents. Int Ophthalmol Clin 1995;35:137–56.
265. Weleber RG, Shults WT. Digoxin retinal toxicity: clinical and electrophysiologic evaluation of a cone dysfunction syndrome. Arch Ophthalmol 1981;99: 1568–72.
266. Baumbach GL, Cancilla PA, Martin-Amat G, et al. Methyl alcohol poisoning. IV. Alterations of the morphological findings of the retina and optic nerve. Arch Ophthalmol 1977;95:1859–65.
267. Eells JT, Makar AB, Noker PE, et al. Methanol poisoning and formate oxidation in nitrous oxide–treated rats. J Pharmacol Exp Ther 1981;217: 57–61.
268. Gilger AP, Potts AM. Studies on the visual toxicity of methanol: the role of acidosis in experimental methanol poisoning. Am J Ophthalmol 1955;39: 63–85.
269. Hayreh MS, Hayreh SS, Baumbach GL, et al. Methyl alcohol poisoning. III. Ocular toxicity. Arch Ophthalmol 1977;95:1851–8.
270. Ingemansson SO. Clinical observations on ten cases of methanol poisoning. Acta Ophthalmol 1984;62:15–24.
271. Martin-Amat G, McMartin KE, Hayreh SS, et al. Methanol poisoning: ocular toxicity produced by formate. Toxicol Appl Pharmacol 1978;45:201–8.
272. Martin-Amat G, Tephly TR, McMartin KE, et al. Methyl alcohol poisoning. II. Development of a model for ocular toxicity in methyl alcohol poisoning using the rhesus monkey. Arch Ophthalmol 1977;95:1847–50.
273. Treichel JL, Murray TG, Lewandowski MF, et al. Retinal toxicity in methanol poisoning. Retina 2004;24:309–12.
274. Fujihara M, Kikuchi M, Kurimoto Y. Methanol-induced retinal toxicity patient examined by optical coherence tomography. Jpn J Ophthalmol 2006;50: 239–41.
275. Frisen L, Malmgren K. Characterization of vigabatrin-associated optic atrophy. Acta Opthalmol Scand 2003;81:466–73.
276. Malmgren K, Ben-Menachem E, Frisen L. Vigabatrin visual toxicity: evolution and dose dependence. Epilepsia 2001;42:609–15.
277. Vobig MA, Klotz T, Staak M, et al. Retinal side-effects of sildenafil [letter]. Lancet 1999;353:375.
278. Vobig MA. Retinal side-effects of sildenafil [letter]. Lancet 1999;353:9162.
279. Zrenner E. No cause for alarm over retinal side-effects of sildenafil. Lancet 1999;353:340–1.
280. Marmor MF, Kessler R. Sildenafil (Viagra) and ophthalmology. Surv Ophthalmol 1999;44:153–62.
281. Marmor MF. Sildenafil (Viagra) and ophthalmology [Editorial]. Arch Ophthalmol 1999;117:518–9.
282. Luu JK, Chappelow AV, McCulley TJ, et al. Acute effects of sildenafil on the electroretinogram and multifocal electroretinogram. Am J Ophthalmol 2001; 132:388–94.
283. Jagle H, Jagle C, Serey L, et al. Visual short-term effects of Viagra: double-blind study in healthy young subjects. Am J Ophthalmol 2004;137:842–9.
284. Jagle H, Jagle C, Serey L, et al. Dose-dependency and time-course of electrophysiologic short-term effects of Viagra: a case study. Doc Ophthalmol 2005;110:247–54.
285. Zoumalan CI, Zamanian RT, Doyle RL, et al. ERG evaluation of daily, high-dose sildenafil usage. Doc Ophthalmol 2008;118:225–31.
286. Cordell WH, Maturi RK, Costigan TM, et al. ERG testing during chronic PDE5 inhibitor administration (ERG-PDEFi) consortium. Arch Ophthalmol 2009; 127:367–73.
287. Grunwald JE, Siu KK, Jacob SS, et al. Effect of sildenafil (Viagra) on the ocular circulation. Am J Ophthalmol 2001;131:751–5.

288. Grunwald JE, Metelitsina T, Grunwald L. Effect of sildenafil citrate (Viagra) on retinal blood vessel diameter. Am J Ophthalmol 2002;133:809–12.
289. McCulley TJ, Luu JK, Marmor MF, et al. Effects of sildenafil citrate on choroidal congestion. Ophthalmologica 2002;216:455–8.
290. Metelitsina TI, Grunwald JE, DuPont JC, et al. Effect of Viagra on the foveolar choroidal circulation of AMD patients. Exp Eye Res 2005;81:159–64.
291. Birch DG, Toler SM, Swanson WH, et al. A double-blind placebo-controlled evaluation of the acute effects of sildenafil citrate (Viagra) on visual function in subjects with early-stage age-related macular degeneration. Am J Ophthalmol 2002;133:665–72.
292. Harris A, Kagemann L, Ehrlich R, et al. The effect of sildenafil on ocular blood flow. Br J Ophthalmol 2008;92:469–73.
293. Tripathi A, O'Donnell NP. Branch retinal artery occlusion: Another complication of sildenafil [letter]. Br J Ophthalmol 2000;84:928.
294. Pomeranz HD, Smith KH, Hart Jr WM, et al. Sildenafil-associated nonarteritic anterior ischemic optic neuropathy. Ophthalmol 2002;109:584–7.
295. Allibhai AZ, Gale JS, Sheidow TS. Central serous chorioretinopathy in a patient taking sildenafil citrate. Ophthalmic Surg Lasers Imaging 2004;35:165–7.
296. Akash R, Hrishikesh D, Amith P, et al. Case report: association of combined nonarteritic anterior ischemic optic neuropathy (NAION) and obstruction of cilioretinal artery with overdose of Viagra. J Ocul Pharmacol Ther 2005;21:315–7.
297. Pomeranz HD, Bhavsar AR. Nonarteritic ischemic optic neuropathy developing soon after use of sildenafil (Viagra): a case report of seven new cases. J Neuroophthalmol 2005;25:9–13.
298. Quiram P, Dumars S, Parwar B, et al. Viagra-associated serous macular detachment. Graefes Arch Clin Exp Ophthalmol 2005;243:339–44.
299. Escaravage GK, Wright JD, Givre SJ. Tadalafil associated with anterior ischemic optic neuropathy. Arch Ophthalmol 2005;123:399–400.
300. Bollinger K, Lee MS. Recurrent visual field defect and ischemic optic neuropathy associated with tadalafil rechallenge. Arch Ophthalmol 2005;123:400–1.
301. Peter NM, Singh MV, Fox PD. Tadalafil-associated anterior ischaemic optic neuropathy. Eye 2005;19:715–7.
302. Hayreh SS. Erectile dysfunction drugs and non-arteritic anterior ischemic optic neuropathy: is there a cause and effect relationship? J Neuroophthalmol 2005;25:295–8.
303. Gedik S, Yilmaz G, Akova YA. Sildenafil-associated consecutive nonarteritic anterior ischaemic optic neuropathy, cilioretinal artery occlusion, central retinal vein occlusion in a haemodialysis patient. Eye 2007;21:129–30.
304. Carter JE. Anterior ischemic optic neuropathy and stroke with use of PDE-5 inhibitors for erective dysfunction: cause or coincidence? J Neurol Sci 2007;262:89–92.
305. Fraunfelder FW, Fraunfelder FT. Central serous chorioretinopathy associated with sildenafil. Retina 2008;28:606–9.

Photic Retinal Injuries: Mechanisms, Hazards, and Prevention

Martin A. Mainster, Patricia L. Turner

Photic retinal injuries are uncommon. Managing them effectively requires knowledge of how intense light interacts with the retina and choroid. Recent advances in retinal imaging have improved our understanding of these interactions.

Photic injuries occur when light is absorbed by tissue chromophores. Melanin and hemoglobin are the most effective retinal light absorbers.[1-3] Light is also absorbed by lipofuscin, macular pigment, and photopigments for visual and nonvisual photoreception.[4,5] Absorption spectra describe how light absorption varies by wavelength. Melanin and lipofuscin absorption increase steadily with decreasing wavelength. Other absorption spectra peak at specific wavelengths.[1,2,4,5]

Optical radiation includes 400–700 nm visible light and shorter wavelength ultraviolet (UV) radiation (UV-C, 100–280 nm; UV-B, 280–320 nm; UV-A, 320–400 nm). The cornea shields the retina from UV radiation below 300 nm.[6] The crystalline lens protects it from most UV-B and UV-A radiation, but crystalline lenses under 30 years of age may transmit a small amount of potentially harmful UV-B radiation.[6-8] Other ocular defense mechanisms against UV radiation and intense visible light include eyebrow shadowing, corneal reflection of light not incident perpendicular to its surface (Fresnel's law), and the pupillary, aversion, squint, and blink responses.[9-11]

Retinal light exposure is specified using parameters including optical energy (joule), exposure (joule/cm^2), power (watt) and irradiance (watt/cm^2).[3] Optical power is high when energy is delivered quickly in brief exposures. Exposure and irradiance are high when optical energy and power are confined to small areas, respectively.

Light can produce beneficial or harmful photomechanical, photothermal, and/or photochemical retinal effects.[12-16]

PHOTOMECHANICAL EFFECTS

The most common signs of acute photomechanical retinal trauma are retinal hemorrhages and/or holes.

Photomechanical mechanisms

Surgical photomechanical effects include photodisruption, photofragmentation, and photovaporization.[16] Photodisruption occurs in Nd:YAG laser capsulotomy and lamellar keratectomy when infrared laser energy ionizes target tissue molecules, producing plasma and a rapidly expanding shock wave that dissects target tissue.[17] Photofragmentation occurs in excimer laser photorefractive keratectomy when ultraviolet laser energy breaks bonds in corneal surface molecules and residual energy volatilizes molecular fragments. Photovaporization occurs in holmium laser sclerostomy and erbium laser phacolysis when rapid water vapor expansion excavates target tissues.

Most accidental photomechanical retinal injuries are caused by very brief laser exposures ranging in duration from a hundred femtoseconds (10^{-15} sec) to microseconds (10^{-6} sec).[18-22] Their very high retinal irradiances (power densities) produce tissue heating and expansion that cause immediate thermomechanical chorioretinal distortion and bleeding. Photovaporization may occur, but retinal irradiances are generally far too low for other photomechanical effects. Most victims experience a brilliant light flash followed by immediate monocular vision loss. An audible sound (pop) and/or momentary pain occur infrequently at the time of the laser accident.

Photomechanical retinal injuries

A small number of photomechanical laser accidents occur each year.[19-22] Most are caused by laboratory research lasers and military rangefinders or target designators.[20-22] Injuries can be prevented by effective laser safety training and proper protective eyewear. Surgical Q-switched and femtosecond laser systems have numerous safeguards that limit high optical irradiances to small, restricted spatial volumes.

Initial vision loss depends on a laser injury's retinal location and associated chorioretinal disruption and bleeding.[21] Blood can spread laterally in subhyaloid, subretinal, or sub-RPE (retinal pigment epithelium) spaces. Chorioretinal scars form and evolve. Vision may improve over days to months. Prognosis is excellent for less severe injuries that do not involve the fovea.

Optical coherence tomography (OCT) and fluorescein angiography are valuable for evaluating, managing, and documenting real and alleged injuries. Anti-inflammatory and neuroprotective drugs for reducing laser damage have been studied experimentally,[23,24] but clinical trials of their efficacy are impractical because injuries are uncommon. Accident victims should be followed for macular holes and choroidal neovascularization that can develop in the months following an injury.[25-29] Macular holes may close and choroidal neovascularization (CNV) may resolve spontaneously but conventional macular hole surgery and CNV therapy are potentially useful when needed.[25-29]

In real laser accidents,

1. the light source is usually known,
2. typical chorioretinal damage occurs,
3. there is an unambiguous temporal relationship between the laser incident and serious visual symptoms,

4. the severity of visual symptoms is commensurate with the extent of retinal damage demonstrable with retinal imaging and examination, and
5. typical chorioretinal remodeling occurs after the injury.[30]

Most laser injuries and noninjurious laser exposures are painless.[30] Eye rubbing after a laser incident can cause painful self-inflicted corneal abrasions, sometimes falsely attributed to the laser exposure.[30–32] Real retinal laser injuries do not cause chronic headache or other somatic complaints, including head, neck or jaw pain.[30]

The ease of laser injury diagnosis is directly proportional to the severity of the laser injury.[30] In ambiguous cases, subtle retinal findings have an excellent visual prognosis. When a retinal laser injury is alleged and objective findings are absent or within normal limits, diagnosis of laser injury should be deferred pending a rigorous review of the patient's retinal findings, ophthalmic and systemic tests, clinical course, and past medical history. Such an analysis may take weeks or even months to perform if there is a complex past medical history. A guideline has been published for this type of analysis.[30]

Pressure from patients or attorneys to reach quick conclusions in alleged but inapparent laser injuries should be resisted.[30,33] There are numerous potential psychiatric, financial or other explanations for complaints of nonorganic origin.[30,33] Differentiating between those origins is challenging, but organic retinal laser injuries do not cause chronic pain, and if a significant visual abnormality is present, it should be reproducible and consistent with a significant chorioretinal abnormality.[30]

PHOTOTHERMAL EFFECTS

The most common signs of acute photothermal retinal trauma are ophthalmoscopically visible photocoagulation burns without hemorrhage or holes.

Photothermal mechanisms

Photocoagulation occurs when intense light is absorbed mostly by melanin in the RPE and choroid. Light energy is converted into heat, increasing the temperature of directly exposed pigmented tissues.[2,3,34] Heat conduction spreads temperature elevation to adjacent sites. Overlying neural retina damaged by heat conduction loses its transparency and becomes visible as a focal white lesion ("burn") because it scatters white fundus illumination light back at an observer. Retinal burns increase in size over time due to postexposure scarring and collateral chorioretinal damage that is not apparent immediately after the exposure.[2]

Standard clinical photocoagulation produces immediately visible burns, with retinal temperature increases exceeding 20 °C.[1] Photomechanical effects occur at roughly three times the laser exposure needed for a visible lesion. Invisible lesions that are apparent only with fluorescein or autofluorescence imaging occur at half to one-quarter of the exposure needed to produce ophthalmoscopically visible lesions. In clinical parlance, "subthreshold" means ophthalmoscopically invisible or "subvisible."[3] Subthreshold photocoagulation can produce beneficial therapeutic effects with low temperature rises that produce minimal or no apparent retinal damage.[35]

Most accidental photothermal retinal injuries are caused by pulsed laser exposures ranging in duration from a microsecond to a few seconds. Retinal irradiance is high enough for photocoagulation but too low for photomechanical effects. The magnitude and duration of chorioretinal temperature elevation determine the severity of a retinal burn, along with lesion size, fundus pigmentation, and chorioretinal sequelae.[3,21] Photothermal and photomechanical retinal injuries are managed similarly. Injuries should be followed for retinal holes and CNV that can develop within a few months of the injury.[27,36]

Photothermal retinal injuries

Industrial and military photothermal laser accidents are less common than photomechanical ones because they require a narrow range of lower retinal irradiances.

Operating room or medical office injuries

Most medical laser accidents go unreported for legal reasons.[30] Indirect ophthalmoscope photocoagulator beams and their reflections are potentially hazardous for many meters. Bystanders should put on protective eyewear before these systems are switched from standby to treatment mode. Protective operating microscope filters should be in place and the laser delivery probe inside a patient's eye before an endoscopic photocoagulator is switched to treatment mode.[37]

Slit-lamp photocoagulators

Slit-lamp photocoagulator operators are protected from back-scattered laser light by optical filters.[38] Laser beam reflections are theoretically hazardous for bystanders up to 2 meters from a flat-surfaced contact lens,[39] so persons within that range should wear laser safety glasses or goggles effective for the laser treatment wavelength. No injury of this type has ever been reported.

Laser pointers and other consumer laser devices

Laser pointers marketed in the United States are regulated by the Food and Drug Administration (FDA).[31,32,40] They are supposed to produce less than 5 mW (milliwatt) of power (Class 3A) and have warning labels cautioning users not to stare into the laser beam. The low cost of laser pointers has made them available to children, adults who do not observe warning labels, and rioters.

Staring deliberately into a laser pointer beam for more than 10 seconds is hazardous and has caused retinal injuries.[31,32,41–43] Brief accidental or inadvertent laser pointer exposures do not cause retinal damage because they are terminated typically in less than 0.25 sec by normal aversion responses to uncomfortable, dazzling light.[31,40] A laser pointer injury occurred in an 11-year-old girl who stared into a red laser pointer beam for more than 10 seconds because her classmates wanted to see if her pupil would constrict.[41] Prominent foveolar pigment mottling occurred in her affected eye, along with an initial decrease in visual acuity to 20/60. Pigment mottling faded and visual acuity normalized over several months.

Powerful "hand-held laser systems" with dangerous output powers ranging from 20 to 1000 mW (Class 3B or 4) can appear identical to laser pointers and be purchased over the Internet. These devices are photocoagulators, not laser pointers. They have already caused serious photothermal retinal injuries.[42,44,45] Lasers in recreational light shows have also caused serious photothermal retinal injuries in bystanders.[46]

PHOTOCHEMICAL EFFECTS

The most common signs of acute photochemical retinal trauma are yellow-white small foveolar lesions in solar and welding arc maculopathy and larger, often extrafoveal lesions in operating microscope and endoilluminator injuries.

Photochemical mechanisms

Accidental photochemical retinal injuries (known as photic retinopathy or retinal phototoxicity) are caused by prolonged intense light exposures that probably would be well tolerated if experienced only momentarily.[5] They occur at chorioretinal temperature elevations too low for photothermal damage, at illuminances far exceeding normal environmental levels, in exposures lasting from seconds to minutes. Optical radiation produces highly reactive oxygen radicals that can damage retinal cell membranes, proteins, carbohydrates, and nucleic acids. The extent of a photochemical retinal injury depends on individual defense mechanisms, the location and area of exposed retina, and the duration, intensity, and spectrum of the light exposure.[5,10,12,47–49]

Photic retinopathy does not occur unless acute cellular damage is so excessive that it acutely overwhelms retinal repair mechanisms.[5,37] People safely undergo bright but much lower irradiances in ophthalmic imaging studies and light therapy for seasonal affective disorder.[12,37,50]

Action spectra characterize how effectively different wavelengths cause a photochemical effect.[51] Photic retinopathy can be divided into photosensitizer- and photopigment-mediated phototoxicities which have different action spectra.[4,5,52]

The hazardousness of photosensitizer-mediated retinal phototoxicity increases rapidly with decreasing wavelength,[5,47] similar to the absorption spectrum of lipofuscin in the RPE which is its primary mediator.[53,54] Thus, UV radiation is much more hazardous than visible light. In an aphakic eye, UV radiation, violet light (400–440 nm) and blue light (440–500 nm) account for 67%, 18%, and 14% of potential retinal phototoxicity, respectively.[55,56] Photosensitizer-mediated phototoxicity is the basis for the international consensus aphakic standard A_λ phototoxicity function used to estimate industrial acute retinal phototoxicity risks.[57]

In an adult phakic eye, the retina has the additional shielding of crystalline lens attenuation of UV radiation and shorter wavelength visible light. That is why the international consensus phakic standard B_λ phototoxicity function peaks at 440 nm in the blue part of the spectrum. The B_λ function is often termed a "blue light hazard" function, even though blue light has far less retinal phototoxicity than violet light or UV radiation.[4,5,57]

The hazardousness of photopigment-mediated retinal phototoxicity[58] peaks around 500 nm (blue-green), similar to the luminous sensitivity of scotopic vision[59] because the photopigment rhodopsin mediates both processes.[5] This type of photic retinopathy requires only 1% of the retinal irradiance needed for photosensitizer-mediated phototoxicity,[10,52,60,61] but experimental studies were performed with highly light-sensitive nocturnal rodents whose primary photopigment is rhodopsin.[5,58,61]

Clinical findings are similar in solar and welding arc maculopathies, as they are in operating microscope and endoilluminator injuries.[5,37]

Photochemical retinal injuries

Solar and welder's maculopathy

Figure 90.1 shows a typical yellow-white solar maculopathy lesion.[62,63] Lesions fade over several weeks, resolving completely or leaving foveolar distortion, pigment mottling or even a macular hole.[62] Welding arc injuries produce similar clinical abnormalities.[5,64,65] Welder's maculopathy is extremely rare but it may be underreported because its transient clinical symptoms may be masked by those of associated photokeratitis.[5,8,66]

Common visual complaints after acute solar or welding arc injury are blurred vision, central scotoma and erythropsia. Post-injury visual acuity may be normal or decreased to the 20/40 to 20/200 range. Visual acuity usually returns to 20/20 to 20/40 over 6 months.[5,62] Fluorescein angiography may be normal but more severe injuries may cause foveal RPE defects.[62,67] The characteristic OCT finding is a well-defined outer retinal hyporeflective space primarily involving the photoreceptor inner and outer segment layers, as shown in Fig. 90.2 for a welding arc

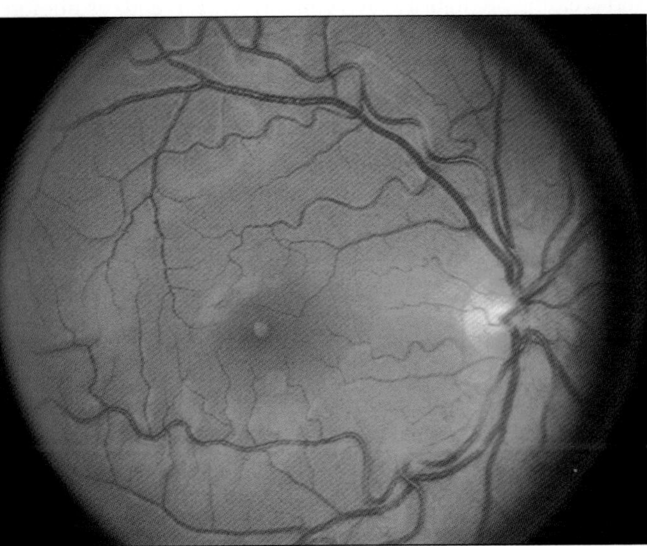

Fig. 90.1 Acute solar maculopathy typically produces a small yellow-white foveolar lesion, as seen in this 15-year-old girl with 20/200 visual acuity. The lesion faded and visual acuity returned to 20/40 in the 3 months following the injury.

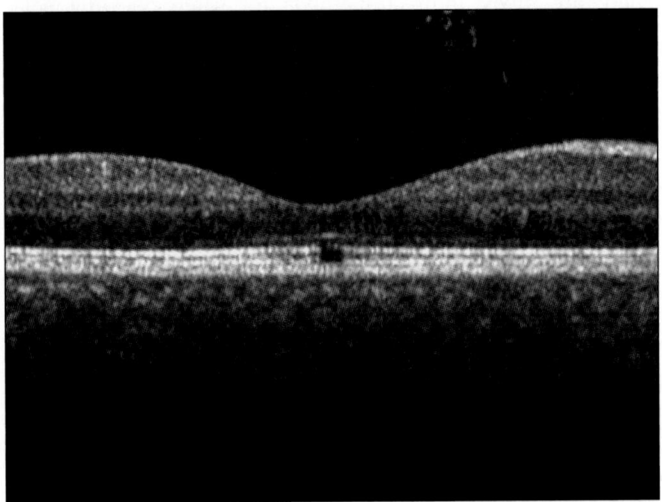

Fig. 90.2 OCT images taken months to years after solar or welding arc injuries usually reveal a well-defined foveolar outer retinal hyporeflective space.[5,65,68–73] This 34-year-old male had been welding since 11 years of age and complained of vision loss for 5 months prior to the OCT study. A horizontal scan through his fovea shows largely normal retinal pigment epithelium (RPE) and external limiting membrane reflective bands but interruption of the Verhoeff's membrane (RPE tight junctions and/or apical processes) as well as the inner/outer-segment junction hyperreflective bands. These OCT findings are consistent with chronic damage to photoreceptor inner- and outer-segment layers.[62] (Courtesy of Suman Pilli, MD, Muralidhar Ogoti, MD, and Vishwanath Kalluri, MD.)

injury.[5,65,68–73] Spectral domain OCT imaging immediately after an injury reveals overlying outer nuclear layer and underlying RPE abnormalities, as shown in Fig. 90.3.

The histopathology of solar retinopathy has been studied in volunteers who stared at the sun monocularly for 10–60 minutes before enucleation for choroidal melanoma.[63,74] Photoreceptor damage included vesiculation and fragmentation of photoreceptor outer segment lamellae, mitochondrial swelling, and nuclear pyknosis.[63,74] Cones appeared more damage-resistant than rods, possibly accounting for good visual outcomes after some injuries.[74] RPE damage was variable.[63,74] Imaging and histopathological data to date do not permit determination of whether solar and welding arc injuries are primarily of RPE and/or photoreceptor origin.

Foveomacular retinitis is a term used to describe foveal abnormalities resembling photic retinopathy. It occurs after blunt ocular trauma and whiplash injury[75–77] and in people with no history of mechanical or photic trauma.[78,79] Outbreaks were reported in military personnel during World War II and again from 1966 to 1973.[80–83] Those incidents were ascribed to solar exposure,[82,84] consistent with reports of solar maculopathy in young people who have been sunbathing but not sungazing.[85,86]

Momentary solar observation is safe or it would be dangerous to look upwards on a bright sunny day. Even at noontime on a clear day, direct solar observation with a 3 mm pupil diameter causes only a 4°C retinal temperature rise, far too low for photocoagulation.[87] Thus, typical solar maculopathy is photochemical not photothermal damage. Conversely, solar observation with a dilated 7 mm pupil produces a 22°C retinal temperature increase, well above the 10°C threshold for retinal photocoagulation.[34,87] Telescope-assisted solar observation produces even higher retinal temperature increases.[87,88]

Solar eclipse observation is particularly hazardous because pupillary dilation can occur and increase retinal irradiance.[88] There are many indirect methods for safely viewing solar eclipses.[88,89] Sungazing injuries have been reported to occur during hypoglycemia, drug abuse, psychosis, and religious rituals.[5,71] Prolonged solar observation causes the most damage, especially with pharmacologically dilated pupils.

Photokeratitis is a common welding arc accident but welder's maculopathy is an unusual event. When welders fail to use appropriate eye protection filters, younger workers are at greater risk for retinal injury because of their clear ocular media. The UV-B window in the crystalline lens discussed previously closes by roughly 30 years of age.[6–8] At younger ages, some highly phototoxic UV-B welding arc radiation may be transmitted to the retina, possibly accounting for welding arc maculopathy and welders' reportedly increased risk of uveal melanoma.[6,8] Photic injuries have also been caused by UV-B radiation and/or short-wavelength visible light from a femtosecond laser plasma[90] and a short-circuiting high-tension electric circuit.[91]

Experimental photic retinopathy is enhanced by elevated body temperature,[58,92,93] so increased body temperature from a hot day, exercise, or fever could increase the risk of retinal phototoxicity, perhaps accounting for the age-old admonishment to protect children with fevers from bright sunlight.[5] Higher chorioretinal pigmentation could increase local chorioretinal temperature rise associated with solar observation, perhaps further increasing the risk of damage. The fovea is at greatest risk for solar damage in direct sungazing, but foveal injuries in young adults who have been sunbathing but not sungazing may occur because of crystalline lens UV-B transmission and/or Henle fiberoptic transmission of short-wavelength photons toward the fovea.[94]

Operating microscope and endoilluminator injuries

Typical operating microscope injuries are oval 0.5–2 disc diameter lesions.[95,96] Damage sites are often inferior to the fovea due to microscope tilt and illumination positioning.[97,98] Fiberoptic endoilluminators can cause comparable lesions elsewhere,[99] as shown in Fig. 90.4. Injuries have occurred in cornea, cataract, glaucoma, and retinal surgery.[95,96,100–102] Photochemical retinal damage is localized primarily to photoreceptors and the RPE as in solar and welder's maculopathies.[103–105]

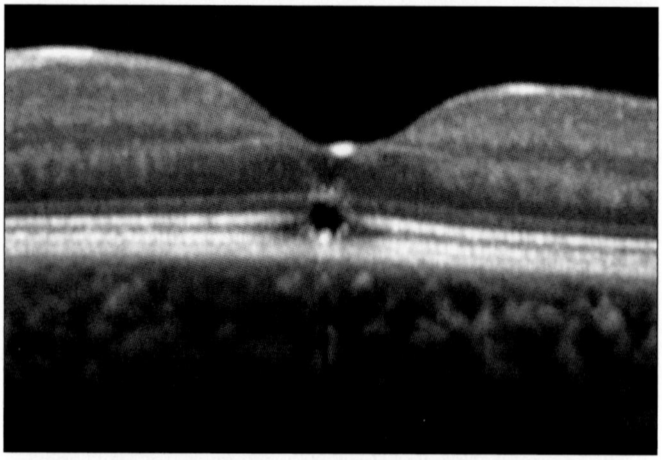

Fig. 90.3 A spectral domain OCT image taken shortly after a solar injury documents the foveolar outer retinal hyporeflective space observed in older lesions and also abnormalities in the overlying outer nuclear layer and underlying retinal pigment epithelium (RPE). These findings are consistent with histopathological evidence of photoreceptor and RPE damage after acute solar maculopathy in human eyes scheduled for enucleation.[74,136] (Courtesy of Giovanni Staurenghi, MD, and Marco Pellegrini, MD.)

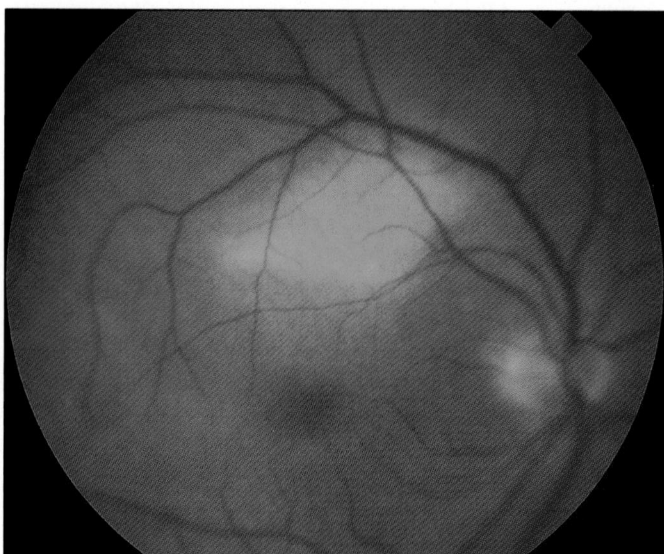

Fig. 90.4 This patient had an endoilluminator lesion after vitrectomy, scleral buckling, and anterior chamber intraocular lens explant. This retinal photograph was taken 4 months postoperatively. The patient's visual acuity was 20/70 preoperatively and 20/50 postoperatively. (Courtesy of Marc M. Whitacre, MD.)

Lesion size, location, and severity determine vision loss from an operating microscope injury. Lesions initially have a yellow-white appearance, sometimes accompanied by a shallow serous neural retinal detachment. This finding resolves rapidly, followed by local RPE atrophy and pigment mottling. Chronic lesions are usually much less apparent ophthalmoscopically than angiographically, as shown in Figs 90.5A and 90.5B, respectively. Figure 90.6A is the OCT image of a 70-year-old female with an operating microscope lesion temporal to her fovea and also central cystoid macular edema (CME) shortly after complicated cataract surgery. The OCT image in Fig. 90.6B taken 3 years later shows chorioretinal scarring at the site of operating microscope illumination,[106] consistent with histopathologic findings in human and animal studies.[103-105] Imaging and histopathological data to date do not permit determination of whether operating microscope and endoilluminator injuries are primarily of RPE and/or photoreceptor origin.

The risk of operating microscope injury is potentially increased by higher body temperature,[92] increased chorioretinal pigmentation (theoretically increasing local light absorption and thermal enhancement of retinal phototoxicity),[5] oxygen administration during surgery (hypothetically increasing retinal

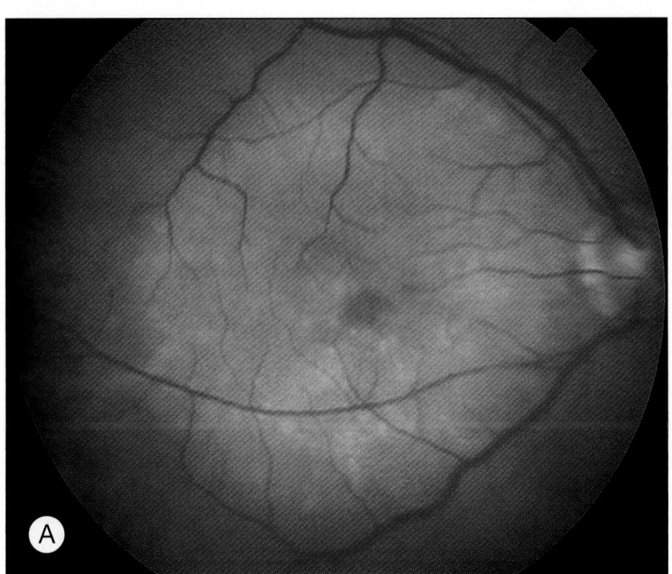

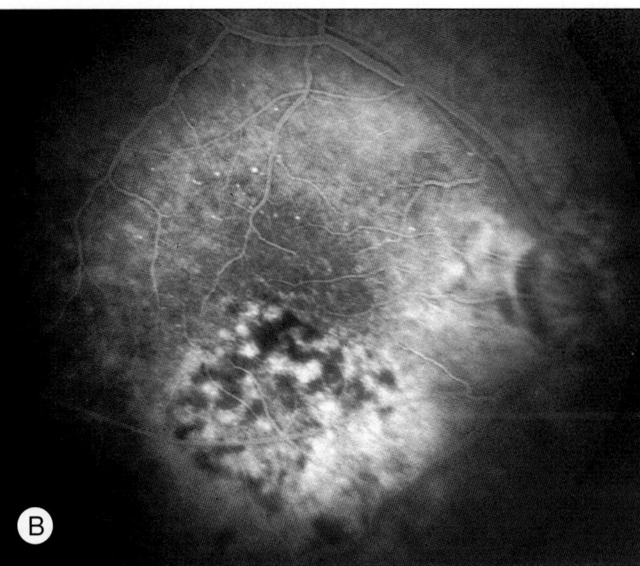

Fig. 90.5 An operating microscope lesion in a 67-year-old male with diabetes who had undergone an intraocular lens exchange operation 1 year earlier. The oval-shaped area of retinal pigment epithelial degeneration inferior to the fovea was not prominent ophthalmoscopically, as shown in the fundus photograph (A), but the lesion was quite apparent in the fluorescein angiogram taken on the same day (B).

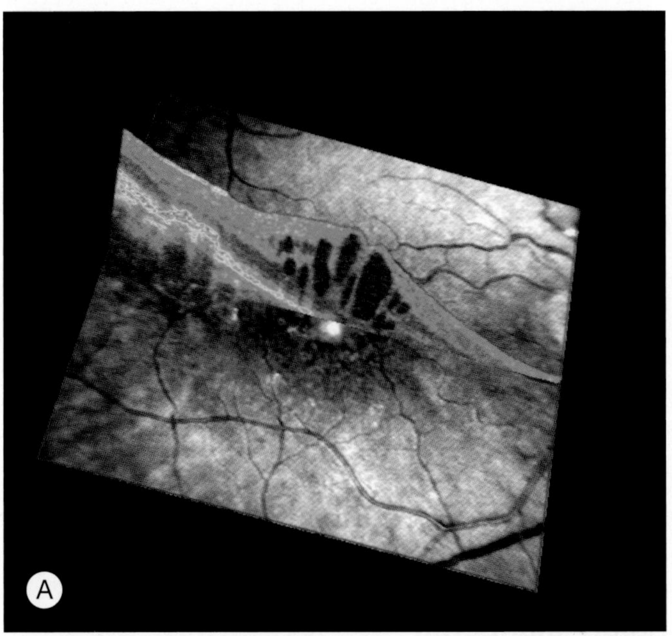

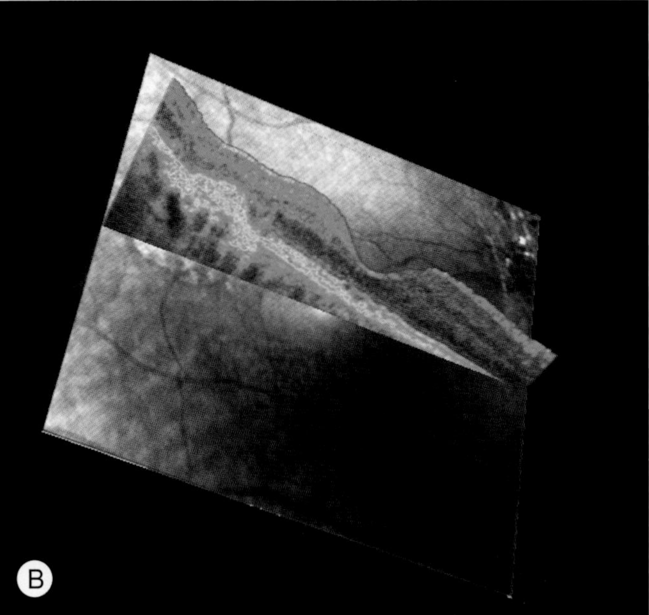

Fig. 90.6 An operating microscope injury in a 70-year-old female who had recently undergone complicated cataract surgery for a partially subluxated crystalline lens due to a tennis ball injury. Initial foveal cystoid macular edema and a serous neural retinal detachment associated with the operating microscope lesion (A) gradually resolved. Prominent chorioretinal scarring (B) is present in the region of the operating microscope lesion 3 years later, long after resolution of the cystoid macular edema. (Courtesy of Richard B. Rosen, MD.)

free radical production),[107] and photosensitizing medications such as hydroxychloroquine, hydrochlorothiazide, furosemide, allopurinol, and the benzodiazepines.[108–110] Diabetes mellitus and hypertension may also increase retinal phototoxicity risks.[111]

Faster cataract surgery reduces the risk of operating microscope injury,[112] as does minimizing operating microscope intensity and discontinuing photosensitizing medications preoperatively when possible.[5,110] Other potentially useful techniques include maintaining patients' eyes in downgaze, using corneal occluders, and avoiding supplemental oxygen use and/or elevated patient core body temperatures.[5,113,114] Operating microscopes produce minimal UV radiation,[115–117] so UV-blocking filters are of little value. One study reported that UV-blocking intraocular lenses (IOLs) reduce postoperative cystoid macular edema,[118] but three subsequent studies refuted that conclusion.[119–121] Reducing operating microscope violet and blue light illumination hypothetically decreases acute retinal phototoxicity risks, but blue light is important for tissue visualization.[5]

Indocyanine green (ICG) is useful for retinal angiography and staining the inner limiting membrane (ILM) during macular hole surgery. ICG fluorescence can persist for months after ICG-assisted vitreoretinal surgery.[122] Visual field defects have been reported after these procedures,[123] as has RPE damage possibly of phototoxic origin.[124] The potential risks and benefits of ILM staining with ICG and alternative vital dyes continue to be evaluated.[125]

Ophthalmoscope and fundus camera exposure

Indirect ophthalmoscopes and fundus cameras produce dazzling exposures and transient afterimages, but there is no evidence that they cause photochemical or thermal retinal injury in routine clinical use.[12,126–129] A 15 minute indirect ophthalmoscope exposure focused on a single retinal area can cause a localized phototoxic injury in an anesthetized rhesus monkey,[92] but that certainly is not a clinical light exposure. No immediate or long-term retinal abnormalities could be detected after similar exposures were attempted in human volunteers with blind eyes or those requiring enucleation.[130] These results are consistent with instrumentation data showing that fundus camera, indirect ophthalmoscope, and scanning laser ophthalmoscope retinal irradiances are lower than experimentally determined damage thresholds.[12,126,127,129,131] Anterior segment slit-lamp photography has been reported to cause photic retinopathy under unusual circumstances.[132]

Sixty-second stabilized retinal exposures accelerated local retinal degeneration in dogs with rhodopsin gene mutations, prompting recommendation that retinal photography and clinical light exposure be minimized in patients with retinitis pigmentosa.[133] Human and canine retinas differ significantly[133] and the experimental exposures were 10 000 times longer than 2 msec clinical fundus camera flashes.[129] Light exposure has never been proven to adversely affect the clinical course of retinitis pigmentosa and even light deprivation does not prevent its progression.[134] No current scientific evidence suggests the need for retinal disease-specific light exposure safety standards.[129] Nonetheless, regardless of a patient's condition, clinical retinal imaging should be performed only when necessary and patient comfort dictates that clinical procedures always be carried out at the lowest clinically effective retinal illumination levels.[12,129]

ENVIRONMENTAL ISSUES

Light and macular degeneration

There has been speculation for almost a century that environmental light exposure may be a risk factor for age-related macular degeneration (AMD).[10,135–138] The retina's high oxygen and light levels increase its vulnerability to oxidative stress which can cause chronic local inflammation.[5] Retinal compensatory internal defenses include photoreceptor disc shedding, and enzymatic and nonenzymatic antioxidants. RPE lipofuscin accumulates with aging because photoreceptor phagocytosis and autophagy of spent intracellular organelles produce undegradable endproducts that are not eliminated effectively.[5] Excessive lipofuscin may compromise RPE cell function, promote angiogenic factor expression or act as a photoinducible generator of reactive oxygen species.[5] Lipofuscin accumulation, phototoxicity, and AMD all involve direct or indirect oxidative damage,[5,54,139] but shared mechanisms do not prove causal relationships.[4]

The retinal phototoxicity-AMD hypothesis conjectures that repetitive acute photic retinopathy from environmental light exposure is a risk factor for AMD. Twelve major epidemiological studies examined this issue over the past three decades: eight studies were population-based and four were case-controlled.[55] Ten of the 12 studies found no link between environmental light and AMD,[55] including a larger second study[140] by the director of the earlier-positive Waterman study.[141] Another critical failure of the phototoxicity-AMD hypothesis is compelling and growing evidence that cataract surgery does not accelerate the development or progression of AMD,[142–146] as it should if light were a significant causative factor in AMD.[55] More than four decades after the discovery of photic retinopathy, there is no experimental or clinical proof that environmental light exposure or repetitive acute phototoxicity is a significant risk factor in AMD.

Sunglasses

Sunglasses are worn for comfort and fashion.[9,147] There is strong evidence that environmental UV exposure plays a significant role in cortical cataractogenesis.[148] Thus, UV-blocking sunglasses and other avoidance strategies may decrease the risk of cataract formation. If environmental light exposure plays any role in AMD in susceptible individuals, then groups that might benefit from wearing sunglasses for retinal protection include lightly pigmented younger people in tropical climates, individuals taking photosensitizing drugs for skin or other systemic diseases, and people suffering from malabsorption syndromes or other conditions contributing to malnutrition.[5]

Sunglass design considers visual comfort and ocular protection.[10] There must be sufficient visible light transmission to permit effective perception of fine detail and color contrast,[9,149] but enough absorption or reflection of optical radiation to provide comfort and protection from UV radiation. Brimmed hats reduce overhead light exposure, but much of eye's UV exposure may come from reflective terrain below or viewing the horizontal sky.[51] Sunglasses are not safe for sungazing and pupillary dilation potentially associated with their use may increase the risk of solar injury.[9,12,89]

Safety standards

Safety standards that affect laser users include the voluntary American National Standard Institute (ANSI) Standards "Safe Use of Lasers" (ANSI Z136.1–2007)[150,151] and "Safe Use of Lasers in Health Care Facilities" (ANSI Z136.3-2005).[152] The ANSI Z136.1 Standard is similar to the International Standard IEC 60825-1.[153] ANSI standards are technically "voluntary," but regulatory groups use them to assess medical laser facility safety and litigants use them to scrutinize purported injuries.[154,155]

Safety standards that affect laser manufacturers in the United States include the FDA's regulatory "Laser Performance Standard" (21 CFR1040).[156] This standard requires manufacturers to equip laser devices with features such as emission indicators and keyed switches. There are also specific standards for ophthalmic devices such as slit lamps and endoilluminators.

ANSI standards define four laser classes.[150,155] Class 1 lasers are considered incapable of causing damaging ocular exposures and do not require control measures. Their maximum power output in the visible spectrum ranges from 0.0004 mW or less for blue or green light to 0.024 mW or less for red light. Class 2, 3a, and 3b lasers produce laser power that is less than 1 mW, between 1 and 5 mW, and between 5 and 500 mW, respectively. Laser pointers are Class 3a devices. Some dangerous Class 3b handheld laser devices are identical in appearance to laser pointers. Class 4 lasers include potentially hazardous industrial, military or medical lasers that generate more than 500 mW of laser power. Safety standards assign control measures to each laser class.[150,152]

Practical considerations

Control measures are designed to decrease the risk of laser accidents.[88,154,155] "Engineering" controls are protective measures built into laser systems such as housings, labels, and interlocks. "Administrative" and "procedural" controls are designed to assure the proper use of potentially hazardous laser systems. They include written protocols for (1) operating, maintaining, and servicing laser systems, (2) assuring proper personnel education and training, and (3) using appropriate protective eyewear.

For an ophthalmic laser facility, the ANSI Z136.3-2005 standard recommends that (1) a "Laser Safety Officer" be given local safety oversight responsibility, (2) a warning sign with the signal word "danger" be displayed on the outside of the closed treatment room door during any laser procedure, (3) personnel wear laser eye protection in the nominal hazard zone where diffuse reflections and stray beams could be hazardous, and (4) operators be trained in the safe use of their laser equipment.[152,154] From a practical perspective, the nominal hazard zone is the treatment or operating room in which a surgical laser is located. The laser safety office is responsible for assuring that (1) protective eyewear is available and used regularly, (2) personnel using lasers are trained properly, and (3) laser safety measures are audited regularly.

CONCLUSION

Light can cause photomechanical (thermomechanical), photothermal (photocoagulation) or photochemical (photic retinopathy) retinal damage. Accidental laser injuries are preventable with protective eyewear. Clinical retinal photocoagulation does not cause chronic pain and neither do accidental retinal laser injuries. Visual abnormalities from an alleged laser injury should be well correlated with chorioretinal abnormalities. Powerful handheld laser devices that appear identical to laser pointers can be retinal photocoagulators. The only common clinical photochemical injuries are solar and welding arc maculopathies and operating microscope and endoilluminator injuries. There is no proven link between environmental light exposure, retinal phototoxicity and AMD. Solar maculopathy can occur with or without sungazing. People under 30 years of age are at greatest risk to photic retinopathy because of the UV-B window in their crystalline lenses.

REFERENCES

1. Mainster MA, White TJ, Allen RG. Spectral dependence of retinal damage produced by intense light sources. J Opt Soc Am 1970;60(6):848–55.
2. Mainster MA. Wavelength selection in macular photocoagulation. Tissue optics, thermal effects, and laser systems. Ophthalmology 1986;93(7):952–8.
3. Mainster MA. Decreasing retinal photocoagulation damage: principles and techniques. Semin Ophthalmol 1999;14(4):200–9.
4. Mainster MA. Violet and blue light blocking intraocular lenses: photoprotection versus photoreception. Br J Ophthalmol 2006;90(6):784–92.
5. Mainster MA, Boulton M. Retinal phototoxicity. In: Albert DM, Miller JW, Blodi BA, et al, editors. Principles and practice of ophthalmology. 3rd ed. London: Elsevier; 2008. ch. 174.
6. Boettner EA, Wolter JR. Transmission of the ocular media. Invest Ophthalmol 1962;1(6):776–83.
7. Barker FM, Brainard GC. The direct spectral transmittance of the excised human lens as a function of age, (FDA 785345 0090 RA). Washington, DC: US Food and Drug Administration; 1991.
8. Mainster MA, Turner PL. Ultraviolet-B phototoxicity and hypothetical photomelanomagenesis: intraocular and crystalline lens photoprotection. Am J Ophthalmol 2010;149(4):543–9.
9. Sliney DH. Eye protective techniques for bright light. Ophthalmology 1983;90(8):937–44.
10. Mainster MA. Light and macular degeneration: a biophysical and clinical perspective. Eye 1987;1(Pt 2):304–10.
11. Stamper DA, Lund DJ, Molchany JW, et al. Human pupil and eyelid response to intense laser light: implications for protection. Percept Mot Skills 2002;95 (3 Pt 1):775–82.
12. Mainster MA, Ham WT Jr, Delori FC. Potential retinal hazards. Instrument and environmental light sources. Ophthalmology 1983;90(8):927–32.
13. Mainster MA. Finding your way in the photoforest: laser effects for clinicians. Ophthalmology 1984;91(7):886–8.
14. Marshall J. Structural aspects of laser-induced damage and their functional implications. Health Phys 1989;56(5):617–24.
15. Mainster MA. Photic retinal injury. In: Ryan SJ, editor. Retina. St Louis: Mosby–Year Book; 1989.
16. Mainster MA. Classification of ophthalmic photosurgery. Lasers Light Ophthalmol 1994;6(2):65–7.
17. Mainster MA, Ho PC, Mainster KJ. Nd: YAG laser photodisruptors. Ophthalmology 1983;(Suppl):45–7.
18. Gabel VP, Birngruber R, Lorenz B, et al. Clinical observations of six cases of laser injury to the eye. Health Phys 1989;56(5):705–10.
19. Thach AB, Lopez PF, Snady-McCoy LC, et al. Accidental Nd:YAG laser injuries to the macula. Am J Ophthalmol 1995;119(6):767–73.
20. Barkana Y, Belkin M. Laser eye injuries. Surv Ophthalmol 2000;44(6):459–78.
21. Mainster MA. Retinal laser accidents: mechanisms, managment and rehabilitation. J Laser Appl 2000;12(1):3–9.
22. Harris MD, Lincoln AE, Amoroso PJ, et al. Laser eye injuries in military occupations. Aviat Space Environ Med 2003;74(9):947–52.
23. Brown J Jr, Hacker H, Schuschereba ST, et al. Steroidal and nonsteroidal antiinflammatory medications can improve photoreceptor survival after laser retinal photocoagulation. Ophthalmology 2007;114(10):1876–83.
24. Shulman S, Belokopytov M, Dubinsky G, et al. Ameliorative effect of PN-277 on laser-induced retinal damage. Graefes Arch Clin Exp Ophthalmol 2009; 247(3):343–8.
25. Ciulla TA, Topping TM. Surgical treatment of a macular hole secondary to accidental laser burn. Arch Ophthalmol. 1997;115(7):929–30.
26. Newman DK, Flanagan DW. Spontaneous closure of a macular hole secondary to an accidental laser injury. Br J Ophthalmol. 2000;84(9):1075.
27. Sasahara M, Noami S, Takahashi M, et al. Optical coherence tomographic observations before and after macular hole formation secondary to laser injury. Am J Ophthalmol 2003;136(6):1167–70.
28. Nehemy M, Torqueti-Costa L, Magalhaes EP, et al. Choroidal neovascularization after accidental macular damage by laser. Clin Experiment Ophthalmol 2005;33(3):298–300.
29. Ying HS, Symons RC, Lin KL, et al. Accidental Nd:YAG laser-induced choroidal neovascularization. Lasers Surg Med 2008;40(4):240–2.
30. Mainster MA, Stuck BE, Brown J, Jr. Assessment of alleged retinal laser injuries. Arch Ophthalmol 2004;122(8):1210–7.
31. Mainster MA, Timberlake GT, Warren KA, et al. Pointers on laser pointers. Ophthalmology 1997;104(8):1213–4.
32. Mainster MA. Blinded by the light – not! Arch Ophthalmol 1999;117(11): 1547–8.
33. Mainster MA, Sliney DH, Marshall J, et al. But is it really light damage? Ophthalmology 1997;104(2):179–80.
34. Mainster MA, White TJ, Tips JH, et al. Retinal-temperature increases produced by intense light sources. J Opt Soc Am 1970;60(2):264–70.
35. Luttrull JK, Musch DC, Mainster MA. Subthreshold diode micropulse photocoagulation for the treatment of clinically significant diabetic macular oedema. Br J Ophthalmol 2005;89(1):74–80.

36. Bernstein PS, Steffensmeier A. Optical coherence tomography before and after repair of a macular hole induced by an unintentional argon laser burn. Arch Ophthalmol 2005;123(3):404–5.
37. Mainster MA, Turner PL. Retinal injuries from light: mechanisms, hazards and prevention. In: Ryan SJ, Hinton DR, Schachat AP, et al, editors. Retina. 4th ed. London: Elsevier; 2006. vol. 2, ch. 109.
38. Mainster MA. Ophthalmic laser surgery: principles, technology, and technique. Trans New Orleans Acad Ophthalmol 1985;33:81–101.
39. Jenkins DL. Hazard evaluation of the coherent model 900 photocoagulator laser system, non-ionizing radiation protection specialty study no. 25-42-0310-79 (NTIS no. ADA 068713). Aberdeen Proving Ground, MD: US Army Environment Hygiene Agency; 1979.
40. Sliney DH, Dennis JE. Safety concerns about laser pointers. J. Laser Applications 1994;6:159–64.
41. Sell CH, Bryan JS. Maculopathy from handheld diode laser pointer. Arch Ophthalmol 1999;117(11):1557–8.
42. Ziahosseini K, Doris JP, Turner GS. Laser eye injuries. Maculopathy from handheld green diode laser pointer. BMJ 2010;340:c2982.
43. Fujinami K, Yokoi T, Hiraoka M, et al. Choroidal neovascularization in a child following laser pointer-induced macular injury. Jpn J Ophthalmol 2010; 54(6):631–3.
44. Wyrsch S, Baenninger PB, Schmid MK. Retinal injuries from a handheld laser pointer. N Engl J Med 2010;363(11):1089–91.
45. Ueda T, Kurihara I, Koide R. A case of retinal light damage by green laser pointer (Class 3b). Jpn J Ophthalmol 2011;55(4):428–30.
46. Boosten K, Van Ginderdeuren R, Spileers W, et al. Laser-induced retinal injury following a recreational laser show: two case reports and a clinicopathological study. Bull Soc Belge Ophtalmol 2011;317:11–6.
47. Ham WT Jr, Mueller HA, Sliney DH. Retinal sensitivity to damage from short wavelength light. Nature 1976;260:153–5.
48. Lawwill T. Three major pathologic processes caused by light in the primate retina: a search for mechanisms. Trans Am Ophthalmol Soc 1982;80:517–79.
49. Sliney DH, Mellerio J, Gabel VP, et al. What is the meaning of threshold in laser injury experiments? Implications for human exposure limits. Health Phys 2002;82(3):335–47.
50. Gallin PF, Terman M, Reme CE, et al. Ophthalmologic examination of patients with seasonal affective disorder, before and after bright light therapy. Am J Ophthalmol 1995;119(2):202–10.
51. Sliney DH. How light reaches the eye and its components. Int J Toxicol 2002;21(6):501–9.
52. van Norren D, Gorgels TG. The action spectrum of photochemical damage to the retina: a review of monochromatic threshold data. Photochem Photobiol 2011;87(4):747–53.
53. Rozanowska M, Jarvis-Evans J, Korytowski W, et al. Blue light-induced reactivity of retinal age pigment. In vitro generation of oxygen-reactive species. J Biol Chem 1995;70(32):18825–30.
54. Boulton M, Rozanowska M, Rozanowski B. Retinal photodamage. J Photochem Photobiol B 2001;64(2–3):144–61.
55. Mainster MA, Turner PL. Blue-blocking IOLs decrease photoreception without providing significant photoprotection. Surv Ophthalmol 2010;55(3): 272–89.
56. Mainster MA. Blue-blocking intraocular lenses and pseudophakic scotopic sensitivity. J Cataract Refract Surg 2006;32(9):1403–4.
57. ACGIH. Threshold Limit Values for chemical substances and physical agents: Biological Exposure Indices. Cincinnati: American Conference of Governmental Industrial Hygienists; 1997.
58. Noell WK, Walker VS, Kang BS, et al. Retinal damage by light in rats. Invest Ophthalmol 1966;5(5):450–73.
59. Griswold MS, Stark WS. Scotopic spectral sensitivity of phakic and aphakic observers extending into the near ultraviolet. Vision Res 1992;32(9): 1739–43.
60. Kremers JJ, van Norren D. Two classes of photochemical damage of the retina. Lasers Light Ophthalmol 1988;2:41–52.
61. Mellerio J. Light effects on the retina. In: Albert DM, Jakobiec FA, editors. Principles and practice of ophthalmology. Philadelphia: W.B. Saunders; 1994;vol. 1.
62. Gass JDM. Stereoscopic atlas of macular diseases. 3rd ed. St Louis: Mosby-Year Book; 1987.
63. Tso MO, La Piana FG. The human fovea after sungazing. Trans Am Acad Ophthalmol Otolaryngol 1975;79(6):OP788–95.
64. Naidoff MA, Slinkey DH. Retinal injury from a welding arc. Am J Ophthalmol 1974;77(5):663–8.
65. Lucas RS, Harper CA, McCombe MF, et al. Optical coherence tomography findings in welder's maculopathy. Retinal Cases Brief Reports 2007;1: 169–71.
66. Magnavita N. Photoretinitis: an underestimated occupational injury? Occup Med (Lond) 2002;52(4):223–5.
67. Kaushik S, Gupta V, Gupta A. Optical coherence tomography findings in solar retinopathy. Ophthalmic Surg Lasers Imaging 2004;35(1):52–5.
68. Steinkamp PN, Watzke RC, Solomon JD. An unusual case of solar retinopathy. Arch Ophthalmol 2003;121(12):1798–9.
69. Charbel Issa P, Fleckenstein M, Scholl HP, et al. Confocal scanning laser ophthalmoscopy findings in chronic solar retinopathy. Ophthalmic Surg Lasers Imaging 2008;39(6):497–9.
70. Chen RW, Gorczynska I, Srinivasan VJ, et al. High-speed ultrahigh-resolution optical coherence tomography findings in chronic solar retinopathy. Retin Cases Brief Rep 2008;2(2):103–5.
71. Jain A, Desai RU, Charalel RA, et al. Solar retinopathy: comparison of optical coherence tomography (OCT) and fluorescein angiography (FA). Retina 2009;29(9):1340–5.
72. Symons RC, Mainster MA, Goldberg MF. Solar maculopathy in a young child. Br J Ophthalmol 2010;94(9):1258–9.
73. Pilli S, Ogoti M, Kalluri V. Fourier-domain optical coherence tomography findings in welder's maculopathy. Ophthalmic Surg Lasers Imaging 2010:1–5. Epub ahead of print, doi: 10.3928/15428877-20100215-93.
74. Hope-Ross MW, Mahon GJ, Gardiner TA, et al. Ultrastructural findings in solar retinopathy. Eye 1993;7 (Pt 1):29–33.
75. Grey RH. Foveo-macular retinitis, solar retinopathy, and trauma. Br J Ophthalmol 1978;62(8):543–6.
76. Kelley JS, Hoover RE, George T. Whiplash maculopathy. Arch Ophthalmol 1978;96(5):834–5.
77. Abebe MT, De Laey JJ. Foveomacular retinitis as a result of ocular contusion. Bull Soc Belge Ophtalmol 1992;243:171–5.
78. Kuming BS. Foveomacular retinitis. Br J Ophthalmol 1986;70(11):816–8.
79. Jacobs NA. Foveomacular retinitis. Br J Ophthalmol 1987;71(7):563.
80. Cordes FC. A type of foveomacular retinitis observed in the U.S. Navy. Am J Ophthalmol 1944;27:803–16.
81. Kerr LM, Little HL. Foveomacular retinitis. Arch Ophthalmol 1966;76(4): 498–504.
82. Ritchey CL, Ewald RA. Sun gazing as the cause of foveomacular retinitis. Am J Ophthalmol 1970;70(4):491–7.
83. Marlor RL, Blais BR, Preston FR, et al. Foveomacular retinitis, an important problem in military medicine: epidemiology. Invest Ophthalmol 1973;12(1): 5–16.
84. Wergel FLJ, Brenner EH. Solar retinopathy foveomacular retinitis. Ann Ophthalmol 1975;7:495–503.
85. Gladstone GJ, Tasman W. Solar retinitis after minimal exposure. Arch Ophthalmol 1978;96(8):1368–9.
86. Yannuzzi LA, Fisher YL, Krueger A, et al. Solar retinopathy: a photobiological and geophysical analysis. Trans Am Ophthalmol Soc 1987;85:120–58.
87. White TJ, Mainster MA, Wilson PW, et al. Chorioretinal temperature increases from solar observation. Bull Math Biophys 1971;33(1):1–17.
88. Sliney DH, Wolbarsht ML. Safety with lasers and other optical sources: a comprehensive handbook. New York: Plenum Press; 1980. p. 1035.
89. Mainster MA. Solar eclipse safety. Ophthalmology 1998;105(1):9–10.
90. Yang X, Jiang F, Song Y, et al. Accidental macular injury from prolonged viewing of a plasma flash produced by a femtosecond laser. Ophthalmology 2010;117(5):972–5.
91. Gardner TW, Ai E, Chrobak M, et al. Photic maculopathy secondary to short-circuiting of a high-tension electric current. Ophthalmology 1982;89(7): 865–8.
92. Friedman E, Kuwabara T. The retinal pigment epithelium. IV. The damaging effects of radiant energy. Arch Ophthalmol 1968;80(2):265–79.
93. Rinkoff J, Machemer R, Hida T, et al. Temperature-dependent light damage to the retina. Am J Ophthalmol 1986;102(4):452–62.
94. Mainster MA. Henle fibers may direct light toward the center of the fovea. Lasers Light Ophthalmol 1988;2:79–86.
95. Fishman GA. Light-induced maculopathy from surgical microscopes during cataract surgery. In: Ernest JT, editor. The 1985 year book of ophthalmology. St Louis: Mosby–Year Book; 1985.
96. Michels M, Sternberg P Jr. Operating microscope-induced retinal phototoxicity: pathophysiology, clinical manifestations and prevention. Surv Ophthalmol 1990;34(4):237–52.
97. Brod RD, Olsen KR, Ball SF, et al. The site of operating microscope light-induced injury on the human retina. Am J Ophthalmol 1989;107(4):390–7.
98. Pavilack MA, Brod RD. Site of potential operating microscope light-induced phototoxicity on the human retina during temporal approach eye surgery. Ophthalmology 2001;108(2):381–5.
99. Michels M, Lewis H, Abrams GW, et al. Macular phototoxicity caused by fiberoptic endoillumination during pars plana vitrectomy. Am J Ophthalmol 1992;114(3):287–96.
100. Khwarg SG, Geoghegan M, Hanscom TA. Light-induced maculopathy from the operating microscope. Am J Ophthalmol 1984;98(5):628–30.
101. Robertson DM, Feldman RB. Photic retinopathy from the operating room microscope. Am J Ophthalmol 1986;101(5):561–9.
102. Mares-Perlman JA, Brady WE, Klein BE, et al. Diet and nuclear lens opacities. Am J Epidemiol 1995;141(4):322–34.
103. Parver LM, Auker CR, Fine BS. Observations on monkey eyes exposed to light from an operating microscope. Ophthalmology 1983;90(8):964–72.
104. Irvine AR, Wood I, Morris BW. Retinal damage from the illumination of the operating microscope. An experimental study in pseudophakic monkeys. Arch Ophthalmol 1984;102(9):1358–65.
105. Green WR, Robertson DM. Pathologic findings of photic retinopathy in the human eye. Am J Ophthalmol 1991;112(5):520–7.
106. Mansour AM, Yunis MH, Medawar WA. Ocular coherence tomography of symptomatic phototoxic retinopathy after cataract surgery: a case report. J Med Case Reports 2011;(1):133.
107. Jaffe GJ, Irvine AR, Wood IS, et al. Retinal phototoxicity from the operating microscope. The role of inspired oxygen. Ophthalmology 1988;95(8): 1130–41.
108. Ferguson J. Photosensitivity due to drugs. Photodermatol Photoimmunol Photomed 2002;18(5):262–9.
109. Long VW, Woodruff GH. Bilateral retinal phototoxic injury during cataract surgery in a child. J Aapos 2004;8(3):278–9.

110. Manzouri B, Egan CA, Hykin PG. Phototoxic maculopathy following uneventful cataract surgery in a predisposed patient. Br J Ophthalmol 2002;86(6):705–6.
111. Khwarg SG, Linstone FA, Daniels SA, et al. Incidence, risk factors, and morphology in operating microscope light retinopathy. Am J Ophthalmol 1987;103(3 Pt 1):255–63.
112. Kleinmann G, Hoffman P, Schechtman E, et al. Microscope-induced retinal phototoxicity in cataract surgery of short duration. Ophthalmology 2002;109(2):334–8.
113. O'Brien DP, Francis IC. The corneal quilt: a protective device designed to reduce intraoperative retinal phototoxicity. Ophthalmic Surg 1994;25(3):191–4.
114. Kraff MC, Lieberman HL, Jampol LM, et al. Effect of a pupillary light occluder on cystoid macular edema. J Cataract Refract Surg 1989;15(6):658–60.
115. Jampol LM, Kraff MC, Sanders DR, et al. Near-UV radiation from the operating microscope and pseudophakic cystoid macular edema. Arch Ophthalmol 1985;103(1):28–30.
116. Keates RH, Genstler DE. UV radiation. Ophthalmic Surg 1982;13(4):327.
117. Sliney DH, Armstrong BC. Radiometric analysis of surgical microscope lights for hazards analyses. Appl Opt 1986;25(12):1882–9.
118. Kraff MC, Sanders DR, Jampol LM, et al. Effect of an ultraviolet-filtering intraocular lens on cystoid macular edema. Ophthalmology 1985;92(3):366–9.
119. Colin J, Ropars YM, Bonissent JF, et al. Cystoid macular oedema and intraocular lenses with ultraviolet filters. J Eur Implant Soc 1987;4:5–10.
120. Clarke MP, Yap M, Weatherill JR. Do intraocular lenses with ultraviolet absorbing chromophores protect against macular oedema? Acta Ophthalmol (Copenh) 1989;67(5):593–6.
121. Komatsu M, Kanagami S, Shimizu K. Ultraviolet-absorbing intraocular lens versus non-UV-absorbing intraocular lens: comparison of angiographic cystoid macular edema. J Cataract Refract Surg 1989;15(6):654–7.
122. Ciardella AP, Schiff W, Barile G, et al. Persistent indocyanine green fluorescence after vitrectomy for macular hole. Am J Ophthalmol 2003;136(1):174–7.
123. Uemura A, Kanda S, Sakamoto Y, et al. Visual field defects after uneventful vitrectomy for epiretinal membrane with indocyanine green-assisted internal limiting membrane peeling. Am J Ophthalmol 2003;136(2):252–7.
124. Engelbrecht NE, Freeman J, Sternberg Jr P, et al. Retinal pigment epithelial changes after macular hole surgery with indocyanine green-assisted internal limiting membrane peeling. Am J Ophthalmol 2002;133(1):89–94.
125. Thompson JT, Haritoglu C, Kampik A, et al. Should indocyanine green be used to facilitate removal of the internal limiting membrane in macular hole surgery. Surv Ophthalmol 2009;54(1):135–8.
126. Delori FC, Parker JS, Mainster MA. Light levels in fundus photography and fluorescein angiography. Vision Res 1980;20(12):1099–104.
127. Delori FC, Pomerantzeff O, Mainster MA. Light levels in ophthalmic diagnostic instruments. Proc Soc Photo Optical Instrum Enginering 1980;229:154–60.
128. Klingbeil U. Safety aspects of laser scanning ophthalmoscopes. Health Phys 1986;1(1):81–93.
129. Mainster MA, Turner PL. Retinal examination and photography are safe: is anyone surprised? Ophthalmology 2010;117(2):197–8.
130. Robertson DM, Erickson GJ. The effect of prolonged indirect ophthalmoscopy on the human eye. Am J Ophthalmol 1979;87(5):652–61.
131. Delori FC, Webb RH, Sliney DH. Maximum permissible exposures for ocular safety (ANSI 2000), with emphasis on ophthalmic devices. J Opt Soc Am A Opt Image Sci Vis 2007;24(5):1250–65.
132. Kohnen S. Light-induced damage of the retina through slit-lamp photography. Graefes Arch Clin Exp Ophthalmol 2000;238(12):956–9.
133. Cideciyan AV, Jacobson SG, Aleman TS, et al. In vivo dynamics of retinal injury and repair in the rhodopsin mutant dog model of human retinitis pigmentosa. Proc Natl Acad Sci U S A 2005;102(14):5233–8.
134. Berson EL. Light deprivation and retinitis pigmentosa. Vision Res 1980;20(12):1179–84.
135. van der Hoeve J. Eye lesions produced by light rich in ultraviolet rays: senile cataract, senile degeneration of the macula. Am J Ophthalmol 1920;3:178–94.
136. Ts'o MO, La Piana FG, Appleton B. The human fovea after sungazing. Trans Am Acad Ophthalmol Otolaryngol 1974;78:OP-677.
137. Mainster MA. Solar retinitis, photic maculopathy and the pseudophakic eye. J Am Intraocul Implant Soc 1978;4(3):84–6.
138. Young RW. A theory of central retinal disease. In: Sears ML, editor. New directions in ophthalmic research. New Haven, CT: Yale University Press; 1981.
139. Margrain TH, Boulton M, Marshall J, et al. Do blue light filters confer protection against age-related macular degeneration? Prog Retin Eye Res 2004;23(5):523–31.
140. McCarty CA, Mukesh BN, Fu CL, et al. Risk factors for age-related maculopathy: the Visual Impairment Project. Arch Ophthalmol 2001;119(10):1455–62.
141. Taylor HR, West S, Munoz B, et al. The long-term effects of visible light on the eye. Arch Ophthalmol 1992;110(1):99–104.
142. Dong LM, Stark WJ, Jefferys JL, et al. Progression of age-related macular degeneration after cataract surgery. Arch Ophthalmol 2009;127(11):1412–9.
143. Chew EY, Sperduto RD, Milton RC, et al. Risk of advanced age-related macular degeneration after cataract surgery in the Age-Related Eye Disease Study: AREDS report 25. Ophthalmology 2009;116(2):297–303.
144. Baatz H, Darawsha R, Ackermann H, et al. Phacoemulsification does not induce neovascular age-related macular degeneration. Invest Ophthalmol Vis Sci 2008;49(3):1079–83.
145. Sutter FK, Menghini M, Barthelmes D, et al. Is pseudophakia a risk factor for neovascular age-related macular degeneration? Invest Ophthalmol Vis Sci 2007;48(4):1472–5.
146. Xu L, Li Y, Zheng Y, et al. Associated factors for age related maculopathy in the adult population in China: the Beijing eye study. Br J Ophthalmol 2006;90(9):1087–90.
147. Sliney DH. Photoprotection of the eye – UV radiation and sunglasses. J Photochem Photobiol B 2001;64(2–3):166–75.
148. Abraham AG, Cox C, West S. The differential effect of ultraviolet light exposure on cataract rate across regions of the lens. Invest Ophthalmol Vis Sci 2011;51(8):3919–23.
149. Rabin JC, Wiley RW, Levine RR, et al. U.S. Army sunglasses: issues and solutions. J Am Optom Assoc 1996;67(4):215–22.
150. American National Standard for the Safe Use of Lasers, ANSI Z136.1-2007. Washington, DC: American National Standards Institute; 2007.
151. Sliney DH, Wolborsht ML. Safety standards and measurement techniques for high intensity light sources. Vision Res 1980;20(12):1133–41.
152. American National Standard for the Safe Use of Lasers in Health Care Facilities, ANSI Z136.3-2005. Washington, DC: American National Standards Institute; 2005.
153. Safety of Laser Products–Part 1: Equipment classification, requirements and user's guide, IEC 60825-1, Ed. 2.0b. Geneva, Switzerland: International Electrotechnical Commission; 2008.
154. Sliney DH, Trokel SL. Medical lasers and their safe use. New York: Springer-Verlag; 1993.
155. Sliney DH, Mainster MA. Ophthalmic laser safety: tissue interactions, hazards and protection. Ophthalmol Clin North Am 1998;11(2):157–64.
156. Performance Standards for Light-Emitting Products, 21CFR1040. Washington, DC: Center for Devices and Radiological Health, United States Food and Drug Administration; 2011.

For additional online content visit http://www.expertconsult.com

Chapter 91

Traumatic Chorioretinopathies

Youxin Chen, Mingwei Zhao, Peng Zhou

EPIDEMIOLOGY

Eye injuries are an important world-wide cause of visual loss, particularly in developing countries. Surveys indicate that there are almost 2.5 million new eye injuries in the United States each year. Of these, between 40 000 and 60 000 patients are diagnosed with trauma-related blindness.[1,2] Ocular trauma is the leading cause of monocular blindness[2] and the affected population tends to be young, with 58% under 30 years of age.[2] Given the potential societal burden, the importance of preventing eye injuries is a point of emphasis in both developed and developing nations.

As noted above, most victims of ocular trauma are in the 18–44 age range.[1,2] Most eye injuries to children occur during athletic or recreational activities.[3,4] In adults, car accidents, work-related injuries and physical assaults are the most commonly reported causes.[5,6] The vast majority of individuals suffering traumatic chorioretinopathies are male (72–90%).[2,6] Blunt injuries account for 51–66% of ocular injuries in both prospective and retrospective studies,[5] with the majority of retinal lesions being unilateral.[1] Previous studies have implicated metal, explosives, and stone as the most common materials contributing to ocular morbidity and blindness in the setting of trauma.[6,7]

The chorioretinopathies described in this chapter are those due to direct or indirect injury to the eye by blunt forces, without scleral rupture. Penetrating injuries are discussed in other chapters (Chapter 110, Surgery for ocular trauma).

CHORIORETINOPATHIES FROM DIRECT OCULAR INJURIES

The blunt force acting on the eye can cause a coup injury at the site of impact, and a contrecoup injury in the opposite part of the eye as a result of shock waves acting at the interface of tissues of different densities. Direct blunt trauma also compresses the eye in the axis of the force and significantly stretches the tissues in the perpendicular plane. This stretching effect may also contribute to indirect injury.[8]

Commotio retinae

The term commotio retinae was first introduced by Berlin[9] in 1873. It is sometimes referred to as Berlin's edema, as Berlin believed that the whitish appearance of the retina was due to extracellular edema. Commotio retinae is a self-limited opacification of the retina secondary to direct blunt ocular trauma, characterized by a transient whitening at the level of the deep sensory retina (Fig. 91.1). Retinal whitening may take hours to develop before it becomes visible ophthalmoscopically.[10] The lesion may involve both the central retina and the periphery.[10]

Commotio retinae has been reproduced in many different animal models in the setting of blunt eye trauma.[11–13] Histopathologic studies of animal models have shown that it is characterized by disruption of the photoreceptor outer segments with associated retinal pigment epithelium (RPE) damage.[10,14–18] and coworkers[19] studied a single human eye with commotio retinae that was enucleated within 24 hours and also demonstrated photoreceptor outer segment disruption and RPE cell injury. Recently, reports[11,20] using optical coherence tomography (OCT) have confirmed that the major site of retinal trauma in commotio retinae appears to be at the level of the photoreceptor outer segment/RPE interface, thus correlating well with the histopathology studies.

Commotio retinae is a common finding after blunt eye trauma and accounts for 9.4% of all post-traumatic fundus changes.[10] Not surprisingly, the vision is more affected when the fovea is involved. No treatment is available or recommended for commotio retinae, other than observation.[10,12]

The severity of commotio retinae may be rated as being in one of two categories: a milder condition or retinal concussion, and a more severe condition or retinal contusion. The division into mild and severe is traditional and clinically useful. Histologic studies, however, do not allow cases to be clearly separated into these two categories.

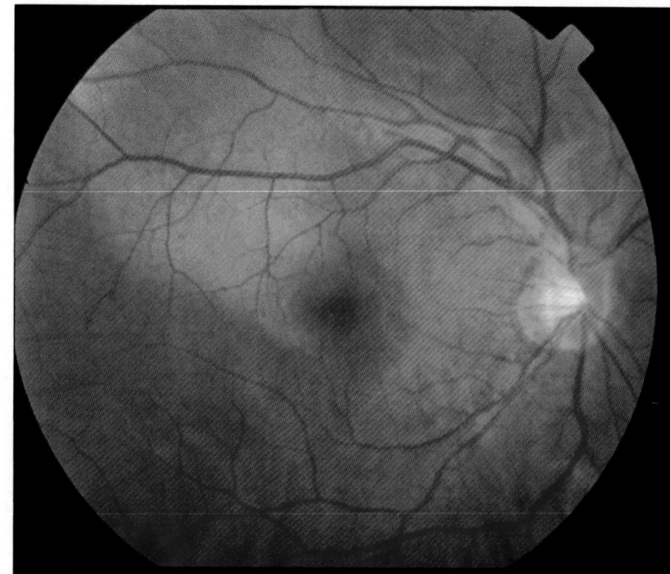

Fig. 91.1 Commotio retina in the macular area. Notice whitish change in the outer retina. (Courtesy of John Payne, MD, Emory University.)

Retinal concussion

Retinal concussion is a milder condition of traumatic retinal opacification. The initial vision is better (usually better than 20/200) and the gray–white change is less dramatic. In addition, the clinical changes are reversible, with vision generally recovering fully with minimal sequelae.[11] On fluorescein angiography (FA) the areas of opaque retina block background choroidal fluorescence. Leakage from the retinal vessels is not observed although mild staining is often noted at the level of the RPE, which generally clears within 24 hours.[10,13] The retinal whitening on ophthalmoscopy also clears spontaneously in a few days.[10,17]

Retinal contusion

In retinal contusion, the retinal whitening is more intense and may be associated with hemorrhages and more persistent visual loss. Visual acuity may be variably affected, from mild to severe, in a fashion that does not correlate with the degree of retinal whitening seen clinically. If the macula is affected, acuity is usually permanently damaged.[21]

In contrast to retinal concussion, more intense staining or leakage is noted at the level of the RPE on FA.[21] Acute pigment epithelial damage leads to permanent pigmented scars in the ensuing weeks.

Choroidal rupture

Choroidal rupture is a tear of the inner choroid and overlying Bruch's membrane and RPE caused by mechanical disruption when the globe is acutely deformed by blunt trauma causing anterior posterior compression, and subsequent horizontal expansion of the eye.[10,22] Choroidal ruptures are noted to be present in approximately 5–10% of blunt ocular trauma cases.[23] During the blunt trauma, the fortified collagenous sclera and the naturally flexible retina are less likely to rupture. However, the relatively inelastic RPE, Bruch's membrane, and choriocapillaris, do rupture.[10,22] Direct choroidal ruptures are relatively uncommon; they tend to be parallel to the ora serrata and are found at the direct site of impact, which is usually anterior to the equator.[10] Indirect choroidal ruptures resulting from compressive injury to the posterior pole of the eye[22] are more common (about 80%),[22,24] with the crescent-shaped tears occurring concentric to the disc because of the tethering or stabilizing effect of the optic nerve.[25] The majority of indirect ruptures occur temporal to the disc and involve the fovea. Many are isolated, but there can be multiple ruptures (Fig. 91.2).[24] Patients with underlying compromise or brittleness of Bruch's membrane, as can be seen in the setting of angioid streaks, are more susceptible to indirect rupture than the normal population.[24]

Choroidal rupture is often associated with intrachoroidal, subretinal, and intraretinal hemorrhage. The associated hemorrhage and accompanying commotio retinae may conceal the presence of the rupture, which may become visible only after the blood clears in 2–3 months.[25] Occasionally they may not be readily evident ophthalmoscopically, and their presence is confirmed after FA or indocyanine green angiography (ICGA). ICGA appears to have an advantage in diagnosis of choroidal rupture as it often highlights broader areas of pathology and disturbance compared to FA.[25] Choroidal ruptures appear as hypofluorescent streaks on ICGA.

In histopathologic studies, Aguilar and Green[22] showed that choroidal rupture is followed by bleeding, fibrovascular tissue proliferation, and RPE hyperplasia. The overlying retina is variably affected, ranging from loss of the outer layers alone to discontinuity affecting the full retinal thickness. Areas of choroidal rupture are noted to heal with a fibroglial response.

Choroidal rupture is associated with a long-term risk of choroidal neovascularization (CNV) with 5–10% of eyes developing CNV.[24,26,27] The development of CNV was most strongly associated with older age, macular location of the choroidal rupture, and a greater length of the choroidal rupture.[24] Neovascularization is a consistent and expected part of the process of scar formation, and in some cases this neovascularization regresses without sequelae.[22] Management approaches for CNV secondary to traumatic choroidal rupture include observation, laser photocoagulation, submacular surgery, photodynamic therapy, and intravitreal anti-vascular endothelial growth factor treatment.[26,28,29]

Visual prognosis after choroidal rupture depends on whether the fovea was affected by the choroidal rupture and on whether late complications such as choroidal neovascularization ensue.[25,26] Most patients with traumatic choroidal rupture do not achieve final VA of 20/40 or better.[24]

Traumatic macular hole

Blunt eye trauma is one of the main causes of secondary macular hole[30] (Fig. 91.3). Traumatic macular holes (TMH) were first described by Knapp in 1869 and by Noyes in 1875.[31]

The exact cause of TMH remains controversial. Ho and associates[32] outlined four basic historical theories regarding its cause: the traumatic theory, the cystic degeneration theory, the vascular theory, and the vitreous theory. Today, it is recognized that the pathogenesis of macular hole formation is a combination of factors, while vitreous traction may play an important role in some cases of TMH formation.[33,34]

Macular holes do not always form immediately after trauma, but may appear after several days. In some cases macular edema and cysts develop, and eventually the roof of the cysts erode leading to the formation of a macular hole.[30] OCT can help to identify alterations that occur before hole formation and may help to explain the pathogenesis of TMH.[35,36]

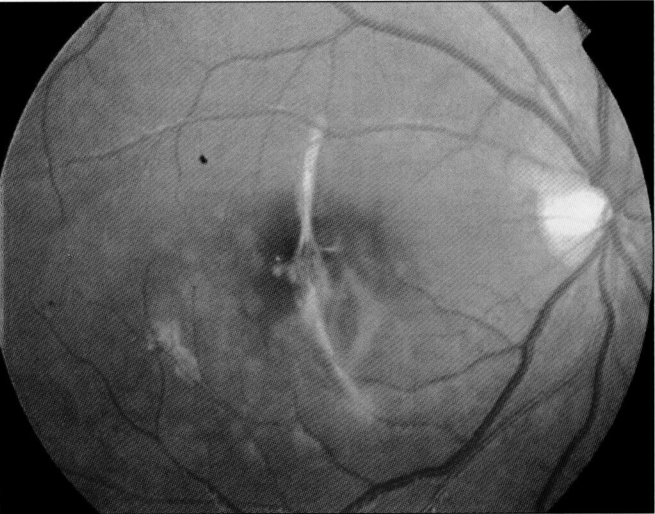

Fig. 91.2 Indirect choroidal rupture after a motor vehicle accident showing the classic crescent shape concentric to the optic disc.

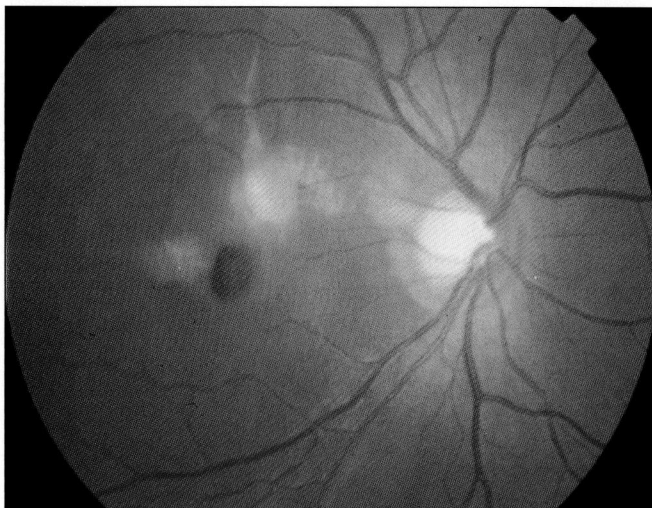

Fig. 91.3 Traumatic macular hole in a 15-year-old boy 4 weeks after being hit by a book during school.

There is no consensus on surgical management for this disease, because some cases demonstrate spontaneous closure of the macular hole and improved visual acuity by 6 months after injury.[31,37] Cases that close spontaneously tend to be in younger patients and in patients with smaller holes (less than 1/3 disc diameter) and without a fluid cuff.[35] Yamada and associates[31] proposed that for young patients with small traumatic macular hole without a fluid cuff, it is probably better to wait at least 6 months from their ocular concussion to allow spontaneous hole closure. Mechanisms of spontaneous TMH closure may include glial cells or RPE cells that proliferate at the margin of the hole and may fill and close the defect.[31]

Traumatic chorioretinal rupture

Goldzieher introduced the term *chorioretinitis plastic sclopetaria*, or the shorter form *chorioretinitis sclopetaria*, in 1901,[38] but now the term *traumatic chorioretinal rupture (TCR)* is deemed to be more acceptable. It refers to a simultaneous break in the retina and choroid resulting from a high-velocity missile passing adjacent to and coming into contact with the globe, entering the orbit without causing a scleral rupture. This injury causes a full-thickness chorioretinal defect and visual loss.[39] Simultaneous retraction of the choroid and retina at the site of the break reveals bare sclera. Two mechanisms have been considered: damage adjacent to the pathway of the high-velocity object is responsible for the direct injury, and the indirect injury is caused by the shock waves transmitted to the globe.[39]

TCR is a rare clinical presentation. Fundus examination may show the chorioretinal defect, bare sclera, pigment proliferation, marked fibrovascular proliferation and scar formation.[40] If the foreign body has come to rest deep in the orbit, the TCR is typically oriented radially.[41] The visual prognosis depends on the extent and location of intraocular injury. Secondary chorioretinal arterial and venous anastomoses have been reported.[42] ICG dye permits visualization of the deeper choroidal vessels and may demonstrate ruptures that are difficult to appreciate clinically.[43]

Despite severe retinal and choroidal injuries in TCR, the patients have a low chance of retinal detachment, as marked proliferation of fibrous tissue causes firm adherence of retina and choroid to the sclera.[40] In addition, the intact posterior hyaloid that is typically present in young patients further mitigates the risk for retinal detachment.[41]

Management includes observation, and rarely requires surgical intervention to repair a retinal detachment or to remove a non-clearing vitreous hemorrhage.[21,41] While confronted with TCR, it is important to make an accurate diagnosis to prevent unwarranted surgical intervention.[40]

TCR is typically caused by gun injuries resulting in retained intraorbital metallic foreign bodies, which are well tolerated and typically have minimal adverse effect on visual prognosis, and as such can be followed up without surgical intervention.[40]

Traumatic retinal pigment epithelial tears

RPE tear is a well-known complication of age-related macular degeneration.[44] But it is also a rare complication after trauma.[45,46] Why? It is thought that the force applied must fit into an extremely narrow window.[46] The force must be sufficiently large so as to cause an RPE tear, but not so large as to cause both the RPE and Bruch's membrane to tear, as in a choroidal rupture. As the elastic torn edge of RPE tends to retract over the adjacent intact RPE, RPE tears are usually prevented from healing, and visual recovery is generally poor.[46]

Biomicroscopy typically demonstrates a hypopigmented area corresponding to RPE loss and exposed Bruch's membrane. A scroll of pigmented RPE is usually noted at the margin of the hypopigmented area.[45] FA demonstrates a window defect in the area of RPE loss with an adjacent area of blocked fluorescence due to the rolled-up RPE (usually with a sharp edge between these regions).[45] OCT is particularly useful in displaying these changes at the level of the RPE.[45] Patients with traumatic RPE tears involving the fovea usually have a poor visual prognosis.[44]

Fok et al.[46] reported spontaneous resolution of traumatic RPE tears in a patient who subsequently had good visual recovery. The mechanisms of resolution in this case included a layer of hypopigmented RPE cells, atrophy of the choriocapillaris, and/or deposition of fibrous tissue.

Traumatic retinal tears and detachments

Ocular contusion may result in numerous types of retinal tears, such as horseshoe tears, operculated holes, macular holes, and retinal dialyses.[47] Dialysis is the most common type of retinal break in the setting of trauma.[48] Contusion leads to direct injury at the site of impact or indirectly as a result of changes in the shape of the eye (anteroposterior shortening followed by equatorial elongation) that may cause peripheral tears immediately, or secondarily following premature separation of the vitreous gel.[10]

Traumatic retinal tears are predominantly located within the vitreous base region. Cox et al.[48] reported that retinal tears were limited to the ora serrata in 59% of cases with traumatic retinal detachments (RD). Only 8% of the traumatic tears were in the equatorial area, whereas approximately 60% of the nontraumatic tears were in the equatorial area. However, Atmaca et al.[49] reported that 34.3% of the eyes with traumatic retinal holes and tears were in the equatorial region.

Johnston reported that 84.4% of the patients with traumatic retinal tears developed rhegmatogenous RD.[50] The presence of RD immediately following injury is extremely rare, and in general RD progress slowly, occurring weeks to months following the trauma.[51] The reason for the slower rate of progression from retinal defect (tear, dialysis) to frank detachment relates to the fact that the vitreous is formed and may be attached in these young patients. For patients developing giant retinal tears following trauma, the progression to detachment is much more rapid, and these types of tears appear to be more common in myopic male patients.[52] Goffstein found that 28% of contusion detachments were myopic, nine times higher than expected.[53]

The treatment of traumatic retinal tears and RD will be discussed in other chapters (Chapter 109, Giant retina tears, and Chapter 110, Surgery for ocular trauma).

Retinal dialyses

Retinal dialysis is a circumferential retinal tear located along its marginal attachment at the ora serrata (Fig. 91.4). Dialyses account for 8–14% of RD.[54] Ocular trauma is widely recognized as an important cause of retinal dialysis, resulting from mechanical disruption of the retina by force transmitted via the vitreous base.[55,56] Dialyses and giant tears caused 69% of traumatic detachments and 6% of nontraumatic detachments.[57] A blow from the fist was the most common mechanism of trauma in these cases.[54,57]

The most common symptoms are visual field loss or vague blurring of vision.[54,55] Other complaints include photopsias, vitreous floaters, or both. Some patients may not have any symptoms at the time of diagnosis.[54] The dialysis-associated RD may develop at the time of injury or months or even years later.[54,57] Because the vitreous in young patients is formed, RD caused by traumatic dialyses advance very slowly, especially in the inferior fundus. Signs of chronicity, such as demarcation lines and intraretinal cysts, are common.[53] In previous reports, the mean size of the traumatic dialyses was 2.4 clock hours as compared to a mean of 1.5 clock hours for the nontraumatic cases.[57]

A defining feature of spontaneous dialysis is its selective localization/involvement of the inferotemporal quadrant,[57] because of developmental asymmetry. However, traumatic dialyses may involve all quadrants. A higher frequency in the superonasal and inferotemporal quadrants has been reported in traumatic dialyses, with an incidence of 16–33.3% and 30.6–72% respectively.[54,57] Weidenthal and Schepens[55] postulated that the nasal peripheral retina has a greater susceptibility to traumatic dialysis secondary to its relatively narrower vitreous base. The inferotemporal quadrant, being the area least protected based on orbital anatomy, remains susceptible to dialysis with temporally directed trauma.[56]

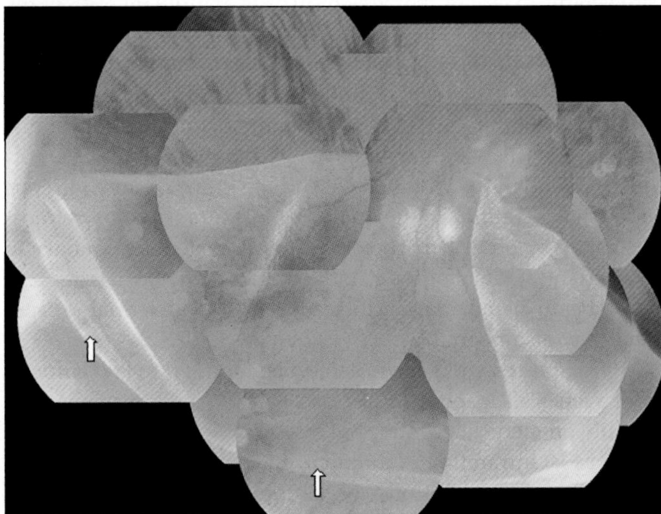

Fig. 91.4 A young man with high myopia developed a giant retinal dialysis and total retinal detachment after blunt trauma. The superior retina has folded downward, exposing bare pigment epithelium in the superior fundus. Arrows show the edge of the folded retina.

Optic nerve avulsion

Optic nerve avulsion is an uncommon yet visually devastating event that usually occurs after nonpenetrating or penetrating ocular trauma, typically when an object intrudes between the globe and the orbital wall and displaces the eye.[58,59] Patients typically describe a sudden loss of vision at the time of the trauma. The loss of vision may be relatively minor or severe, even to the point of no light perception. The avulsion is usually associated with other globe and orbital injuries but may occur as an isolated lesion.[59] It is usually associated with a decelerating injury of significant momentum.[49] Among many different causes, motor vehicle and bicycle accidents are the most common causes, and basketball injuries are the most common sporting injuries.[60]

Both complete and partial (involving only a segment of the optic disc) avulsions have been described. A complete avulsion implies that the optic nerve fibers are disinserted from the retina, choroid, and vitreous and that the lamina cribrosa is retracted from the scleral rim, resulting in a blind eye with a fixed and dilated pupil. Histopathological examination of the enucleated eye may reveal absence of optic nerve fibers from the lamina cribrosa.[59] The diagnosis of optic nerve avulsion is usually apparent if the media is clear. The fundus examination in such cases usually shows an excavation in the optic disc area because of retraction of the optic nerve into its dural sheath.[49] However, the fundus is usually obscured by hyphema or vitreous hemorrhage. Optic nerve avulsion can cause secondary substantial intraocular architectural changes, such as fibroglial scarring in the disc, epiretinal membrane and RD, in long-term follow-up.[61]

Sudden extreme rotation of the globe may be the major mechanism in some cases.[58] Other postulated mechanisms include a sudden marked rise of intraocular pressure that forces the nerve out of the scleral canal or a sudden anterior displacement of the globe.

B-scan ultrasonography has been only variably successful in imaging optic nerve avulsion.[58] A posterior ocular wall defect in the region of the optic disc characterized by a hypoechoic defect may be apparent.[62] A-scan ultrasonography may show a marked widening of the optic nerve suggesting hemorrhage and edema within the nerve sheath.[62] FA may demonstrate normal, delayed, or absent filling of the peripapillary retinal vasculature. In general, ancillary testing, such as CT, MRI, or color Doppler ultrasonography, are unlikely to assist in establishing the diagnosis in the presence of intraocular hemorrhage, although avulsions may be detected in certain cases and these studies may be useful in evaluating comorbid conditions.[58]

There is no known effective medical or surgical treatment for this condition. Final visual outcome is generally poor and dependent on initial post-injury visual acuity. Although administration of high-dose corticosteroids and optic canal decompression have been attempted, these treatments have not proved to be effective.[58] Therefore, early diagnosis is important to spare the patient unnecessary interventions.

CHORIORETINOPATHIES FROM INDIRECT OCULAR INJURIES

Purtscher's retinopathy

Purtscher's retinopathy was first described in 1910 by Otmar Purtscher, in a patient with severe head trauma.[63] Purtscher noted multiple areas of retinal whitening and hemorrhage in the posterior poles of both eyes.[64] The term "Purtscher-like retinopathy" is sometimes used to describe the retinopathy seen in conditions other than trauma, such as acute pancreatitis, fat embolism syndrome, childbirth, connective tissue disorders, and renal failure. Suggested pathophysiological mechanisms have included fat embolization leading to arterial occlusion, angiospasm, or lymphatic extravasation.[64,65]

Patients with Purtscher's retinopathy present with loss of acuity in one or both eyes, ranging from minimal impairment to hand motions visual acuity. Acute fundus abnormalities in Purtscher's retinopathy include Purtscher flecken, cotton-wool spots, retinal hemorrhage, and optic disc swelling (Fig. 91.5). The characteristic Purtscher flecken consists of multiple, discrete areas of retinal whitening in the superficial aspect of the inner retina, between the arterioles and venules. Retinal hemorrhages are often minimal and are typically flame-shaped, but dot and blot hemorrhage may occur. On FA, choroidal fluorescence may be masked by retinal whitening or blood, non-perfusion of the smaller retinal arterioles or capillaries may be seen, and there may be leakage from the retinal vessels in areas of ischemia.[64]

Without treatment, these findings resolve spontaneously within 1–3 months and may be replaced by mottling of the RPE, temporal disc pallor, or attenuation or sheathing of the retinal vessels.[64] Treatment with systemic high-dose steroids may improve visual outcome in some patients but at present there is little evidence to support such treatment.[66–68]

Terson's syndrome

Moritz Litten first described the occurrence of vitreous hemorrhage in association with subarachnoid hemorrhage in 1881.[69] Intraocular hemorrhage secondary to either subarachnoid hemorrhage or subdural hemorrhage is named Terson syndrome after Albert Terson.[70] The reported incidence of Terson syndrome in patients suffering from subarachnoid hemorrhage ranges from 10% to 50%.[71] Terson syndrome is associated with a worse outcome than in patients with subarachnoid hemorrhage but without vitreous hemorrhage.[72]

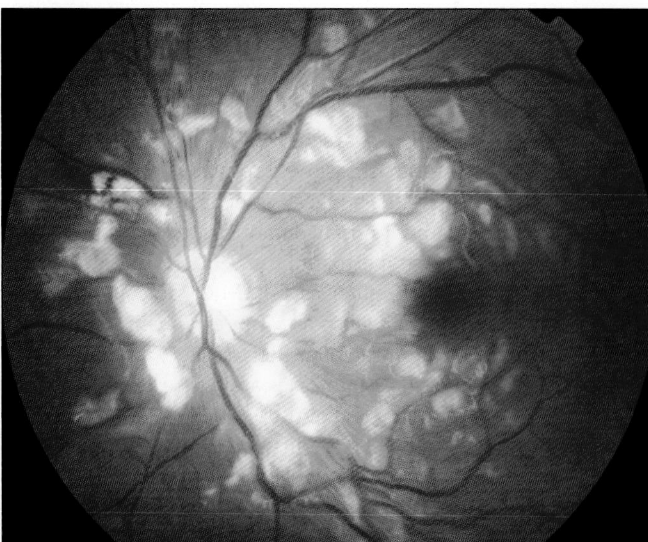

Fig. 91.5 Fundus photograph of the left eye of a 45-year-old man 7 days after a chest trauma. A number of cotton-wool spots and a few superficial hemorrhages provide evidence of Purtscher's retinopathy.

There are two plausible mechanisms for Terson syndrome. One explanation is that the vitreous hemorrhage may derive from ocular blood. The sudden rise in intracranial pressure may lead to a decrease in venous return to the cavernous sinus or obstruct the retinochoroidal anastomoses and central retinal vein, culminating in venous stasis and hemorrhage.[72] Another explanation is that the vitreous hemorrhage may be caused by a large amount of blood entering the subarachnoid space around the optic nerve, subsequently infiltrating the intraocular space through the perivascular space around the central retinal vessels within the optic nerve.[71]

Histopathologic correlation shows that hemorrhages occur in the vitreous, subhyaloid space, sub-internal limiting membrane (ILM), intraretinal, and subretinal spaces, in association with macular holes, retinal detachments, and optic neuropathy. Subhyaloid hemorrhages have a diffuse morphology, whereas sub-ILM are well demarcated. Continuous and noncontinuous blood flow has been observed along optic nerves, within nerve sheaths, and in the subdural and subarachnoid spaces.[73]

Current recommendations in the literature suggest 3–6 months of observation after the acute event, followed by vitrectomy if there is no improvement in visual acuity.[73] Vitrectomy in Terson syndrome usually results in substantial improvement in visual acuity.[74]

Shaken-baby syndrome

Shaken-baby syndrome (SBS) is a type of child abuse especially prevalent in infants under 3 years of age. In 1974, Caffey[75] first reported cases of battered infants presenting with subdural hemorrhage, intraocular bleeding, and metaphyseal fractures.

The mechanism of retinal hemorrhage has not been clarified; however, it is assumed that the acceleration–deceleration causes relative movements of the vitreous body on the one hand and the retina and vessels on the other. Most studies support a link between the extent of retinal hemorrhage and the severity of the trauma suffered and the prognosis.[76]

Ocular examination is critical because up to 90% of babies with SBS display unusual ocular findings. Findings in such cases are typically bilateral but can be asymmetrical. Dilated fundus examination may demonstrate posterior pole retinal hemorrhages, involving any of the layers of the retina. Heavy vitreous hemorrhage, retinal folds, choroidal rupture, and/or retinoschisis may be observed. There may be disc edema secondary to elevated intracranial pressure or indirect optic canal damage and optic sheath hemorrhage. Horseshoe tears and retinal detachment may also be found.[77]

Any suspected child abuse should be reported to law enforcement agencies. Hospital admission of an SBS patient is indicated not only on medical grounds but also to avoid the risk of further abuse. Most intraretinal, subretinal, and preretinal hemorrhages clear spontaneously within 4 weeks after injury. Vitreous hemorrhage may clear or persist longer than a few months. Schisis, choroidal rupture, retinal folds, retinal detachment, and optic nerve trauma may be safely observed until the patient is stabilized and the appropriate surgical strategy is determined. For

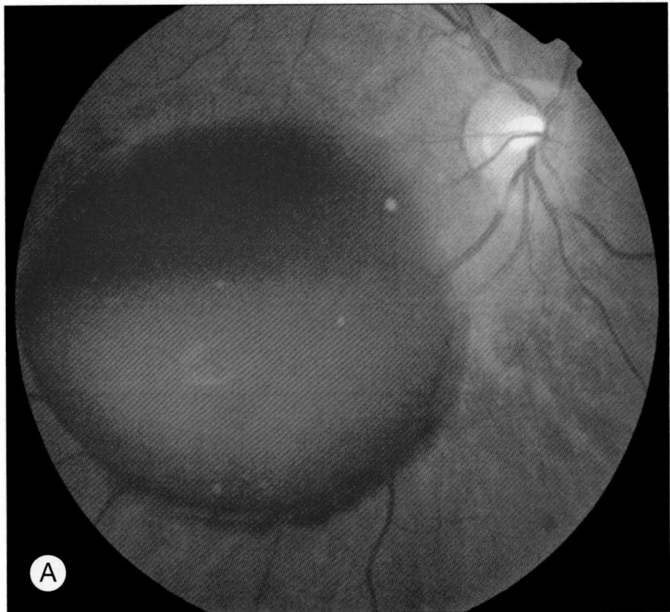

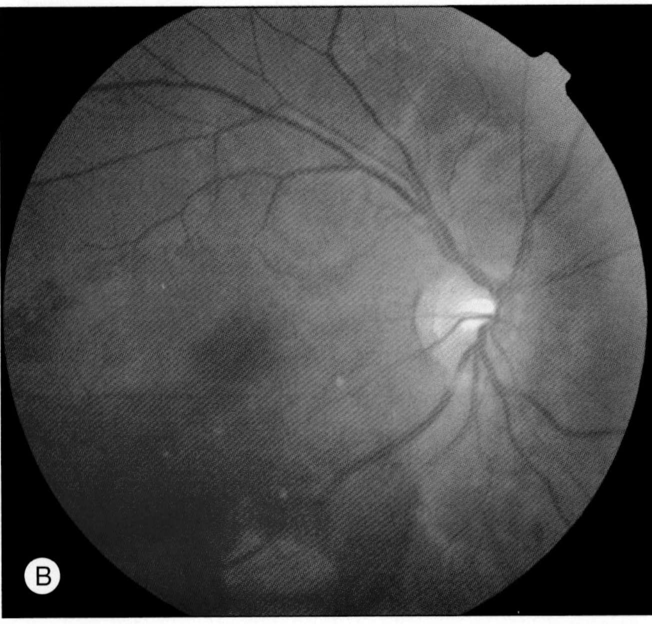

Fig. 91.6 Valsalva retinopathy. Before (A) and 5 minutes after (B) Nd:YAG laser membranotomy. (Courtesy of Dr Qing Chang.)

nonclearing vitreous hemorrhage or subhyaloid hemorrhage overlying the macula, trans-pars plana vitrectomy should be considered, as irreversible visual loss owing to deprivation amblyopia may occur in as little as 4 weeks. Retinal detachment should be repaired with scleral buckling or vitrectomy.[77]

Valsalva retinopathy

Valsalva retinopathy was first described in 1972 by Thomas Duane[78] as a particular form of retinopathy, preretinal and hemorrhagic in nature, secondary to a sudden increase in intrathoracic pressure. Increasing intrathoracic pressure against a closed glottis diminishes venous return to the heart, decreasing stroke volume and subsequently increasing venous system pressure. Valves in the venous system of the head and neck that are not functioning properly may allow the direct transmission of intrathoracic or intra-abdominal pressure into the head and neck. This pressure rise causes a decompensation at the level of the retinal capillary bed resulting in either unilateral or bilateral retinal hemorrhages, which are usually found below the internal limiting membrane, but can occasionally break through to become a subhyaloid or intravitreal hemorrhage.[79]

The anatomic location of the premacular hemorrhage is described as subinternal limiting membrane (ILM), subhyaloid, or a combination of both. Optical coherence tomography (OCT) can be used to distinguish clinically between a subhyaloid and a sub-ILM hemorrhage.[80] Therapeutic options in Valsalva retinopathy include conservative management, surgery (vitrectomy), and Nd:YAG laser membranotomy (Fig. 91.6).

Fat embolism syndrome

Fat embolism syndrome (FES) was first described in 1861 by Zeuker.[81] FES can be a complication of fractures of long bones, such as the femur, and is associated with various neurologic signs including paralysis, tremor, delirium, stupor, and coma. FES has been diagnosed in 5% of all patients with fractures. Clinical features usually commence between 24 and 48 hours after the injury, and the mortality rate has been reported to be as high as 30%.[82] It was suggested that FES is caused by the delayed release of fat droplets from pulmonary fat emboli, by repeated influx of emboli from an inadequately fixed fracture, or by fatty acid hydrolyzed from neutral fat. The pathologic changes in FES are produced by combined mechanical damage induced by fat droplets and biochemical damage induced by fatty acids.[82]

Retinopathy has been reported in 50% of patients with FES and in 4% of patients with long-bone fractures presenting with a subclinical syndrome. Typical lesions consist of cotton-wool spots and flame-like hemorrhages, and are attributed to microvascular injury and microinfarction of the retina. Retinal lesions disappear after a few weeks, although scotomas may persist.[83]

Whiplash retinopathy

Kelley described a slight, grayish retinal haze, a crater-like depression of less than 100 μm in diameter, and a slight disturbance in the pigment epithelium in the fovea following a flexion–extension type of head and neck injury in 1978.[84] The term whiplash maculopathy now refers to an immediate reduction in visual acuity with corresponding development of a foveolar depression and increased thickness of the peripheral retina. Occasionally, there may be small retinal detachments as well.[85] No treatment is required, and in general, the prognosis for normal vision is good.

For online acknowledgments visit **http://www.expertconsult.com**

REFERENCES

1. May DR, Kuhn FP, Morris RE, et al. The epidemiology of serious eye injuries from the United States Eye Injury Registry. Graefes Arch Clin Exp Ophthalmol 2000;238:153–7.
2. Wei Z, Yusheng W. General situation of international eye injury epidemiology. Int J Ophthalmol 2004;4:877–81.
3. Tomazzoli L, Renzi G, Mansoldo C. Eye injuries in childhood: a retrospective investigation of 88 cases from 1988 to 2000. Eur J Ophthalmol 2003;13:710–3.
4. Serrano JC, Chalela P, Arias JD. Epidemiology of childhood ocular trauma in a northeastern Colombian region. Arch Ophthalmol 2003;121:1439–45.
5. Liggett PE, Pince KJ, Barlow W, et al. Ocular trauma in an urban population: review of 1132 cases. Ophthalmology 1990;97:581–4.
6. Chunxia J, Shengyong W, Guibo C. An epidemiological analysis on eye injuries. Chin J Dis Control Prev 2001;5:194–6.
7. Min Wu, Jian Ye. Hospitalized eye injury in a Chinese urban population: a retrospective analysis. Int J Ophthalmol 2010;10:1861–3.

8. Delori F, Pomerantzeff O, Cox MS. Deformation of the globe under high speed impact: its relation to contusion injuries. Invest Ophthalmol 1969;8:290–301.
9. Berlin R. Zur sogenannten. Commotio retinae. Klin Monatsbl Augenheilkd 1873;11:42–79.
10. Youssri AI, Young LH. Closed-globe contusion injuries of the posterior segment. Int Ophthalmol Clin 2002;42:79–86.
11. Sony P, Venkatesh P, Gadaginamath S, et al. Optical coherence tomography findings in commotio retina. Clin Experiment Ophthalmol 2006;34(6):621–3.
12. Viestenz A, Kchle M. Blunt ocular trauma. Part II. Blunt posterior segment trauma. Ophthalmologe 2005;102:89–99.
13. Pulido JS, Blair NP. The blood–retinal barrier in Berlin's edema. Retina 1987;7:233–6.
14. Blight R, Hart JCD. Structural changes in the outer retinal layers following blunt mechanical non-perforating trauma to the globe: an experimental study. Br J Ophthalmol 1977;61:573–87.
15. Blight R, Hart JCD. Histological changes in the internal retinal layers produced by concussive injuries to the globe: an experimental study. Trans Ophthalmol Soc UK 1978;98:270.
16. Sipperly JO, Quigley HA, Hass JDM. Traumatic retinopathy in primates: the explanation of commotio retinae. Arch Ophthalmol 1978;96:2267.
17. Greven CM, Collins AS, Slusher MM, et al. Visual results, prognostic indicators and posterior segment findings following surgery for cataract/lens subluxation-dislocation secondary to ocular contusion injuries. Retina 2002;22:575–80.
18. Itakura H, Kishi S. Restored photoreceptor outer segment in commotio retinae. Ophthalmic Surg Lasers Imaging 2011 Mar 3;42 Online:e29–31.
19. Mansour AM, Green WR, Hogge C. Histopathology of commotio retinae. Retina 1992;12:24–48.
20. Bradley JL, Shah SP, Manjunath V, et al. Ultra-high-resolution optical coherence tomographic findings in commotio retinae. Arch Ophthalmol 2011; 129(1):107–8.
21. Williams DF, Mieler WF, Williams GA. Posterior segment manifestations of ocular trauma. Retina 1990;10:35–44.
22. Aguilar JP, Green WR. Choroidal rupture: a histopathologic study of 47 eyes. Retina 1984;4:269–75.
23. Lavinsky D, Martins EN, Cardillo JA, et al. Fundus autofluorescence in patients with blunt ocular trauma. Acta Ophthalmol 2011;89(1):e89–94.
24. Ament CS, Zacks DN, Lane AM, et al. Predictors of visual outcome and choroidal neovascular membrane formation after traumatic choroidal rupture. Arch Ophthalmol 2006;124:957–66.
25. Kohno T, Miki T, Shiraki K, et al. Indocyanine green angiographic features of choroidal rupture and choroidal vascular injury after contusion ocular injury. Am J Ophthalmol 2000;129:38–46.
26. Francis JH, Freund KB. Photoreceptor reconstitution correlates with visual improvement after intravitreal bevacizumab treatment of choroidal neovascularization secondary to traumatic choroidal rupture. Retina 2011;31: 422–4.
27. Arrim ZI, Simmons IG. Traumatic choroidal rupture. Emerg Med J 2009;26:880.
28. Yadav NK, Bharghav M, Vasudha K, et al. Choroidal neovascular membrane complicating traumatic choroidal rupture managed by intravitreal bevacizumab. Eye 2009;23:1872–3.
29. Harissi-Dagher M, Sebag M, Gauthier D, et al. Photodynamic therapy in young patients with choroidal neovascularization following traumatic choroidal rupture. Am J Ophthalmol 2005;139:726–8.
30. Oehrens AM, Stalmans P. Optical coherence tomographic documentation of the formation of a traumatic macular hole. Am J Ophthalmol 2006;142:866–9.
31. Yamada H, Sakai A, Yamada E, et al. Spontaneous closure of traumatic macular hole. Am J Ophthalmol 2002;134:340–7.
32. Ho AC, Guyer DR, Fine SL. Macular hole. Surv Ophthalmol 1998;42:393–416.
33. Smiddy WE, Flynn Jr HW. Pathogenesis of macular holes and therapeutic implications. Am J Ophthalmol 2004;137:525–37.
34. Li XW, Lu N, Zhang L, et al. Follow-up study of traumatic macular hole. Zhonghua Yan Ke Za Zhi 2008;44:786–9.
35. Takahashi H, Kishi S. Optical coherence tomography images of spontaneous macular hole closure. Am J Ophthalmol 1999;128:519–20.
36. Huang J, Liu X, Wu Z, et al. Comparison of full-thickness traumatic macular holes and idiopathic macular holes by optical coherence tomography. Graefes Arch Clin Exp Ophthalmol 2010;248:1071–5.
37. Chen YJ. Vitrectomy and internal limiting membrane peeling of a traumatic macular hole with retinal folds. Case Report Ophthalmol 2011;2(1):78–83.
38. Goldzieher W. Beitrag zur Pathologie der orbitalen Schussverletzungen. Z Augenheilkd 1901;6:277.
39. Pe'rez-Carro G, Junceda-Moreno C. Dual cause of blindness: chorioretinitis sclopetaria and homonymous hemianopsia. Arch Soc Esp Oftalmol 2006; 81:119–22.
40. Ahmadabadi MN, Karkhaneh R, Roohipoor R, et al. Clinical presentation and outcome of chorioretinitis sclopetaria: A case series study. Injury 2010;41: 82–5.
41. Martin DF, Awh CC, McCuen 2nd BW, et al. Treatment and pathogenesis of traumatic chorioretinal rupture (sclopetaria). Am J Ophthalmol 1994;117: 190–200.
42. Fraser EA, Barr DB. Chorioretinal arterial and venous anastomoses as a result of blunt trauma. Eye 2004;18:336–8.
43. Maguluri S, Hartnett M. Radial choroidal ruptures in sclopetaria. J Am Coll Surg 2003;197:689–90.
44. Shima C, Sakaguchi H, Gomi F, et al. Complications in patients after intravitreal injection of Bevacizumab. Acta Ophthalmol 2008;86:372–6.
45. Chan A, Duker JS, Ko TH, et al. Ultra-high resolution optical coherence tomography of retinal pigment epithelial tear following blunt trauma. Arch Ophthalmol 2006;124:281–3.
46. Fok AC, Lai TY, Wong VW, et al. Spontaneous resolution of retinal pigment epithelial tears and pigment epithelial detachment following blunt trauma. Eye 2007;21:891–3.
47. Dolan BJ. Traumatic retinal detachment. Optom Clin 1993;3:67–80.
48. Cox MS. Retinal breaks caused by blunt nonperforating trauma at the point of impact. Trans Am Ophthalmol Soc 1980;78:414–66.
49. Atmaca LS, Yilmaz M. Changes in the fundus caused by blunt ocular trauma. Ann Ophthalmol 1993;25:447–52.
50. Johnston PB. Traumatic retinal detachment. Br J Ophthalmol 1991;75:18–21.
51. Kennedy CJ, Parker CE, McAllister IL. Retinal detachment caused by retinal dialysis. Aust N Z J Ophthalmol 1997;251:25–30.
52. Nacef L, Daghfous F, Chaabini M, et al. Ocular contusions and giant retinal tears. J Fr Ophthamol 1997;203:170–4 (French).
53. Goffstein R, Burton TC. Differentiating traumatic from nontraumatic retinal detachment. Ophthalmology 1982;89:361–8.
54. Ross WH. Traumatic retinal dialyses. Arch Ophthalmol 1981;99:1371–4.
55. Weidenthal DT, Schepens CL. Peripheral fundus changes associated with ocular contusion. Am J Ophthalmol 1966;62:465–77.
56. Cox MS. Retinal breaks caused by blunt nonperforating trauma at the point of impact. Trans Am Ophthalmol Soc 1980;78:414–66.
57. Hollander DA, Irvine AR, Poothullil AM, et al. Distinguishing features of nontraumatic and traumatic retinal dialyses. Retina 2004;24:669–75.
58. Foster BS, March GA, Lucarelli MJ, et al. Optic nerve avulsion. Arch Ophthalmol 1997;115:623–30.
59. Chaudhry IA, Shamsi FA, Al-Sharif A, et al. Optic nerve avulsion from door-handle trauma in children. Br J Ophthalmol 2006;90:844–6.
60. Anand S, Harvey R, Sandramouli S. Accidental self-inflicted optic nerve head avulsion. Eye 2003;17:646–8.
61. Sturm V, Menke MN, Bergamin O, et al. Longterm follow-up of children with traumatic optic nerve avulsion. Acta Ophthalmol 2010;88:486–9.
62. Sawhney R, Kochhar S, Gupta R, et al. Traumatic optic nerve avulsion: role of ultrasonography. Eye 2003;17:667–70.
63. Purtscher O. Noch unbekannte befunde nach schadeltrauma. Berl Dtsch Ophthalmol Ges 1910;36:294–301.
64. Agrawal A, McKibbin MA. Purtscher's and Purtscher-like retinopathies: a review. Surv Ophthalmol 2006;51:129–36.
65. Trikha S, Tiroumal S, Hall N. Purtscher's retinopathy following a road traffic accident. Emerg Med J 2011;28:453.
66. Wang AG, Yen MY, Liu JH. Pathogenesis and neuroprotective treatment in Purtscher's retinopathy. Jpn J Ophthalmol 1998;42:318–22.
67. Atabay C, Kansu T, Nurlu G. Late visual recovery after intravenous methylprednisolone treatment of Purtscher's retinopathy. Ann Ophthalmol 1993; 25:330–3.
68. Agrawal A, McKibbin M. Purtscher's retinopathy: epidemiology, clinical features and outcome. Br J Ophthalmol 2007;91:1456–9.
69. Litten M. Ueber einige vom allgemein-Klinischen Standpunkt aus interessante Augenveränderungen. Berl Klin Wochenschr 1881;18:23–7.
70. Terson A. De l'hémorrhagie dans le corps vitre au cours del'hémorrhagie cerebrale. Clin Ophthalmol 1900;6:309–12.
71. Sakamoto M, Nakamura K, Shibata M, et al. Magnetic resonance imaging findings of Terson's syndrome suggesting a possible vitreous hemorrhage mechanism. Jpn J Ophthalmol 2010;54:135–9.
72. McCarron MO, Alberts MJ, McCarron P. A systematic review of Terson's syndrome: frequency and prognosis after subarachnoid haemorrhage. J Neurol Neurosurg Psychiatry 2004;75:491–3.
73. Ko F, Knox DL. The ocular pathology of Terson's syndrome. Ophthalmology 2010;117:1423–9.
74. Murjaneh S, Hale JE, Mishra S, et al. Terson's syndrome: surgical outcome in relation to entry site pathology. Br J Ophthalmol 2006;90:512–3.
75. Caffey J. The whiplash shaken infant syndrome. Pediatrics 1974;54:396–403.
76. Matschke J, Herrmann B, Sperhake J, et al. Shaken baby syndrome: a common variant of non-accidental head injury in infants. Dtsch Arztebl Int 2009; 106:211–7.
77. Tang J, Buzney SM, Lashkari K, et al. Shaken baby syndrome: a review and update on ophthalmologic manifestations. Int Ophthalmol Clin 2008;48:237–46.
78. Duane TD. Valsalva hemorrhagic retinopathy. Trans Am Ophthalmol Soc 1972;70:298–313.
79. Tildsley J, Srinivasan S. Valsalva retinopathy. Postgrad Med J 2009;85:110.
80. Shukla D, Naresh KB, Kim R. Optical coherence tomography findings in valsalva retinopathy. Am J Ophthalmol 2005;140:134–6.
81. Zeuker FA. Beitrage zur Anatomie und Physiologie der Lunge. Dresden: J Braunsdorf; 1861.
82. Lee JE, Jea SY, Oum BS, et al. Effect of fat embolism with triolein emulsion on blood–retinal barrier. Ophthalmic Res 2009;41:14–20.
83. Akhtar S. Fat embolism. Anesthesiol Clin 2009;27:533–50.
84. Kelley JS, Hoover RE, George T. Whiplash maculopathy. Arch Ophthalmol 1978;96:834–5.
85. Uebbing C, Miller J, Arnold C, et al. Soccer player whiplash maculopathy. Am J Emerg Med 2010;28:120.e7–8.

Chapter 92

Pregnancy-Related Diseases

Ala Moshiri, Justin C. Brown, Janet S. Sunness

Pregnancy is associated with maternal hormonal, metabolic, hematologic, cardiovascular, and immunologic alterations that can affect the ocular tissues. No significant retinal changes occur in most normal pregnancies. However, pregnancy can be associated with the development of new ocular conditions such as serous retinal detachment related to pre-eclampsia, or with an exacerbation of pre-existing disease processes such as diabetic retinopathy. These ocular changes are usually transient, but can cause permanent visual disability. This chapter presents the current state of knowledge about the relationship between pregnancy and maternal retinal and choroidal disorders. It also includes a brief summary of some considerations regarding diagnostic testing during pregnancy.

RETINAL AND CHOROIDAL DISORDERS ARISING IN PREGNANCY

Pre-eclampsia and eclampsia

Pre-eclampsia typically develops in the second half of pregnancy and is characterized by hypertension, edema, and proteinuria. Eclampsia is pre-eclampsia with convulsions that usually occurs late in pregnancy.

In healthy women pre-eclampsia is generally seen in first pregnancies, with an incidence estimated at 5%. Risk factors for pre-eclampsia include very young or advanced maternal age, multifetal pregnancy, hemolytic disease of the newborn, diabetes mellitus, chronic systemic hypertension, and renal disease.

Pre-eclampsia and eclampsia place the fetus at risk due to placental vascular insufficiency. In the first half of the twentieth century, severe changes in retinal arteriolar caliber were believed to reflect placental vascular insufficiency and to be an indication for pregnancy termination. Therefore, a great deal of attention was paid to retinal findings in pre-eclampsia. With improved medical and obstetrical management of hypertension and other aspects of pre-eclampsia, retinal findings are no longer used to assess this disease. In addition, retinal changes in pre-eclampsia may be significantly less frequent than they were in the past.

Early reports gave an impressive rate of visual disturbances. Scotoma, diplopia, dimness of vision, and photopsias were noted in 25% of patients with severe pre-eclampsia and up to 50% of patients with eclampsia.[1] Recent studies, discussed below, suggest that the rate of visual disturbance has decreased markedly with improved medical management of pre-eclampsia. Although photic stimuli may predispose to seizures in susceptible patients, the benefits of an ophthalmoscopic examination outweigh the small risk of seizure when an examination is indicated.[2]

Pre-eclampsia and eclampsia have been associated with a retinopathy similar to hypertensive retinopathy; serous retinal detachments; yellow, opaque retinal pigment epithelium (RPE) lesions; and cortical blindness. Arterial and venous occlusive disease can also occur and may contribute to visual loss. Early studies of retinal disorders in pre-eclampsia have been discussed in previous reviews.[3]

Retinopathy in pre-eclampsia and eclampsia

Focal or generalized retinal arteriolar narrowing is the most common ocular change seen in pre-eclampsia, but its frequency is declining. Early studies reported arteriolar attenuation in 40–100% of pre-eclamptic patients.[4] A retrospective study of fluorescein angiograms in pre-eclamptic patients by Schreyer identified normal retinal vessel caliber in 16 of 16 patients. In contrast, 4 of 14 patients with pre-existing chronic systemic hypertension had retinal vascular changes.[5] Jaffe prospectively demonstrated a statistically significant difference in arteriolar caliber between 56 study participants with severe pre-eclampsia and 25 healthy controls, but no difference between 17 patients with mild pre-eclampsia and controls.[6] These studies suggest that arteriolar narrowing may be more common in pregnant patients with chronic pre-existing hypertension than those with mild pre-eclampsia. The difference in the reported prevalence of retinopathy between the early and recent literature is probably related to better medical management of pre-eclampsia and its complications.

The cause of retinal arteriolar narrowing seems to be central retinal artery vasospasm suggested by increased central retinal artery blood flow velocity.[7] When present, the retinal arteriolar attenuation associated with pre-eclampsia generally resolves after delivery, presumably due to normalization of central retinal artery blood flow. Other typical hypertensive retinopathy changes such as hemorrhages, cotton-wool spots, lipid deposits, diffuse retinal edema, and papilledema are generally not seen in pre-eclampsia[6] and should raise suspicion about additional concurrent systemic disease. Recently, Gupta and colleagues found that the severity of retinopathy in pre-eclampsia is directly related to the level of placental insufficiency and intrauterine growth retardation. Serum uric acid levels also had a statistically significant correlation with retinopathy in this group, but the meaning of this finding needs further research to investigate possible causation. Interestingly, the severity of retinopathy did not correlate with degree of systolic or diastolic hypertension, suggesting that retinopathy in pre-eclampsia may be independent of systemic blood pressure.[8]

Choroidopathy in pre-eclampsia and eclampsia

Choroidal dysfunction is a common ocular complication of pre-eclampsia and eclampsia that manifests clinically as serous retinal detachments or yellow RPE lesions. The serous retinal detachments usually are bilateral and bullous but occasionally are cystic.[2,9] In the early twentieth century, serous retinal detachments were seen in 1% of severely pre-eclamptic patients and about 10% of eclamptic patients.[10,11] More recently, Saito retrospectively evaluated 31 women with severe pre-eclampsia or eclampsia and found that 40/62 (65%) eyes had serous retinal detachments and 36/62 (58%) had RPE lesions. RPE lesions were usually located in the macular or peripapillary regions, 33/36 (92%) were solitary or grouped, and 3/36 (8%) were large and geographic. After delivery, all serous retinal detachments and RPE lesions resolved. The three eyes with geographic RPE lesions all developed significant chorioretinal atrophy.[12] The apparent historical increase in the incidence of serous detachments and RPE lesions is almost certainly due to improved examination instrumentation and diagnostic testing such as fluorescein angiography.

The etiology of choroidal dysfunction is thought to be ischemia based on fluorescein angiography, limited histopathologic study, the presence of Elschnig spots on resolution[13] and indocyanine green angiography.[14] This is further supported by the observation that posterior ciliary artery blood flow velocity is increased in pre-eclampsia suggesting vasospasm.[7] The primary choriocapillaris ischemia presumably leads to RPE ischemia manifest as yellow opacification and/or fluid pump dysfunction allowing subretinal fluid accumulation.

Although serous retinal detachment and RPE dysfunction can cause marked loss of visual acuity, these changes fully resolve postpartum and most patients return to normal vision within a few weeks. Some patients have residual RPE changes in the macula. Years later, these changes can mimic a macular dystrophy or tapetoretinal degeneration.[15] Rare patients may develop optic atrophy if chorioretinal atrophy is extensive.[16]

Saito has suggested that serous detachments are more specific to pre-eclampsia and eclampsia, whereas retinopathy is seen more often in pre-eclampsia superimposed on pre-existing hypertension.[17] Retinopathy is associated with higher levels of blood pressure than is serous detachment.[18] Although retinopathy was believed to be a reflection of possible placental insufficiency and possible adverse neonatal outcome, serous retinal detachment is not an additional risk factor.[19]

Postpartum serous detachments have been reported in pre-eclamptic patients,[20,21] and there are rare reports of exudative detachments in patients without pre-eclampsia.[22,23] While these serous retinal detachments may be mechanistically distinct, they also resolve over several weeks.

The HELLP syndrome consists of hemolysis, elevated liver enzymes, and low platelets, and it is generally associated with severe pre-eclampsia or eclampsia. Bilateral serous retinal detachments and yellow-white subretinal opacities have been seen in rare patients with this disorder.[24–28]

Other ocular changes seen in pre-eclampsia and eclampsia

Cortical blindness that appears late in pregnancy or shortly after delivery is an uncommon complication of severe pre-eclampsia and eclampsia. The etiology of vision loss may be occipital ischemia in watershed areas from vasospasm,[29–32] possibly related to extracellular hypercalcemia,[33] ischemia from antiphospholipid antibody-related vascular occlusion,[34] vasogenic edema,[35–42] petechial[41] or larger hemorrhages,[42,43] hypertensive encephalopathy,[44,45] ischemia from hypotension during delivery,[46] or as part of a postictal state.[47] Most patients recover normal vision over several weeks. A prospective study by Cunningham showed that 15/15 women with cortical blindness experienced complete recovery over 4 hours to 8 days. CT scanning was obtained in 13/15 and MRI scanning in 5/15 revealing edema and petechial hemorrhages in the occipital cortex.[41]

The presence of large intracranial hemorrhages may portend a worse prognosis in terms of both mortality and visual recovery. Akan evaluated CT scans from 22 patients with neurologic complications from eclampsia and found that 2 of the 3 patients who died had massive intracranial hemorrhages.[42] Drislane found that among 4 patients with severe pre-eclampsia and multifocal cerebral hemorrhages, 1 died and the 3 others developed prolonged cognitive deficits.[43]

Cortical vision loss has been reported in eight patients with HELLP syndrome. One had postictal cortical dysfunction,[47] one had venous sinus thrombosis,[48] two had signs of cortical ischemia or edema,[49,50] and one was idiopathic.[51] Three patients (2.7%) in a prospective evaluation of 107 women diagnosed with HELLP syndrome developed cortical blindness.[52] Retinal arterial and venous occlusions have been reported in patients with pre-eclampsia. These may be a cause of irreversible visual loss and will be discussed later. Other ocular disorders reported associated with pre-eclampsia and eclampsia include ischemic optic neuropathy[53] and optic neuritis,[54,55] ischemic papillophlebitis,[56] peripheral retinal neovascularization,[57] choroidal neovascularization,[58] macular edema,[59] macular ischemia,[60] and a tear of the retinal pigment epithelium.[61] One patient with HELLP syndrome was reported to have developed a vitreous hemorrhage.[62]

Central serous chorioretinopathy

Central serous chorioretinopathy (CSC) is caused by localized RPE dysfunction resulting in the accumulation of subretinal fluid. People between the ages of 20 and 50 years are typically affected and there is an 8:1 male predominance.[63] Pregnancy may predispose some women to CSC. The limited amount of information available concerning CSC in pregnancy makes it difficult to determine whether CSC during pregnancy is typical CSC coincident with pregnancy or if it is a separate disorder possibly related to the hormonal hypercoagulability or hemodynamic changes of pregnancy.

Only a few dozen cases of CSC associated with pregnancy are reported in the medical literature.[64–72] Unlike the serous retinal detachments observed in pre-eclampsia and eclampsia, CSC is generally unilateral. The women were all previously healthy and no cases were associated with pre-eclampsia or eclampsia. No patients had antecedent eye disease other than refractive error. Primiparas and multiparas were both represented. Most of the cases developed in the third trimester and all resolved spontaneously within a few months after delivery. There were no cases of significant visual sequelae.

Pregnancy associated CSC may recur in the context or outside of subsequent pregnancy. CSC recurred in at least two women, always in the same eye, in subsequent pregnancies. One patient had four successive pregnancies with CSC,[70] and one had two successive pregnancies complicated by CSC.[71] There is also one case report of a woman developing CSC 1 month postpartum in two successive pregnancies.[72] However, there is also a report of a woman with CSC in her third pregnancy who did not experience a recurrence during a subsequent pregnancy.[67] So the occurrence of CSC during one pregnancy does not necessarily mean that it will recur with future pregnancies. There is a report of one patient who experienced a recurrence of CSC outside the context of pregnancy.[67]

There is an increased incidence of subretinal white exudates (presumed to be fibrin) in pregnancy-associated CSC (approximately 90%) compared to CSC in males and nonpregnant women (approximately 10%). Sunness reported that 3 of 4 patients with pregnancy-related CSC had subretinal exudates.[67] Gass found that 6/6 cases of pregnancy related CSC had subretinal exudates compared to only 6/50 (12%) of non-pregnancy related cases.[68] However, a recent series of 3 pregnant women with CSC without any exudates has been reported.[73] The cause of this higher prevalence of subretinal exudates in pregnant women is unknown.

Occlusive vascular disorders

An increase in the level of clotting factors and clotting activity occurs during pregnancy.[74] Several pathologic sources of thrombosis and embolic events can also occur. One review of ischemic cerebrovascular disease suggested that pregnancy is associated with a 13-fold increase in the risk of cerebral infarctions compared to nonpregnant women.[75] This increased risk of vaso-occlusive disease may also manifest as retinal or choroidal vascular occlusions.

Retinal artery occlusion

Two cases of unilateral central retinal artery occlusion (CRAO),[76,77] one case of bilateral CRAO,[78] five cases of unilateral branch retinal artery occlusion (BRAO),[79,80] and 3 cases of bilateral multiple BRAO[75] have been reported in association with pregnancy and in the absence of additional risk factors. One case of cilio-retinal artery occlusion has been reported.[81] Three cases of arteriolar occlusion were associated with pre-eclampsia[78,82] and 1 was associated with disc edema.[80] Five of the 12 (42%) cases occurred within 24 hours of delivery, suggesting that this is a particularly susceptible period. Two of the patients with unilateral BRAO also were found to have mild transient protein S deficiency upon further systemic workup.[83]

Blodi reported that multiple retinal arteriolar occlusions were seen within 24 hours after childbirth in four women. Two patients were pre-eclamptic and required cesarean section. One of the two also had evidence of cerebral infarctions. The third patient had hypertension, pancreatitis, and premature labor. The fourth was a previously healthy 16-year-old who had an oxytocin-induced labor and had a generalized seizure 2 hours after delivery. The patients reported decreased vision and all had fundus findings characterized by retinal patches characteristic of ischemia and intraretinal hemorrhages that were similar to Purtscher's retinopathy. After resolution, patients were left with focal arteriolar narrowing and optic disc pallor. The visual acuities ranged from 20/20 to 4/200 and visual field defects were compatible with the areas of occlusion. The authors suggest that complement-induced leukoemboli could have caused the retinal arteriolar occlusions.[82]

At least eight additional cases of pregnancy-associated BRAO have been reported in the literature.[84–90] However, all of these cases had significant additional risk factors for vascular occlusion. Since pregnancy is a common condition, it is difficult to know whether these cases represent true pregnancy associations, multifactorial or synergistic etiologies, or just chance occurrences. One case was associated with intramuscular progestogen therapy for a threatened abortion.[84] Three cases that occurred postpartum were associated with hypercoagulability from protein C[85] or protein S[82,86] deficiency. Two cases were associated with thromboembolic occlusions attributed to mitral valve prolapse[87] and amniotic fluid embolism.[88] The final 2 cases developed BRAO in the first trimester in association with migraine headaches.[89]

Retinal vein occlusion

Retinal vein occlusion associated with pregnancy is exceedingly rare. Only 5 pregnancy-related central retinal vein occlusions (CRVO) have been reported to date[91–93] and we are not aware of any branch retinal vein occlusions. A study of central retinal vein occlusions with diurnal intraocular pressure determination in young adults included a 33-year-old pregnant woman in her third trimester who had unilateral venous dilation and tortuosity with two subretinal hemorrhages and mild foveal edema.[91] Gabsi reported the case of a 27-year-old who was 6 months pregnant when she developed a unilateral CRVO. The authors suggested impaired fibrinolysis after venous stasis as a possible mechanism.[92] A 30-year-old woman presented in the 28th week of her second pregnancy with HELLP syndrome. She developed a unilateral CRVO 10 days after emergency caesarean section.[93] Rahman reported a case of CRVO associated with pre-eclampsia 3 weeks postpartum in a 20-year-old woman.[94] The final case is that of a mild bilateral CRVO that developed early in pregnancy and resolved over several months (J. Wroblewski, personal communication). The paucity of reported cases linking pregnancy to retinal vein occlusion makes the strength of this association suspect.

Disseminated intravascular coagulopathy

Disseminated intravascular coagulopathy (DIC) is an acute pathological process with widespread thrombus formation in small vessels. It can occur in obstetrical complications such as abruptio placentae and intrauterine fetal death that release placental thromboplastin into the maternal circulation and activate the extrinsic coagulation system. This process has a tendency to occlude the posterior choroidal vessels leading to RPE ischemia, dysfunction of the retinal pigment epithelial pump mechanism, and subsequent serous retinal detachments in the macular and peripapillary regions.[95–98] The development of serous retinal detachments in pregnancy, especially late pregnancy, may be an early ocular sign of DIC.[98] We are aware of case reports of only 2 patients in whom DIC caused serous retinal detachments.[95,98] These detachments tend to be bilateral and symptomatic. With recovery from the systemic disorder, vision generally returns to normal with only residual pigmentary change.[97,98] Patel reported a case of bilateral retinochoroidal infarction associated with pre-eclampsia and DIC with permanent vision loss.[99]

Thrombotic thrombocytopenic purpura

Thrombotic thrombocytopenic purpura (TTP) is a rare, idiopathic, acute, systemic coagulopathy characterized by platelet consumption and thrombus formation in small vessels. TTP occurs at any age with a peak incidence in the third decade of life and a female to male preponderance of 3:2. Visual changes occur in approximately 8% of cases[100] due to thrombus formation in the choriocapillaris and secondary RPE ischemia. Clinical findings are usually bilateral and include serous retinal detachments, yellow spots at the level of the RPE, and localized arteriolar narrowing. We are aware of 32 reported cases of TTP in association with pregnancy. Sequelae include RPE pigmentary changes and Elschnig spots with a return to baseline vision over several weeks in most cases.[100-102]

Amniotic fluid embolism

Amniotic fluid embolism is a serious complication of pregnancy with high mortality, second only to pulmonary thromboembolism as a cause of death during pregnancy and the postpartum period. Those patients who survive the initial event usually develop DIC[103] with the potential ocular complications described above. Two patients developed multiple branch retinal arteriolar occlusions, presumably related to particulate material from the amniotic fluid.[104,105] Another patient had massive blood loss from an amniotic fluid embolism leading to severe retinal and choroidal ischemia and blindness in one eye.[106]

Uveal melanoma

Pregnancy is heralded by a hormone-dependent tendency to hyperpigmentation and well-known cutaneous changes like chloasma and an increase in pigmentation of pre-existing nevi owing to increased levels of melanocyte-stimulating hormone in pregnancy.[107] Although estrogen and progesterone may stimulate melanogenesis, there is no evidence that this can cause malignant transformation of melanocytic cells.

A case–control study by Holly et al. found a decreased risk of uveal melanoma for women who had ever been pregnant with an increase in protective effect with more live births. The largest effect was observed between nulliparous and parous women.[108] Others, however, have reported a trend toward a larger-than-expected number of ocular melanomas presenting during pregnancy.[109] There are also a number of anecdotal reports of uveal melanomas presenting or growing rapidly during pregnancy.[110-115] These reports led to speculation that uveal melanoma may be hormone-responsive but two studies have failed to show any estrogen or progesterone receptor expression in ocular melanomas.[113,116] A large retrospective study showed no association of uveal melanoma with the use of oral contraceptives or hormone replacement therapy.[117] It is possible that other hormones may be involved[113] or that tumor growth may be related to pregnancy-associated immune modulation.

Pregnancy-related uveal melanoma does not seem to differ histologically from uveal melanoma not associated with pregnancy. Shields reported that among 10 pregnancy-related choroidal melanomas evaluated after enucleation the tumors did not differ in cell type, mitotic activity, and other features when compared to a matched group of tumors in nonpregnant women.[118]

The treatment of pregnancy-associated uveal melanoma has been described in two studies. Among 16 cases reported by Shields, 10 eyes were enucleated, 4 received plaque radiotherapy during or after pregnancy, and 2 cases were observed. Among 14 of 16 patients who elected to carry the pregnancy to term, all delivered healthy babies with no infant or placental metastases.[118] Romanowska-Dixon reported 8 cases in which there were no treatment-related pregnancy complications. The authors do suggest that brachytherapy is safer towards the end of pregnancy or after delivery.[119]

Childbearing may be associated with improved survival in choroidal melanoma. Egan et al. performed a large prospective cohort study in which death rates from metastasis were 25% higher in nulliparous women and men than in women who had given birth. The protective influence of parity was greatest in the first 3 years of follow-up and increased with the number of live births.[120] These results contradict a small earlier study by the same group that concluded rates of metastasis were not higher among women who reported pregnancies or oral contraceptive use.[121] A much smaller study by Shields also showed similar 5-year survival between pregnant and non-pregnant women with posterior uveal melanoma.[118]

Other changes arising in pregnancy

A choroidal osteoma has been reported that presented in the ninth month of pregnancy with visual loss due to choroidal neovascularization.[122] Cases of acute macular neuroretinopathy,[123,124] Valsalva maculopathy,[125] and cystoid macular edema[126] have been observed in the immediate postpartum period. Placental metastases from orbital rhabdomyosarcoma[127] and primary ocular melanoma have been reported.[128]

PRE-EXISTING CONDITIONS

Diabetic retinopathy

The modern medical, ophthalmologic, and obstetrical management of pregnant diabetic patients has greatly improved the outcome of pregnancy for both the fetus and the mother. Laser photocoagulation has reduced the risk of vision loss from diabetic retinopathy and improved glucose control has improved the likelihood of good fetal outcomes. Well-controlled blood glucose and adequate glycosylated hemoglobin (HbA_{1c}) before conception and throughout the pregnancy may reduce the risk of spontaneous abortion,[129,130] congenital anomalies, and fetal morbidity.[131] A recent study suggested that the severity of diabetic retinopathy may be a significant factor in predicting adverse fetal outcomes, even after correcting for blood glucose control.[132] Another study suggested, however, that blood glucose control may counteract adverse fetal effects associated with maternal retinopathy and nephropathy.[133]

Diabetic women who may become pregnant should establish excellent glucose control before conception, since the major period of fetal organogenesis may take place before the mother is even aware that she is pregnant. In addition, a diabetic woman's retinopathy status should be evaluated and stabilized prior to conception. This is particularly important for patients with severe nonproliferative or proliferative retinopathy because scatter laser photocoagulation may reduce progression during pregnancy.[134] Laser treatment of diabetic macular edema before pregnancy may also be important, although the effects of pregnancy on macula edema have not been adequately studied.

The Diabetes in Early Pregnancy Study (DIEP), a study of 155 insulin-dependent diabetic pregnancies,[135] as well as the data from the Diabetic Control and Complications Trial[136] and the previous data summarized by Sunness,[134] all provide evidence that better metabolic control before pregnancy diminishes the progression of diabetic retinopathy. Recent studies have found a strong correlation between the glycosylated hemoglobin level in the first month and the degree of deterioration once tight metabolic control is achieved.[135] Nerve fiber layer infarctions commonly are associated with the institution of tight metabolic control of chronic hyperglycemic patients. One study described the retinopathy status of 13 patients managed by insulin pump during pregnancy. Two patients who had rapid decrease in the HbA_{1c} level developed acute ischemic changes and ultimately proliferative retinopathy.[136] However, the long-term benefits of adequate blood glucose control outweigh concerns about the transient worsening of retinopathy that has been associated with the sudden imposition of tight metabolic control.[137–139]

The frequency of ophthalmic follow-up of a diabetic patient during pregnancy is determined by her baseline retinopathy status. Guidelines for eye care in diabetic patients recommend that a diabetic woman planning pregnancy within 12 months should be under the care of an ophthalmologist, undergo repeat evaluation in the first trimester, and after that at intervals dependent on the initial findings.[132,140]

Progression of diabetic retinopathy during pregnancy

The interpretation of changes in diabetic retinopathy as being caused by pregnancy is confounded by changes related to blood glucose levels. As medical advances continue to improve glycemic control, changes in blood glucose control that occur at the onset of pregnancy will be minimized and it may be easier to obtain a more direct understanding of the role of pregnancy in the progression of diabetic retinopathy. In the meantime, several mechanisms have been proposed as possible etiologic factors contributing to diabetic retinopathy during pregnancy.

Retinal hemodynamics may play an important role. The increase in cardiac output combined with decreased peripheral vascular resistance during pregnancy[141] have been suggested as pathogenic factors for the development or progression of diabetic retinopathy. Three studies suggest that retinal hyperperfusion may exacerbate pre-existing microvascular damage.[142–144] In contrast, two studies report a reduction in retinal capillary blood flow that may exacerbate ischemia and lead to retinopathy progression.[145,146] Other studies have suggested a possible role for various growth factors found at increased concentrations during pregnancy such as IGF-1,[147] phosphorylated IGF-binding protein,[148] placenta growth factor,[149,150] endothelin-1,[151] and fibroblast growth factor-2.[152] These factors may exert additive or synergistic effects.[153]

Short- and long-term effects of pregnancy on diabetic retinopathy

Since there is a high rate of regression of retinopathy during the postpartum period, one must consider short-term and long-term changes separately. The DCCT research group reported that pregnant women in the conventional treatment group were 2.9 times more likely to progress three or more levels from baseline retinopathy status than nonpregnant women. The odds ratio peaked during the second trimester and persisted as long as 12 months after delivery.[154] One study of short-term effects included 16 women with no retinopathy or nonproliferative retinopathy. Progression during pregnancy was compared to progression between 6 and 15 months postpartum in the same women. The number of microaneurysms showed a rapid increase between the 28th and 35th weeks of pregnancy. Six months postpartum the number of microaneurysms decreased but in most cases remained higher than the baseline level. The number of microaneurysms remained stable over the subsequent 9-month postpartum period.[155]

Three other studies compared short-term progression of retinopathy between separate control groups of nonpregnant women and pregnant women over the same time period. The first compared the course of diabetic retinopathy in 93 pregnant women and 98 nonpregnant women. Progression was observed in 16% of the pregnant group compared to only 6% in the nonpregnant patients. Furthermore, 32% of the nonpregnant group had retinopathy at baseline compared to only 22% of the pregnant cohort. Therefore, one might have expected more progression in the nonpregnant group due to worse baseline disease, making these findings more significant.[156] A second study compared 39 nonpregnant women, 46% of whom had retinopathy at baseline, with 53 pregnant diabetic women, 57% of whom had retinopathy at baseline. In the nonpregnant group the microaneurysms remained stable, streak or blob hemorrhages appeared in three patients (8%), and no nerve fiber layer infarctions developed over 15 months. In the pregnant group, microaneurysms increased moderately, and streak and blob hemorrhages and nerve fiber layer infarctions increased markedly over the same follow-up period. One patient with nonproliferative diabetic retinopathy from the pregnant group developed proliferative retinopathy.[157] In the third study, there were 133 pregnant and 241 nonpregnant women. The groups were statistically equivalent in terms of baseline retinopathy levels. Within each quartile of glycosylated hemoglobin, pregnant women had a greater tendency to have worsening of retinopathy and the nonpregnant women had a greater tendency to have improvement in their level of diabetic retinopathy during the follow-up interval.[158]

There are four studies concerning the long-term effects of pregnancy on diabetic retinopathy. The first included 40 women followed for 12 months postpartum. Among 19 study participants with no retinopathy at baseline, 30% developed mild nonproliferative retinopathy during the second and third trimester. By one year postpartum none had clinically detectable retinopathy. Among the 21 women with retinopathy at baseline, 11 worsened during pregnancy and 2 developed proliferative disease. None of these 11 women had regressed to her initial retinopathy status by 1 year postpartum.[159] The second study reported changes at 12 months postpartum. Among 10 patients with no initial retinopathy who developed mild retinopathy during pregnancy, half experienced total postpartum regression, 30% had partial regression, and 20% had no change. Among 5 patients with initial mild retinopathy who progressed to moderate nonproliferative retinopathy, 40% experienced complete regression, 40% partial regression, and 20% no regression. However, among 12 who progressed from mild initial retinopathy to severe nonproliferative retinopathy, only 17% had total regression, 58% had partial regression, and 25% had no regression. The third study compared 28 diabetic women to 17 nulliparous matched controls over a 7-year period. Only 5 of 26 (19.2%) women who had been pregnant experienced progression of retinopathy compared to 8 of 16 (50%) nulliparous women, suggesting that pregnancy does not affect long-term progression and may even afford a protective effect.[160] A final study of 80 women who had completed at least 1 successful pregnancy found no increase in the risk of proliferative retinopathy later in life compared to matched controls.[161]

Two studies suggest that the number of prior pregnancies does not appear to be a long-term factor in the severity of retinopathy present when duration of diabetes is taken into account.[162,163] In fact, a cross-sectional European study reported lower levels of retinopathy in diabetics with multiple pregnancies compared with women matched for age and duration of diabetes.[164] It is not clear if this improved status was caused by a prolonged period of tight metabolic control and better patient education, or if pregnancy confers a long-term protective effect. Another possibility involves the bias that only women with better metabolic control may have undergone the stress of multiple pregnancies.

The role of baseline retinopathy status, duration of diabetes, and metabolic control

The major determinants of the progression of diabetic retinopathy in a pregnant woman are the duration of diabetes and the degree of retinopathy at the onset of pregnancy.[134,135,157,165–167] Therefore, women with diabetes are strongly encouraged to complete childbearing early in their adult life.[168]

The baseline level of retinopathy at conception is the major risk factor for progression of retinopathy, according to the DIEP. When a logistic regression model was used to separate the influence of diabetes duration (shorter duration being less than 15 years, longer duration being more than 15 years) from the effect of a worse baseline level of nonproliferative diabetic retinopathy, the baseline retinopathy was highly significant but the duration of retinopathy was not. Analysis of patients with moderate or more severe retinopathy in the DIEP showed deterioration (defined as a two-step or more worsening determined on the final scale of the modified Airlie House Diabetic Retinopathy Classification) in 55% of patients with shorter duration and 50% of patients with longer duration of diabetes. However, the rates of development of proliferative retinopathy were 39% of patients with longer duration of diabetes and only 18% of patients with shorter duration of diabetes. The HbA_{1c} level at the beginning of pregnancy was used in the DIEP as a measure of metabolic control. Women with a HbA_{1c} level of 6 standard deviations (SD) or more from the control mean had a statistically significant higher risk of progression of retinopathy compared with patients with a HbA_{1c} baseline level within 2 SD of the control mean.[135]

A longitudinal analysis of the effect of pregnancy on microvascular complications in the Diabetes Control and Complications Trial (DCCT) was recently published. Pregnant women in the intensive treatment group had a 1.63-fold greater risk of retinopathy progression during pregnancy than nonpregnant women, compared to a 2.48-fold greater risk in the conventional treatment group.[154]

A prospective study of 179 pregnancies in 139 women with type-1 diabetes reported a 10% progression rate of retinopathy in women with a duration of diabetes of 10–19 years compared to 0% in women with duration less than 10 years. Furthermore, women with moderate to severe retinopathy experienced progression in 30% of cases compared to only 3.7% with less severe retinopathy.[169]

Lauszus prospectively followed 112 pregnant women with insulin-dependent diabetes and found an association between the severity of retinopathy and poor glycemic control before and after pregnancy. However, no such correlation was found with intensive glycemic control during pregnancy. Those women who had progression of retinopathy during or after pregnancy had an average diabetes onset at age 14 years compared to 19 years in women whose retinopathy remained stable.[170]

The following discussion of the progression of retinopathy during pregnancy is subdivided according to the baseline level of retinopathy present. Many of the studies did not use the more recent classification recommended by the Early Treatment Diabetic Retinopathy Study (ETDRS). Whenever possible, the results have been organized according to this classification.[171]

No initial retinopathy

Sunness summarized nine studies that included 484 diabetic pregnancies with no initial retinopathy. Twelve percent of these patients developed some background change during pregnancy, and one patient (0.2%) developed proliferative retinopathy. In 23 cases with progression for which postpartum follow-up was available, there was some regression of the nonproliferative changes in 57%.[134] The DIEP reported a 10.3% progression to mild nonproliferative diabetic retinopathy for this group of patients.[135] Four other studies of eyes with no initial retinopathy reported progression rates of 0%, 7%, 26%, and 28% respectively.[167,172–174]

A 12-year prospective study of patients with gestational diabetes did not demonstrate an increased risk of diabetic retinopathy.[175] Retinal vascular tortuosity in gestational diabetics has been reported, however, and some degree of tortuosity persisted at 5 months postpartum.[176] There is one case report of a previously healthy nulliparous woman with gestational diabetes diagnosed at 8 weeks' gestation. Glycemic control was instituted and the patient developed bilateral proliferative retinopathy by 31 weeks' gestation. The patient had a markedly elevated HbA1c at initial diagnosis suggesting that she may have been diabetic before becoming pregnant.[177] Puza reported a retrospective review of 100 gestational diabetics and concluded that routine examinations have little utility in these patients.[178]

Mild nonproliferative diabetic retinopathy

In two studies that included 24 pregnant women with fewer than 10 microaneurysms and dot hemorrhages in both eyes, 8% developed additional microaneurysms and 0% developed proliferative retinopathy.[134] A more recent study showed that microaneurysm counts increase during pregnancy, peak at 3 months postpartum, and then decline to baseline levels.[179] The DIEP study found that 18.8% of patients with mild nonproliferative retinopathy showed a 2-step progression on the modified Airlie House classification through the end of pregnancy. Only 6% progressed from mild nonproliferative to proliferative retinopathy.[135] A study that included 7 patients with minimal retinopathy reported progression in only 1 during pregnancy that improved after delivery.[174]

Moderate to severe nonproliferative diabetic retinopathy

The DIEP found that 54.8% of patients with moderate retinopathy showed a two-step progression on the modified Airlie House diabetic retinopathy classification and 29% developed proliferative retinopathy by the end of pregnancy.[135] In addition, 25% of those who developed proliferative retinopathy had high-risk characteristics as defined by the Diabetic Retinopathy Study.[180]

The results of 10 studies published before 1988 that included 259 pregnant women with nonproliferative diabetic retinopathy were summarized by Sunness. The analysis of this information showed that 47% of patients had an increase in the severity of nonproliferative changes during pregnancy. Differences in the scale of measurements of diabetic retinopathy among the studies caused wide variations in progression rates. Most of the studies included mild and moderate retinopathy in the wider group of nonproliferative retinopathy. Only 5% of patients in this analysis developed proliferative retinopathy during pregnancy.[134]

Four studies after 1988 reported progression rates of nonproliferative retinopathy ranging from 12% to 55%.[167,172,173,181] Two of these studies reported rates of proliferative retinopathy development at 8% and 22% during pregnancy.[173,181]

Proliferative retinopathy

Sunness summarized 12 studies, including 122 women with proliferative retinopathy at baseline. Of these 122 women, 46% had some increase in neovascularization that occurred during pregnancy.[134] A more recent study reported a 63% rate of progression in eyes with proliferative retinopathy at baseline.[167]

Optimal treatment of proliferative disease before pregnancy reduces the risk of progression during pregnancy. In the 1988 Sunness review, those patients who had scatter laser photocoagulation before pregnancy showed a 26% rate of progression of their proliferative disease and visual loss compared to 58% of patients without prior treatment. Those patients with complete regression of proliferative disease before pregnancy did not demonstrate progression of proliferative disease during pregnancy.[134] Somewhat different results were found in a later study by Reece. In this analysis, half of the patients with proliferative disease who underwent scatter laser photocoagulation prior to pregnancy required additional scatter treatment during pregnancy. In addition, 65% of patients who had proliferative disease during pregnancy required photocoagulation postpartum. No patient had proliferative disease that did not respond to laser photocoagulation.[182]

Proliferative retinopathy may regress near the end of pregnancy or in the postpartum period. One study found that four out of five women who developed proliferative retinopathy during pregnancy had spontaneous regression to nonproliferative status within 2 months postpartum.[159] In contrast, another study of 8 women with proliferative disease reported no spontaneous regression by 3 months postpartum.[167] The possibility of spontaneous regression is a factor to consider when determining if laser photocoagulation is indicated. Most retina specialists would aggressively treat patients who have high-risk proliferative retinopathy; some retinal specialists would treat one eye or both in cases that are not high risk, given the problem of rapid progression during pregnancy. Figure 92.1 shows the right eye of a 29-year-old diabetic woman who was 25 weeks pregnant at the time of her initial presentation. Figure 92.2 shows the same patient 3 months later. After consideration of high-risk factors such as high initial HbA_{1c} and duration of diabetes, these decisions must be made on a case-by-case basis.

Vitreous hemorrhage during labor and delivery has been reported in a few cases.[183] Currently, no evidence justifies performing a cesarean section on the basis of proliferative retinopathy alone, given the availability of vitrectomy for the treatment of nonclearing vitreous hemorrhage.[134]

Diabetic macular edema in pregnancy

Diabetic macular edema that involves or threatens the fovea is currently treated with anti-VEGF injections, with or without focal laser photocoagulation outside the context of pregnancy in order to reduce the risk of moderate vision loss. Patients who develop macular edema during pregnancy frequently have different prognoses than nonpregnant patients. Spontaneous resolution after pregnancy is a common occurrence and is associated with improvement of visual acuity more frequently than in nonpregnant patients.[181]

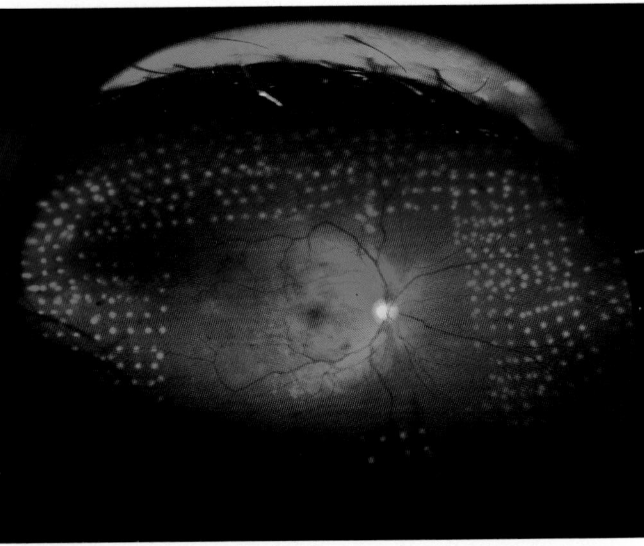

Fig. 92.1 Wide-angle fundus photo shows the right eye of a 29-year-old diabetic woman who was 25 weeks pregnant at the time of her initial presentation. Her fundus exam showed high-risk proliferative diabetic retinopathy in the right eye, and vitreous hemorrhage and tractional retinal detachment involving the fovea in the left eye (not shown). On presentation she had no history of laser in either eye. The image was taken on the day panretinal photocoagulation was initiated in the right eye. She was hospitalized at the time for severe pre-eclampsia, and continued as an inpatient until delivery.

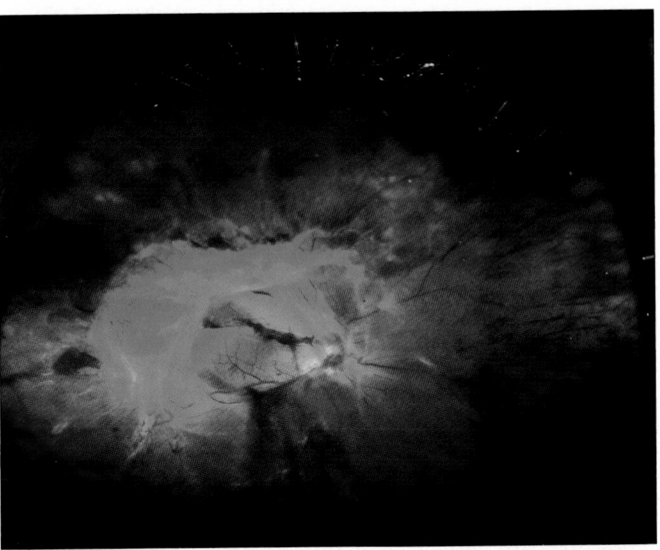

Fig. 92.2 Wide-angle fundus photo of the same patient as Fig. 92.1 showing the right eye 3 months later. She had received additional scatter laser at 29 weeks' gestation, and at 33 weeks' gestation her neovascular tissue appeared to be regressing and no further laser was added. She delivered her baby at 35 weeks' gestation. She presented 3 weeks postpartum with vision loss in the right eye and had progressed to severe traction retinal detachment involving the entire retina despite having had complete laser treatment. Laser scars can be seen on detached retina in the nasal periphery.

Sinclair and Nessler reported that 16 (29%) of 56 eyes of diabetic pregnant women with initial proliferative or nonproliferative retinopathy developed diabetic macular edema during pregnancy. Of these 16 eyes, 14 (88%) had improvement in visual acuity and resolution of macular edema postpartum without laser treatment.[184]

In general, pregnant women with diabetic macular edema should not be treated during pregnancy because of the high rate of spontaneous improvement postpartum. Possible exceptions include cases in which lipid is threatening the fovea or severe progressive macular edema develops early in pregnancy. Due to the lack of adequate safety data regarding the use of anti-VEGF treatments, the authors recommend focal laser photocoagulation in the rare case where treatment during pregnancy is indicated. However, more detailed and systematic study of diabetic macular edema is required to allow scientifically based management recommendations.

Other risk factors for progression of diabetic retinopathy during pregnancy

Nephropathy and systemic hypertension are additional risk factors for the progression of diabetic retinopathy during pregnancy. A well-known association exists between nephropathy and retinopathy in nonpregnant patients. One study in pregnant diabetics showed that 8 of 9 patients in whom macular edema developed during pregnancy had proteinuria of more than 1 g per day.[185] Two studies report elevated systolic blood pressure as a risk factor for the progression of diabetic retinopathy.[167,186] Systolic blood pressure within the normal range but over 115 mmHg has been associated with an increased risk of retinopathy progression among pregnant patients.[172] The DIEP found a 1.3 odds ratio for two-step progression of retinopathy for every 10 mmHg increase in systolic blood pressure.[135]

Diabetic retinopathy and maternal and fetal wellbeing

Advanced diabetic retinopathy has been considered a risk factor for adverse fetal outcomes because it may reflect more widespread systemic disease. Pregnancies associated with nonproliferative diabetic retinopathy may not be at higher risk for adverse fetal outcomes.[187] However, Klein reported an adverse fetal outcome in 43% of 28 women with proliferative retinopathy compared to only 13% of 131 women with nonproliferative retinopathy.[132] Another study of 20 pregnancies of 17 women with proliferative retinopathy reported spontaneous abortion in 2 cases (10%), stillbirth in 1 case (5%), and 3 had major congenital anomalies.[182] Sameshima reported that among 60 pregnant patients with diabetes, the 7 with proliferative retinopathy had a significantly higher incidence of fetal distress.[188] A final study of 26 women with proliferative retinopathy reported serious neonatal morbidity in 19% and mortality in 12%.[189]

One prospective study of 205 women with type-1 diabetes found that low birth weight was associated with retinopathy progression. However, retinopathy progression was not associated with earlier delivery, macrosomia, respiratory distress syndrome, neonatal hypoglycemia, or neonatal death.[190]

Improved medical and obstetrical management has improved the outcome of diabetic pregnancies. In a study of 22 pregnancies complicated by retinopathy and nephropathy in which good glycemic control was present antepartum and throughout pregnancy, there were no infant deaths and only 1 case of mild respiratory distress syndrome.[133] A retrospective study of 482 diabetic pregnancies reported only 3 perinatal deaths, which was statistically equivalent to nonpregnant deliveries over the same period.[191]

Two studies suggest an association between diabetic retinopathy and the development of pre-eclampsia. Hiilesmaa followed 683 consecutive pregnancies with type-1 diabetes and found that retinopathy was a statistically significant independent predictor of pre-eclampsia.[192] A second study looked retrospectively at 65 pregnant type-1 diabetic patients and reported that deterioration of retinopathy occurred more frequently in those with pre-eclampsia (4/8) than those without pre-eclampsia (5/65).[193] Perhaps central retinal artery vasospasm associated with pre-eclampsia exacerbates retinal ischemia.

Toxoplasmic retinochoroiditis

The likelihood of congenital toxoplasmosis occurring in the offspring of a mother with active retinochoroiditis or chorioretinal scars is often a concern. This usually is unfounded, however, since congenital toxoplasmosis in the fetus results only from infection of the mother that occurs during the pregnancy itself. The presence of focal toxoplasmic retinochoroiditis or scars in a patient reflects congenital infection of that patient in essentially all cases and not new infection of the mother.[194]

Therefore the fetus of a woman with active retinochoroiditis or scars should not be at risk for contracting congenital toxoplasmosis. A study of 18 pregnant patients with active toxoplasmosis or scars, some with high stable toxoplasmosis titer, found that no infants developed congenital toxoplasmosis.[195]

A recent retrospective study reported the ocular characteristics of active ocular toxoplasmosis during pregnancy in 9 female patients and compared these attacks with those in the nonpregnant periods. The 9 patients had 10 attacks during pregnancy and 24 attacks while not pregnant. One woman had recurrences during several pregnancies, and in total, 3 female patients had attacks only when pregnant. In general, the severity of the attacks during the pregnant and nonpregnant periods did not differ. They concluded that attacks during pregnancy were not distinctively different in severity, duration, or outcome from the attacks outside pregnancy within their cohort.[196]

Noninfectious uveitis

Uveitis disease activity may be altered during pregnancy and the postpartum period. Rabiah retrospectively evaluated 76 pregnancies of 50 women with noninfectious uveitis. The pregnancies were associated with Vogt–Koyanagi–Harada (VKH) syndrome in 33 women, Behçet disease in 19, and idiopathic uveitis in 24. A worsening of uveitis occurred within the first 4 months of pregnancy in 49/76 (64%) pregnancies and later in pregnancy in 17 (22%). No flare-up occurred in 21 cases (28%). An early pregnancy worsening was typical of VKH and idiopathic uveitis. Postpartum worsening occurred in 38/59 cases (64%) and was characteristic of Behçet disease.[197]

Six patients with preexisting VKH syndrome who improved during pregnancy have been reported.[198–200] All patients had flare-ups of their disease postpartum. Sarcoid uveitis may also improve during pregnancy[200] or develop de novo during the postpartum period.[201] Some authors speculate that elevated endogenous free cortisol levels associated with pregnancy may suppress uveitis.[201,202] However, 2 cases of VKH syndrome arising de novo in the second half of otherwise normal pregnancies have also been reported, with full remission occurring postpartum.[203] The authors have diagnosed two cases of AMPPE during pregnancy, neither of which had atypical features or course of disease. Finally, Rao reported a case of a 28-year-old woman with bilateral macular choroidal neovascularization associated with punctate inner choroidopathy whose pattern of reactivation appeared to follow miscarriage of pregnancy on at least two occasions.[204]

Other retinal disorders

The stress of labor and delivery does not appear to pose a risk for rhegmatogenous retinal detachment in high myopes. This conclusion is based on three studies. The first examined 50 women with high myopia late in pregnancy and again in the first 2 weeks postpartum and reported no postpartum changes.[205] A study of 10 asymptomatic women during 19 pregnancies who gave a history of high myopia, retinal detachment, or retinal holes or lattice degeneration did not develop any new retinal pathology after delivery.[206] The final study examined 42 high myopes and 4 high myopes with previous retinal detachments before and after delivery and documented no progressive retinal changes.[207]

Rapid growth of choroidal hemangiomas has been reported during pregnancy.[208] Another case report described the development of exudative retinal detachments associated with choroidal hemangiomas during pregnancy.[209] The hemangioma may regress postpartum.[210] These changes have been attributed to pregnancy-related hormonal perturbations.

Two previously healthy women developed unilateral endogenous candida endophthalmitis after undergoing surgically induced abortions. One eye underwent vitrectomy and intravitreal amphotericin B injection with a final visual acuity of 20/200. The other eye had a retinal detachment after delayed diagnosis resulting in counting fingers visual acuity.[211]

Retinitis pigmentosa is sometimes characterized by a sudden pregnancy-associated deterioration in visual fields after a period of relative stability. It is difficult to determine whether changes are related to pregnancy or are just coincidental. Five to ten percent of women with retinitis pigmentosa who have been pregnant reported worsening during pregnancy[212,213] and did not return to baseline after delivery.[212] There is one report in the literature of visual field deterioration during pregnancy, which resolved postpartum.[55] One case of pericentral retinal degeneration that worsened during pregnancy has also been reported.[214]

DIAGNOSTIC TESTING AND THERAPY

Fluorescein crosses the placenta and enters the fetal circulation in humans.[215] No reports of teratogenic effects in humans have been reported to the National Registry of Drug-Induced Ocular Side Effects.[134] European investigators have performed research studies involving the administration of fluorescein to 22 pregnant diabetic women and noticed no adverse effects on the fetus.[216] Another study of neonatal outcome of 105 patients who underwent fluorescein angiography (FA) during pregnancy showed no increased rate of adverse neonatal outcomes.[217] This study, however, included only 41 cases of FA during the first trimester, the time when teratogenic effects are more likely to take place and are more severe. Nevertheless, one survey reported that 77% of retinal specialists never perform FA on a patient they know is pregnant.[218] In another survey, 89% of retina specialists who had seen a pregnant woman who required FA withheld testing out of fear of teratogenicity or lawsuit.[219] We recommend that FA in pregnant women can be considered if the results would change the management of a vision-threatening problem and appropriate informed consent is obtained.

Indocyanine green does not cross the placenta, is highly bonded to plasma proteins, and is metabolized by the liver. Reports of only 6 cases of the use of indocyanine green angiography (ICGA) during pregnancy have been published.[220,221] In a survey of 520 retina specialists, 105 had withheld ICGA out of fear of teratogenicity or lawsuit during pregnancy and only 24% thought it was safe to use ICGA in a pregnant patient. The authors suggest that current practice patterns concerning the use of ICGA in pregnancy may be unnecessarily restrictive.[219] Like FA, we recommend that ICGA in pregnant women can be considered if the results would change the management of a vision-threatening problem and appropriate informed consent is obtained.

Photodynamic therapy

Pregnant rats exposed to verteporfin at 40 times the human dose (per kg body weight) have a high incidence of microphthalmia.[222] Accidental exposure to verteporfin for photodynamic therapy during pregnancy has been reported in three cases. Rosen treated a woman with punctate inner choroidopathy with verteporfin and bevacizumab while she was 1–2 weeks pregnant, before the patient knew of her conception. The pregnancy and childbirth were uncomplicated and yielded a healthy term infant who had no abnormality for at least the first 3 months of life.[223] De Santis reported a similar accidental exposure in the third week of pregnancy without any deleterious effects in the patient or child up to 26 months of life.[224] Rodrigues reported a case of accidental exposure to verteporfin in a 45-year-old woman with a 25-week fetus. The pregnancy appeared to be unaffected and the child was healthy, at least through her 16-month follow-up.[225] With regard to PDT during pregnancy, caution is recommended.

Anti-VEGF therapy

Anti-VEGF medications have not been well tested during pregnancy, and at least one report exists describing loss of pregnancy after intravitreal bevacizumab injection.[226] However, an observational case series of four patients treated with bevacizumab in pregnancy for choroidal neovascularization secondary to choroiditis showed different outcomes. Patients received a range of 1–6 injections (mean of 2.6) while pregnant. One patient was treated with five additional injections while breastfeeding. The mean follow-up after the most recent injection was 14 months (range 11–18 months). Visual acuity improved in all patients with a mean of 5.75 lines (range 3–8 lines). All patients delivered healthy full-term infants and had an uneventful prenatal course. All children have remained healthy, exhibiting normal development and growth during infancy.[227] Additional studies with more patients and longer follow-up duration are required to identify any risks associated with anti-VEGF drugs, and until such data become available, caution should be exercised.

CONCLUSION

Information about the effects of pregnancy on the course of retinal disease is limited. In most cases the direct cause of pregnancy effects is only speculative and based on what is known about systemic changes in the mother. As our understanding of the natural course of retinal and choroidal diseases and of the effects of pregnancy on the eye improves, the ophthalmic management of both pregnant and nonpregnant patients will improve.

REFERENCES

1. Dieckmann WJ. The toxemias of pregnancy. 2nd ed. St Louis: Mosby; 1952.
2. Folk JC, Weingeist TA. Fundus changes in toxemia. Ophthalmology 1981;88: 1173–4.
3. Sunness JS, Gass JDM, Singerman U, et al. Retinal and choroidal changes in pregnancy. In: Singerman U, Jampol LM, editors. Retinal and choroidal manifestations of systemic disease. Baltimore: Williams & Wilkins; 1991.
4. Wagener HP. Arterioles of the retina in toxemia of pregnancy. JAMA 1933;101:1380–4.
5. Schreyer P, Tzadok J, Sherman DJ, et al. Fluorescein angiography in hypertensive pregnancies. Int J Gynecol Obstet 1991;34:127–32.
6. Jaffe G, Schatz H. Ocular manifestations of preeclampsia. Am J Ophthalmol 1987;103:309–15.
7. Belfort MA. The effect of magnesium sulphate on blood flow velocity in the maternal retina in mild preeclampsia: a preliminary color flow Doppler study. Br J Obstet Gynaecol 1992;99:641–5.
8. Gupta A, Kaliaperumal S, Setia S, et al. Retinopathy in preeclampsia: association with birth weight and uric acid level. Retina 2008;28:1104–10.
9. Gitter HA, Heuser BP, Sarin LK, et al. Toxemia of pregnancy: an angiographic interpretation of fundus changes. Arch Ophthalmol 1968;80:449–54.
10. Fry WE. Extensive bilateral retinal detachment in eclampsia with complete reattachment. Arch Ophthalmol 1929;1:609–14.
11. Hallum AV. Eye changes in hypertensive toxemia of pregnancy. JAMA 1936; 106:1649–51.
12. Saito Y, Tano Y. Retinal pigment epithelial lesions associated with choroidal ischemia in preeclampsia. Retina 1999;19:262–3.
13. Oliver M, Uchenik D. Bilateral exudative retinal detachment in eclampsia without hypertensive retinopathy. Am J Ophthalmol 1980;90:792–6.
14. Valluri S, Adelberg DA, Curtis RS, et al. Diagnostic indocyanine green in preeclampsia. Am J Ophthalmol 1996;122:672–7.
15. Gass JDM, Pautler SE. Toxemia of pregnancy: pigment epitheliopathy masquerading as a heredomacular dystrophy. Trans Am Ophthalmol Soc 1985;83:114–30.
16. Fry WE. Extensive bilateral retinal detachment in eclampsia with complete reattachment. Arch Ophthalmol 1929;1:609–14.
17. Saito Y, Omoto T, Kidoguchi K, et al. The relationship between ophthalmoscopic changes and classification of toxemia in toxemia of pregnancy. Acta Soc Ophthalmol Jpn 1990;94:870–4.
18. Sadowsky A, Serr DM, Landau J. Retinal changes and fetal prognosis in the toxemias of pregnancy, Obstet Gynecol 1956;8:426–31.
19. Oliver M, Uchenik D. Bilateral exudative retinal detachment in eclampsia without hypertensive retinopathy. Am J Ophthalmol 1980;90:792–6.
20. Bos AM, van Loon AJ, Ameln JG. Serous retinal detachment in preeclampsia. Ned Tijdschr Geneesjd 1999;143:2430–2.
21. Chatwani A, Oyer R, Wong S. Postpartum retinal detachment. J Reprod Med 1989;34:842–4.
22. Bosco JAS. Spontaneous nontraumatic retinal detachments in pregnancy. Am J Obstet Gynecol 1961;82:208–12.
23. Brismar C, Schimmelpfennig W. Bilateral exudative retinal detachment in pregnancy. Acta Ophthalmol 1989;67:699–702.
24. Sanchez JL, Ruiz J, Nanwani K, et al. Retinal detachment in preeclampsia and HELLP syndrome. Arch Soc Esp Oftalmol 2003;78:335–8.
25. Burke JP, Whyte I, MacEwen CJ. Bilateral serous retinal detachments in the HELLP syndrome. Acta Ophthalmol 1989;67:322–4.
26. Karaguzel H, Guven S, Karalezli A, et al. Bilateral serous retinal detachment in a woman with HELLP syndrome and retinal detachment. J Obstet Gynaecol 2009;29:246–8.
27. Mendez-Figueroa H, Davidson C. Bilateral retinal detachments and preeclampsia: thrombotic thrombocytopenic purpura or syndrome of haemolysis, elevated liver enzymes, low platelets? J Matern Fetal Neonatal Med 2010;23:1268–70.
28. Taskapili M, Kocabora S, Gulkilik G. Unusual ocular complications of the HELLP syndrome: persistent macular elevation and localized tractional retinal detachment. Ann Ophthalmol (Skokie) 2007;39:261–3.
29. Yamaguchi K, Fukuuchi Y, Nogawa S, et al. Recovery of decreased local cerebral blood flow detected by the xenon/CT CBF method in a patient with eclampsia. Keio J Med 2000;49:71–4.
30. Neihaus L, Meyer BU, Hoffmann KT. Transient cortical blindness in EHP caused by cerebral vasospasm. Nervenartz 1999;70:931–4.
31. Kesler A, Kaneti H, Kidron D: Transient cortical blindness in preeclampsia with indication of generalized vascular endothelial damage. J Neuroophthalmol 1998;18:163–5.
32. Duncan R, Hadley D, Bone I, et al. Blindness in eclampsia: CT and MRI imaging. J Neurol Neurosurg Psychiatry 1989;52:899–902.
33. Kaplan PW. Reversible hypercalcemic vasoconstriction with seizure and blindness: a paradigm for eclampsia. Clin Electroencephalogr 1998;29:120–3.
34. Branch DW, Andres R, Digre KB, et al. The association of antiphospholipid antibodies with severe preeclampsia. Obstet Gynecol 1989;73:541–5.
35. Do DV, Rismondo V, Nguyen QD. Reversible cortical blindness in preeclampsia. Am J Ophthalmol 2002;134:916–18.
36. Hiruta M, Fukuda H, Hiruta A, et al. Emergency cesarean section in a patient with acute cortical blindness and eclampsia. Masui 2002;51:670–2.
37. Apollon KM, Robinson JN, Schwartz RB, et al. Cortical blindness in severe preeclampsia: CT, MRI, and SPECT findings. Obstet Gynecol 2000;95: 1017–9.
38. Davila M, Pensado A, Rama P, et al. Cortical blindness as symptom of preeclampsia. Rev Esp Anestesiol Reanim 1998;45:189–200.
39. Shieh T, Kosasa TS, Tomai E, et al. Transient blindness in a preeclamptic patient secondary to cerebral edema. Hawaii Med J 1996;55:116–17.
40. Beeson JH, Duda EE. CT scan demonstration of cerebral edema in eclampsia preceded by blindness. Obstet Gynecol 1982;60:529–32.
41. Cunningham FG, Fernandez CO, Hernandez C. Blindness associated with preeclampsia and eclampsia. Am J Obstet Gynecol 1995;172:1291–8.
42. Akan H, Kucac M, Bolat O, et al. The diagnostic value of cranial CT in complicated eclampsia. J Belge Radiol 1993;76:304–6.
43. Drislane FW, Wang AM. Multifocal cerebral hemorrhage in eclampsia and severe preeclampsia. J Neurol 1997;244:194–8.
44. Wijman CA, Beijer IS, van Dijk GW, et al. Hypertensive encephalopathy: does not only occur at high blood pressure. Ned Tijdschr Geneeskd 2002;146: 969–73.
45. Leibowitz HA, Hall PE. Cortical blindness as a complication of eclampsia. Ann Emerg Med 1984;13:365–67.
46. Borromeo CJ, Blike GT, Wiley CW, et al. Cortical blindness in a preeclamptic patient after a cesarean delivery complicated by hypotension. Anesth Analg 2000;91:609–11.
47. Levavi H, Neri A, Zoldan J, et al. Preeclampsia, "HELLP" syndrome and postictal cortical blindness. Acta Obstet Gynecol Scand 1987;66:91–2.
48. Ertan AK, Kujat CH, Jost WH, et al. HELLP syndrome-amausosis in sinus thrombosis with complete recovery. Geburtshilfe Frauenheilkd 1994;54: 646–8.
49. Ebert AD, Hopp HS, Entezami M, et al. Acute onset of blindness during labor: report of a case of transient cortical blindness in association with HELLP syndrome. Eur J Obstet Gynecol Reprod Biol 1999;84:111–3.
50. Crosby ET, Preston R. Obstetrical anesthesia for a parturient with preeclampsia, HELLP syndrome and acute cortical blindness. Can J Anaesth 1998;45: 452–9.
51. Tung CF, Peng YC, Chen Gh, et al. HELLP syndrome with acute cortical blindness. Zhonghua Yi Xue Za Zhi 2001;64:482–5.
52 Erbagci I, Karaca M, Ugur MG, et al. Ophthalmic manifestations of 107 cases with hemolysis, elevated liver enzymes and low platelet count syndrome. Saudi Med J 2008;29:1160–3.
53. Beck RW, Gamel JW, Willcourt RJ, et al. Acute ischemic optic neuropathy in severe preeclampsia. Am J Ophthalmol 1980;90:342–6.
54. Sommerville-Lange LB. A case of permanent blindness due to toxemia of pregnancy. Br J Ophthalmol 1950;34:431–4.
55. Wagener H. Lesions of the optic nerve and retina in pregnancy. JAMA 1934;103:1910–3.
56. Price J, Marouf L, Heine MW. New angiographic findings in toxemia of pregnancy. Ophthalmology 1986;93(Suppl):125.
57. Brancato P, Menchini U, Bandello F. Proliferative retinopathy and toxemia of pregnancy. Ann Ophthalmol 1987;19:182–3.
58. Curi AL, Jacks A, Pevisio C. Choroidal neovascular membrane presenting as a complication of preeclampsia in a patient with antiphospholipid syndrome. Br J Ophthalmol 2000;84:1080.
59. Theodossiadis PG, Kollia AK, Gogas P, et al. Retinal disorders in preeclampsia studied with optical coherence tomography. Am J Ophthalmol 2002;133: 707–9.
60. Shaikh S, Ruby AJ, Piotrowski M. Preeclampsia related chorioretinopathy with Purtscher's-like findings and macular ischemia. Retina 2003;23:247–50.
61. Menchini U, Lanzetta P, Virgili G, et al. Retinal pigment epithelium tear following toxemia of pregnancy. Eur J Ophthalmol 1995;5:139–41.
62. Leff SR, Yarian DR, Masciulli, et al. Vitreous hemorrhage as a complication of HELLP syndrome. Br J Ophthalmol 1990;74:498.
63. Todd KC, Hainsworth DP, Lee LR, et al. Longitudinal analysis of central serous chorioretinopathy and sex. Can J Ophthalmol 2002;37:405–8.
64. Normalina M, Zainal M, Alias D. Central serous choroidopathy in pregnancy. Med J Malaysia 1998;53:439–41.
65. Khairallah M, Nouira F, Gharsallah R, et al. Central serous chorioretinopathy in a pregnant woman. J Fr Ophtalmol 1996;19:216–21.
66. Quillen DA, Gass DM, Brod RD, et al. Central serous chorioretinopathy in women. Ophthalmology 1996;103:72–9.
67. Sunness JS, Haller JA, Fine SL. Central serous chorioretinopathy and pregnancy. Arch Ophthalmol 1993;111:360–4.
68. Gass JD. Central serous chorioretinopathy and white subretinal exudation in pregnancy. Arch Ophthalmol 1991;109:677–81.
69. Fastenberg DM, Ober RR. Central serous choroidopathy in pregnancy, Arch Ophthalmol 1983;101:1055–8.
70. Chumbley LC, Frank RN. Central serous retinopathy and pregnancy. Am J Ophthalmol 1974;77:158–60.
71. Cruysberg JR, Deutman AF. Visual disturbances during pregnancy caused by central serous choroidopathy. Br J Ophthalmol 66:240–1,1982.
72. Bedrossian RH. Central serous retinopathy and pregnancy. Am J Ophthalmol 1974;78:152.
73 Al-Mujaini A, Wali U, Ganesh A, et al. Natural course of central serous chorioretinopathy without subretinal exudates in normal pregnancy. Can J Ophthalmol 2008;43:588–90.
74. Cunningham GF, MacDonald PC, Grant NF. Williams obstetrics. 19th ed. Norwalk, CT: Appleton & Lange; 1993. p. 224–5.
75. Wiebers DO. Ischemic cerebrovascular complications of pregnancy. Arch Neurol 1985;42:1106–13.
76. Ayaki M, Yokoyama N, Furukawa Y. Postpartum CRAO simulating Purtscher's retinopathy. Ophthalmologica 1995;209:37–9.
77. LaMonica CB, Foye GJ, Silberman L. A case of sudden CRAO and blindness in pregnancy. Obstet Gynecol 1987;69:433–5.

78. Lara-Torre E, Lee MS, Wolf MA, et al. Bilateral retinal occlusion progressing to longlasting blindness in severe preeclampsia. Obstet Gynecol 2002;100:940–2.
79. Gull S, Prentice A. BRAO in pregnancy. Br J Obstet Gynaecol 1994;101:77–8.
80. Humayun M, Kattah J, Cupps TR, et al. Papillophlebitis and arteriolar occlusion in a pregnant woman. J Clin Neuroophthalmol 1992;12:226–9.
81. Basu A, Eyong E. Cilioretinal arterial occlusion phenomenon: a rare cause of loss of vision in pregnancy. Eur J Obstet Gynecol Reprod Biol 2008;137: 251–2.
82. Blodi BA, Johnson MW, Gass JD, et al. Purtscher's-like retinopathy after childbirth. Ophthalmology 1990;97:1654–9.
83. Vela JI, Diaz-Cascajosa J, Crespi J, et al. Protein S deficiency and retinal arteriolar occlusion in pregnancy. Eur J Ophthalmol 2007;17:1004–6.
84. Lanzetta P, Crovato S, Pirrachio A, et al. Retinal arteriolar obstruction with progestin treatment of threatened abortion. Acta Ophthalmol Scand 2002; 80:667–9.
85. Nelson ME, Talbot JF, Preston FE. Recurrent multiple branch retinal arteriolar occlusions in a patient with protein C deficiency. Graefes Arch Clin Exp Ophthalmol 1989;227:443–7.
86. Greven CM, Weaver RG, Owen J, et al. Protein S deficiency and bilateral branch retinal artery occlusion. Ophthalmology 1991;98:33–4.
87. Bergh PA, Hollander D, Gregori CA, et al. Mitral valve prolapse and thromboembolic disease in pregnancy: a case report. Int J Gynaecol Obstet 1988;27: 133–7.
88. Kim IT, Choi JB. Occlusions of branch retinal arterioles following amniotic fluid embolism. Ophthalmologica 2002;21:305–8.
89. Brown GC, Magargal LE, Shields JA. Retinal arterial obstruction in children and young adults. Ophthalmology 1981;88:18–25.
90. Chung YR, Kim JB, Lee K, et al. Retinal artery occlusion in a healthy pregnant patient (unilateral BRAO). Korean J Ophthalmol 2008;22:70–1.
91. Chew EY, Trope GE, Mitchell BJ. Diurnal intraocular pressure in young adults with central retinal vein occlusion. Ophthalmology 1987;94:1545–9.
92. Gabsi S, Rekik R, Gritli N, et al. Occlusion of the central retinal vein in a 6-month pregnant woman. J Fr Ophtalmol 1994;17:350–4.
93. Gonzalvo FJ, Abecia E, Pinilla I, et al. Central retinal vein occlusion and HELLP syndrome. Acta Ophthalmol Scand 2000;78:596–8.
94. Rahman I, Saleemi G, Semple D, et al. Pre-eclampsia resulting in central retinal vein occlusion. Eye (Lond) 2006;20:955–7.
95. Bjerknes T, Askvik J, Albrechtsen S, et al. Retinal detachment in association with preeclampsia and abruptio placentae. Eur J Obstet Gynecol Reprod Biol 1995;60:91–3.
96. Cogan DG. Fibrin clots in the choriocapillaris and serous detachment of the retina. Ophthalmologica 1976;172:298–307.
97. Martin VA. Disseminated intravascular coagulopathy. Trans Ophthalmol Soc UK 1978;98:506–7.
98. Hoines J, Buettner H. Ocular complications of disseminated intravascular coagulation (DIC) in abruptio placentae. Retina 1989;9:105–9.
99. Patel N, Riordan-Eva P, Chong V. Persistent visual loss after retinochoroidal infarction in pregnancy-induced hypertension and disseminated intravascular coagulation. J Neuroophthalmol 2005;25:128–3.
100. Benson DO, Fitzgibbons JF, Goodnight SH. The visual system in thrombotic thrombocytopenic purpura. Ann Ophthalmol 1980;12:413–7.
101. Larcan A, Lambert H, Laprevote-Heully MC, et al. Acute choriocapillaris occlusions in pregnancy and puerperium. J Mal Vasc 1985;10:213–19.
102. Coscas G, Gaudric A, Dhermy P, et al. Choriocapillaris occlusion in Moschowitz's disease. J Fr Ophtalmol 1981;4:101–11.
103. Sperry K. Amniotic fluid embolism. JAMA 1986;255:2183–203.
104. Chang M, Herbert WN. Retinal arteriolar occlusions following amniotic fluid embolism. Ophthalmology 1984;91:1634–7.
105. Kim IT, Choi JB. Occlusions of branch retinal arterioles following amniotic fluid embolisms. Ophthalmologica 2000;214:305–8.
106. Fischbein FI. Ischemic retinopathy following amniotic fluid embolization. Am J Ophthalmol 1969;67:351–7.
107. Cunningham GF, MacDonald PC, Grant NF. Williams obstetrics. 19th ed. Norwalk, CT: Appleton & Lange; 1993. p. 215.
108. Holly EA, Aston DA, Ahn DK, et al. Uveal melanoma, hormonal and reproductive factors in women. Cancer Res 1991;51:1370–2.
109. Reese AB. Tumors of the eye. 2nd ed. New York: Hoeber Medical Division, Harper & Row; 1963. p. 366–70.
110. Borner R, Goder G. Melanoblastoma der uvea and schwangerschaft. Klin Monatsbl Augenheilkd 1966;149:684.
111. Frenkel M, Klein HZ. Malignant melanoma of the choroids in pregnancy. Am J Ophthalmol 1966;62:910.
112. Pack GT, Scharnagel IM. The prognosis for malignant melanoma in the pregnant woman. Cancer 1951;4:324.
113. Seddon JM, MacLaughlin DT, Albert DM, et al. Uveal melanomas presenting during pregnancy and the investigation of oestrogen receptors in melanomas. Br J Ophthalmol 1982;66:695.
114. Siegel R, Amslie WH. Malignant ocular melanoma during pregnancy. JAMA 1963;185:542.
115 Lee CS, Yang WI, Shin KJ, et al. Rapid growth of choroidal melanoma during pregnancy. Acta Ophthalmol 2011;89(3):e290–1.
116. Foss AJ, Alexander RA, Guille MJ, et al. Estrogen and progesterone receptor analysis in ocular melanomas. Ophthalmology 1995;102:431–5.
117. Behrens T, Kaerlev L, Cree I, et al. Hormonal exposures and the risk of uveal melanoma. Cancer Causes Control 2010;21:1625–34.
118. Shields CL, Shields JA, Eagle RC, et al. Uveal melamona and pregnancy. A report of 16 cases. Ophthalmology 1991;98:1667–73.
119. Romanowska-Dixon B. Melanoma of choroids during pregnancy:case report. Klin Oczna 2002;104:395–7.
120. Egan KM, Quinn JL, Gragoudas ES. Childbearing history associated with improved survival in choroidal melanoma. Arch Ophthalmol 1999;117:939–42.
121. Egan KM, Walsh SM, Seddon JM, et al. An evaluation of reproductive factors on the risk of metastases from uveal melanoma. Ophthalmology 1993;100: 1160–6.
122. Gass JD. Stereoscopic atlas of macular diseases: a funduscopic and angiographic presentation. 4th ed. St Louis: Mosby; 1997. p. 218–19.
123. Gass JD. Stereoscopic atlas of macular diseases: a funduscopic and angiographic presentation. 4th ed. St Louis: Mosby; 1997. p. 693–5.
124. Gass JDM. Stereoscopic atlas of macular diseases: a funduscopic and angiographic presentation. 3rd ed. St Louis: Mosby; 1987. p. 512–3.
125. Gass JD. Stereoscopic atlas of macular diseases: a funduscopic and angiographic presentation. 4th ed. St Louis: Mosby; 1997. p. 752–4.
126. Gass JDM. Stereoscopic atlas of macular diseases: a funduscopic and angiographic presentation. 3rd ed. St Louis: Mosby; 1987. p. 380–3.
127. Oday MP, Nielsen P, Al Bozom I. Orbital rhabdomyosarcoma metastatic to the placenta. Am J Obstet Gynecol 1994;171:1382–3.
128. Marsh RW, Chu NM. Placental metastasis from primary ocular melanoma: a case report. Am J Obstet Gynecol 1996;174:1654–5.
129. Bendon RW, Mimouni F, Khouri J, et al. Histopathology of spontaneous abortion in diabetic pregnancies. Am J Perinatol 1990;7:207–10.
130. Mills J, Simpson JL, Driscoll SG, et al. Incidence of spontaneous abortion among normal women and insulin-dependent diabetic women whose pregnancies were identified within 21 days of conception. N Engl J Med 1988;319:1617–23.
131. Miller E, Hare JW, Cloherty JP, et al. Elevated maternal hemoglobin A1c in early pregnancy and major congenital anomalies in infants of diabetic mothers. N Engl J Med 1981;304:1331–4.
132. Klein BK, Klein RK, Meuer SM, et al. Does the severity of diabetic retinopathy predict pregnancy outcome? Diabetic Compl 1988;2:179.
133. Jovanovic R, Jovanovic L. Obstetric management when normoglycemia is maintained in diabetic pregnant women with vascular compromise. Am J Obstet Gynecol 1984;149:617–23.
134. Sunness JS. The pregnant woman's eye. Surv Ophthalmol 1988;32:219–38.
135. Diabetes in Early Pregnancy Study Group, Chew EY, James LM, Metzger BE. Metabolic control and progression of retinopathy. Diabetes Care 18:631–7, 1995.
136. Laatikainen L, Teramo K, Hieta-Heikurainen H, et al. A controlled study of the influence of continuous subcutaneous insulin infusion treatment on diabetic retinopathy during pregnancy. Acta Med Scand 1987;221:367–76.
137. The Diabetes Control and Complications Trial Research Group. The effect of intensive diabetes treatment on the progression of diabetic retinopathy in insulin-dependent diabetes mellitus. Arch Ophthalmol 1995;113:36.
138. Chang S, Fuhrmann M, and the Diabetes in Early Pregnancy Study Group. Pregnancy, retinopathy, normoglycemia: a preliminary analysis. Diabetes 1985;34(suppl):39.
139. KROC Collaborative Study Group. Blood glucose control and the evaluation of diabetic retinopathy and albuminuria. N Engl J Med 1984;311:365.
140. Kentucky Diabetic Retinopathy Group. Guidelines for eye care in patients with diabetes mellitus. Arch Intern Med 1989;149:769–70.
141. Cunningham GF, MacDonald PC, Grant NF. Williams obstetrics. 19th ed. Norwalk, CT: Appleton & Lange; 1993. p. 763–807.
142. Chen HC, Newsom RSB, Patel V. Retinal blood flow changes during pregnancy in women with diabetes. Invest Ophthalmol Vis Sci 1994;35:3199–208.
143. Loukovaara S, Kaaja R, Immonen I. Macular capillary blood flow velocity by blue-field entoptoscopy in diabetic and healthy women during pregnancy and the postpartum period. Greafes Arch Clin Exp Ophthalmol 2002;240:977–82.
144. Loukovaara S, Harju M, Kaaja R, et al. Retinal capillary blood flow in diabetic and nondiabetic women during pregnancy and postpartum period. Invest Ophthalmol Vis Sci 2003;44:1486–91.
145. Hellstedt T, Kaaja R, Teramo K, et al. Macular blood flow during pregnancy in patients with early diabetic retinopathy measured by blue-field entoptic stimulation. Graefes Arch Clin Exp Ophthalmol 1996;234:659–63.
146. Schocket LS, Grunwald JE, Tsang AF, et al. The effect of pregnancy on retinal hemodynamics in diabetic versus nondiabetic mothers. Am J Ophthalmol 1999;128:477–84.
147. Lauszus FF, Klebe JG, Bek T, et al. Increased serum IGF-1 during pregnancy is associated with progression of diabetic retinopathy. Diabetes 2002;52: 852–6.
148. Gibson JM, Westwood M, Lauszus FF, et al. Phosphorylated insulin-like growth factor binding protein 1 is increased in pregnant diabetic subjects. Diabetes 1999;48:321–6.
149. Khaliq A, Foreman D, Ahmed A, et al. Increased expression of placenta growth factor in proliferative diabetic retinopathy. Lab Invest 1998;78:109–16.
150. Spirin KS, Saghizadeh M, Lewin SL, et al. Basement membrane and growth factor gene expression in normal and diabetic human retinas. Curr Eye Res 1999;18:490–9.
151. Best RM, Hayes R, Hadden DR, et al. Plasma levels of endothelin-1 in diabetic retinopathy in pregnancy. Eye 1999;13:179–82.
152. Hill DJ, Flyvbjerg A, Arany E, et al. Increased levels of serum fibroblast growth factor-2 in diabetic pregnant women with retinopathy. J Clin Endocrinol Metab 1997;82:1452–7.
153. Castellon R, Hamdi HK, Sacerio I, et al. Effects of angiogenic growth factor combinations on retinal endothelial cells. Exp Eye Res 2002;74:523–35.

154. Diabetes Control and Complications Trial Research Group. Effect of pregnancy on microvascular complications in the diabetes control and complications trial. Diabetes Care 2000;24:1084–91.
155. Soubrane G, Canivet J, Coscas G. Influence of pregnancy on the evolution of background retinopathy: preliminary results of a prospective fluorescein angiography study. In: Ryan JJ, Dawson AK, Little HL, editors. Retinal diseases. New York: Grune & Stratton; 1985. p. 15–20.
156. Ayed S, Jeddi A, Dagfous F, et al. Aspects evolutifs de la retinopathie diabetique pendant la grosse. J Fr Ophtalmol 1992;15:474.
157. Moloney JM, Drury MI. The effect of pregnancy on the natural course of diabetic retinopathy. Am J Ophthalmol 1982;93:745.
158. Klein BK, Mosse SE, Klein R. Effect of pregnancy on progression of diabetic retinopathy. Diabetes Care 1990;13:34.
159. Serup L. Influence of pregnancy on diabetic retinopathy. Acta Endocrinol 1986;277:122.
160. Kaaja R, Sjoberg L, Hellsted T, et al. Long-term effects of pregnancy on diabetic complications. Diabet Med 1996;13:165–9.
161. Hemachandra A, Ellis D, Lloyd CE, et al. The influence of pregnancy on IDDM complications. Diabetes Care 1995;18:950–4.
162. Klein BK, Klein R. Gravity and diabetic retinopathy. Am J Epidemiol 1984;119:564.
163. Lipman MJ, Kranias G, Bene CH, et al. The effect of multiple pregnancies on diabetic retinopathy. Ophthalmology 1993;100:141.
164. Chaturvedi N, Stephenson JM, Fuller JH. The relationship between pregnancy and long-term maternal complications in the EURODIAB IDDM complications study. Diabetic Med 1995;18:950–4.
165. Aiello LM, Rand LI, Briones JC, et al. Nonocular clinical risk factors in the progression of diabetic retinopathy. In: Little HL, Jack RL, Patz A, et al, editors. Diabetic retinopathy. New York: Thieme-Stratton; 1983. p. 21–32.
166. Dibble CM, Kochenour NK, Wocley RJ, et al. Effect of pregnancy on diabetic retinopathy. Obstet Gynecol 1982;59:699.
167. Rosenn B, Miodovnik M, Kranias G, et al. Progression of diabetic retinopathy in pregnancy: association with hypertension. Am J Obstet Gynecol 1992;166: 1214.
168. Beetham WP. Diabetic retinopathy in pregnancy. Trans Am Ophthalmol Soc. 1950;48:205.
169. Temple RC, Aldridge VA, Sampson MJ, et al. Impact of pregnancy on the progression of diabetic retinopathy in type 1 diabetes. Diabet Med 2001;18: 573–7.
170. Lauszus F, Klebe JG, Bek T. Diabetic retinopathy in pregnancy during tight metabolic control. Acta Obstet Gynecol Scand 2000;79:367–70.
171. Early Treatment Diabetic Retinopathy Study Research Group. Fundus photographic risk factors for the progression of diabetic retinopathy. Ophthalmology 1991;98:823.
172. Berk MA, Miodovnik M, Mimouni F. Impact of pregnancy on complications of insulin-dependent diabetes mellitus. Am J Perinatol 1988;5:359.
173. Axer-Sieger R, Hod M, Fink-Cohen S, et al. Diabetic retinopathy during pregnancy. Ophthalmology 1996;103:1815.
174. Lapolla A, Cardone C, Negrin P, et al. Pregnancy does not induce or worsen retinal and peripheral nerve dysfunction in insulin-dependent diabetic women. J Diabetes Complications 1998;12:74–80.
175. Horvat M, MacLean H, Goldberg L, et al. Diabetic retinopathy in pregnancy: a 12-year prospective study. Br J Ophthalmol 1980;64:398.
176. Boone MI, Farber ME, Jovanovic-Peterson L, et al. Increased retinal vascular tortuosity in gestational diabetes mellitus. Ophthalmology 1989;96:251.
177. Hagay Z, Schachter M, Pollack A, et al. Development of proliferative retinopathy in a gestational diabetes patient following rapid metabolic control. Eur J Obstet Gynecol Reprod Biol 1994;57:211.
178. Puza SW, Malee MP. Utilization of routine ophthalmologic examinations in pregnant diabetic patients. J Matern Fetal Med 1996;5:7–10.
179. Hellstedt T, Kaaja R, Teramo L, et al. The effect of pregnancy on mild diabetic retinopathy. Graefes Arch Clin Exp Ophthalmol 1997;235:437–41.
180. Diabetic Retinopathy Study Research Group. Four risk factors for severe visual loss in diabetic retinopathy. Arch Ophthalmol 1979;97:654–5.
181. Stoessel KM, Liao PM, Thompson JT, et al. Diabetic retinopathy and macular edema in pregnancy. Ophthalmology 1991;98:146.
182. Reece E, Lockwood C, Tuck S, et al. Retinal and pregnancy outcomes in the presence of diabetic proliferative retinopathy. J Reprod Med 1994;39:799.
183. Kitzmiller JL, Aiello LM, Kaldany LM, et al. Diabetic vascular disease complicating pregnancy. Clin Obstet Gynecol 1981;24:107.
184. Sinclair SH, Nessler C, Foxman B, et al. Macular edema and pregnancy in insulin-dependent diabetes. Am J Ophthalmol 1984;97:154.
185. Chang S, Fuhrmann M, Jovanovic L, et al. Pregnancy, retinopathy, normoglycemia: a preliminary analysis. Diabetes 1985;34:39A.
186. Teuscher A, Schnell H, Wilson PWF. Incidence of diabetic retinopathy and relationship to baseline plasma glucose and blood pressure. Diabetes Care 1988;11:246–51.
187. Rodman HM, Singerman LJ, Aiello LM, et al. Diabetic retinopathy and its relationship to pregnancy. In: Merkatz IR, Adams PJ, editors. The diabetic pregnancy: a perinatal perspective. New York: Grune & Stratton; 1979. p. 73–91.
188. Sameshima H, Kai M, Kajiya S, et al. Retinopathy and perinatal outcome in diabetic pregnancy. Nippon Sanka Fujinka Gakkai Zasshi 1995;47:1048–54.
189. Lauszus FF, Gron PL, Klebe JG. Pregnancies complicated by diabetic proliferative retinopathy. Acta Obstet Gynecol Scand 1998;77:814–8.
190. McElvy SS, Demarini S, Miodovnik M, et al. Fetal weight and progression of diabetic retinopathy. Obstet Gynecol 2001;97:587–92.
191. Zhu L, Nakabayashi M, Takeda Y. Statistical analysis of perinatal outcomes in pregnancy complicated with diabetes mellitus. J Obstet Gynaecol Res 1997;23:555–63.
192. Hiilesmaa V, Suhonen L, Teramo K. Glycaemic control is associated with preeclampsia but not with pregnancy-induced hypertension in women with type 1 diabetes mellitus. Diabetologia 2000;43:1534–9.
193. Lovestam-Adrian M, Agardh CD, Aberg A, et al. Preeclampsia is a potent risk factor for deterioration of retinopathy during pregnancy in type 1 diabetic patients. Diabet Med 1997;14:1059–65.
194. Perkins ES. Ocular toxoplasmosis. Br J Ophthalmol 1973;57:1–17.
195. Oniki S. Prognosis of pregnancy in patients with toxoplasmic retinochoroiditis. Jpn J Ophthalmol 1983;27:166–74.
196. Braakenburg AM, Rothova A. Clinical features of ocular toxoplasmosis during pregnancy. Retina 2009;29:627–30.
197. Rabiah PK, Vitale AT. Noninfectious uveitis and pregnancy. Am J Ophthalmol 2003;136:91–8.
198. Snyder DA, Tessler HH. Vogt–Koyanagi–Harada syndrome. Am J Ophthalmol 1980;90:69–75.
199. Steahly LP. Vogt–Koyanagi–Harada syndrome and pregnancy. Am J Ophthalmol 1990;22:59–62.
200. Taguchi C, Ikeda E, Hikita N, et al. A report of two cases suggesting positive influence of pregnancy on uveitis activity. Nippon Ganka Gakkai Zasshi 1999;103:66–71.
201. Hyman BN. Postpartum uveitis. Ann Ophthalmol 1976;8:677–80.
202. Scott JS. Immunological diseases and pregnancy. Br Med J 1966;1:1559–67.
203. Friedman Z, Granat M, Neumann E. The syndrome of Vogt–Koyanagi–Harada and pregnancy. Metab Pediatr Ophthalmol 1980;4:147–9.
204. Rao VG, Rao GS, Narkhede NS. Flare up of choroiditis and choroidal neovasculazation associated with punctate inner choroidopathy during early pregnancy. Indian J Ophthalmol 2011;59:145–8.
205. Neri A, Grausbord R, Kremer I, et al. The management of labor in high myopic patients. Eur J Obstet Gynecol Reprod Biol 1985;19:277–9.
206. Landau D, Seelenfreund MH, Tadmor O, et al. The effect of normal childbirth on eyes with abnormalities predisposing to rhegmatogenous retinal detachment. Graefes Arch Clin Exp Ophthalmol 1995;233:598–600.
207. Prost M. Severe myopia and delivery. Klin Oczna 1996;98:129–30.
208. Reese AB. Tumors of the eye. 2nd ed. New York: Hoeber Medical Division, Harper & Row; 1963. p. 366–70.
209. Cohen VM, Rundle PA, Rennie IG. Choroidal hemangiomas with exudative retinal detachments during pregnancy. Arch Ophthalmol 2002;120:862–4.
210. Pitta C, Bergen R, Littwin S. Spontaneous regression of a choroidal hemangioma following pregnancy. Ann Ophthalmol 1979;11:772–4.
211. Chen SJ, Chung YM, Liu JH. Endogenous Candida endophthalmitis after induced abortion. Am J Ophthalmol 1998;125:873–5.
212. Sunness JS. The pregnant woman's eye. Surv Ophthalmol 1988;32:219–38.
213. Yoser SL, Heckenlively JR, Friedman L, et al. Evaluation of clinical findings and common symptoms in retinitis pigmentosa. Invest Ophthalmol Vis Sci 1987;28(Suppl):112.
214. Hayaska S, Ugomori S, Kanamori M, et al. Pericentral retinal degeneration deteriorates during pregnancies. Ophthalmologica 1990;200:72–6.
215. Samples JR, Meyer SM. Use of ophthalmic medications in pregnant and nursing women. Am J Ophthalmol 1988;106:616–23.
216. Soubrane G, Canivet J, Coscas G. Influence of pregnancy on the evolution of background retinopathy: preliminary results of a prospective fluorescein angiography study. In: Ryan SJ, Dawson AK, Little HL, editors. Retinal diseases. New York: Grune & Stratton; 1985.
217. Greenberg F, Lewis RA. Safety of fluorescein angiography during pregnancy. Am J Ophthalmol 110:323–4, 1990 (letter).
218. Halperin LS, Olk RJ, Soubrane G, et al. Safety of fluorescein angiography during pregnancy. Am J Ophthalmol 1990;109:563–6.
219. Fineman MS, Maguire JI, Fineman SW, et al. Safety of indocyanine green angiography during pregnancy: a survey of the retina, vitreous, and macula societies. Arch Ophthalmol 2001;119:353–5.
220. Valluri S, Adelberg DA, Curtis RS, et al. Diagnostic indocyanine green angiography in preeclampsia. Am J Ophthalmol 1996;122:672–7.
221. Iida T, Hagimura N, Otani T, et al. Choroidal vascular lesions in serous retinal detachment viewed with indocyanine green angiography. Nippon Ganka Gakkai Zasshi 1996;100:817–24.
222. US Food and Drug Administration. Visudyne(tm) (verteporfin for injection). [Internet] 2008 [cited 2012 27 Feb]. Available from: www.accessdata.fda.gov/drugsatfda_docs/label/2008/021119s013lbl.pdf.
223. Rosen E, Rubowitz A, Ferencz JR. Exposure to verteporfin and bevacizumab therapy for choroidal neovascularization secondary to punctate inner choroidopathy during pregnancy. Eye (Lond) 2009;23:1479.
224. De Santis M, Carducci B, De Santis L, et al. First case of post-conception Verteporfin exposure: pregnancy and neonatal outcome. Acta Ophthalmol Scand 2004;82:623–4.
225. Rodrigues M, Meira D, Batista S, et al. Accidental pregnancy exposure to verteporfin: obstetrical and neonatal outcomes: a case report. Aust N Z J Obstet Gynaecol 2009;49:236–7.
226. Petrou P, Georgalas I, Giavaras G, et al. Early loss of pregnancy after intravitreal bevacizumab injection. Acta Ophthalmol 2010;88(4):e136.
227. Tarantola RM, Folk JC, Boldt HC, et al. Intravitreal bevacizumab during pregnancy. Retina 2010;30:1405–11.

Optic Disc Anomalies, Pits, and Associated Serous Macular Detachment

Chapter 93

Alfredo A. Sadun, Khizer R. Khaderi

Optic disc pits are congenital excavations of the optic nerve head, usually seen in association with other abnormalities of the optic nerve and peripapillary retina, including large optic nerve head size, large inferior colobomas of the optic disc, and retinal colobomas. These associations gave rise to the hypothesis that optic disc pits develop as a result of incomplete closure of the superior end of the embryonic fissure. Additionally, optic disc pits have been associated with posterior vitreous detachments and, in about half of all cases, with serous retinal detachment. The prevailing theory is that the associated subretinal (and probably intraretinal) fluid derives from liquefied vitreous that passes through the opening created by the optic disc pit.

OPTIC DISC ANOMALIES

A variety of congenital optic disc anomalies challenge the clinical acumen of ophthalmologists, internists, and pediatricians. Since some of these abnormalities are known by various names, it is worthwhile reviewing the general categories.

Megalopapilla

Megalopapilla is a rare anomaly of the optic disc, involving thinning of the nerve fiber across a large optic nerve head, and is often associated with large refractive errors and with midline congenital deformities.[1]

Aplasia

Aplasia of the optic nerve head is extremely rare, and probably represents an extreme form of optic nerve head hypoplasia, and may be associated with the absence or gross maldevelopment of the globe.[1]

Hypoplasia

Optic disc hypoplasia is a congenital underdevelopment of the optic nerve head with a reduced number of axons. Hypoplastic optic discs are often underdiagnosed and may vary in level of development, leading to variable levels of visual acuity and visual field defects.[2]

Cavities in the optic nerve head

Excavated and colobomatous defects of the optic nerve head encompass a spectrum of abnormalities, including tilted discs, peripapillary staphyloma, morning-glory disc anomaly, colobomas, and congenital optic disc pits. Optic disc pits were regarded as atypical colobomas by Grear,[3] who reviewed the subject in 1942.

Optic disc pits should probably be considered one manifestation along a spectrum of cavitary optic disc anomalies. Slusher and coworkers[4] described a family of 35 members spanning five generations with an autosomal dominant pattern of congenital optic disc abnormalities. Remarkably, a myriad of morphologic variations of phenotype were expressed, including optic disc pits, morning-glory syndrome, and coloboma of the optic nerve. One gene defect can result in a variety of optic disc abnormalities; therefore the traditional classification schemes that describe varieties of cavitary optic disc anomalies should be reconsidered.

ANATOMY

A brief review of the anatomy and embryology of the optic nerve head permits a better understanding of these abnormalities.

The retinal ganglion cells of each retina contribute approximately 1.2 million unmyelinated axons that converge at a point approximately 4 mm nasal to the foveola, through which they exit the globe, acquire a myelin sheath, and form the optic nerve. These axons project to various primary visual nuclei in the brain,[5] constitute a fiber tract rather than a nerve, and, as such, have histologic and functional similarities to brain tissue. The optic nerve is enclosed by three meningeal sheaths that are contiguous with the meningeal coverings of the brain. Before exiting the eye, however, the axons of the retinal ganglion cells must converge centripetally, make a sharp turn, traverse the lamina cribrosa, form nerve bundles enclosed by connective tissue septa, and then, once posterior to the lamina cribrosa, become ensheathed by myelin (Fig. 93.1).[6]

Thus, the optic nerve head is remarkable in several respects. Axons deriving from the retina become part of the nerve, go from an unmyelinated to a myelinated state, traverse the sieve-like lamina cribrosa, are partitioned into groups by glial columns, and go from an area of high (intraocular) pressure to relatively low interstitial pressure. Not surprisingly, anomalies of structure at this critical juncture often lead to marked physiologic consequences.[7]

OPTIC DISC PITS

In 1882, Wiethe[8] described abnormalities in both optic discs of a 62-year-old woman. His description of dark-gray depressions in the optic nerve heads was probably the first report of optic disc pits. Since Wiethe's initial description, excavations of the optic nerve head have variously been described as craters, holes, cavities, and, most recently, congenital pits of the optic nerve head.

Studies suggest that optic pits occur in approximately 1 in 10 000 eyes, although there is considerable variance among studies.[3,9] Men and women are equally affected. Approximately 10–15% of optic disc pits are bilateral. Most optic disc pits are nonfamilial; however there are a few reports with an autosomal dominant pattern of inheritance.[10] One such report describes a family for which several members had small iris colobomas, some in combination with the pit, providing insight as to the etiology.[11] About 70% of the pits are on the temporal side of the disc, and about 20% are situated centrally; the remainder are found inferiorly, superiorly, and nasally.[12]

Serous retinal detachments can be associated with optic disc pits. These may occur at any age but are most frequent in early adulthood. However, there have been reports of associated retinal detachment occurring as early as 6 years of age and in patients as old as in the ninth decade of life.[12] Some have suggested that the clinical course differs and leads to better visual acuity in children as spontaneous resolution is the rule.[13,14] Through the analysis of stereoscopic transparencies, it has been proposed that the fluid that enters through the optic disc pit actually travels between the inner and outer layers of the retina to produce a retinal schisis.[15,16] Optical coherence tomography (OCT) has shown such inner retinal schises preceding outer-layer detachment.[17] Following this, detachment of the outer retinal layer may occur as a secondary process.[17] Although no histopathologic studies have confirmed this, the application of OCT has provided compelling evidence for at least two levels of retinal separation (Fig. 93.2).[18] OCT has also been used to demonstrate a marked reduction in thickness of the retinal nerve fiber layer in the quadrant corresponding to the optic nerve pit.[19]

In the series of Brown et al.,[12] most optic disc pits were gray in color, although they varied from yellow to black. Their size can range from minute to large, occupying most of the surface of the optic disc.

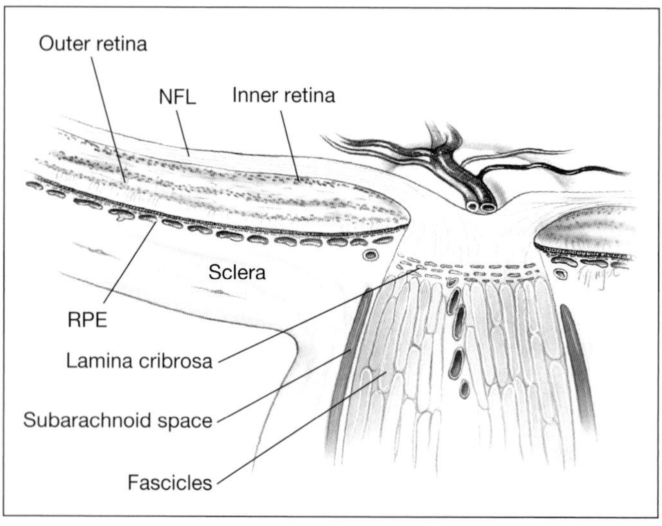

Fig. 93.1 Axial view of optic nerve head and surrounding tissues. Fibers from the retina collect at the optic disc, pass down through the lamina cribrosa, become myelinated, and form fascicles. Note the three parts of the optic nerve: I, anterior portion (retinal); II, midportion (prelaminar or choroidal); III, posterior portion (lamina cribrosa or scleral) at optic nerve head. NFL, nerve fiber layer; RPE, retinal pigment epithelium.

Visual defects

The optic disc pit is most often associated with two types of visual field defect.[20] The first type is typified by arcuate scotomas that probably reflect the absence of the wedge of nerve fibers displaced by the optic disc pit. Larger pits may be associated with large Bjerrum-type scotomas or even altitudinal visual field defects. Nasal or temporal steps are often detectable; less frequently, paracentral scotomas and generalized constriction may be seen.[12] However, Walsh and Hoyt[21] reviewed several studies that demonstrated only an enlarged blind spot as a forme fruste of the visual field defect in association with optic pits.

The second type of visual field defect is that associated with serous detachment of the macula. In 1960 Kranenburg[22] described the association of optic nerve pits and central serous retinopathy. He found that 16 of his 24 patients with optic disc pits had serous detachments of the macula, with corresponding central scotomas or other central visual field changes.

Associated retinal changes

Optic nerve head pits that are centrally located are least likely to be associated with retinal changes. Optic disc pits along the rim of the optic disc are usually seen in association with peripapillary chorioretinal atrophy and retinal pigment epithelium changes (Fig. 93.3). These peripapillary changes may develop over time with or without central serous retinal detachments. In following the development of a serous macular detachment, Walsh and Hoyt[21] described the appearance of what they termed an "occult hole" in the optic nerve head.

Serous detachment of the macula is now known as a common complication of the optic disc pit. The natural history of this complication has been well described by Sobol et al.[23] They followed 15 patients with optic disc pits and macular detachments for an average of 9 years and found that 80% lost vision to 20/200 or worse. The visual loss was generally complete within 6 months of presentation. Long-term macular changes included full-thickness or laminar (through the outer retina) retinal holes,

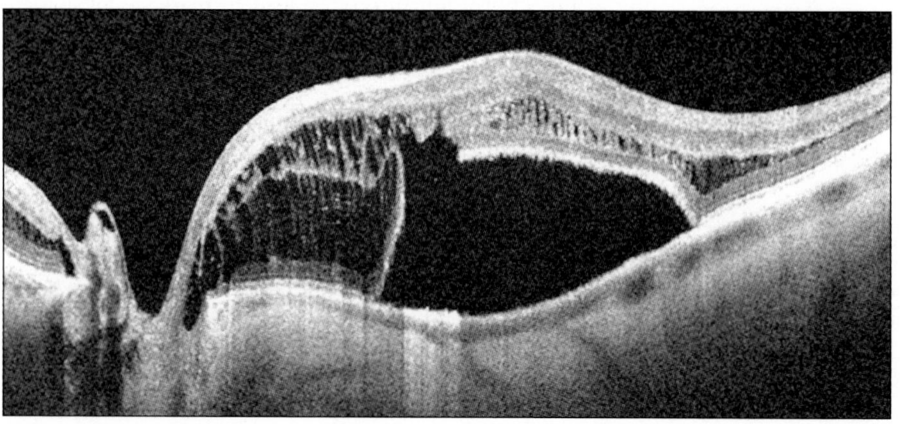

Fig. 93.2 Spectral-domain optical coherence tomography image of optic disc pit maculopathy, with cystoid spaces and schisis in multiple layers as well as subretinal fluid.

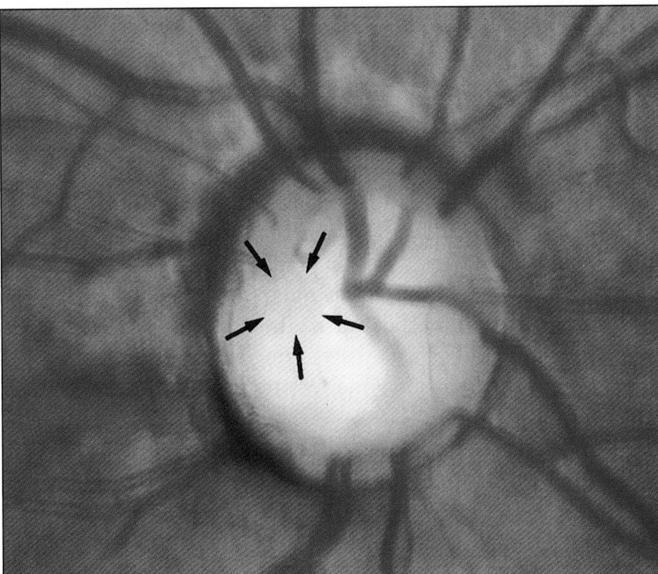

Fig. 93.3 Optic disc pits near the temporal margin are common and are most likely to lead to serous macular detachments (arrows).

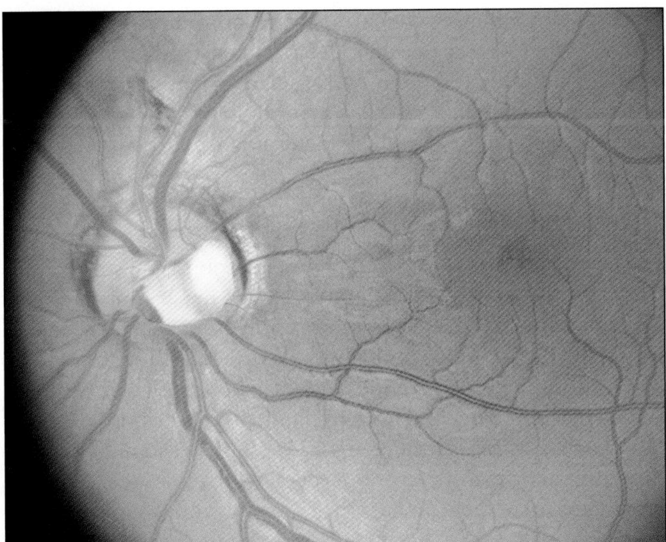

Fig. 93.4 Optic nerve pit. Note overlying gray fibroglial membrane.

retinal pigment epithelium mottling, and general cystic changes of the macula.[23]

Vascular telangiectasis has been reported in connection with intraschistic hemorrhage from a temporal optic disc pit.[24]

A gray fibroglial membrane appears to overlie the pit in many cases (Fig. 93.4). This membrane may be intact or may incompletely cover the pit. The fact that patients with serous macular detachments almost invariably have defects in their diaphanous membrane has prompted theories on how the optic nerve pit leads to the development of serous macular detachment.

MACULAR DETACHMENT

Several investigators have estimated that between 40 and 50% of patients with optic nerve pits have either an associated nonrhegmatogenous, serous retinal detachment or retinal changes suggestive of previous detachment.[12,25] The macular serous detachment (or retinoschisis) seen in association with optic disc pits appears most commonly when the pit is located in the temporal region of the optic disc and in larger pits. Conversely, small pits and those located more centrally are less likely to lead to serous retinal detachments.[12,22]

Appearance of maculopathy

In 1908, Reis[26] described a case of an optic nerve pit with associated maculopathy. However, this association was not taken seriously until Petersen,[27] in 1958, described several patients with what he called crater-like holes in the optic disc; these patients also had a central serous chorioretinopathy. This relationship was firmly emphasized by Kranenburg[22] in 1960, who described 24 cases of optic disc pits. One-third of these patients had serous retinal detachments, and another third had macular changes that he interpreted as reflecting a previous episode of nonrhegmatogenous serous retinal detachment.

Most of the retinal detachments are temporal to the disc and confined between the superior and inferior vascular arcades. Infrequently, a serous retinal detachment is located outside the arcades if the pit is situated on the nasal side of the optic disc. Often, the serous retinal detachment is contiguous with the optic disc, sometimes through a visible isthmus of subretinal fluid.

The serous macular detachments are generally low (less than 1.0 mm in height). The elevated retina often contains cystic regions that have been demonstrated on histologic examination to exist within the inner nuclear layer.[9] Occasionally the cystic areas rupture outward, producing a lamellar macular hole that, unlike idiopathic lamellar macular holes, retains an intact internal limiting membrane.

The variability of the retinal separation is also consistent with an alternative description of the maculopathy proposed by Lincoff and colleagues.[28] In a case report they provide clear OCTs to show a schisis cavity between the inner and outer retina and a larger outer-layer retinal detachment. The two are connected by a hole in the outer layer near the fovea.[28]

Course of associated serous macular detachment

It is difficult to determine the time interval between the beginning of a serous macular detachment and the earliest visual changes, because the patient usually seeks evaluation after symptoms of blurred vision and metamorphopsia occur secondary to foveal involvement. However, Brown and Tasman[29] described one case in which the retinal detachment started at the temporal margin of the optic disc. This serous retinal detachment expanded slowly in a temporal direction until, after several months, it covered the entire macular area. They also described small yellow precipitates seen under the elevated retina late in the course of serous macular detachment.

In analyzing their 15 patients followed over an average of 9 years, Sobol et al.[23] found that most eyes with optic disc pits presented with visual acuities of about 20/40–20/60. However, each patient lost three or more lines of vision within the next 6 months. After 6 months, a few of these patients got worse and even fewer got better. Ultimately, only 20% of the patients maintained visual acuities of better than 20/200.[23] Generally, however, patients with optic disc pits present later in the course of their macular detachments when their visual acuities are already worse than 20/70.[30]

Theories of pathophysiology

By 1960 it was clear that serous macular detachments often occurred as complications of optic disc pits. Ferry[9] had the opportunity to examine histologically two eyes with optic disc pits associated with macular detachments. He suggested that progressive gliosis and "contraction of the retinal elements" contained in the pit produced a traction detachment of the macula. In 1964 Sugar[31] suggested that fluid from the vitreous cavity could enter the subretinal space through a macular hole. However, this is most unlikely because macular holes seen with optic pits are usually lamellar and are only infrequently seen in association with the serous detachment.

It has been reported that fluorescein angiographic examination reveals late hyperfluorescence of the optic disc pit.[25] It was therefore considered possible that blood vessels in this area leaked fluid, which then entered the subretinal space.[25] However, Brown et al.[12] reported that many patients with serous macular detachments had no leakage on their fluorescein angiogram.

Others have speculated that there may be a direct source of fluid from the choroid that penetrates through Bruch's membrane under the macular detachment; it was hypothesized that peripapillary chorioretinal atrophic changes permitted this leakage.[32] However, fluorescein angiographic findings do not support this theory. Moreover, many other diseases produce extensive chorioretinal atrophy that does not lead to serous macular detachment.[12]

A few investigators,[33] including Gass,[34] have suggested that cerebrospinal fluid may leak from the optic nerve subarachnoid space into the optic pit and from there into the subretinal space. However, intrathecal fluorescein injections in humans and in animals and histologic studies have failed to demonstrate any such connection.[9,10,35,36]

Currently, the most widely accepted explanation is that originally proposed by Sugar[37] in 1962 and later endorsed by Brockhurst[38] in 1975. Sugar proposed that fluid from the vitreous leaked through the optic disc pit to fill the subretinal space (Fig. 93.5). In corroboration of this theory, Brown et al.[12] demonstrated that more than three-fourths of patients with optic disc pits and associated serous macular detachments have posterior vitreous detachments. This would allow liquefied vitreous to be contiguous with the optic disc cavity. Moreover, most of the patients in their series who had pits without macular serous elevations did not have posterior vitreous detachments.[12] Additionally, Brown and his colleagues[36] demonstrated experimentally in dogs a direct connection between the posterior vitreous space and the subretinal space via a congenital optic disc pit. Irvine et al.[33] demonstrated in vivo that there is a continuity between the posterior vitreous cavity and the optic nerve subarachnoid space by observing bubbles percolating out of an optic nerve sheath window after pars plana vitrectomy and gas injection.

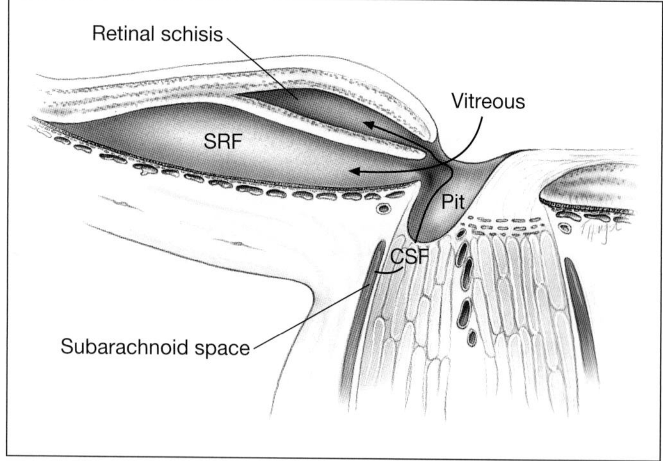

Fig. 93.5 Schematic drawing of axial view of optic nerve head. Various theories describe mechanisms by which fluid enters the subretinal space. Cerebrospinal fluid (CSF) could derive from the subarachnoid space. However, the more widely accepted explanation is that fluid in the vitreous space passes into the optic pit and from there directly into the subretinal space. An optic disc pit located near the margin of the optic nerve head is far more likely to permit fluid to leak subretinally. SRF, Subretinal fluid.

The most recent variation on these theories of pathophysiology is that proposed by Lincoff et al.,[28] who suggest that the primary communication from the optic disc pit is to the retina temporal to the optic disc.[15] Fluid slips under the inner retina, lifting it and the nerve fiber layer up and away from the outer retina. This has been corroborated by OCT[18] and extended to show both this retinal schisis and an outer retinal detachment connected by a hole in the outer retinal layer (Fig. 93.2).

Although the theory of direct vitreous fluid entry via the optic pit into the subretinal space is appealing, it does not explain why serous macular detachments tend to occur first in young adulthood. Brown and Tasman[29] suggest that posterior vitreous detachments may be a precipitating factor. Another possibility is that the impelling factor is macular traction, which occurs with age.

Prognosis

Although the optic nerve head pits, being congenital, are stationary, their associated retinal abnormalities may be progressive. The prognosis for return of vision after serous macular detachment is variable. Walsh and Hoyt[21] described a patient followed between the ages of 14 and 23 years who developed multiple serous macular detachments that remitted to near-normal vision after each episode. A more rigorous study was conducted by Brown et al.[12] in a group of 20 eyes with optic disc pits and serous macular detachments. These eyes were followed for 5 years, untreated. The mean visual acuity at the end of this time was about 20/80. The authors found very little correlation between the visual acuity at the time of detachment and the long-term visual outcome. They also noted that some detachments resolved spontaneously, whereas others persisted for years. Most patients still had some subretinal macular fluid present after 5 years. Other macular changes, as described above, also persisted. Long-term studies confirm the earlier impressions that untreated macular detachments caused by optic disc pits have an overall poor prognosis.[23]

Treatment

Given the rarity of optic disc pits, most studies examining purported treatments are small and nonrandomized, leading to difficulty in coming to a consensus on the best treatment for the associated serous macular detachments. Observation, systemic steroids, optic nerve sheath decompression, and scleral buckling procedures have not been demonstrated to be very effective.[38,39] However, several series have favorably compared the outcome of photocoagulated eyes with untreated eyes in the resolution of the serous macular detachment and in final visual outcome.[33,38–40]

The argon laser procedure was used in most of these series to produce photocoagulation burns in one or several rows between the area of serous retinal detachment and the optic disc. Usually, the burns are only applied to areas of elevated retina. Brockhurst,[38] Gass,[40] and Theodossiadis[41] used similar photocoagulation protocols, and all reported that their patients were likely to have good resolution of the serous detachment to a flat macula.

Combining their results, 15 of the 18 patients in these three series had reattachments of their maculas, as opposed to only 5 of 20 untreated patients in the series of Brown et al.[12] However, the difference in final visual outcome between the treated and untreated groups was less pronounced. The photocoagulated eyes in the three studies had ultimate visual acuities that averaged a little worse than 20/80. This does not compare favorably with the 20/80 final visual outcome in the series of Brown et al. In making a similar comparison, Brown and Tasman[29] concluded that photocoagulation therapy is effective for flattening the retinal detachment, but not for improving final visual outcome.

A macular buckling procedure successfully treated cases of serous detachment in optic disc pit. In such cases, OCT showed a resultant closure of the connection between the pit and a retinal schisis with resolution of the schisis.[42] Multifocal electroretinography was performed in 10 patients with optic disc pit with serous macular detachment before and after treatment with macular buckling procedures.[43] Improvement was measured in all eyes at 12 months, though often this was not accompanied by an increase in visual acuity.[43] Silicon oil has been used successfully in cases of macular hole in association with the optic disc pit.[44]

More recent attempts to combine photocoagulation therapy with posterior vitrectomy and gas–fluid exchange have led to more encouraging long-term visual outcomes.[45] Bonnet[46] looked at 25 eyes with optic disc pits in 24 patients who presented with visual loss due to serous macular detachments. High-magnification biomicroscopy and fluorescein angiography of these eyes revealed evidence of vitreous traction on the retina and on the optic nerve head. Most particularly, Bonnet noted that none of the patients had posterior vitreous detachments at presentation and that in the 2 cases that subsequently developed a posterior vitreous detachment, reattachment of the macula occurred spontaneously. Fluorescein dye was seen to stain the optic nerve head, especially at the pit and temporal margin of the disc. This dye leakage was not seen in cases that underwent surgical peeling of the posterior vitreous face. Moreover, Bonnet observed a small hole in the roof of the optic pit in several cases, and small bubbles of gas passing from the vitreous cavity into the subretinal space via the optic disc pit in a case that underwent vitrectomy and gas injection but not photocoagulation. Hence, Bonnet concluded that macular detachments in optic disc pits have a rhegmatogenous component (at the optic disc), that they are associated with vitreous traction, and that the subretinal fluid comes from the vitreous space via the optic disc pit.[46]

Cox and colleagues[47] looked at three treatment methods. They concluded that the combination of vitrectomy plus gas tamponade plus photocoagulation of the retina temporal to the disc was more effective than vitrectomy and gas or photocoagulation alone. They obtained short-term surgical success in all of their 8 eyes and long-term attachment in 4 out of 8 eyes using the three-part combination therapy.[47] Others have also obtained good anatomic results in optic disc pit with macular detachment using the combination of vitrectomy, air–fluid exchange, and photocoagulation in patients whose final visual acuities averaged 20/60.[48] Various precipitating events may combine with the mechanism described above, leading to macular detachment by vitreous fluid entry into the subretinal space via the optic disc pit.

Novel techniques for treatment of optic disc pit-associated serous macular detachments have been described. Spaide et al.[49] published a case report describing the use of a bent 25-gauge needle to create half-thickness cuts to the retina. This maneuver was combined with a vitrectromy in an attempt to allow intra- and subretinal fluid to escape. This procedure did not use intraocular gas to avoid premature closure of the surgical fenestrations and the posterior hyaloid was left intact. One month after surgery, the patient's visual acuity improved from 8/400 preoperatively to 20/20. Schaal et al.[50] described a similar procedure with the use of a 27-gauge cannula to make three-quarter depth cuts, in combination with a limited preretinal vitrectomy.

Jalil et al.[51] actively drained subretinal fluid with a 42-gauge cannula. This procedure included vitrectomy, induction of posterior vitreous detachment, and internal limiting membrane peel, but without the use of laser photocoagulation around the retinotomy site. Fluid–air exchange followed by internal gas tamponade with 14% C_3F_8 concluded the procedure. The patient's preoperative visual acuity of 1.00 logMAR improved at 8-months follow-up to 0.4 logMAR. Ziahosseini et al.[52] utilized a similar approach with the addition of argon laser to the cannula insertion site.

REFERENCES

1. Sadun AA, Yanoff M. Pathology of the optic nerve. In: Duane TD, Jaeger EA, editors. Biomedical foundations of ophthalmology, vol. 3, Philadelphia: Harper & Row; 1986.
2. Nelson M, Lessell S, Sadun AA. Optic nerve hypoplasia and maternal diabetes mellitus. Arch Neurol 1986;43:20–5.
3. Grear JN Jr. Pits, or crater-like holes in the optic disk. Arch Ophthalmol 1942;28:467–83.
4. Slusher MM, Weaver RG, Greven CM, et al. The spectrum of cavitary optic disc anomalies in a family. Ophthalmology 1989;96:342–7.
5. Sadun AA, Schaecter JD. Tracing axons in the human brain: a method utilizing light and TEM techniques. J Electron Microsc Tech 1985;2:175–86.
6. Hogan MJ, Alvarado JA, Weddell JE. Histology of the human eye: an atlas and textbook, Philadelphia, PA: WB Saunders; 1971.
7. Sadun AA, Currie JN, Lessell S. Transient visual obscurations with elevated optic discs. Ann Neurol 1984;16:489–94.
8. Wiethe T. Ein Fall von angeborener Deformitat der Sehnervenpapille. Arch Augenheilkd 1882;11:4–19.
9. Ferry AP. Macular detachment associated with congenital pit of the optic nerve head: pathologic findings in two cases simulating malignant melanoma of the choroid. Arch Ophthalmol 1963;70:346–57.
10. Kalina RE, Conrad WC. Intrathecal fluorescein for serous macular detachment. Arch Ophthalmol 1976;94:1421.
11. Singerman LJ, Mittra RA. Hereditary optic pit and iris coloboma in three generations of a single family. Retina 2001;21:273–5.
12. Brown GC, Shields JA, Goldberg RE. Congenital pits of the optic nerve head. II. Clinical studies in humans. Ophthalmology 1980;87:51–65.
13. Brodsky MC. Congenital optic pit with serous maculopathy in childhood. J AAPOS 2003;2:150.
14. Yuen CHW, Kaye SB. Spontaneous resolution of serous maculopathy associated with optic disc pit in a child: a case report. J AAPOS 2002;6: 330–1.
15. Lincoff H, Lopez R, Kreissig I, et al. Retinoschisis associated with optic nerve pits. Arch Ophthalmol 1988;106:61–7.
16. Lincoff H, Yannuzzi L, Singerman L, et al. Improvement in visual function after displacement of the retinal elevations emanating from optic pits. Arch Ophthalmol 1993;111:1071–9.
17. Lincoff H, Kreissig I. Optical coherence tomography of pneumatic displacement of optic disc pit maculopathy. Br J Ophthalmol 1998;82:367–72.
18. Krivoy D, Gentile R, Liebmann JM, et al. Imaging congenital optic disc pits and associated maculopathy using optic coherence tomography. Arch Ophthalmol 1996;114:165–70.
19. Myer CH, Rodrigues EB, Schmidt JC. Congenital optic nerve head pit associated with reduced retinal nerve fibre thickness at the papillomacular bundle. Br J Ophthalmol 2003;87:1300–1.
20. Simpson DE. Optic nerve pit. J Am Optom Assoc 1987;58:118–20.

21. Walsh FB, Hoyt WF. Clinical neuro-ophthalmology. 3rd ed. Baltimore, MD: Williams & Wilkins; 1969.
22. Kranenburg EW. Crater-like holes in the optic disc and central serous retinopathy. Arch Ophthalmol 1960;64:912–24.
23. Sobol WM, Boldi CF, Folk JC, et al. Long-term visual outcome in patients with optic nerve pit and serous retinal detachment of the macula. Ophthalmology 1990;97:1539–42.
24. Quinn SM, Charles SJ. Telangiectasis as a cause of intra-schitic haemorrhage in optic disc pit maculopathy. Acta Ophthalmol Scand 2004;82:93–5.
25. Gordon R, Chatfield RK. Pits in the optic disc associated with macular degeneration. Br J Ophthalmol 1969;53:481–9.
26. Reis W. Eine wenig bekannte typische Missbildung am Sehnerveneintritt: umschriebene Grubenbildung auf der Papilla n. optici. Z Augenheilkd 1908; 19:505–28.
27. Petersen HP. Pits or crater-like holes in the optic disc. Acta Ophthalmol 1958;36:345–443.
28. Lincoff H, Schiff W, Krivoy D, et al. Optic coherence tomography of optic disk pit maculopathy. Am J Ophthalmol 1996;122:264–6.
29. Brown GC, Tasman WS. Congenital anomalies of the optic disk. New York: Grune & Stratton; 1983.
30. Theodossiadis GP. Visual acuity in patients with optic nerve pit. Ophthalmology 1991;98:563.
31. Sugar HS. An explanation for the acquired macular pathology associated with congenital pits of the optic disc. Am J Ophthalmol 1964;57:833–5.
32. Wise G, Dollery C, Henkind P. The retinal circulation. New York: Harper & Row; 1971.
33. Irvine AR, Crawford JB, Sullivan JH. The pathogenesis of retinal detachment with morning glory disk and optic pit. Retina 1986;6:146–50.
34. Gass JDM. Serous detachment of the macular secondary to congenital pit of the optic nerve head. Am J Ophthalmol 1969;67:821–41.
35. Brown GC, Shields JA, Patty BE, et al. Congenital pits of the optic nerve head. I. Experimental studies in collie dogs. Arch Ophthalmol 1979;97: 1341–4.
36. Brown GC, Shields JA, Patty BE, et al. Congenital optic pits and serous retinal detachment. Trans Pa Acad Ophthalmol Otolaryngol 1979;32:151–4.
37. Sugar HS. Congenital pits in the optic disc with acquired macular pathology. Am J Ophthalmol 1962;53:307–11.
38. Brockhurst RJ. Optic pits and posterior retinal detachment. Trans Am Ophthalmol Soc 1975;73:264–91.
39. Mustonen E, Varonen T. Congenital pit of the optic nerve head associated with serous detachment of the macular. Acta Ophthalmol 1972;50:689–98.
40. Gass JDM. Stereoscopic atlas of macular diseases. St Louis: Mosby; 1977.
41. Theodossiadis G. Evolution of congenital pit of the optic disk with macular detachment in photocoagulated and nonphotocoagulated eyes. Am J Ophthalmol 1977;84:620–31.
42. Theodossiadis GP, Theodossiadis PG. Optical coherence tomography in optic disk pit maculopathy treated by the macular buckling procedure. Am J Ophthalmol 2001;132:184–90.
43. Theodossiadis G, Theodossiadis P, Lalias J, et al. Preoperative and postoperative assessment by multifocal electroretinography in the management of optic disc pits with serous macular detachment. Ophthalmology 2002;109: 2295–302.
44. Bechmann M, Mueller AJ, Gandorfer A, et al. Macular hole surgery in an eye with an optic pit. Am J Ophthalmol 2001;132:263–4.
45. Pahwa V. Optic pit and central serous detachment. Ind J Ophthalmol 1985;33:175–6.
46. Bonnet M. Serous macular detachment associated with optic nerve pits. Graefes Arch Clin Exp Ophthalmol 1991;229:526–32.
47. Cox MS, Witherspoon CD, Morris RE, et al. Evolving techniques in the treatment of macular detachment caused by optic nerve pits. Ophthalmology 1988;95:889–96.
48. Schatz H, McDonald HR. Treatment of sensory retinal detachment associated with optic nerve pit or coloboma. Ophthalmology 1988;95:178–86.
49. Spaide RF, Fisher Y, Ober M, et al. Surgical hypothesis: inner retinal fenestration as a treatment for optic disc pit maculopathy. Retina 2006;26: 89–91.
50. Schaal KB, Wrede J, Dithmar S. Internal drainage in optic pit maculopathy. Br J Ophthalmol 2007;91:1093.
51. Jalil A, Stavrakas P, Dhawahir-Scala FE, et al. Drainage of subretinal fluid in optic disc pit maculopathy using subretinal 42-gauge cannula: a new surgical approach. Graefes Arch Clin Exp Ophthalmol 2010;248:751–3.
52. Ziahosseini K, Sanghvi C, Muzaffar W, et al. Successful surgical treatment of optic disc pit maculopathy. Eye (Lond) 2009;23:1477–9.

Retina-Related Clinical Trials: A Resource Bibliography

Chapter 94

Barbara S. Hawkins, Usha Chakravarthy

The subspecialty of Retina has probably seen some of the most innovative changes in the field of ophthalmology, largely owing to ground-breaking randomized clinical trials, with several or many centers typically participating, conducted to test novel treatment strategies in the management of diabetes, age-related macular degeneration, and retinal vaso-occlusive disease, among others. In previous decades, large clinical trials of interventions for retinal disorders laid the foundations for evidence-based clinical practice; foremost among these was the Diabetic Retinopathy Study, which was also one of the first initiatives of the National Eye Institute of the USA upon its creation as one of the National Institutes of Health. The Diabetic Retinopathy Study was one of the largest and best-conducted clinical trials of the safety and effectiveness of panretinal photocoagulation in diabetic retinopathy. This trial provided ophthalmologists with the evidence that was needed to show that proliferative diabetic retinopathy could be managed effectively with laser and also demonstrated the potential of the retinal community to generate the evidence base for treatment of retinal disorders through a networked approach. Since the Diabetic Retinopathy Study, the number of clinical trials in retinal disorders has burgeoned, with increasing sponsorship from industry and agencies in other countries. The purpose of this chapter is to provide the retinal specialist with a bibliography of publications in peer-reviewed journals from studies undertaken on the common retinal disorders of diabetes, age-related macular degeneration, and retinal vein occlusion, as well as other retinal disorders for which important clinical trials have been conducted. The organization of the citations is by retinal condition and then by specific randomized clinical trials or sets of trials, with clinical trials that focus on the same condition grouped together. The order of the conditions is chronologic by publication of findings from the first major clinical trial in each condition. Whenever a randomized trial was conducted as part of a larger study, preceded by a pilot study, or continued as an observational study, publications from the pilot study or selected publications from the larger study or observational study have been included in the bibliography for the clinical trial or set of clinical trials.

DIABETIC RETINOPATHY

Findings from several clinical trials of treatment or prevention of diabetic retinopathy are discussed in Chapters 47 (Nonproliferative diabetic retinopathy and diabetic macular edema) and 48 (Proliferative diabetic retinopathy).

Diabetic Retinopathy Study (DRS)

The historical importance of and other information about the DRS are described above. From 1972 through 1975, 1758 patients enrolled at DRS-participating centers.

Diabetic Retinopathy Study Research Group. Preliminary report on effects of photocoagulation therapy. Am J Ophthalmol 1976;81:383–96.

With 1732 patients enrolled and one eye of each patient assigned to photocoagulation, visual acuity of 5/200 or worse at two consecutive examinations 4 months apart was observed in 9% of untreated eyes versus 4% of treated eyes, leading to the decision to halt enrollment of new patients, to disseminate the findings to physicians, and to offer panretinal photocoagulation to all untreated eyes deemed to be at high risk of progression and vision loss.

Diabetic Retinopathy Study Research Group. Photocoagulation treatment of proliferative diabetic retinopathy: the second report of Diabetic Retinopathy Study findings. Ophthalmology 1978;85:82–106.

A detailed analysis of findings for all patients enrolled confirmed that scatter photocoagulation compared to no treatment reduced severe visual acuity loss and reduced the rate of progression to more severe stages of proliferative diabetic retinopathy. Throughout 3 years of follow-up, treated eyes had approximately half the risk of visual acuity of 5/200 or worse at two or more consecutive examinations.

Diabetic Retinopathy Study Research Group. Four risk factors for severe visual loss in diabetic retinopathy: the third report from the Diabetic Retinopathy Study. Arch Ophthalmol 1979; 97:654–5.

The four risk factors were: (1) presence of vitreous or preretinal hemorrhage; (2) presence of new vessels; (3) location of new vessels on or near the optic disc; and (4) severity of new vessels. Risk of severe visual acuity loss increased by the number of factors present.

Diabetic Retinopathy Study Research Group. Photocoagulation treatment of proliferative diabetic retinopathy: a short report of long range results. Diabetic Retinopathy Study (DRS) report number 4. International Congress series no. 500, Diabetes 1979. In: Waldhausl WK, editor. Proceedings of the 10th Congress of the International Diabetes Federation. Amsterdam: Excerpta Medica; 1979. p. 789–94.

Diabetic Retinopathy Study Research Group. Photocoagulation treatment of proliferative diabetic retinopathy: relationship of adverse treatment effects to retinopathy severity. Diabetic Retinopathy Study report no. 5. Dev Ophthalmol 1981;2:248–61.

Diabetic Retinopathy Study Research Group. Diabetic Retinopathy Study report number 6: Design, methods, and baseline results. Invest Ophthalmol Vis Sci 1981;21:149–208.

Diabetic Retinopathy Study Research Group. Diabetic Retinopathy Study report number 7: A modification of the Airlie House classification of diabetic retinopathy. Invest Ophthalmol Vis Sci 1981;21:210–26.

Diabetic Retinopathy Study Research Group. Photocoagulation treatment of proliferative diabetic retinopathy. Clinical application of Diabetic Retinopathy Study (DRS) findings. DRS report number 8. Ophthalmology 1981;88:583–600.

Knatterud GL. Mortality experience in the Diabetic Retinopathy Study. Isr J Med Sci 1983;19:424–8.

Ederer F, Podgor MJ, the Diabetic Retinopathy Study Research Group. Assessing possible late treatment effects in stopping a clinical trial early: a case study. Diabetic Retinopathy Study report no. 9. Control Clin Trials 1984;5:373–81.

Rand LI, Prud'homme GJ, Ederer F, et al. Factors influencing the development of visual loss in advanced diabetic retinopathy: Diabetic Retinopathy Study (DRS) report no. 10. Invest Ophthalmol Vis Sci 1985;26:983–91.

Kaufman SC, Ferris FL, Swartz M, et al. Intraocular pressure following panretinal photocoagulation for diabetic retinopathy: Diabetic Retinopathy report no. 11. Arch Ophthalmol 1987;105: 807–9.

Ferris FL, Podgor MJ, Davis MD, et al. Macular edema in Diabetic Retinopathy Study patients. Diabetic Retinopathy Study report number 12. Ophthalmology 1987;94:754–60.

Kaufman SC, Ferris FL, Seigel DG, et al. Factors associated with visual outcome after photocoagulation for diabetic retinopathy: Diabetic Retinopathy Study report no. 13. Invest Ophthalmol Vis Sci 1989;30:23–8.

Diabetic Retinopathy Study Research Group. Indications for photocoagulation treatment of diabetic retinopathy: Diabetic Retinopathy Study report no. 14. Int Ophthalmol Clin 1987;27: 239–53.

UK Multicentre Controlled Study

This randomized trial of xenon arc photocoagulation for diabetic maculopathy was conducted concurrently with the DRS; initial findings were published shortly after the first publication from the DRS. This multicenter trial was sponsored by the British Diabetic Association and the Wellcome Trust.

Multicentre Controlled Study Coordinating Committee. Photocoagulation treatment of diabetic maculopathy. Interim report of a multicentre controlled study. Lancet 1975;2:1110–3.

Photocoagulation with the xenon arc led to less deterioration in visual acuity than no treatment. Initiation of treatment was recommended before visual acuity was "seriously impaired."

Multicentre Controlled Study Coordinating Committee. Proliferative diabetic retinopathy: treatment with xenon-arc photocoagulation. Interim report of multicentre controlled randomised controlled trial. Br Med J 1977;1:739–41.

Photocoagulation with the xenon arc led to less monocular blindness than no treatment. New vessels on the disc regressed more in treated eyes than in untreated eyes.

Diabetic Retinopathy Vitrectomy Study (DRVS)

The primary goal of the DRVS was to compare early vitrectomy with conventional management of severe vitreous hemorrhage secondary to diabetic retinopathy. Patient accrual began in October 1976 and ended in June 1983. The DRVS was sponsored by the National Eye Institute.

Diabetic Retinopathy Vitrectomy Study Research Group. Two-year course of visual acuity in severe proliferative diabetic retinopathy with conventional management. Diabetic Retinopathy Vitrectomy Study (DRVS) report no. 1. Ophthalmology 1985;92:492–502.

After 2 years of follow-up, visual acuity of eyes assigned to conventional treatment was worse than 5/200 in 45% of eyes with more than four disc areas of new vessels and visual acuity of 10/30 to 10/50 at baseline.

Diabetic Retinopathy Vitrectomy Study Research Group. Early vitrectomy for severe vitreous hemorrhage in diabetic retinopathy. Two-year results of a randomized trial. Diabetic Retinopathy Vitrectomy Study report 2. Arch Ophthalmol 1985;103: 1644–52.

Visual acuity was 10/20 or better in 25% of the early vitrectomy group compared with 15% of the deferral group 2 years after entry.

Diabetic Retinopathy Vitrectomy Study Research Group. Early vitrectomy for severe proliferative diabetic retinopathy in eyes with useful vision. Results of a randomized trial – Diabetic Retinopathy Vitrectomy Study report 3. Ophthalmology 1988; 95:1307–20.

Diabetic Retinopathy Vitrectomy Study Research Group. Early vitrectomy for severe proliferative diabetic retinopathy in eyes with useful vision. Clinical application of results of a randomized trial – Diabetic Retinopathy Vitrectomy Study report 4. Ophthalmology 1988;95:1321–34.

Diabetic Retinopathy Vitrectomy Study Research Group. Early vitrectomy for severe vitreous hemorrhage in diabetic retinopathy. Four-year results of a randomized trial: Diabetic Retinopathy Vitrectomy Study report 5. Arch Ophthalmol 1990;108: 958–64, 1452.

Early Treatment Diabetic Retinopathy Study (ETDRS)

The ETDRS was designed to evaluate the effectiveness of laser photocoagulation and aspirin, together and singly, in delaying or preventing progression of early diabetic retinopathy to more severe stages and blindness and to determine the optimum time to initiate photocoagulation in diabetic retinopathy. This multicenter clinical trial was sponsored by the National Eye Institute. Initiation of the ETDRS was a motivating factor in the development of a new visual acuity chart for use in prospective clinical research studies; see articles that report on the design and evaluation of the chart at the end of the ETDRS bibliography.

Early Treatment Diabetic Retinopathy Study Research Group. Photocoagulation for diabetic macular edema. Early Treatment Diabetic Retinopathy Study report number 1. Arch Ophthalmol 1985;103:1796–806.

Eyes with clinically significant macular edema benefited from focal photocoagulation and were about half as likely to lose three or more lines of vision as eyes assigned to deferral of photocoagulation.

Early Treatment Diabetic Retinopathy Study Research Group. Treatment techniques and clinical guidelines for photocoagulation of diabetic macular edema. Early Treatment Diabetic Retinopathy Study report number 2. Ophthalmology 1987;94:761–74.

Early Treatment Diabetic Retinopathy Study Research Group. Techniques for scatter and local photocoagulation treatment of diabetic retinopathy: Early Treatment Diabetic Retinopathy Study report no. 3. Int Ophthalmol Clin 1987;27:254–64.

Early Treatment Diabetic Retinopathy Study Research Group. Photocoagulation for diabetic macular edema: Early Treatment Diabetic Retinopathy Study report no. 4. Int Ophthalmol Clin 1987;27:265–72.

This report summarizes ETDRS reports number 1 and number 2.

Early Treatment Diabetic Retinopathy Study Research Group. Case reports to accompany Early Treatment Diabetic Retinopathy Study reports 3 and 4. Int Ophthalmol Clin 1987;27:273–334.

Kinyoun J, Barton F, Fisher M et al. Detection of diabetic macular edema: ophthalmoscopy versus photography – Early Treatment Diabetic Retinopathy Study report number 5. Ophthalmology 1989;96:746–51.

Prior MJ, Prout T, Miller D, et al. C-peptide and the classification of diabetes mellitus patients in the Early Treatment Diabetic Retinopathy Study: report number 6. Ann Epidemiol 1993;3:9–17.

Early Treatment Diabetic Retinopathy Study Research Group. Early Treatment Diabetic Retinopathy Study design and baseline patient characteristics. ETDRS report number 7. Ophthalmology 1991;98:741–56.

Early Treatment Diabetic Retinopathy Study Research Group. Effects of aspirin treatment on diabetic retinopathy: ETDRS report number 8. Ophthalmology 1991;98:757–65.

Aspirin (650 mg/day) had no clinically beneficial or harmful effects in patients with retinopathy.

Early Treatment Diabetic Retinopathy Study Research Group. Early photocoagulation for diabetic retinopathy: ETDRS report number 9. Ophthalmology 1991;98:766–85.

Initiation of scatter photocoagulation was recommended for eyes with high-risk proliferative retinopathy. Whenever possible, scatter photocoagulation should be applied after completion of focal laser in eyes with macular edema.

Early Treatment Diabetic Retinopathy Study Research Group. Grading diabetic retinopathy from stereoscopic color fundus photographs – an extension of the modified Airlie House classification. ETDRS report number 10. Ophthalmology 1991;98:786–806.

Early Treatment Diabetic Retinopathy Study Research Group. Classification of diabetic retinopathy from fluorescein angiograms. ETDRS report number 11. Ophthalmology 1991;98:807–22.

Early Treatment Diabetic Retinopathy Study Research Group. Fundus photographic risk factors for progression of diabetic retinopathy: ETDRS report number 12. Ophthalmology 1991;98:823–33.

Severity of intraretinal microvascular abnormalities, hemorrhages and/or microaneurysms, and venous beading were the most important factors in predicting progression to proliferative diabetic retinopathy.

Early Treatment Diabetic Retinopathy Study Research Group. Fluorescein angiographic risk factors for progression of diabetic retinopathy: ETDRS report number 13. Ophthalmology 1991;98:834–40.

Fluorescein leakage, capillary loss and dilation, and various arteriolar abnormalities were associated with progression to proliferative retinopathy.

Early Treatment Diabetic Retinopathy Study Investigators. Aspirin effects on mortality and morbidity in patients with diabetes mellitus: Early Treatment Diabetic Retinopathy Study report 14. JAMA 1992;268:1292–300.

Fong DS, Barton FB, Bresnick GH, et al. Impaired color vision associated with diabetic retinopathy: Early Treatment Diabetic Retinopathy Study report no. 15. Am J Ophthalmol 1999;128:612–7.

Chew EY, Williams GA, Burton TC, et al. Aspirin effects on the development of cataracts in patients with diabetes mellitus: Early Treatment Diabetic Retinopathy Study report 16. Arch Ophthalmol 1992;110:339–42.

Flynn HW, Chew EY, Simons BD, et al. Pars plana vitrectomy in the Early Treatment Diabetic Retinopathy Study. ETDRS report number 17. Ophthalmology 1992;99:1351–7.

Ferris FL. Early photocoagulation in patients with either type I or type II diabetes. Trans Am Ophthalmol Soc 1996;94:505–36.

Patients with type 2 diabetes were more likely to benefit from early scatter photocoagulation than patients with type 1 diabetes based on analysis of data from both the DRS and ETDRS.

Davis MD, Fisher MR, Gangnon RE, et al. Risk factors for high-risk proliferative diabetic retinopathy and severe visual loss: Early Treatment Diabetic Retinopathy Study report no. 18. Invest Ophthalmol Vis Sci 1998;39:233–52.

Early Treatment Diabetic Retinopathy Study Research Group. Focal photocoagulation treatment of diabetic macular edema. Relationship of treatment effect to fluorescein angiographic and other retinal characteristics at baseline: ETDRS report no. 19. Arch Ophthalmol 1995;113:1144–55.

Chew EY, Klein ML, Murphy RP, et al. Effects of aspirin on vitreous/preretinal hemorrhage in patients with diabetes mellitus: Early Treatment Diabetic Retinopathy Study report no. 20. Arch Ophthalmol 1995;113:52–5.

Braun CI, Benson WE, Remaley NA, et al. Accommodative amplitudes in the Early Treatment Diabetic Retinopathy Study. ETDRS report number 21. Retina 1995;15:275–81.

Chew EY, Klein ML, Ferris FL, et al. Association of elevated serum lipid levels with retinal hard exudate in diabetic retinopathy: Early Treatment Diabetic Retinopathy Study (ETDRS) report 22. Arch Ophthalmol 1996;114:1079–84.

Fong DS, Segal PP, Myers F, et al. Subretinal fibrosis in diabetic macular edema. ETDRS report 23. Arch Ophthalmol 1997;115: 873–7.

Fong DS, Ferris FL, Davis MD, et al. Causes of severe visual loss in the Early Treatment Diabetic Retinopathy Study: ETDRS report no. 24. Am J Ophthalmol 1999;127:137–41.

Chew EY, Benson WE, Remaley NA, et al. Results after lens extraction in patients with diabetic retinopathy: Early Treatment Diabetic Retinopathy Study report number 25. Arch Ophthalmol 1999;117:1600–6.

Cusick M, Chew EY, Hoogwert B, et al. and the ETDRS Research Group. Risk factors for renal replacement therapy in the Early Treatment Diabetic Retinopathy Study (ETDRS). ETDRS report no. 26. Kidney International 2004;66:1173–9.

Cusick M, Davis MD, Meleth AD, et al for the Early Treatment Diabetic Retinopathy Study (ETDRS) Research Group. Associations of mortality and diabetes complications in patients with type 1 and type 2 diabetes. Early Treatment Diabetic Retinopathy Study report no. 27. Diabetes Care 2005;28: 617–25.

Barton FB, Fong DS, Knatterud GL, et al. Classification of Farnsworth–Munsell 100-hue test results in the Early Treatment Diabetic Retinopathy Study. Am J Ophthalmol 2004;138: 119–24.

Gangnon RE, Davis MD, Hubbard LD, et al. A severity scale for diabetic macular edema developed from ETDRS data. Invest Ophthalmol Vis Sci 2008;49:5041–7.

Ferris FL, Kassoff A, Bresnick GH, et al. New visual acuity charts for clinical research. Am J Ophthalmol 1982;94:91–6.

Ferris FL, Sperduto RD. Standardized illumination for visual acuity testing in clinical research. Am J Ophthalmol 1982;94: 97–8.

Ferris FL, Freidlin V, Kassoff A, et al. Relative letter and position difficulty on visual acuity charts from the Early Treatment Diabetic Retinopathy Study. Am J Ophthalmol 1993;116:735–40.

Sorbinil Retinopathy Trial (SRT)

The SRT was sponsored by the National Eye Institute and by Pfizer.

Sorbinil Retinopathy Trial Research Group. A randomized trial of sorbinil, an aldose reductase inhibitor, in diabetic retinopathy. Arch Ophthalmol 1990;108:1234–44.

Sorbinil, as administered in the SRT, did not have a clinically important effect on the course of diabetic retinopathy in adults with insulin-dependent diabetes.

Sorbinil Retinopathy Trial Research Group. The Sorbinil Retinopathy Trial: neuropathy results. Neurology 1993;43:1141–9.

Cohen RA, Hennekens CH, Christen WG, et al. Determinants of retinopathy progression in type 1 diabetes mellitus. Am J Med 1999;107:45–51.

Christen WG, Manson JE, Bubes V, et al. Risk factors for progression of distal symmetric polyneuropathy in type 1 diabetes mellitus. Am J Epidemiol 1999;150:1142–51.

Krypton Argon Regression of Neovascularization Study (KARNS)

The KARNS was a multicenter clinical trial with the primary goal of comparing krypton red laser with argon blue–green laser for panretinal photocoagulation with respect to regression of disc neovascularization in diabetic retinopathy.

Singerman LJ, Ferris FL, Mowery RP, et al. Krypton laser for proliferative diabetic retinopathy: the Krypton Argon Regression of Neovascularization Study. J Diab Complications 1988;2: 189–96.

Krypton Argon Regression of Neovascularization Study Research Group. Randomized comparison of krypton versus argon scatter photocoagulation for diabetic disc neovascularization. Ophthalmology 1993;100:1655–64.

Scatter photocoagulation with either krypton red or argon blue–green laser was equally effective in the treatment of proliferative diabetic retinopathy.

Diabetes Control and Complications Trial (DCCT)

The DCCT was a multicenter randomized clinical trial designed to compare intensive with conventional glucose control with respect to development and progression of early vascular and neurologic complications of insulin-dependent diabetes mellitus. The DCCT was sponsored by the National Institute of Diabetes and Digestive and Kidney Diseases, the National Heart, Lung, and Blood Institute, the National Eye Institute, and the National Center for Research Resources (National Institutes of

Health, US Department of Health and Human Services) and various corporate sponsors. A follow-up study of members of the DCCT cohort, the Epidemiology of Diabetes Interventions and Complications (EDIC), was undertaken to assess the long-term effects of intensive and conventional diabetes therapy during the DCCT.

Diabetes Control and Complications Trial Research Group. The Diabetes Control and Complications Trial (DCCT): design and methodologic considerations for the feasibility phase. Diabetes 1986;35:530–45.

Diabetes Control and Complications Trial Research Group. The Diabetes Control and Complications Trial (DCCT): Results of feasibility study. Diabetes Care 1987;10:1–10.

Diabetes Control and Complications Trial Research Group. Feasibility of centralized measurements of glycated hemoglobin in the Diabetes Control and Complications Trial, a multicenter study. Clin Chem 1987;33:2267–71.

Diabetes Control and Complications Trial Research Group. Implementation of a multicomponent process to obtain informed consent in the Diabetes Control and Complications Trial. Control Clin Trials 1989;10:83–96.

Diabetes Control and Complications Trial Research Group. The effect of intensive treatment of diabetes on the development and progression of long-term complications in insulin-dependent diabetes mellitus. N Engl J Med 1993;329: 977–86.

Relative to rates in the conventional treatment arm, intensive therapy reduced onset and progression of diabetic retinopathy by 76% and 54%, respectively, occurrence of nephropathy by 54%, and onset of neuropathy by 60%.

Diabetes Control and Complications Trial Research Group. Expanded role of the dietician in the Diabetes Control and Complications Trial: implications for clinical practice. J Am Diet Assoc 1993;93:758–64, 767.

Diabetes Control and Complications Trial Research Group. Nutrition interventions for intensive therapy in the Diabetes Control and Complications Trial. J Am Diet Assoc 1993;93: 768–72.

Diabetes Control and Complications Trial Research Group. Effect of intensive diabetes treatment on the development and progression of long-term complications in adolescents with insulin-dependent diabetes mellitus: Diabetes Control and Complications Trial. J Pediatr 1994;125:177–88.

In the DCCT cohort of young patients (13–17 years old), intensive control reduced the risk of development and progression of retinopathy compared to conventional treatment by 53% and 70%, respectively.

Diabetes Control and Complications Trial Research Group. A screening algorithm to identify clinically significant changes in neuropsychological functions in the Diabetes Control and Complications Trial. J Clin Exp Neuropsychol 1994;16: 303–16.

Diabetes Control and Complications Trial Research Group. The effect of intensive diabetes treatment on the progression of diabetic retinopathy in insulin-dependent diabetes mellitus. The Diabetes Control and Complications Trial. Arch Ophthalmol 1995;113:36–51.

Intensive therapy significantly reduced the risk of a three-step progression of retinopathy to 12% compared to 54% in the conventional therapy group.

Diabetes Control and Complications Trial Research Group. Progression of retinopathy with intensive versus conventional treatment in the Diabetes Control and Complications Trial. Ophthalmology 1995;102:647–61.

Intensive therapy reduced the risk of development of any retinopathy to 70% from 90% in the conventional treatment arm and also reduced the risk of progression. Intensive therapy was most effective when initiated early after diagnosis of insulin-dependent diabetes mellitus.

Diabetes Control and Complications Trial Research Group. Implementation of treatment protocols in the Diabetes Control and Complications Trial. Diabetes Care 1995;18:361–76.

Diabetes Control and Complications Trial (DCCT) Research Group. Effect of intensive diabetes management on macrovascular events and risk factors in the Diabetes Control and Complications Trial. Am J Cardiol 1995;75:894–903.

Diabetes Control and Complications Trial Research Group. The relationship of glycemic exposure (HbA1c) to the risk of development and progression of retinopathy in the Diabetes Control and Complications Trial. Diabetes 1995;44:968–83.

Diabetes Control and Complications Trial (DCCT) Research Group. Effect of intensive diabetes treatment on nerve conduction in the Diabetes Control and Complications Trial. Ann Neurol 1995;38:869–80.

Diabetes Control and Complications Trial Research Group. Influence of intensive diabetes treatment on quality-of-life outcomes in the Diabetes Control and Complications Trial. Diabetes Care 1996;19:195–203.

Diabetes Control and Complications Trial Research Group. The absence of a glycemic threshold for the development of long-term complications: the perspective of the Diabetes Control and Complications Trial. Diabetes 1996;45:1289–98.

Diabetes Control and Complications Trial Research Group. Lifetime benefits and costs of intensive therapy as practiced in the Diabetes Control and Complications Trial. JAMA 1996;276: 1400–15.

Diabetes Control and Complications Trial Research Group. Pregnancy outcomes in the Diabetes Control and Complications Trial. Am J Obstet Gynecol 1996;174:1343–53.

Diabetes Control and Complications Trial Research Group. Effect of intensive therapy on residual β-cell function in patients with type I diabetes in the Diabetes Control and Complications Trial. Ann Intern Med 1998;128:517–23.

Diabetes Control and Complications Trial Research Group. Early worsening of diabetic retinopathy in the Diabetes Control and Complications Trial. Arch Ophthalmol 1998;116:874–86.

Epidemiology of Diabetes Interventions and Complications (EDIC) Research Group. Design, implementation, and preliminary results of a long-term follow-up of the Diabetes Control and Complications Trial cohort. Diabetes Care 1999;22:99–111.

Epidemiology of Diabetes Interventions and Complications (EDIC) Research Group. Effect of intensive diabetes treatment on carotid artery wall thickness in the Epidemiology of Diabetes Interventions and Complications. Diabetes 1999;48:383–90.

Diabetes Control and Complications Trial/Epidemiology of Diabetes Interventions and Complications Research Group. Retinopathy and nephropathy in patients with type I diabetes four years after a trial of intensive therapy. N Engl J Med 2000;342:381–9.

The intensive therapy group continued to demonstrate a persistent reduction in the risk of progressive retinopathy and nephropathy compared to the conventional therapy group 4 years after the conclusion of the DCCT.

Diabetes Control and Complications Trial Research Group. Effect of pregnancy on microvascular complications in the Diabetes Control and Complications Trial. Diabetes Care 2000;23: 1084–91.

Diabetes Control and Complications Trial (DCCT)/ Epidemiology of Diabetes Interventions and Complications (EDIC) Research Group. Beneficial effects of intensive therapy of diabetes during adolescence: outcomes after the conclusion of the Diabetes Control and Complications Trial (DCCT). J Pediatr 2001;139:804–12.

Diabetes Control and Complications Trial Research Group. Influence of intensive diabetes treatment on body weight and composition of adults with type 1 diabetes in the Diabetes Control and Complications Trial. Diabetes Care 2001;24: 1711–21.

Writing Team for the Diabetes Control and Complications Trial/ Epidemiology of Diabetes Interventions and Complications Research Group. Effect of intensive therapy on the microvascular complications of type 1 diabetes mellitus. JAMA 2002; 287:2563–9.

Diabetes Control and Complications Trials/Epidemiology of Diabetes Interventions and Complications Research Group. Intensive diabetes therapy and carotid intima-media thickness in type 1 diabetes mellitus. N Engl J Med 2003;348: 2294–303.

Writing Team for the Diabetes Control and Complications Trial/Epidemiology of Diabetes Interventions and Complications Research Group. Sustained effect of intensive treatment of type 1 diabetes mellitus on development and progression of diabetic nephropathy: the Epidemiology of Diabetes Interventions and Complications (EDIC) Study. JAMA 2003;290(16): 2159–67.

Lyons TJ, Jenkins AJ, Zheng D, et al. Diabetic retinopathy and serum lipoprotein subclasses in the DCCT/EDIC cohort. Invest Ophthalmol Vis Sci 2004;45:910–8.

Nathan DM, Cleary PA, Backlund JY, et al. for the Diabetes Control and Complications Trial/Epidemiology of Diabetes Interventions and Complications (DCCT/EDIC) Study Research Group. Intensive diabetes treatment and cardiovascular disease in patients with type 1 diabetes. N Engl J Med 2005;353(25): 2643–53.

Steffes M, Cleary P, Goldstein D, et al. Hemoglobin A1c measurements over nearly two decades: sustaining comparable values throughout the Diabetes Control and Complications Trial and the Epidemiology of Diabetes Interventions and Complications Study. Clin Chem 2005;51(4):753–8.

Diabetes Control and Complications Trial/Epidemiology of Diabetes Interventions and Complications Research Group. Prolonged effect of intensive therapy on the risk of retinopathy complications in patients with type 1 diabetes mellitus. Arch Ophthalmol 2008;126(12):1707–15.

Hubbard LD, Sun W, Cleary PA, et al. for the Diabetes Control and Complications Trial/Epidemiology of Diabetes Interventions and Complications Study Research Group. Comparison of digital and film grading of diabetic retinopathy severity in the Diabetes Control and Complications Trial/Epidemiology of Diabetes Interventions and Complications Study. Arch Ophthalmol 2011;129(6):718–26.

UK Prospective Diabetes Study (UKPDS)

Since 1983, the UKPDS investigators have published more than 75 articles to report findings from this prospective study.

United Kingdom Prospective Diabetes Study Group. UK Prospective Study of Therapies of Maturity-Onset Diabetes. I: Effect of diet, sulphonylurea, insulin or biguanide therapy on fasting plasma glucose and body weight over 1 year. Diabetelogia 1983;24:404–11.

United Kingdom Prospective Study Group. United Kingdom Prospective Diabetes Study. III. Prevalence of hypertension and hypotensive therapy in patients with newly diagnosed diabetes. Hypertension 1985;7(Suppl 2):8–13.

United Kingdom Prospective Study Group. United Kingdom Prospective Diabetes Study. IV. Characteristics of newly-presenting type 2 diabetic patients: male preponderance and obesity at different ages. Diabetic Med 1988;5:154–9.

United Kingdom Prospective Diabetes Study Group. United Kingdom Prospective Diabetes Study. VI. Complications in newly diagnosed type 2 diabetic patients and their association with different clinical and biochemical risk factors. Diabetes Res 1990;13:1–11.

United Kingdom Prospective Diabetes Study Group. UK Prospective Diabetes Study (UKPDS): VIII. Study design, progress and performance. Diabetologia 1991;34:877–90.

United Kingdom Prospective Diabetes Study Group. UK Prospective Diabetes Study IX: Relationships of urinary albumin and N-acetylglucosaminidase to glycemia and hypertension at diagnosis of type 2 (non-insulin-dependent) diabetes mellitus and after 3 months diet therapy. Diabetologia 1992;36:835–42.

United Kingdom Prospective Diabetes Study Group. UK Prospective Diabetes Study (UKPDS) XII. Differences between Asian, Afro-Caribbean, and White Caucasian type 2 diabetic patients at diagnosis of diabetes. Diabetic Med 1994;11:670–7.

Kohner EM, Aldington SJ, Stratton IM, et al. United Kingdom Prospective Diabetes Study, 30: Diabetic retinopathy at diagnosis of non-insulin-dependent diabetes mellitus and associated risk factors. Arch Ophthalmol 1998;116:297–303.

United Kingdom Prospective Diabetes Study Group. Intensive blood-glucose control with sulphonylureas or insulin compared with conventional treatment and risk of complications in patients with type 2 diabetes (UKPDS 33). Lancet 1998;352: 837–53.

Over a 10-year period, a 25% risk reduction in microvascular endpoints was observed in the intensive treatment group (median hemoglobin (Hb) A1c 7.0%) compared with the conventional treatment group (median HbA1c 7.9%).

United Kingdom Prospective Diabetes Study (UKPDS) Group. Tight blood pressure control and risk of macrovascular and microvascular complications in type 2 diabetes: UKPDS 38. Br Med J 1998;317:705–13.

Tight blood pressure control (mean, 144/82 mmHg) compared to lesser control (mean, 154/87 mmHg) reduced progression rates of diabetic retinopathy and deterioration of visual acuity.

United Kingdom Prospective Diabetes Study Group. Efficacy of atenolol and captopril in reducing risk of macrovascular and microvascular complications in type 2 diabetes: UKPDS 39. Br Med J 1998;317:713–20.

United Kingdom Prospective Diabetes Study Group. Cost effectiveness of improved blood glucose control in hypertensive patients with type 2 diabetes: UKPDS 40. Br Med J 1998;317: 720–6.

Stratton IM, Kohner EM, Aldington SJ, et al. UKPDS 50: Risk factors for incidence and progression of retinopathy in type II diabetes over 6 years from diagnosis. Diabetologia 2001;44: 156–63.

Of 1216 patients without retinopathy at diagnosis of type 2 diabetes, 22% had developed retinopathy (microaneurysms or worse in both eyes) by 6 years after diagnosis. HbA1c was strongly associated with incidence and, especially, progression of retinopathy. Incidence of retinopathy also was strongly associated with systolic blood pressure. Smoking was associated with a reduced incidence of retinopathy.

Gray A, Clarke P, Farmer A, et al. Implementing intensive control of blood glucose concentration and blood pressure in type 2 diabetes in England: cost analysis (UKPDS 63). Br Med J 2002;325:860–5.

UK Prospective Diabetes Study (UKPDS) Group. Risks of progression of retinopathy and vision loss related to tight blood pressure control in type 2 diabetes mellitus (UKPDS 69). Arch Ophthalmol 2004;122:1631–40.

Stratton IM, Cull CA, Adler AI, et al. Additive effects of glycaemia and blood pressure exposure on risk of complications in type 2 diabetes: a prospective observational study (UKPDS 75). Diabetologia 2006;49:1761–9.

Diabetic Retinopathy Clinical Research Network (DRCR.net)

The DRCR.net investigators have conducted a number of randomized clinical trials and observational studies of diabetic retinopathy. A complete list of publications from the DRCR.net is maintained on the DRCR.net Public Web Site (http://drcrnet.jaeb.org/Publications.aspx [cited 2012 27 Feb]).

Diabetic Retinopathy Clinical Research Network. Diurnal variation in retinal thickening measurement by optical coherence tomography in center-involved diabetic macular edema. Arch Ophthalmol 2006;124:1701–7.

Diabetic Retinopathy Clinical Research Network. Reproducibility of macular thickness and volume using Zeiss optical coherence tomography in patients with diabetic macular edema. Ophthalmology 2007;114:1520–5.

Diabetic Retinopathy Clinical Research Network. A phase 2 randomized clinical trial of intravitreal bevacizumab for diabetic macular edema. Ophthalmology 2007;114(10):1860–7.

Bhavsar AR, Ip MS, Glassman AR for the DRCRnet and the SCORE Study Group. The risk of enophthalmitis following intravitreal triamcinolone injection in the DRCRnet and SCORE clinical trials. Am J Ophthalmol 2007;144:454–6.

Writing Committee for the Diabetic Retinopathy Clinical Research Network. Comparison of the modified Early Treatment Diabetic Retinopathy Study and mild macular grid laser photocoagulation strategies for diabetic macular edema. Arch Ophthalmol 2007;124:469–80.

Bressler NM, Edwards AR, Antoszyk AN, et al. on behalf of the Diabetic Retinopathy Clinical Research Network. Retinal thickness on Stratus optical coherence tomography in people with diabetes and minimal or no diabetic retinopathy. Am J Ophthalmol 2008;145:894–901.

Diabetic Retinopathy Clinical Research Network. A randomized trial comparing intravitreal triamcinolone acetonide and focal/grid photocoagulation for diabetic macular edema. Ophthalmology 2008;115:1447–59.

Scott IU, Bressler NM, Bressler SB, et al. and the Diabetic Retinopathy Clinical Research Network. Agreement between clinician and reading center gradings of diabetic retinopathy severity level at baseline in a phase 2 study of intravitreal bevacizumab for diabetic macular edema. Retina 2008;28: 38–40.

Browning DJ, Altaweel MM, Bressler NM, et al. on behalf of the Diabetic Retinopathy Clinical Research Network. Diabetic macular edema: What is focal and what is diffuse? Am J Ophthalmol 2008;146:649–55.

Diabetic Retinopathy Clinical Research Network. Three-year follow up of a randomized trial comparing focal/grid photocoagulation and intravitreal triamcinolone for diabetic macular edema. Arch Ophthalmol 2009;127(3):245–51.

Bressler NM, Edwards AR, Beck RW, et al. for the Diabetic Retinopathy Clinical Research Network. Exploratory analysis of diabetic retinopathy progression through 3 years in a randomized clinical trial that compares intravitreal triamcinolone acetonide with focal/grid photocoagulation. Arch Ophthalmol 2009; 127(12):1566–71.

Diabetic Retinopathy Clinical Research Network. Observational study of the development of diabetic macular edema following panretinal (scatter) photocoagulation given in 1 or 4 sittings. Arch Ophthalmol 2009;127(2):132–40.

Sun JK, Aiello LP, Stockman M, et al. for the Diabetic Retinopathy Clinical Research Network. Effects of dilation on electronic-ETDRS visual acuity (EVA) in diabetic patients. Invest Ophthalmol Vis Sci 2009;50(4):1580–4.

Diabetic Retinopathy Clinical Research Network Writing Committee. Vitrectomy outcomes in eyes with diabetic macular edema and vitreomacular traction. Ophthalmology 2010;117: 1087–93.

Diabetic Retinopathy Clinical Research Network Writing Committee: Googe J, Brucker AJ, Bressler NM, et al. Randomized trial evaluating short-term effects of intravitreal ranibizumab or triamcinolone acetonide on macular edema after focal/grid laser for diabetic macular edema in eyes also receiving panretinal photocoagulation. Retina 2011;31: 1009–27.

Diabetic Retinopathy Clinical Research Network. Randomized trial evaluating ranibizumab plus prompt or deferred laser or triamcinolone plus prompt laser for diabetic macular edema. Ophthalmology 2010;117:1064–77.

Diabetic Retinopathy Clinical Research Network. Expanded 2-year follow-up of ranibizumab plus prompt or deferred laser or triamcinolone plus prompt laser for diabetic macular edema. Ophthalmology 2011;118:609–14.

Other diabetic retinopathy trials

Chaturvedi N, Sjolie A-K, Stephenson JM, et al. and the EUCLID Study Group. Effect of lisinopril on progression of retinopathy in normotensive people with type 1 diabetes. Lancet 1998;351: 28–31.

Keech AC, Mitchell P, Summanen PA, et al. for the FIELD study investigators. Effect of fenofibrate on the need for laser treatment for diabetic retinopathy (FIELD study): a randomised controlled trial. Lancet 2007;370:1687–97.

Sjolie AK, Klein R, Porta M, et al. for the DIRECT Programme Study Group. Effect of candesartan on progression and regression of retinopathy in type 2 diabetes (DIRECT-Protect 2): a randomised placebo-controlled trial. Lancet 2008;372:1385–93.

Chaturvedi N, Porta M, Klein R, et al. for the DIRECT Programme Study Group. Effect of candesartan on prevention (DIRECT-Prevent 1) and progression (DIRECT-Protect 1) of retinopathy in type 1 diabetes: randomised, placebo-controlled trials. Lancet 2008;372:1394–402.

Stolk RP, Vingerling JR, Cruickshank JK, et al. on behalf of the AdRem project team and ADVANCE management committee. Rationale and design of the AdRem study: Evaluating the effects of blood pressure lowering and intensive glucose control on vascular retinal disorders in patients with type 2 diabetes mellitus. Contemp Clin Trials 2007;28:6–17.

Stolk RP, Thom SAMcG, van Schooneveld MJ, et al. on behalf of the AdRem Project Team and ADVANCE Management Committee. Retinal vascular lesions in patients with Caucasian and Asian origin with type 2 diabetes. Baseline results from the ADVANCE Retinal Measurements (AdRem) study. Diabetes Care 2008;31:708–13.

Beulens JWJ, Patel A, Vingerling JR, et al. on behalf of the AdRem project team and ADVANCE management committee. Effects of blood pressure lowering and intensive glucose control on the incidence and progression of retinopathy in patients with type 2 diabetes mellitus: a randomised controlled trial. Diabetologia 2009;52:2027–36.

Lee CC, Stolk RP, Adler AI, et al. on behalf of the AdRem project team and ADVANCE management committee. Association between alcohol consumption and diabetic retinopathy and visual acuity – the AdRem Study. Diabet Med 2010;27: 1130–7.

Chew EY, Ambrosium WT, Howard LT, et al. for the ACCORD Study Group. Rationale, design, and methods of the Action to Control Cardiovascular Risk in Diabetes Eye Study (ACCORD-EYE). Am J Cardiol 2007;99(Suppl):103i-111i.

ACCORD Study Group and ACCORD Eye Study Group. Effects of medical therapies on retinopathy progression in type 2 diabetes. N Engl J Med 2010;363:233–44.

Ambrosius WT, Danis RP, Goff DC, et al. for the ACCORD Study Group. Lack of association between thiazolidinediones and macular edema in type 2 diabetes. Arch Ophthalmol 2010;128(3):312–8.

Ahmadieh H, Shoeibi N, Entezari M, et al. Intravitreal bevacizumab for prevention of early postvitrectomy hemorrhage in diabetic patients. A randomized clinical trial. Ophthalmology 2009;116:1943–8.

Gillies MC, Simpson JM, Gaston C, et al. Five-year results of a randomized trial with open-label extension of triamcinolone acetonide for refractory diabetic macular edema. Ophthalmology 2009;116:2182–7.

Nguyen QD, Shah SM, Heier JS, et al. for the READ-2 Study Group. Primary end point (six months) results of the Ranibizumab for Edema of the mAcula in Diabetes (READ-2) Study. Ophthalmology 2009;116:2175–81.

Nguyen QD, Shah SM, Khwaja AA, et al. for the READ-2 Study Group. Two-year outcomes of the Ranibizumab for Edema of the mAcula in Diabetes (READ-2) Study. Ophthalmology 2010;117: 2146–51.

Haller JA, Kuppermann BD, Blumenkranz MS, et al. for the Dexamethasone DDS Phase II Study Group. Randomized controlled trial of an intravitreous dexamethasone drug delivery system in patients with diabetic macular edema. Arch Ophthalmol 2010;128(3):289–96.

Mitchell P, Bandello F, Schmidt-Erfurth U, et al. on behalf of the RESTORE study group. The RESTORE Study. Ranibizumab monotherapy or combined with laser versus laser monotherapy for diabetic macular edema. Ophthalmology 2011;118:615–25.

VEIN OCCLUSIONS

Cochrane Systematic Review

Braithwaite T, Nanji AA, Greenberg PB. Anti-vascular endothelial growth factor for macular edema secondary to central retinal vein occlusion. Cochrane Database of Systematic Review 2010, Issue 10, Art. No.: CD007325. DOI: 10.1002/14651858.CD007325.pub2.

Branch Vein Occlusion Study (BVOS)

The BVOS was a multicenter randomized clinical trial sponsored by the National Eye Inistitute and designed to assess in eyes with retinal branch vein occlusion whether scatter photocoagulation with the argon laser could prevent development of neovascularization and peripheral scatter photocoagulation could prevent vitreous hemorrhage, and whether macular photocoagulation would improve visual acuity in eyes with macular edema and visual acuity of 20/40 or worse. BVOS findings are discussed in Chapter 53 Branch retinal vein occlusion.

Finkelstein D, Clarkson J, Diddie K, et al. Branch vein occlusion: retinal neovascularization outside the involved segment. Ophthalmology 1982;89:1357–61.

Branch Vein Occlusion Study Group. Argon laser photocoagulation for macular edema in branch vein occlusion. Am J Ophthalmol 1984;98:271–82.

Argon laser photocoagulation improved visual acuity in eyes with macular edema secondary to retinal branch vein occlusion, macular edema, and visual acuity of 20/40 or worse, with a gain of 2 or more lines of visual acuity in more laser-treated eyes than untreated eyes.

Branch Vein Occlusion Study Group. Argon laser scatter photocoagulation for prevention of neovascularization and vitreous hemorrhage in branch vein occlusion: a randomized clinical trial. Arch Ophthalmol 1986;104:34–41.

Peripheral scatter argon laser photocoagulation decreased the risk of vitreous hemorrhage compared to untreated eyes. In addition, scatter treatment before development of neovascularization was not beneficial; treatment after development of neovascularization was recommended.

Central Vein Occlusion Study (CVOS)

The CVOS included two randomized trials and two observational studies in its design. The goals of the CVOS were: (1) to determine whether photocoagulation therapy could prevent iris neovascularization in eyes with central vein occlusion and evidence of ischemic retina; (2) to assess whether grid photocoagulation could reduce loss of central visual acuity due to macular edema secondary to central vein occlusion; (3) to describe the course and prognosis for eyes with central vein occlusion. Patients were divided into four groups at entry: (1) perfused; (2) nonperfused; (3) indeterminate perfusion; or (4) macular edema. Findings from the CVOS are discussed in Chapter 54 (Central retinal vein occlusion).

Central Vein Occlusion Study Group. Central Vein Occlusion Study of photocoagulation therapy. Baseline findings. Online J Curr Clin Trials 1993,Oct 14; Doc. No. 95.

Central Vein Occlusion Study Group. Baseline and early natural history report. The Central Vein Occlusion Study. Arch Ophthalmol 1993;111:1087–95.

Clarkson JG. Central Vein Occlusion Study: Photographic protocol and early natural history. Trans Am Ophthalmol Soc 1994;92:203–13.

Central Vein Occlusion Study Group. Evaluation of grid pattern photocoagulation for macular edema in central vein occlusion. The Central Vein Occlusion Study Group M report. Ophthalmology 1995;102:1425–33.

Macular grid photocoagulation reduced macular edema but did not provide a better visual acuity outcome than no treatment.

Central Vein Occlusion Study Group. A randomized clinical trial of early panretinal photocoagulation for ischemic central vein occlusion. The Central Vein Occlusion Study Group N report. Ophthalmology 1995;102:1434–4.

Prophylactic panretinal photocoagulation decreased development of angle neovascularization or 2 or more clock-hours of iris neovascularization but did not prevent neovascularization. These findings suggest that photocoagulation should be administered at the time neovascularization is detected.

Central Vein Occlusion Study Group. Natural history and clinical management of central retinal vein occlusion. Arch Ophthalmol 1997;115:486–91.

Standard Care vs COrticosteroid for REtinal Vein Occlusion Study (SCORE)

SCORE is a multicenter study sponsored by the National Eye Institute that includes two randomized trials of intravitreal triamcinolone, one for patients with central vein occlusion and one for patients with branch vein occlusion.

Scott IU, Vanveldhuisen PC, Oden N, et al., SCORE Study Investigator Group. SCORE Study report 1: Baseline associations between cenral retinal thickness and visual acuity in patients with retinal vein occlusion. Ophthalmology 2009;116(3): 504–12.

Scott IU, Blodi BA, Ip MS, et al., SCORE Study Investigator Group. SCORE Study report 2: Interobserver agreement between investigator and reading center classification of retinal vein occlusion type. Ophthalmology 2009;116(4):756–61.

Ip MS, Oden NL, Scott IU, et al., SCORE Study Investigator Group. SCORE Study report 3: Study design and baseline characteristics. Ophthalmology 2009;116(9):1770–7.

Domalpally A, Blodi BA, Scott IU, et al., SCORE Study Investigator Group. The Standard Care vs. Corticosteroid for Retinal Vein Occlusion (SCORE) Study system for evaluation of optical coherence tomograms: SCORE Study report no. 4. Arch Ophthalmol 2009;127(11):1461–7.

Ip MS, Scott IU, VanVeldhuisen PC, et al., SCORE Study Research Group. A randomized trial comparing the efficacy and safety of intravitreal triamcinolone with observation to treat vision loss associated with macular edema secondary to central vein occlusion: Standard Care vs Corticosteroid for Retinal Vein Occlusion (SCORE) Study report no.5. Arch Ophthalmol 2009;127(6): 1101–4.

Scott IU, Ip MS, VanVeldhuisen PC, et al., SCORE Study Research Group. A randomized trial comparing the efficacy and safety of intravitreal triamcinolone with standard care to treat vision loss associated with macular edema secondary to branch retinal vein occlusion: Standard Care vs Corticosteroid for Retinal Vein Occlusion (SCORE) Study report no. 6. Arch Ophthalmol 2009; 127(9):1115–28.

Scott IU, Oden NL, VanVeldhuissen PC, et al., SCORE Study Investigator Group. SCORE Study report 7: Incidence of intravitreal silicone oil droplets associated with staked-on vs luer cone syringe design. Am J Ophthalmol 2009;148(5):725–32.

Oden N, VanVeldhuisen PC, Scott IU, Ip MS, SCORE Study Investigator Group. SCORE Study report 8: Closed tests for all pairwise comparisons of means. Drug Inform J 2010;44: 405–20.

Blodi BA, Domalpally AM, Scott IU, et al. for the SCORE Study Research Group. Standard care vs. corticosteroid for retinal vein occlusion (SCORE) Study system for evaluation of stereoscopic color fundus photographs and fluorescein angiograms. SCORE Study Report 9. Arch Ophthalmol 2010;128(9):1140–5.

Scott IU, VanVeldhuisen PC, Oden NL, for the Standard Care versus COrticosteroid for REtinal Vein Occlusion Study Investigator Group. Baseline predictors of visual acuity and retinal thickness outcomes in patients with retinal vein occlusion: Standard Care versus Corticosteroid for Retinal Vein Occlusion Study report 10. Ophthalmology 2011;118:345–52.

Chan CK, Ip MS, VanVeldhuisen PC, et al. for the SCORE Study Investigator Group. SCORE Study report no. 11. Incidences of neovascular events in eyes with retinal vein occlusion. Ophthalmology 2011;118:1364–72.

Other clinical trials for vein occlusion

Campochiaro PA, Heier JS, Feiner L, et al. for the BRAVO Investigators. Ranibizumab for macular edema following branch retinal vein occlusion. Six-month primary end point results of a phase III study. Ophthalmology 2010;117:1102–12.

Brown DM, Campochiaro PA, Bhisitkul RB, et al. Sustained benefit from ranibizumab for macular edema following branch retinal vein occlusions: 12-month outcomes of a phase III study. Ophthalmology 2011;118:1594–602.

Brown DM, Campochiaro PA, Singh RP, et al for the CRUISE Investigators. Ranibizumab for macular edema following central retinal vein occulusion. Six-month primary end point results of a phase III study. Ophthalmology 2010;117:1124–39.

AGE-RELATED MACULAR DEGENERATION AND OTHER CONDITIONS ASSOCIATED WITH CHOROIDAL NEOVASCULARIZATION

Findings from many of the trials listed below are discussed in Chapters 66 (Neovascular (Exudative or "Wet") Age-Related Macular Degeneration), 67 (Pharmacotherapy of Age-Related Macular Degeneration), 68 (Myopic macular degeneration) 70 (Ocular Histoplasmosis). Because of the numerous trials that have been conducted for these conditions during the past three decades, the clinical trials cited have been subdivided into treatment trials and prevention trials.

TREATMENT TRIALS

Macular Photocoagulation Study (MPS)

The MPS was initiated in 1979 under the sponsorship of the National Eye Institute to evaluate laser photocoagulation for choroidal neovascularization secondary to age-related macular degeneration and ocular histoplasmosis. In addition, small trials of laser photocoagulation for idiopathic choroidal neovascularization were conducted. The MPS Group conducted three multicenter randomized trials of argon laser photocoagulation of extrafoveal choroidal neovascularization (begun in 1979), three trials of krypton laser photocoagulation for juxtafoveal neovascular lesions (begun in 1981), and two trials of laser photocoagulation (with a second randomization of eyes assigned to laser photocoagulation between argon green and krypton red laser) of subfoveal choroidal neovascularization secondary to age-related macular degeneration only (begun in 1985).

Macular Photocoagulation Study Group. Argon laser photocoagulation for senile macular degeneration: results of a randomized clinical trial. Arch Ophthalmol 1982;100:912–8.

After fewer than half the eyes in each treatment arm had been followed for 1 year, severe loss of visual acuity from the baseline levels (loss of six or more lines on a logMar chart) was observed among 25% of laser-treated eyes versus 60% of untreated eyes, the first indication that any treatment for choroidal neovascularization was able to delay or prevent loss of visual acuity.

Macular Photocoagulation Study Group. Argon laser photocoagulation for ocular histoplasmosis: results of a randomized clinical trial. Arch Ophthalmol 1983;101:1347–57.

Laser photocoagulation of extrafoveal choroidal neovascularization was even more effective in eyes with ocular histoplasmosis than in eyes with age-related macular degeneration. By 2 years after enrollment, only 13% of laser-treated eyes versus 46% of untreated eyes had visual acuity 6 or more lines worse than at baseline.

Macular Photocoagulation Study Group. Argon laser photocoagulation for idiopathic neovascularization: results of a randomized clinical trial. Arch Ophthalmol 1983;101:1358–61.

Among a much smaller number of eyes with idiopathic extrafoveal choroidal neovascularization, the findings with respect to severe loss of visual acuity were intermediate between those of the other two MPS trials for extrafoveal lesions.

Macular Photocoagulation Study Group. Changing the protocol: a case report from the Macular Photocoagulation Study. Control Clin Trials 1984;5:203–16.

Macular Photocoagulation Study Group. Recurrent choroidal neovascularization after argon laser photocoagulation for neovascular maculopathy. Arch Ophthalmol 1986;104:503–12.

After more than 80% of the 284 eyes that initially had extrafoveal choroidal neovascularization had been followed for 3 years or more, 59% of eyes with age-related macular degeneration, 30% of eyes with ocular histoplasmosis, and 33% of eyes with idiopathic choroidal neovascularization had recurrent choroidal neovascularization documented at one or more follow-up examinations.

Macular Photocoagulation Study Group. Argon laser photocoagulation for neovascular maculopathy: three-year results from randomized clinical trials. Arch Ophthalmol 1986;104:694–701.

Initial reports of the effectiveness of laser photocoagulation were confirmed with follow-up for 3 years or longer of patients in all three trials for eyes with extrafoveal choroidal neovascularization.

Macular Photocoagulation Study Group. Krypton laser photocoagulation for neovascular lesions of ocular histoplasmosis: results of a randomized clinical trial. Arch Ophthalmol 1987;105: 1499–1507.

The effect of laser photocoagulation of juxtafoveal choroidal neovascular lesions of ocular histoplasmosis was equally dramatic as when used to treat extrafoveal lesions: 6% versus 26% with severe visual acuity loss from baseline by the 3-year examination.

Macular Photocoagulation Study Group. Persistent and recurrent neovascularization after krypton laser photocoagulation for neovascular lesions of ocular histoplasmosis. Arch Ophthalmol 1989;107:344–52.

Blackhurst DW, Maguire MG, the Macular Photocoagulation Study Group. Reproducibility of refraction and visual acuity measurement under a standard protocol. Retina 1989;9:163–9.

Chamberlin JA, Bressler NM, Bressler SB, et al. The use of fundus photographs and fluorescein angiograms in the identification and treatment of choroidal neovascularization in the Macular Photocoagulation Study. Ophthalmology 1989;96:1526–34.

Macular Photocoagulation Study Group. Krypton laser photocoagulation for neovascular lesions of age-related macular degeneration: results of a clinical trial. Arch Ophthalmol 1990;108:816–24.

Three years after enrollment, 49% of laser-treated eyes versus 58% of untreated eyes that enrolled with juxtafoveal neovascular lesions had lost 6 or more lines of visual acuity from baseline. Laser treatment was recommended only for patients without definite hypertension.

Macular Photocoagulation Study Group. Persistent and recurrent neovascularization after krypton laser photocoagulation for neovascular lesions of age-related macular degeneration. Arch Ophthalmol 1990;108:825–31.

Macular Photocoagulation Study Group. Krypton laser photocoagulation for idiopathic neovascular lesions: results of a randomized clinical trial. Arch Ophthalmol 1990;108:832–7.

Bressler SB, Maguire MG, Bressler NM, et al. Relationship of drusen and abnormalities of the retinal pigment epithelium to the prognosis of neovascular macular degeneration. Arch Ophthalmol 1990;108:1442–7.

Large drusen and focal hyperpigmentation were risk factors for development of choroidal neovascularization in the fellow eye. Also, the risk of recurrent neovascularization was nearly three times higher among study eyes after laser treatment of extrafoveal choroidal neovascularization for patients who had large drusen in the fellow eye at baseline compared to those who did not.

Folk JC, Blackhurst DW, Alexander J, et al. Pretreatment fundus characteristics as predictors of recurrent choroidal neovascularization. Arch Ophthalmol 1991;109:1193–4.

Bressler NM, Bressler SB, Alexander J, et al. Loculated fluid: a previously undescribed fluorescein angiographic finding in choroidal neovascularization associated with macular degeneration. Arch Ophthalmol 1991;109:211–5.

Macular Photocoagulation Study Group. Argon laser photocoagulation for neovascular maculopathy: five-year results from randomized clinical trials. Arch Ophthalmol 1991;109:1109–14.

The benefits of laser photocoagulation of extrafoveal choroidal neovascularization due either to age-related macular degeneration or to ocular histoplasmosis and of idiopathic extrafoveal choroidal neovascularization persisted through 5 years of follow-up.

Macular Photocoagulation Study Group. Laser photocoagulation of subfoveal neovascular lesions in age-related macular degeneration: results of a randomized clinical trial. Arch Ophthalmol 1991;109:1220–31.

Despite initially larger losses of visual acuity from baseline among laser-treated than untreated eyes, by 2 years after entry, 21% of laser-treated eyes versus 38% of untreated eyes had visual acuity that was 6 or more lines worse than at baseline.

Macular Photocoagulation Study Group. Laser photocoagulation of subfoveal recurrent neovascular lesions in age-related macular degeneration: results of a randomized clinical trial. Arch Ophthalmol 1991;109:1232–41.

Laser photocoagulation was particularly effective for subfoveal recurrent choroidal neovascularization, with only 10% of laser-treated eyes versus 32% of untreated eyes having visual acuity six or more lines worse at the 2-year examination than at baseline.

Macular Photocoagulation Study Group. Subfoveal neovascular lesions in age-related macular degeneration: guidelines for evaluation and treatment in the Macular Photocoagulation Study. Arch Ophthalmol 1991;109:1242–57.

Fine SL, Wood WJ, Singerman LJ, et al. Laser treatment for subfoveal neovascular membranes in ocular histoplasmosis syndrome: results of a pilot randomized clinical trial. Arch Ophthalmol 1993;111:19–20.

Orr PR, Blackhurst DW, Hawkins BS. Patient and clinic factors predictive of missed visits and inactive status in a multicenter clinical trial. Control Clin Trials 1992;13:40–9.

Macular Photocoagulation Study Group. Five-year follow-up of fellow eyes of patients with age-related macular degeneration and unilateral extrafoveal choroidal neovascularization. Arch Ophthalmol 1993;111:1189–99.

Choroidal neovascularization developed in fellow eyes initially free of such lesions at a rate of approximately 5% per year during 5 years of follow-up.

Macular Photocoagulation Study Group. Laser photocoagulation of subfoveal neovascular lesions of age-related macular degeneration. Updated findings from two clinical trials. Arch Ophthalmol 1993;111:1200–9.

Macular Photocoagulation Study Group. Visual outcome after laser photocoagulation for subfoveal choroidal neovascularization secondary to age-related macular degeneration: the influence of initial lesion size and initial visual acuity. Arch Ophthalmol 1994;112:480–8.

Eyes with lesions larger than 2 disc areas and visual acuity of 20/160 or better had little or no benefit from treatment.

Macular Photocoagulation Study Group. Persistent and recurrent neovascularization after laser photocoagulation for subfoveal choroidal neovascularization of age-related macular degeneration. Arch Ophthalmol 1994;112:489–99.

Macular Photocoagulation Study Group. Laser photocoagulation for juxtafoveal choroidal neovascularization. Five-year results from randomized clinical trials. Arch Ophthalmol 1994;112:500–9.

Macular Photocoagulation Study (MPS) Group. Evaluation of argon green vs krypton red laser for photocoagulation of subfoveal choroidal neovascularization in the Macular Photocoagulation Study. Arch Ophthalmol 1994;112:1176–84.

Macular Photocoagulation Study Group. Laser photocoagulation for neovascular lesions nasal to the fovea. Results from clinical trials for lesions secondary to ocular histoplasmosis or idiopathic causes. Arch Ophthalmol 1995;113:56–61.

Macular Photocoagulation Study Group. The influence of treatment extent on the visual acuity of eyes treated with krypton laser for juxtafoveal choroidal neovascularization. Arch Ophthalmol 1995;113:190–4.

Macular Photocoagulation Study Group. Occult choroidal neovascularization. Influence on visual outcome in patients with age-related macular degeneration. Arch Ophthalmol 1995;114:400–12.

Macular Photocoagulation Study Group. Five-year follow-up of fellow eyes of individuals with ocular histoplasmosis and unilateral extrafoveal or juxtafoveal choroidal neovascularization. Arch Ophthalmol 1996;114:677–88.

Among fellow eyes free of choroidal neovascularization at the time patients enrolled in one of the MPS trials for eyes with ocular histoplasmosis, choroidal neovascularization developed in 9% within 5 years. New choroidal neovascular lesions developed in areas of the macula in which "atypical" histo spots were present earlier in follow-up.

Macular Photocoagulation Study Group. Risk factors for choroidal neovascularization in the second eye of patients with juxtafoveal or subfoveal choroidal neovascularization secondary to age-related macular degeneration. Arch Ophthalmol 1997;115:741–7.

Four independent risk factors were identified: (1) five or more drusen; (2) focal hyperpigmentation; (3) any large drusen; and (4) definite systemic hypertension. Five-year incidence of choroidal neovascularization in second eyes ranged from 7% in eyes with none of these risk factors to 87% of eyes with all four risk factors.

Jefferys JL, Alexander J, Hiner CJ, et al. for the Macular Photocoagulation Study Group. Reproducibility of gradings of retinal photographs of eyes with subfoveal choroidal neovascularization and age-related macular degeneration in the Macular Photocoagulation Study. Ophthalm Epidemiol 2008;15:191–201.

Other trials of laser treatment of choroidal neovascularization and a Cochrane systematic review

Coscas G, Soubrane G, Ramahefasolo C, et al. Perifoveal laser treatment for subfoveal choroidal new vessels in age-related macular degeneration. Results of a randomized clinical trial. Arch Ophthalmol 1991;109:1258–65.

Canadian Ophthalmology Study Group. Argon green vs krypton red laser photocoagulation of extrafoveal choroidal neovascular lesions. One-year results in age-related macular degeneration. Arch Ophthalmol 1993;111:181–5.

Canadian Ophthalmology Study Group. Argon green vs krypton red laser photocoagulation for extrafoveal choroidal neovascularization. One-year results in ocular histoplasmosis. Arch Ophthalmol 1994;112:1166–73.

Virgili G, Bini A. Laser photocoagulation for neovascular age-related macular degeneration. Cochrane Database of Systematic Reviews 2007, Issue 3, Art. No.: CD004763. DOI: 10.1002/14651858. CD004763.pub2.

Trials of photodynamic therapy with verteporfin (Visudyne) and a Cochrane systematic review

Multicenter randomized clinical trials of verteporfin were initiated in 1996 under industry sponsorship to evaluate safety and efficacy for treating subfoveal choroidal neovascularization secondary to age-related macular degeneration. The Verteporfin in Photodynamic Therapy (VIP) trial also investigated the use of verteporfin for subfoveal choroidal neovascularization secondary to pathologic myopia.

Treatment of Age-Related Macular Degeneration with Photodynamic Therapy (TAP) Study Group. Photodynamic therapy of subfoveal choroidal neovascularization in age-related macular degeneration with verteporfin: one-year results of 2 randomized clinical trials – TAP report 1. Arch Ophthalmol 1999;117:1329–45.

After 1 year of follow-up, 67% of eyes with predominantly classic subfoveal lesions assigned to verteporfin compared with 39% of eyes assigned to placebo had lost fewer than 15 letters of visual acuity from baseline.

Treatment of Age-Related Macular Degeneration with Photodynamic Therapy (TAP) Study Group. Photodynamic therapy of subfoveal choroidal neovascularization in age-related macular degeneration with verteporfin: two-year results of 2 randomized clinical trials – TAP report 2. Arch Ophthalmol 2001;119:198–207.

After 2 years of follow-up, 59% of eyes with predominantly classic subfoveal lesions assigned to verteporfin compared with 31% of eyes assigned to placebo had lost fewer than 15 letters of visual acuity from baseline.

Treatment of Age-Related Macular Degeneration with Photodynamic Therapy (TAP) Study Group. Verteporfin therapy of subfoveal choroidal neovascularization in patients with age-related macular degeneration: additional information regarding baseline lesion composition's impact on vision outcomes – TAP report no. 3. Arch Ophthalmol 2002;120:1443–54.

Rubin GS, Bressler NM, Treatment of Age-Related Macular Degeneration with Photodynamic Therapy (TAP) Study Group. Effects of verteporfin therapy on contrast sensitivity: results from the Treatment of Age-Related Macular Degeneration with Photodynamic Therapy (TAP) investigation – TAP report no. 4. Retina 2002;22:536–44.

Treatment of Age-Related Macular Degeneration with Photodynamic Therapy (TAP) Study Group. Verteporfin therapy for subfoveal choroidal neovascularization in age-related macular degeneration: three-year results of an open-label extension of 2 randomized clinical trials – TAP report no. 5. Arch Ophthalmol 2002;120:1307–14.

Bressler SB, Pieramici DJ, Koester JM, et al. Natural history of minimally classic subfoveal choroidal neovascular lesions in the Treatment of Age-Related Macular Degeneration with Photodynamic Therapy (TAP) investigation. Outcomes potentially relevant to management – TAP report no. 6. Arch Ophthalmol 2004;122:325–9.

Verteporfin in Photodynamic Therapy (VIP) Study Group. Photodynamic therapy of subfoveal choroidal neovascularization in pathologic myopia with verteporfin. 1-year results of a randomized clinical trial – VIP report no. 1. Ophthalmology 2001; 108:841–52.

After 1 year of follow-up, 72% of verteporfin-treated eyes compared with 44% of placebo-treated eyes lost fewer than eight letters, with 32% versus 15% improving at least five letters.

Verteporfin in Photodynamic Therapy Study Group. Verteporfin therapy of subfoveal choroidal neovascularization in age-related macular degeneration: two-year results of a randomized clinical trial including lesions with occult with no classic choroidal neovascularization – Verteporfin in Photodynamic Therapy report no. 2. Am J Ophthalmol 2001;131:541–60.

After 2 years of follow-up of patients with lesions composed of occult with no classic choroidal neovascularization who had recent disease progression, 55% of verteporfin-treated eyes compared with 68% of placebo-treated eyes lost at least 15 letters.

Verteporfin in Photodynamic Therapy (VIP) Study Group. Verteporfin therapy of subfoveal choroidal neovascularization in pathologic myopia: 2-year results of a randomized clinical trial – VIP report no. 3. Ophthalmology 2003;110:667–73.

After 2 years of follow-up, 36% of verteporfin-treated eyes compared with 51% of placebo-treated eyes lost at least eight letters on a logMAR visual acuity chart, with 40% versus 13% gaining at least five letters.

Treatment of Age-Related Macular Degeneration with Photodynamic Therapy (TAP) and Verteporfin in Photodynamic Therapy (VIP) Study Groups. Effect of baseline lesion size, visual acuity, and lesion composition on visual acuity changes from baseline with and without verteporfin therapy in choroidal neovascularization secondary to age-related macular degeneration – TAP and VIP report no. 1. Am J Ophthalmol 2003;136:407–18.

Treatment of Age-Related Macular Degeneration with Photodynamic Therapy (TAP) and Verteporfin in Photodynamic Therapy (VIP) Study Groups. Photodynamic therapy of subfoveal choroidal neovascularization with verteporfin. Fluorescein angiographic guidelines for evaluation and treatment – TAP and VIP report no. 2. Arch Ophthalmol 2003;121:1253–68.

Treatment of Age-Related Macular Degeneration with Photodynamic Therapy (TAP) and Verteporfin in Photodynamic Therapy (VIP) Study Groups. Acute severe visual acuity decrease after photodynamic therapy with verteporfin: case reports from randomized clinical trials – TAP and VIP report no. 3. Am J Ophthalmol 2004;137:683–96.

Treatment of Age-Related Macular Degeneration with Photodynamic Therapy (TAP) and Verteporfin in Photodynamic Therapy (VIP) Study Groups. Verteporfin therapy of subfoveal choroidal neovascularization in age-related macular degeneration: meta-analysis of 2-year safety results in three randomized clinical trials: TAP and VIP report no. 4. Retina 2004;24:1–12.

Japanese Age-Related Macular Degeneration Trial (JAT) Study Group. Japanese Age-Related Macular Degeneration Trial (JAT): 1-year results of photodynamic therapy with verteporfin in Japanese patients with subfoveal choroidal neovascularization secondary to age-related macular degeneration. Am J Ophthalmol 2003;136:1049–61.

Wormald R, Evans JR, Smeeth LL, et al. Photodynamic therapy for neovascular age-related macular degeneration. Cochrane Database of Systematic Reviews 2007, Issue 3, Art. No.: CD002030. DOI: 10.1002/14651858.CD002030.pub3.

Submacular Surgery Trials (SST)

The SST was designed to evaluate the safety and effectiveness of surgical removal of subfoveal neovascularization. This set of multicenter randomized trials was sponsored by the National Eye Institute and was preceded by four randomized pilot trials, the SST Pilot Study.

Grossniklaus HE, Green WR, for the Submacular Surgery Trials Research Group. Histopathologic and ultrastructural findings of surgically excised choroidal neovascularization. Arch Ophthalmol 1998;116:745–9.

Submacular Surgery Trials Pilot Study Investigators. Submacular Surgery Trials randomized pilot trial of laser photocoagulation versus surgery for recurrent choroidal neovascularization secondary to age-related macular degeneration. I. Ophthalmic outcomes. Submacular Surgery Trials Pilot Study report number 1. Am J Ophthalmol 2000;130:387–407.

Of 31 patients in the laser treatment arm and 28 patients in the surgery arm with visual acuity measured 2 years after enrollment (89% of 70 patients enrolled in the SST Group R pilot trial), 65% of laser-treated eyes versus 50% of surgery eyes had visual acuity that was better than or no more than one line worse than at baseline.

Submacular Surgery Trials Pilot Study Investigators. Submacular Surgery Trials randomized pilot trial of laser photocoagulation versus surgery for recurrent choroidal neovascularization secondary to age-related macular degeneration. II. Quality of life outcomes. Submacular Surgery Trials Pilot Study report number 2. Am J Ophthalmol 2000;130:408–18.

SF-36 summary scores were similar for both treatment arms throughout 2 years of follow-up in the SST Group R pilot trial and were consistent with those of the general US population of similar age.

Submacular Surgery Trials Research Group. Responsiveness of the National Eye Institute Visual Function Questionnaire to changes in visual acuity: findings in patients with subfoveal choroidal neovascularization. SST report no. 1. Arch Ophthalmol 2003;121:531–9, Erratum 1513.

Submacular Surgery Trials Research Group. Clinical trial performance of community-based compared with university-based practices: lessons from the Submacular Surgery Trials. SST report no. 2. Arch Ophthalmol 2004;122:857–63.

Childs AL, the Submacular Surgery Trials Patient-Centered Outcomes Subcommittee for the Submacular Surgery Trials Pilot Study Investigators. Responsiveness of the SF-36 Health Survey to changes in visual acuity among patients with subfoveal choroidal neovascularization. Am J Ophthalmol 2004;137:373–5.

Sadda SR, Pieramici DJ, Marsh MJ, et al. Changes in lesion size after submacular surgery for subfoveal choroidal neovascularization in the Submacular Surgery Trials Pilot Study. Retina 2004;24:888–99.

Orr PR, Marsh MJ, Hawkins BS, et al. Evaluation of the Traveling Vision Examiner Program of the Submacular Surgery Trials Pilot Study. Ophthalmic Epidemiol 2005;12:47–57.

Submacular Surgery Trials Research Group. Effect of order of administration of health-related quality of life instruments on responses. SST report no. 3. Qual Life Res 2005;14:493–500.

Submacular Surgery Trials Research Group. Health- and vision-related quality of life among patients with choroidal neovascularization secondary to age-related macular degeneration at time of enrollment in randomized trials of submacular surgery. SST report no. 4. Am J Ophthalmol 2004;138:91–108.

Submacular Surgery Trials Research Group. Health- and vision-related quality of life among patients with ocular histoplasmosis or idiopathic choroidal neovascularization at time of enrollment in a randomized trial of submacular surgery. Submacular Surgery Trials report no. 5. Arch Ophthalmol 2005;123:78–88.

Submacular Surgery Trials Research Group. Patients' perceptions of the value of current vision: assessment of preference values among patients with subfoveal choroidal neovascularization – the Submacular Surgery Trials (SST) Vision Preference Value Scale: SST report no. 6. Arch Ophthalmol 2004;122:1856–67.

Submacular Surgery Trials Research Group. Histopathological and ultrastructural features of surgically-excised subfoveal choroidal neovascular lesions: SST report no. 7. Arch Ophthalmol 2005;123:914–21.

Submacular Surgery Trials Research Group. Guidelines for interpreting retinal photographs and coding findings in the Submacular Surgery Trials (SST): SST report no. 8. Retina 2005;25:253–68.

Submacular Surgery Trials Research Group. Surgical removal versus observation for subfoveal choroidal neovascularization, either associated with the ocular histoplasmosis syndrome or idiopathic. I. Ophthalmic findings from a randomized clinical trial: Submacular Surgery Trials Group H Trial. SST report no. 9. Arch Ophthalmol 2004;122:1597–611.

After 2 years of follow-up, 55% of eyes in the surgery arm versus 46% of eyes in the observation arm had visual acuity that was better than or within one line (7 letters) of baseline visual acuity. Within the subgroup of eyes with visual acuity worse than 20/100 at baseline, these percentages were 76%

and 50%, respectively, suggesting that surgery should be considered for such eyes.

Submacular Surgery Trials Research Group. Surgical removal versus observation for subfoveal choroidal neovascularization, either associated with the ocular histoplasmosis syndrome or idiopathic. II. Quality-of-life findings from a randomized clinical trial: SST Group H Trial. SST report no. 10. Arch Ophthalmol 2004;122:1616–28.

Submacular Surgery Trials Research Group. Surgery for subfoveal choroidal neovascularization in age-related macular degeneration: ophthalmic findings. SST report no. 11. Ophthalmology 2004;111:1967–80.

Findings from the SST Group N trial showed no clinically or statistically meaningful difference in ophthalmic outcomes between eyes assigned to surgery and eyes assigned to observation.

Submacular Surgery Trials Research Group. Surgery for subfoveal choroidal neovascularization in age-related macular degeneration: quality-of-life findings. SST report number 12. Ophthalmology 2004;111:1981–92.

Submacular Surgery Trials Research Group. Surgery for hemorrhagic choroidal neovascular lesions of age-related macular degeneration: ophthalmic findings. SST report no. 13. Ophthalmology 2004;111:1993–2006.

Surgery reduced the risk of severe visual acuity loss in the SST Group B trial but the percentage of eyes that achieved stable or improved visual acuity did not differ between the surgery and observation arms. In the absence of any other effective treatment, surgery may be considered in similar eyes with relatively good visual acuity to reduce the risk of severe visual acuity loss.

Submacular Surgery Trials Research Group. Surgery for hemorrhagic choroidal neovascular lesions of age-related macular degeneration: quality-of-life findings. SST report no. 14. Ophthalmology 2004;111:2007–14.

Submacular Surgery Trials Research Group. Comparison of 2D reconstructions of surgically excised subfoveal choroidal neovascularization with fluorescein angiographic features: SST report no. 15. Ophthalmology 2006;113:267–79.

Grossniklaus HE, Wilson DJ, Bressler SB, et al., for the Submacular Surgery Trials Research Group. Clinicopathologic studies of eyes that were obtained postmortem from four patients who were enrolled in the Submacular Surgery Trial: SST report no. 16. Am J Ophthalmol 2006;141:93–104.

Submacular Surgery Trials Research Group. Surgical removal vs observation for idiopathic or ocular histoplasmosis syndrome-associated subfoveal choroidal neovascularization. III. Vision Preference Value Scale findings from the randomized Group H Trial: SST report no. 17. Arch Ophthalmol 2008;126:1626–32.

Submacular Surgery Trials Research Group. Comparison of methods to identify incident cataract in eyes of patients with neovascular maculopathy. Submacular Surgery Trials report no. 18. Ophthalmology 2008;115:127–33.

Submacular Surgery Trials Research Group. Evaluation of minimum clinically meaningful changes in scores on the National Eye Institute Visual Function Questionnaire (NEI-VFQ). SST report no. 19. Ophthalmic Epidemiol 2007;14(4):205–15.

Submacular Surgery Trials Research Group. Incident choroidal neovascularization in fellow eyes of patients with unilateral subfoveal choroidal neovascularization secondary to age-related macular degeneration. SST report no. 20 from the Submacular Surgery Trials Research Group. Arch Ophthalmol 2007;125:1323–30.

Submacular Surgery Trials Research Group. Risk factors for second eye progression to advanced age-related macular degeneration. SST report no. 21. Retina 2009;29:1080–90.

Solomon SD, Dong LM, Haller JA, et al. on behalf of the SST Research Group and the SST Adverse Event Review Committee. Risk factors for rhegmatogenous retinal detachment in the Submacular Surgery Trials. SST report no. 22. Retina 2009;29:819–24.

Trials of radiotherapy for choroidal neovascularization and a Cochrane systematic review

Chakravarthy U, Houston RF, Archer D. Treatment of age-related subfoveal neovascular membranes by teletherapy: a pilot study. Br J Ophthalmol 1993;77:265–73.

Radiation Therapy for Age-Related Macular Degeneration (RAD) Study Group. A prospective, randomized, double-masked trial on radiation therapy for neovascular age-related macular degeneration (RAD Study). Ophthalmology 1999;106:2239–47.

Char DH, Irvine AI, Posner MD, et al. Randomized trial of radiation for age-related macular degeneration. Am J Ophthalmol 1999;127:574–8.

Kobayashi H, Kobayahsi K. Age-related macular degeneration: Long-term results of radiotherapy for subfoveal neovascular membranes. Am J Ophthalmol 2000;130:617–35.

Marcus DM, Sheils WC, Johnson MH, et al. External beam irradiation of subfoveal choroidal neovascularization complicating age-related macular degerneration. One-year results of a prospective, double-masked, randomized clinical trial. Arch Ophthalmol 2001;119:171–80.

Hart PM, Chakravarthy U, Mackenzie G, et al. Visual outcomes in the Subfoveal Radiotherapy Study: A randomized controlled trial of teletherapy for age-related macular degeneration. Arch Ophthalmol 2002;120:1029–38.

AMDRT Research Group. The Age-Related Macula Degeneration Radiotherapy Trial (AMDRT): One year results from a pilot study. Am J Ophthalmol 2004;138:818–28.

Jaakkola A, Heikkonen J, Tommila P, et al. Strontium plaque brachytherapy for exudative age-related macular degeneration. Three-year results of a randomized study. Ophthalmology 2005;112:567–73.

Zambarakji HJ, Lane AM, Ezra E, et al. Proton beam irradiation for neovascular age-related macular degeneration. Ophthalmology 2006;113:2012–9.

Evans JR, Sivagnanavel V, Chong V. Radiotherapy for neovascular age-related macular degeneration. Cochrane Database of Systematic Reviews 2010, Issue 5, Art. No.: CD004004. DOI: 10.1002/14651858.CD004004.pub3.

Trials of anti-VEGF therapy for choroidal neovascularization

Arguably the most important development in the treatment of neovascular age-related macular degeneration, antivascular endothelial growth factor (VEGF) agents have changed the treatment paradigm and the prognosis for this condition. Trials of anti-VEGF agents for neovascular age-related macular degeneration have been sponsored primarily by industry.

V.I.S.I.O.N.

Gragoudas ES, Adamis AP, Cunningham ET, et al. for the VEGF Inhibition Study in Ocular Neovascularization Clinical Trial Group. Pegaptanib for neovascular age-related macular degeneration. N Engl J Med 2004;351:2805–16.

VEGF Inhibition Study in Ocular Neovascularization (V.I.S.I.O.N.) Clinical Trial Group. Pegaptanib sodium for neovascular age-related macular degeneration. Two-year safety results of the two prospective, multicenter, controlled clinical trials. Ophthalmology 2006;113:992–1001.

MARINA

Rosenfeld PJ, Brown DM, Heier JS, et al. for the MARINA Study Group. Ranibizumab for neovascular age-related macular degeneration. N Engl J Med 2006;355:1419–31.

Monthly intravitreal injections of ranibizumab improved visual acuity by 15 or more letters from baseline in approximately one-third of treated eyes and yielded some improvement in almost all eyes so treated.

Kaiser PK, Blodi BA, Shapiro H, et al., for the MARINA Study Group. Angiographic and optical coherence tomographic results of the MARINA study of ranibizumab in neovascular age-related macular degeneration. Ophthalmology 2007;114:1868–75.

Boyer DS, Antoszyk AN, Auh CC, et al. for the MARINA Study Group. Subgroup analysis of the MARINA study of ranibizumab in neovascular age-related macular degeneration. Ophthalmology 2007;114:246–52.

Chang TS, Bressler NM, Fine JT, et al. for the MARINA Study Group. Improved vision-related function after ranibizumab treatment of neovascular age-related macular degeneration. Results of a randomized clinical trial. Arch Ophthalmol 2007;125(11):1460–9.

ANCHOR

Brown DM, Kaiser PK, Michels M, et al. for the ANCHOR Study Group. Ranibizumab versus verteporfin for neovascular age-related macular degeneration. N Engl J Med 2006;355:1432–44.

Brown DM, Michels M, Kaiser PK, et al. for the ANCHOR Study Group. Ranibizumab versus verteporfin photodynamic therapy for neovascular age-related macular degenerantion: Two-year results of the ANCHOR study. Ophthalmology 2009;116:57–65.

Bressler NM, Chang TS, Fine JT, et al. for the Anti-VEGF Antibody for the Treatment of Predominantly Classic Choroidal Neovascularization in Age-Related Macular Degeneration (ANCHOR) Research Group. Improved vision-related function after ranibizumab vs photodynamic therapy. A randomized clinical trial. Arch Ophthalmol 2009;127(1):13–21.

FOCUS

Heier JS, Boyer DS, Ciulla TA, et al. for the FOCUS Study Group. Ranibizumab combined with verteporfin photodynamic therapy in neovascular age-related macular degeneration. Year 1 results of the FOCUS Study. Arch Ophthalmol 2006;124:1532–42.

Antoszyk AN, Tuomi L, Ghung CY, Singh A on behalf of the FOCUS Study Group. Ranibizumab combined with verteporfin photodynamic therapy in neovascular age-related macular degeneration (FOCUS): Year 2 results. Am J Ophthalmol 2008;145:862–74.

ABC Trial

Patel PJ, Chen FK, Rubin GS, et al. Intersession repeatability of visual acuity scores in age-related macular degeneration. Invest Ophthalmol Vis Sci 2008;49:4347–52.

Patel PJ, Chen FK, Rubin GS, et al. Intersession repeatability of contrast sensitivity scores in age-related macular degeneration. Invest Ophthalmol Vis Sci 2009;50:2621–5.

Tufail A, Patel PJ, Egan C, et al. Bevacizumab for neovascular age related macular degeneration (ABC Trial): multicentre randomised double masked study. Br Med J 2010;340:c2459. doi:10.1136/bmh.c2459.

Keane PA, Patel PJ, Ouyang Y, et al. Effects of retinal morphology on contrast sensitivity and reading ability in neovascular age-related macular degeneration. Invest Ophthalmol Vis Sci 2010;51:5431–7.

Patel PJ, Chen FK, Da Cruz L, et al. for the ABC Trial Study Group. Contrast sensitivity outcomes in the ABC Trial: A randomized trial of bevacizumab for neovascular age-related macular degeneration. Invest Ophthalmol Vis Sci 2011;52:3089–93.

Patel PJ, Chen FK, Da Cruz L, et al. Test–retest variability of reading performance metrics using MNREAD in patients with age-related macular degeneration. Invest Ophthalmol Vis Sci 2011;52:3854–9

PIER and other randomized trials of ranibizumab for neovascular age-related macular degeneration

Regillo CD, Brown DM, Abraham P, et al. on behalf of the PIER Study Group. Randomized, double-masked, sham-controlled trial of ranibizumab for neovascular age-related macular degeneration: PIER Study year 1. Am J Ophthalmol 2008;145:239–48.

Rosenfeld PJ, Rich RM, Lalwani GA. Ranibizumab: Phase III clinical trial results. Ophthalmol Clin N Am 2006;19:361–72.

Rosenfeld PJ, Shapiro H, Tuomi L, et al. for the MARINA and ANCHOR Study Groups. Characteristics of patients losing vision after 2 years of monthly dosing in the phase III ranibizumab clinical trials. Ophthalmology 2011;118:523–30.

Comparison of Age-related Macular Degeneration Treatments Trial (CATT)

CATT is sponsored by the National Eye Institute. Patient accrual was completed in December 2009.

Martin DF, Maguire MG, Fine SL. Identifying and eliminating the roadblocks to comparative effectiveness research. N Engl J Med 2010;363:105–7.

CATT Research Group. Ranibizumab and bevacizumab for neovascular age-related macular degeneration. N Engl J Med 2011; 364:1897–908.

Treatment with ranibizumab and bevacizumab yielded similar visual acuity results when administered following the same regimen.

Comparisons of Age-Related Macular Degeneration Treatment Trials (CATT) Research Group. Ranibizumab and bevacizumab for treatment of neovascular age-related macular degeneration. Two-year results. Ophthalmology 2012;119:1388–98.

IVAN Study Investigators. Ranibizumab versus bevacizumab to treat neovascular age-related macular degeneration. One-year findings from the IVAN randomized trial. Ophthalmology 2012;119:1399–411.

Trials of other pharmacologic treatments for choroidal neovascularization

Pharmacological Therapy for Macular Degeneration Study Group. Interferon alfa-2 is ineffective for patients with choroidal neovascularization secondary to age-related macular degeneration. Results of a randomized placebo-controlled clinical trial. Arch Ophthalmol 1997;115:865–72.

Anecortave Acetate Clinical Study Group. Anecortave acetate as monotherapy for treatment of subfoveal neovascularization in age-related macular degeneration. Twelve-month clinical outcomes. Ophthalmology 2003;110:2372–85.

Slakter JS, Bochow T, D'Amico DJ, et al., Anecortave Acetate Clinical Study Group. Anecortave acetate (15 milligrams) versus photodynamic therapy for treatment of subfoveal neovascularization in age-related macular degeneration. Ophthalmology 2006;113:3–13.

Gillies MC, Simpson JM, Penfold P, et al. A randomized clinical trial of a single dose of intravitreal triamcinolone acetonide for neovascular age-related macular degeneration. One-year results. Arch Ophthalmol 2003;121:667–73.

Gillies MC, Simpson JM, Billson FA, et al. Safety of an intravitreal injection of triamcinolone. Results from a randomized clinical trial. Arch Ophthalmol 2004;122:336–40.

Neovascular Age-Related Macular Degeneration, Periocular Corticosteroids, and Photodynamic Therapy (NAPP) Trial Research Group. Periocular triamcinolone and photodynamic therapy for subfoveal choroidal neovascularization in age-related macular degeneration. Ophthalmology 2007;114; 1713–21.

PREVENTION TRIALS

Age-Related Eye Disease Study (AREDS and AREDS 2)

The goal of AREDS, a multicenter prospective study of persons aged 55–80 years, was to assess the clinical course of age-related macular degeneration and age-related cataract. AREDS included a placebo-controlled randomized prevention trial of high-dose vitamin and mineral supplements for patients at risk of age-related macular degeneration and of high-dose vitamin supplement for patients at risk of age-related cataract. Patient accrual began in September 1990 and ended in January 1998. The National Eye Institute sponsored AREDS and currently is sponsoring AREDS 2, a second study to evaluate other supplements.

Age-Related Eye Disease Study Research Group. The Age-Related Eye Disease Study (AREDS): design implications. AREDS report no. 1. Control Clin Trials 1999;20:573–600.

Age-Related Eye Disease Study Research Group. The Age-Related Eye Disease Study (AREDS): a clinical trial of zinc and antioxidants. AREDS report no. 2. J Nutr 2000;130(Suppl): 1516–9.

Age-Related Eye Disease Study Research Group. Risk factors associated with age-related macular degeneration. A case-control study in the Age-Related Eye Disease Study: Age-Related Eye Disease Study report number 3. Ophthalmology 2000;107: 2224–32.

Age-Related Eye Disease Study Research Group. The Age-Related Eye Disease Study (AREDS) system for classifying cataracts from photographs: AREDS report no. 4. Am J Ophthalmol 2001;131:167–75.

Age-Related Eye Disease Study Research Group. Risk factors associated with age-related nuclear and cortical cataract. A case-control study in the Age-Related Eye Disease Study, AREDS report no. 5. Ophthalmology 2001;108: 1400–8.

Age-Related Eye Disease Study Research Group. The Age-Related Eye Diseases Study system for classifying age-related macular degeneration from stereoscopic color fundus photographs: the Age-Related Eye Disease Study report number 6. Am J Ophthalmol 2001;132:668–81.

Age-Related Eye Disease Study Research Group. The effect of five-year zinc supplementation on serum zinc, serum cholesterol, and hematocrit in persons assigned to treatment group in the Age-Related Eye Disease Study: AREDS report no. 7. J Nutr 2002;132:697–702.

Age-Related Eye Disease Study Research Group. A randomized, placebo-controlled clinical trial of high-dose supplementation with vitamins C and E, beta carotene, and zinc for age-related macular degeneration and vision loss. AREDS report no. 8. Arch Ophthalmol 2001;119:1417–36.

With an average follow-up of the 3609 participants of 6.3 years, treatment with zinc alone or zinc in combination with antioxidants reduced the risk of advanced age-related macular degeneration among eyes at highest risk. Antioxidants plus zinc reduced the rate of moderate visual acuity loss.

Age-Related Eye Disease Study Research Group. A randomized, placebo-controlled, clinical trial of high-dose supplementation with vitamins C and E and beta carotene for age-related cataract and vision loss. AREDS report no. 9. Arch Ophthalmol 2001; 119:1439–52.

Clemons TE, Chew EY, Bressler SB, et al. National Eye Institute Visual Function Questionnaire in the Age-Related Eye Disease Study (AREDS). AREDS report no. 10. Arch Ophthalmol 2003; 121:211–7.

Age-Related Eye Disease Study Research Group. Potential public health impact of Age-Related Eye Disease Study results. AREDS report no. 11. Arch Ophthalmol 2003;121:1621–4.

Age-Related Eye Disease Study Research Group. Associations of mortality with ocular disorders and an intervention of high-dose antioxidants and zinc in the Age-Related Eye Disease Study. AREDS report no. 13. Arch Ophthalmol 2004;122:716–26.

Age-Related Eye Disease Study Research Group. Responsiveness of the National Eye Institute Visual Function Questionnaire to progression to advanced age-related macular degeneration, vision loss, and lens opacity. AREDS report no. 14. Arch Ophthalmol 2005;123:1207–14.

Rankin MW, Clemons TE, McBee WL, Age-Related Eye Disease Study (AREDS) Research Group. Correlation analysis of the in-clinic and telephone batteries from the AREDS cognitive function ancillary study. AREDS report no. 15. Ophthalm Epidemiol 2005;12:271–7.

Age-Related Eye Disease Study Research Group. Cognitive impairment in the Age-Related Eye Disease Study. AREDS report no. 16. Arch Ophthalmol 2006;124:537–43.

Age-Related Eye Disease Study Research Group. The Age-Related Eye Disease Study severity scale for age-related macular degeneration. AREDS report no. 17. Arch Ophthalmol 2005; 123:1484–98.

Age-Related Eye Disease Study Research Group. A simplified severity scale for age-related macular degeneration. AREDS report no. 18. Arch Ophthalmol 2005;123:1570–4.

Age-Related Eye Disease Study Research Group. Risk factors for the incidence of advanced age-related macular degeneration in the Age-Related Eye Disease Study (AREDS). AREDS report no. 19. Ophthalmology 2005;112:533–9.

Age-Related Eye Disease Study Research Group. The relationship of dietary lipid intake and age-related macular degeneration in a case-control study. AREDS report no. 20. Arch Ophthalmol 2007;126:671–9.

Age-Related Eye Disease Study Research Group. Centrum use and progression of age-related cataract in the Age-Related Eye Disease Study (AREDS). AREDS report no. 21. Ophthalmology 2006;113:1264–70.

Age-Related Eye Disease Study Research Group. The relationship of dietary carotenoid and vitamin A, E, and C intake with age-related macular degeneration in a case-control study. AREDS report no. 22. Arch Ophthalmol 2007;123:1225–32.

SanGiovanni JP, Chew EY, Agron E, et al for the Age-Related Eye Disease Study Research Group. The relationship of dietary ω-3 long-chain polyunsaturated fatty acid intake with incident age-related macular degeneration. AREDS report no. 23. Arch Ophthalmol 2008;126(9):1274–9.

Chew EY, Sperduto RD, Milton RC, et al. Risk of advanced age-related macular degeneration after cataract surgery in the Age-Related Eye Disease Study. AREDS report 25. Ophthalmology 2009;116:297–303.

AREDS Research Group. Change in area of geographic atrophy in the Age-Related Eye Disease Study. AREDS report number 26. Arch Ophthalmol 2009;127:1168–74.

Forooghian F, Agron E, Clemons TE, et al. for the AREDS Research Group. Visual acuity outcomes after cataract surgery in patients with age-related macular degeneration: Age-Related Eye Disease Study report no. 27. Ophthalmology 2009;116: 2093–100.

Cukras C, Agron E, Klein ML, et al. for the Age-Related Eye Disease Study Research Group. Natural history of drusenoid pigment epithelial detachment in age-related macular degeneration: Age-Related Eye Disease Study report no. 28. Ophthalmology 2010;117:489–99.

Hubbard LD, Danis RP, Neider MW, et al., Age-Related Eye Disease 2 Research Group. Brightness, contrast, and color balance of digital versus film retinal images in the Age-Related Eye Disease Study 2. Invest Ophthalmol Vis Sci 2008;49:3269–82.

Complications of AMD Prevention Trial (CAPT)

CAPT was a multicenter randomized trial designed to evaluate low-intensity laser treatment as a method of preventing vision loss among patients at risk of choroidal neovascularization and other manifestations of advanced age-related macular degeneration due to having large drusen in both eyes. CAPT was sponsored by the National Eye Institute and was preceded by a pilot study, the Choroidal Neovascularization Prevention Trial (CNVPT).

Choroidal Neovascularization Prevention Trial Research Group. Laser treatment in eyes with large drusen: short-term effects seen in a pilot randomized clinical trial. Ophthalmology 1998; 105:11–23.

Although choroidal neovascularization developed with low frequency among both treated and untreated eyes in the Bilateral Drusen Study, it developed in more treated eyes in the Fellow Eye Study: 10 of 59 treated eyes versus two of 59 untreated eyes.

Choroidal Neovascularization Prevention Trial Research Group. Choroidal neovascularization in the Choroidal Neovascularization Prevention Trial. Ophthalmology 1998;105:1364–72.

Kaiser RS, Berger JW, Maguire MG, et al. Laser burn intensity and the risk for choroidal neovascularization in the CNVPT fellow eye study. Arch Ophthalmol 2001;119:826–32.

Choroidal Neovascularization Prevention Trial Research Group. Laser treatment in fellow eyes with large drusen: updated findings from a pilot randomized clinical trial. Ophthalmology 2003;110:971–8.

By 4 years of follow-up, the cumulative incidence of choroidal neovascularization in treated and untreated eyes was similar. The highest risk in treated eyes was during the first 1–2 years after prophylactic laser.

Complications of Age-related Macular Degeneration Prevention Trial Study Group. Complications of Age-related Macular Degeneration Prevention Trial (CAPT): rationale, design and methodology. Clin Trials 2004;1:91–107.

Complications of Age-related Macular Degeneration Prevention Trial Research Group. Baseline characteristics, the 25-item National Eye Institute Visual Functioning Questionnaire, and their associations in the Complications of Age-related Macular Degeneration Prevention Trial (CAPT). Ophthalmology 2004;111:1307–16.

Complications of Age-related Macular Degeneration Prevention Trial Research Group. Laser treatment in patients with bilateral large drusen. Ophthalmology 2006;113:1974–86.

Maguire MG, Alexander J, Fine SL and the Complications of Age-related Macular Degeneration Prevention Trial (CAPT) Research Group. Characteristics of choroidal neovascularization in the Complications of Age-related Macular Degeneration Prevention Trial. Ophthalmology 2008;115:1468–73.

Complications of Age-related Macular Degeneration Prevention Trial (CAPT) Research Group. Risk factors for choroidal neovascularization and geographic atrophy in the Complications of Age-related Macular Degeneration Prevention Trial. Ophthalmology 2008;115:1474–9.

Ying G, Maguire MG, Liu C, et al. for the Complications of Age-related Macular Degeneration Prevention Trial Research Group. Night vision symptoms and progression of age-related macular degeneration in the Complications of Age-related Macular Degeneration Prevention Trial. Ophthalmology 2008;115: 1876–82.

Ying G, Maguire MG, Alexander J, et al. for the Complications of Age-related Macular Degeneration Prevention Trial (CAPT) Research Group. Description of the Age-related Eye Disease Study 9-step severity scale applied to participants in the Complications of Age-related Macular Degeneration Prevention Trial. Arch Ophthalmol 2009;127:1147–51.

Maguire MG, Ying G, McCannel CA. et al. for the Complications of Age-related Macular Degeneration Prevention Trial (CAPT) Research Group. Statin use and the incidence of advanced age-related macular degeneration in the Complications of Age-related Macular Degeneration Prevention Trial. Ophthalmology 2009;116:2381–5.

Ying G, Maguire MG for the Complications of Age-related Macular Degeneration Prevention Trial Research Group. Development of a risk score for geographic atrophy in [the] Complications of Age-related Macular Degeneration Prevention Trial. Ophthalmology 2011;118:332–8.

Other trials of potential preventive treatment for age-related macular degeneration and a Cochrane systematic review

Olk RJ, Friberg TR, Stickney KL, et al. Therapeutic benefits of infrared (810-nm) diode laser macular grid photocoagulation in prophylactic treatment of neoexudative age-related macular degeneration. Two-year results of a randomized pilot study. Ophthalmology 1999;106:2082–90.

Friberg TR, Musch DC, Lim JI, et al. PTAMD Study Group. Prophylactic Treatment of Age-related Macular Degeneration report number 1: 810-nanometer laser to eyes with drusen. Unilaterally eligible patients. Ophthalmology 2006;113:612–22.

Christen WG, Manson JE, Glynn RJ, et al. Beta carotene supplementation and age-related maculopathy in a randomized trial of US physicians. Arch Ophthalmol 2007;125:333–9.

Christen WG, Glynn RJ, Chew EY, et al. Folic acid, pyridoxine, and cyanocobalamin combination treatment and age-related macular degeneration in women. The Women's Antioxidant and Folic Acid Cardiovascular Study. Arch Intern Med 2009;169: 335–41.

Christen WG, Glynn RJ, Chew EY, et al. Vitamin E and age-related macular degeneration in a randomized trial of women. Ophthalmology 2010;117:1163–8.

Owens SL, Bunce C, Brannon AJ, et al. and the Drusen Laser Study Group. Prophylactic laser treatment hastens choroidal neovascularization in unilateral age-related maculopathy: Final results of the Drusen Laser Study. Am J Ophthalmol 2006;141: 276–81.

Parodi MB, VIrgili G, Evans JR. Laser treatment of drusen to prevent progression to advanced age-related macular degeneration. Cochrane Database of Systematic Reviews 2009, Issue 3, Art. No.: CD006537. DOI: 10.1002/14651858.CD006537. pub2.

RETINOPATHY OF PREMATURITY

Initiation of the Multicenter Trial of Cryotherapy for Retinopathy of Prematurity (CRYO-ROP) was stimulated by an increase in the incidence of retinopathy of prematurity following a decline after early clinical trials demonstrated that exposure to 100% oxygen in incubators had been responsible for the epidemic of retinopathy of prematurity in the USA in the 1950s. Increased incidence in the 1970s and 1980s was attributable to advances in neonatal medicine that had increased survival among very-low-birthweight premature infants. CRYO-ROP was designed to determine the safety and efficacy of transscleral cryotherapy of the peripheral retina in selected low-birthweight infants with retinopathy of prematurity and to study the natural history of retinal vessel development and outcome in such children. Following completion of CRYO-ROP, three additional trials were undertaken to evaluate proposed approaches to reduce the complications of retinopathy of prematurity, all with sponsorship by the National Eye Institute, either alone or in collaboration with other institutes of the National Institutes of Health. Findings from these trials are discussed in Chapter 61 (Pediatric retinal vascular diseases) and Chapter 114 (Retinopathy of prematurity).

Multicenter Trial of Cryotherapy for Retinopathy of Prematurity (CRYO-ROP)

Cryotherapy for Retinopathy of Prematurity Cooperative Group. Multicenter trial of Cryotherapy for Retinopathy of Prematurity: preliminary results. Arch Ophthalmol 1988;106:471–9.

Among eyes of infants assigned to cryotherapy, 22% versus 43% of eyes assigned to observation had a posterior retinal detachment, retinal fold involving the macula, or retrolental tissue.

Cryotherapy for Retinopathy of Prematurity Cooperative Group. Multicenter trial of Cryotherapy for Retinopathy of Prematurity: preliminary results. Pediatrics 1988;81:697–706.

This article is a coordinated duplicate publication of the above findings.

Phelps DL, Phelps CE. Cryotherapy in infants with retinopathy of prematurity. A decision model for treating one or both eyes. JAMA 1989;261:1751–6.

Palmer EA. Results of US randomized clinical trial of cryotherapy for ROP (CRYO-ROP). Doc Ophthal 1990;74:245–51.

Cryotherapy for Retinopathy of Prematurity Cooperative Group. Multicenter trial of Cryotherapy for Retinopathy of Prematurity: three-month outcome. Arch Ophthalmol 1990;108:195–204.

Three-month outcomes from the randomized trial for all 260 infants enrolled update the 1988 preliminary report on effectiveness of transscleral cryotherapy. Eyes treated with cryotherapy had reduced risk of posterior retinal detachment, retinal fold involving the macula, or retrolental tissue compared to untreated eyes: 31% versus 51% respectively.

Watzke RC, Robertson JE, Palmer EA, et al. Photographic grading in the Retinopathy of Prematurity Cryotherapy trial. Arch Ophthalmol 1990;108:950–5.

Dobson V, Quinn GE, Biglan AW, et al. Acuity card assessment of visual function in the Cryotherapy for Retinopathy of Prematurity trial. Invest Ophthalmol Vis Sci 1990;31:1702–8.

Cryotherapy for Retinopathy of Prematurity Cooperative Group. Multicenter trial of Cryotherapy for Retinopathy of Prematurity: One-year outcome – structure and function. Arch Ophthalmol 1990;108:1408–16.

After 1 year of follow-up, eyes assigned to transscleral cryotherapy had reduced risk of posterior retinal detachment, retinal fold involving the macula, or retrolental tissue compared to untreated eyes: 26% versus 47%, respectively. Assessment of grating visual acuity using the Teller Acuity Card correlated with retinal findings: 35% of eyes treated with cryotherapy versus 56% of eyes not treated had an unfavorable functional outcome at 1 year.

Palmer EA, Hardy RJ, Davis BR, et al. Operational aspects of terminating randomization in the Multicenter Trial of Cryotherapy for Retinopathy of Prematurity. Control Clin Trials 1991; 12:277–92.

Hardy RJ, Davis BR, Palmer EA, et al. Statistical considerations in terminating randomization in the Multicenter Trial of Cryotherapy for Retinopathy of Prematurity. Control Clin Trials 1991;12:293–303.

Palmer EA, Flynn JT, Hardy RJ, et al. Incidence and early course of retinopathy of prematurity. Ophthalmology 1991;98: 1628–40.

Phelps DL, Brown DR, Tung B, et al. 28-day survival rates of 6676 neonates with birth weights of 1250 grams or less. Pediatrics 1991;87:7–17.

Quinn GE, Dobson V, Barr CC, et al. Visual acuity in infants after vitrectomy for severe retinopathy of prematurity. Ophthalmology 1991;98:5–13.

Gilbert WS, Dobson V, Quinn GE, et al. The correlation of visual function with posterior retinal structure in severe retinopathy of prematurity. Arch Ophthalmol 1992;110:625–31.

Summers G, Phelps DL, Tung B, et al. Ocular cosmesis in retinopathy of prematurity. Arch Ophthalmol 1992;110:1092–7.

Evans MS, Wallace PR, Palmer EA. Fundus photography in infants. J Ophthalm Photo 1993;15:38–9.

Cryotherapy for Retinopathy of Prematurity Cooperative Group. Multicenter trial of Cryotherapy for Retinopathy of Prematurity: 3-year outcome – structure and function. Arch Ophthalmol 1993;111:339–44.

Reynolds J, Dobson V, Quinn GE, et al. Prediction of visual function in eyes with mild to moderate posterior pole residua of retinopathy of prematurity. Arch Ophthalmol 1993;111:1050–6.

Schaffer DB, Palmer EA, Plotsky DF, et al. Prognostic factors in the natural course of retinopathy of prematurity. Ophthalmology 1993;100:230–7.

Cryotherapy for Retinopathy of Prematurity Cooperative Group. The natural ocular outcome of premature birth and retinopathy. Status at 1 year. Arch Ophthalmol 1994;112:903–12.

Dobson V, Quinn GE, Summers CG, et al. Effect of acute-phase retinopathy of prematurity on grating acuity development in the very low birth weight infant. Invest Ophthalmol Vis Sci 1994; 35:4236–44.

Quinn GE, Dobson V, Biglan A, et al. Correlation of retinopathy of prematurity in fellow eyes in the Cryotherapy for Retinopathy of Prematurity study. Arch Ophthalmol 1995;113:469–73.

Dobson V, Quinn GE, Saunders RA, et al. Grating visual acuity in eyes with retinal residua of retinopathy of prematurity. Arch Ophthalmol 1995;113:1172–7.

Dobson V, Quinn GE, Tung B, et al. Comparison of recognition and grating acuities in very-low-birth-weight children with and without retinal residua of retinopathy of prematurity. Invest Ophthalmol Vis Sci 1995;36:692–702.

Cryotherapy for Retinopathy of Prematurity Cooperative Group. Multicenter trial of Cryotherapy for Retinopathy of Prematurity: Snellen visual acuity and structural outcome at 5½ years after randomization. Arch Ophthalmol 1996;114:417–24.

Kivlin JD, Biglan AW, Gordon RA, et al. Early retinal vessel development and iris vessel dilation as factors in retinopathy of prematurity. Arch Ophthalmol 1996;114:150–4.

Quinn GE, Dobson V, Barr CC, et al. Visual acuity of eyes after vitrectomy for retinopathy of prematurity: follow-up at 5½ years. Ophthalmology 1996;103:595–600.

Gilbert WS, Quinn GE, Dobson V, et al. Partial retinal detachment at 3 months after threshold retinopathy of prematurity. Long-term structural and functional outcome. Arch Ophthalmol 1996;114:1085–91.

Quinn GE, Dobson V, Hardy RJ, et al. Visual fields measured with double-arc perimetry in eyes with threshold retinopathy of prematurity from the Cryotherapy for Retinopathy of Prematurity trial. Ophthalmology 1996;103:1432–7.

Dobson V, Quinn GE, Abramov I, et al. Color vision measured with pseudoisochromatic plates at five-and-a-half years in eyes of children from the CRYO-ROP study. Invest Ophthalmol Vis Sci 1996;37:2467–74.

Bartholomew PA, Chao J, Evans JL, et al. Acceptance/use of the teller acuity card procedure in the clinic. Am Orthop J 1996;46: 99–105.

Saunders RA, Donahue ML, Christmann LM, et al. Racial variation in retinopathy of prematurity. Arch Ophthalmol 1997;115: 604–8.

Bremer DL, Palmer EA, Fellows RR, et al. Strabismus in premature infants in the first year of life. Arch Ophthalmol 1998;116: 329–33.

Quinn GE, Dobson V, Kivlin J, et al. Prevalence of myopia between 3 months and 5½ years in preterm infants with and without retinopathy of prematurity. Ophthalmology 1998;105: 1292–300.

Repka MX, Summers CG, Palmer EA, et al. The incidence of ophthalmologic interventions in children with birth weights less than 1251 grams. Results through 5½ years. Ophthalmology 1998;105:1621–7.

Dobson V, Quinn GE, Siatkowski RM, et al. Agreement between grating acuity at age 1 year and Snellen acuity at age 5½ years in the preterm child. Invest Ophthalmol Vis Sci 1999;40: 496–503.

Harvey EM, Dobson V, Tung B, et al. Interobserver agreement for grating acuity and letter acuity assessment in 1- to 5½-year-olds with severe retinopathy of prematurity. Invest Ophthalmol Vis Sci 1997;40:1565–76.

Repka MX, Palmer EA, Tung B, et al. Involution of retinopathy of prematurity. Arch Ophthalmol 2000;118:645–9.

Quinn GE, Dobson V, Siatkowski RM, et al. Does cryotherapy affect refractive error? Results from treated versus control eyes in the Cryotherapy for Retinopathy of Prematurity trial. Ophthalmology 2001;108:343–7.

Cryotherapy for Retinopathy of Prematurity Cooperative Group. Multicenter trial of Cryotherapy for Retinopathy of Prematurity: ophthalmological outcomes at 10 years. Arch Ophthalmol 2001;119:1110–8.

Cryotherapy for Retinopathy of Prematurity Cooperative Group. Effect of retinal ablative therapy for threshold retinopathy of prematurity: results of Goldmann perimetry at the age of 10 years. Arch Ophthalmol 2001;119:1120–5.

Cryotherapy for Retinopathy of Prematurity Cooperative Group. Contrast sensitivity at age 10 years in children who had threshold retinopathy of prematurity. Arch Ophthalmol 2001;119: 1129–33.

Editorial Committee for the Cryotherapy for Retinopathy of Prematurity Cooperative Group. Multicenter Trial of Cryotherapy for Retinopathy of Prematurity. Natural history of ROP: ocular outcome at 5½ years in premature infants with birth weights less than 1251 g. Arch Ophthalmol 2002;120: 595–9.

Hardy RJ, Palmer EA, Dobson V, et al. Risk analysis of prethreshold retinopathy of prematurity. Arch Ophthalmol 2003; 121:1697–701.

Cryotherapy for Retinopathy of Prematurity Cooperative Group. 15-year outcomes following threshold retinopathy of prematurity. Final results from the Multicenter Trial of Cryotherapy for Retinopathy of Prematurity. Arch Ophthalmol 2005;123:311–8.

Cryotherapy for Retinopathy of Prematurity Cooperative Group. Visual acuity at 10 years in Cryotherapy for Retinopathy of Prematurity (CRYO-ROP) Study eyes. Arch Ophthalmol 2006; 124:199–202.

Multicenter Study of Light Reduction in Retinopathy of Prematurity (LIGHT-ROP)

Reynolds JD, Hardy RJ, Kennedy KA, et al. Lack of efficacy of light reduction in preventing retinopathy of prematurity. N Engl J Med 1998;338:1572–6.

Reduced nursery lighting did not decrease the incidence of retinopathy of prematurity compared to normal nursery lighting among premature infants with birth weights of 1250 g or less in this randomized trial.

LIGHT-ROP Cooperative Group. The design of the multicenter study of Light Reduction in Retinopathy of Prematurity (LIGHT-ROP). J Pediatr Ophthalmol Strabismus 1999;36: 257–63.

Kennedy KA, Fielder AR, Hardy RJ, et al. Reduced lighting does not improve medical outcomes in very-low-birth-weight infants. J Pediatr 2001;139:527–31.

Supplemental Therapeutic Oxygen for Prethreshold Retinopathy of Prematurity (STOP-ROP)

STOP-ROP Multicenter Study Group. Supplemental Therapeutic Oxygen for Prethreshold Retinopathy of Prematurity (STOP-ROP), a randomized, controlled trial. I: Primary outcomes. Pediatrics 2000;105:295–310.

Premature infants with prethreshold disease and median pulse oximetry less than 94% saturation were randomly assigned to conventional oxygen with pulse oximetry targeted at 89–94% saturation or supplemental oxygen with pulse oximetry targeted at 96–99% saturation. No substantive difference in rates of progression was found.

Oden NL, Phelps DL, the STOP-ROP Multicenter Study Group. Statistical issues related to early closure of STOP-ROP, a group-sequential trial. Control Clin Trials 2003;24:28–38.

Early Treatment of Retinopathy for Prematurity (ETROP or EARLY-ROP)

Early Treatment for Retinopathy of Prematurity Cooperative Group. Revised indications for the treatment of retinopathy of prematurity. Results of the Early Treatment for Retinopathy of Prematurity randomized trial. Arch Ophthalmol 2003;121: 1684–96.

Early treatment with peripheral retinal ablation reduced unfavorable outcomes with respect to both visual acuity and structure in comparison to standard management of prethreshold retinopathy of prematurity in this randomized trial.

Hardy RJ, Good WV, Dobson V, et al. for the Early Treatment for Retinopathy of Prematurity Cooperative Group. Multicenter trial of early treatment for retinopathy of prematurity: Study design. Control Clin Trials 2004;24:311–26.

Davitt BV, Dobson V, Good WV, et al. for the Early Treatment for Retinopathy of Prematurity Cooperative Group. Prevalence of myopia at 9 months in infants with high-risk prethreshold retinopathy of prematurity. Ophthalmology 2005;112:1564–8.

Repka MX, Tung B, Good WV, et al. Outcome of eyes developing retinal detachment during the Early Treatment for Retinopathy of Prematurity Study (ETROP). Arch Opthalmol 2006;124: 24–30.

VanderVeen DK, Coats DK, Dobson V, et al. for the Early Treatment for Retinopathy of Prematurity Cooperative Group. Prevalence and course of strabismus in the first year of life for infants with prethreshold retinopathy of prematurity. Arch Ophthalmol 2006;124:766–73.

Early Treatment for Retinopathy of Prematurity Cooperative Group. The Early Treatment for Retinopathy of Prematurity Study: structural findings at age 2 years. Br J Ophthalmol 2006;90:1378–82.

Quinn GE, Dobson V, Davitt BV, et al. on behalf of the Early Treatment for Retinopathy of Prematurity Cooperative Group. Progression of myopia and high myopia in the Early Treatment for Retinopathy of Prematurity Study. Findings to 3 years of age. Ophthalmology 2008;115:1058–64.

Early Treatment for Retinopathy of Prematurity Cooperative Group. Final visual acuity results in the Early Treatment for Retinopathy of Prematurity Study. Arch Ophthalmol 2010; 128:663–71.

Early Treatment for Retinopathy of Prematurity Cooperative Group. Visual field extent at 6 years of age in children who had high-risk prethreshold retinopathy of prematurity. Arch Ophthalmol 2011;129:127–32.

Early Treatment for Retinopathy of Prematurity Cooperative Group. Grating visual acuity results in the Early Treatment for Retinopathy of Prematurity Study. Arch Ophthalmol 2011; 129:840–6.

OTHER RETINAL AND RETINA-RELATED CONDITIONS

Collaborative Ocular Melanoma Study (COMS)

The COMS was designed and conducted to evaluate radiotherapy for treatment of choroidal melanoma, either in comparison to enucleation (COMS randomized trial of iodine-125 brachytherapy) or in combination with enucleation (COMS randomized trial of pre-enucleation radiation). Both US and Canadian centers participated in the COMS. In addition, a nonrandomized observational study of small choroidal melanoma was conducted at a subset of COMS centers. A parallel prospective study of quality of life among patients in the brachytherapy trial

(COMS-QOLS) was conducted as well. The COMS was sponsored by the National Eye Institute and the National Cancer Institute, National Institutes of Health, US Department of Health and Human Services. The COMS design and findings are discussed in detail in Chapter 150 (Collaborative Ocular Melanoma Study), which cites most publications from the COMS; only primary outcome publications are cited here.

Collaborative Ocular Melanoma Study Group. The Collaborative Ocular Melanoma Study (COMS) randomized trial of pre-enucleation radiation of large choroidal melanoma. II: Initial mortality findings. COMS report no. 10. Am J Ophthalmol 1998;125:779–96.

Five-year survival rates were 62% for patients assigned to pre-enucleation radiation and 57% for patients who had enucleation only. Five-year rates of death with histopathologically confirmed melanoma were 26% and 28%, respectively.

Collaborative Ocular Melanoma Study Group. The COMS randomized trial of iodine 125 brachytherapy for choroidal melanoma, III: Initial mortality findings. COMS report no. 18. Arch Ophthalmol 2001;119:969–82.

Among the 1317 patients enrolled in this COMS trial, 5-year all-cause mortality rates were 19% among those assigned to enucleation and 18% among those assigned to brachytherapy. Five-year rates of death with confirmed melanoma metastasis were 11% in the enucleation arm and 9% in the brachytherapy arm.

Collaborative Ocular Melanoma Study Group. The Collaborative Ocular Melanoma Study (COMS) randomized trial of pre-enucleation radiation of large choroidal melanoma. IV. Ten-year mortality findings and prognostic factors. COMS report no. 24. Am J Ophthalmol 2004;138:936–51.

Collaborative Ocular Melanoma Study – Quality of Life Study Group. Quality of life after I-125 brachytherapy versus enucleation for choroidal melanoma: 5-year results from the Collaborative Ocular Melanoma Study. COMS-QOLS report no. 3. Arch Ophthalmol 2006;124:226–36.

Collaborative Ocular Melanoma Study Group. The COMS randomized trial of iodine 125 brachytherapy for choroidal melanoma. V. Twelve-year mortality rates and prognostic factors. COMS report no. 28. Arch Ophthalmol 2006;124:1684–93.

Studies of the Ocular Complications of AIDS (SOCA)

In order to address issues regarding treatment of eye involvement, primarily cytomegalovirus retinitis, in patients with the acquired immune deficiency syndrome (AIDS), the National Eye Institute has sponsored SOCA, a clinical trials network. Most of the SOCA clinical trials have been conducted in collaboration with the AIDS Clinical Trials Group. Several of the trials also have had industry sponsorship. Accrual of patients to the first SOCA trial began in March 1990. Clinical applications of SOCA findings are discussed in Chapter 81 (HIV-Associated Infections). A longitudinal observational study (LSOCA) was undertaken by the SOCA investigators to provide information on ocular complications during the HAART era.

Studies of Ocular Complications of AIDS (SOCA) Research Group, in collaboration with the AIDS Clinical Trials Group (ACTG). Studies of Ocular Complications of AIDS foscarnet-ganciclovir cytomegalovirus retinitis trial: 1. Rationale, design, and methods. Control Clin Trials 1992;13:22–39.

Studies of Ocular Complications of AIDS Research Group, in collaboration with the AIDS Clinical Trials Group. Mortality in patients with the acquired immunodeficiency syndrome treated with either foscarnet or ganciclovir for cytomegalovirus retinitis. N Engl J Med 1992;326:213–20.

After 19 months of treatment, the rate of mortality in the ganciclovir group was 77% higher than in the foscarnet group, leading to suspension of the treatment protocol.

Studies of Ocular Complications of AIDS Research Group in collaboration with the AIDS Clinical Trials Group. Foscarnet-ganciclovir cytomegalovirus retinitis trial: 4. Visual outcomes. Ophthalmology 1994;101:1250–61.

At 6 months after randomization, visual outcomes were similar, with 88% of the forscarnet-assigned patients and 93% of the ganciclovir-assigned patients having a best-corrected visual acuity of 20/40 or better.

Studies of Ocular Complications of AIDS Research Group in collaboration with the AIDS Clinical Trials Group. Morbidity and toxic effects associated with ganciclovir or foscarnet therapy in a randomized cytomegalovirus retinitis trial. Arch Intern Med 1995;155:65–74.

Studies of Ocular Complications of AIDS Research Group, in collaboration with the AIDS Clinical Trials Group. Antiviral effects of foscarnet and ganciclovir therapy on human immunodeficiency virus p24 antigen in patients with AIDS and cytomegalovirus retinitis. J Infect Dis 1995;172: 613–21.

Studies of Ocular Complications of AIDS Research Group, in collaboration with the AIDS Clinical Trials Group. Combination foscarnet and ganciclovir therapy vs monotherapy for the treatment of relapsed cytomegalovirus retinitis in patients with AIDS: the Cytomegalovirus Retreatment trial. Arch Ophthalmol 1996;114:23–33.

Combination therapy with foscarnet and ganciclovir decreased the rate of visual field loss and the rate of increase in retinal area involvement.

Studies of Ocular Complications of AIDS Research Group, in collaboration with the AIDS Clinical Trials Group. Clinical vs photographic assessment of treatment of cytomegalovirus retinitis: Foscarnet–Ganciclovir Cytomegalovirus Retinitis Trial report 8. Arch Ophthalmol 1996;114:848–55.

Wu AW, Coleson LC, Holbrook J, et al. Measuring visual function and quality of life in patients with cytomegalovirus retinitis: development of a questionnaire. Arch Ophthalmol 1996;114: 841–7.

Studies of Ocular Complications of AIDS Research Group, in collaboration with the AIDS Clinical Trials Group. Assessment of cytomegalovirus retinitis: clinical evaluation vs centralized grading of fundus photographs. Arch Ophthalmol 1996;114: 791–805.

Studies of Ocular Complications of AIDS Research Group, in collaboration with the AIDS Clinical Trials Group. MSL-109 adjuvant therapy for cytomegalovirus retinitis in patients with acquired immunodeficiency syndrome: the Monoclonal Antibody Cytomegalovirus Retinitis Trial. Arch Ophthalmol 1997;115:1528–36. [Correction in Arch Ophthalmol 1998;116: 296.]

Studies of Ocular Complications of AIDS Research Group, in collaboration with the AIDS Clinical Trials Group. Parenteral cidofovir for cytomegalovirus retinitis in patients with AIDS: the HPMPC Peripheral Cytomegalovirus Retinitis trial. A randomized, controlled trial. Ann Intern Med 1997;126:264–74.

Both low and high doses of cidofovir slowed progression of cytomegalovirus retinitis to medians of 64 and 21 days, respectively.

Studies of Ocular Complications of AIDS (SOCA) Research Group, in collaboration with the AIDS Clinical Trials Group (ACTG). Rhegmatogenous retinal detachment in patients with cytomegalovirus retinitis: the Foscarnet–Ganciclovir Cytomegalovirus Retinitis trial. Am J Ophthalmol 1997;124: 61–70.

Studies of Ocular Complications of AIDS Research Group in collaboration with the AIDS Clinical Trials Group. Foscarnet–Ganciclovir Cytomegalovirus Retinitis Trial: 5. Clinical features of cytomegalovirus retinitis at diagnosis. Am J Ophthalmol 1997;124:141–57.

Studies of Ocular Complications of AIDS Research Group, in collaboration with the AIDS Clinical Trials Group. Cytomegalovirus (CMV) culture results, drug resistance, and clinical outcome in AIDS patients with CMV treated with either foscarnet or ganciclovir. J Infect Dis 1997;176:50–8.

Holbrook JT, Davis MD, Hubbard LD, et al. Risk factors for advancement of cytomegalovirus retinitis in patients with acquired immunodeficiency syndrome. Arch Ophthalmol 2000; 118:1196–204.

Holbrook JT, Meinert CL, Van Natta ML, et al. Photographic measures of cytomegalovirus retinitis as surrogates for visual outcomes in treated patients. Arch Ophthalmol 2001;119: 554–63.

Martin BK, Gilpin AMK, Jabs DA, et al. for the Studies of Ocular Complications of AIDS Research Group. Reliability, validity, and responsiveness of general and disease-specific quality of life measures in a clinical trial for cytomegalovirus retinitis. J Clin Epidemiol 2001;54:376–86.

Studies of Ocular Complications of AIDS Research Group in collaboration with the AIDS Clinical Trials Group. The ganciclovir implant plus oral ganciclovir versus parenteral cidofovir for the treatment of cytomegalovirus retinitis in patients with acquired immunodeficiency syndrome: The Ganciclovir Cidofovir Cytomegalovirus Retinitis Trial. Am J Ophthalmol 2001;131:457–67.

Jabs DA, Gilpin AMK, Min Y-I, et al. for the Studies of Ocular Complications of AIDS Research Group. HIV and cytomegalovirus viral load and clinical outcomes in AIDS and cytomegalovirus retinitis patients: Monoclonal Antibody Cytomegalovirus Retinitis Trial. AIDS 2002;16:877–87.

Holbrook JT, Jabs DA, Weinberg DV, et al. for the Studies of Ocular Complications of AIDS (SOCA) Research Group. Visual loss in patients with cytomegalovirus retinitis and acquired immunodeficiency syndrome before widespread availability of highly active antiretroviral therapy. Arch Ophthalmol 2003; 121:99–107.

Dunn JP, Van Natta M, Foster G, et al for the Studies of Ocular Complications of AIDS Research Group. Complications of ganciclovir implant surgery in patients with cytomegalovirus retinitis. The Ganciclovir Cidofovir Cytomegalovirus Retinitis Trial. Retina 2004;24:41–50.

Jabs DA, Van Natta M, Thorne JE, et al. for the Studies of the Ocular Complications of AIDS Research Group. Course of cytomegalovirus retinitis in the era of highly active antiretroviral therapy. I. Retinitis progression. Ophthalmology 2004;111: 2224–31.

Jabs DA, Van Natta M, Thorne JE, et al. for the Studies of the Ocular Complications of AIDS Research Group. Course of cytomegalovirus retinitis in the era of highly active antiretroviral therapy. 2. Second eye involvement and retinal detachment. Ophthalmology 2004;111:2232–9.

Kempen JH, Min Y-I, Freeman WR, et al. for the Studies of the Ocular Complications of AIDS Research Group. Risk of immune recovery uveitis in patients with AIDS and cytomegalovirus retinitis. Ophthalmology 2006;113:684–94.

Thorne JE, Jabs DA, Kempen JH, et al. for the Studies of Ocular Complications of AIDS Research Group. Incidence of and risk factors for visual acuity loss among patients with AIDS and cytomegalovirus retinitis in the era of highly active antiretroviral therapy. Ophthalmology 2006;113:1432–40.

Thorne JE, Jabs DA, Kempen JH, et al. for the Studies of Ocular Complications of AIDS Research Group. Causes of visual acuity loss among patients with AIDS and cytomegalovirus retinitis in the era of highly active antiretroviral therapy. Ophthalmology 2006;113:1441–5.

Thorne JE, Jabs DA, Kempen JH, et al. for the Studies of Ocular Complications of AIDS Research Group. Incidence of and risk factors for visual acuity loss among patients with AIDS and cytomegalovirus retinitis in the era of highly active antiretroviral therapy. Ophthalmology 2007;114:787–93.

Trials of treatment of posterior uveitis

Callanan DG, Jaffe GJ, Marin DF, et al. Treatment of posterior uveitis with a fluocinolone acetonide implant. Three-year clinical trial results. Arch Ophthalmol 2008;126: 1191–201.

Lowder C, Belfort B, Lightman S, et al. Dexamethasone intravitreal implant for noninfectious intermediate or posterior uveitis. Arch Ophthalmol 2011;129:545–53.

Soheilian M, Ramezani A, Azimzadeh A, et al. Randomized trial of intravitreal clindamycin and dexamethasone versus pyrimethamine, sulfadiazine, and prednisolone in treatment of ocular toxoplasmosis. Ophthalmology 2011;118:134–41.

Silicone Study

The Silicone Study was conducted to compare postoperative tamponade effectiveness of intraocular silicone oil with that of long-acting gas for managing retinal detachment complicated by proliferative vitreoretinopathy. The Silicone Study was sponsored by the National Eye Institute. Clinical application of findings from the Silicone Study is discussed in Chapter 104 (Special adjuncts to treatment).

Azen SP, Irvine AR, Davis MD, et al. The validity and reliability of photographic documentation of proliferative vitreoretinopathy. Ophthalmology 1989;96:352–7.

Lean JS, Stern WH, Irvine AR, et al. Classification of proliferative vitreoretinopathy used in the Silicone Study. Ophthalmology 1989;96:765–71.

Azen SP, Boone DC, Barlow W, et al. Methods, statistical features, and baseline results of a standardized, multicentered ophthalmological surgical trial: the Silicone Study. Control Clin Trials 1991;12:438–55.

Silicone Study Group. Vitrectomy with silicone oil or sulfur hexafluoride gas in eyes with severe proliferative vitreoretinopathy: results of a randomized clinical trial. Silicone Study Report 1. Arch Ophthalmol 1992;110:770–9.

After 24 months of follow-up, more eyes assigned to silicone oil than assigned to sulfur hexafluoride gas had visual acuity of 5/200 or better. Macular attachment was achieved more often in eyes treated with silicone oil.

Silicone Study Group. Vitrectomy with silicone oil or perfluoropropane gas in eyes with severe proliferative vitreoretinopathy: results of a randomized clinical trial. Silicone Study Report 2. Arch Ophthalmol 1992;110:780–92.

McCuen BW, Azen SP, Stern W, et al. Vitrectomy with silicone oil or with perfluoropropane gas in eyes with severe proliferative vitreoretinopathy. Silicone Study Report No. 3. Retina 1993;13:279–84.

Barr CC, Lai MY, Lean JS, et al. Postoperative intraocular pressure abnormalities in the Silicone Study. Silicone Study report 4. Ophthalmology 1993;100:1629–35.

Blumenkranz MS, Azen SP, Aaberg T, et al. Relaxing retinotomy with silicone oil or long-acting gas in eyes with severe proliferative vitreoretinopathy. Silicone Study Report 5. Am J Ophthalmol 1993;116:557–64.

Hutton WL, Azen SP, Blumenkranz MS, et al. The effects of silicone oil removal. Silicone Study Report 6. Arch Ophthalmol 1994;112:778–85.

Abrams GW, Azen SP, Barr CC, et al. The incidence of corneal abnormalities in the Silicone Study. Silicone Study report 7. Arch Ophthalmol 1995;113:764–9.

Cox MS, Azen SP, Barr CC, et al. Macular pucker after successful surgery for proliferative vitreoretinopathy. Silicone Study report 8. Ophthalmology 1995;102:1884–91.

Lean J, Azen SP, Lopez PF, et al. The prognostic utility of the Silicone Study classification system. Silicone Study report 9. Arch Ophthalmol 1996;114:286–92.

Diddie KR, Azen SP, Freeman HM, et al. Anterior proliferative vitreoretinopathy in the Silicone Study. Silicone Study report number 10. Ophthalmology 1996;103:1092–9.

Abrams GW, Azen SP, McCuen BW, et al. Vitrectomy with silicone oil or long-acting gas in eyes with severe proliferative vitreoretinopathy: results of additional and long-term follow-up. Silicone Study report 11. Arch Ophthalmol 1997;115:335–44.

Macular hole trials

Freeman WR, Azen SP, Kim JW, et al. Vitrectomy for the treatment of full-thickness stage 3 or 4 macular holes: results of a multicenter randomized clinical trial. Arch Ophthalmol 1997;115:11–21.

Although more adverse events occurred in eyes treated surgically, those eyes had higher rates of hole closure and improvement in visual acuity than observed eyes.

Tadayoni R, Vicaut E, Devin F, et al. A randomized controlled trial of alleviated positioning after small macular hole surgery. Ophthalmology 2011;118:150–5.

Retinitis pigmentosa

Berson EL, Rosner B, Sandberg MA, et al. A randomized trial of vitamin A and vitamin E supplementation for retinitis pigmentosa. Arch Ophthalmol 1993;111:761–72.

Sandberg MA, Weigel-DeFranco C, Rosner B, et al. The relationship between visual field size and electroretinogram amplitude in retinitis pigmentosa. Invest Ophthalmol Vis Sci 1996;37:1693–8.

Berson EL, Rosner B, Sandberg MA, et al. Clinical trial of docosahexaenoic acid in patients with retinitis pigmentosa receiving vitamin A treatment. Arch Ophthalmol 2004;122:1297–305.

Berson EL, Rosner B, Sandberg MA, et al. Further evaluation of docosahexaenoic acid in patients with retinitis pigmentosa receiving vitamin A treatment: subgroup analyses. Arch Ophthalmol 2004;122:1306–14.

Berson EL, Rosner B, Sandberg MA, et al. Clinical trial of lutein in patients with retinitis pigmentosa receiving vitamin A. Arch Ophthalmol 2010;128:403–11.

Adackapara CA, Sunness JS, DiBernardo CW, et al. Prevalence of cystoid macular edema and stability of OCT retinal thickness in eyes with retinitis pigmentosa during a 48-week lutein trial. Retina 2008;28:103–10.

Index

Page numbers followed by "f" indicate figures, "t" indicate tables, and "b" indicate boxes.

C

E

S